CARDIAC ANESTHESIA

PRINCIPLES AND CLINICAL PRACTICE

SECOND EDITION

CARDIAC ANESTHESIA

PRINCIPLES AND CLINICAL PRACTICE

SECOND EDITION

Editors

FAWZY G. ESTAFANOUS, M.D.

Chairman, Division of Anesthesiology and Critical Care Medicine
Cleveland Clinic Foundation
Cleveland, Ohio

PAUL G. BARASH, M.D.

Professor of Anesthesiology
Yale University School of Medicine
New Haven, Connecticut

J.G. REVES, M.D.

Professor and Chairman
Department of Anesthesiology
Duke University School of Medicine
Durham, North Carolina

LIPPINCOTT WILLIAMS & WILKINS
A **Wolters Kluwer** Company
Philadelphia • Baltimore • New York • London
Buenos Aires • Hong Kong • Sydney • Tokyo

Acquisitions Editor: R. Craig Percy
Developmental Editor: Leah Hayes/Sonya L. Seigafuse
Production Editor: Tony DeGeorge
Manufacturing Manager: Tim Reynolds
Cover Designer: Mark Lerner
Compositor: Maryland Composition
Printer: Maple Press

530 Walnut Street
Philadelphia, PA 19106 USA
LWW.com

Printed in the USA

Library of Congress Cataloging-in-Publication Data

Cardiac anesthesia: principles and clinical practice/edited by Fawzy G. Estafanous, Paul G. Barash, J.G. Reves.—2nd ed.
p. cm.
Includes bibliographical references and index.
ISBN 0-7817-2195-4
1. Anesthesia in cardiology. I. Estafanous, F.G. (Fawzy G.) II. Barash, Paul G. III. Reves, J.G.

RD87.3.H43 C35 2001
617.9′67412—dc21

00-067813

Care has been taken to confirm the accuracy of the information presented and to describe generally accepted practices. However, the authors, editors, and publisher are not responsible for errors or omissions or for any consequences from application of the information in this book and make no warranty, expressed or implied, with respect to the currency, completeness, or accuracy of the contents of the publication. Application of this information in a particular situation remains the professional responsibility of the practitioner.

The authors, editors, and publisher have exerted every effort to ensure that drug selection and dosage set forth in this text are in accordance with current recommendations and practice at the time of publication. However, in view of ongoing research, changes in government regulations, and the constant flow of information relating to drup therapy and drug reactions, the reader is urged to check the package insert for each drug for any change in indications and dosage and for added warnings and precautions. This is particularly important when the recommended agent is a new or infrequently employed drug.

Some drugs and medical devices presented in this publication have Food and Drug Administration (FDA) clearance for limited use in restricted research settings. It is the responsibility of the health care provider to ascertain the FDA status of each drug or device planned for use in their clinical practice.

10 9 8 7 6 5 4 3 2 1

To the pioneers of cardiac anesthesia who had the vision and courage to lead the way for all to follow, to our peers who have made the journey fun, and to our students who make our careers so rewarding

CONTENTS

CONTRIBUTING AUTHORS

Solomon Aronson, M.D., F.A.C.C., F.C.C.P. Professor of Anesthesiology and Critical Care; Chief, Division of Cardiothoracic Anesthesia, University of Chicago, 5841 S. Maryland Avenue, MC 4028, Chicago, Illinois 60637

Darryl Atwell, M.D. Department of Cardiothoracic Anesthesiology, The Cleveland Clinic Foundation, 9500 Euclid Avenue—G30, Cleveland, Ohio 44195

Peter L. Bailey, M.D. Professor of Anesthesiology , University of Rochester; Director, Cardiac Anesthesiology, Strong Memorial Hospital, 601 Elmwood Avenue, Rochester, New York 14642

Jeffrey R. Balser, M.D., Ph.D. Associate Professor of Anesthesiology and Pharmacology, The James Taloe Gwathmey Clinician – Scientist Chair, Vanderbilt University School of Medicine, 2220 Pierce Avenue, 560 MRB II, Nashville, Tennessee 37232

Mark Banoub, M.D. Staff Anesthesiologist, Department of Anesthesiology, St. Vincent Mercy Medical Center, 2409 Cherry Street, Suite 4, Toledo, Ohio 43608

Paul G. Barash, M.D. Professor of Anesthesiology, Yale University School of Medicine, 333 Cedar Street, PO Box 208051, New Haven, Connecticut 06510

Thomas M. Bashore, M.D. Professor of Medicine, Division of Cardiology, Duke University School of Medicine; Director, Fellowship Training Program, Division of Cardiology, Duke University Medical Center, 7624 Duke Hospital North, Durham, North Carolina 27710

Matthew Bigham, M.D. Assistant Professor of Anesthesiology, Washington University School of Medicine, 660 South Euclid Street, St. Louis, Missouri 63110; Attending Anesthesiologist, Department of Cardiothoracic Anesthesia, Barnes-Jewish Hospital, One Barnes-Jewish Plaza, St. Louis, Missouri 63110

Paula M. Bokesch, M.D. Staff Anesthesiologist, Department of Cardiothoracic Anesthesiology, The Cleveland Clinic Foundation, 9500 Euclid Avenue—G30, Cleveland, Ohio 44195

Richard J. Bondy, M.D.C.M., F.R.C.P.(c) Associate Professor of Anesthesia, McGill University Health Center; Staff Anesthesiologist, Royal Victoria Hospital, 687 Avenue Des Pins Ouest, Montreal, Quebec H3A 1A1 Canada

Douglas V. Brown, M.D. Assistant Professor of Anesthesiology, Rush Presbyterian Medical College, Rush Presbyterian – St. Luke's Medical Center, 1653 W. Congress Parkway, Chicago, Illinois 60612

Norbert P. de Bruijn, M.D., F.A.C.C. Professor of Anesthesiology, Duke University; Attending Anesthesiologist, Duke University Medical Center, Erwin Road, Box 3094, Durham, North Carolina 27710

Ira M. Cheifetz, M.D. Assistant Professor of Pediatrics, Duke University Medical Center; Medical Director, Pediatric Intensive Care Unit, Department of Pediatrics, Duke Children's Hospital, Box 3046, Durham, North Carolina 27710

George J. Crystal, Ph.D. Professor of Anesthesiology, Physiology, and Biophysics, University of Illinois College of Medicine, 1740 West Taylor Street, Chicago, Illinois 60612; Director of Research Laboratory, Department of Anesthesiology, Illinois Masonic Medical Center, 836 West Wellington Avenue, Chicago, Illinois 60657

Marc L. Dickstein, M.D. Associate Professor of Anesthesiology, Columbia University College of Physicians and Surgeons; Associate Attending Physician, Division of Cardiothoracic Anesthesia, Columbia-Presbyterian Hospital, 630 West 168 Street, New York, New York 10032

B. Hugh Dorman, M.D., Ph.D. Professor of Anesthesiology, Medical University of South Carolina, 165 Ashley Avenue, Charleston, South Carolina 29425-2207

Michael P. Eaton, M.D. Assistant Professor of Anesthesiology, University of Rochester School of Medicine and Dentistry, 601 Elmwood Avenue, Rochester, New York 14642

John A. Elefteriades, M.D. Professor and Chief, Department of Cardiothoracic Surgery, Yale University School of Medicine, 333 Cedar Street - 121 FMB, New Haven, Connecticut 06520; Attending Physician, Cardiothoracic Surgery, Yale-New Haven Hospital, 20 York Street, New Haven, Connecticut 06510

Fawzy G. Estafanous, M.D. Chairman, Division of Anesthesiology and Critical Care Medicine, The Cleveland Clinic Foundation, 9500 Euclid Avenue, Cleveland, Ohio 44195

Lee A. Fleisher, M.D. Associate Professor of Anesthesiology, Department of Anesthesiology and Critical Care Medicine, The John's Hopkins University; Clinical Director of the Operating Rooms, Department of Anesthesiology and Critical Care Medicine, The John's Hopkins Hospital, 600 North Wolfe Street, Baltimore, Maryland 21287

Peter E. Frasco, M.D. Department of Anesthesiology, Mayo Clinic Scottsdale, 13400 East Shea Boulevard, Scottsdale, Arizona 85259

Sugantha Ganapathy, M.D., F.R.C.A., F.R.C.P.C. Associate Professor of Anesthesia, University of Western Ontario, London, Ontario N6A 5C1; Consultant Anesthesiologist, Department of Anesthesia, London Health Sciences Center, University Campus, 339 Windermere Road, London, Ontario, N6A 5A5 Canada

William J. Greeley, M.D. Professor and Chair, Departments of Anesthesiology and Pediatrics, University of Pennsylvania; Anesthesiologist-in-Chief, Departments of Anesthesiology and Critical Care Medicine, Children's Hospital of Philadelphia, 34th and Civic Center Boulevard, Philadelphia, Pennsylvania 19104

Katherine P. Grichnik, M.D. Assistant Professor of Anesthesiology, Duke University Medical Center, Erwin Road, Durham, North Carolina 27710

Steven R. Gundry, M.D. Professor of Surgery, Loma Linda University; Chief, Cardiothoracic Surgery, Loma Linda University Medical Center, 11175 Campus Street, Loma Linda, California 92354

Raafat S. Hannallah, M.D. Professor of Anesthesiology and Pediatrics, The George Washington University Medical Center; Chairman, Department of Anesthesiology, Children's National Medical Center, 111 Michigan Avenue, NW, Washington, D.C. 20010

Eugene A. Hessel, II, M.D. Professor of Anesthesiology and Cardiothoracic Surgery, University of Kentucky College of Medicine; Director, Cardiothoracic Anesthesia, University of Kentucky Medical Center, 800 Rose Street, Lexington, Kentucky 40536-0293

Thomas L. Higgins, M.D., F.C.C.M., F.A.C.P. Associate Professor of Medicine and Anesthesiology, Tufts University School of Medicine, Fruit Street, Boston, Massachusetts 02111; Director, Adult Critical Care Service, Baystate Medical Center, 759 Chestnut Street, Springfield, Massachusetts 01199

Charles W. Hogue, Jr., M.D. Associate Professor of Anesthesia, Chief, Division of Cardiothoracic Anesthesia, Washington University School of Medicine, 660 South Euclid/Box 8054, St. Louis, Missouri 63110

Frank H. Kern, M.D. Professor of Anesthesia and Pediatrics, Chief, Department of Anesthesia, Duke University Medical Center, Erwin Road, Duke North, Room 5538, Durham, North Carolina 27710

Erik J. Kraenzler, M.D., F.C.C.P. Assistant Professor of Anesthesiology, Ohio State University; Head, Section of General Thoracic Anesthesiology, Department of Cardiothoracic Anesthesiology, The Cleveland Clinic Foundation, 9500 Euclid Avenue, Cleveland, Ohio 44195

Ruth Landau, M.D. Chief, Clinic of Anesthesiology, University Hospital of Geneva, 24 rue Micheli-du-Crest, 1211 Geneva – 4, Switzerland

Michael G. Licina, M.D. Associate Professor of Anesthesiology, Health Science Center of the Ohio State University; Department of Cardiothoracic Anesthesiology, The Cleveland Clinic Foundation, 9500 Euclid Avenue, Cleveland, Ohio 44195

Joseph P. Mathew, M.D. Associate Professor of Anesthesiology, Duke University Medical Center, DUMC 3049, Durham, North Carolina 27710

Gerard McCloskey, M.B., B.Ch. Associate Professor of Anesthesiology, Yale University School of Medicine; Assistant Director of Cardiothoracic Intensive Care Unit, Yale-New Haven Hospital, 333 Cedar Street, PO Box 208051, New Haven, Connecticut 06510

Jon N. Meliones, M.D., F.C.C.M, M.S. Professor of Pediatric Critical Care Medicine; Chief, Medical Director of Children's Services, Duke University Medical Center, Box 3046, Durham, North Carolina 27710

Emad B. Mossad, M.D. Head, Section of Congenital Cardiac Anesthesia, Department of Cardiothoracic Anesthesiology, The Cleveland Clinic Foundation, 9500 Euclid Avenue, Cleveland, Ohio 44195

John M. Murkin, M.D., F.R.C.P.C. Professor of Anesthesiology, University of Western Ontario, London, Ontario N6A 5C1; Director, Department of Cardiac Anesthesiology, University Campus, London Health Sciences Center, 339 Windermere Road, London, Ontario, Canada N6A SA5

Jolie Narang, M.D. Assistant Clinical Professor of Anesthesia, Mt. Sinai School of Medicine, Mount Sinai Hospital, One Gustav Levy Place, New York, New York 10029

Mark F. Newman, M.D. Professor and Vice Chairman; Chief, Division of Cardiothoracic Anesthesiology, Duke Heart Center, DUMC 3094, Durham, North Carolina 27710

Christopher J. O'Connor, M.D. Associate Professor of Anesthesiology, Rush Medical College, Rush-Presbyterian—St. Luke's Medical Center, 1653 West Congress Parkway, Chicago, Illinois 60612

J.G. Reves, M.D. Professor and Chairman, Department of Anesthesiology, Duke University Medical Center, DUMC 3094, Durham, North Carolina 27710

Margaret Roberts-Brown, M.B.A. Department of Cardiothoracic Anesthesiology, The Cleveland Clinic Foundation, 9500 Euclid Avenue, Cleveland, Ohio 44195

Lynda E. Rosenfeld, M.D. Associate Professor of Internal Medicine and Pediatrics, Yale University School of Medicine, 333 Cedar Street, New Haven, Connecticut 06510; Associate Director, Cardiac Electrophysiology Laboratory, Yale- New Haven Hospital, 20 York Street, New Haven, Connecticut 06510

Eliot R. Rosenkranz, M.D. Associate Professor of Surgery, State University of New York at Buffalo; Chief, Cardiothoracic Surgery, The Children's Hospital of Buffalo, 219 Bryant Street, Buffalo, New York 14222

Robert M. Savage, M.D. Department of Cardiothoracic Anesthesiology, The Cleveland Clinic Foundation, 9500 Euclid Avenue, Cleveland, Ohio 44195

Randall M. Schell, M.D. Associate Professor of Anesthesiology, Loma Linda University; Director, Medical Student and Resident Education in Anesthesiology, Loma Linda University Medical Center, 11234 Anderson Street, PO Box 2000, Loma Linda, California 92354

Scott R. Schulman, M.D., F.A.A.P. Assistant Professor of Anesthesiology and Pediatrics, Duke University School of Medicine, The Duke Heart Center, DUMC 3094, Durham, North Carolina 27710

Debra A. Schwinn, M.D. Professor of Anesthesiology, Pharmacology and Cancer Biology, and Surgery, Duke University Medical Center, DUMC 3094, Durham, North Carolina 27710

Jack S. Shanewise, M.D. Associate Professor, Division of Cardiothoracic Anesthesiology, Emory University School of Medicine; Director, Intraoperative Echocardiography, Department of Anesthesiology, Emory University Hospital, 1364 Clifton Road, Atlanta, Georgia 30322

Thomas F. Slaughter, M.D. Assistant Professor of Anesthesiology, Duke University Medical Center, Durham, North Carolina 27710; Department of Anesthesiology, Durham Veterans Affairs Medical Center, 508 Fulton Street, Durham, North Carolina 27705

Richard M. Smiley, M.D., Ph.D. Associate Professor of Anesthesiology, Columbia University, 630 West 168 Street, PH-5, New York, New York 10032; Director, Obstetric Anesthesia, New York Presbyterian Hospital, 622 West 168 Street, New York, New York 10032

Norman J. Starr, M.D. Vice Chairman, Division of Anesthesiology and Critical Care Medicine; Chairman, Department of Cardiothoracic Anesthesiology, The Cleveland Clinic Foundation, 9500 Euclid Avenue, Cleveland, Ohio 44195

Daniel M. Thys, M.D. Professor of Anesthesiology, College of Physicians and Surgeons, Columbia University, New York, New York 10031; Chairman, Department of Anesthesiology, St. Luke's - Roosevelt Hospital Center, 1111 Amsterdam Avenue, New York, New York 10025

Kenneth J. Tuman, M.D. Professor of Anesthesiology, Rush Medical College; Vice-Chairman, Department of Anesthesiology, Rush-Presbyterian — St. Luke's Medical Center, 1653 West Congress Parkway, Chicago, Illinois 60612

Marcella Valente, M.D. Postgraduate, Department of Neurosciences, La Sapienza University, Viole dell'Universita 30, 00185 Rome, Italy; Department of Neuromedicine, Via Atinense 18, 86077 Pozzilli (is), Italy

Susan T. Verghese, M.D. Assistant Professor of Anesthesiology and Pediatrics, The George Washington University Medical Center; Attending Anesthesiologist, Children's National Medical Center, 111 Michigan Avenue, NW, Washington, D.C. 20010

John J. Warner, M.D. Associate in Medicine, Department of Medicine, Division of Cardiology, Duke University Medical Center, 7624 Duke Hospital North, Durham, North Carolina 27710

J. Earl Wynands, M.D. Professor Emeritus, Department of Cardiac Anesthesiology, University of Ottawa Heart Institute, 40 Ruskin Street, H213, Ottawa, Ontario K1Y4W7 Canada

Jean-Pierre Yared, M.D. Staff Anesthesiologist, Cardiothoracic Anesthesiology, The Cleveland Clinic Foundation, 9500 Euclid Avenue, Cleveland, Ohio 44124

PREFACE

We are pleased to offer this second edition of *Cardiac Anesthesia*. As with the prior edition, this text is meant to provide the reader with a detailed reference foundation for the scientific basis and the clinical practice of cardiothoracic anesthesiology. We have changed the format little but have added some new material and changed authorship of some of the chapters. The result, we hope, is a more comprehensive, less redundant, and more practical and current text.

New chapters have been written covering history, physiology, ischemic heart disease, brain protection, surgical devices, minimally invasive surgery, arrhythmia pharmacology, and transesophageal echocardiography (TEE). These chapters address new perspectives and knowledge as well as newly evolving clinical activity. For example, the excellent new chapter on TEE, complete with many color illustrations, will be a vital resource to both the novice resident and fellow and the experienced cardiac anesthesiologist. These new chapters have truly changed and updated the text to make the book reflect state-of-the-art practice.

This book is designed for the resident, fellow, faculty, and practitioner of cardiothoracic anesthesiology as well as other specialists such as cardiologists and cardiac surgeons. In addition, with the increasing societal and professional call for the education of specialists in cardiothoracic anesthesiology, we hope that this text helps fulfill a need to educate these anesthesiology subspecialists. We envision a time when accreditation of a cardiothoracic anesthesiology educational program will come, and, in an effort to formulate a curriculum, we hope that this text will be useful.

As before, we are grateful to the contributors whose labor made the book. We also thank the many staff assistants and others who have helped put this book together, both at the sites of our authors and in the offices of Lippincott Williams & Wilkins.

J. G. Reves, M.D.
Paul G. Barash, M.D.
Fawzy G. Estafanous, M.D.

PREFACE TO THE FIRST EDITION

This book was conceived by the three of us to fill the void that exists between handbooks of cardiac anesthesia and an encyclopedic textbook of the field. From the very outset, our goal was to educate the serious student, whether medical student, resident, fellow, faculty, specialist, or practicing anesthesiologist. We wished to provide the scientific rationale for what we consider to be the safe and effective practice of cardiac anesthesiology. To accomplish this, rather than provide as many possible approaches to topics or issues, we advised our authors to present one or two of the most scientifically sound approaches. It is our hope that our associates in surgery, cardiology, nursing, and perfusion will also find this book of value since we share the same patients.

In reflecting upon the content of this book, we are struck by the amount of knowledge that now constitutes cardiac anesthesiology. What was once a practice based on a cookbook-like list of drug dosages is a full-fledged subspecialty body of comprehensive information within the larger field of anesthesiology. There are clinical and scientific principles and concepts that belong solely in the realm of cardiac anesthesiology such as extracorporeal circulation, transesophageal echocardiography, and the physiology and pharmacology of anticoagulation. In addition, there are areas that are of particular importance to the cardiac anesthesiologist such as cardiac catheterization and invasive cardiology, as well as congential heart disease, all of which enrich the field of cardiac anesthesiology. An impetus for the creation of this book was to provide the educator and student with a useful textbook, and for that reason we have a chapter that deals with the education of all students of cardiac anesthesia.

Our vision of the future is one in which medicine's subspecialization will be increasingly important even as society also demands more primary care providers. As the provision of health care inevitably results in fewer but larger cardiac surgery programs in fewer hospitals with consolidation of specialty services, we believe that there will be an increased need for well-educated cardiac anesthesiologists. Thus the compilation of knowledge and its application in the field of cardiac anesthesiology will enable us to create better practices along with our cardiac surgery and cardiology colleagues. This is what our patients expect and our colleagues demand. In time this will lead inevitably to subspecialty certification in cardiac anesthesia.

We are especially grateful to our contributing authors. They have brought their own original presentation and interpretation of the data upon which our clinical practices are based. Many of them have contributed to the scientific body of knowledge that constitutes the foundation for our practice. They have all labored hard to educate us, and we are the grateful recipients of nights and weekends spent on seemingly endless reviews of original papers, manuscript preparation, and countless revisions. We admire their work.

The authors and editors also want to express their profound gratitude to our respective secretaries and editorial assistants: Beth Grubb, Gail Norup, and Laraine Tuck; and to the editors and publishers of Lippincott: Mary K. Smith, Janet Greenwood, Anne Geyer, and Virginia Barishek. They have helped every step of the way in the preparation and publication of this text.

Fawzy G. Estafanous, M.D.
Paul G. Barash, M.D.
J. G. Reves, M.D.

PART I

FOUNDATIONS OF CARDIAC ANESTHESIA

1

HISTORY OF CARDIAC SURGERY AND ANESTHESIA

EUGENE A. HESSEL, II

> The more extensive a man's knowledge, of what has been done, the greater will be his power of knowing what to do.
> Benjamin Disraeli, 1804–1881

> Those who cannot remember the past are condemned to repeat it.
> Santayana, *Life of Reason*

Why examine our past? First, it tells us of our heritage, of how we got to where we are. Second, it helps us to appreciate what we have today and to place our practice in perspective. Third, it provides clues to the characteristics of successful persons and of the discovery process. Finally, it may inspire us to add to the rich history of our profession. "In the continual remembrance of a glorious past, individuals and nations find their inspiration" (Sir William Osler, 1849–1919).

Cardiac surgery is remarkably young, almost its entire history having occurred in slightly more than the past 100 years, and the most important advances within the lifetimes of currently practicing physicians. Many of the participants are still living or have left personal accounts of these events, and original publications are readily available. The reader may be surprised by how recent in origin are the procedures we take for granted today. In 1936, there was no known surgical treatment for congenital or valvular heart disease. In the spring of 1944, there was no surgical palliation available for cyanotic congenital heart disease. At the start of 1952, open cardiac surgery was not possible. At the start of 1960, there was no satisfactory prosthetic valve available, nor an implantable pacemaker, nor even closed chest massage; and infant heart surgery was very risky. In early 1967, direct coronary artery surgery was a rarity and saphenous vein bypass surgery was unheard of, as was human heart transplantation and surgical therapy for tricuspid atresia or hypoplastic left heart syndrome. Intraortic balloon pumping (IABP), cardioplegia, monitoring of heparin dosing, balloon-tipped pulmonary artery catheters (PACs), high-dose narcotic anesthesia, dopamine, dobutamine, and prostaglandin therapy were not yet available. In 1984, internal mammary artery grafting was not generally practiced, nor was monitoring by pulse oximetry, capnography, or transesophageal echocardiography (TEE). Propofol, aprotinin, amrinone, and adenosine were not available, and nitric oxide was only considered an environmental toxin.

Writing history is always subjective. The author makes decisions as to what is important and what should be included. There is also the problem of priority. Options include who first conceived of a procedure, who first attempted (but failed), who first successfully accomplished the procedure, who first published it, and who popularized the procedure. Often two or more surgeons accomplished a new procedure at almost the same time and possibly (it is often difficult to know for certain) independently and unaware of the other's work. In some secondary sources, the dating is confused because an author has used the date of publication rather than the date of the procedure. In this chapter, the latter was used and the original paper was consulted when there was ambiguity.

Although the history of cardiac anesthesia is inexorably intertwined with that of cardiac surgery, for this chapter the two are dealt with separately so as to emphasize the history of cardiac anesthesia, which has received little attention in the past.

CARDIAC SURGERY

The literature on the history of cardiac surgery is extensive. A number of books (1–3) and articles and book chapters (4–10), are useful, but the recent books by Harris B. Shumacker Jr., *The Evolution of Cardiac Surgery* (11), and by Stephen Westaby with Cecil Bosher, *Landmarks in Cardiac Surgery* (12), are exceptionally informative and are recommended to the inquisitive reader. The book by Shumacker, a pioneer in cardiac surgery, is thoroughly referenced and

E. A. Hessel, II: Department of Anesthesiology and Surgery, University of Kentucky College of Medicine, Lexington, Kentucky 40536

TABLE 1-1. HISTORICAL MILESTONES IN CARDIAC SURGERY[a]

Date	Event	Surgeon	Location	Reference No.
September 9, 1896	Suture closure wound of heart	L Rehn	Frankfurt	11
August 28, 1938	Ligation of patent ductus arteriosus	RE Gross	Children's Hospital, Boston	13
October 19, 1944	Repair of coarctation	C Crafoord	Stockholm	14
November 29, 1944	Blalock-Taussig shunt (subclavian to pulmonary artery)	A Blalock	Johns Hopkins Hospital	15
September 16, 1946	Potts shunt (descending aorta to left pulmonary artery)	WJ Potts	Children's Memorial Hospital, Chicago	16
December 4, 1947	Closed pulmonary valvotomy	TH Sellors	London	17
May 24, 1948	Closed surgical creation of atrial septal defect	A Blalock & CR Hanlon	Johns Hopkins Hospital	18
June 1948	Closed mitral commissurotomy	CP Bailey	Philadelphia	19
		DE Harken	Boston	20
1949	Closed infundibulectomy (right ventricle)	RC Brock	London	21
November 1950	Internal mammary artery implant	A Vineberg	Montreal	22
July 11, 1951	Pulmonary artery banding	WH Muller, JF Dammann Jr	University of California, Los Angeles	23
1950–1952	Closed aortic valvotomy	CP Bailey	Philadelphia	24
April 15, 1952	Open closure of atrial septal defect with aid of atrial well	RE Gross	Children's Hospital, Boston	26
September 2, 1952	Open closure of atrial septal defect with aid of moderate hypothermia	FJ Lewis	University of Minnesota	27
September 11, 1952	Ball valve in descending aorta for aortic regurgitation	CA Hufnagel	Georgetown University, Washington DC	25
October 21, 1952	Open pulmonary valvotomy with aid of right heart bypass	FD Dodril	Detroit	28
May 6, 1953	Open closure of atrial septal defect with aid of heart-lung machine	JH Gibbon Jr.	Philadelphia	29
April 20, 1954	Open closure of ventricular septal defect with aid of cross-circulation	CW Lillehei	University of Minnesota	30,31
March 26–May 1955	First series of open heart surgery with heart-lung machine	JW Kirklin	Mayo Clinic	32
February 25, 1958	Superior vena cava to pulmonary artery shunt (Glenn Shunt)	WWL Glenn	Yale University	33
1958	Senning operation for transposition of great arteries	A Senning	Stockholm	34
1960	Aortic valve replacement with ball valve	D Harken	Boston	35
September 21, 1960	Mitral valve replacement with ball valve	A Starr	Portland, Oregon	36
May 16, 1963	Mustard operation for transposition of great arteries	WT Mustard	Toronto	37
1967	Aorta-coronary saphenous vein bypass	RG Favaloro	Cleveland Clinic	38
December 3, 1967	Human heart transplantation	CN Barnard	Capetown, South Africa	39
1968	Multivessel coronary artery bypass graft	WD Johnson	Milwaukee	40
February 29, 1968	Internal mammary artery-coronary graft[b]	GE Green	New York	41
April 25, 1968	Fontan Procedure	F Fontan	Bordeaux, France	42
May 8, 1975	Arterial switch for transposition of great arteries	AD Jatene	Sao Paulo	43
1979–1981	WI Norwood procedure for hypoplastic left heart syndrome	Norwood	Boston Children's Hospital	44
December 1, 1982	Total artificial heart implantation	WC DeVries	Salt Lake City	45
November 1, 1984	Infant (8-month) heart transplantation	DA Cooley	Texas Heart Institute, Houston	46
November 16, 1985	Neonatal (4-day) heart transplantation	L Bailey	Loma Linda University, California	47

[a] With patient survival.
[b] Others accomplished this earlier, but Green popularized the procedure in United States; see text for details.

provides the insights of a surgeon who was there during most of its development. Westaby is a contemporary British cardiac surgeon; his book is richly illustrated and includes many biographic sketches, anecdotes, vignettes, personal impressions, and quotations from those involved, and well as reprints of 44 original articles of historical import. Unfortunately, it lacks all other references.

Table 1-1 lists some historical milestones in cardiac surgery, and Table 1-2 adds some of the important adjuncts to the development and progress of cardiac surgery. At the same time, other developments were occurring in cardiovascular medicine that had an impact on the practice of cardiac surgery and anesthesia, and some of the more notable of these are listed in Table 1-3.

1896–1928: First Steps and Dogma

Slightly more than 100 years ago, on September 9, 1896, Ludwig Rehn of Frankfurt first successfully sutured a stab wound of the heart (right ventricle) (11). Many consider this to be the beginning of cardiac surgery. Like all "firsts," this accomplishment followed essential work by others. Although operative drainage of pericardial fluid was first suggested by Jean Riolan in 1648, it was not accomplished until the early 1800s, by Francisco Romero of Barcelona and Baron Dominique Jean Larrey of France. In the early 1880s, Block of Danzig and Simplicio Del Vecchio of Italy reported the repair of experimental wounds of the heart (11). However, one of the most prominent surgeons of that

TABLE 1-2. ADJUNCTS TO DEVELOPMENT AND PROGRESS IN CARDIAC SURGERY

Date	Adjunct	Investigator	Institution	Reference No.
1900–1915	Discovery of blood types, blood anticoagulation, storage, and blood transfusion	Landsteiner et al.	Multiple	3,48
1916–38	Discovery of heparin, to commercial production	McLean, Best, et al.	Multiple	49,50
1937–39	Protamine neutralization of heparin	E Chargaff, K Olson	Columbia University	51
		E Jorpes et al.	Stockholm	52
1950	Antifoam for bubble oxygenator	LC Clark Jr.	Antioch College, Ohio	53
January 30, 1957	Epicardial pacemaker for surgical heart block	CW Lillehei	University of Minnesota	54
1957	Use of median sternotomy	OC Julian	Chicago	55
		CW Lillehei et al.	University of Minnesota	56
1957	Moderate hypothermia during cardiopulmonary bypass	WC Sealy	Duke University	57
1959	Use of femoral artery for arterial cannulation	CW Lillehei et al.	University of Minnesota	56
1959	Deep hypothermia with circulatory arrest	CE Drew	London	58
July 1959	Name of *Journal of Thoracic Surgery* changed to *Journal of Thoracic and Cardiovascular Surgery*			
1960	Hemodilution prime	N Zuhdi et al.	Oklahoma	59
August 2, 1965	Deep hypothermia and circulatory arrest without cardiopulmonary bypass for infant surgery	DH Dillard, KA Merendino, H Mohri	University of Washington	60
1970	Introduction of balloon-tipped pulmonary artery catheter	HJC Swan, W Ganz	Los Angeles	61
1973	Cold potassium cardioplegia	WA Gay, PA Ebert[a]	Cornell University	62
1973	Transvenous endocardial biopsy	PK Caves et al.	Stanford University	63
1975	Heparin-protamine monitoring with activated clotting time	BS Bull et al.	Loma Linda University, California	64,65
1976	Prostaglandin therapy of cyanotic newborns	PM Olley et al.	Hospital for Sick Children, Toronto	66
1980	Use of cyclosporin in heart transplantation	N Shumway et al.	Stanford University	67
1987	Use of aprotinin to reduce bleeding	D Royston et al.	London	68,69
1990	Heparin-coated circuits	Multiple	—	70
1991	Use of modified ultrafiltration in infants	MJ Elliott, SK Naik	Hospital for Sick Children, London	71
1992	Epivascular scanning and modified management of atherosclerotic ascending aorta	NT Kouchoukos et al.	Washington University, St. Louis	72
1992–1994	Use of nitric oxide in cardiac surgical patients	Multiple	—	73

[a] Many others contributed to development of cardioplegia; see text for details.

TABLE 1-3. NOTABLE DEVELOPMENTS IN CARDIOVASCULAR MEDICINE

Date	Development	Investigator	Location	Reference No.
April 25, 1953	Structure of DNA proposed (double helix)	JD Watson, FHC Crick	Cambridge	74
1959	Selective coronary angiography	FM Sones	Cleveland Clinic	75
June 6, 1960	Implantable pacemaker for complete heart block	WM Chadack, W Greatbatch	University Buffalo	76
July 9, 1960	Report on closed chest massage	WB Kouwenhoven et al.	Johns Hopkins Hospital	77
1965	Drug treatment of aortic dissection	MW Wheat Jr	Gainesville	78
1966	Transcatheter creation of atrial septal defect	WH Rashkind	Children's Hospital of Philadelphia	79
June 29, 1967	Intraaortic balloon pump in humans	A Kantrowitz	Brooklyn	80
August 27, 1970	Report on balloon-tipped pulmonary artery catheter	HJC Swan, W Ganz, et al.	Los Angeles	61
1976	Report on use of prostaglandins to maintain patency of patent ductus arteriosus in cyanotic neonates	PM Olley et al.	Hospital for Sick Children, Toronto	66
September 16, 1977	Percutaneous transluminal coronary angioplasty	A Gruntzig	Zurich	81
1980–1986	Transcatheter dilitation of pulmonary artery, pulmonary valve, coarctation, mitral valve, aortic valve, and closure of atrial septal defect, patent ductus arteriosis	Multiple	Multiple	82–84
1987	Nitric oxide identified as endothelium-derived relaxing factor	LJ Ignarro et al.	University of California, Los Angeles	85
		S Moncada et al.	Wellcome Lab, UK	86

time, Theodor Billroth, pronounced that "A surgeon who would attempt such an operation [cardiac suture] should lose the respect of his colleagues (7)." Unsuccessful attempts at suturing heart wounds in humans were made by Ansel Cappelen in Norway in 1894 and Guido Farina of Rome in 1896, and in that year Great Britain's Sir Stephen Paget predicted that "surgery of the heart has probably reached the limit set by nature to all surgery; no new method and no new discovery can overcome the natural difficulties that attend a wound of the heart" (7). That same year, Rehn accomplished the "impossible." On September 2, 1902, John H. Gibbon of Philadelphia operated on a moribund patient for a wound of the heart, but the patient died before the wound could be closed (11). Half a century later (1953) his son, John H. Gibbon Jr., would be the first to successfully conduct open heart surgery with the aid of a mechanical heart-lung machine. On September 14, 1902, Luther L. Hill of Montgomery, Alabama, first successfully sutured a cardiac wound in the United States (11). By 1907, Rehn reported 124 such attempts with 40% survival rate (7). This was accomplished in the era before endotracheal intubation, antibiotics, and blood transfusion!

Blood types were first identified by Landsteiner and others in 1900–1902, and blood typing before transfusion was introduced by Ottenberg in 1907. However, satisfactory anticoagulation of the blood with citrate (A. Hustin and L. Agote) and addition of glucose (Rous and Turner), so that it could be bottled and stored to make administration practical, was not introduced until 1915–1916 (3,48).

In 1902, Sir Lauder Brunton of St. Bartholomew's Hospital in London, emboldened by good results with surgical treatment of wounds of the heart and based on autopsy studies and animal experiments, published a paper in *The Lancet* suggesting the possibility of surgical treatment of mitral stenosis. He noted how incapacitating a condition this was and the fact that medical therapy could do nothing to relieve the stenosis. He observed that it was easy to separate the adherent cusps (i.e., fused commissures) at autopsy and advocated consideration of surgically splitting the valve along the adherent contact margins (a procedure later to be called commissurotomy) (87). However, his suggestion was met with strong disapproval in subsequent issues of *The Lancet*, including an editorial, which criticized his failure to completely study the problem experimentally, suggested that such an operation would probably prove fatal and that if it did not its benefits would probably be temporary, and finally pointing out that the prognosis of mitral stenosis depended as much on the condition of the myocardium as on the size of the mitral orifice (7,87). These criticisms stifled further work for the next 20 years.

In 1920, Elliott Cutler and C.S. Beck at the Peter Bent Brigham Hospital in Boston (Harvard), began experiments that led to the first successful operation for mitral stenosis, on May 20, 1923. Unfortunately, their operation was designed to relieve the stenosis by cutting the leaflet (rather than splitting the commissure), assuming that mitral insufficiency was less serious than mitral stenosis. They applied this ill-conceived (in retrospect) procedure in six subsequent patients, the last on April 15, 1928, but none of the patients survived (7,88).

There was one other successful mitral valve operation in that era, which was performed by Henry Souttar in London on May 6, 1925 (87). He use transatrial digital dilitation—a technique that was resurrected by Brock in 1948 and became the standard procedure until it was largely replaced in the mid-1950s by transventricular dilitation using a mechanical dilator. Unfortunately, the patient was found to have considerable mitral regurgitation on initial exploration and benefited minimally from the procedure. However, Souttar was impressed with the information gained from the digital exploration—an appreciation of the reality of stenosis and regurgitation, the mechanical nature of these lesions, and the practicability of their surgical relief (11). However, he did not get another opportunity, because "the physicians declared that it was all nonsense and that the operation was unjustifiable" (7). "It was an article of faith with physicians that the valves were of no importance and that the only thing that mattered was the condition of the cardiac muscle" (7). Successful conquest of mitral stenosis would have to wait 23 more years.

Other notable developments occurred in the first quarter of the 20th century. After extensive laboratory experimentation, Friedrich Trendelenburg of Leipzig first attempted a pulmonary embolectomy with normothermic inflow occlusion (the Trendelenburg procedure) in two patients in 1907–1908, neither of whom survived. Several others attempted this procedure without success until Martin Kirschner of Konigsberg, a student of Trendelenburg, finally succeeded on March 18, 1924 (11). By 1935 about 142 Trendelenburg operations had been reported, with only 9 hospital survivors (89). As described later, this operation played a pivotal role in the subsequent development of the first clinically successful heart-lung machine by John Gibbon Jr.

Following better understanding of the pathophysiology of chronic contrictive pericarditis elucidated by Norman Cheevers of London in 1882 and the German Friedel Pick in 1896, Ludwig Rehn of Frankfurt and Ferdinand Sauerbruch of Berlin both successfully performed pericardiectomies for this condition in 1913 (11). This procedure was applied extensively by Claude Beck of Cleveland, who, based on his observations of vascular adhesions between the pericardium and epicardium in clinical and experimental models of pericarditis, conceived of and developed his various operations to improve collateral blood flow to treat coronary artery disease between 1935 and 1941 (11).

1938–1948: Closed Heart Surgery Comes of Age

The remarkable decade in which closed heart surgery became a therapeutic reality began on August 28, 1938, when a 33-year-old chief resident surgeon at the Children's Hospital in Boston successfully ligated a patent ductus arteriosus (PDA) while his chief, William Ladd, was away on his summer vacation. Robert E. Gross had prepared himself for this endeavor in the experimental laboratory and with 3 years of training in pathology (13,90). As is frequently the case in the history of cardiac surgery, another surgeon had missed the opportunity of this historic first the previous year. John W. Strieder almost obliterated an infected ductus arteriosus on March 16, 1937, in a young woman who did well until she died suddenly 5 days after surgery from acute aspiration after emesis caused by acute gastric dilitation (91).

In October 1944, Clarence Crafoord of Stockholm first successfully resected a coarctation of the aorta in two patients. This was followed by Gross' first success with the same operation in June 1945. Gross may have been unaware of Crafoord's work; both reports were published in the fall of 1945 (14,92).*

Perhaps the most dramatic announcement came in 1945, when Blalock and Taussig of Johns Hopkins Hospital announced their successful creation of a systemic-to-pulmonary artery shunt to palliate tetralogy of Fallot, which was first accomplished on November 29, 1944 (15). The idea for this operation was that of Helen B. Taussig, Chief of Pediatric Cardiology. Although she was the daughter of a Harvard professor, Harvard Medical School did not accept women at that time, so she attended Johns Hopkins Medical School. Again because of her gender she could not obtain an internship at Johns Hopkins (the one position reserved for a woman was given to a classmate), and so she took a cardiology fellowship instead, and eventually was appointed director of the Pediatric Heart Clinic. In the course of caring for children with tetralogy of Fallot, she noted that those who also had a persistent ductus arteriosus did better until it closed off; it then occurred to her that other children with the tetralogy could be helped by surgical creation of a ductus. In about 1938–1939, she took her idea to the leading pediatric cardiac surgeon of that day, Dr. Gross, who allegedly replied, "Madam, I close ductuses, I do not make new ductuses" (10). Taussig had to await the arrival of Alfred Blalock as Chief of Surgery in 1941. Dr. Blalock had been a surgical resident at Johns Hopkins but was not offered a chief residency, so he went to Vanderbilt as their first Surgical Chief Resident and subsequently a faculty member. While there he had attempted (unsuccessfully) to produce pulmonary arteriosclerosis in animals by anastomosing the subclavian artery to the pulmonary artery. When Dr. Taussig approached Dr. Blalock with her idea of creating a ductus to treat tetralogy, Blalock's old experimental procedure came to mind. He then spent 2 years perfecting the operation in the laboratory and testing it in a cyanotic animal model before he was ready to attempt it in a patient

* For an interesting analysis of the reasons for the delay in development of an operation for coarctation and the competition between Robert Gross and Clarence Crafoord, see the article by Dobell (90).

in the fall of 1944. Much of the laboratory work was done by his Afro-American research associate, Vivan Thomas. The first clinical attempt was a success, and in the following year 55 patients underwent the Blalock-Taussig operation, with a mortality rate of 20%. By the end of 1950, they had operated on 1,037 patients, and the mortality rate had fallen to less than 5% (93).*

The first Blalock-Taussig operation was followed 2 years later by the side-to-side descending aorta-to-pulmonary artery anastomosis, performed by Willis J. Potts at the Children's Memorial Hospital in Chicago on September 13, 1946 (16), and the next year by closed pulmonary valvotomy, by T. Holmes Sellors on December 4, 1947 (17), and Russell C. Brock on February 16, 1948 (96), both in London.

Finally, the successful closed treatment of mitral stenosis (closed mitral commissurotomy) was accomplished in 1948—after a latency of about 23 years since the work of Cutler, Allen, and Souttar and 46 years since Sir Lauder Brunton's suggestion was so soundly rejected. The year began with the efforts of H.G. Smithy of Charleston, South Carolina, who performed closed partial mitral valvulectomy (the old Cutler procedure) to palliate mitral stenosis in seven patients between January 30 and June 14, 1948, with five survivors, three of whom improved (97).† On June 10, 1948, after four unsuccessful attempts (the fourth earlier that same day in another hospital), Charles P. Bailey of Philadelphia first successfully incised (with a blade) the fused commissure (and hence the term "mitral commissurotomy"); the female patient did so well that 1 week later he had her travel 1,000 miles by train to be presented at a meeting of the American College of Chest Physicians (19), and she remained well for the next 38 years (98). Dwight Harken, then at Tufts College Medical School in Boston, probably emboldened by his experience of removal of 96 foreign bodies from the heart during World War II (99), successfully incised (with a valvulatome) the commissures of a patient only 6 days later, on June 16, 1948 (20).‡ Six of his first 10 patients died and he almost abandoned the procedure, but his cardiology colleague, Dr. L.B. Ellis, encouraged him to continue, and 14 of the next 15 survived (100). On September 16, 1948, R.C. Brock of Guys Hospital in London successfully accomplished a closed mitral commissurotomy using Souttars' original transatrial finger dilitation technique (101). This became the preferred method until Andrew Logan of Edinburgh introduced the use of the transventricular dilator (Tubbs) in 1954 (102). Logan's method was rapidly adopted as the preferred method of closed mitral commissurotomy and was commonly practiced (including by the author) until the late 1960s and early 1970s, at which time open mitral commissurotomy (i.e., on cardiopulmonary bypass) largely replaced the closed techniques. Transventricular mechanical dilitation was the immediate ancestor of transcatheter balloon dilitation of the mitral valve, which was introduced in the 1980s.*

* For personal recollections of this momentous advance see the articles by Blalock (94) and Taussig (95). For a brief biography of Helen Taussig and her contribution to this operation, see the chapter by Nuland (93).

† It is ironic that Smithy's career abruptly ended later that same year, when he died of aortic stenosis on October 28th at the age of 36 (12).

‡ Perhaps Dr. Harken may be excused if, 41 years later and at the age of 79, he incorrectly stated in his personal recollections the dates of his and Bailey's first successful mitral valve operations (100).

* For a more thorough review of the early history of mitral valve surgery, see the chapter in the book by F. Henry Ellis Jr., (88).

1952–1955: Open Heart Surgery Accomplished

Open heart surgery had not yet been successfully accomplished by the start of 1952. However, on April 15 of that year, Robert E. Gross at the Boston Children's Hospital successfully used his "atrial well" technique to close an atrial septal defect (ASD) (26). This ingenious technique consisted of sewing a soft, plastic, funnel-like device onto the wall of the right atrium, which was then entered. The surgeon was then able to digitally explore the atrial structures and perform a surgical repair working beneath the layer of blood in the well. This method precluded direct vision but in clever hands permitted remarkable results. Using this technique in 1954, Dr. John Kirklin at the Mayo Clinic successfully corrected a partial common atrioventricular (AV) canal (combined atrial and ventricular septal defects) (103).

On September 2, 1952, John F. Lewis and colleagues at the University of Minnesota successfully closed an ASD under direct vision during 5.5 minutes of circulatory arrest (caval inflow occlusion) permitted by moderate surface-induced hypothermia (26°C) (27). By February of 1954 they had used this method 11 times with only 2 deaths; 1 was a patient with a primum ASD who developed surgical complete heart block for which no therapy was then available (104). [Lillehei and colleagues at the University of Minnesota first used an epicardial electrical pacemaker to treat this complication on January 30, 1957 (54).] Henry Swan and colleagues at the University of Colorado also starting using hypothermia and brief periods of circulatory arrest and accomplished open repair of both valvular or infundibular pulmonic stenosis and ASD in 12 patients between February 19 and July 9, 1953, with only one death (105). This method, although it continued to be used for several years for surgical repair of these defects, had the obvious time limitation of about 8 to 10 minutes. There remained the need for a heart-lung machine to support the patient and permit the surgeon time to accomplish complex intracardiac repairs under direct vision. This leads to the remarkable story of John H. Gibbon Jr.*

On October 3, 1930,† during a 1-year surgical research fellowship (immediately after his internship) at the Massachusetts General Hospital under Dr. Edward D. Churchill (studying an animal model of pulmonary embolism), Dr. Gibbon was assigned the task of monitoring a young woman who had suffered a massive pulmonary embolism after a cholecystectomy. The patient was transferred to the operating room, where she was to be observed until she had deteriorated sufficiently to justify an attempt to perform a Trendelenburg operation (closed pulmonary embolectomy). He watched her all night. While observing her distended veins and cyanosis, it occurred to Dr. Gibbon that if he could only remove her venous blood, bypass her heart and lungs, oxygenate the blood and return it to her arterial system, she could be saved. But such technology did not exist, and the patient did not recover from the pulmonary embolectomy that was performed the following morning. Based on this experience, Dr. Gibbon made up his mind to try to develop a heart-lung machine. Over the next 3 years he reviewed previous work in this field and discussed his ambition with numerous colleagues, but no one seemed interested and most experts doubted its feasibility. However, he was not to be discouraged. He obtained a second year of research fellowship with Dr. Churchill in 1934–1935 and, together with his new wife Mary, who had been Dr. Churchill's research assistant, built a heart-lung machine. By the end of the year, they had supported cats for up to 171 minutes of total cardiopulmonary bypass (CPB) (89). He continued his research at the University of Pennsylvania and by 1939 was able to report long-term survivors among cats subjected to total CPB for 10 to 20 minutes (109). Despite interruption by 4 years of military service in World War II and continued skepticism by the medical community, Dr. Gibbon continued his work, now in collaboration with International Business Machines Corporation (IBM), and by the end of 1952 he had developed a heart-lung machine that featured a vertical screen oxygenator and was capable of supporting a human; with this machine he achieved almost 90% survival in dogs (110). Dr. Gibbon first used this heart-lung machine clinically in a 15-month-old child in February 1952, but she died during surgery because she had an undiagnosed PDA instead of the anticipated ASD. However, the next patient, an 18-year-old operated on May 6, 1953, had her ASD successfully closed during 26 minutes of full bypass and 45 minutes of total bypass (29,107,108). Thus after 23 years Dr. Gibbon achieved the goal he first conceived as a resident physician—a goal that had eluded many others. [It is intriguing that just 11 days earlier (April 25, 1953) another monumental development of the 20th century in biomedical science, the description of a proposed structure of DNA (the double helix), was announced by Watson and Crick (74).] Unfortunately, his next two patients, children $5\frac{1}{2}$ years old with ASD operated on in July of that year, both died—one of cardiac arrest before cannulation and the other of unsuspected coexisting ventricular septal defect (VSD) and PDA resulting in excessive blood in the field.* Dr. Gibbon declared a moratorium on further use of his heart-lung machine. The fact that none of the other 12 attempts by five other groups to use total CPB up until this time had succeeded (111) tended to reinforce the attitude of hopelessness.

On March 26, 1954, however, C. Walton Lillehei and his colleagues at the University of Minnesota initiated a remarkable series of direct-vision intracardiac surgery with total CPB using the patient's parent as the "heart-lung machine" (so-called controlled cross-circulation, in which the parent's femoral artery and vein were connected to the patient's arterial and venous system respectively (Fig. 1-1). Between March 1954 and July 1955, 45 patients were operated on using controlled cross-circulation—including 27 patients with VSD, 10 with tetralogy of Fallot, and 5 with AV canal—with 28 survivors (111,112). In his discussion of the report of the first eight VSDs he had closed using cross-circulation Lillehei stated, "The demonstration that right ventricular cardiotomy and septal suture can be successfully performed even in seriously ill patients should dispel much of the discouragement previously prevalent in this field and stimulate further rapid developments in the application of direct vision intracardiac corrective surgery to congenital and acquired cardiac pathology" (31). Lillehei had clearly demonstrated the potential for CPB to permit major open heart surgery once a satisfactory artificial heart-lung machine was available to skillful cardiac surgical teams.

This occurred at the Mayo Clinic (90 miles south of the University of Minnesota). There, under the leadership of John W. Kirklin, the first successful series of patients to undergo intracardiac surgery with the aid of a mechanical pump oxygenator (eight patients, four survivors) was undertaken between March and May of 1955; the heart-lung machine was a Mayo modification of the Gibbon-IBM

* For a biography of John Gibbon and a detailed review of his development of the heart-lung machine, see the book by Romaine-Davis (106).

† This is the date stated by Gibbon's biographer, A. Romaine-Davis (106). Dr. Gibbon, in an historical review published in 1970 (107) and another submitted in 1973 (108), places this event in February of 1931.

* Cardiac surgeons soon learned that an unsuspected patent ductus would cause excessive blood flow into the field during CPB, and they began to routinely look for its presence (and ligate it if present) before proceeding to CPB. This problem can be encountered during adult noncongenital surgery and should be suspected with increased blood return to the left side of the heart (see Chapter 12).

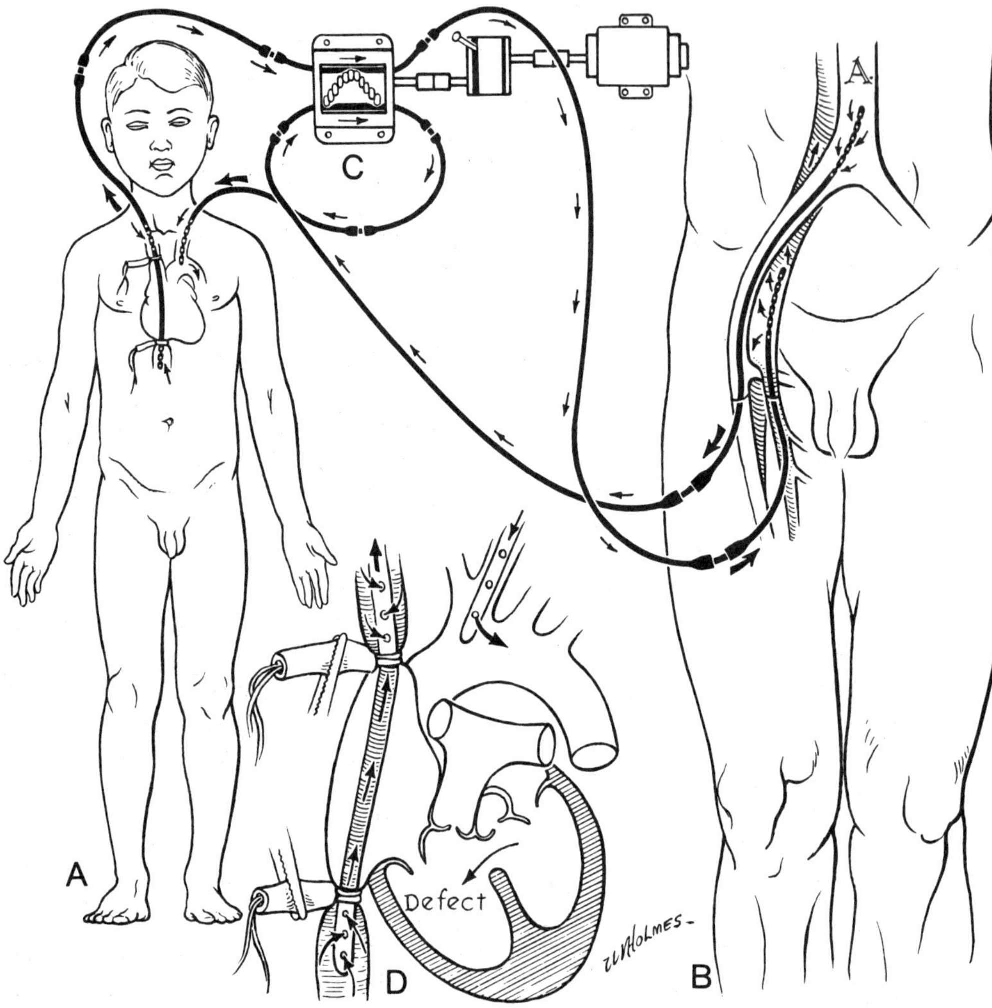

FIGURE 1-1. A depiction of the method of direct-vision intracardiac surgery using extracorporeal circulation by means of controlled cross-circulation used by C. W. Lillehei and his team at the University of Minnesota in 1954 and 1955. **A:** The patient, showing sites of arterial and venous cannulations. **B:** The donor, showing sites of arterial and venous (superficial femoral and great saphenous) cannulations. **C:** The single Sigmamotor pump controlling precisely the reciprocal exchange of blood between the patient and donor. **D:** Close-up of the patient's heart, showing the vena caval catheter positioned to draw venous blood from both the superior and inferior venae cavae during the cardiac bypass interval. The arterial blood from the donor was circulated to the patient's body through the catheter that was inserted into the left subclavian artery. [From Gravelee GP, Davis RF, Utley JR, eds. *Cardiopulmonary bypass: principles and practice.* Baltimore: Williams & Wilkins, 1993: 10 (Fig. 1.2) with permission.]

model, the plans for which had been generously provided by Dr. Gibbon (32).* This was followed by a series of seven cases done by Lillehei at the University of Minnesota (with five survivors), using a simple heart-lung machine of their own design employing a DeWall Bubble Oxygenator, between May 13 and August 9, 1955 (114).† By the fall of that year these two institutions were regularly performing open heart surgery with mechanical heart-lung machines: Kirklin's group had done 40 cases, with 93% survival among their last 14 VSDs (116), and Lillehei's group had done 36 cases with 89% survival in their last 19 cases (114)! Over the span of 4 years the puzzle of open heart surgery had been solved, and many groups followed the next year.*

* For a personal perspective on the beginning of open heart surgery at the Mayo Clinic, see the article by John Kirklin (113).

† For a personal perspective on the beginning of open heart surgery at the University of Minnesota, see the Chapter by C. Walton Lillehei (111) and the article by Warden (115).

* Others have more thoroughly reviewed the early history of the development of CPB (11,12,107,108,111,117–122); Senning has reviewed its development in Stockholm (123) and Cooley its development in Houston (124).

Comroe and Dripps (125) identified 25 bodies of knowledge that were required for the full development of open heart surgery.

As a footnote to the history of the development of the heart-lung machine, it is of interest to note that the first successful use of the machine to perform a pulmonary embolectomy was by Edward Sharp of Johns Hopkins Hospital (on February 17, 1961) and by Denton Cooley in Houston (on April 16, 1961), almost exactly 30 years after John Gibbon first set out to accomplish this goal (11).

In the last half of the 1950s, many groups initiated open heart programs employing CPB, mainly to treat congenital heart disease. A number of important developments occurred. Initially most open heart surgery was performed through a transverse sternotomy bilateral anterior thoracotomy with arterial cannulation of the subclavian artery. By the end of the decade, median sternotomy (55,56) and femoral artery cannulation (56) had replaced earlier approaches. (Why direct cannulation of the ascending aorta was avoided for another 15 years is not obvious). In 1957, Lillehei's group introduced temporary epicardial pacemaking to treat surgical heart block (54). In that same year, Sealy and others (57) introduced moderate hypothermia (approximately 30°C) produced by an efficient heat exchanger as an adjunct to CPB, initially to improve tolerance to low flows. Hypothermia was subsequently adopted by most teams to improve safety of organ preservation and tolerance of hemodilution. In 1959, Charles Drew of London introduced the technique of deep hypothermic (approximately 15°C) circulatory arrest (58).* This was not widely adopted at the time but was reintroduced by David Dillard et al. at the University of Washington and by Brian Barratt-Boyes in Aukland, New Zealand, in the middle and late 1960s for facilitating infant heart surgery, and by Randall Griepp of New York in 1975 for conducting aortic arch surgery. At the end of this decade, Mason Sones at the Cleveland Clinic first accomplished selective coronary angiography (75)—an innovation that would have profound impact on the future of adult cardiac surgery.

The practice of surgery had been affected so greatly by the developments in cardiac surgery that in July 1959, "recognizing the great advances in cardiac surgery," the title of the *Journal of Thoracic Surgery* was changed to the *Journal of Thoracic and Cardiovascular Surgery.*

1960–1970: Open Heart Surgery for Acquired Heart Disease—Prosthetic Heart Valves, Coronary Artery Bypass Surgery, Heart Transplantation

Although many ingenious palliative or reparative procedures for valvular heart disease had been introduced, for many patients a replacement device was needed. Many different devices were introduced with limited success. Even though moderately good short-term success was achieved with aortic valve replacement with prosthetic trileaflet valves (often made of uncoated or coated Teflon fabric or of silicone rubber) that imitated the natural valve, these usually failed after 1 to 2 years. The path to success was initiated by Dwight Harken in 1960 when he successfully replaced the aortic valve in two patients with a caged ball prosthesis implanted in the subcoronary position (35,127) and by Albert Starr of the University of Oregon, who successfully replaced the mitral valve in six of eight patients with a caged ball prosthetic valve between August 1960 and February 1961 (36). This valve was codeveloped with a retired engineer, M. Lowell Edwards (who had come to Dr. Starr in 1958 with a proposal to develop an implantable artificial heart, but who accepted the challenge to start on one valve at a time and ended up with his famous medical products company). Starr and Edwards then developed a caged ball aortic prosthesis featuring a flexible fixation (sewing) ring, which Dr. Starr successfully implanted in eight of ten patients between March and September of 1962 (128). For many years these Starr-Edwards valves were favored by many surgeons and were the standard against which subsequent valves were compared, having been implanted in more than 175,000 patients (12).

Dwight McGoon and his colleagues at the Mayo Clinic provided evidence of the steep learning curve and rapid and dramatic improvement of results with prosthetic replacement of the aortic valve. Their hospital survival rate increased from 45% in 1960 to 85% in mid-1963 (129) and achieved 100% in the first 100 patients in whom they implanted a Starr-Edwards valve in 1963 and 1964 (130)!

Other approaches to valve replacement were introduced but did not receive wide acceptance at the time. Unstented homograft aortic valves were first implanted in the subcoronary position by Donald Ross of London in July 1962 (131) and by Brian Barratt-Boyes of Auckland in August of that same year (132), and Ross introduced his pulmonary autograft procedure (in which the patient's own pulmonary valve was implanted in the subcoronary position of the aortic valve and the pulmonary valve is replaced with a homograft) in 1967 (133).*

A second great breakthrough of the 1960s was the introduction in 1967 of coronary artery bypass grafting (CABG), initially mainly using saphenous vein aortocoronary autografts. This was the first truly effective surgical treatment of coronary artery disease. Innumerable indirect operations had been developed to treat this disease and subsequently discarded because of minimal benefit, beginning with cervical sympathectomy by Jonnesco in 1916 and including the various operations devised by the American Claude Beck

* For an interesting review of Charles Drew and his development of deep hypothermic circulatory arrest, see the article by Dobell (126).

* For a more through review of the development of cardiac valve prostheses, see the book by Lefrak and Starr (134).

between 1935 and 1948 (epicardial abrasion, cardiomyopexy, coronary sinus occlusion, and arterialization of the coronary sinus with a vein graft attached to the descending aorta).*

One of the less rational procedures was bilateral internal mammary artery (IMA) ligation, originated by Fieschi, Zoja, Casa-Bianchi, Battezzati, and others in Italy (11) and popularized in the United States by Glover in the late 1950s. This procedure was laid to rest in 1959 by the negative results of one of the first prospective double-blind clinical studies of a surgical procedure conducted by the group at the University of Washington (136).

The most used indirect technique for treating ischemic heart disease in the early 1960s was implantation of the IMA into the myocardium, a procedure developed by Arthur M. Vineberg of McGill University in Montreal. In 1946 Vineberg demonstrated development of anastomoses between the implanted IMA and the coronary arteries in dogs (137), and in November 1950 he successfully applied this procedure in a human (22). In 1958 he reported his results in 57 patients (138). However, few paid much attention until Sones in 1962 demonstrated, with angiography, coronary collateralization via IMA implants that had been placed 5 to 7 years previously in two patients (139). This led to the widespread application of the procedure. By 1968, the Cleveland Clinic had reported their results in 1,100 patients. An estimated 10,000 to 15,000 IMA implant operations had been performed by 1975, when the procedure was largely abandoned for the bypass procedure without ever having its efficacy conclusively resolved (140–142).

Direct coronary artery surgery in humans began with the performance of coronary endarterectomy by Charles Bailey in October 1956 and by William Longmire and colleagues at the University of California, Los Angeles, in December 1957 (11). In 1963 Effler, at the Cleveland Clinic, modified the technique by eliminating the endarterectomy and simply opening over the stenosis ("endarterotomy") and applying a pericardial patch graft. The Cleveland Clinic used this operation in more than 140 patients between 1962 and 1967 (143). The revolution in direct coronary artery surgery began, however, in May 1967, when Rene Favaloro at the Cleveland Clinic first interposed a segment of saphenous vein (end-to-end and end-to-end) to relieve a stenotic right coronary artery and, before the end of that year, performed his first aortocoronary bypass graft to the right coronary artery (38,144).† In 1968, three other groups began to do this procedure—Kerth and colleagues in San Francisco, Urchell and colleagues in Dallas, and W. Dudley Johnson and colleagues in Milwaukee* (135). However, it was perhaps the presentation of Johnson in the spring of 1969 (40) that had the greatest impact on the widespread use of CABG using the saphenous vein. He suggested and demonstrated that CABG was applicable to most patients with coronary artery disease by placing multiple grafts distal to all disease and targeting the left anterior descending artery, branches of the circumflex, and the posterior descending coronary arteries in addition to the right coronary artery. He emphasized the use of CPB and intermittent aortic cross-clamping (15 minutes or less) to provide a dry, quiet field (40). These concepts revolutionized direct coronary artery surgery. In his prophetic discussion of Johnson's paper, Dr. Frank Spencer stated, "We may have heard a milestone in cardiac surgery today, because for years pathologists, cardiologists and many surgeons have repeatedly stated that the pattern of coronary artery disease is so extensive that direct anastomosis can be done in only 5 to 7 percent of patients. If the exciting data by Dr. Johnson remains valid . . . a total revision of our thinking will be required regarding the feasibility of direct arterial surgery for coronary artery disease" (40). Before the end of the decade more than 180 surgeons were doing CABG, and during the next few years the number of such procedures increased at a rate of 25% to 50% per year, to 54,000 cases in 1975 (135).

In this same decade (1960s), an alternative graft was proposed for CABG, namely the IMA, usually used to anastomose into the left anterior descending coronary artery. This grafting was first successfully accomplished by RH Goetz et al., in the Bronx on May 21, 1960 (146) (without apparent further application), and then by Kolessov of Leningrad in 1964 (147) and Bailey et al. and Read et al. in 1968 (148). Interestingly, Kolessov performed his anastomosis *off-bypass* via a left thoracotomy, employed a 6- to 8-minute period of *trial occlusion* before isolating a segment of the coronary artery for performing the anastamosis, and *administered sublingual nitroglycerin* to his patients every 0.5 to 1 hour intraoperatively and postoperatively to prevent coronary artery spasm (149). After he presented his initial series (five of his first six patients survived) at the Cardiology Society plenum in Leningrad, the plenum adopted the resolution that "the surgical treatment for coronary artery disease was impossible and had no future" (147).

Despite these earlier efforts, it was primarily George E. Green of New York University who championed the use of

* See a catalogue of these various procedures in Table 1 on page 2 in the review by Miller (135).

† An unsuccessful saphenous vein aortocoronary bypass grafting had been done by Sabiston in 1962, and successful grafts had been placed by Garrett and DeBakey in 1964 and by Kahn in 1966, but these were not reported until the 1970s (135) and had no impact on the introduction of CABG surgery.

* Johnson stated that he did his first aortocoronary saphenous vein graft in January 1968, after hearing of the work at Cleveland Clinic (145). Unlike the latter group, which initially did an end-to-end anastomosis between the saphenous vein and the distal coronary artery, Dr Johnson used an end-to-side anastomosis to the distal coronary artery, a technique that was subsequently adopted by the Cleveland Clinic group and most other surgeons.

the IMA graft in the United States. He emphasized the use of CPB and operating on the vented, fibrillating heart, sometimes arrested by aortic cross-clamping and administration of cold (lactated Ringer's solution) cardioplegia. He routinely used high magnification (16×) (41,150). (Interestingly, he never acknowledged the experimental or clinical work of others). Nevertheless, regarding the use of the IMA, Favaloro stated in 1970 that "It is highly doubtful that full clinical application of this procedure will reach a large scale" (139), and most other surgeons discounted or ignored this procedure because it was considered too difficult to perform, the IMA was considered to carry inadequate blood flow, or the operation was thought to be unnecessary. One who immediately recognized its potential, however, was another young surgeon at the Cleveland Clinic, Floyd Loop, who by late 1971 began to use the IMA (but without use of magnification) in significant numbers of patients [Loop, discussion of Green, 1972 (150)].

By 1980, fewer than 15% of surgeons used the IMA (151). This all changed in the mid-1980s, largely because of the long-term follow-up data provided by Loop and his colleagues at the Cleveland Clinic, who documented the dramatically improved patency of the IMA compared with the saphenous vein, especially beyond 5 years (152), as well as improved clinical outcome (153). By the end of that decade (1980s), most surgeons followed Loop's admonition that most patients with left anterior descending artery stenosis should receive an IMA graft whenever technically feasible (153).*

A third great landmark in cardiac surgery in the 1960s occurred on December 3, 1967, when Christiaan Barnard of Capetown, South Africa, performed the first human to human heart transplantation, described in the report on "The Operation," published in the December 30, 1967, issue of the *South African Medical Journal* (39). Unfortunately, the patient died 18 days after the operation. This accomplishment was the culmination of research that began with Alexis Carrel, the "father of vascular surgery" and 1912 Nobel laureate, who performed the first heterotopic heart tansplantation of a puppy's heart into an adult dog's neck. Further development involved many other researchers but especially the group at Stanford under Norman Shumway, who had achieved the first long-term survival (21 to 250 days) of dogs after orthotopically implanted homograft hearts. On January 6, 1968, Shumway's group did their first (and the world's fourth) human-to-human heart transplantation, following up on their extensive research program and initiating their remarkable innovative clinical program in heart transplantation. With inappropriate euphoria about 102 cardiac transplantation operations were performed during the next year by about 60 different teams in 20 countries (154,155). Most patients died as a result of the poorly understood problems of rejection and infection, and the procedure was abandoned by most groups, leaving predominately the Stanford group (Shumway) and a few others—LePetie Hospital in Paris (Cabrol), Grote Schurr Hospital in Capetown (Barnard), and Medical College of Virginia in Richmond (Lower)—to carry on this experiment. It is noteworthy that Shumway, Cabrol, and Barnard had all studied under Lillehei at the University of Minnesota, and Lower had been a trainee of Shumway.*

Although the decade of the 1960s was marked by great strides in adult cardiac surgery, notable advances were also made in the treatment of congenital heart disease. An effective and readily applicable operation for transposition of the great arteries (TGA) was accomplished by William T. Mustard at the Hospital for Sick Children in Toronto on May 16, 1963 (interatrial venous transposition using a pericardial baffle, the so-called Mustard operation) (37). This work was the culmination of a career-long devotion of Dr. Mustard to achieving surgical correction of TGA. After extensive experimental work, in 1952 he attempted to treat TGA with a modified arterial switch operation (leaving the right coronary artery connected to the pulmonary artery) in seven children, using CPB employing a biologic (monkey lung) extracorporeal oxygenator (161). Unfortunately, none survived more than a few hours. This work had been preceded by the development of a palliative procedure for these babies (closed creation of ASD to improve mixing of pulmonary and systemic blood and, hence, improve systemic oxygenation) by Drs. Alfred Blalock and C. Rollins Hanlon of Johns Hopkins Hospital in 1948 (18). In 1957, K. Alvin Merendino at the University of Washington in Seattle almost succeeded in correcting TGA by conceiving of and applying the procedure of total interatrial venous transposition using a baffle made of compressed Ivalon sponge. One patient, operated on March 28, 1957, was alert and talking 3 hours after the operation when she suddenly became apneic, presumably from an air embolism, and died. This operation, except for the material used to construct the baffle, was identical to the subsequent Mustard procedure (162). In 1958, Ake Senning of Stockholm successfully corrected TGA in one of four children with his complex atrial correction using autologous (atrial) tissue (so called Senning operation) (34). Few surgeons could duplicate his success, whereas the Mustard procedure was readily accepted and successful in the hands of many surgeons. However, this procedure was usually done after 6 months to 2 years of age because of the high morbidity and mortality of neonatal surgery in that era, so it was usually preceded by a Blalock-Hanlon procedure. The latter was made obsolete in 1966 by William J. Rashkind of the Children's Hospital of Phila-

* Others have more thoroughly reviewed the history of the surgical management of coronary artery disease (8,135,144,147,148).

* Others have more thoroughly reviewed the history of cardiac transplantation (156–160).

delphia with his balloon septostomy, the beginning of transcatheter or interventional cardiology (79).

In 1965–1967, Drs. David Dillard, K. Alvin Merendino, and Hitoshi Mohri at the University of Washington in Seattle introduced the technique of deep hypothermic (less than 20°C) circulatory arrest using surface cooling and warming without a pump oxygenator for conducting complex operations (e.g., total correction of total anomalous pulmonary venous return, AV canal, and TGA) in infants (60,163). The technique of Horiuchi et al. (164) of Sendi, Japan, had been introduced to the Seattle group by a surgical research fellow from Sendi, Dr. Ichiro Matano, who was working in their laboratory. The Seattle group, under the leadership of another research fellow from Sendi, Dr. Mohri, then modified the technique to permit deeper levels of hypothermia (less than 20°C) and longer duration of circulatory arrest (1 hour), allowing complex surgery (163,165). Deep hypothermic circulatory arrest became a mainstay of complex neonatal surgery for many years and is still practiced in some cases today. However, the pure surface technique of the Seattle group was not readily accepted, and deep hypothermic circulatory arrest did not become common practice until Brian Barratt-Boyes of Aukland, New Zealand, introduced his method in 1969–1970. Barratt-Boyes employed terminal perfusion cooling and rewarming with a pump-oxygenator (166). This also was a modification of a Japanese method of Hikasa et al. of Kyoto (167), and again it was introduced to Barratt-Boyes by visiting Japanese surgeons working in his unit in Aukland.

In the 1960s, CPB became common practice in many hospitals worldwide. Initially many employed Sigmamotor finger pumps, but these were quickly replaced with roller pumps, used by Michael DeBakey for transfusion of blood in 1934. Many employed homemade bubble oxygenators of their own design or copied from DeWall's design (114). In the late 1950s and early 1960s, the rotating disc oxygenator developed by Earle Kay and Fredrick Cross of Cleveland (168) became widely used, but it was subsequently displaced in many centers by unitized plastic disposable bubble oxygenators, such as the Travenol Mini Prime developed by Vincent Gott et al. at the University of Minnesota in 1957 (169), and later by hard shell bubble oxygenators with integral heat exchangers, such as the Bently Temprol Bubble Oxygenator developed by Richard DeWall et al. (170).

In this same decade some other "nonsurgical" developments occurred that were to have a major impact on the practice of cardiovascular medicine. On July 9, 1960, William B. Kouenhaven, a retired electrical engineer, and his colleagues at Johns Hopkins University introduced closed-chest cardiac massage (77). [They discovered the technique serendipitously when they observed an elevation in arterial pressure after the application of external defibrillator paddles to dogs (145)]. On June 6, 1960, William M. Chardack and Wilson Greatbatch, an engineer, implanted the first totally implantable, long-term, battery-powered pacemaking system (76). The unit was subsequently manufactured by Medtronic of Minneapolis. The leads were initially placed epicardially via a thoracotomy, but soon they were placed transvenously, following the work of Parsonet et al. (171) and Siddons et al. (172). The early pacemakers were asynchronous and were used exclusively to treat complete heart block. In 1966, Victor Parsonett et al. of Newark, New Jersey, described implantation of the first implantable R-wave inhibited demand pacemaking system (173). In 1965, Myron Wheat Jr. of Gainesville, Florida, introduced his nonsurgical management of dissecting aortic aneurysm using "anti-impulse" and antihyhypertensive therapy with the use of the antiadrenergic drugs trimethaphan, reserpine, and guanethidine (78). The idea germinated from information communicated to him by colleagues in the Departments of Pharmacology and Veterinary Science, who told him that certain flocks of turkeys were plagued by dissecting aneurysms and that the incidence of this poultry industry problem had been dramatically reduced by the addition of reserpine to the turkeys' feed (78,145).

In June 1967, Adrian Kantrowitz of Brooklyn, New York, first successfully treated a patient with cardiogenic shock with an IABP (80,174). Fifteen years earlier Kantrowitz and his brother Arthur, an engineer, had first introduced the concepts later to be known as "counterpulsation," and in 1961 Spyridon Moulopoulos, Steven Topaz (an engineer), and Willem Kolff of the Cleveland Clinic had conceived of accomplishing this with an IABP (175). Kantrowitz was the first to use it successfully clinically and then to report his dramatic results in a series of 27 patients (174). This was the first successful circulatory assist device, and it was rapidly adopted into the practice of cardiovascular medicine and surgery, where it continues to be applied to this day.*

1970–1980: More Advances

Cardiac surgery was maturing in the 1970s. Perhaps the most notable advance was the introduction of cold potassium cardioplegia and its rapid and widespread acceptance and application in daily practice. In the United States this innovation is commonly attributed to William Gay Jr. and Paul Ebert (62), although numerous workers in many countries were involved in the development and modification of cardioplegia techniques. Although the use of higher concentrations of potassium to *induce cardiac arrest* were first proposed and used by Melrose, Sealy and Young, and others in the 1950s, the concept of administering much lower concentrations of potassium added to ice-cold electrolyte solu-

* For a more detailed history of the IABP, see the chapter by Dehmer et al. (175).

tions in large quantities to not only induce arrest but *preserve myocardial function* was largely novel and quickly replaced other more cumbersome or less reliable techniques. The latter included ischemic arrest (which led to the discovery of ischemic contracture, the so called "stone heart"), topical hypothermia, and continuous coronary perfusion with blood (so effectively practiced by McGoon and his colleagues at Mayo Clinic). An illustration of the explosive acceptance of cold potassium cardioplegia is that in 1975 fewer than 6% of surgeons were using it during CABG, whereas by 1980 almost 92% were employing it (151).*

With improved CPB technology and increased use of deep hypothermic circulatory arrest, infant and neonatal surgery became more successful. In 1975 both Adib Jatene in Sao Paulo (May 8, 1975) (43) and M.H. Yacoub in London (October 30, 1975) (180), apparently independently, succeeded with the anatomic correction ("arterial switch") of transposition of the great vessels, and over the next 10 years this procedure gradually replaced Mustard's operation. The successful implementation of the arterial switch operation was made possible by the application of deep hypothermic circulatory arrest, surgical experience with microvascular techniques that grew out of the development of CABG, the introduction of optical magnification, and the availability of fine monofilament suture material (e.g., Prolene). In the latter part of the same decade, William Norwood of the Boston Children's Hospital developed and successfully applied the first stage of his innovative approach to the problem of hypoplastic left heart syndrome (44). However, one of the most important advances in neonatal cardiac surgery was nonsurgical: the introduction in 1976 by Peter Olley et al., of the Hospital for Sick Children in Toronto, of the use of prostaglandin infusions to maintain the patency of the PDA and, hence, improve oxygenation in neonates with ductal-dependent cyanotic heart disease (66). This largely eliminated the need to emergency cardiac surgery, but more importantly it greatly improved the physiologic condition of these infants when they did come to the operating room (just as had Rashkind's balloon septostomy a decade earlier). This pharmacologic therapy also led to the realization of Helen Taussig's thoughts of 40 years before, that if a method to "prevent the closure of the ductus" could be found "it would be a benefit to cyanotic infants" (95); in that earlier time, she was forced to simply urge her surgical colleagues to create a new ductus.

Notable innovations in prosthetic valves occurred during this decade (134). In the early 1970s, Viking Bjork of Sweden introduced his tilting disc prosthesis (181,182), which became very popular until it was largely supplanted by the St. Jude bileaflet (pyrolytic carbon) valve, which was first implanted the late 1970s and began to be widely used in the 1980s (183). Stent-mounted, glutaraldehyde-preserved heterograft (porcine) valves developed by Alain Carpentier of Paris in the late 1960s became available in the 1970s, first produced commercially by Warren Hancock (184), and bioprotheses began to compete successfully with mechanical valves. In 1976 Shiley laboratories began producing Marion Ionescu's stented valve, which was constructed from glutaraldehyde-preserved bovine pericardium (185).

Two other important innovations of the 1970s that had significant impact on cardiac surgery (and anesthesiology) were nonsurgical. The first occurred in 1970, when H.J.C. Swan, William Ganz, and colleagues at the Cedars-Sinai Medical Center in Los Angeles introduced their balloon-tipped flow-directed PAC (developed in association with and supplied by Lowell Edwards' company) (61). The second was announced in a one-page letter to the editor of *The Lancet* on February 4, 1978, from Andreas Gruntzig of Zurich, who described the first five successful procedures of transluminal dilitation of coronary artery stenosis (percutaneous transluminal coronary angioplasty, or PTCA), performed between September 16–December 20, 1977 (81). As is said, "the rest is history."

Substantial progress in CPB technology was made in the 1970s. Highly efficient, disposable hard shell bubble oxygenators with integrated heat exchangers were introduced by several different manufacturers, including Bently, Harvey, Shiley, and Cobe. Clinically effective disposable membrane oxygenators were introduced by Lande (Edwards Laboratory) and by Kolobow (Sci Med) in the early 1970s, but they were mainly relegated to use in extracorporeal membrane oxygenation (ECMO) to treat respiratory failure. In about 1975, the use of membrane oxygenators for CPB received a boost with the introduction of microporous polypropylene membranes (e.g., Travenol TMO), but by the end of the decade membrane oxygenators were being used in fewer than 20% of cases (186). Microembolization during CPB became recognized as a potentially significant problem, and with it came the introduction of microfiltration. However, one of the most important innovations in CPB technique in this decade was brought about by two papers published in 1975 by Brian Bull (a pathologist) and his colleagues at Loma Linda University in California, who pointed out the limitations of existing heparin protocols and advocated the use of an objective monitor of heparin effect (and its reversal by protamine): the activated clotting time (64,65). Until that time heparin had been administered by various dosing schedules based on the patient's weight and duration of CPB without any monitoring of its effectiveness! Bull's recommendation was quickly adopted by many cardiac surgical teams, and by the end of the decade most used some type of objective monitoring and control of heparinization.

* Others have more thoroughly reviewed the history of cardioplegia and given appropriate credit to the many other contributors to this major change in the conduct of cardiac surgery (176–179).

1980–1990: Cardiac Transplantation Comes of Age, The Pathophysiology of Cardiopulmonary Bypass, Internal Mammary Artery Grafts

Throughout the 1970s only about 30 heart transplantation operations were being performed per year, and many of these were done at Stanford with new innovations and improved results (187). In 1973 the Stanford team introduced transvenous endomyocardial biopsy (63), which greatly improved the accuracy of diagnosis and hence the treatment of rejection. Between 1968 and 1978 the 1-year survival rate among their heart transplantation patients rose from 22% to 65% (157). In 1970, soil samples from the Hardanger Vidda region of Norway were sent to the Sandoz Laboratories, from which the fungus *Tolypocladium inflatum* was isolated. It produced metabolites with weak antifungal properties, but in 1972 Jean-Francois Borel determined that one extract had potent immunosuppressive properties. This was cyclosporin A, the first agent to act selectively on lymphocytes (159). After encouraging results in experimental heart transplantation, the Stanford group began using cyclosporin clinically in December 1980 (67). Between 1980 and 1985 their 1-year survival rate after heart transplantation increased from 63% to 83%, and the 3-year survival rate climbed from 52% to 70%.* This led to a renewed interest in cardiac transplantation, and in 1981 more than 100 such operations were done in a single year, for the first time since 1968. By 1985 ten times that many were done, and by the end of the decade more than 2,400 were performed in a single year worldwide, in more than 200 centers (189). On March 9, 1981, the Stanford group performed the first successful heart-lung transplantation (190); on November 1, 1984, Denton Cooley of Houston performed the first infant (8-month-old) heart transplantation (46); and 1 year later on November 20, 1985, Leonard Bailey of Loma Linda University in California performed the first successful heart transplantation in a neonate (4 days old) (47).

Previously mentioned developments in the 1970s (i.e., PTCA and the use of the IMA) had a major impact on the practice of coronary artery surgery in the 1980s. In 1982, the first total artificial heart was implanted by the group at University of Utah (45). Although this procedure did not work out for its intended purpose, it spurred the development and use of more powerful ventricular arrest devices (compared with the IABP) to treat temporary postoperative cardiac dysfunction and as bridges to heart transplantation. Along with PTCA, there was a beginning growth of interventional catheter-based cardiology, including balloon dilitation of pulmonary artery and valve stenosis, coarctation, and aortic and mitral stenosis; closure of PDA; and attempts at closure of ASD—all designed to reduce the need for conventional cardiac surgery (82–84). On the surgical side, with a more realistic appreciation of the limitations of prosthetic valves, there was a resurgent interest in repair rather than replacement of the mitral valve, especially for mitral regurgitation. This redirection was spearheaded and popularized by Alain Carpentier of Paris, whose work started in the 1970s but began to be widely practiced in the 1980s. Carpentier's introduction of the use of annuloplasty rings facilitated relief of mitral regurgitation in most surgeons' hands (191,192).

Major advances in understanding and improvements in the application of CPB occurred in the 1980s. In 1981, John Kirklin's group at the University of Alabama called attention to the systemic inflammatory reaction induced by CPB as a cause of much of the morbidity associated with cardiac surgery (193); this led to extensive and ongoing investigations into the nature, causes, and ways to modulate the incidence and effects of the inflammatory reaction. Increased interest in the neurologic consequences of CPB was spurred by reports in 1983 of measurements of cerebral blood flow during CPB in humans by L. Henricksen et al. in Copenhagen (194) and by the group at the University of Alabama (195,196). This was followed by more objective and sophisticated studies of the incidence of neurologic and neuropsychometric abnormalities after CPB. The group at Stanford emphasized the potential advantages of alpha-stat management of carbon dioxide and pH levels in arterial blood during hypothermia (197), and by the end of the decade this approach had been adopted by most groups (before that time, most groups employed pH-stat management, which often required the addition of carbon dioxide to the oxygenator). With the development of more efficient membrane oxygenators, and especially with the introduction of hollow fiber technology, the use of membrane oxygenators increased from 20% to 90% during this decade (and to 99% by 1994) in the United States (186). Probably spurred by their use in ECMO and as ventricular assist devices, centrifugal pumps began to supplant roller pumps as arterial pumps during CPB. After the serendipitous discovery of unusually "dry" surgical fields while investigating the use of high-dose aprotinin to reduce the inflammatory response during CPB (198,199), Dave Royston, Willem van Oeveren, Ben Bistrip, Steven Westaby, and others of London and the Netherlands first reported in 1987 the hemostatic benefits of aprotinin for cardiac surgery (68,69). In a few short years, the use of aprotinin or the synthetic antifibrinolytics became ubiquitous in the practice of cardiac surgery. It is of interest that the original characteristic (antiinflammatory) which led to the experiments that revealed aprotinin's hemostatic benefits has now become an additional rationale for the use of aprotinin during CPB.

* For a summary of the remarkable clinical experience with cardiac transplantation at Stanford University, see the article by Robbins et al. (188).

1990–1999: More for Less

The face of cardiac surgery in the 1990s, at least in the United States, was greatly influenced by changes in medical economics and in the "business of medicine" that resulted from the efforts of the Federal government and medical insurance companies to reduce the cost of medical care, the rise in managed care, the commercialization of medical practice, and the open competition among hospitals and practitioners. This contributed to the development of "fast-tracking," the marketing of "minimally invasive" cardiac surgery, and public review and oversight of the surgical results. In New York state, the public disclosure of the results of individual surgeons and hospitals began in 1991 (200)—so called "report-card medicine" (201). This was facilitated by the development of risk stratification systems by the Veterans Administration Hospitals, the Society of Thoracic Surgeons, the Cleveland Clinic, and others in the late 1980s and early 1990s (202), and it had a laudatory affect on the outcome in some regions where hospitals worked together to compare results and help one another improve outcomes [e.g., the Northern New England Cardiovascular Disease Study Group (203)].

Minimally invasive surgery, which includes operating through smaller incisions instead of the usual full sternotomy, performing CABG off-bypass (either through small thoracic incisions or via a median sternotomy), and use of the proprietary Port Access System (Heart Port, Redwood City, CA) has become common practice despite limited objective data to support its benefit in terms of outcome.

Stentless valves were first implanted in 1987 by Dr. Tirone David of Toronto (204); results are beginning to suggest improved left ventricular function and structure, and these devices are receiving more widespread use despite technical demands. Whether they prove to be a better solution to valve replacement remains to be seen.

As pediatric surgeons applied more complicated surgical interventions in smaller infants, concern about the adverse neurologic consequences of prolonged periods of deep hypothermic circulatory arrest were raised, especially by the groups at Boston Children's Hospital (205,206) and Duke University (207). This led to efforts to improve the methods of conducting deep hypothermic circulatory arrest, such as duration of cooling and management of pH, partial carbon dioxide pressure (P_{CO_2}), and hematocrit, or to replace circulatory arrest with low-flow CPB. In 1990 the group at the Hospital for Sick Children in London introduced the use of modified ultrafiltration in infant surgery to reduce fluid overload and possibly to remove inflammatory mediators (71).

Other means to decrease the inflammatory and hematologic effects of CPB were introduced, including the use of heparin-coated circuits in 1990 (70) and the use of leukocyte-removing filters. These methods, as well as modified ultrafiltration, were outgrowths of the interest and studies of the inflammatory response to CPB that began in the previous decade. The merits of these efforts are discussed elsewhere in this book and probably await further investigation. Other refinements or developments in CPB introduced in the 1990s included the use of augmented venous return and the resurgence of "warm bypass" and "warm heart surgery," spearheaded by the surgeons in Toronto (208,209). The advent of warm bypass led to recognition of the potential dangers of cerebral injury from overheating and reassessment of the need, hazards, and benefits of hypothermia, which had been a part of cardiac surgery for almost 50 years. With the continued concern about the neurologic consequences of CPB, in 1992 the Washington University group called attention to the possible role of ascending aortic atherosclerosis and various surgical manipulations involving the ascending aorta and the diagnostic value of ultrasonic interrogation. They suggested ways to modify surgical technique to reduce these risks (72,210). In another area of cerebral protection, the technique of retrograde cerebral perfusion (originally introduced by Mills and Ochsner in 1980 to treat cerebral air embolism) was reintroduced in 1990 by Ueda and colleagues in Japan to improve cerebral tolerance to deep hypothermic circulatory arrest during aortic arch surgery (211). This technique has rapidly gained in popularity, although its benefits are yet to be conclusively proven, as discussed elsewhere in the book.

In the early 1990s, inhaled nitric oxide was added to the armamentarium in treating pulmonary hypertension, although its impact on ultimate outcomes is still being elucidated (73). In fact, the role of excess endogenous nitric oxide in *producing* adverse effects and its modulation may prove to be more important in the future than the addition of nitric oxide to inhaled gases.

CARDIAC ANESTHESIA

The early pioneers in cardiac surgery readily acknowledged the important role played by the anesthesiologists. In his first paper on the systemic-to-pulmonary artery shunt, Blalock mentioned by name the anesthesiologists involved in each case (15), as did Potts (16) and Sellors (17) in their early case reports. In his Harvey Lecture, delivered in November 1945, Blalock offered as proof of the skill of the anesthesiologists who worked with him, Drs. Lamont and Harmel, "that there have been no deaths during the operation on the 55 patients" (94). In referring to his aorta-pulmonary anastamosis operation, Potts stated that "in an operation of this type, expert anesthesia is essential." But perhaps Russell C. Brock (later Lord Brock) expressed it most eloquently in his Alexander Simpson-Smith lecture, given at the Medical Society of London on June 15, 1949, while discussing closed surgery for tetralogy of Fallot: "It is a type of surgery that is not for the lone operator. . . . Teamwork is of course essential in the operating theatre, where in addition to the surgical and nursing assistants, the aneaesthetist plays a part of fundamental importance which deserves a special tribute" (212). On the other hand, the role of anesthesiology in the development of cardiac surgery was virtually ignored in two recent exhaustive books on the history of cardiac surgery authored by Shumacker (11) and Westaby (12).

Little has been written on the history of cardiac anesthesia. Although Meade addressed a section on anesthesia in his book, *A History of Thoracic Surgery,* cardiac anesthesia was not mentioned (1). Keown, in the 1963 edition of his textbook on cardiac anesthesia (213), and Lake, in her textbook on pediatric cardiac anesthesia (214), included brief chapters on the history of cardiac anesthesia, and Arens (215) and Wynands (216) have written articles on the subject. The latter, written by one of the pioneering cardiac anesthesiologists in North America, is a rich review that emphasizes the contributions of Canadian anaesthetists and contains numerous personal memories of the participants as well as of the author. Finally, Arthur Keats, another one of the pioneers in the development of this subspecialty, reflected on his personal perspective on its development in his 1983 Rovenstine Lecture (217). For further information this author has had to search through the cardiac surgery and anesthesia literature and his own personal recollections, leaving much to be desired.

In Table 1-4 are listed some of the notable developments and contributions in cardiac anesthesia.

Early Developments—Anesthesia for Thoracic Surgery

Before cardiac surgery (and hence cardiac anesthesia) could begin, fundamental advances in supporting patients during thoracic surgery had to be accomplished. This history of thoracic anesthesia has been thoroughly reviewed by L. Rendell-Baker (246) and, to a lessor degree, by Meade (1) and Johnson (3). Of course, the pivotal advance was the introduction of anesthesia itself in the late 1840s. However, the next major challenge to thoracic surgery was how to ventilate the patient when the chest was open. Some ingenious approaches were explored, such as placing the patient's head in a positive pressure box [Brauer (1904) and Murphy (1905)] or operating within a negative pressure chamber with only the patient's head outside [Sauerbruch (1904)]; for a while, even into the 1940s, positive-pressure ventilation via a tight-fitting mask was used, particularly for children. The solution, however, was endotracheal ventilation. The first elective oral endotracheal intubation for anesthesia was performed by the Scottish surgeon, William Macewan, in 1878. In 1888, the American surgeon, Joseph O'Dwyer, designed metal endotracheal tubes with a conical tip to occlude the larynx and added a bellows device to provide positive-pressure ventilation. This was first used and advocated as the best means of preventing pulmonary collapse during thoracic surgery by the surgeon Rudolph Matas of New Orleans in about 1899. In 1919 Ivan Magill of Britain introduced blind nasal endotracheal intubation using red rubber (Magill tubes), and in 1926 Arthur Guedel of Indianapolis introduced cuffed endotracheal tubes. Although direct-vision, laryngoscope-aided intubation was slowly adopted in the 1920s, the Miller and Macintosh blades were not introduced until the early 1940s.

In 1924 Ralph Waters at the University of Wisconsin introduced his to-and-fro carbon dioxide absorber using soda lime granules. This was favored by many cardiac anesthesiologists until the mid-1950s, although Brian Sword introduced a circle system with valves and an in-circuit carbon dioxide absorber, removing the cannister from the patient's face, in 1930. Ayre introduced his T-piece in 1937, and G. Jackson Rees his modification in 1950.

The first important new anesthetic agent after ether, chloroform, and nitrous oxide was cyclopropane, which was introduced to clinical anesthesia by Ralph Waters in 1933 and was adopted by many cardiac anesthesiologists as an induction if not a maintenance agent. Its major drawback was its inflammability, which led to its ready replacement when halothane became available in the late 1950s. In 1952, Lucien Morris invented the Copper kettle, which permitted more precise quantitation of anesthetic dosing, and later in that decade the temperature-compensated agent-specific vaporizers (TEC) were introduced by Cyprane Limited of England.

In 1934, John Lundy of Mayo Clinic introduced thiopental into the practice of anesthesia, and for many years it was used for both maintenance and induction. In 1942, Griffith and Johnson of Montreal first used curare, and Stephens used it to facilitate thoracic surgery in 1947. Succinylcholine became available in 1949.

Although mechanical ventilators were developed as early as 1907 (the Draeger Pulmotor), and Crafoord introduced his commercially available Spiropulsator in 1940 and Blease the "pulmoflator" after World War II, the use of ventilators in the operating room was not readily accepted until the late 1950s. "Modern" ICU-type ventilators (e.g., Bennett, Bird) did not appear until the 1960s.

In 1894, Harvey Cushing advocated the recording of pulse rate on an "anesthetic record," and in 1901, he added cuff blood pressures (247).

Although a few recovery rooms were established before World War II and an Anesthesia Study Commission report published in 1947 suggested that they could improve outcome, recovery rooms did not become common until the mid-1950s, and surgical intensive care units, greatly spurred by the advent of open heart surgery, not until the early 1960s (248).*

Early Cardiac Anesthesia

Little is known about the anesthesia provided during early cardiac surgical operations. Ellis, in 1975 (87), reviewed the

* The author acknowledges the informative chapter by the late Rod K. Calverley for much of this background on the development of anesthesiology (249).

TABLE 1-4. NOTABLE CONTRIBUTIONS IN CARDIAC ANESTHESIA

Date	Event	Anesthesiologist	Location	Reference No.
1946	First paper on cardiac anesthesia	MH Harmel, A Lamont	Johns Hopkins Hospital	218
1950	Plastic intravenous cannula	D Massa, JS Lundy, et al.	Mayo Clinic	219
1951	Anesthesia for mitral commissurotomy	KK Keown	Philadelphia	220
1952	Cardiotachoscope	A Himmelstein	New York	221
1954	Esophageal stethescope	C Smith	Hospital for Sick Children, Toronto	222
1956	First textbook on cardiac anesthesia	KK Keown	Philadelphia	223
1957	Anesthesia for cardiopulmonary bypass	EA Gain	University of Alberta	224
		D Mendelsohn et al.	Cleveland	225
		RT Patrick et al.	Mayo Clinic	226
1955	Electroencephalographic monitoring during cardiopulmonary bypass	RA Theye	Mayo Clinic	227
1963	Monitoring left atrial pressure	RA Theye, JW Kirklin	Mayo Clinic	228
1967	First paper on anesthesia for coronary artery surgery (Vineberg procedure)	JE Wynands et al.	Montreal	229
1969	Narcotic (morphine) anesthesia	E Lowenstein et al.	Massachusetts General Hospital	230
1972	Pulmonary artery catheter monitoring during cardiac surgery and cannulation of right internal jugular vein	JM Civetta, JC Gabel	Massachusetts General Hospital	231
1976	Monitoring V_5 lead for detecting myocardial ischemia	JA Kaplan	Emory University	232
1976	Nitroglycerin infusions to treat myocardial ischemia	JA Kaplan	Emory University	233
1978	Founding, Society of Cardiovascular Anesthesiologists	(R Marino, first President)		
1978	High-dose fentanyl anesthesia	TH Stanley et al.	University of Utah	234
1979	First modern American textbook on cardiac anesthesia	J Kaplan (Editor)	Emory University	235
1980	M-mode transesophageal echocardiography monitoring	M Matsumoto, Y Oka	Albert Einstein College of Medicine	236
1981	Pulmonary artery catheter to detect myocardial ischemia	JA Kaplan	Emory University	237
1982	Alpha-stat blood gas management	AK Ream et al.	Stanford University	197
1982	Two-dimensional transesophageal echocardiography monitoring	MK Cahalan, P Kremer, M Roizen	University of California, San Francisco	238,239
1983	Isoflurane steal described	S Reiz	Umea, Sweden	240
1983	Direct measurement of cerebral blood flow during cardiopulmonary bypass	JG Reves et al.	University of Alabama	195
		LH Henricksen et al.	Copenhagen	194
1985	Impact of myocardial ischemia on outcome	S Slogoff, A Keats	Texas Heart Institute	241
1986	Cerebral protection with barbituates	NA Nussemeier, S Slogoff	Texas Heart Institute	242
1987	First issue of the *Journal of Cardiothoracic Anesthesia*	JA Kaplan (Editor)	—	—
1987	Color flow transesophageal echocardiography	NP deBruijn et al.	Duke University	243
1989	Anesthetic agent does not affect outcome	K Tuman et al.	Rush University	244
		S Slogoff, AS Keats	Texas Heart Institute	245
1998	First examination in perioperative transesophageal echocardiography	National Board of Echocardiography	United States of America	—

anesthetic management of Dr. Souttar's patient who underwent mitral commissurotomy in 1925. He stated that anesthesia was administered by a surgeon, Eric Lindsay [although in a letter written to Brian Blades 30 years after the event, Dr. Souttar gives credit to his anaesthetist, Dr. John Challis (7)]. The patient was premedicated with morphine and atropine; induced with a combination of absolute alcohol, chloroform, and ether (ACE); and maintained with ether administered via an endotracheal catheter (? endotrocheal tube), and apparently breathed spontaneously throughout the procedure. Blood pressure was monitored about every 5 minutes (presumably noninvasively).

In 1994, Dobel outlined the anesthetic management of the patient in whom Dr. Gross first ligated a PDA in 1938 (90). Anesthesia was provided by a nurse anesthetist (Betty Lank), who used a tight-fitting adult mask that was shrunk (with alcohol) and strapped to the child's face. Monitoring included a finger on the superficial temporal pulse. The anesthetic agent used was cyclopropane. Blood was available but was not needed (13). For Crafoord's first coarctation repairs, accomplished in 1944, anesthesia consisted of a mixture of cyclopropane and nitrous oxide administered via an airtight endotracheal tube using controlled ventilation provided by a Spiropulsator respirator (14).

Between 1946 and 1950, the first papers on cardiac anesthesia appeared, reviewing the challenging experience of providing anesthesia for severely cyanotic and debilitated children undergoing systemic-to-pulmonary artery shunt operations (218,250–253). Again the words of Lord Brock came to mind: "[These operations] involve considerable anxiety [and] demand the work and attention of an enthusiastic, loyal, and courageous team" (212). It is hard to underestimate the anxiety produced in contemplating anesthetizing for the first time one of these almost moribund children (who often had virtually no exercise tolerance, were bedridden, and suffered repeated hypoxic spells) for this radically new operation. Common themes in these reports included heavy premedication (morphine and scopolamine), induction and maintenance with cyclopropane (with or without a little ether), endotracheal intubation (a few tried mask-only ventilation early in their experience but quickly abandoned it for endotracheal intubation because of problems with maintaining ventilation, despite the concerns about postintubation airway problems in children). Most used controlled ventilation (with or without use of curare). The Waters to-and-fro carbon dioxide absorbing canister closed system was usually used. Monitoring methods were not detailed, nor was fluid management discussed except to warn against fluid overloading. Usually a cannula was placed in the saphenous vein of an ankle, and plasma was administered. In H.M. Harmel and Austin Lamont's report of Blalock's first 103 cases at Johns Hopkins Hospital (patients 10 weeks to 20 years old), the mortality rate was 23% (218). In William McQuiston's report of Potts and Smith's first 236 shunt cases at Children's Memorial Hospital in Chicago, the overall mortality rate was 13%, but that among the 135 patients aged 3 to 16 years in whom a shunt was actually constructed was only 3% (253). These remarkable results were achieved without the benefit of electrocardiographic (ECG) monitoring, arterial and central venous lines and monitoring, pulse oximetry, and end-tidal carbon dioxide monitoring; modern inhalation agents, narcotics, muscle relaxants, and antibiotics; intensive care units, or even recovery rooms. In May 1948, the Chicago group began using mild surface-induced hypothermia ("refrigeration"; rectal temperature, 92° to 93°F) in these cyanotic children and observed decreased incidences of cerebral hypoxia and cerebral death (2% and 1.5%, respectively, compared with 7% and 4% in historical controls) in shunted patients and a reduced mortality rate (14% versus 54%) in those in whom a shunt could not be constructed (253). This was the first clinical use of hypothermia in cardiac surgery, a technique which would reappear on many occasions in the future. Alvin Harris in San Francisco described a somewhat different anesthetic technique in 25 children; he used rectal Avertin (tribromethanol) to induce basal narcosis and maintained the patients with nitrous/oxygen, curare, and morphine sulfate (later to be called "balanced anesthesia") (251). However, this technique did not appear to be well accepted at that time (254).

Robert M. Smith of Boston Children's Hospital (254) and E.M. Papper and Thomas McDermott at Babies Hospital in New York City (255) reviewed the pathophysiology and anesthetic management of patients with ductus arteriosus, coarctation of the aorta, pulmonic stenosis, vascular rings, or tetralogy of Fallot. Papper and McDermott emphasized the benefits of endotracheal intubation [although M.H. Adelman reported his successful use of mask ventilation during surgery for PDAs (256)]. By 1950, the Boston Children's Hospital group (Gross and Smith) reported a mortality rate of 1% in 455 children with PDA and 8.5% in 155 with coarctation (254). The Chicago group (Potts and McQuiston) reported the results in their first 1,000 operations for congenital heart disease as of February 1955 (257): the mortality rate in surgery for isolated pulmonic stenosis (61 patients) was 1.6%, for PDA (347 patients) it was 0%, and for coarctation of the aorta (52 patients) it was 4%. Again, these results were achieved without the "benefits" of modern anesthesia technology.

Between 1951 and 1955, the first papers on providing anesthesia for mitral commissurotomies were published (220,258–262). Moderate premedication including phenobarbital and morphine or meperidine was usually recommended. All groups emphasized the importance of using the lightest possible anesthesia but employed different agents to accomplish this goal. An extreme example of light anesthesia was the technique of C.E. Wasmuth at the Cleveland Clinic. He used nitrous oxide (80% to 50%) in oxygen, supplemented with small amounts of thiopental, morphine, or demerol and local infiltration of the intercostal incision, and insisted that the patients *respond to questioning throughout the procedure* (although they denied pain and had no recall!) (259). All groups employed endotracheal intubation, often with topical anesthesia, but there was considerable controversy as to whether ventilation should be merely assisted (to avoid the possible negative impact of controlled ventilation on right ventricular function) or controlled, and on the pros and cons of using muscle relaxants such as curare (260) or infusions of succinylcholine (262). Two authors recommended use of mechanical ventilators to provide reliable ventilation and "free up the anesthesiologist's hands for other exceedingly important duties" (259, 260). [The Swedes had been using ventilators during cardiac surgery since the late 1930s (14).] In the earliest report Kenneth Keown, who worked with Charles Bailey, advocated running an infusion of procaine throughout the case to reduce arrhythmias (220), but this approach was not adopted by most subsequent authors. Continuous ECG monitoring was employed by all, some using an oscilloscope (258,259). All started large-bore intravenous access and had blood available, including blood pumps and means of giving *intraarterial* transfusions, but all emphasized the need to minimize fluid and blood administration to avoid fluid overload. Keown (220) even advocated removing the venous cannula at the end of the case (if the patient was stable) "to avoid the temptation to give excessive fluids." All patients were extubated at the end of the case but given supplemental oxygen postoperatively. Several groups employed paravertebral or intercostal nerve blocks for postoperative anlagesia. All authors emphasized the need to move or change the patient's position slowly and gently while the patient was still under anesthesia or emerging, to avoid hemodynamic instability.

Perhaps an even more daunting task was the provision of anesthesia for patients with severe aortic regurgitation who were undergoing insertion of a prosthetic ball valve prosthesis in the descending aorta by Dr. Charles Huffnagel of Georgetown University (without benefit of left heart or cardiopulmonary bypass). This was first performed in September 1952 (25). The anesthetic management of these patients was described by John A. O'Donnell and Thomas F. McDermott in 1955 (263). All 42 patients were in medically irreversible congestive heart failure, and 40% had intractable angina pectoris, with 10 to 20 attacks per day not uncommon. After discovering early in their experience that these patients did not tolerate a depth of general anesthesia to permit endotracheal intubation, they thereafter intubated these patients with topical anesthesia, induced very light general anesthesia with a small dose of pentothal, and maintained them on nitrous oxide and oxygen supplemented with intravenous morphine or small amounts of ether. Systolic arterial pressure was kept higher than 100 mm Hg with phenylephrine if needed. Continuous ECG monitoring by oscilloscope and recorder was employed with a cardiologist present, and two 15-gauge intravenous needles were placed. The radial artery was surgically exposed, not for monitoring but to use if needed to withdraw blood to treat extreme hypertension during aortic cross-clamping or to give intraarterial transfusion in the case of catastrophic hemorrage. Blood transfusion replaced blood loss (average, 800 mL), and an electrical defibrillator was always available. The arterial pressure, measured by auscultation in the upper extremities, did not rise as much as anticipated (and in some not at all) with aortic cross-clamping—but we can imagine what the left ventricle would have looked like with TEE monitoring!. There were nine hospital deaths (20%); three patients died during surgery from cardiac arrest or ventricular fibrillation before, during, or after valve insertion, and four died suddenly 5 to 9 days postoperatively after an apparently uncomplicated recovery.

In 1954, S.J. Evelyn and I. Mackay reviewed their anesthestic techniques and results with cardiac anesthesia in 820 cases operated at the Toronto General Hospital (264). Their hospital mortality rates were remarkable: tetralogy of Fallot (shunts; 342 patients), 6%; PDA (133 patients), 0%; coarctation (29 patients), 0%; and mitral valve surgery (260 patients), 6%.

Little has been written about the anesthesia used in the early cases of direct-vision open heart surgery with moderate surface-induced hypothermia. Lewis (104) indicated that anesthesia was induced with pentothal and curare, patients were intubated, and ECG and rectal temperature were monitored. Swan (105) indicated that anesthesia was also induced with pentothal and maintained with cyclopropane and ether, or with ether alone. Robert W. Virtue with Henry Swan in Denver amplified a little on anesthetic management in their 1955 report of their first 100 cases done under hypothermia (265). Monitoring apparently included ECG, electroencephalography (EEG), blood pressure by auscultation (although this was not measured in 12% of cases and could not be obtained in one third of patients cooled to less than 35°C, and in two thirds by 33° to 31°C). Patients were given an "ordinary" anesthesia. Ether was the preferred agent ("second plane, third stage"), supplemented with curare. Virtue and Swan suggested that anesthetizing these patients was a "two-man job," with one anesthesiologist devoting full attention to maintenance of hyperventilation to deliberately achieve a respiratory alkalosis, which they believed reduced the incidence of ventricular fibrillation. [They measured right atrial pH (at the patient's temperature) just before arrest and aimed for it to be greater than 7.5—alpha-stat management!]. Two plastic cannulas were placed in arm veins, and all blood loss was replaced with at least equal amounts of blood. After arrest, 100% oxygen was administered, with nitrous oxide (50%) added if needed. Patients were extubated when they were breathing adequately, apparently often before they awakened. Ventricular fibrillation occurred in 15%, and although two thirds were resuscitated, only 20% survived; in comparison, six of the seven patients who experienced cardiac arrest survived. Postoperative hemorragic shock (compared with cardiac failure) posed a difficult diagnostic problem. Average duration of circulatory arrest was 5 minutes (range, 2 to 10 minutes). Only 1 (3%) of 36 patients with favorable lesions (e.g., secundum ASD, isolated pulmonary valvular or infundibular stenosis) died, whereas 6 (75%) of the 8 with primum ASD or VSD died. Eight of ten patients with tetralogy (undergoing only relief of their pulmonary stenosis) survived.

In 1957 B.A. Sellick in London (266), and in 1959 A.W.

Conn et al. at the Hospital for Sick Children in Toronto (267), reviewed their anesthetic techniques for direct-vision open heart surgery using only hypothermia in detail. Sellick used nitrous oxide with oxygen plus ether and complete relaxation with curare after pentothal and succinylcholine for induction and intubation; Conn et al. used the same agents but without muscle relaxation except for intubation. By 1959 Conn had switched to using halothane. In the paper by Conn et al., a detailed section on monitoring appeared for the first time. Monitoring included a multichannel recorder and oscilloscope, ECG and EEG, and the availability of transducers for direct pressure monitoring, although blood pressure was usually monitored with a Collens oscillometer. They report flooding the surgical field with carbon dioxide to minimize the risk of air embolization. Neither Sellick's nor Conn's group had a single death in their 32 and 63 patients, respectively!

Anesthesia for Early Cardiac Surgery Using Cardiopulmonary Bypass

Few details are known concerning the anesthesia provided for John Gibbon's early cases using CPB. In the dictated operative note about his one successful operation on May 6, 1953, Dr. Gibbon only mentioned that the patient was anesthetized with intravenous pentothal with an endotracheal tube and manual assistance to ventilation. Direct blood pressure readings were made via a needle inserted in the right brachial artery that was connected to a mercury manometer. The veins in both ankles were cannulated for administration of intravenous fluids. The patient was quite light at the conclusion of the operation and *1 hour later, when returned to her bed in the hospital ward,* was awake, recognizing people, and talking (106). According to Anthony Dobell, who was a surgery resident under Dr. Gibbon at that time (and subsequently became chief of cardiac surgery at the Royal Victoria Hospital in Montreal), "A major factor in the deaths of the children was poor ventilation prior to going on cardiopulmonry bypass. There were no physician anesthesiologists at Jefferson at that time and of course mechanical ventilators had not been developed. Some of the children were already moribund by the time they were connected to the heart-lung machine. Thus at Jefferson, lack of expertise in anesthesia, pediatric cardiology and cardiac pathology all played a part in the initial failures" (10).

For Lillehei's early cases of open heart surgery using controlled cross-circulation, anesthesia in the patients was induced with nitrous oxide/cyclopropane and then maintained with pentothal and curare; anesthesia in donors was induced and maintained with pentothal and curare. During CPB, the donors were hyperventilated (two to three times normal values) to induce a respiratory alkalosis and counterbalance the metabolic acidosis that regularly occurred during the low-flow (34 to 40 mL/kg/minute) perfusion of the patient. No mention of monitoring, invasive lines, nor fluid management other than blood administration was made. In the first eight patients who underwent closure of VSDs (5 months to 5 years of age), the average time on CPB was 14 minutes (range, 9 to 28 minutes)! Six patients survived (31). According to Arens, Fred van Bergen and Joe Buckley administered anesthesia to the patient while Jim Matthews and Earl Schultz cared for the father donor for the first successful case (215).

In 1956, just at the time when extracorporeal perfusion was being introduced, Kenneth K. Keown of Hahnemann Medical College, who provided anesthesia for Dr. Bailey, published the first textbook, *Anesthesia for Surgery of the Heart* (223), that provided an insight into the nature of cardiac anesthesia in that era. As a testimony of the teamwork that had developed between cardiac surgeons and cardiac anesthesiologists, he listed the prominent teams practicing at that time (Table 1-5). He also summarized the expected mortality rates for the various procedures done at that time (Table 1-6). He emphasized the role of the anesthesiologist in ensuring that the patient was ready for surgery, the use of checklists for equipment and supplies, and the avoidance of shortcuts. Finally, he listed what he hoped would be coming in the near future: a more ideal inhalation anesthetic (potent, rapid-acting, nonirritating, nonexplosive), mechanical ventilators, arterial lines with partial oxygen pressure (P_{O_2}) and pH measurement, and a practical mechanical heart-lung machine.

Over the next 4 years, several groups reviewed their initial experience in delivering anesthesia care for patients undergoing open heart surgery with the use of mechanical

TABLE 1-5. EARLY CARDIAC SURGERY AND ANESTHESIA TEAMS

Surgeon	Anesthesiologists	Location
CP Bailey	KK Keown	Philadelphia
A Blalock	MH Harmel, A Lamont	Johns Hopkins Hospital
RC Brock	EH Rink, Lucas	London
DB Effler	DE Hale, JF Vijon	Cleveland Clinic
DE Harken	LD Vandam	Boston
CA Hufnagel	TF McDermott	Georgetown University
EB Kay	D Mendelsohn	Cleveland
JW Kirklin	RT Patrick, RA Theye	Mayo Clinic
CW Lillehei	FH Van Bergen	University of Minnesota
DWG Murray	SJ Evelyn	Toronto
WJ Potts	WO McQuiston	Chicago Children's Hospital
TH Sellors	BA Sellick, Brown	London
H Swan	RW Virtue	Denver
R Varco	JJ Buckley	University of Minnesota

Source: Keown KK. *Anesthesia for surgery of the heart.* Springfield, IL: Charles C Thomas, 1956, p. 8.

TABLE 1-6. ESTIMATED MORTALITY RATES ASSOCIATED WITH CARDIAC SURGERY, 1956[a]

Condition	Mortality (%)
Congenital disease	
Tetralogy of Fallot (shunts)	12
Tetralogy of Fallot (Brock-Sellors procedure)	"lower"
Pulmonic stenosis (isolated)	5
Atrial septal defect, secundum	12
Atrial septal defect, primum	60
Atrial septal defect with partial anomalous venous return	12
Patent ductus arteriosus	2.5–3
Aortic stenosis	7
Acquired disease	
Mitral stenosis	7.5
Aortic stenosis	15
Mitral regurgitation	12
Aortic regurgitation	25
Coronary artery surgery (Vineberg, Beck procedures)	20
Pericardiectomy	5

[a] All closed procedures or with moderate hypothermia; none with cardiopulmonary bypass.
Source: Keown KK. *Anesthesia for surgery of the heart.* Springfield, IL: Charles C Thomas, 1956, pp. 13, 14.

heart-lung machines (224–226,268,269). These reports reflected major differences of opinion regarding the optimal oxygenator, flow rates, lung management, control of arterial pressure, need to add carbon dioxide or anesthesic agents to the extracorporeal circuit during surgery, and type of monitoring—items that are still debated 40 years later! The degree of management, intervention, and monitoring ranged from the detailed protocol at the Mayo Clinic (226) to the minimalist approach at Baylor/Texas Children's Hospital in Houston (269). The former resembled modern-day practice: flows were kept at about 2.4 L/minute/m^2 (60 to 200 mL/kg/minute), and ether was administered via a vaporizer on the oxygenator. Intraarterial pressure, venous pressure, rectal temperature, EEG, ECG, *in-line venous saturation*, and arterial blood gases were monitored. Fluid and blood balance was meticulously monitored, and a written, detailed protocol for step-by-step management was published. Vasopressor drugs and resuscitation drugs were prepared and made ready (226). At the other extreme was the practice in Houston (Cooley and Keats). They monitored only one lead of the ECG (and not invasive arterial pressure, venous pressure, EEG, or temperature), ran flows of 35 to 50 mL/kg/minute (adults and infants, respectively), and administered only *d*-tubocurarine during CPB (but with no recall observed!). However, their mean duration of CPB was only 13 minutes (269). Some attributed the amnesia to cerebral hypoperfusion (caused by low arterial carbon dioxide pressure and low flow rates) and found that patients rarely awakened during CPB without anesthesia when flows were 35 to 40 mL/kg/minute but invariably awakened with flows of 60 mL/kg/minute (a situation that was treated with small amounts of barbituates and narcotics) (224). The Mayo Clinic group observed no EEG changes during their high-flow CPB (226), whereas the University of Minnesota group observed severely abnormal EEG changes during their low-flow CPB (268), although no gross neurologic abnormalities were noted afterward. However, their CPB times were also usually very short (average, 14 minutes; range, 8 to 17 for the first seven cases) (114). All favored using minimal possible anesthesia and expected patients to be awake and extubated at the end of the case.

Halothane was first introduced into anesthesia practice in 1957, but there was initial hesitation to use it for cardiac surgery because of concern about its myocardial and respiratory effects. However, the desire to use a potent nonexplosive agent led the groups at Mayo Clinic (270) and Indiana University (271) to explore the use of low concentrations (less than 0.8% to 1.0%) in 50% nitrous oxide for adults and children undergoing open and closed cardiac surgery; they found halothane to be entirely satisfactory. Thereafter, this agent rapidly replaced most others and became the agent of choice for much cardiac surgery until the landmark article by Edward Lowenstein and colleagues at the Massachusetts General Hospital in 1969 (230). Lowenstein et al. indicated that they had used high-dose morphine (0.5 to 3 mg/kg) as the main anesthetic in 1,100 patients because it was devoid of myocardial depression and they considered it to be the agent of choice in patients with minimal cardiac reserve (e.g., end-stage valvular and coronary artery disease). This approach was rapidly adopted by others, and the combination of high-dose narcotics with oxygen and muscle relaxant came to be known as the "cardiac anesthetic." Mainly morphine was used for the next 10 years, until it was replaced by the synthetic narcotics, initially fentanyl in doses of 50 to 100 μg/kg, as popularized in the United States by Theodore H. Stanley of the University of Utah (234). Fentanyl overcame some of the limitations of high-dose morphine, including vasodilation and the need for blood volume expansion.

Anesthesia for Coronary Artery Surgery

In 1967 J. Earl Wynands of Montreal published the first article on the anesthetic management of patients with coronary artery disease undergoing revascularization (Vineberg procedure) (229). This was followed by an article by John F. Viljoen of the Cleveland Clinic, based on his group's experience with 1,500 IMA implant procedures (272). Both authors emphasized the desirability of generous premedication, adequate depth of anesthesia, invasive monitoring of arterial and central venous pressure, frequent measurements of arterial blood gases and serum potassium, and postoperative endotracheal ventilation with adequate analgesia and sedation for 4 to 24 hours and close cardiovascular surveillance in the intensive care unit. Wynands emphasized the importance of maintaining arterial pressures close to baseline and keeping the hematocrit at about 40 percent. In 1970, Wynands reported a hospital mortality rate of only 1.3% in their last 78 patients, despite the fact that one third had angina at rest (273)! Donald Effler, the chief of cardiac surgery at the Cleveland Clinic, attributed much of the improved results to anesthetic management (274). Viljoen advocated intermittent administration of nitroglycerine intramuscularly (272), and in 1976 Joel Kaplan, then at Emory University, introduced the use of nitroglycerine infusions during coronary artery disease (233).

Recognizing the importance of integrating cardiology into the practice of anesthesiology, a symposium on this topic, edited by Arthur Keats, was published in the August 1970 issue of *Anesthesiology* (275).

The 1980s

An article by Allen Ream and colleagues at Stanford in 1982 led to a rethinking of the proper management of PCO_2 and pH during hypothermic CPB (197) and a near-complete shift from pH-stat to alpha-stat management during that decade. A year later, the paper by Sebastian Reiz of Umea, Sweden, raised concern about the risk of coronary steal with isoflurane (240) and led to a flurry of experimental and clinical studies on this topic. Perhaps a more provocative and influential study appeared 2 years later when Stephen Slogoff and Arthur Keats of the Texas Heart Institute in Houston documented the frequency of intaoperative myocardial ischemia during coronary artery surgery and showed that it was associated with postoperative myocardial infarction (241). They also showed that an anesthesiologist (the infamous anesthesiologist #7) can have an impact on the incidence of this problem. This paper helped initiate the intense study of perioperative ischemia, its causes, and methods to prevent it, that continues to the present day. In 1986 another pivotal study came from the Texas Heart Institute in which Drs. Nancy Nussmeier and Slogoff demonstrated that use of high-dose thiopental (to produce isoelectric EEG; average dose, about 40 mg/kg) reduced the rate of postoperative neuropsychiatric dysfunction after open ventricle operations (242). Although the general applicability of this data has been challenged, the study certainly spurred interest in the incidence, cause, and prevention of perioperative neurologic dysfunction. In 1989, two papers occurred side by side, one again from Slogoff and Keats at the Texas Heart Institute and the other from Kenneth Tuman and colleagues at Rush-Presbyterian-St. Luke's Medical Center in Chicago, documenting in large prospective studies (more than 1,000 patients each) what cardiac anesthesiologists had been saying since 1946: that the choice of anesthetic agents does not significantly affect outcome (244,245).

Monitoring

Monitoring receives much attention in modern anesthesia practice, as evidenced by Basic Monitoring Standards and Practice Guidelines, such as those for use of PAC and TEE issued by the American Society of Anesthesiologists. However, as noted previously, in articles on cardiac anesthesia up until the mid-1950s monitoring was rarely mentioned. Obviously these anesthesiologists depended heavily on their five senses, awareness, and clinical accumen (observing, for example, the color of the skin, pupils, and conjunctivae, and keeping a finger on the pulse)—behavior that the modern anesthesiologist could usefully emulate.

The first "new" monitor to be introduced was the ECG. Studies using paper recorders during adult (276) and pediatric surgery (277) were reported by cardiologists in 1939 and 1948. However, apparently ECG monitoring was not commonly practiced (278) until the advent of closed mitral commissurotomy, during which arrhythmias were a major problem and all early reports mentioned use of ECG monitoring. Initially this was accomplished with the use of ordinary diagnostic ECG machines with paper recorders, but in the early 1950s oscilloscopic monitors were introduced to facilitate continuous ECG monitoring (221,258,259). A major advance in ECG monitoring occurred in 1976, when Joel Kaplan advocated the use of the V_5 lead to detect myocardial ischemia in patients with coronary artery disease (232).

In 1954, Dr. Code Smith at the Hospital for Sick Children in Toronto introduced the simple but effective esophageal stethoscope, which was particularly useful in thoracic surgery (222).

With the introduction of CPB in the mid-1950s, sphygmomanometry could no longer provide reliable arterial pressure monitoring, and the use of invasive arterial lines (at least during CPB), not only for pressure monitoring but for arterial blood gas monitoring, was introduced. Initially these were often placed in the radial artery by cutdown by the surgeon, and it was not until the late 1960s that anesthesiologists began to place these lines percutaneously. Blood gas analysis was a difficult and time-consuming process and was infrequently performed until the late 1950s, when Clark, Severinghaus, and Astrup introduced their PO_2, PCO_2, and pH electrodes (279). Even then, it took a few years until blood gas analysis was commonplace.

A major theme of early experiences with surgery using CPB was difficulty in assessing blood volume status and evaluating ventricular function after bypass. Soon thereafter, monitoring of venous pressure (initially from catheters placed in arm veins and external jugular veins, but then from central lines placed via the groin or arm veins or placed directly into the right atrium at time of surgery) was introduced. However, as early as 1963, the Mayo Clinic group called attention to the frequent discrepancies between central venous (right atrial) and left atrial pressure and described placing catheters directly into the left atrium to monitor function and filling of the left side of the heart (228). Subsequent authors emphasized the importance of monitoring left atrial pressure in this manner in cardiac surgical patients (280,281). The monitoring of cardiac patients was revolutionized in 1970, when Swan, Ganz, and colleagues introduce their balloon-tipped PACs (61). The cardiac surgery/anesthesia team at Massachusetts General Hospital was among the first to advocate use of the PAC in cardiac surgery (231). They also introduced percutaneous introduction of the PAC via the internal jugular vein (including use of a "finding needle"), and this rapidly became the approach of choice for most anesthesiologists. (Before this, PACs were usually introduced via the brachial vein, either percutaneoulsy or by cutdown). Joel Kaplan helped to popularize the use of the PAC during cardiac surgery (282) and emphasized its role in the early diagnosis of myocardial ischemia (237) (although the latter is now largely discounted). Not only did the PAC allow estimation of the left atrial pressure, but it also provided access to mixed venous blood for oxygen analysis. In 1972 the PAC was modified to permit the easy monitoring of cardiac output by themodilution. Although the Mayo Clinic group and a few others had monitored cardiac output and identified its prognostic importance and usefulness as a guide to therapy from the dawn of open heart surgery, cardiac output was difficult to measure and was not generally used until thermodilution via PAC became available. And although we think of mixed venous oximetry as a new idea, in 1959 the Johns Hopkins Hospital group identified mixed venous oxygen as their most useful indicator of prognosis after open heart surgery (283). Although cardiac anesthesiologists were among the first and strongest proponents of the use of the PAC, they were also among the first to point out its limitations (284) and to indicate that not all cardiac surgical patients required a PAC (285,286).

The Mayo Clinic group, from the very beginning of their experience in 1955, used EEG monitoring during CPB and advocated its value as a monitor of anesthetic depth as well as integrity of cerebral perfusion (227). Others concurred (287), but early on skepticism was raised (288,289). This debate is still unresolved 40 years later.

Transesophageal Echocardiography

TEE has had a profound effect on the practice of cardiac anesthesiology in the past decade, and anesthesiologists played a key role in the introduction of this modality to the practice of cardiac medicine (290). Paul Barash of Yale was perhaps the first to apply echocardiography in anesthesiology, when he evaluated the effects of halothane on ventricular function in children using transthoracic M-mode echocardiography (291). Transesophageal Doppler was first described in 1971 and transesophageal M-mode in 1976. In 1980, Masayuki Matsumoto, Yasu Oka, and others at Albert Einstein College of Medicine in the Bronx perceived the future of TEE in cardiac anesthesia when they described the use of M-mode TEE for continuous monitoring of left ventricular function in 21 patients during cardiac surgery (236). However M-mode TEE was difficult to apply except by the extremely sophisticated clinician. Although some primitive two-dimensional TEE scanners were described between 1977 and 1980, it was not until Souquet, Schluter, and Hanrath introduced their phased array transducer system mounted on the end of a gastroscope that TEE became a practical reality (292). In the early 1980s, Peter Hanrath brought prototypes to the Mayo Clinic and the University of California in San Francisco (UCSF). A cardiology fellow from Hanrath's group in Germany, P. Kremer, joined anesthesiologists Michael Cahalan and Michael Roizen at UCSF. At the 1982 meeting of the American Society of Anesthesiology, they started the TEE "revolution" when they presented their results in monitoring cardiac and vascular surgery patients with this new TEE probe, describing its usefulness in assessing filling and function of the left ventricle, myocardial ischemia, and intracardiac air (238,239). R.F. Cucchiara and colleagues at the Mayo Clinic described its usefulness in detecting air embolism during neurosurgery (293), while the UCSF group described its superiority over ECG in detecting myocardial ischemia (294). In 1987 Cahalan et al. (295) and Clements and deBruijn at Duke University (296) wrote review articles on the use of TEE in anesthesiology. In 1986, Hewlett-Packard introduced color flow Doppler with TEE, and Norbert deBruijn and colleagues at Duke University reviewed their early experience with this new technology (243). In that same year, pulsed wave Doppler was added to TEE, and in 1989 biplane probes first became available. The Society of Cardiovascular Anesthesiologists has played a key role in the development of perioperative TEE. In conjunction with the American Society of Anesthesiologists they developed the Practice Guidelines for Perioperative TEE in 1996, and in collaboration with the American Society of Echocardiography they helped initiate the first examination in Perioperative TEE, which was administered by the National Board of Echocardiography in 1998. Today TEE is one of the defining characteristics of a cardiac anesthesiologist.

Cardiac Anesthesia Becomes a Subspecialty

It is difficult to identify a precise time when cardiac anesthesia became a subspeciality—in a sense it began with Harmel and Lamont's care of Dr. Blalock's blue babies in late 1944, which led to the first paper on cardiac anesthesia in 1946 (218), or with the publishing of the first textbook on cardiac anesthesia by Keown in 1956 (223). Some could argue that because the subspeciality is not recognized by the American Board of Anesthesiology, nor by the American Board of Medical Specialties, it is not a subspecialty; but most accept its subspecialty status. This is because of the special knowledge, skills, and activities required of anesthesiologists who attend these patients. In the beginning, these aspects consisted of intimate knowledge of the pathophysiology of congenital heart disease and how various anesthetic techniques interact with this pathophysiology (254). Later was added the pathophysiology of valvular heart disease, and finally that of coronary artery disease (273). Next was required knowledge of the entirely new techniques that surgeons used to manage these patients: initially hypothermia, then CPB and all of its nuances including deep hypothermic circulatory arrest, coronary perfusion, cardioplegia, and retrograde cerebral perfusion. In recent years this has included minimally invasive techniques such as Port Access System. "Advanced" monitoring techniques, not usually used in noncardiac anesthesia at the time they were introduced, were on the list of new skills and knowledge required of the cardiac anesthesiologist. These included ECG, EEG, arterial lines, and central venous and left atrial pressure monitoring; next the PAC; and most recently, TEE. Intimate knowledge of blood coagulation and anticoagulation and the administration of blood products (often in large quantities) and of various drugs used to modify coagulation was required. Finally, a thorough understanding of the pathophysiology of abnormal hemodynamic states and manipulation with potent and often novel hemodynamically active agents and mechanical assist devices was required. [In briefly reviewing some of the knowledge and techniques first introduced into and unique to the practice of cardiac anesthesia, it is apparent that much of this was eventually transferred and adopted into the general practice of noncardiac anesthesia].

To gain all of this knowledge and skill, residents began to seek special training (fellowships) in cardiac anesthesia in the 1970s. Programs at Massachusetts General Hospital, Emory University, University of Alabama, Texas Heart Institute, and the Cleveland Clinic, to name only a few, were important "incubators" for future cardiac anesthesiologists. Also, modern encyclopedic textbooks on cardiac anesthesia began to appear, starting with the classic text edited by Joel Kaplan in 1979 (235), and cardiac anesthesiologists began to meet together to share their experience, ideas, and problems. In 1972, the Association of Cardiac Anesthesiologists was founded with B. Dalton as president, Emerson Moffitt as vice president, and Edward Lowenstein as secretary (215). Because this organization limited its membership to 50, in 1978 the Society of Cardiovascular Anesthesiologists was established (Table 1-7) and quickly became a leading society in the entire specialty of anesthesiology, not to mention the subspecialty. In 1987, a new journal appeared devoted to the subspecialty, the *Journal of Cardiothoracic Anesthesia.*

Another somewhat unique characteristic of the subspecialty of cardiac anesthesia was the concept of a team. Brock spoke of this in his previously mentioned lecture in 1949 (212), and Keown listed such teams in 1956 (Table 1-5) (223). The surgeon was no longer able to oversee the whole procedure. Dodds, in his 1961 paper (297), emphasized the role of the anaesthetist in caring for the patient and overseeing perfusion during CPB so that the surgeon could concentrate on the problems involved in correcting the cardiac defects. Cardiac anesthesiologists also continued to care for these patients in the early postoperative period, and cardiac surgery and cardiac anesthesia played important roles in the development of surgical intensive care units (248), and conversely in transferring the practices of intensive care into the operating room.

Although many played invaluable roles in the development of cardiac anesthesia into a subspecialty, it is my personal opinion that much of the credit for the popularity and status of this subspecialty should go to Joel E. Kaplan (originally at Emory University, then Chair of Anesthesiology at Mount Sinai School of Medicine in New York, and now Dean of the School of Medicine in Louisville). He "sold" the importance and value of cardiac anesthesiologists to surgeons and anesthesiologists at various meetings. The textbook he edited, which was first published in 1979, thor-

TABLE 1-7. PRESIDENTS OF SOCIETY OF CARDIOVASCULAR ANESTHESIOLOGISTS

Dates	President	Location
1979	Robert J Marino	New Orleans, Louisiana
1979–1981	Gerald J Reves	University of Alabama (later at Duke University)
1981–1983	Fawzy G Estafanous	Cleveland Clinic
1983–1985	Joel A Kaplan	Emory University (later at Mount Sinai School of Medicine, New York; then University of Louisville)
1985–1987	Paul G Barash	Yale University
1987–1989	George E Burges III	Baton Rouge, Louisiana
1989–1991	J Earl Wynands	University of Ottawa (formerly at McGill University)
1991–1993	John L Waller	Emory University
1993–1995	Alan J Schwartz	Medical College of Pennsylvania
1995–1997	Michael F Roizen	University of Chicago
1997–1999	Richard Davis	University of Oregon
1999–2001	Daniel M Thys	Columbia University

oughly catalogued and covered the knowledge and technical aspects needed and set a standard against which all other texts would be measured. His name almost became synonymous with the PAC (see, for example, the logo on the fourth edition of his textbook and on the journal he edits). He helped introduce intravenous nitroglycerin infusions and monitoring of the V_5 lead to the specialty. In 1987 he started the first journal devoted to cardiac anesthesia. He was the fourth president of the Society of Cardiovascular Anesthesiologists (1983–1985) and, in recognition of his knowledge and skills as a communicator, gave a refresher course lecture on cardiac anesthesia for more than 10 years at the Annual Meeting of the American Society of Anesthesiologists.

Maturation of the Subspecialty

The last two decades have witnessed remarkable growth of our subspecialty in terms of prominence and scientific contributions. Many cardiac anesthesiologists have became chairs of anesthesia departments and a few have been deans or higher officials in various academic centers. Cardiac anesthesiologists play active roles in the Society of Thoracic Surgeons (e.g., leading workshops on neurologic consequences of cardiac surgery), the American Society of Echocardiography, and the American College of Cardiology/American Heart Association (e.g., committee to develop guidelines for perioperative cardiovascular evaluation for noncardiac surgery); serve as associate editors of major anesthesia journals; help produce and edit two modern textbooks on CPB; and organize and direct major annual workshops on CPB and TEE.

Major research contributions have been made and continue to be added in such diverse areas as the pathophysiology of CPB including the systemic inflammation response, neurologic consequences of cardiac surgery, alpha-stat versus pH-stat blood gas management during hypothermia, perioperative myocardial ischemia, molecular cardiovascular medicine, deep hypothermia with or without circulatory arrest in both adults and children, retrograde cerebral perfusion, evaluations of new cardiovascular and anesthetic drugs, changes in coagulation associated with CPB including its monitoring and modulation with drugs, and the application and improvement of information provided by TEE. Cardiac anesthesiologists have made important contributions in the areas of risk assessment (e.g., Higgins) and outcome research (e.g., Mangano and Fleisher). Mangano has been instrumental in initiating large multicenter collaborative research projects (e.g., McSPI) to study outcome and assess methods of improving outcomes in cardiac surgery. Reves, Murkin, Newman, and many others have pioneered in the objective assessment of neurologic effects of CPB. Moffitt elevated to a new level the study of the effects of various anesthetic agents on myocardial ischemia using coronary sinus flow catheters. Cheng has provided objective data on the cost-effectiveness of fast tracking and early extubation. [Interestingly Barash et al. had advocated early extubation as long ago as 1980 (298)].

Finally, cardiac anesthesiologists have been responsive by developing techniques that facilitate new procedures in cardiac surgery, such as minimal access surgery, transmyocardial laser, the Batista operation, valve repair and use of stentless valves, more aggressive neonatal surgery, and fast-tracking.

SUMMING-UP

Several authors have examined the nature of discovery as it applies to medicine in general and to cardiothoracic surgery in particular (125,145,299–302). Comroe's monograph, *Retrospectroscope: Insights into Medical Discovery* (299), is particularly illuminating. Gott identified four common attributes of the great innovators in cardiac surgery: brilliance, determination, creativity, and courage (10). However, when one mentions courage on the part of a surgeon, one must concur with Westaby's comment after reviewing the course of Barney Miller, the first patient to receive a Javik artificial heart: "We should remember that without the consent of many *courageous patients,* the great advances [in cardiac surgery] could not occur" (12).

One of the phenomena frequently noted was the near-simultaneous accomplishment of a new procedure. Crafoord's first coarctation repair was in October 1944, Gross' in July 1945. Sellors' first closed pulmonary valvotomy was in December 1947, while Brock's occurred in February 1948. Bailey's first successful mitral commissurotomy was on June 10, 1948, while Harken's was on June 16. [The latter, on hearing of Bailey's earlier success, rushed to get his case published before Bailey's and was successful in doing so (100).] Smithy had done several mitral valve operations earlier that same year, and Brock did his first case in September. Lewis' first successful closure of an ASD using hypothermia was in September 1952, while Swan did an open pulmonary valvotomy using similar techniques in February of 1953. Kirklin conducted the first series of successful open heart operations with a mechanical heart-lung machine between March and May 1955, while Lillehei, who had been using cross-circulation up until that time, began his series of open heart surgery with a mechanical heart-lung machine between May and August of 1955. Ross first inserted a subcoronary aortic homograft valve in July 1962, and Barratt-Boyes did so in August of the same year. Jateen did the first successful arterial switch operation for TGA in Sao Paulo in May of 1975, and Yacoub did his first in London in October. Some of these surgeons were aware of the others' work, and competition may have played a role. But also it seems that sometimes the time is right for a new procedure to appear. All the pieces of the puzzle are ready to be assembled by the adventuresome, competent, and eager surgeon.

There are a number of relevant observations to be made from a review of the history of cardiac surgery and anesthesiology.

1. Serendipity often comes into play. Examples include the discovery of heparin [McLean was looking for a coagulant (49,50)], protamine reversal of heparin [Chargoff and Olson were trying to prolong the action of heaparin (51)], selective coronary angiography (Sones was performing an aortic root arteriogram when the catheter inadvertently slipped into the coronary artery—and the patient didn't die!), closed chest massage (Kowenhoven and Jude noted a pressure rise when the defibrillator paddles were applied), and aprotinin (while trying to block the inflammatory response to CPB, the investigators noted that the surgical fields were surprisingly dry).
2. There is often a thin line between success and failure. Strieder might have accomplished the first successful ductus closure had not his patient died of sudden gastric aspiration 5 days after surgery, and Merendino might have accomplished the first successful correction of TGA had not his patient suddenly died of an apparent cerebral air embolism several hours postoperatively.
3. Beware of rejecting new ideas and the danger of "conventional wisdom." The early rejection of Brunton's and Souttar's proposal and success with mitral commissurotomy, rejection of Kolessov's and Green's IMA-coronary artery anastomosis, and Gross' rejection of Taussig's proposal to create an artificial ductus are examples.
4. Perserverance is important. Charles Bailey persisted for 3 years before he achieved a successful mitral commissurotomy. Mustard devoted 10 years to conquering TGA. Vineberg demonstrated the validity of his operation in the laboratory in 1946 and performed the operation clinically and published his results throughout the 1950s, but it was not until Sones demonstrated function of these implants in the early 1960s that Vineberg's work was accepted. Most impressively, John Gibbon pursued his quest for 23 years until he solved the challenge of CPB.
5. Do not get discouraged if you do not get to train where you want to. Helen Taussig was rejected for an internship at Johns Hopkins, and Alfred Blalock was rejected for a chief residency by the same institution. (The institution then had the wisdom to bring both of them back on its faculty.)
6. Youth does not preclude innovative success and in fact tends to encourage it. McLean was a medical student when he discovered heparin (49,50), and Gross was a surgery resident when he first successfully ligated a PDA. Gibbon constructed his first successful heart-lung machine while still in training. Kirklin, Lillehei, and Starr were in their mid-thirties and barely out of their training when they started making their monumental contributions. [Conversely, Lowell Edwards and William Kouwenhoven were retired engineers when they made their important contributions].
7. Laboratory work is important in providing a foundation for clinical success. Most of the great clinical advances, such as ligation of PDA, resection of coarctation, creation of the subclavian-to-pulmonary artery shunt, IMA implantation, and artificial valves, were preceded by extensive laboratory investigation. Further, as pointed out by Comroe, many of these clinical advances were dependent on basic science research, much of which had no apparent practical application at the time that it was performed (125).
8. Interaction with those in other disciplines and other countries is also important. Wheat's application of anti-adrinergic therapy for aortic dissection was inspired by communication with pharmacologists and veterinary science specialists. Dillard's and Barratt-Boyes' development of techniques for deep hypothermic circulatory arrest arose from input from surgeon-scientists from Japan who were working in their units.
9. Competetion can spur success—witness Crafoord and Gross, Harken and Bailey, Swan and Lewis, and Kirklin and Lillehei.
10. A creative environment stimulates success. The Johns Hopkins Hospital under Alfred Blalock was an early example. From this environment also came Bahnson, Cooley, McGoon, Sabistan, and Spencer. Another dramatic example is the University of Minnesota in the early 1950s under the leadership of its chairman of surgery, Owen Wangensteen. In that environment over the course of 5 years, Dennis attempted the first open heart surgery using a heart-lung machine, Lewis first closed an ASD with hypothermia, Lillehei introduced cross-circulation and with it first successfully closed a VSD and repaired a tetralogy of Fallot, Campbell successfully used a biologic (dog lung) oxygenator, and DeWall introduced his bubble oxygenator. Trainees at the University of Minnesota at that time included Barnard, Shumway, and Gott (303). A similarly productive environment was subsequently established by Shumway at Stanford with its impressive research and clinical program in heart transplantation.
11. Consider reexamining the staus quo, the "standard of care"—examples include hypothermia, cold cardioplegia, and prolonged intubation.
12. Reexamine discarded ideas and methods. Examples are potassium cardiac arrest, mitral annuloplasty, off-pump CABG, radial artery grafts, homograft valves, and the Ross procedure.
13. Reassess but don't necessarily abandon a sound procedure because of early failure. After his first five attempts at correction of tetralogy failed, Kirklin waited a year and tried again, this time with 80% success. Harken

and Brock almost quit doing mitral commissurotomies when they had a series of early deaths, but immediately thereafter almost all of their patients survived. Four of Starr's first five aortic valve replacement patients died. After the prosthesis was modified, nine of the next ten survived.
14. Finally, we all "stand on the shoulders of giants."

Lest we become overly impressed with the accomplishments and outcome with current cardiac surgery and anesthesia, some of the remarkably good results of our predecessors should be recalled. In their 1956 report of their first 1,000 cases of surgery for congenital heart disease at Chicago's Memorial Children's Hospital, Potts and McQuiston (surgeon and anesthesiologist, respectively) reported no deaths among 347 children (age 28 days to 16 years) undergoing closure of a PDA (257). In 1959 Conn reported 63 consecutive secundum ASDs closed with the aid of hypothermia and inflow occlusion at the Hospital for Sick Children in Toronto without a fatality (267). In 1970 Wynands reported only 1 death in their last 78 patients undergoing a Vineberg procedure in Montreal, even though one third had rest angina and this operation did not result in immediate improvement in coronary perfusion (273). But perhaps most striking of all was the report by Dwight McGoon and Emerson Moffitt, respectively surgeon and anesthesiologist at the Mayo Clinic, of their first 100 aortic valve replacements with a Starr-Edwards valve, done between February 1993 and December 1994 with no deaths (130). This was of course before the availability of CABG, cardioplegia, PACs, and TEE—and the patients were usually extubated in the operating room!

In closing this brief history of cardiac surgery and anesthesia, if we wonder what it has all been about, we need only listen to Lord Brock: "These operations . . . are tiring and anxious procedures involving much care, responsibility and hard work. Fortunately they have their happier side and we are in large part recompensated for the long and difficult hours by seeing the almost miraculous change in the children themselves and in witnessing the joy and relief of the parents when they see their children running about happily and without effort like other children" (212). The modern anesthesiologist is perhaps jaded by daily miracles that go unrecognized. To really appreciate what the cardiac anesthesiologist does, it may be necessary to have been a physician, as Lord Brock was 4 years before he made the statement quoted, when medicine and surgery had nothing to offer most patients with heart disease. And if we are content with what we are able to do today and accept some obstacles as unsolvable, let us contemplate the closing paragraph in Kirklin's article on the occasion of the 25th anniversary of open heart surgery at the Mayo Clinic: "We could, of course . . . rejoice in our accomplishments, and accept the idea that nature sets certain limits to everything, including cardiac surgery. Billroth expressed such a view in 1897 when he said that cardiac surgery had reached the limits set by nature. Those in 1954 who urged aborting the pump-oxygenator effort must have had a similar notion. Not the passage of time but the efforts of many people have proven the idea to be wrong at both points in time. I believe that acceptance of such an idea today would also be wrong" (113).

ACKNOWLEDGEMENT

The author gratefully acknowledges the opportunities, challenges, and inspiration provided to him by Drs. K. Alvin Merendino and Thomas F. Hornbein of the University of Washington and Dr. Fawzy G. Estafanous of the Cleveland Clinic.

REFERENCES

1. Meade RH. *A history of thoracic surgery.* Springfield, IL: Charles C Thomas Publisher, 1961.
2. Liss RS. *The history of heart surgery in the United States (1938–1960).* Zurich: Juris Druck + Verlag, 1967.
3. Johnson SL. *The history of cardiac surgery 1896–1955.* Baltimore: The Johns Hopkins University Press, 1970.
4. Clowes GHA. The historical development of the surgical treatment of heart disease: *Symposium on the Heart, American Association for the History of Medicine 32nd Annual Meeting, May 22, 1959.* New York: Plenum Press, 1960.
5. Blalock A. Cardiovascular surgery, past and present. *J Thorac Cardiovasc Surg* 1966;51:153.
6. Harken DE, Curtis LE. Heart surgery: legend and a long look. *Am J Cardiol* 1967;19:393.
7. Litwak RS. The growth of cardiac surgery: historical notes. *Cardiovascular Clinics* 1971;3:5.
8. Brewer LA III. Open heart surgery and myocardial revascularization: historical notes. *Am J Surg* 1981;141:618.
9. Kirklin JW. Technical and scientific advances in cardiac surgery over the past 25 years. *Ann Thorac Surg* 1990;49:26.
10. Gott VL. And it happened during our lifetime. . . . *Ann Thorac Surg* 1993;55:1057.
11. Shumacker HB Jr. *The evolution of cardiac surgery.* Bloomington, IN: Indiana University Press, 1992.
12. Westaby S, Bosher C. *Landmarks in cardiac surgery.* Oxford: Isis Medical Media, 1997.
13. Gross RE, Hubbard JP. Surgical ligation of a patent ductus arteriosus. *JAMA* 1939;112:729.
14. Crafoord C, Nylin G. Congenital coarctation of the aorta and its surgical treatment. *J Thorac Surg* 1945;14:347.
15. Blalock A, Taussig HB. The surgical treatment of malformations of the heart in which there is pulmonary stenosis or pulmonary atresia. *JAMA* 1945;138:189.
16. Potts WJ, Smith S, Gibson S. Anastomosis of the aorta to a pulmonary artery: certain types in congenital heart disease. *JAMA* 1946;132:627.
17. Sellors TH. Surgery of pulmonary stenosis: a case in which the pulmonary valve was successfully divided. *Lancet* 1948;1:988.
18. Blalock A, Hanlon CR. The surgical treatment of complete transposition of the aorta and the pulmonary artery. *Surg Gynecol Obstet* 1950;90:1.
19. Bailey CP. The surgical treatment of mitral stenosis (mitral commissurotomy). *Dis Chest* 1949;15:377.

20. Harken DE, Ellis LB, Ware PF, et al. The surgical treatment of mitral stenosis: I. Valvuloplasty. *N Engl J Med* 1948;239:801.
21. Brock RC, Campbell M. Infundibular resection or dilitation for infundibular stenosis. *Br Heart J* 1950;12:403.
22. Vineberg A, Miller G. Internal mammary coronary anastomosis in the surgical treatment of coronary artery insufficiency. *Can Med Assoc J* 1951;64:204.
23. Muller WH Jr, Dammann JF Jr. The treatment of certain congenital malformations of the heart by the creation of pulmonic stenosis to reduce pulmonary hypertension and excessive pulmonary blood flow: a preliminary report. *Surg Gynecol Obstet* 1952;95:213.
24. Bailey CP, Romirez HPR, Larzelene HB. Surgical treatment of aortic stenosis. *JAMA* 1952;150:1647.
25. Hufnagel CA, Harvey WP. The surgical correction of aortic regurgitation: preliminary report. *Bull Georgetown Univ Med Center* 1953;6:3.
26. Gross RE, Watkins E Jr, Pomeranz AA, et al. A method for surgical closure of interauricular septal defects. *Surg Gynecol Obstet* 1953;96:1.
27. Lewis FJ, Taufic M. Closure of atrial septal defects with aid of hypothermia: experimental accomplishments and the report of one successful case. *Surgery* 1953;33:52.
28. Dodrill FD. Experience with the mechanical heart. *JAMA* 1954; 154:299.
29. Gibbon JH Jr. Application of a mechanical heart and lung apparatus to cardiac surgery. *Minn Med* 1954;37:171.
30. Warden HE, Cohen M, Read RC, et al. Controlled cross circulation for open intracardiac surgery: physiologic studies and results of creation and closure of ventricular septal defects. *J Thorac Surg* 1954;28:331.
31. Lillehei CW, Cohen M, Warden HE, et al. The results of direct vision closure of ventricular septal defects in eight patients by means of controlled cross circulation. *Surg Gynecol Obstet* 1955; 43:1980.
32. Kirklin JW, Dushane JW, Patrick RT, et al. Intracardiac surgery with the aid of a mechanical pump-oxygenator system (Gibbon type): report of eight cases. *Proc Staff Meetings Mayo Clinic* 1955;30:201.
33. Glenn WWL. Circulatory bypass of the right side of the heart: IV. Shunt between superior vena cava and distal right pulmonary artery: report of clinical application. *N Engl J Med* 1958; 259:117.
34. Senning A. Surgical correction of transposition of the great vessels. *Surgery* 1959;45:966.
35. Harken DE, Soroff HS, Taylor WJ, et al. Partial and complete prosthesis in aortic insufficiency. *J Thorac Cardiovasc Surg* 1960; 40:744.
36. Starr A, Edwards ML. Mitral replacement: clinical experience with a ball-valve prosthesis. *Ann Surg* 1961;154:726.
37. Mustard WT. Successful two-stage correction of transposition of the great vessels. *Surgery* 1964;55:469.
38. Favaloro RG. Saphenous vein autograft replacement of severe segmental coronary artery occlusion. *Ann Thorac Surg* 1968;5: 334.
39. Barnard CN. The operation: a human cardiac transplant. An interim report of a successful operation performed at Groote Schuur Hospital, Cape Town. *S Afr Med J* 1967;41:1271.
40. Johnson WD, Flemma RJ, Lepley D, et al. Extended treatment of severe coronary artery disease: a total surgical approach. *Ann Surg* 1969;170:460.
41. Green GE, Stertzer SM, Reppert EH. Coronary arterial bypass grafts. *Ann Thorac Surg* 1968;5:443.
42. Fontan F, Baudet E. Surgical repair of tricuspid atresia. *Thorax* 1971;26:240.
43. Jatene AD, Fontes VF, Paulista DP, et al. Anatomic correction of transposition of the great vessels. *J Thorac Cardiovasc Surg* 1976;72:364.
44. Norwood WI, Lang P, Castaneda AR, et al. Experience with operations for hypoplastic left heart syndrome. *J Thorac Cardiovasc Surg* 1981;82:511.
45. DeVries WC, Anderson JL, Joyce LD, et al. Clinical use of the total artificial heart. *N Engl J Med* 1984;310:273.
46. Cooley DA, Frazier DH, VanBuren CT, et al. Cardiac transplantation in an 8 month old female infant with subendocarial fibroelastosis. *JAMA* 1986;256:1326.
47. Bailey LL, Nehlsen-Cannarella SL, Doroshow RW, et al. Cardiac allotransplantation in newborns as a therapy for hypoplastic left heart syndrome. *N Engl J Med* 1986;315:949.
48. Leonard KA, Davey RJ. Principles of transfusion medicine. In: Lake CL, Moore RA, eds. *Blood: hemostasis, transfusion, and alternatives in the perioperative period.* New York: Raven Press, 1995:231.
49. Couch NP. About heparin, or . . . Whatever happened to Jay McLean? *J Vasc Surg* 1989;10:1.
50. Baird RJ. "Give us the tools. . . . " The story of heparin—as told by sketches from the likes of William Howell, Jay McLean, Charles Best and Gordon Murray. *J Vasc Surg* 1990;11:4.
51. Chargaff E, Olson KB. Studies on the chemistry of blood coagulation: IV. Studies on the action of heparin and other anticoagulants: the influence of protamine on the anticoagulant effect in vitro. *J Biol Chem* 1937;122:153.
52. Jorpes E, Edman P, Thaning T. Neutralization of action of heparin by protamine. *Lancet* 1939;237:975.
53. Clark LC Jr, Gollan F, Gupta VB. The oxygenation of blood by gas dispersion. *Science* 1950;111:85.
54. Weirich WL, Paneth M, Gott VL, et al. Control of complete heart block by use of an artificial pacemaker and a myocardial electrode. *Circ Res* 1958;6:410.
55. Julian OC, Lopez-Belio M, Dye WS, et al. The median sternal incision in intracardiac surgery with extracorporeal circulation: a general evaluation of its use in heart surgery. *Surgery* 1957; 42:753.
56. Lillehei CW, Cardozo RH. Use of median sternotomy with femoral artery cannulation in open cardiac surgery. *Surg Gynecol Obstet* 1959;108:707.
57. Sealy WC, Brown IW, Young WG Jr. A report on the use of both extracorporeal circulation and hypothermia for open-heart surgery. *Ann Surg* 1958;147:603.
58. Drew CE, Anderson IM. Profound hypothermia in cardiac surgery: report of three cases. *Lancet* 1959;1:748.
59. Zuhdi N, McCollough B, Carey J, et al. Double-helical reservoir heart-lung machine: designed for hypothermic perfusion; primed with 5% glucose in water; inducing hypothermia. *Arch Surg* 1961;82:166.
60. Dillard DH, Mohri H, Hessel EA, et al. Correction of total anomalous pulmonary venous drainage in infants using hypothermia and total circulatory arrest. *Circulation* 1967;35[Suppl I]:I-105.
61. Swan HJC, Ganz W, Forrester J, et al. Catheterization of the heart in man with use of a flow-directed balloon-tipped catheter. *N Engl J Med* 1970;283:447.
62. Gay WA Jr, Ebert PA. Functional, metabolic, and morphologic effects of potassium induced cardioplegia. *Surgery* 1973;74:284.
63. Caves PK, Stinson EB, Graham AF, et al. Percutaneous transvenous endomyocardial biopsy. *JAMA* 1973;225:288.
64. Bull BS, Korpmon RA, Huse WM, et al. Heparin therapy during extracorporeal circulation: I. Problems inherent in existing heparin protocols. *J Thorac Cardiovasc Surg* 1975;69:674.
65. Bull BS, Huse WM, Brauer FS, et al. Heparin therapy during extracorporeal circulation: II. The use of a dose-response curve

to individualize heparin and protamine dosage. *J Thorac Cardiovasc Surg* 1975;69:685.

66. Olley PM, Coceani F, Bodach E. E-type prostaglandins: a new emergency therapy for certain cyanotic congenital heart malformations. *Circulation* 1976;53:728.
67. Oyer PE, Stinson EB, Jamieson SW, et al. [Shumway's group]. One year experience with cyclosporin-A in clinical heart transplantation. *Heart Transplant* 1982;1:285.
68. Royston D, Bidstrup BD, Taylor KM, et al. Effect of aprotinin on need for blood transfusion after repeat open-heart surgery. *Lancet* 1987;2:1289.
69. Van Oeveren W, Jansen NJG, Bidstrup BP, et al. Effects of aprotinin on hemostatic mechanisms during cardiopulmonary bypass. *Ann Thorac Surg* 1987;44:640.
70. Gravlee GP. Heparin-coated cardiopulmonary bypass circuits. *J Cardiothorac Vasc Anesth* 1994;8:213.
71. Naik SK, Knight A, Elliott M. A prospective randomized study of a modified technique of ultrafiltration during pediatric open-heart surgery. *Circulation* 1991;84[Suppl III]:III-422.
72. Wareing TH, Davila-Roman VG, Barzilai B, et al. Management of the severely atherosclerotic ascending aorta during cardiac operations: a strategy for detection and treatment. *J Thorac Cardiovasc Surg* 1992;103:453.
73. Steudel W, Hurford WE, Zapol WM. Inhaled nitric oxide: basic biology and clinical applications. *Anesthesiology* 1999;91:1590.
74. Watson JD, Crick FHC. A structure for deoxyribose nucleic acid. *Nature* 1953;171:737.
75. Sones FM Jr, Shirey EK, Proudfit L, et al. Cine-coronary arteriography. *Circulation* 1959;20:773(abst).
76. Chardack WM, Gage AA, Greatbatch W. A transistorized implantable pacemaker for the long-term correction of complete heart block. *Surgery* 1960;48:643.
77. Kouwenhoven WB, Jude JR, Knickerbocker GG. Closed-chest cardiac manage. *JAMA* 1960;173:1064.
78. Wheat MW, Palmer RF, Bartley TD, et al. Treatment of dissecting aneurysms of the aorta without surgery. *J Thorac Cardiovasc Surg* 1965;50:364.
79. Rashkind WJ, Miller WW. Creation of an atrial septal defect without thoracotomy: a palliative approach to complete transposition of the great arteries. *JAMA* 1966;196:173.
80. Kantrowitz A, Tjonneland S, Freed PS, et al. Initial clinical experience with intraaortic balloon pumping in cardiogenic shock. *JAMA* 1968;203:113.
81. Gruntzig A. Transluminal dilitation of coronary-artery stenosis. *Lancet* 1978;2:263.
82. Rashkind WJ. Transcatheter treatment of congenital heart disease. *Circulation* 1983;67:71.
83. McKay RG, Safian RD, Lock JE, et al. Balloon dilitation of calcific aortic stenosis in elderly patients: postmortem, intraoperative, and percutaneous valvuloplasty studies. *Circulation* 1986;74:119.
84. Rocchini AP. Transcatheter closure of atrial septal defects: past, present, future [Editorial comment]. *Circulation* 1990;82:1044.
85. Ignarro LJ, Buga GM, Wood KS, et al. Endothelium-derived relaxing factor produced and released from artery and vein is nitric oxide. *Proc Natl Acad Sci USA* 1987;84:9265.
86. Palmer RMJ, Ferrige AG, Moncada S. Nitric oxide release accounts for the biologic activity of endothelium-derived relaxing factor. *Nature* 1987;327:524.
87. Ellis RH. The first trans-auricular mitral valvotomy: an account to mark the fiftieth anniversary of the operation. *Anaesthesia* 1975;30:374.
88. Ellis FH Jr. Development of mitral valve surgery. In: Ellis FH Jr. *Surgery for acquired mitral valve disease.* Philadelphia: WB Saunders, 1967:3.
89. Gibbon JH Jr. Artificial maintenance of the circulation during experimental occlusion of the pulmonary artery. *Arch Surg* 1937;34:1105.
90. Dobell ARC. The ductus and the coarctation. *Ann Thorac Surg* 1994;57:246.
91. Graybiel A, Strieder JW, Boyer NH. An attempt to obliterate the patent ductus arteriosus in a patient with subacute bacterial endocarditis. *Am Heart J* 1938;15:621.
92. Gross RE. Surgical correction for coarctation of the aorta. *Surgery* 1945;18:673.
93. Nuland SB. A triumph of twentieth-century medicine: Helen Taussig and the blue-baby operation. In: Nuland SB. *Doctors.* New York: Vintage Books, 1988:422.
94. Blalock A. Physiopathology and surgical treatment of congenital cardiovascular defects: Harvey Lecture, November 15, 1945. *Bull N Y Acad Med* 1946;22:57.
95. Taussig HB. On the evaluation of our knowledge of congenital malformations of the heart: The T. Duckett Jones Memorial Lecture. *Circulation* 1965;31:768.
96. Brock RC. Pulmonary valvotomy for the relief of congenital pulmonary stenosis: a report of three cases. *BMJ* 1948;1:1121.
97. Smithy HG, Boone JA, Stallworth JM. Surgical treatment of constrictive valvular disease of the heart. *Surg Gynecol Obstet* 1950;90:175.
98. Gonzalez-Levine L, Bailey CP, Harken DE. The dawn of the modern era of mitral valve surgery. *Ann Thorac Surg* 1992;53:916.
99. Harken DE. Foreign bodies in, and in relation to the thoracic blood vessels and heart: I. Techniques for approaching and removing foreign bodies from the chambers of the heart. *Surg Gynecol Obstet* 1946;83:117.
100. Harken DE. The emergence of cardiac surgery: I. Personal recollections of the 1940's and 1950's. *J Thorac Cardiovasc Surg* 1989;98:805.
101. Baker C, Brock RC, Campbell M. Valvotomy for mitral stenosis: report of six successful cases. *BMJ* 1950;1:1283.
102. Logan A, Turner K. Surgical treatment of mitral stenosis with particular reference to the transventricular approach with a mechanical dilator. *Lancet* 1959;2:874.
103. Kirklin JW, Daugherty GW, Burchell HB, et al. Repair of the partial form of persistent common atrioventricular canal: so-called ostium primum type atrial septal defect with interventricular communication. *Ann Surg* 1955;142:858.
104. Lewis JF, Varco RL, Taufic M. Repair of atrial septal defects in man under direct vision with the aid of hypothermia. *Surgery* 1954;36:538.
105. Swan H, Zeavin I, Blount SG Jr, et al. Surgery by direct-vision in the open heart during hypothermia. *JAMA* 1953;153:1081.
106. Romaine-Davis A. *John Gibbon and his heart-lung machine.* Philadelphia: University of Pensylvania Press, 1991.
107. Gibbon JH Jr. Development of heart-lung apparatus. *Rev Surg* 1970;24:231.
108. Gibbon JH Jr. The development of the heart-lung apparatus. *Am J Surg* 1978;135:608.
109. Gibbon JH Jr. The maintenance of life during experimental occlusion of the pulmonary artery followed by survival. *Surg Gynecol Obstet* 1939;91:138.
110. Miller BJ, Gibbon JH Jr, Fineberg C. An improved mechanical heart and lung apparatus: its use during open cardiotomy in experimental animals. *Med Clin North Am* 1953;37:1603.
111. Lillehei CW. Historical development of cardiopulmonary bypass in Minnesota. In: Gravelee GP, Davis RF, Kurusz M, eds. *Cardiopulmonary bypass: principles and practice,* 2nd Ed. Baltimore: Lippincott Williams & Wilkins, 2000:3.
112. Lillehei CW, Cohen M, Warden HE, et al. The direct-vision intracardiac correction of congenital anomalies by controlled

cross circulation: results in thirty-two patients with ventricular septal defects, tetralogy of Fallot and atrioventricularis communis defects. *Surgery* 1955;38:11.
113. Kirklin JW. Open-heart surgery at the Mayo Clinic: the 25th anniversary. *Mayo Clinic Proc* 1980;55:339.
114. Lillehei CW, DeWall RA, Read RC, et al. Direct vision intracardiac surgery in man using a simple, disposable artificial oxygenator. *Dis Chest* 1956;29:1.
115. Warden HE. C Walton Lillehei: Pioneer cardiac surgeon. *J Thorac Cardiovasc Surg* 1989;98:833.
116. Kirklin JW, Donald DE, Harshbarger HG, et al. Studies in extra-corporeal circulation: I. Applicability of Gibbon-type pump oxygentor to human intracardiac surgery: 40 cases. *Ann Surg* 1956;144:2.
117. Hewitt RL, Creech O Jr. History of the pump oxygenator. *Arch Surg* 1966;93:680.
118. Utley JR. Early development of cardiopulmonary bypass. *Perfusion* 1986;1:1.
119. Melrose DG. A history of cardiopulmonary bypass. In: Taylor KM, ed. *Cardiopulmonary bypass.* Baltimore: Williams & Wilkins, 1986:1.
120. Livesey SA, Lennox SC. Historical aspects. In: Kay PH, ed. *Techniques in extracorporeal circulation.* Boston: Butterworth Heinemann, 1992:1.
121. Castillo JE, Bocchieri KA, Fyman P, et al. Historical aspects of cardiopulmonary surgery. In: Casthely DA, Bergman D, eds. *Cardiopulmonary bypass: physiology related complications and pharmacology.* Mount Kisco, NY: Futura Publishing, 1991:1.
122. Galletti PM, Mora CT. Cardiopulmonary bypass: the historical foundation, the furure promise. In: Mora CT, ed. *Cardiopulmonary bypass: principles and techniques of extracorporeal circulation.* New York: Springer-Verlag, 1995:3.
123. Senning A. Developments in cardiac surgery in Stockholm during the mid and late 1950's. *J Thorac Cardiovasc Surg* 1989;98:825.
124. Cooley DA. Recollections of early development and later trends in cardiac surgery. *J Thorac Cardiovasc Surg* 1989;98:817.
125. Comroe JH Jr, Dripps RD. Ben Franklin and open heart surgery. *Circ Res* 1974;35:661.
126. Dobell ARC, Bailey JS. Charles Drew and the origins of deep hypothermic circulatory arrest. *Ann Thorac Surg* 1997;63:1193.
127. Harken DE, Taylor WJ, Lefemine AA, et al. Aortic valve replacement with a caged ball valve. *Am J Cardiol* 1962;9:292.
128. Starr A, Edwards ML, McCord CW, et al. Aortic valve replacement: clinical experience with a semirigid ball-valve prosthesis. *Circulation* 1963;27:779.
129. McGoon DC, Moffitt EA. Total prosthetic reconstruction of the aortic valve. *J Thorac Cardiovasc Surg* 1963;46:162.
130. McGoon DC, Pestana C, Moffitt EA. Decreased risk of aortic valve surgery. *Arch Surg* 1965;91:779.
131. Ross DN. Homograft replacement of the aortic valve. *Lancet* 1962;2:487.
132. Barratt-Boyes BG. Homograft aortic valve replacement in aortic incompetence and stenosis. *Thorax* 1964;19:131.
133. Ross DN. Replacement of aortic and mitral valves with a pulmonary autograft. *Lancet* 1967;2:956.
134. Lefrak EA, Starr A. *Cardiac valve prostheses.* New York: Appleton-Century-Crofts, 1979.
135. Miller DW Jr. A short history of myocardial revascularization. In Miller DW Jr. *The practice of coronary artery bypass surgery.* New York: Plenum Medical Book Co., 1982:1.
136. Cobb LA, Thomas GJ, Dillard DH, et al. An evaluation of internal-mammary-artery ligation by a double-blind technique. *N Engl J Med* 1959;260:1115.
137. Vineberg AM. Development of an anastomosis between the coronary vessels and a transplanted internal mammary artery. *Can Med Assoc J* 1946;55:117.
138. Vineberg A. Coronary vascular anastomosis by internal mammary artery implantation. *Can Med Assoc J* 1958;78:871.
139. Favaloro RG. History. In: Favalora RG. *Surgical treatment of coronary arteriosclerosis.* Baltimore: Williams & Wilkins, 1970: 1.
140. Dobell ARC. Arthur Vineberg and the internal mammary implantation procedure. *Ann Thorac Surg* 1992;53:167.
141. Shrager JB. The Vineberg procedure: the immediate forerunner for coronary artery bypass grafting. *Ann Thorac Surg* 1994;57: 1354.
142. Thomas JL. The Vineberg legacy: Internal mammary artery implantation from inception to obsolescence. *Tex Heart Inst J* 1999;26:107.
143. Effler DB, Favaloro RG, Groves LK. Coronary artery surgery utilizing saphenous vein graft techniques: clinical experience with 224 operations. *J Thorac Cardiovasc Surg* 1970;59:147.
144. Favaloro RG. Landmarks in the development of coronary artery bypass surgery. *Circulation* 1998;98:466.
145. Spencer FC. Intellectual creativity in thoracic surgeons. *J Thorac Cardiovasc Surg* 1983;86:163.
146. Goetz RH, Rohman M, Haller JD, et al. Internal mammary coronary artery anastomosis: a non suture method employing tantalum rings. *J Thorac Cardiovasc Surg* 1961;41:378.
147. Mueller RL, Rosengart TK, Isom DW. The history of surgery for ischemic heart disease. *Ann Thorac Surg* 1997;63:869.
148. Connolly JE. The history of coronary artery surgery. *J Thorac Cardiovasc Surg* 1978;76:733.
149. Kolessov VI. Mammary artery-coronary artery anastomosis as method of treatment for angina pectoris. *J Thorac Cardiovasc Surg* 1967;54:535.
150. Green GE. Internal mammary artery-to-coronary artery anastomosis: three-year experience with 165 patients. *Ann Thorac Surg* 1972;14:261.
151. Miller DW Jr, Ivey TD, Bailey WW, et al. The practice of coronary artery bypass surgery in 1980. *J Thorac Cardiovasc Surg* 1981;81:423.
152. Lytle BW, Loop FD, Cosgrove DM, et al. Long-term (5 to 12 years) serial studies of internal mammary artery and saphenous vein coronary bypass grafts. *J Thorac Cardiovasc Surg* 1985;89: 248.
153. Loop FD, Lytle BW, Cosgrove DM, et al. Influence of the internal-mammary-artery graft on the 10-year survival and other cardiac events. *N Engl J Med* 1986;314:1.
154. Kantrowitz A, Haller JD, eds. Symposium on human heart transplantation. *Am J Cardiol* 1968;22:760.
155. Haller JD, Cerruti MM. Heart transplantation in man: a compilation of cases, January 1, 1967 to October 23, 1968. *Am J Cardiol* 1968;22:840.
156. McGregor CGA, Oyer PE, Shumway NE. Heart and heart-lung transplantation. *Prog Allergy* 1986;38:346.
157. Lansman SL, Ergin MA, Griepp RB. History of cardiac transplantation. In: Wallwork J, ed. *Heart and heart-lung transplantation.* Philadelphia: WB Saunders, 1989:3.
158. Reitz BA. The history of heart and heart-lung transplantation. In: Baumgartner WA, Reitz BA, Archuff SC. *Heart and heart-lung transplantation.* Philadelphia: WB Saunders, 1990:1.
159. Patterson C, Patterson KB. The history of heart transplantation. *Am J Med Sci* 1997;314:190.
160. Di Bardino DJ. The history and development of cardiac transplantation. *Tex Heart Inst J* 1999;26:198.
161. Mustard WT, Chute AL, Keith JD, et al. A surgical approach to transposition of the great vessels with extracorporeal circuit. *Surgery* 1954;36:39.
162. Merendino KA, Jesseph JE, Herron PW, et al. Interatrial venous transposition: a one-stage intracardiac operation for the conversion of complete transposition of the aorta and pulmonary artery

to corrected transposition. Theory and clinical experience. *Surgery* 1957;42:898.
163. Mohri H, Hessel EA II, Nelson RJ, et al. Use of Rheomacrodex and hyper-ventilation in prolonged circulatory arrest under deep hypothermia induced by surface cooling: method for open heart surgery in infants. *Am J Surg* 1966;112:241.
164. Horiuchi T, Koyamada K, Matano I, et al. Radical operation for ventricular septal defect in infancy. *J Thorac Cardiovasc Surg* 1963;46:180.
165. Mohri H, Dillard DH. *Hypothermia for cardiovascular surgery.* New York: Igaku-Shoin, 1981.
166. Barratt-Boyes BG, Simpson MN, Neutze JM. Intracardiac surgery in neonates and infants under deep hypothermia. *Circulation* 1970;61[Suppl III]:III-71.
167. Hikasu Y, Shrotani H, Satomura K, et al. Open heart surgery in infants with an aid of hypothermia anesthesia. *Arch Jap Chir* 1967;36:495.
168. Cross FS, Kay EB. Direct vision repair of intracardiac defects utilizing a rotating disc reservoir-oxygenator. *Surg Gynecol Obstet* 1957;104:711.
169. Gott VL, Sellers RD, DeWall RA, et al. A disposable unitized plastic sheet oxygenator for open heart surgery. *Dis Chest* 1957; 32:615.
170. DeWall RA, Najafi H, Roden T. A hard-shell temperature controlling disposable blood oxygenator: use in clinical open heart surgery. *JAMA* 1966;197:1061.
171. Parsonnet V, Zucker IR, Asa MM. Preliminary investigation of the development of a permanent implantable pacemaker utilizing an intracardiac dipolar electrode. *Clin Res* 1962;10:391.
172. Siddons H, Davies JG. A new technique for internal cardiac pacing. *Lancet* 1963;2:1204.
173. Parsonnet V, Zucker R, Gilbert L, et al. Clinical use of an implantable standby pacemaker. *JAMA* 1966;196:104.
174. Kantrowitz A, Krankauer JS, Rosenbaum A, et al. Phase-shift balloon pumping in medically refractory cardiogenic shock. *Arch Surg* 1969;99:739.
175. Dehmer GJ, Starek PJF, Norfleet EA. History of intra-aortic balloon pump therapy. In: Maccioli GA, ed. *Intra-aortic balloon pump therapy.* Baltimore: Williams & Wilkins, 1997:1.
176. Roe BB. A history of clinical cardioplegia. In: Engelman RM, Levitsky S, eds. *A textbook of clinical cardioplegia.* Mount Kisco, NY: Futura Publishing, 1982:1.
177. Kirklin JW. Historical developments in myocardial management during cardiac surgery. In: Engelman RM, Levitsky S, eds. *A textbook of cardioplegia for difficult clinical problems.* Mount Kisco, NY: Futura Publishing, 1992:1.
178. Cordell AR. Milestones in the development of cardioplegia. *Ann Thorac Surg* 1995;60:793.
179. Shiroishi MS. Myocardial protection: the rebirth of potassium-based cardioplegia. *Tex Heart Inst J* 1999;26:71.
180. Yacoub MH, Radley-Smith R, Hilton CJ. Anatomic correction of complete transposition of the great arteries and ventricular septal defect in infancy. *BMJ* 1976;1:1112.
181. Bjork VO. The central flow tilting disc valve prosthesis (Bjork-Shiley) for mitral valve replacement. *Scand J Thorac Cardiovasc Surg* 1970;4:15.
182. Bjork VO, Holmgren A, Olin C, et al. Clinical and hemodynamic results of aortic valve replacement with the Bjork-Shiley tilting disc valve prosthesis. *Scand J Thorac Cardiovasc Surg* 1971;5:177.
183. Nicoloff DM, Emery RW, Arom KV, et al. Clinical and hemodynamic results with the St. Jude Medical cardiac valve prosthesis: a three-year experience. *J Thorac Cardiovasc Surg* 1981; 82:674.
184. Hannah H, Reis RL. Current status of porcine heterograft prosthesis: a 5 year appraisal. *Circulation* 1976;54[Suppl III]:III-27.
185. Ionescu MI, Tandon AP, Mary DAS, et al. Heart valve replacement with the Ionescu-Shiley pericardial xenograft. *J Thorac Cardiovasc Surg* 1977;73:31.
186. Voorhees MC, Brian BF. Blood-gas exchange devices. In: Stammers AH, ed. *Cardiopulmonary bypass: emerging trends and continued practices. Int Anesthesiol Clin* 1996;34:29.
187. Kaye MP. The registry of the International Society of Heart Transplantation: Fourth Official Report—1987. *J Heart Transpl* 1987;6:63.
188. Robbins RC, Barlow CW, Oyer PE, et al. Thirty years of cardiac transplantation at Stanford University. *J Thorac Cardiovasc Surg* 1999;117:939.
189. Kriett JM, Kaye MP. The registry of the International Society for Heart Transplantation: Seventh Official Report—1990. *J Heart Transplant* 1990;9:323.
190. Reitz BA, Wallwork JL, Hunt SA, et al. Heart-lung transplantation: successful therapy for patients with pulmonary vascular disease. *N Engl J Med* 1982;306:557.
191. Carpentier A, Chauvaud S, Fabiani JM, et al. Reconstructive surgery of mitral valve incompetence: ten year appraisal. *J Thorac Cardiovasc Surg* 1980;79:338.
192. Carpentier A. Cardiac valve surgery: the "French Connection." *J Thorac Cardiovasc Surg* 1983;86:323.
193. Chenoweth DE, Cooper SW, Hugli TE, et al. Complement activation during cardiopulmonary bypass. *N Engl J Med* 1981; 304:497.
194. Henriksen L, Hjelms E, Lindeburgh T. Brain hyperperfusion during cardiac operations: cerebral blood flow measured in man by intra-arterial injection of xenon-133. Evidence suggestive of intra-operative microembolism. *J Thorac Cardiovasc Surg* 1983; 86:202.
195. McKay RD, Reves JG, Karp RB, et al. Effects of cardiopulmonary bypass on cerebral blood flow. *Anesth Analg* 1983;62: 274(abst).
196. Govier AV, Reves JG, McKay RD, et al. Factors and their influence on regional cerebral blood flow during nonpulsatile cardiopulmonary bypass. *Ann Thorac Surg* 1984;38:592.
197. Ream AK, Reitz BA, Silverberg G. Temperature correction of PCO_2 and pH in estimating acid-base status: an example of the emperor's new clothes? *Anesthesiology* 1982;56:41.
198. Royston D. High-dose aprotinin therapy: a review of the first five-years experience. *J Cardiothorac Vasc Anesth* 1992;6:76.
199. Westaby S. Aprotinin in perspective. *Ann Thorac Surg* 1993; 55:1033.
200. Burack JH, Impellizzeri P, Hormel P, et al. Public reporting of surgical mortality: a survey of New York State cardiac surgeons. *Ann Thorac Surg* 1999;68:1195.
201. Green J, Wintfeld N. Report cards on cardiac surgeons: assessing the New York State approach. *N Engl J Med* 1995;332:1229.
202. Chassin MR, Itannan E, Spencer FC. Measuring and improving the outcomes of coronary artery bypass graft surgery: New York's experience. In: Kaplan JA, ed. *Cardiac anesthesia,* 4th ed. Philadelphia: WB Saunders, 1999:1347.
203. O'Connor GT, Plume SK, Olmstead EM, et al. A regional intervention to improve the hospital mortality associated with coronary artery bypass surgery. *JAMA* 1996;275:841.
204. David TE, Pollick C, Bos J. Aortic valve replacement with stentless porcine aortic bioprosthesis. *J Thorac Cardiovasc Surg* 1990; 99:113.
205. Newburger JW, Jonas RA, Wernousky G, et al. A comparison of the perioperative neurologic effects of hypothermic circulatory arrest versus low-flow cardiopulmonary bypass in infant heart surgery. *N Engl J Med* 1993;329:329.
206. Bellinger DC, Jonas RA, Rappaport LA, et al. Developmental and neurologic status of children after heart surgery and hypo-

thermic circulatory arrest or low-flow cardiopulmonary bypass. *N Engl J Med* 1995;332:549.
207. Greeley WJ, Kern FH, Ungerleider RM, et al. The effects of hypothermic cardiopulmonary bypass and total circulatory arrest on cerebral metabolism in neonates, infants and children. *J Thorac Cardiovasc Surg* 1991;101:783.
208. Lichtenstein SV, Ashe FA, Dalati EL, et al. Warm heart surgery. *J Thorac Cardiovasc Surg* 1991;101:269.
209. Cook DJ. Changing temperature management for cardiopulmonary bypass. *Anesth Analg* 1999;88:1254.
210. Beique FA, Joffe D, Tousignant G, et al. Echocardiography-based assessment and management of atherosclerotic disease of the thoracic aorta. *J Cardiothorac Vasc Anesth* 1998;12:206.
211. Ueda Y, Miki S, Kusuhara F, et al. Surgical treatment of aneurysm or dissection involving the ascending aorta and aortic arch, utilizing circulatory arrest and retrograde cerebral perfusion. *J Cardiovasc Surg* 1990;31:553.
212. Brock RC. The surgery of pulmonic stenosis: The Alexander Simpson-Smith Lecture. *BMJ* 1949;2:399.
213. Keown KK. *Anesthesia for surgery of the heart,* 2nd ed. Springfield, IL: Charles C Thomas, 1963.
214. Lake CL. History of pediatric cardiac anesthesia. In: Lake CL. *Pediatric cardiac anesthesia,* 3rd ed. Stanford, CT: Appleton & Lange, 1998:1.
215. Arens JF. Three decades of cardiac anesthesia. *Mt Sinai J Med* 1985;52:516.
216. Wynands JE. History of cardiac anaesthesia: the contribution of Canadian anaesthetists to the evolution of cardiac surgery. *Can J Anaesth* 1996;43:518.
217. Keats AS. Cardiovascular anesthesia: perceptions and perspectives. The Rovenstine Lecture, 1983. *Anesthesiology* 1984;60:467.
218. Harmel MH, Lamont A. Anesthesia in the surgical treatment of congenital pulmonic stenosis. *Anesthesiology* 1946;7:477.
219. Massa DJ, Lundy JS, Faulconer A, et al. A plastic needle. *Proc Staff Meetings Mayo Clinic* 1950;25:413.
220. Keown KK, Grove DD, Roth HS. Anesthesia for commissurotomy for mitral stenosis: preliminary report. *JAMA* 1951;146:446.
221. Himmelstein A, Scheiner M. The cardiotachoscope. *Anesthesiology* 1952;13:62.
222. Smith C. An endo-esophageal stethoscope. *Anesthesiology* 1954;15:566.
223. Keown KK. *Anesthesia for surgery of the heart.* Springfield, IL: Charles C Thomas, 1956.
224. Gain EA. Anaesthetic experiences using extracorporeal circulation for open heart surgery. *Can Anaesth Soc J* 1957;4:419.
225. Mendelsohn D, MacKrell TN, MacLachlan MA, et al. Experiences using the pump-oxygenator for open cardiac surgery in man. *Anesthesiology* 1957;18:223.
226. Patrick RT, Theye RA, Moffitt EA. Studies in extracorporeal circulation: V. Anesthesia and supportive care during intracardiac surgery with the Gibbon-type pump-oxygenator. *Anesthesiology* 1957;18:673.
227. Theye RA, Patrick RT, Kirklin JW. The electro-encephalogram in patients undergoing open intracardiac operations with the aid of extracorporeal circulation. *J Thorac Surg* 1957;34:709.
228. Kirklin JW, Theye RA. Cardiac performance after open intracardiac surgery. *Circulation* 1963;28:1061.
229. Wynands JE, Sheridan CA, Kelkar K. Coronary artery disease and anaesthesia: experience in 120 patients for revascularization of the heart. *Can Anaesth Soc J* 1967;14:382.
230. Lowenstein E, Hallowell P, Levine FH, et al. Cardiovascular response to large doses of intravenous morphine in man. *N Engl J Med* 1969;281:1389.
231. Civetta JM, Gabel JC. Flow directed-pulmonary artery catheterization in surgical patients: indications and modification of technique. *Ann Surg* 1972;176:753.
232. Kaplan JA, King SB. The precordial electrocardiographic lead (V_5) in patients who have coronary-artery disease. *Anesthesiology* 1976;45:570.
233. Kaplan JA, Dunbar RW, Jones EL. Nitroglycerin infusion during coronary-artery surgery. *Anesthesiology* 1976;45:14.
234. Stanley TH, Webster LR. Anesthetic requirements and cardiovascular effects of fentanyl-oxygen and fentanyl-diazapam-oxygen anesthesia in man. *Anesth Analg* 1978;57:411.
235. Kaplan JA, ed. *Cardiac anesthesia.* Philadelphia: WB Saunders, 1979.
236. Matsumoto M, Oka Y, Strom J, et al. Application of transesophageal echocardiography to continuous intraoperative monitoring of left ventricular performance. *Am J Cardiol* 1980;46:95.
237. Kaplan JA, Wells PH. Early diagnoses of myocardial ischemia using the pulmonary artery catheter. *Anesth Analg* 1981;60:789.
238. Cahalan MK, Kremer P, Schiller NB, et al. Intraoperative monitoring with two dimensional transesophageal echocardiography. *Anesthesiology* 1982;57:A-153(abst).
239. Roizen MF, Kremer P, Cahalan M, et al. Monitoring with transesophageal echocardiography: patients undergoing supraceliac aortic occlusion. *Anesthesiology* 1982;57:A-152(abst).
240. Reiz S, Balfors E, Sorensen MB, et al. Isoflurane: a powerful coronary vasodilator in patients with coronary artery disease. *Anesthesiology* 1983;59:91.
241. Slogoff S, Keats AS. Does perioperative myocardial ischemia lead to postoperative myocardial infarctions? *Anesthesiology* 1985;62:107.
242. Nussmeier NA, Arlund C, Slogoff S. Neuropsychiatric complicatons after cardiopulmonary bypass: cerebral protection by a barbituate. *Anesthesiology* 1986;64:165.
243. deBruijn NP, Clements FM, Kisslo JA. Intraoperative color flow mapping: initial experience. *Anesth Analg* 1987;66:386.
244. Tuman KJ, McCarthy RJ, Spiess BD, et al. Does choice of anesthetic agent significantly affect outcome of coronary artery srugery? *Anesthesiology* 1989;199.
245. Slogoff S, Keats AS. Randomized trial of primary anesthetic agents on outcome of coronary artery bypass operations. *Anesthesiology* 1989;70:179.
246. Rendell-Baker L. History of thoracic anesthesia. In: Mushin WW, ed. *Thoracic anesthesia.* Philadelphia: FA Davis, 1963:598.
247. Shephard DAE. Harvey Cushing and anaethesia. *Can Anaesth Soc J* 1965;12:431.
248. Hilberman M. The evolution of intensive care units. *Crit Care Med* 1975;3:159.
249. Calverley RK. Anesthesia as a specialty: past, present, future. In: Barash PG, Cullen BF, Stoelting RK, eds. *Clinical anesthesia,* 3rd ed. Philadelphia: Lippincott-Raven, 1997:3.
250. Rink EH, Helliwell PJ, Hutton AM. Anaesthesia for operations for the relief of congenital pulmonary stenosis. *Guys Hosp Rep* 1948;97:48.
251. Harris AJ. The management of anesthesia for congenital heart operations in children. *Anesthesiology* 1950;11:328.
252. McQuiston WO. Anesthetic problems in cardiac surgery in children. *Anesthesiology* 1949;10:590.
253. McQuiston WO. Anesthesia in cardiac surgery: observations on three hundred and sixty-two cases. *Arch Surg* 1950;61:892.
254. Smith RM. Circulatory factors affecting anesthesia in surgery for congenital heart disease. *Anesthesiology* 1952;13:38.
255. Papper EM, McDermott F. Anesthesia in cardiac surgery. *Surg Clin North Am* 1952;32:655.
256. Adelman MH. Anesthesia in surgery of the patent ductus arteriosus. *Anesthesiology* 1948;9:42.
257. Potts WJ, McQuiston WO, Baffes TG. Causes of death in

one thousand operations for congenital heart disease. *Arch Surg* 1956;73:508.
258. Artusio JF Jr. Anesthetic management of the rheumatic cardiac for mitral valvulotomy. *Bull N Y Acad Med* 1953;29:684.
259. Wasmuth CE. Anesthesia for mitral commissurotomy. *Cleve Clin Q* 1953;171:737.
260. Preston FS. Anaesthesia for mitral valvotomy. *Br J Anaesth* 1953; 25:299.
261. Pender JW. Anesthesia for mitral commissurotomy. *Anesthesiology* 1953;14:77.
262. Little DM, Sutton GC. Succinylcholine-nitrous oxide anaesthesia for mitral commissurotomy. *Can Anaesth Soc J* 1955;2:156.
263. O'Donnell JA, McDermott F. Anesthetic problems of surgical correction of aortic insufficiency. *Anesthesiology* 1955;16:343.
264. Evelyn SJ, Mackay I. Anesthetic for cardiac surgery. *Anesth Analg* 1954;33:186.
265. Swan H, Virtue RW, Blount SG Jr, et al. Hypothermia in surgery: analysis of clinical cases. *Ann Surg* 1955;142:382.
266. Sellick BA. A method of hypothermia for open heart surgery. *Lancet* 1957;1:443.
267. Conn AW, Allan D, Junkin CI. Anaesthesia with hypothermia for closure of atrial septal defects in children. *Can Anaesth Soc J* 1959;6:327.
268. Mathews JH, Buckley JJ, Van Bergen FH. Acute effect of low-flow extracorporeal circulation on cerebral physiology. *Anesthesiology* 1957;18:169(abst).
269. Keats AS, Kurosu Y, Telford J, et al. Anesthetic problems in cardiopulmonary bypass for open heart surgery: experiences with 200 patients. *Anesthesiology* 1958;19:501.
270. Dawson B, Theye RA, Kirklin JW. Halothane in open cardiac operations: a technique for use with extracorporeal circulation. *Anesth Analg* 1960;39:59.
271. Taylor C, Stoelting VK. Halothane (fluothane) anaesthesia for pediatric cardiac surgery. *Can Anaesth Soc J* 1961;8:247.
272. Viljoen JF. Anaesthesia for internal mammary implant surgery. *Anaesthesia* 1968;23:515.
273. Wynands JE, Sheridan CA, Batra MS, et al. Coronary artery disease. *Anesthesiology* 1970;33:260.
274. Effler DB. Anesthesia in revascularization surgery: a new advance [Editorial]. *J Thorac Cardiovasc Surg* 1968;56:163.
275. Keats AS, ed. Symposium on cardiology and anesthesiology. *Anesthesiology* 1970;33:125.
276. Feil H, Rossman PL. Electrocardiographic observations in cardiac surgery. *Ann Intern Med* 1939;13:402.
277. Ziegler RF. The cardiac mechanism during anesthesia and operation in patients with congenital heart disease and cyanosis. *Bull Johns Hopkins Hosp* 1948;33:237.
278. Smith RM, Wiley HP. Evaluation of electocardiography during congenital heart surgery. *Anesthesiology* 1957;18:398.
279. Severinghaus JW, Astrup PB. pH and acid-base balance measurements. *Int Anesth Clin* 1999;37:55.
280. Fishman NH, Hutchinson JC, Roe BB. Controlled atrial hypertension: a method for supporting cardiac output following open-heart surgery. *J Thorac Cardiovasc Surg* 1966;52:777.
281. Sarin CL, Yalav E, Clement AJ, et al. The necessity for measurement of left atrial pressure after cardiac surgery. *Thorax* 1970; 75:185.
282. Waller JL, Johnson SP, Kaplan JA. Usefulness of pulmonary artery catheter during aortocoronary bypass surgery. *Anesth Analg* 1982;61:221(abst).
283. Boyd AD, Tremblay RE, Spencer FC, et al. Estimation of cardiac output soon after intracardiac surgery with cardiopulmonary bypass. *Ann Surg* 1959;150:613.
284. Pace NL. A critique of flow-directed pulmonary arterial catheterization. *Anesthesiology* 1977;47:455.
285. Mangano DT. Monitoring pulmonary arterial pressure in coronary artery disease. *Anesthesiology* 1980;53:364.
286. Tuman KJ, McCarthy RJ, Spiess BD, et al. Effects of pulmonary artery catheterization on outcome in patients undergoing coronary artery surgery. *Anesthesiology* 1989;70:199.
287. Stephen CR, Bourgeois-Gavardin M, Dent S, et al. Anesthetic management in open-heart surgery: electroencephalographic and metabolic findings in 81 patients. *Anesth Analg* 1959;38: 198.
288. Coons RE, Keats AS, Cooley DA. Significance of electro-encephalographic changes occurring during cardiopulmonary bypass. *Anesthesiology* 1959;20:804.
289. Davenport HT, Arfel G, Sanchez FR. The electroencephalogram in patients undergoing open heart surgery with heart-lung machine. *Anesthesiology* 1959;20:674.
290. Seward JB. Tranesophageal echocardiography: past, present, future. In: Freeman WK, Seward JB, Khandheria, et al. *Transesophageal echocardiography.* Boston: Little, Brown, 1994:1.
291. Barash PG, Glanz S, Katz JD, et al. Ventricular function in children during halothane anesthesia: an echocardiographic evaluation. *Anesthesiology* 1978;49:79.
292. Schluter M, Langenstein BA, Polster J, et al. Transesophageal cross-sectional echocardiography with a phased array transducer system: technique and initial clinical results. *Br Heart J* 1982; 48:67.
293. Cucchiara RF, Nugent M, Seward JB, et al. Air embolism in upright neuro-surgical patients: detection and localization by two-dimensional transesophageal echocardiography. *Anesthesiology* 1984;60:353.
294. Smith JS, Cahalan MF, Benfiel DJ, et al. Intraoperative detection of myocardial ischemia in high-risk patients: electrocardiography versus two-dimensional transesophageal echocardiography. *Circulation* 1985;72:1015.
295. Cahalan MK, Litt L, Botvinick EH, et al. Advances in noninvasive cardiovascular imaging: implication for the anesthesiologist. *Anesthesiology* 1987;66:356.
296. Clements FM, deBruijn NP. Perioperative evaluation of regional wall motion by transesophageal two-dimensional echocardiography. *Anesth Analg* 1987;66:249.
297. Dodds WA, Graves HB, Nixon JE, et al. The anaesthetist's role in open heart surgery. *Can Anaesth Soc J* 1961;8:239.
298. Barash PG, Lescovich F, Katz JD, et al. Early extubation following pediatric cardiothoracic operation: a viable alternative. *Ann Thorac Surg* 1980;29:228.
299. Comroe JH Jr. *Retrospectroscope: insights into medical discovery.* Meno Park, CA: VonGher Press, 1977.
300. Gibbon JH Jr. The inquiring mind [Editorial]. *Ann Surg* 1949; 130:137.
301. Blalock A. The nature of discovery. *Ann Surg* 1956;144:289.
302. Shires GT. The fourth surgical renaissance? *Ann Surg* 1980; 192:269.
303. Gott VL. C Walton Lillehei: pioneer cardiac surgeon. *J Thorac Cardiovasc Surg* 1989;98:833.

Cardiac Anesthesia: Principles and Clinical Practice, Second Edition, edited by Fawzy G. Estafanous, Paul G. Barash, and J.G. Reves. Lippincott Williams & Wilkins, Philadelphia © 2001.

2

PRINCIPLES OF CARDIOVASCULAR PHYSIOLOGY

GEORGE J. CRYSTAL

An understanding of basic principles of cardiovascular physiology is essential for effective and safe patient management in the perioperative period. This information provides a theoretical rationale for the use of drugs and interventions to maintain and optimize the patient's vital organ function.

A primary role of the circulation is to provide sufficient blood flow to satisfy the metabolic demands of the body tissues. The individual factors and relationships determining tissue blood flow are summarized in Fig. 2-1. Tissue blood flow is dependent on activity of both the heart and blood vessels; aortic pressure, one primary determinant of tissue blood flow, is the product of cardiac output and total peripheral resistance, whereas local vascular resistance, the other primary determinant of tissue blood flow, is a function of local vasomotor tone. An appreciation of the relationships presented in Fig. 2-1 is essential for even the most rudimentary understanding of cardiovascular physiology. A major portion of this chapter is devoted to clarifying them.

Additional information on topics presented in the chapter or on related topics can be obtained from the suggested reading list at the end of the chapter.

CARDIAC PHYSIOLOGY

Control of Cardiac Output

Cardiac output (CO) is the volume of blood pumped to the body tissues per minute. It is equal to the product of heart rate (HR) and stroke volume (SV) (Fig. 2-2). Normal values for CO are 5 to 6 L/minute in a 70-kg man, with an HR of 60–80 beats/minute and an SV of 60 to 90 mL/beat. CO varies in proportion to the work demand and oxygen needs of the body.

HR is normally determined by the rhythmic, spontaneous depolarizations of the pacemaker cells located in the sinoatrial (SA) node. The rate of these depolarizations is modulated by the autonomic nervous system. Sympathetic stimulation increases activity of the SA node, whereas parasympathetic stimulation (vagus nerve) decreases its activity.

SV is the difference between end-diastolic volume and end-systolic volume (Fig. 2-2). It is augmented by increases in end-diastolic volume (Starling's law) and in myocardial contractility; it is decreased by increases in afterload. These factors are discussed in detail later in this chapter.

The sarcomere is the basic functional unit of the myocardium (Fig. 2-3). The ultrastructural arrangement of the thick (myosin) and thin (actin) myofilaments within sarcomeres and their interaction can explain much of the mechanical behavior of the cardiac muscle. Cardiac muscle contraction is initiated by an increase in intracellular calcium, which results in the formation of cross-bridges between the adjacent actin and myosin filaments. This process tends to draw the thin myofilaments and the Z lines toward the center of the sarcomere. This is the fundamental basis of the sliding filament mechanism for muscle contraction.

The relation between resting sarcomere length and the level of developed tension was originally defined in isolated skeletal muscle fibers (Fig. 2-4). Developed tension is a direct function of the number of cross-bridges pulling in parallel, and therefore of the amount of overlap between the thin and thick filaments before activation. Tension development (and myofilament overlap) is maximum at an intermediate sarcomere length and minimum at either extreme.

The length-tension relation provides a basis for Starling's law of the heart, which states that the strength of contraction of the intact heart is proportional to the initial length of the cardiac muscle fibers—that is, the end-diastolic volume (*preload*). This can be demonstrated with the use of a cardiac function curve, which is a plot of ventricular performance (e.g., SV) as a function of ventricular end-diastolic volume or an index thereof, such as ventricular end-diastolic pressure or pulmonary capillary wedge pressure (Fig. 2-5, top, right). *In vivo*, the cardiac muscle fibers are stretched by venous inflow. Normally, the volume in the ventricle before

G. J. Crystal: Departments of Anesthesiology and of Physiology and Biophysics, University of Illinois College of Medicine, Chicago, Illinois, and Department of Anesthesiology, Illinois Masonic Medical Center, Chicago, Illinois 60657

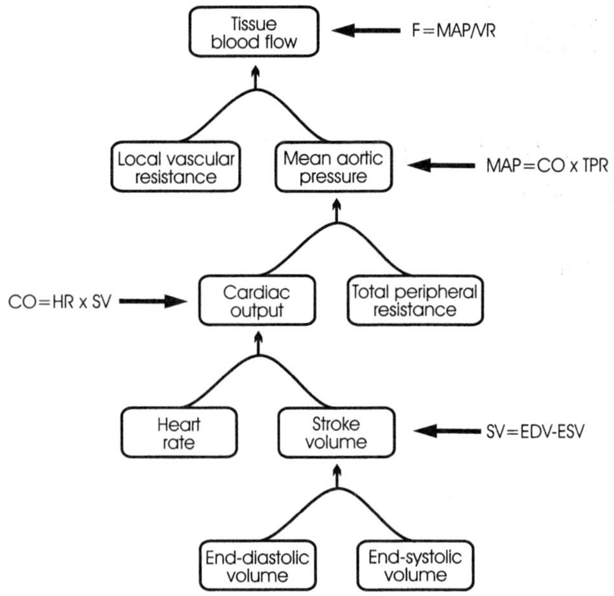

FIGURE 2-1. The cardiac and peripheral vascular factors that determine tissue bloow flow and their interrelationships. (Modified from Rothe CF. Cardiodynamics. In: Selkurt EE. *Physiology.* Boston: Little, Brown, 1971, with permission.)

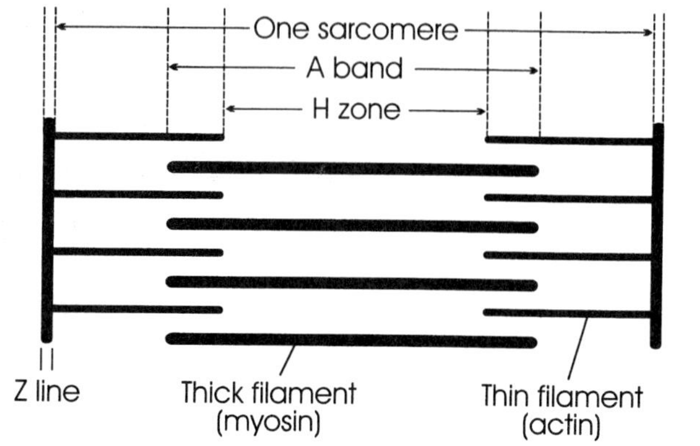

FIGURE 2-3. Contractile machinery and ultrastructure of the cardiac cell. (Modified from Braunwald E, Ross J Jr, Sonnenblick EH. *Mechanisms of contraction of the normal and failing heart.* Boston: Little, Brown, 1976, with permission.)

contraction (the preload) sets the sarcomere to a suboptimal length; the active tension that can be developed from that length is only about 20% of maximum. Increases in end-diastolic volume due to enhanced venous return cause an improvement in ventricular performance.

Venous return is augmented by conditions associated with reduced peripheral vascular resistance. These include the opening of an arteriovenous fistula and conditions that mimic it, such as fever (marked dilation of cutaneous beds), pregnancy, or exercise. Other factors affecting venous return are presented in Fig. 2-5 (bottom, left). Rapid, significant reductions in total blood volume reduce the venous return. At any given total blood volume, venous return is a function of the distribution of blood between the intrathoracic and extrathoracic compartments. For example, the assumption of an upright posture, because of the force of gravity, tends to increase extrathoracic volume at the expense of intratho-

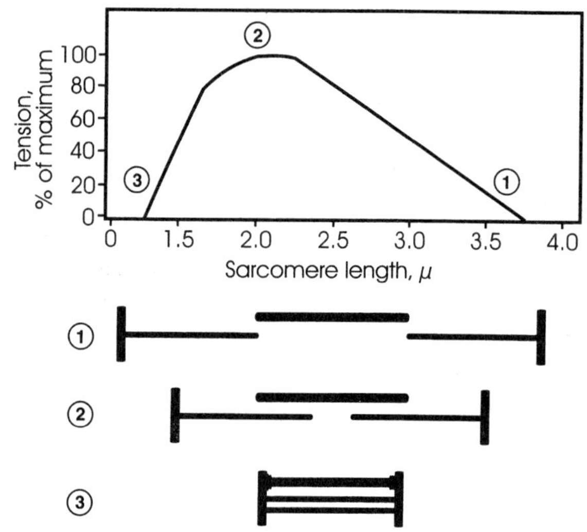

FIGURE 2-4. Tension development as a function of sarcomere length and myofilament overlap. (Modified from Braunwald E, Ross J Jr, Sonnenblick EH. *Mechanisms of contraction of the normal and failing heart.* Boston: Little, Brown, 1976, with permission.)

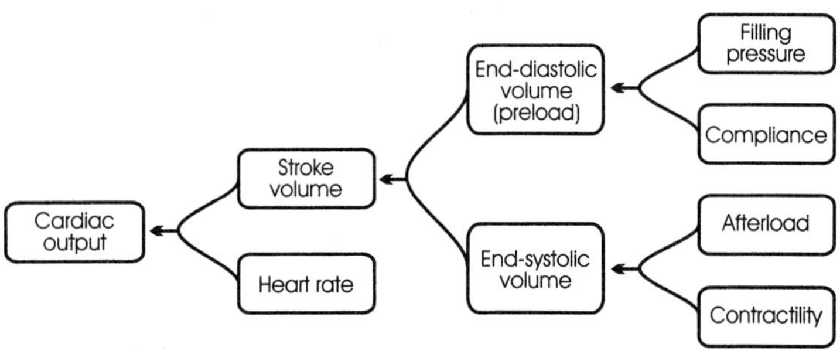

FIGURE 2-2. Determinants of cardiac output.

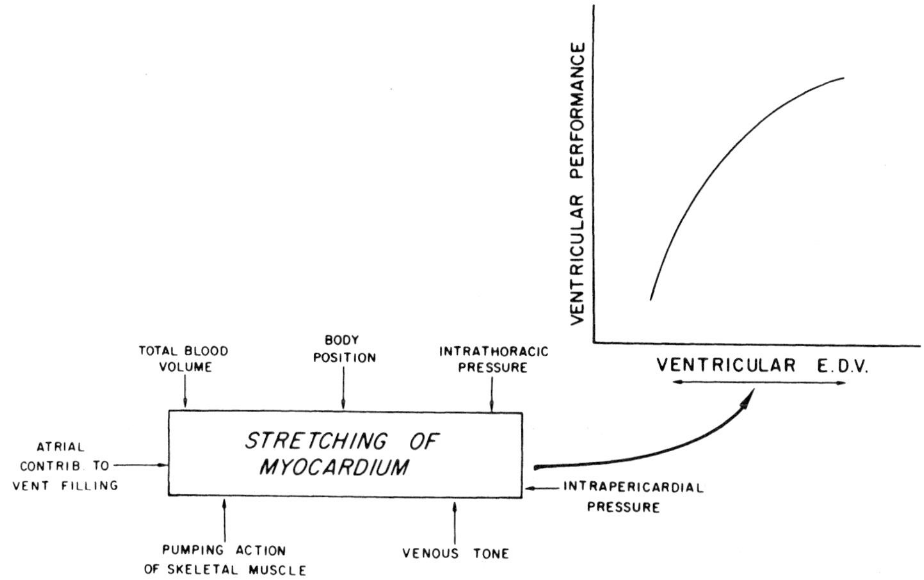

FIGURE 2-5. Top, right: Diagram of a cardiac function curve, relating ventricular end-diastolic volume (EDV) (i.e., stretching of the myocardium) to ventricular performance. **Bottom, left:** Major factors determining the magnitude of EDV. (From Braunwald E, Ross J Jr, Sonnenblick EH. *Mechanisms of contraction of the normal and failing heart.* Boston: Little, Brown, 1976, with permission.)

racic volume, thereby reducing venous return. An elevation of intrathoracic pressure, as occurs during positive-pressure ventilation, pneumothorax, or opening of the chest, has a similar effect. The systemic veins are endowed with smooth muscle in their walls, and they respond to humoral and neural stimuli. Sympathetic nerve stimulation produces venoconstriction, which augments venous return, whereas drugs that interfere with adrenergic nerve function (e.g., ganglionic blockers) and drugs that act directly to relax venous smooth muscle (e.g., nitrates) have the opposite effect. Extravascular compression of veins by contracting muscle increases venous return during exercise. Atrial contraction normally makes a relatively minor contribution to ventricular filling, but it becomes more important at high HRs, when the time available for passive filling of the ventricles is limited. Increases in pericardial pressure, such as occur in cardiac tamponade, limit ventricular filling and SV.

The relation between ventricular volume and pressure during diastole is termed *compliance.* A stiff or noncompliant ventricle demonstrates impaired diastolic filling and a reduced SV. This condition is associated with a variety of pathologic states, including ischemia, healing or healed myocardial infarction, hypertrophy, and constrictive pericarditis.

Contractility reflects the ability of the myocardium to perform mechanical work at a given preload. It can be shown graphically by a family of cardiac function curves (Fig. 2-6, bottom, left). Changes in contractility can aug-

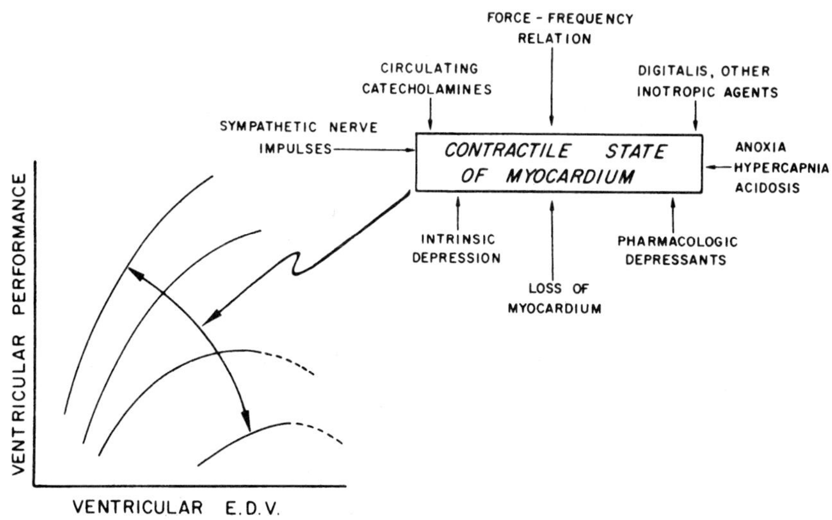

FIGURE 2-6. Top, right: Diagram showing major factors affecting myocardial contractility. **Bottom, left:** Family of cardiac function curves demonstrating the effect of contractility on ventricular performance. (From Braunwald E, Ross J Jr, Sonnenblick EH. *Mechanisms of contraction of the normal and failing heart.* Boston: Little, Brown, 1976, with permission.)

ment cardiac performance (positive inotropic effect) or decrease it (negative inotropic effect). Movement of an entire curve upward or downward signifies a positive or a negative inotropic effect, respectively. Examples of positive inotropic factors are circulating catecholamines and the cardiac sympathetic nerves; examples of negative inotropic factors are severe anoxia or acidosis, pharmacologic depressants (e.g., anesthetics), and loss of myocardium (e.g., myocardial infarction) (Fig. 2-6, top, right).

Afterload may be defined as the tension, force, or stress in the ventricular wall during ventricular ejection. In accordance with the law of Laplace, afterload is directly related to intraventricular pressure and size and inversely related to its wall thickness. Because of changing size and pressure, afterload varies continuously during ventricular ejection. For this reason, it is difficult to quantify with precision. Aortic pressure for the left ventricle and pulmonary artery pressure for the right ventricle usually provide a reasonable estimate of afterload *in vivo*. In isolated heart preparations, in which preload, inotropic state, and beating rate are controlled, increases in afterload cause reductions in left ventricular output (i.e., SV) (Fig. 2-7). In the intact circulation, this impairment to cardiac performance may be avoided when the level of contractility is high or when venous return and preload increase sufficiently. This is demonstrated in Fig. 2-8, which indicates an almost constant SV when normal hearts are exposed to increased afterload (outflow resistance), but a marked decrease in SV when failing hearts are faced with the same condition. Afterload-reducing vasodilating drugs (e.g., nitroprusside) improve cardiac function in patients with heart failure, but they have minimal effect in normal patients.

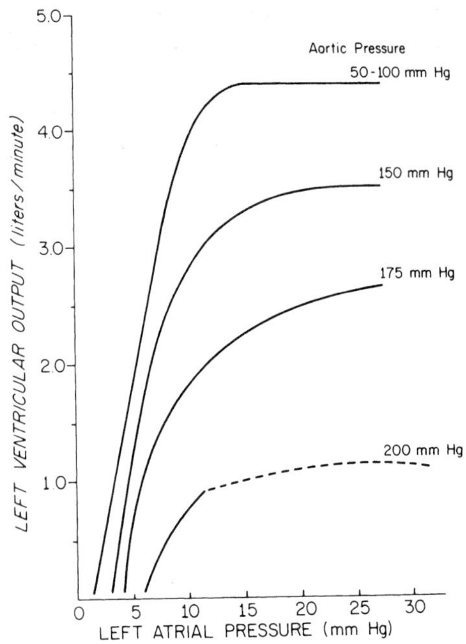

FIGURE 2-7. Left ventricular output as a function of left atrial pressure (i. e., filling pressure), plotted at several aortic pressures (afterloads). The increases in aortic pressure cause progressive reductions in left ventricular output at each filling pressure. (From Sagawa K. Analysis of the ventricular pumping capacity as function of input and output pressure loads. In: Reeve EB, Guyton AC, eds. *Physical bases of circulatory transport: regulation and exchange.* Philadelphia: WB Saunders, 1967, with permission.)

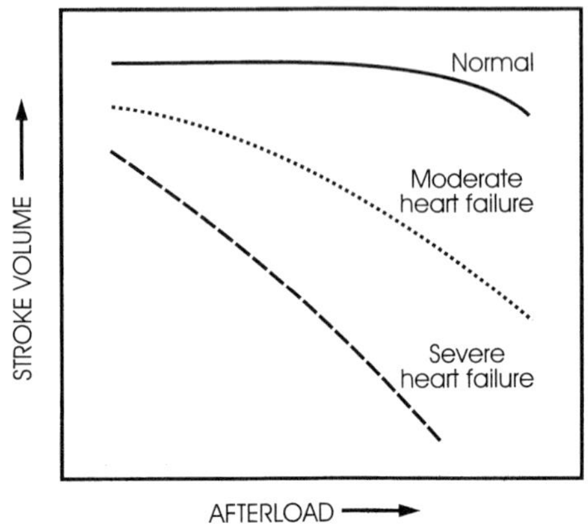

FIGURE 2-8. Effect of increased afterload on stroke volume in normal and compromised hearts. (Modified from Cohn JN, Franciosa JA. Vasodilator therapy of cardiac failure. *N Engl J Med* 1977; 297:27, with permission.)

Events of the Cardiac Cycle

The events of the cardiac cycle are shown in Fig. 2-9. At "O" the heart valve opens, and at "C" it closes. The salient points of this figure are the following: (a) Atrial systole begins after the P wave of the electrocardiogram; ventricular systole begins near the end of the R wave and ends just after the T wave. (b) When ventricular pressure exceeds aortic pressure, the aortic valve opens and ventricular ejection begins. (c) The amount of blood ejected by the ventricle (i.e., the SV) is about 65% of the end-diastolic volume; this is termed the *ejection fraction*. (d) About 80% of ventricular filling is passive; that is, it occurs before atrial systole. (e) Events on the right side of the circulation are similar to those on the left side, but they are somewhat asynchronous. Right atrial systole precedes left atrial systole, and contraction of the right ventricle begins after that of the left. However, because pulmonary arterial pressure is less than aortic pressure, right ventricular ejection precedes left ventricular ejection.

The Ventricular Pressure-Volume Loop

Figure 2-10 presents the relation between ventricular pressure and volume during a cardiac cycle. A similar plot (with a reduced pressure range) could be generated for the right ventricle. For the normal left ventricle (solid lines), diastolic

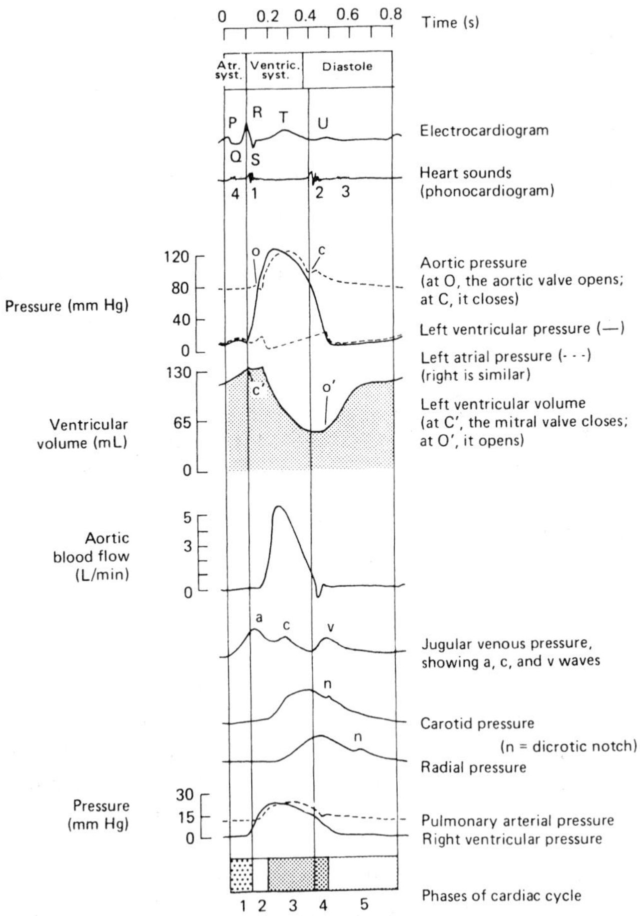

FIGURE 2-9. Events of a cardiac cycle. The phases of the cardiac cycle are identified at the bottom as follows: 1, atrial systole; 2, isovolumetric ventricular contraction; 3, ventricular ejection; 4, isovolumetric relaxation; 5, ventricular filling. (From Ganong WF. *Review of medical physiology,* 19th ed. Stamford, CT: Appleton & Lange, 1999, with permission.)

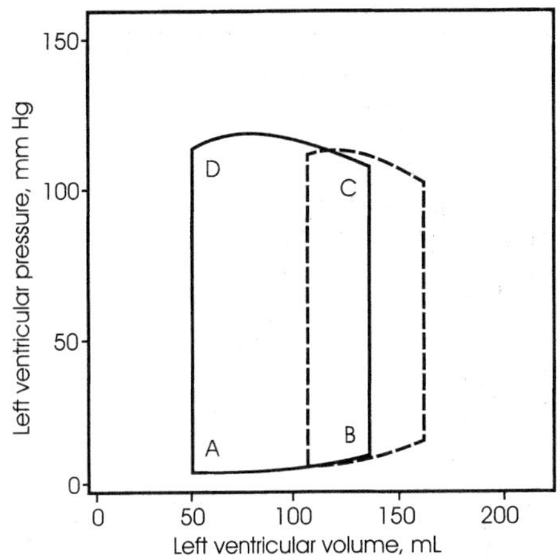

FIGURE 2-10. Pressure-volume loop of the cardiac ventricle. A–B, Diastolic filling; B–C, isovolumetric contraction; C–D, systolic ejection; D–A, isovolumetric relaxation. A plot for a normal ventricle is shown by the solid line, and one for a failing ventricle by the dashed line.

filling starts at A and ends at B, when the mitral valve closes. The increase in ventricular pressure during this period of filling reflects the compliance of the ventricular wall. During isovolumetric contraction (B to C), pressure increases steeply while volume remains constant. At C, ventricular pressure rises to a level that exceeds aortic pressure, the aortic valve opens, and blood is ejected. Ventricular ejection (systole) continues until the ventricular pressure falls below the aortic pressure and the aortic valve closes (D). What follows is the period of isovolumetric relaxation (D to A), which is characterized by a sharp decrease in pressure and no change in volume. The mitral valve opens at A, thus completing one cardiac cycle. Effects of variations in loading conditions and contractile state can be demonstrated with the use of the pressure-volume relation. In Fig. 2-10, the dashed lines show the effect of heart failure (i.e., decreased contractility) on the pressure-volume relation. The area within the pressure-volume loop represents the mechanical work of the heart.

HEMODYNAMICS AND SYSTEMIC VASCULAR CONTROL

Pressure Changes in Systemic and Pulmonary Circulations

The heart comprises two parallel pumps, each consisting of an atrium and a ventricle. The right side of the heart supplies the pulmonary circulation, where exchange of oxygen and carbon dioxide occurs in the lung alveoli; the left side of the heart supplies the systemic circulation, which carries oxygenated blood to the body tissues. Figure 2-11 compares the pressure changes as blood flows through the series-coupled components of the systemic and pulmonary circulations—from the large arteries to the arterioles, capillaries, and veins. Important features of this figure are the following: (a) The pressure developed by the right ventricle is approximately one sixth that by the left ventricle. This results in a smaller workload for the right ventricle, which is in keeping with its much thinner wall. (b) Although pressure in the ventricles falls almost to zero during diastole, pressure is maintained in the large arteries. This is possible because a portion of the energy released by cardiac contraction during systole is stored in the distensible large arteries. During diastole, the elastic recoil of the vessels converts this potential energy into forward blood flow, which ensures that capillary flow is continuous throughout the cardiac cycle. (c) The most severe drop in pressure occurs in the arterioles; for this reason, they are often termed the *resistance vessels.* The diameter of the arteriole is regulated by the contractile activity of the smooth muscle contained in its wall. Variations in arteriolar diameter are a primary determinant of local blood flow and capillary hydrostatic pressure.

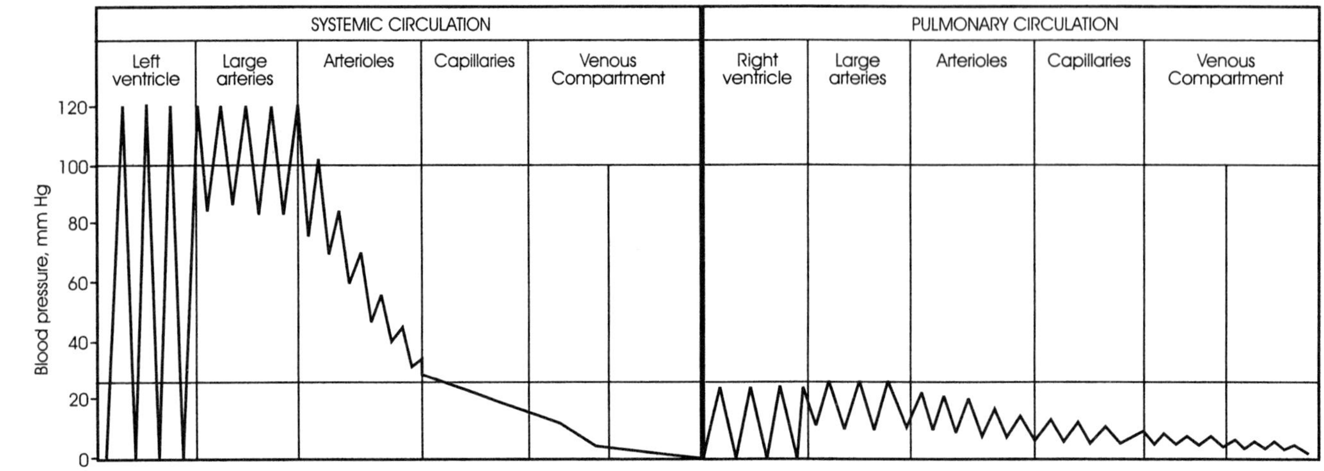

FIGURE 2-11. Pressure changes as blood flows through the series-coupled components of the systemic and pulmonary circulations. (Modified from Folkow B, Neil E. *Circulation.* New York: Oxford University Press, 1971, with permission.)

Determinants of Blood Flow: Poiseuille's Law

Blood flow (F) is a function of the arteriovenous pressure gradient (Pa − Pv) and local vascular resistance (VR), according to the equation:

$$F = (Pa - Pv) \div VR \qquad [2\text{-}1]$$

This is analogous to Ohm's law in an electrical circuit. Because arterial and venous blood pressures are normally well maintained within narrow limits by homeostatic mechanisms, tissue blood flow usually varies inversely as a function of vascular resistance.

Poiseuille performed studies that yielded an equation describing resistance to flow (R) in a straight, rigid tube of length l and radius r:

$$R = \eta 8l/r^4 \qquad [2\text{-}2]$$

where η is the viscosity. Of note, flow resistance varies inversely with tube radius (r) raised to the fourth power. Therefore, small changes in tube radius cause large changes in resistance.

Because the length of blood vessels *in situ* is fixed, geometric changes in blood flow resistance occur through variations in vessel radius. These adjustments are the result of contraction or relaxation of the smooth muscle investing the arterioles. Chemical factors that are linked to the metabolic activity of the tissue (e.g., adenosine) modulate vascular resistance so that blood flow (and oxygen delivery) is commensurate with the prevailing local oxygen demands.

Blood Viscosity

Viscosity is the internal friction resulting from the intermolecular forces operating within a flowing liquid. The term *internal friction* emphasizes that as a fluid moves within a tube, laminae in the fluid slip on one another and move at different speeds. This produces a velocity gradient in a direction perpendicular to the wall of the tube. This velocity gradient is termed the *shear rate.* In the circulation, shear rate is directly correlated with rate of blood flow. An intuitive understanding of the term viscosity can be gained from the experiment shown in Fig. 2-12. In this experiment, a homogeneous fluid is confined between two closed spaced, parallel plates (analogous to playing cards). Assume that the area of each plate is A, the distance between the plates is Y, and the bottom plate is stationary. If a tangential force (a shear stress) is applied to the upper plate, that plate moves with velocity V in the direction of the applied force, and a

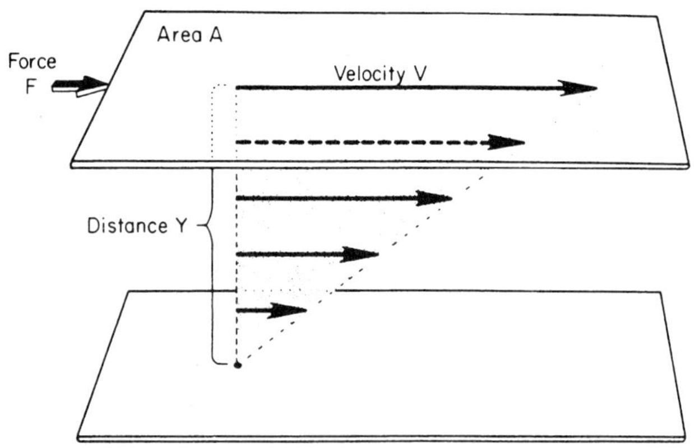

FIGURE 2-12. Relation between shear stress and shear rate when a fluid is sheared between two parallel plates. Details are included in the text. (From Fahmy NR. Techniques for deliberate hypotension: haemodilution and hypotension. In: Enderby GEH, ed. *Hypotensive anaesthesia.* Edinburgh, Scotland: Churchill-Livingstone, 1985, with permission.)

velocity gradient (or shear rate) is developed in the fluid. Viscosity is defined as the factor of proportionality relating shear stress and shear rate for the fluid.

$$\text{Viscosity} = \text{Shear stress} \div \text{Shear rate} \qquad [2\text{-}3]$$

Newton assumed that viscosity was a constant property of a particular fluid and independent of shear rate. Fluids that demonstrate this behavior are termed *Newtonian.* The units of viscosity are dynes per second per square centimeter, or poise.

The viscosity of blood varies as a direct function of hematocrit (Fig. 2-13): the greater the hematocrit, the more friction there is between successive layers. Plasma is a Newtonian fluid, even at high protein concentrations. However, because blood consists of erythrocytes suspended in plasma, it does not behave like a homogeneous Newtonian fluid; the viscosity of blood increases sharply with reductions in shear rate (Fig. 2-13). This non-Newtonian behavior of blood has been attributed to changes in the behavior of erythrocytes at low flow rates: (a) Erythrocytes lose their axial position in the stream of blood (Fig. 2-14). (b) Erythrocytes lose their ellipsoidal shape. (c) Erythrocytes form aggregates; this tendency toward aggregation appears to depend on the plasma concentration of large protein molecules (e.g., fibrinogen), which form cell-to-cell bridges. (d) Erythrocytes adhere to the endothelial walls of microvessels. Figure 2-15 demonstrates that non-Newtonian behavior is localized *in vivo* on the venous side of circulation because of its lower shear rates, but that this behavior can be blunted or abolished by hemodilution.

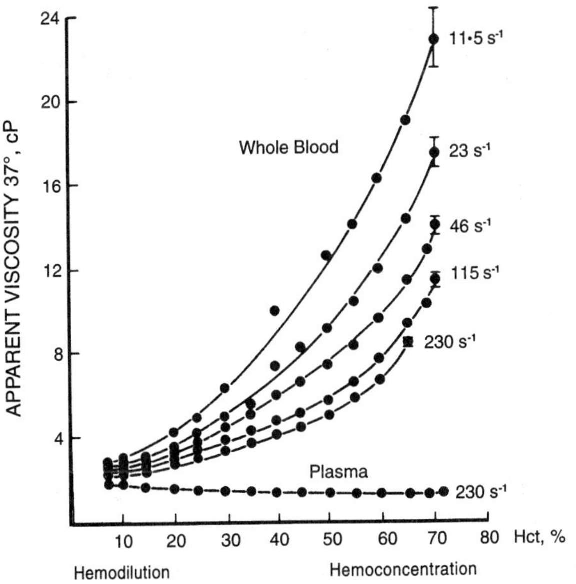

FIGURE 2-13. Viscosity of whole blood at various hematocrits as a function of shear rate. Hematocrit was varied by the addition of dextran and packed red blood cells. Viscosity increases with hematocrit, and these increases are greatest at the lower shear rates. (Modified from Messmer K. Hemodilution. *Surg Clin North Am* 1975;55:662, with permission.)

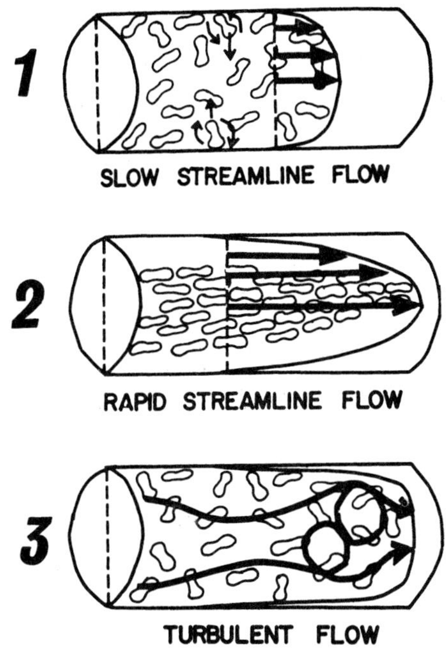

FIGURE 2-14. Diagram representing various features of streamline and turbulent flow. (From Keele CA, Neil E. *Samson Wright's applied physiology.* London: Oxford University Press, 1971, with permission.)

The tendency for an increased hematocrit to increase the blood viscosity is attenuated when blood flows through tubes of capillary diameter (Fig. 2-16). Because erythrocytes are normally very deformable and have a diameter similar to that of the capillary, they can squeeze through the vessel lumen in single file with minimal extra force required. Therefore, the rate at which erythrocytes pass through the capillary has little influence on blood viscosity there; viscosity remains close to that of plasma.

Blood viscosity varies inversely with temperature. This is an important consideration during hypothermic cardiopulmonary bypass. After circulatory arrest, the shear stress required to reinitiate flow and to break up red cell aggregates is likely to be high. Additional rheologic benefit may be gained by a further decrease in hematocrit.

Turbulent Flow

A condition of Poiseuille's law is that flow must be laminar. Above a critical flow rate, the laminae break down into eddies that move in all directions. Such flow is said to be *turbulent* (Fig. 2-14). The tendency for turbulence is given by the Reynolds number (Re):

$$\text{Re} = \text{VD}\rho/\eta \qquad [2\text{-}4]$$

where V = linear velocity, D = diameter, ρ = density,

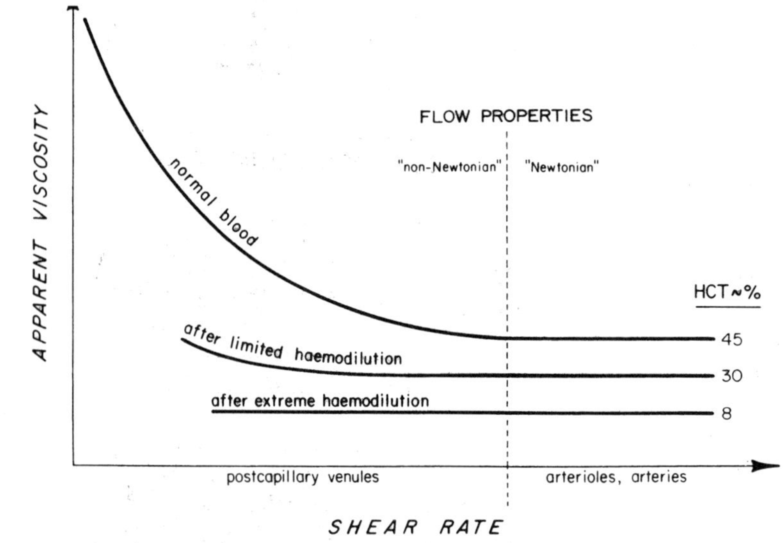

FIGURE 2-15. Graphic representation of the level of blood viscosity in the various vascular compartments. Under normal condition (hematocrit = 45%), viscosity increases in postcapillary venules because of reduced shear rate. Hemodilution can blunt or even eliminate this regional variation in viscosity. (From Messmer K, Sunder-Plassman L. Hemodilution. *Prog Surg* 1974; 12:208, with permission.)

and η = viscosity. Re is dimensionless because it is the ratio of inertial and cohesive forces. The former tend to disrupt the stream, whereas the latter tend to maintain them. In long straight tubes, turbulence occurs when Re exceeds a value of approximately 2,000. However, the critical Re *in vivo* is much less because of pulsatile flow patterns and complicated vascular geometries. When flow is turbulent, a greater portion of the total fluid energy is dissipated as heat and vibration; therefore the pressure drop is greater than what would be predicted from the Poiseuille equation (Fig. 2-17). The vibrations associated with turbulent flow can often be heard as a murmur during physical examination.

Major Vessel Types: Structure and Function

The various vessel types have structural and geometric features (Fig. 2-18) that correlate with their functional characteristics and roles within the circulation (Fig. 2-19). The

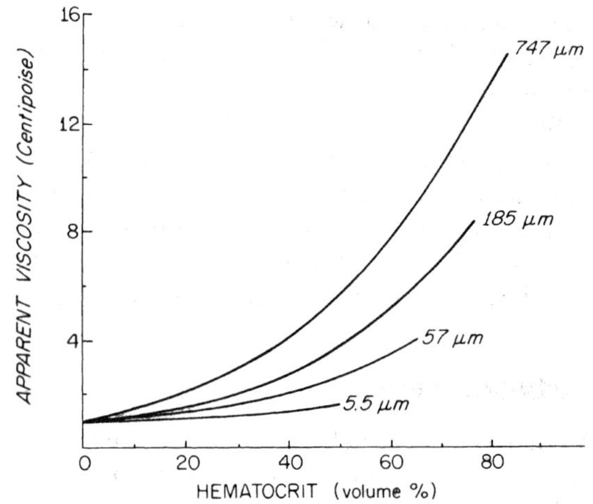

FIGURE 2-16. The effect of hematocrit on viscosity of blood in tubes of varying radius. In wide tubes, increasing the hematocrit raises viscosity; in narrow tubes, it has no effect. (From Feigl EO. Physics of the cardiovascular system. In: Ruch TC, Patton HD, ed. *Physiology and biophysics II: circulation, respiration, and fluid balance.* Philadelphia: WB Saunders, 1974, with permission.)

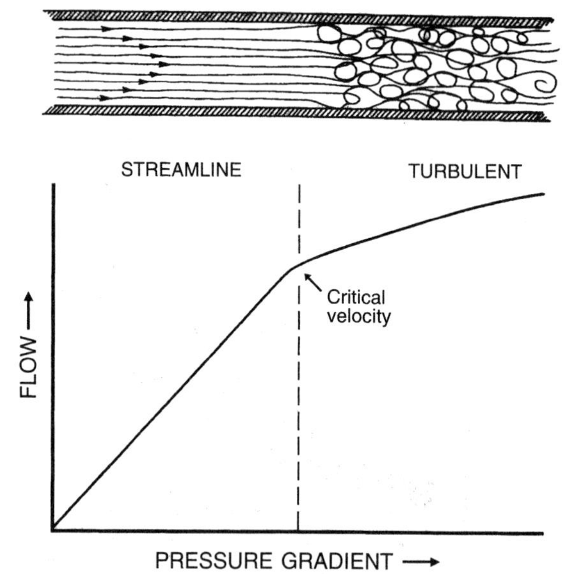

FIGURE 2-17. The linear relation between pressure gradient and flow. Beyond a critical velocity, turbulence begins and the relation between pressure and flow is no longer linear. (From Feigl EO. Physics of the cardiovascular system. In: Ruch TC, Patton HD, ed. *Physiology and biophysics II: circulation, respiration, and fluid balance.* Philadelphia: WB Saunders, 1974, with permission.)

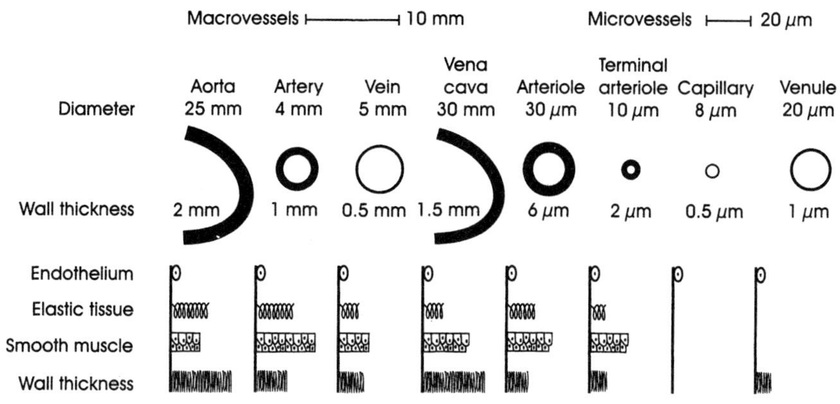

FIGURE 2-18. Dimensions and structural attributes of the various vessel types. (Modified from Berne RM, Levy MN. *Principles of physiology.* St. Louis: CV Mosby, 1990, with permission.)

large conduit arteries are predominantly elastic structures, allowing them to convert intermittent CO into continuous peripheral flow. Because the cross-sectional area of these vessels is small, the velocity of flow in them is high. The resistance to flow in the arteries is small, and therefore the pressure drop is also small. The arterioles and the terminal arterioles have significant smooth muscle in their walls, which permits active changes in vascular diameter and modulation of local vascular resistance and blood flow. The capillaries have a very large aggregrate cross-sectional area (which decreases the flow velocity) and a thin wall, two features that favor blood-tissue exchange. The veins and venules have the greatest volume, which makes them an appropriate site for blood storage.

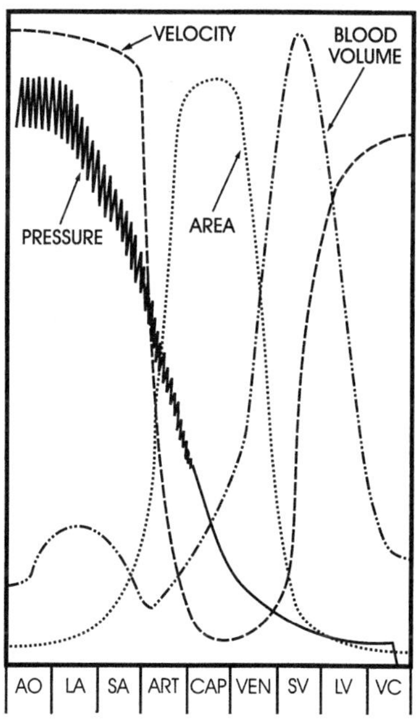

FIGURE 2-19. Velocity, cross-sectional area, blood volume, and pressure within the various vessel types. AO, aorta; LA, large arteries; SA, small arteries; ART, arterioles; CAP, capillaries; VEN, venules; SV, small veins; LV, large veins; VC, vena cavae. (Modified from Berne RM, Levy MN. *Principles of physiology.* St. Louis: CV Mosby, 1990, with permission.)

Factors Influencing the Balance Between Capillary Filtration and Absorption: Mechanisms of Edema

Mechanisms of capillary-tissue fluid exchange are portrayed in Fig. 2-20. Because the capillary wall is highly permeable to water and to almost all the solutes of the plasma (with the exception of the plasma proteins), it acts like a porous filter through which protein-free plasma moves by bulk flow under the influence of a hydrostatic pressure gradient. Transcapillary filtration is defined by the equation:

$$\text{Fluid filtration} = C_F \times [(P_{cap} - P_{IF}) - (\Pi_{cap} - \Pi_{IF})] \quad [2\text{-}5]$$

where C_F = capillary filtration coefficient, P_{cap} = capillary hydrostatic pressure, P_{IF} = interstitial fluid hydrostatic pressure, Π_{cap} = capillary oncotic pressure Π_{IF} = interstitial fluid oncotic pressure. P_{cap} and Π_{IF} are forces of filtration. P_{cap} is determined by arterial pressure, venous pressure, and the ratio of postcapillary to precapillary resistance. Increases in each of these parameters raise the value for P_{cap}. P_{cap} is approximately 35 mm Hg at the arterial end of the capillaries and approximately 15 mm Hg at the venous end. Π_{IF} is a result of plasma proteins that have passed through the capillary wall and is normally very low compared to P_{cap}. Therefore, P_{cap} is normally the major force of filtration. P_{IF} and Π_{cap} are forces favoring absorption. P_{IF} is determined by the volume of fluid and the distensibility of the interstitial space and is normally almost equal to zero. Π_{cap} is caused by the plasma proteins (most predominantly albumin) and has a value of approximately 25 mm Hg. Π_{cap} is normally the major force for absorption. *The direction and magnitude of capillary bulk flow is essentially a function of the ratio of P_{cap} to Π_{cap}.* Filtered fluid that reaches the extravas-

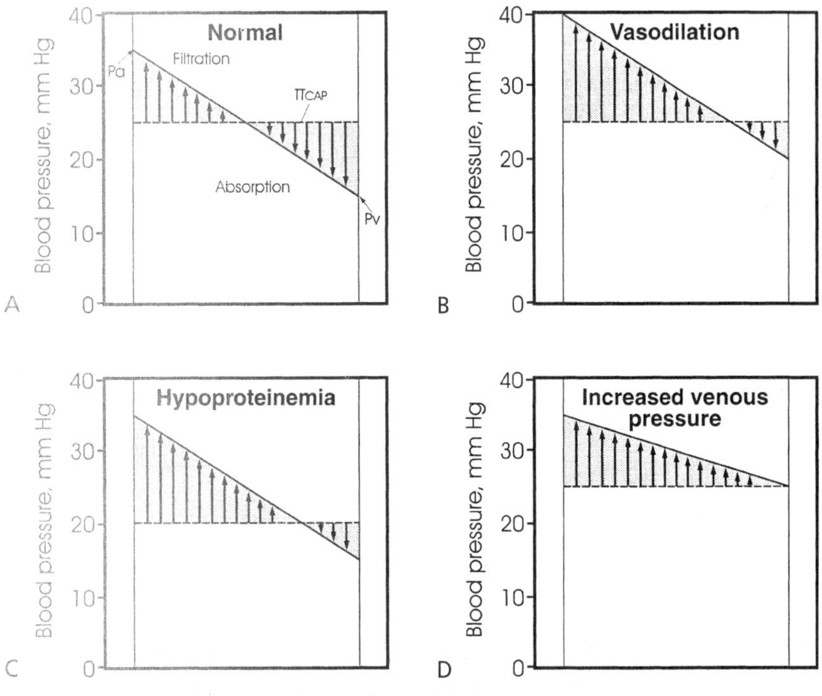

FIGURE 2-20. Mechanisms of capillary-tissue fluid exchange: **A** depicts normal condition, while **B–D** depict conditions favoring edema. Upward arrows indicate filtration, and downward arrows indicate absorption. The area of the shaded triangles reflects the magnitude of filtration and absorption under each condition. (Modified from Friedman JJ. Microcirculation. In: Selkurt EE, ed. *Physiology.* Boston: Little, Brown, 1971, with permission.)

cular spaces is returned to the circulatory system via the lymphatic network. Under normal conditions (Fig. 2-20, panel A), filtration dominates at the arterial end of the capillary, and absorption at the venous end, because of the gradient of hydrostatic pressure; there is a small net filtration, which is compensated by lymph flow. Edema is a condition of excess accumulation of fluid in the interstitial space. It occurs when net filtration exceeds drainage via the lymphatics. This can be caused by (a) increased capillary pressure, (b) decreased plasma protein concentration, (c) accumulation of osmotically active substances in the interstitial space, (d) increased capillary permeability, or (e) inadequate lymph flow. Conditions resulting in edema are diagramatically depicted in Fig. 2-20, panels B through D.

Baroreceptor Control of the Circulation

Arterial blood pressure is maintained within narrow limits by a negative feedback system. The major components of this system are as follows (Fig. 2-21): (a) an afferent limb composed of the baroreceptors in the carotid and aortic arch and their respective sensory nerves, the glossopharyngeal and vagus nerves; (b) the cardiovascular centers in the medulla, which receive and integrate the sensory information; and (c) an efferent limb composed of the sympathetic nerves to the heart and blood vessels and the parasympathetic (vagus) nerves to the heart. Figure 2-22 presents the neural relationships of the arterial baroreceptor reflex. The baroreceptors are stimulated by stretch of the vessel wall, which results from an increase in transluminal pressure. Impulses originating in the baroreceptors tonically inhibit discharge of the sympathetic nerves to the heart and blood vessels and tonically facilitate discharge of the vagus nerves to the heart. A rise in arterial pressure reduces baroreceptor afferent activity, resulting in further inhibition of the sympathetic nerves and facilitation of the vagus nerves. This produces vasodilation, venodilation, and reductions in SV, HR, and CO, which tend to normalize arterial pressure. A decrease in arterial pressure has opposite effects. The cardio-

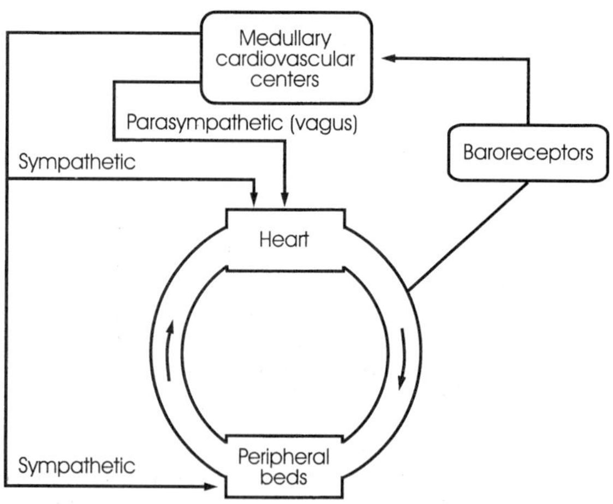

FIGURE 2-21. Diagram of arterial baroreceptor reflex loop. (Modified from Rothe CF, Friedman JJ. Control of the cardiovascular system. In: Selkurt EE, ed. *Physiology.* Boston: Little, Brown, 1971, with permission.)

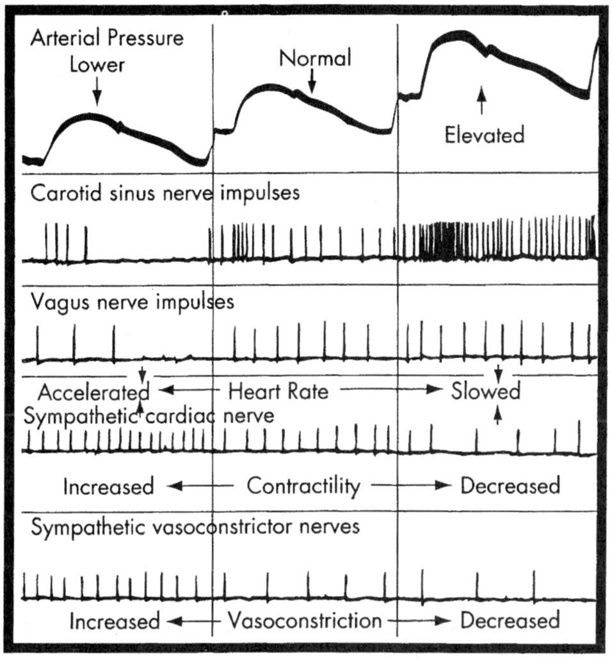

FIGURE 2-22. Effect of changes in arterial pressure on carotid sinus nerve discharge and impulse rate of efferent nerves. (Modified from Rushmer RF. *Cardiovascular dynamics,* 3rd ed. Philadelphia: WB Saunders, 1970, with permission.)

vascular centers in the medulla are also under the influence of neural factors arising in the arterial chemoreceptors, hypothalamus, and cerebral cortex, and of local changes in the partial pressures of carbon dioxide and oxygen (PCO_2 and PO_2, respectively). Anesthetics have been demonstrated to inhibit baroreceptor control of the cardiovascular system, although this effect seems to vary from agent to agent (1). This effect may be either an advantage or a disadvantage, depending on the clinical circumstances. For example, an agent that preserves baroreflex function would be advantageous in the presence of a systemic circulatory stress, such as hypovolemia. On the other hand, an agent that blunts baroreflex function would be advantageous in the clinical management of coronary artery disease, where reflex tachycardia (and increased myocardial oxygen demand) would be undesirable.

TISSUE OXYGEN TRANSPORT

Oxygen serves as an electron acceptor in oxidative phosphorylation, permitting production of adenosine triphosphate (ATP) along efficient aerobic pathways. The high-energy phosphate bonds of ATP provide energy for functional and biochemical processes within the cell, such as the contraction of muscle proteins or the metabolic activity of enzymes.

The cardiovascular system acts in concert with the respiratory system to transport oxygen from the environmental air to tissue mitochondria. Oxygen transport is composed of a series of steps, each corresponding to a transport process with a PO_2 cost, the so-called *oxygen cascade* (Fig. 2-23). The objective of the oxygen transport system is to maintain PO_2 in the vicinity of all mitochondria at 0.1 mm Hg, which is the level required for unimpaired O_2 use (Fig. 2-24). The only function of higher PO_2 values is to provide for diffusion of oxygen to mitochondria remote from capillaries.

The amount of oxygen carried from the lungs to tissues by circulating blood—that is, the convective systemic oxygen delivery (DO_2), is given by the equation:

$$DO_2 = CO \times CaO_2 \qquad [2\text{-}6]$$

where CO is cardiac output in liters per minute and CaO_2 is the arterial oxygen content in volume percent (vol%). The determinants of CO have already been discussed. What follows is a discussion of the factors affecting CaO_2.

Oxygen Carriage in the Blood: Oxyhemoglobin Dissociation Curve

CaO_2 comprises oxygen bound to hemoglobin and oxygen dissolved in plasma. The human hemoglobin molecule is composed of two basic portions. The protein or globin portion is made up of identical polypeptide chains: two α and two β chains. The polypeptide chains are folded and assembled as a tetramer. Each of these chains contains one heme group, which serves as an iron-containing, reversible carrier of one molecule of oxygen. Therefore, each molecule of hemoglobin can bind four molecules of oxygen. The amount of oxygen bound is a function of hemoglobin concentration (Hb), the oxygen saturation of hemoglobin (SaO_2), and the oxygen carrying capacity for hemoglobin (1.39 mL O_2 per gram of hemoglobin), according to the equation:

$$O_2 \text{ bound} = Hb \times SaO_2 \times 1.39 \qquad [2\text{-}7]$$

SaO_2 is a function of PO_2 and the oxyhemoglobin dissociation curve (Fig. 2-25). The sigmoid shape of this curve reflects the fact that the four binding sites on a given hemoglobin molecule interact with each other. When the first site has bound a molecule of oxygen, the binding of the next site is facilitated, and so forth. The result is a curve that is steep up to a PO_2 of 60 mm Hg and then becomes more shallow, approaching 100% saturation asymptotically. At a PO_2 of 100 mm Hg to which human arterial blood is equilibrated, the hemoglobin saturation (SaO_2) is approximately 97%; at 40 mm Hg, a typical value for the mixed venous oxygen tension ($P\bar{v}O_2$) in a resting person, the saturation is about 75%.

The shape of the oxyhemoglobin dissociation curve has important physiologic implications. The flatness of the curve beyond a PO_2 of 80 mm Hg ensures a relatively con-

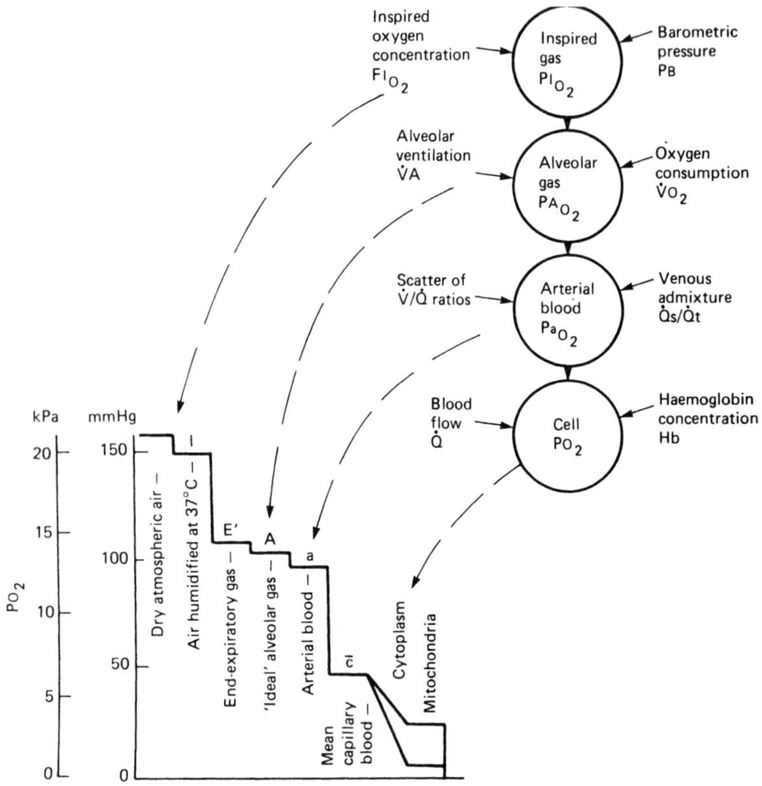

FIGURE 2-23. On the left is the oxygen cascade, with partial oxygen pressure (PO_2) decreasing from the level in the ambient air to the level in the mitochondria. On the right are listed the factors influencing PO_2 at various steps in the cascade. (From Nunn JF. *Nunn's applied respiratory physiology.* Oxford: Butterworth Heinemann, 1993, with permission.)

stant oxyhemoglobin saturation for arterial blood despite wide variations in alveolar oxygen pressure. The steep portion of the curve between 20 and 60 mm Hg permits unloading of oxygen from hemoglobin at relatively high PO_2 values, which allows the delivery of large amounts oxygen into the tissue by diffusion.

The oxygen binding properties of hemoglobin are influenced by a number of factors, including pH, PCO_2, and

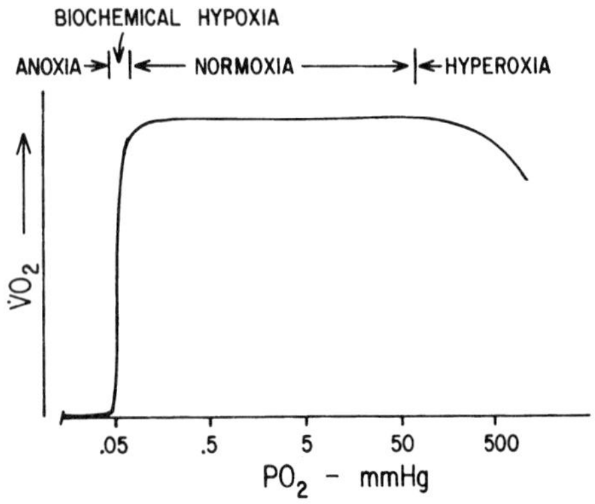

FIGURE 2-24. Oxygen consumption $\dot{V}O_2$ of isolated mitochondria as a function of partial oxygen pressure (PO_2). (From Honig CR. *Modern cardiovascular physiology.* Boston: Little, Brown, 1981, with permission.)

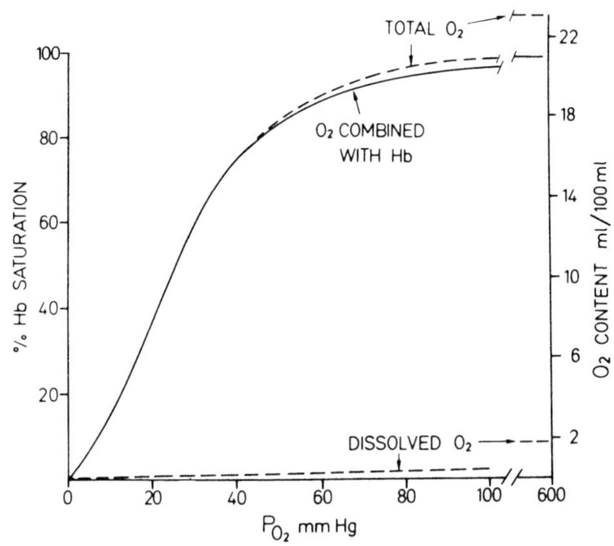

FIGURE 2-25. The oxyhemoglobin dissociation curve. The oxygen content of blood has two components: oxygen binding to hemoglobin follows an S-shaped curve up to full saturation; the amount of oxygen in solution increases linearly with the partial oxygen pressure (PO_2) without limit. (From West JB. *Respiratory physiology: the essentials.* Baltimore: Williams & Wilkins, 1974, with permission.)

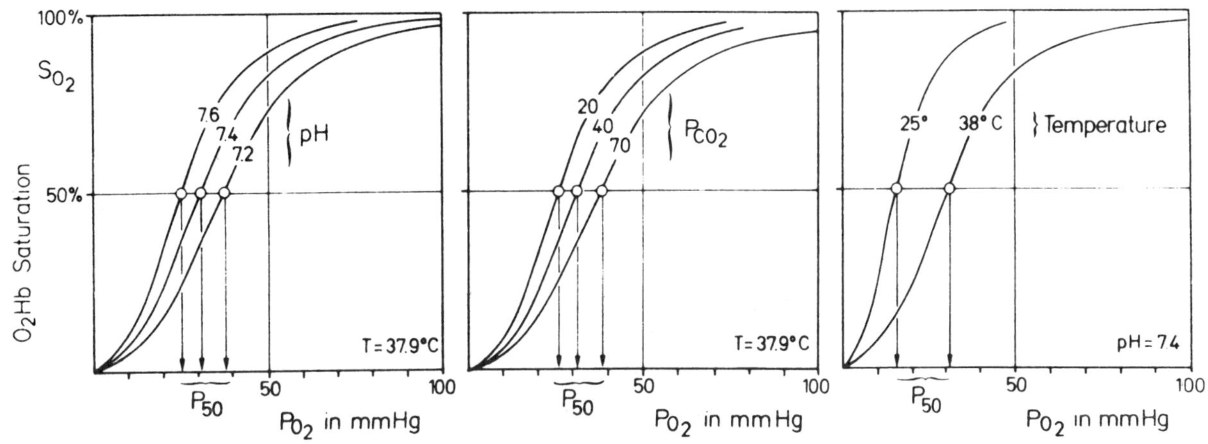

FIGURE 2-26. Effects of variations in pH, partial carbon dioxide pressure (P_{CO_2}), and temperature on the oxyhemoglobin dissociation curve. (From Weibel ER. *The pathway for oxygen.* Cambridge, MA: Harvard University Press, 1984, with permission.)

temperature (Fig. 2-26). These factors cause shifts of the oxyhemoglobin dissociation curve to the right or left without changing the slope of the curve. For example, an increase in temperature or a decrease in pH, such as may occur in active tissues, decrease the affinity of hemoglobin for oxygen and shift the oxyhemoglobin dissociation curve to the right. Therefore, a higher P_{O_2} is required to achieve a given saturation, which facilitates unloading of oxygen at the tissue. To quantify the extent of a shift in the oxyhemoglobin dissociation curve, the so-called P_{50} is used; this is the P_{O_2} required for 50% saturation. The P_{50} of normal adult hemoglobin at 37°C and normal pH and P_{CO_2} is 26 to 27 mm Hg.

The compound 2,3-diphosphoglycerate (2,3-DPG) is an intermediate in anaerobic glycolysis (the biochemical pathway by which red blood cells produce ATP) that binds to hemoglobin. Increases in intraerythrocytic 2,3-DPG concentration reduce the affinity of hemoglobin for oxygen (i.e, they shift the oxyhemoglobin dissociation curve to the right), whereas decreases have an opposite effect. Several factors have been found to influence the red cell 2,3-DPG concentration. For example, after storage in a blood bank of only 1 week, the 2,3-DPG concentration is one-third normal, resulting in a shift to the left of the oxyhemoglobin dissociation curve. On the other hand, conditions associated with chronic hypoxia, such as living at high altitude or chronic anemia, stimulate production of 2,3-DPG, causing a rightward shift of the oxyhemoglobin dissociation curve.

Dissolved oxygen is linearly related to P_{O_2} (Fig. 2-25). At 37°C it is defined by the equation:

$$O_2 \text{ dissolved} = 0.003 \text{ vol\%/mm Hg} \times P_{O_2}(\text{mmHg}) \qquad [2\text{-}8]$$

Dissolved oxygen normally accounts for only 1.5% of total oxygen, but this contribution increases when the bound component is reduced during hemodilution. Because hemoglobin is essentially saturated at a P_{O_2} of 100 mm Hg, increases in Pa_{O_2} to levels greater than 100 mm Hg increase the Ca_{O_2} by raising the dissolved oxygen component.

Characteristic Values for Parameters of Oxygen Delivery

For an individual with normal values for Hb (15 g/100 mL), Pa_{O_2} (100 mm Hg), $P\bar{v}_{O_2}$ (40 mm Hg), and CO (5 L/minute):

$$Ca_{O_2} = (15 \times 0.97 \times 1.39) + (0.003 \times 100) = 20.5 \text{ vol\%}$$

$$D_{O_2} = (5{,}000 \times 20.5/100) = 1{,}025 \text{ mL/minute}$$

$$C\bar{v}_{O_2} = (15 \times 0.75 \times 1.39) + (0.003 \times 40) = 15.8 \text{ vol\%}$$

and the arteriovenous oxygen difference $(Ca_{O_2} - C\bar{v}_{O_2})$

$$= (20.5 - 15.8) = 4.7 \text{ vol\%}.$$

$C\bar{v}_{O_2}$ is mixed venous oxygen content.

Diffusion of Oxygen to Tissues: Capillary-to-Cell Oxygen Delivery

The final step in the delivery of oxygen to tissue mitochondria is diffusion from the capillary blood. According to the law of diffusion, this process is determined by the capillary-to-cell P_{O_2} gradient and the diffusion parameters, capillary surface area and blood-cell diffusion distance. In 1919, Krogh formulated the capillary recruitment model to describe the processes underlying oxygen transport in tissue (2). The basic model was later expanded and refined (3). Although Krogh's model is limited by multiple simplifying assumptions, it has value as a tool for appreciating the role

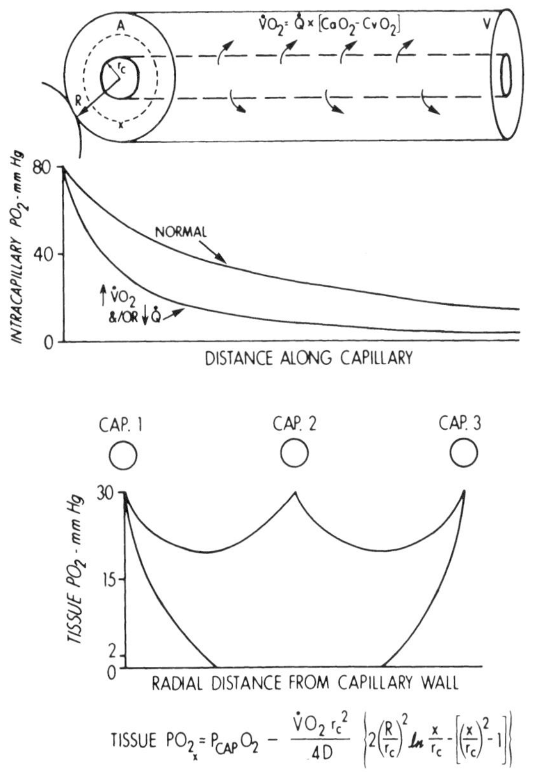

FIGURE 2-27. Longitudinal and radial oxygen gradients within tissue in accordance with the Krogh cylinder model. Details are provided in the text. $\mathring{V}O_2$, oxygen consumption; $\dot{Q}$, blood flow; $[CaO_2 - C\bar{v}O_2]$, arteriovenous oxygen content difference; r_c, capillary radius; R, tissue cylinder radius; A, arterial end of capillary; V, venous end of capillary; x, point within tissue cylinder; $Pcapo_2$, oxygen tension of capillary blood; D, diffusion coefficient for oxygen. (From Honig CR. *Modern cardiovascular physiology.* Boston: Little, Brown, 1981, with permission.)

of vascular control mechanisms in the transport of oxygen to tissue.

The model consists of a single capillary and the surrounding cylinder of tissue that it supplies (Fig. 2-27). Two interrelated oxygen gradients are involved: a longitudinal gradient within the capillary, and a radial oxygen gradient extending into the tissue. Most oxygen in capillary blood is bound to hemoglobin and cannot leave the capillary. This bound oxygen is in equilibrium with the small amount of oxygen dissolved in the plasma. The consumption of oxygen by the tissue ($\mathring{V}O_2$) creates a transcapillary gradient for oxygen. Diffusion of oxygen into the surrounding tissue shifts the equilibrium between bound and dissolved oxygen, so that more oxygen is released from hemoglobin. By this mechanism, oxygen dissociation from hemoglobin is controlled by $\mathring{V}O_2$.

The longitudinal oxygen gradient within the capillary is created by the extraction of oxygen by tissue as blood passes from the arterial to the venous end of the capillary. The arteriovenous oxygen difference is equivalent to the ratio of $\mathring{V}O_2$ to blood flow (Fick equation). An increase in $\mathring{V}O_2$ or a decrease in blood flow (or both) steepens the longitudinal oxygen gradient. Proportional changes in $\mathring{V}O_2$ and blood flow are required to maintain the longitudinal oxygen gradient constant.

A corresponding value for capillary PO_2 (PcO_2) can be estimated from the value for capillary O_2 content, taking into account the Hb and the oxyhemoglobin dissociation curve. The shape of the longitudinal gradient in PO_2 within the capillary is approximately exponential because of the influence of the oxyhemoglobin dissociation curve. The PcO_2 is the driving force for diffusion of O_2 into the tissue. Because PcO_2 is minimal at the venous end of the capillary, the mitochondria in this region are most vulnerable to oxygen deficits.

At the bottom of Fig. 2-27 is Krogh's original equation for estimating PO_2 at a specific point (x) in the surrounding tissue cylinder. This equation was later simplified to provide a value for mean tissue PO_2 (PtO_2) (3):

$$\text{Mean } PtO_2 = PcO_2 - A(\mathring{V}O_2 \times r^2/4D) \quad [2\text{-}9]$$

where PcO_2 is blood oxygen tension at a midway point in the capillary, A is a constant representing the relation between capillary radius and tissue cylinder radius, $\mathring{V}O_2$ is oxygen consumption of the tissue cylinder, r is the radius of the tissue cylinder (half of the intercapillary distance), and D is the oxygen diffusion coefficient. The value for r is determined by the number of capillaries perfused with red blood cells per volume of tissue and is controlled by the precapillary sphincters. The favorable influence of capillary recruitment on tissue PO_2 is evident in the Fig. 2-27 (lower panel). If only capillaries 1 and 3 are open, the diffusion distance is so large that PO_2 falls to zero toward the center of the tissue cylinder. The low tissue PO_2 causes relaxation of the precapillary sphincter controlling capillary 2. Perfusion of capillary 2 decreases the diffusion distance and increases tissue PO_2 to an adequate level throughout the tissue.

Mean PtO_2 is a reflection of the overall balance between oxygen supply and demand within a particular tissue. An increase in blood flow without a change in oxygen demand (i.e., luxuriant perfusion) raises the mean PtO_2, whereas a reduction in blood flow without a change in oxygen demand lowers it. If mean PtO_2 falls below a critical level, $\mathring{V}O_2$ becomes impaired. Measurements of mean PtO_2 have been obtained in laboratory animals in various tissues, including the myocardium and skeletal muscle, by use of a polarographic technique involving bare-tipped platinum electrodes (4,5). The invasiveness of this technique has curtailed the use of mean PtO_2 measurements in patients. Measurements of local venous PO_2 provide an approximation for average end-capillary PO_2, and although they neglect the radial PO_2 gradient, they generally show a reasonable correlation to mean PtO_2 (6).

Oxygen Consumption and Other Measurable Variables *In Vivo*

In a clinical setting, there are several methods to measure $\dot{V}O_2$ of the whole body (7,8): (a) oxygen loss or replacement into a closed breathing system, (b) subtraction of expired from inspired volume of oxygen, and (c) use of the Fick principle.

The first method, oxygen loss or replacement into a closed breathing system, is the most fundamental, is well validated, and has an accuracy well in excess of clinical requirements. However, it is cumbersome and requires meticulous attention to detail to be used safely during intensive care. The second method, subtraction of expired from inspired volume of oxygen, is a difficult and potentially inaccurate method to determine $\dot{V}O_2$. The major problem is that $\dot{V}O_2$ is a small number that is calculated as the difference between two large numbers.

Under steady state conditions, the Fick equation can be used to calculate systemic $\dot{V}O_2$:

$$\dot{V}O_2 = CO \times (CaO_2 - C\bar{v}O_2) \quad [2\text{-}10]$$

In this technique, CO is usually measured by thermodilution using a Swan-Ganz catheter situated in the pulmonary artery. Samples of blood are collected from an artery and from the pulmonary artery (mixed venous sample) and analyzed for oxygen content. Using the normal values for CO and ($CaO_2 - C\bar{v}O_2$) described earlier, systemic $\dot{V}O_2$ can be calculated:

$$\dot{V}O_2 = 5{,}000 \times 4.7/100 = 235 \text{ mL/minute} \quad [2\text{-}11]$$

The Fick technique is popular in the intensive care setting, probably because the necessary arterial and pulmonary artery catheters are frequently already placed in critically ill patients. An important advantage of this method is that it also provides a measurement of DO_2 (Eq. 2-6), which permits analysis of the relation between DO_2 and $\dot{V}O_2$. A drawback of the Fick technique is that it excludes $\dot{V}O_2$ of the lungs. Although this component is negligible in the case of normal lungs, simultaneous measurements of $\dot{V}O_2$ by the Fick and gasometric methods indicate that it may be significant (as much as 20% of total $\dot{V}O_2$) in critically ill patients (9). It has been proposed that the increased $\dot{V}O_2$ in the lung is related to production of the superoxide free radical and, in turn, the hydroxyl free radical, hydrogen peroxide, and hypochlorous acid (10).

The oxygen extraction ratio (EO_2), as a percentage, is defined by the equation:

$$EO_2 = (CaO_2 - C\bar{v}O_2) \div CaO_2 \quad [2\text{-}12]$$

Combining equations and rearranging terms, it can be demonstrated that EO_2 is also equal to the ratio of $\dot{V}O_2$ to DO_2 and, therefore, reflects the balance between systemic oxygen demand and delivery. Measurements of EO_2, as well as of $P\bar{v}O_2$, are frequently used clinically to assess the overall adequacy of DO_2 in critically ill patients (11–13).

Critical Oxygen Delivery

At rest, DO_2 greatly exceeds $\dot{V}O_2$ (in our examples, they are 1,025 and 235 mL/minute, respectively); therefore EO_2 is relatively modest (approximately 25%), resulting in a substantial reserve for increased EO_2. This results in a biphasic relation between DO_2 and $\dot{V}O_2$ (Fig. 2-28) (14). At normal or high levels of DO_2, $\dot{V}O_2$ is constant and independent of DO_2 (Fig. 2-28, panel A). As DO_2 is gradually reduced, an increased EO_2 maintains the $\dot{V}O_2$ (panel B). Eventually a point is reached at which EO_2 cannot increase adequately. Below this threshold, the so-called critical DO_2, $\dot{V}O_2$ is limited by the supply of oxygen. In anesthetized dogs, the critical DO_2 was found to be approximately 10 mL/minute/kg (15). The normal biphasic DO_2-$\dot{V}O_2$ relationship has been demonstrated in patients without respiratory failure undergoing coronary artery bypass surgery (16), whereas a direct linear relationship between DO_2 and $\dot{V}O_2$ has been demonstrated in patients with acute adult respiratory distress syndrome (17,18), implying a pathologic impairment to tissue extraction of oxygen in these patients. A decrease in DO_2 can follow a reduction in any one of its major factors

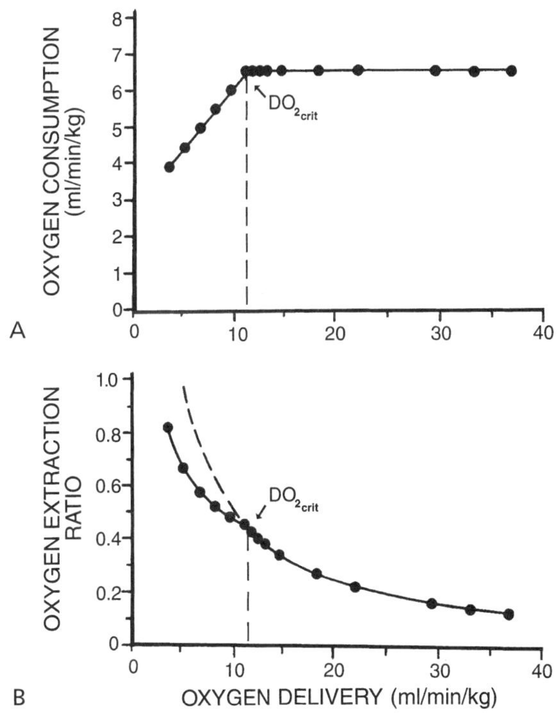

FIGURE 2-28. Changes in systemic oxygen consumption (**A**) and oxygen extraction ratio (**B**) during progressive reduction in oxygen delivery. An increased oxygen extraction ratio maintains oxygen consumption at a constant level until oxygen delivery is lowered to a critical value (DO_{2crit}). The dashed line demonstrates the theoretical increase in oxygen extraction required to maintain oxygen consumption for levels of oxygen delivery below DO_{2crit}. (Modified from Schumacker PT, Cain SM. The concept of critical oxygen delivery. *Intensive Care Med* 1987;13;223, with permission.)

TABLE 2-1. INTERORGAN VARIATION IN BASELINE VALUES FOR BLOOD FLOW, OXYGEN CONSUMPTION, ARTERIOVENOUS OXYGEN DIFFERENCE, AND OXYGEN EXTRACTION IN THE AVERAGE HUMAN

Organ	Blood Flow (mL/min/100 g)	Oxygen Consumption (mL/min/100 g)	Arteriovenous O_2 Differences (vol%)	O_2 Extraction (%)
Left ventricle	80	8	14	70
Brain	55	3	6	30
Liver	85 }	2	6	30
Gastrointestinal tract	40 }			
Kidneys	400	5	1.3	6.5
Muscles	3	0.15	5	25
Skin	10	0.2	2.5	12.5
Rest of body	3	0.15	4.4	22

(Hb, SaO_2, or CO) or a small reduction in more than one of these factors, such as may occur in critical illness. Old terminology referred to the conditions of hypoxia resulting from reductions in Hb, SaO_2, and CO, as anemic, hypoxic, and stagnant hypoxia, respectively.

Equations 2-6, 2-10, and 2-12 can be applied to individual tissues by substituting local blood flow for CO and local venous oxygen measurements for mixed venous oxygen measurements. The individual body tissues vary widely with respect to the relation between baseline DO_2 and VO_2, and therefore also in their baseline EO_2 (Table 2-1). For example, in the left ventricle baseline EO_2 is 70% to 75%, whereas in the kidney it is 5% to 10%. The high baseline EO_2 of the left ventricle renders it extremely dependent on changes in blood flow to maintain adequate oxygen transport.

DETERMINANTS OF MYOCARDIAL OXYGEN DELIVERY AND CONSUMPTION

Control of Coronary Blood Flow

Blood flow to the myocardium, like that to other vascular beds, is a function of the arteriovenous pressure gradient and the local vascular resistance. In the left ventricular wall, coronary vascular resistance is determined by the throttling effect caused by extravascular compressive forces during systole and by active changes in the tone of arteriolar smooth muscle (Fig. 2-29). The mechanical impediment to coronary blood flow is most prominent in the subendocardial layers of the left ventricular wall. This factor means that blood flow in the left coronary circulation occurs predominantly during diastole, rather than during systole, as is the case elsewhere, including the right coronary circulation. The pressure gradient for blood flow in the left ventricular wall is approximated by the difference between aortic diastolic pressure and left ventricular end-diastolic pressure. Local metabolic mechanisms predominate in the active control of coronary vasomotor tone. These mechanisms provide a close coupling between coronary blood flow and myocardial oxygen demand, which serves to maintain myocardial PO_2 (and coronary sinus PO_2) an an almost constant level. Adenosine, a breakdown product of ATP, is a potent endogenous vasodilator that is thought to play a central role in the metabolic regulation of coronary perfusion. However, other chemical factors may also contribute, including oxygen, hydrogen ions, carbon dioxide, and nitric oxide (released from the vascular endothelium). The term *autoregulation* refers to the intrinsic capability of the coronary circulation to maintain a relatively constant coronary blood flow over a wide range of perfusion pressures, by metabolic and/or myogenic mechanisms. A myogenic response refers to the intrinsic tendency of vascular smooth muscle to contract in response to increased distending pressure and to relax in response to decreased distending pressure. The higher tissue pressures in the subendocardium result in a reduced autoregulatory capability in the subendocardium compared with the subepicardium. This contributes to the greater vulnerability of that region to infarction during coronary insufficiency. The coronary arterioles are endowed with α- (constricting) and β_2- (dilating) adrenergic receptors and with muscarinic receptors, and they are supplied by sympathetic and parasympathetic (vagus) nerves. These autonomic pathways normally play a secondary role in coronary vascular regulation.

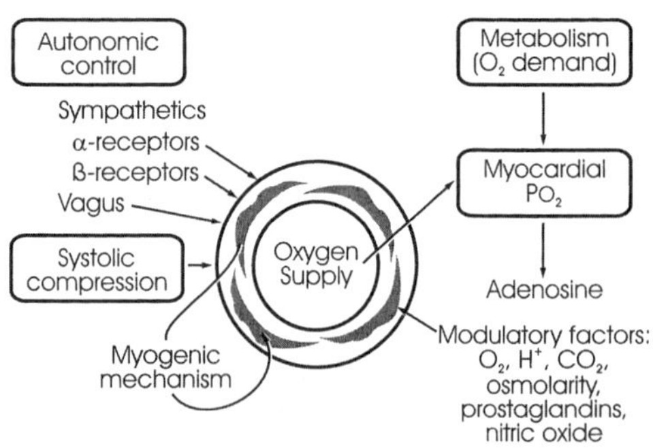

FIGURE 2-29. Factors influencing coronary vascular resistance. (Modified from Rubio R, Berne RM. *Progress in cardiovascular diseases.* New York: Grune & Stratton, 1975;18:105, with permission.)

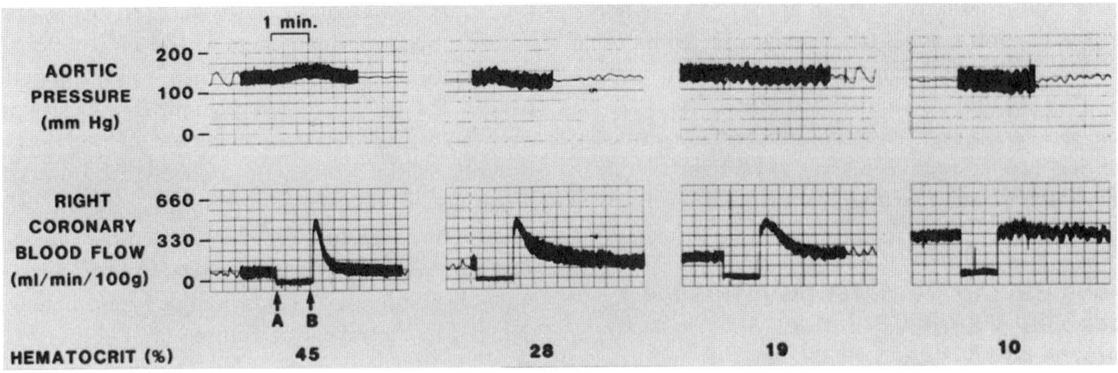

FIGURE 2-30. Coronary reserve assessed by analysis of the reactive hyperemia response in the right coronary circulation of a dog. Graded hemodilution was associated with a progressive diminution of this response. (From Crystal GJ, Kim S-J, Salem MR. Right and left ventricular O_2 uptake during hemodilution and β-adrenergic stimulation. *Am J Physiol* 1993:265:H1769, with permission.)

Coronary Reserve Assessed by Analysis of the Reactive Hyperemic Response

The transient increase in blood flow above the control rate that follows an interval of arterial occlusion is termed a *reactive hyperemia* (Fig. 2-30). The temporal characteristics of this response have been explained by the concept that metabolites produced in the ischemic tissue first dilate the resistance vessels and then are washed out during reperfusion. A coronary occlusion of 60 seconds is usually required to maximally dilate the coronary circulation and therefore to assess the coronary reserve. Longer occlusions only increase the duration of the reactive hyperemic response. Coronary reserve in the normal right and left ventricular walls is appreciable (500% to 600%), but it is reduced in a variety of conditions, including left ventricular hypertrophy, coronary obstruction, and hemodilution (19) (Fig. 2-30). A diminished coronary reserve renders the myocardium more vulnerable to ischemia secondary to increases in cardiac work or reductions in perfusion pressure.

Determinants of Myocardial Oxygen Consumption

The heart is a continuously active organ that normally depends almost exclusively on aerobic metabolism to meet its energy demands. Although the heart constitutes less than 0.5% of the weight of the body, it accounts for approximately 7% of the body's basal oxygen consumption. The utilization of substrates by the heart depends on their availability as well as the heart's nutritional status and hormonal influences. Various substrates—including glucose, fatty acids, lactate, pyruvate, acetate, ketone bodies, and amino acids—can serve as energy sources, although under physiologic conditions glucose and fatty acids are the major substrates. The most important determinants of myocardial oxygen consumption are contractility, HR, and wall tension (Fig. 2-31). Other points worthy of mention are the following: (a) Wall tension is directly proportional to the pressure and radius of the heart and inversely proportional to the wall thickness (law of Laplace); the area beneath the left ventricular pressure pulse per minute, the time-tension index (TTI), bears a direct relation to myocardial oxygen consumption. (b) When external work (pressure × SV) is considered, pressure work has a much greater oxygen cost than does flow work. Muscle shortening *per se* has only a small influence on myocardial oxygen consumption.

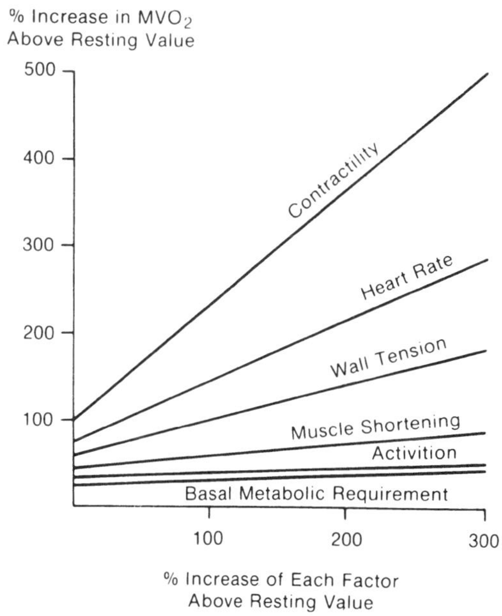

FIGURE 2-31. Determinants of myocardial oxygen consumption. (From Marcus ML. *The coronary circulation in health and disease*. New York: McGraw-Hill, 1983, with permission.)

(c) Basal metabolism reflects ATP-requiring processes not directly related to contraction, such as activity of cell membrane Na^+,K^+-ATPase for maintaining the ionic environment, and other cellular processes such as protein synthesis. (d) The oxygen cost of activation comprises two components: electrical activation, and release and uptake of calcium by the sarcoplasmic reticulum.

Conditions Having Detrimental Influence on Myocardial Oxygen Balance: Mechanisms of Myocardial Ischemia

When the vasodilator reserve of the coronary bed is limited by a proximal stenosis (or by hypoxemia or anemia), the myocardium, especially the subendocardium, becomes vulnerable to ischemia (i.e., oxygen demands exceeding oxygen delivery). The factors tending to promote this condition are presented on Fig. 2-32. An increase in HR is especially detrimental to oxygen delivery/demand balance because it decreases coronary blood flow (via a shortening of the diastolic period) while also increasing myocardial oxygen demand. An increase in preload also reduces coronary blood flow by compromising the pressure gradient, and it increases myocardial oxygen demand via an increase in wall tension. Although an increase in aortic pressure tends to augment coronary blood flow by increasing driving pressure, it also increases myocardial oxygen demand via an increase in wall tension. Therefore, its net effect depends on the balance between these factors. Under conditions of restricted coronary vasodilator reserve, the most favorable hemodynamic situation is characterized by a low HR and preload, a normal aortic pressure, and a normal to moderate inotropic state (20).

In the early 1970s, Hoffman and Buckberg (21) proposed the endocardial viability ratio (EVR) as an index to detect subendocardial ischemia. The EVR reflects the relationship between indices of oxygen supply (blood flow) and oxygen demand in subendocardium. The diastolic pressure-time index (DPTI) is used an index for blood flow to subendocardium. This index is based on the proposition that blood flow to the subendocardium occurs primarily during diastole and therefore is dependent on the integrated pressure difference between the aorta and left ventricle. The time-tension index (TTI) is used as an estimate for oxygen demand in the subendocardium:

$$EVR = DPTI/TTI \qquad [2\text{-}13]$$

A normal value for EVR is 1.0 or greater. An EVR lower than 0.7 is considered to reflect subendocardial ischemia. The reliability of EVR as an index for detecting subendocardial ischemia intraoperatively is open to debate. Marcus (22) has criticized EVR on the basis that DPTI does not take into account a host of factors, including pathologic changes (e.g., cardiac hypertrophy), drugs, and neural stimuli, that have potential independent effects on the transmural distribution of left ventricular perfusion, and that TTI ignores important determinants of myocardial oxygen demand (e.g., changes in contractility and ventricular wall thickness, such as occurs in hypertrophy).

Two other indices are used clinically as estimates of myocardial oxygen demand. The rate-pressure product (RPP) is obtained by multiplying the systolic arterial pressure (SAP) by the HR:

$$RPP = SAP \times HR \qquad [2\text{-}14]$$

The triple index (TI) adds an estimate of left ventricular end-diastolic volume, the pulmonary capillary wedge pres-

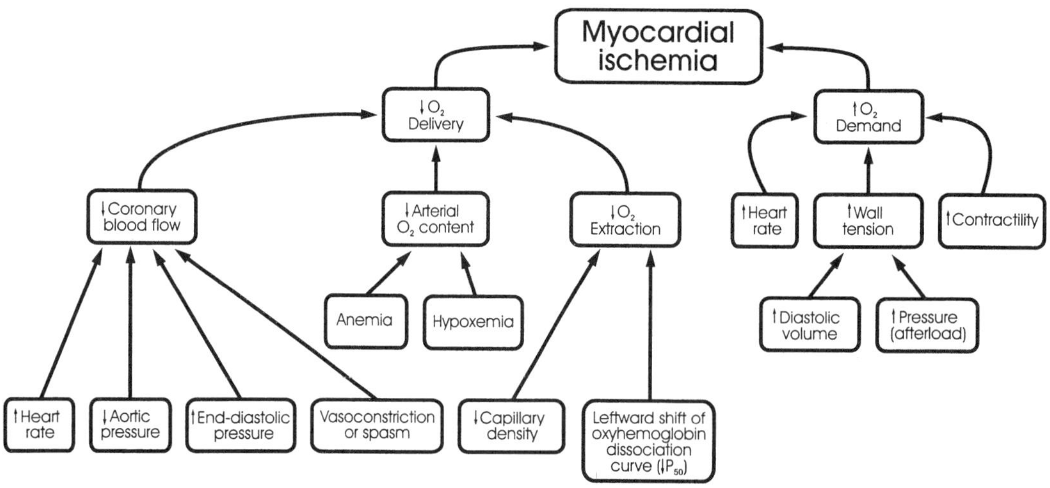

FIGURE 2-32. Conditions having detrimental influence on myocardial oxygen balance: mechanisms of myocardial ischemia.

sure (PCWP), to the index of myocardial oxygen demand:

$$TI = SAP \times HR \times PCWP \qquad [2\text{-}15]$$

Determinants of Coronary Steal

Coronary steal refers to the phenomenon in which small-vessel dilation and an increase in flow to an area of already well-perfused myocardium leads to a decrease in flow to another area of myocardium with borderline perfusion and limited coronary reserve. Coronary steal can occur between two arteries connected by collateral vessels (intercoronary steal) or from subendocardium to subepicardium distal to a coronary stenosis (transmural steal). A schematic diagram demonstrating the hemodynamic basis of vasodilator-induced intercoronary steal is shown in Fig. 2-33. Under the control condition (panel A) in this hypothetical situation, (a) the left anterior descending coronary artery (LAD) is completely occluded, and the myocardium in its perfusion territory receives flow via collateral vessels originating at the circumflex artery (CX); (b) the CX has a significant stenosis; (c) collateral flow to the LAD bed is equal to antegrade flow to the CX bed; and (d) resistance vessels in the LAD bed are maximally dilated, so blood flow in this region is pressure-dependent. On the other hand, resistance vessels in the CX bed retain a significant vasdilator reserve capacity. Coronary steal occurs (panel B) when a vasodilator, either a drug or a physiologic factor such as hypercapnia, reduces vascular resistance in the distal CX bed, which increases the rate of blood flow through the CX. This steepens the pressure drop within this artery, resulting in a reduced pressure at the source of the collateral vessels and a decrease in collateral flow to the pressure-dependent LAD bed.

Transmural steal occurs because the subepicardium has a greater capacity for autoregulation than does the subendocardium. This is probably the result of the higher tissue pressures in the subendocardium. Coronary steal can precipitate myocardial ischemia if the decrease in flow is not accompanied by a proportional decrease in myocardial oxygen demand.

Nitric Oxide: Its Source, Release, and Functions in the Cardiovascular System

In 1980, Furchgott and Zawadzki observed that acetylcholine-induced relaxation of isolated arterial segments required an intact endothelium (23). This observation led to their conclusion that acetylcholine was acting on the muscarinic receptors located on the endothelial membrane to cause release of a vasodilating substance, which they termed endothelium-derived relaxing factor (EDRF). In 1987, EDRF was identified as nitric oxide (NO) (24). It is now known that NO is a ubiquitous molecule that has important roles in the circulation system and elsewhere, including roles in immunologic reactions and as a neurotransmitter in the central nervous system (24).

Figure 2-34 shows the signal-transduction pathway for endothelium-derived NO.

NO is a free radical produced in the vascular endothelium from the amino acid L-arginine in a reaction requiring the constitutive enzyme nitric oxide synthase (NOS) (24). NOS activity is stimulated by increases in intracellular calcium concentration, which occur in response to the interaction of a chemical agent in the blood (e.g., bradykinin, acetylcholine) with its specific membrane receptor or by increases in shear stress. Constitutive NOS produces small

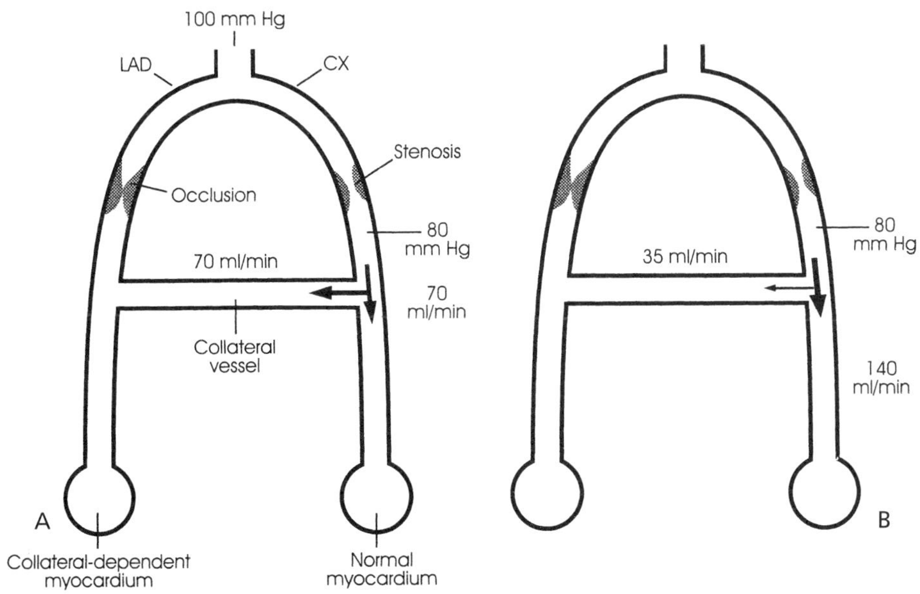

FIGURE 2-33. Mechanism of coronary steal. **A:** Control condition. **B:** Vasodilator-induced coronary steal.

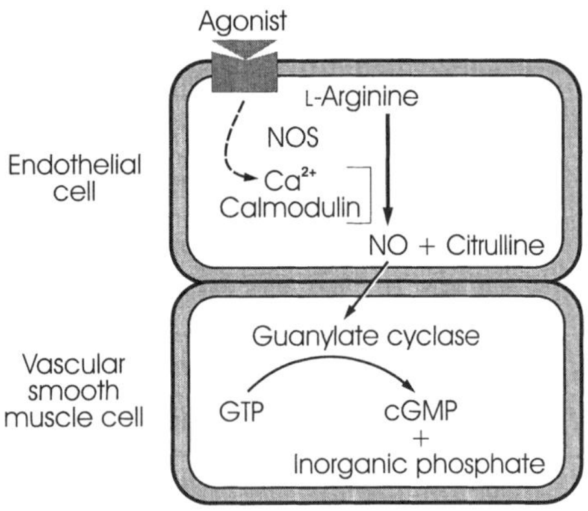

FIGURE 2-34. Diagram showing the signal-transduction pathway for endothelium-derived nitric oxide.

quantities of NO (picomoles) over short periods (seconds). Endothelium-derived NO diffuses into the underlying vascular smooth muscle, where it stimulates production of cyclic guanosine monophosphate (cGMP), thereby causing vascular relaxation. In the circulation, NO is rapidly scavenged by hemoglobin. Inhibitors of NOS have been shown to produce hypertension in animals, implying that basally released NO maintains a tonic vasodilator tone in the systemic resistance vessels (25).

NO has important physiologic roles in the circulation, in addition to its vasodilating effect. It is a potent inhibitor of platelet aggregation and adhesion to the endothelial surface (24,26). Furthermore, platelets that do aggregrate release serotonin and adenosine diphosphate, which in turn act on the endothelium to cause massive release of NO, resulting in vasodilation and a flushing out of the developing thrombus. NO also inhibits leukocyte activation and proliferation of vascular smooth muscle cells. Recent evidence suggests that constitutive NOS is normally expressed in tissues other than the vascular endothelium, including the endocardial endothelium, myocytes, and neurons in the myocardium (27,28).

NO may influence cardiac function indirectly by affecting vascular tone and directly by influencing the cGMP pathway in the myocytes themselves. With respect to the indirect mechanisms, coronary endothelial dysfunction may impair cardiac function by compromising coronary blood flow and oxygen delivery. Furthermore, changes in peripheral arterial tone may influence cardiac function via variations in ventricular afterload, whereas changes in peripheral venous tone and capacitance may alter cardiac function via variations in preload (Starling mechanism). Evidence for the former mechanism are the decreases in SV and CO that characteristically accompany the peripheral vasoconstriction caused by NOS inhibitors (25).

Studies in various *in vitro* cardiac preparations have demonstrated that both endogenous NO and NO donors may have direct cGMP-mediated negative inotropic actions (27,28). However, results obtained *in vivo* suggest that these actions do not apply to the normal, *in situ* heart exposed to physiologically relevant levels of NO (29). NO release from the vascular endothelium is inhibited in a number of pathologic conditions, including atherosclerosis, diabetes mellitus, and hypercholesterolemia (30). Vascular endothelial dysfunction may promote coronary vasospasm.

A second isoform of NOS, so-called inducible NOS, has been identified (24,31,32). Inducible NOS is not normally present and has no physiologic role, but it is expressed after stimulation by microbial products (e.g., endotoxin) or by inflammatory mediators, including the cytokines, interleukin-1 (IL-1), IL-2, IL-6, and tumor necrosis factor. Activity of inducible NOS is not sensitive to calcium concentration. Inducible NOS was originally described in macrophages but subsequently identified in the vascular endothelium, vascular smooth muscle, and myocardial cells. Inducible NOS is generally activated by induction of transcription over several hours. It can produce large quantities of NO (nanomoles) over extended periods (hours). It can have cytotoxic effects either directly or via reaction with superoxide anion (O_2^-) to form peroxynitrite ($OONO^-$), which is a potent oxidant capable of causing significant cellular damage. Formation of peroxynitrite has been demonstrated in tissue during inflammation, hypoxia-reoxygenation, and ischemia-reperfusion (33,34). The expression of inducible NOS is inhibited by glucocorticoids. The inducible NOS isoform is responsible for the uncontrolled, excessive vasodilation associated with septic shock, and it may be involved in acute myocarditis, dilated cardiomyopathy, and cardiac transplant rejection (31,32).

The vasodilating effects of sodium nitroprusside and nitroglycerin have been explained by their ability to provide exogenous NO (35). Inhaled NO has been shown to be a potent and selective pulmonary vasodilator that may have a role in the treatment of adult respiratory distress syndrome, pulmonary hypertension, and asthma (36,37).

REFERENCES

1. Segard JL, Bosnjak ZJ, Hopp FA Jr, et al. Cardiovascular effects of general anesthetics. In: Covino BJ, Fozzard HA, Rehder K, et al., eds. *Effects of anesthesia.* Bethesda, MD: American Physiological Society, 1985:149.
2. Krogh A. The number and distribution of capillaries in muscles with calculations of the oxygen pressure head necessary for supplying the tissue. *J Physiol (London)* 1919;52:409.
3. Kety SS. Determinants of tissue oxygen tension. *Fed Proc* 1957; 16:666.
4. Crystal GJ, Weiss HR. V_{O_2} of resting muscle during arterial hypoxia: role of reflex vasoconstriction. *Microvasc Res* 1980;20: 30.
5. Crystal GJ, Downey HF, Bashour FA. Small vessel blood and total coronary blood volume during intracoronary adenosine infusion. *Am J Physiol* 1981;241:H194.
6. Tenny SM. Theoretical analysis of the relationship between venous blood and mean tissue oxygen pressure. *Respir Physiol* 1975; 20:283.

7. Nunn JF, Makita K, Royston B. Validation of oxygen consumption measurements during artificial ventilation. *J Appl Physiol* 1989;67:2129.
8. Makita K, Nunn JF, Royston B. Evaluation of metabolic measuring instruments for use in critically ill patients. *Crit Care Med* 1990;18:638.
9. Smithies MN, Royston B, Makita K, et al. Comparison of oxygen consumption measurements: indirect calorimetry versus the reversed Fick method. *Crit Care Med* 1991;19:1401.
10. Webster NR, Nunn JF. Molecular structure of free radicals and their importance in biological reactions. *Br J Anaesth* 1988;60:98.
11. Astiz ME, Rackow EC, Kaufman B, et al. Relationship of oxygen delivery and mixed venous oxygenation and to lactate acidosis in patients with sepsis and acute myocardial infarction. *Crit Care Med* 1988;16:655.
12. Pinsky MR. Assessment of adequacy of oxygen transport in the critically ill. *Appl Cardiopulm Pathophysiol* 1990;3:271.
13. Levy PS, Chavez RP, Crystal GJ, et al. Oxygen extraction ratio: a valid indicator of transfusion need in limited coronary vascular reserve? *J Trauma* 1992;32:769.
14. Schumacker PT, Cain SM. The concept of critical oxygen oxygen delivery. *Intensive Care Med* 1987;13:223.
15. Cain SM. Oxygen delivery and uptake in dogs during anemic and hypoxic hypoxia. *J Appl Physiol* 1977;42:228.
16. Shibutani K, Komatsu T, Kubal K, et al. Critical level of oxygen delivery in anesthetized man. *Crit Care Med* 1983;11:640.
17. Danek SJ, Lynch JP, Weg JG, et al. The dependence of oxygen uptake on oxygen delivery in the adult respiratory distress syndrome. *Am Rev Respir Dis* 1980;122:387.
18. Mohsenifar Z, Goldbach P, Tachkin DP, et al. Relationship between O_2 delivery and O_2 consumption in the adult respiratory distress syndrome. *Chest* 1983;84:267.
19. Crystal GJ, Kim S-J, Salem MR. Right and left ventricular O_2 uptake during hemodilution and β-adrenergic stimulaton. *Am J Physiol* 1993;265:H1769.
20. Hug CC Jr, Shanewise JS. Anesthesia for adult cardiac surgery. In: Miller RD, ed. *Anesthesia,* 4th ed, vol 2. New York: Churchill Livingstone, 1994:1757.
21. Hoffman JIE, Buckberg GD. Regional myocardial ischemia: causes, prediction and prevention. *Vasc Surg* 1974;8:115.
22. Marcus ML. *The coronary circulation in health and disease.* New York: McGraw-Hill, 1983.
23. Furchgott RF, Zawadzki JV. Obligatory role of endothelial cells in the relaxation of arterial smooth muscle by acetylcholine. *Nature (London)* 1980;288:373.
24. Moncada S, Palmer RMJ, Higgs EA. Nitric oxide: physiology, pathophysiology, and pharmacology. *Pharmacol Rev* 1991;43:109.
25. Crystal GJ, Zhou X, Halim AA, et al. Nitric oxide does not modulate whole-body oxygen consumption in anesthetized dogs. *J Appl Physiol* 1999;86:1944.
26. Vanhoutte PM, Scott-Burden T. The endothelium in health and disease. *Tex Heart Inst J* 1994;21:62.
27. Shah AM, Grocott-Mason RM, Pepper CB, et al. The cardiac endothelium: cardioactive mediators. *Prog Cardiovasc Dis* 1996;39:263.
28. Kelly RA, Balligand J-L, Smith TW. Nitric oxide and cardiac function. *Circ Res* 1996;79:363.
29. Crystal GJ, Gurevicius J. Nitric oxide does not modulate myocardial contractility acutely in in situ canine hearts. *Am J Physiol* 1996;270:H1568.
30. Searle NR, Sahab P. Endothelial vasomotor regulation in health and disease. *Can J Anaesth* 1992;39:838.
31. Birks EJ, Yacoub MH. The role of nitric oxide and cytokines in heart failure. *Coron Artery Dis* 1997;8:389.
32. De Belder AJ, Ramdomski MW, Martin JF, et al. Nitric oxide and the pathogenesis of heart muscle disease. *Eur J Clin Invest* 1995;25:1.
33. Lefer AM, Lefer DJ. Pharmacology of the endothelium in ischemia-reperfusion and circulatory shock. *Ann Rev Pharmacol Toxicol* 1993;33:71.
34. Xie Y-W, Wolin MS. Role of nitric oxide and its interaction with superoxide in the suppression of cardiac muscle mitochondrial respiration: involvement in response to hypoxia/reoxygenation. *Circulation* 1996;94:2580.
35. Anderson TJ, Meredith IT, Ganz P, et al. Nitric oxide and nitrovasodilators: similarities, differences, and potential interactions. *J Am Col Cardiol* 1994;24:555.
36. Conti CR. Nitric oxide as a therapeutic agent. *Clin Cardiol* 1994;17:227.
37. Lowson SM, Rich GF, McArdle PA, et al. The response to varying concentrations of inhaled nitric oxide in patients with acute respiratory distress syndrome. *Anesth Analg* 1996;82:574.

SUGGESTED READINGS

Braunwald E, Ross J Jr, Sonnenblick EH. *Mechanisms of contraction of the normal and failing heart.* Boston: Little, Brown, 1976.

Edwards JD, Shoemaker WC, Vincent J-L, eds. *Oxygen transport: principles and practice.* London: WB Saunders, 1993.

Feigl EO. Coronary physiology. *Physiol Rev* 1983;63:1.

Honig CR. *Modern cardiovascular physiology.* Boston: Little, Brown, 1981.

Nunn JF. *Nunn's applied respiratory physiology.* Oxford: Butterworth-Heinemann, 1993.

Weibel ER. *The pathway for oxygen.* Cambridge: Harvard University Press, 1984.

Cardiac Anesthesia: Principles and Clinical Practice, Second Edition, edited by Fawzy G. Estafanous, Paul G. Barash, and J.G. Reves. Lippincott Williams & Wilkins, Philadelphia © 2001.

3

CARDIAC PHARMACOLOGY

DEBRA A. SCHWINN

The cardiovascular system consists of a complex array of pipes (vessels), flexible tubing (smooth muscle capable of constriction and relaxation), flow restrictors (venous and cardiac valves), and a mechanical pump (myocardium). Because of the many functions of the cardiovascular system, its chemical modulation by drugs is diverse, with sites of action distributed over vast physical locations and spanning numerous receptor systems. Ultimately, however, distinct individual receptors bind drugs (both agonists and antagonists) and mediate expected clinical responses. Therefore, basic principles of receptor pharmacology are presented briefly to provide a foundation for discussing individual cardiovascular medications. Once these principles are established, the discussion turns to perioperative chronic cardiac medications, followed by intraoperative acute cardiac medications, and finally ends with protocols for drug therapy within specific clinical situations. Antiarrhythmic drugs and cardiopulmonary resuscitation protocols are discussed separately in Chapters 4 and 5. Because cardiovascular pharmacology is a vast discipline, whenever possible only pertinent reviews are cited, enabling the reader to delve further while providing the broadest and simplest overview possible.

NEUROTRANSMITTERS AND RECEPTORS

Autonomic Nervous System

The autonomic nervous system is composed of a complex intertwining of nerves, sensory and effector arcs, and brain modulation of impulses. Peripheral stimuli such as pain, pressure, temperature, and touch, as well as stimuli of more specialized senses such as taste, smell, hearing, and sight, are processed at various levels of the nervous system. The major central sites of integration, processing, and transport of nervous system impulses include the brain, spinal cord, and peripheral nerves. In addition to local effects, the cardiovascular system is modulated closely via the autonomic nervous system. A rich network of peripheral nerves innervate vessels and myocardial tissue to maintain the constant integrated function of blood flow. An example of the protective complexity of autonomic regulation can be illustrated by a patient who is frightened of having blood drawn. In this situation, mental stress occasionally mediates acute venodilation (and/or vasodilation), resulting in an abrupt decrease in effective circulating blood volume; this may decrease brain blood flow in the standing position, produce "starry sky" vision momentarily in the patient, and sometimes result in the patient fainting to the floor. Ironically, the prone/supine position thus attained is protective because major organs (particularly the brain) are able to be perfused despite relative hypovolemia, because gravitationally mediated venous pooling does not occur in the new position.

Sympathetic and Parasympathetic Nervous Systems

The autonomic nervous system consists of two major components: the sympathetic nervous system and the parasympathetic nervous system (Fig. 3-1). Major efferents of both the sympathetic and the parasympathetic nervous system originate in the brain, travel in the anterolateral columns of the spinal cord (albeit each at different levels), and use acetylcholine (ACh) as the neurotransmitter at the level of the ganglion, but they utilize different neurotransmitters at the neuroeffector junction located in the target tissue. Specifically, efferent sympathetic fibers (which travel predominantly in thoracolumbar regions of the spinal cord) operate with norepinephrine as the neurotransmitter at the effector junction. Parasympathetic efferents (which travel predominantly in cervical and sacral regions of the spinal cord) utilize ACh as the neurotransmitter at both the ganglion and the neuroeffector junction.

Neurotransmitters

Neurotransmitters classically convert electrical energy (in the form of waves of depolarization propagated along a nerve fiber) into chemical information. Neurotransmitters are used at two discrete locations along efferent autonomic

D. A. Schwinn: Departments of Anesthesiology, Pharmacology/Cancer Biology, and Surgery, Duke University Medical Center, Durham, North Carolina 27710

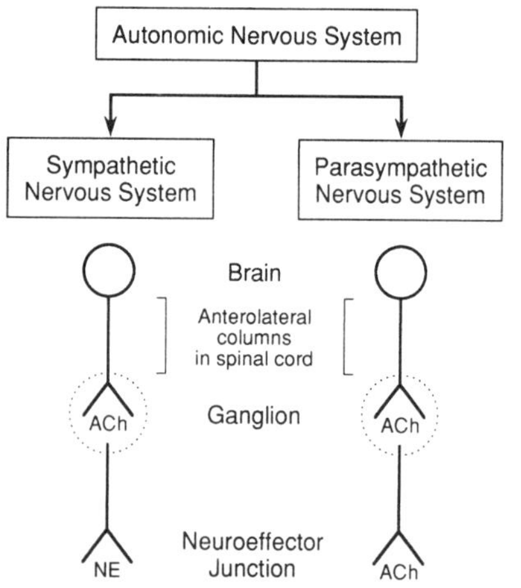

FIGURE 3-1. Autonomic nervous system. The autonomic nervous system is composed of two major components: the sympathetic nervous system and the parasympathetic nervous system. Efferent nerve fibers for both sympathetic and parasympathetic components generally originate in the brain, traverse the spinal cord, use acetylcholine (ACh) as a neurotransmitter at the ganglion, and are distinguished by the neurotransmitter at the neuroeffector junction (norepinephrine for the sympathetic fibers and ACh for the parasympathetic fibers).

nerves: at the ganglion and at the neuroeffector junction in the target tissue. As exemplified by the neuroeffector junction of the sympathetic nervous system, the neurotransmitter norepinephrine is synthesized in the nerve terminal and stored in vesicles (Fig. 3-2). Upon nerve stimulation, vesicles containing norepinephrine are mobilized to the plasma membrane where granules are released, resulting in norepinephrine entering the synaptic cleft. Neurotransmitters may then stimulate presynaptic receptors or postsynaptic receptors, or be degraded by enzyme systems such as catechol-*O*-methyltransferase (COMT, which methylates a hydroxyl group), and monoamine oxidase (MAO, which catalyzes oxidative deamination of catecholamines), or be taken up by local tissues. Although this simplistic picture has existed for many years, more recent evidence suggests that neurotransmitters stored in vesicles are not homogeneous. In addition to norepinephrine (in terminal sympathetic fibers) and ACh (in terminal parasympathetic fibers), adenosine triphosphate (ATP) has been shown to be present (1). Hence, ATP may modulate the response to sympathetic or parasympathetic nerve stimulation. In the case of sympathetic innervation to arteries, release of ATP along with norepinephrine may augment the classic norepinephrine-induced vasoconstrictor response to sympathetic stimulation by binding to

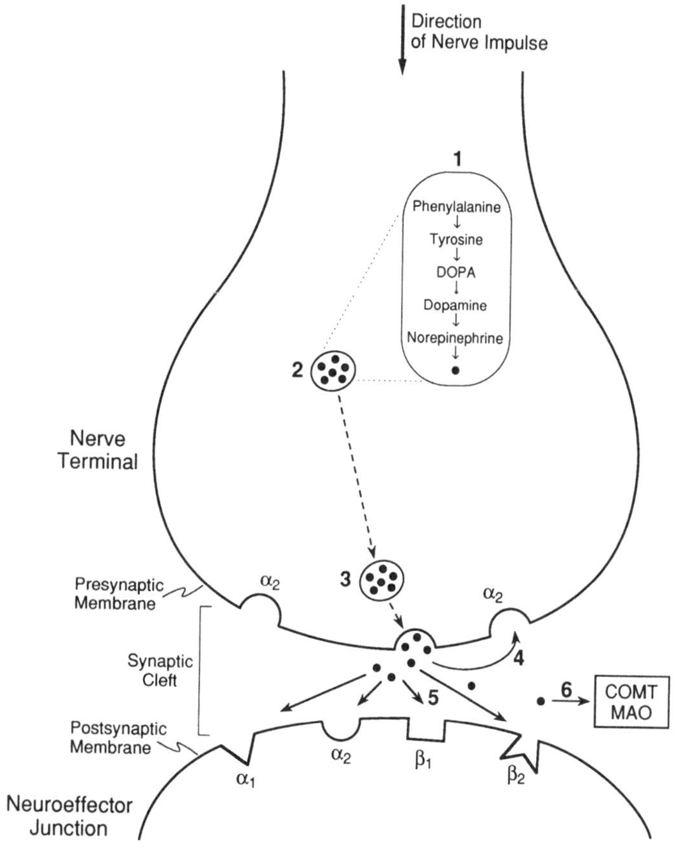

FIGURE 3-2. Components of a sympathetic nerve terminal. **1:** The neurotransmitter norepinephrine (*NE*) is synthesized in sympathetic nerve terminals. **2:** Neurotransmitters are stored in vesicles. **3:** With nerve stimulation, vesicles are mobilized to the plasma membrane where granules are released, resulting in NE entering the synaptic cleft. **4:** Neurotransmitters may stimulate presynaptic receptors. **5:** Neurotransmitters may stimulate postsynaptic receptors. **6:** Neurotransmitters may be degraded by enzyme systems such as catechol-*O*-methyltransferase (*COMT*) and monoamine oxidase (*MAO*).

purinergic P_{2Y} receptors and mediating enhanced vasoconstriction.

Synaptic Cleft

The synaptic cleft contains both presynaptic (nerve terminal) and postsynaptic neuroeffector membranes. Electromicrographs of postsynaptic membranes reveal topology consisting of many invaginations, thereby multiplying the potential surface area affected by a single innervating nerve. The small space between pre- and postsynaptic membranes (which makes up the synaptic cleft) is rich with waves of neurotransmitters and enzyme systems. Receptors that bind neurotransmitters are present both presynaptically and postsynaptically. Typically, presynaptic receptors modulate the release (or reuptake) of neurotransmitters, whereas postsynaptic receptors mediate the desired effect in the target tissue. Many classes of receptors are present on postsynaptic membranes. In addition to receptors, activation of ion channels in the postsynaptic membrane (either via receptor systems or directly) is another potential mechanism by which the target tissue is activated or inhibited.

Receptors

General Receptor Concepts

The concept that drugs interact with distinct receptors to mediate alterations of physiologic responses is well ingrained in clinicians today. However, the existence of receptors is a relatively recent discovery. Although many individuals were ultimately involved in elucidating the concept of receptors, contributions made by three individuals are reviewed briefly here because these investigators used drugs and concepts familiar to the practicing anesthesiologist.

Claude Bernard (1813–1878) is generally credited with the concept that circulating substances produce selective effects on end-organ systems. In a now classic experiment, Bernard ligated the main artery in one hindlimb of a frog then administered the muscle relaxant curare intravenously; flaccid paralysis resulted in all extremities except the one with the ligated vessel. Stimulation of the paralyzed hindlimb resulted in movement of the unparalyzed limb, effectively demonstrating separation of sensory and motor components of the nervous system. Paul Erhlich (1854–1915) then refined the concept of receptors by invoking selectivity of effect with his now famous phrase "agents cannot act unless they are bound." J.N. Langley (1852–1926) extended Bernard's work by showing that nicotine and curare have mutually antagonistic effects on the same "receptive substance" that is neither nerve nor muscle. In the case of nicotine and curare, this receptive substance was later found to be the neuromuscular junction. It is Langley's phrase, "receptive substance," that ultimately led to the name "receptor." Many researchers have since refined the definition of "receptor." Currently, receptors are described as proteins that bind a single class (or subclass) of hormones and/or drugs. Receptor subtypes can also be defined by virtue of their agonist potency series, binding of selective antagonists, second-messenger pathways, and/or distinct gene structures.

Signal Transduction

Receptors are located in two major areas of the cell: the membrane and the cytoplasm. Steroid and thyroid hormones are examples of very large lipophilic molecules that pass easily through the lipid cell membrane to interact with receptors located in the cytoplasm, ultimately interacting with deoxyribonucleic acid (DNA) located in the nucleus to modulate synthesis and expression of their own and other receptor systems. However, the vast majority of clinically available drugs and endogenous hormones are hydrophilic and cannot easily pass through the lipid cell membrane. Hence, most receptor systems important to clinicians are excitable membrane-bound proteins. Because the ligand (endogenous hormone or exogenous drug) binds receptor on the extracellular surface, but physiologic responses occur secondary to second-messenger activation in the cytoplasm of the cell, a mechanism of notifying the cytoplasm of receptor occupancy is important; this process is referred to as "signal transduction." One common motif of transmembrane receptor signal transduction is interaction of the activated receptor with an intermediary guanine nucleotide protein (G protein), which then (after hydrolysis of guanosine 5′-triphosphate [GTP] to guanosine 5′-diphosphate to provide energy) interacts and activates (or inhibits) a second-messenger system (Fig. 3-3). This results in initiation of a

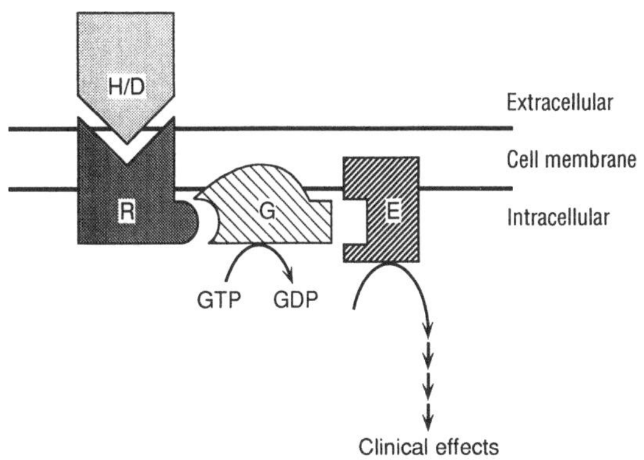

FIGURE 3-3. Signal transduction of transmembrane receptors. Hydrophilic endogenous hormones (*H*) or exogenous drugs (*D*) bind to the extracellular surface of transmembrane receptors (*R*). The activated receptor then interacts with a cytoplasmic intermediary guanosine nucleotide protein (G protein) (*G*). Hydrolysis of guanine triphosphate (*GTP*) to guanosine diphosphate (*GDP*) provides the energy required for the G protein to interact with the effector molecule (*E*). Effector molecule activation (or inhibition) leads to a cascade of chemical reactions within the cell, ultimately leading to the observed clinical effects.

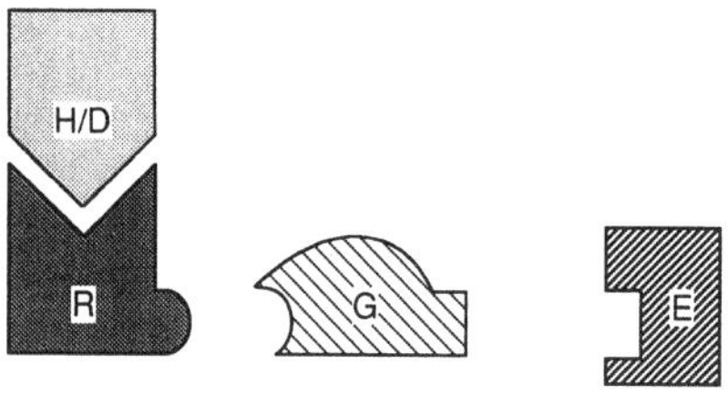

RECEPTOR	G PROTEIN	EFFECTOR	2ND MESSENGER
βAR	G_s	Stimulates adenylyl cyclase	↑ cAMP
α_2AR	G_i	Inhibits adenylyl cyclase	↓ cAMP
α_1AR	G_q	Phospholipase C	↑ Phospholipid hydrolysis (IP_3, DAG)

FIGURE 3-4. Components of the signal transduction pathway for adrenergic receptors. When stimulated by endogenous hormones (*H*) or exogenous drugs (*D*), individual receptors (*R*) couple to G proteins (*G*), activate or inhibit effector systems (*E*), and produce second messengers. The specific G proteins, effectors, and second-messenger systems involved with each classic adrenergic receptor subtype are shown here. (IP, inositol trisphosphate; DAG, diacylglycerol.)

cascade of chemical reactions within the cell, which ultimately leads to the desired clinical effect. In the case of the β-adrenergic receptor (AR), β-AR agonists (isoproterenol, epinephrine, norepinephrine, and dopamine) activate the stimulatory G protein, G_s, which stimulates the enzyme adenylyl cyclase, resulting in the production of 3′,5′,-cyclic adenosine monophosphate (cAMP) in the cell. Figure 3-4 illustrates general classes of G proteins, effector molecules, and second messengers for the "classic" ARs (β_1, β_2, α_1, and α_2), an important transmembrane G-protein–coupled receptor family for cardiovascular homeostasis. Reviews on G proteins and G-protein–coupled receptors are available (2–4).

In addition to transmembrane G-protein–coupled receptors, ligand-gated ion channels are another important receptor system in cell membranes. Here, ion channels are coupled to distinct macromolecular protein complexes containing several distinct receptors and binding sites for modulating ions. *N*-Methyl D-aspartate and γ-aminobutyric acid (GABA) receptors are examples of ligand-gated receptors. In each of these cases, a chloride channel is coupled to several receptors within a larger complex; for example, in the GABA receptor complex, distinct receptors for benzodiazepam and alcohol exist as part of a larger macromolecule. G-protein–coupled and ligand-gated receptors of importance to the anesthesiologist have been reviewed (5,6). Although ligand-gated receptor systems are needed to induce the anesthetic state and for some cardiovascular responses, G-protein–coupled receptors mediate most cardiovascular responses and hence are the primary focus of this chapter.

Not all cardiovascular drugs work via transmembrane receptors; compounds such as nitric oxide (NO) produce vascular relaxation via stimulation of guanylyl cyclase in the endothelium and smooth muscle. Many agents previously thought to act directly on arterial smooth muscle actually cause relaxation of smooth muscle via activation of NO. In addition, a separate class of drugs that inhibit enzyme systems are useful as cardiovascular drugs. An example of an enzyme-inhibiting drug important in cardiovascular homeostasis is provided by phosphodiesterase inhibitors, which inhibit breakdown of cyclic nucleotides. Because β-ARs ultimately mediate myocardial inotropy via activation of the enzyme adenylyl cyclase, resulting in increased production of cAMP within the myocardial cell, a Type III phosphodiesterase inhibitor, which inhibits the breakdown of cAMP, will augment this response. Such interactions demonstrate the critical need to understand signal transduction pathways of individual receptors to ultimately understand the mechanism of action of many cardiovascular drugs.

Ligand-receptor Interactions

Ligand (or drug) concentration at a receptor site depends on many factors. Such factors include the first-pass phenomenon (liver metabolism, which can dramatically decrease the final plasma concentration of orally administered drugs), volume of distribution, metabolism (particularly increased metabolism with chronic exposure or decreased metabolism from missing enzymes), elimination (potentially altered in various disease states), and pharmacokinetic parameters. Therefore, pharmacokinetics can be broadly defined as "what the body does to the drug"; in a corollary statement, pharmacodynamics can be defined as "what the drug does to the body." General pharmacokinetic and pharmacodynamic concepts have been reviewed extensively in general anesthesiology textbooks and hence will not be discussed in this chapter. Of note, genetic polymorphisms (single nucleotide changes in genomic DNA that often encode a single amino acid base change in receptors) are increasingly being found to modulate end-organ responsiveness to drugs. This new area is called pharmacogenomics.

Classic receptor theory describes interactions between ligands and receptors. The reader is referred to an excellent book on ligand binding (7) for a more detailed approach to classic ligand-receptor interactions. In transmembrane receptor systems, the ligand is usually a hydrophilic drug, such as a catecholamine. Binding of the catecholamine to the receptor is actually an intermediate event between ligand "floating free" in the extracellular fluid both before and after binding. In classic receptor theory, no drug effect is detected before binding to the receptor, effects are detectable once ligand and receptor are bound, then drug effect terminates as the ligand dissociates from the receptor. Rate of binding of ligand to receptor increases as ligand and receptor concentrations increase. Hence, binding follows the law of mass action. Furthermore, a series of association and dissociation parameters can be established for any ligand and receptor. Association constants are the reciprocal of dissociation constants. Dissociation kinetics for receptor binding can be described using classic models such as the Michaelis-Menten enzyme kinetics. Mathematically, this is expressed as

$$[D] + [R] \rightleftarrows [DR] \qquad [3\text{-}1]$$

where $[D]$ equals concentration of drug, $[R]$ equals concentration of receptor, and $[DR]$ equals concentration of drug-receptor complex. At equilibrium, the dissociation constant (or kd) can be defined mathematically as

$$k_d = \frac{[D][R]}{[DR]} \qquad [3\text{-}2]$$

When 50% of receptors are occupied, the k_d concentration equals the administered dose. A low k_d value indicates that lower drug concentrations are required to occupy 50% of receptors; hence, the drug has a high affinity for the receptor. High k_d values indicate that far higher concentrations of the administered ligand are required to occupy 50% of receptors; hence, the drug has a low affinity for the receptor.

At a molecular level, the binding of agonist (a drug that activates) and receptor was initially interpreted to initiate a change in receptor protein conformation; hence, the change from an inactive (R) to an activated (R^*) state was thought to require ligand binding. More recent experiments using transgenic animals suggest spontaneous conversion from R to R^* occurs instead. In most tissues, the concentration of R^* represents a small fraction of total overall receptor. However, baseline receptor responses are known to differ between tissues, suggesting that the absolute concentration of R^* (and hence spontaneous conversion rates between R and R^*) may be tissue dependent. Therefore, instead of agonists causing conversion from R to R^*, it is now thought that agonists simply stabilize the R^* state. This new way of thinking about receptors has implications in defining antagonists. An antagonist is a drug that prevents agonist binding and therefore prevents receptor activation. A neutral antagonist binds equally to R and R^* and does not affect the equilibrium between R and R^* present in any given tissue. However, a new class of compounds, inverse agonists, binds preferentially to R and stabilizes this configuration; these drugs can be thought of as "superantagonists" that bring the system to a true basal state, or zero receptor activation. The use of inverse agonist drugs may be clinically important in tissues in which higher concentrations of spontaneous R^* exist. Many classic "antagonists" have now been tested and found to be inverse agonists rather than neutral antagonists. For example, "inverse efficacy" of common β-AR antagonists has been determined as follows: timolol $\geq$ propranolol $>$ alprenolol $\geq$ pindolol $>$ labetalol $>$ dichloroisoproterenol. Because inverse agonists may have theoretical advantages in treating certain diseases (such as seizures and congestive heart failure), clinicians should critically evaluate recent pharmacologic data before using an antagonist to distinguish whether the drug is an antagonist or an inverse agonist. For more information on the concept of R and R^*, the reader is directed to a recent review (8).

In clinical medicine, it is often difficult to measure actual ligand-receptor interactions. Fortunately, because agonist occupancy of a receptor by a drug elicits an evoked response (or prevents an evoked response in the case of an antagonist), it is possible to measure a clinical response. However, when contemplating receptor evaluation using clinical responses, it is critical to consider several points. The first is that maximum clinical effects may be produced by an agonist when only a small portion of receptors is occupied. Second, the evoked clinical response may not be linear with regard to the number of receptors occupied. Third, not every drug that binds evokes the maximal clinical response (i.e., some drugs are agonists but less efficacious than others [partial agonists]; by definition, inverse agonists have zero efficacy while antagonists have near-zero efficacy). Therefore a strict correlation between clinical responses and receptor occupancy cannot be attained. This does not make clinical pharmacodynamic data useless. On the contrary, drugs are used primarily for their clinical effects and not for their ability to bind a certain receptor. However, researchers must be cautious in their description of clinical events. For example, a dose-response curve measuring changes in blood pressure with a vasopressor describes vascular or receptor responsiveness and not receptor binding. With these principles and caveats in mind, it is now possible to examine in more detail mechanisms involved in ligand binding to receptors and therefore learn about receptor structure at a molecular level.

Molecular Structure of G-protein–coupled Receptors

Since the advent of molecular biology, discrete segments of DNA (genes) have been discovered that encode many transmembrane G-protein–coupled receptors. This has greatly facilitated the analysis of overall receptor structure and function. Ligand binding can now be thought of in terms of detailed molecular receptor structure-activity relationships, instead of diagrams. In general, G-protein–coupled receptors are proteins consisting of approximately 400 to 450 amino acids. Seven stretches of hydrophobic amino acids orient these transmembrane receptors with an extracellular amino terminus, seven transmembrane stretches, and an intracellular carboxyl terminus (shown in schematic form in Fig. 3-5. Sugar moieties in the amino terminus give rise to the characteristic glycoprotein nature of these receptors.

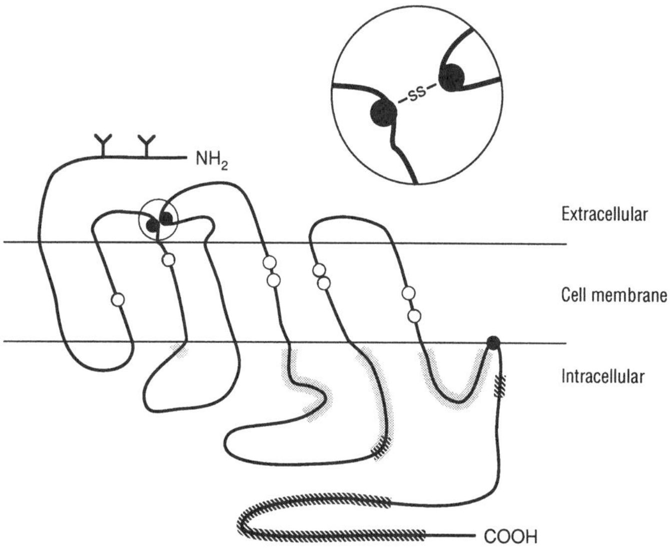

FIGURE 3-5. Schematic drawing representing overall topology of G-protein–coupled receptors. An extracellular amino terminus (*NH_2*), intracellular carboxyl terminus (*COOH*), and seven stretches of hydrophobic amino acids span the cell membrane as shown. Sugar moieties (*Y*) in the amino terminus give rise to the characteristic glycoprotein nature of these receptors. Boxed regions in the large intracellular loop and carboxyl terminus indicate regions of the receptor that when phosphorylated by various enzymes appear to modulate receptor function. Cysteine residues (•) appear to stabilize the receptor via sulfhydryl bonds (—S═S—) into a three-dimensional ligand-binding pocket. Charged groups in hydrophilic ligands are stabilized by counterions in the form of charged side-chain groups of hydrophobic transmembrane amino acids (these are depicted as a • located as they are found in the β-adrenergic receptor).

In terms of ligand binding, one must remember that transmembrane receptors have three-dimensional (3D) structures. Cysteine residues stabilize (via sulfhydryl bonds) a 3D binding pocket in the receptor with access from the extracellular surface. Charged hydrophilic ligands are stabilized by counterions residing in the receptor ligand-binding pocket as charged side-chain groups of hydrophobic transmembrane amino acids. G-protein coupling involves intracellular domains of transmembrane receptors, specifically the third intracellular loop, initial portions of the carboxyl terminus, and possibly the second intracellular loop. Regions in the large third intracellular loop and carboxyl terminus have also been found to be phosphorylated by various enzymes; this phosphorylation appears to modulate (desensitize) receptor function. Experimental evidence documenting the function of each region of transmembrane receptors can be found in reviews describing the β-AR as a model for structure and function properties of G-protein–coupled receptors (9–11).

Adrenergic Receptors

Most currently available drugs used to rapidly modulate the cardiovascular system (heart and vessels) mediate their action via ARs. Although ARs are far from the only receptors of significance in the cardiovascular system, the overwhelming preponderance of currently available drugs for acutely mediating vasoconstriction and increased myocardial inotropy in the perioperative setting are direct or indirect AR agonists. Hence, the ARs are described in some detail before describing the mechanism of action of cardiovascular drugs. As time progresses, more selective AR and non-AR agonists and antagonists will become increasingly valuable, ultimately giving the cardiac anesthesiologist more flexibility in choosing appropriate cardiovascular drugs for a given patient.

ARs were first described and divided into α and β types by Ahlquist in his landmark manuscript in the *American Journal of Physiology* in 1948 (12). By 1967, Lands had subdivided β-ARs into β_1 and β_2 subtypes (13,14), and by the mid-1970s α-ARs had been subdivided into α_1 and α_2 (Fig. 3-6). These four subtypes are referred to in this chapter as the "classic" AR subtypes; properties of most acute AR-mediated cardiovascular drugs are based on these subtypes. ARs mediate physiologic responses in many tissues; however, only their predominant cardiovascular properties are presented in this chapter. To delve further into other properties of AR subtypes (including gluconeogenesis, glycogenolysis, and sedation), the reader is referred to a classic general textbook (15) on ARs. Classically, ARs have the following locations and properties: α_1-ARs are located postsynaptically and mediate vasoconstriction; α_2-ARs, when located presynaptically, inhibit norepinephrine release, and when located postsynaptically, mediate vasoconstriction and venoconstriction; β_1-ARs are located predominantly in the heart and mediate increased myocardial chronotropy and inotropy; and β_2-ARs are located predominantly in the lungs and vessels and mediate bronchodilation and vasodilation, respectively. Evidence suggests that β_2-ARs are clearly located in the human myocardium as well and mediate myocardial inotropy. These properties of AR subtypes conveniently explain most of the clinical cardiovascular actions of AR drugs and are used in the following sections to describe mechanisms of action of various cardiovascular agents. However, most AR agonists and antagonists available today are not very subtype selective. For example, dopamine alone can activate dopamine receptors (of which five have now been cloned) as well as all AR subtypes (depending on the

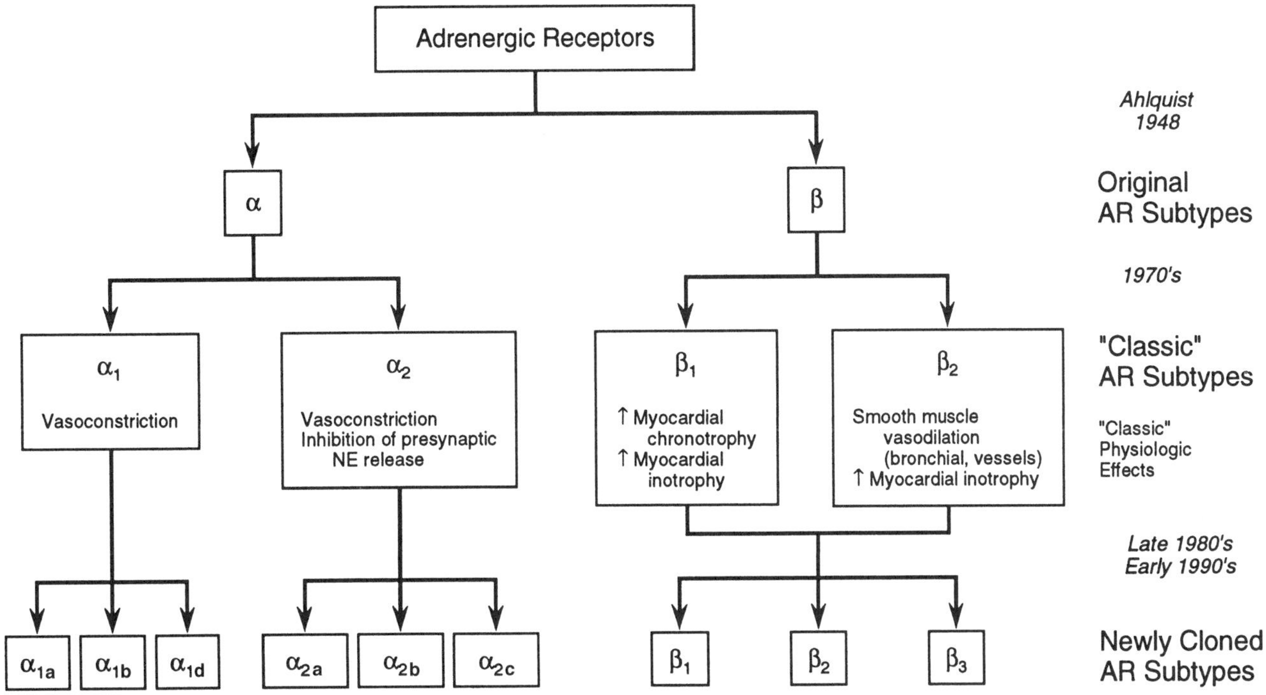

FIGURE 3-6. History of adrenergic receptor subtypes. Individual adrenergic receptor subtypes are listed historically, along with associated cardiovascular responses to activation.

dose used). In addition, there has been an explosion recently in the number of AR subtypes identified and cloned using genetic techniques. By the late 1980s and early 1990s, at least nine AR subtypes (three α_1-ARs: α_{1a}, α_{1b}, and α_{1d}; three α_2-ARs: $\alpha 2_a$, $\alpha 2_b$, and $\alpha 2_c$; and three β-ARs: β_1, β_2, and β_3) had been discovered, described, and complementary DNAs cloned (Fig. 3-6). The ability to express a cloned receptor gene in a cell previously not containing the receptor enables a researcher to study individual receptor subtypes and analyze their signal transduction properties. Because multiple ARs are usually expressed simultaneously in various tissues, the ability to study individual subtypes greatly enhances the understanding of molecular pharmacology of ARs. This should eventually lead to more selective compounds for use in the operating room.

PERIOPERATIVE CHRONIC CARDIAC MEDICATIONS

Cardiovascular drugs take two predominant forms. The first are cardiovascular medications administered chronically (frequently as oral preparations) before surgery, and the second are medications acutely administered (usually as intravenous agents) immediately preoperatively in an acute setting of the coronary care unit, intraoperatively, and/or postoperatively. After a very brief review of myocardial oxygen supply and demand (discussed in more detail in Chapters 2 and 5) in order to facilitate understanding the principles of medical management of ischemic heart disease preoperatively, common classes of chronic preoperative medications will be analyzed for their mechanism of action and potential interactions with anesthetics. The next section deals with acute cardiovascular management.

Ischemia Basics: Myocardial Oxygen Supply and Demand

Understanding the rationale underlying administration of various chronic cardiovascular medications for the treatment of hypertension and/or ischemic heart disease requires a brief review of basics of myocardial oxygen supply and demand. As shown in Fig. 3-7, key determinants of myocardial oxygen demand are increased heart rate, increased afterload (mean arterial blood pressure), increased wall tension (resulting from volume loading of the left ventricle), and increased contractility. Key determinants of myocardial oxygen supply are coronary blood flow (local metabolic effects, autoregulation, and coronary vascular tone), decreased heart rate (to give more time for diastolic coronary perfusion), increased diastolic blood pressure (to give a higher overall coronary perfusion pressure), and the oxygen-carrying capacity of the blood. Because heart rate appears on both sides of the equation, this parameter is clearly important in potentially causing or reducing myocardial ischemia in the presence of flow-restricting lesions of the coronary arteries.

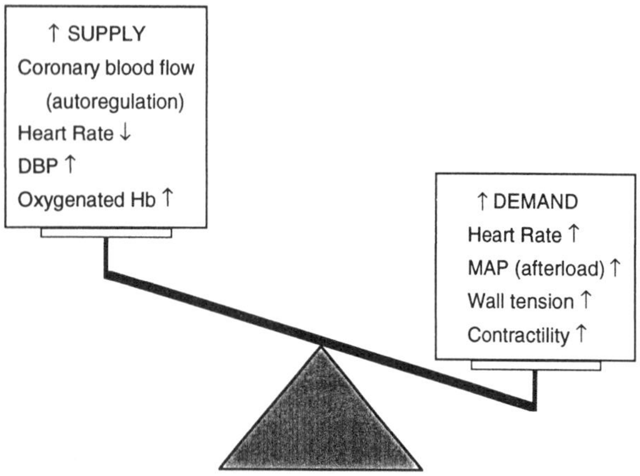

FIGURE 3-7. Myocardial oxygen supply and demand. Key determinants of myocardial oxygen supply and demand are listed. (HR, heart rate; DBP, diastolic blood pressure; Hb, hemoglobin; MAP, mean arterial pressure.)

By increasing heart rate, myocardial oxygen demand increases while supply decreases, potentially mediating myocardial ischemia. However, decreased heart rate generally decreases myocardial oxygen demand and increases coronary perfusion time, hence favoring oxygen supply to the myocardium, particularly the left ventricular subendocardium, which cannot receive coronary blood flow during systole because of compression of intramyocardial coronary vessels. Changing one cardiovascular parameter frequently also changes another parameter (e.g., decreased heart rate also increases time for venous return, potentially increasing ventricular volume and wall tension—a process that may oppose other beneficial effects of decreased heart rate). Hence, understanding complex interactions in the cardiovascular system is necessary for rational therapy of ischemic heart disease. A solid grasp of basic principles of myocardial supply and demand usually enables prediction of the multiplicity of potential responses for a given cardiovascular manipulation, thus facilitating intervention with various drug modalities.

Chronic Medical Therapy for Heart Disease

Many myocardial diseases can be treated chronically. Therefore, when patients with myocardial disease come to the operating room, they are frequently taking several oral medications. Cardiovascular diseases that may require chronic therapy include congestive heart failure, hypertension, and myocardial ischemia. Other concurrent diseases, such as chronic renal failure and diabetes mellitus, often require additional medication. The most common preoperative chronic medications used for cardiovascular diseases include digitalis, diuretics, coronary vasodilators such as nitrates, β-AR antagonists, calcium channel antagonists, and drugs targeting the renin-angiotensin system (angiotensin-converting enzyme [ACE] inhibitors and angiotensin II receptor antagonists). Mechanisms of action for each of these agents are presented below as well as potential interactions (if any) with anesthetic agents. Because many of these drugs can also be given intravenously acutely, some topics presented in this section are also referred to later in the chapter.

Pharmacologic Agents

Digitalis

Digitalis has been in clinical use for more than 200 years. A member of the larger family of cardiac glycosides, digitalis was originally derived from the plant foxglove. It was not until the late 1920s, however, that its positive inotropic effects were first discovered. The potential benefit of digoxin therapy in patients with chronic heart failure results from both an overall increased myocardial inotropic state and resulting decreases in ventricular pressures (16,17). Most recent evidence suggests that positive inotropic effects of digitalis glycosides result from altered excitation-contraction coupling. In humans, calcium enters myocardial cells via slow calcium channels during the plateau phase of the myocardial action potential, a process that triggers the release of intracellular calcium from the sarcoplasmic reticulum and results in activation of contractile proteins. In general, many excitable cell-membrane proteins are responsible for calcium entry into myocardial cells; these include a slow calcium channel, fast calcium channel, nonspecific cation channel, sodium-calcium exchanger, Na-K-ATPase, sodium-hydrogen exchanger, sarcoplasmic-reticulum ATP-dependent calcium pump, and the ryanodine-sensitive sarcoplasmic-reticulum calcium-release channel. Na-K-ATPase activity mediates the active transport of sodium and potassium ions against their respective concentration gradients. Cardiac glycosides bind to the extracellular surface of the α subunit of myocardial Na-K-ATPase and inactivate this enzyme system. Blockade of Na-K-ATPase prevents the pumping of sodium and potassium against their concentration gradients, leading to increased sodium-calcium exchange. The resulting increase in intracellular calcium activates the slow calcium channel and is therefore thought to mediate increased myocardial inotropy. Interestingly, genes encoding four distinct forms of this α subunit vary considerably in their ability to bind digitalis (18), perhaps accounting for some of the variability seen in the effectiveness of digitalis therapy and possibly toxicity. A more detailed account of this mechanism of action of digitalis glycosides can be found in other articles (16,19). In one study, inhibition of Na-K-ATPase by digitalis preparations was shown to have effects on neurotransmitter exocytosis and neuronal catecholamine transport systems in the heart as well (20). One of the most potentially life-threatening side effects of digitalis therapy is arrhythmia. This may seem ironic, because digitalis is classically used to treat atrial fibrillation by slowing ventricular response to rapid atrial rates (see Chapter 4). However, increased intracellular calcium concentrations mediating digitalis-induced increases in inotropy may also lead to arrhythmias. In addition to side effects directly attributable to inhibition of the sodium pump by inhibiting Na-K-ATPase (such as changes in membrane depolarizations, conduction, automaticity, and excitability), delayed afterpotentials and mechanical aftercontractions have been demonstrated with digitalis and may lead to ventricular arrhythmias. Because atrial tissue depends on the entry of the slow inward current of calcium for depolarization, increased digitalis concentrations and associated increases in intracellular calcium may slow depolarization and result in sinus exit block. Atrioventricular (AV) block may also result from accumulation of potassium inside the cell and sodium outside the cell. Bolus infusion of digoxin has been shown to induce epicardial coronary artery vasoconstriction, a process not mediated via activation of coronary α-ARs and easily reversible by nitrate therapy (21). Massive digitalis overdoses may lead to widespread inhibition of Na-K-ATPase, even in noncardiac tissues; this may result in extracellular hyperkalemia, a process that may slow conduction and lead to reentrant arrhythmias. Effects of digitalis on chemoreceptors in the area postrema of the medulla in the central nervous system mediate the anorexia, nausea, and vomiting frequently associated with digitalis toxicity. Poor correlation between clinical symptoms and the presence of toxic digitalis levels makes clinical detection of toxicity difficult. Clearly serum digoxin concentrations should be followed regularly; patients with congestive heart failure receiving digoxin therapy have been shown to have serum concentrations of approximately 1.4 ng/mL (1.8 nmol/L), whereas toxicity is generally present at levels two to three times this amount (17,22). A 50% mortality rate is associated with digoxin concentrations of 6 ng/mL, and serum concentrations of more than 20 ng/mL are usually fatal unless prompt therapy with the specific digoxin antibody (Fab) is administered (see reference 23 for details concerning Fab administration and effectiveness).

In addition to decreases in renal function and overdosing regimens, digoxin serum concentrations are affected by several drugs. Digitalis levels have been reported to be acutely elevated with administration of quinidine at least partly as a result of displacement of digitalis-binding sites in tissues. β-AR antagonists and succinylcholine may increase the likelihood of digitalis-induced arrhythmias; in the case of β-AR antagonists, both β-AR antagonists and digitalis preparations decrease AV conduction, and this property gives rise to potential increases in arrhythmias (despite that β-AR antagonists do not interfere with digitalis inotropic effects). Succinylcholine has the propensity for increasing serum potassium levels acutely, which in turn can increase digitalis arrhythmias. Procainamide, an antiarrhythmic agent that can be used to treat digitalis toxicity, also has the potential in the presence of disturbances of AV conduction to cause asystole or ventricular fibrillation. Because hypercalcemia predisposes to digitalis arrhythmias, acute bolus administration with calcium intraoperatively must be done with caution in patients receiving chronic digitalis therapy. Several agents have the potential for increasing serum levels by decreasing renal clearance of digitalis; they include calcium channel antagonists, spironolactone, amiloride, and triamterene. Both hyperkalemia and hypokalemia may aggravate digitalis toxicity. On the other hand, some drugs are able to enhance the metabolism of digitalis preparations (and hence decrease serum digitalis levels) by increasing hepatic microsomal enzyme activity. These agents include phenylbutazone, phenobarbital, phenytoin, and rifampin. Interestingly, calcium channel–blocking drugs may attenuate the effectiveness of inotropic responses seen with digitalis. However, β-AR antagonists do not abolish the inotropic action of digitalis on heart muscle. Although it is not relevant for acute intraoperative management, one should note that aminoglycoside antibiotics decrease absorption of digitalis oral doses.

In light of potential toxicity associated with digitalis glycosides, it may be surprising that controversy exists regarding the effectiveness of digitalis therapy in patients with congestive heart failure in the absence of atrial arrhythmias (24). Although many measures of myocardial function (both invasive and noninvasive) document increased myocardial inotropy with digitalis therapy even in the absence of atrial arrhythmias, clinical response appears to depend somewhat on the type of congestive failure present. For example, patients with dilated cardiomyopathy, impaired systolic function, and an associated S_3 gallop frequently benefit from digitalis therapy, whereas patients with elevated myocardial filling pressure but relatively preserved systolic function do not (16).

A question is frequently raised regarding administration of digitalis on the morning of surgery. Because digitalis toxicity is related to plasma concentration, the digitalis level should be evaluated preoperatively in patients receiving oral digitalis preparations. The presence or absence of a clinical history of nausea and vomiting should be established because these can be symptoms of digitalis toxicity, even in the face of "normal" therapeutic digitalis serum concentrations. There is probably no harm in administering the patient's usual dose of digitalis on the day of surgery as long as no evidence of toxicity is present. However, if the serum digitalis concentration is elevated, it is prudent to hold the morning dose on the day of surgery. Perhaps instead of worrying whether digitalis glycosides should be given on the day of surgery, one should concentrate on keeping the extracellular (serum) potassium concentration in the normal range perioperatively in patients receiving digitalis, to prevent arrhythmias associated with this drug.

Coronary Vasodilators: Nitrates

Nitrates have been used as therapy for ischemic heart disease since the late 1800s. Sublingual nitroglycerin tablets have been (and remain) the mainstay of medical therapy for acute coronary artery insufficiency, only recently being replaced by sublingual spray nitroglycerin and longer acting preparations, such as nitropaste and nitropatches. Nitroglycerin, the active ingredient in dynamite, was invented by Alfred Nobel, who ultimately endowed the Nobel Prize. Nobel himself had angina in his later life and was required by his physician to take nitroglycerin internally—an irony not lost on him (25). Anesthesiologists have used nitrovasodilators such as nitroglycerin and sodium nitroprusside for more than 20 years. The mechanism of action of these compounds, however, has only recently been described. Increased interest in and understanding of the vital role of the endothelium in vascular processes has lead recently to the description of an endogenous nitrovasodilator, first called endothelium-derived relaxing factor and now known as NO (25–31). Nitroglycerin (and other organic nitrates) penetrate the endothelium, where they act as the substrate for formation of NO. NO then binds to the NO receptor, which is an iron group in the enzyme guanylate cyclase. NO binding to this iron-containing heme group causes a 3D change that results in the production of 3′,5′-cyclic guanosine monophosphate (cGMP) from GTP (25). cGMP then acts as the second messenger responsible for producing relaxation of vascular smooth muscle.

Nitrovasodilators act on different arterial beds, with sodium nitroprusside affecting predominantly systemic vasculature (particularly arteries and arterioles) and nitroglycerin acting on venous capacitance vessels. With increasing doses, these relatively selective effects disappear. Because these effects are clearly demonstrated with acute intravenous administration of sodium nitroprusside and nitroglycerin, this aspect of nitrate therapy is examined in more detail in the acute vasodilator therapy section of this chapter. However, sublingual or topical administration of nitrates for acute anginal episodes is addressed in this section. Beneficial effects of nitroglycerin therapy for acute angina result predominantly from the effects of nitrates on coronary arteries. Specific coronary artery effects of nitrates include dilation of epicardial (conduit) coronary arteries, dilation of coronary collaterals, reversal and prevention of coronary spasm and vasoconstriction, and (perhaps most importantly) dilation of atherosclerotic coronary artery stenosis, including those with eccentric lesions (32,33). Hence, an overall redistribution of myocardial blood flow to areas of ischemia occurs. In addition, acute venodilation may result in decreased venous return, lower ventricular volumes, and therefore lower wall tension; the net result decreases myocardial oxygen consumption. Although decreased ventricular volume may be beneficial, it may also decrease cardiac output (see Starling's law described in the discussion under Intraoperative Acute Cardiac Medications), so nitroglycerin should be administered cautiously. Even sublingual administration of nitrates may occasionally result in syncope secondary to acute venodilation.

Sublingual nitroglycerin is rapidly absorbed from the sublingual mucosa with onset of action within 2 to 5 minutes, maximal effect at 3 to 15 minutes, and little remaining activity after 30 minutes. All nitrate esters produce the same physiologic effects as nitroglycerin, with varying onset and duration depending on the preparation. Nitroglycerin and nitrate esters are rapidly metabolized in the liver by the enzyme glutathione organic nitrate reductase, and metabolites have no residual cardiovascular activity. Longer acting nitrate preparations (and duration of action) include oral nitroglycerin (4 to 6 hours); 2% nitroglycerin ointment (3 to 6 hours); isosorbide dinitrate—sublingual (1.5 to 3 hours), oral (4 to 6 hours), and chewable (2 to 3 hours); and oral pentaerythritol tetranitrate (3 to 5 hours) (34). Although nitrate therapy is usually well tolerated, the most frequent side effects include dizziness, headaches, and postural hypotension. Virtually no interactions occur with preoperative nitrates and anesthetic agents as long as adequate volume status is maintained. Indeed, because tolerance to nitrate therapy is a fairly common phenomenon, abruptly stopping nitrate therapy may result in acute myocardial ischemia. Therefore, nitrate therapy should be continued perioperatively in patients already receiving these medications. Potential side effects of acute administration of nitrates intraoperatively are addressed in more detail in the acute vasodilator therapy section further on.

β-Adrenergic Receptor Antagonists

As stated in the earlier discussion under Adrenergic Receptors, most currently available drugs used to rapidly modulate the cardiovascular system (heart and vessels) mediate their action via ARs. The predominant ARs in human myocardium are β-ARs, both β_1 and β_2 subtypes. β_3-ARs are also present in the heart where they couple to Gi and initiate negative inotropic responses. α_1-ARs also exist in human myocardium and provide increases in inotropy to a much lesser degree. Although β_1-AR agonists are classically thought to mediate increases in inotropy and chronotropy, and β_2-AR agonists to mediate smooth-muscle relaxation (both bronchial and vascular), it is now clear that both β_1-AR and β_2-AR subtypes are important in mediating myocardial inotropic responses and increases in heart rate to both exogenous and endogenous catecholamines and to synthetic catecholamine derivatives. Because increases in both inotropic state and heart rate increase myocardial oxygen demand (a condition not well tolerated in patients with coronary artery disease), β-AR antagonists are frequently used therapeutically to decrease overall myocardial oxygen demand and hence to decrease frequency of angina attacks.

Because β-AR antagonists inhibit responses to endogenous catecholamines, and because many anesthetic agents (particularly the inhalation agents) are known to depress myocardial function, it is theoretically possible to predict that withholding β-AR antagonists preoperatively might provide a more stable course intraoperatively. This hypothesis came to the fore in the early 1970s, and generally anesthesiologists held the morning dose of β-AR antagonists. However, instead of improving intraoperative stability, acutely withholding β-AR antagonists preoperatively was found to increase the incidence of myocardial ischemia and infarction. We now know that chronic administration of β-AR antagonists up-regulates β-ARs. Hence, in the presence of antagonists, β-AR number actually increases. Because the half-life of most β-AR antagonists in the early 1970s was approximately 3 to 6 hours, holding the morning dose in effect resulted in almost no β-AR antagonist concentration during surgery. Because many stimulating events occur during surgery (including intubation, incision, sternotomy, and extubation), the resulting surge in endogenous catecholamines during these stressful events resulted in rapid activation of more than the normal number of myocardial β-ARs. Acute increases in myocardial inotropic state resulted, often precipitating angina and myocardial infarction. This syndrome was recognized many years ago, and it is now routine to continue β-AR antagonists throughout the perioperative period. If β-AR antagonists need to be discontinued, the patient should be monitored closely during gradual tapering of the dose for at least 1 to 2 weeks.

Structurally, β-AR agonists and antagonists are very similar. The basic structure consists of a benzene ring and an ethylamine side chain (34). β-AR antagonists bind to the receptor and prevent its activation. For β-AR agonists and antagonists, the levo stereoisomer has much greater affinity for the receptor and is considered the active form; however, the dextro isomer binds weakly and has all of the usual β-AR antagonist properties. Interestingly, most clinical preparations are mixtures of both isomers. In recent years β_1-AR–selective antagonists have been developed; these include metoprolol, atenolol, esmolol, and acebutolol, bucindolol, carvedilol, and bisoprolol (35). β-AR–cardioselective drugs have particular advantages in patients with reactive airway diseases and diabetes mellitus, because β_2-ARs are present in the bronchi and in the liver, where they mediate glycogenolysis and gluconeogenesis. By using β_1-AR–selective antagonists, acute asthma is less likely to be precipitated, and recovery from insulin-induced hypoglycemia may be more rapid. However, β_1-AR–selective antagonists currently available tend to be only relatively selective, sometimes as little as one order of magnitude. In addition, few β_1-AR–selective antagonists remain selective at higher doses. Hence, extreme caution should be used in administering β-AR antagonists to patients with asthma, even relatively β_1-AR–selective antagonists. Other medical conditions in which β-AR antagonists should be avoided include sinus bradycardia, greater than first-degree conduction block, cardiogenic shock, and overt cardiac failure (although low-dose β-AR antagonists have been used for some forms of congestive heart failure). Treatment with β-AR antagonists may mask the symptoms of hyperthyroidism.

Table 3-1 lists several commonly used β-AR antagonists, their relative β-AR subtype selectivity, and dosing information. A rapid-acting β-AR antagonist with a short half-life, esmolol, is now available intravenously. Hence, rapid titration of β-AR antagonist effects can be performed using a continuous infusion of esmolol intraoperatively. In general, the cardiovascular effects of β-AR antagonists include decreased resting and exercise heart rate, decreased resting and exercise blood pressure, decreased resting and exercise cardiac output, and decreased contractility. The presence or absence of intrinsic sympathetic activity can slightly modify these effects, as can concurrent therapy with an α-AR antagonist. Hence, when β-AR antagonists are administered acutely intravenously or for the first time orally, careful monitoring of blood pressure and cardiac output should occur. Concurrent use of β-AR antagonists and calcium channel antagonists may lead to severe hypotension, although ironically this combination is frequently used in patients with myocardial ischemia and angina. The advantage of using β-AR antagonists is that resulting decreases in heart rate, blood pressure, cardiac output, and contractility in general decrease myocardial oxygen consumption and therefore decrease angina frequency. Noncardiac side effects such as general malaise and impotence occasionally limit the use (or patient compliance) of β-AR antagonist therapy. However, despite these caveats, β-AR antagonists remain one of the major classes of drugs in the armamentarium of the cardiovascular clinician.

One of the most interesting developments in the use of β-AR antagonists is their effectiveness in preventing death. This occurs in the post–myocardial infarction patient and also in patients with congestive heart failure (36,37). Although at first it seems paradoxical that an agent with negative inotropic properties would be given to patients with heart failure, these drugs have been shown to be effective presumably due to changes in β-ARs associated with congestive heart failure. During congestive heart failure, elevated systemic catecholamine levels result in desensitization (or dampening) of β-AR function. Use of low-dose β-AR antagonists prevents desensitization and improves congestive heart failure class. Often initiation of β-AR antagonist therapy requires hospitalization and careful slow titration of drug (36).

Calcium Channel Antagonists

Calcium is a major component in excitation-contraction coupling in both myocardial cells and vascular smooth muscle. Calcium fluxes into these cells (via calcium channels) mediate calcium-induced calcium release from the sarcoplasmic reticulum; this rapidly mobilized calcium from internal stores is critically important for muscle contraction. Contraction is mediated via actin/myosin interactions, facilitated by the troponin calcium complex; in vascular smooth muscle, calmodulin replaces troponin in this important role. Calcium channel antagonists have been used extensively

TABLE 3-1. COMMON β ADRENERGIC RECEPTOR (BETA-AR) ANTAGONISTS

Generic Name	Trade Name	Relative β-AR Subtype Receptor Selectivity	Usual Adult Dose[a,b,c]	Maximum Adult Dose[a,b,c]
Acebutolol[d]	Sectral	β_1-AR	200–800 mg total (PO) (q.d. or b.i.d. dosing)	1200 mg total (PO) (q.d. or b.i.d. dosing)
Atenolol	Tenormin	β_1-AR	50–100 mg q.d. (PO) 5–10 mg (IV)	200 mg q.d. (PO)
Betaxolol	Kerlone		5–30 mg q.d. (PO)	
Bisoprolol	Zebeta (Ziac; in combination with HTCZ)	β_1-AR	2.5–5.0 mg q.d. (PO)	40 mg (PO)
Bucindolol		Nonselective	12.5 q 12 hr (PO) ×3 then titrate upward	100 mg bid (PO)
Cartrolol[f]	Cartrol		2.5–5.0 mg q.d. (PO)	
Carvedilol	Coreg	β_1-AR	3.125 mg b.i.d. (PO) ×2 weeks, then ↑ to 6.25 mg b.i.d as tolerated	25 mg b.i.d. (PO)
Esmolol	Brevibloc	(β_1-AR)	25–200 $\mu g \cdot kg^{-1} \cdot min^{-1}$ (IV)	300 $\mu g \cdot kg^{-1} \cdot min^{-1}$ (IV)
Metoprolol	Lopressor	β_1-AR	100–450 mg q.d. (PO) 5–15 mg (IV)	450 mg q.d. (PO)
Metoprolol	Toprol-XL	β_1-AR	50–200 mg q.d. (PO)	450 mg q.d. (PO)
Nadolol	Corgard	Nonselective	40–80 mg q.d. (PO)	160–320 mg q.d. (PO)
Penbutolol[d]	Levatol		20 mg q.d. (PO)	
Pindolol[d]	Visken	Nonselective	5–30 mg b.i.d. (PO)	60 mg/d total (PO)
Propranolol	Inderal	Nonselective	40–160 mg b.i.d. (PO) 0.5–2 mg (IV)[e]	640 mg/d total (PO) 4–5 mg (IV)[e]
Propranolol LA	(Inderol LA)	Nonselective	80–160 mg q.d. (PO)	
Sotolol	Betapace		120 mg b.i.d. (PO)	160 mg b.i.d. (PO)
Timolol	Blocadren, Timoptic (eye drops)	Nonselective	10–20 mg b.i.d. (PO)	60 mg/d total (PO)
Xamoterol[f]		β_1-AR	0.2–1.5 mg/kg IV for arrhythmias (over 5 min)	

[a] *Note:* This is not a complete list of β-AR drugs. q.d., once daily; b.i.d., twice daily; t.i.d., three times daily; q.i.d., four times daily; PO, oral dose; IV, intravenous dose; (β_1-AR), β_1-AR selective but less so than other β_1-AR selective agents; HCTZ, hydrochlorothiazide; FDA, Food and Drug Administration. Does not reflect doses for patients with renal or hepatic impairment, or other drug-drug interaction that might affect exact dose for a given patient.
[b] Doses should always be checked on individual package inserts before administering drugs.
[c] Titrate carefully to heart rate and cardiac output.
[d] ISA, intrinsic sympathomimetic action (slight β_1-AR stimulation).
[e] Doses for treatment of hypertension and ischemic heart disease only are listed (dose is less for treating essential tremor, hypertrophic subaortic-stenosis, and pheochromocytoma).
[f] Not FDA approved as of 1/2000.

over the years by cardiologists for the treatment of hypertension and ischemic heart disease. In some institutions, calcium antagonists replaced β-AR antagonists and diuretics as first-line drug therapy in the treatment of hypertension and/or angina; however, more recent concern regarding a possible increase in mortality associated with this class of drugs has dampened initial enthusiasm (38,39). Many patients with cardiovascular disease scheduled for surgery, however, will be receiving calcium channel antagonists chronically (40). General properties of calcium channels must be reviewed for a full understanding of this class of drugs.

Three basic types of ion channels exist: receptor operated, ligand gated, and voltage gated. Receptor-operated ion channels are channels distinct from membrane receptors; yet upon activation of the receptor by ligand, the channel is activated (usually via intermediate guanine nucleotide proteins or via second messengers). Ligand-gated channels are larger macromolecules containing the ion channel surrounded by protein structures that contain binding sites for various ligands. Voltage-gated ion channels, however, depend on cell-membrane potential changes to activate opening and closing of these channels. Many types of voltage-operated calcium channels exist. Three general types of voltage-gated calcium channels include the L type (long-lasting inward calcium current), T type (transient inward calcium current), and N type (found in sensory neurons). Calcium channel antagonists act on voltage-sensitive calcium channels by decreasing entry of calcium during phase 2 of the action potential of fast-response cells (slow calcium channels) and during phase 0 of the action potential of slow-response cells in sinuatrial and AV nodes (36). Dihydropyridines (a major class of calcium channel antagonists represented by nifedipine) bind to L-type calcium channels and not to T or N types (41). Although initial animal experiments suggested that T-type calcium channel blockade might be beneficial, there is no evidence this is the case in humans, so the first drug in this class (mibefradil) was recently withdrawn from the market.

L-type calcium channel antagonists can be divided into two general groups: those selective for voltage-operated slow calcium channels and those nonselective for these same channels. Most of the currently available calcium channel antagonists are selective for voltage-operated slow calcium channels; these include phenylalkylamines (verapamil), benzothiazepines (diltiazem), and dihydropyridines (nifedipine, nicardipine, nimodipine, isradipine, and several others not available currently in the United States). Table 3-2 lists several commonly used calcium antagonists, their relative mechanisms of action at the calcium channel, and dosing information. Although both verapamil and diltiazem block voltage-gated slow calcium channels, this is a frequency-dependent block. Dihydropyridines, on the other hand, are able to block voltage-gated slow calcium channels at rest. This may account for some of their differing clinical properties, with diltiazem and verapamil having more negative chronotropic inotropic actions than nifedipine and other dihydropyridines (see further on). Further division of calcium antagonists according to the exact location of their ligand-binding site within the calcium channel has been suggested.

Three general clinical effects are apparent with calcium antagonists. These include effects on ventricular function, myocardial electrophysiology, and vascular smooth muscle (42). Interestingly, the three oldest clinically available calcium antagonists (verapamil, diltiazem, and nifedipine) can be stratified according to their differing effects on these three tissues; they therefore provide good models for understanding the effects of calcium channel antagonists in general. Because reflex responses clearly influence the effect of calcium antagonists in the presence of an intact nervous system, the net response in humans is presented here whenever possible. In general, dihydropyridines such as nifedipine mediate predominantly vascular effects such as peripheral vascular vasodilation (including a spasmolytic effect on cerebral vessels) and pulmonary artery vasodilation with minimal myocardial effects. This selectivity is increasingly apparent with newer dihydropyridine calcium antagonists such as isradipine. Verapamil and diltiazem therapy also results in some vasodilation (diltiazem far less than verapamil), but significantly less than that seen with the dihydropyridines. However, all calcium channel antagonists to date cause coronary artery dilation (in normal and constricted coronary arteries) and have important anticoronary

TABLE 3-2. SELECTED CALCIUM CHANNEL ANTAGONISTS

General Class	Drug Class	Example Drug (Trade Name)	Mechanism of Action at the Calcium Channel[a,b]	Recommended Daily Oral Dose[b]
Group A	Phenylalkylamines	Verapamil (Calan, Isoptin)	Frequency-dependent block of calcium channels[a]	90–360 mg[d]
Group A	Benzothiazepines	Diltiazem (cardizem)	Frequency-dependent block of calcium channels[c]	120–360 mg
Group A	Dihydropyridines			
	Amlodipine	Norvasc		2.5–10 mg
	Felodipine	Plendil SR		2.5–20 mg
	Isradipine	DynaCirc CR		5–20 mg
	Nicardipine	Cardene SR		60–90 mg
	Nifedipine GITS	Procardia XL		30–90 mg
		Adalat CC		
	Nisoldipine	Sular		20–40 mg
Group B	Piperazines	Cinnarizine	Nonselective blockade of slow calcium channels	
		Flunarizine		
		Lidoflazine		
Group B	Other types	Phenylamine	Nonselective blockade of slow calcium channels	
		Perhexiline		
		Bepridil	Bepridil also attaches to smooth-muscle calmodulin	

Note: q.d., once daily; b.i.d., twice daily; t.i.d., three times daily; q.i.d., four times daily; PO, oral dose; IV, intravenous dose; SR, sustained-release formulation; q4h, every 4 hours.
[a] Calcium channel antagonists in Group A are selective for slow calcium channels, while those in Group B are nonselective for slow calcium channels.
[b] Dose for hypertension and ischemic heart disease is given. Doses for other therapies (*i.e.*, arrhythmias) may vary. Doses should always be checked on individual package inserts before administering drug.
[c] Voltage-gated slow calcium channels. *Note:* Calcium channel antagonists may also block postsynaptic $alpha_2$-adrenergic receptors.
[d] Verapamil can also be given intravenously (2–10 mg) for the acute therapy of supraventricular arrhythmias; careful monitoring of blood pressure is required.

artery spasm properties. Verapamil and diltiazem both mediate electrophysiologic effects on the heart by altering the kinetics of slow calcium currents in excitable tissues. Because the myocardial tissues most dependent on slow calcium currents include the sinoatrial and AV nodes, these regions are therefore most affected by calcium channel antagonists. The net result includes modest prolongation of the AH interval in clinical doses, no effect on sinus node recovery time or sinuatrial conduction time in the absence of preexisting sinus node disease (however, verapamil and diltiazem prolong these times in the presence of such disease), and prolongation of refractory periods of the AV node. Hence, verapamil and diltiazem are useful for treating supraventricular arrhythmias. Interestingly, because calcium channel antagonists affect slow calcium channels and not fast calcium channels, their general effects are not readily apparent by monitoring the QRS complex via surface electrocardiography. All three calcium channel antagonists mediate negative inotropic effects, with dihydropyridines having the least and verapamil having the most after intracoronary injection *in vivo.* In healthy and ischemic myocardium, administration of calcium channel antagonists impairs left ventricular relaxation when given via intracoronary injection, yet ironically improves left ventricular relaxation when given intravenously (due to effects of decreased myocardial afterload and sympathetic response). Decreases in cardiac output and myocardial inotropy are still present in spite of this improved ventricular relaxation. Hence, calcium channel antagonists should be used with caution in patients with impaired ventricular function. This potentially negative side effect is highly beneficial in the treatment of ischemic heart disease where decreases in myocardial inotropic state can decrease myocardial oxygen demand and hence relieve ischemia. Potential mechanisms for reduced myocardial oxygen consumption with calcium channel antagonists have been reviewed elsewhere (41,42).

When one considers the mechanism of action of various calcium channel blockers described, many of the side effects of these drugs become readily apparent (41). In general, calcium antagonists are contraindicated in severe left ventricular dysfunction (ejection fraction less than 30%), hypotension (systolic arterial blood pressure less than 90 mm Hg), sick sinus syndrome and second- or third-degree AV conduction block (without concurrent functioning artificial pacemaker in place), and atrial flutter or fibrillation in the presence of an accessory conduction bypass tract. Because dihydropyridines have far fewer negative inotropic effects compared with verapamil and diltiazem, this class of calcium channel antagonists might theoretically be able to be used cautiously in patients with heart failure. Side effects of calcium antagonist drugs include dizziness (frequently from decreased blood pressure), occasional elevation of liver enzymes, first-degree heart block, and transient bradycardia (occasionally progressing to further heart block), prolongation of the PR interval on the electrocardiogram, heart failure, and pulmonary edema. Because calcium channel antagonists are metabolized by the liver, liver failure or decreased hepatic blood flow can aggravate the potential side effects of these drugs.

Many interactions between calcium channel antagonists and other drugs occur. One of the most noteworthy is the interaction with digoxin; calcium channel antagonists increase serum digoxin concentrations probably secondary to reduced renal clearance. Cimetidine increases serum levels of verapamil, diltiazem, and dihydropyridines possibly as a result of effects on liver blood flow. Concurrent use of β-AR antagonists and calcium channel antagonists may lead to severe hypotension. Verapamil may potentially increase serum theophylline levels. Hence, one must consider potential interactions of calcium channel antagonists and other medications given chronically perioperatively or acutely intraoperatively.

Both general anesthetics and calcium channel antagonists are myocardial depressants, potentiate the development of AV block, and produce varying degrees of vasodilation (albeit via different mechanisms)(41); hence, considerable potential for drug interactions exists between these two types of drugs. One obvious potential effect of calcium channel antagonists during anesthesia is exaggerated hypotension, because these agents can theoretically block calcium entry via voltage-sensitive L-type calcium channels in vascular smooth muscle. In fact, this issue has been hotly debated over recent years. Sympathetic α agonists (including endogenous epinephrine and norepinephrine) act at the level of vascular smooth muscle via calcium mobilization and influx (43). In addition, verapamil binds to both α_1-ARs and α_2-ARs, where it acts as an antagonist. Calcium channel antagonists, which are structural analogs of verapamil, such as D600, D591, fendiline, and prenylamine, also bind to α_2-ARs (but not α_1-ARs), whereas other structurally unrelated calcium channel blockers such as diltiazem and nifedipine do not bind to α-ARs (44). However, in more physiologic models using arterial and venous rings, diltiazem and verapamil preferentially inhibit α_2-AR–mediated contraction (45,46). Despite these potential interactions between calcium antagonists and α-ARs at the level of receptor binding and second messengers, very little difference in α-adrenergic responsiveness is seen in patients receiving calcium channel antagonists chronically preoperatively compared with patients not receiving these drugs, either awake or after fentanyl anesthesia (47,48). In fact, it is a general observation that most patients receiving chronic calcium channel antagonist therapy have very stable intraoperative and postoperative courses. This may result from the absence of inhalation anesthetics (narcotic-based and sedative-hypnotic–based anesthetics are commonly used during cardiac surgery), although the addition of an inhalation agent does not seem to perturb this stability. More likely, aggressive fluid therapy prevents most clinical manifestations of vasodilation potentially aggravated with the combination of calcium channel antagonists and anesthetics; even depressed myocardial function (in an otherwise healthy patient with good ventricular function) can be used as an advantage, because decreases in myocardial inotropy also decrease myocardial oxygen consumption, a situation that may alleviate ongoing myocardial ischemia in the presence of fixed coronary lesions. However, caution should be used in administering calcium channel antagonists to patients with poor ventricular function, particularly during anesthesia, due to the potential for additive myocardial depression.

β-AR antagonists may also potentiate the negative inotropic effects of calcium channel antagonists and general anesthetics. However, because β-AR antagonists and calcium channel antagonists are two of the drugs most commonly administered cardiovascular to patients chronically to relieve angina, many patients coming for cardiac surgery are receiving both of these agents. As previously stated, β-AR antagonists should not be discontinued preoperatively because of the risk of precipitating acute myocardial ischemia. The same argument has been used for calcium channel antagonists, because recent studies demonstrate that abrupt withdrawal of calcium channel antagonists in patients with ischemic heart disease is associated with severe myocardial ischemia in 5% to 20% of patients, with an increase in affinity of α_2-AR agonists as a potential mechanism. Hence, most cardiac anesthesiologists continue both β-AR antagonists and calcium channel antagonists throughout the perioperative period. Clearly, individual evaluation of each patient in this situation is essential.

Renin-Angiotensin-Aldosterone System Drugs

In addition to β-AR antagonists, calcium channel antagonists, and diuretics, ACE inhibitors have emerged as valuable therapeutic modalities in the treatment of hypertension and congestive heart failure. The renin-angiotensin system is an important pathway in the maintenance of blood pressure via the pressor hormone angiotensin II (49,50). Briefly, the renin-angiotensin pathway begins in the liver, where the precursor substrate angiotensinogen is generated. Angiotensinogen is then cleaved by renin (secreted from the juxtaglomerulus apparatus in the kidney in response to decreased arterial blood pressure or decreases in sodium delivery to the macula densa) to form angiotensin I, a relatively physiologically inert substance. However, when angiotensin I passes through the lungs, the last two amino acids are cleaved from the peptide by the enzyme dipeptidyl carboxypeptidase (or ACE) to form the eight–amino acid active compound angiotensin II. ACE also inactivates circulating bradykinin, a potent endogenous circulating vasodilator agent (49). Hence both activation of a pressor hormone and inhibition of a dilator hormone are accomplished almost simultaneously. A final amino acid is cleaved from angiotensin II by the enzyme aminopeptidase to form angiotensin III, a compound that acts predominantly on the adrenal cortex. The feedback loop is completed when angiotensin II itself acts on the adrenal cortex to stimulate the release of aldosterone, a compound that then acts on the kidney to expand volume, retain sodium, and suppress further renin release from the juxtaglomerulus apparatus.

Although classically the renin-angiotensin system has involved many organs (as described), more recently all components of the system have been found in locations such as vascular smooth muscle, myocardium, brain, uterus, and salivary gland (49,51). These "local systems" may have a role in mediating specific local physiologic responses, a process that when more completely understood may prove highly significant.

Angiotensin II acts at several sites, the most important of which is arteriolar smooth muscle, where it stimulates contraction, a process that ultimately results in increased systemic vascular resistance (SVR) and increased blood pressure. Interestingly, angiotensin II has little effect on veins in physiologic doses; however, at higher concentrations (e.g., during disease states or exogenous drug administration), this hormone may cause venoconstriction. Other organs affected by angiotensin II include the heart (increases contractility and heart rate presumably via direct stimulation of angiotensin II sites and has a possible role in myocyte growth in hypertrophy), adrenal cortex (stimulates release of aldosterone), adrenal medulla (stimulates release of catecholamines), brain (stimulates adrenergic pathways in the brain responsible for control of blood pressure), kidney (interacts with prostaglandins in interstitium, increases glomerular hydraulic pressure, and aids in sodium reabsorption), and several other organs to a lesser extent (liver, spleen, and salivary glands) (49,51,52).

Angiotensin-Converting Enzyme Inhibitors. ACE inhibitors include captopril, enalapril, lisinopril, pentopril, ramipril, alacepril, and quinapril (Table 3-3) (53–55). From the effects of angiotensin II on various organs, the response to ACE inhibitors can be predicted. Specifically, decreases in blood pressure (secondary to decreased SVR), blunted cardiac responses (and sympathetic responses in general) to decreased blood pressure (no heart rate, cardiac output, or myocardial contractility changes—except for lisinopril, which slightly decreases cardiac output), and some venodilation (53). These are all valuable in the treatment of heart failure by decreasing afterload and preload while having minimal cardiac effects per se. In fact, in the patient with congestive heart failure, cardiac output increases secondary to vasodilation (decreased afterload) provided by ACE inhibitors. However, acute decreases in blood pressure may decrease effective circulating blood volume and result in renal hypoperfusion; ACE inhibitor therapy has been associated with acute renal failure, particularly in patients with underlying renal disease. Therefore, careful attention to fluid status should occur when ACE inhibitors are administered. However, some beneficial renal responses are seen when ACE inhibitors are used for the therapy of essential

TABLE 3-3. RENIN-ANGIOTENSIN SYSTEM DRUGS

Drug	Trade Name	Recommended Total Oral Daily Dose Range[a]	Dose Frequency[b]
A. SELECTED ANGIOTENSIN-CONVERTING ENZYME (ACE) INHIBITORS			
Alacepril	—	50 mg	q.d.
Benazepril	Lotensin	5–20 mg	q.d.-b.i.d.
Captopril	Capoten	12.5–150 mg	b.i.d.-t.i.d.
Enalapril	Vasotec	2.5–20 mg	q.d.-b.i.d.
Fosinopril	Monopril	5–20 mg	q.d.-b.i.d.
Lisinopril	Zestril Prinivil	5–20 mg	q.d.
Moexipril	Univasc	7.5–15 mg	q.d.-b.i.d.
Perindopril	Aceon	4 mg	q.d.
Quinapril	Accupril	5–20 mg	q.d.-b.i.d.
Ramipril	Altace	1.25–10 mg	q.d.-b.i.d.
Trandolapril	Mavik	1–4 mg	q.d.
B. SELECTED ANGIOTENSIN II RECEPTOR (TYPE AT_1) ANTAGONISTS			
Candesartan	Atacand	16–32 mg	q.d.
Eprosartan	Teveten	600 mg	q.d.
Irbesartan	Avapro	150–300 mg	q.d.
Losartan	Cozaar	50–100 mg	q.d.
Telmisartan	Micardis	40–80 mg	q.d.
Valsartan	Diovan	80–320	q.d.

[a] Doses should always be checked on individual package inserts before administering drug. ACE inhibitor doses should be decreased in the presence of renal impairment.
[b] q.d., once daily; b.i.d., twice daily; t.i.d., three times daily.
Source: Adapted from Siragy H. Angiotensin II receptor blockers: review of the binding characteristics. *Am J Cardiol* 1999;84:3S.

hypertension, including reduction of renal vascular resistance, enhancement of renal blood flow, enhancement of glomerular filtration rate, acute natriuresis, increased free-water clearance, spared potassium loss, and decreased urinary protein excretion (54). Further examination reveals that afferent and efferent glomerular arterioles are dilated by ACE inhibitors. Therefore, the gradient of pressure from afferent to efferent arterioles required to actually increase long-term glomerular filtration rate does not exist, effectively preventing glomerular hyperfiltration. If glomerular hyperfiltration continues chronically, it can theoretically lead to glomerular sclerosis; therefore, this action on the kidney may one day result in the expansion of the use of ACE inhibitors from hypertension and congestive heart failure (the current indication) to diabetes for the treatment of diabetic renal disease or other conditions in which glomerular hyperfiltration is a problem (51,55). However, ACE inhibitors may also inhibit the ability to increase glomerular filtration rates in response to acute volume overload. This may be significant in the perioperative period, as acute changes in circulating blood volume intraoperatively are frequently compensated for by effective diuresis over the ensuing days and weeks. Theoretically, the inability to effectively increase glomerular filtration rate in the presence of ACE inhibitors may decrease the ability of the kidney to respond as rapidly to acute volume loads presented in the perioperative period; fluid overload may therefore be a potential problem postoperatively.

Side effects of ACE inhibitor therapy include proteinuria (secondary to membranous glomerulopathy presumably from the sulfhydryl group on the captopril molecule, in patients with underlying renal disease only), neutropenia (occurs most frequently in patients with complicated hypertension), and to a lesser extent rash, varying degrees of taste loss, angioedema, and cough (51,52). Overall, ACE inhibitors are very well tolerated over time (although patients should be followed after starting these drugs, for proteinuria and neutropenia), but they should not be given to patients with bilateral renal disease or only one kidney. In these renal disease conditions, normal autoregulatory mechanisms are not present and severe renal failure and/or malignant hypertension may result from the initiation of ACE inhibitor therapy (49).

Angiotensin II Type 1 Receptor Antagonists. In addition to ACE inhibitors, several direct angiotensin II receptor antagonists, including candesartan cilexetil, irbesartan, losartan, telmisartan, and valsartan are currently approved by the Food and Drug Administration (FDA) for the treatment of hypertension. All antagonize the angiotensin II type 1 (AT1) receptor and therefore block a number of angiotensin II effects—vasoconstriction, renal sodium reabsorption, aldosterone and vasopressin secretion, sympathetic activation, and vascular/cardiac hyperplasia and hypertrophy. Such blockade is effective whether angiotensin II is produced systemically in the circulation or locally via ACE or non-

ACE–dependent pathways in tissues. Also blockade of angiotensin II–induced feedback regulation of renin release occurs, resulting in increased angiotensin II levels. With the AT1 receptor blocked, angiotensin II is therefore able to activate the angtiotensin type 2 (AT2) receptor with beneficial effects in the cardiovascular system such as vasodilation, antiproliferative actions, and apoptosis (50,56,57).

The renin-angiotensin system is activated during anesthesia and surgery as part of the "stress response" to noxious stimuli (intubation, surgical incision, cardiopulmonary bypass). Other hormones involved in the stress response include catecholamines, antidiuretic hormone, cortisol, endorphins, glucagon, growth hormone, glucose, lactate, and pyruvate (52). Administration of sodium nitroprusside to induce hypotension activates the renin-angiotensin system (two-fold increases in renin activity as well as catecholamine levels) in a manner similar to that seen during anesthesia and surgery, suggesting that hypotensive episodes may provide a stimulus for renin release (52). Acute renin release can thus be viewed as a protective mechanism for the maintenance of blood volume during hypotension. However, activation of renin secretion secondary to other stimuli (e.g., incision) may provide examples of exaggerated responses that may not be protective and may be potentially harmful because acute increases in afterload and blood volume may place additional burdens on patients with impaired myocardial function. Increases of both renin and angiotensin II levels during cardiopulmonary bypass occur, and they persist for up to 24 hours; an association of this response and the potential for postoperative hypertension in the cardiac surgery patient has been suggested but not clearly demonstrated. In aortic surgery, cross-clamping of the aorta is a potent stimulus to renin release. Decreased renal perfusion occurs with elevated renin release; therefore, an association of acute elevations of renin and the incidence of renal failure during aortic surgery has been hotly debated.

The use of ACE inhibitors during anesthesia and surgery has been controversial. As with most cardiovascular drugs, most anesthesiologists continue preoperative chronic medications up to the time of surgery and reinstitute therapy as soon as possible after surgery to promote hemodynamic stability and myocardial performance (particularly in the face of myocardial ischemia or congestive heart failure). This is the general trend with ACE inhibitors. However, over the years, some reports in the literature have suggested that ACE inhibitors given preoperatively do not enhance hemodynamic stability during the intraoperative period. These reports have generally involved healthy patients in whom hypotension occurred more frequently and was more prolonged after induction; one study reported an association with preoperative ACE inhibitors and decreases in cerebral blood flow compared with patients who received either a β-AR antagonist or a placebo (55). Hypotension in the intraoperative period in patients receiving ACE inhibitors may be associated with blunting of sympathetic responses seen with ACE inhibitors in general. Although this effect is advantageous in patients with cardiac disease, blunting of sympathetic responses in otherwise healthy patients could interfere with the normally vigorous sympathetic response to anesthetic induction, intubation, and surgical stimulation. However, in these same patients, careful attention to volume status can prevent many potential hypotensive episodes. Because blunting of the sympathetic response with other agents (e.g., narcotics such as fentanyl) has been found to be advantageous for a smooth anesthetic course (despite that "sympatholysis" is controversial in anesthesia in general), ACE inhibitors are still routinely given preoperatively in patients receiving these drugs chronically. Interestingly, a few early reports suggest that ACE inhibitors may have renal protective effects in the setting of nonpulsatile cold cardiopulmonary bypass. However, because of the general association of ACE inhibitors and renal failure in patients with underlying renal disease, it may be prudent to discontinue ACE inhibitors in patients in whom the surgical procedure could incur renal injury (e.g., in abdominal aortic aneurysm surgery).

Aldosterone Antagonists. It is important to note that neither ACE inhibitors nor angiotensin II receptor antagonists effectively block aldosterone production. Because the entire renin-angiotensin-aldosterone system is elevated with heart failure and some forms of hypertension, blockade of this part of the system is also important. Spironolactone, a diuretic with aldosterone-blocking properties (see Diuretics for its action as a diuretic) has recently been shown to decrease mortality by 30% in patients with severe heart failure (58). For years physicians assumed that treatment with an aldosterone-blocking agent in conjunction with an ACE inhibitor was relatively contraindicated because of the potential for serious hyperkalemia. However, treatment with the aldosterone-receptor blocker spironolactone at a daily dose of 12.5 to 25 mg in conjunction with standard doses of an ACE inhibitor, a loop diuretic, and in many cases digoxin is pharmacologically effective and well tolerated, leads to decreased atrial natriuretic peptide (ANP) levels, and does not result in serious hyperkalemia (58). Hence, it can be expected that more patients with heart failure will be receiving spironolactone therapy when they come for surgery.

Diuretics

Diuretics enhance urine flow. In 1958 chlorothiazide became the first orally effective diuretic and represented one of the first synthetic drugs to be used in clinical medicine. Since then, several classes of diuretics with varying chemical structures and mechanisms of action have been discovered and utilized clinically. To understand the mechanism of action of each class of diuretics, a brief review of renal anatomy and physiology is necessary.

The kidney is a vital organ that maintains extracellular

fluid homeostasis by regulating sodium reabsorption (and accompanying water) as urine passes along the nephron. Blood supplied by the renal arteries is filtered by glomeruli to form urine (blood minus high-molecular-weight proteins and blood cells), which then passes through various portions of the nephron (first the proximal tubule, followed by descending and thick ascending loop of Henle, distal convoluted tubule, and finally the collecting tubule). Specialized polarized epithelial cells lining the nephron are equipped with specific ion transporters on the luminal (urine-side) and basolateral (blood-side) membranes. Each region of the nephron exhibits different mechanisms for salt and water reabsorption. A brief synopsis of each of these is presented to facilitate an understanding of the site (and mechanism) of action of classes of diuretics, thereby promoting rational selection and use of more than one diuretic when indicated. Diuretics must be present in the urine to act; hence, diseases of the kidney that impair glomerular filtration frequently make diuretics less effective because access to their site of action may be impaired. More detailed references regarding the mechanism of diuretic action are cited in the References(59,60) and summarized in Table 3-4.

The proximal tubule reabsorbs 60% to 70% of filtered sodium and water. Sodium is cotransported into the proximal tubule cell with substances such as glucose, amino acids, and phosphate. The basolateral membrane maintains a low urine-to-proximal tubule cell sodium balance by pumping sodium ions out of the cell and into the blood via an Na-K-ATPase. Bicarbonate also has a major role in this process, because it is transported across the basolateral membrane with three sodium molecules. Water in the proximal tubule cell is broken down by carbonic anhydrase to form hydrogen and hydroxide; this hydroxide molecule then combines with carbon dioxide (present from the breakdown of carbonic acid in the urine, then crossing the membrane into the proximal tubule cell) to form the bicarbonate, which is cotransported from the cell across the basolateral membrane with three sodium molecules. As part of the bicarbonate system, hydrogen is also transported from the cell to the urine lumen via sodium-hydrogen proton exchange. The net removal of sodium bicarbonate and water generates a concentration gradient favoring chloride reabsorption, which in turn generates a lumen-positive potential favoring sodium reabsorption (59). Carbonic anhydrase inhibitors (e.g., acetazol-

TABLE 3-4. SITES AND MECHANISMS OF ACTION OF VARIOUS DIURETICS

Class of Diuretic	Example	Site of Action in Nephron	Mechanism(s) of Action
Carbonic anhydrase inhibitors	Acetazolamide	Proximal tubule	Blocks movement of sodium into the proximal tubule
		Collecting tubule	
Osmotic agents	Mannitol	Glomerulus	Has osmotic effect
Xanthines	Aminophylline	Glomerulus	Increases vascular perfusion of glomerulus
		Proximal tubule (minor)	Unknown mechanism
m-Sulfamoylbenzoic acids	Furosemide	Thick ascending loop of Henle	Binds to and inhibits Na^+-K^+-$2Cl^-$ cotransporter; furosemide at very high concentrations may inhibit the basolateral K^+-Cl^- cotransporter
	Bumetanide Piretanide		
Phenoxyacetic acids (mercurial)	Merbaphen	Thick ascending loop of Henle	Binds to and inhibits Na^+-K^+-$2Cl^-$ cotransporter
Phenoxyacetic acids (nonmercurial)	Ethacrynic acid (l-cysteine form) (−) Indacrinone		Ethacrynic acid may inhibit the basolateral K^+-Cl^- cotransporter
Aminopyrazolinones	Muzolimine	Thick ascending loop of Henle	Inhibits K^+-Cl^- cotransporter
Pyrazine carboxamides	Amiloride	Proximal tubule	Blocks sodium-proton exchange at supraclinical concentrations
		Collecting tubule	
			Inhibits luminal sodium channel
Chloride channel blockers		Thick ascending loop of Henle	Inhibits basolateral chloride channels
Benzothiazides	Thiazides	Proximal tubule	Has saluretic effects, poorly characterized
	Hydrothiazides	Distal convoluted tubule	Inhibits Na^+-Cl^- cotransporter
	Metolazone	Distal convoluted tubule	Inhibits Na^+-Cl^- cotransporter
Pteridine	Triamterene	Collecting tubule	Inhibits luminal sodium channel
Spirolactones	Spironolactone	Collecting tubule	Inhibits aldosterone receptor

amide) block the movement of sodium into proximal tubule cells and indirectly inhibit sodium-proton exchange. This results in an elevated proximal cell pH level, a lowered urine luminal pH level, and increased delivery of sodium and bicarbonate to more distal segments of the nephron. Amiloride blocks sodium-proton exchange in the proximal tubule but at supraclinical levels. Osmotic agents such as mannitol also act at the proximal tubule. Although the diuretic effects of xanthines (e.g., coffee and tea) appear to result from an increase in vascular perfusion of the glomerulus, they may also have some effect in the proximal tubule. Finally, the saluretic effects of thiazides may be due to a poorly characterized effect on the proximal tubule.

The next major site of solute and water reabsorption along the nephron is the thick ascending limb of the loop of Henle. Here, Na^+-K^+-$2Cl^-$ cotransport occurs on the luminal surface of the cell, by energy derived from Na-K-ATPase on the basolateral surface of the cell. This results in a higher than equilibrium concentration of potassium and chloride in the cell, thus facilitating potassium and chloride exodus via a basolateral cotransporter. Potassium also leaves the cell on the luminal surface, and chloride on the basolateral surface, resulting in a transepithelial positive potential, which ultimately facilitates paracellular sodium reabsorption. Hence, sodium is reabsorbed in the ascending limb of the loop of Henle by cotransport and via paracellular mechanisms. Many diuretics act in this region of the nephron. m-Sulfamoylbenzoic acids (furosemide, bumetanide, and piretanide) and phenoxyacetic acids (both mercurial [merbaphen] and nonmercurial [ethacrynic acid Bl-cysteine form N and B-N indacrinone]) bind to and inhibit the Na^+-K^+-$2Cl^-$ cotransporter, specifically at the chloride site. The result is increased delivery of sodium out of the thick ascending limb and a decrease in the medullary interstitial osmotic gradient; this has the ultimate effect of interfering with both the diluting and concentrating mechanisms of the kidney. Aminopyrazolinones (muzolimine), ethacrynic acid, and furosemide (at very high concentrations) may also act in the thick ascending loop of Henle by inhibiting the basolateral K^+-Cl^- cotransporter, which ultimately inhibits the Na^+-K^+-$2Cl^-$ cotransporter secondary to high intracellular concentrations of potassium and chloride. In addition, chloride channel blockers may act as diuretics by inhibiting chloride flux across the basolateral membrane.

In the distal convoluted tubule, sodium and chloride are reabsorbed via a neutral luminal sodium chloride cotransporter. Na-K-ATPase activity, potassium and chloride fluxes occur at the basolateral membrane. Two predominant diuretics act at the distal convoluted tubule: thiazides and metolazone. Each inhibits sodium chloride reabsorption by binding to and inhibiting the sodium-chloride cotransporter on the luminal surface. The net result is increased sodium-chloride excretion and impaired ability to dilute urine.

The final site of diuretic action in the nephron is the collecting tubule. Here, a luminal sodium channel in principal cells (i.e., the predominant cell type in the collecting tubule) provides entry of sodium while an Na-K-ATPase on the basolateral membrane provides an exit for sodium. In addition, potassium fluxes exist across both luminal and basolateral membranes. Pteridines (triamterene) and pyrazine carboxamides (amiloride) appear to block the sodium channel on the luminal surface competitively. In addition, aldosterone stimulates potassium secretion, sodium reabsorption, and proton secretion in the collecting duct via an intracellular aldosterone receptor, an effect that is blocked by spirolactones (spironolactone). The net result of each of these diuretics is a decreased transepithelial potential difference in the collecting tubule, which decreases potassium excretion. The other type of cell in the collecting tubule, the intercalated cell, pumps protons from the cell to the lumen via a proton-translocating ATPase as part of a process catalyzed by carbonic anhydrase. In this cell, bicarbonate is exchanged for chloride at the basolateral membrane, resulting in a chloride flux across the basolateral membrane. Because of these pathways, carbonic anhydrase inhibitors have some effects in the collecting tubule in addition to their predominant effects in the proximal tubule.

Because so many patients receive chronic diuretic therapy, it is necessary to understand each drug's mechanism and site of action. It is thereby possible to tailor therapy to increase urine flow if needed. Clearly, combinations of diuretics that act at different sites increase the probability of an effective response. Although diuretics are known to interact with several drugs, such as nonsteroidal antiinflammatory drugs (inhibition of prostaglandin synthesis may blunt the effects of loop diuretics), lithium (sodium depletion from diuretics may enhance proximal reabsorption of lithium potentially leading to toxic levels), and endogenous lipids (long-term therapy with thiazide diuretics may increase total cholesterol and low-density and very low-density lipoproteins), there are few if any known interactions between diuretics and anesthetic agents. Acute treatment of cardiac failure and pulmonary edema can be enhanced using diuretics as part of treatment strategies. Chronic therapy with diuretics may lead to a depletion of potassium, which could become significant in relation to arrhythmias during treatment of ischemic heart disease, particularly in patients receiving digitalis (see the preceding discussion). In addition, chronic therapy with diuretics may lead to decreased effective blood volume, a situation that may be unmasked only after anesthesia induction. Hence, careful regard for fluid status and potassium level is required whenever a patient has been on diuretics preoperatively.

Summary of Chronic Cardiovascular Drug Interactions with Anesthetic Agents

Digitalis, nitrates, β-AR antagonists, calcium channel antagonists, ACE inhibitors, and diuretics represent the six most common drugs administered chronically to patients with myocardial disease. Each has been described in detail, including potential interactions with anesthetic agents and other drugs used in the perioperative period. This section simply serves to coalesce a few major points regarding the effects of these drugs on perioperative management. Although few serious interactions are thought to occur with nitrates, β-AR antagonists, and diuretics, fluid status must be carefully monitored with these agents. Side effects such as hypotension from venodilation or low effective circulating volume can be avoided, and myocardial function can be optimized (particularly with β-AR antagonists) in this manner. In addition, the potential for hypotension in patients receiving ACE inhibitors and calcium channel antagonists has been described in detail. As with nitrates, β-AR antagonists, and diuretics, careful attention to fluid status and optimization of myocardial preload is essential. The remaining drug, digitalis, has a potential for causing arrhythmias during the perioperative period. As mentioned in the discussion of digitalis, rapid changes in serum potassium concentration may lead to arrhythmias in the drug's presence. Therefore it is necessary to keep careful control of serum potassium concentration during anesthesia and surgery in patients receiving chronic digitalis preparations. In general, careful monitoring and management of patients receiving chronic cardiovascular medications are essential so that the beneficial effects of these drugs (prevention of myocardial ischemia and hypertension as well as increases in myocardial inotropy) may be preserved while potential side effects are prevented. Careful titration of clinical effects in patients receiving such agents is a large part of the "art" of cardiac anesthesiology.

INTRAOPERATIVE ACUTE CARDIAC MEDICATIONS

The cardiovascular anesthesiologist is an expert in anesthetizing critically ill patients with cardiovascular disease. This includes administering vasoactive drugs, manipulating SVR and myocardial inotropy, and managing acute side effects of pharmacologic agents. Although part of this regimen may include management of cardiopulmonary bypass, intraaortic balloon counterpulsation and ventricular assist devices, and severe valvular heart disease physiology, these topics are addressed in other chapters (Chapters 14, 15, and 20). Here, we concentrate on medications available to the cardiac anesthesiologist for acute administration in the operating room. Rational use of these drugs requires not only a firm grasp of concepts of myocardial oxygen supply and demand (see brief review in discussion under Perioperative Chronic Cardiac Medications and in Chapter 2) but also a thorough understanding of Starling's law, venous return, myocardial inotropy, heart rate, and SVR. Hence each of these areas is reviewed briefly before a detailed analysis of each clinically available acute cardiovascular drug potentially used during cardiothoracic surgery. A more detailed presentation of cardiac physiology is presented in Chapter 2.

Cardiac Physiology Important in Drug Therapy

Starling's Law

The heart is essentially a pumping muscle. Information learned from skeletal muscle physiologists in the early part of the 20th century was important in ultimately understanding the mechanism of action of myocardial muscle pumping. Hill (61) provided evidence that the velocity of shortening of skeletal muscle is inversely related to the magnitude of tension development (or stretch) of the muscle. Hence, when skeletal muscle is stretched more tonically (usually by attaching weights passively), the resulting shortening occurs more slowly, once the muscle is stimulated. By altering the tonic stretch and then stimulating skeletal muscle, force-velocity curves could be established. More recently, this concept has been extended to myocardial muscle. Although skeletal muscle contractile activity can be enhanced by recruitment of additional muscle fibers, the number of cardiac cells that are activated remains fixed for each contraction. Myocardial contractility can therefore be altered by changes in either resting fiber length or intrinsic inotropic state. Unlike skeletal muscle, however, increasing stretch (or preload) does not change the velocity of shortening of myocardium, although it does alter the overall force developed. In other words, the more cardiac muscle is stretched, the more force can be generated without a change in velocity of force. This relationship is frequently called the Frank-Starling relationship, or Starling's law.

Figure 3-8 demonstrates Starling's law of the heart in clinical terms. Stretch of myocardial ventricular muscle is related to ventricular wall tension, which is related closely to ventricular volume, or filling. (Left ventricular filling is frequently highlighted, because the left ventricle provides the work of pumping blood systemically. This convention does not mean that right ventricular pumping to the lungs is not important, rather that alterations in left ventricular function [including failure] are far more frequent. All of the following statements apply with equal validity to the right ventricle.) Left ventricular filling can be thought of in terms of absolute volume (i.e., left ventricular end-diastolic volume), or in more easily measurable terms as left ventricular end-diastolic pressure, pulmonary artery occlusion pressure (PAOP), or central venous pressure (CVP). Each measurement provides an indication of left ventricular filling (in the absence of lung disease), and PAOP and CVP can be measured using a pulmonary artery catheter or central venous catheter. Myocardial ventricular muscle shortening results in forward flow of blood. This forward flow is frequently designated "left ventricular output" and can be described in terms of left ventricular stroke volume or cardiac

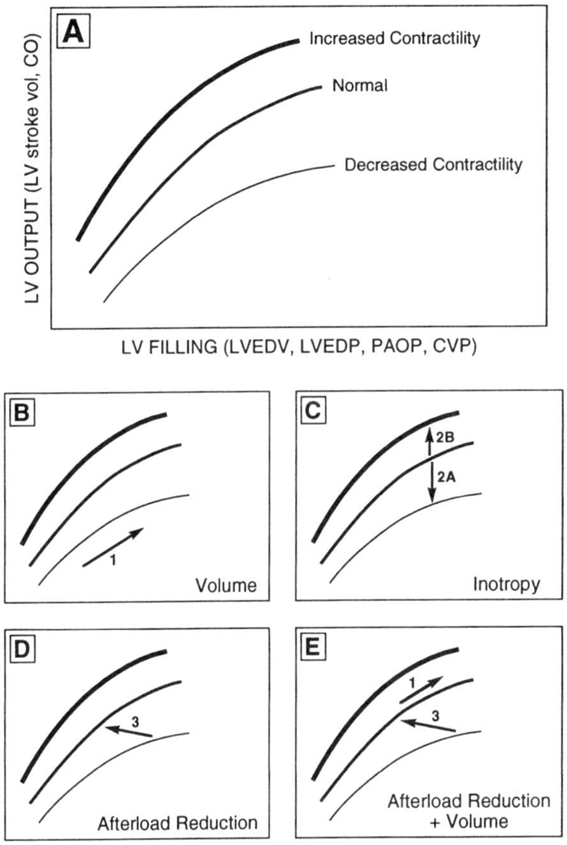

FIGURE 3-8. Starling's law of the heart. When more cardiac muscle is stretched, more force is able to be generated without a change in velocity of force. Stretch of myocardial ventricular muscle is related to ventricular wall tension, which is related closely to ventricular volume, or filling. Hence the x axis is labeled left ventricular filling. Left ventricular end-diastolic volume (*LVEDV*) or more indirect pressure measurements such as left ventricular end-diastolic pressure (*LVEDP*), pulmonary artery occlusion pressure (*PAOP*), or central venous pressure (*CVP*) could also be used on the x-axis as markers for ventricular filling. Left ventricular output is shown on the y-axis; other measures of this phenomenon include left ventricular stroke volume and cardiac output (*CO*). Normal, failing (decreased contractility curve), and stimulated (increased contractility) myocardium all have different Starling curves. **A:** These concepts are shown in general schematic form. **B–E:** The effects of various manipulations (volume, increases, and decreases in inotropy, afterload reduction, and combined afterload reduction with volume, respectively) are demonstrated on location on each of these Starling curves.

output. As can be seen in Fig. 3-8A, the more left ventricular filling occurs, the more left ventricular output increases (to the point at which myocardial muscle begins to become overstretched and mechanical damage occurs). In an increased inotropic state or with contractility (as is frequently seen during exercise or during an episode of fear), a new Starling curve occurs, which roughly parallels the original (normal) curve but is shifted upward and to the left. Hence, in the presence of increases in contractility, more forward blood flow is possible at a lower ventricular filling volume. In heart failure, the opposite situation occurs. Myocardial pump failure frequently results from intrinsic decreases in contractility, and in this case, the Starling curve is shifted downward and to the right. This means that higher filling volumes are required to achieve the same cardiac output compared with a nonfailing heart. Starling's law is extremely significant in the perioperative period in patients with cardiovascular disease, because manipulation of ventricular volume is frequently possible (Fig. 3-8B). However, one should never overfill the heart, because overdistention of the myocardium can rapidly result in mechanical injury to myofibrils, potentially leading to further heart failure.

Venous Return

Venous return can be described simply as blood return to the heart. The cardiovascular system consists of the heart and vessels; therefore, the vasculature has a major function in determining the amount of blood in the heart at any given time. Because ventricular volume is critical in ultimately determining ventricular output (Starling's law), vascular tone actually plays a significant role in ultimately determining cardiac output. In general, arterial resistance is an important determinant of blood pressure, and veins can be thought of as capacitance vessels. Hence, venodilation (dilation of veins of all sizes) can result in blood pooling, potentially decreasing blood returned to the heart for pumping to the body. A common example of the effectiveness of acute venous pooling occurs when someone faints. If the individual is standing just before fainting, acute venodilation causes blood to pool in the lower extremities (due to gravity), acutely decreasing venous blood returning to the heart. Therefore the left ventricle has less volume and is forced to operate at the lower end of the Starling curve; less forward flow of blood to the body is the result. Reduced forward flow means decreased organ perfusion (particularly in the brain), and the person faints. Because of the effects of gravity, fainting to the floor actually increases venous return to the heart (since blood is no longer pooling only in the legs) and acutely increases cardiac output by moving back up the Starling curve; hence, end organs such as the brain are now perfused, which promotes awakening. In spite of this example, decreased venous return is not always bad. In a failing ventricle, left ventricular volumes may be quite elevated to the point of producing pulmonary edema and myocardial ischemia. Venodilation may acutely decrease ventricular volume and thus relieve symptoms of pulmonary edema and myocardial ischemia. Several cardiovascular medications are both venodilators and vasodilators. The effect of such agents on venous return to the heart should always be remembered. Undesired decreases in venous return can frequently be avoided during administration of cardiovascular drugs with venodilatory properties by concurrent administration of intravenous fluids.

Myocardial Inotropy and Systemic Vascular Resistance

Myocardial inotropy refers to the intrinsic ability of myocardial cells to contract vigorously. In more scientific terms, increases in inotropy are characterized by an increase in the velocity of shortening of the unloaded muscle. Although not characterized fully, increases in inotropy are thought to be related to increased availability of calcium within myocardial cells, facilitating actin-myosin interactions at the level of the sarcomere to produce more effective contraction (see Myocardial Inotropic Agents for more details regarding actin-myosin interactions). Myocardial failure is frequently associated with decreased inotropic states, whereas exercise and therapeutic interventions with catecholamines increase inotropic states. This is distinct from Starling's law, which states that increases in volume produce more effective contraction. In fact, changes in inotropic state result in totally new Starling curves (Fig. 3-8C), with increases in inotropy leading to greater contractility at the same left ventricular filling pressure compared with "normal" (new Starling curve displaced upward and to the left), and decreases in inotropy resulting in lower contractility for a given filling pressure (new Starling curve displaced downward and to the right). Hence, increases in left ventricular volume can still lead to more effective ventricular contraction even in heart failure (up to a point), but the degree of effectiveness of volume therapy depends on the location of the Starling curve itself, which is intimately related to the inotropic state. This is a critical point for deciding on potential therapeutic interventions.

One other factor is important in cardiovascular homeostasis (and forward blood flow by the heart), besides Starling's law, venous return, and inotropic state. This is the concept of afterload, which refers to resistance to forward flow presented to the heart by the vasculature. All things being equal, it is easier to pump blood forward against a mean arterial pressure (MAP) of 60 mm Hg rather than 100 mm Hg. It is also easier to pump 3 L rather than 5 L of blood forward at a fixed MAP. Arterial resistance is one of the prime determinants of blood pressure and (in the absence of other constricting lesions such as coarctation of the aorta) afterload presented to the heart. SVR is a calculated number that takes into account MAP, cardiac output, and ventricular filling (as measured indirectly by atrial pressure). Because most intraoperative measurements of cardiac output (CO) utilize thermodilution methods via pulmonary arterial catheters, right ventricular cardiac output and hence right atrial pressures (RAP) are utilized in this calculation. Because right and left ventricles should be pumping the same volume of blood forward at any given time, this is a valid number to use to calculate SVR. The equation for SVR is

$$\mathrm{SVR} = \frac{(\mathrm{MAP} - \mathrm{RAP})}{\mathrm{CO}} \times 80 \text{ dyne·cm·second}^{-5} \qquad [3\text{-}3]$$

Normal SVR values range between 900 and 1,200 dyne·cm·second^{-5}. If the values are not multiplied by 80, then the units are described as Wood units. It is useful to calculate SVR during clinical situations, because low cardiac output can occur from decreases in inotropic state or from elevated SVR (increased afterload). If an elevated SVR is the cause of myocardial failure, then careful titration of arterial vasodilating agents concurrently administered with intravenous fluids can be effective therapy.

Heart Rate

One last parameter is critical in ultimately determining the amount of blood ejected from the heart. This is heart rate. Cardiac output is determined by stroke volume (the amount of blood ejected with each beat [determined by the four variables described above]) multiplied by the heart rate. Therefore, the higher the heart rate rises, the more blood can be ejected from the heart. (This is true unless the heart rate climbs to higher than 120 beats per minute, because at this point, there may be insufficient time in diastole to enable the ventricle to fill completely, and stroke volume begins to decrease.) An appropriate rhythm is also important. Sinus rhythm provides coordinated atrial, then ventricular, ejection. Because atrial ejection of blood into the ventricles can provide up to 20% of overall ventricular filling, sinus rhythm is essential for optimal cardiac output. Atrial and ventricular arrhythmias disturb this delicate coordination and therefore impair optimal cardiac output. Consequently, arrhythmias must be controlled as much as possible with antiarrhythmic drugs (see Chapter 4), particularly in patients with ventricular failure.

General Therapeutic Interventions with Cardiovascular Drugs

With an understanding of Starling's law, venous return, inotropy, heart rate, and afterload, rational clinical application of cardiovascular drugs can be accomplished. Although only general principles of cardiovascular drug therapy are presented in this discussion, descriptions of specific drugs follow and more detailed management schemes are presented in the final section of this chapter. For the sake of this discussion, heart rate is assumed to be stable at 70 to 100 beats per minute with sinus rhythm. Once a stable heart rate is established, general principles of cardiovascular drug therapy are shown in Fig. 3-8B–E. Before any cardiovascular drugs are given to a patient, it is imperative that the anesthesiologist, or clinician, ensure the volume status of the left ventricle is optimal. Figure 3-8B demonstrates that even in heart failure with decreased contractility (with the resulting depressed Starling curve), volume therapy can still be effective in improving left ventricular output (*arrow 1*). It is imperative that volume status (and hence ventricular filling) be checked repeatedly, because abrupt changes in vascular resistance, body temperature, and drug therapy will continue to change ventricular filling. As a general rule, before every intervention in a patient with cardiovascular disease, volume status should be quickly reassessed and optimized. Once volume status is ensured, then drug therapy can begin. As shown in Fig. 3-8C, heart failure decreases inotropic state and hence contractility, moving the patient to a different (lower) Starling curve (*arrow 2A*); exercise and drugs with positive inotropic properties (e.g., catecholamines) move the Starling curve upward (*arrow 2B*). Frequently in clinical medicine, a patient with heart failure requires inotropic drug therapy to move from a Starling curve with decreased contractility up to the "normal" curve. Hence, for a given filling volume, the treated failing heart is able to generate more forward blood flow (or cardiac output). A third general therapy for failing hearts is afterload reduction, particularly in the setting of high SVR. As briefly described and demonstrated in Fig. 3-8D, careful administration of vasodilating agents can actually move a patient from a myocardial failure Starling curve to a normal curve in this setting (*arrow 3*). Although inherent contractility is not improved by vasodilating agents alone, effective contractility is improved (because it is easier to eject the same volume against a lower resistance). However, vasodilating agents also decrease blood flow to the venous circulation and thereby decrease venous return to the heart, so the patient now operates on a lower aspect of the new normal Starling curve. Finally, Fig. 3-8E demonstrates that once afterload reduction is applied (*arrow 3*), volume can be added (*arrow 1*) to move to a better position along the new Starling curve.

Myocardial Inotropic Agents

Myocardial inotropy refers to the intrinsic ability of myocardial cells to contract vigorously. Cellular mechanisms for increasing myocardial contractility relate predominantly to the availability of calcium to the contractile apparatus. This includes binding of calcium to troponin C, a conformational change in tropomyosin (which is bound to the troponin complex) such that a space between actin and myosin occurs, and finally, cross-bridging of actin and myosin filaments. During diastole, calcium is rapidly sequestered in the cell and actin and myosin cross-bridging is reduced, facilitating relaxation of the myocardium. Myocardial inotropic agents act in general by either increasing intracellular calcium or increasing sensitivity of contractile proteins to calcium. Inotropic agents described in this section are predominantly used to treat congestive heart failure, cardiogenic shock, and occasionally severe hypotension. Agents that increase myocardial inotropy also increase myocardial oxygen consumption, potentially exacerbating imbalances between myocardial oxygen supply and delivery. Therefore, inotropic agents should be used with extreme caution in patients with ischemic heart disease. However, in the case of severe congestive heart failure or cardiogenic shock, improving forward blood flow created by increasing intrinsic myocardial contractility may improve arterial blood pressure (including diastolic blood pressure), lead to improved coronary artery perfusion, and so relieve myocardial ischemia. In addition to effects on the heart, many positive inotropic agents have effects on the peripheral vasculature. Therefore, a thorough knowledge of potential benefits and side effects of each of these inotropic agents is essential in order for the cardiovascular clinician to make appropriate decisions regarding acute therapy. Three general classes of myocardial inotropic agents are currently available for intravenous therapeutic intervention. These include catecholamines (both endogenous and synthetic derivatives), sympathomimetics (predominantly phenylisopropylamines), and phosphodiesterase inhibitors. Each is described in detail later. For more information, the reader is guided to several reviews (62–73) on myocardial inotropic agents.

Catecholamine-Mediated Inotropic Agents

Catecholamines are the major type of inotropic agent available for clinical use today. Each catecholamine drug structure is characterized by the presence of a catechol ring moiety, catechol hydroxyl groups, and side chains of varying length and composition. Figure 3-9 illustrates the structure of several catecholamines, both endogenous (dopamine, norepinephrine, and epinephrine) and synthetic (isoproterenol and dobutamine). By understanding the basic tenets of receptor action (shown in Fig. 3-3 and described in the discussion under Signal Transduction), it is possible to understand the cellular mechanisms of each of these agents. Most catecholamines that act to increase myocardial inotropy mediate their action via stimulation of myocardial β-ARs (both β_1 and β_2). Although α_1-ARs have been shown in various models to have positive inotropic effects in the heart, this effect is relatively minor compared with β-AR stimulation in normal myocardium; this discussion therefore focuses on the effects of myocardial β-AR stimulation. Drug binding to myocardial β-ARs activates the stimulatory G protein, G_s, which results in activation of the enzyme adenylyl cyclase. Adenylyl cyclase catalyzes the production of cAMP from ATP, a reaction that initiates a cascade of reactions within the cell (including protein phosphorylation and increased calcium availability via slow membrane-bound calcium channels), ultimately leading to the physiologic effect of increased myocardial contractility. Although endogenous circulating catecholamines are capable of acutely stimulating myocardial β-ARs (as demonstrated by acute increases in myocardial inotropy during exercise or fright when rapid endogenous catecholamine release occurs), exogenous administration of catecholamines provides higher drug levels and hence potentially greater degrees of inotropic support. When catecholamines are administered at clinical doses, they have clear effects on peripheral vessels. Most currently available catecholamine drugs stimulate α-ARs and β-ARs; hence, increases in blood pressure mediated via increased SVR (via α-AR stimulation) are not an uncom-

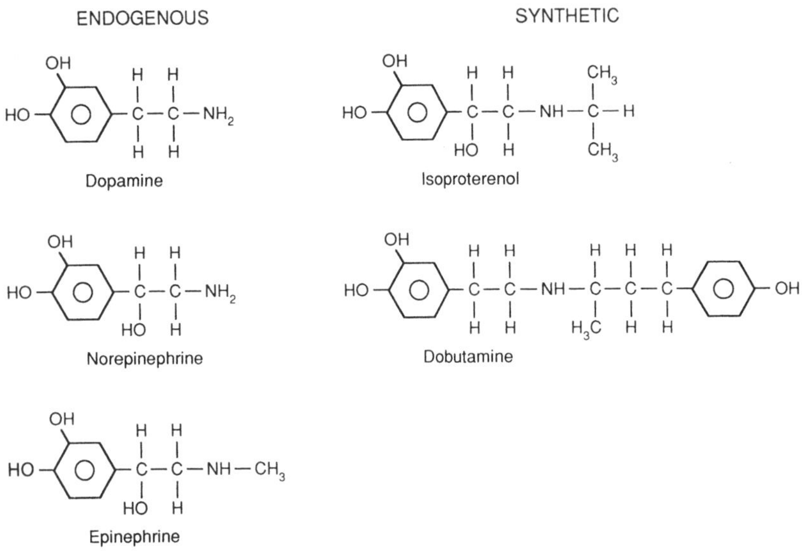

FIGURE 3-9. The chemical structures of catecholamines. Endogenous catecholamines include dopamine, norepinephrine, and epinephrine, and clinically used synthetic catecholamine derivatives include isoproterenol and dobutamine. The chemical properties of each drug are described in detail in the text.

mon finding at higher doses for many of these agents. Properties of each catecholamine-derived inotropic agent are described in detail in the following sections. Table 3-5 lists the properties and doses of currently available inotropic agents.

Endogenous Catecholamines. Endogenous catecholamines include norepinephrine, epinephrine, and dopamine. Norepinephrine is the postganglionic neurotransmitter in the sympathetic nervous system, and epinephrine is secreted from the adrenal medulla as part of the stress response. Dopamine is found predominantly in the central nervous system, although receptors and nerve endings have been found for dopamine at several other clinically important sites in the periphery. The pathway for synthesis of endogenous catecholamines is important clinically. Briefly, the amino acid phenylalanine is the starting point. This compound is hydroxylated on the phenyl ring to form tyrosine; a second hydroxylation on the phenyl ring forms the compound dopa. Acid decarboxylation forms dopamine from dopa, β-hydroxylation forms norepinephrine from dopamine, and the addition of a methyl group on the side chain of norepinephrine then forms epinephrine. Actions of endogenous catecholamines include peripheral stimulatory action on smooth muscle (e.g., blood vessels supplying skin and mucous membranes) and glands, peripheral inhibitory action on other types of smooth muscle (e.g., gastrointestinal tract, bronchial tree, blood vessels to skeletal muscle), cardiac excitatory action (e.g., increases in heart rate and force of contraction), metabolic actions (e.g., increased glycogenolysis and release of free fatty acids), endocrine actions (e.g., modulation of insulin, renin, and pituitary hormone secretion), and central nervous system actions (e.g., increased wakefulness and decreased appetite). Many of these responses have teleologic significance, because they are part of the fight-or-flight response, preparing the body to escape or fight an attacker. Most of the sites of action of these effects are at ARs distributed throughout the body. ARs are described earlier in this chapter, and the reader is referred to the discussion under Neurotransmitters and Receptors for further information. Because most of the currently available inotropic agents act via myocardial β-ARs and peripheral α-ARs, only the four classic AR subtypes (α_1, α_2, β_1, β_2) are addressed in the following descriptions of each catecholamine drug.

Epinephrine. Epinephrine is a potent α-AR and β-AR agonist, but effects on β-ARs predominate at lower doses. In the heart, epinephrine is a potent stimulant of myocardial inotropy, has significant arrhythmogenic potential, and increases stroke volume, coronary blood flow, and heart rate. Intravenous injection of epinephrine results in vasoconstriction, particularly in the skin and kidneys while vessels to skeletal muscles dilate. Increases in blood pressure mediated by intravenous administration of epinephrine are mediated predominantly by constriction of small arterioles and precapillary sphincters (although some constriction occurs on large arteries and veins); a characteristically higher systolic blood pressure than diastolic blood pressure is produced, and thus a widening of the pulse pressure. Because epinephrine acts directly on ARs (instead of indirectly by releasing norepinephrine from the nerve terminal), repeated bolus doses of epinephrine generally mediate continued increases in blood pressure.

Epinephrine is used as therapy in several clinical situations, including cardiopulmonary resuscitation (CPR), asthma, anaphylaxis, shock, and heart failure. As can be seen in Table 3-5, the dose and route of administration of epinephrine depends on the clinical condition being treated. In CPR, 1-mg bolus doses are common, given intravenously, via the endotracheal tube or directly into the ventri-

TABLE 3-5. POSITIVE INOTROPIC DRUGS

Drug (Trade Name)	Catecholamine Receptor Activation α_1	α_2	β_1	β_2	Dopamine	Noncatecholamine Mechanism	Drug Doses and Suggested Intravenous Infusion Schemes
Epinephrine (Adrenalin)	+ + +	+ + + (High dose)	+ +	+ + (Low dose)	−	No	Infusion: 1 mg/250 mL (4 μg/mL), start 2–4 μg/min or 0.01–0.03 μg · kg^{-1} · min^{-1} (max 0.1–0.3 μg/kg/min) CPR: 0.5–1 mg IV or ETT Asthma: 0.3–0.5 mg s.c.; 1 μg/min IV
Norepinephrine (Levophed)	+ + +	+ + +	+	Little	−	No	Infusion: 1 mg/250 mL (4 μg/mL), start 2 μg/min or 0.01–0.03 μg · kg^{-1} · min^{-1} (max 0.1 μg · kg^{-1} · min^{-1})
Dopamine (Intropin)	+ +	+ (High dose)	+ +	+ (Low dose)	+ + +	No[a,b]	Infusion: 200 mg/250 mL (800 μg/mL) or 400 mg/250 mL (1600 μg/mL)
	Direct and indirect actions: (1) NE 2° metabolism *via* hydroxylation of alpha carbon, (2) inhibition of NE reuptake, (3) promotion of NE release						2–5 μg · kg^{-1} · min^{-1}— ↑ renal blood flow (dopamine effects, some beta effects) 5–10 μg · kg^{-1} · min^{-1}— ↑ HR and cotractility, beta effects 10–20 μg · kg^{-1} · min^{-1}— vasoconstriction (alpha effects predominate)
Isoproterenol (Isuprel)	−	−	+ + +	+ + +	−	No	Infusion: 1 mg/250 mL (4 μg/mL), 0.01–0.1 μg · kg^{-1} · min^{-1} (keep HR <120) Arrythmogenic; use in status asthmaticus, complete heart block
Dobutamine (Dobutrex)	Little	Little	+ + +	+ +	−	No[a]	Infusion: 250 mg/250 mL (1000 μg/mL), 2–15 μg · kg^{-1} · min^{-1}
	Direct and minimal indirect effects						
Dopexamine	−	−	Little	+ + +	+ +	No[a]	Infusion: 1–10 μ · kg^{-1} · min^{-1}
	Both direct and indirect effects						
Ephedrine	+	+	+	+	−	No[b]	Bolus: 50 mg/10 mL (5 mg/mL), 10–25 mg IV boluses effect lasts 10–15 min, ↑ CO ↑ SVR ↑ HR
	Both direct and indirect effects						
Denopamine	Antag	−	+ +	−	−	No	Oral administration
Amrinone (Inocor)	−	−	−	−	−	Yes	Loading dose: 0.75 mg/kg IV (maximum up to 3 mg/kg in CHF) Infusion: 2–10 μg · kg^{-1} · min^{-1} IV (higher infusion rates have been used in CHF)
	Phosphodiesterase inhibitor, ↑ cAMP in heart, Pheripheral vasodilator, ↑ inotrophy (additive to other types)						
Milrinone	−	−	−	−	−	Yes	Bolus: 50–75 μg/kg IV bolus Oral administration
	Similar to amrinone, but more potent inotropy						
Calcium chloride	−	−	−	−	−	Yes	Bolus: 1 g/10 mL (100 mg/mL), 2–4 mg/kg IV boluses

Note: Do not give inotropes in same IV line as HCO_3^- or alkaline solutions, because these drugs will be inactivated (by autooxidation). Doses should always be checked on individual package inserts before administering drug. α_1, α_2, β_1, β_2, adrenergic receptor subtypes (the catecholamine receptors); antag, antagonist; −, no effect; +, positive effect; 2°, secondary to; cAMP, cyclic adenosine monophosphate; CHF, congestive heart failure; CPR, cardiopulmonary resuscitation; ETT, endotracheal tube; HR, heart rate; IV, intravenous; max, maximum; NE, norepinephrine; SC, subcutaneous; CO, cardiac output; SVR, systemic vascular resistance.

[a] Blocks reuptake of norepinephrine from the nerve terminal.

[b] Promotes the release of norepinephrine from the nerve terminal.

cle. In asthma, as well as for allergic reactions, epinephrine can be administered subcutaneously or intravenously. Prevention of urticaria and treatment of anaphylaxis and asthma may be partly attributable to an increase in cAMP in mast cells, which then stabilizes these cells and prevents further degranulation. Relaxation of bronchial smooth muscle by epinephrine (via stimulation of β_2-ARs) is important in the treatment of asthma. Epinephrine is also useful in treating cardiac failure. Doses of 0.01 to 0.03 $\mu g \cdot kg^{-1} \cdot minute^{-1}$ provide low-dose epinephrine effects in which β-AR agonist effects predominate. However, at a higher dose range (maximum 0.1 $\mu g \cdot kg^{-1} \cdot minute^{-1}$), vasoconstrictive α-AR effects tend to predominate. This is potentially useful in the setting of hypotensive cardiac failure, in which positive inotropic and some vasoconstrictive effects are desired. Because epinephrine has been shown to mediate renal artery constriction, this agent should perhaps be avoided in patients with renal failure. Renal failure is not an absolute contraindication to epinephrine however, because in the long run, severe hypotension may be more detrimental to renal function than acute therapy with epinephrine in which renal perfusion pressure is reestablished.

Epinephrine can be administered via intravenous, subcutaneous, or pulmonary routes. Because it is rapidly conjugated and oxidized in gastrointestinal mucosa and liver, oral administration of epinephrine does not provide therapeutic drug levels. Subcutaneous administration of epinephrine slows absorption significantly, enabling beneficial effects to last longer and potential side effects to be minimized; this route has proved useful in the treatment of asthma. Epinephrine is rapidly metabolized in the liver and other tissues by the enzymes COMT and MAO; these metabolites are excreted in the urine. Therefore, epinephrine should be used with extreme caution in patients on MAO inhibitor medication for symptoms of depression. In addition, epinephrine is taken up by sympathetic neurons. Epinephrine administration may result in serious side effects, the most serious being cerebral hemorrhage (from an acute elevation of blood pressure) and cardiac arrhythmias (usually ventricular arrhythmias including ventricular fibrillation). Cardiac arrhythmias occur at a lower epinephrine dose in the presence of inhalation anesthetics (74). However, when used properly, epinephrine can be a safe and lifesaving drug for acute use in patients with cardiopulmonary arrest, heart failure, bronchospasm, and hypersensitivity reactions.

Norepinephrine. Norepinephrine, structurally similar to epinephrine (Fig. 3-9), is the endogenous postganglionic neurotransmitter for the sympathetic nervous system. In addition, norepinephrine constitutes 10% to 20% of the catecholamine content of the adrenal medulla and is secreted in more than 95% of pheochromocytomas. Norepinephrine stimulates predominantly α-ARs, although stimulation of β_1-ARs also occurs to a lesser extent; very little stimulation of β_2-ARs occurs with norepinephrine (see Table 3-5). From this information, most of the cardiovascular effects of norepinephrine can be derived. Blood pressure increases with intravenous administration of norepinephrine, primarily based on significant increases in SVR (α-AR stimulation without opposing β_2-AR stimulation). Because of the rise in SVR, heart rate actually tends to decrease with norepinephrine administration, due to reflex vagal pathways that overcome direct stimulation of myocardial β_1-ARs. Norepinephrine stimulation of myocardial β_1-ARs mediating increases in contractility does occur, so norepinephrine is considered a positive inotropic agent, particularly at low doses in which β-AR effects are not overcome by peripheral α-AR effects. The cardiac effects of norepinephrine in the intact animal or patient include increases in stroke volume and coronary blood flow (in the absence of coronary vasospasm), significant arrhythmogenic potential (although less than epinephrine or isoproterenol), little overall change in cardiac output, and potential decreases in heart rate. Compared with epinephrine, in which increases in blood pressure result predominantly from increases in heart rate and cardiac output with a mild concurrent decrease in SVR (due to vascular β_2-AR stimulation), norepinephrine increases blood pressure predominantly via vasoconstriction.

As listed in Table 3-5, the usual clinical dose range for intravenous norepinephrine is 0.01 to 0.1 $\mu g \cdot kg^{-1} \cdot minute^{-1}$. Like epinephrine, norepinephrine is easily oxidized and is metabolized by enzyme systems such as COMT and MAO and taken up by sympathetic neurons; therefore, norepinephrine should be used with extreme caution in patients on MAO inhibitor medication. Norepinephrine decreases renal artery blood flow (with little or no change in glomerular filtration rate), in addition to mesenteric, splanchnic, and hepatic blood flow in humans. Because norepinephrine does not bind well to β_2-ARs, low-dose administration does not result in decreased SVR as it does with epinephrine. Hence, low-dose norepinephrine can be used for its vasoconstrictive properties and titrated to effect. Because norepinephrine is so effective at increasing SVR, it should only be administered centrally (or very proximally in a large peripheral vein) to avoid severe tissue necrosis and sloughing resulting from potential extravasation of the drug at the site of administration. Cardiac output must also be monitored closely when norepinephrine is used, because blood pressure increases predominantly due to increased SVR can be detrimental to forward blood flow from the heart and in some circumstances may contribute to myocardial failure. However, when cardiac output is normal (or well supported with inotropic agents), hypotension can be treated effectively with norepinephrine.

Dopamine. Dopamine is the immediate metabolic precursor of norepinephrine and epinephrine and is a central nervous system and peripheral neurotransmitter. In addition to stimulating dopamine receptors, dopamine binds to and activates ARs (both α-ARs and β-ARs) (75). Indirect effects include inhibition of norepinephrine reuptake at the nerve terminal, release of norepinephrine at the nerve terminal, and metabolism by hydroxylation of the α carbon to form norepinephrine. The primary cardiovascular effects of intravenously administered dopamine are dose dependent (Table 3-5) (75). At relatively low intravenous doses (1 to 3 $\mu g \cdot kg^{-1} \cdot minute^{-1}$), dopamine stimulates predominantly dopamine receptors, which mediate renal and mesenteric arterial relaxation (76). Although increases in both renal blood flow and sodium excretion occur with dopamine administration, it is not clear that increases in renal blood flow are the sole cause of enhanced diuresis and natriuresis; dopamine may also inhibit tubular solute reabsorption directly. At moderate to high intravenous doses (3 to 10 $\mu g \cdot kg^{-1} \cdot minute^{-1}$), dopamine is classically thought to directly stimulate predominantly β-ARs, thus accounting for its positive inotropic effects. Evidence suggests that the exact mechanism of dopamine-mediated positive inotropic responses in this dose range actually depend on conversion of dopamine to norepinephrine (77). At high intravenous doses (10 to 15 $\mu g \cdot kg^{-1} \cdot minute^{-1}$), α-AR stimulation becomes apparent and vasoconstriction results, reversing potential renal perfusion benefits seen at lower doses. Because of its unique effects on renal artery blood flow, as well as positive inotropic effects, dopamine is a useful drug clinically. It has been used effectively in heart failure and in various hypotensive states, including septic shock. Although controversial, dopamine has been used in low doses potentially to offset renal artery vasoconstrictive effects of other concurrently administered positive inotropic agents. Dopamine receptors exist in the central nervous system; however, dopamine administration does not result in central nervous system effects because intravenous dopamine cannot cross the blood-brain barrier. Dopamine is a substrate for both COMT and MAO; consequently, it is ineffective when administered orally and is rapidly metabolized by the liver and other tissues when administered intravenously. Dopamine should therefore be used with extreme caution in patients on MAO inhibitor medication for symptoms of depression. For more detailed reviews on dopamine as a positive inotrope, the reader is referred to several of the general references on inotropic agents listed at the beginning of this discussion, as well as three review articles on dopamine, dobutamine, and dopexamine administration in children and adults (78–80). In contrast to dopamine, which is an endogenous neurohormone that binds and activates all dopamine receptor subtypes (DA1–DA5), recent development of a highly selective DA1 receptor agonist (fenoldopam) have proven to be clinically useful. This new drug is described below.

Synthetic Catecholamines. Although epinephrine, norepinephrine, and dopamine are endogenous catecholamines, many other catecholamine drugs have been synthesized by changing side groups of these basic molecules (Fig. 3-9). Hence, synthetic catecholamine derivatives have many of the same properties as those found in endogenous catecholamines. As positive inotropic agents, they increase myocardial oxygen consumption and have varying effects on the peripheral vasculature. The three most commonly used synthetic catecholamine derivatives are isoproterenol, dobutamine, and dopexamine; the new DA1 receptor vasoactive agonist, fenoldopam, is also now gaining in popularity. Each of these agents is examined below.

Isoproterenol. Isoproterenol is a synthetic catecholamine derivative (see Fig. 3-9). It is the only clinically available drug with pure β-AR agonist activity. Therefore, isoproterenol causes a decrease in peripheral vascular resistance (via β_2-ARs) concurrent with increases in heart rate and myocardial contractility (and hence, cardiac output via both β_1-ARs and β_2-ARs). Because of its direct effects on stimulation of heart rate, isoproterenol is indicated in the treatment of severe heart block and in conduction abnormalities resulting in severe life-threatening bradycardia. Isoproterenol is also useful in various low-cardiac-output states, because it stimulates increases in myocardial inotropy. Intravenous administration of isoproterenol begins with 2 to 4 μg/minute and is titrated to effect (see Table 3-5). As with other catecholamines, isoproterenol is rapidly metabolized in the liver and other tissues by the enzyme COMT; however, it is not well metabolized by MAO and is not taken up by sympathetic neurons to the same extent as epinephrine and norepinephrine. Fluids should be administered concurrently with isoproterenol to maintain myocardial preload secondary to the vasodilatory properties of this drug. Another side effect of isoproterenol administration is significant arrhythmogenic potential (equal to that seen with epinephrine). Indeed, it is this potential side effect that limits the use of isoproterenol in asthma despite excellent bronchodilatory effects of β_2-AR stimulation (as can be seen in its use in status asthmaticus); more selective β_2-AR agonists (such as terbutaline and salbutamol) tend to be used in asthma instead. Interestingly, isoproterenol has been shown to stimulate secretion of ANP from atria (81), a process that is dependent on calcium influx through voltage-sensitive calcium channels as well as calcium release from the sarcoplasmic reticulum; this process is inhibited in the presence of calcium channel antagonists. Because ANP mediates vasodilation, this may add to the vasodilation already seen with isoproterenol from direct β_2-AR agonist activity in vascular beds.

Dobutamine. Dobutamine is similar in structure to dopamine except for the addition of a bulky aromatic group (Fig. 3-9). Dobutamine is primarily a direct-acting β-AR agonist, relatively selective for the β_1-AR subtype. Minimal indirect effects of preventing reuptake of norepinephrine at the nerve terminal are also seen. Dobutamine is more effective in providing positive inotropic effects than increases in heart rate (although increases in sinus node automaticity are apparent with dobutamine). Notably, dobutamine does not bind to dopamine receptors and therefore does not provide the increases in renal blood flow seen with dopamine. In typical clinical concentrations of dobutamine (2 to 15 $\mu g \cdot kg^{-1} \cdot minute^{-1}$), positive inotropic responses are seen with modest increases in heart rate and little change in SVR (despite some α-AR agonist properties of the drug). However, in patients receiving β-AR antagonist therapy, cardiac output does not change and SVR increases with dobutamine administration. Nevertheless, in marked contrast to other catecholamines, higher doses of dobutamine in general do not cause large increases in blood pressure due to increasing vasoconstriction. In patients with pure myocardial pump failure, this may be an advantage. On the other hand, in patients with combined myocardial failure and vasodilation, an additional vasopressor may be required in conjunction with dobutamine. Positive inotropic effects are seen in patients with right ventricular failure when dobutamine is administered, and this therapy is considered by some to be better than nitroprusside and volume. Although both isoproterenol and dobutamine are agonists at the β_1-AR subtype, increases in heart rate are clearly higher with isoproterenol than dobutamine, even when reflex tachycardia secondary to isoproterenol vasodilation is taken into account. In some patients, however, dobutamine may increase heart rate profoundly, although this side effect can be minimized by decreasing the dose of the infusion. This property of dobutamine is often used diagnostically in stress echocardiography studies designed to explore myocardial reserve and determine whether hibernating myocardium exists after myocardial ischemia/infarction. In more practical therapeutic situations, some clinicians use combinations, such as dopamine and dobutamine simultaneously, to achieve clinical benefits while minimizing side effects, such as tachycardia, for any single agent. The chemical structure of dobutamine (which is missing the β-hydroxyl group thought to confer selectivity for β_1-ARs) may have some effect in this regard. Dobutamine is metabolized somewhat differently from other catecholamines in that although it is rapidly metabolized in the liver, different enzyme systems (glucuronic acid and not COMT or MAO) are involved. Because the chemical structure of dobutamine is similar to that of both epinephrine and isoproterenol, dobutamine is also capable of inducing ventricular dysrhythmias, but to a lesser extent than the other two agents. In summary, dobutamine has some advantageous properties compared with other inotropic agents and therefore may be the inotropic agent of choice in selected patients. For more details regarding dobutamine therapy in adults and children, the reader is referred to several excellent reviews (78,82–84).

Dopexamine. Dopexamine, a synthetic analog of dopamine, has potent β_2-AR and dopamine agonist properties and little or no β_1-AR and α-AR activity, and dopexamine inhibits reuptake of catecholamines at the nerve terminal (75,79,85–88). Because of its potent β_2-AR agonist properties, dopexamine causes vasodilation (similar to isoproterenol); dopexamine has no demonstrable venous effects. This feature can be beneficial in unloading the heart and thus enhancing forward flow of blood, particularly in congestive heart failure. Effects of dopexamine on the heart include direct β_2-AR stimulation of heart rate and positive inotropy, indirect increases in heart rate from β_2-AR–mediated vasodilation, and effects of norepinephrine release at the nerve terminal, which include β_1-AR and β_2-AR increases in heart rate and inotropy. Interestingly, dopexamine has more marked direct positive inotropic effects in healthy myocardium and fewer vasodilatory effects; most inotropic effects in patients with heart failure appear to be manifest from effects of decreased afterload (from decreased SVR) and heart rate increases, and not direct increases in myocardial inotropy. Because of dopamine and β_2-AR agonism, renal artery dilation occurs with resultant increases in renal blood flow. Some dispute exists about whether increases in renal artery blood flow actually occur secondary to renal artery dilation or simply secondary to increases in cardiac output in some patients (76,80). Dopexamine is metabolized in the liver (methylation and sulfation) and taken up into the tissues via extraneuronal catecholamine uptake mechanisms. Although dopexamine produces atrial tachycardia (mostly from reflex tachycardia secondary to vasodilation or increases in dose directly), it shows no propensity for development of ventricular arrhythmias either with halothane administration or ischemia. In fact, there have even been some suggestions that dopexamine may have a class 1–like antiarrhythmic effect (86). Most of the clinical experience with dopexamine exists for short-term therapy of congestive heart failure; evaluation of long-term therapy with this compound remains to be completed.

Fenoldopam. Fenoldopam mesylate is a new DA1 receptor selective agonist that causes both systemic and renal arteriolar vasodilation. In hypertensive patients, fenoldopam rapidly decreases blood pressure, increases renal blood flow, and maintains or improves the glomerular filtration rate. Hence, it has been used to treat hypertension, particularly acute elevations of blood pressure requiring an intravenous agent. Because of its beneficial renal effects, fenoldopam has been suggested to be a new agent of choice to prevent or minimize renal damage often associated with hypertensive states either as a sole agent or in combination with other catecholamine drugs. Because fenoldopam provides overall vasodilation, it is important to choose a dose that increases renal artery blood flow without systemic hypotension. This "renal" dose has been found to be 0.05 to 0.10 $\mu g \cdot kg^{-1} \cdot min^{-1}$. Higher doses (0.1 to 0.3 $\mu g \cdot kg^{-1} \cdot min^{-1}$) provide systemic antihypertensive effects. The reader is referred to recent reviews on fenoldopam for more detail (88–92).

Sympathomimetics. Sympathomimetics have many of the same properties as catecholamines but do not contain the catecholamine moiety in their structure. Phenylisopropylamines are such a class of compounds, which stimulate α-ARs and β-ARs and are powerful central nervous system stimulants but do not have the same chemical structure as catecholamines. Amphetamines, methamphetamine, ephedrine, denopamine, mephentermine, metaraminol, hydroxyamphetamine, phenylephrine, and methoxamine are all phenylisopropylamines. However, because ephedrine and denopamine are the only clinically used phenylisopropylamines with significant β-AR agonist properties (and hence provide positive inotropic support), they are discussed here. Phenylisopropylamines such as phenylephrine and methoxamine, which activate primarily α-ARs, are covered under Vasoconstrictors.

Ephedrine. Although catecholamine and phosphodiesterase inhibitors provide rapid changes in cardiac output, they are almost all administered via an intravenous infusion and usually used in critically ill patients. Most patients with and without cardiovascular disease coming to the operating room, however, do not require inotropic support for a long time. Hence, ephedrine has become a common drug (administered by intravenous bolus) in the perioperative period, used specifically to increase blood pressure predominantly by increasing cardiac output. Ephedrine is a naturally occurring compound found in several plants. It was used in China for more than 2,000 years before being introduced into Western medicine in 1924. Ephedrine has both direct effects (stimulation of myocardial β-ARs) and indirect effects (release of norepinephrine from the nerve terminal). It therefore has a mixture of properties. Because both ephedrine and norepinephrine stimulate β-ARs, the primary effect of ephedrine is to increase cardiac output, and hence blood pressure, by stimulation of myocardial β-ARs. However, because norepinephrine also activates α-ARs, some vasoconstriction can be seen with ephedrine, primarily due to its secondary effect of release of norepinephrine at the nerve terminal. Taking into account both mechanisms of action, the overall effect of ephedrine administration is to increase cardiac output, increase heart rate, and increase SVR. These effects are most striking when parasympatholytic agents have been administered, effectively preventing reflex responses in the heart.

Ephedrine is administered as an intravenous bolus of 5 to 10 mg (Table 3-5), and its clinical effect lasts for approximately 10 to 15 minutes. One unique feature of phenylisopropylamines in general is that they are effective when administered orally. Ephedrine is not a substrate for metabolism by the enzyme COMT, and only a small amount is oxidatively deaminated by MAO in humans; most of the ephedrine is excreted unchanged. Two asymmetric carbon atoms exist in the ephedrine molecule, creating the possibility of several isomers; only *l*-ephedrine and racemic forms are used clinically. Because ephedrine increases blood pressure primarily by increasing heart rate and cardiac output, it is considered the drug of choice in clinical situations in which blood pressure increases are required but vasoconstriction is not desired—for example, during pregnancy and cesarean section surgery (93). As with any drug that increases myocardial inotropy, myocardial oxygen consumption is increased, and therefore ephedrine can precipitate myocardial ischemia in patients with coronary artery disease. Hence, like all catecholamines and positive inotropic agents, it should be used with extreme caution in patients with cardiovascular disease.

Denopamine. Denopamine is unique in having selective β_1-AR agonist and an α_1-AR antagonist properties (94–96). It is used clinically as an oral positive inotropic agent, particularly in patients with congestive heart failure. Denopamine mediates direct positive inotropic effects via myocardial β_1-AR stimulation and also decreases SVR via α_1-AR antagonist properties, providing afterload reduction and effective forward flow from the heart. The net cardiovascular effects are positive inotropic ones with little change in blood pressure. Denopamine also causes concentration-dependent relaxation in canine coronary, mesenteric, and renal arteries. Although not yet widely used in the United States, denopamine promises to provide effective therapy for patients in congestive heart failure. Therefore, in the future, anesthesiologists may encounter patients maintained on chronic oral denopamine in the operating room for heart surgery and various other noncardiac surgeries.

Phosphodiesterase Inhibitors. Phosphodiesterase inhibitor drugs provide myocardial inotropy via a mechanism different from those of catecholamines and sympathomimetics. Although stimulation of β-ARs results in the production of cAMP, this product is rapidly inactivated by metabolism by phosphodiesterases in the cell. Phosphodiesterase inhibitors therefore act by preventing the breakdown of cAMP, prolonging its effectiveness and augmenting its physiologic response. Because endogenous circulating catecholamines provide a basal level of cAMP production, phosphodiesterase inhibitors given alone are effective in producing increases in myocardial inotropy. However, when β-ARs are stimulated with β-AR agonists such as isoproterenol, epinephrine, dopamine, or norepinephrine, one can see how adding a phosphodiesterase inhibitor (which inhibits the breakdown of cAMP), will have synergistic effects. In addition to positive inotropic properties, phosphodiesterase inhibitors cause vasodilation. Hence, they are "inodilators," inotropic agents that also reduce afterload. Three phosphodiesterase inhibitors have been used clinically: amrinone, milrinone, and enoximone. Each of these is reviewed below. The reader is referred to several review articles on this class of drugs (64,71,97–102).

Amrinone. The phosphodiesterase inhibitor amrinone was the initially used clinical positive inotropic agent in this class. In addition to positive inotropy, amrinone has potent vasodilatory effects (potentially profound decreases in SVR). When amrinone is administered clinically, its vasodilatory effects are immediately apparent, whereas approximately 10 to 15 minutes must pass before positive inotropic effects become appreciable. Because amrinone acts via phosphodiesterase inhibition, its inotropic and vasodilator effects are not reversed by AR blocking drugs or by norepinephrine depletion from the nerve terminal. This combination of vasodilation and positive inotropy is useful in heart failure, in which combined afterload reduction and inotropic support provide more effective forward flow of blood from the heart. However, because positive inotropic drugs in general increase myocardial oxygen consumption, and because vasodilation can decrease diastolic blood pressure and hence decrease coronary blood flow, amrinone has the potential for exacerbating myocardial ischemia in the presence of coronary artery disease. This potential side effect can be minimized or avoided with careful fluid management and vasopressor therapy when required, to increase diastolic blood pressure and improve coronary perfusion. Interestingly, administration of amrinone to patients with severe congestive heart failure has been shown to improve myocardial performance while decreasing myocardial oxygen consumption by 30%.

Amrinone is administered as a bolus loading dose (1.5 mg/kg for 2 to 3 minutes), followed by continuous intravenous infusion at 2 to 10 $\mu g \cdot kg^{-1} \cdot minute^{-1}$ (Table 3-5). The maximum suggested daily dose of amrinone should not exceed 10 $mg \cdot kg^{-1}$. In the presence of congestive heart failure however, up to 3 $mg \cdot kg^{-1}$ is considered an acceptable loading dose; experience by a few investigators suggests that short-term infusion rates can be increased to 20 $\mu g \cdot kg^{-1} \cdot minute^{-1}$ in patients with congestive heart failure with careful monitoring. Monitoring of CVP and cardiac output is essential when amrinone therapy is contemplated. Although bolus doses of amrinone can be injected directly into an infusion line containing glucose, a slow reaction with glucose occurs over 24 hours; therefore, long-term intravenous infusions of amrinone should not be mixed in glucose-containing solutions. Amrinone ampules should be protected from light and stored at room temperature. Furosemide precipitates with amrinone; therefore, they should not be administered in the same intravenous line. In addition to hypotension, potential side effects of amrinone therapy include thrombocytopenia in 2% to 3% of patients, and to a far lesser degree gastrointestinal upset, myalgia, fever, hepatic dysfunction, and ventricular irritability. Because amrinone solution contains metabisulfite, it is contraindicated in patients with allergy to sulfonamides.

Because of tonic stimulation of β-ARs from circulating resting levels of catecholamines, phosphodiesterase inhibitors can provide positive inotropic effects when administered as the sole agent. However, concurrent administration of a catecholamine-derived inotropic agent and a phosphodiesterase inhibitor provides much more effective positive inotropic effects than either agent by itself. Because catecholamine inotropic agents stimulate β-ARs, cAMP levels in the cell rise acutely. Concurrent administration of a phosphodiesterase inhibitor then prevents the breakdown of cAMP, greatly enhancing effectiveness of the catecholamine-derived inotropic agent. This is one reason for amrinone's high effectiveness when added to other inotropic regimens and its importance in the armamentarium of the cardiac anesthesiologist.

Milrinone. Milrinone, a 2-methyl,5-carbonitrile derivative of amrinone, is a phosphodiesterase inhibitor that can be administered either intravenously or orally. Milrinone has nearly 20 times the inotropic potency of amrinone and does not cause fever or thrombocytopenia. Like amrinone, milrinone has vasodilator properties. Vasodilation also occurs in the coronary artery bed, resulting in increased coronary blood flow. When administered to patients with congestive heart failure, milrinone reduces ventricular filling pressures by 30% to 40%. Milrinone is a unique phosphodiesterase compound in that it can be administered orally for a long term (Table 3-5) and therefore could be administered to patients with congestive heart failure on an outpatient basis. However, a recent multicenter study has found that despite its beneficial hemodynamic actions, long-term therapy with oral milrinone increases morbidity (hypotension, syncope) and mortality (28% increase in overall mortality, 34% increase in cardiovascular mortality), compared with other agents in patients with severe congestive heart failure; the mechanism for these severe effects is not known. Although not promising for long-term therapy, short-term administration of milrinone in the operating room has been proven to be of benefit.

Enoximone. Enoximone is an imidazole derivative that is also a phosphodiesterase inhibitor. Although enoximone has positive inotropic properties, it has more vasodilator effects than either amrinone or milrinone. Because enoximone is a relatively new phosphodiesterase inhibitor drug (experience with this drug has occurred in Europe), more studies are needed before its final role among other inotropic agents is established.

Calcium Chloride. Because calcium ions are ultimately involved in improved excitation-contraction coupling in the heart, and calcium channels exist in myocardium, exogenous administration can be useful in the acute management of heart failure. Great controversy exists regarding the long-term effectiveness of calcium chloride, and indeed potential harmful side effects of calcium overload in ischemic myocardial cells leading to cell injury and death are known to occur. These questions have led to recent restrictions in the use of calcium chloride in CPR. However, acute bolus administration of calcium chloride is generally thought effective for short-term treatment of myocardial pump failure. Calcium is particularly useful after cardiopulmonary bypass if the heart begins to dilate and fail, because rapid increases in myocardial inotropy from calcium chloride administration lasts for the necessary minutes required to start another more definitive intravenous positive inotropic agent. In this setting, the overwhelming benefit of short-term calcium administration in preventing myocardial injury from acute ventricular dilation offsets any potential negative effects of the drug. However, caution should be used in administering calcium, because it has been shown to attenuate epinephrine's β-AR effects in postoperative heart surgery patients (103), and high doses have been associated with pancreatic cellular injury in the same patient population (104).

Calcium chloride is usually administered intravenously from a 10-mL prefilled syringe containing 100 mg/mL calcium chloride (1 g total); this syringe contains 13.6 mEq of calcium. The usual dose for acute calcium chloride therapy is 2 to 4 mg/kg, a dose that may be repeated approximately every 10 minutes. Although calcium comes in three clinical formulations—calcium chloride, calcium gluceptate, and calcium gluconate—calcium chloride is preferred in adults because it results in predictably higher levels of ionized calcium. In addition to positive inotropic effects, calcium chloride has variable effects on the vasculature but most frequently causes vasoconstriction. Hence, in patients with healthy hearts, calcium chloride administration causes a predictable rise in blood pressure secondary to its positive inotropic and vasoconstrictive properties.

Calcium-Sensitizing Agents

Although most inotropic drugs currently used in clinical medicine utilize the β-AR signal transduction pathway, either by direct receptor activation or indirect actions via second messengers, a new class of drugs has recently become available that acts more directly on actin/myosin filaments. These drugs sensitize the myocardium to the actions of calcium and are hence called calcium-sensitizing agents. It is interesting to note that recent evidence suggests that shortening deactivation occurs in the myocardium (105). This concept suggests that a "rapid change of length applied during isometric contraction of skeletal or cardiac muscle may result in redeveloped tension less than appropriate for the new length because of 'deactivation' of the contractile system."(105) Reduced tension developed from this process is associated with reduced affinity of troponin C for Ca^{2+}; remaining calcium is then sequestered into the sarcoplasmic reticulum and not immediately available for the next contraction. Hence, this process potentially provides inconsistencies in the Frank-Starling relationship, particularly notable in disease states with high afterload, and suggests that calcium-sensitizing agents may be clinically applicable. Currently available calcium-sensitizing agents include pimobendan, levosimendan, and MCI-154 (106,107). Calcium-sensitizing action of these agents predominates during the early phase of myocardial contraction and therefore avoids problems associated with impaired lusitropy (relaxation that results from calcium-sequestering action), which is common with other inotropic agents. Although these agents have not been used extensively, they will be used more frequently during the next few years, particularly as the incidence of congestive heart failure increases with the predicted aging population. For further information on this class of agents, the reader is referred to two recent reviews on the subject (106,107).

Vasodilators

In addition to positive inotropic agents, another method of improving forward blood flow from the heart includes afterload reduction. By decreasing mean arterial blood pressure (and SVR), the heart has less resistance against which to pump. Although afterload reduction alone does not change intrinsic myocardial contractility, *effective* contractility is improved (because it is easier to eject the same volume against a lower resistance). Vasodilating agents cause relaxation of arterial smooth muscle, resulting in decreases in SVR. This effect is important in hypertension as well as myocardial afterload reduction. Although vasodilating agents work predominantly on arterial smooth muscle, they frequently also have some venodilating capability. Therefore, careful titration of fluids must accompany administration of vasodilating agents to prevent decreases in venous return, ultimately resulting in less effective myocardial contraction (Starling's law). Vasodilation can be accomplished by several mechanisms. Nitrate vasodilators such as sodium nitroprusside and hydralazine activate endothelium relaxing factor now known to be NO to produce arterial smooth muscle relaxation (29–31). In addition, hydralazine interferes with calcium transport in vascular smooth muscle, ganglionic blockers block nerve impulses to arterial smooth muscle and hence prevent arterial vasoconstriction, and α-AR antagonists block vasoconstriction at the level of the AR. Less common agents include inhaled NO, intravenous ANP, endothelin (ET) antagonists, and an older intravenous drug, diazoxide. Table 3-6 lists vascular effects and doses for each intravenous vasodilator and venodilator discussed. All clinically available vasodilators provide effective arterial relaxation in clinical concentrations and can be used effectively by the cardiac anesthesiologist (108,109).

Sodium Nitroprusside. Sodium nitroprusside was introduced into clinical medicine in the United States in 1974 and is one of the most commonly used vasodilators in the perioperative period. As described in detail under Coronary Vasodilators: Nitrates, the mechanism of action of nitrates such as sodium nitroprusside has only recently been elucidated. Briefly, nitrates penetrate the endothelium, where they act as substrates for the formation of NO. NO then binds to the NO receptor, which is an iron group in the enzyme guanylate cyclase. NO binding to this iron-contain-

TABLE 3-6. VASODILATOR AND VENODILATOR DRUGS

Drug (Trade Name)	Vasodilation	Venodilation	Mechanism of Action	Drug Doses and Suggested Intravenous Infusion Schemes
Diazoxide (Hyperstat)	+ + + +	−	Direct smooth muscle relaxation	Bolus: 300 mg/20 mL (15 mg/mL), 150–300 mg rapid IV bolus
Fenoldopam	+ + + +	−	DA1 receptor agonist	Infusion: 0.05–0.1 $\mu g \cdot kg^{-1} \cdot min^{-1}$ (renal dose) 0.1–0.3 $\mu g \cdot kg^{-1} min^{-1}$ (vasodilation)
Hydralazine (Apresoline)	+ + + +	+	Activation of nitric oxide	Bolus: 2.5–5 mg boluses, titrate to effect on blood pressure, lasts approx 2–4 h, rare side-effect: lupus-like syndrome
Trimethaphan (Arfonad)	+ + +	+ + +	Ganglionic blockade	Infusion: 500 mg/500 mL D5W (1 mg/mL), start at 0.5 $\mu g \cdot kg^{-1} \cdot min^{-1}$ and titrate to effect Bolus: 1 mg/mL, 1–2 mg IV bolus (duration approx. 2 min)
Pentolinium (Ansolysen)	+ + +	+ + +	Ganglionic blockade	Bolus: 10 mg/mL, 0.03–0.1 $mg \cdot kg^{-1}$ IV bolus
Phentolamine (Regitine)	+ +	+	α-AR antagonist	Bolus: 5 mg IV bolus for hypertension 5–10 mg in 10 mL saline injected locally for catecholamine extravasation
Nitroglycerin (Nitrobid, Nitrostat, Tridil)	+	+ + + +	Activation of nitric oxide	Infusion: 50 mg/250 mL D5W (200 µg/mL), start at 0.5 $\mu g \cdot kg^{-1} \cdot min^{-1}$ and titrate to effect
Sodium nitroprusside (Nipride, Nitropress)	+ + + +	+ +	Activation of nitric oxide	Infusion: 50 mg/250 mL D5W (200 µg/mL), start at 0.5 $\mu g \cdot kg^{-1} \cdot min^{-1}$, titrate to effect Cyanide toxicity[a] 1.5 $mg \cdot kg^{-1}$ over 1–3 h = max acute dose, 0.5 $mg \cdot kg^{-1} \cdot h^{-1}$ max chronic dose (8 $\mu g \cdot kg^{-1} \cdot min^{-1}$)

Note: Doses should always be checked on individual package inserts before administering drug. −, no effect; +, positive effect; approx, approximately; D5W, dextrose 5% in water; IV, intravenous; max, maximum.
[a] Treatment of cyanide toxicity: (a) Suspect it (especially when metabolic acidosis is present). (b) Discontinue sodium nitroprusside. (c) If hemodynamics are stable, administer the specific cyanide antagonist thiosulfate (150 mg/kg intravenously over 15 min; thiosulfate is a sulfur donor, so it converts cyanide to thiocyanate). (d) Alternative therapy when hemodynamics are unstable is slow intravenous infusion of sodium nitrate, 5 mg/kg (converts hemoglobin to methemoglobin, which acts as an antidote to cyanide by converting cyanide cyanmethemoglobin (see text for potential problems to this approach).

ing heme group causes a 3D change that results in the production of cGMP from guanine triphosphate (25). cGMP then acts as the second messenger responsible for producing relaxation of vascular smooth muscle by activating calcium-binding proteins, which then bind calcium and thereby reduce the intracellular calcium concentration. Nitrovasodilators act on different arterial beds, with sodium nitroprusside affecting predominantly systemic vasculature (particularly arteries and arterioles). Sodium nitroprusside is most effective when background sympathetic tone is high—that is, when vasoconstriction is present. With increasing doses, these relatively selective effects disappear; hence, sodium nitroprusside mediates venodilation at higher doses.

As listed in Table 3-6, sodium nitroprusside infusions usually begin at 0.5 $\mu g \cdot kg^{-1} \cdot minute^{-1}$ and are titrated to effect (blood pressure decrease secondary to decreasing SVR). Clinical effects are apparent within 1 to 2 minutes of administration; rapid waning of effects occurs upon discontinuation. Nitroprusside should be mixed with dextrose-containing solutions only and wrapped to prevent light from catalyzing breakdown products and cyanide release (110,111). It is critically important to infuse fluids during therapy with sodium nitroprusside, because acute vasodilation in the absence of intravenous fluid infusion may decrease myocardial preload acutely and therefore decrease cardiac output. Concurrent fluid administration also dampens any reflex tachycardia caused by acute vasodilation. The net effect on the heart when preload is maintained is an increase in stroke volume secondary to diminished vascular impedance to forward flow. Sodium nitroprusside also dilates coronary arteries. Because coronary arteries with restrictive lesions do not dilate normally, nitroprusside has long been known to potentially cause redistribution of blood flow from potentially ischemic areas of the myocardium to normal areas (a process called coronary steal). However, decreases in myocardial oxygen consumption resulting from decreased afterload frequently offset this potential disadvantage. Because nitroprusside severely attenuates the normal hypoxic vasoconstrictor response in the lungs, it may cause shunting at the level of the lung, potentially contributing to hypoxia. However, this effect is rapidly reversed upon discontinuation of nitroprusside.

The ferrous ion in nitroprusside reacts rapidly with sulfhydryl-containing compounds in red blood cells to form cyanide (111), a product that is rapidly converted to thiocyanate by the liver and excreted by the kidneys (or by hemodialysis in renal failure). Signs of cyanide toxicity include increased mixed venous O_2, increasing dose requirements (tachyphlaxis) and metabolic acidosis. Cyanide toxicity can occur when conversion to thiocyanate by the liver is impaired (as in liver failure) or is overwhelmed by rapid or excessive administration of sodium nitroprusside. Cyanide interferes with oxygen transport in the final steps of the electron-transport chain and hence prevents tissue utilization of oxygen. Guidelines for safe administration of sodium nitroprusside have been established to prevent the risk of cyanide toxicity. The suggested maximum acute dose of sodium nitroprusside is 1.5 $mg \cdot kg^{-1}$ administered for 1 to 3 hours. Guidelines for maximal chronic administration of nitroprusside are 0.5 $mg \cdot kg^{-1} \cdot hour^{-1}$ or 8 $\mu g \cdot kg^{-1} \cdot minute^{-1}$. If cyanide toxicity does occur, treatment includes the following steps: (a) Suspect cyanide toxicity, particularly in the presence of metabolic acidosis, (b) discontinue sodium nitroprusside administration, and (c) a cyanide antidote kit is commercially available. If the patient is hemodynamically stable, administer the specific cyanide antagonist sodium thiosulfate intravenously (150 $mg \cdot kg^{-1}$ for 15 minutes); because thiosulfate is a sulfur donor, it provides the substrate for the enzyme rhodanase to convert cyanide to thiocyanate, which can then be excreted (112). However, thiosulfate itself in very high concentrations can cause toxicity. If the patient is hemodynamically unstable, alternative therapy is a slow intravenous infusion of sodium nitrate (5 $mg \cdot kg^{-1}$). This compound converts hemoglobin to methemoglobin, which acts as an antidote to cyanide by converting cyanide to cyanomethemoglobin. The problem with this approach is that methemoglobin is hemoglobin with iron in the ferric (oxidized) form and not the ferrous (reduced) form. Because the ferric form of iron cannot carry oxygen (because it cannot combine with oxygen), the oxyhemoglobin dissociation curve is shifted to the left. It is possible to convert methemoglobin to hemoglobin with the reducer methylene blue (1 $mg \cdot kg^{-1}$) if necessary. Despite the risk of cyanide toxicity, sodium nitroprusside is in general a very safe compound when used in the appropriate clinical dose range. It provides rapid, effective, and easily reversible arterial vasodilation and is therefore a very useful drug for the clinician, particularly during the perioperative period.

Hydralazine. Hydralazine produces arterial smooth-muscle vasodilation in a manner similar to the organic nitrates, as described for sodium nitroprusside and covered in detail under Coronary Vasodilators: Nitrates. In addition, hydralazine appears to inhibit calcium transport in smooth muscle; this may augment vasodilation from the other, more classical method. Although hydralazine has been available for more than 30 years, with the advent of β-AR antagonists to minimize tachycardia side effects, it is regaining popularity. Hydralazine has minimal effects on capacitance veins and hence does not result in postural hypotension. Acute decreases in SVR mediated by hydralazine result in increased heart rate, stroke volume, and cardiac output in spite of decreased overall blood pressure. Because hydralazine is frequently administered as an intravenous bolus (2.5- to 5-mg bolus) (Table 3-6), has an onset of action of within 10 to 15 minutes after intravenous injection, and has antihypertensive effects that last 2 to 4 hours, it provides a convenient alternative antihypertensive drug to sodium nitroprusside in the perioperative (particularly postoperative) period. With the advent of fenoldopam, this may become less important during the next 5 years. Hydralazine is useful on the inpatient hospital ward because it can also be given by intramuscular injection or orally and therefore frequently does not require an intensive care unit setting. Hydralazine is a useful drug for treatment of severe hypertension during pregnancy, but it should always be administered with fluids, because drastic decreases in blood pressure may occur secondary to the relative intravascular volume depletion in some diseases associated with pregnancy, such as preeclampsia. When given orally, hydralazine has a rather large first-pass phenomenon, where it is acetylated in the liver. Therefore, patients who are "slow acetylators" should be given lower doses of oral hydralazine because they tend to have higher overall plasma levels. Parenteral administration of hydralazine bypasses this phenomenon, with acetylation phenotype having little effect on plasma drug concentration. One significant potential side effect (occurs in less than 10% of patients) of hydralazine is development of a lupus-like syndrome. This usually occurs only after 2 months of therapy or with large amounts of drug and disappears within 6 months of stopping the drug. Although not used during heart surgery as often as sodium nitroprusside, hydralazine is a highly useful drug for treatment of hypertension during the perioperative period in patients with cardiac disease who are having noncardiac surgery.

Ganglionic Blockers: Trimethaphan, Pentolinium. Ganglionic blockers such as trimethaphan and pentolinium are now seldom used during the perioperative period, but they have proved to be useful vasodilating agents through the years. Pentolinium is a bisquaternary ammonium compound first used in the mid-1950s, and trimethaphan is a sulfonium ganglionic-blocking agent that was available soon thereafter. Almost all of the pharmacologic properties of these drugs can be attributed to ganglionic blockade of both sympathetic and parasympathetic fibers. Ganglionic blockade has the following effects: vasodilation and hypotension on arterioles; dilation, venous pooling, decreased venous return, and resultant decreased cardiac output on veins; tachycardia on the heart; mydriasis on the iris; cycloplegia on ciliary muscle; reduced tone and motility in the gastrointestinal tract; urinary retention in the bladder; and anhydrosis on sweat glands. In spite of these wide-ranging side effects, ganglionic blockers provide rapid, effective, and easily reversible arterial vasodilation in the setting of cardiac surgery. Bolus intravenous injections of trimethaphan (1 to 2 mg) (Table 3-6) have a duration of approximately 2 minutes; continuous infusion is therefore recommended for continuing therapy. However, rapid desensitization limits the duration of ganglionic blocker therapy. Ganglionic blockers such as trimethaphan are potent noncompetitive inhibitors of pseudocholinesterase and can approximately double the duration of paralysis produced by the usual dose of succinylcholine (113). In addition, the mydriasis resulting from ganglionic blockade may make it difficult to judge the depth of a narcotic- or sedative-based anesthesia. Perhaps ganglionic blocker agents such as trimethaphan will be relegated to use when severe hypertension is unresponsive to more conventional therapies, such as sodium nitroprusside.

α-Adrenergic Receptor Antagonists

Many compounds have been shown to be α-AR antagonists (selective for either α_1-AR or α_2-AR subtypes), but few are available clinically for acute intravenous application in the operating room. α_1-AR selective antagonists such as prazosin, terazosin, doxazosin, and tamsulosin are particularly popular orally administered drugs initially used for long-term treatment modalities of hypertension, and more recently for prostatic hyperplasia. Because this section is limited to acute vasodilating agents, the reader is referred to a review (114) for details of these drugs. Nonselective α-AR antagonists such as phenoxybenzamine are also available in oral form and are quite useful in the preoperative treatment of pheochromocytoma. However, phentolamine is the only drug in this category that is readily available for intravenous use during surgery in the Unites States. Most clinical effects of α-AR antagonists stem directly from the fact that baseline arterial vascular tone in humans results from tonic stimulation of α-ARs. Postsynaptic α_1-ARs and α_2-ARs mediate vasoconstriction, whereas presynaptic α_2-ARs inhibit the release of norepinephrine from the nerve terminal. Treatment with phentolamine blocks α-AR–mediated vasoconstriction, with a resulting decrease in SVR. Because α-ARs are present in veins, phentolamine therapy also results in some venodilation. Most of the side effects of phentolamine are directly attributable to acute decreases in SVR, such as potentially severe hypotension. Because most clinically available drugs used acutely to increase blood pressure in the presence of hypotension are α_1-AR agonists, phentolamine therapy should be approached cautiously. As with other vasodilating agents, acute decreases in SVR result in increases in heart rate, cardiac output, and stroke volume. Careful titration of fluid status is necessary with phentolamine therapy to maintain preload and optimize cardiac output. Phentolamine has been used through the years during cardiopulmonary bypass to decrease hypertension as rewarming occurs. Although sodium nitroprusside is also useful in this regard, there is still a place for phentolamine in the armamentarium of the cardiac anesthesiologist. A newer α_1-AR antagonist used extensively in Europe is urapidil (115). This drug is α_{1a}-subtype selective and is therefore important in human coronary and resistance vessel vasodilation (116). Once FDA approved, this drug may provide selective vasodilation to splanchnic and coronary circulations and may therefore be beneficial in the perioperative period and in the intensive care unit.

Diazoxide. Diazoxide is structurally similar to thiazide diuretics (see discussion under Pharmacologic Agents and Table 3-4), has potent antidiuretic effects, and directly relaxes arterial smooth muscle. In contrast to sodium nitroprusside, diazoxide has virtually no effects on venous capacitance vessels. Resulting cardiovascular effects are those predicted for acutely decreased SVR, such as reflex tachycardia and increased cardiac output. Administration of intravenous fluids or intrinsic potent antidiuretic effects may dampen cardiovascular responses to diazoxide; however, antidiuretic effects can be reversed with concurrent administration of potent diuretics. Diazoxide is frequently administered acutely as a rapid intravenous bolus (150 to 300 mg) (Table 3-6), most commonly in the emergency room for the treatment of malignant hypertension. Diazoxide is rarely used in the operating room and is contraindicated for hypertension resulting from aortic coarctation, arteriovenous shunts, aortic dissection, intracerebral hemorrhage, and acute pulmonary edema. The availability of sodium nitroprusside, and more recently fenoldopam, has decreased the use of diazoxide significantly in recent years.

Less Common and Experimental Vasodilating Agents

Atrial Natriuretic Peptide. Over the last several years, new vasodilating agents have become available. ANP and inhaled NO are two new compounds that although not now universally available for clinical purposes, may be used by cardiac anesthesiologists. ANP is a 28–amino acid hormone secreted by the atria (and to a lesser extent the ventricles) in response to atrial stretch or tachycardia (117,118). ANP secretion results rapidly in vasodilation and natriuresis. Levels of ANP have been found to be elevated in congestive heart failure, hypertension, hyperthermia, and renal failure. Administration of synthetic ANP to humans results in decreased blood pressure secondary to decreases in SVR, as well as a brisk natriuresis. The mechanism of ANP-induced smooth-muscle vasodilation of both endogenous and synthetic ANP appears to be mediated by ANP receptors with stimulation of cGMP by guanylate cyclase (117,118). In addition, ANP infusions appear to decrease overall sympathetic tone (119) and mediate/augment β-AR–induced vasodilation (120). Because a drug with both vascular relaxation and natriuresis would be useful in treating patients with cardiac disease in the operating room, one day ANP infusions may have a place in cardiac anesthesiology.

Nitric Oxide. NO is an old drug. Recent interest in the role of the endothelium in vascular responses and the discovery that endothelium relaxing factor is NO, an important second messenger, have resurrected this drug. NO binds to guanylate cyclase and activates the conversion of guanine triphosphate to cGMP, the compound ultimately is responsible for smooth-muscle relaxation. Inhaled NO is of interest to the cardiovascular clinician because inhalation promotes pulmonary vascular dilation (121). Because NO is bound to the ferrous form of iron in hemoglobin, it is rapidly inactivated during transit through the pulmonary circulation, thereby minimizing the profound systemic vascular relaxation that often complicates NO administration. Although still considered experimental at many institutions, NO is often inhaled in concentrations starting at 2 to 10 ppm and increased to 80 ppm as clinically indicated. It is important to have an accurate method to measure end-tidal NO because of the profound clinical activity of this compound. Although technically considered experimental, the use of inhaled NO has become very routine during heart and lung transplantation and in patients with severe right ventricular failure. It can be administered chronically in the intensive care unit (122,123), although care must be taken to monitor its effects over time carefully.

Venodilators: Nitroglycerin. Venodilators provide relaxation of veins. Because venous capacitance is important in venous return, and hence preload of the ventricles, venodilators play an important role in cardiovascular medicine. Venodilators play a major role in congestive heart failure because they can acutely unload the left ventricle, minimizing pulmonary edema. This same mechanism explains partly how venodilators relieve acute myocardial ischemia in the failing heart, because high ventricular filling pressures increase wall tension and therefore increase myocardial oxygen consumption. Many vasodilators have venodilator properties, particularly at high concentrations. However, one drug commonly used by cardiac anesthesiologists for the treatment of ischemic heart disease is primarily a venodilator; this drug is nitroglycerin.

Intravenous nitroglycerin is one of the mainstays of cardiovascular medicine. The mechanism of action of nitroglycerin is similar to those of other nitrate compounds and is described under Coronary Vasodilators: Nitrates and Sodium Nitroprusside. Nitroglycerin penetrates the endothelium, where it acts as the substrate for formation of NO. NO then binds to the NO receptor, which is an iron group in the enzyme guanylate cyclase, causing a 3D change that results in the production of cGMP from guanine triphosphate (25). cGMP then acts as the second messenger responsible for producing relaxation of vascular smooth muscle. Intravenous nitroglycerin dilates venous capacitance vessels and has several effects on coronary arteries (dilation of epicardial coronary arteries, dilation of coronary collaterals, reversal and prevention of coronary vasospasm, and dilation of atherosclerotic coronary artery stenoses (32,33). The starting dose of intravenous nitroglycerin is 0.5 $\mu g \cdot kg^{-1} \cdot minute^{-1}$ (Table 3-6), but this dose can be rapidly increased and titrated to effect (relief of ischemia, decreased ventricular filling pressures, or decreased blood pressure). At higher concentrations, nitroglycerin does have some systemic vascular vasodilatory properties, albeit minimal ones (124). Because acute venodilation produced by nitroglycerin may result in decreased venous return, acute decreases in cardiac output may occur; therefore, nitroglycerin therapy should be administered cautiously and with careful attention to fluid status. Many of the common side effects of nitrates in general (e.g., headache, postural hypotension, dizziness, and weakness) are avoided when nitroglycerin is administered during anesthesia.

Nitroglycerin is metabolized in the liver; two molecules of reduced glutathione react with each molecule of nitroglycerin to form one inorganic nitrite ion, glyceryl dinitrate, and oxidized glutathione. Nitrite is able to oxidize iron in the ferrous state, which is present in hemoglobin, to the ferric state, producing methemoglobin (125). Methemoglobin produces a functional anemia (because it is unable to carry oxygen) and can shift the oxygen-hemoglobin dissociation curve to the left. However, because several enzyme systems in the body are able to reduce methemoglobin, methemoglobinemia becomes a problem only at extremely high doses of nitroglycerin. Because of rapid metabolism, intravenous nitroglycerin has a half-life of 1 to 3 minutes. With prolonged administration (more than 8 hours), tolerance can develop to intravenous nitroglycerin, with attenuation of peripheral arterial dilation (120). Reversal of nitroglycerin tolerance has been accomplished with *N*-acetylcysteine (200 $mg \cdot kg^{-1}$ orally), a sulfhydryl-containing compound. Of interest to the cardiac anesthesiologist, intravenous nitroglycerin has been associated with dose-related prolongation of bleeding time, a process found not to be associated with platelet function, aggregation, or vascular-platelet interactions, but with vasodilation and increased venous capacitance (126). It may be prudent, therefore, to limit the dose of nitroglycerin in patients who are bleeding after cardiac surgery.

Because cardiac anesthesiologists strive to provide adequate myocardial oxygen supply and minimize myocardial oxygen demand, nitroglycerin has proved a very useful drug. By decreasing ventricular preload (hence decreasing wall tension and myocardial oxygen consumption), having minimal effects on SVR and therefore blood pressure (hence maintaining coronary artery perfusion pressure), and dilating coronary arteries (hence increasing myocardial oxygen delivery), nitroglycerin has earned its well-deserved position as a ubiquitous and one of the most commonly used cardiovascular drugs in patients with ischemic heart disease.

Endothelin Receptor Antagonists

ET is a recently discovered endogenous polypeptide that when bound by its receptor on the endothelium, mediates potent vasoconstriction. This protein has been isolated, purified, and cloned (127), and receptors for several subtypes have also been isolated and cloned (128). ETs are actually a family of acidic, 21–amino acid peptides named ET-1, ET-2, and ET-3. Pre-pro-ET is cleaved proteolytically to form pro-ET, and finally mature ET. The structure of ET-1 is a twisted loop held together by two disulfide bridges. Binding of ET to ET receptors activates inositol phosphate hydrolysis, leading to mobilization of intracellular calcium. At high concentrations, ET is clearly a potent vasoconstrictor, but when administered at low doses, it may have transient vasodilatory effects before vasoconstriction begins. In addition to vasoconstrictor properties, ET has positive inotropic effects, decreases renal blood flow, and stimulates the release of hormones such as ANP and aldosterone. ETs are thought to be part of the active ingredients in snake venom and therefore may have caused Cleopatra's death when she subjected herself to snake bites. Recent evidence suggests that increased levels of ET may play a role in the development of heart failure (129,130). Several ET receptor antagonists are currently being developed for the treatment of hypertension and should be marked soon in the United States (131,132). A recent study using epoprostenol (formerly called prostacyclin), a compound which has been shown to alter pulmonary handling of ET-1, showed improvement in patients with hypertension (133). This study supports the idea that ET receptor antagonists (as well as other drugs that modify the ET axis) should be beneficial in the therapy of hypertension.

Etanercept. The recent explosion in understanding of mechanisms underlying heart failure has resulted in new drugs designed to prevent this detrimental process. Etanercept (Enbrel) is a new soluble p75 tumor necrosis factor receptor (so TNF antagonist) that can be administered intravenously. Recent clinical studies suggest this drug is safe and well tolerated in patients with New York Heart Association class III heart failure (134). TNF antagonists therefore can be expected to play an increasing role in the treatment and prevention of heart failure in the future. The interaction of this class of drugs and surgical stress remains to be determined.

Vasoconstrictors

The final category of drugs important in cardiovascular regulation is vasoconstrictors. As a group, vasoconstrictors have predominant effects on arteries and arterioles, causing an increase in SVR. In general, pure vasoconstrictors have very little effect on β-ARs and therefore minimal effects on the heart, particularly because these agents are often administered to correct hypotension. If hypertension is generated by acute increases in SVR by vasoconstrictor agents, then reflex bradycardia and decreased cardiac output (secondary to acutely increased afterload) are seen. Some vasoconstrictors have secondary effects such as release of norepinephrine from the nerve terminal; these compounds, therefore, have some β-AR effects as well. It is critically important that whenever vasoconstrictor agents are utilized, careful monitoring of fluid status and cardiac output must occur. This should prevent inappropriate treatment of hypotension with vasoconstrictor agents when fluid resuscitation or myocardial inotropy support might be more appropriate.

Several types of compounds have vasoconstrictor properties. The most commonly used vasoconstrictors are sympathomimetics, particularly phenylisopropylamines or isopropylamines. However, catecholamines such as norepinephrine (and also epinephrine and dopamine at high concentrations) are potent vasoconstrictors. Newer agents, such as ET (see description of ET under Endothelin Receptor Antagonist section), are also potent vasoconstrictors and may play increasing roles in cardiovascular management in the future. Currently utilized drugs are described further.

Sympathomimetics

Most clinically available vasoconstrictor agents are sympathomimetics, such as phenylisopropylamines or isopropylamines. These compounds differ from catecholamines structurally in subtle ways, for example, having less than two hydroxyl groups on the benzene moiety and other alterations of side groups. Included in this noncatecholamine family are phenylephrine, methoxamine, ephedrine, denopamine, metaraminol, amphetamine, methamphetamine, and mephentermine. In general, phenylisopropylamines and isopropylamines stimulate α-ARs and β-ARs and are powerful central nervous system stimulants but do not have the same chemical structure as catecholamines. Phenylisopropylamines and isopropylamines are metabolized by the enzyme COMT; many are also metabolized by MAO (with the exception of amphetamine and ephedrine). Because many of these compounds have secondary effects of release of norepinephrine at the nerve terminal, they should be avoided in patients receiving MAO inhibitor medication. Phenylephrine is a direct-acting agent with very few secondary effects, so it can be used safely in this patient population. Because ephedrine and denopamine are phenylisopropylamines with significant β-AR properties, they are positive inotropic agents and therefore described in detail in the discussion of sympathomimetics under Myocardial Inotropic Agents; the reader is referred there for information regarding ephedrine and denopamine. The remaining phenylisopropylamines and isopropylamines have significant α-AR stimulation properties and therefore act as potent vasoconstrictors. However, only phenylisopropylamines and isopropylamines, which can be administered parenterally (via either intramuscular or intravenous injection), are considered here.

Phenylephrine. Phenylephrine has a chemical structure virtually identical to that of epinephrine (Fig. 3-9), lacking a hydroxyl group only at position 4 on the benzene ring. However, agonist-binding properties of phenylephrine are significantly different from those of epinephrine. Phenylephrine is a pure α_1-AR agonist at clinical concentrations; it binds α_2-ARs only at extremely high concentrations and β-ARs in concentrations approximately 10 times the clinical concentration. Hence, phenylephrine is the most selective α_1-AR agonist available clinically. Increases in SVR secondary to α_1-AR stimulation are the primary effect of phenylephrine, although in the absence of parasympatholytic agents such as atropine, reflex bradycardia may be seen. Vasoconstriction occurs in most vascular beds (renal, splanchnic, cutaneous, and limbs) at the level of the arteriole, but coronary artery perfusion is increased. This may result from increased diastolic perfusion pressure generated by phenylephrine providing improved coronary artery driving pressure. Large epicardial coronary arteries have relatively high concentrations of α_1-ARs, with less present in distal coronary branches; the opposite is true of α_2-ARs (124). Phenylephrine stimulation of α_1-ARs results in epicardial coronary artery constriction and constriction of normal distal coronary vascular beds. This effect increases perfusion pressure across concentric coronary stenoses, potentially providing a potential "antisteal" effect. However, phenylephrine can constrict coronary vessels with ectopic stenoses, potentially eliciting myocardial ischemia. In general, increases in diastolic perfusion pressure provide increased coronary artery blood flow, even in the presence of occlusive lesions. In addition to acute therapy in patients with cardiovascular disease, phenylephrine is available in several other formulations, most notably as an integral ingredient in nasal and ophthalmic decongestants. It is also quite useful as a vasoconstricting agent in combination with local anesthetic administration.

Phenylephrine is frequently administered in bolus form (50 to 100 μg) intravenously (Table 3-7); clinical effects are apparent within 1 minute and may last 5 to 20 minutes. When continued administration of vasopressors is required, phenylephrine can be administered as a continuous intravenous infusion at rates of 20 to 40 μg/minute (0.5 to 1.0 $\mu g \cdot kg^{-1} \cdot minute^{-1}$). The *l* form is the active one. Whenever phenylephrine or other vasoconstrictors are used, careful monitoring of fluid balance and cardiac output is required to ensure that vasoconstriction is not used to treat hypotension instead of more appropriate therapies such as fluid resuscitation or inotropic support.

TABLE 3-7. VASOCONSTRICTOR DRUGS

Drug (Trade Name)	Catecholamine Receptor Activation α_1	α_2	β_1	β_2	Drug Doses and Suggested Intravenous Infusion Schemes
Phenylephrine (Neosynephrine)	+++	+	− (Little at very high doses)	−	Bolus: 3 mg/30 mL (100 μg/mL), 50–100 μg IV boluses Infusion: 10 mg/250 mL (40 μg/mL), start at 20–40 μg/min or 0.5–1 $\mu g \cdot kg^{-1} \cdot min^{-1}$ 10–100 $\mu g \cdot kg^{-1} \cdot min^{-1}$
Methoxamine (Vasoxyl)	++	+	−	−	Bolus: 20 mg/mL, 2–10 mg IV bolus
Ephedrine	+	+	+	+	Bolus: 50 mg/10 mL (5 mg/mL), 5–10 mg IV boluses effect lasts 10–15 min, ↑ CO ↑ SVR ↑ HR
	Both direct and indirect (NE release) effects				
Metaraminol (Aramine)	+	+	+	+	Bolus: 100 μg IV bolus IM: 10 mg/mL, 2–10 mg IM, effects lasts approx 1.5 h Infusion: 20–200 mg/500 mL (40–400 μg/mL), 20–500 $\mu g \cdot kg^{-1} \cdot min^{-1}$
	Similar to ephedrine initially[a]				
Mephentermine (Wyamine)	+	+	+	+	IM: 15–30 mg/mL, 15–45 mg IM, effects lasts up to 4 h
	Similar to ephedrine				
Norepinephrine[b] (Levophed)	+++	+++	+	Little	Infusion: 1 mg/250 mL (4 μg/mL), start 2 μg/min or 0.01–0.03 $\mu g \cdot kg^{-1} \cdot min^{-1}$ (max 0.1 $\mu g \cdot kg^{-1} \cdot min^{-1}$)

Note: Doses should always be checked on individual package inserts before administering drug. α_1, α_2, β_1, β_2, adrenergic receptor subtypes (the catecholamine receptors); −, no effect; +, positive effect; IM, intramuscular; IV, intravenous; max, maximum; CO, cardiac output; SVR, systemic vascular response; HR, heart rate; NE, norepinephrine.
[a] Metaraminol replaces norepinephrine in storage vesicles in the nerve terminal. Because it is a false transmitter (one tenth as effective at the α_1-adrenergic receptors as norepinephrine), after approximately 5 hours, hypotension can result.
[b] Other catecholamines with vasoconstrictor properties at high concentrations include epinephrine and dopamine (see Table 3-5)

Methoxamine. Methoxamine is an isopropylamine-type compound and a potent α_1-AR agonist with mild α_2-AR properties. Methoxamine shares many properties with phenylephrine (increases in SVR, increases in blood pressure, no myocardial β-AR activation, potential for reflex bradycardia, and vasoconstriction of many vascular beds), but it has one major difference. Once bolus methoxamine is administered (2 to 10 mg) intravenously, the clinical effect is rapidly apparent and lasts significantly longer than phenylephrine (60 to 90 minutes). This is advantageous in some settings, such as after surgical removal of a pheochromocytoma, but may last too long to be clinically useful in other settings. Methoxamine does have slightly more propensity to induce bradycardia compared with phenylephrine and, in contrast to epinephrine, slows AV conduction in the heart and does not provoke cardiac arrhythmias. Although not used frequently in the perioperative period any longer, methoxamine is still quite a useful drug and a significant part of a cardiac anesthesiologist's range of options for vasoconstrictors.

Less Common Phenylisopropylamines. Metaraminol and mephentermine are older vasoconstrictor agents that are no longer commonly used. Each acts directly as an α_1-AR agonist, has secondary effects of releasing norepinephrine at the nerve terminal, and has effects that may last several hours. The pressor response is mediated by these agents predominantly by increases in SVR but also by some increases in cardiac output. Administration is accomplished via intramuscular injection (metaraminol and mephentermine) or by slow intravenous infusion (metaraminol) (Table 3-7). Metaraminol has one additional interesting characteristic. It can replace norepinephrine in storage vesicles in the nerve terminal, where it acts as a false transmitter (one tenth as effective as α_1-ARs compared with norepinephrine). Hence, after approximately 5 hours, hypotension can result from metaraminol therapy. Metaraminol and mephentermine are primarily of historical interest.

Catecholamines

Several catecholamines, both endogenous and synthetic, are vasoconstrictors. The most striking example is norepinephrine, in which α-AR stimulation predominates over β-AR stimulation. However, compounds such as epinephrine and dopamine also have significant vasoconstrictor properties when administered at extremely high doses. The reader is referred to the discussion under Catecholamine-Mediated Inotropic Agents for details regarding the mechanism of action and clinical properties of each drug.

PROTOCOLS FOR CIRCULATORY SUPPORT

After reviewing transmitters and receptors, basic cardiovascular physiology pertinent to drug therapy, chronic perioperative cardiac medications, and intraoperative acute cardiac medications, we now discuss "practical" cardiovascular pharmacology. In considering therapy for patients with cardiovascular diseases, three caveats are immediately apparent. First, each of the two protocols presented assumes normal myocardial valves. If valvular heart disease is present, treatment protocols may be significantly altered; the reader is referred to Chapter 20 for management of these patients. Second, serum electrolytes should be within normal laboratory guideline values and the hematocrit appropriate for the clinical situation. Third, one must always check for signs of myocardial ischemia before undertaking any therapy. Electrocardiographic changes (elevation or depression of the ST segment), chest pain in an awake patient, acute changes in PAOPs, and the new onset of a V wave in the patient who is awake or anesthetized may all indicate acute myocardial ischemia. As described in the discussion under Perioperative Chronic Cardiac Medications, basic principles of myocardial oxygen supply and demand must be used as a guide to initial therapy of acute ischemia. Key determinants of myocardial oxygen demand are increased heart rate, increased afterload (mean arterial blood pressure), increased wall tension (resulting from volume loading of the left ventricle), and increased contractility. Key determinants of myocardial oxygen supply are coronary blood flow (local metabolic effects and autoregulation), decreased heart rate (to give more time for diastolic coronary perfusion), increased diastolic blood pressure (to give a higher overall coronary perfusion pressure), and the oxygen-carrying capacity of the blood. By optimizing myocardial oxygen supply and minimizing myocardial oxygen demand, ischemia can be treated. Intravenous nitroglycerin (to improve coronary blood flow and acutely unload dilated ventricles), sublingual nifedipine (if coronary vasospasm is suspected), increases in blood pressure (to increase diastolic coronary perfusion pressure), decreases in heart rate (to increase coronary perfusion time and decrease myocardial oxygen consumption), and morphine (to decrease pain and hence myocardial oxygen consumption) may all be used as therapy. If these measures are inadequate and severe ischemia persists, notification of the surgeon and rapid initiation of cardiopulmonary bypass may be necessary. Positive inotropic agents always increase myocardial oxygen consumption, whereas vasoconstrictors may increase both myocardial oxygen supply (by increasing diastolic blood pressure) and myocardial oxygen consumption (by increasing afterload). By aiming for stable hemodynamic parameters such as normal to slow heart rate, normal or slightly elevated blood pressure, and normal to slightly decreased myocardial contractility, one can optimize myocardial oxygen supply and minimize demand and therefore minimize the risk of acute intraoperative myocardial ischemia.

Hypotension and hypertension are common hemodynamic aberrations requiring therapy in patients with cardiovascular disease. Although myocardial ischemia must be immediately recognized and treated in this patient population, ironically treatment modalities for myocardial ischemia frequently rely on resolution of hypotension and/or hypertension. Therefore, general protocols for evaluating the underlying causes of hypotension and hypertension as well as appropriate drug therapies are presented. Each protocol assumes a good understanding of concepts such as Starling's law, preload, venous return, afterload, contractility, heart rate, and venous return (see discussion under Cardiac Physiology Important in Drug Therapy). All of the steps in each protocol must be done quickly and sequentially before and after each intervention, because hemodynamic changes occur rapidly in patients with cardiovascular disease, particularly in the setting of cardiac surgery and cardiopulmonary bypass. Because hypotension is a far more common condition and has many more potential sources, it is presented first. Again, each protocol assumes the absence of valvular pathology and the ability to monitor CVP and perform cardiac output measurement (e.g., presence of a pulmonary artery catheter).

Protocol 1: Hypotension

Hypotension in patients with cardiac disease is a common clinical scenario with many potential sources (see Protocol 1 flow diagram). When hypotension is first identified, it is imperative that all vasodilating anesthetic agents (i.e., volatile anesthetics) be discontinued until the hypotension has resolved. The first hemodynamic parameter to monitor in the presence of hypotension is heart rate. If the heart rate is extremely low or is no longer sinus rhythm (e.g., heart block; see Chapter 4 for correct diagnosis of bradyarrhythmias), then atrial or AV sequential pacing may provide coordinated contraction of the atrium and ventricle at an increased heart rate (e.g., heart rate of 90 beats/minute); this therapy alone may be enough to resolve hypotension, particularly in the initial post–cardiopulmonary bypass period. Atropine (0.4 to 1.0 mg intravenous) is sometimes administered to patients with hypotension and severe sinus bradycardia, but this drug should generally be avoided in patients with myocardial ischemia, because uncontrolled rapid heart rates (which may precipitate myocardial ischemia) may result. If the heart rate is very rapid in the presence of hypotension, the rhythm should be evaluated carefully. Ventricular fibrillation with no blood pressure clearly requires immediate defibrillation and CPR. If a supraventricular tachycardia or ventricular tachycardia is present, cardioversion should be seriously considered. If cardioversion is unsuccessful in the presence of a rhythm such as atrial fibrillation with a rapid ventricular response, therapy with antiarrhythmic agents should be considered (see Chapter 4). Sinus tachycardia may simply be a reflex due to hypovolemia. Therefore, upon resolution of a severely slow or rapid heart rate, presence of a normal heart rate, or presence of a rapid sinus tachycardia, the next step should be evaluation of myocardial preload.

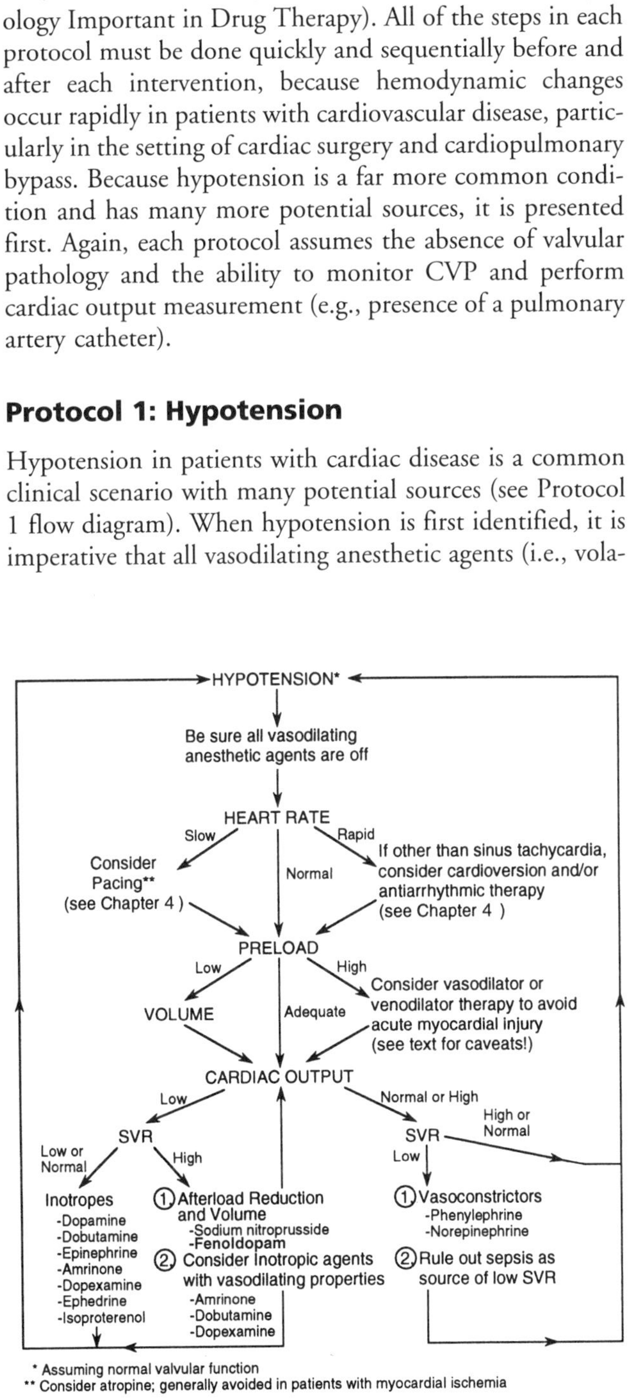

PROTOCOL 1.

Myocardial preload refers to the filling of the ventricles. Venous return and overall fluid balance are important determinants of myocardial preload. Because according to Starling's law, increased stretch of the myocardial provides more efficient forward flow of blood from the heart (see discussion under Cardiac Physiology Important in Drug Therapy), preload is a significant determinant of blood pressure. However, one must not overfill the heart, because acute ventricular dilation can injure myocardial tissue and abruptly and drastically decrease myocardial contractility. Because preload is critically dependent on venous return, which is dependent on venous (and arterial) tone, any vascular changes can potentially alter myocardial preload. Hence, it is absolutely critical that preload be reassessed frequently, particularly before and after any intervention, whether with volume, pacing, or pharmacologic agents. If in the presence of hypotension, preload is low, then volume in the form of intravenous fluids (or blood components when indicated) should be administered. Because many measurements of volume are made from the right side of the heart, in acute right ventricular failure it is possible to have high right-sided filling pressures reflected on the CVP but low left ventricular preload. Therefore, one must assess left ventricular preload using the PAOP (see Chapter 8), left atrial pressure catheter, or transesophageal echocardiography (see

Chapter 8) if there is a question in this regard. In the presence of very high ventricular preload, it is necessary to consider vasodilator (or venodilator) therapy to avoid acute myocardial injury from overdistention. However, giving vasodilators to a patient who is already hypotensive may aggravate the hypotension and therefore may not be the therapy of choice. Improving myocardial contractility may be a far more effective therapy. However, frequently a combination of acutely unloading the ventricle with concurrent administration of inotropic agents may be a solution for this problem. Hence, evaluation of cardiac output is the logical next step.

Cardiac output is an important branch point in the therapy of hypotension. If cardiac output is normal or high, the next step is determination of the calculated SVR. If SVR is low in the face of normal or high cardiac output, vasoconstrictor agents such as phenylephrine and norepinephrine are the agents of choice. It is necessary to rule out the presence of sepsis at this point, because decreased SVR with normal to elevated cardiac output is a common manifestation of sepsis. If SVR is normal or high (or once vasoconstrictor agents are given in the low SVR branch point), one must return to the beginning of the protocol and reassess each hemodynamic parameter.

If cardiac output is low, SVR should be calculated. If SVR is low or normal in the face of adequate heart rate and preload, hypotension is solely attributable to myocardial pump failure. Positive inotropic agents such as dopamine, dobutamine, epinephrine, amrinone, or ephedrine (in less critically ill patients) are appropriate therapies in the face of pure myocardial pump failure. If SVR is high, however, two potential problems may exist. In the presence of severely elevated SVR, myocardial failure may simply be due to acutely elevated afterload with no problems with intrinsic myocardial contractility. In this case, one must decrease the afterload with vasodilating agents such as sodium nitroprusside (concurrent with volume replacement). Then cardiac output should be reevaluated. If decreased cardiac output is solely due to an elevated SVR, once SVR is normalized with concurrent volume replacement, cardiac output should return to normal. If cardiac output is still depressed, inotropic support is required. If myocardial pump failure is suspected in the presence of an elevated SVR, then from the beginning, an inotropic agent with vasodilating properties, such as amrinone or dobutamine, could be considered. As with every branch point of this decision tree, once a therapy is instituted, hemodynamic parameters should be quickly reassessed from the beginning of the protocol to gauge effectiveness of therapy and/or before another intervention is contemplated.

Protocol 2: Hypertension

Hypertension in patients with cardiac disease is another common clinical situation with many potential sources (see

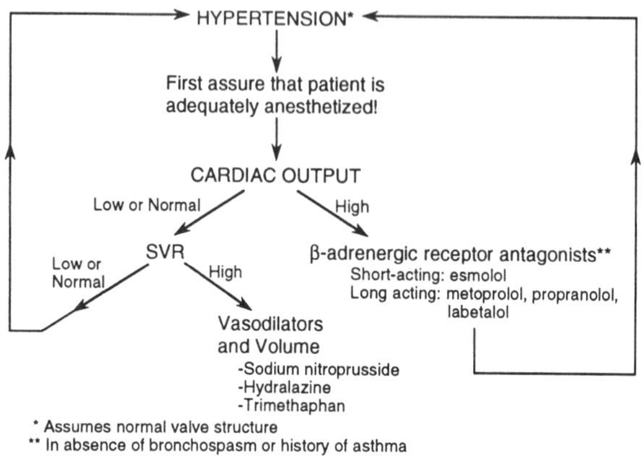

PROTOCOL 2.

Protocol 2 flow diagram). The first step in the treatment of hypertension is to ensure that the patient is adequately anesthetized. Frequently simply deepening the level of anesthesia is sufficient to resolve hypertensive episodes in this patient population. However, in many situations, anesthesia is adequate but hypertension persists. In this setting, the most important hemodynamic variable to check is cardiac output. Often after coronary revascularization surgery, when the heart is provided with oxygen more abundantly than ever before in recent history, the response (particularly in young otherwise healthy patients) by healthy myocardium may be an acutely increased cardiac output. Although this makes separation from cardiopulmonary bypass relatively easy, it can become a problem by provoking hypertension and if allowed to continue, may eventually lead to high-output myocardial failure. Hence, if an extremely high cardiac output is present (i.e., 8 to 10 L/minute or more), it is prudent to decrease myocardial contractility with β-adrenergic antagonists. β-AR antagonists should not be used (or short-acting agents used with extreme caution) in patients with a history of bronchospasm or asthma. Esmolol is a short-acting β-AR antagonist given by infusion; longer acting agents include metoprolol, propranolol, and labetalol.

If in the presence of hypertension, cardiac output is low or normal, then SVR should be calculated. If SVR is elevated, vasodilators such as sodium nitroprusside, hydralazine, trimethaphan, or fenoldopam are appropriate therapies administered concurrently with volume. If a low or normal SVR is found, the anesthetic state and cardiac output should be reassessed, because hypertension is rarely manifest in the presence of a low to normal cardiac output and low to normal SVR. As for every branch point of the decision tree, once a therapy is instituted, hemodynamic parameters should be quickly reassessed from the beginning of the protocol to gauge effectiveness of therapy and/or before another intervention is contemplated.

CONCLUSION

Cardiovascular pharmacology provides challenges to every clinician, because effective therapy requires an intimate knowledge of cardiovascular physiology, receptor pharmacology, and clinical medicine. Therefore, this chapter has reviewed neurotransmitters and receptors, basic cardiovascular physiology pertinent to drug therapy, chronic perioperative cardiac medications, intraoperative acute cardiac medications, and "practical" cardiovascular pharmacology. Patients with cardiovascular disease provide challenges to the anesthesiologist, whether they come to the operating room for cardiac or noncardiac surgery. Armed with an understanding of basic cardiovascular principles and an intimate knowledge of cardiovascular drugs, the anesthesiologist can make a great difference in medical management of these patients. Although rational cardiovascular drug therapy is essential, an understanding of when to use such agents is far more important and part of the art of anesthesiology.

REFERENCES

1. Lincoln J, Burnstock G. Neural-endothelial interactions in control of local blood flow. In: Warren JB, ed. The endothelium: an introduction to current research. New York: Wiley-Liss, 1990:21.
2. Morris AJ, Malbon CC. Physiological regulation of G protein–linked signaling. *Physiol Rev* 1999;79:1373.
3. Meij JT. Regulation of G protein function: implications for heart disease. *Mol Cell Biochem* 1996;157:31.
4. Somlyo AP, Wu X, Walker LA, et al. Pharmacomechanical coupling: the role of calcium, G-proteins, kinases and phosphatases. *Rev Physiol Biochem Pharmacol* 1999;134:201.
5. Berkowitz DE, Schwinn DA. New advances in receptor pharmacology. *Curr Opin Anaesth* 1991;4:486.
6. Franks NP, Lieb WR. Which molecular targets are most relevant to general anaesthesia? *Toxicol Lett* 1998;100:1.
7. Limbird LE. *Cell surface receptors: a short course on theory and methods.* Boston: Martinus Nijhoff Publishing, 1986.
8. Strange PG. G-Protein coupled receptors: conformations and states. *Biochem Pharmacol* 1999;58:1081.
9. Schwinn DA, Caron MG, Lefkowitz RJ. The β-adrenergic receptor as a model for molecular structure-function relationships in G protein–coupled receptors. In: Fozzard HA, Jennings RB, Katz AM, et al., eds. *The heart and cardiovascular system,* 2nd ed. New York: Raven Press, 1992:1657.
10. Schoneberg T, Schultz G, Gudermann T. Structural basis of G protein–coupled receptor function. *Mol Cell Endocrinol* 1999; 151:181.
11. Lefkowitz RJ, Caron MG. Adrenergic receptors: models for the study of receptors coupled to guanine nucleotide regulatory proteins. *J Biol Chem* 1988;263:4993.
12. Ahlquist RP. A study of adrenotropic receptors. *Am J Physiol* 1948;153:586.
13. Lands AM, Arnold A, McAuliff JP, et al. Differentiation of receptor systems activated by sympathomimetic amines. *Nature* 1967;214:597.
14. Lands AM, Luduena FP, Buzzo HJ. Differentiation of receptors responsive to isoproterenol. *Life Sci* 1967;6:2241.
15. Insel PA. *Adrenergic receptors in man.* New York: Marcel Dekker Inc, 1987.
16. Demers C, McKelvie RS, Yusuf S. The role of digitalis in the treatment of heart failure. *Coron Artery Dis* 1999;10:353.
17. Terra SG, Washam JB, Dunham GD, et al. Therapeutic range of digoxin's efficacy in heart failure: what is the evidence? *Pharmacotherapy* 1999;19:1123.
18. Shull MM, Lingrel JB. Multiple genes encode the human Na^+,K^+-ATPase catalytic subunit. *Proc Natl Acad Sci USA* 1987;84:4039.
19. Akera T, Ng Y-C. Minireview: digitalis sensitivity of Na^+,K^+-ATPase myocytes and the heart. *Life Sci* 1991;48:97.
20. Kranzhofer R, Haass M, Kurz T, et al. Effect of digitalis glycosides on norepinephrine release in the heart: dual mechanism of action. *Circ Res* 1992;68:1628.
21. Indolfi C, Piscione F, Russolillo E, et al. Digitalis-induced vasoconstriction of normal and atherosclerotic epicardial coronary arteries. *Am J Cardiol* 1991;68:1274.
22. Pentel PR, Salerno DM. Cardiac drug toxicity: digitalis glycosides and calcium-channel and β-blocking agents. *Med J Aust* 1990;152:88.
23. Smith TW. Review of clinical experience with digoxin immune Fab (ovine). *Am J Emerg Med* 1991;9:1.
24. Hauptman PJ, Kelly RA. Digitalis. *Circulation* 1999;99:1265
25. Snyder SH, Bredt DS. Biological roles of nitric oxide. *Sci Am* 1992;May:68.
26. Johns RA. EDRF/nitric oxide: the endogenous nitrovasodilator and a new cellular messenger. *Anesthesiology* 1991;75:927.
27. Moncada S, Palmer RMJ, Higgs EA. Nitric oxide: physiology, pathophysiology and pharmacology. *Pharm Rev* 1991;43:109.
28. Hughes MN. Relationships between nitric oxide, nitroxyl ion, nitrosonium cation and peroxynitrite. *Biochim Biophys Acta* 1999;1411:263.
29. Tousoulis D, Davies GJ, Toutouzas PC. Vasomotion of coronary arteries: from nitrates to nitric oxide. *Cardiovasc Drugs Ther* 1999;13:295.
30. Gruetter CA, Gruetter DY, Lyon JE, et al. Relationship between cyclic guanosine 38:58-monophosphate formation and relaxation of coronary arterial smooth muscle by glyceryl trinitrate, nitroprusside, nitrite and nitric oxide: effects of methylene blue and methemoglobin. *J Pharm Exp Ther* 1981;219:181.
31. Moncada S, Palmer RMJ, Higgs EA. Nitric oxide: the endogenous regulator of vascular tone. In: Warren JB, ed. *The endothelium: an introduction to current research.* New York: Wiley-Liss, 1990:1.
32. Leopold JA, Loscalzo J. New developments in nitrosovasodilator therapy. *Vasc Med* 1997;2:190.
33. Parker JD, Parker JO. Nitrate therapy for stable angina pectoris. *N Engl J Med* 1998;338:520.
34. Olsen EG, Hamilton SF, Thadani U. Beta-adrenergic antagonists. In: Abrams J, Pepine CJ, Thadani U, eds. Medical therapy of ischemic heart disease: nitrates, beta blockers, and calcium antagonists. Boston: Little, Brown and Company, 1992: 137.
35. Gonzalez Maqueda I. Treatment of chronic stable angina with carvedilol: a multiple-action neurohormonal antagonist. A review of clinical trials. *J Int Med Res* 1998;26:107.
36. Teerlink JR, Massie BM. Beta-adrenergic blocker mortality trials in congestive heart failure. *Am J Cardiol* 1999;84:94R.
37. Carson PE. Beta blocker treatment in heart failure. *Progr Cardiovasc Dis* 1999;41:301.
38. Lubsen J. The calcium channel antagonist debate: recent developments. *Eur Heart J* 1998;19:I3.

39. Epstein M. The calcium antagonist controversy: the emerging importance of drug formulation as a determinant risk.
40. Epstein M. Calcium antagonists and renal protection: emerging perspectives. *J Hypertens* 1998;16[Suppl]:S17
41. Abernethy DR, Schwartz JB. Calcium-antagonist drugs. *N Engl J Med* 1999;341:1447.
42. Kern MJ. Perspective: the cellular influences of calcium antagonists on systemic and coronary hemodynamics. *Am J Cardiol* 1992;69:3B.
43. Smiley RM, Kwatra MM, Schwinn DA. New developments in adrenergic receptor pharmacology: molecular mechanisms and clinical relevance. *J Cardiovasc Anesth* 1998;12:80.
44. Motulsky JH, Snavely MD, Hughes RJ, et al. Interaction of verapamil and other calcium channel blockers with α_1- and α_2-adrenergic receptors. *Circ Res* 1983;52:226.
45. Cavero I, Shepperson N, Lefevre-Borg F, et al. Differential inhibition of vascular smooth muscle responses to α_1- and α_2-adrenoceptor agonists by diltiazem and verapamil. *Circ Res* 1983; 52[Suppl]:69.
46. Kenny D, Pelc LR, Brooks HL, et al. Calcium channel modulation of α_1- and α_2-adrenergic pressor responses in conscious and anesthetized dogs. *Anesthesiology* 1990;72:874.
47. Massagee JT, McIntyre RW, Kates RA, et al. Effects of preoperative calcium entry blocker therapy on α-adrenergic responsiveness in patients undergoing coronary revascularization. *Anesthesiology* 1987;67:485.
48. Schwinn DA, McIntyre RW, Hawkins BS, et al. α_1-Adrenergic responsiveness during coronary artery bypass surgery: effect of preoperative ejection fraction. *Anesthesiology* 1988;69:206.
49. Frohlich ED. Angiotensin converting enzyme inhibitors: present and future. *Hypertension* 1989;13:I125.
50. Luzier AB, DiTusa L. Underutilization of ACE inhibitors in heart failure. *Pharmacotherapy* 1999;19:1296.
51. Melby JC. Angiotensin-converting enzyme in cardiovascular and adrenal tissues and implications for successful blood pressure management. *Am J Cardiol* 1992;69:2C.
52. Mirenda JV, Grissom TE. Anesthetic implications of the renin-angiotensin system and angiotensin-converting enzyme inhibitors. *Anesth Analg* 1991;72:667.
53. Frishman WH. Comparative pharmacokinetic and clinical profiles of angiotensin-converting enzyme inhibitors and calcium antagonists in systemic hypertension. *Am J Cardiol* 1992;69: 17C.
54. Banas JS. Effects of inhibitors of angiotensin-converting enzyme on regional hemodynamics. *Am J Cardiol* 1992;69:40C.
55. Williams GH. Converting-enzyme inhibitors in the treatment of hypertension. *N Engl J Med* 1988;319:1517.
56. Siragy H. Angiotensin II receptor blockers: review of the binding characteristics. *Am J Cardiol* 1999;84:3S
57. Colson P, Ryckwaert F, Coriat P. Renin angiotensin system antagonists and anesthesia. *Anesth Analg* 1999;89:1143.
58. Pitt B, Zannad F, Remme WJ, et al. The effect of spironolactone on morbidity and mortality in patients with severe heart failure. *N Engl J Med* 1999;341:709.
59. Breyer J, Jacobson HR. Molecular mechanisms of diuretic agents. *Annu Rev Med* 1990;41:265.
60. Lant A. Diuretics drugs: progress in clinical pharmacology. *Drugs* 1986;31:40.
61. Hill AV. Heat of shortening and dynamic constants of muscle. *Proc R Soc London Ser* 1938; B230:163.
62. Cheng EY. Vasopressors and inotropes. *Anesth Rev* 1989;16: 17.
63. Siegl PKS. Overview of cardiac inotropic mechanisms. *J Cardiovasc Pharmacol* 1986;8:S1.
64. Notterman DA. Inotropic agents: catecholamines, digoxin, amrinone. *Crit Care Clin* 1991;7:583.
65. Coodley E. Newer drug therapy for congestive heart failure. *Arch Intern Med* 1999;159:1177.
66. Colucci WS, Wright RF, Braunwald E. New positive inotropic agents in the treatment of congestive heart failure: mechanism of action and recent clinical developments. *N Engl J Med* 1986; 314:290.
67. Grupp G. Selective updates on mechanisms of action of positive inotropic agents. *Mol Cell Biochem* 1987;76:97.
68. Stanford GG. Use of inotropic agents in critical illness. *Surg Clin North Am* 1991;71:683.
69. Merin RG. Basic physiology and pharmacology of cardiovascular function. *J Cardiac Surg* 1990;5:266.
70. Endoh M. The effects of various drugs on the myocardial inotropic response. *Gen Pharmacol* 1995;26:1.
71. Colucci WS. Positive inotropic/vasodilator agents. *Cardiol Clin* 1989;7:131.
72. Butterworth J. Selecting an intrope for the cardiac surgery patient. *J Cardiothorac Vasc Anesth* 1993;7:26.
73. Schlepper M, Thormann J, Kremer P, et al. Present use of positive inotropic drugs in heart failure. *J Cardiovasc Pharmacol* 1989;14:S9.
74. Sumikawa K, Ishizaka N, Suzaki M. Arrhythmogenic plasma levels of epinephrine during halothane, enflurane, and pentobarbital anesthesia in the dog. *Anesthesiology* 1983;58:322.
75. Ghosh S, Gray B, Oduro A, et al. Dopexamine hydrochloride: pharmacology and use in low cardiac output states. *J Cardiothorac Vasc Anesth* 1991;5:382.
76. Szerlip HM. Renal-dose dopamine: fact and fiction. *Ann Intern Med* 1991;115:153.
77. Brown L. Pharmacological responses to dopamine in isolated guinea-pig cardiovascular tissues: mechanisms of action. *Arch Int Pharmacodyn Ther* 1990;308:47.
78. Bhatt-Mehta V, Nahata MC. Dopamine and dobutamine in pediatric therapy. *Pharmacotherapy* 1989;9:305.
79. Bennett ED. Dopexamine: much more than a vasoactive agent. *Crit Care Med* 1998;26:1621.
80. Power DA, Duggan J, Brady HR. Renal-dose (low-dose) dopamine for the treatment of sepsis-related and other forms of acute renal failure: ineffective and probably dangerous. *Clin Exp Pharmacol Physiol* 1999;26[Suppl]:S23.
81. Schiebinger RJ, Baker MZ, Linden J. The effect of adrenergic and muscarinic cholinergic agonists on atrial natriuretic peptide secretion by isolated rat atria: a potential role of the autonomic nervous system in modulating atrial natriuretic peptide secretion. *J Clin Invest* 1987;80:1687.
82. Majerus TC, Dasta JF, Bauman JL, et al. Dobutamine: ten years later. *Pharmacotherapy* 1989;9:245.
83. Leier CV, Binkley PF. Parenteral inotropic support for advanced congestive heart failure. *Prog Cardiovasc Dis* 1998;41:207.
84. Kaul S. Dobutamine echocardiography for determining myocardial viability after reperfusion: experimental and clinical observations. *Eur Heart J* 1995;16[Suppl]:M17.
85. Foulds RA. Clinical development of dopexamine hydrochloride and an overview of its hemodynamic effects. *Am J Cardiol* 1988; 62:41C.
86. Boachie-Ansa G, Kane KA, Parat JR. The cardiac electrophysiologic effects of dopexamine under normal and simulated ischaemic conditions. *J Mol Cell Cardiol* 1989;21:S23.

87. Bennett ED. Dopexamine: much more than a vasoactive agent. *Crit Care Med* 1998;26:1621.
88. Ghosh S, Gray B, Oduro A, et al. Dopexamine hydrochloride: pharmacology and use in low cardiac output states. *J Cardiothorac Vasc Anesth* 1991;5:382.
89. Mathur VS, Swan SK, Lambrecht LJ, et al. The effects of fenoldopam, a selective dopamine receptor agonist, on systemic and renal hemodynamics in normotensive subjects. *Crit Care Med* 1999; 279:1832.
90. Oparil S, Aronson S, Deeb GM, et al. Fenoldopam: a new parenteral antihypertensive: consensus roundtable on the management of perioperative hypertension and hypertensive crises. *Am J Hypertens* 1999;12:653.
91. Frishman WH, Hotchkiss H. Selective and nonselective dopamine receptor agonists: an innovative approach to cardiovascular disease treatment. *Am Heart J* 1996;132:861.
92. Post JB IV, Frishman WH. Fenoldopam: a new dopamine agonist for the treatment of hypertensive urgencies and emergencies. *J Clin Pharmacol* 1998;38:2.
93. Morgan P. The role of vasopressors in the management of hypotension induced by spinal and epidural anaesthesia. *Can J Anaesth* 1994;41:404.
94. Aikawa J, Koike K, Takayanagi I. Vascular smooth muscle relaxation by α_1-adrenoceptor blocking action of denopamine in isolated rabbit aorta. *J Cardiovasc Pharmacol* 1991;17:440.
95. Inamasu M, Totsuka T, Ikeo T, et al. β_1-Adrenergic selectivity of the new cardiotonic agent denopamine in its stimulating effects on adenylate cyclase. *Biochem Pharmacol* 1987;36: 1947.
96. Endoh M. The effects of various drugs on the myocardial inotropic response. *Gen Pharmacol* 1995;26:1.
97. Shipley JB, Tolman D, Hastillo A, et al. Milrinone: basic and clinical pharmacology and acute and chronic management. *Am J Med Sci* 1996;311:286.
98. Goenen M. Historical perspectives and update of amrinone. *J Cardiovasc Anesth* 1989;3:15.
99. Baim DS. Effect of phosphodiesterase inhibition on myocardial oxygen consumption and coronary blood flow. *Am J Cardiol* 1989;63:23A.
100. Makela VHM, Kapur PA. New drugs for the treatment of heart failure: amrinone and milrinone. *Semin Anesth* 1988;7:92.
101. Packer M, Carver JR, Rodeheffer RJ, et al. Effect of oral milrinone on mortality in severe chronic heart failure. *N Engl J Med* 1991;325:1468.
102. Remme WJ. Vasodilator therapy for heart failure. Early, late, or not at all? *Circulation* 1993;87:IV97.
103. Zaloga GP, Strickland RA, Butterworth JF, et al. Calcium attenuates epinephrine's β-adrenergic effects in postoperative heart surgery patients. *Circulation* 1990;81:196.
104. Castillo CR, Harringer W, Warshaw AL, et al. Risk factors for pancreatic cellular injury after cardiopulmonary bypass. *N Engl J Med* 1991;325:382.
105. Leach JK, Priola DV, Grimes LA, et al. Shortening deactivation of cardiac muscle: physiological mechanisms and clinical implications. *J Investig Med* 1999;47:369.
106. Teramura S, Yamakado T. Calcium sensitizaers in chronic heart failure: inotropic interventions-reservation to preservation. *Cardiologia* 1998;43:375.
107. Nielsen-Kudsk JE, Aldershvile J. Will calcium sensitizers play a role in the treatment of heart failure? *J Cardiovasc Pharamcol* 1995;26:S77.
108. Kirsten R, Nelson K, Kirsten D, et al. Clinical pharmacokinetics of vasodilators. Part I. *Clin Pharmacokinet* 1998;34:457.
109. Kirsten R, Nelson K, Kirsten D, et al. Nitroprusside and urapidil, and vasodil in general: clinical pharmacokinetics of vasodilators. Part II. *Clin Pharmacokinet* 1998;35:9.
110. Ikeda S, Schweiss JF, Frank PA, et al. *In vitro* cyanide release from sodium nitroprusside. *Anesthesiology* 1987;66:381.
111. Arnold WP, Longnecker DE, Epstein RM. Photodegradation of sodium nitroprusside: biologic activity and cyanide release. *Anesthesiology* 1984;61:254.
112. Vesey CJ, Krapez JR, Variey JG, et al. The antidotal action of thiosulfate following acute nitroprusside infusion in dogs. *Anesthesiology* 1985;62:415.
113. Sklar GS, Lanks KW. Effects of trimethaphan and sodium nitroprusside on hydrolysis of succinylcholine *in vitro*. *Anesthesiology* 1977;47:31.
114. Sever PS. α_1-Blockers in hypertension. *Curr Med Res Opin* 1999;15:95.
115. Dooley M, Goa KL. Urapidil. A reappraisal of its use in the management of hypertension. *Drugs* 1998;56:929.
116. Rudner XL, Berkowitz DE, Booth JV, et al. Subtype specific regulation of human vascular α_1-adrenergic receptors by vessel bed and age. *Circulation* 1999;100:2336.
117. McIntyre RW, Schwinn DA. Atrial natriuretic peptide. *J Cardiothorac Anesth* 1989;3:91.
118. Chinkers M, Garbers DL, Chang M-S, et al. A membrane form of guanylate cyclase is an atrial natriuretic peptide receptor. *Nature* 1989;338:78.
119. Abramson BL, Ando S, Notarius CF, et al. Effect of atrial natriuretic peptide on muscle sympathetic activity and its reflex control in human heart failure. *Circulation* 1999;99:1810.
120. Papadopoulos CL, Kokkas B, Kotridis P, et al. Effect of the β_1-blocker/β_2-agonist celiprolol on atrial natriuretic peptide plasma levels in hypertensive patients. *Cardiovasc Drugs Ther* 1998;12:345.
121. Steudel W, Hurford WE, Zapol WM. Inhaled nitric oxide: basic biology and clinical applications. *Anesthesiology* 1999;91: 1090
122. Ullrich R, Lorber C, Roder G, et al. Controlled airway pressure therapy, nitric oxide inhalation, prone position, and extracorporeal membrane oxygenation (ECMO) as components of an integrated approach to ARDS. *Anesthesiology* 1999;91:1577.
123. Dent CL, Perez Fontan JJ. Long-term therapy for pulmonary hypertension in children. *Curr Opin Pulm Med* 1999;5: 390.
124. Mustafa SS, Rivers RJ, Frame MDS. Microcirculatory basis for nonuniform flow delivery with intravenous nitroprusside. *Anesthesiology* 1999;91:723.
125. Curry SC, Arnold-Capell P. Nitroprusside, nitroglycerin, and angiotensin-converting enzyme inhibitors. *Crit Care Clin* 1991; 7:555.
126. Lichtenthal PR, Rossi EC, Louis G, et al. Dose-related prolongation of the bleeding time by intravenous nitroglycerin. *Anesth Analg* 1985;64:30.
127. Yanagisawa M, Kurihara H, Kimura S, et al. A novel potent constrictor peptide produced by vascular endothelial cells. *Nature* 1988;332:411.
128. Hiroshi A, Hori S, Aramori I, et al. Cloning and expression of a cDNA encoding an endothelin receptor. *Nature* 1990;348: 730.
129. Cohn JN. Is there a role for endothelin in the natural history of heart failure? *Circulation* 1996;94:604.
130. Sam F, Colucci WS. Role of endothelin 1 in myocardial failure. *Proc Assoc Am Physicians* 1999;111:417.
131. Barton M, Luscher TF. Endothelin antagonists for hypertension and renal disease. *Curr Opin Nephrol Hypertens* 1999;8: 549.

132. Miyauchi T, Katsutoshi G. Heart failure and endothelin receptor antagonists. *Trends Pharmacol Sci* 1999;20:210.
133. Langleben D, Barst RJ, Badesch D, et al. Continuous infusion of epoprostenol improves the net balance between pulmonary endothelin-1 clearance and release in primary pulmonary hypertension. *Circulation* 1999;99:3266.
134. Deswal A, Bozkurt B, Seta Y, et al. Safety and efficacy of a soluble p75 tumor necrosis factor receptor (enbrel, etanercept) in patients with advanced heart failure. *Circulation* 1999;99:3224.
135. Moser M. *Clinical management of hypertension,* 4th ed. Caddo, OK: Professional Communications Inc, 1999:240.

Cardiac Anesthesia: Principles and Clinical Practice, Second Edition, edited by Fawzy G. Estafanous, Paul G. Barash, and J.G. Reves. Lippincott Williams & Wilkins, Philadelphia © 2001.

4

PHARMACOLOGIC MANAGEMENT OF ARRHYTHMIAS

JEFFREY R. BALSER

Arrhythmias are a significant source of morbidity in the period surrounding major surgical procedures, and arrhythmia management strategies in perioperative patients are distinctive. Although arrhythmia management in surgical patients is influenced heavily by the clinical literature in nonsurgical patients, recent evidence linking arrhythmias to the length of hospital stay and the cost of surgery has motivated new clinical investigation specifically aimed at the perioperative period. At the same time, our emerging understanding of the relevant molecular targets for manipulating cardiac excitability is rapidly expanding the range of options for antiarrhythmic therapy.

This chapter first reviews the basic molecular pharmacology of cardiac excitability (Electropharmacology and Molecular Targets section), with specific emphasis on the latest discoveries that are unraveling the molecular targets of antiarrhythmic agents. The section provides a framework for understanding how pharmacologic modulation of specific molecular targets in turn alters cardiac excitability. In the sections that follow, clinical management strategies for perioperative supraventricular arrhythmias and ventricular arrhythmias are discussed in the context of this molecular framework.

ELECTROPHARMACOLOGY AND MOLECULAR TARGETS

Ion Channel Mechanisms

The antiarrhythmic agents act primarily through suppressing the activity of cardiac ion channels. These drug targets fall into three general classes based on the cation they principally conduct: sodium (Na), calcium (Ca), and potassium (K) channels. As shown in Fig. 4-1, these distinct classes of cation channels possess striking structural homology and are members of a common gene family. This structural similarity among the antiarrhythmic drug targets underlies much of the "class overlap" exhibited by most of the commonly used agents.

Given the substantial overlapping clinical effects of most antiarrhythmic agents, it is more useful to classify them according to their ion channel targets (Table 4-1) (1). With an increasing understanding of ion channels as antiarrhythmic drug targets, the classic drug "classes" originally based on *in vivo* electrophysiologic effects (the electrocardiogram [ECG])(2) are now thought of as discrete functional activities resulting directly from blocking specific ion channel targets. The classification scheme provided (Table 4-1) is not exhaustive and emphasizes the commercially available antiarrhythmic agents available for use in intravenous form. Although a detailed discussion of the functional effects of suppressing particular ion channel targets follows, it should be noted that many agents fall under multiple categories. Hence, many antiarrhythmic drugs that block Na channels and slow cardiac conduction (the so-called local anesthetics) also block Ca channels and K channels at therapeutically relevant concentrations, and therefore have the potential for myriad unwanted electrophysiologic side effects (e.g., negative inotropic effects and the long-QT syndrome). As an extreme case, although traditionally grouped as a class III agent, it is clear that amiodarone has electropharmacologic effects linked to suppression of all three classes of ion channels.

Drug effects on the surface ECG can be predicted from their effects on the cardiac action potential, which in turn results from activity toward the members of the specific ion channel classes. The action potential represents the time-varying transmembrane potential of the myocardial cell during the cardiac cycle. In this context, the ECG should be viewed as the temperospatial average of the action potentials arising from all myocardial cells and is skewed toward the activity of the left ventricle due to its greater overall mass. Figure 4-2 examines some of the principal ion channel currents that compose the cardiac action potential, as well as linkages between the action potential and the surface ECG.

The trajectory of the cardiac action potential is divided

J.R. Balser: Departments of Anesthesiology and Pharmacology, Vanderbilt University School of Medicine, Nashville, Tennessee 37232-6602

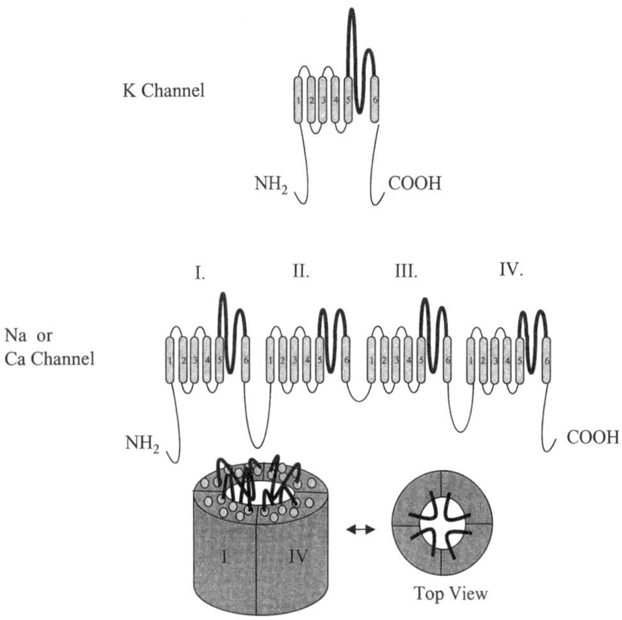

FIGURE 4-1. Schematic depiction of the topology of the three principle voltage-gated cation channels. **Top:** Predicted transmembrane topology of the largest family of voltage-gated K channels (known as Shaker), with six transmembrane repeats. The channel assembles as a tetrad of four identical domains. **Middle:** Topology of the voltage-gated Na and Ca channels, which are translated as a single four-domain protein, each domain resembling a single subunit of the putative K channel. **Bottom:** Three-dimensional schematic emphasizing the tetrad structure of the voltage-gated ion channels. The extracellular sequences connecting the fifth and sixth membrane spanning regions in each domain (*shown in bold*) partly line the ion channel pore and are known as P loops (for ion permeation). (From Balser JR. Structure and function of the cardiac sodium channels. *Cardiovasc Res* 1999; 42:328, with permission.)

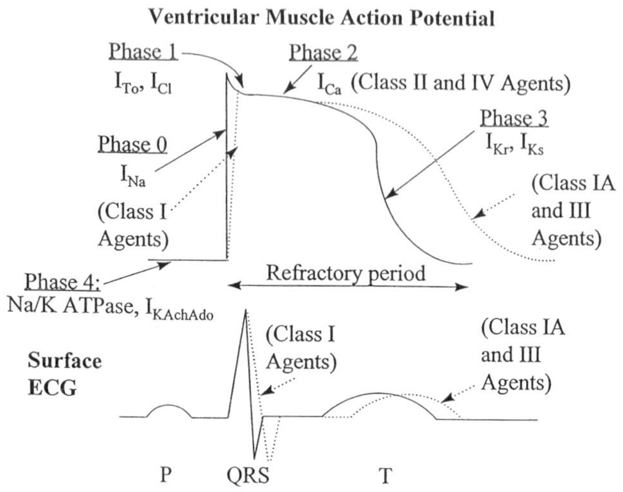

FIGURE 4-2. The action potential in ventricular muscle and its temporal relationship with the surface electrocardiogram (ECG). The QRS interval is related to the rate of upstroke of the action potential, which partly determines the rate of impulse conduction through the ventricular myocardium. The QT interval is related to the length of the action potential (the absolute refractory period). The phases of the action potential are indicated, as are the major ionic currents that flow during each phase. The dotted lines indicate anticipated effects on the action potential and ECG when drugs suppress either the Na current (class IA or IB) or the K current (class IA or III). (From Balser JR. Perioperative management of arrhythmias. In: Barash PG, Fleisher, LA, Prough DS, eds. *Problems in anesthesia,* 2nd ed, vol 10. Philadelphia: Lippincott–Raven Publishers, 1998:199, with permission.)

TABLE 4-1. ANTIARRHYTHMIC AGENTS PRINCIPALLY USED IN ANESTHESIOLOGY AND CRITICAL CARE, LISTED BY THEIR MOLECULAR TARGET

Receptor	Class[a]	Drugs
Na and K Channels	IA	Procainamide, quinidine disopyramide, amiodarone,
Na Channels	IB	Lidocaine, phenytoin, mexiletine,[b] tocainide[b]
β Receptors	II	Esmolol, amiodarone, propranolol, atenolol, sotalol[b]
K Channels	III	Bretylium, ibutilide, sotalol,[b] dofetilide[b]
Ca Channels	IV	Verapamil, diltiazem, amiodarone

[a] Classification by functional effect according to the Vaughan Williams scheme is also provided (from Vaughan Williams EM. A classification of antiarrhythmic actions reassessed after a decade of new drugs. *J Clin Pharmacol* 1984;24:129).
[b] Only available commercially in oral form.
Source: From Balser JR. Perioperative management of arrhythmias. In: Barash PG, Fleisher LA, Prough DS, eds. *Problems in anesthesia,* 2nd ed, vol 10. Philadelphia: Lippincott–Raven Publishers, 1998:199, with permission.

into five distinct phases, which reflect changes in the predominant ionic current flowing during the cardiac cycle (Fig. 4-2). These ionic currents arise from movement of cations through the ion channels down their electrochemical gradients. Because Na^+ and Ca^{2+} ion concentrations are much higher outside the cell than inside, these ions move inwardly through their respective channels to depolarize the cell membrane. Conversely, the K^+ ion concentration is higher inside the cell than outside, so these ions move outwardly through K channels to repolarize the cell membrane back to its resting potential. "Phase 0" is the initial period of depolarization, which describes the rapid upstroke of the cardiac action potential. In the atria and ventricles, this depolarization is produced by sodium current (I_{Na}) through Na channels. The rate of upstroke of the action potential determines the rate of impulse conduction through ventricular tissue and therefore generally determines the length of the QRS complex on the surface ECG. Hence, drugs that suppress Na current (class I agents, Fig. 4-2, Table 4-1) in the ventricle slow myocardial conduction and prolong the QRS complex.

In atrioventricular (AV) and sinoatrial (SA) nodal cells, phase 0 is produced by calcium current (I_{Ca}) through L-type Ca channels. Because I_{Ca} activates more slowly than I_{Na}, the upstroke of the SA and AV nodal action potential is delayed, and conduction velocity through the AV node is relatively slow (and modulates the PR interval). This difference in phase 0 among the cardiac tissues importantly determines drug selection for many arrhythmia syndromes. For example, during supraventricular arrhythmias, atrial impulses may be generated at rates exceeding 400 beats/minute. In this setting, slowing conduction through the AV node via Ca channel blockade is of primary importance to limit the rate of ventricular stimulation, thus preventing ventricular fibrillation. At the same time, conduction velocity in atrium and ventricle is determined by I_{Na} rather than I_{Ca}, so blocking Ca channels does not slow conduction in these tissues. Hence, Ca channel blockade slows the ventricular response to atrial tachycardia but usually does not terminate arrhythmias arising in either the atrium or the ventricle.

β-Blockers (Table 4-1) also suppress I_{Ca} and thus slow conduction in the SA and AV node and prolong the PR interval. Therefore, like Ca channel blockers, these agents are useful for slowing the ventricular rate during rapid atrial arrhythmias (AV nodal blockade), for slowing the SA node firing rate during sinus tachycardia, and for terminating those supraventricular arrhythmias that involve either the SA or the AV node in a reentrant pathway. In contrast, Na channel–blocking drugs are more useful for terminating arrhythmias that arise in atrial or ventricular muscle where Na current defines tissue conduction velocity. Although β-blockers are useful for chronic management of ventricular arrhythmias, the molecular mechanisms are not well defined and may involve voltage-gated ion channels only indirectly. The most important effect of I_{Ca} suppression in ventricular muscle is manifest in the action potential plateau (phase 3), as discussed further.

The later phases of the action potential (phases 1, 2, and 3, see Fig. 4-2) inscribe repolarization. Transient outward K current (I_{To}) and anion current through chloride channels produce the rapid "notch" of early repolarization (phase 1). This is followed by a long plateau (phase 2) of depolarization that is maintained by I_{Ca}, and then terminated (phase 3) by the rapid (I_{Kr}) and slow (I_{Ks}) components of delayed rectifier K current. The duration of the action potential (and hence, the QT interval on the ECG) is determined by a delicate balance between these and many other smaller inward and outward currents. Drugs that reduce I_{Ca}, namely those with class II or class IV activity (Table 4-1), abbreviate the action potential plateau, shorten the QT interval, and reduce the inward movement of Ca^{2+} into the cardiac cell, causing a negative inotropic effect. Conversely, agents with class IA or III activity block outward K current, prolonging the action potential and the QT interval on the ECG. Because Na channels require a recovery period at the resting membrane potential to once again be activated, drugs that prolong the action potential also serve to prolong the refractory period of the cardiac cell (Fig. 4-2). The electrophysiologic manifestations of QT prolongation may be either therapeutic or arrhythmogenic, as discussed under Automaticity and Arrhythmias.

Phase 4 is the period in which the action potential is fully repolarized (Fig. 4-2) and manifests properties in SA and AV nodal tissue that are again distinctive from those in atrial and ventricular muscle. In cardiac muscle, the resting potential is maintained near the potassium equilibrium potential of -90 mV (E_K) by voltage-gated potassium channels active near the resting membrane potential and by the Na-K-ATPase. Conversely, in nodal cells, inward pacemaker currents cyclically depolarize the resting membrane potential to "threshold" potentials near -60 mV, allowing the spontaneous firing of action potentials. Activation of the adenosine A_1 receptor results in activation of the outward potassium current $I_{KAch,Ado}$ (3). This effect of adenosine hyperpolarizes the cell membrane to a value approaching E_K. Because atrial and ventricular tissue already rests near E_K, adenosine has little or no effect in these tissues. However, in SA and AV nodal tissue, adenosine hyperpolarizes the cell, reducing the likelihood of firing an action potential, thus slowing or blocking conduction. Adenosine also slows nodal conduction by inhibiting I_{Ca} through reducing 3′,5′-cyclic adenosine monophosphate (cAMP).

These transient and specific effects make adenosine a choice agent for terminating supraventricular tachycardias (SVTs) that involve SA or AV node reentrant pathways, and it is therefore possible to classify supraventricular arrhythmias according to their response to adenosine (Table 4-2) (4). SVT due to reentry in atrial tissue, such as atrial flutter or fibrillation, responds to adenosine with transient slowing of the ventricular response rate but does not terminate. Similarly, atrial tachycardias that result from enhanced phase 4 depolarization will transiently slow but rarely cease. Atrial tachycardia due to cAMP-mediated triggered activity in the SA node is a rare exception, in which adenosine-mediated inhibition of adenylate cyclase sometimes terminates the arrhythmia (4).

Conversely, SVTs that use the AV nodal tissue as a substrate for reentry are terminated by bolus adenosine administration (Table 4-2). Junctional tachycardias, common during the surgical period, also sometimes convert to sinus rhythm in response to adenosine. Ventricular arrhythmias exhibit no response to adenosine because these rhythms originate in tissues distal to the AV conduction pathway. This allows one to distinguish wide-complex SVTs (the R-R interval transiently increases with adenosine) from ventricular tachycardia (no R-R interval change). However, adenosine administration in this setting (treatment with long-acting AV-nodal–blocking agents), through vasodilation, can compromise preload during ventricular tachycardia, and is not recommended.

Reentry and Arrhythmias

Reentry is a mechanism that may precipitate a wide variety of supraventricular and ventricular arrhythmias and implies

TABLE 4-2. THE RESPONSE OF COMMON SUPRAVENTRICULAR TACHYARRHYTHMIAS TO ADENOSINE

SVT	Mechanism	Adenosine Response
AV nodal reentry	Reentry within AV node	Termination
AV reciprocating tachycardias (orthodromic and antidromic)	Reentry involving AV node and accessory pathway (WPW)	Termination
Intraatrial reentry	Reentry in the atrium	Transiently slows ventricular response
Atrial flutter/fibrillation	Reentry in the atrium	Transiently slows ventricular response
Other atrial tachycardias	Abnormal automaticity	Transient suppression of the tachycardia
	cAMP-mediated triggered activity	Termination
AV junctional rhythms	Variable	Variable

Note: AV, atrioventricular; IV, intravenous; SVT, supraventricular tachyarrhythmia; WPW, Wolff-Parkinson-White; cAMP, cyclic adenosine monophosphate
Source: From Balser JR. Perioperative management of arrhythmias. In: Barash PG, Fleisher LA, Prough DS, eds. *Problems in anesthesia,* 2nd ed, vol 10. Philadelphia: Lippincott–Raven Publishers, 1998:201, with permission.

the existence of a pathological circus movement of electrical impulses around either an anatomic (e.g., Wolff-Parkinson-White syndrome) or functional (e.g., myocardial ischemia) loop. Fibrillation, in either the atrium or the ventricle, is believed to involve multiple coexistent reentrant circuits of the functional type. These reentrant loops may result from disparities in either the repolarization rates or the conduction rates between healthy and ischemic myocardium, or even from refractory period differences between epicardial and endocardial layers (5).

Unfortunately, our understanding of reentry and its pharmacologic termination by ion channel current suppression is incomplete. Drugs may terminate reentry through at least two mechanisms. Agents that suppress currents responsible for phase 0 of the action potential (I_{Na} in atrium and ventricle, I_{Ca} in the SA and AV node, Table 4-1) may slow or block conduction in a reentrant pathway and thus terminate an arrhythmia. Alternatively, by prolonging the action potential, drugs with K-channel–blocking activity (Table 4-1) prolong the refractory period of cells in a reentrant circuit and thus "block" impulse propagation through the circuit. In clinical trials, agents operating through this latter mechanism have proven more successful in suppressing fibrillation in both the atrium (6) and the ventricle (7).

At the same time, clinical trials have shown that suppression of I_{Na} may exacerbate ventricular arrhythmias (8). A useful model system for understanding how Na channel blockade may augment reentry rests in our emerging understanding of an inherited idiopathic ventricular arrhythmia known as the "Brugada" syndrome (9). Patients with the Brugada syndrome have an abnormal ECG pattern that includes ST-segment elevation in the right precordial leads (resembling an ischemic pattern, Fig. 4-3) and a right bundle-branch block. These patients experience unanticipated cardiac arrest due to ventricular fibrillation. It was recently shown that a kindred of patients with the Brugada syndrome carry mutations in the gene encoding the cardiac Na channel (*SCN5A* on chromosome 3) that leads in some cases to a loss of Na channel function (10). Moreover, treatment of these patients with a potent sodium channel blocker (flecainide) worsens the ST-segment elevation. A proposed mechanism to explain this phenomenon rests in the understanding that repolarization rates differ between the endocardium and epicardium. Suppression of I_{Na} in the epicardial layer worsens this heterogeneity (Fig. 4-3), augmenting the substrate for reentry (11).

Automaticity and Arrhythmias

Automaticity refers to abnormal depolarization of atrial or ventricular muscle cells during periods of the action potential normally characterized by repolarization (phases 2 or 3) or rest (phase 4). A pathologic process such as ischemia may

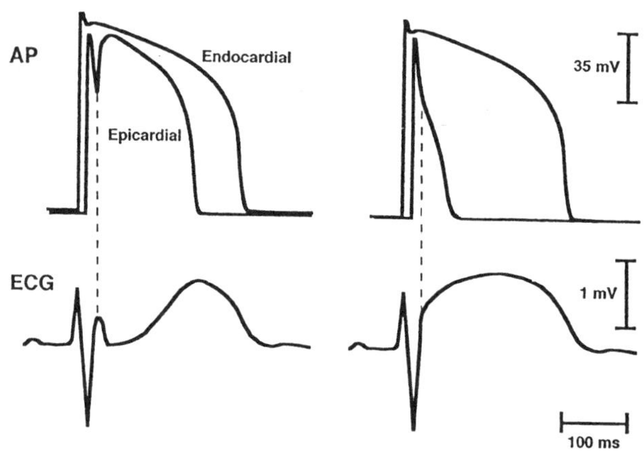

FIGURE 4-3. Hypothesized linkage between distinct epicardial and endocardial action potential morphologies in the right ventricular outflow tract and the Brugada electrocardiogram (ECG) phenotype. **Top:** Epicardial and endocardial action potential morphologies are shown under normal conditions (*left*) and under conditions where the Na current in the epicardium is markedly reduced (*right*). Loss of I_{Na} may drastically shorten the epicardial AP duration, augmenting transmural heterogeneity and allowing ST-segment elevation in the surface ECG. (From Alings M, Wilde A. "Brugada" syndrome: clinical data and suggested pathophysiological mechanism. Circulation 1999;99:666, with permission.)

cause an increase in the rate of phase 4 depolarization and may induce the ventricular tachycardias seen in the days following myocardial infarction (12). More striking depolarizations that occur during phase 2 or 3 (early afterdepolarization [EAD]) or phase 4 (delayed afterdepolarization [DAD]) are known as triggered automaticity.

Studies over the last decade have identified some of the key molecular substrates that underlie triggered automaticity. Although K-channel blockade is highly effective for treating certain arrhythmias in the atrium and ventricle, delaying repolarization (manifest as prolongation of the QT interval) may at the same time provoke ventricular arrhythmias in 2% to 10% of patients. Low serum potassium concentrations, slow heart rates, and K-channel blocking (class IA or III) drugs synergistically induce EAD formation *in vitro* (13) and provoke a polymorphic ventricular tachycardia known as torsade de pointes *in vivo* (14). Recent studies have revealed mutations in a number of cardiac ion channels that are responsible for subtypes of the congenital long-QT syndrome, inherited conditions in which the QT interval is prolonged, and the risk for sudden death from torsade de pointes is increased (15). In all cases, the ion channel mutations linked to the long-QT syndrome produce a functional phenotype that prolongs cardiac repolarization. At least six inherited long-QT mutations have been identified in *SCN5A,* the gene encoding the cardiac Na channel (16,17). These genetic lesions, denoted *LQT3* mutations to indicate their chromosome 3 loci, consistently produce a "gain-of-function" phenotype—that is, the mutation inhibits closing or "inactivation" of the channel that would normally occur during the action potential plateau (Fig. 4-4) (18). Hence, excess inward (depolarizing) current flows during the action potential plateau, delaying repolarization, provoking EAD formation, and prolonging the QT interval.

Loss-of-function mutations have also been identified in the genes of patients with inherited forms of the long-QT syndrome (15). These mutations have been localized to three genes (*HERG, KVLQT1,* and *KCNE1*) (19–21) that encode transmembrane proteins underlying the major ionic currents comprising phase 3 repolarization (Fig. 4-2: I_{Kr}, I_{Ks}). I_{Kr} in particular plays an important role in repolarization at slow heart rates (22), and low potassium concentrations reduce the magnitude of I_{Kr} (23). Further, I_{Kr} is a target of many drugs with class IA or III activity, and block of this current underlies the QT-prolonging effect of most of these agents (24). Hence, the proarrhythmic features of drug therapy with repolarization-prolonging agents appear to be acquired manifestations of the same molecular mechanisms involved in certain forms of the congenital long-QT syndrome (25). More recently, mutations have been identified in the protein substituents of I_{Kr} (MirP1)(26) and I_{Ks} (MinK) (27) that do not cause excessive QT prolongation unless patients are exposed to K-channel–blocking drugs. These silent mutations "sensitize" the cardiac cell to K-channel blockade and provide a pharmacogenetic rationale for the idiosyncratic proarrhythmic response of certain patients to QT-prolonging drugs (28).

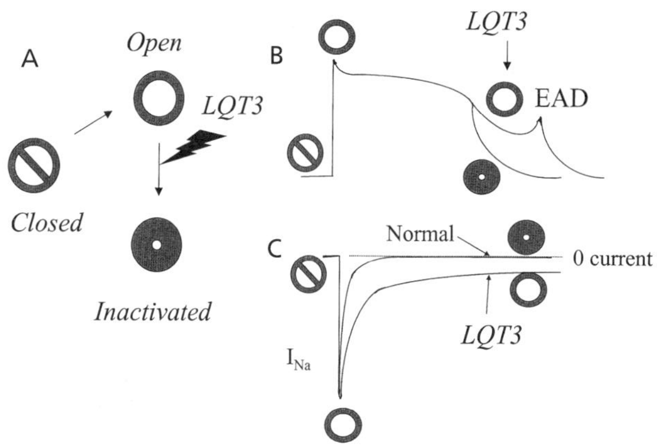

FIGURE 4-4. A mutation in the Na channel induces the long-QT syndrome. **A:** During the cardiac cycle, Na channels transition from the closed to open conformational state during the beginning of the action potential, allowing inward Na^+ ion flux. During the plateau phase, the channels inactivate and conduction normally ceases. LQT3 mutations damage the inactivation gate. **B:** The cardiac action potential under conditions where Na channel inactivation is normal (normal repolarization) or impaired (delayed repolarization). The LQT3 mutations prevent inactivation and thereby induce action potential prolongation and early afterdepolarization (EAD) formation. **C:** Na currents normally open only transiently and then fully inactivate. With a LQT3 mutation, some of the channels remain open during the action potential plateau, allowing persistent inward current that prolongs repolarization and predisposing to EAD formation (**B**) and torsade de pointes.

DADs are a less understood form of triggered automaticity that are most common during conditions of intracellular Ca overload. Although many conditions induce intracellular Ca overload, commonly recognized clinical entities are digitalis toxicity, excess catecholamine states (exercise, acute myocardial infarction, perioperative stress), and heart failure (29). Digitalis toxicity produces Ca overload indirectly; Na overload is induced by direct inhibition of the Na-K pump, and high intracellular Na inhibits the normal Ca extrusion from the cell by the Na-Ca exchanger (30). Catecholamines induce Ca overload directly by increasing I_{Ca} through L-type Ca channels (31), which are up-regulated through protein kinase A via cardiac β_1-receptor stimulation (32). In heart failure, the disorder in Ca^{2+} homeostasis may result from altered expression of a number of signaling molecules, including increased expression of the Ca^{2+}/calmodulin-dependent protein kinase (CaMK) (33). Arrhythmias provoked by DADs should therefore be responsive to maneuvers aimed at lowering intracellular Ca, such as Ca channel blockade (1). Moreover, recent studies suggest that CaMK facilitates EAD and DAD formation when the action potential is prolonged (34,35) and in the future may prove to be a valuable drug target for managing triggered arrhythmias.

SUPRAVENTRICULAR ARRHYTHMIAS

Acute Management of Perioperative Supraventricular Arrhythmias

A cascade of adverse physiologic phenomena can precipitate SVT in critically ill or anesthetized patients. Hence, the management of the surgical patient who suddenly develops SVT requires an organized approach. The immediate focus should not be on heart-directed pharmacologic therapies, but on the patient as a whole. SVT is among the anesthesiologist's most valuable warning signs, often foreshadowing life-threatening conditions that may be correctable. These include hypoxemia (O_2 saturation), hypoventilation (end-tidal CO_2), hypotension (absolute or relative hypovolemia due to bleeding, anaphylaxis, and so on), light anesthesia, electrolyte abnormalities (K^+ or Mg^{2+}), or cardiac ischemia (heart rate, nitroglycerin).

Patients with narrow complex tachycardias who are dangerously hypotensive (e.g., a systolic blood pressure of less than 80 mm Hg) require immediate synchronous DC cardioversion to prevent the life-threatening complications of hypoperfusion, such as central nervous system or cardiac ischemia. Although some patients may only respond transiently to cardioversion in this setting (or not at all), a brief period of sinus rhythm may provide valuable time for correcting the reversible causes of SVT (discussed earlier) and/or instituting pharmacologic therapies. In less urgent cases, adenosine may be administered as a 6-mg intravenous bolus (repeated with 12 mg if no response). In practice, the SVTs most commonly seen in the perioperative period (such as atrial fibrillation, Table 4-2) do not involve the AV node in a reentrant pathway, and AV nodal block by adenosine will therefore produce only transient slowing of the ventricular rate. Nonetheless, for tachycardias that are regular and wide complex, adenosine may be useful in identifying and converting the SVT (Table 4-2). The vasodilating effects of adenosine, like the vasodilating intravenous β-blockers or Ca channel blockers during ventricular tachycardia may invite hemodynamic collapse from reduced preload.

Patients with underlying structural heart disease are at greatest risk for developing either supraventricular or ventricular arrhythmias during the induction of anesthesia secondary to hypotension, autonomic imbalance, or airway manipulation (36). In addition, during cardiac or major vascular surgery, patients may experience SVT during dissection of the pericardium, placement of atrial sutures, or insertion of the venous cannulas required for cardiopulmonary bypass. If hemodynamically unstable SVT occurs during open thoracotomy, the surgeon should attempt open synchronous cardioversion. However, in patients with critical coronary lesions or severe aortic stenosis, SVT may be refractory to cardioversion and provoke a malignant cascade of ischemia and worsening arrhythmias that requires the institution of cardiopulmonary bypass. Hence, early preparation for cardiopulmonary bypass is recommended before inducing anesthesia in those cardiac surgery patients at exceptionally high risk for SVT and consequent hemodynamic deterioration.

Ventricular rate control is the mainstay of therapy for SVT that does not require immediate DC cardioversion. The advantages of slowing the ventricular rate during SVT are two-fold. First, lengthening diastole serves to enhance left ventricular filling, thus enhancing stroke volume and improving hemodynamic stability. Second, slowing the ventricular rate reduces myocardial oxygen consumption and lowers the risk of cardiac ischemia. Intraoperatively, rate control is readily achieved with one of a variety of AV nodal blockers (agents with class II or class IV activity, Table 4-1). Among the i.v. β-blockers, esmolol has ultrarapid elimination properties that render it titratable on a minute-to-minute basis (37), allowing meaningful dose adjustments during periods of surgery that provoke changes in hemodynamic status (e.g., bleeding and abdominal traction). Although esmolol is largely β_1 selective and generally well tolerated by patients with chronic obstructive lung disease, the drug has obligatory negative inotropic effects that may not be well tolerated in patients with severe left ventricular dysfunction. Both i.v. verapamil and IV diltiazem are Ca channel blockers that are less titratable than esmolol but nonetheless provide rapid slowing of the ventricular rate in SVT within minutes. The agents are therapeutically equivalent for purposes of AV nodal blockade (38), but i.v. diltiazem has less negative inotropic action and is preferable in patients with heart failure (39,40). Intravenous digoxin slows the ventricular response during SVT through its vagotonic effects but should be temporally supplemented with other agents due to its slow onset (approximately 6 hours) (41).

Paroxysmal SVT (PSVT) due to reentrant circuits that involve accessory pathways (congenital electrical connections between the atrium and ventricle that bypass the AV node) pose caveats in the management of SVT. During sinus rhythm, forward (antegrade) conduction through the accessory pathway may produce ventricular preexcitation on the ECG (known as Wolff-Parkinson-White syndrome) with a short PR interval (less than 0.12 seconds), a slurred QRS upstroke (delta wave) and a wide QRS complex. During PSVT, when the conduction circuit is antegrade through the AV node and retrograde through the accessory bundle, the QRS complex will be narrow; however, in 5% to 10% of cases, the conduction is antegrade through the accessory bundle, producing a wide QRS complex that may be confused with ventricular tachycardia. Normally, PSVT does not provoke a marked deterioration in hemodynamic status. However, 10% to 35% of patients with Wolff-Parkinson-White syndrome eventually develop atrial fibrillation, and an episode of PSVT sometimes precipitates atrial fibrillation. In this case, the rapid rate of atrial excitation (more than 300 impulses/minute), normally transmitted to the ventricle after considerable "filtering" by the AV nodal system, may instead be transmitted to the ventricle via the accessory bundle at a rapid rate. The danger of inducing ventricular fibrillation in this scenario is exacerbated by treatment with classic AV nodal–blocking agents (digoxin, Ca channel blockers, β-blockers, adenosine) because they reduce the accessory bundle refractory period. Hence, although vagal maneuvers or adenosine are useful for converting the PSVT in Wolff-Parkinson-White syndrome to sinus rhythm, Wolff-Parkinson-White syndrome patients who experience atrial fibrillation should not receive AV nodal blockers. Rather, i.v. procainamide, which slows conduction over the accessory bundle, is the drug of choice for treating atrial fibrillation in this condition (42).

Chemical Cardioversion of Supraventricular Tachycardias

Efforts to chemically convert SVT to sinus rhythm in the operating room should be aimed at those patients who cannot tolerate (or do not respond to) rate control therapy or who fail DC cardioversion and remain hemodynamically unstable. In patients who are hemodynamically stable and rate controlled in SVT, the risk-benefit ratio of chemical cardioversion should be carefully weighed. The 24-hour rate of spontaneous conversion to sinus rhythm for recent-onset perioperative SVT exceeds 50%, and many patients who develop SVT under anesthesia will remit spontaneously before or during emergence. Moreover, most of the antiarrhythmic agents with chronic activity against atrial arrhythmias have limited efficacy when used for rapid chemical cardioversion. Although 50% to 80% efficacy rates are cited for many i.v. antiarrhythmic drugs in uncontrolled studies, these findings are largely an artifact of high placebo rates of conversion. For example, the efficacy of i.v. procainamide for conversion of SVT has not been established in placebo-controlled trials (6). Moreover, a placebo-controlled trial of patients with atrial fibrillation recently found a 60% 24-hour conversion rate for patients in the placebo arm, statistically indistinguishable from that of patients treated with i.v. amiodarone (68%) (43). Although improved rates of chemical cardioversion are seen with high doses of i.v. amiodarone (about 2 g/day)(44), the potential for undesirable side effects in the perioperative setting requires further study.

Although the most effective agents for converting atrial fibrillation are K-channel blockers that prolong atrial repolarization, the use of these agents is hampered by the proarrhythmic risk inherent in coexistent prolongation of ventricular repolarization (manifest as QT prolongation). Ibutilide, a rapid-acting antiarrhythmic, produced an astounding 31% rate of conversion in nonsurgical patients with atrial fibrillation, with a mean time from treatment to conversion of 27 minutes (45). Unfortunately, an 8% incidence of torsade de pointes was reported (15 of 180 ibutilide-treated subjects), and the risk/benefit ratio for IV ibutilide use in perioperative SVT remains unestablished. Intraoperative elective DC cardioversion in an otherwise stable patient with SVT also carries risks (ventricular fibrillation, asystole, stroke). Moreover, the underlying factors provoking SVT during or shortly after surgery are likely to persist beyond the time of cardioversion, inviting recurrence (36). A recent trial of post–coronary artery bypass graft (CABG) patients with SVT (mainly atrial fibrillation) did find that low-energy DC cardioversion (utilizing indwelling atrial pacing leads) was 80% effective and minimized sedation requirements, but the rate of recurrence within 1 minute was nearly 50% (46). Hence, when elective DC cardioversion is considered, it may be prudent to first establish a therapeutic level of an antiarrhythmic agent that maintains sinus rhythm (e.g., procainamide and amiodarone), with a view to preventing SVT recurrence following electrical cardioversion.

Management of Postoperative Supraventricular Arrhythmias

SVT occurs after cardiac surgery with an incidence of 15% to 40% and primarily consists of atrial fibrillation (47–49). SVT may also occur after a wide range of noncardiac surgeries (e.g., gastrointestinal procedures, vascular surgery, and neurosurgery) (50,51). In cardiac surgery patients, preoperative atrial fibrillation and advanced age are consistently identified as the most important risk factors. The number of procedures (i.e., valve replacement plus CABG), preoperative congestive heart failure, chronic pulmonary disease, and surgical factors including cross-clamp time, bicaval venous cannulation, and pulmonary vein venting have also been implicated as independent risk factors. Although the incidence and risk factors for SVT after noncardiac surgeries are not as well documented, pneumonectomy procedures have a 20% risk of SVT (52) and appear to be associated with elevated right heart pressures (with no right ventricle enlargement or fluid overload) (53).

The morbidity of SVT after cardiac surgery appears to differ from that of noncardiac surgery. Studies of cardiac surgery patients with SVT have not detected increased mortality but consistently identify a 1- to 3-day increase in hospital stay (47,48). In addition, SVT after cardiac surgery is correlated with an increased rate of stroke (3.3% versus 1.4%, $p < .005$), ventricular tachycardia or fibrillation (tachycardia 9.2% versus fibrillation 4.0%, $p < .005$), and need for a permanent pacemaker (3.7% versus 1.6%, $p < .0005$) (48). In contrast, SVT after noncardiac surgery has been linked to high mortality rates (25% to 50%) (50–52,54). It is unclear whether SVT after noncardiac surgery actually contributes to this excess mortality or whether it foreshadows a high mortality risk due to decreased organ reserve and/or a generally debilitated state.

For postsurgical SVT, the goal of acute therapy is usually ventricular rate control because a safe and effective means of chemical cardioversion has not been demonstrated (55). Paradoxically, it appears that certain rate control agents may additionally effect conversion to sinus rhythm. In a trial of 57 nonsurgical patients comparing IV magnesium to IV verapamil for recent-onset SVT (primarily atrial fibrillation and flutter), 15 of 26 (58%) magnesium-treated patients were in sinus rhythm versus only 7 of 31 (23%) verapamil-treated patients after 4 hours ($P < .01$) (56). By 24 hours, the rate of conversion was similar (50% to 60%) in the two treatment groups. A trial comparing a 24-hour infusion of IV amiodarone (5-mg/kg bolus, 10 mg/kg infusion) to high-dose IV magnesium (2.6-g bolus, followed by a 1.75-g/hour infusion) in 42 medical and surgical intensive care unit patients with SVT found a higher rate of conversion for magnesium at 4 hours (60% versus 44%), 12 hours (72% versus 50%), and 24 hours (78% versus 50%) (57). Finally, β blockade may have benefits that extend beyond ventricular rate control. A study comparing esmolol to verapamil in nonsurgical patients found that 50% of esmolol-treated patients with new onset atrial fibrillation or flutter converted to sinus rhythm, whereas only 12% of those receiving verapamil converted ($P < .03$) (58). Similarly, a recent study comparing IV esmolol to IV diltiazem for ventricular rate control in general surgical intensive care unit patients with SVT found that after 2 hours of treatment, 59% of the esmolol-treated patients converted to sinus rhythm versus only 33% of patients treated with diltiazem ($p < .05$) (50). This difference may partly reflect unopposed catecholamines, a potential etiologic factor in postoperative SVT, and may not apply to the well-anesthetized intraoperative patient with SVT.

Because SVT in surgical patients is usually delayed until postoperative days 2 to 4, various postoperative prophylaxis regimens have been evaluated. Recent studies suggest that prophylactic administration of a number of drugs typically used to slow AV nodal conduction may also significantly reduce the incidence of postoperative atrial fibrillation. Although a metaanalysis of 12 studies involving cardiac surgery patients found no benefit to the prophylactic use of digoxin, a significant benefit was detected for β blockade (atrial fibrillation incidence reduced from 20.2% to 9.8%, $P < .001$) or combined therapy with β blockade and digoxin (from 29.4% to 2.2%, $P < .001$) (59). Notably, these studies did not control for preoperative β-blocker therapy, so the degree to which postoperative therapy in the treatment arms mitigated SVT primarily through suppressing β-blocker withdrawal is unclear. Nonetheless, most patients who undergo cardiac surgery do receive preoperative β blockade, so low-dose β-blocker prophylaxis in the early postoperative period is generally recommended after patients wean from inotropic support.

Several recent perioperative trials suggest that prophylactic administration of IV magnesium reduces the incidence of SVT after either cardiac or noncardiac thoracic surgery (Table 4-3). One-time low-dose postoperative magnesium supplementation (2 g $MgCl_2$) is an effective means to reduce the incidence of ventricular arrhythmias after cardiac surgery but may have limited value for suppressing atrial fibrillation (60,61). Although ventricular arrhythmias commonly occur in the immediate postoperative period, the incidence of postoperative SVT rises after the first postoperative day (62,63). Hence, SVT suppression requires higher magnesium doses and more prolonged administration (Table 4-3). Although serum levels of more than 4 mEq/L may suppress deep tendon reflexes (higher levels suppress ventilation), the doses required for SVT suppression have been well tolerated. In patients free of renal failure, serum levels generally remain below 3 mEq/L (64). One adverse effect linked to high-dose postoperative magnesium therapy has been an increased requirement for temporary pacing due to the AV nodal blockade (61). This approach to SVT prophylaxis appears promising but is not in widespread use and deserves additional study in larger patient groups.

The antiarrhythmic agents most effective against atrial fibrillation prolong repolarization in the atrium and ventricle (class IA or III activity, Table 4-1). These agents have a property termed reverse use-dependence; that is, they prolong repolarization more at slow heart rates than at rapid rates (65). For example, in an animal model, sotalol was significantly more effective at preventing the induction of atrial fibrillation while in sinus rhythm at 60 beats/minute than at terminating the arrhythmia at an atrial cycle length of 300 beats/minute (66). Hence, the antiarrhythmic agents currently available are more effective for prevention of SVT or maintaining sinus rhythm following DC cardioversion than for chemically converting SVT to sinus rhythm.

It is therefore not surprising that clinical trials have identified a number of antiarrhythmic agents that prevent postoperative SVT when administered prophylactically. In a recent prospective, randomized, placebo-controlled study of 255 cardiac surgery patients (67), low-dose oral sotalol (80 mg twice of day, first dose immediately before surgery) administered throughout the postoperative period reduced the incidence of SVT after cardiac surgery from 46% to 26% ($p = .0012$). These findings support earlier trials (68) suggesting that low sotalol doses (160 mg/day or less) are effective and have an incidence of hemodynamic intolerance indistinguishable from placebo. Nonetheless, patients with poor left ventricular function (ejection fraction of less than 40%) are poorly represented in the available studies (68), and it remains unclear whether oral sotalol (which also has β-blocking activity) is more effective than some of the more traditional low-dose β-blockade regimens (e.g., propranolol) (69). Low-dose oral amiodarone prophylaxis was recently evaluated in a prospective, randomized placebo-controlled trial of 124 cardiac surgical patients, including a number of patients with controlled congestive heart failure (New York Heart Association class 2.4 $\pm$ 0.9) (70). Patients received 600 mg/day of amiodarone for 7 days preopera-

TABLE 4-3. PUBLISHED CLINICAL TRIALS THAT EXAMINE IV MAGNESIUM AS PROPHYLAXIS FOR POSTOPERATIVE ATRIAL FIBRILLATION

Study	Intervention	Patients	% Patients with afib	Complications	Comments
Fanning et al., 1991 (5)	$MgSO_4$ POD 0: 0.5 g/hr POD 1–3: 0.125 g/hr	Total: 99 CAB	Placebo: 28% Drug: 14% P = NS	None	Mg^{2+} reduced number of afib events from 42 to 12 ($p < .02$)
Colquhoun et al., 1993 (27)	$MgCl_2$ 50 mmol infusion over 48 h	Total: 130 CAB	Placebo: 37.5% Drug: 16.7% $P = .013$	- 3 mg-treated pts. had VF - 1 death in Mg group from MI	None
Wistbacka et al., 1995 (14)	$MgSO_4$ Preop: 4 g; POD 0: 12 g/d; POD 1: 5.5 g/d. Placebo: 4 g Mg^{2+} × 1	Total: 81 CAB	Placebo: 45% Drug: 24% $P = .063$	17.5% vs. 5.3% rate of bradycardia requiring transient pacing	1) Placebo: 4 g Mg^{2+} 2) Mg^{2+} reduced number of afib events from 41 to 19 ($P < .01$)
Nurozler et al., 1996 (28)	$MgSO_4$ 200 mEq for 5 days postop (pending)	Total: 50 CAB	Placebo: 20% Drug: 4%	None	Excluded patients with poor LV function
Terzi et al., 1996 (29)	$MgSO_4$ *POD 0: 4 g* POD 1, 2: 2 g/d	Total: 194 noncardiac thoracic	Placebo: 27% Drug: 11% $P = .008$	None	Excluded patients with an MI in prior 6 months

Note: IV, intravenous; LV, left ventricular; MI, myocardial infarction; NS, not significant; afib, atrial fibrillation; CAB, coronary artery bypass.
Source: From Balser JR. Pro: all patients should receive pharmacologic prophylaxis for atrial fibrillation after cardiac surgery. *J Cardiothorac Vasc Anesth* 1999;13:98, with permission.

tively, and then 200 mg/day from the time of surgery until discharge from the hospital. The incidence of postoperative atrial fibrillation was 53% in the placebo arm and 25% among amiodarone-treated patients ($P = .003$). A reduction in hospital cost was also identified in amiodarone-treated patients (\$26,491 ± \$23,837 versus \$18,375 ± \$13,863, $P = .03$). Although amiodarone, like sotalol, has β-blocking properties, it appears to be well tolerated in patients with congestive heart failure, and adverse hemodynamic side effects have not been identified during low-dose therapy in cardiac surgical patients (70).

Among the class IA or III antiarrhythmic compounds with the potential to prevent fibrillation after surgery, amiodarone is the least associated with proarrhythmia (less than 2% torsade de pointes) (71). However, retrospective studies have linked high-dose preoperative amiodarone therapy with acute pulmonary toxicity after cardiac (72,73) and noncardiac (74) thoracic surgical procedures. In the recent prospective trials, no acute pulmonary complications have been linked to low-dose oral preoperative therapy (70,75), and prophylactic IV amiodarone therapy initiated postoperatively has not been associated with pulmonary toxicity in small single-center trials (reviewed in reference 76). The expense and potential for low-incidence side effects with antiarrhythmic drug prophylaxis of large cardiac surgical patient populations suggest that risk/benefit analyses from multicenter trials are needed. Nonetheless, antiarrhythmic prophylaxis should be considered in selected patients at high risk for hemodynamic or ischemic complications from postoperative SVT.

VENTRICULAR ARRHYTHMIAS

General Classification of Ventricular Arrhythmias

Ventricular arrhythmias may be subdivided according to their morphology but are less distinctive in their response to antiarrhythmic drug therapies (Table 4-4). Nonsustained ventricular tachycardia (NSVT) is defined as three or more premature ventricular contractions (PVCs) that occur at a rate exceeding 100 beats/minute and last 30 seconds or less without hemodynamic compromise. These arrhythmias are routinely seen in the absence of cardiac disease and as discussed further (Suppressing Postoperative Ventricular Arrhythmias) may not require drug therapy in the perioperative period. Conversely, in patients with structural heart disease, these nonsustained rhythms do predict subsequent life-threatening ventricular arrhythmias (77), and particular antiarrhythmic drug therapies in patients with structural heart disease and NSVT may either worsen (encainide, flecainide)(8) or improve (amiodarone)(78) survival.

Sustained ventricular tachycardias generally fall into one of two categories: monomorphic and polymorphic. In monomorphic ventricular tachycardia, the amplitude of the QRS complex remains constant while in polymorphic ven-

TABLE 4-4. CLASSIFICATION OF VENTRICULAR ARRHYTHMIAS BASED ON MORPHOLOGY

Arrhythmia	Common Substrate	Usual IV Therapy
PVCs, nonsustained VT (<30 sec)	Normal ventricle postsurgical	None unless associated with ischemia or hypotension
Sustained monomorphic VT (>30 sec or hemodynamically unstable)	Prior myocardial infarction or structural heart disease	Procainamide,[a] amiodarone, or lidocaine
(a) Polymorphic VT with normal QT (b) Ventricular fibrillation	Acute ischemia, infarction, idiopathic cardiomyopathy	Amiodarone, procainamide, or lidocaine
Polymorphic VT with prolonged QT (Torsades de Pointes)	Congenital, acquired complication of drug therapy[b]	Magnesium, pacing, lidocaine or phenytoin, consider amiodarone

Note: IV, intravenous; VT, ventricular tachycardia.
[a] Procainamide may be the preferred agent for stable monomorphic VT in patients with normal ejection fractions (reference 80).
[b] See Table 4-5
Source: Modified from Balser JR. Perioperative management of arrhythmias. In: Barash PG, Fleisher LA, Prough DS, eds. *Problems in anesthesia,* 2nd ed, vol 10. Philadelphia: Lippincott–Raven Publishers, 1998:209, with permission.

tricular tachycardia the QRS morphology continually changes. The best understood mechanism for monomorphic ventricular tachycardia is formation of a reentrant pathway around scar tissue from a healed myocardial infarction (79). Although lidocaine has traditionally been the primary drug therapy for all sustained ventricular arrhythmias, a recent study of 29 patients with hemodynamically stable monomorphic ventricular tachycardia found termination within 24 hours was more common with IV procainamide therapy (12 of 15 patients) than with IV lidocaine (3 of 14; $p < .01$) (80).

In contrast, the therapeutic approach for polymorphic ventricular tachycardia depends critically on whether the QT interval during a prior interval of sinus rhythm was prolonged. Polymorphic VT in the setting of a normal QT interval usually occurs in a setting of structural heart disease, although idiopathic cases are seen (81). Its pharmacologic management is poorly defined, but is similar to that of monomorphic ventricular tachycardia or ventricular fibrillation (Table 4-4). Polymorphic ventricular tachycardia in the setting of a prolonged QT interval, otherwise known torsade de pointes, arises from triggered automaticity (EAD formation) in a setting of prolonged repolarization (81). As discussed previously (under Automaticity and Arrhythmias), a predisposition to torsade de pointes may be inherited but is more often an acquired complication of therapy with drugs that prolong the QT interval. In addition to QT-prolonging antiarrhythmic drugs (class IA or III), a number of other medications may evoke QT prolongation and torsade de pointes (Table 4-5).

The management of torsade de pointes differs markedly from other forms of ventricular tachycardia (Table 4-4) and includes intravenous magnesium sulfate and maneuvers aimed at increasing the heart rate (atropine, isoproterenol, or temporary ventricular pacing). When antiarrhythmic therapy is deemed necessary, agents devoid of K-channel–blocking properties such as lidocaine or phenytoin (Table 4-1) usually are chosen to avoid further prolongation of the QT interval (82). In practice, it may be relatively unclear whether an observed episode of polymorphic ventricular tachycardia is related to QT-interval prolongation. In such cases, magnesium and Na channel–blocking agents may be administered empirically. Among the antiarrhythmic agents that prolong the QT interval, the incidence of torsade de pointes is lowest with amiodarone (83); hence, IV amiodarone is a rational alternative therapy for refractory polymorphic ventricular tachycardia of unclear etiology.

Suppressing Postoperative Ventricular Arrhythmias

NSVTs occur in nearly 50% of patients after cardiac and major vascular surgeries but do not influence early or late mortality in patients with preserved left ventricular function (84–86). In addition, nearly 2% of patients experience sustained ventricular tachycardia or ventricular fibrillation after cardiac surgery (84,87,88), and low cardiac output following CABG (requiring pressor support) has been identified as an independent predictor of life-threatening ventricular tachycardia/fibrillation within 72 hours of surgery (89). In most cases, symptoms of postoperative ischemia are not ap-

TABLE 4-5. QT-PROLONGING DRUGS

Antiarrhythmics	Quinidine, procainamide, disopyramide, sotalol, amiodarone, ibutilide, dofetilide
Antipsychotics	Haloperidol, risperidone
Antihistamines	Terfenadine, astemizole
Antifungal	Ketoconazole, fluconazole, itraconazole
Antibiotics	Trimethoprim-sulfamethoxasole, pentamidine, erythromycin
Antidepressants	Amitriptyline, imipramine, doxepin
Phenothiazines	Chlorpromazine, thioridazine
GI	Cisapride

Source: From Murray KT, Roden DM, *personal communication,* 1999.

parent, although one trial did identify saphenous vein graft failure at angiography in three of seven patients experiencing unanticipated ventricular tachycardia/fibrillation, suggesting subclinical graft occlusion is a frequent etiology of postoperative ventricular tachycardia/fibrillation (87). After aortic valve replacement, a retrospective analysis found that patients who died unexpectedly had an elevated incidence of NSVT on their postoperative ECG (44%) compared with survivors (10%, $p < .05$) (90). Nonetheless, the incidence NSVT after aortic valve replacement approaches 50% (91), and the role for electrophysiologic diagnostic evaluation in this population has not been clarified.

There are few studies available to guide therapeutic decision making for patients with ventricular arrhythmias in the early postoperative period. Although NSVT has not been linked to increased morbidity or mortality after cardiopulmonary bypass, unstable patients with marginal perfusion may deteriorate with recurrent episodes of NSVT (problematic ventricular pacing or intraaortic balloon counterpulsation) and may benefit from suppression with lidocaine (92) or β blockade (84,85). In addition, repletion of postbypass hypomagnesemia (2g $MgCl_2$ intravenously) reduces the incidence of NSVT after cardiac surgery (60) and is now standard at most centers. A retrospective evaluation recently identified a survival benefit with electrophysiologically guided prophylaxis in post-CABG patients with low ejection fraction who survived an episode of sudden cardiac death (93), although a definitive role for prophylactic antiarrhythmic drug therapy in this setting has not been evaluated prospectively. A recent multicenter trial (CABG Patch Trial) found no survival advantage with implantation of a cardiac defibrillator in high-risk patients (those with low ejection fractions) at the time of elective cardiac surgery (94). Hence, identification of effective strategies for preventing ventricular arrhythmias after thoracic surgery is an ongoing challenge.

Drug Selection for Acute Management of Ventricular Fibrillation

The necessity to treat life-threatening arrhythmias in the operating room is self-evident, and in this setting, the risks of drug therapy would appear to be small. However, there is little objective evidence to support the notion that IV antiarrhythmic therapy improves survival during cardiac arrest. Hence, the most important first maneuvers in patients who experience ventricular fibrillation intraoperatively are nonpharmacologic and are nearly the same as those utilized in hemodynamically destabilizing SVT: rapid defibrillation (versus synchronous cardioversion in SVT) and correction of reversible etiologies (hypoxemia, hypercarbia, ischemia, electrolytes, and so on).

In the realm of pharmacologic intervention, there are no human clinical studies available to suggest that IV lidocaine, the putative Na-channel blocker most often used during cardiac arrest, promotes the conversion of sustained ventricular tachycardia or fibrillation to sinus rhythm during either in-hospital or out-of-hospital cardiac arrest. This paucity of clinical data is underscored by emerging evidence that K-channel blockade is a more effective pharmacologic strategy for suppressing or converting life-threatening ventricular arrhythmias. In the ESVEM trial (7), nonsurgical patients with sustained ventricular arrhythmias were managed with one of seven different antiarrhythmic drugs and monitored by Holter or electrophysiologic testing. Most of the agents were either Na-channel or mixed Na-channel/K-channel blockers. However, patients receiving oral sotalol, a compound with β blockade and potassium-channel–blocking activity, had the lowest incidence of arrhythmia and sudden death during multiyear follow-up. Intravenous sotalol is not commercially available and therefore does not have a role in the acute management of cardiac arrest. IV amiodarone has both K-channel–blocking and β-blocking properties and is effective against recurrent life-threatening ventricular tachycardia and ventricular fibrillation refractory to other therapies. A multicenter trial evaluated 273 patients with various types of cardiac disease who were experiencing refractory ventricular tachyarrhythmias (95). After failing three other standard IV antiarrhythmic therapies (lidocaine, procainamide, and bretylium), 40.3% of patients placed on IV amiodarone were arrhythmia-free at 24 hours. A concurrent multicenter trial found that IV bretylium and IV amiodarone were equally effective for suppressing recurrent sustained ventricular tachycardia or fibrillation in hospitalized patients with heart disease who were refractory to both IV lidocaine and IV procainamide, and that amiodarone was better tolerated hemodynamically (96). Although successful use of IV amiodarone in postoperative ventricular arrhythmia management has been reported (97,98), placebo-controlled trials in surgical populations (either intraoperative or postoperative) are not yet available. It should be recognized that amiodarone has noncompetitive α and β blockade effects, so that rapid IV loading may exacerbate hemodynamic instability during the initial (rapid) loading phase in patients with severe left ventricular dysfunction. In these cases, systemic perfusion may be maintained during the initial bolus with additional pressors, and occasionally intraaortic balloon counterpulsation (97). If time permits, the negative inotropic effects of IV amiodarone are also mitigated by slowing the infusion.

ACKNOWLEDGMENT

Salary support provided by the Established Investigator Award of the American Heart Association.

REFERENCES

1. Task Force of the Working Group on Arrhythmias of the European Society of Cardiology. The Sicilian Gambit: a new approach

to the classification of antiarrhythmic drugs based on their actions on arrhythmogenic mechanisms. *Circulation* 1991;84:1831.
2. Vaughan Williams EM. A classification of antiarrhythmic actions reassessed after a decade of new drugs. *J Clin Pharmacol* 1984; 24:129.
3. Belardinelli L, Isenberg G. Isolated atrial myocytes: adenosine and acetylcholine increase potassium conductance. *Am J Physiol* 1983;244:H737.
4. Engelstein ED, Lippman N, Stein KM, et al. Mechanism-specific effects of adenosine on atrial tachycardia. *Circulation* 1994;89: 2645.
5. Lukas A, Antzelevitch C. Differences in the electrophysiological response of canine ventricular epicardium and endocardium to ischemia: role of the transient outward current. *Circulation* 1993; 88:2903.
6. Roden DM. Ibutilide and the treatment of atrial arrhythmias. *Circulation* 1996;94:1499.
7. Mason JW. A comparison of seven antiarrhythmic drugs in patients with ventricular tachyarrhythmias. Electrophysiologic Study versus Electrocardiographic Monitoring Investigators. *N Engl J Med* 1993;329:452.
8. Echt DS, Liebson PR, Mitchell LB, et al. Mortality and morbidity in patients receiving encainide, flecainide, or placebo. *N Engl J Med* 1991;324:781.
9. Brugada P, Brugada J. Right bundle-branch block, persistent ST segment elevation and sudden cardiac death: a distinct clinical and electrocardiographic syndrome. A multicenter report. *J Am Coll Cardiol* 1992;20:1391.
10. Chen Q, Kirsch GE, Zhang D, et al. Genetic basis and molecular mechanism for idiopathic ventricular fibrillation. *Nature* 1998; 392:293.
11. Alings M, Wilde A. "Brugada" syndrome: clinical data and suggested pathophysiological mechanism. *Circulation* 1999;99:666.
12. Zipes DP. Cardiac electrophysiology: promises and contributions. *J Am Coll Cardiol* 1989;13:1329.
13. Roden DM, Hoffman BF. Action potential prolongation and induction of abnormal automaticity by low quinidine concentrations in canine Purkinje fibers. Relationship to potassium and cycle length. *Circ Res* 1985;56:857.
14. Roden DM, Woosley RL, Primm K. Incidence of clinical features of the quinidine associated long QT syndrome. Implications for patient care. *Am Heart J* 1986;111:1088.
15. Priori SG, Barhanin J, Hauer RN, et al. Genetic and molecular basis of cardiac arrhythmias: impact on clinical management parts I and II. *Circulation* 1999;99:518.
16. Wang Q, Shen J, Splawski I, et al. *SCN5A* mutations associated with an inherited cardiac arrhythmia, long QT syndrome. *Cell* 1995;80:805.
17. Balser JR. Structure and function of the cardiac sodium channels. *Cardiovasc Res* 1999;42:327.
18. Bennett PB, Yazawa K, Naomasa M, et al. Molecular mechanism for an inherited cardiac arrhythmia. *Nature* 1995;376:683.
19. Wang Q, Curran ME, Splawski I, et al. Positional cloning of a novel potassium channel gene: *KVLQT1* mutations cause cardiac arrhythmias. *Nat Genet* 1996;12:17.
20. Curran ME, Spawski I, Timothy KW, et al. A molecular basis for cardiac arrhythymia: *HERG* mutations cause long QT syndrome. *Cell* 1995;80:795.
21. Splawski I, Tristani-Firouzi M, Lehmann MH, et al. Mutations in the hminK gene cause long QT syndrome and suppress I_{Ks} function. *Nat Genet* 1997;17:338.
22. Jurkiewicz NK, Sanguinetti MC. Rate-dependent prolongation of cardiac action potentials by a methanesulfonanilide class III antiarrhythmic agent: specific block of rapidly activating delayed rectifier K^+ current by dofetilide. *Circ Res* 1995;76:351.
23. Sanguinetti MC, Jurkiewicz NK. Role of external Ca^{2+} and K^+ in gating of cardiac delayed rectifier K^+ currents. *Pflugers Arch* 1992;420:180.
24. Roden DM. Current status of class III antiarrhythmic therapy. *Am J Cardiol* 1993;72:44B.
25. Sanguinetti MC, Jiang C, Curran ME, et al. A mechanistic link between an inherited and an acquired cardiac arrhythmia: HERG encodes the I_{Kr} potassium channel. *Cell* 1995;81:299.
26. Abbott GW, Sesti F, Splawski I, et al. MiRP1 forms I_{Kr} potassium channels with HERG and is associated with cardiac arrhythmia. *Cell* 1999;97:175.
27. Wei J, Yang I, Tapper A, et al. *KCNE1* polymorphism confers risk of drug-induced long QT syndrome by altering kinetic properties of I_{Ks} potassium channels. *Circulation* 1999;100:I-495.
28. Roden DM. Taking the "idio" out of "idiosyncratic": predicting torsade de pointes [Editorial]. *Pacing Clin Electrophysiol* 1998; 21:1029.
29. Beuckelmann DJ, Nabauer M, Erdmann E. Intracellular calcium handling in isolated ventricular myocytes from patients with terminal heart failure [Comments]. *Circulation* 1992;85:1046.
30. Wit AL. Triggered activity. In: Podrid PJ, Kowey PR, eds. *Cardiac arrhythmia: mechanisms, diagnosis, and management.* Baltimore, MD: Williams & Wilkins, 1995:70.
31. Reuter H. Localization of beta adrenergic receptors, and effects of noradrenaline and cyclic nucleotides on action potentials, ion currents and tension in mammalian cardiac muscle. *J Physiol* 1974;242:429.
32. Kameyama M, Hoffmann F, Trautwein W. On the mechanism of β-adrenergic regulation of the Ca channel in the guinea-pig heart. *Pflugers Arch* 1985;405:285.
33. Hoch B, Meyer R, Hetzer R, et al. Identification and expression of δ-isoforms of the multifunctional Ca^{2+}/calmodulin-dependent protein kinase in failing and nonfailing human myocardium. *Circ Res* 1999;84:713.
34. Wu Y, MacMillan LB, McNeill RB, et al. CaM kinase augments cardiac L-type Ca^{2+} current: a cellular mechanism for long QT arrhythmias. *Am J Physiol* 1999;276:H2168.
35. Wu Y, Roden DM, Anderson ME. Calmodulin kinase inhibition prevents development of the arrhythmogenic transient inward current. *Circ Res* 1999;84:906.
36. Waldo AL, Henthorn RW, Epstein AE, et al. Diagnosis and treatment of arrhythmias during and following open heart surgery. *Med Clin North Am* 1984;68:1153.
37. Das G, Ferris J. Esmolol in the treatment of supraventricular tachyarrhythmias. *Can J Cardiol* 1988;4:177.
38. Rowland E, McKenna WJ, Gulker H, et al. The comparative effects of diltiazem and verapamil on atrioventricular conduction and atrioventricular reentry tachycardia. *Circ Res* 1983;52:163.
39. Chew C, Hecht H, Colett J, et al. Influence of severity of ventricular dysfunction on hemodynamic responses to intravenously administered verapamil in ischemic heart disease. *Am J Cardiol* 1981;47:927.
40. Walsh RW, Porter CB, Starling MR, et al. Beneficial hemodynamic effects of intravenous and oral diltiazem in severe congestive heart failure. *J Am Coll Cardiol* 1984;3:1044.
41. Tisdale JE, Padhi ID, Goldberg AD, et al. A randomized, double-blind comparison of intravenous diltiazem and digoxin for atrial fibrillation after coronary artery bypass surgery. *Am Heart J* 1998; 135:739.
42. Wellens HJJ, Smeets JLRM, Rodriguez LM, et al. Atrial fibrillation in Wolff-Parkinson-White syndrome. In: Falk RH, Podrid PJ, eds. Atrial fibrillation: mechanisms and management. New York: Raven Press, 1992:333.
43. Galve E, Rius T, Ballester R, et al. Intravenous amiodarone in treatment of recent-onset atrial fibrillation: results of a randomized, controlled study. *J Am Coll Cardiol* 1996;27:1079.
44. Kochiadakis GE, Igoumenidis NE, Solomou MC, et al. Efficacy

of amiodarone for the termination of persistent atrial fibrillation. *Am J Cardiol* 1999;83:58.
45. Stambler BS, Wood MA, Ellenbogen KA, et al. Efficacy and safety of repeated intravenous doses of ibutilide for rapid conversion of atrial flutter or fibrillation. *Circulation* 1996;94:1613.
46. Liebold A, Wahba A, Birnbaum DE. Low-energy cardioversion with epicardial wire electrodes: new treatment of atrial fibrillation after open heart surgery. *Circulation* 1998;98:883.
47. Mathew JP, Parks R, Savino JS, et al. Atrial fibrillation following coronary artery bypass graft surgery. *JAMA* 1996;276:300.
48. Cresswell LL, Scheussler RB, Rosenbloom M, et al. Hazards of postoperative atrial arrhythmias. *Ann Thorac Surg* 1993;56:539.
49. Leitch JW, Thomson D, Baird DK, et al. The importance of age as a predictor of atrial fibrillation and flutter after coronary artery bypass grafting. *J Thorac Cardiovasc Surg* 1990;100:338.
50. Balser JR, Martinez EA, Winters BD, et al. Beta-adrenergic blockade accelerates conversion of postoperative supraventricular tachyarrhythmias. *Anesthesiology* 1998;89:1052.
51. Goldman L. Supraventricular tachyarrhythmias in hospitalized adults after surgery. *Chest* 1978;73:450.
52. Krowka MJ, Pairolero PC, Trastek VF, et al. Cardiac dysrhythmia following pneumonectomy: clinical correlates and prognostic significance. *Chest* 1987;91:490.
53. Amar D, Roistacher N, Burt M, et al. Clinical and echocardiographic correlates of symptomatic tachydysrhythmias after noncardiac thoracic surgery. *Chest* 1995;108:349.
54. Brathwaite D, Weissman C. New onset atrial arrhythmias are associated with increased mortality after noncardiothoracic surgery. *Anesthesiology* 1996;85:A266.
55. Balser JR. Pro: all patients should receive pharmacologic prophylaxis for atrial fibrillation after cardiac surgery. *J Cardiothorac Vasc Anesth* 1999;13:98.
56. Gullestad L, Birkeland K, Molstad P, et al. The effect of magnesium versus verapamil on supraventricular arrhythmias. *Clin Cardiol* 1993;16:429.
57. Moran JL, Gallagher J, Peake SL, et al. Parenteral magnesium sulfate versus amiodarone in the therapy of atrial tachyarrhythmias: a prospective, randomized study. *Crit Care Med* 1995;23:1816.
58. Platia EV, Michelson EL, Porterfield JK, et al. Esmolol versus verapamil in the acute treatment of atrial fibrillation or atrial flutter. *Am J Cardiol* 1989;63:925.
59. Kowey PR, Taylor JE, Rials SJ, et al. Metaanalysis of the effectiveness of prophylactic drug therapy in preventing supraventricular arrhythmia early after coronary artery bypass grafting. *Am J Cardiol* 1992;69:963.
60. England MR, Gordon G, Salem M, et al. Magnesium administration and dysrhythmias after cardiac surgery. *JAMA* 1992;268:2395.
61. Wistbacka JO, Koistinen J, Karlqvist KE, et al. Magnesium substitution in elective coronary artery surgery: a double-blind clinical study. *J Cardiothorac Vasc Anesth* 1995;9:140.
62. Aranki SF, Shaw DP, Adams DH, et al. Predictors of atrial fibrillation after coronary artery surgery: current trends and impact on hospital resources. *Circulation* 1996;94:390.
63. Olshansky B. Management of atrial fibrillation after coronary bypass graft. *Am J Cardiol* 1996;78(8A):27.
64. Fanning WJ, Thomas CS, Roach A, et al. Prophylaxis of atrial fibrillation with magnesium sulfate after coronary artery bypass grafting. *Ann Thorac Surg* 1991;52:529.
65. Hondeghem LM, Snyders DJ. Class III antiarrhythmic agents have a lot of potential but a long way to go: reduced effectiveness and dangers of reverse use dependence. *Circulation* 1990;81:686.
66. Villemaire C, Talajic M, Nattel S. Mechanisms by which sotalol prevents atrial fibrillation at doses that fail to terminate the arrhythmia. *Circulation* 1997;96:I-236.
67. Pfisterer ME, Kloter-Weber UC, Huber M, et al. Prevention of supraventricular tachyarrhythmias after open heart operation by low-dose sotalol: a prospective, double-blind, randomized, placebo-controlled study. *Ann Thorac Surg* 1997;64:1113.
68. Suttorp MJ, Kingma JH, Peels HOJ, et al. Effectiveness of sotalol in preventing supraventricular tachyarrhythmias shortly after coronary artery bypass grafting. *Am J Cardiol* 1991;68:1163.
69. Suttorp MJ, Kingma JH, Tjon Joe Gin RM, et al. Efficacy and safety of low- and high-dose sotalol versus propranolol in the prevention of supraventricular tachyarrhythmias early after coronary artery bypass operations. *J Thorac Cardiovasc Surg* 1990;100:921.
70. Daoud EG, Strickberger SA, Man KC, et al. Preoperative amiodarone as prophylaxis against atrial fibrillation after heart surgery. *N Engl J Med* 1997;337:1785.
71. Lazzara R. Amiodarone and torsade de pointes. *Ann Intern Med* 1989;111:549.
72. Mickleborough LL, Maruyama H, Mohamed S, et al. Are patients receiving amiodarone at increased risk for cardiac operations? *Ann Thorac Surg* 1994;58:622.
73. Greenspon AJ, Kidwell GA, Hurley W, et al. Amiodarone-related postoperative adult respiratory distress syndrome. *Circulation* 1991;84:407.
74. Van Mieghem W, Coolen L, Malysse I, et al. Amiodarone and the development of ARDS after lung surgery. *Chest* 1994;105:1642.
75. Dimopoulou I, Marathias K, Daganou M, et al. Low-dose amiodarone-related complications after cardiac operations. *J Thorac Cariovasc Surg* 1997;114:31.
76. Balser JR. The rational use of intravenous amiodarone in the perioperative period. *Anesthesiology* 1997;86:974.
77. Kuchar DL, Thorburn CW, Sammel NL. Prediction of serious arrhythmic events after myocardial infarction: signal-averaged electrocardiogram, Holter monitoring, and radionuclide ventriculography. *J Am Coll Cardiol* 1987;9:531.
78. Singh SN, Fletcher RD, Fisher SG, et al. Amiodarone in patients with congestive heart failure and asymptomatic ventricular arrhythmia. *N Engl J Med* 1995;333:77.
79. Mandel WJ. Sustained monomorphic ventricular tachycardia. In: Podrid PJ, Kowey PR, eds. *Cardiac arrhythmia: mechanisms, diagnosis, and management.* Baltimore, MD: Williams & Wilkins, 1995:919.
80. Gorgels APM, van den Dool A, Hofs A, et al. Comparison of procainamide and lidocaine in terminating sustained monomorphic ventricular tachycardia. *Am J Cardiol* 1996;78:43.
81. El-Sherif N. Polymorphic ventricular tachycardia. In: Podrid PJ, Kowey PR, eds. *Cardiac arrhythmia: mechanisms, diagnosis, and management.* Baltimore, MD: Williams & Wilkins, 1995:936.
82. Priori SG, Diehl L, Schwartz PJ. Torsade de pointes. In: Podrid PJ, Kowey PR, eds. *Cardiac arrhythmia: mechanisms, diagnosis, and management.* Baltimore, MD: Williams & Wilkins, 1995:951.
83. Mattioni TA, Zheutlin TA, Dunnington C, et al. The proarrhythmic effects of amiodarone. *Prog Cardiovasc Dis* 1989;31:439.
84. Abedin Z, Soares J, Phillips DF, et al. Ventricular tachyarrhythmias following surgery for myocardial revascularization. *Chest* 1977;72:426.
85. Smith RC, Leung JM, Keith FM, et al. Ventricular dysrhythmias in patients undergoing coronary artery bypass graft surgery: incidence, characteristics, and prognostic importance. *Am Heart J* 1992;123:73.
86. O'Kelly B, Browner WS, Massie B, et al. Ventricular arrhythmias in patients undergoing noncardiac surgery. *JAMA* 1992;268:217.
87. Topol EJ, Lerman BB, Baughman KL, et al. De novo refractory

ventricular tachyarrhythmias after coronary revascularization. *Am J Cardiol* 1986;57:57.
88. Kron I, DiMarco J, Harman P, et al. Unanticipated postoperative ventricular arrhythmias. *Ann Thorac Surg* 1984;38:317.
89. Elami A, Merin G, Flugelman MY, et al. Usefulness of late potentials on the immediate postoperative signal-averaged electrocardiogram in predicting ventricular tachyarrhythmias early after isolated coronary artery bypass grafting. *Am J Cardiol* 1994;74:33.
90. Santinga JT, Kirsh MM, Flora JD, et al. Factors relating to late sudden death in patients having aortic valve replacement. *Ann Thorac Surg* 1980;29:249.
91. Michel PL, Mandagout O, Vahanian A, et al. Ventricular arrhythmias in aortic valve disease before and after aortic valve replacement. *Acta Cardiol* 1992;47:145.
92. King FG, Addetia AM, Peters SD, et al. Prophylactic lidocaine for postoperative coronary artery bypass patients, a double-blind, randomized trial. *Can J Anaesth* 1990;37:363.
93. Kaul TK, Fields BL, Riggins LS, et al. Ventricular arrhythmia following successful myocardial revascularization: incidence, predictors and prevention. *Eur J Cardiothorac Surg* 1998;13:629.
94. Bigger JT Jr. Prophylactic use of implanted cardiac defibrillators in patients at high risk for ventricular arrhythmias after coronary artery bypass graft surgery. Coronary Artery Bypass Graft Patch Trial Investigators [comments]. *N Engl J Med* 1997; 337:1569.
95. Levine JH, Massumi A, Scheinman MM, et al. Intravenous amiodarone for recurrent sustained hypotensive ventricular tachyarrhythmias. *J Am Coll Cardiol* 1996;27:67.
96. Kowey PR, Levine JH, Herre JM, et al. Randomized, double-blind comparison of intravenous amiodarone and bretylium in the treatment of patients with recurrent hemodynamically destabilizing ventricular tachycardia or fibrillation. *Circulation* 1995; 92:3255.
97. Installe E, Schoevaerdts JC, Gadisseux P, et al. Intravenous amiodarone in the treatment of various arrhythmias following cardiac operations. *J Thorac Cardiovasc Surg* 1981;81:302.
98. Perry JC, Knilans TK, Marlow D, et al. Intravenous amiodarone for life-threatening tachyarrhythmias in children and young adults. *J Am Coll Cardiol* 1993;22:95.

Cardiac Anesthesia: Principles and Clinical Practice, Second Edition, edited by Fawzy G. Estafanous, Paul G. Barash, and J.G. Reves. Lippincott Williams & Wilkins, Philadelphia © 2001.

5

DIAGNOSTIC AND INTERVENTIONAL CARDIAC CATHETERIZATION

JOHN J. WARNER
THOMAS M. BASHORE

Over the past two decades there has been a tremendous increase in the number of cardiac catheterizations performed in the United States. The number in 1996 exceeded 1.5 million and had increased more than three-fold since 1979 (1). During this time the development of percutaneous therapeutic procedures for coronary, valvular, and congenital heart disease has been phenomenal. It is estimated that more than 600,000 patients will receive a percutaneous, nonoperative cardiac intervention in the United States this year. There are now more than 2,000 cardiac catheterization laboratories in the United States. This chapter summarizes the indications, techniques, and risks associated with both diagnostic and interventional cardiac catheterization procedures.

HISTORY OF CARDIAC CATHETERIZATION

Werner Forssmann performed the first human cardiac catheterization on himself in 1929 (2). He inserted a urethral catheter into his own antecubital vein, advanced it into the right side of his heart, and confirmed the position with a chest radiograph. Interest in cardiac catheterization increased in the 1940s and 1950s, led by the work of Cournard and Richards at Bellevue Hospital in New York. In 1956 Forssmann, Cournard, and Richards received the Nobel Prize in Medicine for their pioneering work in the field. Catheterization of the left side of the heart continued to present a formidable challenge, with descriptions of risky transbronchial and transthoracic direct puncture of the left atrium and the left ventricle (LV). In 1953, Seldinger described the technique of arterial needle puncture with catheter exchange over a guidewire (3). This basic technique remains the standard today, and its simplicity has made retrograde catheterization of the left heart commonplace.

In 1962, Sones and Shirey described a reliable method for selective catheterization and arteriographic visualization of the coronary arteries (4). This technique involved catheter insertion via a brachial artery cutdown. In 1967, Judkins and Amplatz developed preformed catheters for selective coronary arteriography from the femoral artery approach (5). Modifications of these preformed catheters remain in widespread use today.

Right-sided heart catheterization was simplified in 1970 when Swan and Ganz introduced a balloon-tipped flow-directed catheter that allowed catheterization of the right heart without the use of fluoroscopy (6). During this same decade the technique of coronary angioplasty was first promoted by Gruntzig (7). This procedure revolutionized the treatment strategies for ischemic heart disease and launched the field of interventional cardiology. Interventional cardiology now offers effective percutaneous treatment for selected cases of valvular, congenital, and ischemic heart disease. Currently, there continues to be an explosion of technology directed toward improving the immediate and late outcomes of these procedures. With novel percutaneous techniques come increased risks, including life-threatening complications. Optimal care for patients undergoing these high-risk procedures requires the cooperative efforts of cardiologists, cardiac anesthesiologists, and cardiac surgeons.

INDICATIONS FOR CARDIAC CATHETERIZATION

The indications for cardiac catheterization continue to expand and evolve, due in part to improvement in the catheterization technique itself and also to therapeutic options now available because of advances in cardiac surgery and interventional cardiology. The increased number of therapeutic options and their applicability to a larger population of patients have lowered the threshold for defining specific cardiac anatomic information through cardiac catheterization. Several indications for catheterization remain controversial. In an effort to address the changing role of cardiac catheterization, the American College of Cardiology and the American Heart Association have formulated guidelines

J. J. Warner and T. M. Bashore: Department of Medicine, Division of Cardiology, Duke University, Durham, North Carolina 27710

TABLE 5-1. INDICATIONS FOR CARDIAC CATHETERIZATION

1. Evaluation of patients with valvular or congenital heart disease before cardiac surgery
2. Infective endocarditis with evidence of coronary embolization
3. Evaluation of patients with hypertrophic cardiomyopathy and angina when knowledge of coronary anatomy might affect therapy or when cardiac surgery is planned
4. Evaluation of patients with disease affecting the aorta when knowledge of coronary artery involvement is necessary for management (e.g., aortic dissection or aneurysm)
5. Evaluation of patients with suspected coronary artery disease in the following situations:
   a. Unstable angina
   b. Angina refractory to medical therapy
   c. High-risk findings on noninvasive testing
   d. Suspected Prinzmetal angina variant
   e. Patients resuscitated from sudden cardiac death or who have ventricular arrhythmias
   f. Patients with known or suspected coronary artery and high-risk or equivocal noninvasive test results undergoing noncardiac surgery
6. Evaluation of patients with congestive heart failure in the following situations:
   a. Systolic dysfunction with angina, regional wall motion abnormalities, or reversible ischemia on scintigraphic images when revascularization is being considered
   b. Before cardiac transplantation
   c. Congestive heart failure secondary to mechanical complications of myocardial infarction
7. Evaluation of patients with acute myocardial infarction in the following situations:
   a. Coronary angiography coupled with the intent to perform primary percutaneous transluminal coronary angioplasty
   b. Patient within 36 hours after an acute myocardial infarction complicated by cardiogenic shock
   c. Patient with spontaneous or inducable ischemia during recovery from infarction

for the use of cardiac catheterization and coronary angiography (8). Although these guidelines are not absolute, they do illustrate some of the more common indications for cardiac catheterization (Table 5-1). The risks involved with cardiac catheterization must be weighed against the potential benefit of the information obtained for each individual. The overall mortality risk of diagnostic cardiac catheterization is about 0.1%, and most patients can be studied safely in the outpatient setting. Patients at increased risk for complications during cardiac catheterization include those with complex congenital heart disease, critical aortic stenosis, pulmonary hypertension, severe chronic obstructive pulmonary disease, renal insufficiency, severe LV dysfunction, severe cerebrovascular or peripheral vascular disease, or advanced age. These higher-risk patients should be monitored carefully after the procedure.

With few exceptions, diagnostic cardiac catheterization is indicated for all adult patients who are to undergo cardiac surgery. In patients with valvular or congenital heart disease, cardiac catheterization provides confirmatory and complementary data to echocardiography and Doppler studies of valvular function. Some patients (e.g., younger patients with well-defined lesions such as a secundum atrial septal defect or active endocarditis) may not require preoperative cardiac catheterization. Catheterization also allows definition of coronary anatomy and quantification of the hemodynamic consequences of the valvular dysfunction, which are data not routinely obtainable by echocardiography. This is particularly relevant in congenital heart disease, where the severity of associated pulmonary hypertension is extremely important to determine suitability for surgical repair. In addition, angiography provides complementary data regarding valvular regurgitation for comparison with Doppler echocardiographic data. We believe these studies are complementary in making therapeutic decisions for almost all patients with valvular or congenital heart disease. The risk/benefit ratio of preoperative cardiac catheterization in adult patients with valvular heart disease remains weighted heavily in favor of preoperative cardiac catheterization (9).

The most frequent indication for adult cardiac catheterization is in the identification and definition of the severity of coronary artery disease. Coronary angiography remains the reference standard for defining the presence and severity of coronary disease. Patients with unstable or crescendo angina are at increased risk for acute myocardial infarction (MI) and should undergo coronary arteriography. These lesions are dynamic, and noninvasive functional studies may not only be unsafe but may also fail to identify coronary lesions with unstable morphology (e.g., ulcerated plaque, presence of thrombus). Patients with recurrent angina after MI also require cardiac catheterization, because these patients have unstable lesions and are at increased risk for reinfarction. In addition, patients at high risk after MI, such as those with congestive heart failure, life-threatening ventricular arrhythmias, or mechanical complications (e.g., ventricular septal defect, mitral regurgitation), will benefit from cardiac catheterization because surgical repair may be indicated.

Patients with stable angina in whom a noninvasive functional study indicates a high probability of severe coronary disease should undergo cardiac catheterization. Coronary artery bypass grafting (CABG) has been shown to decrease mortality, compared with medical therapy, in patients with multivessel coronary disease, especially in association with depressed LV function, and in patients with significant disease of the left main coronary artery (10,11). Therefore, patients with a noninvasive exercise test suggesting extensive coronary disease should be invasively studied. These include patients with an early positive exercise test (i.e., positive in stage 1 or at a heart rate of less than 100 beats/minute), those with ST-segment depression greater than 2 mm, and those with angina associated with hypotension during exercise. In patients undergoing radionuclide exercise testing, a large reversible perfusion defect on radionuclide imaging or a substantial decrease (10 or more ejection fraction points) with exercise radionuclide-gated blood pool imaging indicates significant myocardial ischemia and warrants coronary arteriography.

As more people undergo noninvasive screening for coronary artery disease, the incidence of suspected coronary disease in asymptomatic patients increases. Asymptomatic myocardial ischemia does occur in patients with coronary disease and has adverse prognostic implications consistent with the extent of anatomic disease (12,13). Therefore, patients with early positive or diffusely abnormal noninvasive exercise tests, regardless of symptoms, should undergo coronary arteriography. No noninvasive study is perfectly sensitive or specific for coronary disease, and coronary arteriography also defines those patients who have a false-positive exercise result, thus avoiding erroneous diagnoses and unnecessary treatment.

Cardiac catheterization can be potentially valuable for patients with known or suspected heart disease before major noncardiac surgery. Most of the perioperative risk information can be obtained, however, from the patient's history and noninvasive exercise testing. Cardiac catheterization may provide valuable information in the patient who is unable to undergo noninvasive exercise testing. Pharmacologic "stress" tests using dobutamine, adenosine, or dipyridamole are noninvasive alternatives that are also available for those patients who are unable to exercise.

Despite an extensive body of literature, the routine use of cardiac catheterization after MI remains controversial (14–19). Systemic intravenous thrombolytic agents are now widely used in attempts to recanalize the acute infarct vessel during acute ST-segment elevation MI. These agents have been proved effective in decreasing mortality, limiting infarct size, improving LV function, and angiographically recanalizing the occluded artery in approximately 75% of patients (20–24). Routine coronary arteriography and angioplasty performed acutely after the administration of thrombolytic agents has not been shown to provide a survival advantage or improvement in LV function compared with these same procedures performed on a delayed, elective basis (24,25). Routine invasive study in conjunction with the use of intravenous thrombolytic agents was associated with a high frequency of bleeding complications. We currently reserve emergency coronary arteriography for patients with suspected persistent coronary occlusion after intravenous administration of thrombolytic agents and for those in whom intravenous thrombolytic agents are contraindicated. Although infarct-related artery patency remains imperfectly defined based on noninvasive clinical criteria, patients who have persistent chest discomfort, persistent ST-segment elevation, cardiogenic shock, or persistent hemodynamic instability after receiving intravenous thrombolytic agents for acute MI should undergo emergency cardiac catheterization (26). Patients with non–ST-segment elevation MI or unstable angina should be considered for emergency cardiac catheterization if they exhibit episodes of recurrent spontaneous ischemia, recurrent arrhythmias, or evidence of shock.

Patients with continued occlusion of the infarct vessel are thus identified and taken for immediate coronary arteriography. In patients with suitable anatomy, percutaneous transluminal coronary angioplasty (PTCA) is employed to restore infarct vessel patency. In patients with unsuitable or high-risk anatomy, emergency CABG may be preferable.

Patients who are not candidates for intravenous systemic thrombolytic agents (those with a history of severe bleeding, recent surgery, or stroke) are candidates for acute emergency cardiac catheterization and intervention. Immediate PTCA during acute MI, often referred to as primary PTCA, is successful in restoring infarct artery patency in more than 90% of cases in laboratories where it is frequently used (27–33). This approach has the advantage of a markedly lower risk of stroke or intracranial hemorrhage than thrombolysis and should be used, if available, in patients at high risk for these complications. Elderly patients and those with preexisting symptomatic cerebrovascular disease or severe hypertension are at increased risk for both hemorrhagic and nonhemorrhagic stroke and should receive primary PTCA if it can be accomplished without delay (34).

There is significant debate as to which strategy should be the preferred choice in acute MI: thrombolysis or primary angioplasty. Primary angioplasty is limited by the time required to get patients into the catheterization laboratory and by its availability only at large centers. Thrombolytic therapy is limited by lower infarct artery patency rates compared with primary PTCA and by bleeding complications. To date, the six largest randomized, prospective trials have individually failed to show a distinct advantage for either strategy in mortality, LV function, or need for subsequent intervention (27–32). A metaanalysis of ten trials illustrated what had been seen with many of the smaller trials (33). Primary angioplasty, when accomplished successfully, appears to provide a small short-term advantage over thrombolytic therapy. At 30 days, these trials all show a trend toward lower mortality, less reinfarction, and lower rates of disabling stroke in patients who receive PTCA versus thrombolysis. When end points were combined, there was a 2% mortality advantage for the PTCA strategy. Total stroke (0.7% versus 2%) and hemorrhagic stroke (0.1% versus 1.1%) were markedly lower when PTCA was the initial strategy. The Global Use of Strategies to Open Occluded Arteries in Acute Coronary Syndromes (GUSTO) IIb primary angioplasty substudy showed similar improvements in a composite end point of death, reinfarction, and disabling stroke at 30 days (9.6% versus 13.7%). However, at 6 months there was no statistical difference between groups in the incidence of the composite end point (32). Outcomes following primary angioplasty for acute myocardial infarction continue to improve as more patients receive coronary artery stents and aggressive antiplatelet therapy with IIb/IIIa inhibitors.

At present, the evidence for widespread primary PTCA for acute MI is not conclusive. Future research will more clearly define which patients stand to benefit most from primary PTCA and which patients are at highest risk for life-threatening complications or stroke when given thrombolytic therapy. Until these facts are known, the emphasis should be on restoring brisk antegrade coronary flow as quickly and safely as possible, because time to reperfusion remains overwhelmingly the strongest predictor of improved survival (21,22).

Another area of controversy is the routine delayed performance of cardiac catheterization in patients who have had clinically uncomplicated courses after MI. Four large randomized, prospective trials have addressed this issue, assigning patients to either an "invasive" strategy of routine predischarge coronary angiography and revascularization or a "conservative" strategy in which cardiac catheterization and revascularization was performed only for recurrent spontaneous or exercise-induced ischemia (18,35–37). These studies showed that routine coronary angiography and revascularization does not reduce the incidence of death or reinfarction or produce an improvement in LV function compared with the more conservative, ischemia-guided approach. These observations have led some to recommend a conservative, noninvasive approach for patients with an uncomplicated course after receiving intravenous thrombolytic therapy for acute MI. This approach recommends coronary arteriography only for patients with spontaneous or exercise-induced ischemia, those with a mechanical complication of MI, and those who have clinical indicators suggesting a high risk of recurrent MI or death (Table 5-2). Proponents of a more invasive approach, in which all infarction survivors undergo routine predischarge coronary arteriography, believe that cardiac catheterization contributes more reliable prognostic information than does noninvasive testing and that routine coronary arteriography followed by selective use of noninvasive studies is the most efficient and cost-effective method of identifying patients who may benefit from coronary revascularization (14). In support of this argument is the fact that up to two thirds of patients treated in the "conservative" arms of these trials eventually underwent coronary angiography within 6 weeks after randomization.

Although controversy exists about the preferred initial strategy, the overwhelming majority of patients in the United States who sustain a MI do undergo cardiac catheterization. Seventy-eight percent of ST-segment elevation MI patients in the GUSTO III trial underwent angiography, and 88% patients with a non–ST-segment elevation MI received angiography in the Platelet Glycoprotein IIb/IIIa in Unstable Angina: Receptor Suppression using Integrelin Therapy (PURSUIT) trial (38,39). In today's managed care–based environment, the controversy surrounding these two divergent approaches is likely to shift from efficacy, which to date appears equivalent, to cost-effectiveness.

TABLE 5-2. CLINICAL PREDICTORS OF HIGH RISK FOR RECURRENT MYOCARDIAL INFARCTION OR DEATH AFTER ACUTE MYOCARDIAL INFARCTION

Congestive heart failure
Arterial hypotension
Recurrent ischemia
Malignant arrhythmia more than 24 hours after onset of chest pain
Mechanical complication (mitral regurgitation, ventricular septal defect)

TECHNIQUE OF CARDIAC CATHETERIZATION

Advances in catheter design, x-ray equipment, and radiographic contrast agents have improved the safety of diagnostic cardiac catheterization and have permitted the development of therapeutic transcatheter procedures. These advances allow cardiac catheterization to be applied to the most acutely ill patients during acute MI and have also allowed the procedure to be commonly performed on a less costly outpatient basis.

Cardiac catheterization can be performed via either brachial, radial, or femoral artery vascular access. Most centers prefer the femoral technique, reserving alternative techniques for patients with severe aortic or iliac disease. The original technique, the Sones brachial technique, involved a cutdown of the brachial vessel with direct catheter insertion (4). The Sones catheter is retrogradely advanced via the brachial artery to the aorta. Selective intubation of both coronaries can be achieved with this one catheter, and left ventriculography can be performed with it as well. When the catheter is removed, vascular repair at the cutdown site is required. Because of the smaller caliber of the brachial artery compared with the femoral artery, vascular occlusion is a more frequent complication with this technique.

Cardiac catheterization can also be performed via the brachial artery using a percutaneous approach without vascular cutdown (40). The Seldinger technique is used to gain access to the brachial artery, and a small-caliber vascular sheath (usually 5F or 6F) is inserted and flushed with heparin. Small-caliber catheters with preformed Judkins curves can be used for selective coronary arteriography via this percutaneous brachial approach. Hemostasis after catheter removal is achieved by direct compression of the puncture site. Despite anticoagulation with heparin, occlusion of the brachial vessels or their downstream branches remains a risk.

Cardiac catheterization is most frequently performed by a percutaneous catheter insertion approach from the femoral artery. A local anesthetic agent is infiltrated, and the common femoral artery is punctured just below the inguinal ligament. The Seldinger technique is employed: the femoral artery is entered with a thin-walled needle; then a flexible guidewire is inserted through the needle into the vessel lumen. The needle is removed, leaving the guidewire in place, and then a catheter or vascular sheath is inserted into

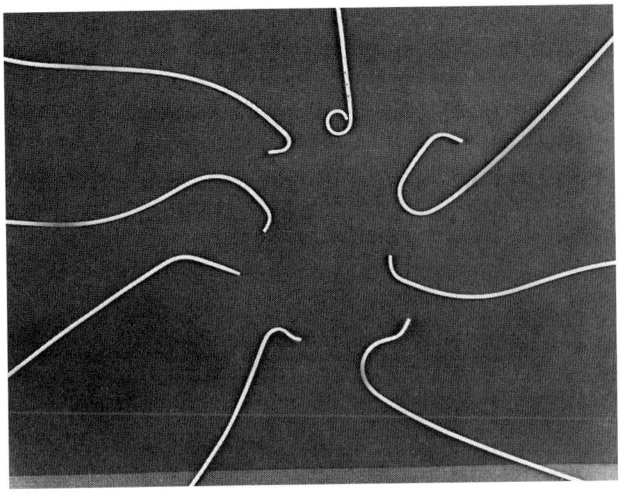

FIGURE 5-1. Diagnostic catheters commonly used during cardiac catheterization. *From the top, proceeding clockwise:* pigtail catheter used for left ventriculography, Judkins left coronary catheter, Judkins right coronary catheter, Amplatz left coronary catheter, Amplatz right coronary catheter, multipurpose coronary catheter, coronary artery bypass graft catheter, internal mammary artery catheter. (From Davidson CJ, Harrison JK. Basic catheter techniques. In: Bashore TM, ed. *Invasive cardiology: principles and techniques.* Toronto: BC Decker, 1990: 121, with permission.)

the vessel over the guidewire. The left side of the heart is then retrogradely catheterized with introduction of the catheters over a long (175 cm; 0.035-inch diameter) guidewire. Left ventriculography is commonly performed using a pigtail catheter with multiple side holes. Selective coronary arteriography is achieved with the use of preformed arteriographic catheters (Fig. 5-1). Catheters with Judkins curves can be used in most patients for selective coronary arteriography. Whereas the Judkins left coronary catheter often intubates the left main coronary artery when the catheter is simply advanced, the Judkins right coronary catheter requires more manipulation and torquing of the catheter to selectively engage the right ostium. The Judkins right coronary catheter can also be used to selectively engage the majority of venous bypass grafts or the internal mammary arteries. In patients with large ascending aortic roots, or in cases where there is anomalous origin of the coronary ostia, a variety of alternative catheters are available.

Multiple radiographic projections of the coronary arteries are routinely obtained, usually with hand injection of radiographic contrast material. The goal is to obtain orthogonal views of the coronary arteries, because eccentric atherosclerotic stenoses may be missed unless adequate views are obtained (Fig. 5-2).

There is growing enthusiasm for left heart catheterization via the radial artery approach. This technique was developed in an attempt to reduce the vascular complications and patient discomfort that plague the femoral and brachial techniques (41). The hand has a dual arterial supply connected across the palmar arch. As long as the ulnar artery is sufficient to provide collateral supply to the radial artery in the event of radial artery occlusion, there is minimal risk of an ischemic complication. In addition, the more superficial puncture site is more easily compressed than either the femoral or brachial site. Finally, the procedure is more comfortable for patients, because they can be ambulatory within 1 hour after the procedure and only the wrist and hand need be immobile during removal of the sheath, eliminating the need for prolonged bed rest.

In our laboratory, we perform radial artery catheterization by introducing a 20-gauge needle into the radial artery after an Allen test has confirmed sufficient collateral flow through the ulnar artery circulation. We then introduce a flexible 0.025-inch guidewire through the 20-gauge needle and advance it to the ascending aorta. A 5F, 6F, or 7F sheath is placed into the radial arery over the guidewire. We administer verapamil and heparin through the side port of the sheath as it is introduced to prevent painful vasospasm and prevent thrombotic complications. Traditional catheters or specialized radial catheters can be used to perform routine angiography and PTCA via the radial technique. Because most coronary interventions can now be performed through 6F or 7F catheters, this approach is appropriate for both diagnostic angiography and coronary angioplasty. Once the procedure is completed, the sheath is immediately withdrawn and digital compression is applied. A variety of wristband-type devices are available to assist with achieving hemostasis. Although this procedure currently is used at relatively few centers, the initial results with both diagnostic coronary angiography and coronary angioplasty show a promising decrease in entry-site complications with acceptable rates of procedural success (42).

Although right-sided heart catheterization is not routinely necessary in patients with isolated coronary disease, it is an essential component of the cardiac catheterization data in patients with valvular or congenital heart disease and in those patients with suspected pulmonary hypertension (43). Right-sided heart catheterization provides hemodynamic data, cardiac output, vascular resistance measurements, and intracardiac shunt determinations. Catheterization of the right side of the heart may be performed by the Seldinger technique via either the femoral, iliac, jugular, or subclavian veins. It is most commonly performed with a balloon-tipped, flow-directed catheter. The pulmonary capillary wedge pressure can be measured with this catheter as well. This measurement accurately reflects the left atrial pressure in most patients, although the phasic waveforms may be damped and are temporally delayed compared to those obtained by direct left atrial measurements. In patients with pulmonary vascular disease, however, the pulmonary capillary wedge pressure may not always reflect left atrial pressure. In these instances, transseptal catheterization of the left atrium must be performed (44,45).

Transseptal catheterization of the left atrium is per-

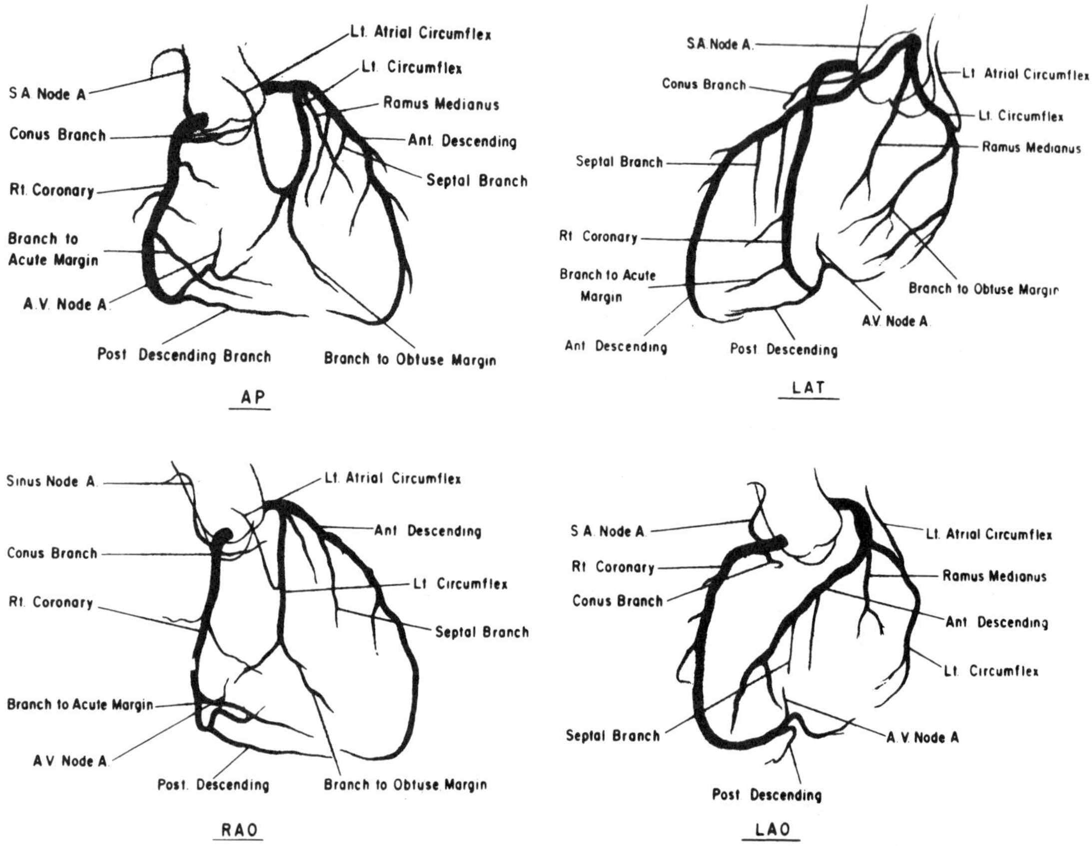

FIGURE 5-2. Illustration of coronary anatomy in commonly used projections. *From the top left, proceeding clockwise:* anteroposterior projection, lateral projection, left anterior oblique projection, right anterior oblique projection. (From Abrams HL, Adams DF. The coronary arteriogram: structural and functional aspects. *N Engl J Med* 1969;281:1276, with permission.)

formed from the right femoral vein, using a specially designed catheter (Mullins or Brockenbrough catheter). The catheter is first positioned in the right atrium (RA), and a thin, long transseptal needle is then inserted through the catheter's length to its tip. The position of the catheter tip is monitored by biplane fluoroscopy, and the tip is manipulated posteriorly toward the fossa ovalis. Monitoring of pressure via the needle lumen is mandatory. With pressure and fluoroscopic monitoring, the transseptal needle is advanced through the intraatrial septum. Once the left atrial pressure is confirmed, the catheter is advanced over the needle into the left atrium.

Percutaneous endomyocardial biopsies can be also obtained during cardiac catheterization (46–48). Biopsies are performed via the internal jugular or femoral vein. With the internal jugular approach, a preformed Caves-Schultz bioptome is inserted into the RA. It is manipulated with counterclockwise rotation, under fluoroscopic or echocardiographic guidance, across the tricuspid valve to the right side of the intraventricular septum. Monitoring the intracardiac electrocardiogram may also be used to confirm that the tip of the bioptome is in the right ventricle (RV). From the femoral approach, a long, curved sheath is inserted into the femoral vein and is manipulated across the tricuspid valve and directed toward the intraventricular septum. A flexible bioptome is then inserted through the sheath. Multiple biopsies, about 2 mm in diameter, can be obtained with either technique. Endomyocardial biopsies are useful for monitoring rejection in heart transplant recipients and may be used to diagnose acute myocarditis or cardiac toxicity in patients receiving chemotherapy (e.g., Adriamycin). Endomyocardial biopsies may also be obtained in efforts to define the cause of a dilated cardiomyopathy; however, biopsies in this situation are diagnostic in only about 5% of cases (49).

Catheterization techniques in patients with prosthetic heart valves offer a unique challenge. Although porcine or Starr-Edwards valves may be safely crossed with small-diameter catheters in a retrograde fashion, the tilting disk valvular prostheses (e.g., St. Jude, Medtronic Hall and Lillehei-Kastor) should not be crossed with a guidewire or catheter. If these disk valves are crossed, severe, acute valvular insufficiency may result. Of even greater importance, the catheter may become entrapped, with the disk acting as a one-way valve.

COMPLICATIONS OF CARDIAC CATHETERIZATION

Although older and acutely ill patients are currently safely undergoing diagnostic coronary catheterization, the incidence of major morbidity and mortality associated with these diagnostic studies remains low and is probably declining (Table 5-3) (50–52). The largest series examining complications of diagnostic coronary arteriography is from the Society of Coronary Angiography and Interventions Registry (50). Their latest report describes the complications in 59,792 patients who underwent selective coronary arteriography in 1990. The overall incidence of complications was 1.7%. The rate of arteriography-related death was 0.11%, unchanged from their previous series of more than 200,000 patients.

These same investigators also developed a multivariate model which identified 12 variables that predict major complications in patients undergoing elective diagnostic cardiac catheterization (51). Patients who were in a moribund condition before catheterization were at highest risk (a ten-fold increase) for a major complication, followed by patients with shock (a six-fold increase), patients within 24 hours of MI (a four-fold increase), and patients with renal insufficiency or a cardiomyopathy (a three-fold increase). Patients with aortic or mitral valve disease had a risk of major complication 2.5 times higher than that of the total population. Patients with left main coronary artery disease had a two-fold increased risk of major complications (51). The elderly were also at increased risk.

These risks of cardiac catheterization in patients with coronary artery disease may not be completely applicable to patients with valvular heart disease. The Veterans Administration Cooperative Study on Valvular Heart Disease reported the complications of cardiac catheterization in 1,559 patients with significant valvular disease (Table 5-3) (53). The complication rate was higher in this population than in the Society of Coronary Angiography and Interventions Registry, although the characteristics of the two populations were substantially different. Women were excluded from the Veterans Administration study, and the mortality figures included all deaths occurring within 90 days after cardiac catheterization; the Registry's mortality figures included only periprocedural deaths (within 24 hours). Reporting of late complications was encouraged but not monitored. Predictors of major complications in the Veterans Administration report were a history of hypertension or a diagnosis of aortic stenosis. The need for transseptal catheterization was associated with an increased incidence of cardiac tamponade, and the use of a brachial approach was associated with an increased risk of arterial thrombosis.

There have been several conflicting reports concerning the incidence of complications in patients studied by the brachial versus the femoral approach. The overall rate of complications appears to be similar, but the types of complications differ. Arterial thrombosis or distal embolization occurs more frequently in patients studied by the brachial approach, whereas bleeding complications are more common with the femoral approach. Early reports from radial artery catheterization series show low incidences of both thrombosis and embolization, with a bleeding risk that approaches zero (52). It is clear that experience of the operator is important, and whichever method is more frequently used by the operator will be associated with less risk. Because of ease of use, most procedures are now performed from the femoral vessels.

TABLE 5-3. RISKS OF DIAGNOSTIC CARDIAC CATHETERIZATION (%)

Parameter	Society of Coronary Angiography Study[a]	Veterans Administration Study[b]
No. of catherizations	59,792	1,559
Population	All diagnostic studies	Valvular disease
Risk		
Death	0.11	0.19
Myocardial infarction	0.05	0.19
Neurologic deficit	0.07	0.32
Arrhythmia	0.38	2.0
Vascular	0.43	1.5
Contrast reaction	0.37	1.8
Perforation	0.03	0.3
Other	0.54	2.5
Total	1.7	6.9

[a] From Noto TJ, Johnson LW, Krone R, et al. Cardiac catheterization 1990: a report of the Registry of the Society for Cardiac Angiography and Interventions. *Cathet Cardiovasc Diagn* 1991; 24:75.
[b] From Folland ED, Oprian C, Giacomini J, et al. Complications of cardiac cathetrization and angiography in patients with valvular heart disease. *Cathet Cardiovasc Diagn* 1989;19:15.

CORONARY ARTERIOGRAPHY

Defining the extent and severity of coronary disease is a major goal in adult patients undergoing cardiac catheterization. Traditionally, cine angiograms were taken on 35-mm film at a rate of 30 frames per second during the hand injection of radiographic contrast material. With the rapid progress in digital technology, many laboratories are now making the transition to digital acquisition and archiving systems, eliminating the need to develop and store cine films. The advantages of a digital catheterization laboratory include on-line review, the ability to use quantitative computer analysis and manipulate image properties, flicker-free images at low frame rates, and the ability to transfer studies between catheterizaton laboratories. Images can be viewed on inexpensive personal computers rather than expensive cine film projectors and can be read at various stations throughout the hospital, office, or operating rooms.

At the beginning of coronary arteriograms, patients are usually given intravenous heparin (e.g., 2,000 units). The aortic pressure is monitored via the fluid-filled catheter lumen, which is connected to a transducer located on the catheterization table. After selective cannulation of the coronary ostia, aortic pressure is noted. If there is ostial disease, a damped pressure tracing may occur (Fig. 5-3). If this occurs, the catheter is withdrawn to just outside the ostium, and "flush" injections are recorded to define the severity of the ostial coronary disease. If severe ostial coronary disease does not exist, the catheter is positioned in the ostium of the coronary and selective injections of 3 to 10 mL of contrast agent are performed.

Low-osmolar, nonionic contrast medium is now used in most catheterization laboratories for coronary arteriography and interventions. Nonionic contrast medium is better tolerated and results in fewer allergic reactions, less nausea, fewer arrhythmias, and less hypotension during coronary arteriography than does high-osmolar, ionic contrast medium (54,55). The cost of nonionic contrast medium exceeds the cost of the ionic contrast agents by a ratio of about 10 : 1, however, and there remains an ongoing debate as to

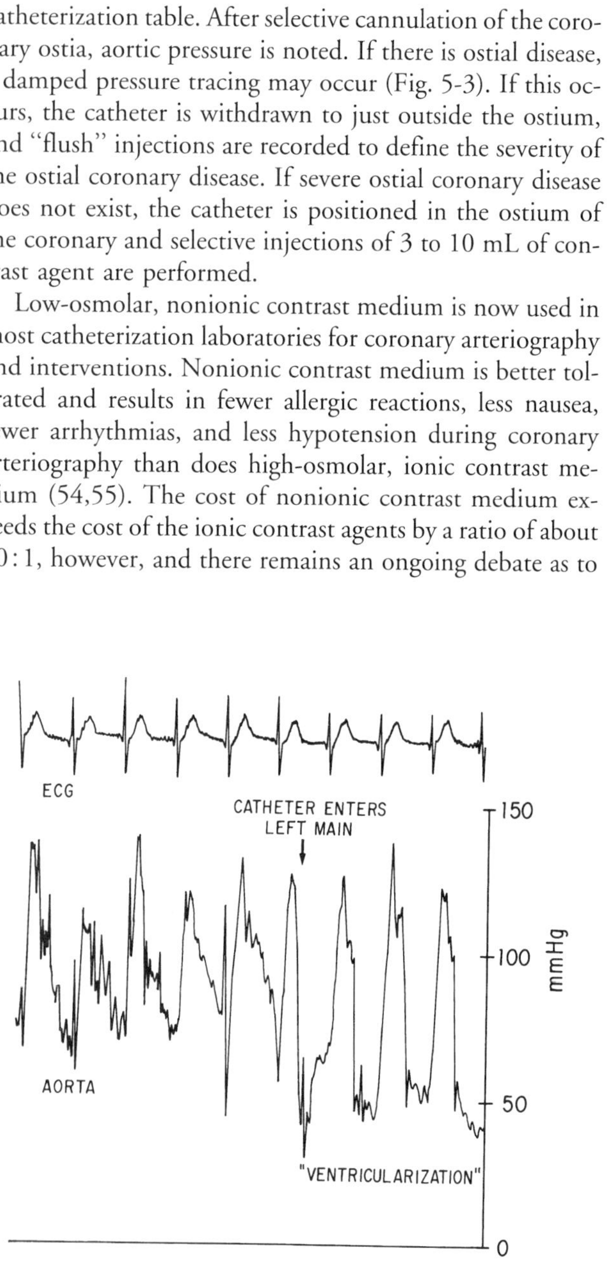

FIGURE 5-3. Aortic and coronary artery pressure measured through the fluid-filled lumen of the coronary catheter. Note the "ventricularized" pressure once the coronary catheter engages the left coronary ostium. This type of ventricularized pressure suggests ostial coronary artery stenosis. (From Davidson CJ, Harrison JK. Basic catheter techniques. In: Bashore TM, ed. *Invasive cardiology: principles and techniques.* Toronto: BC Decker Inc., 1990:123, with permission.)

whether the markedly improved comfort felt by the patient with the use of nonionic contrast medium warrants this cost differential. Although most studies show no difference in the incidence of serious complications, there are clearly some high-risk patients who will derive a benefit from the use of nonionic contrast medium. These include patients with congestive heart failure, those with a previous contrast reaction, those with an unstable coronary syndrome, and possibly those with renal insufficiency. Although most small trials have failed to show decreased nephrotoxicity with newer, lower-osmolar agents, the largest randomized trial to date reported a three-fold greater incidence of nephrotoxicity with a high-osmolar, ionic contrast dye (56,57). Patients with baseline renal insufficiency (creatinine greater than 2.0 mg/dL) are at greatest risk for contrast nephropathy. Pre-treatment with hydration and n-acetylcysteine appears to reduce the risk of contrast nephrotoxicity.

NORMAL CORONARY ANATOMY

Multiple angulated views of the coronary arteries are required to completely define the extent and severity of the coronary disease. Figure 5-4 outlines the normal coronary anatomy. The left main coronary artery usually bifurcates into the left anterior descending coronary artery (LAD) and the left circumflex coronary artery. It occasionally trifurcates, with the large middle branch, the ramus intermedius or optional diagonal artery, supplying the anterolateral wall of the LV. The left circumflex coronary travels posteriorly in the atrioventricular (AV) groove, giving off marginal branches while supplying the lateral and posterior walls of the LV. It is these marginal branches that are bypassed at the time of surgery, because the left circumflex itself lies in the epicardial fat of the AV groove and is usually surgically inaccessible. The LAD gives off septal perforators and diagonal branches (to the anterolateral wall) before ending at or beyond the ventricular apex. Coronary "dominance" is defined by the vessel that supplies the posterior descending artery. This is the right coronary in about 85% of people. If the right coronary artery supplies the posterior descending vessel and gives rise to posterolateral branches to the inferolateral LV, then the system is called right-dominant. If the circumflex coronary artery supplies the posterior descending vessel, it is a left-dominant coronary system. A codominant system exists if the right coronary artery supplies the posterior descending vessel but provides no further posterolateral branches to the LV.

Coronary anomalies are occasionally encountered, but most are clinically insignificant. Rarely, when the left coronary artery arises from the right sinus of Valsalva and courses between the aorta and pulmonary artery (PA), the slit-like origin of the left coronary artery may result in ischemia during exertion. A coronary anomaly seen in children and in adults is origin of the left main coronary artery from the PA (Bland-White-Garland syndrome) (58). In this anom-

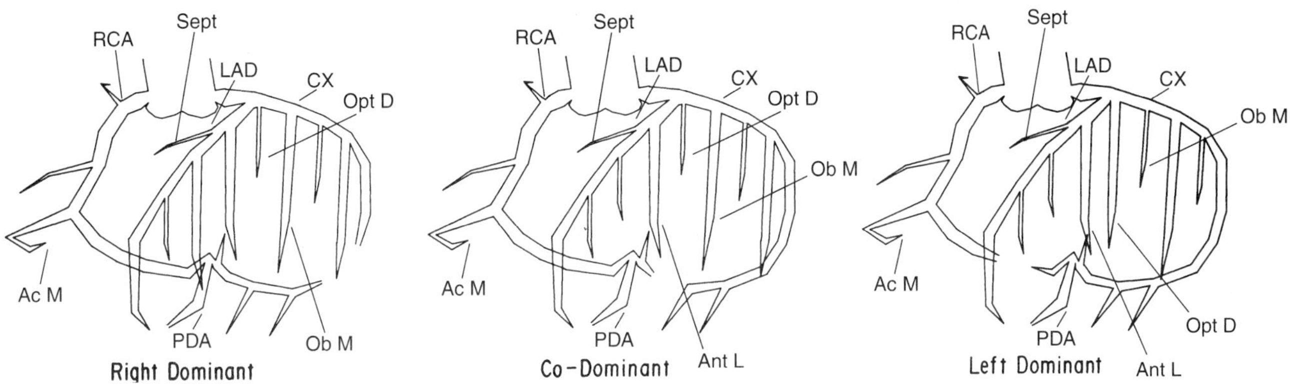

FIGURE 5-4. The definition of coronary dominance. Diagrams of coronary anatomy demonstrating right-dominant, left-dominant, and codominant coronary anatomy based on the origin of the blood supply to the posterior diaphragmatic surface of the left ventricle. RCA, right coronary artery; LAD, left anterior descending artery; CX, circumflex artery; PDA, posterior descending artery; Ac M, acute marginal artery; Ant L, anterolateral (diagonal) arteries; Opt D, optional diagonal artery; Ob M, obtuse marginal arteries; Sept, septal perforator artery. (From Davidson CJ, Bashore TM. Coronary arteriography. In: Sabiston DC Jr, Spencer FC, eds. *Surgery of the chest.* Philadelphia: WB Saunders, 1990:1663, with permission.)

aly, the left coronary artery receives collateral flow from the right coronary artery. Coronary "steal" into the low-pressure PA may result in ischemia, MI, ischemic cardiomyopathy, and sudden death. Similarly, coronary fistulas may rarely cause myocardial ischemia because of the pathophysiology of coronary steal.

Coronary lesion severity is usually interpreted through visual estimates of the percent diameter stenosis of the lesion compared with an adjacent segment of apparently normal vessel. The projection showing the greatest degree of narrowing is used. Lesions with greater than 50% diameter stenosis are usually interpreted as significant. There is significant variability among readers (Fig. 5-5). In addition, angiographically "normal" segments may frequently represent regions of diffuse coronary disease.

On-line quantitative coronary angiography computer al-

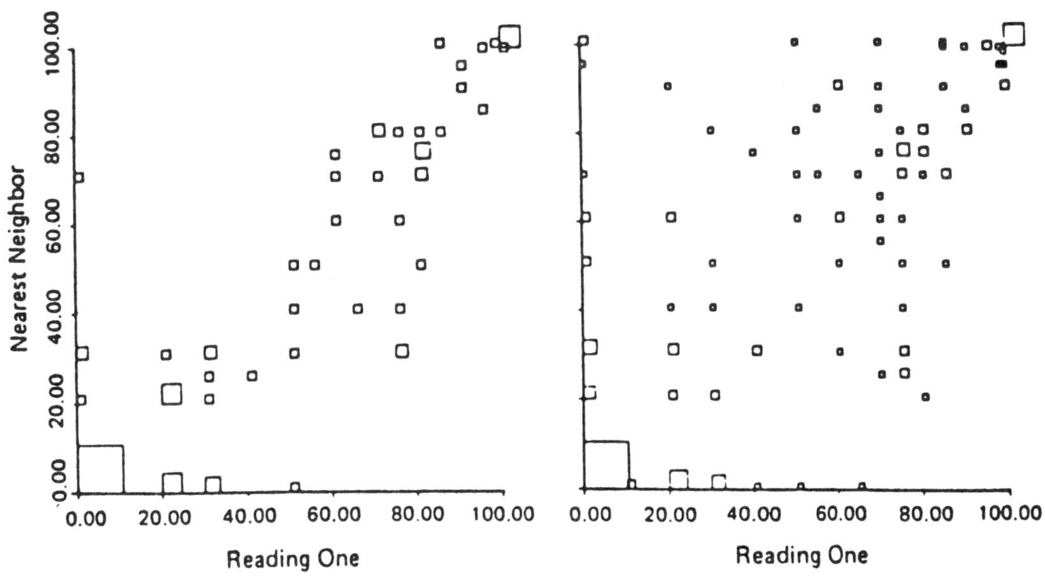

FIGURE 5-5. Intraobserver **(left panel)** and interobserver **(right panel)** variability of coronary artery stenosis severity, from the Coronary Artery Surgery Study. Note the significant variability, especially between observers, in visually estimating the severity of coronary stenosis **(right panel)**. (From Kennedy JW, Fisher LD, Killip T. Coronary angiography quality control in the CASS study. In: Bond MG, Insull W, Glogov S, et al., eds. *Clinical diagnoses of atherosclerosis: quantitative methods of evaluation.* New York: Springer-Verlag, 1982:475, with permission.)

gorithms employing digital edge detection are now available to define vessel diameter in stenotic and normal segments. This technology is useful in measuring lesion length and vessel diameter, variables that are important when choosing equipment for coronary interventions. Quantitative angiography is also an important research tool in defining long-term angiographic results after percutaneous coronary interventions or drug or diet therapy. As the knowledge of vessel disease has evolved, it is clear that angiographic measures of lesion severity are always limited. Intravascular ultrasound has further confirmed that extensive disease, dissection, and thrombus may be overlooked by contrast radiographic methods.

LEFT VENTRICULOGRAPHY

Left ventriculography is used to define LV systolic function and to assess the severity of mitral regurgitation, if present. Usually a pigtail catheter with multiple side holes is placed retrogradely across the aortic valve into the LV. Right anterior oblique (30° of rotation) and left anterior oblique (60° of rotation) are commonly used projections. (These views can be simultaneously performed when biplane radiographic equipment is available.) Contrast medium is injected via a power injector (usually 35 to 40 mL of contrast agent, at a rate of 10 to 15 mL/second) in order to opacify the LV cavity. The images are recorded on cine film or as a digital loop. The end-diastolic and end-systolic contours of the LV are traced, and the LV ejection fraction is calculated using standard methods (59). These methods assume that the shape of the ventricle resembles a prolated ellipse.

Regional segmental wall motion can also be defined. Figure 5-6 depicts the commonly used definitions. If there is reduced motion in a wall segment, hypokinesia is present; if no wall motion occurs, akinesia is present; if the wall bulges outward during systole, dyskinesia is present. A variety of quantitative methods have been used to define regional wall motion. One popular method uses 100 equally spaced chords perpendicular to the centerline between the end-diastolic and end-systolic contours (60). The lengths of these chords are normalized by the perimeter of the LV and compared with those obtained from a population of normal control subjects. Chords more than 1 standard deviation below normal are considered abnormal, and these data can be plotted in histogram format (Fig. 5-7).

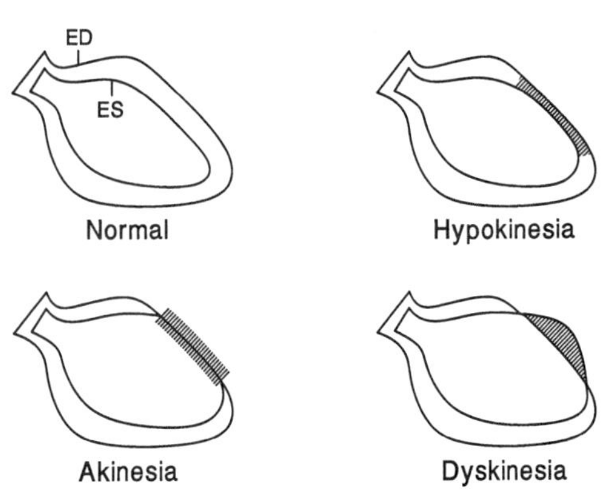

FIGURE 5-6. Definitions of regional left ventricular wall motion. The end-diastolic (ED) and end-systolic (ES) contours are drawn, and abnormalities of regional wall motion are defined as shown.

TABLE 5-4. DEFINITION OF VALVULAR REGURGITATION USING ANGIOGRAPHY

0	No regurgitation
1+	Trace regurgitation
2+	The proximal chamber never becomes as opacified as the distal chamber
3+	The proximal chamber becomes as opacified as the distal chamber
4+	The proximal chamber becomes more opacified than the distal chamber

Mitral regurgitation severity is usually graded on a standard semiquantitative scale from 0 to 4+ (61). The angiographic grade of mitral regurgitation depends on factors such as left atrial size, in addition to the actual volume of the regurgitant flow. In this scheme, 3 + regurgitation is present when left atrial opacification equals LV opacification at some point in the cycle. Regurgitation of 4 + implies that the left atrium is more opacified than the LV at some point, whereas 2+ and 1+ regurgitation represent subjectively less opacification of the left atrium (Table 5-4).

VALVULAR HEART DISEASE

In the catheterization laboratory, valvular regurgitation and valvular stenosis are defined by angiographic and hemodynamic measurements, respectively. Valvular regurgitation or insufficiency is defined by the injection of contrast medium into the chamber just distal to the valve in question (i.e., into the aorta in aortic insufficiency). The degree of contrast medium refluxing back into the proximal chamber defines the severity of the valvular insufficiency. The angiographic severity of valvular insufficiency is graded on the same semiquantitative scale as that described for mitral regurgitation. Valvular regurgitation grades of 3+ or 4+ are usually considered severe.

Valvular stenosis severity, on the other hand, is defined by measuring the pressure gradient across the valvular orifice and the flow across the valve. In modern catheterization laboratories, the pressure gradient across the valve can be measured very accurately. The flow across the valve, which is derived from measurement of the cardiac output, is more

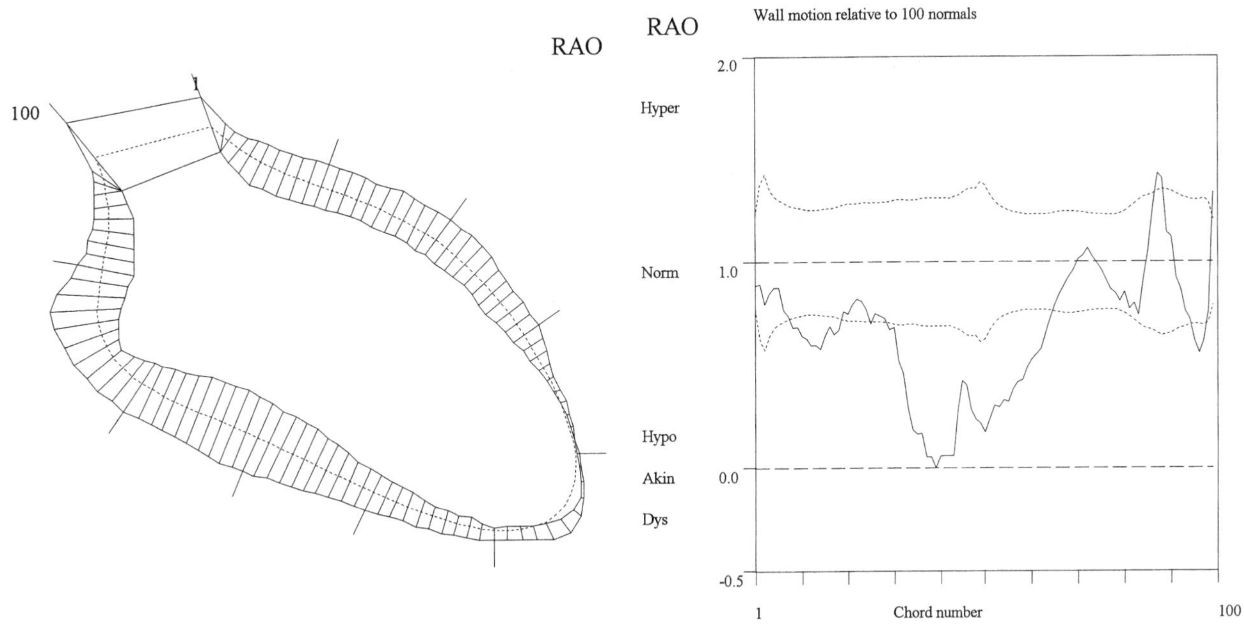

FIGURE 5-7. Centerline method of regional wall motion analysis. A centerline is drawn between the end-diastolic and end-systolic left ventricular endocardial contours, and 100 chords are constructed perpendicular to the centerline. Motion along each chord is normalized to the end-diastolic perimeter length, yielding a shortening fraction. This measurement of wall motion *(solid line)* is compared with the mean ± 1 standard deviation in 100 normal patients *(dotted lines).*

difficult to determine and can lead to errors in valve area determinations if not done carefully. Valve areas are calculated from the modified Gorlin equation (62):

$$\text{Valve area} = \frac{\text{Cardiac output}/(\text{HR} \times \text{FI})}{\text{K}\sqrt{\text{Mean pressure gradient}}} \qquad [5\text{-}1]$$

where HR is heart rate, FI is flow interval (length of either systole or diastole, depending on the valve) across the valve per beat, and K is an empirically derived constant. For practical purposes, one can also estimate the valve area by using the Hakki formula:

$$\text{Valve area} = \frac{\text{Cardiac output}}{\sqrt{\text{Mean gradient}}} \qquad [5\text{-}2]$$

Thus, valve area measurements are directly affected by cardiac output measurements. Cardiac output can be determined by the Fick principle or by thermodilution or angiographic output measurements. The Fick method is usually the most accurate, but it requires measurement of oxygen (O_2) consumption with a metabolic cart, or assumes O_2 consumption either from a series of lookup tables or from equating it to 125 mL/m^2 body surface area. A thermodilution output may be used, but it may be inaccurate in patients with extremes in output or in those with significant tricuspid valve regurgitation (56). Finally, angiographic outputs are required when significant insufficiency and stenosis of a valve coexist. However, angiographic outputs may be the least accurate because they are calculated from estimates of ventricular volume based on the ventricular shape's being a prolated ellipse (rarely the case) and because of the requirement for correction for x-ray divergence and magnification of the resultant image.

Aortic valve areas of 0.7 cm^2 or less and mitral valve areas of 1.5 cm^2 or less are usually considered indicative of significant valve stenosis. Valve area calculations for the right-sided valves are less well established, and the pressure gradient alone is usually reported. Peak-to-peak pressure gradients of 50 mm Hg or more are considered indicative of significant pulmonic valve stenosis. A mean pressure gradient of 5 mm Hg or more across the tricuspid valve indicates significant tricuspid valve stenosis.

CARDIAC OUTPUT MEASUREMENTS

Cardiac output can be determined by a number of techniques. Indicator-dye curves are cumbersome and poor at low output or in the presence of valvular regurgitation. The Fick method is the most accurate method of cardiac output measurement, but it requires measurement of the mixed venous (MV) and systemic arterial blood O_2 saturation. The MV O_2 saturation represents an average value of blood entering the RA. Blood enters the RA from three sources with widely disparate O_2 saturations; the superior vena cava (SVC), the inferior vena cava (IVC), and the coronary sinus.

An approximate SVC saturation is 75%, whereas the IVC saturation is 5% to 7% higher due to highly saturated blood from the renal vein entering the IVC. Coronary sinus O_2 saturations are in the 40% to 50% range. Adequate mixing from these three sources does not occur until the PA. In the absence of a known central cardiac shunt, a sample from the PA is used as the MV O_2 saturation. If a shunt is suspected, the MV O_2 saturation is estimated from the SVC and IVC saturations. The following formula is used, reflecting the predominance of SVC flow over IVC flow:

$$\text{MV } O_2 \text{ saturation} = \frac{3\,(\text{SVC saturation}) + \text{IVC saturation}}{4} \qquad [5\text{-}3]$$

In addition to MV and arterial saturations, O_2 consumption must be determined.

$$\text{Fick cardiac output (L/minute)} = \frac{O_2 \text{ consumption (ml/minute)}}{10 \times (\text{Arterial } O_2 \text{ vol\%} - \text{MV } O_2 \text{ vol\%})} \qquad [5\text{-}4]$$

The Fick principle is shown schematically in Fig. 5-8. The flow through an organ (in this case the lungs) can be determined if one knows how many O_2 molecules are attached to red blood cells entering and leaving the lung and how many molecules were consumed. The amount of hemoglobin-containing oxygen can be determined by multiplying the hemoglobin concentration (in milligrams per deciliter) by 1.36 times the O_2 saturation. The units of oxygen content are in volume percent (vol%).

Thermodilution cardiac output measurements are also commonly used, and they are the best alternative when the patient is receiving inspired O_2, which makes Fick methods inaccurate. The thermodilution method is similar to other indicator-dilution techniques except that temperature is measured rather than density (such as is used with green dye methods). Indicator-dilution methods result in the plot of a curve wherein the area under the curve is smallest when cardiac output is greatest. In low-output states, appearance of the indicator (cold water with thermodilution) can be delayed, and the area appears greater than actual, resulting in a factitiously high number. Conversely, with tricuspid regurgitation, there is mixing of the indicator back in the RA and the curve may be strung out, giving falsely low output readings (63).

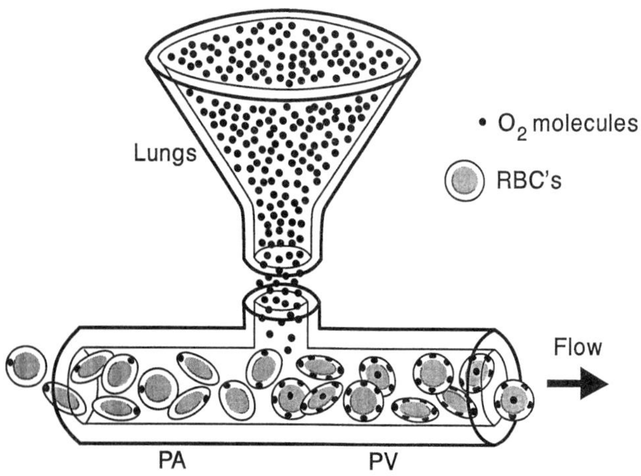

FIGURE 5-8. The Fick principle. If the amount of oxygen (O_2) consumed (delivered by the lungs) is known and the O_2 content of the red blood cells (RBCs) entering and the RBCs leaving the pulmonary bed is defined, then the rate at which the RBCs travel through the lungs (the cardiac output) can be determined. PA, pulmonary artery; PV, pulmonary vein. (From Bashore TM, Davidson CJ. Cardiac catheterization, angiography, and balloon valvuloplasty. In: Sabiston DC Jr, Spencer FC, eds. *Surgery of the chest.* Philadelphia: WB Saunders, 1990:1005, with permission.)

Angiographic cardiac output assumes that the ventricular shape can be modeled by a prolated ellipsoid. This allows for calculation of volume using the formula:

$$\text{Volume} = \frac{4\pi}{3} \cdot \frac{D_S}{2} \cdot \frac{D_L}{2} \cdot \frac{L}{2} \qquad [5\text{-}5]$$

where D_S is the diameter in short-axis view, D_L is the diameter in long-axis view, and L is the long axis of the ventricle. The diameters are not directly measured but are calculated from knowledge of the area (A):

$$D = \frac{4A}{\pi L} \qquad [5\text{-}6]$$

Because all of the volume data can be derived by knowledge of the area within the ventriculogram silhouette, the procedure is referred to as the area-length method. The absolute values require determination of a correction factor to allow for magnification produced by the x-ray system. Cardiac output can then be determined by first determining the stroke volume per beat (LV end-diastolic minus end-systolic volume) and multiplying by the heart rate:

$$\text{Angiographic cardiac output} = (\text{EDV} - \text{ESV}) \times \text{HR} \qquad [5\text{-}7]$$

where EDV is end-diastolic volume in milliliters, ESV is end-systolic volume in milliliters and the difference is one stroke volume (SV), HR is heart rate in beats per minute.

In patients with aortic and/or mitral regurgitation, calculation of the regurgitant fraction (RF) represents an estimate of the amount of the ejected volume that is regurgitated and therefore does not contribute to the true forward cardiac output. The regurgitant fraction is defined as:

$$\text{RF} = \frac{\text{Angiographic stroke volume} - \text{Forward stroke volume}}{\text{Angiographic stroke volume}} \qquad [5\text{-}8]$$

where forward stroke volume is the cardiac output determined by the Fick, indicator-dilution, or thermodilution techniques. The thermodilution technique cannot be used in the presence of concomitant tricuspid regurgitation.

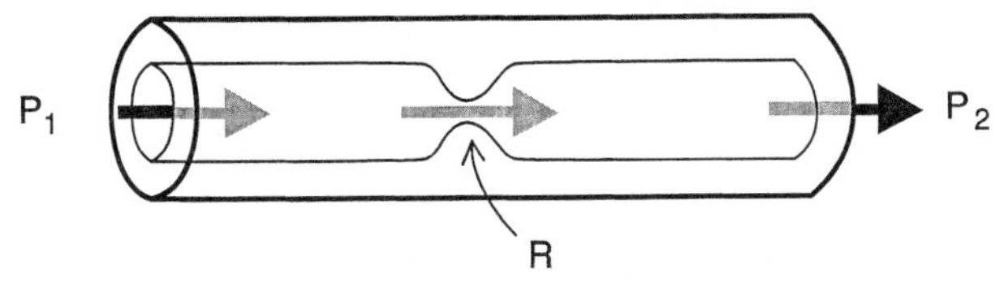

$$\text{Flow} \;\alpha\; \frac{P_1 - P_2}{R} \qquad R = \frac{\bar{m}P_1 - \bar{m}P_2}{C.O.}$$

FIGURE 5-9. Ohm's law for the vascular system. The flow through a tube increases with increased pressure drop across the tube and decreases with increased resistance in the tube. Rearranging the equation allows calculation of resistance. (From Bashore TM, Davidson CJ. Cardiac catheterization, angiography, and balloon valvuloplasty. In: Sabiston DC Jr, Spencer FC, eds. *Surgery of the chest.* Philadelphia: WB Saunders, 1990:1004, with permission.)

RESISTANCE MEASUREMENTS

Resistance is clinically measured in catheterization laboratories using the analogy to Ohm's law. Figure 5-9 outlines this method. The method assumes that constant pressure (nonphasic) is present on each side of a resistance. Flow is directly proportional to the pressure drop across the resistance and inversely proportional to the degree of resistance:

$$\text{Flow} = \frac{\text{Mean pressure proximal} - \text{Mean pressure distal}}{\text{Resistance}}$$

Rearranging, then, resistance is a function of the pressure drop divided by flow (cardiac output):

$$\text{Resistance} = \frac{\text{Mean pressure proximal} - \text{Mean pressure distal}}{\text{Cardiac output}}$$

Since this relationship assumes constant pressure, the mean pressures are used. Therefore, to determine pulmonary resistance (PVR):

$$\text{PVR} = \frac{\text{Mean PAP} - \text{Mean PCWP}}{\text{Cardiac output}} \qquad [5\text{-}9]$$

where PAP is the pulmonary artery pressure and PCWP is the pulmonary capillary wedge pressure.

By the same logic, systemic resistance is equal to the mean aortic pressure minus the mean right atrial pressure divided by cardiac output. When the pressure is measured in mm Hg and the cardiac output in L/minute, the result is expressed in Wood units. Multiplying by 80 produces results in dynes·cm·sec^{-5}. Table 5-5 lists normal values.

TABLE 5-5. NORMAL VALUES FOR RESISTANCE MEASUREMENTS

Measurement	dyne · sec · cm^{-5}	Wood Units
Total pulmonary resistance	205 ± 51	2.5 ± 1.0
Pulmonary vascular resistance	67 ± 30	1 ± 0.5
Systemic vascular resistance	1170 ± 270	15 ± 3.5

INTRACARDIAC SHUNTS

Because few use indocyanine green dye curves anymore, estimation of the degree of shunting in patients with intracardiac defects is most commonly accomplished by oximetry measurements. A modification of the Fick principle described earlier is used to define a shunt. The method is described in this section. Oximetric values are used to determine the shunt size.

It is important to appreciate that blood entering the RA has a variety of saturations. IVC blood is highly oxygenated, owing to renal vein flow (the kidneys extract relatively little oxygen relative to flow). SVC blood contains flow from the upper extremities and flow from the lower extremities (via azygous blood) as well. A small amount of coronary sinus flow also enters the RA that is quite desaturated, owing to the high extraction ratio in the coronary bed. As blood reaches the RA and RV, mixing occurs, and this mixing becomes more complete once the PA is reached. Because of the heterogeneity of blood reaching the RA, interpretation of a single RA saturation value must be done with caution.

To help normalize for all these variable saturations, an MV value is determined by Eq. 5-3. Because of the variability in the saturations found in the RA, Table 5-6 outlines the minimal change required to diagnose a true step-up in O_2 content from the SVC to the RA (atrial left-to-right shunt), from the RA to the RV (ventricular left-to-right shunt), or from the RV to the PA (e.g., patent ductus).

In a patient without a shunt, the MV saturation should be the same as the RV and PA saturations. Using the Fick equation, pulmonary blood flow (PBF) is a function of the O_2 consumption divided by the O_2 content in the pulmo-

TABLE 5-6. MINIMUM VARIABILITY IN OXYGEN CONTENT REQUIRED TO DETECT A SHUNT

Shunt	Sampling Sites	Minimal Change in Oxygen Content (vol %)	Minimal Change in Oxygen Saturation (%)
PDA	RV to PA	0.5	5
VSD	RA to RV	0.9	7
ASD	MV to RA	1.9	11

Note: PDA, patent ductus arteriosus; VSD, ventricular septal defect; ASD, atrial septal defect; RV, right ventricle; RA, right atrium; MV, mixed venous.

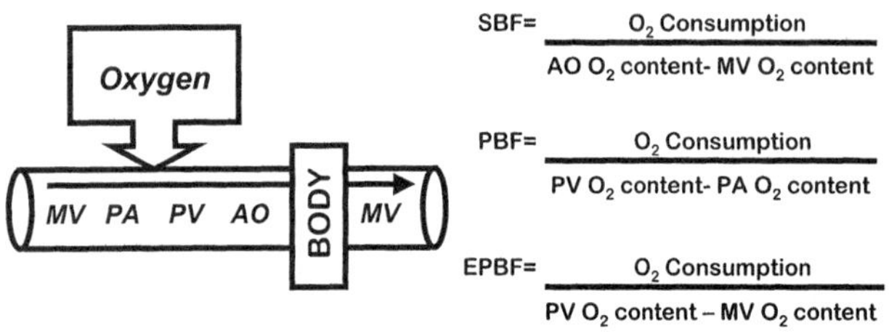

FIGURE 5-10. Calculations of the various blood flows using the Fick principle. SBF, systemic blood flow; EPBF, effective pulmonary blood flow; PBF, pulmonary blood flow; MV, mixed venous; PV, pulmonary vein; PA, pulmonary artery; AO, aorta. If there is no shunt, then the saturations of MV = PA and PV = AO. All of the equations for SBF, EPBF, and PBF are therefore equal.

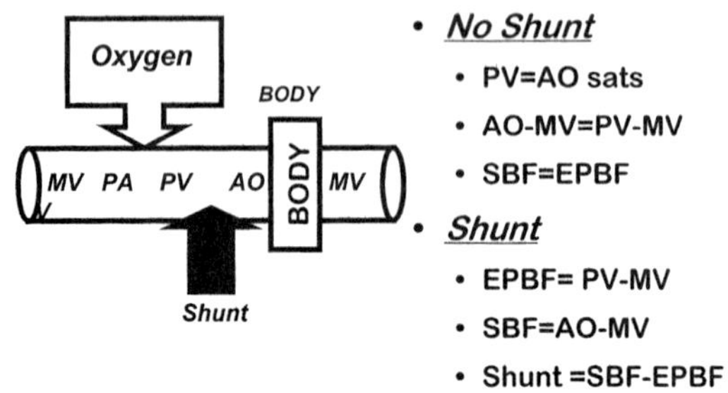

FIGURE 5-12. Calculation of right-to-left intracardiac shunts. EPBF, effective pulmonary blood flow; SBF, systemic blood flow; MV, mixed venous; PV, pulmonary vein; AO, aorta. As in the previous figures, when a right-to-left shunt occurs, the SBF is increased. The EPBF still represents what the flow was before any shunt occurred (see Fig. 5-10). The SBF equation now represents systemic flow including the shunt. The difference between the SBF and the EPBF is the magnitude of the shunt.

nary vein (PV) minus the O_2 content in the PA:

$$\text{PBF} = \frac{O_2 \text{ consumption}}{(\text{PV } O_2 \text{ content } - \text{ PA } O_2 \text{ content}) \times 10}$$

To simplify the concept, consider the abbreviations of PV and PA for their respective O_2 contents (Fig. 5-10). Thus:

$$\text{PBF} = \frac{O_2 \text{ consumption}}{\text{PV} - \text{PA}} \qquad [5\text{-}10]$$

If there is no left-to-right shunt, the PA O_2 content should equal the MV content. Therefore, the cardiac output derived from the O_2 consumption/PV-PA equation would be the same as that derived from the O_2 consumption/PV-MV equation.

Effective pulmonary blood flow (EPBF) uses the equation:

$$\text{EPBF} = \frac{O_2 \text{ consumption}}{\text{PV} - \text{MV}} \qquad [5\text{-}11]$$

This represents the normal pulmonary blood flow with no shunt.

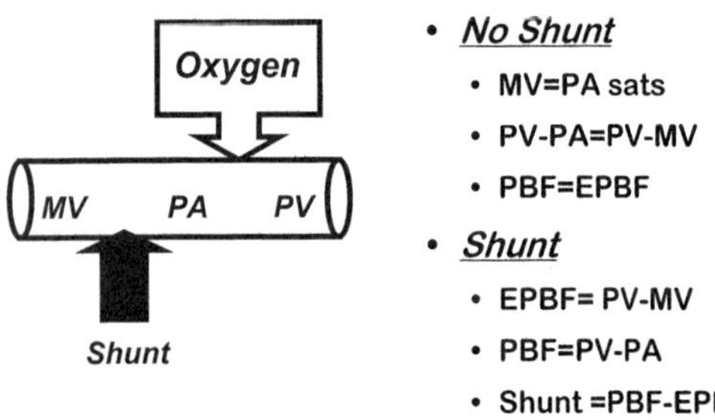

FIGURE 5-11. Calculation of left-to-right intracardiac shunts. EPBF, effective pulmonary blood flow; PBF, pulmonary blood flow; MV, mixed venous; PV, pulmonary vein; PA, pulmonary artery. When a left-to-right shunt occurs, the PBF is increased. The EPBF represents what the flow was before any shunt occurred (see Fig. 5-10). The PBF equation now represents the flow in the presence of the left-to-right shunt. The difference betwee the PBF and the EPBF is the magnitude of the shunt.

Systemic blood flow (SBF) represents flow across the systemic bed in much the same manner as the PBF represents flow across the pulmonary bed. In the absence of any shunt, the EPBF, the SBF, and the PBF should all be the same.

Now note what happens when a left-to-right shunt is present (Fig. 5-11). Oxygenated blood causes the PA O_2 content and the pulmonary flow to be higher. Since EPBF represents what the flow would have been without a shunt, the difference between PBF and EPBF is the size of the left-to-right shunt.

Calculation of a right-to-left shunt is based on the same principle (Fig. 5-12). As before, if there is no shunt, EPBF and SBF are equal. The EPBF again represents the baseline state with no shunt. If deoxygenated venous blood is shunted to the left heart circulation, the aorta O_2 content decreases and the calculated SBF increases. The difference between the newly calculated SBF and the EPBF therefore represents the size of the shunt.

One easy way to determine the shunt size using only the blood saturations is as follows.

Since the shunt ratio (PBF/SBF) is often the most desired value to be determined, note that

$$\text{PBF} = \frac{O_2 \text{ Consumption}}{(\text{PV } O_2 \text{ content } - \text{ PA } O_2 \text{ content}) \times 10}$$

$$\text{SBF} = \frac{O_2 \text{ Consumption}}{(\text{PV } O_2 \text{ content } - \text{ MV } O_2 \text{ content}) \times 10}$$

When the ratio of PBF/SBF is set in place, O_2 consumption, hemoglobin, and the correction factors cancel out, and one is left with:

$$\frac{\text{PBF}}{\text{SBF}} = \frac{\text{PV saturation } - \text{ MV saturation}}{\text{PV saturation } - \text{ PA saturation}} \qquad [5\text{-}12]$$

For example, if a patient has a PA saturation of 80%, a PV saturation of 99%, and a MV saturation of 70%, the shunt ratio would be 2.1 : 1, according to the calculation:

$$\frac{0.99 - 0.60}{0.99 - 0.80} = \frac{0.39}{0.19} = 2.1$$

INTERVENTIONAL CARDIOLOGY

Introduction and History

Whereas cardiac catheterization was once thought of as a strictly diagnostic procedure, over the past two decades effective transcatheter treatments for coronary, valvular, and congenital heart disease have been developed. In 1968, percutaneous transcatheter balloon septostomy of the atrial septum was described by Rashkind and Miller (64). The technique remains in use today for infants with transposition of the great vessels. In 1977, Andreas Gruntzig described percutaneous coronary balloon angioplasty (7). This technique was initially confined to proximal, discrete stenoses in patients with single-vessel coronary disease. In the 1980s, catheter-based balloon valvuloplasty for patients with pulmonic, aortic, or mitral valve stenosis was introduced. Over the past 15 years, advances in catheter and guidewire design and improvements in radiographic imaging systems have fueled the explosion of percutaneous coronary interventional procedures. Presently, with few exceptions, distal, complex coronary lesions in patients with multivessel disease can now be successfully dilated. In addition to these coronary interventions, selected cases of valvular and congenital heart disease can now be effectively treated using percutaneous catheter-based techniques.

HISTORY OF ANGIOPLASTY

Improvements in arteriographic techniques in the 1960s led to the first successful attempts at dilation of atherosclerotic peripheral arterial narrowings. Dotter and colleagues described a technique in which a system of rigid dilators were passed over a guidewire and through stenoses in the iliac or femoral arteries, thereby successfully enlarging the lumen and improving antegrade blood flow (65). This technique was limited in its applicability because of the trauma exerted by these rigid, large-caliber dilators on the arterial inner lumen and at the vascular insertion site. In the 1970s, Gruntzig and colleagues introduced the technique of dilation of atherosclerotic narrowing using a balloon-tipped catheter in place of the rigid dilators (66,67). The deflated balloon catheter could be placed via a much smaller vascular puncture. Once across the stenosis, the balloon could be expanded to a predetermined size. This technique, the basis for current angioplasty procedures, was first applied to the peripheral and renal arteries before coronary stenoses were reported in 1977 (7,68). The initial coronary angioplasty catheters consisted of a balloon-tipped catheter with a short segment of flexible wire attached to the balloon tip (the wire leader) to help guide the device through the stenosis. This technology was feasible only for dilation of discrete proximal stenoses. Smaller-profile catheter shafts and balloons and the development of thin steerable guidewires with balloon catheters designed to be delivered over these wires made even the most complex, distal coronary lesions approachable with angioplasty.

The past decade has witnessed an explosion of new device development in interventional cardiology, currently dominated by the development of the coronary artery endovascular stent. After the development of percutaneous balloon angioplasty, a host of controversial devices were studied. These include atherectomy devices (transluminal extraction catheter [TEC], directional coronary atherectomy [DCA] devices), heated balloons, laser balloons, lasers themselves, and rotational atherectomy burrs for plaque removal. As of this writing, the only devices in major use are percutaneous balloon angioplasty, rotational atherectomy, and coronary stents.

The term "stent" came from work by Dotter in 1969 describing the percutaneous placement of coiled wire grafts in canine femoral and popliteal arteries (69). The modern concept of a balloon-mounted stent was promoted by Palmaz and colleagues in 1985 (70). In 1986, Jacques Puel delivered the first coronary stent, a self-expanding stent, in humans; this was followed shortly by U.S. phase I trials of the Palmaz-Schatz and Gianturco-Roubin stents in 1987 (71). Coronary stents have provided marked improvement in the rate of restenosis seen with balloon angioplasty and have almost eliminated the need for emergency CABG for abrupt closure. The development of coronary stents and several new devices designed to overcome challenges associated with high-risk lesions has made the overwhelming majority of coronary stenoses approachable for percutaneous intervention.

INDICATIONS FOR PERCUTANEOUS TRANSLUMINAL CORONARY ANGIOPLASTY

As technology and pharmacologic therapy during angioplasty continue to improve procedural outcomes, the indications for PTCA remain in evolution. Most coronary lesions can be approached percutaneously. In patients with symptomatic coronary disease, where revascularization is deemed important, PTCA is a reasonable alternative if suitable anatomy exists. Almost all patients with unprotected (nongrafted) left main coronary artery disease should be referred for CABG. Although angioplasty and stenting of the left main artery can be performed with a high success rate in the setting of an acute MI, elective left main percutaneous revascularization has been associated with increased rates of cardiac death is the first year of follow-up (72,73). Elective left main angioplasty should be reserved for those patients who are critically ill with an acute MI and for patients for whom CABG is deemed unacceptable.

The decision to refer a patient with single or multivessel coronary artery disease for angioplasty or CABG requires consideration of many patient and angiographic variables. The primary focus in the decision analysis should be the likelihood of long-term success with percutaneous intervention. The American College of Cardiology/American Heart Association (ACC/AHA) Task Force created a classification of lesion morphology designed to predict both procedural success and risk of complication with balloon angioplasty (Table 5-7) (74). This classification is widely used, and although the guidelines are not absolute, they do stress the importance of lesion morphology and location to the success of percutaneous revascularization techniques.

Several randomized trials have compared CABG with PTCA in patients with symptomatic coronary disease (75,76). In patients who were eligible to receive either strategy, the risks of death and MI, both short-term and long-term, were similar. Patients receiving PTCA did require significantly more revascularization. Diabetic patients in the Bypass Angioplasty Revascularization Investigation (BARI) study appeared to derive a mortality benefit from CABG at 5 years. This benefit has not been consistently reproducible in other studies, although there is mounting evidence that diabetic patients are at increased risk for restenosis after coronary artery stenting (76–78).

TABLE 5-7. LESION-SPECIFIC CHARACTERISTICS OF TYPE A, B, AND LESIONS[a]

Type A lesions—high success >85%, low risk
Discrete (<10 mm)
Concentric
Readily accessible
Nonangled segment, <45°
Smooth contour
Little or no calcification
Less than totally occlusive
Nonostial in location
No major branch involvement
Absence of thrombus
Type B lesions—moderate success (60%–85%), moderate risk
Tubular (10–20 mm length)
Eccentric
Moderate tortuosity of proximal segment
Moderately angulated segment, 45°–90°
Irregular contour
Moderate to heavy calcification
Total occlusions <3 mo old
Ostial in location
Bifurcation lesions requiring double guidewires
Some thrombus present
Type C lesions—low success (<60%), high risk
Diffuse (>2 cm)
Excessive tortuosity of proximal segment
Extremely angulated segments >90°
Total occlusion >3 mo old
Inability to protect major side branches
Degenerated vein grafts with friable lesions

[a] American Heart Association/American College of Cardiology classification of lesion type.
Source: From Ryan TJ, et al. Guidelines for percutaneous transluminal angioplasty. *J Am Coll Cardiol* 1988;12:529, with permission.

Most patients with single-vessel disease are referred for percutaneous intervention, provided lesion anatomy is suitable and the patient is symptomatic while taking medications. In patients with multivessel disease, an initial percutaneous strategy is acceptable provided all lesions are approachable and the patient understands that repeat procedures may be required. There currently is a trend toward surgical intervention in patients with multivessel disease, especially if the proximal LAD is involved. If complete revascularization can be accomplished only with a surgical approach, then patients undergoing elective procedures are usually referred for surgical intervention.

Diabetic patients with mutivessel disease should be considered for CABG unless the surgical morbidity and mortality risk is unacceptable, because they may derive a mortality benefit and are at increased risk of restenosis after percutaneous revascularization (76–78). All of the current data comparing percutaneous revascularization, CABG, and medical therapy were obtained in the era of balloon angioplasty, performed without the use of coronary stents, alternative devices, or optimal pharmacologic therapy during and after the intervention. Several large, randomized trials nearing completion should more clearly define this long-standing issue.

ANGIOPLASTY PROCEDURE AND EQUIPMENT

Pharmacologic Treatment Accompanying Coronary Interventions

Before any percutaneous coronary reascularization procedure, patients are treated with aspirin to prevent platelet aggregation and coronary thrombosis during the procedure. Because more than 50% of patients receive coronary stents, patients are pretreated with one of two regimens designed to prevent stent thrombosis (79–81). Ticlopidine and clopidigrel both block adenosine diphosphate–induced platelet aggregation and have been shown to lower the rate of stent thrombosis when given in combination with aspirin. The widespread use of ticlopidine has been complicated by low but clinically significant rates of neutropenia, thrombocytopenia, and thrombotic thrombocytopenic purpura, and its use has dropped dramatically. Use of clopidogrel avoids these side effects, and the dru is better tolerated by patients, predominantly because of less gastrointestinal intolerance (81). If ticlopidine (250 mg twice daily) and aspirin (325 mg once daily) are used, a 2- to 4-week regimen is given (80). Patients receiving clopidigrel and aspirin should receive a 300 mg loading dose followed by a daily 75-mg dose for 4 weeks (81). Use of these agents results in a lower rate of stent thrombosis with less bleeding, compared with previous regimens using combinations of aspirin, warfarin, and low-molecular-weight heparin.

After arterial sheath placement, patients receive high-dose intravenous heparin during the procedure. Heparin is administered to achieve an activated clotting time (ACT) longer than 300 seconds if heparin is to be used alone or longer than 200 seconds if heparin is used in conjunction with a glycoprotein IIb/IIIa receptor inhibitor.

Glycoprotein IIb/IIIa receptor antagonists given at the time of coronary intervention have been shown to reduce acute ischemic events, mainly reinfarction, and to reduce target vessel revascularization (TVR), or clinical restenosis, at 6 months (82–85). The initial data suggest that patents at highest risk derive the majority of the benefit of these agents. These patients include those with acute MI, unstable angina, saphenous vein graft interventions, angiographically present thrombus, and multivessel interventions.

The Evaluation of Platelet IIb/IIIa Inhibitor for Stenting (EPISTENT) trial showed a 50% reduction in death or MI at 6 months in patients randomly assigned to receive the IIb/IIIa receptor antagonist abciximab (ReoPro) and coronary stent placement, compared with those receiving a coronary stent without IIb/IIIa inhibition. This trial encompassed a broad group of patients and demonstrated less angiographic and clinical restenosis in patients receiving IIb/IIIa inhibition (85). Although these results require confirmation, the enthusiasm for these agents during coronary intervention is growing. More research will determine which patients and which drugs are most beneficial and most cost-effective.

Once anticoagulation is achieved with heparin and/or a platelet glycoprotein IIb/IIIa receptor inhibitor, the ACT is monitored hourly. After the procedure, sheaths are removed 4 hours after administration of the last dose of heparin, or when the ACT is less than 175 seconds. Early removal of access sheaths, even while glycoprotein IIb/IIIa receptor antagonists are still infusing, has been shown to reduce groin complications.

In addition to anticoagulants, patients usually receive combinations of narcotics and benzodiazepines for sedation. As for diagnostic coronary arteriography, many patients routinely receive diphenhydramine before PTCA to help prevent contrast agent reactions. Patients with a known prior reaction to contrast agents also receive intravenous steroids and histamine H_2 antagonists for 24 hours before the procedure.

Angioplasty Equipment and Technique

Tremendous advances have taken place in angioplasty equipment over the past decade (62). Angioplasty equipment continues to evolve, making more lesions approachable with percutaneous techniques and increasing the acute angiographic success rate of the procedure. Newer technology has involved balloon-over-the-wire systems (66). A guidewire is placed across the coronary stenosis, and then a balloon catheter is advanced over the guidewire and positioned across the coronary stenosis (Fig. 5-13). Guidewires themselves have developed into sophisticated pieces of angioplasty equipment. The goal of the angioplasty guidewire is to be torquable and steerable yet have a soft, flexible, atraumatic tip so as not to damage the coronary endothelium. Standard quidewires are 0.14 inch in diameter. Guidewires also have different degrees of tip flexibility. Although relatively stiff guidewire tips are required in certain cases, such as when attempting to cross total occlusions, they also increase the risk of endothelial damage and coronary dissection. Tip stiffness depends on the morphology of the inner portion of the guidewire. Guidewires are also available with a slick, hydrophilic coating. This coating enhances the ability of the guidewire to traverse tortuous anatomy and cross tight stenoses, but it also increases the risk of endothelial disruption and dissection because the tip can more easily penetrate the endothelium or disrupt an atherosclerotic plaque.

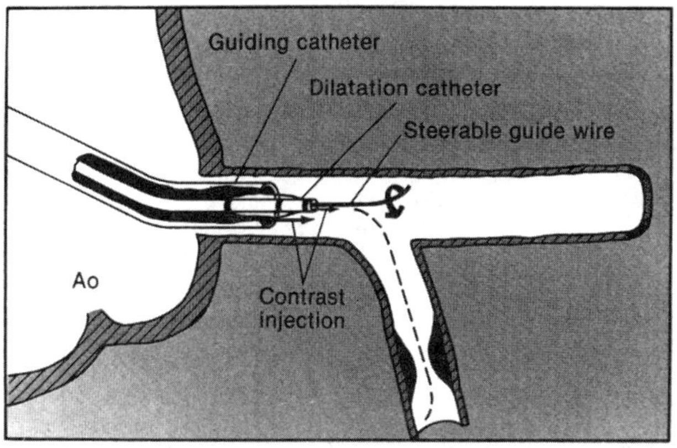

FIGURE 5-13. Movable guidewire coronary angioplasty system. The guide catheter is shown positioned in the left main coronary artery. The balloon angioplasty catheter (dilatation catheter) is illustrated just beyond the guiding catheter tip. The steerable guidewire is directed through and beyond the area of coronary stenosis. The balloon angioplasty catheter is then advanced over the guidewire and positioned across the area of stenosis. The positions of the guidewire and the balloon angioplasty catheter are monitored by contrast injection through the guiding catheter. (From Baim DS. Coronary angioplasty. In: Grossman W, Baim DS, eds. *Cardiac catheterization, angiography and intervention.* Philadelphia: Lea & Febiger, 1991, with permission.)

Balloon catheter technology has also advanced (Fig. 5-14). Two major areas of interest have been the catheter-balloon profile and compliant versus noncompliant balloon materials. Smaller catheter-balloon profiles have allowed even critical coronary lesions to be crossed. Catheter shaft diameters now have been reduced to 0.021 inch. The balloons come wrapped on the catheter shaft and are prepared by aspiration of the residual air in the balloon-catheter

FIGURE 5-14. A typical balloon angioplasty dilatation catheter. The balloon is advanced over a guidewire placed into the central lumen through the top port. Contrast material delivered into the balloon lumen through the bottom side port inflates the balloon. The balloon is positioned using radiopaque markers, here a central marker, attached to the balloon catheter. (Courtesy of SCIMED Life Systems, Inc., Boston Scientific Corporation, Maple Grove, MN.)

lumen. Negative pressure is left on the balloon after aspiration to keep the profile as low as possible. In addition, balloon materials have been developed that are thinner and yet still capable of withstanding enough pressure to dilate most coronary stenoses. Noncompliant balloon materials have been developed to allow high-pressure balloon dilations (more than 8 atm) without increasing balloon diameter significantly. These balloons are useful for fibrotic or calcified coronary stenoses, where high pressure may be required to adequately dilate the stenosis and assist in optimal stent deployment against the vessel wall. Oversizing of the balloon relative to the native vessel diameter may occur at high pressures when compliant balloon materials are used. This oversizing is associated with a greater incidence of significant vessel dissection and reduced acute success. The noncompliant balloon materials enable the operator to use even higher pressures (up to 20 atm) without increasing balloon diameter significantly.

Another key component of the angioplasty equipment is the guide catheter. The goal of the guide catheter is to provide support for the coronary angioplasty equipment and to be atraumatic to the coronary ostium. Guide catheters come preformed in configurations common to diagnostic coronary catheters. However, they have stiffer shafts and large internal lumens. This may be achieved by using a woven steel mesh in the wall of the guide catheter shaft. The tips are made of softer plastic but must be radiopaque so that the guide catheter tip position can be visualized easily. This is critical in maintaining proper guide tip position and support while avoiding migration of the guide tip down into the coronary lumen. Extra-support guiding catheters have a more pronounced curve, allowing the catheter shaft to rest against the wall of the aorta opposite the coronary ostium. This allows the catheter tip to remain firmly seated in the ostium and to resist moving out of the ostium if tortuosity or calcified, tight stenoses are encountered by the guidewire, balloon catheter, or stent delivery system. Adequate guiding catheter support is particularly critical for procedures in which large or stiff devices are used.

As devices, balloons, and stent delivery systems with smaller profiles have been developed, smaller guide catheters have been developed and used more frequently. Currently, all commercially available coronary balloon dilatation catheters and stent delivery systems can be delivered through a 6F guide catheter. These catheters are particularly advantageous for the brachial or radial approach. The disadvantages of smaller catheters are the reduced support they provide for delivery of the angioplasty catheter to challenging coronary locations and the inability of the guide catheter lumen to accommodate angioplasty catheters with larger shafts (perfusion balloon catheters (PBCs), atherectomy devices, and thrombectomy devices) should a change in strategy be required during the procedure. They also limit the quality of angiographic imaging, because adequate contrast material may not be able to be injected around the angioplasty catheter, which occupies the majority of a 6F lumen, to opacify the coronary lumen. Larger coronary devices, such as atherectomy devices, require 9F and 10F guide catheters. These larger guide catheters introduce a significant risk of vascular trauma.

ACUTE COMPLICATIONS OF PERCUTANEOUS TRANSLUMINAL CORONARY ANGIOPLASTY

The risks of coronary angioplasty include all the problems associated with diagnostic cardiac catheterization, and then some. The major acute problem is acute closure, which occurs in about 5% of all procedures. The risk of vascular damage after angioplasty is significantly greater than that after diagnostic catheterization. Guide catheters cause larger vascular punctures than diagnostic catheters do. The systemic anticoagulation that accompanies routine percutaneous coronary interventions also adds to the risk of bleeding complications. Vascular injuries secondary to angioplasty include greater frequency of hematoma formation, formation of a femoral artery pseudoaneurysm or arteriovenous fistula, retroperitoneal bleeding, arterial thrombosis, and embolic phenomena leading to ischemia of the affected extremity. The reduced risk of stent thrombosis with ticlopidine or clopidigrel and aspirin and the use of IIb/IIIa receptor blockers in most high-risk cases has virtually eliminated the need for postprocedural heparin infusions and delayed sheath removal. These two important alterations in postprocedural care have led to a reduction in anticoagulation-related groin complications.

A rare complication of PTCA is coronary rupture or perforation. This may occur if grossly oversized angioplasty balloons are used, but it is more of a risk with related techniques such as atherectomy and laser angioplasty. Ventricular tachycardia or fibrillation may occur during balloon inflations and periods of ischemia. These events are rarely fatal. Treatment consists of electrical cardioversion or defibrillation along with balloon deflation and restoration of coronary flow. Severe bradycardia may occur and may be significant, especially during right coronary angioplasty, and it is more common when ionic contrast media are used. Bradycardia can usually be overcome with atropine or a temporary venous pacemaker inserted into the RV.

Coronary lesion characteristics have been shown to influence the acute procedural success rates for percutaneous interventions (74) (Table 5-7). Although improvements in angioplasty equipment, alternative percutaneous devices, and operator experience have increased the acute procedural success rate to 90% to 95% in many high-volume centers, the major procedural obstacle in percutaneous coronary interventions remains abrupt vessel closure. The majority of abrupt closures occur during the catheterization procedure (86). Closures outside the catheterization laboratory most commonly occur within the first 6 hours. Immediate repeat catheterization in an effort to restore coronary flow is required in this situation. Therefore, all patients must be monitored closely for at least 24 hours after a coronary intervention, and immediate 24-hour availability of catheterization facilities is mandatory.

Abrupt coronary closure after PTCA most often results from coronary dissection with an intimal flap occluding the vessel lumen. Small intimal dissections are the main pathologic findings after successful angioplasty (87,88). Intracoronary thrombus, with or without coronary dissection, may also result in abrupt vessel closure. When abrupt closure is encountered, most lesions can be recrossed and treated with successful angioplasty or stent placement. Glycoprotein IIb/IIIa receptor inhibition may also reduce the incidence of abrupt closure and should be considered in patients with lesion characteristics that suggest an increased risk of abrupt closure. If the occlusion cannot be retreated successfully, and emergency CABG is required, vessel patency and hemodynamic stability may often be restored after the lesion has been crossed with a guidewire and a PBC has been placed across the lesion (89) (Fig. 5-15). The balloon is left deflated, and the perfusion balloon is left in place during transport to the operating room. The perfusion catheter is withdrawn after the institution of cardiopulmonary bypass.

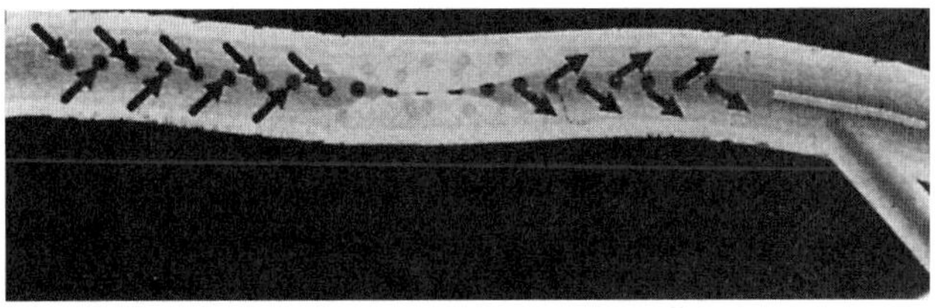

FIGURE 5-15. Illustration of the autoperfusion principle employed by the perfusion balloon catheters. Blood proximal to the stenosis enters the upstream side holes in the catheter and then exits the catheter distal to the coronary stenosis. (From Stack RS. Percutaneous transluminal coronary angioplasty. In: Sabiston DC Jr, Spencer FC, eds. *Surgery of the chest.* Philadelphia: WB Saunders, 1990: 1039, with permission.)

RESTENOSIS AFTER PERCUTANEOUS REVASCULARIZATION

Despite improvements in equipment, improved operator technique, and directed pharmacotherapy in the catheterization laboratory, unacceptable restenosis still dominates any discussion of success of percutaneous interventions. Although the use of coronary artery stents and the administration of glycoprotein IIb/IIIa blockade to patients at risk for restenosis has markedly lowered the average rate of restenosis across the board, most authors still report rates of 15% to 30% (83–85,90). Approximately 25% of percutaneous interventions involve previously treated lesions.

Angiographic restenosis is defined as a stenosis of at least 50% of the vessel diameter at the site of a previous intervention. Restenosis usually occurs within 6 months after the angioplasty procedure and is most likely multifactorial. Many proposed mechanisms exist, including vessel recoil (both acute and chronic), thrombus at the injury site, medial smooth muscle cell proliferation, and hyperplasia of the neointima (91). Stents have addressed much of the problem with recoil, and the larger lumens obtained at the time of stenting have allowed more tolerance of intimal thickening. There is still, however, much to be learned and accomplished to reduce the neointimal hyperplasia that plagues one fourth of patients receiving coronary interventions.

Patient and lesion risk factors for restenosis are listed in Table 5-8 (92–99). The degree of residual stenosis after coronary intervention is also strongly predictive of the risk of restenosis. A residual stenosis of greater than 30% carries at least a 10% higher risk of restenosis than does a residual stenosis of 20% or less (97).

The advent of the coronary stent and improved pharmacologic therapy has markedly reduced the risk of restenosis over the past decade. However, there remains much to be done to target the 15% to 30% of patients still affected by this problem. Many device strategies that have been developed to target this problem are discussed individually in the next section.

TABLE 5-8. RISK FACTORS FOR RESTENOSIS

Patient
Diabetes
Unstable angina
Lesion anatomy
Saphenous vein grafts
Smaller vessel diameter
Ostial location
Left anterior descending artery
Increased degree of baseline stenosis
Chronic occlusion
Longer lesion length

PERCUTANEOUS CORONARY INTERVENTION DEVICES

Coronary Artery Stents

The introduction of the coronary stent is the most significant advance in interventional cardiology since balloon angioplasty was initiated 22 years ago. Well over 50% of patients who undergo a percutaneous coronary interventional procedure receive a stent (100). The popularity of coronary stents in the angioplasty laboratory is due to many favorable stent characteristics: (a) Stents are easy to use and have decreased procedure time compared with conventional balloon angioplasty (PTCA). (b) The availability of stent deployment for abrupt or threatened closure has markedly reduced both the incidence of and complications resulting from these events. (c) Even in the setting of the most complex lesion morphology, stents produce predictable and favorable acute angiographic results.

Beyond the initial appeal of a favorable angiographic result, stents have also been shown to reduce the incidence of restenosis when compared with PTCA (100–103). This reduction seems to depend on achieving a larger initial lumen diameter. Stenting results in more late loss of diameter than does PTCA, due either to vessel remodeling or intimal hyperplasia. However, this late loss is more than overcome by the greater initial lumen gain achieved with stenting. Trials with complete angiographic follow-up have shown an angiographic restenosis rate of approximately 15% in patients receiving stents, about one half of the rate seen with PTCA. Many trials do not employ angiographic follow-up, instead reporting TVR as a surrogate end point. Trials of stenting versus PTCA have consistently shown a reduction (although somewhat variable) in TVR and in a composite end point of reinfarction and mortality in favor of stenting. In the EPISTENT trial, in which both PTCA and stent patients received aggressive antiplatelet therapy including the IIb/IIIa inhibitor abciximab, a 6-month incidence of death or MI of 5.6% in patients receiving stents was found, compared with 7.8% in those treated with PTCA alone (103). At 6 months, TVR was 8.7% in the stent group and 15.4% in the PTCA group.

These impressive clinical results have sparked a dynamic industry with new and innovative stent designs, applications, and delivery systems. The available stents are usually divided into two categories based on the method of expansion: balloon expandable and self-expanding. The majority of stents are balloon expandable (Fig. 5-16). Metal stents, usually made from stainless steel, are preloaded on a deflated angioplasty balloon catheter. The balloon catheter has markers on each end, with the stent positioned between the markers. There is significant variability in angiographic visibility of stents, due in part to the thickness of the metal struts and the composition of the metal alloy. Once the stent is positioned at the site of a lesion, the balloon is inflated, expanding the metal stent into position. The stent is then dilated to high pressure (12 to 20 atm) with a noncompliant balloon, which grows little in diameter with increasing pressure. This expands the stent fully and ensures that it is completely apposed against the vessel wall. The result is then assessed by angiography or intravascular ultrasound. If the results are not optimal, higher pressure or a larger balloon is employed. Many delivery systems now have a stent mounted on a high-pressure balloon, eliminating the need for postdilation with an additional balloon.

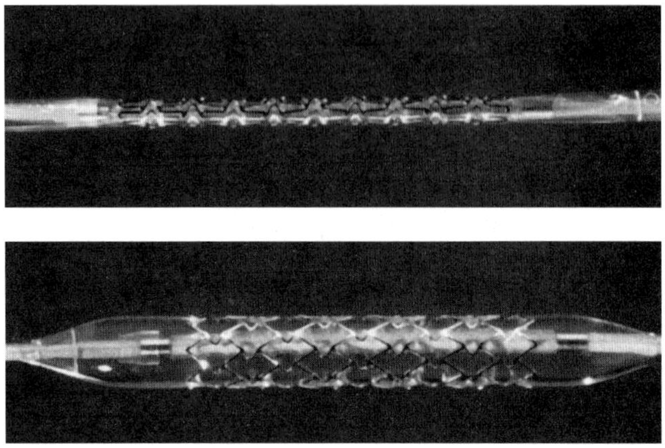

A

B

FIGURE 5-16. The SCIMED NIR balloon expandable intracoronary stent. **A:** The stent in the collapsed state is shown preloaded on a deflated angioplasty balloon. **B:** The stent in its expanded state after inflation of the angioplasty balloon. (Courtesy of SCIMED Life Systems, Inc., Boston Scientific Corporation, Maple Grove, MN.)

Self-expanding stents are designed to expand to a predetermined size (Fig. 5-17). They are delivered to the site of

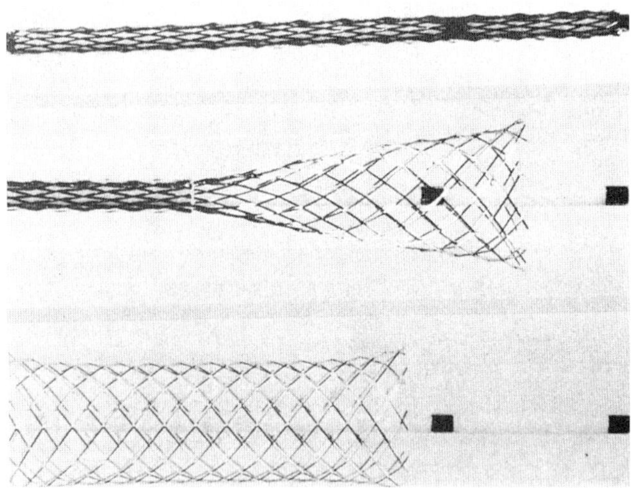

FIGURE 5-17. A self-expanding stent, the Schneider Wallstent, is shown in stages of delivery. **Top:** Fully covered by a sheath. **Middle:** The sheath is partially withdrawn, allowing the stent to be released. **Bottom:** The sheath is completely withdrawn and the stent fully delivered.

a stenosis covered by a sheath. Once in positioned, the sheath is withdrawn, deploying the stent. The newer self-expanding stents are made of nitinol (nickel-titanium alloy). Nitinol is a unique metal alloy, which exists in two crystalline phases (104). Stents of nitinol are heated until its crystal structure assumes a parent, or austenitic, phase. The alloy is then rapidy cooled to a separate crystal phase, called the martensitic phase. In this phase, the alloy can be compressed into a tube with a narrow profile. Once in the body, the sheath is removed, and the stent is exposed to body temperature. The nitinol then reverts back to the parent, or austenitic, crystal phase and is restored to its initial shape and diameter.

Anticoagulation during coronary stenting is maintained with heparin with or without a glycoprotein IIb/IIIa receptor inhibitor. All patients should be pretreated with aspirin (325 mg) and either ticlopidine (500 mg) or clopidogrel (300 mg) before the procedure. After the procedure, patients should receive one of two regimens to prevent stent thrombosis while the stent is incorporated into the endothelium of the vessel wall: (a) aspirin plus ticlopidine (250 mg twice daily) for 2 weeks or (b) aspirin plus clopidogrel (75 mg once daily) for 4 weeks. These regimens have been shown to reduce stent thrombosis and to minimize bleeding complications (79–81).

New developments continue to make coronary stents more flexible and lower profile, enabling more lesions to be reached. In addition, the pharmacotherapy surrounding stenting is rapidly evolving. There is growing evidence that aggressive platelet inhibition with glycoprotein IIb/IIIa receptor inhibitors improves clinical outcomes in many patients receiving coronary stents. In the future, stents may be used as devices to deliver drugs, gene therapy, or radiation, all of which hold promise to improve outcomes.

Perfusion Balloon Catheter

The PBC was a major development in balloon angioplasty and remains important in selected scenarios in the interventional laboratory (89). This catheter has multiple side holes in the catheter shaft, both immediately proximal to and distal to the angioplasty balloon (Fig. 5-15). Once the lesion is crossed with the PBC, the balloon is inflated to dilate the lesion and the guidewire is withdrawn back into the guide catheter to allow distal coronary autoperfusion via the catheter side holes and the central angioplasty catheter lumen. The catheter lumen delivers about 60 mL of blood per minute to the coronary bed distal to the inflated balloon. The guide catheter is withdrawn from the coronary ostium to facilitate the autoperfusion, and heparinized saline is flushed via the angioplasty catheter lumen every 3 minutes to ensure patency.

The PBC was at one time critical for procedures complicated by dissection or abrupt closure. Long inflations were necessary to tack up intimal flaps, allowing stabilization of dissected lesions. The advent of the coronary stent has decreased the need for PBCs; however, they remain useful for treatment of vessels that are too small or otherwise unsuitable for stenting, and for patients who are unable to tolerate the myocardial ischemia induced with routine balloon inflations. The PBC remains the standard for maintaining coronary perfusion in the setting of a complication requiring emergency CABG.

Laser Angioplasty

Laser-assisted coronary angioplasty was developed to treat the eccentric and calcified atherosclerotic plaque that accompanies many high-risk coronary stenoses. The most extensively evaluated coronary laser system, the excimer laser, directly ablates atherosclerotic plaque by transmitting high-intensity pulses of ultraviolet light directly to the plaque. The transmitted energy denatures proteins within the plaque and effectively melts away or vaporizes atherosclerotic debris. The coronary lesion is first crossed with a guidewire, and a small laser wire is passed across the stenosis. Saline is infused into the target vessel while the laser is activated. This minimizes plasma or vapor bubble formation, which is thought to produce plaque and tissue disruption and dissection. Almost all laser angioplasty cases require adjunctive balloon angioplasty or coronary stent placement to achieve an acceptable angiographic result.

Although the technique is theoretically appealing, clinical results of laser angioplasty have been disappointing. Procedural success rates are similar to those seen with PTCA of complex stenoses, but laser-assisted angioplasty results in more coronary dissections and perforations with no improvement in angiographic or clinical restenosis (105–107). There is still enthusiasm for laser-assisted angioplasty in chronic total occlusions, although several trials have failed to show improvements in angiographic or clinical outcome. An eccentric laser wire is currently in use that allows most of the laser energy to be directed at the bulk of the atherosclerotic plaque rather than at other, nondiseased portions of the vessel wall. It is hoped that this strategy will reduce the vascular complications while improving outcome with more tailored debulking of the atheroclerotic plaque. There is also enthusiasm for use of this strategy in the treatment of in-stent restenosis. Randomized trials of laser-assisted angioplasty for in-stent restenosis versus balloon angioplasty and other debulking strategies are currently underway.

Coronary Atherectomy

A variety of different devices now exist to perform percutaneous coronary atherectomy. These devices offer advantages over balloon angioplasty in specific anatomic situations. Like laser angioplasty, they are technically more challenging and therefore are associated with a high incidence of procedure-related complications. They are also more expensive

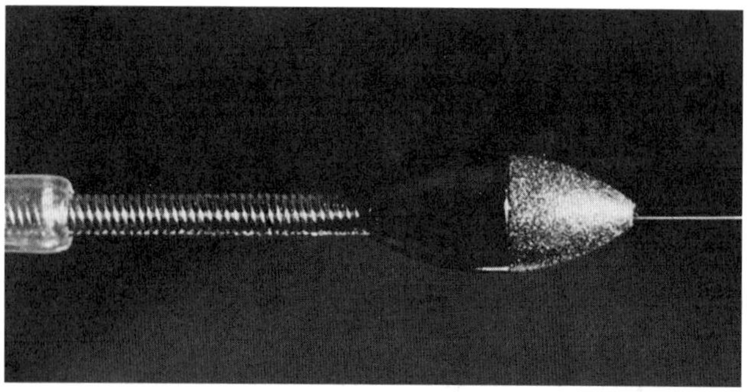

FIGURE 5-18. A rotational atherectomy burr. Diamond chips are embedded into a metal tip, which is attached to a drive shaft. The tip is rotated at 160,000 to 200,000 rpm and advanced across a plaque, debriding it into small atheromatous particles. (From Reisman M. Guide to Rotational Atherectomy. Seattle: Physicians Press, 1997:2, with permission.)

than standard angioplasty procedures. Although they afford improved acute results in certain coronary lesions, these devices have failed to reduce the incidence of coronary artery restenosis.

Rotational Atherectomy

The rotational atherectomy (Rotablator) catheter (Fig. 5-18) consists of an elliptical metal tip attached to a flexible metal shaft. The tip, or burr, is impregnated with diamond chips, making it very abrasive. A motor attached to the catheter shaft rotates the burr at speeds of 160,000 to 200,000 rpm (108). As the catheter is advanced across a stenosis, the burr debrides the atherosclerotic plaque producing atheromatous particles, the majority of which are smaller than 15 μm. Theoretically, this debris is too small to cause cause capillary obstruction. Burr sizes of 1.5 to 2.5 mm may be used, and adjunctive balloon angioplasty is required in most cases.

Most operators use rotational atherectomy in the setting of heavily calcified lesions or ostial stenoses, or to debulk atheromata seen with in-stent restenosis. Although observational studies have suggested that rotational atherectomy may be useful in these settings, randomized trial data have been less impressive. Clinical complications are similar to those seen with conventional balloon angioplasty, whereas angiographic complications including dissection, abrupt closure, and perforation may be more common (109,110). Up to 6% of patients have a significant rise in creatine phosphokinase, myocardial type (CPK-MB) isoenzyme levels (more than two times normal) after the procedure. Restenosis rates with rotational atherectomy in the absence of coronary stenting range from 42% to 62% in most studies. It remains to be seen whether rotablator atherectomy performed with coronary stenting will improve on these disappointing rates of restenosis. Operator technique and experience seem to be particularly important with rotational atherectomy, because angiographic results and clinical outcomes are more widely varied than those seen with other devices or strategies.

Directional Coronary Atherectomy

Figure 5-19 shows a schematic diagram of the DCA catheter. The distal, working end of the catheter consists of a metal cylinder with a slot in one side. There is a rotating, concave blade within the cylinder and a small angioplasty balloon 180° opposite the open slot in the cylinder. The conical hollow end of the cylinder is used to collect the shaved-off material. The device requires a large (9F or 10F) guide catheter and is advanced over a 0.014-inch coronary

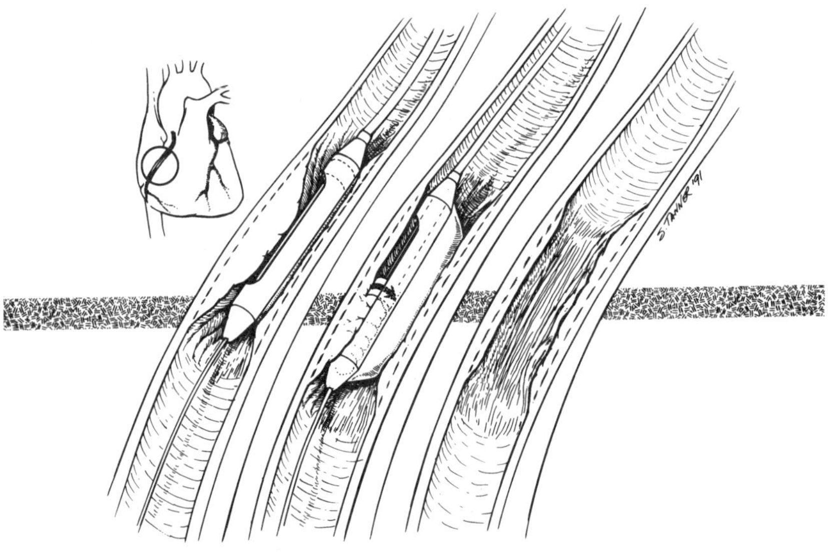

FIGURE 5-19. Illustration of the mechanism of directional coronary atherectomy (DCA). Starting from the left, the catheter is positioned across a stenosis. The balloon opposite the slot of the metal cylinder is inflated. The rotating cutting blade is advanced forward through the cylinder to shave off the plaque and force it into the conical tip of the device. The catheter is then withdrawn. (Courtesy of Richard S. Stack, Duke University Medical Center.)

guidewire. Once across the coronary lesion, the catheter is "directional" in that rotation of the catheter can be used to direct the cutting slot toward eccentric plaque within the coronary. Once the device is positioned properly, the balloon opposite the cutting slot is inflated (under low pressure, 10 to 30 psi) to force the cutting slot against the coronary plaque. The motor device unit is turned on, rotating the concave cutting blade within the cylinder, and the blade is slowly advanced forward, shaving off the plaque within the cutting slot and forcing it into the conical reservoir at the catheter tip. Several cuts are usually required, with the cutting slot rotated to a different position each time. After six to eight cuts, the device must be withdrawn out of the body and the plaque within the reservoir removed. Directional atherectomy can produce some of the best acute angiographic results achieved with percutaneous coronary interventions, although many patients require adjunctive balloon angioplasty to achieve an acceptable angiographic result.

The limitations of DCA relate to the stiff characteristics of this catheter and its relatively bulky size. The guide catheters are extra stiff and can dissect coronary ostia, resulting in proximal coronary closure. In addition, use of the 9F or 10F guide catheter leads to increased vascular trauma and groin complications. The stiffness of the DCA catheter itself allows only proximal coronary lesions to be readily treated. In addition, small-caliber left main coronary arteries or minor degrees of plaque in the left main coronary artery can cause problems when trying to get the DCA device into the LAD or circumflex coronary artery. Once in proper position, the device itself may be almost occlusive and may cause severe ischemia when applied to proximal lesions in vessels jeopardizing a large territory of myocardium.

The initial enthusiasm generated for DCA has been tempered by the long-term follow-up review of several multicenter, randomized trials (111–113). The Coronary Angioplasty Versus Excisional Atherectomy Trial (CAVEAT-1) trial reported larger luminal diameters and a trend toward reduction in restenosis, primarily confined to the proximal LAD, in patients treated with DCA versus conventional PTCA (111). At 6 months, however, the incidence of death or MI was higher in the atherectomy group (8.6% versus 4.6%). CAVEAT-II randomly assigned symptomatic patients with saphenous vein bypass graft stenoses to DCA or PTCA (112). Atherectomy was again associated with improved angiographic success and luminal diameters, but not with improved rates of restenosis at 6 months. The most recent study, the Balloon versus Optimal Atherectomy Trial (BOAT), compared a strategy of "optimal" atherectomy (aimed at producing a residual stenosis of less than 20% by aggressive debulking and dilatation) versus PTCA with coronary stent backup for a suboptimal angiographic result (113). The BOAT study again demonstrated improved angiographic success rates with DCA. Clinical events, including mortality, were similar, with DCA holding a slight edge in angiographic restenosis at a cost of increased in CPK-MB fraction elevations in the DCA group. Currently, enthusiasm for DCA has waned, owing primarily to the unacceptably high incidence of ischemic complications without a consistent reduction in the rate of clinical restenosis.

Transluminal Extraction Catheter

The Transluminal Extraction Catheter (InterVentional Technologies, San Diego, CA) consists of a pair of stainless steel blades aligned in a conical configuration and connected to a hollow torque-tube (114). The catheter is delivered over an extra-stiff guidewire placed across a coronary stenosis. An external motor rotates the blades at 750 rpm while the catheter is advanced across the lesion (Fig. 5-20). As the catheter is advanced, suction is also applied to the central lumen of the catheter, removing excised debris.

As with the DCA device, the limitations of the TEC primarily arise from its stiff, bulky characteristics. These catheters also require a 10F, very stiff guide catheter, which increases the risk of coronary ostium dissections and vascular complications at the femoral artery puncture site. Perforation when negotiating bends in the vessel is also a serious risk with the TEC.

These limitations have contributed to the declining use of the TEC, which is now almost exclusively reserved for degenerated saphenous vein bypass grafts and lesions comprising large amounts of thrombus. These lesions are often friable, and embolization of this material into the distal coronary bed is common with conventional angioplasty techniques. The TEC offers the theoretic opportunity to remove this debris, although clinical results have been disappointing. Use of the TEC in native coronary arteries has resulted in unacceptably high rates of abrupt vessel closure, dissection, coronary perforation, and late vessel occlusion (114,115). Its use in saphenous vein grafts is associated with

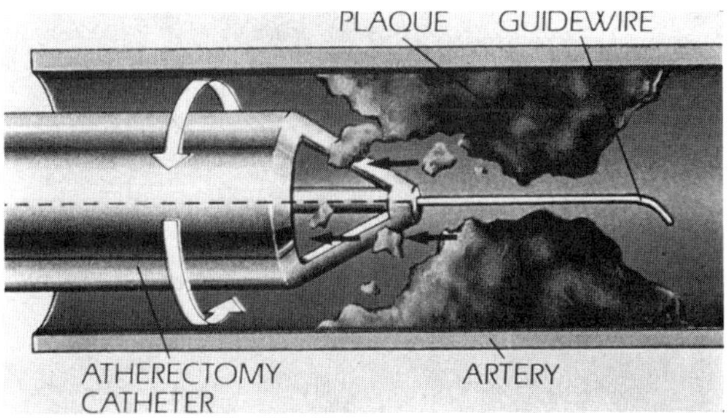

FIGURE 5-20. The transluminal extraction catheter (TEC). A guidewire is positioned across the area of narrowing, and the rotating conical head is advanced across the stenosis. During the procedure, suction is applied to the inner lumen of the catheter for removal of debris. (From Stack RS, Califf RM, Phillips HR, et al. New interventional technology. *Am J Cardiol* 1988;62:12F, with permission.)

distal embolism in up to 17% of cases, and restenosis rates are in the 50% range. These values are not different from those seen with conventional balloon angioplasty. Such limitations have dampened the enthusiasm for the TEC and made it very much a niche device for high-risk lesions where the potential benefit of reducing distal embolization outweighs the risk of other complications.

Alternative Devices for Intracoronary Thrombus

The presence of intracoronary thrombus is accompanied by higher rates of adverse clinical and angiographic events, including abrupt closure, procedural failure, distal embolization, restenosis, and periprocedural MI (116–118). Several new devices are under investigation to address this important problem.

The Possis AngioJet Rheolytic Thrombectomy System (Possis Medical, Minneapolis, MN) is a 5F catheter with two lumens, a large lumen for guidewire passage and debris aspiration and a smaller lumen carrying saline under high pressure to a stainless steel loop at at the tip of the catheter (Fig. 5-21). Pressurized saline is projected through small holes in the distal loop retrogradely toward an aspiration port at the end of the larger lumen. These high-pressure saline jets create an area of low pressure through the Venturi effect, leading to a vortex that draws in adjacent thrombus. Once inside the vortex, the thrombus is fragmented and aspirated through the end hole of the larger lumen (119).

The PercuSurge Guardwire (PercuSurge, Santa Rosa, CA) is a hollow guidewire connected to a distal balloon. The balloon is inflated during a coronary intervention performed over the hollow guidewire. After the intervention and before the distal balloon is deflated, an aspiration catheter removes

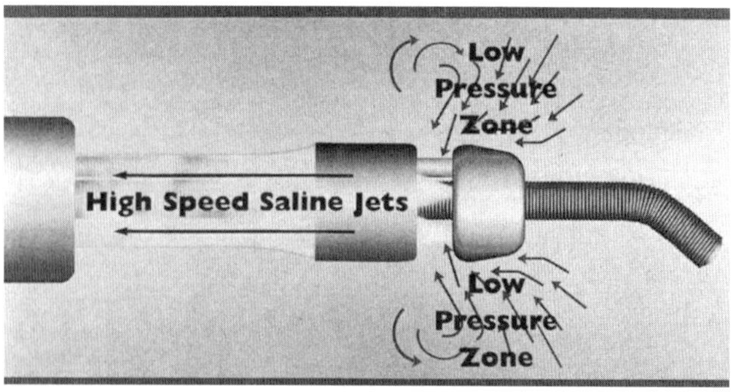

FIGURE 5-21. The Possis AngioJet Rheolytic Thrombectomy System. High-pressure saline jets are directed retrogradely from the catheter tip producing a zone of low pressure through the Bernoulli effect. This vacuum draws in adjacent thrombus into the saline jets, where it is fragmented and aspirated through a catheter lumen. (From Sharafuddin MJ, Hicks ME, Jenson, et al. Rheolytic thrombectomy with use of the AngioJet-F105 catheter: preclinical evaluation of safety. *J Vasc Interv Radiol* 1997:8:939 and Possis Medical, Minneapolis, MN, with permission.)

atherosclerotic and thrombotic debris, preventing distal embolization (120).

Ultrasound energy can also be applied to the problem of intracoronary thrombus. Elastic tissue such as a blood vessel wall is relatively resistant to ultrasound, whereas thrombus can be fragmented by ultrasound energy. The Acolysis (Angiosonics, Morrisville, NC) coronary ultrasound thrombolysis device fits into a 7F sheath over a standard 0.14-inch guidewire and has shown promise in registry data.

All of these devices have demonstrated initial results that exceed those seen with atherectomy performed for removal of thrombus. Large randomized trials of each of these stat-egies in multiple clinical settings will determine wheter they offer an improvement over conventional therapy.

INTRACORONARY RADIATION

One of the more promising strategies for reducing restenosis is intracoronary radiation. Both beta and gamma radiation systems are in clinical trials, both for in-stent restenosis and for *de novo* coronary stenoses. Radioisotopes can be delivered as seeds affixed to a wire that is placed across a coronary stenosis for 5 to 10 minutes with beta radiation emmitters or for 15 to 30 minutes for gamma emmitters. Studies are also underway using a beta-emitting solution to inflate an angioplasty balloon and deliver the radiation dose to the vessel wall. Another promising strategy is radioisotope coating of coronary stents.

After promising results at 6 months of follow-up, the longer-term results of studies of catheter-based radiation therapy are just becoming available (121,122). The most complete study to date, from Teirstein et al. at the Scripps Clinic, reported 2-year follow-up in 55 patients with restenosis after previous PTCA treated with gamma radiation (iridium 192) or placebo (121). Angiographic restenosis at 6 months was 54% in the control group and 17% in the irradiated group. At 2 years, TVR occurred in 45% of control patients versus 15% of irradiated patients. Early intravascular ultrasound results at 6 months showed a marked reduction in neointima formation with some suppression of chronic artery contracture, or remodeling. Many questions remain regarding the long-term effects of coronary radiation, the optimal radiation dose, and the preferred type and delivery method of intracoronary radiation.

INTRAAORTIC BALLOON PUMP SUPPORT FOR HIGH-RISK PERCUTANEOUS TRANSLUMINAL CORONARY ANGIOPLASTY

Improvements in percutaneous coronary interventional devices and the development of coronary artery stents have markedly shortened procedure times. Prolonged ischemia is now rare and has allowed many patients with severe LV dysfunction the option of percutaneous revascularization. Intraaortic balloon pump (IABP) counterpulsation has proved beneficial in these cases, improving coronary perfusion pressure to the nonischemic coronary bed, decreasing myocardial O_2 demand, reducing LV afterload, and providing hemodynamic stability (123,124). The IABP is inserted into one femoral artery and angioplasty is performed via the other. Counterpulsation needs to be discontinued only for brief periods while inserting or exchanging guide catheters. IABP counterpulsation is also extremely beneficial in cases of primary angioplasty during acute MI, especially when the MI is accompanied by pulmonary edema or hypotension. IABP support after primary angioplasty or rescue angioplasty (after unsuccessful thrombolysis) was shown to prevent infarct artery occlusion (123,125). Although coronary artery stents have markedly reduced periinfarct artery occlusion, intraaortic balloon counterpulsation is still of enormous benefit in critically ill patients in the setting of acute infarction. The 8F that are now available should reduce the bleeding complications and limb ischemia that were associated with the larger systems.

PERCUTANEOUS BALLOON VALVULOPLASTY

Balloon Pulmonic Valvuloplasty

Balloon valvuloplasty of valvular pulmonic stenosis has been shown to be extremely effective and is now considered the procedure of choice for these patients (126–128). Patients with pulmonic stenosis may complain of dyspnea on exertion and fatigue. They may also develop signs of RV hypertrophy and failure leading to increased venous pressures and peripheral edema. Patients often remain asymptomatic until RV failure ensues. Patients with greater than 50 mm Hg peak systolic gradient across the valve are generally considered candidates for balloon pulmonic valvuloplasty.

Clinically, valvular pulmonary stenosis results from congenital fusion of the valve leaflets. The leaflets themselves are relatively normal, but the fused commissures lead to the characteristic domed appearance of the valve during systole (Fig. 5-22). This domed appearance can be identified during angiography of the RV outflow tract or on two-dimensional echocardiography. This type of valvular anatomy responds dramatically to balloon dilation. Less frequently, pulmonic stenosis may be caused by more rigid, thickened, deformed valve leaflets, so-called "dysplastic" valves. These valves lack the domed appearance. The heavily thickened valve leaflets can be identified on angiography or echocardiography in distinction to the fine, thin leaflets of a normal pulmonic valve. Reduction in the severity of pulmonic stenosis can be accomplished with balloon therapy, but success (almost uniform with the classic domed valves) is lower with dysplastic valves (129,130).

Hypertrophy of the RV outflow area can result in dynamic outflow obstruction during systolic ejection, thereby contributing to the severity of the pressure gradient between the RV and PA, which needs to be determined before balloon dilation. RV outflow tract obstruction may develop or worsen transiently after successful balloon dilation and relief of the valvular stenosis. This phenomenon largely resolves after a day or so. Intravenous β-blockers (e.g., metoprolol) or calcium channel blockers (e.g., verapamil) provide relief of severe outflow obstruction.

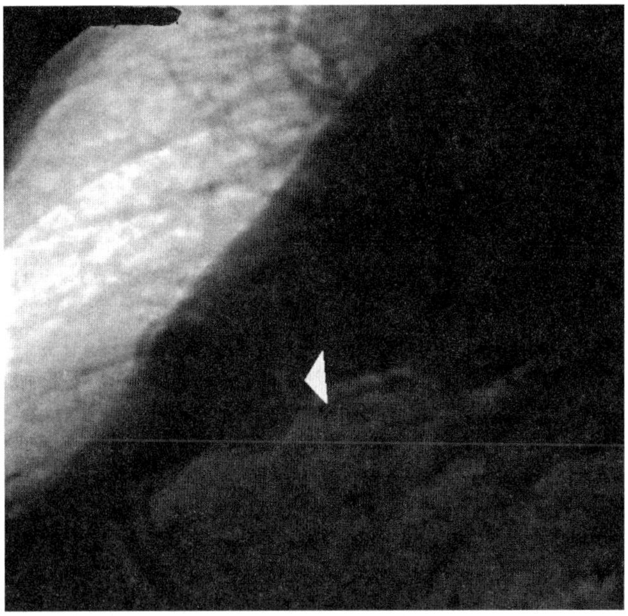

FIGURE 5-22. Lateral projection of a right ventricular outflow tract angiogram in an adult with severe pulmonary valve stenosis. The arrow points out the classic "domed" appearance of the fused commissures of the valve during systole. Also note the significant poststenotic dilatation of the main pulmonary artery in the top right corner of the photograph.

Balloon catheters of 1.4 to 1.6 times the pulmonic valve annulus are required to effectively dilate the pulmonic valve. In adults, this may require the use and simultaneous inflation of two balloons. The high degree of elasticity in the PA allows gross overdilation of this vessel without vascular rupture. This is especially important when dilation of dysplastic valves is attempted, because these valves often require aggressive overdilation for successful relief of the valvular stenosis. Actual balloon dilation results in a transient drop in blood pressure and often also causes reflex bradycardia after stretching of the PA.

Balloon valvuloplasty of the pulmonic valve results in dramatic reduction of the pulmonic valvular pressure gradient. This pressure gradient often improves further with time, as RV infundibular obstruction regresses. The long-term results after successful balloon dilation are excellent, with sustained relief of the ventricular stenosis. Valvular restenosis is uncommon and probably represents an inadequate acute result rather than true restenosis. After balloon dilation, as with surgical valvulotomy for valvular pulmonic stenosis, many patients are left with pulmonic valvular insufficiency. This does not cause a clinical problem acutely or on short-term follow-up, because the RV is more capable of handling volume rather than pressure loads.

Balloon Aortic Valvuloplasty

There are few indications for balloon valvuloplasty for adults with aortic stenosis (131). Balloon valvuloplasty to treat aortic stenosis was initially described in 1986, and it was hoped that it would be an alternative to valve replacement for these patients, most of whom are at increased surgical risk and are elderly with comorbid illnesses. The initial enthusiasm for this procedure has now been replaced by the realization that it is largely ineffective and probably does not favorably influence the dismal natural history of this disease in adults (132). This is less true in childhood and adolescence, where commissural fusion plays a larger role in the stenosis and excellent intermediate-term results (5 years) are common.

The pathology of the aortic valve largely determines the ineffectiveness of balloon dilation of aortic stenosis. In adults, the overwhelming majority of the cases are caused by idiopathic degenerative calcific disease of the valve, with the calcium virtually weighing down the cusps. Bicuspid and rheumatic aortic stenoses are also encountered in adults, and these disease processes often have superimposed calcium deposition as well. Therefore, most of the valvular obstruction is secondary to the thickened, stiff, fibrotic and calcific leaflets themselves, with fusion of commissures contributing in only a minority of patients. For this reason, balloon dilation of adult patients with aortic stenosis has minimal morphologic effects (133). Cracking of the calcific leaflet plaques, stretching of the aortic annulus, and commissural tearing result in early improvement in valve mobility.

Aortic valvuloplasty is usually performed by a retrograde approach via the femoral artery (Fig. 5-23). Large arterial sheaths (10F to 14F) are required. The balloon is introduced over a guidewire retrogradely positioned across the stenotic valve. The stenotic valve is dilated by hand inflation of a contrast-saline mixture. After balloon deflation and withdrawal, repeat measurements of the aortic pressure gradient and cardiac output, as well as aortography to reassess the severity of aortic insufficiency, are made. Single, double, and triple balloon combinations have been described, all with similar acute hemodynamic results.

Balloon aortic valvuloplasty results in about a 50% reduction in aortic valve gradient and a 50% acute increase in aortic valve area (134). Unfortunately, restenosis of the aortic valve occurs quickly. In one study, 75% of patients demonstrated restenosis by 6 months (135). Clinical follow-up reveals a dismal outcome. At 6 months, 60% have recurrent symptoms, and at 1 year, the survival rate is 50%. The 3-year survival rate is only 7% (131). It should be noted that the status of LV function, rather than the severity of

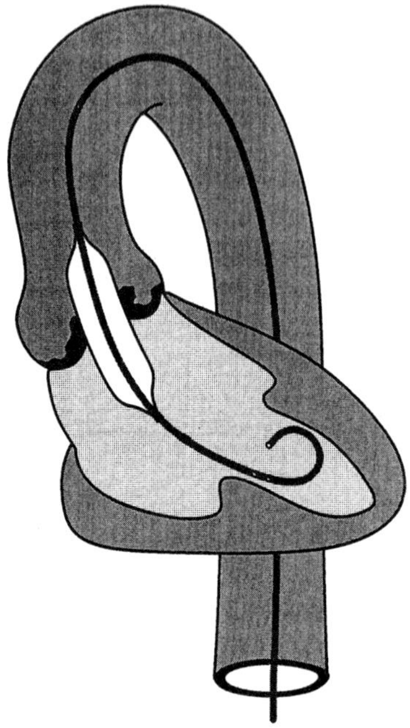

FIGURE 5-23. Procedure of balloon aortic valvuloplasty. The balloon valvuloplasty catheter is positioned retrogradely across the aortic valve. (From Bashore TM, Davidson CJ. Cardiac catheterization, angiography, and balloon valvuloplasty. In: Sabiston DC Jr, Spencer FC, eds. *Surgery of the chest.* Philadelphia: WB Saunders, 1990:1025, with permission.)

valvular stenosis, most importantly affects prognosis. Complications after aortic valvuloplasty are common, and the procedure-related mortality rate approaches 5% (134).

Because of the high incidence of restenosis at 6 months, poor long-term outcome, and a high complication rate, balloon aortic valvuloplasty is currently reserved (a) for severely symptomatic elderly patients with normal LV function (LV ejection fraction greater than 45%) who are not otherwise candidates for aortic valve replacement, (b) as a temporizing measure for patients with cardiogenic shock, or (c) as a stabilizing measure for patients who require urgent, extensive noncardiac surgery. In the adolescent and child, commissural fusion can be opened by the procedure, and percutaneous balloon aortic valvuloplasty remains an option.

Balloon Mitral Commissurotomy

Percutaneous balloon mitral commissurotomy (BMC), also known as balloon mitral valvuloplasty, is an effective alternative to the surgical treatment of selected cases of mitral stenosis (136). Since Kanji Inoue performed the first balloon mitral valvotomy in 1984, the popularity of this technique has increased and understanding of the variables favoring a successful procedural outcome has expanded.

As with most valvular disease, echocardiography plays a critical role in the selection of patients with valvular morphology amenable to balloon dilation. The degree of mitral

TABLE 5-9. ECHOCARDIOGRAPHIC GRADING OF MITRAL VALVE CHARACTERISTICS IN RHEUMATIC MITRAL STENOSIS[a]

Grade	Mobility	Subvalvular Thickening	Thickening	Calcification
1	Highly mobile valve with only leaflet tips restricted	Minimal thickening just below mitral leaflets	Leaflets near normal in thickness (4–5 mm)	Single area of increased echo brightness
2	Leaflet middle and base portions have normal mobility	Thickening of chordal structures extending up to one third of chordal length	Midleaflets normal, considerable thickening of margins (5–8 mm)	Scattered areas of brightness confined to leaflet margins
3	Valve continues to move forward in diastole, mainly from the base	Thickening extending to distal third of chords	Thickening extending through entire leaflet (5–8 mm)	Brightness extending into midportion of leaflets
4	No or minimal forward movement of leaflets in diastole	Extensive thickening and shortening of all chordal structures, extending down to papillary muscles	Considerable thickening of all leaflet tissue (>8—10 mm)	Extensive brightness throughout much of leaflet tissue

[a] The total echocardiographic score is derived from an analysis of mitral leaflet mobility, valvular and subvalvular thickening, and calcification, each graded from 0 to 4 according to the above criteria. This allows for a total score of 0 to 16.

leaflet mobility and the extent of leaflet thickening affect the outcome of patients undergoing surgical commissurotomy, so it is not surprising that these factors also affect the outcome of percutaneous BMC. Early investigators examined the prognostic value of multiple echocardiographic and clinical variables in the first 22 patients to undergo BMC (137). After considering leaflet mobility, thickening, and calcification, as well as the degree of thickening of the subvalvular apparatus, they devised a semiquantitative echocardiographic score for assessing the degree of mitral valve deformity and pliability (Table 5-9). They and other investigators found that a high total echo score (higher than 8) was predictive of a poor acute hemodynamic result and also predicted higher restenosis rates (138,139).

Echocardiography is a critical component of the preprocedure assessment. Transthoracic echocardiography (TTE) is used to determine the extent of valvular and subvalvular deformity and to exclude the presence of other coexisting valvular disease. Transesophageal echocardiography (TEE) is important to exclude the presence of left atrial thrombi and to evaluate the thickness and morphology of the interatrial septum. Left atrial thrombi are a contraindication to BMC because the balloon catheter may dislodge the thrombus and result in systemic embolization.

The presence of significant mitral stenosis and the absence of significant mitral regurgitation (greater than 2+ by Sellers' classification; Table 5-4) should be confirmed by diagnostic cardiac catheterization before BMC is performed. BMC may be accomplished with one or two polyethylene balloons (140) or with a single latex Inoue catheter, now the more popular system worldwide (136).

Both procedures usually require the performance of transseptal left atrial catheterization. With the polyethylene double-balloon technique, two guidewires are placed through the transseptal catheter and directed through the stenotic mitral valve orifice, finally resting in the LV. A balloon catheter (usually 15 to 20 mm in diameter, depending on annulus size) is then inserted over each guidewire and manipulated into the mitral orifice. The two balloons are simultaneously inflated to their maximum diameter with a saline and contrast mixture until the waist in the balloons is relieved (Fig. 5-21).

The latex Inoue balloon catheter has several advantages over the polyethylene double-balloon technique. The Inoue balloon has a curved shaft and an inner steering wire, which facilitates placement of the balloon through the stenotic mitral valve orifice. In addition, its hourglass shape "locks" the balloon's position within the valve orifice during balloon inflation (Fig. 5-24). The Inoue balloon also allows stepwise dilation of the mitral valve through a range of balloon diameters by simply injecting calibrated amounts of the contrast-saline mixture into the balloon catheter, obviating multiple-catheter manipulations and exchanges.

Favorable acute, intermediate, and now long-term results have made BMC the procedure of choice for patients with favorable valvular anatomy. Patients treated with successful BMC have similar or improved outcomes as those treated with either open or closed surgical commissurotomy (141,142). The definition of a successful acute result varies from series to series. Most centers define BMC success either as a final valve area greater than 1.5 cm^2 or as an improvement in the valve area or gradient by 50%, with either value accompanied by 2+ or less angiographic mitral regurgitation. Complications of BMC include embolic events, hemopericardium leading to cardiac tamponade, and severe mitral regurgitation. Mortality in most recent series was less than 1%.

Two studies with late follow-up have been published.

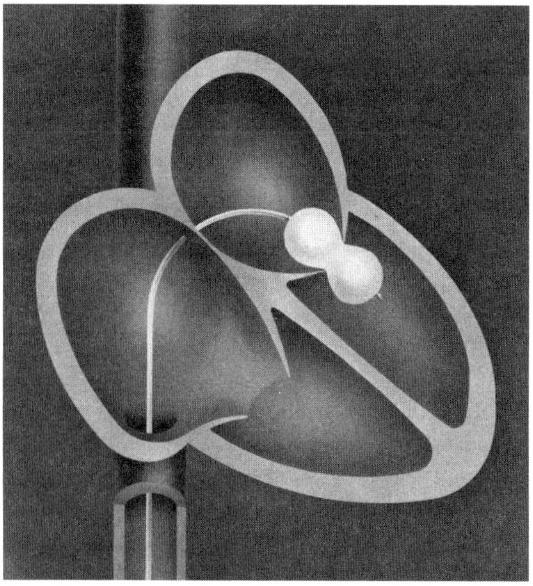

FIGURE 5-24. Technique of balloon mitral commissurotomy with the Inoue balloon-catheter system. A single, steerable balloon catheter system is inserted across the intraatrial septum and positioned across the mitral valve. The hourglass shape of the balloon serves to trap the mitral annulus in the waist of the balloon. (Courtesy of Toray Inc., Tokyo, Japan.)

Iung et al. reported the results of 1,024 patients undergoing BMC in France (143). Procedural success was obtained in 89% of patients. Procedural failure due to 3+ or 4+ mitral regurgitation was 3.4%, with the remainder of procedural failures caused by inadequate valve area. At a mean follow-up of 49 months, 12% of patients with a successful immediate result required mitral valve surgery or a repeat BMC. The mortality rate in this group was 5%. In those patients with a poor initial result, the mortality rate was 14.3% and 66% required subsequent mitral valve surgery.

Hernandez et al. reported similar results, with echocardiographic follow-up, in 561 patients undergoing BMC (144). Procedural success was achieved in 78% of patients, while severe mitral regurgitation occurred in 4%. At a median follow-up of 39 months, 69% of patients were free of major events (cardiac death, mitral surgery, repeat BMC, or declining functional status). In patients with good procedural results, freedom from major events ranged from 72% to 88%, when grouped by echo characteristics. Echocardiographic score, postprocedural mitral valve area, and mitral regurgitation were independent predictors of event-free survival. Echocardiographic score was an independent predictor of restenosis, and a mitral valve area of 1.8 cm^2 or greater was a negative predictor of restenosis.

These results highlight a 15-year experience with BMC. In young patients with favorable valvular anatomy by echocardiography, BMC is clearly the procedure of choice. Elderly patients and patients with higher echo scores may also derive a significant benefit from the procedure but are at higher risk for complications and restenosis. The emphasis in all patients should be on improving valve area as much as possible while avoiding mitral regurgitation, because these variables more significantly correlate with long-term prognosis.

INTERVENTIONAL CARDIOLOGY IN CONGENITAL HEART DISEASE

The field of interventional cardiology and congenital heart disease is an exciting area of investigation and seems like a new field. However, interventional cardiology began in the 1960s, when Rashkind described the first percutaneous balloon atrial septostomy for critically ill infants with transposition of the great arteries (145). This procedure is still widely used today. A catheter is inserted via either the internal jugular vein or the femoral vein into the RA and then across the foramen ovale into the left atrial chamber. The balloon catheter is then inflated with a mixture of contrast and saline to a diameter of 10 to 15 mm. The balloon is then withdrawn abruptly through the intraatrial septum to create a large defect in the atrial septum. This increases atrial mixing, improving cardiac output and systemic oxygenation. This continues to allow critically ill infants to survive surgical correction. Presently, arterial switch is available even in infancy. These patients, palliated with balloon septostomy, then undergo complete repair with arterial switch before discharge from the hospital.

Balloon Valvuloplasty and Congenital Valvular Stenosis

As previously discussed, congenital pulmonic valvuloplasty is effectively treated with balloon dilation of the valve. As in adults, balloon valvuloplasty for congenital pulmonic stenosis in children is almost uniformly successful except in cases of severe valvular dysplasia or when the stenosis is actually caused by obstruction in the RV outflow tract.

As opposed to balloon aortic valvuloplasty in the adult patient, aortic stenosis can be effectively palliated in children with percutaneous balloon valvuloplasty (146–148). The difference lies in the pathology between aortic stenosis in children and in adults. In children, aortic stenosis is predominantly caused by bicuspid or unicuspid stenosis of the valve. Surgical incision to improve the degree of stenosis has previously been the treatment of choice. The surgical results have enabled many children to have adequate valvular function for decades before requiring valve replacement. Aortic stenosis valvuloplasty in children and adolescents with bicuspid aortic valves can be effectively treated with balloon valvuloplasty in many cases. The mechanism of improvement is similar, in that commissural splitting of the valve occurs with balloon dilation. In children an anterograde septal approach is frequently used to insert the balloon catheters. This avoids the use of large sheaths and catheters in the arterial system and therefore avoids the risk of severe arterial injury. Single- or double-balloon catheters are positioned across the valve from the femoral vein via transseptal puncture.

Congenital mitral stenosis is rarely amenable to balloon dilation (149). Unlike rheumatic mitral valve stenosis, commissural fusion is uncommon, and stenosis results from chordal fusion or from abnormal chordal attachments. The parachute-type mitral valve (single papillary muscle), for example, produces conical fusion of the subvalvular apparatus. Severe acute mitral regurgitation may result from attempted dilation of these valves in the majority of these patients.

Percutaneous Treatment of Coarctation of the Aorta

Controversy continues regarding the optimal treatment for coarctation of the aorta (150). Balloon angioplasty is effective in reducing the pressure gradient and degree of stenosis in aortic coarctation. Balloon angioplasty of the aorta is technically not difficult. The problem relates more to the risk of the procedure and long-term complications from the trauma created by balloon dilation. Balloon angioplasty of the aorta may create large intimal tears that may extend into the deeper layers of the aortic wall (151). In the extreme case, this may cause aortic rupture and death. This is uncommon, but the deep intimal and medial injury coupled with long-term aortic pressure may cause aneurysm formation at the site of previous balloon dilation. Balloon-expandable stents have also been used in conjunction with balloon angioplasty for coarctation (152). This technique holds promise because lower inflation pressures can be used, with less resultant trauma to the vessel wall, and dissections can be covered with stents, stopping their potential progression. Although this technique is theoretically attractive, there is concern regarding the consequences of side-branch occlusion, limitations in growth of stented segments in children and young adults, and perturbations in flow through a nonpulsatile segment of the aorta.

Balloon Angioplasty and Stent Placement for Venous and Pulmonary Artery Stenosis

A congenital stenosis of the systemic and pulmonary veins as well as the branch PAs has posed difficult problems that may be attacked in the catheterization laboratory. Surgical attempts at correcting these stenoses have been disappointing. Many stenoses in the more distal segments of the PAs also are not reachable surgically. These types of PA stenoses are not uncommon in patients with left-to-right shunts that are native or surgically created (e.g., patients with tetralogy with previous Blalock-Taussig or Potts shunts). Balloon dilation has been effective in relieving the stenosis in many cases (153,154). In the PA the tremendous elasticity of this vessel requires gross overdilation to two to three times the normal vessel diameter. Despite overdilation, recoil is not infrequent, leading to only moderate improvement in the stenosis even immediately after balloon dilation. For this reason, metallic intravascular stents have been successfully employed (155). The most effective stents have been the balloon-expandable Palmaz stents. These stents are preloaded onto an angioplasty balloon catheter and delivered through a long sheath to the site of stenosis.

Closure Devices

Various devices are now available or under investigation for closure of the intravascular or even intracardiac defects. The simplest of these devices are metallic intravascular coils or detachable balloons that can be used to close unwanted vessels (156). For example, many patients with Eisenmenger's syndrome or reduced PBF develop large systemic-to-pulmonary collaterals. These large, friable vessels can cause fatal hemoptysis. These types of events can be very difficult to control. Percutaneous techniques now exist to selectively catheterize the vessel. Once the vessel is selectively engaged, a metal coil may be delivered through the catheter lumen to the vessel. It is simply pushed out the end of the catheter with a guidewire, leaving the coil in place in the vessel. The metallic coil contains some Dacron mesh as well, which results in rapid thrombosis of the vessel. This simple technique can be employed rapidly, with lifesaving consequences.

Closure of intracardiac defects is more complex. Since the late 1970s, devices have been under investigation for closure of patent ductus, atrial septal defects, and ventricular septal defects (157–160) (Fig. 5-25). The most promising are the double-umbrella-type devices. With this technology, the defect is crossed with a catheter. The catheter contains a special metal cylinder at its distal end. The defect is sized, and a device of appropriate size is chosen. The device is then preloaded into the cylindrical pod on the end of the catheter. The catheter is delivered across the defect, and the distal umbrella is pushed out of the end of the catheter and expanded. The expanded arms are then pulled back against the defect and, while they are held in this position, the external catheter cylinder is withdrawn to release the proximal umbrella arms. This allows the defect to be entrapped within the two sets of opposing arms. The device is then released from the catheter and the catheter is withdrawn from the body. These devices become endothelialized within 2 to 3 months. The greatest risk with this device is improper positioning and embolization of the device. These types of devices are currently under investigation and hold great promise for nonoperative closure of these congenital defects.

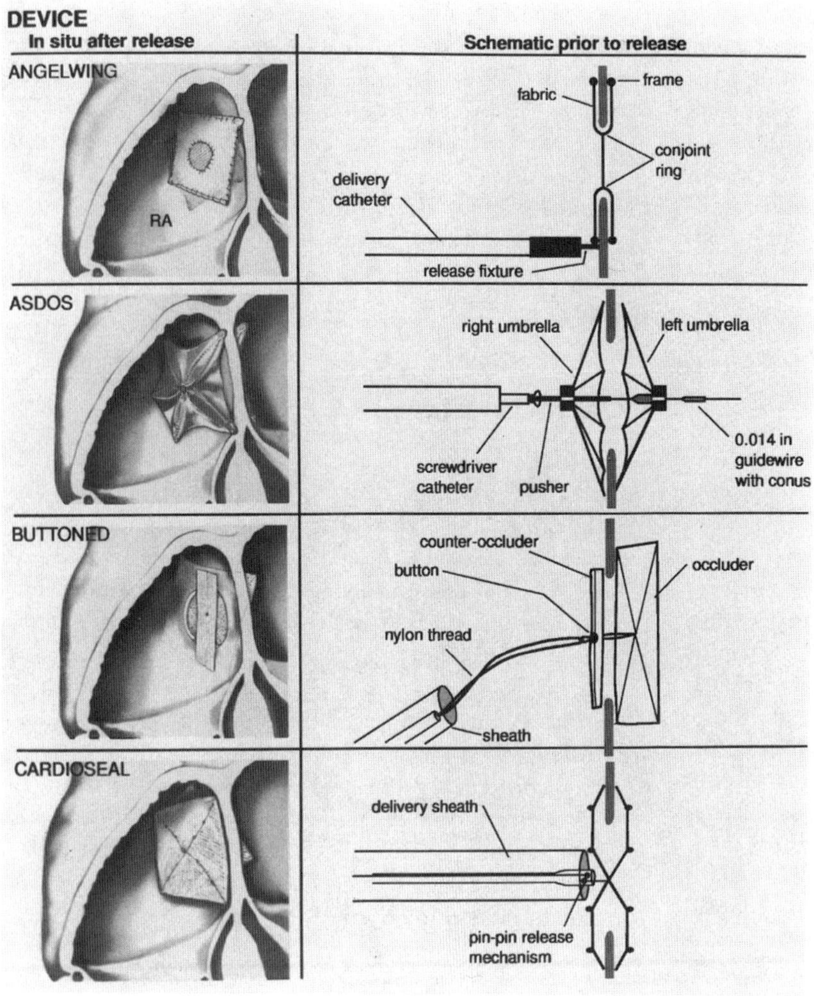

FIGURE 5-25. Representative atrial septal defect (ASD) closure devices. A schematic of the more popular ASD occluder devices is shown with their release mechanisms outlined. (From Latson LA. Per-catheter ASD closure. *Pediatr Cardiol* 1998;19:86.)

REFERENCES

1. American Heart Association. On-Line statistics. 1999.
2. Warren JV. Fifty years of invasive cardiology. *Am J Med* 1980; 69:10.
3. Seldinger SI. Catheter replacement of the needle in percutaneous arteriography. *Acta Radiol* 1953;39:368.
4. Sones FM, Shirey EK. Cine coronary arteriography. *Mod Concepts Cardiovasc Dis* 1962;21:735.
5. Judkins MP. Selective coronary arteriography: Part I. A percutaneous transfemoral technique. *Radiology* 1967;89:815.
6. Swan HJC, Ganz W, Forrester J, et al. Catheterization of the heart in man with use of a flow-directed balloon-tipped catheter. *N Engl J Med* 1970;283:447.
7. Gruntzig A. Transluminal dilatation of coronary-artery stenosis. *Lancet* 1978;1:263.
8. ACC/AHA Guidelines for Coronary Angiography: a report of the American College of Cardiology/American Heart Association Task Force (Committee on Coronary Angiography). *J Am Coll Cardiol* 1998;32:1756.
9. Rahimtoola SH. The need for cardiac catheterization and angiography in valvular heart disease is not disproven. *Ann Intern Med* 1982;97:433.
10. Kirklin JW, Akins CW, Blackstone EH, et al. Guidelines and indications for coronary artery bypass graft surgery: a report of the American College of Cardiology/American Heart Association Task Force on Assessment of Diagnostic and Therapeutic Cardiovascular Procedures (Subcommittee on Coronary Artery Bypass Graft Surgery). *J Am Coll Cardiol* 1991;17:543.
11. Nwasokwa ON, Koss JH, Friedman GH, et al. Bypass surgery for chronic stable angina: predictors of survival benefit and strategy for patient selection. *Ann Intern Med* 1991;114:1035.
12. Gottlieb SO, Gottlieb SH, Achuff SC, et al. Silent ischemia on Holter monitoring predicts mortality in high-risk postinfarction patients. *JAMA* 1988;259:1029.
13. Cohn PF. Silent myocardial ischemia. *Ann Intern Med* 1988; 109:312.
14. Kulick DL, Ramimtoola SH. Risk stratification in survivors of acute myocardial infarction: routine cardiac catheterization and angiography is a reasonable approach in most patients. *Am Heart J* 1991;121:641.
15. Topol EJ, Holmes DR, Rogers WJ. Coronary angiography after thrombolytic therapy for acute myocardial infarction. *Ann Intern Med* 1991;114:877.
16. Gunnar RM, Bourdillon PDV, Dixon DW, et al. ACC/AHA guidelines for the early management of patients with acute myocardial infarction. *Circulation* 1990;82:664.
17. Feit F, Mueller HS, Braunwald E, et al. Thrombolysis in Myocardial Infarction (TIMI) Phase II trial: outcome comparison

of a "conservative strategy" in community versus tertiary hospitals. *J Am Coll Cardiol* 1990;16:1529.
18. The TIMI Study Group. Comparison of invasive and conservative strategies after treatment with intravenous tissue plasminogen activator in acute myocardial infarction. *N Engl J Med* 1989; 320:618.
19. Muller DWM, Topol EJ, Ellis SG, et al. Determinants of the need for early acute intervention in patients treated conservatively after thrombolytic therapy for acute myocardial infarction. *J Am Coll Cardiol* 1991;18:1594.
20. Gruppo Italiano per lo Studio Della Streptochi-nasi Nell'Infarto Miocardio (GISSI). Long-term effects of intravenous thrombolysis in acute myocardial infarction: final report of the GISSI study. *Lancet* 1987;2:871.
21. ISIS-2 [Second International Study of Infarct Survival] Collaborative Group. Randomized trial of intravenous streptokinase, oral aspirin, both, or neither among 17,187 cases of suspected acute myocardial infarction: ISIS-2. *Lancet* 1988;2:349.
22. The GUSTO Angiographic Investigators. The effects of tissue plasminogen activator, streptokinase, or both on coronary-artery patency, ventricular function, and survival after acute myocardial infarction. *N Engl J Med* 1994;329:1616.
23. Simoons ML, Serruys PW, Van Den Brand ML, et al. Early thrombolysis in acute myocardial infarction: limitation of infarct size and improved survival. *J Am Coll Cardiol* 1986;7:717.
24. Topol EJ, Califf RM, George BS, et al. A randomized trial of immediate versus delayed elective angioplasty after intravenous tissue plasminogen activator in acute myocardial infarction. *N Engl J Med* 1987;317:581.
25. The TIMI Research Group. Immediate vs delayed catheterization and angioplasty following thrombolytic therapy for acute myocardial infarction. *JAMA* 1988;260:2849.
26. Califf RM, O'Neill WW, Stack RS, et al. Failure of simple clinical measurements to predict perfusion status after intravenous thrombolysis. *Ann Intern Med* 1988;108:658.
27. Gibbons RJ, Holmes DR, Reeder GS, et al. Immediate angioplasty compared with the administration of a thrombolytic agent followed by conservative treatment for myocardial infarction. *N Engl J Med* 1993;328:685.
28. Zijlistra F, de Boer MJ, Hoorntje JCA, et al. A comparison of immediate coronary angioplasty with intravenous streptokinase in acute myocardial infarction. *N Engl J Med* 1993:328:680.
29. Grines CL, Browne KF, Marco J, et al. A comparison of immediate angioplasty with thrombolytic therapy for acute myocardial infarction. *N Engl J Med* 1993;328:673.
30. Ribeiro EE, Silva LA, Carneiro R, et al. Randomized trial of direct coronary angioplasty versus intravenous streptokinase in acute myocardial infarction. *J Am Coll Cardiol* 1993;22:376.
31. Every NR, Parsons LS, Hlatky M, et al. A comparison of thrombolytic therapy with primary coronary angioplasty for acute myocardial infarction. *N Engl J Med* 1996;335:1253.
32. The GUSTO IIb Substudy Investigators. A clinical trial comparing primary coronary angioplasty with tissue plasminogen activator for acute myocardial infarction. *N Engl J Med* 1997; 336;1621.
33. Weaver WD, Simes RJ, Betriu A, et al. Comparison of primary coronary angioplasy and intravenous thrombolytic therapy for acute myocardial infarction: a quanitative review. *JAMA* 278; 23:2093.
34. Mahaffey KW, Granger CB, Sloan MA, et al. Risk factors for in-hospital nonhemorrhagic stroke in patients treated with thrombolysis: results from GUSTO-I. *Circulation* 97;8:757.
35. Boden WE, O'Rourke RA, Crawford MH, et al. Outcomes in patients with acute non-Q wave myocardial infarction randomly assigned to an invasive as compared with a conservative management strategy. *N Engl J Med* 1998;338:1785.
36. Anderson HV, Cannon P, Stone PH, et al. One-year results of the Thrombolysis in Myocardial Infarction (TIMI) IIIB clinical trial: a randomized comparison of tissue-type plasmingen activator versus placebo and early invasive versus early conservative strategies in unstable angina and non-Q wave myocardial infarction. *J Am Coll Cardiol* 1995;26:1643.
37. SWIFT (Should We Intervene Following Thrombolysis) Trial Study Group. SWIFT trial of delayed intervention versus conservative treatment after thrombolyis with anistreplase in acute myocardial infarction. *BMJ* 302;6776:555.
38. The GUSTO III Investigators. A comparison of reteplase with alteplase for acute myocardial infarction. *N Engl J Med* 1997; 337:1118.
39. The PURSUIT Trial Investigators. Inhibition of platelet glycoprotein IIb/IIIa with eptifibatide in patients with acute coronary syndromes. *N Engl J Med* 1998;339:436.
40. Pepine CJ, Von Gunten C, Hill JA, et al. Percutaneous brachial catheterization using a modified sheath and new catheter system. *Cathet Cardiovasc Diagn* 1984;10:637.
41. Campeau L. Percutaneous radial artery approach for coronary angiography. *Cathet Cardiovasc Diagn* 1989;16:3.
42. Kiemeneij F, Laarman GJ, Odekerken D, et al. A randomized comparison of percutaneous transluminal coronary angioplasty by the radial, brachial and femoral approaches: the ACCESS study. *Am J Cardiol* 29;6:1269.
43. Roberts WC. Reasons for cardiac catheterization before cardiac-valve replacement. *N Engl J Med* 1982;306:1291.
44. Weiner RI, Maranhoe V. Development and application of transseptal left heart catheterization. *Cathet Cardiovasc Diagn* 1988;15:112.
45. O'Keefe JH, Vlietstra RE, Hanley PC, et al. Revival of the transseptal approach for catheterization of the left atrium and ventricle. *Mayo Clin Proc* 1985;60:790.
46. Mason JW. Techniques for right and left ventricular endomyocardial biopsy. *Am J Cardiol* 1978;41:887.
47. Deckers JW, Hare JM, Baughman KL. Complications of transvenous right ventricular endomyocardial biopsy in adult patients with cardiomyopathy: a seven-year survey of 546 consecutive diagnostic procedures in a tertiary referral center. *J Am Coll Cardiol* 1992;19:43.
48. Anderson JL, Marshall HW, Allison SB. The femoral venous approach to endomyocardial biopsy: comparison with internal jugular and transarterial approaches. *Am J Cardiol* 1984;53:833.
49. Chow LC, Dittrich HC, Shabetari R. Endomyocardial biopsy in patients with unexplained congestive heart failure. *Ann Intern Med* 1988;109:535.
50. Noto TJ, Johnson LW, Krone R, et al. Cardiac catheterization 1990: a report of the Registry of the Society for Cardiac Angiography and Interventions. *Cathet Cardiovasc Diagn* 1991;24:75.
51. Laskey W, Boyle J, Johnson LW, et al. Multivariable model for prediction of risk of significant complication during diagnostic cardiac catheterization. *Cathet Cardiovasc Diagn* 1993;30:185.
52. Johnson LW, Lozner EC, Johnson S, et al. Coronary arteriography 1984–1987: a report of the Registry of the Society for Cardiac Angiography and Interventions. Results and complications. *Cathet Cardiovasc Diagn* 1989;17:5.
53. Folland ED, Oprian C, Giacomini J, et al. Complications of cardiac catheterization and angiography in patients with valvular heart disease. *Cathet Cardiovasc Diagn* 1989;17:15.
54. Davidson CJ, Mark DB, Pieper KS, et al. Thrombotic and cardiovascular complications related to nonionic contrast media during cardiac catheterization: analysis of 8,517 patients. *Am J Cardiol* 1990;65:1481.
55. Davidson CJ, Hlatky M, Morris KG, et al. Cardiovascular and renal toxicity of a nonionic radiographic contrast agent after cardiac catheterization. *Ann Intern Med* 1989;110:119.

56. Schwab ST, Klatky MA, Pieper KS, et al. Contrast nephrotoxicity: a randomized controlled trial of a nonionic and an ionic radiographic contrast agent. *N Engl J Med* 1989;320:149.
57. Rudnick MR, Goldfarb S, Wexler L, et al. Nephrotoxicity of ionic and nonionic contrast media in 1196 patients: a randomized trial. *Kidney Int* 1995;47:254.
58. Sabiston DC, Pelargonio S, Taussig HB. Myocardial infarction in infancy: the surgical management of a complication of congenital origin of the left coronary artery from the pulmonary artery. *J Thorac Cardiovasc Surg* 1960;40:321.
59. Sandler H, Dodge HT. The use of single plane angiocardiograms for the calculation of left ventricular volume in man. *Am Heart J* 1968;75:325.
60. Sheehan FH, Bolson EL, Dodge HT, et al. Advantages and applications of the centerline method for characterizing regional ventricular function. *Circulation* 1986;74:293.
61. Sandler H, Dodge HT, Hay RE, et al. Qualitation of valvular insufficiency in man by angiocardiography. *Am Heart J* 1963; 65:501.
62. Gorlin R, Gorlin SG. Hydraulic formula for calculation of the area of the stenotic mitral valve, other cardiac valves, and central circulatory shunts. *Am Heart J* 1951;41:1.
63. Van Grondelle A, Ditchey RV, Groves BM, et al. Thermodilution method overestimates low cardiac output in humans. *Am J Physiol* 1983;245:H690.
64. Rashkind WJ, Miller WW. Transposition of the great arteries: results of palliation by balloon atrioseptostomy in thirty-one infants. *Circulation* 1968;38:453.
65. Dotter CT, Judkins MP. Transluminal treatment of arteriosclerotic obstruction: description of a new technique and a preliminary report of its application. *Circulation* 1964;30:654.
66. Gruntzig A, Kumpe DA. Technique of percutaneous transluminal angioplasty with the Gruntzig balloon catheter. *Am J Radiol* 1979;132:547.
67. Gruntzig A, Vetter W, Meier B, et al. Treatment of renovascular hypertension with percutaneous transluminal dilation of a renal-artery stenosis. *Lancet* 1978;1:801.
68. Gruntzig AR, Senning A, Siegenthaler WE. Nonoperative dilatation of coronary-artery stenosis. *N Engl J Med* 1979;301:61.
69. Dotter CT. Transluminally placed coil spring end arterial tube grafts: long term patency in canine popliteal artery. *Invest Radiol* 1969;4:329.
70. Palmaz JC, Sibbit RR, Reuter SL, et al. Expandable intraluminal graft: a preliminary study. *Radiology* 1985;156:73.
71. Puel J, Joffre F, Rousseau H, et al. Endo-protheses coronariennes auto-expansives dans le prevention des restenoses apres angioplasie transluminale. *Arch Mal Coeur Vaiss* 1987;8:1311.
72. Marso SP, Steg G, Plokker T, et al. Catheter-based reperfuson of unprotected left main stenosis during an acute myocardal infarction (the ULTIMA experience). *Am J Cardiol* 1999;83: 1513.
73. Ellis S, Tamai H, Nobuyoshi M, et al. Contemporary percutaneous treatment of unprotected left main coronary stenoses: initial results from a multicenter registry analysis 1994–1996. *Circulation* 1997;96:3867.
74. Ryan TJ, Faxon DP, Gunnar RM, et al. Guidelines for percutaneous transluminal coronary angioplasty: a report of the American College of Cardiology/American Heart Association Task Force on Assessment of Diagnostic and Therapeutic Cardiovascular Procedures (Subcommittee on Percutaneous Transluminal Coronary Angioplasty). *J Am Coll Cardiol* 1988;12:529.
75. King SB, Lembo NJ, Weintraub WS, et al. A randomized trial comparing coronary angioplasty with coronary artery bypass surgery. *N Engl J Med* 1994;331:1044.
76. The Bypass Angioplasty Revascularization Investigation (BARI) Investigators. Comparison of coronary bypass surgery with angioplasty in patients with multivessel disease. *N Engl J Med* 1996;335:217.
76. Barsness GW, Peterson ED, Ohman EM, et al. Relationship between diabetes mellitus and long-term survival after coronary artery bypass and angioplasty. *Circulation* 1997;96:2551.
77. Elizi S, Kastrati A, Pache J, et al. Diabetes mellitus and the clinical and angiographic outcome after coronary stent placement. *J Am Coll Cardiol* 1998;32:1866.
78. Abizaid A, Kornowski R, Mintz GS, et al. The influence of diabetes mellitus on acute and late clinical outcomes following coronary stent implantation. *J Am Coll Cardiol* 1998;32:584.
79. Leon MB, Baim DS, Popma JJ, et al. A clinical trial comparing three anti-thrombotic regimens after coronary artery stenting. *N Engl J Med* 1998;339:1665.
80. Berger PB, Bell MR, Hasdai D, et al. Safety and efficacy of ticlopidine for only 2 weeks after successful intracoronary stent placement. *Circulation* 1999;99:248.
81. Moussa I, Oetgen M, Roubin G, et al. Effectiveness of clopidogrel and aspirin versus ticlopidine and aspirin in preventing stent thrombosis after coronary stent implantation. *Circulation* 1999;99:2364.
82. The EPIC Investigators. Use of a monoclonal antibody directed at the platelet glycoprotein IIb/IIIa receptor in high-risk coronary angioplasty. *N Engl J Med* 1994;330:956.
83. Topol EJ, Califf RM, Weisman HF, et al. Randomized trial of platelet IIb/IIIa integrin for reduction of clinical restenosis: results at 6 months. *Lancet* 1994;343:881.
84. The Epilog Investigators. Platelet glycoprotein IIb/IIIa receptor blockade and low-dose heparin during percutaneous coronary revascularization. *N Engl J Med* 1997;336:1689.
85. The EPISTENT Investigators. Randomized placebo-controlled and balloon-angioplasty-controlled trial to assess safety of coronary stenting with use of platelet glycoprotein-IIb/IIIa blockade. *Lancet* 1998;352:87.
86. De Feyter PJ, van Den Brand M, Jaarman GJ, et al. Acute coronary artery occlusion during and after percutaneous transluminal coroary angioplasty: frequency, prediction, clinical course, management and follow-up. *Circulation* 1991;83:927.
87. Baughman KL, Pasternak RC, Fallon JT, et al. Transluminal coronary angioplasty of postmortem human hearts. *Am J Cardiol* 1981;48:1044.
88. Tenaglia AN, Buller CE, Kisslo KB, et al. Mechanisms of balloon angioplasty and directional coronary atherectomy as assessed by intracoronary ultrasound. *J Am Coll Cardiol* 1992;20: 685.
89. Hinohara T, Simpson JB, Phillips HR, et al. Transluminal intracoronary reperfusion catheter: a device to maintain coronary perfusion between failed coronary angioplasty and emergency coronary bypass surgery. *J Am Coll Cardiol* 1988;11:977.
90. Dangas V, Fuster V. Management of restenosis after coronary interventions. *Am Heart J* 1996;132:428.
91. Mintz GS, Kent KM, Pichard AAD, et al. Intravascular ultrasound insights into mechanisms of stenosis formation and restenosis. *Cardiol Clin* 1997;15:17.
92. Van Belle E, Bauters C, Hubert E, et al. Restenosis rates in diabetic patients: a comparison of coronary stenting and balloon angioplasty in native coronary vessels. *Circulation* 1997;96: 1454.
93. Rupprerecht HJ, Brennecke R, Bernhard G, et al. Analysis of risk factors for restenosis after PTCA. *Cathet Cardiovasc Diagn* 1990;19:151.
94. Bourassa MG, Lesperance J, Eastwood C, et al. Clinical, physiologic, anatomic and procedural factors predictive of restenosis after percutaneous transluminal coronary angioplasty. *J Am Coll Cardiol* 1991;18:368.
95. Foley DP, Melkert R, Serruys PW, et al. Influence of coronary

vessel size on renarrowing process and late angiographic outcome. *Circulation* 1994;90:1239.

96. Akiyama T, Moussa I, Reimers B, et al. Angiographic and clinical outcome following coronary artery stenting of small vessels: a comparison with coronary stenting of large vessels. *J Am Coll Cardiol* 1998;32:1610.
97. Hirshfield JWJ, Schwartz JS, Jugo R, et al. Restenosis after coronary angioplasty: a multivariate statistical model to relate lesion and procedural variables to restenosis. *J Am Coll Cardiol* 1993;21:6.
98. Puma JA, Sketch MHJ, Tcheng JE, et al. Percutaneous revascularization of chronic total occlusions: an overview. *J Am Coll Cardiol* 1995;26:1.
99. Violoaris AG, Melkert R, Serruys PW. Long term luminal renarrowing after successful elective coronary angioplasty of total occlusions: a quantitative analysis. *Circulation* 1995;91:2140.
100. ACC Expert Consensus Document on Coronary Artery Stents. *J Am Coll Cardiol* 1998;32:171.
101. Macaya C, Serruys PW, Ruygrok P, et al. Continued benefit of coronary stenting versus balloon angioplasty: one-year clinical follow-up of BENESTENT trial. *J Am Coll Cardiol* 1996;27: 255.
102. Fischman DL, Leon MB, Baim DS, et al. A randomized comparison of coronary-stent placement and balloon angioplasty in the treatment of coronary artery disease. Stent Restenosis Study (STRESS) investigators. *N Engl J Med* 1994;331:496.
103. Randomized comparison of implaantation of heparin-coated stents with balloon angioplasty in selected patients with coronary artery disease (Benestent II) *Lancet*α98:352:673.
104. Schetky LM. Shape-memory alloys. *Sci Am* 1979;241:74.
105. Litvack F, Eigler N, Margolis J, et al. Percutaneous excimer coronary angioplasty: results in the first consecutive 3,0000 patients. The ELCA investigators. *J Am Coll Cardiol* 1994;23:323.
106. Baumbach A, Bittl JA, Fleck E, et al. Acute complications of excimer laser coronary angioplasty: a detailed analysis of multicenter results. *J Am Coll Cardiol* 1994:23:1305.
107. Stone GW, de Marchena E, Dageforde D, et al. Prospective, randomized, multicenter comparison of laser-facilitated balloon angioplasty versus stand-alone balloon angioplasty in patients with obsructive coronary artery disease. *J Am Coll Cardiol* 1997; 30:1714.
108. Fourrier JL, Bertrand ME, Auth DC, et al. Percutaneous coronary rotational angioplasty in humans: preliminary report. *J Am Coll Cardiol* 1980;14:1278.
109. Bertrand ME, Van Belle E. Rotational atherectomy. In: Topol EJ, ed. *Textbook of interventional cardiology,* 3rd ed. Philadelphia: WB Saunders, 1999:523.
110. Reifart N, Vandormael M, Krajar M. Randomized comparison of angioplasty of complex coronary lesions at a single center: excimer laser, rotational atherectomy, and balloon angioplasty comparison (ERBAC) study. *Circulation* 1997;96:91.
111. Topol EJ, Leya F, Pinkerton CA, et al. A comparison of directional atherectomy with coronary angioplasty in patients with coronary artery disease. *N Engl J Med* 1993;329:221.
112. Holmes DRJ, Topol EJ, Califf RM, et al. A muticenter, randomized trial of coronary angioplasty versus directional atherectomy for patients with saphenous vein bypass graft lesions. CAVEAT-II investigators. *Circulation* 1995;91:1966.
113. Baim DS, Cutlip DE, Sharma SK, et al. Final results of the balloon vs optimal atherectomy trial (BOAT). *Circulation* 1998; 97:322.
114. Annex BH, Sketch MHJ, Stack RS. Transluminal extraction coronary atherectomy. *Cardiol Clin* 1994;12:611.
115. Sketch MHJ, Davidson CJ, Yeh W, et al. Predictors of acute and long-term outcome with transluminal extraction atherectomy: the New Approaches to Coronary Intervention (NACI) registry. *Am J Cardiol* 1997;80:68K.
116. Khan MM, Ellis SG, Aguirre FV. Does intracoronary thrombus influence the outcome of high risk percutaneous coronary angioplasty? Clinical and angiographic outcomes in a large multicenter trial. EPIC Investigators. *J Am Coll Cardiol* 1998;31:31.
117. Violaris AG, Melkert R, Herrman JPR. Role of angiographically identifiable thrombus on long-term luminal renarrowing after coronary angioplasty: a qualitative angiographic analysis. *Circulation* 1996;93:889.
118. Lincoff AM, Popma JJ, Ellis SE, et al. Abrupt vessel closure complicating coronary angioplasty: clinical, angiographic and therapeutic profile. *J Am Coll Cardiol* 1992;19:926.
119. Sharafuddin MJ, Hicks ME, Jenson ML, et al. Rheolytic thrombectomy with use of the AngioJet-F105 catheter: preclinical evaluation of safety. *J Vasc Interv Radiol* 1997;8:939.
120. Carlino M, De Gregorio J, DiMario C, et al. Prevention of distal embolization during saphenous vein graft lesion angioplasty: experience with a new temporary occlusion and aspiration system. *Circulation* 1999;99:3221.
121. Teirstein PS, Massullo V, Jani S, et al. Two-year follow-up after catheter-based radiotherapy to inhibit coronary restenosis. *Circulation* 1999;99:243.
122. Meerkin D, Tardif JC, Crocker IR, et al. Effects of intracoronary β-radiation therapy after coronary angioplasty. *Circulation* 1999;99:1660.
123. Lincoff AM, Popma JJ, Ellis SG, et al. Percutaneous support devices for high risk or complicated coronary angioplasty. *J Am Coll Cardiol* 1991;17:770.
124. Aguire FV, Kern MJ, Bach R, et al. Intraaortic balloon pump support during high-risk coronary angioplasty. *Cardiology* 1994; 84:175.
125. Ohman EM, George BS, White CJ, et al. Use of aortic counterpulsation to improve sustained coronary artery patency during acute myocardial infarction: results of a randomized trial. *Circulation* 1994;90:792.
126. Kan JS, White RI Jr, Mitchell SE, et al. Percutaneous balloon valvuloplasty: a new method for treating congenital pulmonary valve stenosis. *N Engl J Med* 1982;307:540.
127. Kan JS, White RI, Mitchell SE, et al. Percutaneous transluminal balloon valvuloplasty for pulmonary valve stenosis. *Circulation* 1984;69:554.
128. Rao PS, Fawzy ME, Solymar L, et al. Long-term results of balloon pulmonary valvuloplasty of valvar pulmonic stenosis. *Am Heart J* 1988;115:1291.
129. Marantz PM, Huhta JC, Mullins CE, et al. Results of balloon valvuloplasty in typical and dysplastic pulmonary valve stenosis: Doppler echocardiographic follow-up. *J Am Coll Cardiol* 1988; 12:476.
130. DiSessa TG, Alpert BS, Chase NA, et al. Balloon valvuloplasty in children with dysplastic pulmonary valves. *Am J Cardiol* 1987;60:405.
131. Lieberman EB, Bashore TM, Hermiller JB, et al. Balloon aortic valvuloplasty in the elderly: the final chapter. *J Am Coll Cardiol* 1995:26:1522.
132. O'Keefe JH, Vlietstra RE, Bailey KR, et al. Natural history of candidates for balloon aortic valvuloplasty. *Mayo Clin Proc* 1987;62:986.
133. Isner JM, Samuels DA, Slovenkai GA, et al. Mechanism of aortic balloon valvuloplasty: fracture of valvular calcific deposits. *Ann Intern Med* 1988;108:377.
134. NHLBI Balloon Valvuloplasty Registry Participants. Percutaneous balloon aortic valvuloplasty: acute and 30 day follow-up results in 674 patients from the NHLBI Balloon Valvuloplasty Registry. *Circulation* 1991;84:2383.
135. Harrison JK, Davidson CJ, Leithe ME, et al. Serial left ventricu-

lar performance evaluated by cardiac catheterization before, immediately after and at 6 months after balloon aortic valvuloplasty. *J Am Coll Cardiol* 1990;16:1351.
136. Inoue K, Feldman T. Percutaneous transvenous mitral commissurotomy using the Inoue balloon catheter. *Cathet Cardiovasc Diagn* 1993;28;119.
137. Wilkins GT, Weyman AE, Abaseal VM, et al. Percutaneous balloon dilatation of the mitral valve: an analysis of echocardiographic variables related to outcome and the mechanism of dilation. *Br Heart J* 1988;60:299.
138. Davidson CJ, Bashore TM, Mickel M, et al., for the NHLBI Balloon Valvuloplasty Registry Participants. Balloon mitral commissurotomy after previous surgical commissurotomy. *Circulation* 1992;86:91.
139. Nobuyoshi M, Hamasaki N, Kimura T, et al. Indications, complications, and short-term clinical outcome of percutaneous transvenous mitral commissurotomy. *Circulation* 1989;80:782.
140. Zaibag MA, Kasab SA, Ribeiro PA, et al. Percutaneous double-balloon mitral valvotomy for rheumatic mitral-valve stenosis. *Lancet* 1986;1:757.
141. Turi ZG, Neyes VP, Raju BS, et al. Percutaneous balloon versus surgical closed commissurotomy for mitral stenosis: a prospective, randomized trial. *Circulation* 1991;83:1179.
142. Reyes VP, Raju BS, Wynne J, et al. Percutaneous balloon valvulolasty compared with open surgical commissurotomy for mitral stenosis. *N Engl J Med* 1994;331:961.
143. Iung B, Garbarz E, Michaud P, et al. Late results of percutaneous mitral commissurotomy in a series of 1024 patients. *Circulation* 1999;99:3272.
144. Herandez R, Banuelos C, Alfonso F, et al. Long-term clinical and echocardiographic follow-up after percutaneous mitral valvuloplasty with the Inoue balloon. *Circulation* 1999;99:1580.
145. Lock JE, Keane JF, Fellows KE. The use of catheter intervention procedures for congenital heart disease. *J Am Coll Cardiol* 1986; 7:1420.
146. Beekman RH, Rocchini AP, Crowley DC, et al. Comparison of single and double balloon valvuloplasty in children with aortic stenosis. *J Am Coll Cardiol* 1988;12:480.
147. Choy M, Beekman RH, Rocchini AP, et al. Percutaneous balloon valvuloplasty for valvar aortic stenosis in infants and children. *Am J Cardiol* 1987;59:1010.
148. Sholler GF, Keane JF, Perry SB, et al. Balloon dilation of congenital aortic valve stenosis: results and influence of technical and morphological features on outcome. *Circulation* 1988;78: 351.
149. Kveselis DA, Rocchini AP, Beekman R, et al. Balloon angioplasty for congenital and rheumatic mitral stenosis. *Am J Cardiol* 1986;57:348.
150. Lock JE, Bass JL, Amplatz K, et al. Balloon dilation angioplasty of aortic coarctations in infants and children. *Circulation* 1983; 68:109.
151. Harrison JK, Sheikh KH, Davidson CJ, et al. Balloon angioplasty of coarctation of the aorta evaluated with intravascular ultrasound imaging. *J Am Coll Cardiol* 1990;15:906.
152. Ebeid MR, Prieto LR, Latson LA. Use of balloon-expandable stents for coarctation of the aorta: initial results and intermediate-term follow-up. *J Am Coll Cardiol* 1997;30:1853.
153. Lock JE, Castaneda-Zuniga WR, Fuhrman BP, et al. Balloon dilation angioplasty of hypoplastic and stenotic pulmonary arteries. *Circulation* 1983;67:962.
154. Hoekenga DE, Stevens GF, Ball WS. Percutaneous angioplasty for peripheral pulmonary stenosis in an adult. *Am J Cardiol* 1987;59:188.
155. O'Laughlin MP, Mullins CE. Balloon dilation and stenting of hypoplastic pulmonary arteries: a new area of cooperation between interventional pediatric cardiologists and cardiac surgeons. *Texas Heart Inst J* 1992;19:185.
156. Terry PB, White RI, Barth KH, et al. Pulmonary arteriovenous malformations: physiologic observations and results of therapeutic balloon embolization. *N Engl J Med* 1983;308:1197.
157. Lock JE, Cockerham JT, Keane JF, et al. Transcatheter umbrella closure of congenital heart defects. *Circulation* 1987;75:593.
158. Rashkind WJ, Mullins CE, Hellenbrand WE, et al. Nonsurgical closure of patent ductus arteriosus: clinical application of the Rashkind PDA occluder system. *Circulation* 1987;75:583.
159. O'Laughlin MP, Bricker JT, Mullins CE, et al. Transcatheter closure of residual atrial septal defect following cardiac transplantation. *Cathet Cardiovasc Diagn* 1993;28:162.
160. Lock JE, Block PC, McKay RG, et al. Transcatheter closure of ventricular septal defects. *Circulation* 1988;78:361.

Cardiac Anesthesia: Principles and Clinical Practice, Second Edition, edited by Fawzy G. Estafanous, Paul G. Barash, and J.G. Reves. Lippincott Williams & Wilkins, Philadelphia © 2001.

PART II

THE CARDIAC SURGERY PATIENT: GENERAL CONSIDERATIONS

6

PREOPERATIVE ANESTHETIC EVALUATION

DARRYL ATWELL
EMAD B. MOSSAD

Despite the medical advances made in the past century in our understanding of the pathophysiology of cardiovascular disease, it continues to remain a leading cause of death throughout the world. In the year 2000, 100 million patients will undergo surgery worldwide; one third of those patients will be older than 65 years of age and will have two or more cardiovascular risk factors (1). A significant number of these patients will suffer from perioperative myocardial infarctions (MIs) that will significantly affect their survival as well as health care costs. More specifically, mortality rates among those patients with coronary disease who suffer perioperative MIs has been reported to be as high as 80%, with a cost of up to $12,000 per patient (2,3). With the increasing complexity and new advances being made in cardiac surgery, (e.g., off-pump revascularization, minimally invasive surgery) along with increases in life expectancy, these figures are expected to escalate. Therefore, a challenge remains for medical caretakers to find the appropriate methods to detect and modify risk factors while concomitantly reducing adverse outcome and cost in this subset of patients.

Attempts have been made to devise risk stratification methods for accurate prediction and evaluation of the risks of mortality and morbidity in cardiac and noncardiac surgical patients (4). More than 20 years ago, the Framingham study attempted to create a profile that would identify persons at risk for coronary artery disease (CAD) and therefore in need of preventive care. In 1992 Higgins et al. devised standardized criteria for comparing outcomes in relation to preoperative conditions (5). They identified a specific clinical severity scoring system based on the preoperative risk factors of patients undergoing myocardial revascularization surgery (Table 6-1). Other mechanisms to reduce adverse outcomes have included the increasing use of preoperative tests and perioperative monitoring. Whatever mechanisms are used, the goal of the preoperative assessment is to prepare and optimize the patient for cardiac surgery. As part of this preparation, the anesthesiologist attempts to identify factors that may put the patient at risk for an adverse outcome and then makes the appropriate interventions to curtail adverse consequences of these risks.

This chapter discusses preoperative assessment of the cardiac patient and focuses on the factors that cause increased morbidity and mortality, diagnostic tests, and preoperative drug therapy.

HISTORY AND PHYSICAL EXAMINATION

History

When the anesthesiologist first visits the patient who is scheduled for cardiac surgery, the diagnosis is usually established, and the results of multiple tests are already available for evaluation. Nevertheless, the preoperative assessment that begins with a routine history and physical examination of the patient is the cornerstone of anesthetic management. First, a thorough history of the present illness should be taken, with the focus on manifestations of cardiac disease. Not to be forgotten are routine questions concerning other systems that can affect surgical outcome, medications, allergies, previous surgeries, and previous anesthetics.

Angina pectoris was first described as a clinical syndrome more than 200 ago. However, only recently has it been recognized as a common and important clinical entity (6,7). Words that have been commonly used to describe the pain of angina include chest tightness, heaviness, dullness, and even strangling. Most frequently, it occurs in an area about the size of a clenched fist in the anterior chest. However, it may radiate to arm, neck, jaw, or back. Typically, it occurs during strenuous activity or emotion, with a duration of 5 to 15 minutes, and is relieved by rest or nitroglycerin; angina that occurs with rest or lasts for longer periods usually indicates more complex CAD or an evolving MI (8). This symptom occurs when there is imbalance between myocardial oxygen supply and demand and indicates an underperfused myocardium. Angina pectoris must be differentiated from chest pain that can occur with other clinical entities, such as esophageal reflux, pulmonary disease, musculoskeletal disease, and peptic ulcer disease.

D. Atwell and E. B. Mossad: Department of Cardiothoracic Anesthesiology, The Cleveland Clinic Foundation, Cleveland, Ohio 44195

TABLE 6-1. CLINICAL SEVERITY SCORING SYSTEM

Preoperative Factors	Score
Emergency case	6
Serum creatinine	
≥1.6 and ≤1.8 mg/dL	1
≥1.9 mg/dL	4
Severe left ventricular dysfunction	3
Reoperation	
Operative mitral valve insufficiency	3
Age ≥65 and ≤74 years	1
Age ≥75	2
Prior vascular surgery	2
Chronic obstructive pulmonary disease	2
Anemia (hematocrit ≥0.34)	2
Operative aortic stenosis	1
Weight ≤65 kg	1
Diabetes	1
Cerebrovascular disease	1

Source: Higgins TL, Estafanous FG, Loop FD, et al. Stratification of morbidity and mortality outcome by preoperative risk factors in coronary artery bypass patients. *JAMA* 1992;267:2344.

TABLE 6-2. SEVERITY OF CARDIOVASCULAR DISEASE

Class	New York Heart Association	Canadian Cardiovascular Society
I	Cardiac disease without limits on physical activity	Ordinary activity does not cause angina; angina with prolonged or strenuous activity
II	Slight limitation of physical activity; ordinary activity causes fatigue	Slight limitation of ordinary activity; limits on walking stairs, climbing uphill, cold
III	Marked limitation of physical activity; comfortable at rest	Marked limitation of physical activity, one flight of stairs or walking one to two blocks
IV	Inability to carry on any physical activity, angina at rest	Unable to carry on any activity without discomfort; angina at rest

Source: Mangano DT. Preoperative assessment of cardiac risk. In: Kaplan J, ed. *Cardiac anesthesia*. Philadelphia: WB Saunders, 1993.

Although it can have varying presentations and is associated with a variety of different conditions, angina can have prognostic significance depending on its type. Typically, angina is classified into three types: stable, unstable, and variant. Stable angina is the classic case that has been previously described. It is very specific for patients with CAD and therefore indicates that these patients are at higher risk for development of cardiac complications than the general population (9).

Unstable angina, which is sometimes called crescendo angina, is defined as (a) new-onset angina within the past 2 months; (b) worsening angina with increasing frequency, intensity, or duration that is less responsive to rest or medications; or (c) angina lasting longer than 30 minutes and is associated with ST or T-wave changes (10). Variant angina typically occurs at rest with ST-segment changes. The perioperative risk of patients with variant angina is unknown. However, because this syndrome is associated with a greater incidence of conduction abnormalities and dysrhythmias, it would not be surprising if patients with this angina had a greater incidence of perioperative cardiac morbidity. In fact, it has been demonstrated that patients with any angina have increased operative complications including MI and death (11).

Despite the clinical significance of angina, it is probably a late manifestation in the sequelae of CAD. Many patients show ischemic changes with the absence of symptoms. This so-called silent ischemia occurs in more than half of patients with chronic stable angina, especially in the diabetic and elderly populations (12). Silent myocardial ischemia is now recognized as a marker of morbidity; studies have shown that 20% to 30% of asymptomatic postinfarction patients have silent ischemia on exercise stress testing (6). In addition, Mangano et al. found that perioperative silent myocardial ischemia is very common. Up to 40% of patients in their study demonstrated ischemia in the postoperative period. This ischemia was silent in 97% of the patients studied and was an important predictor of postoperative cardiac events (13).

Finally, in the history there should be some assessment of the overall cardiac function in relation to symptoms. Two standardized systems exist that associate symptoms with severity of myocardial disease. They are the New York Heart Association Functional Classification and the Canadian Cardiovascular Society Functional Classification (Table 6-2). These scoring systems provide additional insight into the functional capacity of the patient and concomitantly the increase risk for adverse perioperative outcome.

Physical Examination

A complete physical examination with emphasis on the cardiovascular system should be performed on each patient. The examination should encompass everything from routine items, such as airway evaluation, to the examination of the other systems that can affect outcome. It is now well known that clinical signs can be used to evaluate myocardial function and therefore potentially to make an assessment of risk (Table 6-3). Patients with evidence of congestive

TABLE 6-3. PHYSICAL FINDINGS ASSOCIATED WITH INCREASED PERIOPERATIVE RISK

Arrhythmias
Murmurs (indicative of aortic stenosis)
Third or fourth heart sounds
Jugular venous distention
Cardiomegaly
Peripheral edema

heart failure (CHF), as exhibited by jugular venous distention, S_3 gallop, or evidence of pulmonary edema, have increased risk factors for perioperative cardiac morbidity (14). Murmurs can be indicative of valvular abnormalities, the most ominous being aortic stenosis. The potential predictive value of findings on physical examination makes these findings an important part of every anesthetic evaluation but paramount in the patient undergoing cardiac surgery.

PREOPERATIVE RISK FACTORS

Several factors have been identified as significant preoperative risk factors and therefore potential predictors of outcome after cardiac surgery. As previously mentioned, in a retrospective study of 5,051 patients Higgins et al. identified such factors and attempted to assign a score to patients that could predict mortality and morbidity. A follow-up prospective study proved the validity of the scoring system; that is, a patient's preoperative score based on presenting risk factors could be used to predict not only expected mortality and morbidity but also length of hospital stay, cost, and likelihood of early discharge from the intensive care unit (Fig. 6-1) (15). Based on the history and physical examination, the anesthesiologist can determine which factors are germane to the patient. In addition, identification of these factors gives the opportunity to implement any special perioperative management or studies to minimize the risks. The most important preoperative risk factors to be considered are now described.

Cigarette Smoking

The negative health effects of cigarette smoking are well known today. It is a major risk factor in the development of atherosclerosis, and there is a strong correlation between smoking and the occurrence of major coronary events (16). Ironically, it is the one risk factor that the population can most control.

Nicotine and carbon monoxide are the components of cigarettes that adversely effect the cardiovascular system. Carbon monoxide competes with oxygen to bind with hemoglobin; the product is carboxyhemoglobin (COHgb), which is incapable of carrying oxygen. In addition, COHgb interferes with the release of oxygen to the tissues. The result is decreased oxygen delivery at the tissue level. The myocardium, with its particularly high oxygen extraction ratio, would be at considerable risk. Carbon monoxide is also thought to have a negative inotropic effect secondary to interference with mitochondrial function and muscle contraction (17). Additionally, in patients with CAD, COHgb causes no increase in coronary flow as it does in patients without CAD, and coronary sinus O_2 tensions decrease significantly (17). Furthermore, carbon monoxide effects platelet number and function: platelet survival time is decreased, and there is increased platelet aggregation and disruption of endothelium. These factors play a definitive role in the accelerated rate of atherosclerosis seen in smokers.

Nicotine is known to have a sympathetic effect that results in vasoconstriction of coronary and peripheral vascular beds, leading to increase blood pressure and heart rate (HR). The sum of the cardiovascular effects of smoking, in addition to its effect on the respiratory, immune, and other systems, puts these patients at greater risk for adverse events compared with controls.

Age

As a result of medical advances, life expectancy has increased dramatically over the past century. In the United States the rate of rise in the population of persons older than 55 years of age is more than double that of those younger than 55. Over the next 50 years, persons 65 years and older may constitute up to 20% of the population (18). As the population becomes older, more cardiac procedures will be performed on these patients. It is in this milieu that anesthesiologists, surgeons, and cardiologists must work.

In general, physiologic age is a better indicator of risk than chronologic age. In other words, a patient's overall functional status is more important than absolute age. However, the fact that increasing age of the patient is still associated with higher morbidity and mortality has been recog-

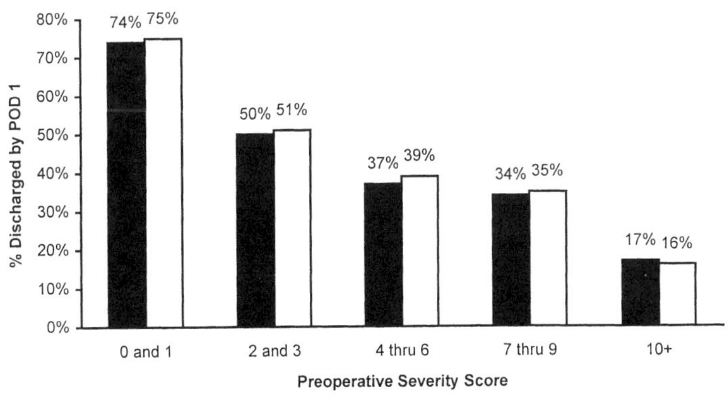

FIGURE 6-1. Three fourths of low-risk coronary artery bypass graft (CABG) patients can be expected to leave the intensive care unit (ICU) by the first postoperative day (POD). In contrast, very few high-risk patients can be expected to have a short stay. Percent discharged by preoperative score. (*solid squares*, all CABG; (*open squares*, isolated CABG. (Adapted from Higgins TL. Safety issues regarding early extubation after coronary artery bypass surgery. *J Cardiothorac Vasc Anesth* 1995;9:24, with permission.)

nized for many years. The Coronary Artery Surgery Study (CASS) reported a 5.2% mortality rate among patients older than 65 years of age, compared with 1.9% in younger patients. Several studies have shown left ventricular (LV) dysfunction to correlate with increasing age and operative mortality (19). LV dysfunction can be the beginning of a "low output" syndrome that can lead to a sequelae of infection, pulmonary insufficiency, sternal dehiscence, and mediastinitis, all of which are associated with death within the first several postoperative weeks (20). Additionally, the elderly have an increased propensity for multiple chronic diseases, slower metabolism, and a decreased reserve capacity of their organ systems to respond to stress (21). As a result, they may have altered responses to many anesthetic medications, and the doses should be altered accordingly. Despite the aforementioned risks, major cardiac procedures can still be performed on this subset of patients with acceptable outcome. Therefore, the predictive value of age as a risk factor is difficult to assess.

Peripheral Vascular and Cerebral Vascular Disease

There is a common association between peripheral and cerebral vascular disease and CAD. Hertzer et al. reported in a prospective study of 1,000 patients presenting for aortic, lower extremity, or carotid reconstruction that 30% of these patients had severe or inoperable CAD (22). In fact, in patients with cerebrovascular disease who are recovering from a cerebral infarct or transient ischemic attack, the leading cause of death is MI. In addition to CAD, peripheral vascular disease is often associated with a high incidence of diabetes, hypertension, and renal dysfunction, all of which place the patient at a higher perioperative risk. Patients with peripheral vascular disease are at risk for aortic or femoral dissection during cannulation, and they are more vulnerable to embolization during cardiopulmonary bypass (CPB). Postoperatively, these patients are at risk for mesenteric ischemia, and peripheral vascular disease may prevent the use of intraaortic balloon counterpulsation when needed. Because of the importance of ischemic heart disease in both of these subsets of patients, simultaneous angiography of the coronary arteries, carotids, and aorta seems prudent. This will assist in the evaluation of the extent of disease and the prioritizing of treatment.

Hypertension

Hypertension is known to be associated with an increased incidence of mortality in surgical patients. After CAD, hypertension is the leading cause of ischemic heart disease, secondary to LV hypertrophy and the resulting imbalance in myocardial oxygen supply and demand. This and other complications from hypertension, including CHF, renal disease, peripheral vascular disease, and CAD, give it its relative importance as a risk factor. Currently, large numbers of hypertensive patients are admitted to surgery with their blood pressure well controlled by diet and medical therapy, which decreases the complications related to hypertension. However, hypertensive individuals, controlled and uncontrolled, are more vulnerable to blood pressure fluctuations during anesthesia and postoperatively (23). A large number of CAD patients are hypertensive preoperatively, as are some of the patients with valvular disease. Understanding and assessing the pathophysiology of hypertension helps the anesthesiologist to better manage these patients and results in a lower incidence of ischemia and morbidity.

The preoperative evaluation of hypertensive patients should take into consideration the following:

1. Severity and duration of hypertension, because the preoperative levels of systolic blood pressure are predictors of the risk (23)
2. Presence of primary disease, (e.g., renal stenosis, catecholamine-secreting tumor) (23)
3. Presence of undiagnosed disease that can cause hypertension, (e.g., arteriovenous [AV] shunt) (24)
4. Extent of effect of hypertension on target organ, such as cardiac hypertrophy and renal dysfunction
5. Possible effects and interactions with antihypertensive therapy (25)
6. Adequacy of cerebral circulation and history of stroke
7. Most important, the pathophysiology of hypertension (24)

Almost all anesthetic agents, premedications, and muscle relaxants have hemodynamic effects that can significantly alter the blood pressure. Moreover, hypertensive patients are usually treated with more than one drug, which can cause variable interactions and significant hemodynamic changes. Therefore, anesthesia that is managed according to the hemodynamic characteristics of hypertension will be safer and accompanied by minimal complications.

Angina

As previously discussed, angina pectoris is part of the classic syndrome of patients presenting with cardiac disease. More specifically, angina is a sensitive and specific indicator of patients with CAD (9). It would seem reasonable that patients with unstable angina (i.e., emergency patients) would have a greater risk of perioperative complications, especially because these patients have an associated increased incidence of MIs and dysrhythmias. However, studies to prove such an assumption have been lacking. In fact even those patients with stable angina have not had this symptom listed as a perioperative risk factor in many studies. Nonetheless, because of its diagnostic significance in CAD, patients with angina should receive special consideration.

Previous Myocardial Infarction

MI is a risk after general anesthesia and surgery. The risk is relatively low, reportedly between 0.1% and 0.7% (26,27). Several studies have shown that patients with a previous MI have a greater incidence of perioperative MI with a greater mortality rate (26–28). The initial data showed reinfarction rates to be as high as 37% when the surgery was performed in the first 3 months after MI (26,27). The incidence of reinfarction was shown to decrease with the passage of time, to 16% at 4 to 6 months after MI, and down to 5% if longer than 6 months after MI. More recently, Rao et al. showed that the incidence of reinfarction can be significantly reduced to an overall rate of 1.9% (28). The reduced infarction rate was attributed to greater awareness of perioperative risk, advancements in anesthetic management and monitoring, and aggressive intervention to maintain hemodynamic stability.

Previous MI should be documented by an increase in cardiac enzymes and electrocardiographically by the presence of a Q wave if the infarction is transmural or by persistent ST elevation if the infarction is subendocardial. Patients who have experienced silent MI have the same risks as patients with diagnosed MI.

Congestive Heart Failure

Many diseases involving the cardiovascular system, including hypertension, diabetes, acute MI, and valvular disease, have CHF as a complication. Patients with CHF compensate by increasing sympathetic tone and circulating blood volume to maintain blood pressure. Pulmonary edema may occur with signs of right ventricle failure such as an S_3 gallop and jugular venous distention.

Several studies have shown CHF to be a major risk factor for perioperative morbidity (28–30). Untreated CHF correlates with a 5-year 50% mortality rate (31). Cooperman et al. reported a 33% incidence of cardiovascular complications in patients with CHF, compared with an 8% incidence in those with no failure. Further, Rao et al. reported a higher rate of reinfarction with CHF that is evidenced by rales, increased jugular venous pressure, pitting edema, or high pulmonary capillary wedge pressure (28).

CHF is often associated with LV dysfunction. In patients with CAD, evidence of LV failure correlates with poor prognosis. These patients may have a more difficult time being weaned from CPB and have a greater need for intraaortic balloon counterpulsation and inotropic support (32).

Diabetes Mellitus

Of the patients undergoing coronary artery bypass graft surgery (CABG), 7% to 11% are diagnosed diabetics. Diabetics have an increased incidence of cardiovascular disease compared with nondiabetics, as well as an increased incidence of hypertension, atherosclerosis, renal disease, and vascular diseases (33,34). In addition, they have a greater risk of perioperative MIs of extensive size and have a decreased rate of survival (35). The perioperative mortality rate from a variety of causes, including pneumonia, wound infection, renal failure, and cerebral infarct, is greater for diabetics than for controls (36). In addition, many diabetics manifest autonomic dysfunction that accounts for impairment of the circulatory reflexes and results in labile blood pressure perioperatively and may require more vasoactive support (37). Autonomic dysfunction has been implicated in silent ischemia and MI; the implications of these entities have been previously discussed.

Diabetics' blood sugar levels should be controlled perioperatively. Hyperglycemia should be anticipated from the stress of surgery and from CPB. Because of their problems with microcirculation secondary to hyperglycemia, diabetics have traditionally had difficulty with wound healing. Wallace et al. showed that poor perioperative control of glucose was associated with an increased incidence of mediastinitis and wound infection (38). In addition to delaying wound healing, hyperglycemia is associated with worse outcomes in patients with neurologic complications.

Race and Gender

Despite the enormous strides made in recent decades, race and gender continue to be major issues that plague this society. Therefore, it should not be surprising that they both substantially influence the health status, access to health care, and quality of care rendered to female and nonwhite patients of this country (39). A multitude of studies have shown with great consistency that there is a disparity in the diagnosis, treatment, and consequently outcome of cardiovascular diseases between white males and their black and female counterparts (40–45). Most disturbingly, the majority of these studies controlled for variables such as age, Medicare, insurance status, income, disease severity, and concomitant morbid conditions that may have made these findings statistically insignificant (39). One such study by Whittle et al., completed in a Veterans Administration hospital (to eliminate access bias), showed the rate of cardiac catheterization was 19.3% for whites and 11.8% for blacks (41). For having percutaneous transluminal coronary angioplasty (PTCA) performed, the rate was 1.8% for whites versus 0.8% for blacks. Five percent of whites but only 1.6% of blacks underwent CABG. Similarly, Ayanian et al. showed substantial differences in rates of revascularization with PTCA or CABG for white males compared with their black and female counterparts (41). Among men and women, blacks were less likely than whites to receive a revascularization procedure; for PTCA the rates were 19% and 12% for whites and blacks, respectively; for CABG, they were 39% and 29%. Additionally, in each of the hospitals surveyed for this study, whites were significantly more likely than blacks to proceed from angiography to a revascularization procedure. Even more astonishingly, the CASS study documented that physicians were less likely to recommend CABG to blacks than to whites despite equivalent numbers of diseased arteries and more severe angina among blacks (45).

In terms of gender, the data is not quite as clear; factors such as smaller body surface area, smaller coronary vessels, and greater preoperative severity scores have been reported to explain differences in outcome. Alternatively, there have been studies controlling outcome for preoperative comorbidity that suggest gender itself is an independent risk for worse outcome (46). In a multivariate analysis of data from Emory University, female gender remained as a risk factor for mortality; the authors ascertained that the risk factor assessment did not account for biologic differences between men and women (46).

The extent to which overt or subtle racism and sexism determine these results may not be able to be quantified; however, they do suggest the existence of race- and sex-related inequities in our health care system. These inequities are in part responsible for making race and gender independent risk factors for patient with cardiovascular disease.

PREOPERATIVE DIAGNOSTIC TESTS

Electrocardiogram

The technology of electrocardiography (ECG) is almost 100 years old; however, preoperative and intraoperative ECG was not used until the late 1960s. Since then, ECG has become a powerful clinical tool that can provide information about myocardial ischemia, injury, and infarction; hypertrophy; and arrhythmias. As with any laboratory test, it must be integrated into the clinical picture, and if it does not conform, its interpretation should be carefully reevaluated or the tracing repeated (47). Additionally, there are limitations to routine ECG monitoring. There are a number of clinical entities that can imitate ECG changes seen in ischemia and MI. They include Wolff-Parkinson-White syndrome, LV and right ventricular hypertrophy, idiopathic hypertrophic subaortic stenosis, left bundle branch block, chronic obstructive pulmonary disease (COPD), central nervous system disorders, hypothermia, and acute pulmonary embolism.

Perioperatively, certain leads or combinations of leads are highly useful for specific purposes. Lead II is the most sensitive for arrhythmia monitoring, because P waves are normally most prominent in this lead. The detection of ischemic changes or infarction varies with the area studied. Leads II, III, and aVF are preferable for inferior or diaphragmatic lesions; leads I, aVL, V_5, and V_6 for lateral lesions; and leads V_1 through V_4 for anterior lesions. Posterior myocardial ischemia or MI can be detected either by reciprocal changes in the anterior leads or by an esophageal lead ECG.

Traditionally, the diagnosis of MI using ECG was related to the location and the extent of the lesion, be it epicardial, endocardial, or transmural. Clinically, the distinction was made on the basis of the presence or absence of Q waves in the 12-lead ECG. It is now recognized that there is no clear relation between the extent of necrosis into the thickness of the ventricular wall and the presence or absence of a Q wave (48,49). As a result, these terms have been replaced by the terms Q-wave and non–Q-wave MI, respectively (50). However, for an anatomic understanding of ECG changes with these entities, the former terms are still useful.

Endocardial infarction commonly occurs in patients with LV hypertrophy, obstructive CAD, and hypotension from cardiac and noncardiac causes (51). The QRS complex may be normal. The Q-T interval is either normal or prolonged. The ST-segment vector is directed away from the center of generalized endocardial injury. Madias et al. noted the following other characteristic ECG patterns: (a) ST-segment depression in the limb and precordial leads, (b) deep symmetric inversion of T waves in some or all precordial leads with similar changes in limb leads, (c) transient reduction on R-wave amplitude, and (d) slight ST-segment elevation in aVR (52).

Conversely, in patients with transmural infarction three distinguishable zones of myocardium exist: a central core of necrosis, a surrounding zone of ischemic injury, and a peripheral zone of injury (47). It is the central core that produces the characteristic Q waves seen in the leads overlying the infarct and identifies a transmural infarct (47). In 80% to 87% of cases, the hallmark diagnosis of transmural infarction is the presence of a pathologic Q wave; the wave at first increases in size, as does the area of necrosis, and over years it regresses as the scar from the infarct shrinks. Nevertheless, Q waves may be absent when a transmural infarct is present, for example in a posterior infarct. Other characteristic ECG changes of a transmural infarct include Q waves with a duration longer than 0.04 seconds and more than 25% of amplitude of the R wave in the same lead, and transient ST elevation that is followed temporally by T-wave inversion.

Studies have been performed in which routine frequent 12-lead ECG monitoring or Holter monitoring has been used to detect large percentages of ischemia before and on arrival at the operating room. Slogoff and Keats, in their studies, diagnosed ischemia on arrival at the operating room and before induction of anesthesia in 18.8%, 26.5%, 27.5%, and 29.3% of patients about to undergo CABG (53–56). They postulated that this high incidence represented the same phenomenon as silent myocardial ischemia, which is known to be associated with CAD in nonsurgical patients (54). Meanwhile, the SPI Research Group reported an incidence of ischemia of only 4% before induction of anesthesia in similar groups of patients (57). The difference between these results was challenged by Lowenstein and

McPeek (58). Some of the differences may be attributed to different methods of detecting ischemia.

Slogoff and Keats used a standard preoperative 12-lead ECG recording, and tracings were obtained for analysis every 2 minutes (56). Further use of Holter monitors with computer-analyzed tapes confirmed a high incidence of myocardial ischemia similar to that reported by Slogoff and Keats (57,59,60). However, these studies did not demonstrate a strong relation between the incidence of preoperative ischemia and perioperative hemodynamic abnormalities, although they demonstrated a high incidence of postoperative ischemia after CABG. This should focus attention on surgical factors and interoperative myocardial protection as important factors. There is currently no practical substitute for routine preoperative ECG recording. However, the preoperative use of routine Holter monitoring may be feasible and may provide more updated information to the practicing anesthesiologist. In addition, both the ECG and Holter monitor are important determinants of preoperative arrhythmias and the increased risk of developing potentially fatal rhythms.

Exercise Stress Testing

Background

The link between exercise and alteration of the ECG has been known for almost 100 years. Goldhammer and Scherf were the first to apply exercise testing to patients with angina in 1933 (61). In the ensuing years, Masters standardized stress testing, and his work has served as the foundation for modern theory. Since then, exercise testing has developed into a powerful clinical tool whose usefulness is considered for (a) diagnosis; (b) severity of disease, risk assessment, and prognosis in patients with known CAD; (c) risk assessment of patients early after MI; and (d) risk assessment of specific clinical populations identified by gender, age, other cardiac disease, or prior coronary revascularization (62). The prognostic and predictive value of exercise testing in these clinical situations remains a hotly debated topic.

Exercise testing provides a controlled situation to assess the effects of increase myocardial oxygen demand due to progressive increases in work by treadmill or cycle ergometer devices. Evidence of ischemia results in both clinical symptoms and ECG changes. In addition, exercise testing can be combined with echocardiography and radionuclear medicine to provide more specific information about ventricular function. Several protocols are available that vary in their number of stages, degree of work,and duration. Most commonly used is the Bruce protocol, which consists of five 3-minute stages that vary in speed and grade. A baseline ECG is performed, and the patient continues to exercise until the test end points are met. The most commonly used end point is a percentage of predicted maximum HR. However, there are multiple indications for termination of the test, including clinical symptoms such as angina, dizziness, or syncope; ECG changes; hypotension or hypertension; and technical difficulties.

Physiology

Exercise causes a compensatory increase in cardiac output (CO). The two determinants of CO are HR and stroke volume (SV). During exercise, the HR can increase up to three-fold secondary to sympathetic stimulation and decrease in vagal tone. Secondary to increases in preload, SV also increases but not to the same degree as HR. The increased preload causes an increased tension in myocardial fibers and, consequently, increased contractility to further augment CO. In the periphery, there are seemingly contrasting effects of exercise to increase preload and thus CO; there is a vasodilatory response in working muscles and an increased resistance in renal and mesenteric beds (63). The overriding response is a decrease in systemic vascular resistance. Despite this decrease, there is an increase in systolic and mean blood pressure due to the marked increase in CO.

There is an increased oxygen requirement for the heart in an exercising body. To accommodate this, minute ventilation and oxygen delivery rise during exercise. In addition, CO can increase to several times its resting value to further augment oxygen delivery. As previously mentioned, HR can triple secondary to increases in sympathetic tone, and therefore HR plays a greater role in the increases in CO seen. The increase in CO results in an increase in coronary blood flow. Therefore, the ability of the coronary vessels to vasodilate to accommodate this increase flow is paramount for the exercising heart to get adequate perfusion. In addition to delivering less blood because of obstruction, stenotic vessels have a reduced ability to vasodilate and may even be vasospastic, therefore possibly precipitating exercise-induced ischemia. The response to such events during work, including signs and symptoms of ischemia, dysrhythmias, and other prototypical ECG changes, provides the basis for exercise stress testing. This information can be used by the anesthesiologist as a guideline to assist in caring for the patient undergoing cardiovascular surgery, during which similar stresses will be encountered.

Results and Interpretation

Interpretation of the exercise test is usually in a standard format that includes exercise capacity and clinical, hemodynamic, and ECG responses. Test conclusions are limited to one of three categories: (a) positive for ischemia, (b) negative for ischemia, and (c) inconclusive or nondiagnostic for ischemia. Despite this format, the test does not provide absolute answers in all subjects tested as to the presence or absence of ischemic disease. In fact, a review by Philbrick et al. of 33 patients showed a range of sensitivity of 33% to

88%, with a specificity range of 41% to 100% (64). As a result, all information available about the patient must be used to make an accurate clinical assessment.

The ECG response consistent with a positive exercise test is classically a 1-mm (0.1 mV) horizontal or downsloping depression that persists for 80 msec beyond the J junction in any lead during exercise. Other ECG findings specific for ischemia include ST-segment depression of 0.2 mV, ST-segment elevation of 0.1 mV, and U-wave inversion. ST-segment depression is associated with subendocardial ischemia, whereas elevation suggests transmural ischemia. Pseudonormalization of T waves (inverted at rest and becoming upright with exercise) may be a marker for ischemia (65). Exercise-induced hypotension, angina, S_3, S_4, or murmur in conjunction with the aforementioned ECG changes gives greater credence to the diagnosis.

Echocardiology

Two-dimensional (2D) echocardiography is a noninvasive modality that provides anatomic and physiologic information by real-time imaging of the heart in multiple tomographic planes (66). When it is used in combination with Doppler technology, calculations of pressure gradients and intracardiac pressures and flows can be made, and information can be gained about regurgitant lesions and the systolic and diastolic function of the heart. Over the past 30 years, echocardiography has been gaining wider acceptance for the perioperative diagnosis, assessment, and management of cardiac disease. This section reviews 2D and Doppler echocardiography and their uses for evaluation of ventricular performance.

Two-dimensional Echocardiography

A standard echocardiographic examination includes, M-mode, 2D, and color flow Doppler imaging. M-mode echocardiography provides a single-dimensional view of the heart plotted against time. A strip chart depiction of the cardiac structures is generated as they move during the cardiac cycle (Fig. 6-2). Estimates about chamber dimension wall thickness, ejection fraction, and fiber shortening can be made, as can an evaluation of valve structure. With the advent of 2D echocardiography, the information provided by M-mode is often supplementary. However, when measurements include a temporal component, M-mode may detect more subtle changes than 2D echocardiography because it is updated more frequently.

2D echocardiography is based on the detection of reflected ultrasonic sound waves in the range of 2.5 to 10 MHz. A piezoelectric crystal inside a transducer oscillates at a rapid frequency to generate and receive the sound waves. Reflected waves return to the transducer and are processed to create an image. As the sound waves travel through tissues of different densities, they are reflected or echoed back to the transducer accordingly, or are refracted if they are transmitted into the tissue. The time for the wave to be generated and received is measured, and, in conjunction with knowledge of the speed of sound, the depth of an object can be calculated. The intensity of the reflected waves determines

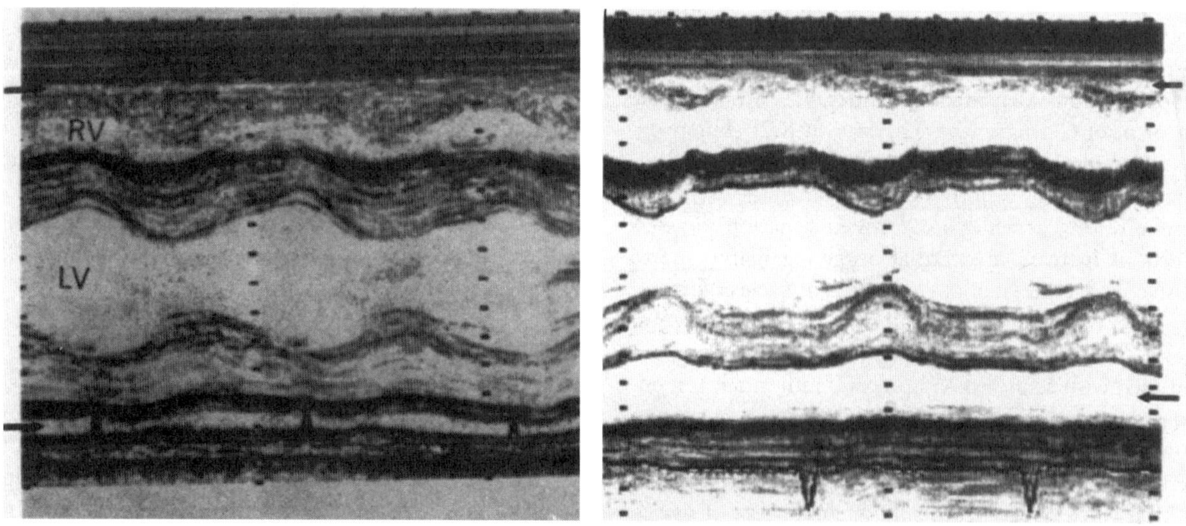

FIGURE 6-2. M-mode echocardiographic tracing from two patients with pericardial effusion. In the left a small echo-free space is seen between the epicardium and pericardium both anteriorly and posteriorly *(arrows)*. On the right, the effusion is larger *(arrows)*. LV, left ventricle; RV, right ventricle. (From Brockinton GM, et al. Echocardiography in pericardial diseases. In: Melvin Marcus, et al., eds. *Cardiac imaging: a companion to Braunwalds' heart disease.* Philadelphia: WB Saunders, 1991, with permission.)

the intensity of the object being studied. Multiple ultrasound images of aligned segments are summated to created a cross-sectional image or 2D echocardiogram (67).

In contrast to M-mode echocardiography, in which temporal manifestations of any structure lying parallel to the beam are assessed, 2D echocardiography simultaneously scans an entire field by recording individual lines; this scanning is done either manually, by physically rotating a single crystal, or electronically, by stimulating a row of crystals so that the resultant waves are slightly out of phase with one another (linear phased-array transmission) (8,68). This produces a real-time image of the heart. Initially, scanning was performed transthoracically. Now, in addition to transthoracic scanning, transesophageal images can be acquired by placing the transducer into the esophagus of the patient. With the probe in such close contact with the heart and with the avoidance of chest wall and lung structures, higher-quality images can be obtained. Biplanar and omniplane probes exist for transesophageal echocardiograms. The biplanar probe has a second 2D plane that is perpendicular to the transverse plane used in single 2D probes. In the omniplane probe, the transducer can rotate 180° to obtain multiple myocardial images. The result with either is a powerful perioperative diagnostic tool that can give comprehensive pictorial and calculated information about myocardial anatomy and performance (Fig. 6-3).

Doppler Echocardiography

Doppler echocardiography is used in conjunction with 2D echocardiography to attain hemodynamic information about the heart. It operates on the principle of the "Doppler effect," which is used to explain how the speed of a moving object can be calculated. In the heart the moving objects,

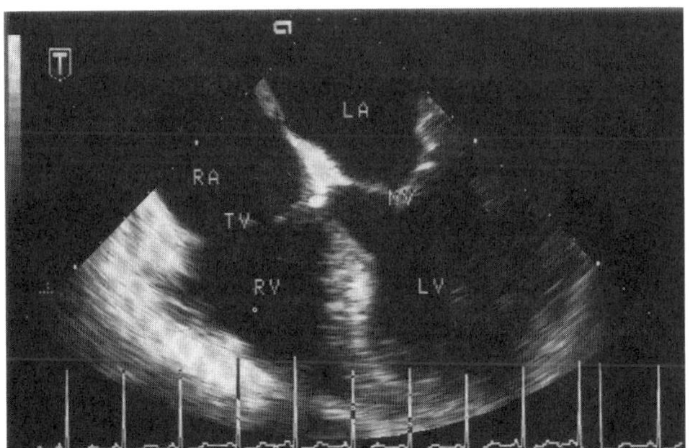

FIGURE 6-3. Two-dimensional echocardiogram that shows four-chamber view of the heart. LA, left atrium; RA, right atrium; LV, left ventricle; MV, mitral valve; RV, right ventricle; TV, tricuspid valve; IVC, inferior vena cava. (From Konstadt S, et al. Transesophageal echocardiography. In: Kaplan JA, ed. *Cardiac anesthesia.* Philadelphia: WB Saunders, 1993, with permission.).

red blood cells, reflect sound waves that are transmitted by a transducer, and the phase shift between the transmitted and reflected waves can be used to calculate the velocity of flow of blood through a structure. This allows for the calculation of many hemodynamic variables, including pressure gradients, intracardiac pressures, volumetric flow, valve areas, and diastolic filling.

Currently, three techniques are used in Doppler echocardiology: pulsed-waved, continuous-wave, and color flow imaging. In pulsed-wave Doppler, a single transducer emits and receives a short burst of ultrasound waves that are delivered at a certain frequency. By analyzing the frequency shift of the reflected waves, blood flow parameters can be determined at precise locations within the heart. Pulse-wave Doppler is best suited for examining instantaneous velocities, the degree of valvular regurgitation, and intracardiac shunts. Contrastingly, continuous-wave Doppler uses continuous emission and receiving of ultrasound waves; high blood flow velocities can be measured accurately at the expense of precise location. Continuous-wave Doppler is the preferred technique when evaluating high-velocity jets and for measuring gradients and intracardiac pressures (Fig. 6-4). With color flow Doppler, blood flow in the heart may be seen in color in real time (Fig. 6-5). This type of Doppler imaging uses three colors (red, blue, and green), individually or in combination, to represent a picture element. By convention, blood flow toward the transducer is seen as red, and flow directed away from the transducer is seen as blue. When flow is turbulent, green is added to give a mosaic pattern. Color flow Doppler can be used for accurate assessment of the severity of valvular regurgitation and the size of intracardiac shunts.

Assessment of Ventricular Function

With the ever-growing prevalence of CAD and its relation to ischemia and infarct, the perioperative use of echocardiography as a monitor to evaluate ventricular function is becoming more popular. The literature is filled with examples that show an association between ischemia and wall motion abnormalities. Consequently, the use of echocardiography to monitor ventricular function can be valuable. More specifically, echocardiography can be used to give both a qualitative and a quantitative assessment of ventricular function.

Wall motion during systole can be used to estimate ventricular function. Normally, the endocardial surfaces move to a central point and ventricular wall thickness increases. With ischemia or infarct, areas of the ventricle do not move appropriately, or the wall thickness does not increase and may actually become thinner. 2D echocardiography had been shown to be a sensitive indicator of systolic wall motion abnormalities (SWMAs). Additionally, it has been shown that SWMAs may be more sensitive indicators of myocardial ischemia than ECG changes, as well as better

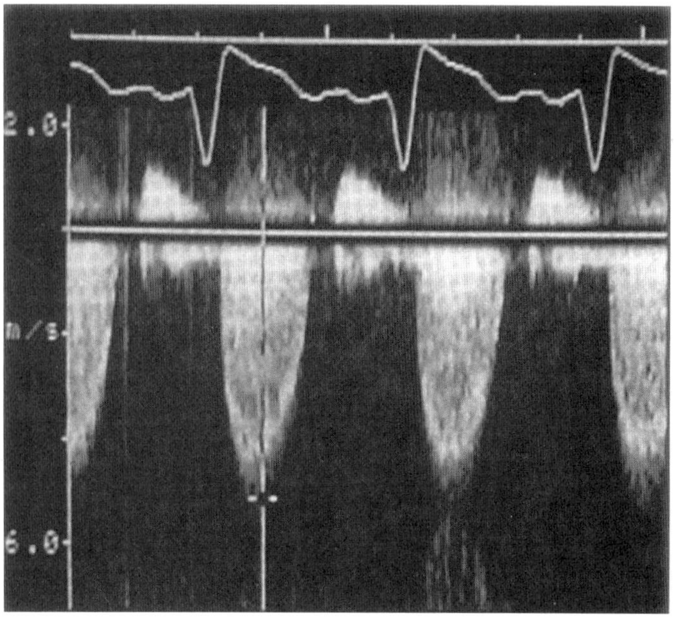

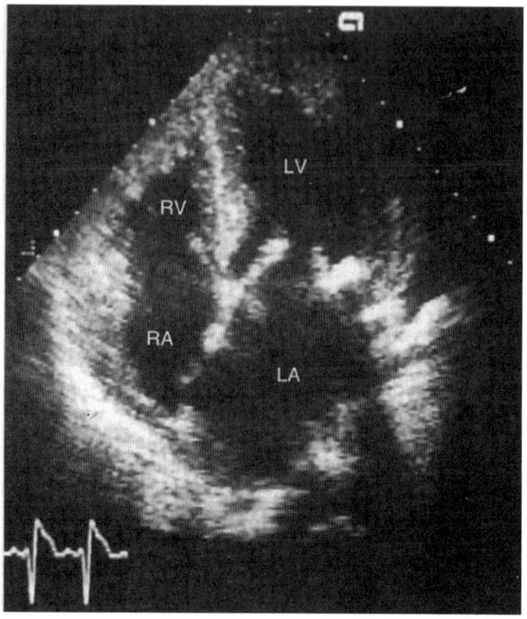

FIGURE 6-4. Continous wave Doppler ultrasonography.

predictors of progression to MI (54). In fact, what most data have revealed is that the positive predictive value of SWMAs for adverse outcome is low but the negative predictive value is high. In other words, the absence of wall motion abnormalities can be associated with a good outcome (68).

Normal wall motion is defined by the degree of systolic wall thickening; at the midpapillary region, normal wall thickening is represented by a 30% to 50% thickening of the myocardium (69). Four types of abnormal wall motion have been described: hypokinesis, hyperkinesis, akinesis, and dyskinesis. Hypokinesis and hyperkinesis refer to the presence of less than normal and greater than normal ventricular motion, respectively. Akinesis indicates the absence of motion, and a dyskinetic ventricle is one that has a paradoxic outward movement of the wall. The American Society of Echocardiography has divided the LV into 16 segments for segmental examination in the short-axis view (Fig. 6-6). This view is advantageous because the coronary distribution for the segment being evaluated can be identified.

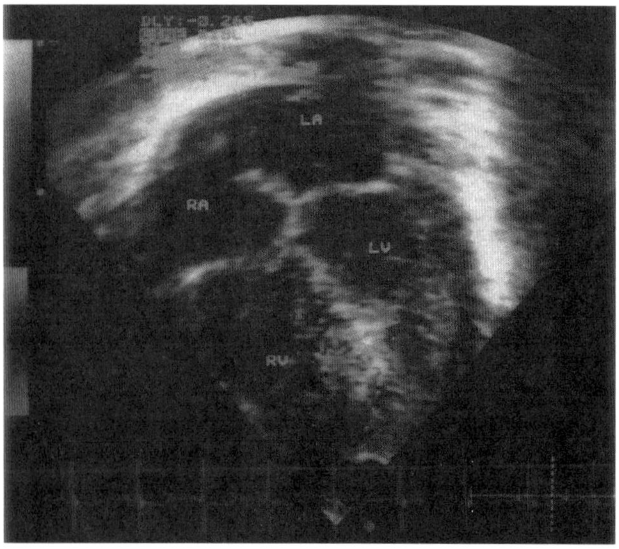

FIGURE 6-5. Color flow Doppler ultrasonogram illustrating ventricular septal defect. (From Czer LC, et al. Transesophageal and epicardial color flow Doppler echocardiography surgical repair of valvular, ischemic, and congenital heart disease. In: Kaplan JA, ed. *Cardiac anesthesia.* Philadelphia: WB Saunders, 1993, with permission.)

Quantitative assessment of ventricular function can be made using 2D and M-mode echocardiography through the ability of these modes to measure changes in ventricular cavity size. Calculations of ejection fraction, fractional shortening, SV, and CO can be made based on estimates of ventricular volumes. The accuracy of these measurements depends on an image quality that shows good definition of the endocardial border and reproducible transducer positioning. Again, the short-axis view at the midpapillary muscle level is one that is reliably reproduced. Clements et al. showed good correlation between transesophageal echocardiography and radionuclide angiography for ventricular volume measurements (70). However, the problem with the use of transesophageal echocardiography intraoperatively to make these measurements is the length of time needed in an atmosphere of constantly changing hemodyamic variables.

In summary, echocardiography is a perioperative test that can reveal pertinent information in patients undergoing car-

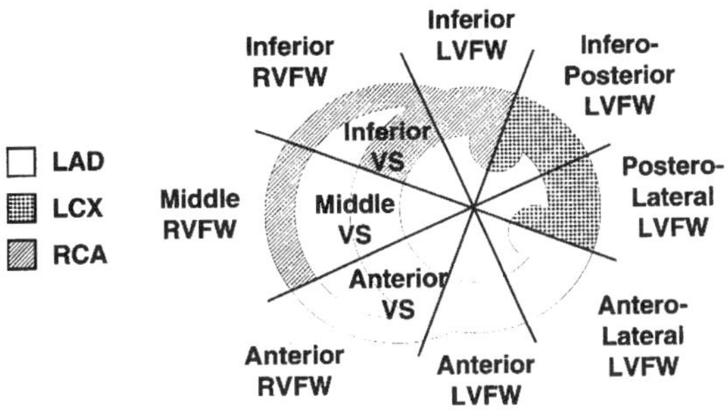

FIGURE 6-6. Midpapillary short-axis transesophageal view to show segmental nomenclature and coronary flow distribution. LAD, left anterior descending coronary artery; LCX, left circumflex coronary artery; RCA, right coronary artery; VS, ventricular septum; LVFW and RVFW, left and right ventricular free wall. (From Kato M, et al. Does transesophageal echocardiography improve postoperative outcome in patients undergoing coronary artery bypass surgery? *J Cardiothorac Vasc Anesth* 1993;7:285, with permission.)

diac surgery. It can be used to diagnose acute myocardial problems, to assess ventricular function, and as a monitor of wall motion abnormalities. Intraoperatively, it has been shown to be a sensitive indicator of ischemia. In the future, echocardiography may be seen as a viable option to other monitors such as the ECG and pulmonary artery catheters to decide optimal perioperative care for these high-risk patients. Its effect on patient outcome is still largely unknown.

Magnetic Resonance Imaging

Since its inception in 1946 by Bloch et al. and Purcell et al., nuclear magnetic resonance (NMR) imaging (MRI) has developed into a proven clinical modality for the examination of molecular structures (71,72). In cardiovascular medicine, its use has been extended into the generation of three-dimensional images of the heart and great vessels. Continuing technologic advances will allow MRI to become a routine test in the evaluation of patients with cardiovascular disease.

The basis of NMR lies in the evaluation of the spin angular momentum of nuclei in an object; that is, the outcome of the rotational motion of the nucleus about its own axis (73). The hydrogen nucleus is most commonly used in NMR. The spinning nuclei generate magnetic fields, the strengths of which are expressed as magnetic moments. When exposed to external magnetic fields, which are perpendicular to one another, one field will rotate with the same frequency as the nuclear spins; the natural frequency of the nuclear spin is called its resonance. The difference in resonance frequencies, as seen in NMR spectrum, gives information about molecular structure or chemical composition. The accumulation of multiple resonance frequencies results in the formation of an image (Fig. 6-7).

Development of the standard spin-echo images as previously described is a continuous process; therefore signals must be gated to the cardiac cycle. The beating heart in a magnetic field can make the QRS complex difficult to obtain, because it has induced potentials in the leads. In addition, arrhythmias and respiratory motion can affect the quality of image acquisition. The development of "ultrafast" cine and spin-echo sequences permits images to be obtained in the span of a single held breath on standard MRI imaging equipment (74,75).

NMR's ability to acquire information noninvasively makes it quite appealing. Its value for assessing LV volume, LV masses, and aortic aneurysms has been well documented.

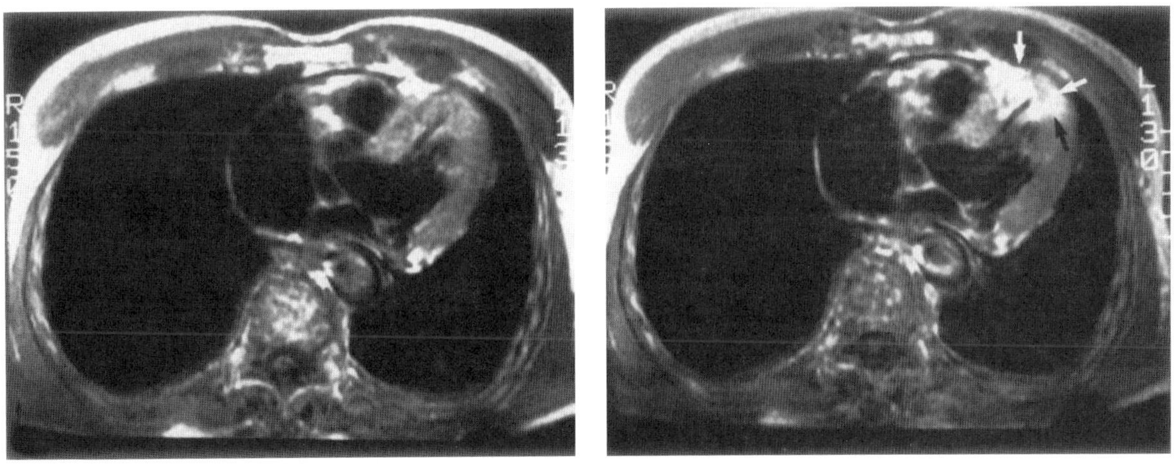

A B

FIGURE 6-7. Magnetic resonance imaging examination in a 58-year-old man 7 days after anterior infarction. **A:** Spin-echo image without contrast. **B:** After-contrast image shows marked enhancement *(arrows)* in the anterior wall and septum. (From Rumberger JA. MRI, CT and PET of the heart and great vessels. In: Giuliani ER, et al., eds. *Mayo Clinical practice of cardiology.* St Louis: Mosby, 1996, with permission.)

Improved techniques allow coronary angiography to be performed, including accurate assessment of bypass graft course and patency. A noninvasive analysis of myocardial metabolism which is independent of external tracers has also been demonstrated (76,77). NMR may also detect ischemic insults to the heart, since prolonged ischemia affects proton relaxation parameters; increased signal intensities in ischemic regions appear to be associated with lipid accumulation, edema, and fibrosis (8). With continued improvements in scanning techniques and wider clinical applications, the use of NMR use as a major diagnostic tool in the assessment of cardiac patients appears to be very promising.

Nuclear Imaging

Nuclear cardiology imaging techniques have developed dramatically in the past decade and now have several applications in the assessment of cardiovascular disease. The following section describes the theory, pharmaceuticals, equipment, and techniques currently used in nuclear imaging.

Principles of Radionuclide Imaging

The basis of nuclear imaging is the detection of photons generated by radioisotopes that have been injected into a patient. Photons are units of electromagnetic energy that can have many forms but for imaging studies are most often in the form of gamma rays. A gamma camera is used to detect the emitted photons. A problem arises in that not all of the generated photons leave the patient; more often, the photons are scattered by intervening tissues or bone. This scattering can result in inaccuracies in the detection of the original photon location. Additionally, tissues may absorb photons. This involves destruction of the photon and a transfer of energy to the patient, which renders the photon undetectable. Isotopes with the highest energy have the least chance for scatter or absorption of their respective photons and therefore the greatest chance for detection. Similarly, materials with higher atomic numbers, such as bone and calcium, absorb more photons than those with low atomic numbers, such as water and soft tissue. These principles eventually determine the attenuation of tissues.

Detector Equipment and Isotopes

The two radioisotopes most commonly used in nuclear imaging are technetium 99m (^{99m}Tc) and thallium 201 (^{201}Tl). ^{99m}Tc is formed from molybdenum 99. It has a relatively short half-life (6 hours) compared with ^{201}Tl, and it emits photons with a 140-keV peak. ^{201}Tl is produced in a cyclotron and has a half-life of 73 hours. The majority of the photons emitted from ^{201}Tl (93%) are in the 69- to 83-keV range. There are additional photon emissions at 135 and 167 keV. The properties of ^{99m}Tc make it a far more desirable isotope to use. It is less expensive, and its short half-time results in less radiation exposure to the patient. Additionally, its higher-energy photons lead to less scatter and absorption and therefore better image quality.

Two devices exist for photon detection in nuclear imaging: the single and multiiodide crystal cameras. Both work on the principle of converting the gamma rays emitted from photons into visible light by a sodium iodide crystal. The light is then directed to a photomultiplier tube, which converts it to an electrical signal and generates an image. The more common single camera has one large sodium crystal with several photomultiplier tubes. Contrastingly, the multiiodide camera has one photomulitplier for several crystals. To eliminate scatter, a lead collimator with holes covers the iodide crystals and allows only those photons striking it at a proper angle to be detected. The effectiveness of the gamma camera and therefore the quality of image depend on the efficiency of the crystal, the photomuliplier, and the collimator.

Imaging Techniques

Radionuclide Angiography

Assessment of ventricular function and myocardial perfusion can be achieved by imaging a tracer as it passes through the circulation. Radionuclide angiography involves imaging ^{99m}Tc-labeled blood cells as they distribute through the blood volume. Labeled cells have a biologic half-life of about 20 hours, and the usable blood pool activity of ^{99m}Tc is about 6 hours (78). Images are formed by ECG-gating. Data collected during the same frame of successive cardiac cycles are added together; this results in a series of images of the great chambers and vessels, each taken at a particular point in the cardiac cycle (79). Wall motion of the LV at rest can then be assessed in several views, including the anterior, lateral, and left anterior oblique projections.

Exercise radionuclide angiography may be performed with the use of a supine or semirecumbent bicycle. The exercise is divided into 3-minute stages, and acquisition usually takes 2 minutes. With exercise, only the left anterior oblique view is obtained. The image is divided into segments that correspond with coronary artery distribution. The septal segments are perfused by the left anterior descending coronary artery, the inferior segment by the right coronary artery, and the lateral segments by the circumflex artery (80). Radionuclide angiography yields accurate information regarding the heart, including LV and right ventricular ejection fractions, regional wall motion, volume, and LV filling and output. Ventricular functions and volumes are particularly accurate in serial measurements because imaging conditions are essentially unchanged, and no assumption of ventricular geometry is required.

Thallium Imaging

^{201}Tl can be used to evaluate the response of the coronary circulation during stress and, therefore, the significance of

CAD. Because stenotic vessels have limited vascular reserve in response to stress, the normal resting homogeneous pattern of coronary perfusion can be altered and made heterogeneous (8). ^{201}Tl, which has an affinity for myocardial cells and undergoes a regional distribution and then redistribution, can be used to examine coronary perfusion. Regions of the myocardium that are supplied by significantly stenosed vessels do not increase their blood flow during exercise; these areas appear as defects on the initial ^{201}Tl scan. Over time, thallium equilibrates with the blood and myocardial washout (redistribution) occurs. Subsequently, further uptake occurs in areas that were previously hypoperfused, and initial defects resolve with time; this indicates areas of viable myocardium. Areas of infarct, however, demonstrate no further uptake of ^{201}Tl and persist as defects on imaging (Fig. 6-8).

Image acquisition occurs with either planar imaging or tomography. Planar imaging is very similar to what was previously described for radionuclide angiography imaging. The use of tomography has a theoretic advantage of fewer superimposed layers and less background activity. In single-photon emission computed tomographic imaging (SPECT), a gamma camera rotates around the patient while taking a series of images. These images are then reconstructed by computer to give a three-dimensional view of the myocardium. It appears that SPECT is superior to planar imaging for detection of previous MI, diagnosis of multiple-vessel CAD, and detection of mild CAD (81). Both planar and tomographic ^{201}Tl imaging can also be used to assess lung and right ventricular uptake. Increase in lung uptake immediately after exercise is indicative of left-sided heart failure and has a strong correlation with left main CAD (82).

As discussed previously, ^{201}Tl is not the ideal agent for imaging because of its long half-life and the low-energy photons that it emits, which result in low-resolution images with marked attenuation in soft tissues. This had led to the introduction of other isotopes, such as ^{99m}Tc, in the hope of obtaining higher-quality images. Included in the ^{99m}Tc family of isotopes are teboroxime, tetrofosmin, and sestamibi. Of these, sestamibi has been most widely used and studied. After injection, sestamibi is taken up by myocardial mitochondria; it undergoes little tissue washout or redistribution. This quality makes this agent ideal for evaluation of acute MI and unstable angina. The myocardium at risk can be assessed without any delay in reperfusion therapy. Compared with ^{201}Tl, ^{99m}Tc-sestamibi imaging is superior in the detection of single-vessel CAD and may be combined with a first-pass study to assess global LV function.

Positron Emission Tomography

Positron emission tomography (PET) allows the measurement of metabolic activity and regional myocardial perfusion by tracing compounds that have been labeled with positron-emitting isotopes. Most commonly, fluorodeoxyglucose (FDG) is used for metabolic analysis in combination with nitrogen-13 ammonia or oxygen-15 water, which are both used for perfusion analysis. Carbon-11 acetate is used to assess oxidative metabolism and consumption. Under ischemic conditions, the myocardial tissue switches to glucose as an energy source instead of fatty acids (83). Therefore, a region of myocardium that persistently uptakes FDG in combination with decreased perfusion tracer can be deemed viable but with decreased function. In such cases, improved myocardial function may return with revascularization (Fig. 6-8). With this approach, myocardial viability can be detected with a sensitivity in the range of 78% to 85% and a specificity of 78% to 92% (84). However, there have been no conclusive studies that justify PET's increased cost for its potentially greater diagnostic accuracy. In addition, some studies have shown that there is not always a correlation between flow-metabolism mis-

A,B

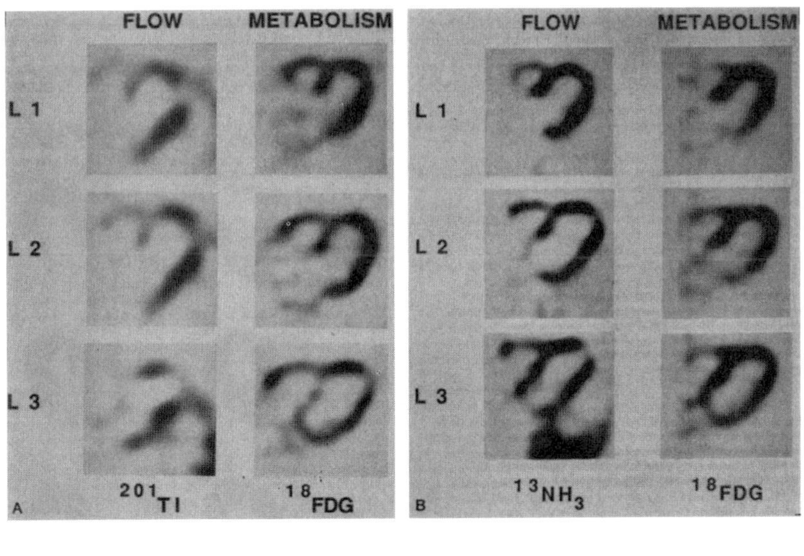

FIGURE 6-8. Thallium imaging and positron emission tomography. **Panel A:** 24-Hour redistribution thallium 201 images with corresponding fluorodeoxyglucose (FDG) metabolic images. Thallium images show extensive perfusion defects but well-preserved glucose metabolism indicating residual myocardial viability. **Panel B:** Ammonia perfusion and FDG metabolic images in the same patient 2 months after coronary artery bypass grafting. Perfusion has markedly improved in septal, inferior, inferolateral, and anteroapical regions of the ventricle. Ejection fraction improved from 16% to 26%. (From Luu M, et al. Delayed recovery of revascularized myocardium after referral for cardiac transplantation. *Am Heart J* 1990;199;668, with permission.)

match and infarcted tissue, which could hamper the accuracy of PET scanning (85).

Pharmacologic Stress Agents

In patients who cannot exercise, pharmacologic stress is a viable alternative for evaluation of the coronary circulation. The three agents primarily used are dipyridamole, adenosine, and dobutamine. Dipyridamole is an indirect vasodilator that acts by blocking adenosine uptake and transport into cells, therefore increasing adenosine availability at the receptor site. Adenosine is a direct coronary vasodilator that causes inappropriate flow distribution; normal vessels vasodilate to increase flow, while stenosed vessels have no reserve and do not vasodilate. The overall effect is coronary steal from hypoperfused areas of myocardium to induce ischemia. Perfusion differences are evaluated by SPECT, as previously described. Both dypyridamole and adenosine are very safe agents, but adenosine seems to have a more pronounced side effect profile that is less tolerated by patients, including headache, flushing, hypotension, and dyspnea. Other major side effects for both agents include angina, ST-segment changes, MI, AV block, and bronchospasm. Adenosine is also contraindicated in patients with history of bronchospasm, those with borderline hypertension, and those taking methylxanthines or dipyridamole.

Dobutamine, a synthetic catecholamine, acts directly on β_1-receptors and results in increased inotropic and chronotropic effects on the myocardium. It is titrated in a stepwise fashion to a target HR of 85% of the maximal predicted HR. The overall effects are an increase in coronary blood flow and myocardial ischemia because of increase oxygen demands. In fact, coronary vessels probably become vasospastic because of their altered endothelium due to CAD despite the fact that dobutamine causes vasodilatation through β_1-receptor stimulation. Dobutamine seems to be a safe and reasonable alternative for perfusion scintigraphy in those patients who have contraindications for dipyridamole or adenosine.

Prognosis

Nuclear cardiology imaging has made significant contributions to the diagnosis of CAD and the assessment of myocardial perfusion. In addition, it has added diagnostic value in its ability to predict future cardiac events. Overall there is a high predictive value of the test, regardless of the technique used to acquire images (Table 6-4). A review by Brown of several studies that included a total of 3,594 patients showed the overall rate of cardiac events in patients with normal myocardial perfusion studies to be 0.9% (86). Macheocourt et al. found even a lower rate, with an annual mortality rate of 0.1% (87). These results may have great clinical and economic implications in the future as myocardial imaging may decrease the need for more invasive methods to examine CAD.

TABLE 6-4. SENSITIVITY AND SPECIFICITY OF RADIONUCLIDE IMAGING METHODS

Test	Sensitivity	Specificity
Exercise		
Planar thallium	82	88
Planar sestamibi	84	83
Spect thallium	90	80
Spect sestamibi	90	93
Adenosine/Dipyridamole		
Planar thallium	82	75
Spect thallium	89	78
Dobutamine		
Spect thallium	82	73

Cardiac Catheterization

Cardiac catheterization is a comprehensive test that is routinely performed in almost all patients undergoing heart surgery (88,89). Anesthesiologists managing heart patients must be capable of interpreting cardiac catheterization results and correlating the information available regarding the coronary circulation, valvular function, myocardial performance, and congenital abnormalities.

Coronary angiography reveals the anatomy of the coronary vessels, the sites and extent of stenoses and occlusions, and the extent of the collateral circulation (90–94).

Ventriculography is a valuable method of defining ventricular function and assessing regional wall motion. It enables segmental evaluation of the ventricle, to differentiate normal segments from areas of transmural damage or ischemia, and to correlate these findings with the status of the coronary circulation (95). As previously described with 2D echocardiography, wall motion is usually described as (a) normal, (b) reduced (reduced amplitude or velocity of contraction), (c) dyskinetic (paradoxic motion), or (d) aneurysmal (aneurysmal dilation with defined margins or undefined motion of the wall) (96,97). The terms hypokinesis (reduced motion) and akinesis (absent motion) are also used. Ventriculography enables the measurement of end-systolic and end-diastolic volumes (98,99). Also, with ventriculography the velocity of circumferential fiber shortening, mean ejection rate, wall thickness, hypertrophy, LV mass, LV stress, and segmental wall abnormalities can be identified and assessed. Latent ventricular dysfunction can also be assessed by inducing myocardial ischemia (100,101).

Measurements of the pressure gradients and visualization of the movements of valvular leaflets and the amount of regurgitation fractions allow evaluation of the function and size of the valve area before surgery. Pressure measurements in the various chambers of the heart and the great vessels and observation of the direction of blood flow and degrees of shunts during ventriculography reveal the congenital heart defects. In addition, ventriculography allows assessment of ventricular function by measurement or calculation of the ejection fractions, which together with the degree of synergy are a good indicator of the cardiac index. Cardiac catheterization also facilitates the measurement of hemodynamic parameters, including CO, O_2 consumption, and O_2 saturation in different chambers and coronary sinus flow.

Anesthesiologists should familiarize themselves with the sites of cannulation for cardiac catheterization, which can be either the brachial artery (Sones technique) or the femoral vessels (Jedkins technique). Occasionally, the radial vessels distal to brachial cannulation have a decreased pulse and are not very reliable for arterial pressure measurements, particularly when repeated catheterizations are performed at the same site.

Catheterization of the femoral vessels can be complicated by subcutaneous hematoma and, rarely, by significant blood loss that can decrease preoperative hematocrit levels.

Anesthesiologists should also familiarize themselves with the catheterization laboratories in their institutions and coordinate triaging mechanisms with the cardiologists, in case they are needed for resuscitation or during transportation of emergency patients in the catheterization laboratory. Standardization of monitoring equipment, monitoring lines, and transducers in both operating rooms and the catheterization laboratory facilitates the transport of patients and shortens the time of preoperative preparation for emergency surgery.

PREOPERATIVE DRUG THERAPY

Patients undergoing cardiac surgery are usually receiving multiple-drug therapy. Their drugs may include digitalis, coronary dilators, drugs that decrease myocardial O_2 consumption, antihypertensive agents, antiarrhythmic drugs, and drugs that are used for treatment of CHF. Not infrequently, patients are also using drugs that inhibit platelet function and decrease clotting. The effects of these drugs on hemodynamics, electrolytes, and clotting mechanisms must be carefully assessed by the anesthesiologist.

Most drugs used in the treatment of the cardiac conditions should be continued until the day of surgery. Exceptions generally include drugs that increase the incidence of bleeding (e.g., aspirin) and diuretic therapies. However, in many instances the half-lives of the antiplatelet and anticoagulant drugs are long, and it is more realistic to manage the anticipated side effects.

Antihypertensives

As early as 1929, Sprague reported a mortality rate of 30% in hypertensive patients undergoing surgery (102). It has since been shown that the risks of anesthesia and surgery to patients experiencing hypertensive emergencies as well as patients with uncontrolled hypertension are serious and include higher incidences of myocardial ischemia, MI, and cerebral hemorrhage (103). The close association between CAD, hypertension, and myocardial hypertrophy explains the high risk of these perioperative complications in these patients. Cessation of antihypertensive therapy renders the patient more vulnerable to fluctuations of the blood pressure during and after the induction of anesthesia. Therefore, it would be prudent for patients to continue taking medication for their hypertension preoperatively.

Calcium Channel Antagonists

Calcium antagonists remain among the most commonly used agents for angina and hypertension. They work by selectively inhibiting the normal Ca^{2+} influx via "slow" channels into cells (104). Cardiac and vascular smooth muscle contain relatively small amounts of endoplasmic Ca^{2+}, so they are more dependent than skeletal muscle on Ca^{2+} influx and therefore more sensitive (104). The result is less calcium available for the excitation-contraction coupling process. This causes a peripheral vasodilation and a negative inotropic effect. A sympathetic reflex results to counteract these effects and maintain CO.

The cardiovascular effects of calcium antagonists include chronotropic, dromotropic, inotropic, and vasodilatory effects. Each of these must be considered by the anesthesiologist when caring for the cardiac patient. The negative chronotropic and dromotropic effects of calcium antagonists on the heart cause depression of SA-node rate of discharge, prolongation of AV-node refractoriness, and slowing of AV-node conduction (105). The significance of these effects can be accentuated in patients receiving β-blocker therapy.

Concurrent therapy with β-blockers and calcium channel blockers has an additive myocardial depressant effect, which should not be underestimated, particularly in patients with impaired myocardial function and especially when inhalational anesthetics are used. In addition, there is evidence that concurrent use of calcium channel blockers and β-blockers can cause second- and third-degree AV block (106). The additive bradycardic effect of calcium channel blockers and potent opioids is more apparent when a muscle relaxant free of cardiovascular effect (e.g., vecuronium) is used for induction of anesthesia. This bradycardia is readily reversed by atropine (107). In contrast to β-blockers, previous administration of calcium channel blockers does not protect patients from tachycardia, hypertension, or perioperative ischemia (108).

The use of calcium channel blockers can also be a contributing factor in hypotension during induction because of both their myocardial depressant and their vasodilatory effects. This hypotension can be severe in patients who are receiving diuretics (hypovolemic) and have a depressed baroreceptor reflex and in whom a low systemic vascular resistance is further decreased by hemodilution. The hypotension caused by calcium channel blockers does not respond to calcium administration but responds to larger-than-usual doses of α-pressors. There is evidence that α_1-pressors such as phenylephrine are more effective than a combined α_1- and α_2-pressor such as norepinephrine (109).

Administration of calcium channel blockers to patients receiving digitalis therapy can cause a precipitous rise of serum digitalis levels during the first week of calcium channel blocker therapy. Despite all these possible side effects and interactions, it is still commonly agreed that calcium channel blocker therapy should be maintained until the day of surgery and the anesthesia management should plan to minimize such side effects.

Angiotensin-Converting Enzyme Inhibitors

The renin-angiotensin system plays a role in the control of blood pressure and water homeostasis. Activation of this system results in the formation of angiotensin I (AGI), which is later converted to angiotensin II (AGII). As one of the most potent vasoactive substances released during CPB, AGII can have detrimental effects on patients, including disruption of oxygen utilization of splanchnic organs and vasoconstriction of macrovasculature and microvasuclature (110,111). In addition, AGII augments the release and action of other endogenous vasoconstrictors, such as catecholamines and endothelin, and also inhibits the synthesis of vasodilators from vascular endothelium, such as nitric oxide and prostacyclin (112,113). Angiotensin-converting enzyme inhibitors (ACEIs) block the synthesis of AGII and thereby attentuate the previously mentioned mechanisms that may be deleterious in heart failure. As a result, it has become accepted, at least in theory, that the use of ACEIs can improve outcome in patients undergoing cardiovascular surgery. However, Rady et al. showed no difference in the incidence of organ dysfunction, nosocomial infection, length of intubation, length of intensive care unit stay, or death between patients treated with ACEIs versus controls. Despite these findings, because of their potential benefits ACEIs are continued perioperatively. Multiple studies have demonstrated that ACEIs can reduce mortality in CHF (114). Additionally, the use of ACEIs has been extended in the early phase of MI to prevent ventricular muscle remodeling and cardiac failure as well as premature death (115,116). Use of ACEIs prevents AGII-related vasoconstriction and AGII-stimulated activation of the sympathetic nervous system.

The ACEIs are effective in the treatment of both essential and renovascular forms of hypertension with minimal side effects. There is now speculation that they may aid in the treatment of hypertension that occurs after CPB. Blank et al. showed good correlation between plasma renin and intraoperative mean arterial blood pressures in patients undergoing CPB. Both renin and AGII levels have been shown to be increased during and after CPB, and their elevated levels justifies the use of perioperative ACEIs to ameliorate pathology caused by the activation of the renin-angiotensin system (117). There is new evidence to suggest that, in patients undergoing procedures involving aortic cross-clamping, ACEIs may be beneficial in protecting renal function. The role of the renin-angiotensin system in decreasing intraoperative renal blood flow and causing renal failure are well known; therefore, further investigations into the usefulness of ACEIs in aortic surgery are warranted.

It is recommended that ACEI therapy be continued during the perioperative period. However, there are some reports of refractory hypotension and hemodynamic instability during anesthesia and surgery in patients taking ACEIs. This may be seen in CPB procedures where there are significant blood losses or third-space losses and with the use of longer-acting agents. It may be unreasonable to discontinue longer-acting preparations (e.g., enalapril) in these patients *in lieu* of other antihypertensive agents.

β-Adrenergic Blockers

As a class, β-adrenergic blocking drugs are one of the major pharmacotherapeutic advances of the 20th century. They have a variety of uses in cardiovascular medicine, including treatment of angina pectoris, hypertension, arrhythmias, thyrotoxicosis, hypertrophic cardiomyopathy, and myocardial infarct (to reduce size, risk of mortality, and rates of reinfarction). Other clinical syndromes for which they are currently used include migraine headache, open-angle glaucoma, anxiety states, delirium tremens, gastrointestinal bleeding, and subarachnoid hemorrhage. As a consequence of their widespread therapeutic application, a thorough understanding of β-adrenergic blocking agents is necessary to adequately care for the patient who presents for cardiothoracic surgery.

All β-blocking agents competitively block the effects of both endogenously and exogenously administered catecholamines at the β-adrenergic receptors (118). Receptor number and confirmation can be regulated by various pathophysiologic and pharmacologic conditions. Upregulation or increased number of receptors, which may result in increased sensitivity to agonists, occurs with thyrotoxicosis and acute β-blocker withdrawal (119). Conversely, downregulation or decrease in receptor number, leading to decreased agonist sensitivity, occurs with CHF, hypothyroidism, and aging (119). In addition, continuous exposure to high levels of catecholamines may desensitize β-receptors rendering them ineffective.

Despite having the same mechanism of action, these agents vary greatly in their pharmacokinetic properties, activity, and side effects. In general, the overall cardiovascular effects of β-blockers include decreases in both resting and exercise HR, blood pressure, CO, and contractility (120).

Differences in β-blockers begin with routes of elimination. Those metabolized by the liver (propranolol, timolol, metoprolol, pindolol, acebutolol, and labetolol) tend to have a short elimination half-life. Because these β-blockers decrease liver blood flow, the drugs metabolized by the liver may have prolonged elimination half-lives when administered concurrently. Nadolol, atenolol, and sotalol are excreted by the kidney and tend to have longer half-lives. Esmolol is hydrolyzed by plasma cholinesterase and is the shortest-acting β-blocker.

Relative selection of β receptor subtypes is the next difference among this class of drugs. β-Blockers such as propranolol act at both β_1- and β_2-receptor subtypes. Selective β_1-receptor antagonism occurs with esmolol, metoprolol, acebutolol, and atenolol. However, with increasing concentrations of the drug, β_2-receptors are also blocked. Selective antagonism of the β-receptors may be advantageous in patients with COPD and in those with hypertension, secondary to the β_2-mediated dilation of the bronchioles and peripheral vasculature, respectively. In addition to nonselective β-blockade, labetolol had the added characteristic of being an α-blocker as well. Further still, other β-blockers, including acebutolol and pindolol, have intrinsic sympathomimetic activity; these drugs can activate the receptor as well as block it. Some investigators have claimed that intrinsic sympathomimetic activity protects against myocardial depression, asthma, and peripheral vascular complications (119). However, the data supporting these claims are still inconclusive.

Patients taking β-blockers should continue their medication up to and throughout the perioperative period. The stresses of surgery, intubation, and emergence from anesthesia are associated with increases in HR and blood pressure and, consequently, disruption of myocardial metabolism. β-Blockade diminishes the stress response during surgery, blunts the response to intubation, and improves the myocardial oxygen supply-demand ratio (121). Abrupt withdrawl of β-blockers has been reported to result in unstable angina, MI, and even death (122). Rarely, patients encounter side effects of β-blockers, including hypotension, pulmonary edema, and heart block (119). Preoperatively, patients are frequently taking both β-blockers and calcium slow channel blockers. These drugs have an additive effect and therefore are better tolerated orally than intravenously, but they can prolong AV conduction, leading to complete heart block (123). Finally, in patients with COPD, β-blockers must be used cautiously for fear of intraoperative bronchospasm.

Digitalis

Although digitalis compounds have been used for 20 years, questions still remain about their safety and mechanism of action. Their actions can be summarized into three primary effects: (a) direct myocardial stimulation to enhance contractility and automaticity; (b) increase in vagal tone that causes bradycardia, decreased atrial refractoriness, and delayed atrioventricular conduction; and (c) increased risk of arrythmias secondary to calcium-dependent afterdepolarizations (124). The two primary uses for digitalis are for CHF and for cardiac arrythmias. In mild to moderate heart failure (class I and II), digoxin is no longer considered mandatory in the treatment regimen; in severe failure, triple therapy with diuretics, ACEIs, and digoxin has become standard practice (125). Digoxin increases contractility and decreases myocardial oxygen consumption in the failing heart. It has been shown to lessen effort intolerance and to reduce morbidity (126).

Digitalis is effective in the treatment of atrial fibrillation or flutter and occasionally for the treatment of acute supraventricular tachycardia. Patients with CHF in combination with these arrthymias appear to respond best. Digitalis should be used cautiously in patients with AV nodal heart block, because it may precipitate complete heart block. The margin between the therapeutic level of digoxin and levels that cause digitalis toxicity is narrow. Factors altering its activity include electrolyte disturbances, pulmonary function, renal function, and sympathetic discharge. Hypokalemia, acute hypoxemia, and right-sided heart failure caused by cor pulmonale all sensitize the myocardium to the potential toxic effects of digitalis therapy. Enhanced sympathetic tone decreases digoxin's effect on the SA and AV nodes. Patients should continue their digitalis therapy throughout the perioperative period. The serum digoxin level should be assessed 24 hours preoperatively, and undertreatment or toxicity should be corrected. Preoperative prophylactic digitalization may be beneficial in improving LV performance postoperatively in patients with CAD or cardiomyopathy (127).

Nitrates

Organic nitrates have been used in the management of patients with ischemic heart disease for more than 100 years; their first reported use was by Murrell in 1879! (128). Since then, it has been shown that nitrates can be effective antianginals and antiischemics that can relieve anginal attacks and, when taken prophylactically, prolong exercise tolerance (129). Yusef et al. showed that organic nitrates used in acute MI led to a 35% reduction in mortality (130). Additionally, nitroglycerin used intraoperatively can improve signs of ongoing myocardial ischemia. Corait et al. showed that a nitroglycerin infusion improved ST-segment depression in patients undergoing noncardiac surgery, compared with controls (131).

The major mechanism of action of the nitrates is relaxation of vascular smooth muscle; this occurs primarily in venous circulation, but at higher concentrations virtually all vascular beds are affected (132). It had previously been thought that this vasodilation would increase coronary perfusion to balance myocardial oxygen supply and demand, accounting for the therapeutic effects of nitrates. It has since been observed that other coronary vasodilators do not predictably relieve anginal symptoms; only when peripheral vasodilation is present are nitrates efficacious (133,134). Their overall effect is a decrease in cardiac chamber size, preload, and afterload, which leads to decrease in myocardial oxygen consumption. In addition, it has been shown that nitrates have antiplatelet effects and consequently a potential antithrombotic effect that may benefit in unstable angina.

Many patients who present for cardiac surgery are already receiving nitrate therapy. Prophylactic use of nitrates has not been shown to decrease the incidence of myocardial ischemia nor to effect outcome. However, because of their proven efficacy in the treatment of ischemic heart disease, hypertension, and angina, their continued use perioperatively is desirable. Tolerance has been reported with all preparations of nitrates and can be minimized by judicious use and nitrate-free periods. Nitrates undergo renal metabolism; toxicity can develop from excess cyanide or thiocyanate accumulation, and therefore they should be used cautiously in patients with renal failure.

CONCLUSION

This chapter discusses the most significant risk factors and the most commonly used diagnostic tests and preoperative drug therapies for the cardiac surgical patient. A smooth induction and successful anesthesia begins with a thorough preoperative evaluation that results in a well informed and less apprehensive patient. The goal of the preoperative evaluation is to optimize the patient's status and to determine what interventions can be made to ensure the best possible outcome.

REFERENCES

1. Mangano DT. Adverse outcomes after surgery in the year 2001: a continuing odyssey. *Anesthesiology* 1998;88:561.
2. Tarhan S, Moffitt E, Taylor WF, et al. Myocardial infarction after general anesthesia. *JAMA* 1972;220:1451.
3. Hamson, DC. Cost containment in medicine: why cardiology? *Am J Cardiol* 1985;56:10C.
4. Estafanous FG, Mossad E. Anesthesia evaluation. In: Estafanous FG, ed. *Cardiac anesthesia: principles and practice.* Philadelphia: JB Lippincott, 1994:161.
5. Higgins TL, Estafanous FG, Loop FD, et al. Stratification of morbidity and mortality outcome by preoperative risk factors in coronary artery bypass patients. *JAMA* 1992;267:2344.
6. Marcus ML. Effects of cardiac hypertrophy on the coronary circulation. In: Marcus ML, ed. *The coronary circulation in health and disease.* New York: McGraw-Hill, 1983.
7. Wilson WS, Criley JM, Ross RS. Dynamics of left ventricular emptying in hypertrophic subaortic stenosis: a cineangiographic and hemodynamic study. *Am Heart J* 1967;73:4.
8. Mangano DT. Preoperative assessment of cardiac risk. In: Kaplan J, ed. *Cardiac anesthesia.* Philadelphia: WB Saunders, 1993.
9. Diamond GA, Forrester JS. Analysis of probability as an aid in the clinical diagnosis of coronary artery disease. *N Engl J Med* 1979;300:1350.
10. Coronary Artery Surgery Study (CASS). *Manual of operations 11: data collection and storage, collaborative studies in coronary artery surgery.* Washington, DC: National Heart, Lung, and Blood Institute, prepared by CASS Coordinating Center, University of Washington, Seattle, 1978.
11. Kennedy JW, Kaiser GC, Fisher LD, et al. Clinical and angiographic predictors of operative mortality from CASS. *Circulation* 1981;63:793.
12. Martin D, Hensley FA, Chambers CE, et al. The cardiac patient. In: Hensley FA, Martin D, ed. *A practical approach to cardiac anesthesia.* Boston: Little, Brown, 1995.
13. Mangano DT, Browner WS, Hollenburg M. Association of perioperative myocardial ischemia with cardiac morbidity and mortality in men undergoing non-cardiac surgery. *N Engl J Med* 1990;323:1781.
14. Grover FL, Hammermeister KE, Burchfiel C, et al. Initial report of the Veterans' Administration preoperative risk assessment study for cardiac surgery. *Ann Thorac Surg* 1990;50:12.
15. Higgins TL. Quantifying risk and assessing outcome in cardiac surgery. *J Cardiothoracic Vasc Anesth* 1998;12:330.
16. Nicod P, Rehr P, Winniford MD, et al. Acute systemic and coronary hemodynamic and serologic responses to cigarette smoking in long-term smokers with atherosclerotic coronary artery disease. *J Am Coll Cardiol* 1984;4:964.
17. Pearce AC, Jones RM. Smoking and anesthesia: preoperative abstinence and perioperative morbidity. *Anesthesiology* 1984;61:576.
18. U.S. Department of Health and Human Services: The National Institute on Aging Macroeconomic Demographic Model. *Population Estimates,* 1984:59.
19. Wilson K, Krieger KH, Lazenby D, et al. Isolated coronary artery bypass grafting in one hundred consecutive octogenarian patients. *J Thorac Cardiovasc Surg* 1991;102:532.
20. Ross J. Myocardial ischemia. In: Rosen MR, Hoffman BF, eds. *Cardiac therapy.* Boston: Martinus Nijhoff, 1983.
21. Roberts A, Woodhall D, Conti R, et al. Mortality, morbidity, and cost-accounting related to coronary artery bypass graft surgery in the elderly. *Ann Thorac Surg* 1985;39:426.
22. Hertzer NR, Beven EG, Young JR, et al. Coronary artery disease in peripheral vascular patients. *Ann Surg* 1984;199:223.
23. Estafanous FG. Preoperative hypertension. In: Estafanous FG, ed. *Anesthesia and the heart patient.* Boston: Butterworth, 1989.
24. Tarazi RC, Gifford RW. Systemic arterial pressure. In: Sodeman WA and Sodeman TM, eds. *Pathologic physiology: mechanisms of disease,* 5th ed. Philadelphia: WB Saunders, 1974.
25. Veterans' Administration Cooperative Study on Antihypertensive Agents. Effects of treatment on morbidity in hypertension: results in patients with diastolic blood pressure averaging 90 through 114 mmHg. *JAMA* 1970;213:1143.
26. Tarhan S, Moffitt EA, Taylor WF, et al. Myocardial infarction after general anesthesia. *JAMA* 1972;220:1451.
27. Steen PA, Tinker JH, Tarhan S. Myocardial reinfarction after anesthesia and surgery. *JAMA* 1978;239:2566.
28. Rao TL, Jacobs KH, EL-Etr AA. Reinfarction following anesthesia in patients with myocardial infarction. *Anesthesiology* 1983;59:499.
29. Goldman L. Multifactorial index of cardiac risk in noncardiac surgical procedures. *J Cardiothorac Vasc Anesth* 1987;1:237.
30. Cooperman M, Pflug B, Martin EW Jr, et al. Cardiovascular risk factors in patients with peripheral vascular disease. *Surgery* 1987;84:505.

31. Mangano DT. Preoperative assessment of the patients with ischemic heart disease. In: Mangano DT, ed. *Preoperative cardiac assessment.* Philadelphia: JB Lippincott, 1990.
32. Christakis GT, Weisel RD, Fremes SE, et al. Coronary artery bypass grafting in patients with poor ventricular function. *J Thorac Cardiovac Surg* 1992;103:1083.
33. Kannel WB, McGee DL. Diabetes and cardiovascular risk factors: The Framingham Study. *Circulation* 1979;59:8.
34. Arvan S, Singal K, Knapp R, et al. Subclinical left ventricle abnormalities in young diabetics. *Chest* 1988;93:1031.
35. Rennart G. Saltz-Rennart H, Wanderman K, et al. Size of acute myocardial infarcts in patients with diabetes mellitus. *Am J Cardiol* 1985;55:1629.
36. Salomon N, Page S, Okies E, et al. Diabetes mellitus and coronary artery bypass. *J Thorac Cardiovasc Surg* 1983;85;264.
37. Burgos LG, Ebert TJ, Asiddao C. Increased intraoperative cardiovascular morbidity in diabetics with autonomic neuropathy. *Anesthesiology* 1989;70:591.
38. Wallace LK, Starr NJ, Leventhal MJ, et al. Hyperglycemia on ICU admission after CABG is associated with increased incidence of mediastinitis of wound infection. Presented Sept. 1996 American Society of Anesthesiologists, New Orleans. *Anesthesiology* 1996;85:A286.
39. Geiger HJ. Race and health care: an American dilemma? *N Engl J Med* 1996;335:815.
40. Peterson ED, Wright SM, Daley J, et al. Racial variation in cardiac procedure use and survival following acute myocardial infarction in the Department of Veterans Affairs. *JAMA* 1994; 271:1175.
41. Ayanian JZ, Udvarhelyi IS, Gatsonis CA, et al. Racial differences in the use of revascularization procedures after coronary angiography. *JAMA* 1993;269:2642.
42. Whittle J, Conigliaro J, Good CB, et al. Racial differences in the use of invasive cardiovascular procedures in the Department of Veterans Affairs medical system. *N Engl J Med* 1993;329: 621.
43. Goldberg K, Hartz AJ, Jacobsen S, et al. Racial and community factors influencing coronary artery bypass graft surgery rates for all 1986 Medicare patients. *JAMA* 1992;267:1473.
44. Udvarhelyi IS, Gastonis C, Epstein AM, et al. Acute myocardial infarction in the Medicare population: process of care and clinical outcomes. *JAMA* 1992;268:2530.
45. Maynard C, Fisher LD, Passamani ER, et al. Blacks in the Coronary Artery Surgery Study (CASS): race and clinical decision making. *Am J Public Health* 1986;76:1446.
46. Koch CG, Higgins TL, Capdeville M, et al. The risk of coronary artery sugery in women: a matched comparison using preoperative severity of illness scoring. *J Cardiothorac Vasc Anesth* 1996; 10:839.
47. Gau TG. Electrocardiography: a standard electrocardiography and vectorcardiography. In: Giuliani ER, et al., eds. *Mayo Clinic practice of cardiology,* 3rd ed. St. Louis: Mosby, 1996.
48. Savage RM, Wager GS, Idea RE, et al. Correlation of postmortem anatomic findings with electrocardiograph changes in patients with myocardial infarction: retrospective study of patients with typical anterior and posterior infarcts. *Circulation* 1977; 55:279.
49. Rain H, Risen V, Romppanen T, et al. Changes in the QRS complex and ST segment in transmural and subendocardial infarctions: a clinicopathologic study. *Am Heart J* 1979;98:176.
50. Rowlands DJ. Role of clinical presentation and ECG. *Int J Cardiol* 1999;68[Suppl 1]: S35.
51. Hurst JW. Abnormalities of the S-T segment: part II. *Clin Cardiol* 1997;20:595.
52. Madias JE, Chahine RA, Gorlin R, et al. A comparison of transmural and nontransmural acute myocardial infarction. *Circulation* 1974;49:498.
53. Slogoff S, Keats AS. Randomized trial of primary anesthetic agents on outcome of coronary artery bypass operations. *Anesthesiology* 1989;70:179.
54. Slogoff S, Keats AS. Does perioperative myocardial ischemia lead to postoperative myocardial infarction? *Anesthesiology* 1985; 62:107.
55. Slogoff S, Keats AS. Further observations on perioperative myocardial ischemia. *Anesthesiology* 1986;65:539.
56. Slogoff S, Keats AS. Does chronic treatment with calcium entry blocking drugs reduce the perioperative myocardial ischemia? *Anesthesiology* 1988;68:676.
57. Knight AA, Hollenburg M, London MJ, SPI Research Group. Perioperative myocardial ischemia: importance of the preoperative ischemic pattern. *Anesthesiology* 1988;68:681.
58. Lowenstein E, McPeek B. Capitalizing on research findings that appear to conflict. *Anesthesiology* 1988;68:668.
59. Yousif H, Davies G, Westaby S, et al. Preoperative myocardial ischemia: its relation perioperative infarction. *Br Heart J* 1987; 58:9.
60. Wilton NCT, Luckoff C, Sachdev V, et al. Silent preoperative myocardial ischemia in surgical patients with ischemic heart disease. *Anesthesiology* 1987;67:A591(abst).
61. Goldhammer S, Schert D. Elektrokardiographische untersuchungen bei kranker mit angina pectori. *Z Klin Med* 1933;122: 134.
62. Gibbons RJ, Balady GJ, Beasley JW, et al. ACC/AHA Guidelines for exercise testing: a report of the American College of Cardiology/American Heart Association Task Force on Practice Guidelines. *J Am Coll Cardiol* 1997;30:260.
63. Bardsley WT, Mankin HT, Miller TD. Electrocardiography B: exercise testing. In: Giuliani ER, et al., eds. *Mayo Clinic practice of cardiology,* 3rd ed. St. Louis: Mosby, 1996.
64. Philbrick JT, Horwitz RI, Feinstein AR. Methodologic problems of exercise testing for coronary artery disease: groups, analysis and bias. *Am J Cardiol* 1980;46:807.
65. Lavie CJ, Oh JK, Mankin HT, et al. Significance of T-wave pseudonormalization during exercise: a radionuclide angiographic study. *Chest* 1988;94:512.
66. Tajik AJ, Seward JB, Hagler DJ, et al. Two-dimensional realtime ultrasonic imaging of the heart and great vessels: technique, image orientations, structure identification and validation. *Mayo Clin Proc* 1978;53:271.
67. Mamby SA. Echocardiography A: Two-dimensional echocardiography. In: Giuliani ER, et al., eds. *Mayo Clinic practice of cardiology,* 3rd ed. St. Louis: Mosby, 1996.
68. Skeehan TM, Thys DM. Monitoring the cardiac surgical patient. In: Hensley FA, Martin DE, eds. *A practical approach to cardiac anesthesia,* 3rd ed. Boston: Little, Brown, 1995.
69. Clements F. Monitoring ventricular function in the OR: impact on clinical outcome. In: Giuliani ER, et al., eds. *Mayo Clinic practice of cardiology,* 3rd ed. St. Louis: Mosby, 1996:167.
70. Clements FA, Harpole DH, Quill T, et al. Estimation of left ventricular volume and ejection fraction by two-dimensional transesophageal echocardiography: comparison of short axis imaging and simultaneous radionuclide angiography. *Br J Anaesth* 1990;64:331.
71. Bloch F. Nuclear induction. *Phys Rev* 1946;70:460.
72. Purcell EM, Torrey HC. Resonance absorption by nuclear magnetic moments in a solid. *Phys Rev* 1946;69:37.
73. Talagala SL, Wolf GL. Principles of nuclear magnetic resonance. In: Melvin Marcus, et al., eds. *Cardiac imaging: a companion to Braunwald's heart disease.* Philadelphia: WB Saunders, 1991.
74. Matthaei D, Hassse A, Henrich D, et al. Cardiac and vascular

imaging with a MR snapshot technique. *Radiology* 1990;177: 527.
75. Henrich D, Haase A, Matthaei D. 3D-Snapshot flash NMR imaging of the heart. *Magn Reson Imaging* 1990;8:377.
76. Neubauer S, Krahe T, Schindler R, et al. ^{31}P magnetic resonance spectroscopy in dilated cardiomyopathy and coronary artery disease: altered cardiac high-energy phosphate metabolism in heart failure. *Circulation* 1992;86:1810.
77. Yabe T, Mitsunami K, Intubushi T, et al. Quantitative measurements of cardiac phosphorus metabolites in coronary artery disease by ^{31}P magnetic resonance spectroscopy. *Circulation* 1995; 92:15.
78. Gibbons RJ, Raymond J. Nuclear cardiology. In: Giuliani ER, et al., eds. *Mayo Clinic practice of cardiology*, 3rd ed. St. Louis: Mosby, 1996.
79. Berger HJ, Zaret BL. Nuclear cardiology. *N Engl J Med* 1981; 305:855.
80. Behrenbeck T, Christian T, Mullan B. Nuclear cardiology and stress testing. In: Murphy JG, ed. *Mayo Clinic cardiology review*. Armonk, NY: Futura, 1997.
81. Ritchie JL, Williams DL, Harp G, et al. Transaxial tomography with thallium-201 for detecting remote myocardial infarction: comparison with planar imaging. *Am J Cardiol* 1982;50:1236.
82. Bingham JB, Strauss HW, Pohost GM, et al. Mechanism of lung uptake of Tl-201. *Circulation* 1978;58[Suppl 2]:62.
83. Marshall RC, Tillisch JH, Phelps ME, et al. Identification and differentiation of resting myocardial ischemia and infarction in man with positron computed tomography ^{18}F-labelled, fluorodeoxyglucose and ^{13}N-ammonia. *Circulation* 1983;67:766.
84. Tamaki N, Yonekura Y, Yamashita K, et al. Positron emission tomography using fluorine-18 deoxyglucose in evaluation of coronary artery bypass grafting. *Am J Cardiol* 1989;64:860.
85. vom Dahl J, Eitzman DT, Al-Aouar ZR, et al. Relation of regional function, perfusion, and metabolism in patients with advanced coronary artery disease undergoing surgical revascularization. *Circulation* 1994; 90:2356.
86. Brown KA. Prognostic value of thaliium-201 myocardial perfusion imaging: a diagnostic tool comes of age. *Circulation* 1991; 83:363.
87. Macheocourt J, Longere P, Fagret D, et al. Prognostic value of thallium-201 single photon emission computed tomographic myocardial perfusion imaging according to extent of myocardial defect: study in 1926 patients with follow-up at 33 months. *J Am Coll Cardiol* 1994;23:1096.
88. Sones RM, Shirley EK. Cine coronary arteriography. *Mod Concepts Cardiovasc Dis* 1962;31:735.
89. Judklins MP. Selective coronary artery catherterization via femoral approach. *Radiology* 1967;89:1040.
90. White CW. Physiologic assessment of coronary artery stenosis severity. *Trends Cardiovasc Med* 1991;1:70.
91. Vita JA, Treasure CB, Nabel EG, et al. Coronary vasomotor response to acetylcholine relates to risk factors for coronary artery disease. *Circulation* 1990;81:491.
92. Mock MB, Ringqvist I, Fisher ID, et al. Survival of medically treated patients in the CASS registry. *Circulation* 1982;66:562.
93. Little WC, Constantinescu M, Applegate RJ, et al. Can coronary angiography predict the site of subsequent myocardial infarction in patients with mild to moderate coronary artery disease? *Circulation* 1988;78:1157.
94. Mizuno K, Horiuchi K, Matui H, et al. Role of coronary collateral vessels during transient coronary occlusion during angioplasty assessed by hemodynamic, electrocardiographic and metabolic changes. *J Am Coll Cardiol* 1988;12:624.
95. Bove AA, Kreulen TH, Spann JF. Computer analysis of left ventricular dynamic geometry in man. *Am J Cardiol* 1978;41; 1239.
96. Sheehan FH, Stewart DK, Dodge HT, et al. Variability in the measurement of regional left ventricular wall motion from contrast angiograms. *Circulation* 1983;68:550.
97. Nissen Se, Booth D, Waters J, et al. Evaluation of left ventricular contractile pattern by intravenous digital subtraction ventriculography: comparison with cineangiography and assessment of interobserver variability. *Am J Cardiol* 1983;52;1293.
98. Dodge HT, Snadler H, Ballew DW, et al. Use of biplane angiocardiography for the measurement of left ventricular volume in man. *Am Heart J* 1960;60:762.
99. Wynne J, Green LH, Mann T, et al. Estimation of left ventricular volumes in man from biplane cineangiograms filmed in oblique projections. *Am J Cardiol* 1978;41:726.
100. Scroeder JS, Bolen Jl, Quint RA, et al. Provocation of coronary spasm with ergonovine maleate: new test with results in 57 patients undergoing coronary arteriography. *Am J Cardiol* 1977; 40:487.
101. Heupler FA Jr, Proudfit WL, Razavi M, et al. Ergonovine maleate provocative test for coronary arterial spasm. *Am J Cardiol* 1978;41:631.
102. Sprague HB. The heart in surgery: an analysis of the results of surgery on cardiac patients during the last ten years at the Massachusetts General Hospital. *Surg Gynecol Obstet* 1929;49: 54.
103. Estafanous FG. Hypertension in the surgical patient: management of blood pressure and anesthesia. *Cleve Clin J Med* 1989; 56:385.
104. Fleckenstein A. Specific pharmacology of calcium in myocardium, cardiac pacemakers, and vascular smooth muscle. *Ann Rev Pharmacol Toxicol* 1977;17:149.
105. Reves JG, Kissin I, Lell W, et al. Calcium entry blockers: uses and implications for anesthesiologists. *Anesthesiology* 1982;57: 504.
106. Benaim ME. Asystole after verapamil. *Br Med J* 1972;2:169.
107. Starr NJ, Sethna DH, Estafanous FG. Bradycardia and asystole following the rapid administration of sufentanil with vecuronium. *Anesthesiology* 1986;64:521.
108. Chung F, Houston PL, Cheng CH, et al. Calcium channel blockade does not offer adequate protection from perioperative myocardial ischemia. *Anesthesiology* 1989;69:343.
109. McGrath JC. Evidence for more than one type of post-junctional alpha-adrenoceptor. *Biochem Pharmacol* 1982;31:467.
110. Boldt J, Schindler E, Harter K, et al. Influence of intravenous administration of angiotensin-converting enzyme inhibitor undergoing cardiac surgery. *Anesth Analg* 1995;80:480.
111. Bottcher M, Behren EA, Christensen H, et al. ACE inhibitor premedication attenuates sympathetic responses during surgery. *Br J Anaesth* 1994;72:633.
112. Lyons D, Webster J, Benjamin N. Adrenergic sympathetic constrictor action in humans. *Circulation* 1995;91:1457.
113. Greenwald L, Becker RC. Expanding the paradigm of the renin-angiotensin system and angiotensin converting enzyme inhibitors. *Am Heart J* 1994;128:997.
114. Braunwald E. ACE inhibitors: a cornerstone of the treatment of heart failure. *N Engl J Med* 1991;325:351.
115. Bonarjee VVS, Cartensen S, Caidalh K, et al. Attenution of left ventricular dilatation after myocardial infarction by early initiation therapy. *Am J Cardiol* 1993;72:1004.
116. Ball SG. The acute infarction ramipril efficacy study investigators: effect of ramipril on mortality and morbidity of survivors of acute myocardial with clinical evidence of heart failure. *Lancet* 1993;342:821.
117. Mirenda JV, Grissom TE. Anesthetic implications of the renin angiotensin system and angiotesin-converting enzyme inhibitors. *Anesth Analg* 1991;72:667.
118. Wood, AJ. Adrenoreceptor blocking agents. In: Wood AJ, ed.

Drugs and anesthesia: pharmacology for *anesthesiologists.* Baltimore: Williams & Wilkins, 1990.

119. Frishman WH. Beta-adrenergic blockade. *Cardiology* 1985;72: 280.
120. Schwinn DA. Cardiac pharmacology. In: Estafanous FG, et al. eds. *Cardiac anesthesia: principles and practice.* Philadelphia: JB Lippincott, 1994.
121. Cucchiara RF, Benefiel DJ, Matteo RS, et al. Evaluation of esmolol in controlling increases in heart rate and blood pressure during tracheal intubation in patients undergoing carotid endarterectomy. *Anesthesiology* 1986;65:528.
122. Olsson HG, Miller RR, Amsterdam EA, et al. The propranolol rebound phenomenon: acute and catastrophic exacerbation of symptoms and death following the abrupt cessation of larger doses of propranolol in coronary artery disease. *Am J Cardiol* 1975;35:165.
123. Graham RM. Adrenergic receptors: structure and function. *Cleve Clin J Med* 1990;7:480.
124. Roden DM, Woosley RL. Antiarrythymic drugs. In: Wood AJ, ed. *Drugs and anesthesia: pharmacology for anesthesiologists.* Baltimore: Williams & Wilkins, 1990.
125. Marcus FI, Opie LH, Sonnenblick EH, et al. Digitalis and acute inotropes. In: Opie LH, ed. *Drugs for the heart.* Philadelphia: WB Saunders, 1995.
126. Kelly RA, Smith TW. Digoxin in heart failure: implications of recent trials. *J Am Coll Cardiol* 1993;22[Suppl A]:107A.
127. Pinaud MJ, Blanloei Y, Souron RJ. Preoperative prophylactic digitilization of patients with coronary artery disease: a randomized echocardiographic and hemodynamic study. *Anesth Analg* 1983;62:865.
128. Murrell W. Nitroglycerin as a remedy for angina pectoris. *Lancet* 1879:80.
129. Aronow WS. Management of stable angina. *N Engl J Med* 1973; 289:516.
130. Yusef S, MacMahon S, Collin R, et al. Effect of intravenous nitrates on mortality in acute myocardial infarction: an overview of the randomized trials. *Lancet* 1988;2:1088.
131. Coriat P, Daloz M, Bousseau D, et al. Prevention of intraoperative myocardial ischemia during noncardiac surgery with intravenous nitroglycerin. *Anesthesiology* 1984;61:193..
132. Abrams J. Mechanism of action of the organic nitrates in the treatment of myocardial ischemia. *Am J Cardiol* 1992;70:30B.
133. Ganz W, Marcus HS. Failure of intracoronary nitroglycerin to alleviate pacing-induced angina. *Circulation* 1972;46:880.
134. DeCoster PM, Chierchia S, Davies G, et al. Dual effects of nitrates on the coronary and peripheral circulation in exercise induced ischemia in chronic stable angina. *Circulation* 1986; 74[Suppl II]:137.

Cardiac Anesthesia: Principles and Clinical Practice, Second Edition, edited by Fawzy G. Estafanous, Paul G. Barash, and J.G. Reves. Lippincott Williams & Wilkins, Philadelphia © 2001.

7

ELECTROCARDIOGRAPHIC MONITORING

DANIEL M. THYS
JOLIE NARANG

The intraoperative use of the electrocardiogram (ECG) has markedly developed over the last several decades (1). Originally, this monitor was used during anesthesia for the detection of arrhythmias in high-risk patients. However, more recently, its importance as a standard monitor has been recognized, and its use during the conduct of any anesthesia is now recommended (2). Beyond its usefulness for the intraoperative recognition of arrhythmias, one of the major indications for ECG monitoring is the intraoperative diagnosis of myocardial ischemia (3).

NORMAL ELECTRICAL ACTIVITY

P Wave

Under normal circumstances, the sinoatrial (SA) node has the most rapid spontaneous depolarization rate and is, therefore, the dominant cardiac pacemaker (Fig. 7-1). From the SA node, the impulse spreads through the right and left atria. Conducting tracts can conduct the impulse to the atrioventricular (AV) node, but they are not essential. On the ECG, depolarization of the atria is represented by the P wave (Fig. 7-2). The initial depolarization involves primarily the right atrium and occurs predominantly in an anterior, inferior, and leftward direction. Subsequently, it proceeds to the left atrium, located in a more posterior position.

PR Interval

Once the depolarization has reached the AV node, a delay is observed. The delay permits contraction of the atria and supplemental filling of the ventricular chambers. On the ECG it is represented by the PR interval.

D. M. Thys: Department of Anesthesiology, College of Physicians and Surgeons, Columbia University, and Department of Anesthesiology, St. Luke's–Roosevelt Hospital Center, New York, New York 10025

J. Narang: Department of Anesthesia, Mt. Sinai School of Medicine and Mt. Sinai Hospital, New York, New York 10029

QRS Complex

After passage through the AV node, the electrical impulse is conducted along the ventricular conduction pathways consisting of the common bundle of His, the left and right bundle branches, the distal bundle branches, and the Purkinje fibers. The QRS complex represents the progress of the depolarization wave through this conduction system. After terminal depolarization, the ECG should normally return to baseline.

ST Segment and T Wave

Repolarization of the ventricles begins at the end of the QRS complex and consists of the ST segment and T wave. Whereas ventricular depolarization occurs along established conduction pathways, ventricular repolarization is a prolonged process occurring independently in every cell. The T wave represents the uncanceled potential differences of ventricular repolarization. The junction of the QRS complex and the ST segment is called the J junction. The T wave is sometimes followed by a small U wave, the origin of which is unclear. An inverted U wave has been associated with several clinically significant conditions, such as hypertension, coronary artery disease, valvular heart disease, and certain metabolic disorders. There may be an association between exercise or rest-related U-wave inversion and significant stenosis of the left anterior descending artery or the left main coronary artery.

LEAD SYSTEMS

Standard Limb and Precordial Leads

The small electrical currents produced by the electrical activity of the heart spread throughout the body, which behaves as a volume conductor, allowing the surface ECG to be recorded at any site. The standard leads are bipolar leads because they measure differences in potential between pairs of electrodes. The electrodes are placed on the right arm, the left arm, and the left leg. The leads are formed by the

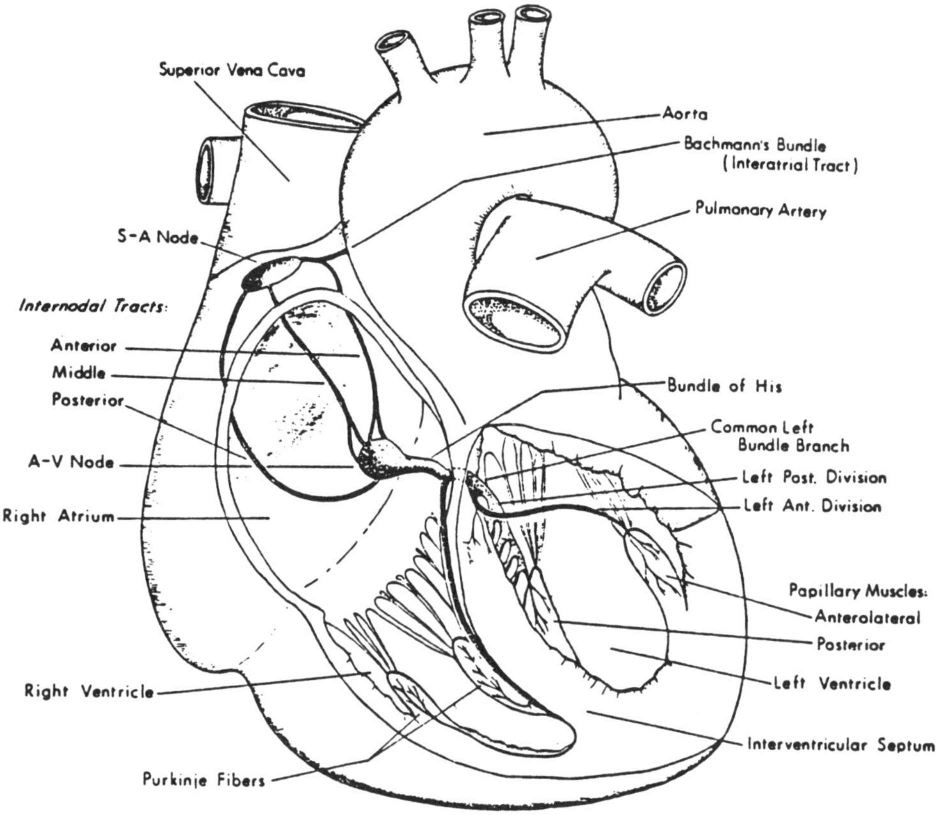

FIGURE 7-1. Schematic representation of distribution of the specialized conductive tissues in the atria and ventricles, showing the impulse-forming and conducting system of the heart. (From Lipman BS, Dunn M, Marsie E. *Clinical electrocardiography,* 7th ed. Chicago: Year Book, 1984. Copyright 1984 by Year Book Medical Publishers, Inc., Chicago. With permission.)

imaginary lines connecting the electrodes, and the polarities correspond to the conventions of Einthoven's triangle (Fig. 7-3). They are labeled leads I, II, and III. If the three electrodes of the standard leads are connected through resistances of 5,000 ohms each, a common central terminal with zero potential is obtained (Fig. 7-4). When this common electrode is used with another active electrode, the potential difference between them represents the actual potential. On a standard 12-lead ECG, three unipolar limb leads are usually recorded: aVR, aVL, and aVF. The "a" indicates that they are augmented limb leads and were obtained using Goldberger's modification (Fig. 7-5). In this modification, the resistors are removed from the lead wires and the explor-

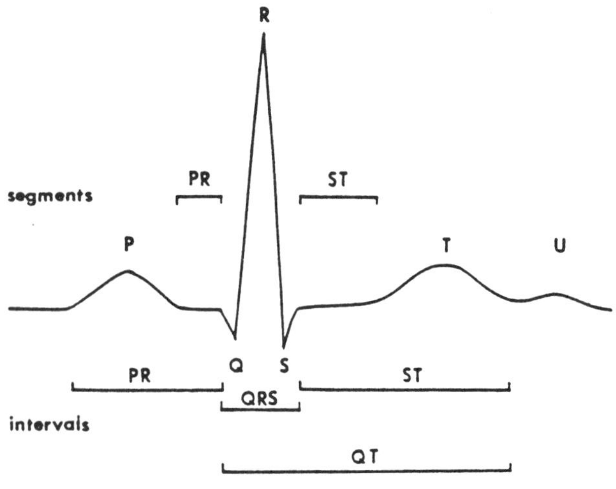

FIGURE 7-2. Electrocardiographic segments and intervals. (From Thys DM, Kaplan JA. *The ECG in anesthesia and critical care.* New York: Churchill Livingstone, 1987, with permission.)

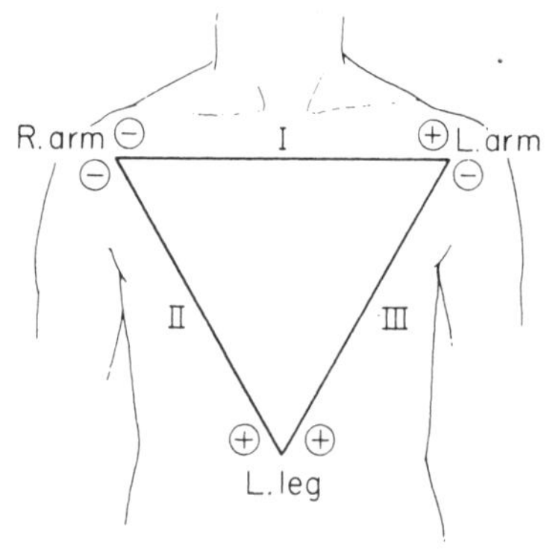

FIGURE 7-3. Einthoven's triangle. (From Thys DM, Kaplan JA. *The ECG in anesthesia and critical care.* New York: Churchill Livingstone, 1987, with permission.)

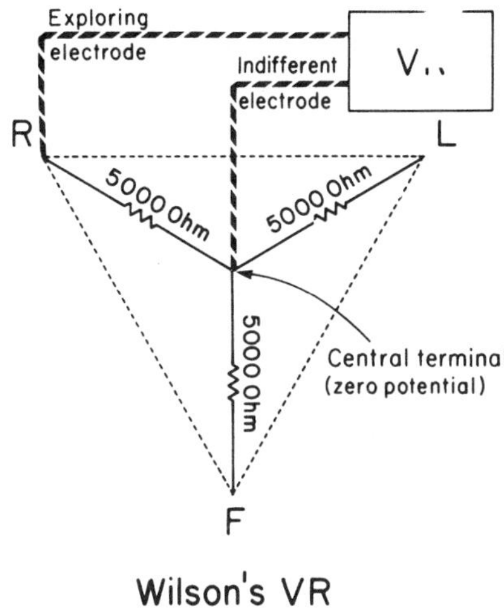

FIGURE 7-4. Wilson's unipolar lead (VR). (From Thys DM, Kaplan JA. *The ECG in anesthesia and critical care.* New York: Churchill Livingstone, 1987, with permission.)

ing electrode is disconnected from the central terminal. It results in larger ECG deflections.

Additional information on the heart's electrical activity is obtained by placing electrodes closer to the heart or around the thorax. In the precordial lead system, the neutral electrode is formed by the standard leads and an exploring electrode is placed on the chest wall. The ECG is normally recorded with the exploring electrode in one or more of six precordial positions. They are indicated by the letter "V" followed by a numeral from 1 to 6 indicating the location of the electrode on the chest wall (Fig. 7-6).

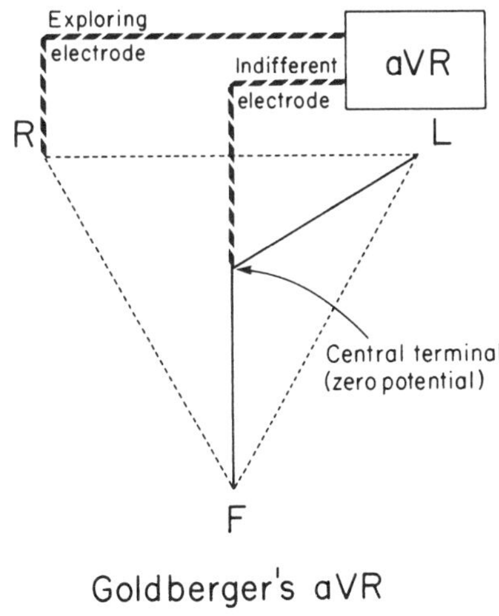

FIGURE 7-5. Goldberger's unipolar lead (aVR). (From Thys DM, Kaplan JA. *The ECG in anesthesia and critical care.* New York: Churchill Livingstone, 1987, with permission.)

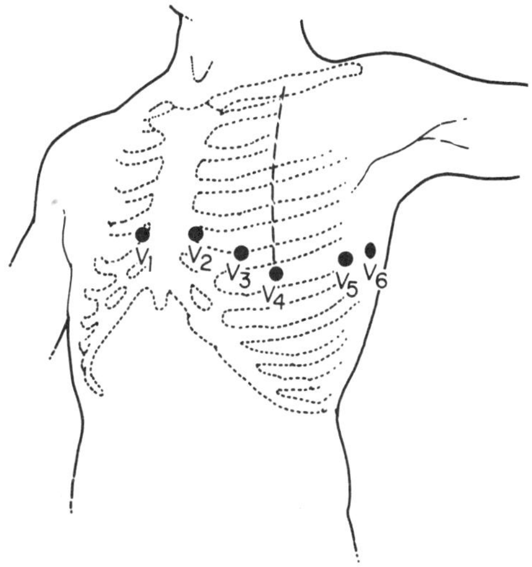

FIGURE 7-6. Anatomic locations of the precordial unipolar leads. Occasionally right-sided precordial leads are recorded as well. They are labeled V_3R, V_4R, and so forth, and their locations correspond to the left-sided leads but on the right side of the chest. (From Thys DM, Kaplan JA. *The ECG in anesthesia and critical care.* New York: Churchill Livingstone, 1987, with permission.)

Electrocardiographic Monitoring Systems

Three-Electrode System

As the name implies, this system uses only three electrodes to record the ECG. In such a system, the ECG is observed along one bipolar lead between two of the electrodes while the third electrode serves as a ground. A selector switch allows the user to alter the designation of the electrodes. Three ECG leads can be examined in sequence without changing the location of the electrodes. Although the three-electrode system has the advantage of simplicity, its use is limited in myocardial ischemia because it provides a narrow picture of myocardial electrical activity.

Modified Three-Electrode System

Numerous modifications of the standard bipolar limb lead system have been developed. Some of these are displayed in Fig. 7-7. They are used in an attempt to maximize P-wave height for the diagnosis of atrial arrhythmias or to increase the sensitivity of the ECG for the detection of anterior myocardial ischemia. In clinical studies, these modified three-electrode systems have been shown to be as sensitive or more sensitive than the standard V_5 lead system for the intraoperative diagnosis of ischemia (4).

CS_5 Lead (Central Subclavicular). The central subclavicular lead is particularly well suited for the detection of anterior myocardial wall ischemia. The right-arm (RA) electrode is placed under the right clavicle, the left-arm (LA)

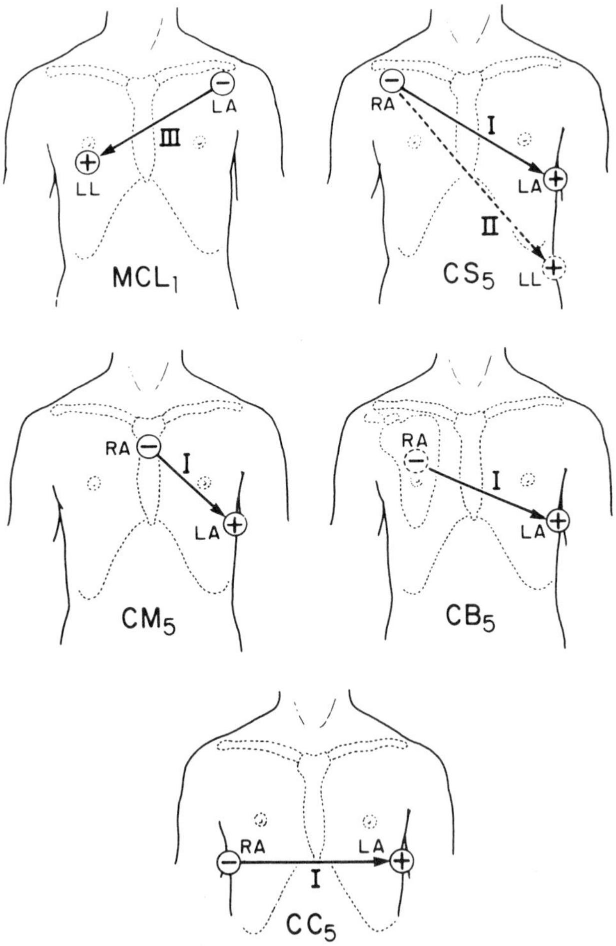

FIGURE 7-7. Modified bipolar limb systems. (From Thys DM, Kaplan JA. *The ECG in anesthesia and critical care.* New York: Churchill Livingstone, 1987, with permission.)

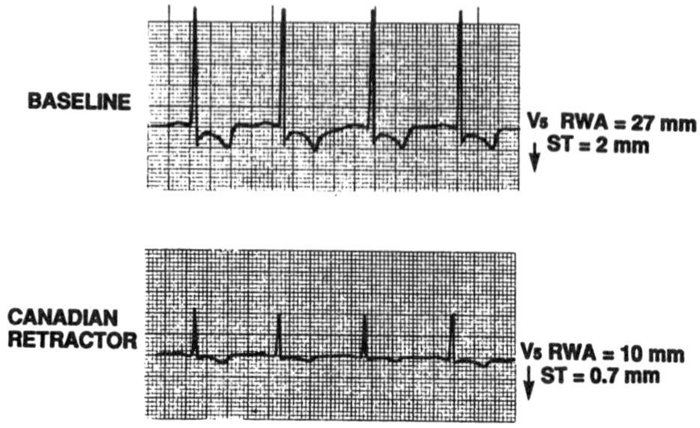

FIGURE 7-8. Changes in the electrocardiogram after placement of a Canadian sternal retractor. Reduction in V_5 R-wave amplitude (RWA) is accompanied by a comparable reduction in ST-segment depression (↓ST). In both tracings, 10 mm = 1 mV. (From Mark JB, Chien GL, Steinbrook RA, et al. Electrocardiographic R-wave changes during cardiac surgery. *Anesth Analg* 1992;74:26, with permission.)

electrode is placed in the V_5 position, and the left-leg electrode is in its usual position to serve as a ground. Lead I is selected for detection of anterior wall ischemia, and lead II can be selected for monitoring inferior wall ischemia or for the detection of arrhythmias. If a unipolar precordial electrode is unavailable, this CS_5 bipolar lead is the most effective and easiest alternative to a true V_5 lead for monitoring myocardial ischemia.

CB_5 Lead (Central Back Lead). This lead is useful for the detection of ischemia and supraventricular arrhythmias, as was demonstrated in a study comparing CB_5 and V_5 in patients with closed and open chests (5). The P wave was 90% larger than in lead V_5, while a good correlation between ventricular deflections of CB_5 and V_5 leads was noted. CB_5 is obtained by placing the RA electrode over the center of the right scapula and the LA electrode in the V_5 position. The lead selector switch should be on lead I. The CB_5 lead may be used in patients with ischemic heart disease who are susceptible to the development of arrhythmias during the perioperative period.

When using modified bipolar limb leads, the operator should be aware that in certain aspects they differ significantly from true unipolar precordial leads. The modified precordial leads usually show a greater R-wave amplitude than standard precordial leads do, and this can result in amplification of the ST-segment response. Therefore, the criteria for diagnosing myocardial ischemia (described later) may need to be adjusted when modified bipolar leads are used. It has been shown during exercise stress testing that normalization of the degree of ST-segment depression to the height of the R wave increases the sensitivity and specificity of ECG for the recognition of myocardial ischemia (6). In an intraoperative study, Mark et al. noted that during cardiac surgery placement of a Canadian sternal retractor was associated with a reduction in V_5 R-wave amplitude from 15 ± 1 to 10 ± 1 mm (7). Simultaneously, V_5 S-wave amplitude and absolute ST-segment deviation were reduced from 3.5 ± 0.4 to 1.7 ± 0.3 mm and from 0.50 ± 0.04 to 0.39 ± 0.05 mm, respectively (Fig. 7-8). The authors concluded that their results support the proposal that inclusion of an R-wave gain factor may improve perioperative ECG monitoring.

Five-Electrode System

The use of five electrodes allows recording of the six standard limb leads (I, II, III, aVR, aVL, aVF) as well as one precordial unipolar lead. Generally, the unipolar lead is placed in the V_5 position, along the anterior axillary line in the fifth intercostal space (Fig. 7-9). With the addition of only two electrodes to the ECG system, up to seven different leads can be monitored simultaneously. Therefore, one can

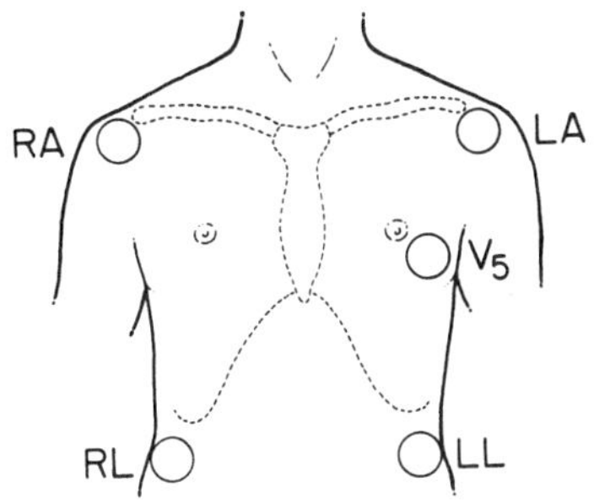

FIGURE 7-9. Standard placement of the five electrodes in a five-electrode system.

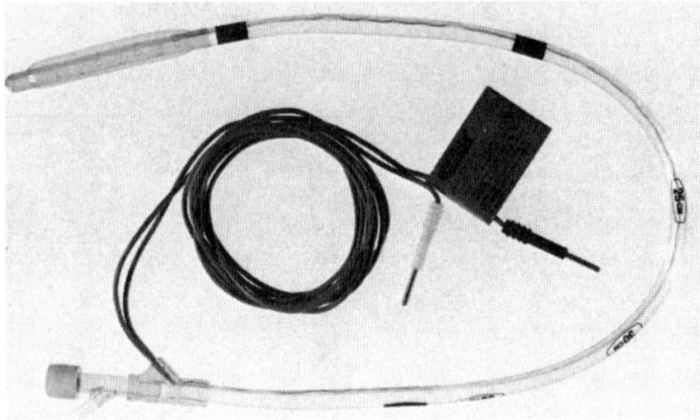

FIGURE 7-10. The Portex cardioesophagoscope. The electrocardiograph (ECG) wires are attached to lead I of the ECG monitor. (From Thys DM, Kaplan JA. *The ECG in anesthesia and critical care.* New York: Churchill Livingstone, 1987, with permission.)

monitor several areas of the myocardium for ischemia or establish a differential diagnosis between atrial and ventricular arrhythmias.

In 1976, Kaplan and King suggested monitoring lead V_5 as the leading choice for the detection of intraoperative ischemia (8). London et al. demonstrated that in high-risk patients undergoing noncardiac surgery, by using a single lead the greatest sensitivity was obtained with lead V_5 (75%), followed by lead V_4 (61%) (9). Combining leads V_4 and V_5 increased the sensitivity to 90%, whereas with the combination of standard leads II and V_5 the sensitivity was only 80%. They also suggested that if three leads (II, V_4, V_5) could be examined simultaneously, the sensitivity would rise to 98%.

Invasive Electrocardiography

The electrical potentials of the heart can be measured not only from a surface ECG but also from body cavities adjacent to the heart (esophagus or trachea), or from within the heart itself.

Esophageal Electrocardiography. The concept of esophageal ECG is not new, and numerous studies have demonstrated the usefulness of this approach in the diagnosis of complicated arrhythmias (Fig. 7-10). A prominent P wave is usually displayed in the presence of atrial depolarization, and its relation to the ventricular electrical activity can be examined (Fig. 7-11). The esophageal electrodes are incorporated into an esophageal stethoscope and welded to conventional ECG wires. To observe a bipolar esophageal ECG, the electrodes are connected to the RA and LA terminals and lead I is selected on the monitor. In one study of 20 cardiac patients, 100% of atrial arrhythmias were correctly diagnosed with the esophageal lead (using intracavitary ECG as the standard), whereas lead II led to a correct diagnosis in 54% of the cases, and V_5 in 42% of the cases (Fig. 7-12) (10). Additionally, the esophageal ECG may be helpful in the detection of posterior wall ischemia because of its proximity to the posterior aspect of the left ventricle (Fig. 7-13). To minimize the risk of esophageal burn injury, an electrocautery protection filter capable of filtering radiofrequencies greater than 20 kHz should be inserted between the ECG cable and the esophageal lead.

Intracardiac Electrocardiography. For many years, long central venous catheters filled with saline have been used to record the intracardiac ECG. More recently, Chatterjee et al. described the use of a modified balloon-tipped flotation catheter for recording intracavitary electrograms (Fig. 7-14) (11). The multipurpose pulmonary artery catheter that is presently available has all the features of a standard pulmonary artery catheter. In addition, three atrial and two ventricular electrodes have been incorporated into the catheter. These electrodes allow the recording of intracavitary ECGs and the establishment of atrial or AV pacing. The diagnostic capabilities with this catheter are great because atrial, ventricular, or AV nodal arrhythmias and conduction blocks can be demonstrated. The large voltages obtained from the intracardiac electrodes are relatively insensitive to electrocautery interference and therefore are useful for intraaortic balloon pump triggering (12). Other pulmonary artery catheters have ventricular and atrial ports, which allow passage of pacing wires. These catheters too can be used for diagnostic purposes or for therapeutic interventions (pacing).

Endotracheal Electrocardiography. The endotracheal ECG allows monitoring of the ECG when it is impractical or impossible to monitor the surface ECG. The endotracheal ECG consists of a standard endotracheal tube in which two electrodes have been embedded (Fig. 7-15). This device may be most useful for the diagnosis of atrial arrhythmias in pediatric patients (13). The same safety precautions as for esophageal ECG should be followed.

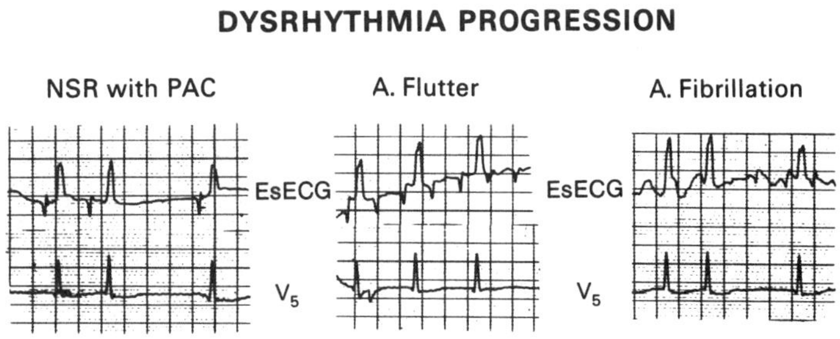

FIGURE 7-11. The esophageal electrocardiogram (EsECG) is shown on top and compared with a V_5 lead on the bottom. During cannulation of the heart, the patient progressed from normal sinus rhythm (NSR) to atrial fibrillation. PAC, premature atrial contraction. (From Kates RA, Zaidan JR, Kaplan JA. Esophageal lead for intraoperative electrocardiographic monitoring. *Anesth Analg* 1982;61:781, with permission.)

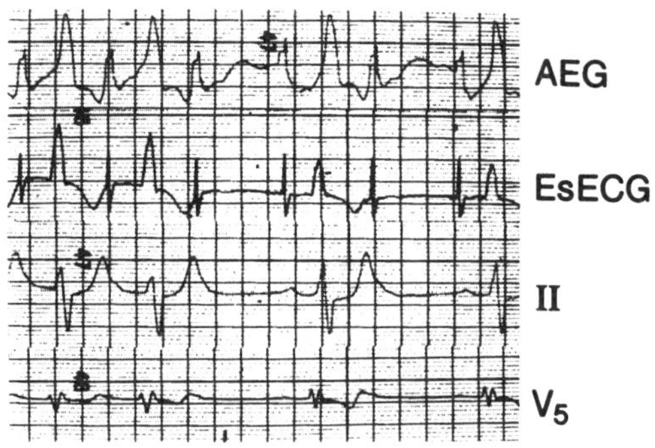

FIGURE 7-12. Four electrocardiographic leads are demonstrated in a patient after cardiopulmonary bypass. The patient progressed from a normal sinus rhythm with first-degree heart block to a Mobitz Type II block. The type of bradycardia was misdiagnosed from leads II and V_5 as sinus bradycardia, whereas the AEG and EsECG show the heart block. AEG, atrial ECG; EsECG, esophageal ECG. (From Kates RA, Zaidan JR, Kaplan JA. Esophageal lead for intraoperative electrocardiographic monitoring. *Anesth Analg* 1982;61:781, with permission.)

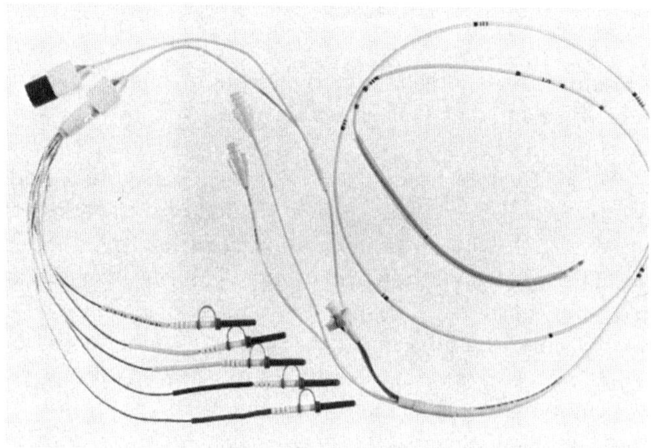

FIGURE 7-14. The multipurpose pacing Swan-Ganz catheter. Three atrial and two ventricular electrodes can be seen. (From Thys DM, Kaplan JA. *The ECG in anesthesia and critical care.* New York: Churchill Livingstone, 1987, with permission.)

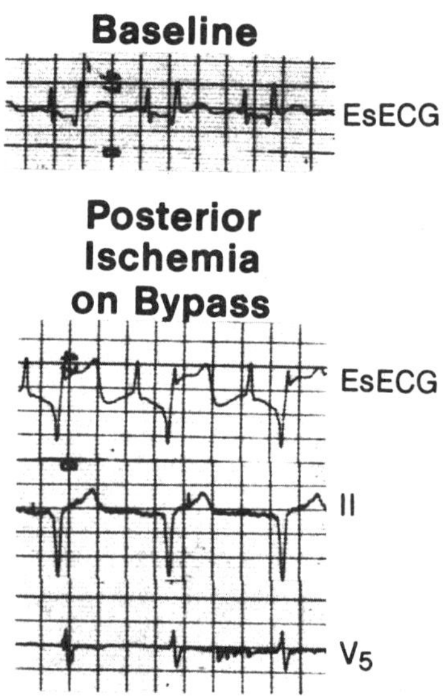

FIGURE 7-13. Posterior myocardial ischemia during cardiopulmonary bypass diagnosed on the esophageal electrocardiographic (EsECG) lead but not seen on leads II and V_5. The baseline EsECG is shown at the top. (From Kates RA, Zaidan JR, Kaplan JA. Esophageal lead for intraoperative electrocardiographic monitoring. *Anesth Analg* 1982;61:781, with permission.)

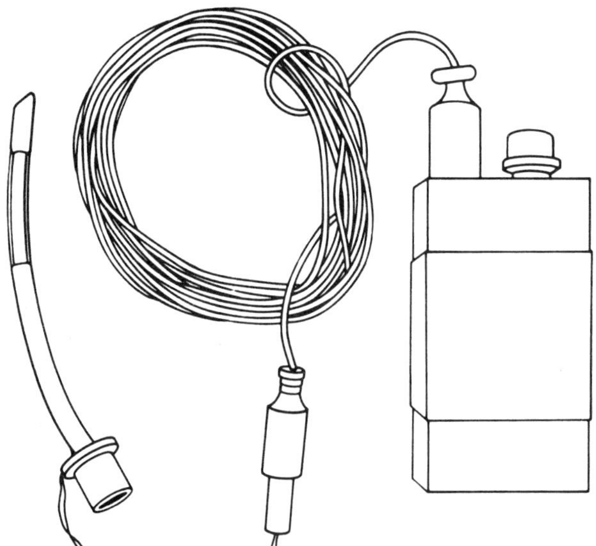

FIGURE 7-15. The endotracheal electrocardiographic system.

DISPLAY, RECORDING, AND INTERPRETATION

The American Heart Association has published instrumentation and practice standards for ECG monitoring in special care units (14). Many of the principles delineated in these standards are also applicable to intraoperative monitoring, and the interested reader is referred to them for detailed information.

Basic Requirements

The function of the ECG monitor is to detect, amplify, display, and record the ECG signal. The ECG is usually displayed on an oscilloscope, and several monitors now offer nonfade storage oscilloscopes to facilitate wave recognition. All ECG monitors for use in patients with cardiac disease should also have paper recording capabilities. The recorder is needed to make accurate diagnoses of complex arrhythmias and to allow careful analysis of all the ECG waveforms. In addition, the recorder allows one to differentiate real ECG changes from oscilloscope artifacts.

Oscilloscope Displays

Most modern oscilloscopes are high-resolution monochrome or color monitors, similar to those used in computer technology. They frequently allow considerable flexibility in screen configuration, including waveform positions, colors, and sweep speeds. The norm in modern technology is to display three ECG channels simultaneously. These usually consist of two limb leads and one unipolar precordial lead. In addition to the waveforms, average heart rates and optional arrhythmia and ST-segment information are displayed in alphanumeric format (see later discussion).

Standard Electrocardiogram Recordings

The ECG is normally recorded on special paper consisting of grids of horizontal and vertical lines. Distances between vertical lines represent time intervals, whereas distances between horizontal lines represent voltages. The lines are 1 mm apart, with every fifth line intensified. The speed of the paper is standardized to 25 mm/second. Therefore, on the horizontal axis 1 mm = 0.04 second and 0.5 cm = 0.20 second. On the vertical axis, 10 mm represents 1 mV. On every recording, a 1 cm = 1 mV calibration mark should indicate that the ECG is appropriately calibrated. The user should follow the manufacturer's recommended calibration procedure for each monitoring episode. Strip chart recorders that are part of an ECG monitoring system should meet all the standards for time-base accuracy, frequency response, and linearity proposed for conventional ECG recording systems (15,16).

Artifacts

Patient

The electrical signal that is generated by the heart and monitored by the ECG is a very weak signal, amounting to only 0.5 to 2 mV at the skin surface. It is therefore imperative that the skin be prepared optimally, to avoid signal loss at the skin-electrode interface. Hair should be removed from the electrode sites with scissors and shavers. The skin should be cleaned with alcohol and free of all dirt. It is advised to abrade the skin lightly to remove part of the stratum corneum, which can be a source of high resistance to the measured voltages. To avoid the problem of muscle artifact, electrodes should be placed over bony prominences whenever possible. Muscle movement, in the form of shivering, can produce significant ECG artifact.

Electrodes and Leads

Loose electrodes and broken leads can produce a variety of artifacts that may simulate arrhythmias, Q waves, or inverted T waves. Pregelled, disposable silver or silver chloride electrodes are usually used in the operating room. The technical standards for such electrodes have been published by the American Association for the Advancement of Medical Instrumentation (17). All the electrodes must be moist, uniform, and not out of date. Needle electrodes should be avoided because of the risk of thermal injury. Some ECG monitors have built-in cable testers that enable a lead to be tested by connecting the cable's distal end into the monitor. A high resistance causes a large voltage drop, indicating that the lead is faulty. The main source of artifact from ECG leads is loss of the integrity of the lead insulation. This results in picking up other electrical fields in the operating room, such as the 60-Hz alternating current from lights and currents from the electrocautery device. Any damaged ECG lead should be discarded for this reason. Lead movement can also result in artifact.

Operating Room Environment

Many pieces of equipment found in the operating room emit electrical fields that can interfere with the ECG: 60-Hz power lines for lights, electrosurgical equipment, cardiopulmonary equipment, and defibrillator discharges. Most of this interference can be minimized by proper shielding of the cables and leads of the cardiogram, although to date the interference created by the electrosurgical equipment cannot be reliably filtered without distortion of the ECG. Electrocautery is the most significant source of interference on the ECG in the operating room, and it usually completely obliterates the ECG tracing. Analysis of the electrocautery has identified three component frequencies. The radiofrequency between 800 and 2,000 kHz constitutes most of the interference, coupled with 60-Hz AC frequency and 0.1- to 10-Hz low-frequency noise from intermittent contact of the electrosurgical unit with the patient's tissues. Preamplifiers may be modified to suppress radiofrequency interference, but these filter circuits are still not widely available in the operating room.

Other causes of ECG artifacts in the operating room environment have been reported. Intraoperative monitoring of somatosensory evoked potentials has been known to simulate pacemaker spikes (18). They are caused by incorporation in certain monitors of a pacer enhancement circuit. This problem can be eliminated by disabling the circuit. Artifactual spikes have been noted to coincide with the drip rate in the drip chamber of a warming unit (19). The spikes were probably related to the generation of static electricity from water droplets. Use of an automated percutaneous lumbar discectomy nucleotome has been reported to simulate supraventricular tachycardia related to a mechanical interference (20).

Monitoring System

All ECG monitors use filters to narrow the bandwidth in an attempt to reduce environmental artifacts. The high-frequency filters reduce distortions from muscle movement, 60-Hz electrical current, and electromagnetic interference from other electrical equipment (21). The low-frequency filters ensure a more stable baseline by reducing respiratory and body movement artifacts, as well as those resulting from poor electrode contact. The American Heart Association recommends that a flat frequency response be obtained at a bandwidth of 0.05 to 100 Hz (14). The 100-Hz high-frequency limit ensures that tracings are of sufficient fidelity to assess QRS morphology and accurately evaluate rapid rhythms such as atrial flutter. The low-frequency limit of 0.05 Hz allows accurate representation of slower events such as P- and T-wave morphology and ST-segment excursion.

Most modern ECG monitors allow the operator a choice between several bandwidths. The actual filter frequencies tend to vary among manufacturers. One manufacturer (Hewlett-Packard, Andover, MA) allows a choice between a diagnostic mode with a bandwidth of 0.05 to 130 Hz for adults and 0.5 to 130 Hz for neonates, a monitoring mode with a bandwidth 0.5 to 40 Hz for adults and 0.5 to 60 Hz for neonates, and a filter mode with a bandwidth of 0.5 to 20 Hz.

The importance of bandwidth selection on the detection of perioperative myocardial ischemia was recently evaluated by Slogoff et al. (22). They simultaneously used five ECG systems: an Alpha 14 Model Series 3200 Cardule (Spacelabs, Redmond, WA) with bandwidths of 0.05 to 125 Hz or 0.5 to 30 Hz; a MAC II ECG (Marquette Electronics, Milwaukee, WI) with 0.05 to 40 Hz or 0.05 to 100 Hz; and a Holter recorder (Del Mar, Cincinatti, OH) at 0.1 to 100 Hz. The ST-segment positions with the three systems using the lower filter limit recommended by the American Heart Association (0.05 Hz) were similar, whereas on the Spacelabs machine (0.5 to 30 Hz) they were consistently more negative. The ST-segment displacement on the Holter was consistently less negative and less positive. In at least one automatic ST-segment analysis system (Hewlett-Packard), the lower-frequency filter (0.05 Hz) is automatically activated when the ST analyzer is turned on.

INDICATIONS

Diagnosis of Arrhythmias

Arrhythmias are common during surgery, and their causes are numerous. Bertrand et al. (23) reported an 84% incidence of supraventricular and ventricular arrhythmias in 100 patients during surgery. They are most common during endotracheal intubation or extubation and occurred more frequently in patients with preexisting cardiac disease. The major factors contributing to the development of perioperative arrhythmias are as follows:

1. Anesthetic agents. Halogenated hydrocarbons, such as halothane or enflurane, are known to produce arrhythmias, probably by a reentrant mechanism (24). Halothane has also been shown to sensitize the myocardium to endogenous and exogenous catecholamines. Drugs that block the reuptake of norepinephrine, such as cocaine and ketamine, can facilitate the development of epinephrine-induced arrhythmias.
2. Abnormal arterial blood gases or electrolytes. Hyperventilation is known to reduce serum potassium levels (25). If the preoperative potassium concentration is low, it is possible to reduce serum potassium into the 2 mEq/L range and thus precipitate severe cardiac arrhythmias. Electrolyte disturbances associated with cardiopulmonary bypass can also lead to intraoperative arrhythmias.
3. Endotracheal intubation. This may be the most common cause of arrhythmias during surgery, and it is often associated with hemodynamic alterations.
4. Reflexes. Vagal stimulation may produce sinus bradycardia and allow ventricular escape mechanisms to occur. In vascular surgery, these reflexes may be related to traction on the peritoneum or direct pressure on the vagus nerve during carotid surgery. Stimulation of the carotid sinus can also lead to arrhythmias.
5. Central nervous system stimulation and dysfunction of the autonomic nervous system.
6. Preexisting cardiac disease. Angelini et al. showed that patients with known cardiac disease have a much higher incidence of arrhythmias during anesthesia than patients without known disease (26).
7. Central venous cannulation. The insertion of catheters or wires into the central circulation often leads to arrhythmias.
8. Surgical manipulation of the cardiac structures. Arrhyth-

mias are often noted during insertion of atrial sutures or placement of venous bypass cannulas.

Once an arrhythmia is recognized, it is important to determine whether it produces a hemodynamic disturbance, what type of treatment is required, and how urgently treatment should be instituted. Treatment should be initiated promptly if the arrhythmia results in marked hemodynamic impairment. Additionally, treatment should be instituted if the arrhythmia is a precursor of a more severe arrhythmia (e.g., frequent multifocal premature ventricular contractions [PVCs] with R-on-T phenomenon can lead to ventricular fibrillation) or if the arrhythmia may be detrimental for the patient's underlying cardiac disease (e.g., tachycardia in a patient with mitral stenosis). For the detection of rhythm disturbances, the standard limb lead II is preferred, because it usually displays large P waves.

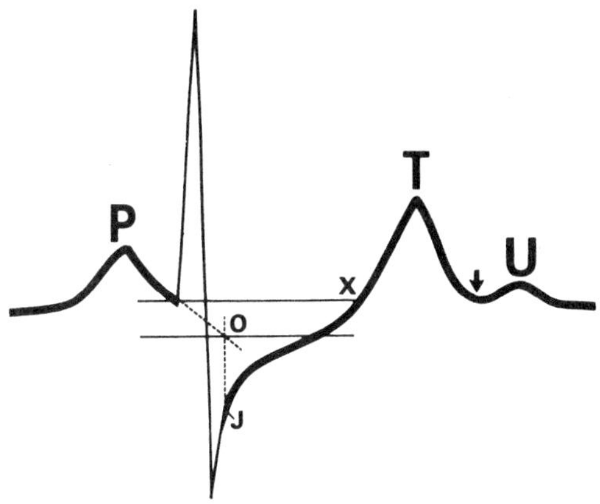

FIGURE 7-16. Diagram illustrating methods of measuring (1) true and false ST-segment depression, and (2) the degree of horizontality of the ST segment. (1) The line of the sloping PR segment is continued until it meets, at point O, a vertical line drawn from the junction of the QRS complex and ST segment. Distance O-J indicates the true amount of ST-segment depression. (2) A horizontal line drawn from the beginning of the QRS deflection is continued until it meets the T wave at point X. Distance Q-X is expressed as a percentage of the QT interval (measured from the beginning of the QRS complex to the end of the T wave at the arrow). Q-X is greater than 50% of Q-T in most true-positive tests. (From Schamroth L. *The ECG of coronary artery disease.* Oxford: Blackwell, 1984, with permission.)

Diagnosis of Ischemia

Factors that predispose to the development of perioperative ischemia include the presence of preexisting coronary artery disease and perioperative events that affect the myocardial oxygen balance. A number of perioperative clinical studies have found a high incidence of ECG evidence of ischemia (20% to 80%) in patients with coronary artery disease undergoing cardiac or noncardiac surgery (27,28). In the anesthetized patient, the detection of ischemia by ECG becomes even more important because the hallmark symptom of angina is not available.

In recent years, it has also become evident that a significant number of patients experience asymptomatic or "silent" ischemia (29). Ischemia is manifested by characteristic ECG signs of myocardial ischemia in the absence of angina and is not necessarily associated with changes in hemodynamics or heart rate. Among patients with chronic stable angina who have ST-segment depression during exercise, ambulatory ECG monitoring during daily life identifies transient ambulant ischemic episodes in approximately 40% to 50%. In these patients, silent ischemic episodes account for about 75% of all ambulant ischemic episodes (30).

The ECG changes occurring during myocardial ischemia are often characteristic and can be detected with careful ECG monitoring. Although the ECG criteria for ischemia were established in patients undergoing exercise stress testing, they may also be applied to anesthetized patients (Fig. 7-16). These criteria are (a) horizontal or downsloping ST-segment depression of 0.1 mV, (b) ST-segment elevation of 0.1 mV in a non–Q-wave lead, (c) slowly upsloping ST-segment depression of 0.2 mV (all measured from 60 to 80 msec after the J point) (Fig. 7-17) (31). Okin et al. studied the relation of the time after the J point at which ST depression is measured to the magnitude of ST-segment depression during peak exercise (32). They found that a positive exercise ECG (0.1 mV or more of additional horizontal or downsloping ST-segment depression at the end of exercise) had a specificity of 96% for coronary artery disease when ST-segment depression was measured at either the J point or J + 60 msec. There were no differences in sensitivity of ECG criteria at the J point or J + 60 msec. However, at J + 60 msec there were significant differences in ST-segment depression at peak exercise among normal subjects, patients with clinical angina, and patients with documented coronary artery disease.

It is also commonly believed that monitoring for intraoperative myocardial ischemia is unnecessary in neonates. Whereas ECG lead systems for adults are concerned with the detection of ischemia as well as arrhythmias, neonatal ECG monitoring has focused on arrhythmia recognition

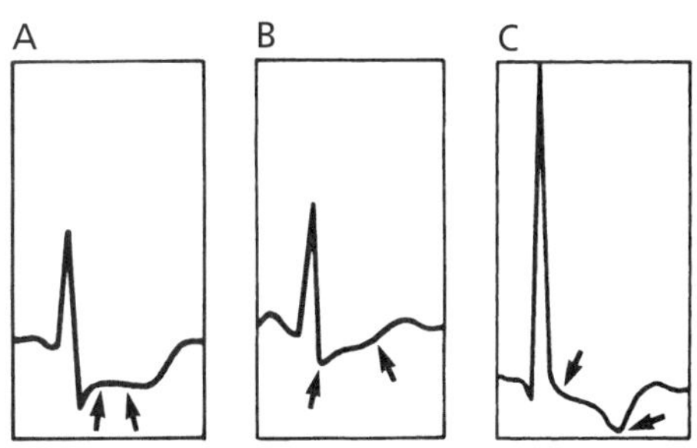

FIGURE 7-17. A: Horizontal ST segment. **B:** Upsloping ST segment. **C:** Downsloping ST segment. The arrows indicate the beginning and end of the ST segment.

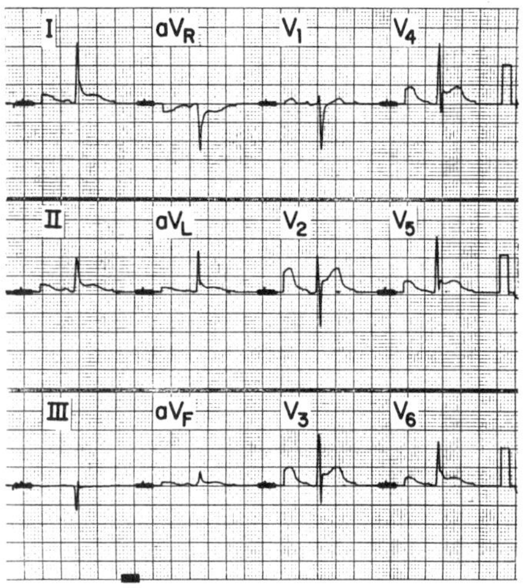

FIGURE 7-18. Acute pericarditis in a patient in the early postoperative period after coronary artery bypass grafting. The ST origins are elevated above the baseline defined by the TP segment, and the PR segments are depressed. (From Thys DM, Kaplan JA. *The ECG in anesthesia and critical care.* New York: Churchill Livingstone, 1987, with permission.)

alone. Some studies, however, suggest that the neonatal heart is more susceptible to ischemia than the adult heart (33). They have demonstrated the importance of calibrated ECG monitoring in neonates with congenital heart disease.

Although ST-segment analysis provides sensitive information about myocardial ischemia, in about 10% of patients underlying ECG abnormalities hinder the analysis. Such abnormalities include hypokalemia, digitalis administration, left bundle branch block, Wolff-Parkinson-White syndrome, left ventricular hypertrophy with strain, and acute pericarditis (Fig. 7-18). In these patients other diagnostic modalities, such as transesophageal echocardiography (TEE), should be considered.

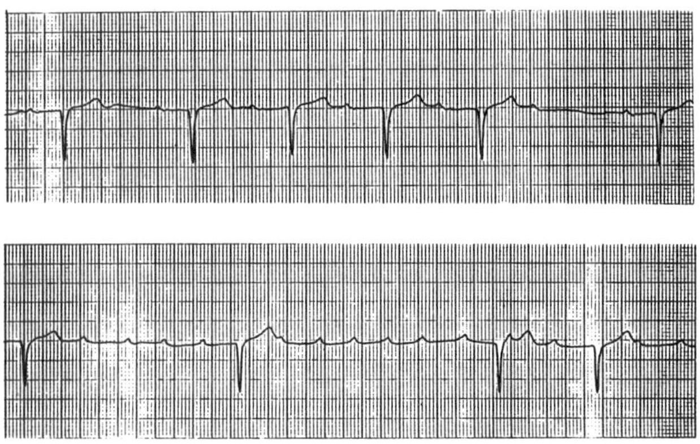

FIGURE 7-19. Top: Second-degree atrioventricular (AV) block (Mobitz Type I), which 1 hour later progressed to a third-degree AV block **(bottom)**. (From Thys DM, Kaplan JA. *The ECG in anesthesia and critical care.* New York: Churchill Livingstone, 1987, with permission.)

Diagnosis of Conduction Defects

Conduction defects can also occur during surgery. They can result from passage of the pulmonary artery catheter through the right ventricle, or they can be a manifestation of myocardial ischemia. Because high-grade conduction defects (second- and third-degree AV blocks) often have deleterious effects on hemodynamic performance, their intraoperative recognition is important (Fig. 7-19).

AUTOMATIC RECORDING

Holter monitoring has been used by a number of anesthesiologists to document the perioperative incidence of arrhythmias and ischemia. In Holter monitoring, ECG information from one or two bipolar leads is recorded by a miniature magnetic tape recorder. Up to 48 hours of ECG signals can be collected. Subsequently, the tape is processed by a playback system and the ECG signals are analyzed. On most modern systems the playback unit includes a dedicated computer for rapid analysis of the data and automatic recognition of arrhythmias. A significant limitation of traditional Holter monitoring in the perioperative period is that recordings are usually analyzed and interpreted retrospectively. A real-time Holter monitor not only records specific ECG segments for later playback but also analyzes the rhythm and ST segment in real time and alerts the user to acute perturbations (34). The application of Holter monitoring is, as of yet, primarily limited to the research environment.

The Q-Med device (Q-Med Inc., Clark, NJ) is a small continuous ECG recording device that has been used in patients undergoing cardiac and noncardiac surgery (35,36). The device not only records the ECG signals but also performs an automatic analysis of the ECG tracing and sounds an alarm when ischemic changes are recognized. Abnormal events are selectively stored and are subsequently retrievable.

COMPUTER-ASSISTED ELECTROCARDIOGRAM INTERPRETATION

Modern monitoring equipment is highly computerized, and most of the physiologic information is manipulated, analyzed, and stored in digital format. Therefore, an early step in data collection involves the conversion of analog signals (time-variable voltages of amplitudes) into the digital format with an analog-to-digital converter. Once in the digital format, the physiologic information can readily be subjected to a variety of analyses. In ECG, the most common analyses, besides rate calculations, are related to arrhythmia recognition and the detection of myocardial ischemia.

Arrhythmias

There is little doubt that during prolonged visual observation of the ECG on the oscilloscope, certain arrhythmias will go undetected. This was clearly demonstrated by Romhilt et al., who showed that coronary care unit nurses failed to detect serious ventricular arrhythmias in 84% of their patients (37). Computers have, therefore, been designed for the automatic detection of arrhythmias in an attempt to increase the detection of abnormal rhythms. Using an early preprocessing algorithm called AZTEC, a computer accurately detected 78% of ventricular ectopic beats. It measured QRS width, offset, amplitude, and area to classify complexes in morphologic families (38). In a prospective evaluation of such a system, it was found that the computer accurately detected 95.4% of ventricular premature beats but only 82.4% of supraventricular premature beats.

Other systems have depended on QRS recognition and cross-correlation with stored QRS complexes (39). In cross-correlation, each detected QRS complex is compared with a list of previously detected complexes. If a complex does not correlate more closely than 0.9 with a previously stored complex, it is considered to have a new configuration and is added to the list (Fig. 7-20). A number of points of the complex, such as PR interval and ST segment, are stored as a template for future comparison. Whenever a new complex matches an existing template, it is averaged into that template so that each template represents a running average of all complexes of a particular configuration (40). Each template is defined as normal, abnormal, or questionable, according to previously defined criteria. The American Heart Association has published several parameters that need to be tested to permit a meaningful understanding of a system's values and limitations and to allow a reasonable comparison among systems (14).

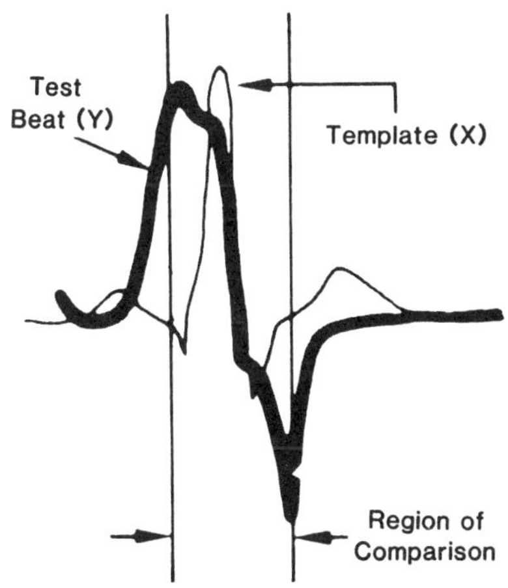

FIGURE 7-20. Computerized "template" of the underlying normal QRS complex (*X*) and an ectopic complex termed a "test beat" (*Y*). Beat Y is matched to beat X by the computer during the region of comparison by cross-correlation algorithms. (From Morganroth J. Ambulatory Holter electrocardiography. *Ann Intern Med* 1985;102:73, with permission.)

Myocardial Ischemia

Several computer programs for on-line detection of ischemia and analysis of ST segments are available commercially. Each manufacturer uses different analysis techniques, and not all the algorithms are in the public domain.

In one system (Marquette Electronics), an ST learning phase begins by observing the first 16 beats, in all leads, for the dominant normal or paced shape. The shapes are correlated using a selected number of points on each of the active, valid lead waveforms. An algorithm searches for leads in the fail or artifact mode to determine the number of valid leads used in the analysis. The algorithm also makes all leads positive to enable totaling the sum of the points on the valid leads. This sum is used in determining a peak or fiducial point. The fiducial point is used as a point of reference on the QRS. A template is formed from selected points around the fiducial point for each ECG lead. As each beat is analyzed, its template is compared with templates of previous beats. If the template correlates within 75% of a previously stored shape, it is deemed a match and is classified as an existing shape. If there is no match, it becomes a new shape. On the 17th beat, the dominant normal QRS shape or paced shape is determined. The algorithm then searches for an additional 16 beats that correlate with the dominant template. With the 18th beat a process called incremental averaging is initiated. The incremental averaging is a method of tracking positive or negative changes occurring on the waveform. These changes are tracked for each of the valid leads. The changes may be physiologic, such as ST-segment changes caused by ischemia, or they may be related to artifact caused by high-frequency noise. The tracking of the changes is achieved by allowing only a 0.1-mm adjustment, either positive or negative, from the previous shape of each beat. On the 32nd beat, the product of the incrementally averaged templates becomes the learned ST template. Until ST is relearned, all changes in the QRS shape are tracked against this learned template. The isoelectric point and ST points are determined during the learning phase and are based on the width of the QRS shape. The isoelectric point is placed 40 msec before the onset of the QRS, and the ST point is placed 60 msec past the offset of the QRS measurement. The isoelectric point provides the point of reference for determining the ST-segment measurement. The technique of incremental averaging is well suited to a continuous input with slow changes. However, it links the speed at which changes occur in the template to the heart rate (41). This system was recently evaluated intraoperatively in patients undergoing cardiac surgery (42). The device monitored three selected leads and displayed the absolute values of the ST segment as a line. Upward deflection of the trend line indicated worsening ischemia, whereas a downward trend reflected return of the ST segment toward the isoelectric line. The authors concluded that once the device was clinically accepted, the awareness of ischemic changes was heightened among participating anesthesiologists and therapeutic interventions were more rapidly instituted.

Other systems differ from the one just described in various ways. In the Hewlett-Packard system, a period of 15 seconds is analyzed first, and the ST displacement is determined on five "good" beats. These displacements are ranked, and the median value is determined. This eliminates the influence of occasional PVCs and ensures that a representative beat is selected. The objective of this procedure is to obtain a representative beat rather than an average template. The measurement point for the ST segment can be selected as the R wave + 108 msec (default), the J point + 60 msec, or the J point + 80 msec. ST values and representative complexes are stored at 1-minute resolution for the most recent 30-minute trend, and at 5-minute resolution for the preceding 7.5-hour trend. In a third system (Spacelabs), a composite ST-segment waveform is developed every 30 seconds and compared with a reference tracing acquired during an initial learning period. The isoelectric and ST points can be manually adjusted to any location on the ECG tracing or automatically set to predetermined values.

In recent years, a few comparisons of the various ST-segment analysis systems have been conducted. They have also been compared with other techniques for the intraoperative diagnosis of myocardial ischemia. Ellis et al. compared ST-segment analysis systems (Hewlett-Packard and Marquette) with standard ECG and TEE (43). They observed that monitors of intraoperative myocardial ischemia often do not agree with each other. Although ST-segment monitoring showed good agreement with the standard ECG, neither had the sensitivity of TEE. Leung et al. compared ST-segment trend monitoring (Hewlett-Packard, Marquette, and Datex) with Holter monitoring in 94 patients undergoing coronary artery bypass grafting (44). They observed sensitivities for the detection of ischemia of 75%, 78%, and 69%, respectively. They identified small R-wave morphology, baseline drift, and conduction abnormalities as conditions that contributed to the inaccuracy.

To better define the role of QRS morphology on automated ST-segment analysis, London et al. (45) bench-tested a commercially available ECG monitor (PC2 Bedside Monitor, ECG software version 6.05.16, Spacelabs) using an ECG simulator (M311 Fogg System, Aurora, CO). Using seven different QRS shapes, they noted subtle errors in placement of the J point for each of the QRS shapes. In two QRS shapes, the isoelectric point was displaced onto the upstroke of the R-wave, leading to erroneous ST-segment values. Because each manufacturer uses distinct analysis algorithms, differences in results are to be expected, and the authors suggested that common testing standards should be developed. They believe that the factors leading to differences between manufacturers are the location of the fiducial point or points and the number of measurement points that are being used.

TREATMENT OF ARRHYTHMIAS

The diagnosis and treatment of arrhythmias can be simplified by using the following six questions as a checklist when looking at an ECG display and attempting to decide whether treatment is necessary (46):

1. What is the heart rate?
2. Is the rhythm regular?
3. Is there one P wave for each QRS complex?
4. Is the QRS complex normal?
5. Is the rhythm dangerous?
6. Does the rhythm require treatment?

Some common intraoperative arrhythmias to which the six questions should be applied are as follows.

Sinus Bradycardia

The pacemaker site is in the sinus node, but the rate is slower than normal (Fig. 7-21). Etiologic factors include drug effects, acute inferior myocardial infarction, hypoxia, vagal stimulation, and high sympathetic blockade. Sinus bradycardia accounts for 11% of intraoperative arrhythmias.

1. Heart rate. This is 40 to 60 beats/minute (if the patient is receiving chronic β-blocker therapy, it is less than 50 beats/minute).
2. Rhythm. The rhythm is regular, except for occasional escape beats from other pacemaker sites.
3. P:QRS. There is a 1:1 relation between the P waves and the QRS complexes.
4. QRS complex. This is normal.
5. Significance. Heart rates slower than 40 beats/minute are poorly tolerated, even in healthy patients, and should

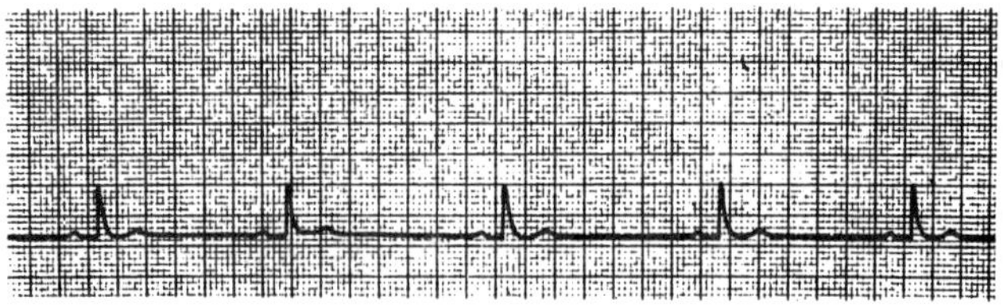

FIGURE 7-21. Sinus bradycardia with an intrinsic rate of about 45 beats/minute. Also notice that the patient has a mild sinus arrhythmia with variations in heart rate associated with respirations. (From Kaplan JA, Thys DM. Electrocardiography. In: Miller R, ed. *Anesthesia,* 3rd ed. New York: Churchill Livingstone, 1990, with permission.)

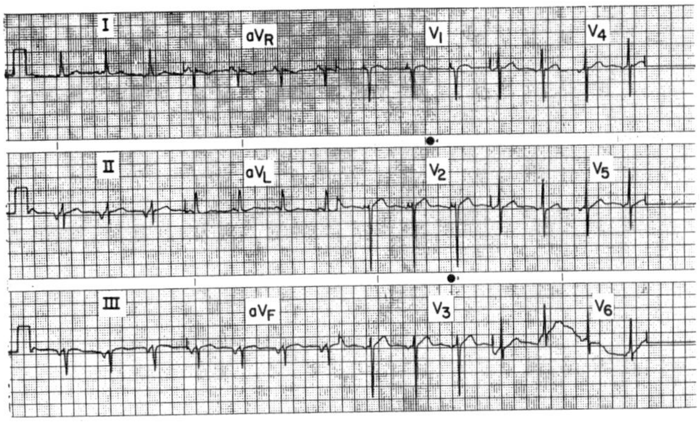

FIGURE 7-22. Ectopic atrial rhythm in a patient with left axis deviation. The rhythm is also termed coronary sinus rhythm. Note the inverted P waves in leads II, III, and aVF. (From Thys DM, Kaplan JA. *The ECG in anesthesia and critical care.* New York: Churchill Livingstone, 1987, with permission.)

be evaluated on the basis of their effect on cardiac output. Treatment is recommended if hypotension, ventricular arrhythmias, or signs of poor peripheral perfusion are observed. A sinus bradycardia may be part of the sick sinus syndrome, in which sinus node dysfunction can precipitate bradycardias, heart block, tachyarrhythmias, or alternating bradytachyarrhythmias (Fig. 7-22) (47).

6. Treatment. Usually none is necessary, but a progression from atropine (0.4 to 2 mg IV) to ephedrine (5 to 25 mg IV) to isoproterenol (1 to 4 mg IV) to temporary transvenous pacemaker insertion may be necessary for severe or refractory sinus bradycardia.

Sinus Tachycardia

The pacemaker site is in the sinus node, but the rate is faster than normal (Fig. 7-23). Sinus tachycardia is the most commonly occurring arrhythmia in the perioperative period. It occurs with such frequency that it is not included in most incidence studies. Common causes include pain, inadequate anesthesia, hypovolemia, fever, hypoxia, hypercarbia, heart failure, and drug effects.

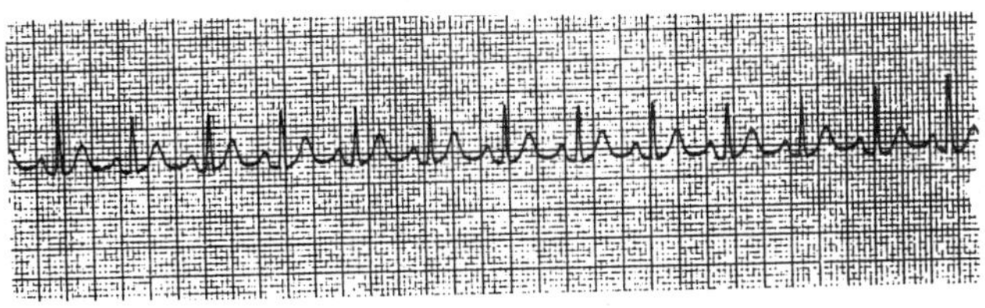

FIGURE 7-23. Sinus tachycardia with an intrinsic rate greater than 100 beats/minute. (From Kaplan JA, Thys DM. Electrocardiography. In: Miller R, ed. *Anesthesia,* 3rd ed. New York: Churchill Livingstone, 1990, with permission.)

1. Heart rate. The rate is greater than 100 beats/minute and can reach 170 beats/minute, which may be seen with a severe episode of hyperpyrexia.
2. Rhythm. This is regular.
3. P:QRS. The relation is 1:1.
4. QRS complex. This complex is normal. There may be associated ST-segment depression with severe increases in heart rate and resulting myocardial ischemia.
5. Significance. Prolonged tachycardias in patients with underlying heart disease can precipitate congestive heart failure owing to the increased myocardial work required. The tachycardia decreases coronary perfusion time, which can cause secondary ST–T-wave changes and can precipitate angina pectoris in patients with coronary artery disease. A major diagnostic problem is encountered when the heart rate is 150 beats/minute, because this is a common rate for a sinus tachycardia, a paroxysmal atrial tachycardia (PAT), or an atrial flutter with a 2:1 block. These three arrhythmias can sometimes be separated by the use of carotid sinus massage, intravenous administration of edrophonium, or atrial or esophageal ECG leads to identify more accurately the P waves on the ECG.
6. Treatment. The underlying disorder should be treated. If necessary, while determining the cause, esmolol or propranolol should be used in patients with ischemic heart disease who develop ST-segment changes to prevent further myocardial ischemia.

Sinus Arrhythmia

The pacemaker impulse arises from the SA node, but the arrhythmia is manifested by alternating periods of slower and faster heart rates (Fig. 7-24). The PR interval is normal, as is the QRS complex. Most commonly but not invariably, the rate increases with inspiration and decreases with expiration. It occurs more often in children than in adults.

1. Heart rate. The rate is 60 to 100 beats/minute.
2. Rhythm. The rhythm is irregular.
3. P:QRS. The relation is 1:1.
4. QRS complex. The complex is normal.
5. Significance. This is a normal finding.
6. Treatment. No treatment is necessary.

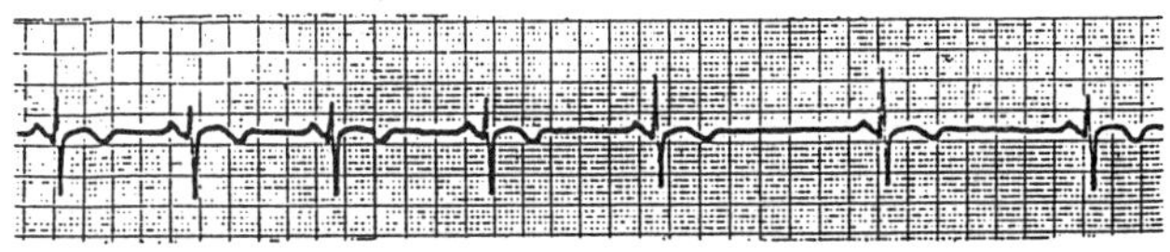

FIGURE 7-24. Sinus arrhythmia. Note the normal PR interval and QRS complex. (From Kaplan JA, Thys DM. Electrocardiography. In: Miller R, ed. *Anesthesia,* 3rd ed. New York: Churchill Livingstone, 1990, with permission.)

Premature Atrial Contraction

An ectopic pacemaker site in either the left or the right atrium initiates the premature atrial contraction (PAC) (Fig. 7-25). The shape of the P wave is abnormal and possibly inverted. The PR interval may be shorter or longer than normal, depending on the site of the ectopic focus and the refractoriness of the AV nodal pathway. The PAC spreads not only through the AV node and ventricular conduction system but also, in a retrograde fashion, reaches the SA node, thus resetting the sinus pacemaker. The interval from the PAC to the next sinus beat is therefore a normal sinus cycle (i.e., no compensatory pause). The absence of a compensatory pause is a major feature distinguishing PACs from PVCs. Occasionally, PACs may find part of the ventricular conduction system refractory. In that case, they will travel down an aberrant pathway and create an abnormal QRS complex. They are then called PACs with ventricular aberration and can easily be confused with PVCs. Because the recovery period of the right ventricular conduction system outlasts that of the left, the most common form of aberration appears as a right bundle branch block. Helpful points in separating a PAC with aberration from a PVC are the following: (a) there is a preceding P wave, usually abnormally shaped; (b) the QRS complex has a right bundle branch block configuration; (c) there is an rsR′ in V_1; and (d) the initial vector forces are identical with the preceding beat (they are usually the opposite with a PVC). Other characteristics of PACs are as follows:

1. Heart rate. Heart rate is variable, depending on the frequency of PAC.
2. Rhythm. The rhythm is irregular.
3. P:QRS. The relation is usually 1:1. The P waves have various shapes and may even be lost in the QRS or T waves. Occasionally, the P wave is so early as to find the ventricle refractory, and a nonconducted beat occurs.
4. QRS complex. This is usually normal, unless there is ventricular aberration.
5. Significance. In one study PACs represented 10% of all intraoperative arrhythmias. They have little clinical significance, but frequent PACs may lead to other more serious supraventricular arrhythmias or may be a sign of digitalis intoxication.
6. Treatment. Treatment is rarely necessary, but digitalis, β-blockers, or verapamil may be considered if hemodynamic function is impaired.

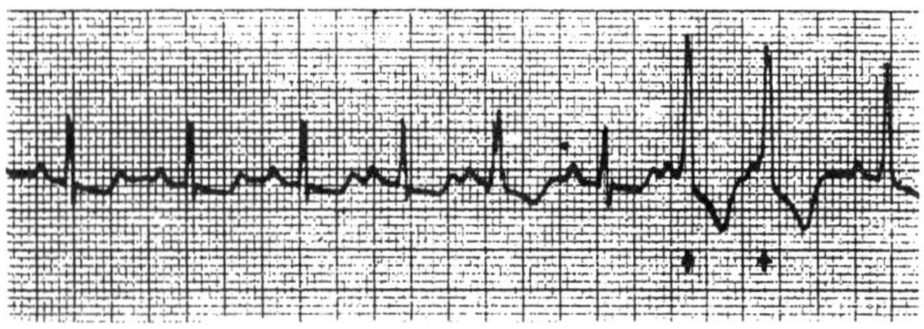

FIGURE 7-25. Electrocardiographic tracing with multiple premature atrial contractions. The fourth beat shows no aberration, while the fifth beat shows partial aberration and the seventh and eighth beats *(arrows)* show marked aberration. (From Kaplan JA, Thys DM. Electrocardiography. In: Miller R, ed. *Anesthesia,* 3rd ed. New York: Churchill Livingstone, 1990, with permission.)

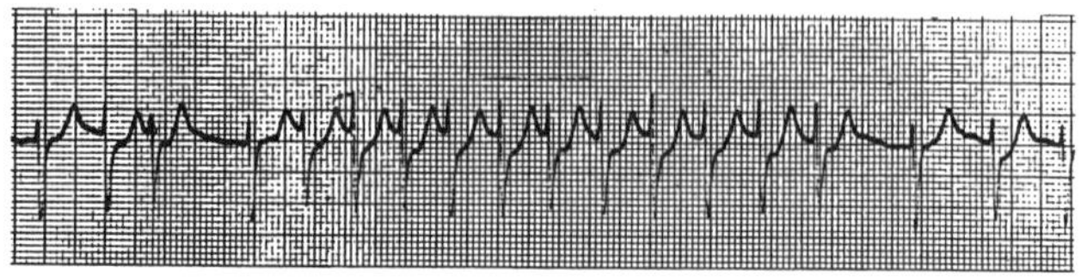

FIGURE 7-26. Paroxysmal atrial tachycardia. (From Kaplan JA, Thys DM. Electrocardiography. In: Miller R, ed. *Anesthesia,* 3rd ed. New York: Churchill Livingstone, 1990, with permission.)

Paroxysmal Atrial Tachycardia

A run of rapidly repeated supraventricular premature beats from a site other than the SA node characterizes PAT (Fig. 7-26). The inclusion of tachycardias originating in the AV node allows for the useful classification of paroxysmal supraventricular tachycardias (SVT) (Fig. 7-27). The rhythm is usually abrupt in both its onset and its termination.

1. Heart rate. The heart rate is 150 to 250 beats/minute.
2. Rhythm. The rhythm is usually regular, unless the impulse originates from multiple atrial foci.
3. P:QRS. There is a 1:1 relation, although the P wave is often hidden in the QRS complex or T wave.
4. QRS complex. Generally normal, but ST–T-wave changes indicative of ischemia may be noted. Aberration of ventricular conduction may occur, thus complicating

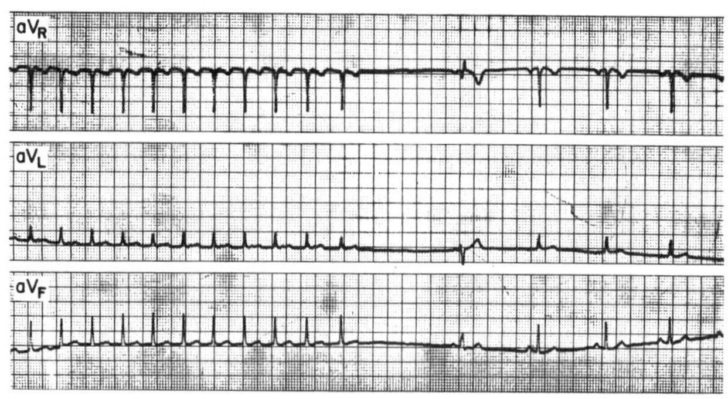

FIGURE 7-27. Paroxysmal supraventricular tachycardia with P waves visible in the ST segment. Vagal tone induced by carotid sinus massage resulted in momentary slowing, interruption of the reentrant circuit, and termination of the tachycardia. This was followed by an escape complex and then by restitution of sinus rhythm. (From Thys DM, Kaplan JA. *The ECG in anesthesia and critical care.* New York: Churchill Livingstone, 1987, with permission.)

the differential diagnosis with ventricular tachycardia. SVT may also be confused with sinus tachycardia, atrial flutter, and atrial fibrillation. In differentiating these rhythms, carotid sinus massage and edrophonium (5 to 10 mg IV) may be used to slow the rate. Esophageal ECG leads, to define atrial activity more accurately, may also be helpful.

5. Significance. Paroxysmal SVT can be seen in 5% of normal young adults and in patients with Wolff-Parkinson-White syndrome or other aberrant conduction pathway syndromes. During anesthesia, it constitutes 2.5% of all arrhythmias, and it has been associated with intrinsic heart disease, systemic illness, thyrotoxicosis, digitalis toxicity, pulmonary embolism, and pregnancy. Under anesthesia, it can be precipitated by changes in the autonomic nervous system, drug effects, or volume shifts and can produce severe hemodynamic deterioration. At times the PAT may be associated with AV block, owing to the fast atrial rate and slow AV conduction. PAT with 2:1 block represents digitalis intoxication in many patients.
6. Treatment. This arrhythmia must often be treated because of its rapid rate and associated poor hemodynamic function. Several steps can be taken to treat this arrhythmia:
   a. Vagal maneuvers such as carotid sinus massage, which should be applied only to one side.
   b. Adenosine, in adults, as a rapid intravenous bolus of 6 mg, followed by 12 mg one minute later if the SVT persists.
   c. Verapamil (5 to 10 mg IV), which terminates AV nodal reentry successfully in about 90% of cases.
   d. Esmolol (1 mg/kg bolus and 50 to 200 $mg \cdot kg^{-1} \cdot min^{-1}$ infusion), which has been shown to be effective.
   e. Propranolol in 0.5-mg IV bolus doses.
   f. Edrophonium in 5- to 10-mg IV bolus doses.
   g. Phenylephrine (100 mg IV bolus) if the patient is hypotensive.
   h. Intravenous digitalization with one of the short-acting digitalis preparations: ouabain (0.25 to 0.5 mg IV) or digoxin (0.5 to 1.0 mg IV).
   i. Rapid overdrive pacing, in an effort to capture the ectopic focus.
   j. Cardioversion with appropriate synchronization.

Atrial Flutter

Atrial flutters represent a faster discharge from an irritable focus in the atria than does a rapid atrial tachycardia (Fig. 7-28). Because it is so fast, it is usually associated with AV block. Classic sawtooth flutter waves (F waves) are usually present. The characteristics of atrial flutter are as follows:

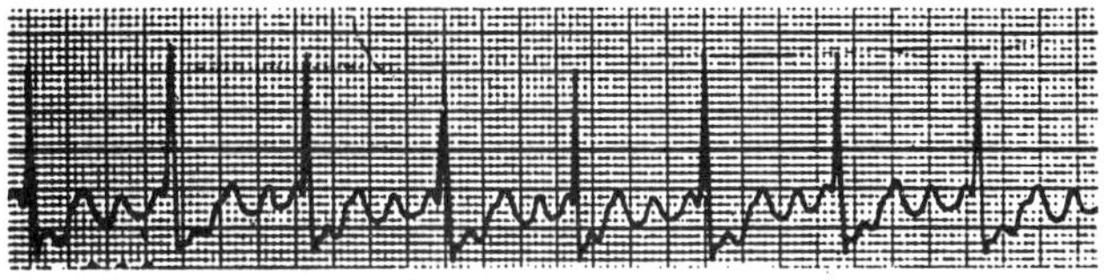

FIGURE 7-28. Classic sawtoothed flutter waves (F waves) are seen in this patient with atrial flutter. (From Kaplan JA, Thys DM. Electrocardiography. In: Miller R, ed. *Anesthesia,* 3rd ed. New York: Churchill Livingstone, 1990, with permission.)

1. Heart rate. The atrial heart rate is 250 to 350 beats/minute with a ventricular rate of about 150 beats/minute.
2. Rhythm. The atrial rhythm is regular. The ventricular rhythm may be regular if a fixed AV block is present or irregular if a variable block exists.
3. P:QRS. Usually there is a 2:1 block with an atrial rate of 300 beats/minute and a ventricular rate of 150 beats/minute, but it may vary between 2:1 and 8:1. F waves are best seen in leads V_1 or II or the esophageal lead.
4. QRS complex. This is normal. T waves are lost in the F waves.
5. Significance. It usually indicates the presence of severe heart disease. It is seen with increased incidence in patients with coronary artery disease, mitral valve disease, pulmonary embolism, hyperthyroidism, cardiac trauma, malignant cancers of the heart, and myocarditis.
6. Treatment.
   a. The initial treatment of choice, synchronous direct current cardioversion with very low voltages (10 to 40 W-sec), which is effective in more than 90% of cases (48).
   b. Rapid atrial pacing, which effectively terminates atrial flutter in many patients and results in a return to sinus rhythm or atrial fibrillation with a slow ventricular rate.
   c. Esmolol (1 mg/kg IV bolus).
   d. Verapamil (5 to 10 mg IV).
   e. Digitalis with or without propranolol.

Atrial Fibrillation

Atrial fibrillation is an excessively rapid and irregular atrial focus with no P waves appearing on the ECG but instead a fine fibrillatory activity called F waves (Fig. 7-29). This

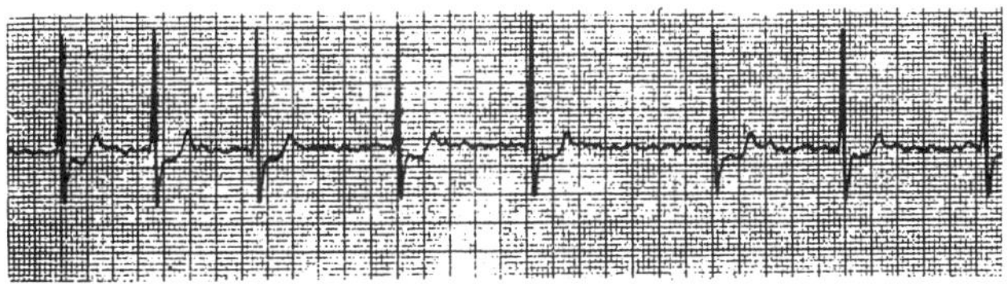

FIGURE 7-29. Atrial fibrillation with fine fibrillatory activity. Note the irregularly irregular pattern of the QRS complexes. (From Kaplan JA, Thys DM. Electrocardiography. In: Miller R, ed. *Anesthesia,* 3rd ed. New York: Churchill Livingstone, 1990, with permission.)

is the most irregular rhythm: it is called "irregularly irregular" and may be associated with a pulse deficit. The characteristics are as follows:

1. Heart rate. The atrial rate is 350 to 500 beats/minute, and the ventricular rate is between 60 and 170 beats/minute.
2. Rhythm. The rhythm is irregularly irregular.
3. P : QRS. P wave is absent and is replaced by F waves or no obvious atrial activity at all.
4. QRS complex. This is normal.
5. Significance. The etiologic factors of atrial fibrillation are similar to those of atrial flutter. This rhythm is almost invariably associated with significant cardiac disease. The clinical significance and treatment of atrial fibrillation are also similar to those of atrial flutter, except for two important considerations. The loss of an atrial kick secondary to inefficient contraction of the atria reduces ventricular filling and may significantly compromise cardiac output. In addition, atrial fibrillation may lead to the formation of atrial thrombi with resultant pulmonary and systemic embolization.
6. Treatment. Digitalis is most commonly used to slow the ventricular rate on a chronic basis. Esmolol is very effective in the perioperative period and may lead to a higher rate of conversion to sinus rhythm than verapamil.

Junctional Rhythms

The AV node itself shows no intrinsic phase 4 depolarization; therefore, cells in the node cannot act as pacemakers (Fig. 7-30). Ectopic activity, however, may be initiated from sites just above and below the node. It would make sense to consider these arrhythmias as AV junctional in nature. The resultant P wave is abnormal and, depending on the position of the ectopic pacemaker, may be very close to, buried in, or after the QRS complex. Depending on the rate of fire of the ectopic pacemaker, the resultant rhythm will be nodal premature; nodal quadrigeminy, trigeminy, or bigeminy; nodal rhythm; or nodal tachycardia.

1. Heart rate. The rate is variable, 40 to 180 beats/minute (nodal bradycardia to tachycardia).
2. Rhythm. Rhythm is regular.
3. P : QRS. This relation is 1 : 1, but there are three varieties.
   a. High-nodal rhythm: the impulse reaches the atrium before the ventricle; therefore, the P wave precedes the QRS but has a shortened PR interval (less than 0.1 second)
   b. Midnodal rhythm: the impulse reaches the atrium and the ventricle at the same time. The P wave is lost in the QRS.
   c. Low-nodal rhythm: the impulse reaches the ventricle first and then the atrium, so that the P wave follows the QRS complex.
4. QRS complex. This is normal, unless altered by the P wave.
5. Significance. Junctional rhythms are common under anesthesia (about 20%), especially with halogenated anesthetic agents. The junctional rhythms frequently decrease blood pressure and cardiac output by about 15% but can reduce it up to 30% in patients with heart disease (49).
6. Treatment. Usually no treatment is required, and the rhythm reverts spontaneously. If hypotension and poor perfusion are associated with the rhythm, treatment is indicated. Atropine, ephedrine, or isoproterenol can be used in an effort to increase the activity of the SA node so that it will take over as the pacemaker. A small dose of succinylcholine (10 mg IV) may cause a nodal rhythm to revert to a sinus rhythm during anesthesia with halothane or enflurane. This probably works as a result of the effect of succinylcholine as a sympathetic ganglionic stimulator. In some cases, propranolol may correct the rhythm disturbance if it has resulted from sympathetic stimulation.

Premature Ventricular Contractions

PVCs result from ectopic pacemaker activity arising from below the AV junction (Fig. 7-31). The PVC originates in and spreads through the myocardium or ventricular conducting system, resulting in a wide (0.12-second), bizarre QRS complex. The ST segment usually slopes in the direc-

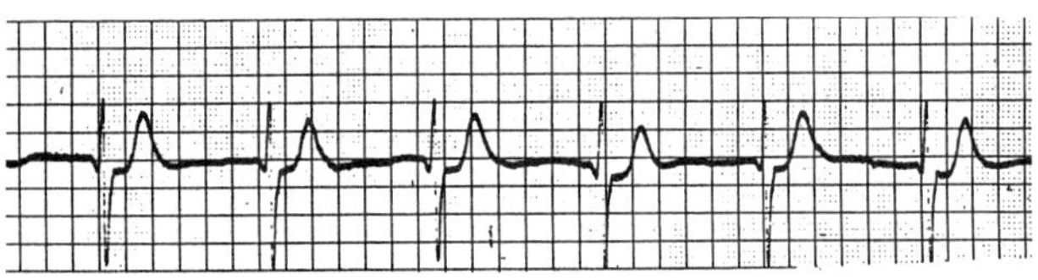

FIGURE 7-30. Junctional rhythm. Note that the P waves are buried in the QRS complex. (From Kaplan JA, Thys DM. Electrocardiography. In: Miller R, ed. *Anesthesia,* 3rd ed. New York: Churchill Livingstone, 1990, with permission.)

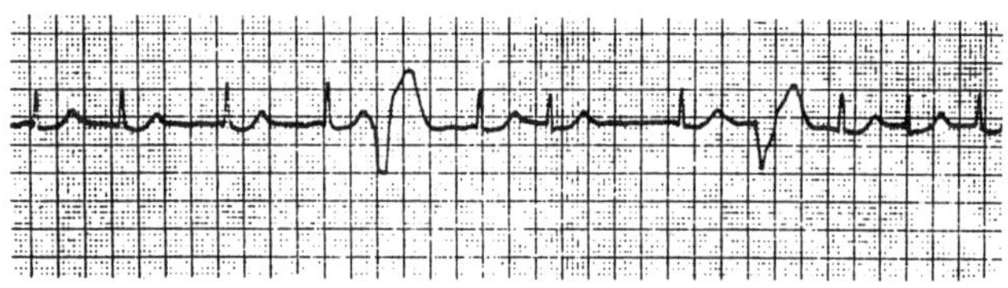

FIGURE 7-31. Premature ventricular contractions are identified by the fact that they are premature, have a wide QRS complex, and have an ST segment that slopes in the opposite direction. They may also have a compensatory pause. (From Kaplan JA, Thys DM. Electrocardiography. In: Miller R, ed. *Anesthesia,* 3rd ed. New York: Churchill Livingstone, 1990, with permission.)

tion opposite to the main deflection of the QRS complex. There is no P wave associated with a PVC, but retrograde depolarization of the atria or blocked sinus beats may obscure the diagnosis.

The most significant entity in the differential diagnosis is PAC with aberrant ventricular conduction. The distinction should be made whenever possible. Although a PAC normally reaches the SA node and resets the sinus rhythm, such an occurrence is rare when the ectopic pacemaker is in the ventricle. Therefore, a PVC blocks the next depolarization from the SA node, but the following sinus beat occurs on time. The result is a compensatory pause, consisting of the interval from the PVC to the expected normal QRS, which is blocked at the AV node, plus a normal sinus interval. PVCs are common during anesthesia, accounting for 15% of observed arrhythmias. They are much more common in anesthetized patients with preexisting cardiac disease. Other than heart disease, known etiologic factors include electrolyte and blood gas abnormalities, drug interactions, brain stem stimulation, and trauma to the heart.

1. Heart rate. The heart rate depends on the underlying sinus rate and frequency of the PVCs.
2. Rhythm. The rhythm is irregular.
3. P:QRS. There is no P wave with the PVCs.
4. QRS complex. This is wide and bizarre with a width of more than 0.12 seconds.
5. Significance. The new onset of PVCs must be considered life-threatening, because in certain clinical situations it may progress to ventricular tachycardia or fibrillation. These situations include coronary artery insufficiency, myocardial infarction, digitalis toxicity with hypokalemia, and hypoxemia. PVCs are more likely to lead to fibrillation if they are multiple, multifocal, or bigeminal, or if they occur near the vulnerable period of the preceding ventricular depolarization (the R-on-T phenomenon) (50).
6. Treatment. The first step is to correct any underlying abnormalities such as decreased serum potassium or low arterial oxygen tension. Lidocaine is then usually the treatment of choice, with an initial bolus dose of 1.5 mg/kg. Recurrent PVCs can be treated with a lidocaine infusion of 1 to 4 mg/minute; additional therapy can be supplied with esmolol, propranolol, bretylium, procainamide, quinidine, verapamil, disopyramide, atropine, or overdrive pacing.

Ventricular Tachycardia

Ventricular tachycardia is a run of rapidly repeated ectopic beats arising from the ventricle, which are potentially life-threatening (Fig. 7-32). Diagnostic criteria include the presence of fusion beats, capture beats, and AV dissociation. The characteristics of ventricular tachycardia are as follows:

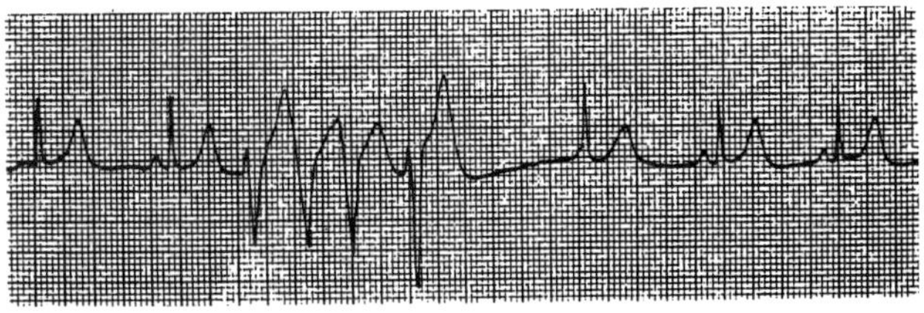

FIGURE 7-32. Three or more premature ventricular contractions (PVCs) in a row is defined as a run of ventricular tachycardia. A fusion beat, capture beat, or atrioventricular (AV) dissociation seen on the trace helps make the specific diagnosis of ventricular tachycardia. (From Kaplan JA, Thys DM. Electrocardiography. In: Miller R, ed. *Anesthesia,* 3rd ed. New York: Churchill Livingstone, 1990, with permission.)

1. Heart rate. The heart rate is 100 to 200 beats/minute.
2. Rhythm. Usually it is regular, but it may be irregular if the ventricular tachycardia is paroxysmal.
3. P:QRS. No fixed relation exists, because ventricular tachycardia is a form of AV dissociation in which the P waves can be seen marching through the QRS complex.
4. QRS complex. The complex is wide, more than 0.12 seconds in width.
5. Significance. Acute onset is life-threatening and requires immediate treatment.
6. Treatment. Lidocaine and/or immediate cardioversion is usually required. Recurrent episodes may require therapy with any or all of the drugs listed for the treatment of PVCs.

Ventricular Fibrillation

Ventricular fibrillation is an irregular rhythm resulting from a rapid discharge of impulses from one or more foci in the ventricles (Fig. 7-33). The ventricular contractions are erratic and are represented on the ECG by bizarre patterns of various sizes and configurations. P waves are not seen. Important causes of the arrhythmia include myocardial ischemia, hypoxia, hypothermia, electric shock, electrolyte imbalance, and drug effects. The characteristics are as follows:

1. Heart rate. The heart rate is rapid and grossly disorganized.
2. Rhythm. The rhythm is totally irregular.
3. P:QRS. None is seen.
4. QRS complex. This is not present.
5. Significance. There is no effective cardiac output, and life must be sustained by artificial means such as external cardiac massage.
6. Treatment. Cardiopulmonary resuscitation must be initiated immediately, and then defibrillation must be performed as rapidly as possible. External defibrillation should be performed with a DC defibrillator, using 200

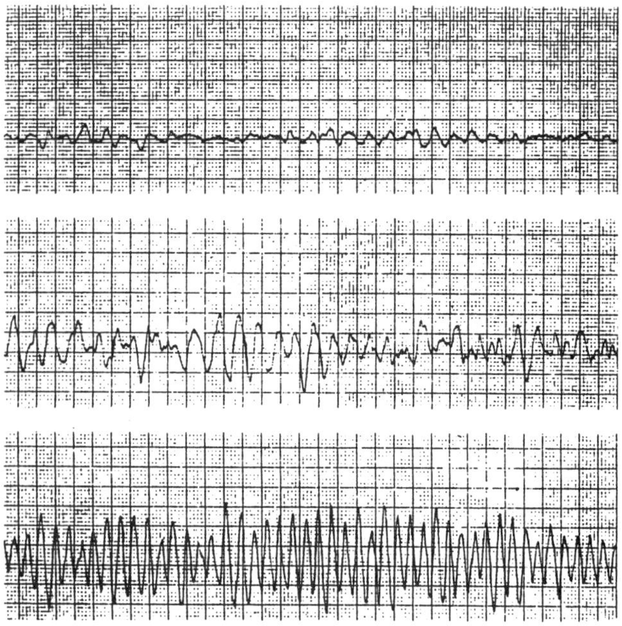

FIGURE 7-33. Ventricular fibrillation can occur in a very fine, moderate, or coarse pattern, as demonstrated on this electrocardiogram. (From Kaplan JA, Thys DM. Electrocardiography. In: Miller R, ed. *Anesthesia,* 3rd ed. New York: Churchill Livingstone, 1990, with permission.)

to 400 W-sec. Supportive pharmacologic therapy may include propranolol, bretylium, or lidocaine. In some instances, epinephrine is used to coarsen the fibrillation in an attempt to defibrillate the patient.

CONCLUSIONS

The ECG should be monitored in all patients undergoing anesthesia for cardiac surgery. Although it does not provide information on the heart's mechanical function, it allows the detection of electrical disturbances that can profoundly affect this function. Today, with the judicious use of selected lead combinations, most arrhythmias and ischemic events can be precisely diagnosed intraoperatively. However, this diagnostic activity is time-consuming, and there is considerable evidence that many intraoperative ECG changes go undetected. There is little doubt that future technologic developments will facilitate the intraoperative recognition of ECG disturbances and, one hopes, improve patient outcome.

REFERENCES

1. Thys DM, Kaplan JA. *The ECG in anesthesia and critical care.* New York: Churchill Livingstone, 1987.
2. Narang J, Thys DM. Electrocardiographic monitoring. In: Ehrenwerth J, Eisenkraft JB, eds. *Anesthesia equipment: principles and applications.* Malvern, PA: Mosby-Year Book, 1992:284.
3. Skeehan TM, Thys DM. Monitoring the cardiac surgical patient. In: Hensley FA, Martin DE, eds. *The practice of cardiac anesthesia.* Boston: Little, Brown, 1990.
4. Griffin RM, Kaplan JA. Comparison of ECG V_5, CS_5, CB_5, and II by computerized ST segment analysis. *Anesth Analg* 1986;65: S1(abst).
5. Bazaral MG, Norfleet EA. Comparison of CB_5 and V_5 leads for intraoperative electrocardiographic monitoring. *Anesth Analg* 1981;60:849.
6. Hollenberg M, Mateo G, Massie BM, et al. Influence of the R-wave amplitude on exercise-induced ST depression: need for a "gain factor" correction when interpreting a stress electrocardiogram. *Am J Cardiol* 1985;56:13.
7. Mark JB, Chien GL, Steinbrook RA, et al. Electrocardiographic R-wave changes during cardiac surgery. *Anesth Analg* 1992;74: 26.
8. Kaplan JA, King SB. The precordial electrocardiographic lead (V_5) in patients who have coronary artery disease. *Anesthesiology* 1976;45:570.
9. London MJ, Hollenberg M, Wong MG, et al. Intraoperative myocardial ischemia: localization by continuous 12 lead electrocardiography. *Anesthesiology* 1988;69:232.
10. Kates RA, Zaidan JR, Kaplan JA. Esophageal lead for intraoperative electrocardiographic monitoring. *Anesth Analg* 1982;61:781.
11. Chatterjee K, Swan HJC, Ganz W, et al. Use of a balloon-tipped flotation electrode catheter for cardiac monitoring. *Am J Cardiol* 1975;36:56.
12. Lichtenthal PR. Multipurpose pulmonary artery catheter. *Ann Thorac Surg* 1983;36:493.
13. Mylrea KC, Calkins JM, Carlson J, et al. ECG lead with the endotracheal tube. *Crit Care Med* 1983;11:199.
14. Mirvis DM, Berson AS, Goldberger AL, et al. Instrumentation and practice standards for electrocardiographic monitoring in special care units. *Circulation* 1989;79:464.
15. Pipberger HV, Arzbaecher RC, Berson AS, et al. American Heart Association Committee Report. Recommendations for standardization of leads and of specifications for instruments in electrocardiography and vectorcardiography. *Circulation* 1975;52:11.
16. Sheffield LT, Berson AS, Bragg-Remschel D, et al. The Task Force of the Committee on Electrocardiography and Cardiac Electrophysiology of the Council on Clinical Cardiology. Recommendations for standards of instrumentation and practice in the use of ambulatory electrocardiography. *Circulation* 1985;71; 626A.
17. Association for the Advancement of Medical Instrumentation. *American national standards for pregelled disposable electrodes (EC12-1983).* Arlington, VA: ANSI/AAMI, 1984.
18. Legatt AD, Frost EAM. ECG artifacts during intraoperative evoked potential monitoring. *Anesthesiology* 1989;70:559.
19. Paulsen AW, Pritchard DG. ECG artifact produced by crystalloid administration through blood/fluid warmer sets. *Anesthesiology* 1988;69:803.
20. Lampert BA, Sundstrom FD. ECG artifacts simulating supraventricular tachycardia during automated percutaneous lumbar discectomy. *Anesth Analg* 1988;67:1096.
21. Arbeit SR, Rubin IL, Gross H. Dangers in interpreting the electrocardiogram from the oscilloscope monitor. *JAMA* 1970;211: 453.
22. Slogoff S, Keats ASS, David Y, et al. Incidence of perioperative myocardial ischemia detected by different electrocardiographic systems. *Anesthesiology* 1990;73:1074.
23. Bertrand CA, Steiner NV, Jameson AG, et al. Disturbances of cardiac rhythm during anesthesia and surgery. *JAMA* 1971;216: 1615.

24. Atlee JL, Rusy BF. Ventricular conduction times and AV nodal conductivity during enflurane anesthesia in dogs. *Anesthesiology* 1977;47:498.
25. Edwards R, Winnie AP, Ramamurthy S. Acute hypocapneic hypokalemia: an iatrogenic anesthetic complication. *Anesth Analg* 1977;56:786.
26. Angelini L, Feldman MI, Lufschonowski R, et al. Cardiac arrhythmias during and after heart surgery: diagnosis and management. *Prog Cardiovasc Dis* 1974;16:469.
27. Sonntag H, Larsen R, Hilfiker O, et al. Myocardial blood flow and oxygen consumption during high-dose fentanyl anesthesia in patients with coronary artery disease. *Anesthesiology* 1982;56:416.
28. Coriat P, Harari A, Daloz M, et al. Clinical predictors of intraoperative myocardial ischemia in patients with coronary artery disease undergoing non-cardiac surgery. *Acta Anaesthesiol Scand* 1982;26:287.
29. Coy KM, Imperi GA, Lambert CR, et al. Silent myocardial ischemia during daily activities in asymptomatic men with positive exercise response. *Am J Cardiol* 1987;59:45.
30. Pepine CJ. Is silent ischemia a treatable risk factor in patients with angina pectoris? *Circulation* 1990;82[Suppl 2]:135.
31. Chaitman BR, Hanson JS. Comparative sensitivity and specificity of exercise electrocardiographic lead systems. *Am J Cardiol* 1981;47:1335.
32. Okin PM, Bergman G, Kligfield P. Effect of ST segment measurement point on performance of standard heart rate-adjusted ST segment criteria for the identification of coronary artery disease. *Circulation* 1991;84:57.
33. Bell C, Rimar S, Barash P. Intraoperative ST segment changes consistent with myocardial ischemia in the neonate: a report of three cases. *Anesthesiology* 1989;71:601.
34. Dodds TM, Delphin E, Stone G, et al. Detection of perioperative myocardial ischemia using Holter with real-time ST segment analysis. *Anesth Analg* 1988;67:890.
35. Levin RI, Cohen D, Frisbie W, et al. Potential for real-time processing of the continuously monitored electrocardiogram in the detection, quantitation, and intervention of silent myocardial ischemia. *Cardiol Clin* 1986;4:735.
36. Clements FM, McCann RL, Levin RI. Continuous ST-segment analysis for the detection of perioperative myocardial ischemia. *Crit Care Med* 1988;16:710.
37. Romhilt DW, Bloomfield SS, Chai TC, et al. Unreliability of conventional electrocardiographic monitoring of arrhythmia detection in coronary care units. *Am J Cardiol* 1973;31:457.
38. Oliver GE, Nolle FM, Wolff GA, et al. Detection of premature ventricular contractions with a clinical system for monitoring electrocardiographic rhythms. *Comput Biomed Res* 1971;4:523.
39. Shah PM, Arnold JM, Haberen NA, et al. Automatic real-time arrhythmia monitoring in the intensive coronary care unit. *Am J Cardiol* 1977;39:701.
40. Morganroth J. Ambulatory Holter electrocardiography: choice of technique and clinical uses. *Ann Intern Med* 1985;102:73.
41. London MJ. Monitoring for myocardial ischemia. In: Kaplan JA, ed. *Vascular* anesthesia. New York: Churchill Livingstone, 1991:249.
42. Kotter GS, Kotrly KJ, Kalbfleisch JH, et al. Myocardial ischemia during cardiovascular surgery as detected by an ST segment trend monitoring system. *J Cardiothorac Anesth* 1987;1:190.
43. Ellis JE, Shah MN, Briller et al. A comparison of methods for the detection of myocardial ischemia during non-cardiac surgery: automated ST-segment analysis systems, electrocardiography, and transesophageal echocardiography. *Anesth Analg* 1992;75:764.
44. Leung JM, Voskanian A, Bellows WH, et al. Automated electrocardiograph ST-segment trending monitors: accuracy in detecting myocardial ischemia. *Anesth Analg* 1998;87:4.
45. London MJ, Ahlstrom LD. Validation testing of the Spacelabs PC2 ST-Segment Analyzer. *J Cardiothorac Vasc Anesth* 1995;9:684.
46. Kaplan JA, Thys DM. Electrocardiography. In: Miller R, ed. *Anesthesia,* 3rd ed. New York: Churchill Livingstone, 1990.
47. Slapa WJ. The sick sinus syndrome. *Am Heart J* 1976;92:648.
48. Glassman E. Direct current cardioversion. *Am Heart J* 1971;82:128.
49. Haldemann G, et al. Haemodynamic effects of transient atrioventricular dissociation in general anesthesia. *Br J Anaesth* 1972;44:159.
50. Cranefeld PF. Ventricular fibrillation. *N Engl J Med* 1973;289:732.

Cardiac Anesthesia: Principles and Clinical Practice, Second Edition, edited by Fawzy G. Estafanous, Paul G. Barash, and J.G. Reves. Lippincott Williams & Wilkins, Philadelphia © 2001.

8

HEMODYNAMIC AND RELATED MONITORING

JOSEPH P. MATHEW
MARK F. NEWMAN

Few operative procedures rival the complexity, invasiveness, and alteration of normal physiology observed during cardiac surgery. Many vital organ systems are influenced by the utilization of cardiopulmonary bypass (CPB), necessitating comprehensive monitoring of the systems most affected. Clearly the anesthesia practitioner participating in cardiac surgical procedures must fully understand the sophisticated monitoring techniques that are commonly, if not universally, applied to the care of these patients.

CARDIOVASCULAR MONITORING

Arterial Blood Pressure Monitoring

The measurement of arterial blood pressure is a critical part of patient monitoring during cardiac surgery. In general, techniques for measuring blood pressure fall into two major categories: indirect (occlusive cuff devices) and direct (arterial cannulation and pressure transduction) methods. These differ in essentially every aspect, particularly in the physical process being monitored and in the level of invasiveness. Both have advantages and disadvantages, which tend to direct their use to particular classes of patients and procedures. In almost every cardiac surgical case, direct arterial cannulation is the method of choice for monitoring blood pressure. The wide range and rapid changes in blood pressure observed even in the usual course of such operations make continuous transduction and display of this variable necessary. However, there are many ways in which blood pressure monitoring can yield spurious information. The anesthesiologist must therefore acquire sufficient understanding of the characteristics of all of these monitoring devices to become the arbiter of discrepancies. A brief description of noninvasive as well as direct, invasive blood pressure determination serves to provide the basis for making such interpretive decisions.

Noninvasive Techniques

All indirect methods of blood pressure determination rely on the Riva-Rocci sphygmomanometer (1). This technique consists of inflating a pneumatic bladder or cuff around a peripheral artery to the point of occluding blood flow, then sensing a sequence of physical changes occurring in or around the artery as the occlusion pressure is released.

Manual Methods

The simplest technique is an intermittent estimate using auscultation of Korotkoff sounds, which are a complex set of audible frequencies resulting from turbulent blood flow and shock waves, created as external occluding pressure on a major artery is reduced (2). The pressure at which the first sound (phase I) is heard is usually taken as the systolic value. The sound character changes, becoming muffled (phases II to IV), and finally is inaudible (phase V). Diastolic pressure is recorded at phase IV or V.

The primary shortcoming of auscultatory techniques is the reliance on blood flow to generate the Korotkoff sounds. Pathologic or iatrogenic causes of decreased peripheral blood flow, such as cardiogenic shock or the use of vasopressors, can result in delayed sound generation and a significant underestimation of blood pressure (3). Moreover, low compliance of the tissues underlying the cuff, encountered in a shivering patient, will require an excessively high occluding pressure and can produce a falsely elevated blood pressure determination (2).

Automatic Methods

Automated noninvasive blood pressure devices provide some advantages that have resulted in expanded use of this technology in many areas of medical care. The technique most commonly incorporated in automated noninvasive blood pressure is the oscillometric principle. In this method, oscillations in cuff pressure resulting from arterial pulsation

J. P. Mathew: Department of Anesthesiology, Duke University Medical Center, Durham, North Carolina 27710
M. F. Newman: Division of Cardiothoracic Anesthesiology, Department of Anesthesiology, Duke Heart Center, Durham, North Carolina 27710

during deflation are sensed by the device and are used to determine arterial blood pressure values. Systolic blood pressure is commonly designated as the point at which pressure oscillations are first detected. Mean blood pressure is the point at which the amplitude of oscillations is maximal. Although the method by which diastolic pressures is derived is proprietary to the various manufacturers, diastolic pressure is frequently calculated using the following equation:

$$\text{mean pressure} = (\text{systolic pressure} + [2 \times \text{diastolic pressure}]) / 3$$

The slope of the declining rate of oscillations has also been employed in determining the diastolic blood pressure. When compared to the radial artery pressure, oscillometry tends to overestimate blood pressure during hypotension and to underestimate blood pressure during hypertension. An improperly sized oscillometric blood pressure cuff also introduces significant error. Use of a cuff width that is larger than one half to two thirds the circumference of the mid upper arm results in a lower pressure reading. Similarly, a cuff that is too small results in a pressure reading that is higher than the true pressure.

In using automated noninvasive blood pressure devices, care must be taken that the automated inflation-deflation cycling of the cuffs not occur so frequently as to limit perfusion of the distal extremity. Rare cases of ulnar nerve paresthesia, superficial thrombophlebitis, and compartment syndrome have been reported to result from automated noninvasive blood pressure cuffs repeatedly inflating in the presence of an artifact-producing condition, such as involuntary muscle tremors or shivers (4).

Despite these problems, multiple studies have suggested that the oscillometric technique correlates well with the direct arterial approach and provides an acceptable measurement of blood pressure (5–7). Thus, a suitable role for noninvasive blood pressure measurement techniques may be as a backup to a direct arterial pressure monitor or as an additional source of data when this primary technique is questioned.

Other automated noninvasive blood pressure devices incorporate the Doppler principle to determine blood flow distal to the cuff or to detect motion of the arterial wall itself. Both provide acceptable blood pressure data (8,9). However, in addition to suffering from the general problems of auscultatory techniques, they also require significant attention to the placement and stability of the ultrasound detector. Dislodgment of the transducer leads to a sudden loss of information. Therefore, widespread use of these devices has not occurred.

Invasive Techniques

Despite its invasive nature and potential risks, direct arterial cannulation with continuous-pressure transduction is the accepted standard for blood pressure monitoring during cardiac surgical procedures. In addition, arterial catheters solve another universally accepted requirement in these patients: the need for repeated sampling of arterial blood for blood gas or other analyses. Fortunately, experience with this technique has demonstrated its value and safety, so its use does not present a serious risk of adverse outcome for these patients.

Technique for Percutaneous Radial Artery Cannulation

Several peripheral arteries are available for percutaneous cannulation, but by far the most popular is the radial artery. This is because of its accessibility and the presence of collateral circulation to the hand and because of extensive experience in its use and safety (10,11).

As with any procedural skill, percutaneous arterial cannulation is best learned by observing and emulating the methods of other, more experienced personnel. From the individual elements of this collected array of practiced techniques, it is possible to compile one's own method that results in the greatest overall success. With this in mind, the following technique for cannulation of the radial artery is given.

Exposure of the radial artery is optimized by gentle dorsiflexion and securing of the wrist across a pad. The artery is palpated along its course over several centimeters to the point at which it enters the flexor retinaculum. The area should be prepared widely with multiple layers of antiseptic solution. Local anesthetic (typically 1% lidocaine) solution should be injected intradermally using a small (25-gauge) needle. A wheal that blanches the skin, as well as a generous subcutaneous infiltration on either side of the artery, has several advantages. First, satisfactory local anesthesia is imperative in this and all invasive monitoring techniques. Also, the anesthetic solution may prevent arterial spasm at the time of puncture. Finally, the dermis becomes somewhat softened, and the volume of the subcutaneous space is expanded, increasing the control over the catheter in the tissues. A nick in the anesthetized skin wheal with a large (16- to 18-gauge) hypodermic needle will further enhance the entry of the catheter. A 20-gauge Teflon catheter first should be checked for smooth movement of the catheter over the stylet. Many commercial catheters come encased in a plastic sleeve that can be inserted into the stylet hub and act as a reservoir for the blood that pulses out when the artery is entered. The catheter is introduced at a fairly steep angle (typically 30°) to the skin (Fig. 8-1A). When the stylet pierces the vessel and blood begins to flow vigorously into the stylet hub and reservoir, the angle of the catheter should be decreased somewhat (typically to 10°). At this point, carefully advancing the stylet another half mm may ensure that the catheter tip is within the lumen of the vessel. The catheter is then gently slipped off the stylet and into the artery (Fig. 8-1B).

Puncturing the back wall of the artery with the stylet is not a serious error. Studies have shown no influence of arterial puncture technique (single-wall versus transfixion)

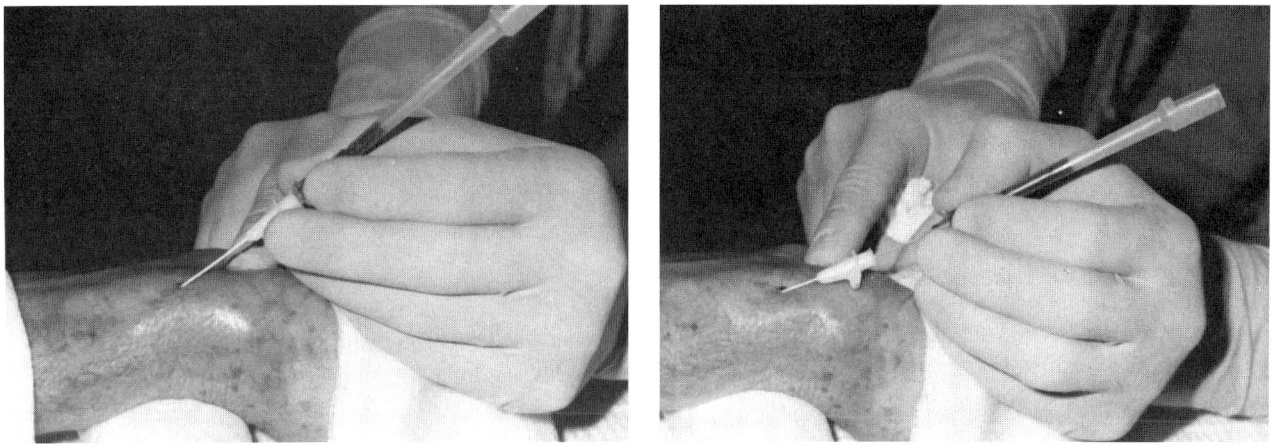

A B

FIGURE 8-1. Percutaneous radial artery cannulation. **A:** The catheter assembly is inserted at a 30-° angle to puncture the artery. **B:** The angle is then decreased to 10° and the catheter advanced off the needle.

on the incidence of postcannulation arterial thrombosis (12–14). In case of transfixion, the stylet should be retracted into the catheter, and the catheter slowly pulled back until pulsatile blood flow is restored. Then the cannula usually can be advanced into the artery but difficulty may arise if the tip of the plastic catheter is bent or frayed. The catheter should never be advanced against a resistance in the artery, as this may lead to intimal damage of the artery and subsequent thrombosis. If one is unsuccessful in passing the catheter, repeated attempts can be made, but excessive punctures of the artery increase the risk of damage to the vessel. If the catheter appears to be in the lumen of the artery but there is difficulty in advancing further into the vessel, a sterile guidewire may be passed up the artery to direct insertion. Some arterial cannulation kits have integrated stylet-guidewire–catheter assemblies for this purpose. Once the catheter is fully advanced into the vessel lumen, occlusive pressure is held transiently on the proximal artery to limit blood loss and the stylet is removed. A narrow-bore, low-compliance pressure tubing is then fastened to the catheter; an appropriate sterile dressing is applied, and the apparatus is securely taped to the wrist.

Alternative Arterial Cannulation Sites

Ulnar Artery. The ulnar artery is often an appropriate alternate choice if the radial arteries are unavailable for catheterization, particularly if it appears to be the nondominant arterial supply to the hand (see complications further in this chapter). The considerations and techniques for its cannulation are the same as those for the radial artery.

Femoral Artery. Use of the femoral artery offers particular advantages under certain circumstances in cardiac surgical procedures. It is a safely cannulated, large, superficial artery that provides excellent access to the central arterial tree. Femoral artery catheters are sometimes placed in anticipation of a later need for an intraaortic balloon pump and act as quick-access sites for this device. However, in the presence of an intraaortic balloon pump, further monitoring of femoral arterial blood pressure is of little value, because the physiologic parameters of interest exist proximal to the balloon. Femoral artery cannulation is accomplished using a percutaneous technique just below the inguinal ligament. A short (7.5-cm) catheter is placed directly, or a longer (15-cm) catheter is inserted over a guidewire. Femoral artery catheters have a record of safety similar to that for other sites (15), although there may be a slightly higher risk of infectious complications with this approach than for the radial arterial site (16–18).

Brachial Artery. Because the brachial artery has no parallel collateral blood supply route, its use carries a theoretically higher risk of distal ischemic complications. However, studies have demonstrated the safety of this technique in intraoperative (19), and even long-term outpatient settings (20,21). Short, small-gauge catheters are recommended when the brachial artery is used.

Axillary Artery. When more peripheral locations are inaccessible (22), or when pressure monitoring must extend over protracted periods (16,23), the axillary artery can be used as a cannulation site. A 15-cm-long, 20- or 18-gauge Teflon catheter is placed using a Seldinger guidewire technique. It is preferable to use the left axillary artery, because it has a decreased risk of carotid artery obstruction or embolization. However, vertebral artery impingement may occur on either side. Advantages of this approach include increased patient comfort and mobility during long-term monitoring, and the ability to insert large, secure cannulas that can be used for hemodialysis outflow (23). Potential complications include infections, bleeding, and nerve plexus injury, but these are infrequent (16,23–25).

Dorsalis Pedis and Posterior Tibial Arteries. The dorsalis pedis artery is an acceptable choice for cannulation under most circumstances, although it is absent in up to one eighth of the population (26). Together with the posterior tibial artery and its branches, the dorsalis pedis artery forms the same loop collateral circulation for the foot as the radial and ulnar arteries do for the hand, thus allowing for its safe cannulation (27). The posterior tibial artery is a similarly useful vessel for arterial pressure monitoring. Catheters placed in this artery are less susceptible to kinking on dorsiflexion of the foot than in the dorsalis pedis artery, and they may be particularly valuable in neonates and infants (28).

Superficial Temporal Artery. This vessel provides an arterial monitoring site that originates at the aortic arch, but it is not a branch of a subclavian artery. The superficial temporal artery is palpable between the lateral margin of the maxilla and the superior-anterior edge of the pinna. Randel and colleagues (28) have reported the safety of cannulating this artery in a series of 21 neonates. However, the risks of ischemia of the scalp and face, as well as the possibility of cerebral embolization by flushing air or particulate matter retrograde to the carotid artery, have been described (29) and should be kept in mind when considering this site for pressure monitoring.

Analysis of Blood Pressure Signal

An electromechanical transduction system, which consists of fluid-filled tubing and electrical strain gauge, is used to derive a pressure waveform from direct intravascular cannulas, either intraarterial or intravenous. Many such transducer systems incorporate an automatic mechanism for continuous, slow (1 to 3 mL/hour) flushing with saline, sometimes heparinized at a concentration of 1 U/mL. Recently, saline alone has been preferred at many institutions because saline appears to be as effective as heparin in maintaining catheter patency (30) and because of the association of heparin-containing flush solutions with heparin-induced thrombocytopenia (31). A final component of the pressure transduction system is a spring-loaded valve that allows periodic, high-pressure flushing after blood sampling.

The accuracy with which a transducer system measures arterial pressure is dependent on many complex and interrelated physical factors (2,32–34). Sufficient understanding of the dynamic response of transducer systems, however, can be gained by the comprehension of only two parameters. The first is the *natural frequency* (f_n) of the integrated pressure-monitoring apparatus—the frequency at which the system will resonate or "ring" (system oscillation). Physiologic frequencies occurring near f_n are spuriously amplified by the system. Therefore, it is preferable that the f_n of the pressure transducing system exceed the maximum frequency that exists in a blood pressure signal (typically 20 Hz) (2). The second parameter is the *damping coefficient* (ζ), which describes the tendency of the apparatus to retard oscillations through viscous and frictional forces (rate at which the system comes to rest). The mechanical characteristics of the system that combine to produce these variables are given in the following equations: (35)

$$f_n = \frac{d}{8}\sqrt{\frac{3}{\pi L \rho V_d}}$$

$$\zeta = \frac{16n}{d^3}\sqrt{\frac{3LV_d}{\pi \rho}}$$

where d equals tubing diameter, L equals tubing length, ρ equals density of the fluid, V_d equals transducer fluid volume displacement, and n equals viscosity of the fluid.

In clinical practice, f_n and ζ can be calculated using the "fast-flush" procedure. After a rapid system flush, resonant waves are created in the pressure tracing (Fig. 8-2). The natural frequency is calculated by dividing the paper speed in millimeters per second by the number of millimeters between resonant wave peaks. The damping coefficient is calculated by division of the amplitudes of any two successive resonant wave peaks and applying the chart shown in Fig. 8-2. From the equations above, it can be seen that both natural frequency and the damping coefficient are affected by the stiffness (elasticity) of the system, the mass of the fluid in the system, and the friction in the system created by fluid movement. The addition of extension tubing or more compliant tubing to the pressure monitoring system therefore tends to lower the natural frequency (underdamped system) with a resulting overshoot of the pressure waveforms (35). Likewise, an overdamped system (as produced by catheter kinking, thrombus formation, or air bubbles) tends to underestimate the systolic blood pressure. Diastolic blood pressure is also affected but is more resistant to deficiencies in the dynamic response. For accurate repro-

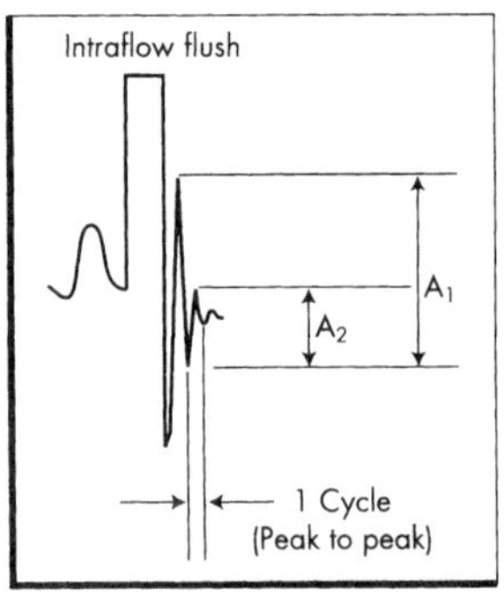

Amplitude Ratio (A_2/A_1)	Damping Coefficient
.9	.034
.8	.071
.7	.113
.6	.160
.5	.215
.4	.280
.3	.358
.2	.456
.1	.591
.05	.690

$$fn = \frac{\text{Paper speed, } mm/sec}{\text{1 cycle, } mm}$$

$$\text{Damping coefficient} = \frac{\text{Ln (Ratio)}}{\sqrt{\pi^2 + (\text{Ln [Ratio]}^2)}}$$

FIGURE 8-2. "Fast-flush" method of determining the dynamic response of a pressure monitoring system. In an optimal system, a fast-flush procedure produces an undershoot followed by a small overshoot and then a return to the waveform. Ratio = A_2/A_1. (From Gardner RM. Direct blood pressure measurement—dynamic response requirements. *Anesthesiology* 1981;54:227, with permission.)

duction of pressures, the natural frequency of the measuring system should be more than 30 Hz and the damping coefficient should be 0.6. However, a larger natural frequency allows for a greater range in the damping coefficient. In an optimal system, a "fast-flush" produces an undershoot followed by a small overshoot and then a return to the arterial waveform. Commercial devices are available that allow fine-tuning of system damping (36).

Baseline drift of the transducer's electrical circuits can occur, which requires periodic checks and re-zeroing. Proper placement of the transducer relative to the patient's position (usually at the level of the right atrium) is necessary for the correct interpretation of pressure data. These factors are clearly more significant during the measurement of low-pressure parameters, such as central venous pressure (CVP).

Improper damping and calibration account for a large percentage of the errors in direct arterial pressure monitoring. Another cause of these errors is the automated numeric display of pressure values on the monitor screens. The algorithm usually implemented in these monitors simply determines the maxima and minima that are present in the waveform and displays these as the systolic and diastolic values, respectively. Resonance and artifactual amplification in an underdamped system are usually not recognized automatically and result in an erroneous pressure display. Moreover, low-frequency variation in blood pressure caused by ventilation and diastolic blood pressure augmentation produced by an intraaortic balloon pump may not be accounted for in the numeric presentation. Therefore, the use of strip-chart recordings of pressure waveforms is often a requirement for accurate blood pressure interpretation.

Arterial pulse pressure undergoes a natural amplification during transit through the arterial tree (Fig. 8-3). Accurately measured radial arterial systolic pressure is normally greater, and diastolic pressure lower, than that found in the central aorta. However, after CPB, it has been demonstrated in adults (37) and pediatric patients (38) that systolic and mean radial artery pressures are significantly lower than corresponding central aortic values. This phenomenon is thought to result from transient vascular resistance changes induced by CPB.

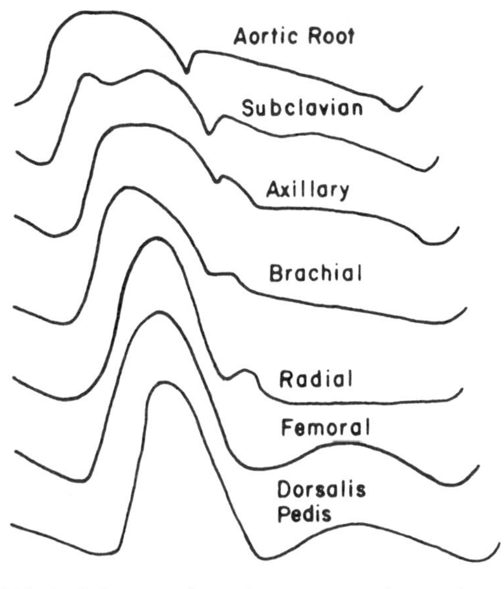

FIGURE 8-3. Pulse waveform changes occurring as the monitoring site moves from the central circulation to the periphery due to forward wave propagation and wave reflection. In the periphery, systolic pressure is higher and diastolic and mean pressures are lower. After cardiopulmonary bypass, this phenomenon is often reversed, with lower pulse pressure measured at peripheral sites. (From Bedford RF. Invasive blood pressure monitoring. In: Blitt CD, ed. *Monitoring in anesthesia and critical care medicine.* New York: Churchill Livingstone, 1985:50, with permission.)

Complications of Arterial Cannulation

Invasive arterial pressure monitoring carries with it the risk of limiting blood flow in that vessel and causing distal ischemia. Because the risk of this complication is diminished by the presence of collateral blood supply, it is appropriate to take steps to ensure the adequacy of reserve perfusion. The Allen test (39) has become a popular technique for bedside assessment of ulnar artery patency before radial artery cannulation. In this test, the examiner compresses both radial and ulnar arteries while the patient alternately flexes and extends the fingers, causing the hand to be relatively exsanguinated. Releasing the ulnar artery occlusion and timing the return of original rubor indicates the results of the test. Normally, full blushing is complete at 7 seconds; 8 to 14 seconds is a borderline result; and 15 seconds is considered abnormal. However, the predictive value of this test has been questioned. Many reports reviewing permanent ischemic sequelae noted normal Allen test results before these catheterizations (40–43). Moreover, cannulations performed in spite of abnormal Allen test results developed no ischemic complications (11,13,44). Other authors have found the Allen test to be useful and have encouraged its implementation to assess arterial blood flow to the hand (12,45). While the clinician must minimize the chances of significant distal ischemia from radial artery monitoring, it appears that the Allen test cannot be relied upon to predict this adverse outcome.

Arterial thrombus formation is a complication of cannulation and can occur even after decannulation. The incidence of thrombosis increases with duration of catheterization (10,44) and catheter size (18 gauge versus 20 gauge) (46). Teflon catheters cause significantly less radial artery thrombosis than those made of polypropylene (47,48). In a study of 1,699 patients, Slogoff et al. (11) found a 25% incidence of diminished arterial flow after removal of percutaneous radial artery catheters. Abnormal flow was correlated only with the presence of hematoma at the site, female gender, and the use of CPB. Despite acute flow reductions or occlusions in the radial artery as a result of cannulation, the great majority of vessels recanalized over a period of days or weeks. Thus, the incidence of serious ischemic complications is low (0% to 4%) (11,12,40,49).

Cardiac Filling Pressure Monitoring

Cardiac filling pressures are an integral part of hemodynamic monitoring during a cardiac surgical procedure, not only because of the obvious influence that they exert on overall cardiac function but also because filling pressures change dramatically during institution of and emergence from CPB. The controversy in cardiac surgery is not whether to monitor filling pressures, but from what location in the circulatory system these data should be derived, because the feasible techniques not only offer different information but also carry different patient risk characteristics and expenses. Noninvasive methods of obtaining filling pressure data are limited to techniques employing ultrasound and will be discussed later in this chapter. Invasive methods of obtaining filling pressure data that are currently available to the anesthesiologist include monitoring of central venous pressure (CVP) and pulmonary artery pressure. Either requires access to a central vein, customarily accomplished by cannulation of the internal jugular vein. Another useful source of filling pressure data is direct left atrial pressure (LAP) monitoring, which almost always requires surgical intervention in the open chest.

Central Venous Pressure Monitoring

Strictly speaking, CVP is the blood pressure at the junction of the venae cavae and the right atrium. It represents the driving force for filling the right side of the heart. The large veins of the thorax, abdomen, and proximal lower extremities form a compliant reservoir for a sizable percentage of the total blood volume. CVP therefore reflects intravascular volume status and the intrinsic tone of these vessels. The functional capacity of the right side of the heart is another determinant of CVP. Thus, CVP monitoring is utilized for assessment of blood volume as well as function of the right side of the heart.

CVP monitoring can be accomplished using an aqueous fluid-filled manometer connected via stopcock to a running fluid line. However, valuable information exists in the waveform of the CVP, which can be observed most easily by electronic transduction and display. A typical CVP trace is generated by the normal sequence of mechanical events in the cardiac cycle (Fig. 8-4). The *a* wave is a positive deflection caused by atrial contraction and coincides with the P wave on the electrocardiogram (ECG). The smaller *c* wave, which follows the onset of the QRS complex on the ECG results from the increase in right atrial pressure that occurs with bowing of the closed tricuspid valve during isovolumic right ventricular contraction. The *x* descent follows this wave as the atrium relaxes and the tricuspid valve is pulled downward by right ventricular contraction. A late, positive *v* wave reaches its peak just after the T wave on the ECG as blood accumulates in the right atrium from the venae

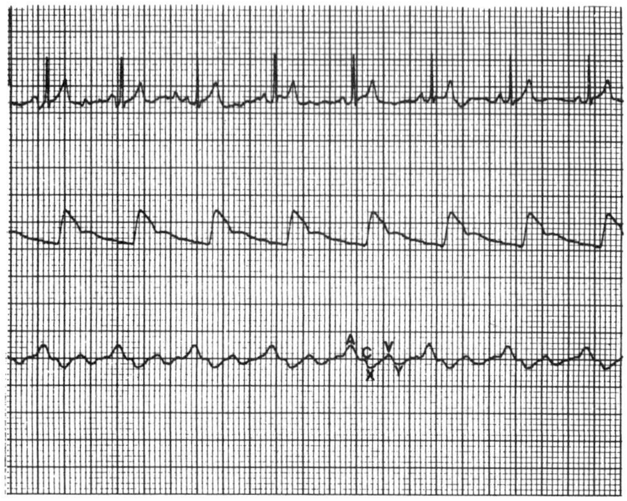

FIGURE 8-4. Central venous pressure waves (*lower trace*) with their temporal relationship to the electrocardiogram (*upper trace*) and arterial pressure waveform (*middle trace*). See text for description of the *a, c,* and *v* waves, and *x* and *y* descents.

cavae. Finally, when the tricuspid valve opens, right atrial pressure decreases, producing the *y* descent.

Several pathophysiologic conditions may be diagnosed or confirmed by examination of the CVP waveform. Atrial fibrillation results in ineffective atrial contraction, and therefore an absence of the *a* wave. Giant (cannon) *a* waves occur when the atrium contracts against a closed tricuspid valve and can assist in diagnosing dysrhythmias such as heart blocks or nodal rhythms (Fig. 8-5). Tricuspid regurgitation from ventricular overfilling or failure causes a distortion and increased size of the *v* wave (50).

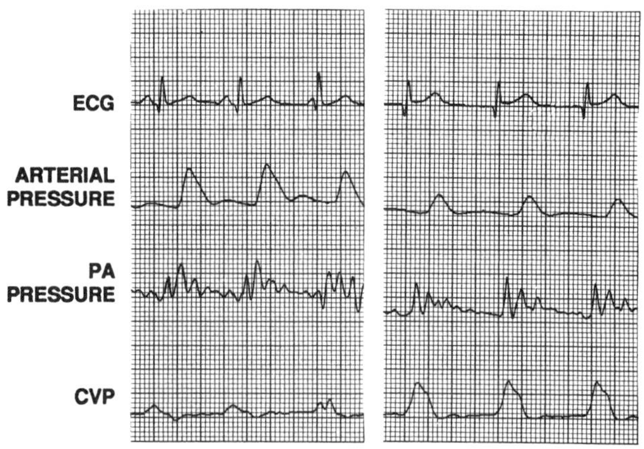

FIGURE 8-5. Development of a nodal rhythm. The last cardiac cycle in the *left panel* shows the beginning of this dysrhythmia. The central venous pressure (CVP) trace at this beat starts to demonstrate an abnormality. In the *right panel* the nodal rhythm is established, and the CVP has a giant "cannon" *a* wave. Note the arterial and pulmonary artery hypotension caused by the lack of atrial contribution to ventricular filling.

The value recorded for CVP is typically a single reading of the mean value of the wave at end-exhalation. Ventilation, either spontaneous or controlled, has a significant effect on CVP and should be accounted for in the interpretation of these data. CVPs measured at end-expiration provide the most accurate estimate of central volume regardless of whether the patient is breathing spontaneously or with positive pressure ventilation. Trends in the CVP during anesthesia and surgery are useful in determining the extent of fluid or blood loss and in guiding replacement therapy. The response of the CVP to fluid boluses in turn can provide information regarding overall fluid volume status, venous compliance, and the function and efficiency of the right side of the heart.

Pulmonary Artery Pressure Monitoring

The introduction of the flow-directed pulmonary artery catheter (PAC) three decades ago represented a significant advance in our ability to define and monitor the hemodynamic status of a patient. With this catheter, pulmonary artery pressures as well as CVP can be easily measured. The pulmonary capillary wedge pressure (PCWP) or pulmonary artery occlusion pressure under most circumstances provides an accurate estimate of the diastolic filling (preload) of the left heart. This inference is based on the proportionality of pulmonary artery pressures with LAP and left ventricular end-diastolic pressure (LVEDP) (Fig. 8-6).

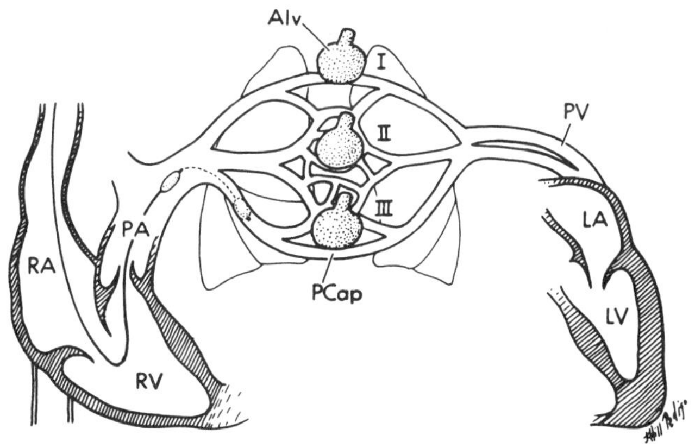

FIGURE 8-6. The course of a pulmonary artery catheter (PAC) through the right side of the heart and its normal position in a proximal pulmonary artery. With the balloon inflated, the PAC floats (*dotted line*) to the "wedge" position, in this case to a segment of zone 3 lung. (RA, right atrium; RV, right ventricle; PA, pulmonary artery; PCap, pulmonary capillary; Alv, alveolus; PV, pulmonary vein; LA, left atrium; LV, left ventricle; PAEDP, pulmonary artery end-diastolic pressure; PWP, pulmonary capillary wedge pressure; PVP, pulmonary venous pressure; LAP, left atrial pressure; LVEDP, left ventricular end-diastolic pressure; 1, 2, and 3, zones of pulmonary vasculature as described by West.) (From Vender JS. Pulmonary artery catheter monitoring. In: Barash PG, ed. *Cardiac monitoring.* Philadelphia: WB Saunders, 1988:743, with permission.)

If left ventricular compliance is normal, LVEDP can be used as an indicator of left ventricular end-diastolic volume, the best overall measure of preload. In the absence of an abnormal pressure gradient across the mitral valve or elevated airway pressures, LAP and pulmonary venous pressure (PVP) reflect LVEDP. LAP may be greater than the LVEDP in patients with mitral stenosis or left atrial myxoma but lower than LVEDP in patients with a stiff ventricle, premature closure of the mitral valve (e.g., acute aortic insufficiency), or when LVEDP is more than 25 mm Hg.

In the absence of elevated airway pressures, such as positive end-expiratory pressure (PEEP), PCWP can in turn be used as an estimate of PVP and LAP. By "wedging" the catheter tip in a small pulmonary artery, the phasic blood flow and pressure in that artery and all distal branches cease, leaving a static column of blood between the catheter tip and the pulmonary veins and left atrium. Thus, this fraction of the pulmonary vascular bed becomes a simple conduit, essentially extending the catheter tip to the left heart, and can therefore approximate LAP. However, a major consideration in these relationships is the influence of alveolar pressure (PA) on the capillary bed. The pulmonary vasculature has been described as a group of zones (1, 2, and 3) based on the relationships among pulmonary artery pressure, PVP, and PA (51). The PAC must be in a pulmonary segment within zone 3, in which PVP exceeds PA, for the capillary conduit to be completely open and capable of transmitting blood pressure information (see Fig. 8-6). In the supine position, a large portion of the lung will be in zone 3. However, significant increases in PA caused by PEEP may "convert" an area of zone 3 to zone 2 or zone 1, resulting in discrepancies between PCWP and LAP. Lorzman et al., reported that the PCWP to LAP correlation was lost when PEEP exceeded 10 cm H_2O (52). Several studies of simultaneous PCWP and direct LAP in cardiac surgical patients have shown a good correlation between these measurements (53,54), except when LAP exceeds 15 mm Hg, during which time PCWP may be a poor predictor of LAP (55).

Pulmonary artery diastolic pressure (PAD), typically 1 to 4 mm Hg more than PCWP, is very often used as a substitute for PCWP. It should be remembered that PAD is measured during phasic pulmonary artery blood flow and is therefore subject to the influences of pulmonary vascular impedance on the pressure wave. Pulmonary vascular resistance, normally low, is increased by hypoxemia, hypercarbia, and hypothermia, as well as many forms of chronic lung disease. Under these conditions, PAD may not correlate well with PCWP. Also, tachycardia will limit the time for diastolic "runoff" of blood flow, so at a high heart rate (more than 120 beats/minute), PAD may exceed PCWP (56).

In contrast to the generally strong agreement of PAD and PCWP with LAP, there is ample evidence to suggest that CVP is an unreliable index of left ventricular filling pressure (57–62). CVP not only is influenced by the pulmonary impedance parameters just described but also is largely determined by the functional capacity or contractility of the right side of the heart. Thus, only in situations in which left heart function is believed to match that of the right side of the heart and there is no condition suggesting grossly abnormal pulmonary vascular resistance should the CVP be trusted as the sole indicator of overall cardiac filling pressures. For cases in which this degree of normality exists, PACs are probably not needed (63).

Indications for Pulmonary Artery Pressure Monitoring
The indications for placement of a PAC thus center on the presence of significant left ventricular dysfunction or the suspicion that dysfunction may develop or be uncovered as a result of the planned surgical procedure or an ongoing medical condition. Cardiac surgery patients frequently either possess or attain such substantial left ventricular dysfunction. Similarly, known or suspected lung disease that could affect the pulmonary vasculature is considered an indication for pulmonary artery pressure monitoring. Again, many patients undergoing cardiovascular surgery have coexisting parenchymal pulmonary disease.

By virtue of its ability to indicate changes in left ventricular compliance and thus diastolic function, the PAC was thought to be useful in detecting myocardial ischemia in patients (64). Although initial studies pointed to a role for PAC in detecting myocardial ischemia, subsequent studies have highlighted the limitations of pulmonary artery pressure monitoring in this arena (65,66). Tuman and colleagues examined outcome variables in a series of 1,094 patients undergoing coronary artery bypass graft surgery, matched for preoperative risk factors, who did or did not receive PAC monitoring perioperatively (66). They found no influence of the use of PACs on such variables as in-hospital mortality, postoperative myocardial infarction rates, and length of stay in the intensive care unit. However, assignment to PAC or non-PAC groups was not randomized. Moreover, 7% of the non-PAC patients had a PAC placed during the study because, in the opinion of the anesthesiologist, a clinical need for more comprehensive monitoring existed. It is therefore unclear what influence the continuation of CVP monitoring only might have had on outcome results in these patients. In contrast, Connors et al. (67) recently reported that pulmonary artery catheterization was associated with increased 30-day mortality and resource utilization. This study has been subject to significant criticism because of the failure of the investigators to specify treatment algorithms, define or control the indications for a PAC, and account for the variations in PAC data interpretation. Multiple studies have demonstrated deficiencies in the ability of the patient care team to accurately interpret the PAC data (68,69).

The American Society of Anesthesiologists has developed *Practice Guidelines for Pulmonary Artery Catheterization* after reviewing a total of 860 clinical trials, controlled observational studies, uncontrolled case reports, and individual reports (70). Although the data indicated a change in therapy as a result of PAC monitoring in 30% to 62% of all cases, these studies demonstrated no effect on mortality. The task force developing these guidelines recommended that pulmonary artery catheterization should be considered in surgical settings associated with an increased risk of complications caused by hemodynamic instability. The risk of developing hemodynamic compromise was to be based on the interrelationship between patient status, surgical procedure, and practice setting. In this document, competence in PAC placement was related to experience and the quality of initial training, as well as the frequency of procedure performance after training. A recent consensus conference determined that conclusive data showing benefit or harm were lacking yet reaffirmed the likely worth of PACs (71). Clearly, prospective, randomized, and adequately controlled studies are necessary to determine whether PACs reduce morbidity and mortality. Until then, the decision to use PAC monitoring during cardiac surgery rests on the clinical judgment of the physician, who must consider and weigh all facets of this process in the context of the patient's physical condition (Table 8-1).

TABLE 8-1. INDICATIONS FOR PULMONARY ARTERY CATHETERIZATION IN CARDIAC SURGERY

Left ventricular dysfunction (present or anticipated)
Dilated cardiomyopathy
Valvular heart disease
Ventricular aneurysm
Severe ischemic heart disease
Global or regional dysfunction
Recent myocardial infarction
Ischemia-related valve dysfunction
Idiopathic hypertrophic subaortic stenosis
Severe pulmonary disease
Pulmonary hypertension
Pulmonary emboli

Technique for Internal Jugular Vein Cannulation

The complex and invasive nature of central venous cannulation for any filling pressure monitoring raises the question of the proper timing for catheter placement. In patients presenting for cardiac surgery, many of whom have ischemic heart disease, the cardiovascular consequences of stimulation, either from pain or anxiety, may be detrimental. For this reason, some authors suggest that pulmonary artery catheterization in cardiac surgical patients be performed only after induction of anesthesia (72). Although some investigators have shown that central venous cannulation (including the placement of PACs) in the awake patient can result in unwanted increases in heart rate and blood pressure (73), other studies fail to confirm these findings (74–76). Moreover, judicious preoperative sedation and the use of adequate anesthesia and or β-adrenergic blockade largely avoids the problem. Therefore, the many benefits of cardiac filling pressure monitoring for anesthesia induction and the dubious contraindications to its establishment in the awake state seem to advocate its preinduction implementation.

The locations and techniques for placing central venous cannulas are numerous. Among anesthesiologists especially a popular site for this procedure is the internal jugular vein (IJV) (77). The reasons for this preference are related to its consistent, predictable anatomic location within palpable landmarks; its short, straight (right IJV), valveless course to the superior vena cava and right atrium; and its position at the patient's head providing easy access by the anesthesiologist in most intraoperative settings. Finally, the success rate for its use exceeds 90% in most series of adults (78). External jugular veins may also be used, but because of their more tortuous course, the success rate in passing a large catheter centrally via this route is less than for the IJV. Other locations for central venous cannulation, such as the subclavian veins, also have advantages and proponents (79). The right IJV is used here as the example of a technique for placement of central venous catheters.

Careful positioning of the patient for IJV cannulation is necessary, not only to afford the greatest chance of success of the procedure but also for optimal patient comfort. For the right IJV, the patient's head should be turned to the left and the neck slightly extended. A small pillow rest at the left of the patient's head may allow for greater relaxation of neck musculature and reduced anxiety. Placement of the patient in the Trendelenburg position is beneficial particularly when there is evidence that the patient is hypovolemic.

Most descriptions of the position of the IJV in adult patients focus on the relationship of the IJV to the sternocleidomastoid muscle. A typical approach starts at the apex of the triangle formed by the two heads of the sternocleidomastoid muscle as the insertion site, with the needle directed toward the ipsilateral nipple. This is generally a useful guide; however, a patient's body habitus (obesity, short neck) can obscure or distort the usual association of the IJV and sternocleidomastoid muscle. An undistorted anatomic relationship is that between the IJV and the carotid artery (80). In the neck, both of these vessels, along with the vagus nerve, are enclosed in the fibrous carotid sheath that allows no separation of its contents. At the point of emergence of this sheath from the thoracic inlet, the IJV is positioned laterally and slightly anteriorly to the carotid artery. Moving cephalad, the IJV maintains a lateral position but swings posteriorly, crossing behind the carotid artery at the level of the thyroid cartilage. The most commonly used IJV cannulation techniques use an insertion site caudad to the thyroid cartilage. Palpation of the carotid artery at the level of the cricoid cartilage defines the position of the IJV (just lateral and anterior to the carotid) in every instance. All approaches based on sternocleidomastoid muscle anatomy (central, posterior, anterior) converge on this location of the IJV. In this approach the edges of the carotid artery should be well defined. Thus, having the patient transiently lift the head to tense and more clearly distinguish the sternocleidomastoid muscle is counterproductive as well as inconvenient for the patient. Instead, full relaxation of the muscles of the neck should be encouraged at the outset to provide easy and complete palpation and definition of the carotid artery.

In performing any type of central venous cannulation, attention to sterility is essential. The chosen insertion site should be prepared widely and scrubbed gently with multiple layers of povidone iodine or another antiseptic solution. Most central venous catheter kits include a sterile fenestrated paper drape, which should be applied lightly and centered over the puncture site. At this juncture, it is particularly important to communicate with the patient, because the drape may contribute to unwanted anxiety. Supplemental oxygen administration via nasal cannulas not only may be therapeutic but also may offer a psychologic advantage by allaying any fears of "smothering." Maximal barrier precautions (e.g., gloves, gown, drape, and mask) are recommended to decrease the risk of bacterial colonization (81).

The significance of an excellent local anesthetic preparation of the cannulation site for any central venous catheterization cannot be overemphasized. The arguments favoring preinduction placement of these monitoring devices depend largely on this aspect of the procedure. It is not unreasonable to use the entire allotment of local anesthetic solution, usually 50 mg (5 mL of 1%) lidocaine, found in most sets for IJV cannulation. If a 25-gauge needle is used and the anesthetic is injected slowly in a mildly sedated patient, the intradermal skin wheal can often be established without being noticed by the patient (Fig. 8-7A). A large skin wheal is advised so an area of anesthetized skin will be available for later suturing of the catheter. The ¾-inch 25-gauge needle is then inserted toward the predetermined IJV location and aspirated gently. Several milliliters of anesthetic solution are slowly injected in the subcutaneous tissue, after having extracted the needle slightly if blood had been aspirated. In nonobese patients, the length of this needle may be sufficient to pierce the IJV. Changing to a 1½–inch 22-gauge needle may be necessary to locate the IJV and to anesthetize the entire tract to the skin.

Keeping in mind the orientation of the "finder" needle, a 1¾–inch 18-gauge catheter-over-needle assembly is used to cannulate the IJV. A small skin nick in the anesthetic wheal may make this step easier and cause less discomfort to the patient. Also, gentle countertraction on the skin with one's nondominant hand makes for a smoother puncture (Fig. 8-7B). This larger slightly less sharp needle may not puncture the encasing sheath as easily as the smaller finder needle, and when it does, its force may cause it to quickly pierce both walls of the IJV. Thus, extracting the needle slowly with gentle aspiration is advised, demonstrating that a perceived "miss" with no blood return on insertion is actually a "hit."

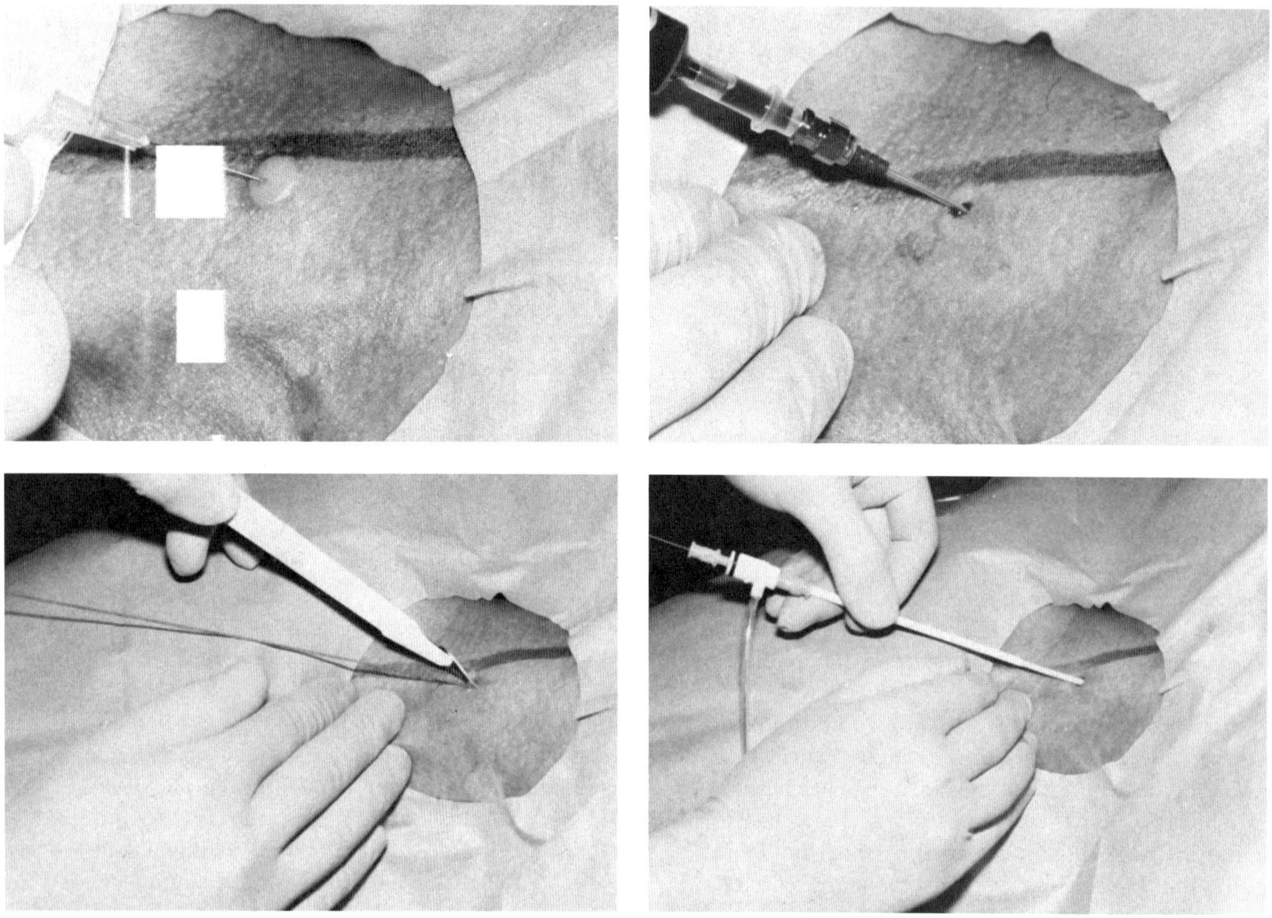

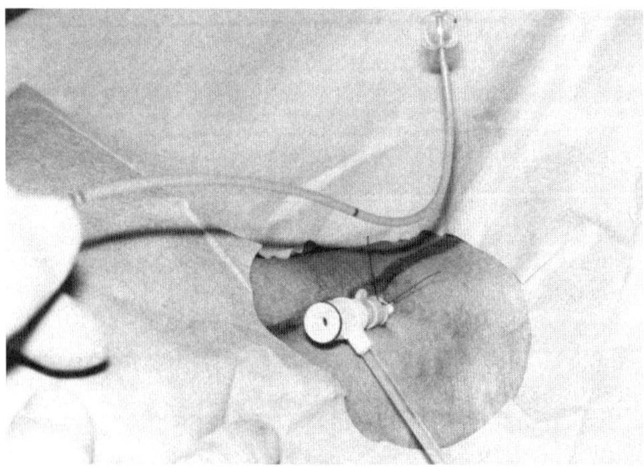

FIGURE 8-7. Technique for cannulation of the right internal jugular vein (IJV). **A:** The right side of the neck has been sterilely prepared and draped. The patient's head is to the left of the photograph, and the line on the neck indicates the position of the palpated carotid artery. Local anesthetic is injected subdermally, raising a large wheal that blanches the skin. **B:** An 18-gauge needle-catheter assembly punctures the IJV located lateral and slightly anterior to the carotid artery. **C:** Enlarging the puncture site slightly with a no. 11 scalpel blade to accommodate the larger introducer used for a pulmonary artery catheter (PAC). **D:** The introducer sheath and dilator assembly are inserted using the wire guide. Note the countertraction applied with the nondominant hand to prevent the skin from "bunching" and distorting the insertion tract. **E:** The introducer is in place and the PAC balloon is tested before insertion. The PAC has been passed through the sterile sheath. Note the curve of the PAC pointing the tip at an "11 o'clock" position. Maintaining this orientation during insertion facilitates the passage through the anteriorly located tricuspid valve.

With the needle in the IJV, the catheter is advanced carefully into the vessel and the needle is removed. Covering the tip of the catheter with one's thumb limits the risk of air entrainment. One should attach the syringe to the catheter and aspirate to ensure free blood return. If this maneuver fails, careful adjustment of the catheter while aspirating and having the patient perform a gentle Valsalva maneuver may be necessary to properly place the cannula.

A small amount of blood should flow from the catheter when the syringe is removed. If not, a slight increase in the Trendelenburg angle should be used so air embolization may be avoided. At this point, measurement of the pressure in the catheter is strongly advised and can be accomplished either by using an electronic pressure transduction system or by attaching a short piece of noncompliant, fluid-filled tubing to the catheter and observing a change in the fluid level with respiration. A Seldinger guidewire, typically having a J-shaped end or a soft flexible straight end, is inserted in the cannula. The wire should advance easily into the IJV with little resistance and the ECG should be continuously monitored to observe dysrhythmias (82). The 18-gauge catheter is then removed, leaving the guidewire in place.

Technique of Central Venous Pressure Catheter Placement

For CVP monitoring, a 20- to 30-cm single-lumen or multilumen catheter is chosen. The skin nick at the puncture site should be enlarged to accommodate the size of the catheter used (Fig. 8-7C) and a dilator employed to enhance the passage of the CVP catheter. One should be particularly careful to ensure that control of the guidewire is never lost. This is done by leaving a sufficient amount of wire extending beyond the length of the catheter. The catheter should be inserted smoothly, holding firm countertraction on the skin. Failure to stabilize the skin against the pressure of the advancing catheter can result in "bunching" of the skin, distortion of the established tract to the IJV, damage to the catheter tip, and significant discomfort for the patient. Gently twisting the catheter during insertion also may help to avoid these problems.

With the catheter inserted to the appropriate distance (typically 18 to 20 cm to reach the junction of the superior vena cava and right atrium), the wire is gently extracted and the catheter is connected to the monitoring tubing. The system is aspirated to remove any air before use. Securing the catheter is usually done with a suture passed behind the puncture site in the original skin wheal. Placing an occlusive dressing on the site completes the procedure. Studies evaluating the application of antimicrobial ointments to the catheter site have yielded contradictory findings (81). The use of polyantibiotic ointments that are not fungicidal may significantly increase the rate of *Candida* infections (83).

Technique of Pulmonary Artery Catheter Placement

For placement of PACs, the right IJV is again preferred by most anesthesiologists. Cannulation of the right IJV for PAC placement is similar to that for CVP monitoring up through the step of inserting the guidewire into the IJV. Modern PAC introducer kits contain an 8.5- or 9.0-French, 15-cm Teflon sheath introducer with a side-port adapter for infusion of fluids. A dilator stylet placed through the adapter and sheath allows for smooth insertion of this larger cannula. This apparatus is passed over the guidewire into the IJV, and the dilator and wire are extracted. Excellent local anesthesia, adequate enlargement of the skin nick, and a careful gentle insertion technique are essential to this step of the procedure (Fig. 8-7D). Because the PAC is a longer more cumbersome catheter, attention to maintaining a wide sterile field is necessary. In most situations, an assistant is needed to handle the nonsterile aspects of PAC placement.

Modern PACs are available in various sizes (typically 7.0 to 7.5 French for adults) and often incorporate additional diagnostic or therapeutic features. All have a distal port for pulmonary artery pressure monitoring, a proximal port (typically at the 30-cm mark) for CVP monitoring or intravenous fluid infusion, and a balloon at the catheter tip for flow-directed placement. This balloon should be inflated with no more than 1.5 mL of air. The syringe included with the PAC is usually restricted to this maximum inflation volume. Special PACs include extra venous-infusion ports, the capacity to measure right ventricular ejection fraction, fiberoptic bundles for blood oxygen saturation measurement, ultrasonic crystals for continuous cardiac output measurement, a lumen for passage of a ventricular pacing wire, or externally mounted electrodes for ventricular and atrial pacing or ECG recording.

Regardless of which PAC is chosen, all lumina are flushed and the distal port is connected to a transducer system with a continuous waveform display and preferably a strip-chart recorder. The catheter is passed through a sterile plastic sheath before being inserted in the introducer. The balloon is tested by inflation to the full 1.5-mL volume and should inflate evenly without becoming eccentric. Although the PAC is a flexible catheter, most are manufactured with a slight stiffness over the distal 10 cm in the shape of a gentle curve. This curve is helpful in directing the catheter, particularly from more awkward insertion sites such as the left IJV.

The PAC is inserted through the valved port of the introducer to approximately 20 cm. As it is inserted in a right IJV cannula, the curvature of the PAC should be oriented such that it points just leftward of the true anterior (the "11 o'clock" position as viewed from the head) (Fig. 8-7E). The balloon is then inflated, and the catheter is advanced toward the right atrium and tricuspid valve. At this point, ECG monitoring for dysrhythmias (and arterial pressure monitoring to note their significance) is essential, because premature ventricular complexes are often seen during PAC insertion and may require intervention. The location of the tip of the PAC is determined by identifying the characteristic pressures of the cardiac chambers and vessels encountered (Fig. 8-8). Typically, the tricuspid valve is encountered at 35 to 45 cm from a right IVJ approach, and the wide pulse of the right ventricular trace is observed. The pulmonic valve is crossed at the 45- to 55-cm mark, and the higher diastolic pressure of the pulmonary artery is noted, typically with some additional high-frequency artifact from catheter "fling." Although the right ventricle and pulmonary artery traces are usually easily distinguished, they may be confused when large respiratory variation is present, adding significant artifacts to the pressure traces. An observation that can often solve this dilemma is noting that just before the rapid pressure upswing of the next systole, the diastolic pressure in the pulmonary artery is decreasing (because of

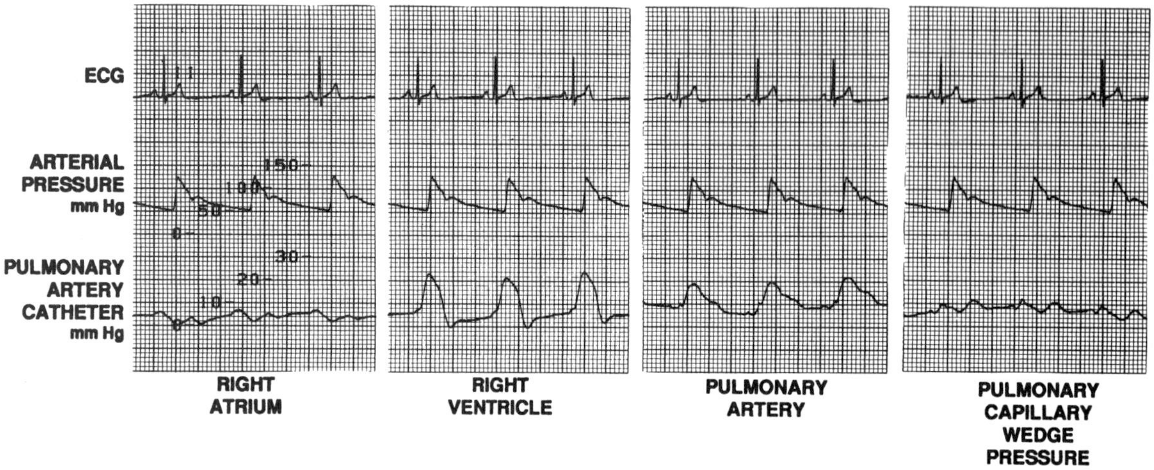

FIGURE 8-8. Characteristic waveforms encountered during normal passage of the pulmonary artery catheter. Note the progressive increase in diastolic pressure in the right ventricle, as opposed to a decrease during diastole in the pulmonary artery pressure. Note also the mild respiratory variation in all of these pressures.

continued forward blood flow and a closed pulmonic valve), whereas in the right ventricle, pressure at end-diastole is increasing (with progressive right ventricular filling and atrial contraction).

If the pulmonary artery waveform is not observed after the catheter is inserted to 60 cm, it is likely that coiling in the right ventricle has occurred, which predisposes to catheter knotting. Careful extraction after balloon deflation, redirecting (twisting), and readvancing of the catheter are employed to avoid this complication. The catheter is advanced further through the pulmonary artery until the "wedge" position is reached (usually at 50 to 60 cm), with a lower mean pressure and loss of much of the pulsatile character seen in the pulmonary artery. The balloon is then deflated, and the pulmonary artery waveform should be restored. Repeated inflation of the balloon should demonstrate the PCWP only at the full extent of the inflation (or shortly afterward as the balloon is gently guided by forward blood flow into the wedge position). Wedging at lower balloon inflation volumes not only predisposes to "overwedged" traces (see below) and erroneous data but also increases the risk of pulmonary artery rupture. PACs often migrate distally during the course of their use, and they may need to be periodically checked (by x-ray film or by careful balloon inflation) and pulled back as appropriate (84). Adjustment of the catheter position is made possible by the sterile protective sleeve covering the PAC outside of the introducer, although it is debatable whether this device offers significant protection from contamination (85)

The natural curve of the catheter and the course defined by its passage through the right side of the heart place the catheter tip most frequently in the arteries to the right middle or lower lobe of the lung (86). This is fortunate, because this location is likely to represent zone 3 pulmonary vasculature and therefore provides a useful PCWP measurement. Whenever possible, a chest x-ray film should be obtained to confirm the satisfactory position of the catheter.

Measurement of Pulmonary Artery Pressure

Although the PAC can provide information that may be invaluable to the care of the critically ill patient, there are several pitfalls in the measurement and interpretation of these data that can make the PAC a counterproductive and even hazardous tool. Inflation of the catheter balloon for PCWP measurement is done "blindly" and the catheter position can only be estimated by observing the pulmonary artery pressure trace. The waveform can be distorted by artifacts altering the expected normal progression of the pulmonary artery pulse wave to the "wedge" trace. This confusion can result in erroneous information or dangerous overinflation of the balloon (87).

The effects of PAC movement during the cardiac cycle can result in significant high-frequency artifacts in the displayed waveform. The low natural frequency f_n and resonance amplification of these necessarily long catheters are responsible for these erroneous data. Automated numeric display monitors are generally not to be trusted to interpret these waveforms accurately, and monitoring of pulmonary artery pressure and PCWP is performed optimally by examining a strip-chart recording of these pressures. The mode of ventilation (spontaneous or controlled) also must be accounted for in interpreting the effects of respiratory variation on pulmonary artery pressures and the appropriate information chosen at end-exhalation.

If the PAC balloon is inflated excessively, overwedging

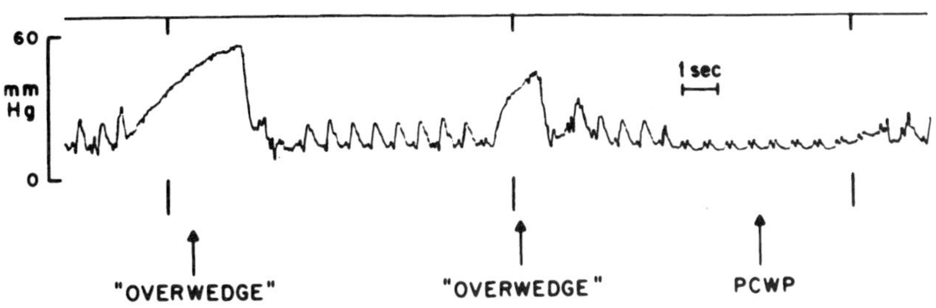

FIGURE 8-9. Pulmonary artery pressure tracing that demonstrates overwedging patterns with balloon inflation. When such a pressure tracing is obtained, the pulmonary artery catheter should be withdrawn until a normal transition from pulmonary artery to pulmonary capillary wedge pressure (PCWP) is seen. (Reprinted with permission from Barash PG, et al. Catheter-induced pulmonary artery perforation. Mechanisms, management, and modifications. J Thorac Cardiovasc Surg 1981;82:5)

can occur. This is generally the result of the overfilled balloon either herniating over the tip of the catheter or driving the tip into the wall of the pulmonary artery. An overwedged trace appears as a ramplike increase in pressure and loss of pulsatile character (Fig. 8-9). Often, it is a failure to recognize the PCWP trace that results in overinflation. The presence of a significant *v* wave, for example, as a result of mitral regurgitation, can cause the PCWP tracing to resemble the normal pulmonary artery waveform, and the unsuspecting clinician may continue to inflate the balloon after the wedge position has been obtained. Careful attention to subtle changes in the waveforms during PCWP measurement is thus required to avoid this error.

Alternative Central Venous Cannulation Sites

External Jugular Vein

Besides the IJVs, either external jugular vein may be cannulated for central venous access. The smaller and more tortuous external jugular vein is cannulated with an 18-gauge catheter in a fashion similar to that for a peripheral vein. A guidewire is then passed into the central circulation. This wire should be of the J-type with a small radius of curvature of the J, as these have been found to be advanced more successfully. Because the external jugular vein is a superficial vessel, its cannulation carries less risk of damage to neck anatomy. However, the presence of two sets of venous valves, the acute angle at which the external jugular vein joins the subclavian vein, and the compressive effects of the overlying clavicle may impede catheter placement. Moreover, the large sheath introducers for PACs should be inserted carefully, as there is risk of this stiff introducer tearing the vein at its juncture with the subclavian vein.

Subclavian Vein

The subclavian vein still enjoys popularity as a site for central venous access (79). The fact that the point of insertion is in a broad flat area of the chest makes it ideal for use in chronic central venous cannulation by affording increased patient comfort and longevity of the occlusive dressing. The infraclavicular approach to this vein is the most commonly taught technique (88). Beginning in the skin and subcutaneous tissue inferior to the clavicle, a 16-gauge needle is advanced medially toward the sternal notch so that it passes behind the clavicle just lateral to the curvature at its midpoint. The angle of the needle should be low (tangential to the ribs, if possible) to avoid perforation of the pleura. Passage of a guidewire and catheter is done in the usual fashion. If the neck veins are unavailable for PAC placement, the left subclavian vein is the best alternative choice, because its course to the superior vena cava offers a more gradual angle than does the right subclavian vein. The subclavian artery is posterior to the vein and in line with this approach. Its puncture may result in significant hemothorax or hemomediastinum because it is difficult to apply direct occlusive pressure to this artery.

Antecubital Veins

The basilic and cephalic veins provide the least risk of complications in central venous catheterization. However, the difficulty in reliably passing these catheters into the superior vena cava makes them a less popular technique in routine practice. Studies report meager success rates, ranging from 25% to 67% with passage through the basilic vein generally providing greater success (89). Moreover, an increased risk of thrombosis and thrombophlebitis may accompany long-term cannulation of these vessels.

Complications of Central Venous Cannulation

Complications of central venous cannulation are infrequent but can result in serious morbidity (Table 8-2). They may be divided into (a) complications of the puncture and insertion technique and (b) those relating to the catheter itself. Trauma to structures adjacent to the targeted vein is the most commonly recognized error during the cannulation process. Punctures of the carotid artery (1.9% to 3.6% incidence) (90–92), the pleural cavity, and the brachial plexus or stellate ganglion are seen during IJV cannulation. Subclavian vein catheterization can result in subclavian artery puncture, pleural injury, and damage to the thoracic duct (left-sided approaches).

Entrainment of air during catheter placement can be avoided with careful cannulation technique, but it may also occur if the catheter becomes disconnected later. Catheter shearing and embolization of fragments are serious compli-

TABLE 8-2. COMPLICATIONS OF CARDIAC FILLING PRESSURE MONITORING

Complications of central venous cannulation
Arterial puncture
Carotid artery
Subclavian artery
Hematoma, hemothorax, chylothorax
Mediastinal, pleural effusion
Pneumothorax
Nerve injury
Brachial plexus
Stellate ganglion (Horner's syndrome)
Emboli
Air
Catheter shearing
Complications of catheter insertion
Cardiac perforation
Dysrhythmias, heart block
Knotting
Tricuspid, pulmonic valve injury
Complications of catheter presence
Thrombosis, thromboembolism
Infection
Sepsis
Endocarditis
Dysrhythmias
Pulmonary artery rupture
Pulmonary infarction
Valve trauma

cations sometimes seen with catheter-through-the-needle sets. Dysrhythmias are occasionally noted when the guidewire or central venous catheter is advanced too far into the right atrium or right ventricle and are typically self-limited when these objects are withdrawn. Infectious complications may involve a superficial inflammation at the insertion site or a more serious contamination of the catheter with the possibility of generalized sepsis. The presence of infection requires removal of the catheter.

Complications of Pulmonary Artery Catheterization

Clearly, PAC use is associated with various potential complications that must be considered in the decision to implement this type of cardiac monitoring. One study of 211 PACs placed in an intensive care ward found a 51% incidence of complications when all problems, major and minor, were considered (93). In 4% of cases, the complications were considered life-threatening, and two PACs (0.9%) were thought to result in the demise of patients. As mentioned above, in a study with significant methodological limitations, Connors et al. (67) demonstrated an association between pulmonary artery catheterization and increased mortality, as well as resource utilization. However, in a review of 6,245 undergoing pulmonary artery catheterization, Shah et al. (90) reported extremely low rates of morbidity resulting from the PAC itself.

Tachydysrhythmias

Studies have reported a 17% to 78% incidence of premature ventricular complexes during PAC insertion or removal (94,95). However, only 3% of these dysrhythmias required intervention other than manipulation of the catheter to eliminate the mechanical irritation (90). Although premature ventricular complexes rarely may progress to ventricular tachycardia, most are transient and have been shown not to cause significant morbidity.

Complete Heart Block

Case reports of PAC passage causing complete heart block in patients with preexisting left bundle-branch block have led to suggestions that temporary pacing catheters be used prophylactically in this population (96). The incidence of new right bundle-branch block in patients undergoing pulmonary artery catheterization ranges from 3% to 6% (97). Morris et al. (98) reported 82 PAC placements in 47 patients with either chronic or newly diagnosed left bundle-branch block. There were five episodes of complete heart block in the chronic left bundle-branch block group, but each of these occurred either before the PAC was placed or after it was removed. Two episodes of complete heart block occurred in patients with new left bundle-branch block, but neither could be attributed to the presence of the PAC. The authors concluded that PAC placement was associated with a very low risk of complete heart block in patients with left bundle-branch block and that temporary transvenous pacing was unnecessary.

Although the risk of complete heart block is very low, the capacity to provide temporary pacing during placement of the PAC in patients with left bundle-branch block is still recommended. In this setting, the use of a PAC with a port through which a pacing wire can be passed (Paceport) is not an effective strategy because induction of complete heart block typically occurs during passage of the PAC and not after the PAC is properly positioned. Proper positioning of the pacing port within the right ventricle is a prerequisite for ventricular capture. Temporary percutaneous pacing (e.g., Zoll pacemaker), on the other hand, is an effective option in patients with left bundle-branch block. Alternatively, the PAC may be advanced beyond the atrium only when the chest has been surgically opened and the capacity to pace epicardially becomes available.

Infectious Complications

Catheter-related infections are a well-recognized complication of all types of invasive hemodynamic monitoring. Colonization at the insertion site, IJV cannulation, and duration of catheterization have been associated with a greater incidence of PAC-related infection. The overall incidence of PAC colonization ranges from 5.9% to 29.1% but only about 1% of PACs cause catheter-related bacteremia or candidemia, with 50% of the bloodstream infections originating from contamination of a hub or infusate (99). Organisms commonly producing bloodstream infections include coagulase-negative staphylococci (33%), *Staphylococcus aureus* (30%), enteric Gram-negative bacilli (20%), and yeasts (16%). Bacteremias caused by *Enterobacter* species, *Serratia marcescens,* or nonaeruginosa pseudomonads should suggest contamination of an infusate (99).

Catheter Knotting

This is a rare complication but when it occurs is a difficult problem to solve and can add significantly to patient morbidity (100). Predisposing factors for development of PAC kinks and knots include excessive catheter insertion and coiling in the right ventricle. Incomplete inflation of the balloon during insertion may increase the chance of the catheter passing around a papillary muscle or chordae tendineae (100). The most effective therapy for this PAC knotting is an awareness of these risk factors and early recognition of the problem (damped pulmonary artery pressure trace or difficulty in flushing the distal lumen), with subsequent confirmation by chest x-ray films. If knotting is highly suspected during a cardiac surgical procedure, a small right atriotomy by the surgeon can be advised to confirm and remedy the situation. If the knot has not already been drawn tightly, it may be untied under fluoroscopy using a combination of intravascular snares (101). Otherwise, removal under direct surgical exposure of the venous cannulation site may be required (102).

Pulmonary Artery Rupture

The most devastating complication of PAC use is rupture of a pulmonary artery. Fortunately, this is an uncommon event (0.2% to 0.5%)(92,103) because its occurrence carries an extremely high mortality (41%) (104). Pulmonary artery rupture can be caused by tip perforation of the vasculature, eccentrically inflated balloon driving an exposed catheter tip through the artery, or balloon inflation disrupting the pulmonary artery (105,106). Hardy et al., studying cadaveric specimens, determined that the pressure required to rupture the pulmonary artery was well within the range of pressures normally exerted by balloon inflation when the patient's age exceeded 60 years (107). Advanced age, hypothermia, pulmonary hypertension, female gender, radiation therapy to the area (e.g., breast cancer), and deviations from standard insertion techniques have been associated with a greater risk of perforation (104,106).

The hallmark of pulmonary artery rupture is hemoptysis, which may occur acutely in small amounts or as massive exsanguination. Signs in less obvious cases include hypoxia, hypotension, bronchospasm, or pulmonary artery air emboli. A chest x-ray film may show infiltration around the catheter tip. Injection of radiopaque dye through the pulmonary artery port will help differentiate pulmonary infarction from pulmonary artery rupture by demonstrating extravasation into the pulmonary parenchyma in cases of rupture. Treatment of pulmonary artery rupture depends on the rate of blood loss and the cardiorespiratory stability of the patient. Unless required for CPB, anticoagulation should be reversed. Steps should be taken to lower pulmonary artery pressure. Ventilatory support requirements range from oxygen supplementation to endobronchial intubation to protect the unaffected lung. Only after selective bronchial intubation should the patient be turned laterally to place the bleeding lung up to decrease effective pulmonary artery pressure at that site (105). PEEP may be used to tamponade the bleeding site (108). In severe cases, emergency surgical intervention is required, with procedures ranging from simple vascular repair to pneumonectomy. In the setting of CPB, conservative management strategies have been associated with a high incidence (45%) of secondary and often fatal hemorrhage when compared to patients having surgical control of bleeding (104). The best treatment for this potentially catastrophic complication, however, is prevention, which is achieved by adhering to general guidelines for safe balloon inflation (Table 8-3).

TABLE 8-3. GUIDELINES FOR PULMONARY ARTERY CATHETER BALLOON INFLATION

Never use fluid to inflate balloon
Never use more than the recommended inflation volumes
Always inflate balloon slowly, watching trace for signs of an "early" or "over" wedge pressure trace that might signify peripheral migration of the catheter tip
Withdraw pulmonary artery catheter several centimeters just before instituting cardiopulmonary bypass
Be particularly aware of the risk of pulmonary artery rupture in elderly and female patients

Left Atrial Pressure Monitoring

As a monitor of cardiac filling pressure, LAP monitoring is considered separately, primarily because of its method of placement, which is typically via direct cannulation in an open surgical field. Access to the left atrium is accomplished by passing a thin catheter through a secure purse-string suture in the right superior pulmonary vein, although a transseptal approach from the right atrium has been described (109). The catheter is then brought out through the infraxiphoid chest wall and securely connected to a closed pressure monitoring system. This technique affords a more definitive assessment of left ventricular filling pressure, because the confounding variables associated with the pulmonary vasculature are avoided. LAP monitoring is particularly useful in patients undergoing cardiac valve surgery, in whom left ventricular compliance and pulmonary vascular changes occurring as a result of the valve disease can make PCWP measurements significantly inaccurate.

This direct access to the left chambers of the heart carries the obvious risk of air and particulate embolization to the systemic circulation. LAP monitoring systems therefore require very close attention to proper management of periodic or continuous saline flushes. Also, removal of these lines can result in catheter shearing or mediastinal bleeding (110). This risk of bleeding generally dictates the removal of the LAP catheter before removing the mediastinal drainage tubes.

CARDIAC OUTPUT MONITORING

Cardiac output is the total blood flow generated by the heart, and in a healthy adult at rest, it ranges from 5 to 6 L/minute. In combination with the measurement of arterial and venous pressures, determination of cardiac output allows the computation of other useful hemodynamic parameters, such as systemic vascular resistance, which can assist greatly in the management of cardiac surgical patients in both the intraoperative and postoperative periods.

Fick Cardiac Output Measurement

Measurement of flow in any fluid system can be performed by injecting a measurable indicator into the flow stream and determining the changes in its concentration at various points. This principle, first proposed for practical use by the German physiologist Adolph Fick in 1870, states that flow is directly proportional to the amount of a substance entering a stream of flow during the measurement period, divided by the difference between the concentrations of the substances at upstream and downstream measurement sites:

$$\text{Flow} = \frac{\text{Indicator Amount/Time}}{\text{Downstream-Upstream Indicator Concentration Difference}}$$

Fick described a means to determine blood flow by measuring overall oxygen uptake and content in blood. In this case, oxygen is the indicator whose uptake in the lungs and extraction by the tissues cause a difference in its content in arterial and venous blood. The direct Fick method is limited by (a) errors in sampling and analysis of the oxygen, (b) changing cardiac output over the usual 2- to 3-minute sampling time, and (c) changes in the respiratory conditions. Moreover, cumbersome equipment (exhaled gas collection bag) is required to accurately measure the oxygen consumption, and blood gases must be analyzed from invasively sampled arterial and mixed venous (preferably pulmonary artery) sites. However, provided that steady-state hemodynamic conditions are present, the Fick method yields highly reproducible measurements of cardiac output (111,112).

The development of continuous respiratory gas analysis using infrared and mass spectroscopy, as well as continuous arterial and mixed venous oximetry, has rekindled an interest in Fick's methodology for cardiac output measurement during anesthesia and in the intensive care unit. In the differential Fick partial rebreathing method, carbon dioxide elimination and the change in end-tidal CO_2 in response to a change in ventilation (rebreathing) is used to calculate cardiac output.

$$Q = \frac{\Delta VCO_2}{S\Delta ETCO_2}$$

where *Q* equals pulmonary capillary blood flow, $V\text{CO}_2$ equals CO_2 elimination rate, *S* equals slope of CO_2 dissociation curve, and $ETCO_2$ equals end-tidal CO_2.

This partial rebreathing method assumes the constancy of cardiac output, partial pressure of mixed venous CO_2, end-tidal arterial CO_2 gradient, and intrapulmonary shunt. Additionally, the intrapulmonary shunt is estimated using the inspired concentration of oxygen and the pulse oximeter–derived oxygen saturation and added to the pulmonary capillary blood flow to determine cardiac output. Although good correlation ($r = 0.8$) with thermodilution cardiac output has been demonstrated in patients *after* cardiac surgery (113), the accuracy of this method in patients undergoing sternotomy for CPB has not been established. Surgical manipulation in the open chest, extensive changes in ventilation, and effects of hypothermia and rewarming on CO_2 elimination are potential sources of error.

Indicator Dilution Cardiac Output Measurement

The indicator dilution method is a variant of the Fick technique in which a known amount of a substance is injected into the bloodstream, and its concentration change is measured at a downstream location. The Stewart-Hamilton equation (114,115) relates these quantities to blood flow:

$$Q = \frac{I}{C_I(t)dt}$$

where Q equals cardiac output, I equals amount of indicator, $C_I(t)dt$ equals change in indicator concentration over time.

In this method, computers are used to calculate the area under the concentration curve and quickly generate a cardiac output. However, continuous withdrawal of arterial blood is required to plot the concentration curve, and an indicator dye, such as indocyanine green, can gradually build up with repeated injections.

Thermodilution Cardiac Output Measurement

The introduction of thermal indicators (iced or room temperature saline or dextrose in water) by Fegler in 1954 (116) and the incorporation of thermistors in the tips of standard flow-directed PACs have vastly improved the facility of measuring cardiac output. Cardiac output determination is immediately available when pulmonary artery catheterization is implemented, and it can be performed repeatedly with a nontoxic, nonaccumulating, nonrecirculating indicator. Because of its ease of implementation and long clinical experience, the thermodilution technique has become the standard means of clinical cardiac output determination.

For thermal indicators, the Stewart-Hamilton equation becomes:

$$Q = \frac{V_I\,(T_B - T_I)\,K_1K_2}{T_B(t)dt}$$

where Q equals cardiac output (L/min), V_I equals volume of the injectate (ml), T_B equals blood temperature, T_I equals injectate temperature, K_1 equals density factor, K_2 equals computation constant, $T_B(t)dt$ equals change in blood temperature over time.

The constant K_1, is a function of the specific gravity and heat of both the injectate and blood. K_1 does not change significantly with the use of D5W or normal saline as the injectate and shows little variation as hematocrit is changed from 52 to 30. The computation constant K_2, which adjusts the units to liters per minute and is a function of catheter size (dead space), rate of heat change in transit, rate of injection, and (usually) injectate volume, is entered manually by the operator into the cardiac output computer. It is essential, therefore, that the constants are the correct value for the particular catheter and injectate characteristics and that the chosen injection technique be adhered to during measurements; otherwise, significant errors in derived cardiac output may occur.

Most thermodilution systems automatically measure injectate temperature. This is a useful feature that corrects for occasional variability in T_I but requires close attention to ensure that the additional thermistor at the injection port does not become disconnected. If disconnection occurs, T_I is read as room temperature, and when using an iced injectate, the $T_B - T_I$ term is erroneously low, resulting in artificially decreased cardiac output values. Finally, it is useful to have a display of the temperature curve during the injection. This display allows the user to detect artifact in the curve that may occur from baseline temperature drift or recirculation peaks from intracardiac shunts, both of which cause errors in the measurement. This detection is particularly important early after separation from CPB because variability in baseline pulmonary artery blood temperature occurring at this time can underestimate cardiac output (Fig. 8-10) (117).

Studies comparing thermodilution cardiac output determination to controlled *in vitro* measurements (118) and to other *in vivo* techniques (119) have demonstrated a 3% to 13% variability in its overall accuracy. This variance is primarily the result of discrepancies between the injection technique or injectate characteristics and the computation constant. Therefore, multiple cardiac output determinations are generally performed to reach an average value. Measurements done in triplicate have been shown to improve the confidence limits of the value nearly two-fold (120). It would be expected that the use of a large volume of colder injectate, which results in the largest temperature curve area, would add to the precision of the integral term

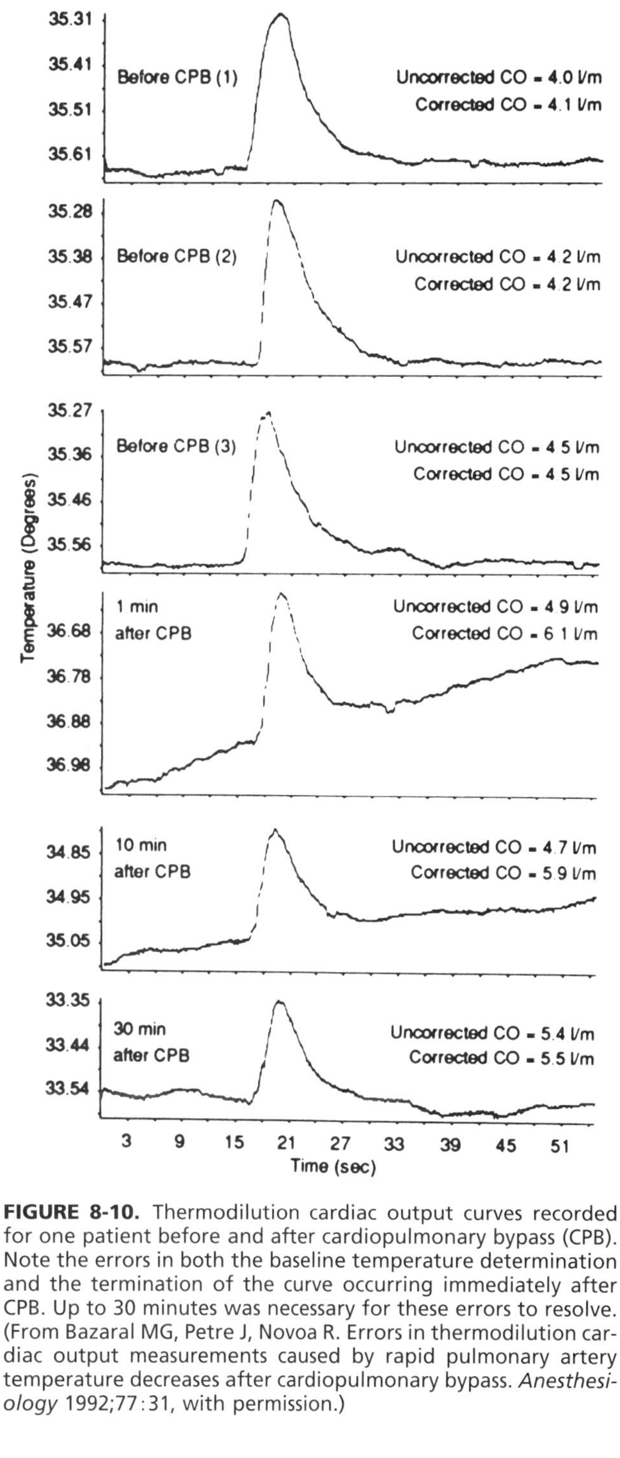

FIGURE 8-10. Thermodilution cardiac output curves recorded for one patient before and after cardiopulmonary bypass (CPB). Note the errors in both the baseline temperature determination and the termination of the curve occurring immediately after CPB. Up to 30 minutes was necessary for these errors to resolve. (From Bazaral MG, Petre J, Novoa R. Errors in thermodilution cardiac output measurements caused by rapid pulmonary artery temperature decreases after cardiopulmonary bypass. *Anesthesiology* 1992;77:31, with permission.)

of the cardiac output equation. While it is true that 10-mL injectate volumes improve the reproducibility of cardiac output values, studies have shown little if any added precision with the use of iced versus room temperature injectate (118,121). Moreover, cardiac dysrhythmias and bradycardia have been shown to result from the rapid injection of iced indicator (122,123). The effects of respiration on instantaneous cardiac output can be standardized by making repeated injections during the same phase of the respiratory cycle (typically end-exhalation).

Continuous Cardiac Output Monitoring

Thermodilution Cardiac Output

Although cardiac output determination by the bolus thermodilution technique has become the "gold standard," it is not ideal in critically ill patients because information is obtained intermittently and triplicate measurements can lead to substantial volume loading. Stochastic system identification techniques pioneered by Yelderman (124) have led to the development of a continuous cardiac output PAC that incorporates a heating filament in the right atrial position. When the filament is turned on and off, the resulting temperature fluctuations in the pulmonary artery are recorded. These temperature fluctuations and the thermal input energy are incorporated into the numerator of a modified Stewart-Hamilton equation to calculate the cardiac output. In a group of 122 intensive care unit patients, excellent correlation ($r = 0.94$) was obtained with bolus thermodilution (125). High levels of variability in blood temperature, commonly seen immediately after CPB, may decrease the accuracy of this method. The higher cost of these catheters has also prevented their widespread use.

Doppler Ultrasound

The Doppler principle applied to clinical ultrasound technology provides the capacity to quantify blood flow velocity. This has stimulated the development of devices designed to monitor cardiac output on a continuous basis. A detailed description of the Doppler principle and the technology surrounding its use in monitoring is in the Transesophageal Echocardiography section. The various methods of Doppler-derived cardiac output differ in the anatomic location from which the blood flow measurements are obtained. However, all techniques require that several steps be completed: (a) A value for the cross-sectional area of a main outflow vessel (ascending aorta, descending aorta, or main pulmonary artery) ($Area_{Ao}$) must be obtained or estimated using a normogram; (b) an ultrasonic transducer is placed in a position such that its beam falls in a line closely parallel to the direction of blood flow through that vessel; (c) the ultrasound device must integrate measured blood flow velocity over the period of ejection (T_{ej}) to determine an average velocity value (V_{avg}) for each heart beat; and (d) V_{avg}, $Area_{Ao}$, T_{ej}, and heart rate (HR) are multiplied to derive cardiac output (CO in the following equation):

$$CO = (V_{avg})\,(Area_{Ao})\,(T_{ej})\,(HR)$$

The shape of the flow velocity waveform has also been used to assess left ventricular filling and contractility, as well as systemic vascular resistance (126). Prospective studies in patients undergoing cardiac (127) and orthopedic (128) surgery indicate that stroke volume, rather than cardiac output, may be a more sensitive indicator of impending hemodynamic compromise.

Transesophageal Doppler Cardiac Output

The best acoustic window to the ascending aorta that is closely in line with the direction of its blood flow is the top of the thorax at the suprasternal notch. The total cardiac output (minus coronary artery blood flow) can be assessed from this vantage point. The diameter of the aortic root is measured using standard precordial echocardiographic imaging, but it also may be estimated from a nomogram using the patient's height and weight. However, the use of a suprasternal probe is at best an intermittent cardiac output monitor.

In an effort to provide continuous measurements of cardiac output using Doppler techniques, an ultrasound transducer fitted to the tip of a standard esophageal stethoscope has been developed that determines blood flow velocity in the descending thoracic aorta. Obviously, some form of calibration is needed to account for blood flow distributed to the head and upper extremities and for the significant angle of incidence between the Doppler signal and descending aortic flow. This is accomplished using a suprasternal probe built into the same unit that provides a value for total cardiac output at the same moment that the esophageal probe reports descending aortic flow. The suprasternal probe is then removed, and the stored proportionality factor is used to infer the cardiac output measurement from the constantly monitored esophageal transducer. Of course, this assumes that this blood flow relationship remains constant over the range of cardiac output reported—an unwarranted premise, given the autoregulation of cerebral blood flow.

Initial comparisons of the esophageal approach for cardiac output measurement (CO_{ed}) to thermodilution tech niques (CO_{td}) demonstrated only fair correlation ($r = 0.67$) (129). However, cases studied later in the investigation showed improved agreement ($r = 0.85$), possibly indicating a progressive familiarization for proper instrument use. Another study using esophageal Doppler-derived cardiac output during cardiac surgery reported that tracking of cardiac output trends by the esophageal instrument was generally good (multiple regression analysis $R^2 = 0.95$), but the absolute difference between CO_{ed} and CO_{td} was significant in many cases (130). Common causes for these differences include deviations in the angle of incidence between the Doppler probe and blood flow, as well as fluctuations in the proportionality constant during surgery in response to changes in sympathetic tone and anesthetic depth (131).

Transtracheal Doppler Cardiac Output

A Doppler device has also been incorporated into a modified endotracheal tube to assess flow velocity and the cross-sectional area of the ascending aorta. Data from a study in non–cardiac surgery patients suggested limited accuracy ($r = 0.84$, mean percentage error of 12.4%) combined with a difficult learning curve and a requirement for frequent repositioning of the probe (132).

Pulmonary Artery Doppler Cardiac Output

A more invasive but nonetheless continuous monitor of cardiac output is available in Doppler-equipped PACs. These instruments operate on the same principle as those that derive blood flow from the aorta, except that the main pulmonary artery is the conduit that is interrogated for total cardiac output. New technology in this area of development has resulted in probes that continually measure main pulmonary artery diameter ultrasonically as well as measure a space-averaged blood flow velocity in the main pulmonary artery. Several assumptions are made in this computation, such as the angle of incidence of the Doppler beam with the blood flow vector, as well as a circular main pulmonary artery. Segal et al. (133) reported reasonable correlation of Doppler pulmonary artery cardiac output (CO_{dpa}) in humans with simultaneous thermodilution measurements ($r = 0.76$). However, the average bias of $-0.13 + 0.79$ L/minute could result in errors approaching 2 L/minute or more than 30% of actual cardiac output in patients.

Tissue Perfusion Monitoring

Mixed Venous Oxygen Saturation

Venous oxygen saturation (SvO_2) is possibly a more comprehensive measure of cardiac performance than cardiac output itself, because it reflects whether or not cardiac output is adequate to meet overall metabolic needs. It is a representation of the balance between total body oxygen supply and demand. However, several other important factors influence SvO_2, which must be accounted for when this measurement is interpreted. These factors can easily be understood by deriving the formula for SvO_2:

$$SvO_2 = SaO_2 - \frac{VO_2}{1.34\ (CO)(Hb)}$$

Thus, SvO_2 is a function of (a) the level of arterial oxygen saturation SaO_2, (b) the rate of oxygen consumption VO_2, (c) the cardiac output CO, and (d) the concentration of hemoglobin Hgb. The amount of oxygen physically dissolved in blood at normal FIO_2 is considered to be a negligible factor in this equation at normal atmospheric pressures.

Improvements in reflective photometric oximetry techniques and advances in fiberoptic design have resulted in incorporation of this technology within a PAC, providing the capability of continuously determining mixed venous oxygen saturation. A specialized computer connected to this PAC measures and displays trends in SvO_2. These devices take advantage of multiwavelength technology and reflection intensity algorithms that avoid measuring reflectance from a wall of the pulmonary artery. They also incorporate both *in vitro* and *in vivo* methods of calibration to provide accurate SvO_2 data.

An advantage of SvO_2 monitoring is its ability to provide continuous assessment of cardiac performance, by allowing an immediate quantitative appraisal of the influence of a physiologic event or intervention on the cardiovascular system. Its disadvantage is that multiple independent parameters have equal influence in determining SvO_2. Rapid changes in hemoglobin level, arterial oxygenation, or oxygen consumption quickly dissociate SvO_2 from cardiac output. Even as a general index of the oxygen-delivery–to–oxygen-consumption ratio, SvO_2 has pitfalls. In septic shock or in the presence of anatomic arteriovenous shunts, SvO_2 monitoring clearly loses diagnostic value (134). Moreover, the addition of SvO_2 measurement capability adds greatly to the cost of the PAC itself.

This mixture of advantages and disadvantages of SvO_2 monitoring has led to many studies of its clinical usefulness and cost-effectiveness. An early study in cardiac surgical patients demonstrated the sensitivity of decreased SvO_2 in predicting parallel changes in cardiac output (135). A 5% decrease in SvO_2 had an 86% chance of being associated with a significant lowering of cardiac output. A subsequent study in a similar cardiac surgical patient population in the postoperative period reported a poorer correlation of SvO_2 and cardiac output (136). This probably resulted from instability of other factors involved in the SvO_2 equation, such as hemoglobin level (resolution of intraoperative hemodilution) and oxygen consumption (shivering after hypothermic CPB). It should also be remembered that because blood flow exhibits regional differences, a normal SvO_2 level does not necessarily imply adequate perfusion in every organ system. Although the most hemodynamically unstable patients might benefit from this technology, significant benefit and cost-effectiveness of this catheter have yet to be documented (137).

Gastric Tonometry

The determination of intramucosal PCO_2 has been used to assess splanchnic perfusion and to estimate the prognosis of critically ill patients (138). Conventional gastric tonometry has been shown to be an unreliable manual method that takes too long to permit the early detection of mesenteric hypoperfusion. Furthermore, intramucosal pH, calculated using the serum bicarbonate value, may not be accurate because of an ischemia-induced impairment of the CO_2-bicarbonate buffer. Newer techniques incorporating a fiberoptic sensor (139,140) allow rapid determination of intramucosal P_{CO_2}, but studies demonstrating its efficacy in patients undergoing cardiac surgery are currently lacking.

Transesophageal Echocardiography

Although the original purpose of transesophageal imaging was simply to enhance cardiac diagnostic efforts by overcoming the limitations in image quality of the standard precordial position, transesophageal echocardiography (TEE) has gained significant popularity in anesthesiology—particularly in cardiac surgical procedures—as a platform for stable, continuous, noninvasive, high-quality intraoperative monitoring of global and regional cardiac function. Moreover, Doppler technology and color-flow imaging, which allow detailed examinations of valvular function, intracardiac shunts, and diastolic function, has further established TEE as an important tool in modern anesthesia practice. In the near future, contrast echocardiography may enhance our intraoperative diagnostic capabilities by providing an assessment of myocardial perfusion. Three-dimensional (3D) echocardiography linked to virtual reality heart models offers the potential for dramatic changes in the diagnosis and surgical management of cardiac disease. However, successful implementation of TEE requires a clear understanding of the principles and methodology of echocardiography.

Cardiac Imaging

Physics of Ultrasound

Sound energy behaves according to the principles of longitudinally propagating waves, with alternating compression and rarefaction of the transmitting medium. Ultrasound is defined as sound whose frequency exceeds the maximum audible frequency of 20,000 Hz. In clinical applications, ultrasound frequencies in the range of several million Hertz (megahertz) are used.

To produce ultrasound with these frequencies, special piezoelectric crystals are used. These materials have the property of mechanically expanding when stimulated by an electrical potential. With removal of the applied voltage, the crystal returns to its previous shape. The energy of this mechanical process is then propagated as ultrasound through the surrounding medium. Most crystals used in echocardiography are designed to produce frequencies ranging from 2.5 to 15 MHz.

The principal characteristic of ultrasound that forms the basis of its use in imaging is its reflection from surfaces encountered in its path. A surface can be defined as the interface between two media of differing acoustic impedance, which is determined by the density and velocity of

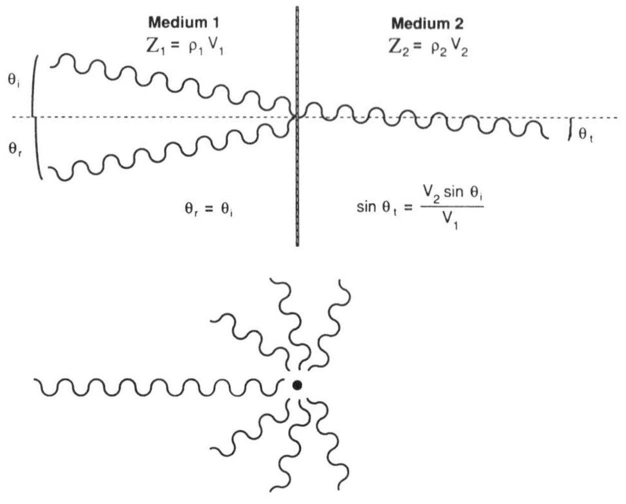

FIGURE 8-11. Behavior of a sound wave contacting surfaces of various sizes. **Upper panel:** Specular reflection caused by a surface that is large in comparison to the wavelength. The angle of incidence θ_i equals the angle of reflection θ_r. The intensity of the reflected wave is a function of the difference in acoustic impedance (Z) between the media forming the surface. Acoustic impedance of a material is the product of its density (ρ) and the velocity of sound conduction (V). **Lower panel:** Scattering of a wave occurs when the reflecting surface is small in comparison to its wavelength. The angles of reflection are many and unpredictable.

sound conductance of the individual materials. If the surface is large with respect to the wavelength of the sound then the reflection is specular, or mirror-like (Fig. 8-11, *upper panel*), and the angle of reflection is equal to the angle of incidence of the wave.

If, on the other hand, the reflecting surface is small in comparison to the sound wavelength, specular reflection is not observed, but the waveform is scattered, with only a small portion of its energy being reflected to the source (Fig. 8-11, *lower panel*). Irregularities in a large surface also can act as individual small surfaces and cause significant scattering of the ultrasound beam. Using higher frequency, shorter wavelength ultrasound enhances the desirable specular reflection.

When the reflected ultrasonic waves reach the transducer, an energy transfer process that is the inverse of sound transmission results. An electrical signal proportional to the received sound intensity is generated by the piezoelectric crystal and can be detected by the imaging system circuits. As noted, a reflected wave indicates that a surface exists between different media. Knowing the velocity of the ultrasound (V), the time (t) required for transmission and reflection determines the distance (d) of the surface from the transducer:

$$d = (V\,t)\,/\,2$$

The reflected ultrasound waves thus determine the location of the surfaces of objects in the field being examined.

Ultrasound Instrumentation

Most intraoperative ultrasound transducers are constructed as an array of small crystal elements. With this design, a number of advantages are realized. By controlling the timing of electrical impulses to the individual elements, the ultrasound waves can be created in such a way that the resulting wave front can be purposefully steered in a direction other than perpendicular to the plane of the transducer face. This process forms the basis of electronic phased-array two-dimensional (2D) ultrasound scanning. Typically, a 1-msec pulse of ultrasound is transmitted, after which the transducer is placed in the receive or "listen" mode for 250 msec. This process can thus be repeated several thousand times per second, providing sufficient time for reflected sound "interrogations" to be made in numerous directions.

Because of the attenuation of ultrasound during its transit through tissues, objects at greater distances will return diminished signals relative to those of nearer objects, even though their surfaces may be equally distinct. To correct for this problem, circuits within the imaging system allow selective amplification of late-arriving, more distant signals. This time-gain compensation is usually provided by series of slide potentiometers that allow the user to make these adjustments easily and improve image clarity.

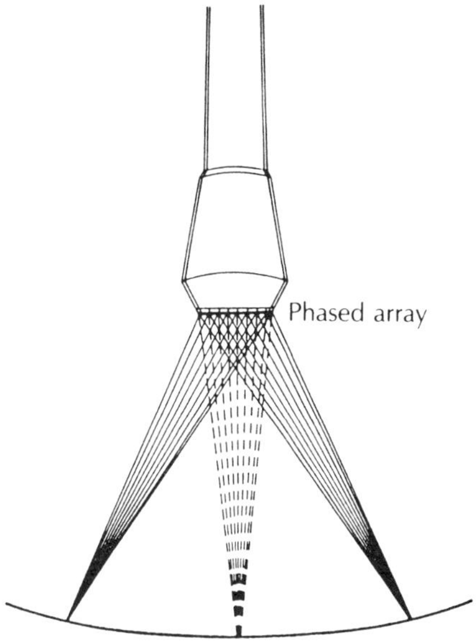

FIGURE 8-12. A phased-array two-dimensional scanner that uses multiple elements to steer the transmission as well as focus the reception of the ultrasound beam. (From de Bruijn NP, Clements FM. *Transesophageal echocardiography.* Boston: Little, Brown and Co, 1991, with permission.)

Imaging Systems

Today the vast majority of clinical echocardiographic monitoring is done using 2D scanning. 2D ultrasound scanning represents a significant advance in complexity and sophistication of ultrasound technology, because it provides a recognizable image of the objects being examined. In essence, 2D imaging consists of multiple interrogations performed over a sweeping arc of scan lines. The resulting information is displayed on a video screen as a series of lines emanating radially from a single location, with the intensities of the surfaces along the lines indicated by a particular brightness or "gray level." The time needed for performing an entire sweep of the sector arc is sufficiently short that the resulting image is considered a still frame of a moving object. Moreover, the 2D scan can be repeated 30 to 60 times per second so the resulting video image is seen by the human eye as a continuous, real-time monitor, with essentially all movement of the examined objects displayed. Modern scanners use phased-array technology that takes advantage of the ability of multielement transducers to electronically "steer" the beam across the scan area (Fig. 8-12).

Transesophageal Approach in Echocardiography

Diagnostic echocardiographic examinations are often limited by the presence of only a few "acoustic windows" into the mediastinum, because adjacent anatomic structures, such as bone and lung, present significant obstacles to the conduction of ultrasound. Common pathologic states, such as obesity and emphysema, compound this already difficult problem. Because of these limitations, the transesophageal approach became an attractive means of improving the quality of imaging in selected circumstances. Esophageal placement of the ultrasound transducer results in its close proximity to the heart, separated only by the soft tissues of the mediastinum, thereby avoiding the problems of image degradation. The additional advantage of TEE is its ability to provide stable views of the heart for protracted periods. In an intraoperative setting, TEE thus becomes a continuous monitor of the cardiovascular system.

Most 2D TEE devices use the smaller phased-array transducer developed by Schluter (141). The transducer, typically 1.2 × 1.0 × 3.0 cm, is placed at the tip of a standard 110-cm-long flexible gastroscope (Fig. 8-13). The distal 10 cm of the shaft is particularly flexible and can be retroflexed and anteflexed through approximately 100°. Multiplane technology allows for axial rotation of the imaging plane from 0° to 180°, providing a variety of echocardiographic views.

Although TEE is often used in awake patients with mild sedation and topical oropharyngeal anesthesia, it is even more easily applied during general anesthesia. Only after securing the anesthetized patient's airway by tracheal intubation should the TEE device be placed. Gastric air that may have been introduced previously should be evacuated.

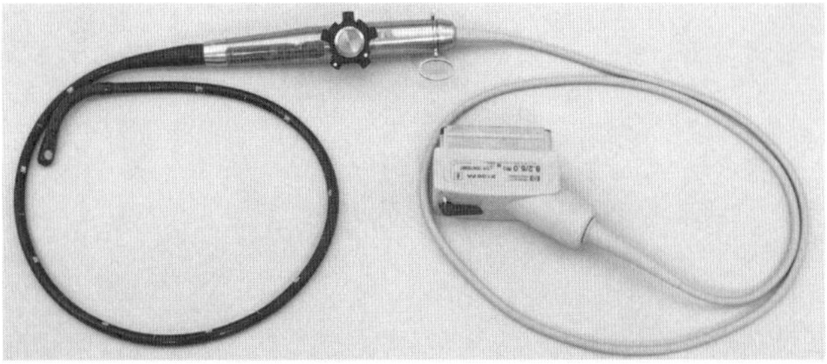

FIGURE 8-13. Transesophageal echocardiography probe. The transducer element is fitted into the tip of a modified gastroscope and can be steered by manipulating the wheels in the handle. Axial rotation from 0° to 180° permits multiplane imaging.

A water-soluble acoustic jelly is usually placed in the oropharynx or on the tip of the orally introduced transducer. The presence of the endotracheal tube tends to push the larynx down over the esophagus, and this may require gentle lifting of the mandible in order to open the posterior pharynx. Alternatively, a laryngoscope can be used to expose the opening of the esophagus. A bite block should be used to protect both the patient's teeth and the TEE probe. Once the device has passed the upper pharynx, its positioning is guided by observing the ultrasound image. Very few risks are associated with TEE use. Pharyngeal trauma is avoided by careful attention to gentle placement of the instrument. The transducer generates some heat, but the problem of thermal injury to the esophagus has been avoided by incorporation of a thermistor within the transducer that guards against overheating. TEE is contraindicated in patients with esophageal pathology including stricture, masses, varices, diverticulum, and recent upper esophageal or gastric surgery.

Various imaging planes may be obtained from the transesophageal position using multiplane TEE. In recognition of the increasing complexity related to the use of intraoperative TEE, the American Society of Echocardiography and the Society of Cardiovascular Anesthesiologists have developed *Guidelines for Performing a Comprehensive Intraoperative Multiplane Transesophageal Examination* (142). A TEE examination based on a series of 20 anatomically referenced cross-sectional images (Fig. 8-14) and the nomenclature (Fig. 8-15) that constitutes a comprehensive intraoperative

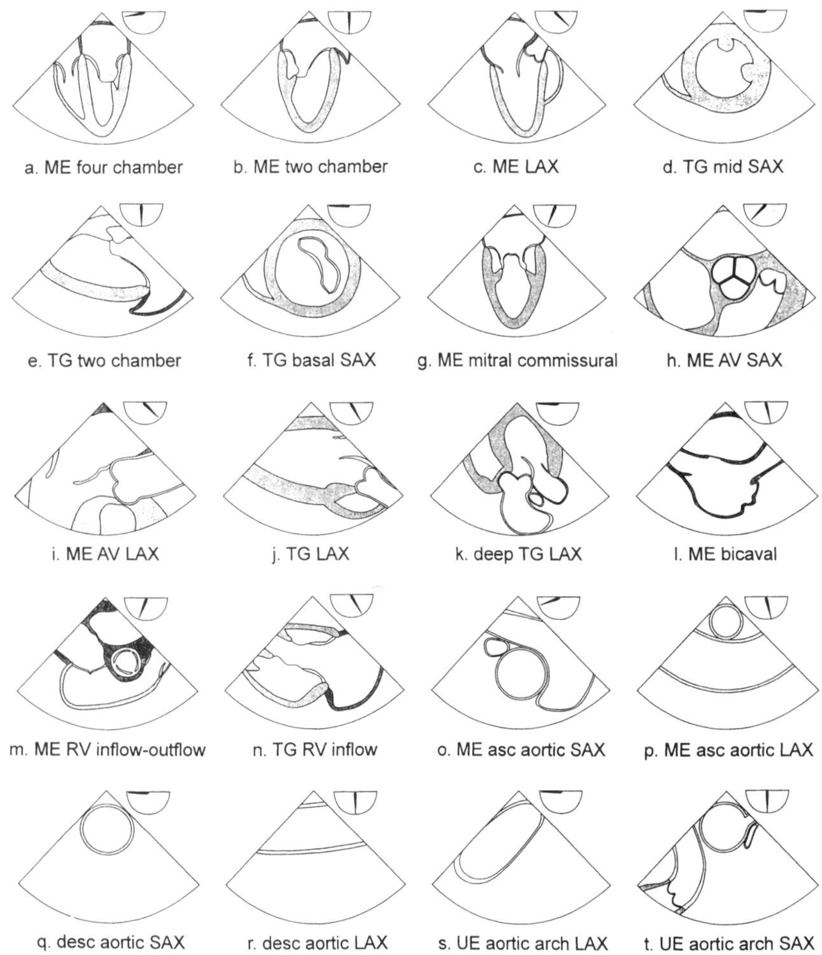

FIGURE 8-14. Cross-sectional images that constitute a comprehensive intraoperative transesophageal echocardiography examination. (ME, midesophageal; LAX, long axis; TG, transgastric; SAX, short axis; AV, aortic valve; RV, right ventricle; asc, ascending; desc, descending; UE, upper esophageal.) (From Shanewise JS, Cheung AT, Aronson S, et al. ASE/SCA guidelines for performing a comprehensive intraoperative multiplane transesophageal echocardiography examination: recommendations of the American Society of Echocardiography Council for Intraoperative Echocardiography and the Society of Cardiovascular Anesthesiologists Task Force for Certification in Perioperative Transesophageal Echocardiography. *Anesth Analg* 1999;89:870, with permission.)

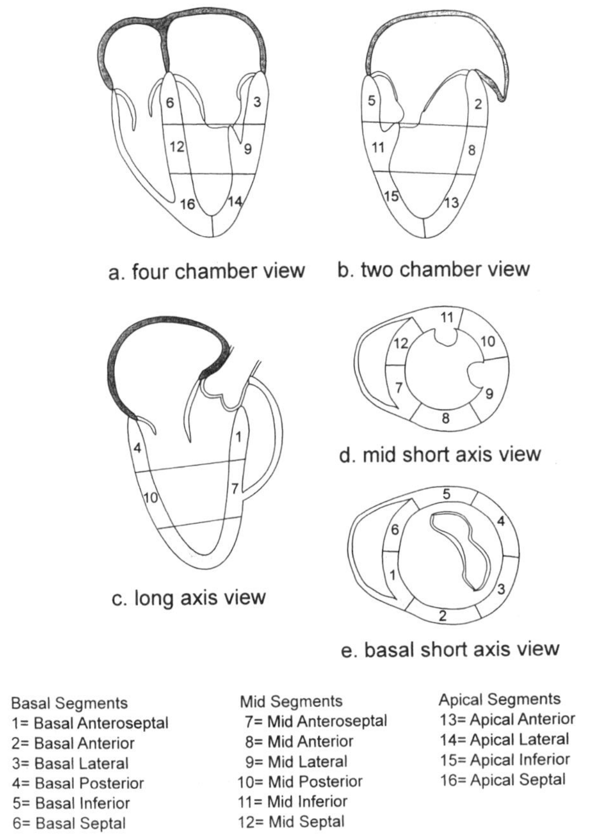

FIGURE 8-15. Sixteen-segment model of the left ventricle. (From Shanewise JS, Cheung AT, Aronson S, et al. ASE/SCA guidelines for performing a comprehensive intraoperative multiplane transesophageal echocardiography examination: recommendations of the American Society of Echocardiography Council for Intraoperative Echocardiography and the Society of Cardiovascular Anesthesiologists Task Force for Certification in Perioperative Transesophageal Echocardiography. *Anesth Analg* 1999;89:870, with permission.)

multiplane examination are described. A systematic and complete approach to the intraoperative TEE examination is required to ensure that unanticipated or clinically important findings are not overlooked. Routine performance of a comprehensive examination also provides for a rapid expansion of operator knowledge and experience.

Clinical Uses of Transesophageal Echocardiography

Global Cardiac Function

Like other important cardiac monitors, TEE provides a means of assessing overall cardiac performance by allowing the clinician to evaluate the global function of the heart, with the focus usually on the left ventricle. With the advent of multiplane TEE, both long-axis and short-axis imaging planes should be employed to assess overall contractility. Intraoperatively, the transgastric mid-short-axis view is chosen for this type of monitoring, because the approximately circular view of the left ventricular cavity is best suited to computations of area changes. By obtaining 2D images at end-diastole (ED) and at end-systole (ES), it is possible to outline left ventricular cavity areas using the tracing features built into most ultrasound imaging systems. Automated border detection features may also be employed to generate continuous end-diastolic and end-systolic areas. A cross-sectional area (A) measurement is computed, and area ejection fraction (EF_{area}) can be derived using the following equation:

$$EF_{area} = \frac{(A_{ED} - A_{ES})(100\%)}{A_{ED}}$$

Echocardiographic measurements have been shown to predict overall left ventricular ejection fraction as estimated from angiograms performed at cardiac catheterization (143,144). In patients with adequate image quality, short-axis fractional area change also correlated well with ejection fraction by radionuclide studies ($r = 0.92$) (145,146).

Cardiac Preload

In addition to providing an estimate of global cardiac function, TEE has been useful in assessing left ventricular volume. Typically, end-diastolic area is used as an approximation of left ventricular preload. Immediately after cardiac surgery, the correlation between end-diastolic area obtained from a single cross-sectional short-axis TEE image and those obtained by scintigraphy is only fair ($r = 0.72$) (147). The accuracy of TEE in measuring left ventricular volume is improved by increasing the number of cross-sectional images obtained (148) and by evaluating the end-diastolic area in multiple planes (149). When compared with more traditional hemodynamic parameters for measuring left ventricular volume such as PAD, CVP, and heart rate changes, TEE appears to provide a more sensitive and reliable method for detecting intraoperative hypovolemia (150,151). TEE-based assessment of left ventricular volume is also superior in the intensive care unit (152). It should be remembered that the transgastric mid-short-axis view does not provide a good estimate of right ventricular volume and a reliance on this imaging plane alone in guiding volume replacement can lead to right ventricular distension.

Regional Cardiac Function

In what has become a classic work, Tennant et al. (153) demonstrated an immediate decrease in the force of contraction in hearts after occlusion of a coronary artery, proving that the cardiac function is exquisitely sensitive to levels of perfusion. Detection of regional cardiac dysfunction in response to acute ischemia is desirable and readily monitored by echocardiography. Moreover, the occurrence of regional wall motion abnormalities (RWMA) with the onset of acute ischemia has been found to precede the development of characteristic electrocardiographic changes (Fig. 8-

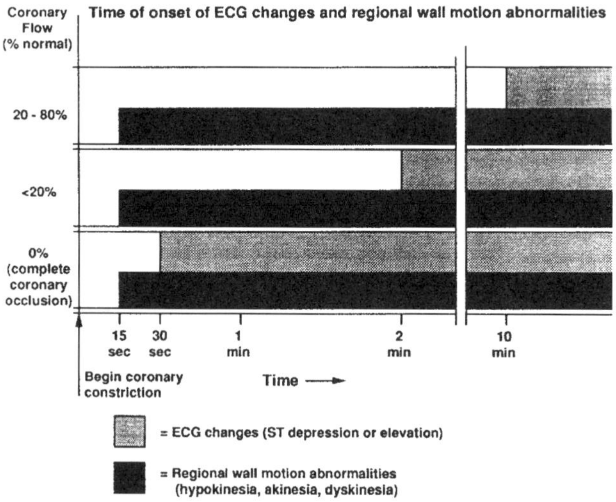

FIGURE 8-16. Temporal relationship between acute coronary constriction and the onset of electrocardiogram and regional wall motion abnormalities. (From Clements FM, de Bruijn NP. Perioperative evaluation of regional wall motion by transesophageal two-dimensional echocardiography. *Anesth Analg* 1987;66:249, with permission.)

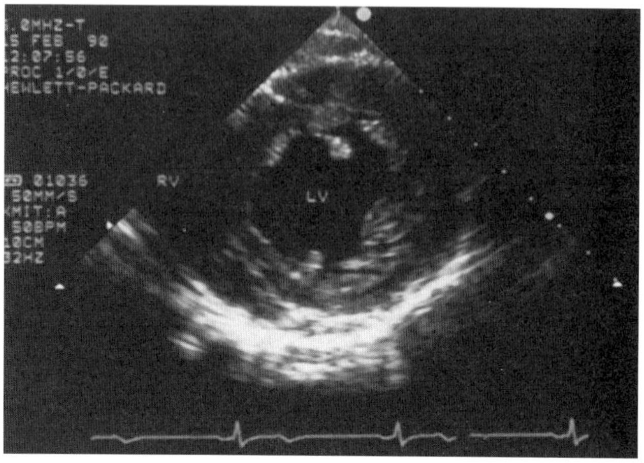

FIGURE 8-17. Transgastric mid short-axis image of the heart. (RV, right ventricle; LV, left ventricle.)

16). Waters et al. (154) noted RWMA after 50% reduction in coronary blood flow, whereas ECG changes were not apparent until flow reduction reached 75%. Similarly, Battler et al.(155) reported a dissociation in onset of RWMA versus ECG changes in graded reductions in coronary blood flow in conscious animals. The differences in time of onset were most apparent when partial coronary artery stenoses were applied.

In clinical investigations, Smith et al.(156) studied a group of patients undergoing major vascular surgery who were considered to be at high risk of perioperative ischemia. Intraoperative episodes of RWMA were present in 100% of those patients who later developed myocardial infarction postoperatively. ECG changes were seen during surgery in only one third of this subset of patients. A similar examination of the RWMA episodes diagnosed by TEE was performed by Leung et al. (157) in 50 patients undergoing coronary artery bypass surgery. They found that RWMA episodes occurring in the post-CPB period were predictive of postoperative adverse cardiac outcomes.

Clinically, the transgastric mid-short-axis view is commonly used to monitor for myocardial ischemia because it represents segments of myocardium supplied by all three major coronary arteries (Fig. 8-17). Although ideal for assessing ischemia resulting from epicardial artery occlusion, this view may not reflect ischemia involving the more peripheral coronary arteries and arterioles. As a result of monitoring only one imaging plane, basilar, apical, or right ventricular ischemia may go undiagnosed. The advent of multiplane technology mandates the use of multiple imaging planes in monitoring for ischemia. Studies have shown that monitoring the long-axis view of the left ventricle in addition to a short-axis view will increase detection of ischemia by approximately 40% (158,159).

Operator experience, resulting in a poor quality image or "echo dropout" of segments, can lead to misinterpretation of a specific RWMA. Errors may also result from attempts to grade oblique views. A paced rhythm or the presence of a left bundle branch block may alter the timing of ventricular contraction, resulting in the impression of regional dysfunction. Rotational changes in the position of the heart, particularly during the respiratory and cardiac cycle, may also distort the TEE image. Finally, not all myocardium found to be dysfunctional by echocardiographic monitoring is necessarily ischemic. A "tethering" phenomenon has been described, by which areas of healthy myocardium adjacent to ischemic regions may show decreased systolic function due to simply being attached to the truly hypoperfused areas (160).

London et al. (161) have reported poor specificity of intraoperative TEE-diagnosed RWMAs as a predictor of adverse cardiac outcome in patients undergoing noncardiac surgical procedures. This study also demonstrated a discordance between ECG and TEE in monitoring for ischemic changes. Temporal overlap with these two monitoring modalities was present in only 5 of 19 patients. Comunale et al.(162) in a study of 351 patients undergoing coronary artery bypass graft surgery similarly demonstrated a low (17%) concordance between ECG and TEE evidence of ischemia. In contrast to the findings of London et al. (161), these investigators demonstrated that TEE was twice as predictive as ECG in identifying patients who have myocardial infarction. Thus, the presence of cardiac dysfunction, either global or regional, does not absolutely indicate an ischemic etiology. Other hemodynamic factors, such as afterload, heart rate, and the effects of anesthetic or vasoactive drugs, can play a significant role in altering the functional profile from one moment to the next. In the setting of coronary artery bypass graft surgery, RWMAs diagnosed by TEE appear to be predictive of adverse outcome.

A caveat in the use of echocardiographic techniques is the reliance on qualitative evaluation of images. Unlike other intraoperative cardiac monitors that provide numeric results and have well-established ranges of normal values, TEE monitoring currently requires a subjective interpretation, which is possible only after a period of supervised training of the observer. Terminology used to score cardiac ultrasound images reflects the qualitative nature of these assessments. A decrease in regional function is evaluated as mild, moderate, or severe hypokinesis and is further identified by its location within the ventricle. Absence of movement is termed akinesis while outward systolic bulging or thinning of the ventricular wall is designated dyskinesia. Moreover, these descriptions must be applied with respect to a baseline examination of the particular patient to diagnose an intraoperative change in function. This step is often best accomplished by recording TEE images on videotape at selected periods to facilitate a quick review of the patient's previous status. Imaging systems that incorporate digital storage or "cine-loop" feature offer simultaneous observation of moving images recorded at separate times.

A quantitative approach to echocardiographic analysis of regional cardiac function has been a goal of investigators for a number of years. Today, the need for a more objective treatment of this information is even more apparent during TEE examinations in the intraoperative setting, where rapid changes in a patient's cardiovascular status and the effects of therapeutic intervention are most effectively followed with quantitative trendable information.

A serious impediment to the routine use of any presently available quantitative analysis scheme in echocardiography is the requirement for a significant amount of user interaction. The operator commonly must trace cardiac outlines (endocardial or epicardial edges) on a frozen video image for measurements to be made. This consumes too much time to be a practical part of intraoperative monitoring with TEE. Computer analysis and image processing in echocardiography also constitute a well-established field of research, and on-line automatic computerized image recognition and processing could ultimately solve this problem (163). However, progress in this area has been restrained by the lack of a mathematically clear, comprehensive understanding of the interaction of ultrasound with biologic tissue. Efforts of echocardiograph manufacturers have begun to make marginal progress in solving this problem (164). However, improvements in overall image quality by enhanced TEE technology, and the further development of powerful, portable computer resources, may finally allow implementation of the complex algorithms needed to replicate objectively what the observer's eye and brain subjectively perform.

Cardiac Anatomy

TEE can be used to visualize anatomic abnormalities of the heart and to evaluate their potential influence on the conduct of a cardiac surgical procedure. The widespread use of intraoperative TEE is the primary reason for the advancement of surgical techniques such as valve repair. The midesophageal long-axis views (Fig. 8-18) offer excellent perspectives of the mitral, tricuspid, and aortic valves, thus permitting diagnosis of the presence and severity of various pathologic changes including calcification, myxomatous degeneration, chordal rupture, and endocarditis. Inspection of the left atrial cavity is very easy using TEE, because this is the closest cardiac chamber to the esophageal transducer. Cardiac myxomas, which most frequently occur in the left atrium, can therefore easily be diagnosed with this monitoring technique. Thrombus formation in the atrium, seen in patients with chronic atrial fibrillation or in the left ventricle after large myocardial infarction, is another type of cardiac mass that can be assessed using echocardiography.

Aortic Atherosclerosis

The close anatomic relationship between the esophagus and the aorta also allows for high-resolution images of the aortic intima. The potential for embolization from aortic atheromatous plaques during CPB has led to the frequent use of TEE to define the nature and severity of aortic atherosclerotic disease. Many studies have demonstrated the correlation between the severity of aortic atheromatous disease and postoperative stroke (165,166). Although most of the aortic arch and descending thoracic aorta is clearly imaged with TEE, epiaortic scanning is better than TEE in detecting plaque in the ascending aorta (167). Palpation of the aorta clearly underestimates the presence and severity of atherosclerosis (167,168).

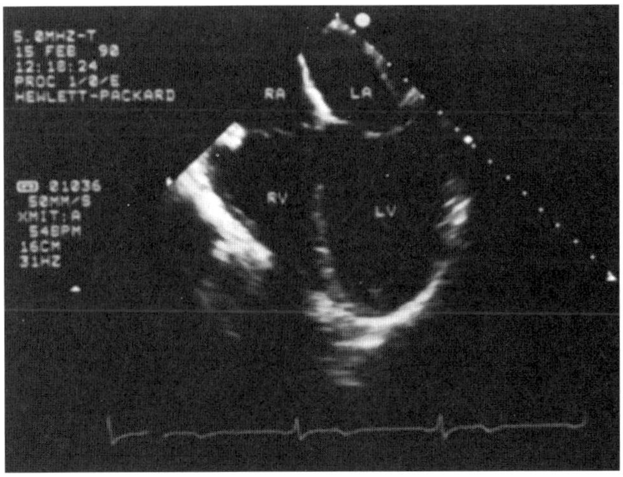

FIGURE 8-18. Midesophageal four-chamber image of the heart. (RA, right atrium; LA, left atrium; RV, right ventricle; LV, left ventricle.)

Intracardiac Air

Open-chamber cardiac surgical procedures necessarily result in intracardiac air introduction. The extreme difference in acoustic impedance between air and blood causes air bubbles to be strongly reflective of ultrasound. Exceptionally small bubbles (2 to 100 mm) can be visualized by echocardiography, making this technique a most sensitive means of diagnosing air bubbles in the circulation (Fig. 8-19). The incidence and severity of air emboli diagnosed by TEE in patients undergoing various types of cardiac surgical procedures has been addressed (169). Not surprisingly, air was present in a much greater percentage of patients undergoing open-chamber procedures (74%) than undergoing extracardiac operations (12%). Interestingly, there was no association of the severity of air emboli and postoperative focal neurologic abnormalities, although detailed prospective neuropsychiatric testing was not performed. Neurologic sequelae after cardiac surgery can be quite subtle. It is therefore possible to speculate that using TEE to determine and direct the process of air evacuation after cardiac surgery may have a positive effect on efforts to minimize neurologic complications.

Myocardial Perfusion

The intense reflectivity of air-filled bubbles has been put to use safely as a "contrast agent" in echocardiography. The first generation of commercially developed contrast agents were limited to air-filled agents such as sonicated albumin that were, by necessity, administered directly into the coronary arterial circulation for an assessment of myocardial perfusion. The second-generation agents, currently being developed, feature high-molecular-weight gasses that make them less diffusible than the air-filled agents. The newer agents also are stable, require less preparation, and cross the pulmonary circulation in good concentration, thus permitting standard intravenous administration.

Myocardial contrast echocardiography has improved endocardial border delineation and wall motion visualization. Studies have also demonstrated that myocardial contrast echocardiography can identify the site and extent of acute myocardial infarction. In combination with dobutamine or vasodilators such as adenosine, myocardial contrast echocardiography can aid in the detection of coronary artery disease and quantify myocardial perfusion (170). In the operating room, myocardial contrast echocardiography has been applied principally to assess the adequacy of cardioplegia administration. As harmonic imaging technology is adapted to the operating room, myocardial contrast echocardiography will become a valuable tool in the diagnosis and monitoring of patients with coronary artery disease (Fig. 8-20).

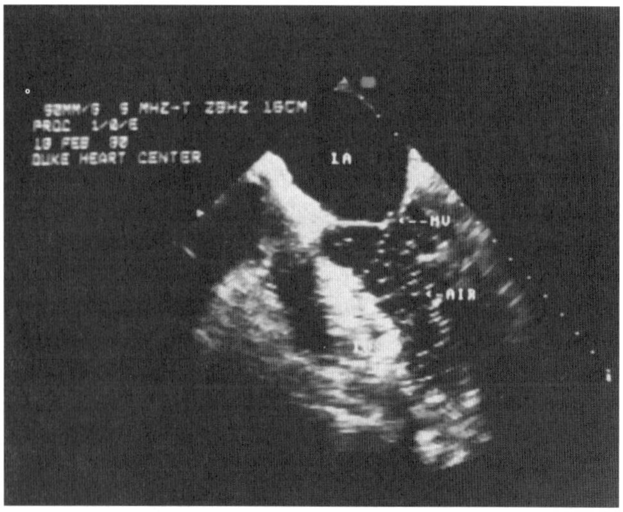

FIGURE 8-19. Midesophageal four-chamber image of the left ventricle (*LV*) and the left atrium (*LA*) demonstrating the appearance of intracavitary air bubbles in the LV just below the mitral valve (*MV*).

Cardiac Surgery

TEE is a vital component of cardiac monitoring during the newer cardiac surgical procedures. It could be argued that many of these surgeries can not be performed without the availability of intraoperative TEE. Positioning of catheters in the aorta and the coronary sinus during minimally invasive surgery mandates the use of TEE (171). Similarly, TEE-detected intracardiac air is an end point during transmyocardial laser revascularization. Finally, monitoring for myocardial ischemia with multiplane imaging is vital during coronary grafting without CPB, particularly when ischemic preconditioning is practiced.

Doppler Ultrasound

An extension of the diagnostic and monitoring capabilities of clinical ultrasound is the measurement of blood flow velocities using the Doppler principle. Improvements in ultrasound processing technology, particularly color-flow imaging and its incorporation in TEE devices, have provided facility for visualizing Doppler-derived blood flow information.

Basic Principles

The Doppler principle takes its name from the Austrian mathematician and physicist, Johann Christian Doppler, who presented the principle by using an erroneous suggestion to describe his idea that the movement of stars relative to Earth caused their altered coloration (172). One of his critics, Buys Ballot, while seeking to disprove this theory, performed an experiment that verified the principle. He placed a trumpeter on a train moving past an observer who was trained to recognize perfect musical pitch. Other stationary trumpets were placed nearby and played the same note to provide a reference. As the train approached, the pitch of the trumpet moving toward the observer was per-

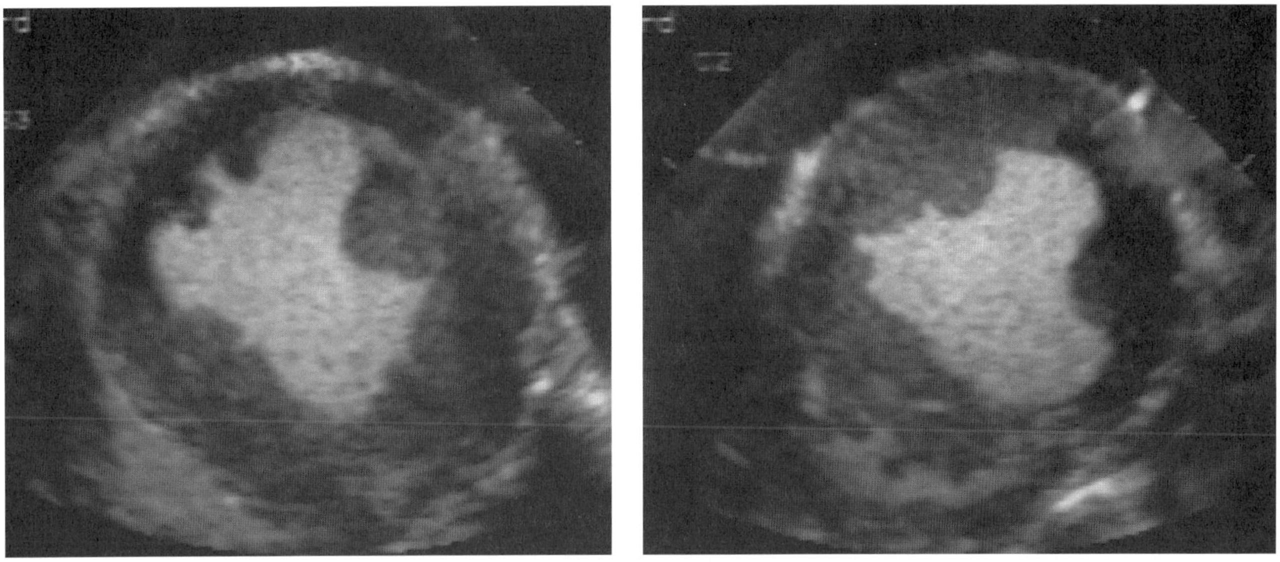

FIGURE 8-20. Transthoracic contrast echocardiography demonstrating occlusion (*dark areas*) of the left anterior descending (*left panel*) and circumflex (*right panel*) coronary arteries. (Photo courtesy of S. Kaul, MD.)

ceived to be higher than that of the stationary trumpets. As the train went by, the pitch heard immediately dropped below the reference note (173).

In Doppler ultrasound measurement of blood flow, the transducer instrument is both the source of sound energy and the "observer," or receiver, of the frequency-shifted reflected sound. The moving objects that reflect the ultrasound are red blood cells. Figure 8-21 demonstrates this effect for blood cells moving toward the transducer. Movement away from the transducer results in a lower reflected frequency compared with that originally emitted. Another difference in this application from the classic example is that there are many millions of these objects (red blood cells) whose potentially different velocities are assessed simultaneously. Thus, a variable set of reflected frequencies is actually returned to the transducer, particularly when blood flow loses its laminar characteristics and becomes turbulent.

To use this frequency-shift phenomenon, one must have a means of quantifying the velocities represented by the frequency changes. Fortunately, a relatively simple equation fulfills this requirement. The original Doppler equation to predict the reflected frequency can be rearranged for the velocity (V) of the object(s):

$$V = \frac{(c)\ (f_r)}{(2f_t)\ (\cos\ \theta)}$$

where c equals speed of sound in blood, f_r equals frequency of the reflected sound wave, f_t equals frequency of the transmitted sound wave, θ equals the angle between the sound wave direction and the direction of blood flow.

All of these factors are known or measured during a Doppler examination, with the exception of the angle of incidence θ, which must be estimated. Every effort should be made to align the ultrasound beam as parallel to the flow vector as possible so that $\theta = 0$. Generally, angles greater than 25° yield clinically unacceptable quantitative estimates of velocity (174). Much of the error in the techniques using Doppler is the result of an inability to optimize or standardize this alignment angle.

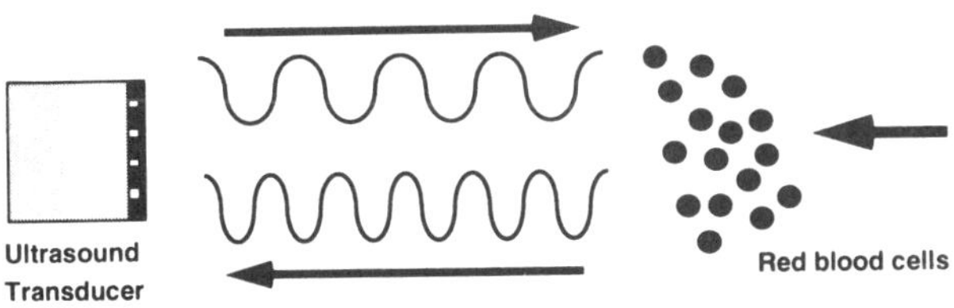

FIGURE 8-21. Example of the Doppler effect resulting from red blood cells traveling toward the transducer at the left. A burst of ultrasound is sent into the tissue at a given frequency and is reflected off the red cells moving toward the transducer at a higher frequency. This is a positive Doppler shift.

Doppler Instrumentation

Continuous-Wave Doppler. To this point, the discussion of Doppler techniques has assumed that the velocity of measurement is uninterrupted. In fact, the continuous-wave Doppler does provide constant blood flow information by using separate transmit and receive transducer elements (Fig. 8-22). Normal blood flow velocity in humans does not exceed 1.5 m/sec. However, in pathologic conditions

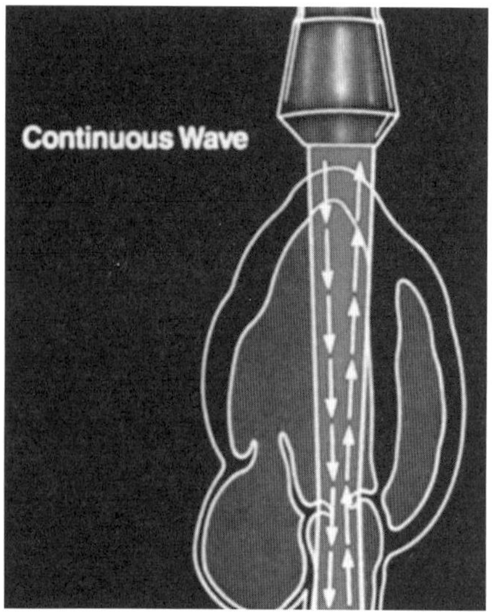

FIGURE 8-22. Continuous-wave Doppler blood flow measurement using separate transmit and receive transducers allows measurement of very high velocities but provides no localization along the path of the beam. (From Kisslo J. *An introduction to Doppler echocardiography.* London: Medi-Cine, 1987, with permission.)

such as aortic stenosis, a jet of blood flow can exceed 5 m/sec. Continuous-wave Doppler can measure a limitless range of blood flow velocities, making it very useful in quantifying these jets. The main disadvantage of continuous-wave Doppler is its inability to determine the anatomic position from which the abnormal jet arises. In other words, continuous-wave Doppler has no capacity for range discrimination but displays a mix of velocity data from all points along its beam.

Pulsed Wave Doppler. A more common technique for providing range (location) information for the velocity being measured is pulsed wave Doppler. In this method, short bursts or pulses of ultrasound are emitted by a single transducer, which then switches to a "listen" mode and waits for a returning signal (Fig. 8-23). Thus, velocity information from a specific site is available, and the remainder of the returning Doppler signal outside of this "gate" is ignored. This allows the possibility for the ultrasound system to perform standard imaging during the intervening time, which is a great advantage because one can "see" where the pulsed wave Doppler sampling is taking place within the field of view.

The major disadvantage of pulsed wave Doppler techniques is that the maximum measurable velocity is limited. The reason for this problem is a phenomenon called aliasing, in which high velocities appear negative. Aliasing is the result of a mismatching of the Doppler frequency shift being measured and the rate at which pulsed wave samples are repeated.

Color-Flow Imaging. Doppler color-flow imaging is a valuable enhancement in Doppler echocardiography, providing real-time images of blood flow velocity in two dimensions superimposed on a standard 2D echocardiogram. This allows an immediate and relatively straightforward identification and qualitative assessment of many intracardiac lesions that affect blood flow patterns. Color-flow imaging is the product of very sophisticated high-speed electronic processing, which separates Doppler frequency shift information obtained from reflected ultrasound signals from multiple points along most or all of the scan lines of a 2D ultrasound image. In essence, color-flow systems perform multigated pulsed wave Doppler analyses on literally hundreds of sample volumes over a 2D space. To present a recognizable display of the direction and velocity of these many individual flow measurements, a color scheme is used. Typically, blood flow directed toward the transducer is red, whereas flow away is blue. The velocity is indicated by the shade of the color, with higher velocities causing the red hue to become lighter or even turn yellow and blue colors to reach a light cyan appearance. Because of the use of pulsed wave Doppler methods with a necessarily low-pulse repetition frequency, aliasing occurs to a significant degree in color-flow imaging. However, aliasing is actually somewhat advantageous in this method, because it has the effect of "wrapping" the color around to the opposite hue (bright red aliases immediately to bright blue), creating a "mosaic" color pattern when high-velocity turbulent flows are imaged. This makes abnormal blood flow jets more recognizable, because these are most likely to attain velocities high enough to cause aliasing.

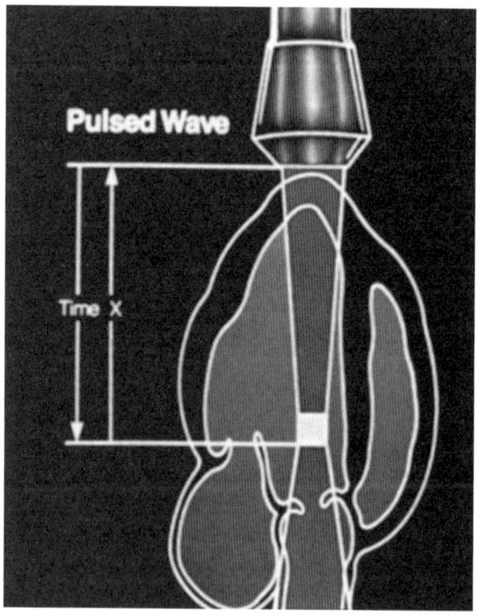

FIGURE 8-23. Pulsed wave Doppler blood flow measurement allows localization and focusing of discrete "sample volumes" for velocity interrogation but is limited to a maximum measurable velocity. (From Kisslo J. *An introduction to Doppler echocardiography.* London: Medi-Cine, 1987, with permission.)

Clinical Applications of Doppler Ultrasound

Hemodynamic Data. Cardiac output can be readily calculated with Doppler imaging by measuring the flow across a valve:

$$CO = (TVI)\ (CSA)\ (HR)$$

where CO equals cardiac output, TVI equals time velocity integral of the flow across the valve, CSA equals cross-sectional area of the valve, and HR equals heart rate.

The transgastric long-axis view (Fig. 8-14) allows good alignment between the Doppler beam and blood flow through the valve. Thus, cardiac output measurements at the level of the aortic annulus are reliable (175,176). Accurate estimation of the annular diameter of atrioventricular valves is the primary source of error when cardiac output is derived from flow across these valves.

Systolic pulmonary artery pressures also can be derived from continuous-wave assessment of tricuspid regurgitant flow: (177)

$$PAS = (4)\ (V_{Reg})^2 + RAP$$

where PAS equals pulmonary artery systolic pressure, V_{Reg} equals peak velocity of tricuspid regurgitant jet, and RAP equals right atrial pressure.

Valvular Function. Aortic valvular stenosis is easily measured using the Bernoulli or the continuity equations (178). Mitral valve areas can be derived using the pressure half-time or proximal isovelocity surface area methods (179). Color-flow Doppler imaging also provides a rapid assessment of the degree of valvular regurgitation. The popularity of cardiac valve repair is greatly assisted by the ability of color-flow imaging to provide intraoperative assessment of the effectiveness of this surgery and by allowing immediate revision of the procedure if necessary. Sheikh et al. (180) found that the presence of persistent valvular abnormality as demonstrated by intraoperative Doppler color-flow imaging in patients undergoing valve operations was significantly related to adverse postoperative outcome.

Congenital Heart Disease. Doppler color-flow imaging is also extremely valuable during repair of congenital cardiac defects. Several investigations have documented the usefulness of color-flow imaging in this setting (181,182). The ability to measure stroke volumes at multiple levels also permits the calculation of shunt fraction (Q_p/Q_s) (183).

Clinical Utility of Transesophageal Echocardiography

In 1996, *Practice Guidelines for Perioperative Transesophageal Echocardiography* was published by the American Society of Anesthesiologists (184). After a review of 558 studies considered relevant to the perioperative setting, recommendations for performing TEE were made based on the strength of supporting evidence or expert opinion that TEE improves clinical outcome. Category I indications are supported by the strongest evidence or expert opinion and TEE is frequently useful in improving clinical outcomes. Category II indications are supported by weaker evidence and TEE may be useful in improving clinical outcomes. In contrast, category III indications have little scientific support and are infrequently useful in improving outcome (Table 8-4).

TABLE 8-4. INDICATIONS FOR PERIOPERATIVE TRANSESOPHAGEAL ECHOCARDIOGRAPHY

Category I

- Evaluation of acute, persistent, and life-threatening hemodynamic disturbances in which ventricular function and its determinants are uncertain and have not responded to treatment
- Valve repair
- Congenital heart surgery requiring cardiopulmonary bypass
- Hypertrophic obstructive cardiomyopathy repair
- Endocarditis when preoperative testing was inadequate or extension of infection is suspected
- Aortic valve function in repair of aortic dissections with possible aortic valve involvement
- Evaluation of pericardial window procedures
- Preoperative use in unstable patients with suspected thoracic aortic aneurysms, dissection, or disruption who need to be evaluated quickly
- Use in intensive care unit for unstable patients with unexplained hemodynamic disturbances, suspected valve disease, or thromboembolic problems

Category II

- Valve replacement
- Repair of cardiac aneurysms
- Removal of cardiac tumors
- Detection of foreign bodies
- Detection of air emboli
- Intracardiac thrombectomy
- Pulmonary embolectomy
- Suspected cardiac trauma
- Repair of thoracic aortic dissections without suspected aortic valve involvement
- Detection of aortic atheromatous disease
- Evaluation of pericardiectomy, pericardial effusions, or pericardial surgery
- Evaluation of anastomotic sites during heart and/or lung transplantation
- Monitoring placement and function of assist devices
- Perioperative use in patients with increased risk of myocardial ischemia or infarction
- Perioperative use in patients with increased risk of hemodynamic disturbances
- Preoperative use in unstable patients with suspected thoracic aortic aneurysms, dissection, or disruption

Category II

- Evaluation of myocardial perfusion, coronary artery anatomy, or graft patency
- Repair of cardiomyopathies other than hypertrophic obstructive cardiomyopathy
- Uncomplicated endocarditis during noncardiac surgery
- Monitoring for emboli during orthopedic procedures
- Assessment of repair of thoracic aortic injuries
- Uncomplicated pericarditis
- Evaluation of pleuropulmonary diseases
- Monitoring of cardioplegia delivery
- Monitoring placement of intraaortic balloon pumps, automatic implantable cardiac defibrillators, or pulmonary artery catheters

Source: From Practice guidelines for perioperative transesophageal echocardiography. A report by the American Society of Anesthesiologists and the Society of Cardiovascular Anesthesiologists Task Force on Transesophageal Echocardiography. *Anesthesiology* 1996;84:986, with permission.

CENTRAL NERVOUS SYSTEM MONITORING

Neurologic monitoring during CPB is nearly as old as extracorporeal circulation itself, with electroencephalographic (EEG) monitoring used by colleagues of Kirklin and Cooley (185,186). Advances in the surgical and anesthetic management of the cardiac patient during the last 35 years have significantly reduced perioperative morbidity and mortality. The decline in cardiac morbidity and mortality has directed resources toward reducing neurologic and neuropsychologic complications, which can affect up to 60% of patients undergoing CPB (187). This focus on neurologic outcome has placed many new and old neurologic monitors at the forefront of investigation, with the goal of early detection of central or peripheral neurologic derangement.

Electrophysiologic Monitoring

Electroencephalography

Intraoperative EEG has proved to be of significant value in cerebrovascular surgery, but its usefulness during CPB remains controversial (188–190). The EEG is a recording of localized spontaneous electrical activity of the brain limited to detection of events occurring within a small area surrounding a recording electrode. Measurements of somatosensory evoked potentials (SSEPs) and the EEG have repeatedly shown that electrode position changes of 2 cm from the site of maximal activity will reduce the measured electrical activity by 80% (191). Adjacent cortex overshadows distant cortical activity, requiring that multiple recording electrodes be used to ensure EEG monitoring of all areas of the cortex.

Signal Acquisition

Meticulous recording technique is essential to an interpretable EEG in or out of the operating room. Standard placement of EEG electrodes improves correlation between EEG activity and cortical activity and allows reproducibility and comparison of the EEG data. Precise placement of electrodes by nasion, inion, head circumference, and distance between the ears using the 10-20 electrode system of the International Federation (192) facilitates symmetric placement of electrodes, allowing similar amplitudes at baseline that facilitate computer processing of signals (Fig. 8-24).

The operating room is a hostile electrical environment, making the selection and application of EEG electrodes even more important. Leakage currents from electrical devices, ground-loop interference, and electrocautery interruption can make recording and interpreting the EEG data difficult or impossible. Even though modern EEG monitors, specifically designed for the operating room, are relatively immune to many of the artifacts of the environment, the impedance of the electrodes must be kept low (less than 5 kohms). Ten-mm Ag-AgCl cup electrodes attached with

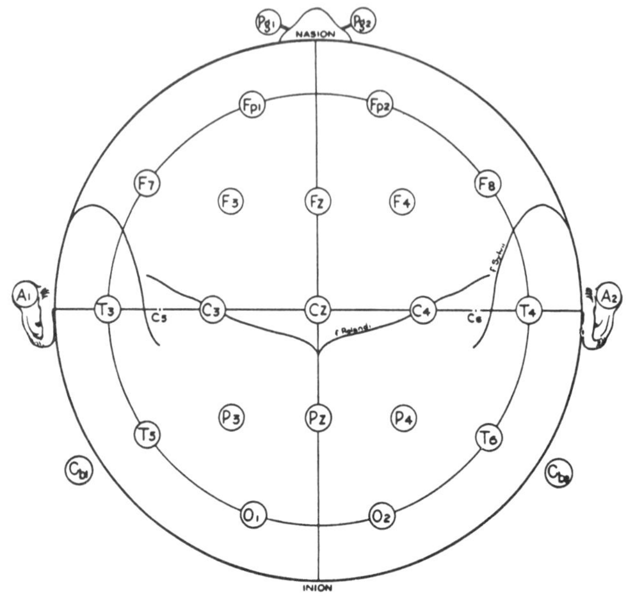

FIGURE 8-24. The 10-20 electrode system of the International Federation. (From Jasper HH. The ten-twenty electrode system of the International Federation. *Electroenceph Clin Neurophysiol* 1958;10:371, with permission.)

collodion, filled with salt gel, and sealed with collodion and gauze are the gold standard. Conductive pastes can be used to secure electrodes but often decrease long-term success. Stick-on electrodes with a saline gel pellet and Ag-AgCl disc are convenient but are limited to areas without hair.

The EEG is generated from pyramidal cells of the cerebral cortex with voltage fluctuations resulting primarily from postsynaptic potentials. Surface electrodes can detect the simultaneous electrical activity of many cells, but the cortical voltage falls rapidly to only 1/20 of its actual value at a distance of 2.5 cm. Thus, two or four recording channels improve the value of EEG monitoring by increasing the area monitored and allowing the detection of electrical asymmetry, often the first indication of cerebral dysfunction (193). Sixteen channels provides even greater information but are only useful if an electroencephalographer is available to continuously record and interpret the EEG.

The voltages obtained in an EEG are expressed in microvolts (μV) compared with the millivolts (mV) for signals obtained from ECG, further emphasizing the necessity of low impedance in the recording electrodes. Waveforms obtained on the EEG records are described in terms of frequency, amplitude, distribution, regularity, and specific patterns. Beta rhythm (13 to 30 Hz) is the dominant rhythm in alert patients with eyes open, and it is increased by sedation levels of barbiturates and benzodiazepines. Alpha rhythm (8 to 13 Hz) is seen during awake states with eyes closed or under moderate levels of anesthesia. Theta rhythm (4 to 8 Hz) is common during anesthesia and drowsiness. Delta waves (1 to 4 Hz) are normally seen during deep sleep or deep anesthesia. The presence of delta waves during wakefulness or light anesthesia is suggestive of pathology.

The use of anesthetic agents produces characteristic EEG changes. Therefore, when EEG monitoring is used, the maintenance of stable anesthetic levels is critical. EEG changes cannot be correlated with surgical or physiologic interventions unless anesthetic levels have been invariable. The only exception to this approach in cardiac surgery is the production of burst suppression or isoelectric EEG during CPB using anesthetic agents. Without large doses of cerebral depressants, EEG "slowing" (decreased amplitude of alpha or beta waves and/or increased amplitude of theta or delta waves) is pathologic. Although this pattern is not specific to the type of injury (hypoxia, hypoglycemia, hypothermia, and extreme hypotension), it is highly specific for cortical malfunction of some cause.

Analysis Methods

Although a 16-channel strip-chart EEG recording is used to evaluate patients undergoing carotid endarterectomy (194) in some centers (Fig. 8-25), lack of any proven benefit, significant cost, technical difficulty, and personnel requirements makes the routine use of EEG difficult during cardiac surgery. On the other hand, two-channel and four-channel machines utilizing stick-on Ag-AgCl electrodes on the forehead and mastoid (FA-A1 and FP-2-A2) can be used by a single anesthesiologist without excessive cost or personnel. A drawback is that electrodes must be placed where convenient (areas without hair) rather than given optimal placement, as afforded by the Ag-AgCl disc electrodes previously described.

To facilitate analysis, attempts are made to process EEG data and generate useful displays that can be analyzed effectively on line. Power spectral analysis converts information from a time domain (frequency versus time) to a frequency domain (plot of power against frequency) for a given segment of the EEG (epoch of time) (195). The compressed spectral array displays serial power spectra plotted one above the other to give a "mountain and valley" representation of EEG pattern (Fig. 8-26). Computers using fast Fourier transformation can simultaneously plot power spectra for several channels. Although instantaneous changes may take several epochs of time to recognize, data loss is not great, unless frequency components are averaged.

Density-modulated spectral array involves the same EEG

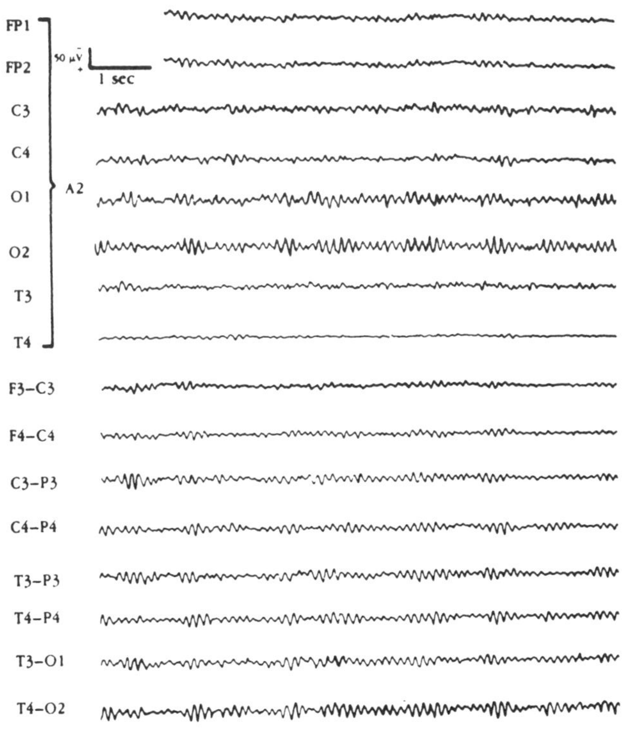

FIGURE 8-25. Normal 16-channel electroencephalograph. (From Grundy BL. Electrophysiologic monitoring: electroencephalography and evoked potentials. In: Newfield P, Cottrell JE, eds. *Neuroanesthesia: handbook of clinical and physiologic essentials,* 2nd ed. Boston: Little, Brown and Company, 1991, with permission.)

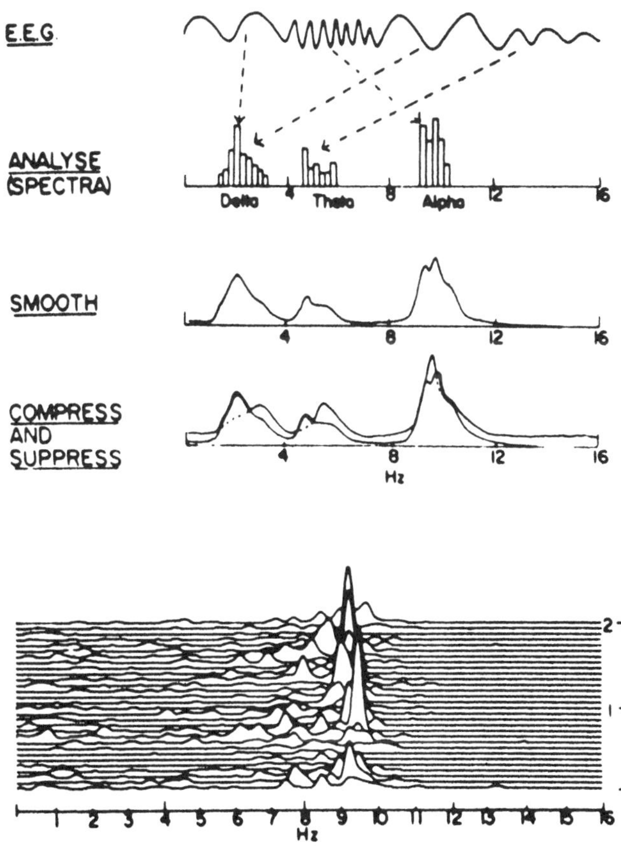

FIGURE 8-26. Power spectral analysis converting raw electroencephalograph to compressed spectral array. (From Stockard JJ, Bickford RG. The neurophysiology of anaesthesia. In: Gordon E, ed. *A basis and practice of neuroanaesthesia,* 2nd ed. New York: Excerpta Medica, 1981, with permission.)

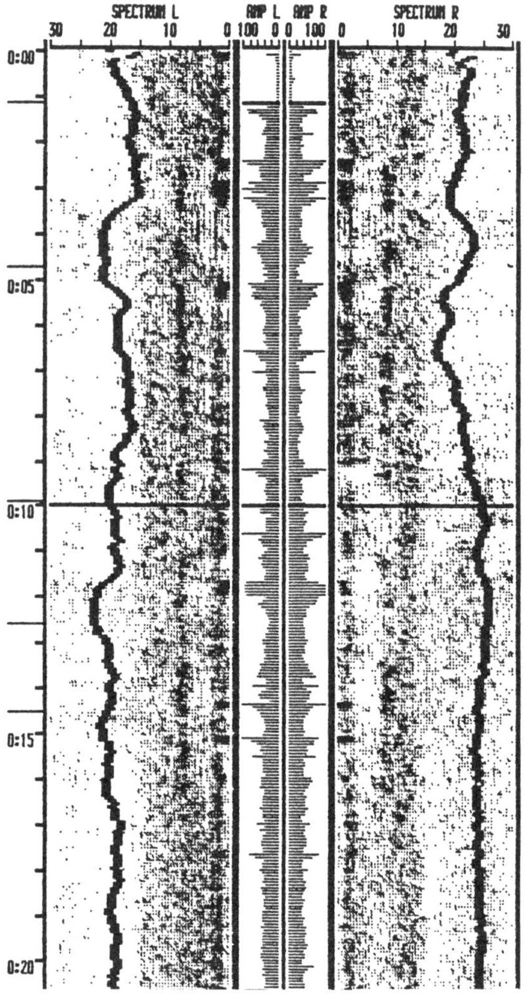

FIGURE 8-27. Density spectral array.

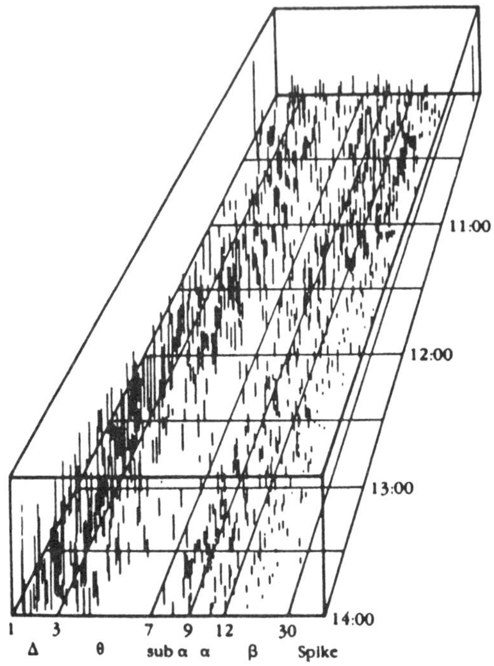

FIGURE 8-28. A single-channel presentation of aperiodic analysis, noting the frequency ranges of electroencephalograph rhythms. (From Grundy BL. Electrophysiologic monitoring: Electroencephalography and evoked potentials. In: Newfield P, Cottrell JE, eds. *Neuroanesthesia: handbook of clinical and physiologic essentials,* 2nd ed. Boston: Little, Brown and Company, 1991, with permission.)

analysis but a different display (Fig. 8-27). The proposed advantage is lower data loss in the peaks and valleys. Aperiodic analysis is a distinct type of EEG processing in which each wave of the analog EEG is converted to a vertical line whose height is proportional to the amplitude of the wave. A 3D display represents time, frequency, and amplitude (Fig. 8-28). This analysis method produces more complete data, but with less time compression and therefore less trend observation. The bispectral index is a new technique of EEG processing employing bispectral analysis to generate a single number that correlates with hypnosis (196). Bispectral analysis has been used solely to assess the adequacy of anesthesia, but few studies describe the bispectral index during cardiac surgery and hypothermic CPB.

Regardless of the analysis method used, access to raw EEG data must be maintained so electrical interference and other artifacts can be identified. Advancing technology in this field continues to allow more on-line determination of power, relative power, and different wave frequencies, which may allow for early intervention and thus prevention of neurologic or neuropsychologic sequelae.

Significance of Electroencephalographic Monitoring

The significance of EEG monitoring during CPB remains a hotly debated topic (197). Despite improvement in intraoperative EEG technology, data show no reasonable correlation between EEG abnormalities and neuropsychologic outcome (189,198). This lack of correlation between EEG findings and neurologic or neuropsychologic outcome was thought to be related to the mechanism of injury. Small emboli commonly seen during CPB may cause injury to areas too small to have significant impact on the larger area monitored by surface EEG electrodes. This argument, although reasonable in nature, is contradicted by data from the study of Edmonds et al.(190). They noted that an increase in relative low-frequency power occurring over 5 minutes during rewarming was a significant predictor of cerebral cortical dysfunction (disorientation). Treatment of these abnormalities by raising perfusion pressure significantly decreased disorientation after CPB.

Despite the finding of Edmonds et al. (190), the predictive value of the EEG at current technology levels remains questionable. Furthermore, the absence of a unique ischemic pattern on the EEG necessitates additional monitoring to identify the cause of EEG slowing. Reliably predicting neurologic or neuropsychologic outcome may rest with newer forms of cerebral flow or cerebral oxygenation monitoring or with a combination of new and old monitors.

Evoked Potentials

SSEPs are electrical responses of the nervous system to known sensory stimulation. When a sensory pathway is at risk during surgery, evoked potentials can be used to monitor neurologic function and reduce the risk of neurologic injury (Fig. 8-29) (199). The SSEP has been evaluated as a mean of assessing neurologic wellness during CPB (200). Unfortunately, SSEPs evaluate only a select portion of the central nervous system and therefore would not be expected to predict central nervous system outcome. Monitoring SSEPs of the upper extremities may help identify patients at risk of brachial plexus injury (201). Early detection may allow an intervention that could reverse these deficits.

The greatest value of the SSEP in cardiothoracic surgery appears to be during surgery on the descending thoracic aorta. SSEPs of the posterior tibial nerve provide information on the ischemic stress to the spinal cord, allowing for early detection and intervention to remedy potential insults. Unfortunately the false-negative rate in these patients is high due to the significant lag time from the onset of ischemia to the detection of changes, slow response to interventions, and monitoring of the posterior column only (possibly missing anterior spinal artery and therefore motor nerve injury).

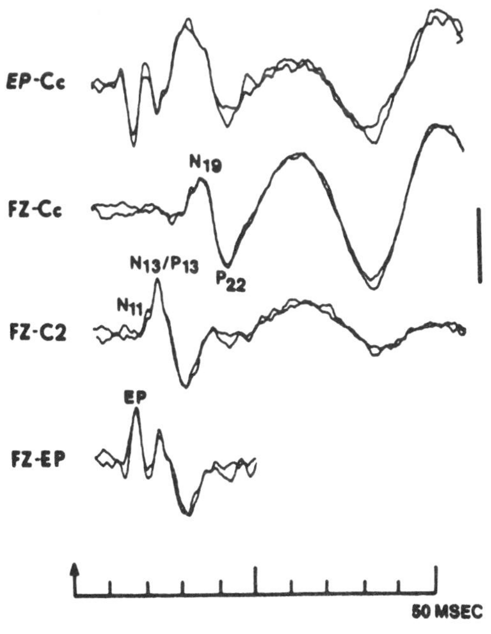

FIGURE 8-29. Short-latency somatosensory evoked potentials produced by stimulation of the median nerve at the wrist. (From Chippa KH, Ropper AH. Evoked potentials in clinical medicine. *N Engl J Med* 1982;306:1205, with permission.)

Despite these obvious difficulties, the potential benefit outweighs the cost and risk in this particular patient population.

Cerebral Blood Flow and Blood Flow Velocity

Cerebral Blood Flow

Xenon-133 (^{133}Xe) measurement of cerebral blood flow is a well-validated technique (202). ^{133}Xe washout techniques, as described by Mckay et al.(203), Govier et al.(204), and colleagues (205–207), have been used to measure the effects of CPB and interventions during CPB on cerebral blood flow. This has allowed a clearer understanding of cerebral blood flow autoregulation during CPB, identified groups at risk of losing autoregulation, and questioned the mechanism by which some anesthetics may provide cerebral protection (208,209). Unfortunately, cerebral blood flow during CPB has not proven to be as predictive of neurologic dysfunction in patients undergoing CPB as it has for CEA patients (204). This may relate to the lack of continuous recording or may point to factors other than changes in flow as the primary source of neurologic deficits. Therefore, despite its continued usefulness as a research tool, measurement of cerebral blood flow during CPB is not a predictor of neurologic or cognitive deficits after CPB.

Transcranial Doppler

Measurement of cerebral blood flow velocity in the middle cerebral artery during CPB is a noninvasive technology that has blossomed during the last 15 years (Fig. 8-30). The

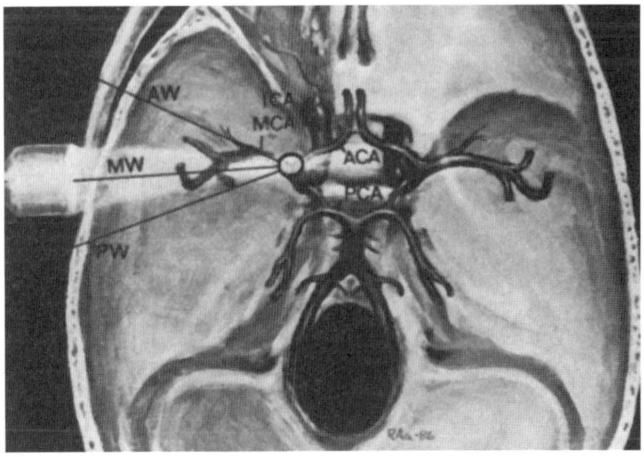

FIGURE 8-30. View of the circle of Willis demonstrating the insonation pathway for transcranial Doppler from the different temporal windows. (AW, anterior window; MW, middle window; PW, posterior window; MCA, middle cerebral artery; ACA, anterior cerebral artery; PCA, posterior cerebral artery.) (From Aaslid R. The Doppler principle applied to measurement of blood flow velocity in the cerebral arteries. In: Aaslid R, ed. *Transcranial Doppler sonography.* New York: Springer-Verlag New York, 1986, with permission.)

technique consists of focusing the ultrasound beam through the temporal window at the circle of Willis. The vessel is identified by direction of flow, spatial relation to the other signals, and compression of inflow vessels. A head strap and locking mechanism allow for continuous monitoring of cerebral blood flow velocities through the middle cerebral artery, which carries a large percentage of cerebral flow. This technique also allows for detection of middle cerebral artery emboli occurring during high-risk periods of cardiac surgery (Fig. 8-31) (210). Computer analysis allows for continuous detection and recording of these events, with recent studies showing an ability to differentiate between air and particulate matter (211).

Cerebral emboli detected with transcranial Doppler occur primarily with manipulation of the aorta (e.g., cross-clamp placement and removal), suggesting a role for aortic atheromatous debris in the embolization (212). Gaseous emboli are commonly detected upon initiation of CPB and during the initial phases of cardiac ejection after CPB, particularly in patients undergoing open-chamber procedures (213). The number of microemboli detected during surgery has been related to neuropsychologic function (214) and cerebral injury manifested by an increase in the serum levels of the glial protein, S100β (215). Unfortunately, the threshold of transcranial Doppler derived flow velocity or emboli count at which neurologic or neuropsychologic deficits occur is not defined. Most studies show no correlation between blood flow velocity and neurologic outcome (216).

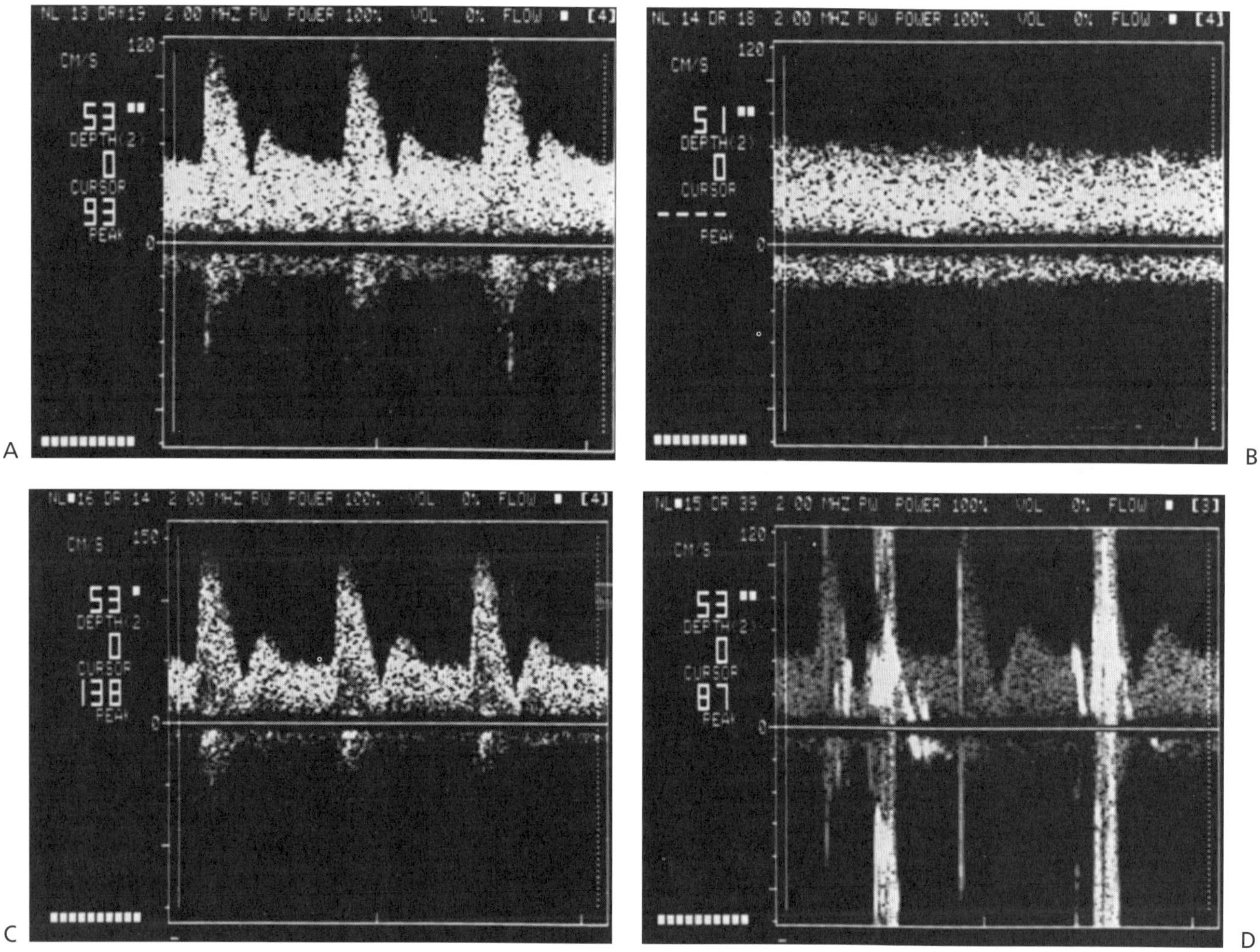

FIGURE 8-31. **A** and **B:** Spectral display of Doppler signal shortly before the institution of cardiopulmonary bypass and during steady-state cardiopulmonary bypass. **C** and **D:** Spectral display of Doppler signal at baseline and at release of aortic cross-clamp after aortic valve replacement, demonstrating probable embolic event signified by increased signal intensity. (From Newman M, Frasco P, Kern F, et al. Central nervous system dysfunction after cardiac surgery. In: Karp RB, Laks H, Wechsler AS, eds. *Advances in cardiac surgery,* vol 3. St. Louis: Mosby–Year Book, 1992, with permission.)

Furthermore, transcranial Doppler derived velocity is a poor correlate of cerebral blood flow during hypothermic CBF (217).

Despite these shortcomings, the noninvasive ability to measure cerebral blood flow velocity and detect cerebral emboli perioperatively is of potential value in cardiac surgery. Large studies correlating MCA emboli with neurologic and neuropsychologic outcome after CPB are necessary to determine the role of this monitor in predicting post-CPB central nervous system dysfunction.

Cerebral Oxygenation Monitoring

Jugular Bulb Saturation

Jugular venous saturation ($Sjvo_2$) is measured by retrograde placement of a catheter through the IJV into the jugular bulb. Blood is withdrawn through this catheter and analyzed for pH, Po_2, and hemoglobin saturation. Saturation can also be measured continuously with a fiberoptic catheter but the accuracy of these measurements has been questioned (218). $Sjvo_2$ is related to oxygen extraction and cerebral metabolic rate, and would theoretically predict cerebral ischemia. Jugular venous desaturation occurs in 23% of patients during rewarming from CPB, but the significance of this desaturation is not yet known and a correlation between jugular desaturation and neurologic or neuropsychologic outcome has not been demonstrated (219). Focal cerebral injury may not be detected by techniques such as $Sjvo_2$ because of the admixture of blood from healthy and injured tissue at the level of the jugular bulb. Further evaluation with techniques allowing continuous measurement is needed to determine any correlation between $Sjvo_2$ and neurologic or cognitive outcome.

Near-Infrared Spectroscopy

Reflectance cerebral oximetry involves near-infrared (NIR) photons projected into the skin over the forehead (Fig. 8-32). After scattering by skin, scalp, skull, dura, and brain, some fraction of the projected photons return to the skin surface. By measuring the quantity of returning photons as a function of wavelength, one can characterize the spectral absorption of the underlying tissue and make sequential determinations of the average regional hemoglobin oxygen saturation (trended rSO_2 index). Near-infrared spectroscopy (NIRS) has been promoted as a technique for neurologic monitoring for many years. The technique has been limited by the utilization of "trends from baseline," as opposed to absolute values. These "trends from baseline" are often difficult data from which to make clinical decisions, thus limiting the usefulness of NIRS to clinicians. Application of internal algorithms to better assess and determine regional saturation have enhanced the utility of the devices,

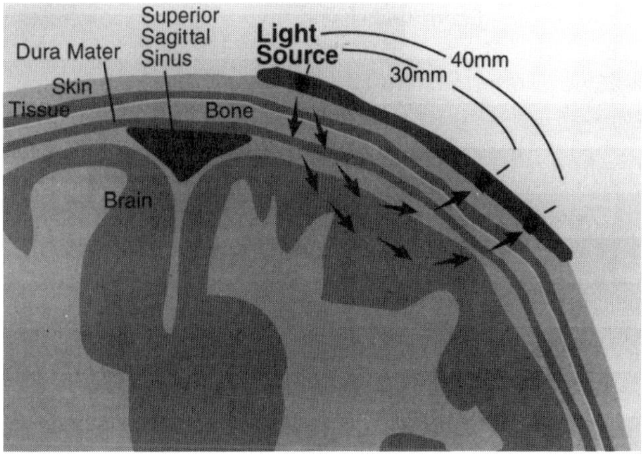

FIGURE 8-32. Diagrammatic representation of the infrared light source and receivers on the cranium of an adult subject monitored with a cerebral oximeter. Infrared light penetrates the scalp, cranium, and cerebral parenchyma and returns to the receivers. One receiver is affected by attenuation in the superficial tissue and the other by attenuation in both the superficial and deep tissues. (From Edmonds HL. Detection and treatment of cerebral hypoxia key to avoiding intraoperative brain injuries. *Anesthesia Patient Safety Foundation Newsletter* 1999;14:25, with permission.)

but questions have remained as to the tissue that is actually measured as well as the accuracy of the data (220). Studies evaluating the association between declines in regional saturation during CPB and postoperative cognitive dysfunction have been promising but have only recently demonstrated statistically significant correlations with neurocognitive or cost outcomes data in small numbers of patients (221–223).

A number of controversies surrounding the currently available FDA-approved device (Somanetics INVOS 4100) have been delineated by Edmonds (224).

- Absolute versus relative measurement is an important concept because values obtained are based on an assumption of the path length of the photons generated and returned to sensors. Dual detectors limit but do not eliminate this difficulty. Recent human studies using a prototype NIR capable of path length determination by phase-modulated light (225), produced results similar to the spatially resolved system currently available for clinical use (226).
- Scattering may be wavelength dependent (227); therefore, the current technology uses a signal quality index to alert the clinician that the absolute value may be suspect.
- The lack of consistent association between jugular bulb saturation $Sjvo_2$ and rSO_2 has led to criticism of the cerebral oximeter. This inconsistency, especially during CPB may be explained by a number of factors including measurement of different cerebral regions, the fact that rSO_2 is a venous weighted average as opposed to a measurement of venous blood only, and the inability of $Sjvo_2$ to

completely determine areas of hypoperfusion due to the large venous admixture of returning blood.

- Reports of normal rSO_2 values obtained from dead subjects (228,229) have further questioned the reliability of the cerebral oximeter. However, Maeda et al.(230) have reported that the oxygen saturation of venous blood samples taken at autopsy ranged from 0.3% to 95%. Maeda et al. concluded that oximetric profiles reflected the circumstances of death and postmortem oximetry was of limited value. It is not difficult to imagine that any monitor used for assessment in inappropriate situation may not yield usable results.
- The ratio of cerebral venous to arterial blood is not constant, and changes in this ratio would result in changes in the value measured. However, trend values can still be followed and desaturation corrected.
- Dual wavelength technology cannot measure carboxyhemoglobin or methemoglobin and can result in either overestimation or underestimation, as with pulse oximetry (231).

The cerebral oximeter can be viewed as an indicator of the adequacy of global perfusion as assessed by saturation in a small region. Marked ischemia in distant regions could obviously occur with no substantial change in monitored values. However, if hypoperfusion plays a secondary role after embolization in determining neurological outcome, or a primary role, then determination of the adequacy of global/regional perfusion could be of benefit. Like most new technologies, early experience with cerebral oximetry has produced mixed result with a series of anecdotal and retrospective efficacy reports (197,232,233). A randomized, prospective, interventional study is needed to determine the value of NIRS because its ease of use and interpretation make it a monitor that could reach mainstream practice and improve outcome.

Biochemical Markers of Cerebral Injury

The release into the circulation of proteins of neuronal, glial and endothelial cell origin in response to injury offers, at least in theory, the potential for rapid diagnosis and early intervention with neuroprotective agents. Of the biochemical markers studied, the S100 protein has received the most interest. Recent reports have described encouraging correlations between perioperative levels of S100 and cerebral emboli as well as neurocognitive outcome (234,235). This and other markers hold substantial promise in assessing the efficacy of perioperative neuroprotection strategies or identifying those patients that would benefit from aggressive postoperative treatment strategies.

REFERENCES

1. Riva-Rocci S. Un nuovo sfigmomanometro. *Gazetta Medica di Torino* 1896;47:981.
2. Gorback MS. Considerations in the interpretation of systemic pressure monitoring. In: Lumb PD, Bryan-Brown CW, eds. *Complications in critical care medicine.* Chicago: Mosby–Year Book, 1988:296.
3. Cohn JN. Blood pressure measurement in shock. *JAMA* 1967; 199:118.
4. Celoria G, Dawson JA, Teres D. Compartment syndrome in a patient monitored with an automated blood pressure cuff. *J Clin Monit* 1987;3:139.
5. Davis RF. Clinical comparison of automated auscultatory and oscillometric and catheter-transducer measurements of arterial pressure. *J Clin Monit* 1985;1:114.
6. Yelderman M, Ream AK. Indirect measurement of mean blood pressure in the anesthetized patients. *Anesthesiology* 1979;50: 253.
7. Borow KM, Newburger JW. Noninvasive estimation of central aortic pressure using the oscillometric method for analyzing systemic artery pulsatile blood flow: comparative study of indirect systolic, diastolic, and mean brachial artery pressure with simultaneous direct ascending aortic pressure measurements. *Am Heart J* 1982;103:879.
8. Kazamias TM, Gander MP, Franklin DL, et al. Blood pressure measurement with Doppler ultrasonic flowmeter. *J Appl Physiol* 1971;30:585.
9. Zahed B, Sadove MS, Hatano S, et al. Comparison of automated Doppler ultrasound and Korotkoff measurements of blood pressure of children. *Anesth Analg* 1971;50:699.
10. Mandel MA, Dauchot PJ. Radial artery cannulation in 1,000 patients: precautions and complications. *J Hand Surg* 1977;2: 482.
11. Slogoff S, Keats AS, Arlund C. On the safety of radial artery cannulation. *Anesthesiology* 1983;59:42.
12. Cederholm I, Sorensen J, Carlsson C. Thrombosis following percutaneous radial artery cannulation. *Acta Anaesthesiol Scand* 1986;30:227.
13. Davis FM, Stewart JM. Radial artery cannulation. A prospective study in patients undergoing cardiothoracic surgery. *Br J Anaesth* 1980;52:41.
14. Jones RM, Hill AB, Nahrwold ML, et al. The effect of method of radial artery cannulation on postcannulation blood flow and thrombus formation. *Anesthesiology* 1981;55:76.
15. Ersoz CJ, Hedden M, Lain L. Prolonged femoral artery catheterization for intensive care. *Anesth Analg* 1970;49:160.
16. Gurman GM, Kriemerman S. Cannulation of big arteries in critically ill patients. *Crit Care Med* 1985;13:217.
17. Singh S, Nelson N, Acosta I, et al. Catheter colonization and bacteremia with pulmonary and arterial catheters. *Crit Care Med* 1982;10:736.
18. Soderstrom CA, Wasserman DH, Ransom KJ, et al. Infected false femoral artery aneurysms secondary to monitoring catheters. *J Cardiovasc Surg* 1983;24:63.
19. Barnes RW, Foster EJ, Janssen GA, et al. Safety of brachial arterial catheters as monitors in the intensive care unit—prospective evaluation with the Doppler ultrasonic velocity detector. *Anesthesiology* 1976;44:260.
20. Moran KT, Halpin DP, Zide RS, et al. Long-term brachial artery catheterization: ischemic complications. *J Vasc Surg* 1988; 8:76.
21. Mann S, Jones RI, Millar-Craig MW, et al. The safety of ambulatory intra-arterial pressure monitoring: a clinical audit of 1000 studies. *Int J Cardiol* 1984;5:585.
22. Yacoub OF, Bacaling JH, Kelly M. Monitoring of the axillary arterial pressure in a patient with Buerger's disease requiring

clipping of an intracerebral aneurysm. *Br J Anaesth* 1987;59:1056.
23. Adler DC, Bryan-Brown CW. Use of the axillary artery for intravascular monitoring. *Crit Care Med* 1973;1:148.
24. Brown M, Gordon LH, Brown OW, et al. Intravascular monitoring via the axillary artery. *Anaesth Intensive Care* 1985;13:38.
25. Bryan-Brown CW, Kwun KB, Lumb PD, et al. The axillary artery catheter. *Heart Lung* 1983;12:492.
26. Huber JF. The arterial network supplying the dorsum of the foot. *Anat Rec* 1941;80:373.
27. Youngberg JA, Miller ED. Evaluation of percutaneous cannulations of the dorsalis pedis artery. *Anesthesiology* 1976;44:80.
28. Randel SN, Tsang BH, Wung JT, et al. Experience with percutaneous indwelling peripheral arterial catheterization in neonates. *Am J Dis Child* 1987;141:848.
29. Bull MJ, Schriner RL, Garg BG, et al. Neurologic complications following temporal artery catheterization. *J Pediatr* 1980;96:1071.
30. Stephens LC, Haire WD, Tarantolo S, et al. Normal saline versus heparin flush for maintaining central venous catheter patency during apheresis collection of peripheral blood stem cells (PBSC). *Transfus Sci* 1997;18:187.
31. Garrelts JC. White clot syndrome and thrombocytopenia: reasons to abandon heparin I.V. lock flush solution. *Clin Pharm* 1992;11:797.
32. Geddes LA. *Cardiovascular devices and their applications.* New York: John Wiley and Sons, 1984.
33. Prys-Roberts C. Invasive monitoring of the circulation. In: Saidman LJ, Smith NT, eds. *Monitoring in anesthesia,* 2nd ed. Boston, MA: Butterworth, 1984:79.
34. Gardner RM. Direct blood pressure measurement—dynamic response requirements. *Anesthesiology* 1981;54:227.
35. Boutros A, Albert S. Effect of the dynamic response of transducer-tubing system on accuracy of direct blood pressure measurement in patients. *Crit Care Med* 1983;11:124.
36. Abrams JH. Damping devices in clinical practice. In: Cerra FB, ed. *Perspectives in critical care,* vol 1. St. Louis, MO: Quality Medical Publishers, 1988:133.
37. Stern DH, Gerson JI, Allen FB, et al. Can we trust the direct radial artery pressure immediately after cardiopulmonary bypass? *Anesthesiology* 1985;62:557.
38. Gallagher JD, Moore RA, McNicholas KW, et al. Comparison of radial and femoral arterial blood pressures in children following cardiopulmonary bypass. *J Clin Monit* 1985;1:168.
39. Allen EV. Thromboangiitis obliterans: methods of diagnosis of chronic obstructive lesions distal to the wrist with illustrative cases. *Am J Med Sci* 1929;178:237.
40. Wilkins RG. Radial artery cannulation and ischaemic damage: a review. *Anaesthesia* 1985;40:896.
41. Baker RJ, Chunprapaph B, Nyhus LM. Severe ischemia of the hand following radial artery catheterization. *Surgery* 1976;80:449.
42. Mangano DT, Hickey RF. Ischemic injury following uncomplicated radial artery catheterization. *Anesth Analg* 1979;58:55.
43. Thompson SR, Hirshberg A. Allen's test reexamined [Letter]. *Crit Care Med* 1988;16:915.
44. Bedford RF, Wollman H. Complications of percutaneous radial-artery cannulation: an objective prospective study in man. *Anesthesiology* 1973;38:228.
45. Meyer RM, Katele GV. The case for a complete Allen's test. *Anesth Analg* 1983;62:947.
46. Bedford RF. Radial artery function following percutaneous cannulation with 18- and 20-gauge catheters. *Anesthesiology* 1977;47:37.
47. Bedford RF. Percutaneous radial artery cannulation—increased safety using Teflon catheters. *Anesthesiology* 1975;42:219.
48. Kim JM, Arakawa K, Bliss J. Arterial cannulation: factors in the development of occlusion. *Anesth Analg* 1975;54:836.
49. Russell JA, Joel M, Hudson RJ, et al. Prospective evaluation of radial and femoral artery catheterization sites in critically ill adults. *Crit Care Med* 1983;11:936.
50. Mark JB. Patterns of valvular heart disease. In: Mark JB. *Atlas of cardiovascular monitoring.* New York: Churchill Livingstone, 1998:287.
51. West JB, Dollery CT, Naimark A. Distribution of blood flow in isolated lung: relation to vascular and alveolar pressures. *J Appl Physiol* 1964;19:713.
52. Lorzman J, Powers SR, Older T, et al. Correlation of pulmonary wedge and left atrial pressures. A study in the patient receiving positive end expiratory pressure ventilation. *Arch Surg* 1974;109:270.
53. Humphrey CB, Gibbons JA, Folkerth TL, et al. An analysis of direct and indirect measurements of left atrial filling pressure. *J Thorac Cardiovasc Surg* 1976;71:643.
54. Lappas D, Lell WA, Gabel JC, et al. Indirect measurement of left atrial pressure in surgical patients—pulmonary-capillary wedge pressure and pulmonary-artery diastolic pressures compared with left atrial pressure. *Anesthesiology* 1973;38:394.
55. Walston A, Kendall ME. Comparison of pulmonary wedge and left atrial pressure in man. *Am Heart J* 1973;86:159.
56. Vender JS. Pulmonary artery catheter monitoring. In: Barash PG, ed. *Cardiac monitoring.* Philadelphia: WB Saunders, 1988:743.
57. Forrester JS, Diamond G, McHugh TJ, et al. Filling pressures in right and left sides of the heart in acute myocardial infarction. A reappraisal of central-venous pressure monitoring. *N Engl J Med* 1971;285:190.
58. Civetta JM, Gabel JC. Flow-directed pulmonary artery catheterization in surgical patients: indications and modification of technique. *Ann Surg* 1972;176:753.
59. Swan HJC. Central venous pressure monitoring is an outmoded procedure of limited practical value. In: Ingelfinger FJ, Ebert RV, Finland M, et al., eds. *Controversies in internal medicine.* Philadelphia: WB Saunders, 1974:185.
60. Samii K, Conseiller C, Viars P. Central venous pressure and pulmonary wedge pressure. A comparative study in anesthetized surgical patients. *Arch Surg* 1976;111:1122.
61. Bell H, Stubbs D, Pugh D. Reliability of central venous pressure as an indicator of left atrial pressure. A study in patients with mitral valve disease. *Chest* 1971;59:169.
62. Toussaint GP, Burges JH, Hampson LG. Central venous pressure and pulmonary capillary wedge pressure in critical surgical illness. A comparison. *Arch Surg* 1974;109:265.
63. Bashein G, Johnson PW, Davis KB, et al. Elective coronary bypass surgery without pulmonary artery catheter monitoring. Anesthesiology 1985;63:451.
64. Kaplan JA, Wells PH. Early diagnosis of myocardial ischemia using the pulmonary arterial catheter. *Anesth Analg* 1981;60:789.
65. Van Daele ME, Sutherland GR, Mitchell MM, et al. Do changes in pulmonary capillary wedge pressure adequately reflect myocardial ischemia during anesthesia? A correlative preoperative hemodynamic, electrocardiographic, and transesophageal echocardiographic study. *Circulation* 1990;81:865.
66. Tuman KJ, McCarthy RJ, Spiess BD, et al. Effect of pulmonary

artery catheterization on outcome in patients undergoing coronary artery surgery. *Anesthesiology* 1989;70:199.
67. Connors AF, Speroff T, Dawson NV, et al. The effectiveness of right heart catheterization in the initial care of critically ill patients. *JAMA* 1996;276:889.
68. Iberti TJ, Daily EK, Leibowitz AB, et al. Assessment of critical care nurses' knowledge of the pulmonary artery catheter. *Crit Care Med* 1994;22:1674.
69. Gnaegi A, Feihl F, Perret C. Intensive care physicians' insufficient knowledge of right-heart catheterization at the bedside: time to act? *Crit Care Med* 1997;25:213.
70. Practice guidelines for pulmonary artery catheterization. A report by the American Society of Anesthesiologists Task Force on pulmonary artery catheterization. *Anesthesiology* 1993;78:380.
71. Pulmonary Artery Catheter Consensus conference: consensus statement. *Crit Care Med* 1997;25:910.
72. Dzelzkalns R, Stanley TH. Placement of the pulmonary arterial catheter before anesthesia for cardiac surgery: a stressful, painful, unnecessary crutch. *J Clin Monit* 1985;1:197.
73. Lunn JK, Stanley TH, Webster LR, et al. Arterial blood pressure and pulse-rate responses to pulmonary and radial arterial catheterization prior to cardiac and major vascular operations. *Anesthesiology* 1979;51:265.
74. Waller JL, Zaidan JR, Kaplan JA, et al. Hemodynamic responses to preoperative vascular cannulation in patients with coronary artery disease. *Anesthesiology* 1982;56:219.
75. Quintin L, Whalley DG, Wynands JE, et al. The effects of vascular catheterization upon heart rate and blood pressure before aorto-coronary bypass. *Can Anaesth Soc J* 1981;28:244.
76. Streisand JB, Clark NJ, Pace NL. Placement of the pulmonary artery catheter before anesthesia for cardiac surgery: safe, intelligent, and appropriate use of invasive hemodynamic monitoring. *J Clin Monit* 1985;1:193.
77. Sanford TJ. Internal jugular vein cannulation versus subclavian vein cannulation. An anesthesiologist's view: the right internal jugular vein. *J Clin Monit* 1985;1:58.
78. Tyden HE. Cannulation of the internal jugular vein—500 cases. *Acta Anaesthesiol Scand* 1982;26:485.
79. Hoyt DB. Internal jugular vein cannulation versus subclavian vein cannulation. A surgeon's view: the subclavian vein. *J Clin Monit* 1985;1:61.
80. Horrow JC, Metz S, Thickman D, et al. Prior carotid surgery does not affect the reliability of landmarks for location of the internal jugular vein. *Anesth Analg* 1987;66:452.
81. Pearson ML. Guidelines for prevention of intravascular device-related infections. *Am J Infect Control* 1996;24:262.
82. Royster RL, Johnston WE, Gravlee GP, et al. Arrhythmias during venous cannulation prior to pulmonary artery catheter insertion. *Anesth Analg* 1985;64:1214.
83. Flowers RH III, Schwenzer KJ, Kopel RF, et al. Efficacy of an attachable subcutaneous cuff for the prevention of intravascular catheter-related infection. A randomized, controlled trial. *JAMA* 1989;261:878.
84. Johnston WE, Royster RL, Choplin RH, et al. Pulmonary artery catheter migration during cardiac surgery. *Anesthesiology* 1986; 64:258.
85. Heard SO, Davis RF, Sherertz RJ, et al. Influence of sterile protective sleeves on the sterility of pulmonary artery catheters. *Crit Care Med* 1987;15:499.
86. Benumof JL, Saidman LJ, Arkin DB, et al. Where pulmonary artery catheters go: intrathoracic distribution. *Anesthesiology* 1977;46:336.
87. Schmitt EA, Brantigan CO. Common artifacts of pulmonary artery and pulmonary artery wedge pressures: recognition and interpretation. *J Clin Monit* 1986;2:44.
88. Borja AR, Hinhaw JR. A safe way to perform infraclavicular subclavian vein catheterization. *Surg Gynecol Obstet* 1970;130: 673.
89. Webre DR, Arens JF. Use of cephalic and basilic veins for introduction of central venous catheters. *Anesthesiology* 1973;38:389.
90. Shah KB, Rao TLK, Laughlin S, et al. A review of pulmonary artery catheterization in 6,245 patients. *Anesthesiology* 1984;61: 271.
91. Davies MJ, Cronin KD, Domaingue CM. Pulmonary artery catheterisation. An assessment of risks and benefits in 220 surgical patients. *Anaesth Intensive Care* 1982;10:9.
92. Sise MJ, Hollingsworth P, Brimm JE, et al. Complications of the flow-directed pulmonary artery catheter: a prospective analysis in 219 patients. *Crit Care Med* 1981;9:315.
93. Horst HM, Obeid FN, Vij D, et al. The risks of pulmonary artery catheterization. *Surg Gynecol Obstet* 1984;159:229.
94. Damen J. Ventricular arrhythmias during insertion and removal of pulmonary artery catheters. *Chest* 1985;88:190.
95. Coulter TD, Wiedemann HP. Complications of hemodynamic monitoring. *Clin Chest Med* 1999;20:249.
96. Thomson IR, Dalton BC, Lappas DG, et al. Right bundle-branch block and complete heart block caused by the Swan-Ganz catheter. *Anesthesiology* 1979;51:359.
97. Sprung CL, Elser B, Schein RM, et al. Risk of right bundle-branch block and complete heart block during pulmonary artery catheterization. *Crit Care Med* 1989;17:1.
98. Morris D, Mulvihill D, Lew WY. Risk of developing complete heart block during bedside pulmonary artery catheterization in patients with left bundle-branch block. *Arch Intern Med* 1987; 147:2005.
99. Mermel LA, Maki DG. Infectious complications of Swan-Ganz pulmonary artery catheters. Pathogenesis, epidemiology, prevention, and management. *Am J Respir Crit Care Med* 1994; 149:1020.
100. Fibuch EE, Tuohy GF. Intracardiac knotting of a flow-directed balloon-tipped catheter. *Anesth Analg* 1980;59:217.
101. Dumesnil JG, Proulx G. A new nonsurgical technique for untying tight knots in flow-directed balloon catheters. *Am J Cardiol* 1984;53:395.
102. Michel L, Installe E, Joucken K. Knotting of intracardiac flow-directed balloon catheter. Simple surgical method of removal. *Chest* 1983;83:147.
103. McDaniel DD, Stone JG, Faltas AN, et al. Catheter-induced pulmonary artery hemorrhage. Diagnosis and management in cardiac operations. *J Thorac Cardiovasc Surg* 1981;82:1.
104. Urschel JD, Myerowitz PD. Catheter-induced pulmonary artery rupture in the setting of cardiopulmonary bypass. *Ann Thorac Surg* 1993;56:585.
105. Muller BJ, Gallucci A. Pulmonary artery catheter induced pulmonary artery rupture in patients undergoing cardiac surgery. *Can Anaesth Soc J* 1985;32:258.
106. Barash PG, Nardi D, Hammond G, et al. Catheter-induced pulmonary artery perforation. Mechanisms, management, and modifications. *J Thorac Cardiovasc Surg* 1981;82:5.
107. Hardy JF, Morissette M, Taillefer J, et al. Pathophysiology of rupture of the pulmonary artery by pulmonary artery balloon-tipped catheters. *Anesth Analg* 1983;62:925.
108. Scuderi PE, Prough DS, Price JD, et al. Cessation of pulmonary artery catheter-induced endobronchial hemorrhage associated with the use of PEEP. *Anesth Analg* 1983;62:236.
109. Wolpowitz A. Trans-septal monitoring of left atrial pressure

after cardiac surgery. An alternative method. *S Afr Med J* 1978; 53:185.

110. Akl BF, Pett SB, Wernly JA, et al. Unusual complication of direct left atrial pressure monitoring line. *J Thorac Cardiovasc Surg* 1984;88:1033.
111. Selzer A, Sudrann RB. Reliability of the determination of cardiac output in man by means of the Fick principle. *Circ Res* 1958;6:485.
112. Thomasson B. Cardiac output in normal subjects under standard basal conditions: the repeatability of measurements by the Fick method. *Scand J Clin Lab Invest* 1957;9:365.
113. Osterlund B, Gedeon A, Krill P, et al. A new method of using gas exchange measurements for the noninvasive determination of cardiac output: clinical experiences in adults following cardiac surgery. *Acta Anesthesiol Scand* 1995;39:727.
114. Stewart GN. Researches on the circulation time and on the influences which affect it. IV. The output of the heart. *J Physiol* 1897;22:159.
115. Hamilton WF, Moore JW, Kinsman JM, et al. Studies on the circulation. IV. Further analysis of the injection method, and changes in hemodynamics under physiologic and pathological conditions. *Am J Physiol* 1932;99:534.
116. Fegler G. Measurement of cardiac output in anesthetized animals by a thermodilution method. *Q J Exp Physiol* 1954;39: 153.
117. Bazaral MG, Petre J, Novoa R. Errors in thermodilution cardiac output measurements caused by rapid pulmonary artery temperature decreases after cardiopulmonary bypass. *Anesthesiology* 1992;77:31.
118. Bilfinger TV, Lin CY, Anagnostopoulos CE. In vitro determination of accuracy of cardiac output measurements by thermal dilution. J Surg Res 1982;33:409.
119. Levett JM, Replogle RL. Thermodilution cardiac output: a critical analysis and review of the literature. J Surg Res 1979;27: 392.
120. Stetz CW, Miller RG, Kelly GE, et al. Reliability of the thermodilution method in the determination of cardiac output in clinical practice. *Am Rev Respir Dis* 1982;126:1001.
121. Nelson LD, Anderson HB. Patient selection for iced versus room temperature injectate for thermodilution cardiac output determinations. *Crit Care Med* 1986;13:182.
122. Weisel RD, Berger RL, Hechtman RB. Current concepts in measurement of cardiac output by thermodilution. *N Engl J Med* 1975;292:682.
123. Nishikawa T, Dohi S. Slowing of heart during cardiac output measurement by thermodilution. Anesthesiology 1982;57:538.
124. Yelderman M. Continuous measurement of cardiac output with the use of stochastic system identification techniques. *J Clin Monit* 1990;6:322.
125. Yelderman M. Continuous cardiac output by thermodilution. *Int Anesth Clin* 1993;3:127.
126. Singer M, Allen MJ, Webb AR, et al. Effects of alterations in left ventricular filling, contractility, and systemic vascular resistance on the ascending aortic blood velocity waveform of normal subjects. *Crit Care Med* 1991;19:1138.
127. Mythen MG, Webb AR. Perioperative plasma volume expansion reduces the incidence of gut mucosal hypoperfusion during cardiac surgery. *Arch Surg* 1995;130:423.
128. Sinclair S, James S, Singer M. Intraoperative intravascular volume optimisation and length of hospital stay after repair of proximal femoral fracture: randomised controlled trial. *BMJ* 1997;315:909.
129. Freund PR. Transesophageal Doppler scanning versus thermodilution during general anesthesia. An initial comparison of cardiac output techniques. *Am J Surg* 1987;153:490.
130. Mark JB, Steinbrook RA, Gugino LD, et al. Continuous noninvasive monitoring of cardiac output with esophageal Doppler ultrasound during cardiac surgery. *Anesth Analg* 1986;65:1013.
131. Perrino AC. Cardiac output monitoring by echocardiography; should we pass on Swan-Ganz catheters? *Yale J Biol Med* 1993; 66:397.
132. Perrino AC, O'Connor T, Luther M. Transtracheal Doppler cardiac output monitoring: comparison to thermodilution during noncardiac surgery. *Anesth Analg* 1994;78:1060.
133. Segal J, Gaudiani V, Nishimura T. Continuous determination of cardiac output using a flow-directed Doppler pulmonary artery catheter. *J Cardiothorac Vasc Anesth* 1991;5:309.
134. Norfleet EA, Watson CB. Continuous mixed venous oxygen saturation measurement: a significant advance in hemodynamic monitoring? *J Clin Monit* 1985;1:245.
135. Waller JL, Kaplan JA, Bauman DI, et al. Clinical evaluation of a new fiberoptic catheter oximeter during cardiac surgery. *Anesth Analg* 1982;61:676.
136. Magilligan DJ, Teasdall R, Eisinminger R, et al. Mixed venous oxygen saturation as a predictor of cardiac output in the postoperative cardiac surgical patient. *Ann Thorac Surg* 1987;44:260.
137. Cariou A, Monchi M, Dhainaut JF. Continuous cardiac output and mixed venous oxygen saturation monitoring. *J Crit Care* 1998;13:198.
138. Gutierrez G, Palizas F, Doglio G, et al. Gastric intramucosal pH as a therapeutic index of tissue oxygenation in critically ill patients. *Lancet* 1992;339:195.
139. Knichwitz G, Rotker J, Brussel T, et al. A new method for continuous intramucosal Pco2 measurement in the gastrointestinal tract. *Anesth Analg* 1996;83:6.
140. Knichwitz G, Rotker J, Mollhoff T, et al. Continuous intramucosal P_{CO_2} measurement allows the early detection of intestinal malperfusion. *Crit Care Med* 1998;26:1550.
141. Schluter M, Langenstein BA, Polster J, et al. Transesophageal cross-sectional echocardiography with a phased-array transducer system. Technique and initial clinical results. *Br Heart J* 1982; 48:67.
142. Shanewise JS, Cheung AT, Aronson S, et al. ASE/SCA guidelines for performing a comprehensive intraoperative multiplane transesophageal echocardiography examination: recommendations of the American Society of Echocardiography Council for Intraoperative Echocardiography and the Society of Cardiovascular Anesthesiologists Task Force for Certification in Perioperative Transesophageal Echocardiography. *Anesth Analg* 1999; 89:870.
143. Ren JF, Panidis IP, Kotler MN, et al. Effect of coronary bypass surgery and valve replacement on left ventricular function: assessment by intraoperative two-dimensional echocardiography. *Am Heart J* 1985;109:281.
144. Epperlein S, Wittlich N, Mohr-Kahaly S, et al. Echocardiographic on-line volumetry using acoustic quantification—comparison with manual echocardiographic analysis and cineventriculography. *Z Kardiol* 1994;83:658.
145. Clements FM, Harpole DH, Quill T, et al. Estimation of left ventricular volume and ejection fraction by two-dimensional transesophageal echocardiography: comparison of short-axis imaging and simultaneous radionuclide angiography. *Br J Anesth* 1990;64:331.
146. Yvorchul KJ, Davies RA, Chan KL. Measurement of left ventricular ejection fraction by acoustic quantification and comparison with radionuclide angiography. *Am J Cardiol* 1994;74:1052.
147. Weiss JI, Eaton LW, Kallman CH, et al. Accuracy of volume

determination by two-dimensional echocardiography: defining requirements under controlled conditions in the ejecting canine left ventricle. *Circulation* 1983;67:889.
148. Urbanowicz JH, Shaaban JM, Cohen NH, et al. Comparison of transesophageal echocardiographic and scintigraphic estimates of left ventricular end-diastolic volume index and ejection fraction in patients following coronary artery bypass grafting. *Anesthesiology* 1990;72:607.
149. Krebs W, Klues HG, Steinert S, et al. Left ventricular volume calculations using a multiplanar transesophageal echoprobe; in vitro validation and comparison with biplane angiography. *Eur Heart J* 1996;17:1279.
150. Leung JM, Levine EH. Left ventricular end-systolic cavity obliteration as an estimate of intraoperative hypovolemia. *Anesthesiology* 1994;81:1102.
151. Cheung AT, Savino JS, Weiss, SJ, et al. Echocardiographic and hemodynamic indexes of left ventricular preload in patients with normal and abnormal ventricular function. *Anesthesiology* 1994; 81:376.
152. Fontes ML, Bellows W, Ngo L, et al. Assessment of ventricular function in critically ill patients: limitations of pulmonary artery catheterization. *J Cardiothorac Vasc Anesth* 1999;13:521.
153. Tennant R, Wiggers CJ. Effects of coronary occlusion on myocardial contraction. *Am J Physiol* 1935;112:351.
154. Waters DD, da Luz P, Wyatt HL, et al. Early changes in regional and global left ventricular function induced by graded reductions in regional coronary perfusion. *Am J Cardiol* 1977;39: 537.
155. Battler A, Froelicher VF, Gallagher KP, et al. Dissociation between regional myocardial dysfunction and ECG changes during ischemia in the conscious dog. *Circulation* 1980;62:735.
156. Smith J, Cahalan M, Benefiel DJ, et al. Intraoperative detection of myocardial ischemia in high-risk patients: electrocardiography versus two-dimensional transesophageal echocardiography. *Circulation* 1985;72:1015.
157. Leung JM, O'Kelly B, Browner WS, et al. Prognostic importance of postbypass regional wall-motion abnormalities in patients undergoing coronary artery bypass graft surgery. *Anesthesiology* 1989;71:16.
158. Shah PM, Kyo S, Matsumura M, et al. Utility of biplane transesophageal echocardiography in left ventricular wall motion analysis. *J Cardiothorac Vasc Anesth* 1991;5:316.
159. Rouine-Rapp K, Ionescu P, Balea M, et al. Detection of intraoperative segmental wall-motion abnormalities by transesophageal echocardiography: the incremental value of additional cross-sections in the transverse and longitudinal planes. *Anesth Analg* 1996;83;1141.
160. Lima JA, Becker LC, Melin JA, et al. Impaired thickening of non-ischemic myocardium during acute regional ischemia in the dog. *Circulation* 1985;71:1048.
161. London MJ, Tubau JF, Wong MG, et al. The "natural history" of segmental wall motion abnormalities in patients undergoing noncardiac surgery. *Anesthesiology* 1990;73:644.
162. Comunale ME, Body SC, Ley C, et al. The concordance of intraoperative left ventricular wall-motion abnormalities and electrocardiographic S-T segment changes: association with outcome after coronary revascularization. *Anesthesiology* 1998;88: 945.
163. Skorton DJ, Collins SM, Kerber RE. Digital image processing and analysis in echocardiography. In: Collins SM, Skorton DJ, eds. *Cardiac imaging and image processing.* New York: McGraw-Hill, 1986:171.
164. Mor-Avi V, Godoy IE, Lang RM. Color kinesis: new technique or just another display of acoustic quantification? *Echocardiography* 1999;16:95.
165. Marschall K, Kanchuger M, Kessler K, et al. Superiority of transesophageal echocardiography in detecting aortic arch atheromatous disease: identification of patients at increased risk of stroke during cardiac surgery. *J Cardiothorac Vasc Anesth* 1994; 8:5.
166. Roach GW, Kanchuger M, Mangano CM, et al. Adverse cerebral outcomes after coronary bypass surgery. Multicenter study of Perioperative Ischemia Research Group and the Ischemia Research and Education Foundation Investigators. *N Engl J Med* 1996;335:1857.
167. Davila-Roman VG, Phillips KJ, Daily BB, et al. Intraoperative transesophageal echocardiography and epiaortic ultrasound for assessment of atherosclerosis of the thoracic aorta. *J Am Coll Cardiol* 1996;28:942.
168. Davila-Roman V, Barzilai B, Wareing TH, et al. Intraoperative ultrasonographic evaluation of the ascending aorta in 100 consecutive patients undergoing cardiac surgery. *Circulation* 1991; 84:III47.
169. Topol EJ, Humphrey LS, Borkon AM, et al. Value of intraoperative left ventricular microbubbles detected by transesophageal 2-dimensional echocardiography in predicting neurologic outcome after cardiac operations. *Am J Cardiol* 1985;56:773.
170. Kaul S. Myocardial contrast echocardiography. 15 years of research and development. *Circulation* 1997;96:3745.
171. Clements F, Wright SJ, deBruijn N. Coronary sinus catheterization made easy for Port-Access minimally invasive cardiac surgery. *J Cardiothorac Vasc Anesth* 1998;12:96.
172. Doppler JC. Uber das farbige Licht der Doppelsterne. *Abhandlungen der Koniglishen Bohmischen Gesellschaft der Wissenschaften* 1842;2:465.
173. Kisslo J, Adams DB, Belkin RN. *Doppler color flow imaging.* New York: Churchill Livingstone, 1988.
174. Kisslo J, Adams DB, Marks DB, eds. *Basic Doppler echocardiography.* New York: Churchill Livingstone, 1986.
175. Darmon PL, Hillel Z, Mogtader A, et al. Cardiac output by transesophageal echocardiography using continuous-wave Doppler across the aortic valve. *Anesthesiology* 1994;80:796.
176. Perrino AC, Harris SN, Luther MA. Intraoperative determination of cardiac output using multiplane transesophageal echocardiography: a comparison to thermodilution. *Anesthesiology* 1998;89:350.
177. Vasquez de Prada JA, Ruano J, Martin-Duran R, et al. Noninvasive determination of pulmonary arterial systolic pressure by continuous-wave Doppler. *Int J Cardiol* 1987;16:177.
178. Blumberg FC, Pfeifer M, Holmer SR, et al. Quantification of aortic stenosis in mechanically ventilated patients using mutiplane transesophageal Doppler echocardiography. *Chest* 1998; 114:94.
179. Rifkin RD, Harper K, Tighe D. Comparison of proximal isovelocity surface area method with pressure half-time and planimetry in evaluation of mitral stenosis. *J Am Coll Cardiol* 1995;26: 458.
180. Sheikh KH, de Bruijn NP, Rankin JS, et al. The utility of transesophageal echocardiography and Doppler color flow imaging in patients undergoing cardiac valve surgery. *J Am Coll Cardiol* 1990;15:363.
181. Hagler DJ, Tajik AJ, Seward JB, et al. Intraoperative two-dimensional Doppler echocardiography. A preliminary study for congenital heart disease. *J Thorac Cardiovasc Surg* 1988;95:516.
182. Bengur AR, Li JS, Herlong JR, et al. Intraoperative transesophageal echocardiography in congenital heart disease. *Semin Thorac Cardiovasc Surg* 1998;10:255.

183. Sabry AF, Reller MD, Silberbach GM, et al. Comparison of four Doppler echocardiographic methods for calculating pulmonary-to-systemic shunt flows in patients with ventricular septal defect. *Am J Cardiol* 1995;75:611.
184. Practice guidelines for perioperative transesophageal echocardiography. A report by the American Society of Anesthesiologists and the Society of Cardiovascular Anesthesiologists Task Force on Transesophageal Echocardiography. *Anesthesiology* 1996;84:986.
185. Theye RA, Patrick R, Kirklin JW. The electroencephalogram in patients undergoing open intracardiac operations with the aid of extracorporeal circulation. *J Thorac Surg* 1957;34:709.
186. Coons RE, Keats AS, Cooley DA. Significance of electroencephalographic changes occurring during cardiopulmonary bypass. *Anesthesiology* 1959;20:208.
187. Shaw PJ, Bates D, Cartlidge NEF, et al. Early neurological complications of coronary artery bypass surgery. *Br Med J (Clin Res)* 1985;291:1384.
188. Levy WJ. Monitoring of the electroencephalogram during cardiopulmonary bypass. *Anesthesiology* 1992;76:876.
189. Bashein G, Nessly ML, Bledsoe SW, et al. Electroencephalography during surgery with cardiopulmonary bypass and hypothermia. *Anesthesiology* 1992;76:878.
190. Edmonds HL, Griffiths LK, Van der Laken J, et al. Quantitative electroencephalographic monitoring during myocardial revascularization predicts postoperative disorientation and improves outcome. *J Thorac Cardiovasc Surg* 1992;103:555.
191. Allison T. Calculated and empirical evoked-potential distributions in human recordings. In: Otta DA, ed. *Multidisciplinary perspectives in event-related brain potential research.* Washington: US Environmental Protection Agency, 1978.
192. Jasper HH. The ten-twenty electrode system of the International Federation. *Electroenceph Clin Neurophysiol* 1958;10:371.
193. Grundy BL, Sanderson AC, Webster MW, et al. Hemiparesis following carotid endarterectomy: comparison of monitoring methods. *Anesthesiology* 1981;55:462.
194. Sundt TM, Sharbrough FW, Piepgras DG, et al. Correlation of cerebral blood flow and electroencephalographic changes during carotid endarterectomy with results of surgery and hemodynamics of cerebral ischemia. *Mayo Clin Prog* 1981;56:533.
195. Stockard J, Bickford R. The neurophysiology of anaesthesia. In: Gordon E, ed. *A basis and practice of neuroanaesthesia,* 2nd ed. Amsterdam: Excerpta Medica, 1981.
196. Sebel PS. Central nervous system monitoring during open heart surgery: an update. *J Cardiothorac Vasc Anesth* 1998;12:3.
197. Edmonds HL, Rodriguez RA, Audenaert SM, et al. The role of neuromonitoring in cardiac surgery. *J Cardiothorac Vasc Anesth* 1996;10:15.
198. Levy WJ. Quantitative analysis of EEG changes during hypothermia. *Anesthesiology* 1984;60:291.
199. Grundy BL, Nelson PB, Doyle E, et al. Intraoperative loss of somatosensory evoked potentials predicts loss of spinal cord function. *Anesthesiology* 1982;57:321.
200. Dolman J, Silvay G, Zappulla R, et al. The effect of temperature, mean arterial pressure, and cardiopulmonary bypass flows on somatosensory evoked potential-latency in man. *Thorac Cardiovasc Surg* 1986;34:217.
201. Hickey C, Gugino LD, Aglio LS, et al. Intraoperative somatosensory evoked potential monitoring predicts peripheral nerve injury during cardiac surgery. *Anesthesiology* 1993;78:29.
202. Spahn DR, Quill TJ, Hu WC, et al. Validation of 133Xe clearance as a cerebral blood flow measurement technique during cardiopulmonary bypass. *J Cereb Blood Flow Metab* 1992;12:155.
203. McKay RD, Reves JG, Karp RB, et al. Effects of cardiopulmonary bypass on cerebral blood flow. *Anesth Analg* 1983;62:245.
204. Govier AV, Reves JG, McKay RD, et al. Factors and their influence on regional cerebral blood flow during nonpulsatile cardiopulmonary bypass. *Ann Thorac Surg* 1984;38:592.
205. Croughwell N, Smith LR, Quill T, et al. The effect of temperature on cerebral metabolism and blood flow in adults during cardiopulmonary bypass. *J Thorac Cardiovasc Surg* 1992;103:549.
206. Rogers AT, Prough DS, Roy RC, et al. Cerebrovascular and cerebral metabolic effects of alterations in perfusion flow rate during hypothermic cardiopulmonary bypass in man. *J Thorac Cardiovasc Surg* 1992;103:363.
207. Aladj LJ, Croughwell N, Smith LR, et al. Cerebral blood flow autoregulation is preserved during cardiopulmonary bypass in isoflurane-anesthetized patients. *Anesth Analg* 1991;72:48.
208. Croughwell N, Lyth M, Quill TJ, et al. Diabetic patients have abnormal cerebral autoregulation during cardiopulmonary bypass. *Circulation* 1990;82[Suppl 5]:IV407.
209. Newman MF, Croughwell ND, White WD, et al. Pharmacologic electroencephalographic suppression during cardiopulmonary bypass: a comparison of thiopental and isoflurane. *Anesth Analg* 86:246.
210. Van der Linden J, Casimir AH. When do cerebral emboli appear during open heart operations? A transcranial Doppler study. *Ann Thorac Surg* 1991;51:237.
211. Smith JL, Evans DH, Bell PR, et al. A comparison of four methods for distinguishing Doppler signals from gaseous and particulate emboli. *Stroke* 1998;29:1133.
212. Barbut D, Hinton RB, Szatrowski TP, et al. Cerebral emboli detected during bypass surgery are associated with clamp removal. *Stroke* 1994;25:2398.
213. Braekken SK, Russell D, Brucher R, et al. Cerebral microembolic signals during cardiopulmonary bypass surgery. Frequency, time of occurrence, and association with patient and surgical characteristics. *Stroke* 1997;28:1988.
214. Pugsley W, Klinger L, Paschalis C, et al. The impact of microemboli during cardiopulmonary bypass on neuropsychological functioning. *Stroke* 1994;25:1393.
215. Grocott HP, Croughwell ND, Amory DW, et al. Cerebral emboli and serum S100 during cardiac operations. *Ann Thorac Surg* 1998;65:1645.
216. Von Reutern GM, Hetzel A, Birnbaum D, et al. Transcranial Doppler ultrasonography during cardiopulmonary bypass in patients with severe carotid stenosis or occlusion. *Stroke* 1988;19:674.
217. Grocott HP, Amory DW, Lowry E, et al. Transcranial Doppler blood flow velocity versus ^{133}Xe clearance cerebral blood flow during mild hypothermic cardiopulmonary bypass. *J Clin Monit Comput* 1998;14:35.
218. Trubiano P, Heyer EJ, Adams DC, et al. Jugular venous bulb oxyhemoglobin saturation during cardiac surgery: accuracy and reliability using a continuous monitor. *Anesth Analg* 1996;82:964.
219. Croughwell ND, Frasco P, Blumenthal JA, et al. Warming during cardiopulmonary bypass is associated with jugular bulb desaturation. *Ann Thorac Surg* 1992;53:827.
220. Brown R, Wright G, Royston D. A comparison of two systems for assessing cerebral venous oxyhaemoglobin saturation during cardiopulmonary bypass in humans. *Anaesthesia* 1993;48:697.
221. Yao FF, Tseng CC, Braverman JM, et al. Cerebral oxygen desaturation is associated with prolonged lengths of stay in the intensive care unit (ICU) and hospital. *Anesthesiology* 1999;91:A123.

222. Yao FF, Tseng CC, Boyd WC, et al. Cognitive dysfunction following cardiac surgery is associated with cerebral oxygen desaturation, *Anesthesiology* 1999;91:A73.
223. Newman MF, Lowry E, Croughwell ND, et al. Near-infrared spectroscopy (Invos 3100A) and cognitive outcome after cardiac surgery. *Anesth Analg* 1997;84:S111.
224. Edmonds HL. Detection and treatment of cerebral hypoxia key to avoiding intraoperative brain injuries. *Anesthesia Patient Safety Foundation Newsletter* 1999;14:25.
225. Levy WJ, Carpenter J, Fairman RM, et al. The calibration and validation of a phase-modulated near-infrared cerebral oximeter. *Anesthesiology* 1998;89:A539.
226. Henson LC, Calalang C, Temp JA, et al. Accuracy of a cerebral oximeter in healthy volunteers under conditions of isocapnic hypoxia. *Anesthesiology* 1998;88:58.
227. Benaron DA, Stevenson DK. Resolution of near infrared time-of-flight brain oxygenation imaging. *Adv Exp Med Biol* 1994; 345:609.
228. Schwarz G, Litscher G, Kleinert R, et al. Cerebral oximetry in dead subjects. *J Neurosurg Anesthesiol* 1996;8:189.
229. Muellner T, Schramm W, Kwasny O, et al. Patients with increased intracranial pressure cannot be monitored using near-infrared spectroscopy. *Brit J Neurosurg* 1998;12:136.
230. Maeda H, Fukita K, Oritani S, et al. Evaluation of post-mortem oxymetry in fire victims. *Forensic Sci Int* 1996;81:201.
231. Sprung J, Bourke DL, Mackenzie CF, et al. Chronic methemoglobinemia: improving hemoglobin saturation monitoring during anesthesia. *J Clin Monit* 1994;10:267.
232. Austin EH, Edmonds HL, Auden SM, et al. Benefit of neurophysiologic monitoring for pediatric cardiac surgery. *J Thorac Cardiovasc Surg* 1997;114:707.
233. BhaskerRao B, VanHimbergen D, Edmonds HL, et al. Evidence for improved cerebral function after minimally invasive bypass surgery. *J Card Surg* 1998;13:27.
234. Kilminster S, Treasure T, McMillan T, et al. Neuropsychological change and S-100 protein release in 130 unselected patients undergoing cardiac surgery. *Stroke* 1999;30:1869.
235. Croughwell ND, Reves JG, White WD, et al. Cardiopulmonary bypass time does not affect cerebral blood flow. *Ann Thorac Surg* 1998;65:1226.

Cardiac Anesthesia: Principles and Clinical Practice, Second Edition, edited by Fawzy G. Estafanous, Paul G. Barash, and J.G. Reves. Lippincott Williams & Wilkins, Philadelphia © 2001.

9

INTRAOPERATIVE ECHOCARDIOGRAPHY

ROBERT M. SAVAGE
SOLOMON ARONSON
JACK S. SHANEWISE
EMAD B. MOSSAD
MICHAEL G. LICINA

Intraoperative echocardiography (IOE) has become an integral, if not defining, aspect of the discipline and practice of cardiovascular anesthesia (1). Nationwide this is reflected by the increasing numbers of cardiac surgery programs in which this diagnostic and monitoring capability is part of the anesthetic management of cardiac surgery patients. In addition, echocardiography training and education is demanded by residents and fellows and viewed as an important component of their postgraduate training in cardiac anesthesia. The Society of Cardiovascular Anesthesiologists (SCA) has further emphasized the importance of echocardiography by developing the Perioperative Echocardiography Certification Examination, which was recently placed under the auspices of the National Board of Echocardiography (2). IOE provides a more definitive quality of care for our patients and offers the cardiovascular anesthesiologist greater involvement in perioperative decision making as well as increased interdisciplinary interaction in patient care and research. It challenges the anesthesiologist to combine the skills of critical care specialist and diagnostic echocardiographer in the most crucial of circumstances. This chapter provides an overview of IOE and its impact on the clinical practice and discipline of cardiovascular anesthesia. The synopsis of IOE, including its historical background and the principles of ultrasound, will be followed by a discussion of its definition, indications/contraindications, technical considerations in performance of the comprehensive study, and the overall organization of a cohesive IOE service. We will then focus on the recommended guidelines and standardized nomenclature for performing a comprehensive examination and proceed with a more in-depth examination of the clinical applications of ultrasound in the operating room and its future potential directions.

R. M. Savage, E. B. Mossad, and M. G. Licina: Department of Cardiothoracic Anesthesiology, The Cleveland Clinic Foundation, Cleveland, Ohio 44195.

S. Aronson: Department of Anesthesiology and Critical Care, University of Chicago, Chicago, Illinois 60637.

J. S. Shanewise: Division of Cardiovascular Anesthesiology and Critical Care, Emory University School of Medicine, Atlanta, Georgia 30322.

HISTORICAL PERSPECTIVES

The first reported use of echocardiography in the operating room was in 1971 by Side and Gosling who utilized transesophageal continuous-wave (CW) Doppler to demonstrate thoracic aortic flow (3). Epicardial M mode was subsequently reported by Johnson et al. (4) in 1972 to show the success of an open mitral commissurotomy. In 1976, Frazin et al.(5) demonstrated the ability to accurately measure the aortic valve (AV) and left atrium (LA) diameter as well as the velocity of opening of the mitral valve (MV) using a transducer passed into the esophagus on a thin coaxial cable (5). In the late 1970s, Hisanaga et al. (6) introduced two-dimensional (2D) transesophageal imaging incorporating a rotating transducer on a gastroscope. Peter Hanrath first developed a 2D transducer prototype that was placed on a flexible gastroscope shaft. Using this imaging probe, Cahalan and Schiller demonstrated changes in segmental wall motion during cardiac surgical procedures (7). The phenomenal potential for clinical application was recognized by Topol et al. (8) and is now used in all centers performing cardiac surgery to identify previously unidentified cardiac lesions, to ensure the success of valve repair and revascularization procedures, and to reduce perioperative complications.

PHYSICS OF ULTRASOUND

Basic Principles of Ultrasound

To understand the principles of image acquisition and interpretation, an understanding of the basic physics of ultrasound is essential. Sound that is above the audible range of the human ear is referred to as ultrasound and has a fre-

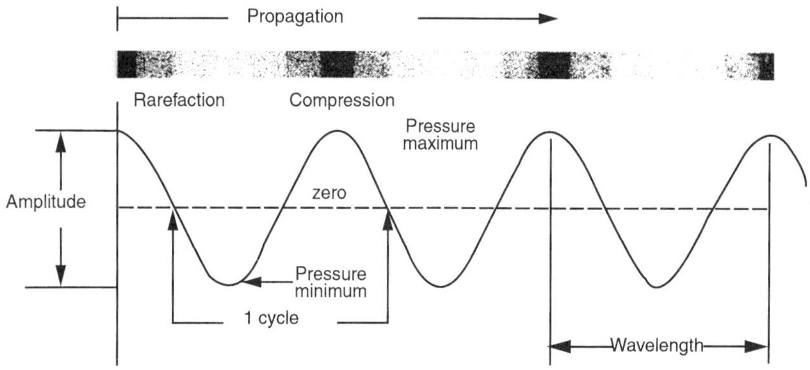

FIGURE 9-1. Properties of sound waves.

quency of more than 20,000 cycles/second or 20 kHz (8). The ultrasound used for transesophageal echocardiography (TEE) usually has a frequency between 3 and 7 million cycles/second (3 to 7 MHz). Sound waves possess the properties of frequency (cycles/second), wavelength (mm), propagation velocity (1,540 m/second in blood), and amplitude (decibels), as illustrated in Fig. 9-1. The velocity of propagation of sound waves in tissue (roughly 1,540 m/second) is essentially constant and equal to the product of the frequency and length of the sound wave.

C (velocity of sound in tissue) =

$$\lambda \text{ (wavelength)} \times \text{F (frequency)}$$

$$\lambda \text{ (mm)} = 1.540 \text{ mm/second/F (cycles/second)}$$

Thus, frequency and wavelength are inversely related. Although shorter wavelengths provide a greater ability to distinguish between two objects in close proximity (resolution), they do so at the expense of their diminished ability to penetrate tissue depth. As sound passes through a homogenous substance, it travels in a linear fashion. However, when the sound wave reaches an interface between two tissues with differing densities (acoustic impedances), part of the sound beam is reflected back to the source. The amount of reflection is dependent on the differences in the acoustic impedances of the two tissues. Structures that are less than 1 wavelength lead to a scattering of the sound beam. Scattering from blood cells is the origin of the Doppler signal in conventional echocardiography. Some of the sound waves may not be reflected directly back toward their origin but may simply be deflected (refracted) from a straight passage through tissue. Because ultrasound energy is absorbed as it passes through tissue in the form of heat, the overall amplitude of the sound wave becomes diminished or attenuated. Attenuation is related to frequency, with lower frequency wavelengths having greater penetrating ability than higher frequency sound waves because of less reflection and scattering. The depth of penetration for image formation is approximately 200 wavelengths. If deeper structures require visualization, using a lower frequency transducer is necessary. Ultrasound interrogation involving dense tissues, such as bone, or those that contain air, such as lung, are not possible because of the reflection and scattering of sound waves.

Transducers

Ultrasound transducers use piezoelectric crystals to both generate and receive ultrasound waves (Fig. 9-2). These crystals have the ability to expand and compress when an electrical current is administered. Conversely, when a piezoelectric crystal receives an ultrasound wave, a high-frequency electrical current is generated. Even though the crystal functions in the receiver mode approximately 99% of the time, it is referred to as a transducer. Currently, available transducers are quite sensitive and can detect a received wavelength signal that is less than 1% of the initially transduced signal. Knowing the velocity of ultrasound in tissue

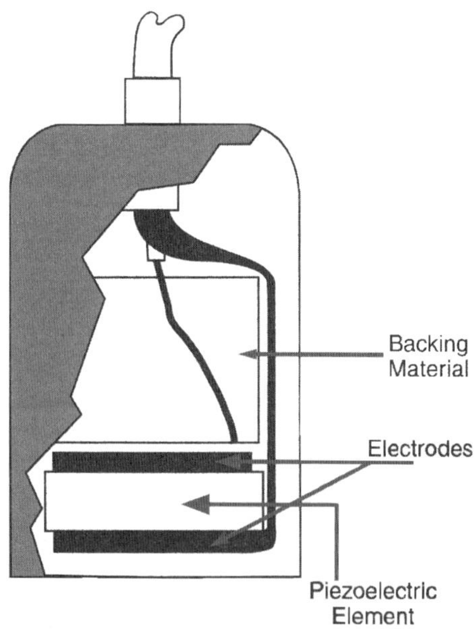

FIGURE 9-2. Ultrasound transducer construction.

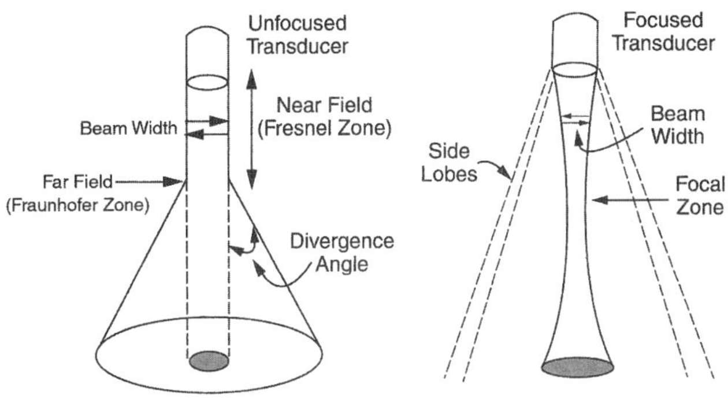

FIGURE 9-3. Focused and unfocused transducer.

and the time between the ultrasound transmission and reception, the image distance from the transducer is determined. Most transducers consist of multiple piezoelectric crystals arranged so that the overall beam may be focused or steered electronically by altering the sequence of activation. CW Doppler uses a pair of piezoelectric crystals, one continuously in the transducer mode and one in the receiver mode. Pulsed repetition frequency (PRF) Doppler employs a single crystal that transmits and waits to receive the return signal before transmitting again. The signal formed by multiple piezoelectric crystals is referred to as a beam and may be either unfocused or focused (Fig. 9-3). The unfocused beam travels in a columnar fashion in its near-field zone, whose length is directly proportional to the diameter of the transducer and inversely related to the wavelength ($F_n = D^2/4\ \lambda$). A 5-MHz transducer with a 5-mm diameter has a near-field distance equal to 20.8 cm.

$$\lambda = c/f = 1.54/5\ \text{MHz} = 0.3\ \text{mm})$$

$$F_n = D^2/4\ \lambda$$

$$F_n = D^2/4\ \lambda = 5\ \text{mm} \times 5\ \text{mm}/4 \times 0.3\ \text{mm} = 20.8\ \text{cm}$$

Distal to the near field, the beam diverges in a manner that is directly proportional to the wavelength and inversely related to the transducer diameter (divergence angle equals 1.22 λ/D). Beams may be focused by either making the transducer surface concave or by electronically focusing the beam by the crystal activation sequence. The resulting beam has a lateral width and height. The dispersion of the beam beyond the near field results in "side lobes" with reflected signals being interpreted as originating from the main beam. The ability to distinguish two points in space is referred to as resolution. Such distinction may be either in the axial dimension (oriented along the length of the ultrasound beam), lateral (side-to-side resolution), or elevational (resolution along the beam thickness), as illustrated in Fig. 9-3. Of the three different types of resolution, axial is the most precise. Lateral resolution is dependent on the width of the generated beam. The narrower the beam, the better the lateral resolution. The greater the distance from the transducer, the less the lateral resolution, resulting in blurring at greater depths of field.

Ultrasound Instruments and Imaging Modalities

A-, B-, or M-Mode Echocardiography

Cardiac ultrasound imaging modalities may be thought of in terms of one-dimensional (A, B, or M mode) or 2D echocardiography. More recently, three-dimensional (3D) echo has been introduced into the clinical setting. Single-dimension echo A or B mode has only the capability to determine (a) the distance between the transducer and the reflective interface and (b) the intensity of the reflected ultrasound. In A mode, this intensity is noted by the height of the electric signal on the oscilloscope. In B mode, "brightness," mode echo depicts the intensity of reflection by varying degrees of brightness of the reflected point. M-mode echocardiography provides a time or motion mode so that B mode is provided with a time reference. In B mode or M mode, a single crystal is used. The depth of imaging is determined by the time it takes for ultrasound to travel to and from the object being investigated. The frequency with which a transmission may be repeated is refereed to as the PW. The typical m-mode pulse-repetition frequency is up to 3,800 times per second. Such a pulse-repetition frequency permits the evaluation of rapidly moving structures such as valve leaflets or small vegetations on cardiac structures.

2D Echocardiography

2D image generation results from rapid and repetitive scanning along multiple B-mode lines in a fan-shaped sector. This results in a sweeping of the ultrasound beam across an image plane and occurs at a rate of up to 60 times per second, resulting in a "real-time" lifelike image of the heart and its internal structures. The beam may be steered or swept along an imaging plane either mechanically or electronically as used in current phased-array transducers.

Doppler Effect

Doppler echocardiography is derived from the change in frequency (Doppler shift) resulting from the scattering of ultrasound signals after contacting moving cellular blood components. Such moving objects will alter the frequency of the wavelength according to the direction the blood is moving. If it is moving toward the transducer, the frequency is increased. It is moving away, the frequency is reduced. The difference between the received "scattered" frequency (F_s) and the originally transmitted frequency (F_t) is referred to as the Doppler shift and is characterized by the relation:

$$\text{Doppler Shift (v)} = c(F_s - F_t)/2F_t\ (\cos\theta)$$

where v is the Doppler shift, c is the propagation velocity in tissue (1,540 m/second), and θ is the intercept angle between the ultrasound beam and direction of flow. The most accurate measurement occurs when this intercept angle is 0° (cos 0 = 1) compared to 90° when the cos 90 = 0. Because an intercept angle of less than 20° results in a less than 6% error, interrogation angles of less than 20° are considered acceptable in clinical practice. The information received by the ultrasound transduced is displayed via fast Fourier analysis in a spatial mode that incorporates measurements of both time and velocity.

Continuous-Wave Doppler

CW Doppler uses two ultrasound crystals in the transducer head in a mode with one continuously transmitting and one simultaneously receiving. Given the larger pulse-repetition frequency of the continuous measurement mode, larger Doppler shifts may be measured. However, given the lack of pulse gating, determination of the depth of these higher potential velocities cannot be determined. Higher velocity blood flows, such as those associated with turbulent flow across stenotic or regurgitant valve lesions, are particularly well suited for measurement using this Doppler mode.

Pulsed Wave Doppler

In PW Doppler, the transducer emits a burst of ultrasound and then turns off. The receiver mode is then gated open corresponding to a particular depth of interrogation. A complete cycle of transmission-waiting-receiving is called the pulse-repetition frequency. The greater the depth of interrogation, the longer the waiting period. Therefore, the deeper the interrogation, the lower is the pulse-repetition frequency and the maximal velocity that may be measured. To interrogate at a certain depth (D), time must be permitted for the ultrasound burst to travel to and from the depth, which is equal to 2(D). The time gate (delay) between transmission and reception is expressed in the relation $T_d = 2D/Vc$. As the depth increases, eventually the frequency of sampling will be insufficient to measure the particular Doppler shift. When the Doppler frequency shift is greater than half the sampling frequency, an ambiguous signal appears, which is going in the opposite direction to the interrogated flow. This is referred to as aliasing. The maximum measurable frequency shift is no more than half of the pulse-repetition frequency and is referred to as the Nyquist limit. A similar phenomena is seen in the western movies when the frame rate of the movie camera is exceeded by the velocity of the movement of the wagon wheels, resulting in the appearance of a wheel rotating in reverse direction.

Color Flow Doppler

Color flow (CF) Doppler is based on PW Doppler in that multiple sample volumes are evaluated along each sampling line. Usually up to eight ultrasound bursts are determined along each sample line, with velocities being encoded in color (red being indicative of flow toward the transducer and blue away). As with PW Doppler, if the blood flow velocity, being interrogated exceeds half the pulse-repetition frequency for that particular depth, aliasing of the color signal will occur. This is visualized as an immediate change from red to blue, or color aliasing, as the interface where the blood flow velocity exceeds the established maximal measurable velocity (Nyquist limit). Each of the following parameters may affect the Nyquist limit or the maximal measurable velocity of flow: (a) depth of interrogation sector, (b) width of interrogation sector, (c) scan line density, and (d) density of ultrasound bursts per scan line. Shifting each of these parameters in addition to shifting the baseline in the direction away from the flow will optimize the signal and reduce aliasing.

High Frame Rate Doppler

Some of the newer ultrasound platforms provide a high pulse-repetition frequency mode. In high pulse-repetition frequency mode, sampling does not wait for a specific distance gate. By sampling in multiples of two, three, or four times the usual PW mode, higher velocities may be measured but with the potential artifact of ambiguity or image appearance at multiples or fractions of the true depth.

Contrast Echocardiography

Myocardial contrast echocardiography (MCE) is a diagnostic technique that uses an ultrasound contrast agent and adapted ultrasound systems to enhance ultrasound imaging. Early MCE applications employed contrast solutions containing relatively large bubbles, which were injected into the venous circulation to demonstrate gross anatomic abnormalities. Currently, contrast solutions are available containing smaller and more stable microbubbles approximately the size of red blood cells. Presently, several commercially produced contrast agents are undergoing evaluation (Table 9-1). In general, the mean diameter of the microspheres is smaller than that of red blood cells (10 μm). This enables agents to behave as intravascular tracers. The ultrasound technology available for contrast agent detection and quantitation has evolved greatly in the past few years. Contrast echocardiography is a diagnostic tool used for assessing intracardiac structures (Table 9-2). When contrast is employed to image intracardiac shunts, right heart valvular incompetence, and/or pericardial effusions, hand-agitated saline (or blood or both) is used. The agitated solution, which serves to produce ultrasound reflectors, creates relatively large microcavitations (40 to 50 μ in diameter). These microbubbles are unstable and do not last long after mixed in solution. More recently, microbubbles produced by commercial processes have resulted in smaller more stable tracer agents. These agents when injected intravenously, cross the pulmonary circulation and allow enhancement of left-sided structures. In addition to left-sided valvular incompetence,

TABLE 9-1. COMMERCIALLY PRODUCED ULTRASOUND CONTRAST AGENTS

Company	Agent	Characteristics	Stage Of Testing
Mallinckrodt/MBI	Albunex	Sonicated human serum albumin	Approved (FDA) 1994
Mallinckrodt/MBI	Optison	Perfluoropropane-filled sonicated albumin	Approved
Dupont	Infinity	Nondiffusable gas	Phase III
Schering AG	Levovist	Saccharide-based	Phase III
Schering AG	SHU 454	Saccharide-based	Approved (Europe) 1991
Schering AG	SHU 563-A		Preclinical
Bracco	BR-1	Nondiffusable gas	Phase I
IMARx	Aerosomes MRX-115	Liposomes	Phase I
Alliance	Imagent US/AFO 145	Nondiffusable gas	Preclinical
Sonus	Echogen	Phaseshift technology	Phase III

Note: FDA, Food And Drug Administration.

TABLE 9-2. APPLICATION OF INTRAOPERATIVE CONTRAST ECHO

Identify intracardiac structures
Enhance endocardial border detection
Enhance Doppler signal
Cardioplegia distribution
Perfusion assessment

their use has been shown to be valuable for enhancing endocardial borders and therefore regional wall motion assessment. Despite increased resolution afforded by higher frequency TEE transducers, approximately 5% to 10% of the time adequate regional wall motion interpretation is not possible during surgical imaging. Erb et al.(9) demonstrated that the use of contrast intraoperatively with TEE enables endocardial border visualization 70% of the time when regions were not visualized without contrast. MCE will also enhance Doppler interrogation when inadequate spectral envelopes are problematic. Because the ultrasound contrast agents behave as surrogate red blood cells, they create an excellent Doppler signal enhancer. Finally, the direct, real-time interpretation of cardioplegic distribution and myocardial function reserve are applications of contrast combined with stress echocardiography that enable the surgeon and anesthesiologist to assess the adequacy of myocardial protection and surgical revascularization. Both of these applications are discussed further.

INTRAOPERATIVE ECHOCARDIOGRAPHY

IOE, consisting of both TEE and epicardial/epivascular echocardiography (EPE), is a rapidly expanding technical application of ultrasound in the operating room. It permits visualization and evaluation of the structure and function of the heart and thoracic aorta. In noncardiac surgery, IOE is utilized to evaluate and monitor the patient's underlying cardiac function and to detect unrecognized cardiovascular disease. In cardiac surgery, IOE provides a method of confirming or redefining the preoperative diagnosis, which guides the surgical approach and management. Hemodynamic management by the anesthesia care team is enhanced by IOE.

IOE Indications, Contraindications, Limitations, and Safety

Using an evidenced-based analysis of the literature regarding the effectiveness of TEE in the perioperative setting, the Joint American Society of Anesthesiologists–SCA Task Force on Transesophageal Echocardiography developed practice guidelines for the use of TEE (10). Current indications for IOE include its general monitoring and diagnostic applications (Table 9-3) as well as surgery-specific indications (Table 9-4). Intraoperative TEE may be safely performed in most patients. As with any monitoring technique, though, there are associated complications and limitations (Tables 9-5 and 9-6). Included among the limitations are the inability to pass the TEE probe (less than 2%), and inability to obtain an optimal diagnostic image or angle of interrogation for determination of Doppler-derived gradients across the ventricular outflow. However, probably the greatest challenge for the anesthesiologist involved in IOE is the maintenance of clinical vigilance of the patient while performing the IOE study. Weinger et al. (11) have suggested that overall vigilance may be reduced when an inexperienced anesthesiologist is performing the IOE. Learning to safely and efficiently incorporate IOE into the overall workload of the anesthesiologist is an essential part of the training in intraoperative patient management. The contraindications of TEE probe placement are those associated with esophageal or gastric disease (e.g., esophageal strictures, recent surgery, or cancer). Relative contraindications include previous gastroesophageal surgery, surgery in the sitting position, small body size, hiatal hernia, a Zenker diverticulum, esophageal varices, a Barrett esophagus, previ-

TABLE 9-3. INDICATIONS

Monitoring	Diagnostic
Myocardial ischemia	Valve dysfunction
Segmental thickening	Structural abnormalities
Regional wall motion	Severity and mechanism
Preload assessment	Congenital heart disease
Ventricular volume	Aortic vascular disease
Ventricular compliance	Dissection
Global LV function	Aneurysm
Gross estimation	Pseudoaneurysm
dP/dt	Rupture
Fractional area of change	Coronary artery disease
Ejection fraction	Complications
Cardiac output	Ischemia or infarction
Myocardial air	Ventricular dysfunction
Open cardiac procedure	Ventricular septal
Neurosurgical procedure	Defects
	Ruptured papillary
	Muscle
	Pseudoaneurysm
	Aneurysm
	Thrombi
	RV infarction
	Difficulty weaning from CPB
	Hypotension
	Endocarditis

Note: LV, left ventricular; RV, right ventricular; CPB, cardiopulmonary bypass.

TABLE 9-5. COMPLICATIONS AND CONTRAINDICATIONS OF TRANSESOPHAGEAL ECHO

Complications	Contraindications
Patient vigilance reduced	Extensive esophageal or gastric disease
Esophageal injury	Esophageal varices
Gastrointestinal bleeding	Barrett's esophagus
Vocal cord pariesis	Zenker's diverticulum
Dysrythmias	Esophageal irradiation
Seizures	Oropharyngeal abscess (airway unprotected)
Aspiration	Oropharyngeal trauma
Cardiac arrest	Small body surface area
Lip injury	
Hoarseness	
Bacteremia	

ous mediastinal radiation, and oropharyngeal trauma (12). In small children, it is necessary to use an appropriate size probe to avoid compression of the airway or pulmonary artery (PA). To avoid unnecessary risks of infections, routine cleaning and sterilization guidelines must be closely followed (see Chapter 32, Practice Management).

The incidence of complications involving IOE is extremely low. The most notable of which are esophageal trauma (e.g., perforation, submucosal pouches, mucosal

TABLE 9-4. PERIOPERATIVE SURGERY-SPECIFIC INDICATIONS

Cardiovascular Surgery	Noncardiac Surgery	Critical Care Unit
Congenital heart surgery	Higher risk thoracic surgery	Hypotension
Valvular surgery	Pulmonary hypertension	Source of emboli
HOCM surgery	RV dysfunction	Valvular disease
High risk myocardial revascularization	Ischemic heart disease or CHF	
Cardiac mass removal	Higher risk peripheral vascular surgery	
Intracardiac tumor	Abdominal aortic aneurysms	
Intracardiac thrombi	Liver transplantation	
Thoracic aortic surgery	Ischemic heart disease or CHF	
Aneurysm		
Aortic dissection		
Traumatic aortic disruption		
Pulmonary embolectomy		
Surgical procedures for CHF		
Heart transplantation		
LVAD or BiVAD placement		
Dor procedure		
MV repair		
Aneurysmectomy		
Surgery for endocarditis		
Surgery for pericardial disease		
Cardiac tamponade		
Constrictive pericarditis		
Lung transplantation		
Hemodynamic instability		
Difficulty weaning CPB		
Hypotension		

Note: HOCM, hypertrophic obstructive cardiomyopathy; CHF, congestive heart failure; LVAD, left ventricular atrial defect; MV, mitral valve; CPB, cardiopulmonary bypass; RV, right ventricular; BiVAD.

TABLE 9-6. LIMITATIONS OF TRANSESOPHAGEAL ECHO

Training and personnel
Capital equipment requirements
Inadequate Doppler angulation
Misdiagnosis
  Artifact production
  Technical examination
    Doppler angulation
    Imaging plane
  Interpretation

tears), Mallory-Weiss tears at the gastroesophageal junction, vocal cord paresis, and postextubation aspiration. In a report of 10,419 TEE procedures performed in awake patients, significant complications occurred in only 0.18% (13). However, included among these complications was one death secondary to esophageal perforation, in a patient with an unsuspected neoplasm, and one patient with an esophageal hematoma.

Technical Considerations

Transesophageal Echocardiography

Anatomic Considerations. The esophagus extends from the posterior pharynx, at its narrowest point, to the stomach and is approximately 25 to 30 cm long (Fig. 9-4). In the mediastinum, it passes immediately behind the tracheal and left main bronchus and contacts the posterior surface of the LA and left ventricle (LV). Due to the overlap of the air-filled trachea and esophagus, there is a "blind spot" where TEE cannot visualize the ascending aorta due to this acoustic mismatch. At the level of the left main bronchus, the aorta lies anterior to the esophagus. It then descends lateral and posterior to the esophagus at the level of the diaphragm.

Probe Insertion. Before each examination, the TEE probe should be inspected for any potential defects in the protective insulated casing and the controls manipulated to ensure the ability to properly perform the study. The TEE probe consists of five distinct sections including the ultrasound platform connector, cable, control handle, fiberoptic shaft, and the probe head with the rotating ultrasound transducer. It is also of benefit to plug the probe into the machine to ensure that the probe properly interfaces with the ultrasound platform. Some centers routinely use a bite block to reduce the damage inflicted on the probe by dental trauma. In the event of an inability to remove the probe from the esophagus, it should be advanced back into the stomach, straightened, and then withdrawn. After the placement of copious lubricating gel in the posterior pharynx, the TEE probe may be inserted by either direct visualization with a laryngoscope and passage into the esophagus or by inserting the thumb into the mouth behind the teeth and thrusting the mandible upward and inserting the probe with the rotating transducer element facing anteriorly and the probe tip gently anteflexed. Although there is a gentle resistance, it is imperative that the operator not force the probe. Noticeable loss of resistance usually indicates that the probe has passed the constrictor muscles and entered the esophagus. In many patients, passage of the probe is not possible and epicardiac or epivascular echocardiography is necessary.

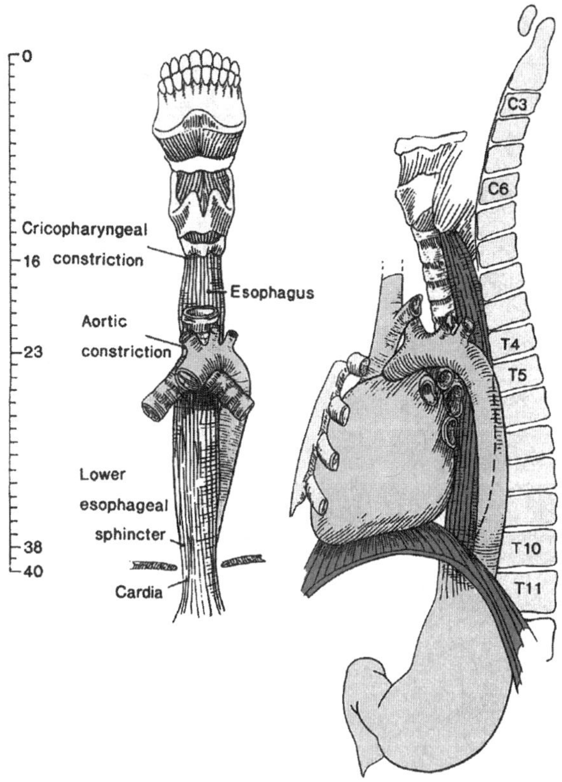

FIGURE 9-4. Diagram of esophagus. The TEE probe is placed in the midesophagus which is posterior to the heart. When the probe is placed in the stomach, it lies inferior and to the left ventricle. If the TEE probe is in the upper esophagus, it lies directly posterior to the trachea, creating the TEE "blind spot" in which portions of the ascending aorta are not visualized.

Epicardial or Epivascular Echocardiography

Although TEE usually provides a satisfactory image for obtaining the necessary clinical information, there are some circumstances in which EPE is indicated. Due to the "blind spot" of the transesophageal window caused by the interposition of the tracheal between the esophagus and ascending aorta, direct application of a sterile sleeved "transthoracic" imaging probe is occasionally necessary to determine the optimal location for cannula placement. If there are significant protruding atheroma in the ascending aorta at the customary site of arterial cannulation, an alternative site such as the axillary or femoral artery may be used for arterial access to minimize the incidence of stroke. Other common indications, however, include the inability to achieve an acceptable angle of interrogation (less than 20°) for determination of transvalvular gradient (aortic stenosis) or subvalvular gradient in patients with hypertrophic cardiomyopathy. In minimally invasive cardiac surgery, EPE imaging may be utilized to assist the surgeon in localizing the coronary arteries (particularly when intramyocardial) and documenting revascularized distal coronary flow, using either CF or PW Doppler or the newer ultrasonic contrast agents.

A transthoracic imaging probe (3.5 to 5 MHz for epicardial imaging or more than 7 MHz for epiaortic imaging) is inserted into a sterile plastic sleeve with a latex tip, into which 3 to 5 mL of imaging gel has been placed. After the probe is fit snugly into the gel-filled receptacle, sterile rubber bands are placed externally to maintain a standoff 1.5- to 2-cm column of gel. This permits optimal near-field imaging. Imaging planes for EPE are similar to those used in transthoracic. In addition to the standard imaging planes, the aortic superior vena cava sulcus may be accessed for determining aortic and LV outflow tract (LVOT) gradients.

IOE Service Requirements

One of the most important issues surrounding IOE is the development of an integrated echocardiography service that provides the patient with the necessary expertise regardless of the time of day. There must be a number of requirements fulfilled to satisfy this goal (Table 9-7). The most important among these is the availability of a competent echocardiographer for emergent IOE studies. The IOE evaluation cannot detract from the overall anesthetic or hemodynamic care of the patient. In circumstances in which a second opinion is indicated or there is hemodynamic instability or respiratory insufficiency, immediate expert backup should be available. For such a service to function, there should be sufficient numbers of ultrasound imaging platforms and probes to support the clinical activity. Capabilities for providing a written IOE report, the ability to retrieve the recorded study for clinical review, and ongoing quality assurance are necessary to optimally serve the potential patient requirements. Rafferty et al. (14) have reported on their program, which includes a peer review of every study to ensure that the study was retrievable, the correct diagnosis was made, the study was recorded in a standardized fashion, and the report was correctly copied and present in the patient's chart (see Chapter 32, Practice Management).

TABLE 9-7. INTRAOPERATIVE SERVICE REQUIREMENTS

Personnel
- Adequate cardiac anesthesia service staffing
- Competently echo–trained cardiovascular anesthesiologists
- Immediate consultative expertise (cardiologists or anesthesiologists)
- Technical support
  - Sonographer
  - Record keeping
  - Library retrieval
  - Probe cleaning and sterilization

Equipment
- Sufficient resources for clinical caseload
- Echo-Doppler platforms capabilities matched for caseload
- Daily maintenance and cleaning
- Long-term maintenance umbrella
- Backup systems available

Patient continuity of care for each patient
- Incorporate long-term care physician into decision making
- Availability of previous echo studies and related data

Quality assurance program
- Technical aspects of study (record, retrievability, and so on)
- Professional
  - Comprehensive study
  - Correct diagnosis
  - Appropriate management decisions
- Patient outcome

Confidence of hospital system
- Surgeons
- Cardiologists
- Referring physicians

Note: One of the most important issues surrounding intraoperative echo is the development of an integrated comprehensive echo service that provides the patient with the necessary expertise irrespective of the time of day. There must be a number of requirements fulfilled to satisfy the development of an integrated comprehensive echo service.

Training

The professional discipline of the individual performing the IOE study is not as important as his or her training and possession of the skills necessary to competently perform the study. In 1990, the American College of Cardiology and the American Society of Echocardiography (ASE) provided guidelines for training in TEE and established levels of performance depending on the supervised experience and assimilation of the technical and cognitive skills (Tables 9-8 and 9-9) necessary to be a competent echocardiographer (15). Competence in IOE may be accomplished by a dedicated period of training during the cardiac anesthesia fellowship or in a postgraduate training experience. At our institution, training is integrated between the Cardiology Imaging Service and the Department of Cardiothoracic Anesthesia. Training includes dedicated time performing transthoracic studies and TEE in the nonoperative setting (16). A cohesive relation between cardiology and cardiac anesthesia serves the dual purpose of promoting the anesthesiologist's understanding of echocardiographic principles and the cardiologist's understanding of operating room physiology and pharmacology.

Examination Certification for Perioperative TEE

The SCA developed a certification examination for perioperative TEE, which was transferred under the administrative umbrella of the National Board of Echocardiography with appropriate representation by cardiovascular anesthesiologists. The purpose of this examination is to permit the dedicated student an opportunity to demonstrate their knowl-

TABLE 9-8. IOE COGNITIVE SKILLS

Knowledge of appropriate indications, contraindications, and risks of TEE
Understanding of differential diagnostic considerations in each clinical case
Knowledge of the physical principles of image formation and data acquisition as well as a working knowledge of the echocardiographic instrument and all controls affecting the quality of the data displayed
Knowledge of normal tomographic cardiovascular anatomy and alterations in anatomy resulting from acquired and congenital heart diseases
Knowledge of normal cardiovascular hemodynamics and fluid dynamics
Knowledge of alterations in cardiovascular hemodynamics and blood flow resulting from acquired and congenital heart diseases
Understanding of the component techniques for echocardiography and TEE, including which methods to use to investigate specific clinical questions
Understanding the intraoperative environment including the stages of cardiopulmonary bypass and their associated hemodynamic alterations
Knowledge of the pharmacology of medications utilized intraoperatively and their hemodynamic effects
Understanding of the surgical interventions and their consequences
Ability to distinguish "adequate from inadequate" echocardiographic data, to distinguish an "adequate from an inadequate" TEE examination, and to determine the necessity for epicardial imaging
Understanding of other cardiovascular diagnostic methods for correlation with TEE findings
Understanding the rationale for surgical decisions based on echocardiographic data
Ability to communicate examination results to patient, other health care professionals, and medical record

Note: IOE, intraoperative echocardiography; TEE, transesophageal echocardiography.
Source: From Guidelines for physician training in transesophageal echocardiography: recommendations of the American Society of Echocardiography Committee for Physician Training in Echocardiography, with permission.

edge in perioperative echocardiography (2). It is important to keep in mind, however, that IOE credentialing is a hospital-based responsibility. Although organizations may provide general guidelines, it is ultimately the responsibility of health care providers in an institution to develop their own guidelines and standards that meet their clinical requirements and best serve their patients.

Requirement of a Comprehensive Intraoperative Study

The intraoperative study, involving both cardiac or noncardiac surgery, includes a number of components (Table 9-10). It begins with a thorough preoperative review of the patient's chart and diagnostic studies. Specific diagnostic questions are identified that must be addressed by the intraoperative study. In noncardiac surgery, the initial compre-

TABLE 9-9. IOE TECHNICAL SKILLS

Proficiency in performing a complete standard echocardiographic examination, using all echocardiographic modalities relevant to the case
Proficiency in safely passing the TEE transducer into the esophagus and stomach and in adjusting probe position to obtain the necessary tomographic images and Doppler data
Proficiency in operating correctly the echocardiographic instrument, including all controls affecting the quality of the data displayed
Proficiency in recognizing abnormalities of cardiac structure and function as detected from the transesophageal and transgastric windows, in distinguishing normal from abnormal findings, and in recognizing artifacts
Proficiency in recognizing abnormalities of cardiac structure and function as detected from the epicardial imaging planes
Proficiency in performing qualitative and quantitative analysis of the echocardiographic data
Proficiency in producing a cogent written report of the echocardiographic findings and their clinical implications

Note: TEE, transesophageal echocardiography; IOE, intraoperative echocardiography.
Source: From Guidelines for physician training in transesophageal echocardiography: recommendations of the American Society of Echocardiography Committee for Physician Training in Echocardiography, with permission.

TABLE 9-10. COMPREHENSIVE IOE EXAMINATION COMPONENTS

- Review of history and physical
- Review of previous cardiovascular studies
  - Echocardiographic
  - Cardiac catheterization
  - Other cardiac imaging studies
    - Nuclear
    - MRI
- Identify issues that must be addressed
  - Patient defined
  - Procedure specific
- Machine setup, ECG, and probe safety check
- Probe insertion and documentation
- Issue-specific examinations
- Comprehensive examination
  - All chambers
  - All valve structures
  - Major vascular structures
    - Thoracic aorta
    - Inferior and superior vena cave
- Record of comprehensive study
  - Preliminary report in chart
  - Final report to database and electronic record
- Communication
  - Direct to primary surgeon
  - Primary care notification of variances
- Repeat of comprehensive examination
  - Progressive stages of surgery
  - Change in patient's condition
    - Physiologic Alteration
- Equipment maintenance
  - Appropriate platform shut down
  - Equipment cleaning and sterilization

Note: IOE, intraoperative echocardiography; MRI, magnetic resonance imaging; ECG, electrocardiogram.

hensive diagnostic study serves as an ultimate preoperative screening test and is followed by actively directed monitoring. Depending on the expertise of the echocardiographer, the depth of the examination may vary. Some diagnostic issues may require greater expertise. In the setting of cardiac surgery, the diagnostic portion of the study is divided between the presurgery and postsurgery studies with the probe being left in a monitoring position during the intervals. The purpose of the presurgery study is to confirm or refine the preoperative diagnosis, as well as determine the mechanism, severity, and underlying etiology. It also serves as a baseline of cardiac function for comparison with any subsequent clinical events. If the surgical procedure involves cardiopulmonary bypass (CPB), IOE is instrumental in developing the cannulation, perfusion, and myocardial protection strategy. If there are significant differences from the preoperating room studies, every attempt should be made to explain the variance. This would include altering the loading conditions (in mitral or aortic regurgitation) or improving perfusion pressures (in unsuspected segmental wall motion abnormalities). If there are new diagnostic conclusions, the patient's cardiologist should be included in the surgical decision-making process. Not only is this in the best interest of patient care, but it also enhances the role of the cardiac anesthesiologist as a perioperative physician.

After the patient has been safely anesthetized, an orogastric tube is placed in the stomach and its contents are removed. The TEE probe is placed and the study is initiated. It is very important that the anesthesiologist involved in performing the intraoperative study develop an ongoing scanning routine in which his or her vigilance is focused between the patient's airway, breathing, hemodynamic assessment, surgical field, and the IOE study that they are performing. If this scanning routine is interrupted and the physician develops "target fixation," the patient's care may potentially be compromised. Learning this skill is as important as developing competence in echocardiography. In performing a comprehensive examination, each physician develops a routine of performing a study that includes a complete structural and Doppler evaluation of all cardiac chambers, valves, and the aorta. Most echocardiographers address the most urgent diagnostic first. This is due to (a) the time constraints of the surgeon's need to finalize a plan, (b) the available electrocautery free period, and (c) the potential for patient hemodynamic instability to interrupt the study. The most significant finding of any intraoperative study may not be the primary indication for the study (17). Consequently, it is very important that such a goal-oriented approach be followed by a comprehensive evaluation. After the intraoperative study has been completed, the echocardiographer records the findings in the patient's chart and ensures the retrievability of the clinical study. The significant findings of the study should be communicated directly to the surgeon performing the procedure.

The purpose of the postsurgical study is to confirm the success of the procedure, assess the patient's cardiac function, and exclude any unanticipated complications. IOE may identify the causes of hemodynamic instability. The success of the surgical procedure is confirmed before administration of protamine and decannulation. It is optimally performed under "street conditions" to ensure that abnormalities are not missed due to altered hemodynamic conditions. It is advantageous to leave the TEE probe in place after successful separation from CPB in the event of post-CPB deterioration of the patient's condition.

Technique and Nomenclature Guidelines for the Comprehensive Examination

The SCA and the ASE formed a writing group to create guidelines for performing an intraoperative examination and to develop recommended nomenclature that was acceptable to both societies (18). These guidelines provide a common understanding of the knowledge and technical skills necessary to perform a complete study and provide a framework for scientific communication. This encourages both the development of quality documentation and overview for study completeness and the multicenter collaboration regarding patient care issues.

Although every patient is somewhat unique in their body habitus and cardiac orientation in the chest cavity, the utilization of multiplane imaging transducers has facilitated the recognition of imaging planes that are commonly employed in evaluation of cardiovascular structure. There are five possible manipulations of the TEE probe to obtain the necessary imaging (Fig. 9-5). Included among these possibilities are probe advancement or withdrawal within the esophagus, turning the probe to the patient's right (clockwise) or left (counterclockwise), flexing the probe anteriorly (anteflex-

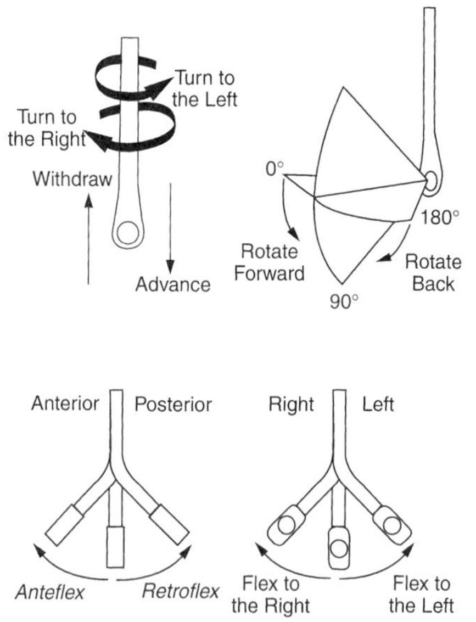

FIGURE 9-5. Potential manipulations of the transesophageal echocardiography probe.

TABLE 9-11. ASE-SCA IMAGING NOMENCLATURE

Imaging Window	Imaging Plane Nomenclature	Angle Rotation (degrees)	Structures Imaged
Upper Esophageal (20–25 Cm)	Aortic Arch LAX (s)	0°	Aortic arch, (L) Brachiocephalic V
	Aortic Arch SAX (t)	90°	Aortic Arch, (L) Brachiocephalic V, PA, PV
Mid Esophageal (30–40 Cm)	Four Chamber (a)	0°–20°	LA, LV, RA, RV, MV, TV, IAS, IVS
	Mitral Commissural (g)	60°–70°	LA, LV, MV
	Two Chamber (b)	80°–100°	LA, LV, LAA, MC, CS
	LAX (c)	120°–160°	LA, LV, AV, LVOT, MV, Ascending Aorta
	RV Inflow-outflow (m)	60°–90°	RA, RV, TV, RVOT, PA, PV
	AV SAX (h)	30°–60°	AV, IAS, Coronary Ostia, LVOT, PV
	AV LAX (i)	120°–160°	AV, LVOT, Ascending Aorta, (R) PA
	Bicaval (l)	80°–110°	RA, SVC, IVC, IAS, LA
	Ascending Aorta SAX (o)	0°–60°	Ascending Aorta, SVC, PA, (R) PA
	Ascending Aorta LAX (p)	100°–150°	Ascending Aorta, (R) PA
	Descending Aorta SAX (q)	0°	Descending Thoracic Aorta, (L) Pleura space
	Descending Aorta LAX (r)	90°–110°	Descending Thoracic Aorta, (L) Pleura Space
Transgastric (40–45 Cm)	Basal SAX (f)	0°–20°	MV, LV, TV, RV
	Mid SAX (d)	0°–20°	Pap Muscle, LV, RV
	Two Chamber (e)	80°–100°	MV, Chordae, Pap Muscle, LA, LV, CS
	LAX (j)	90°–120°	LVOT, AV, MV
	RV Inflow (n)	100°–120°	TV, Chordae, Pap Muscle, RA, RV,
Deep Transgastric (45–50 Cm)	LAX (k)	0°–20° (anteflexion)	LVOT, AV, Ascending Aorta, Arch

Note: LAX, long axis; SAX, short axis; RV, right ventricle; AV, aortic valve; LA, left atrium; LV, left ventricle; RA, right atrium; MV, mitral valve; TV, tricuspid valve; LVOT, left ventricular outflow tract; RVOT, right ventricular outflow tract; SVC, superior vena cava; PA, pulmonary artery.

ion) or posteriorly (retroflexion), flexing the probe to the right or left, and axial transducer rotation from 0° toward 180° (forward) or in the opposing direction (backward).

There are four echocardiographic windows used in TEE: (a) the upper esophageal (UE), (b) midesophageal (ME), (c) transgastric (TG), and (d) deep transgastric (TG). Each probe location occurs at an increasing distance from the incisors, with ranges within 5 to 10 cm depending on the patient's body habitus. There are 20 cross-sectional imaging views (Fig. 8-14A-T), which are dependent on probe depth and probe manipulations discussed earlier (Table 9-11) (18). Each imaging view (e.g., ME AV short-axis) is characterized by the probe position, imaging plane, the major anatomic structure in the image, and orientation of the imaging plane (either long axis [LAX] or short axis [SAX]). Imaging view designations that do not include an anatomic structure imply that the LV is visualized.

The ultrasound platform has an instrumentation panel that varies from corporate vendor but consists of similar settings or adjustments. Most TEE probes can take images at multiple frequencies (3.5 to 7 MHz). Higher imaging *frequency* transducers provide better resolution, due to a smaller wavelength size, but have a shorter depth of penetration. The lower *frequency* transducers provide a better depth of imaging but at the expense of less resolution. The *transmit focus* adjusts the near-field imaging depth for maximal definition at any one frequency. If the anatomic structure being imaged is close to the probe head transducer (LA, MV, or AV), a higher frequency transducer setting may be used and the structure is placed in the center of the image with the transmit focus set at the appropriate depth. The image *gain* adjusts the intensity of the image, whereas the dynamic range setting adjusts the gray scale (compression). The gain and compression settings are adjusted so that the blood is black and is easily distinguishable from the gray tissue. The *time gain compensation* settings adjust the gain at specific depths, whereas the *lateral gain control* settings adjust the gain settings at specific angle sectors in the image. As previously discussed, *CF Doppler* is a color designated collection of PW signals along an individual sector line. The CF Doppler settings are adjusted low enough that any noise, due to excessive gain, is eliminated. Decreasing the depth or width of the CF Doppler interrogation sector increases the frame rate and maximal velocity that may be measured (Nyquist limit) before aliasing occurs.

Nomenclature.

Left Ventricle. The LV chamber is divided into three levels extending from mitral annulus to apex and are referred to as the basal, mid, and apical levels (Fig. 9-6). The upper two levels of the heart (basal and mid) are divided into six circumferential segments. The apical level is divided into four segments resulting in a total of sixteen ventricular segments (18). The six circumferential segments of the basal and mid levels are called the anteroseptal, anterior, lateral, posterior, inferior, and septal (referring to inferoseptal) segments (Fig. 9-6). The four apical segments are the anterior, lateral, inferior, and septal. As illustrated in Fig. 9-7, the

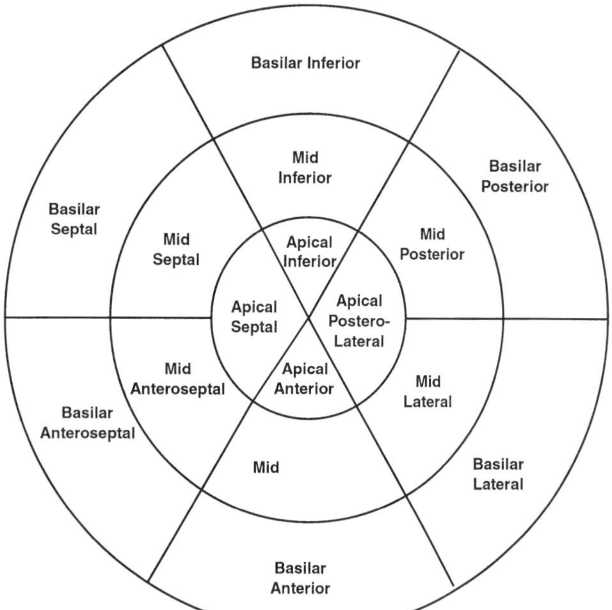

FIGURE 9-6. Six circumferential segments.

segments of the LV may be individually assessed using four imaging planes or views (ME four chamber, ME two chamber, ME LAX, and TG SAX). The ME four-chamber view (Fig. 8-14A) is obtained by positioning the transducer in the midesophagus at the level of the MV and directing the imaging plane through the center of the valve and the apex. The transducer angle is then rotated forward from 0° up toward 20°, when the AV or LVOT are no longer in view and the tricuspid valve (TV) is visualized at its maximum diameter. The ME two-chamber view (Fig. 8-14B) is established by rotating the transducer further forward to approximately 90° where the right atrium (RA) and right ventricle (RV) are no longer visualized. The ME LAX imaging view

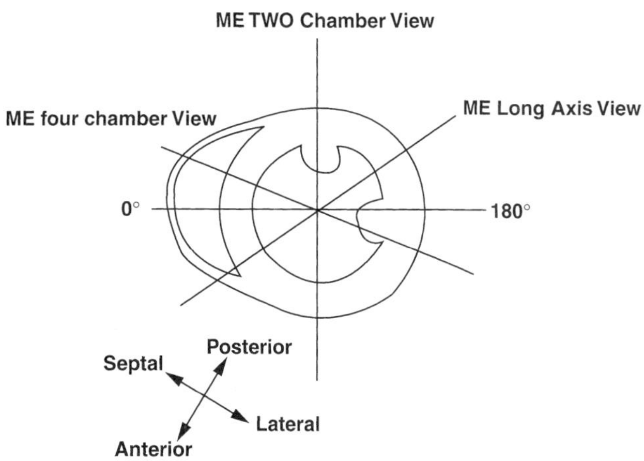

FIGURE 9-7. Four apical segments. Imaging planes utilized in assessment of LV function (18).

(Fig. 8-14C) is obtained by rotating the transducer further forward to somewhere between 110° and 150° where the LVOT, AV, and proximal ascending aorta are visualized. The TG views are obtained by advancing the TEE probe further into the stomach and anteflexing the tip of the probe until a symmetrically circular image of the LV is established (Figs. 8-14D and 8-14F). The levels of the SAX (basal, mid, and apical) are visualized by advancing the probe and applying varying degrees of anteflexion. With the ME SAX view centered on the screen, the transducer angle is rotated forward to approximately 80°, resulting in the TG two-chamber view (Fig. 8-14E). To visualize the apical cavity without foreshortening the image, the transducer probe may need to be retroflexed somewhat. As illustrated in Fig. 9-8, each segment is perfused by the right coronary artery, the left anterior descending artery, or the left circumflex coronary artery. While each patient's coronary circulation varies somewhat, there are generalities regarding individual coronary perfusion beds. The left anterior descending artery typically peruses the anterior two thirds of the interventricular septum and varying amounts of the LV free wall (anterior and lateral). In addition, depending on its length, variable areas of the inferoseptal apex may be supplied by the left anterior descending coronary artery. The left circumflex coronary artery coronary artery usually supply the lateral and posterior walls. The right coronary artery supplies the RV, the inferior LV, and the inferior one third of the interventricular septum depending on which coronary artery is dominant or supplies the posterior descending coronary artery. The posterior descending coronary artery arises from the right coronary artery in 85% of patients. It originates from the left circumflex coronary artery in approximately 8% of patients, whereas in the remaining 7% of patients there is no dominant posterior descending coronary artery. If the right coronary artery is unusually dominant, it may also supply a significant portion of the posterior wall of the LV.

Right Ventricle. The RV is a crescentic chamber composed of the RV free wall, septum, and the RV outflow tract. The examination of the RV is performed beginning with the ME four-chamber view and then turning the probe to the patient's right until the TV is positioned in the center of the screen. With less muscle mass and nonconcentric shape, the force of contraction of the RV does not appear as vigorously as that of the LV. Hence, detection of RV segmental wall motion abnormalities is more difficult. Rotating the transducer forward toward 60° to 75° displays the RV outflow tract along with the pulmonic valve (PV) and main PA. The ME RV inflow-outflow view (Fig. 8-14M) is developed from the TG mid-SAX view by rotating the probe clockwise until the RV is positioned in the center of the screen with the inferior RV wall in the near field of the image. If the transducer angle is rotated forward between 60° and 100°, the RV outflow tract may be imaged. This view is particularly useful in patients undergoing the Ross procedure to visualize the integrity of the PV homograft.

Left Atrium and Right Atrium. Examination of the atria begins from the ME four-chamber view. Reducing the depth of field to 10 to 14 cm and turning the probe to the left places the LA in the center of the imaging sector. The LA is visualized in its entirety by withdrawing and advancing the probe. Upon probe withdrawal, the superior LA structures are visualized including the LA appendage and the left pulmonary veins (lower and upper). CF Doppler confirms the pulmonary venous inflow. The ridge between the pulmonary veins and the LA appendage may give the appearance of an echogenic mass and has often been referred to as the "Coumadin ridge" due to the number of patients who have been anticoagulated suspecting a LA thrombus in this locale. The LA appendage is multilobed and has an irregular surface due to the pectinate muscles that comprise its inner surface. Utilizing CF Doppler at lower aliasing velocities may help distinguish artifact from true LA appendage structure. The right pulmonary veins are visualized by turning the probe clockwise to the patient's right at a more superior level of the LA.

The RA is visualized by further turning the probe to the right placing the RA in the center of the screen. The superior and inferior aspects of the RA are visualized by advancing and withdrawing the probe. The coronary sinus is inferior and posteriorly located in the RA just above the TV. The extent of the coronary sinus may be visualized by turning the probe counterclockwise, keeping it in the center of the imaging sector. This is an excellent view for guiding the placement of the retrograde coronary sinus catheter and for visualizing the anomalous insertion of a persistent left-sided superior vena cava into the coronary sinus. The coronary sinus SAX may be visualized by rotating the transducer angle forward 90° to 110° maintaining the central screen position of the coronary sinus.

The interatrial septum may be examined beginning at the ME four-chamber view at an image depth that maximizes the septal image. The septum is composed of the fossa ovalis and the septal limbus superiorly and inferiorly where it attaches to the atrioventricular cushion. The presence of an interatrial shunt may be detected by injecting an agitated mixture of 7 mL of saline, 2.75 mL of blood, and 0.25 mL of air put in solution by an agitation process using two 10-mL syringes connected by a three-way stopcock. After injection of this mixture intravenously, upon release of 30 cm H_20 positive airway pressure, a shunt exists between the left side and the right side of the heart if micro air bubbles appear on the left side of the heart within 5 cardiac cycles. CF Doppler at low aliasing velocities may also detect interatrial shunting.

Mitral Valve Apparatus. The MV is a complex structure consisting of the valvular apparatus (valve leaflets) and tensor apparatus (chordal structures, papillary muscles, ventricular free wall extending between the base of the papillary muscle insertion and the fibrous MV annulua). All of these components are essential for the proper function of the MV and play an important role in the performance of the LV (Fig. 9-8). During systole, the leaflets come together along a "line of coaptation." This line extends anteriorly to the anterolateral commissure and posteriorly to the posteromedial commissure (Fig. 9-9). Each leaflet corresponds to a similarly named PM. The posterior leaflet consists of three scallops: lateral, middle, and medial. The anterior leaflet (comprising 60% to 70% of the total MV area and 30% of the annular circumference) may be, for purely descriptive purposes, divided into the corresponding lateral, middle, and medial thirds. The chordae extend from the head of the PM to the mitral leaflet. The chordae are classified as primary (attached to the leaflet tip), secondary (attached to the belly of the leaflet), and tertiary (attached to base of leaflet or annulus). There is usually a dominant posterior chordal structure referred to as a "stay" or "stabilizing" chordae. Interruption of the tertiary or posterior "stay" chordae has a profound impact on the maintenance of nor-

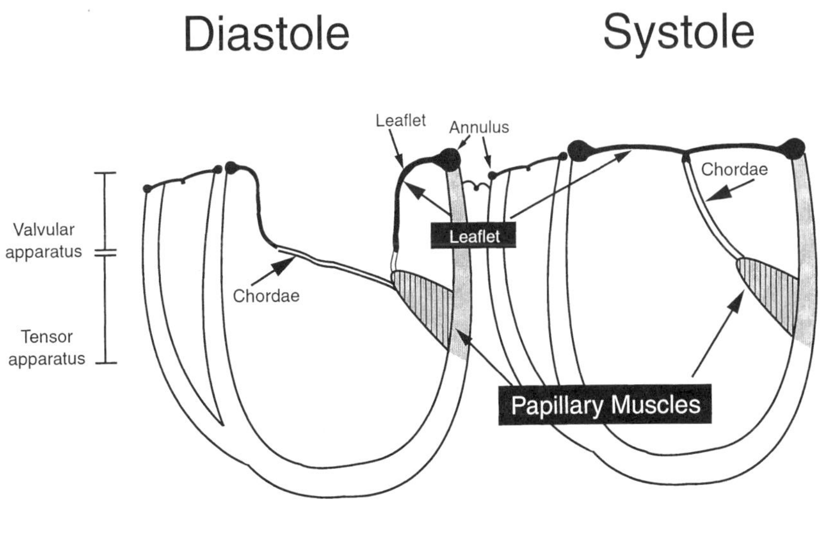

FIGURE 9-8. Mitral valve structure. The mitral valve apparatus consists of the valvular apparatus and tensor apparatus. The tensor apparatus is composed of the chordae, papillary muscle, and ventricular wall which is attached to the fibrour skeleton of the heart at the mitral annulus.

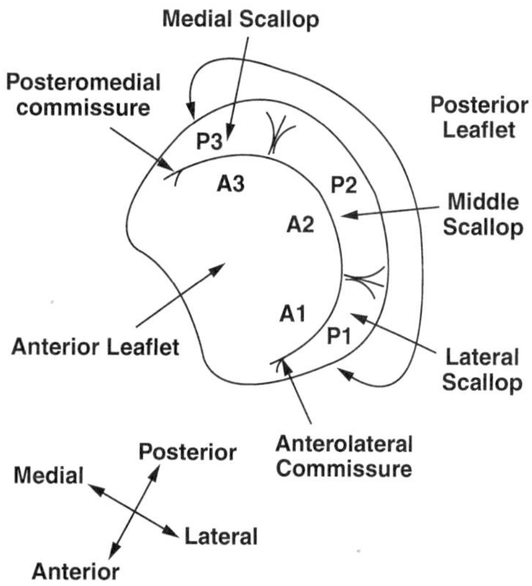

FIGURE 9-9. American Society of Echocardiography–Society of Cardiovascular Anesthesiologists nomenclature of the segmental structure of the mitral valve (18).

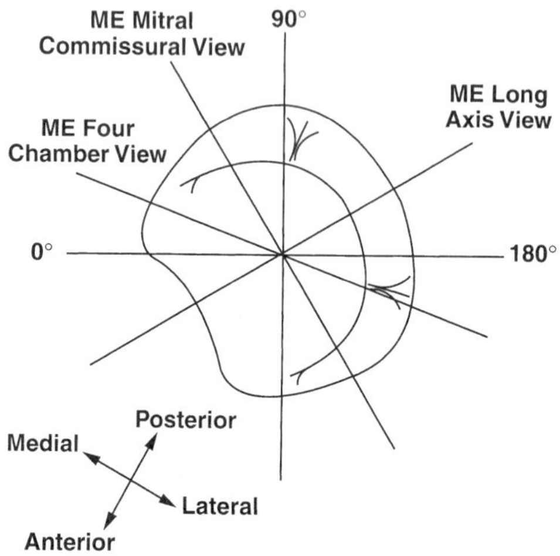

FIGURE 9-11. Midesophageal imaging planes utilized in assessment of the mitral valve segmental (18).

mal LV geometry and overall ventricular function. There are between one and five heads of a PM. The chordae that arise from the (antero) lateral PM extend to the (antero) lateral halves of the posterior and anterior MV leaflets, whereas the chordae from the (postero) medial PM extend to the corresponding halves of the mitral leaflets. Although some surgical mitral repair centers refer to the structures of the MV by the anatomic nomenclature, others use a shorthand nomenclature system. As illustrated in Fig. 9-9, the Carpentier classification divides the posterior MV leaflet into P1, P2, and P3 corresponding to the lateral, middle, and medial scallops (20). The Duran classification (Fig. 9-10) uses a P1, PM, and P2 in referring to the same scallops, respectively (21). The middle scallop is further subdivided into the PM1 and PM2, corresponding to the portion of the middle scallop that receives chordae from the anterolateral PM (PM1) or the posteromedial PM (PM2). In the Carpentier classification scheme (Fig. 9-9), the anterior MV leaflet is subdivided into the A1, A2, and A3 corresponding to the lateral, middle, and medial portions of the leaflet. The Duran classification (Fig. 9-10) simply divides the anterior leaflet into the A1 and A2 portions corresponding to the areas subtended by the corresponding chordal attachments from the anterolateral (A1) and posteromedial PMs. The anterolateral commissure is referred to as the C1 and the posteromedial as the C2. The corresponding PMs are referred to as PM1 (anterolateral) or PM2 (posteromedial). The terminology, which was agreed upon by both the ASE and the SCA nomenclature committees, incorporates the anatomic or Carpentier classification and will be used for purposes of this discussion, recognizing the valuable contribution that the Duran system provides for those involved in MV surgery.

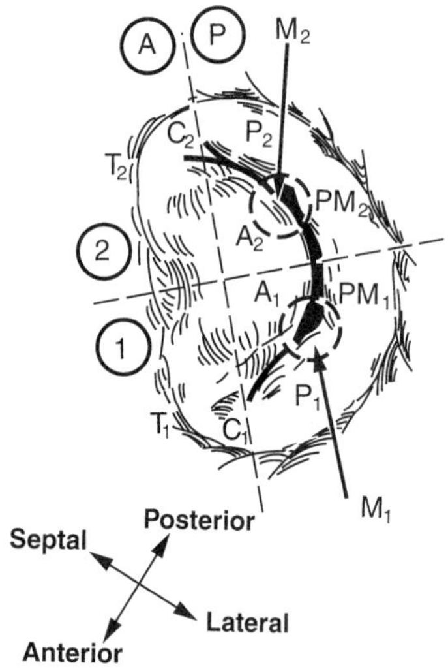

FIGURE 9-10. Duran classification of the mitral valve surgical anatomy.

As illustrated in Fig. 9-11, the MV is examined using five views (ME four-chamber, MV commissural view, ME two-chamber, ME LAX, and TG SAX views). Beginning with the ME four-chamber image (Fig. 9-12), the anterior MV leaflet is to the left of the screen. The image plane cuts across the medial (A3) and the middle (A2) or A1 (lateral) segments (the latter depending on the degree of transducer rotation). The posterior MV leaflet is visualized on the screen's right. The image plane cuts through the lateral (P1) scallop. This imaging view is used to clearly demonstrate prolapse or flail of the corresponding sections of the mitral leaflets. Advancing the transducer angle forward to approximately 45° to 60° produces the ME mitral commissural view (Fig. 9-13). Commonly this view is referred to as the

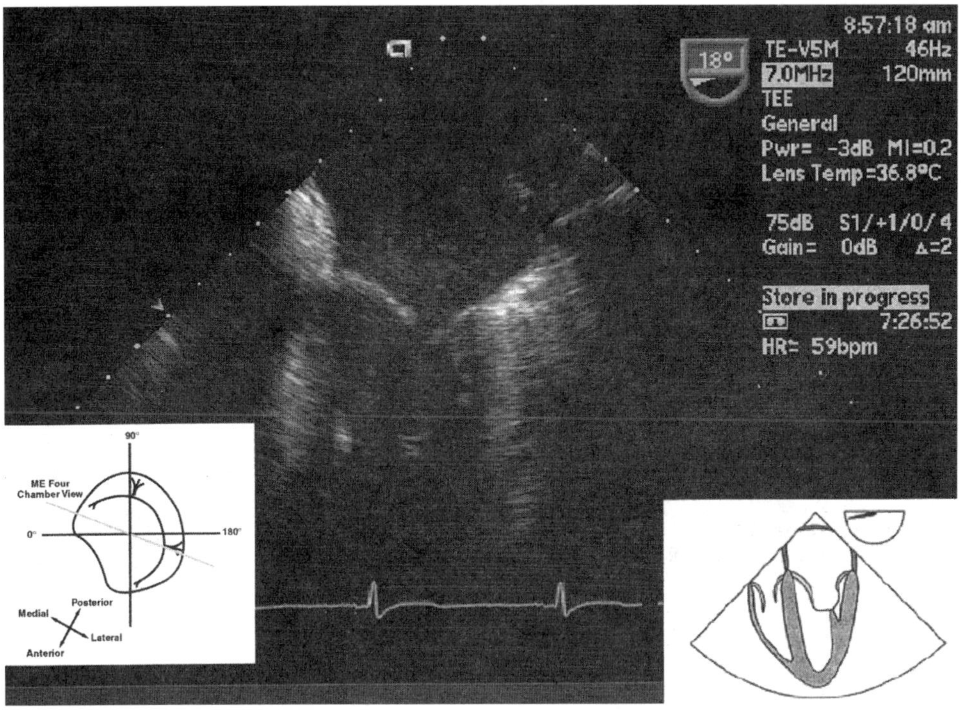

FIGURE 9-12. Midesophageal four-chamber image.

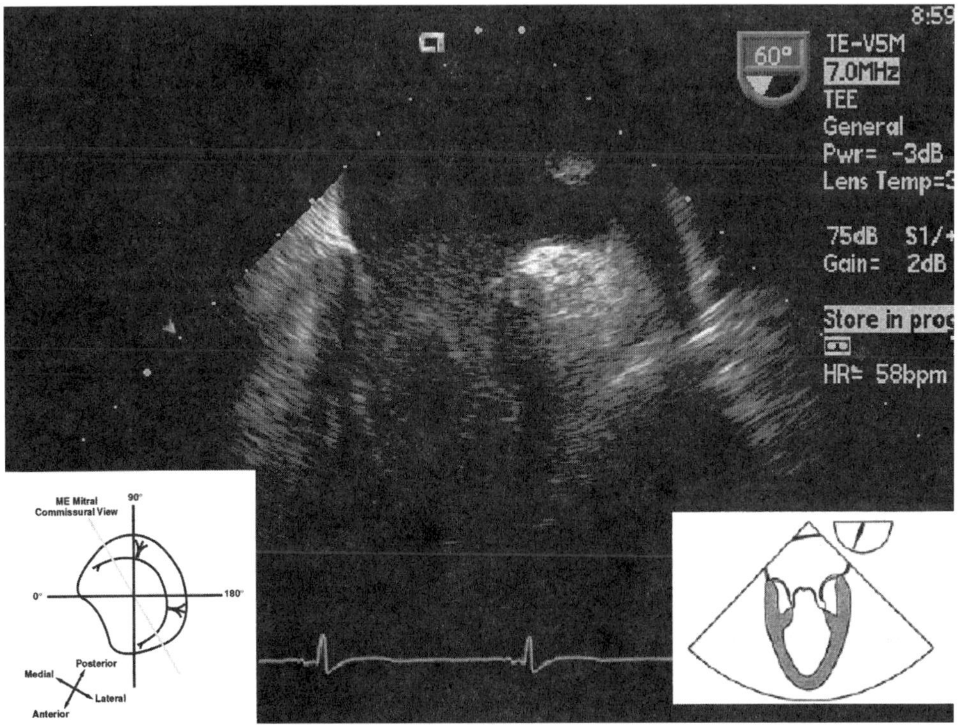

FIGURE 9-13. Midesophageal commissural image of the mitral valve.

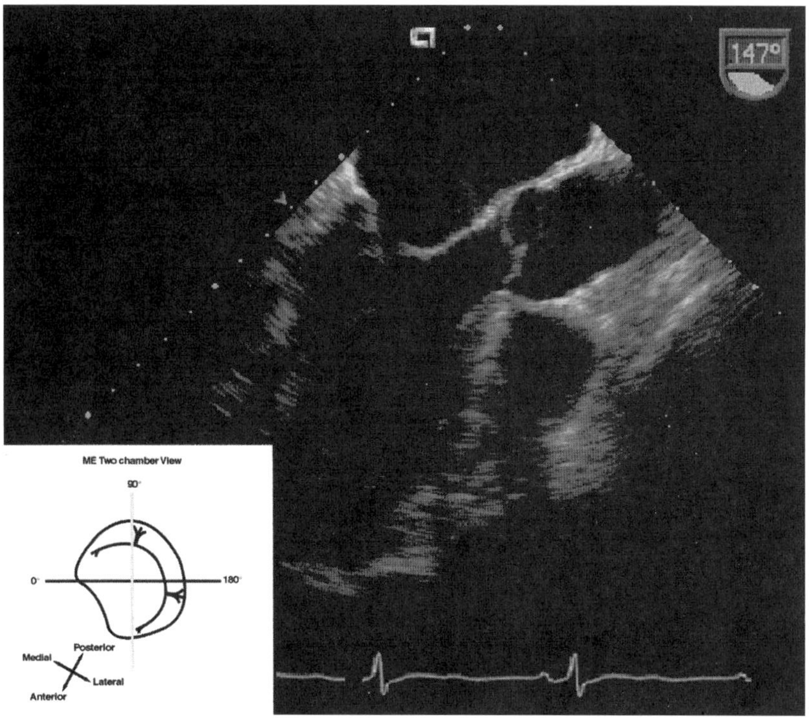

FIGURE 9-14. Midesophageal long-axis image of the mitral valve.

"trap door" or "seagull" image. As illustrated in Fig. 9-13, the medial (P3) scallop is visualized on the screen's left, and the lateral (P1) scallop on the right with the anterior MV leaflet (usually A2) in the middle forming the intermittently seen "trap door" or "head of the seagull." Rotating the angle to 120° to 150° provides the ME LAX view of the MV with the anterior MV leaflet (A1 and A2) segment on the screen's right and the middle (P2) scallop of the posterior MV leaflet on the left (Fig. 9-14). CF Doppler is commonly employed in each of these imaging planes to detect regurgitant systolic flow or turbulent diastolic flow.

The transducer angle is then rotated back to the neutral 0° and the probe is advanced into the stomach (while both anteflexing and leftward flexing the probe) to obtain basal SAX view of the LV and MV (Fig. 9-15). This permits a TG basal SAX view of the MV that is parallel to the annulus and perpendicular to the LAX of the LV. In this image (TG basal SAX), the posterior leaflet is to the right and the anterior MV leaflet is to the left, as illustrated in Fig. 9-15. CF Doppler interrogation of the MV in this imaging view will permit precise localization of the origin of the regurgitant jet and direct the surgeon to the exact point of surgical engagement (see Mitral Valve Repair section). The TG two-chamber view is obtained by rotating the transducer forward to 75° to 90° with visualization of the longitudinal structures of both the anterolateral and posteromedial PMs. This view is particularly useful during MV homograft placement when the numbers of PM heads, the length of the primary and secondary chordae, and annulus size determinations are essential to the correct sizing of the homograft.

Aortic Valve and Root. The AV apparatus (root) is not a single anatomic structure but is comprised of the aortic annulus, valve cusps, the Valsalva sinus, the sinotubular ridge, and the proximal ascending aorta (Fig. 9-16). The architectural orientation of the annulus is further supported by the structural support of the LVOT lying just inferior to the valve. There are three valve leaflets that are individually attached to the Valsalva sinus having structural suspension from the superior aspects of the sinus. The cusps are named for the coronary artery, which may or may not arise from the corresponding sinus of Valsalva. The more anterior of the cusps is the right coronary cusp. The noncoronary cusp is directly adjacent to the interatrial septum. The left coronary cusp gives rise to the left main coronary artery. The three coronary cusps coapt during diastole at an interface called the AV commissure. Each AV cusp has a central nodule of Arantius, which serves as a point of coaptation. The commissural surface of each coronary cusp also coapts with an adjacent coronary cusp along a surface referred to as the lunula. The comprehensive examination of the aortic root is accomplished with four imaging views: (a) ME AV SAX, (b) ME AV LAX, (c) TG LAX, and (d) deep TG LAX (Fig. 8-14H through K).

Beginning in the ME four-chamber imaging view, the probe is withdrawn until the AV is visualized and positioned

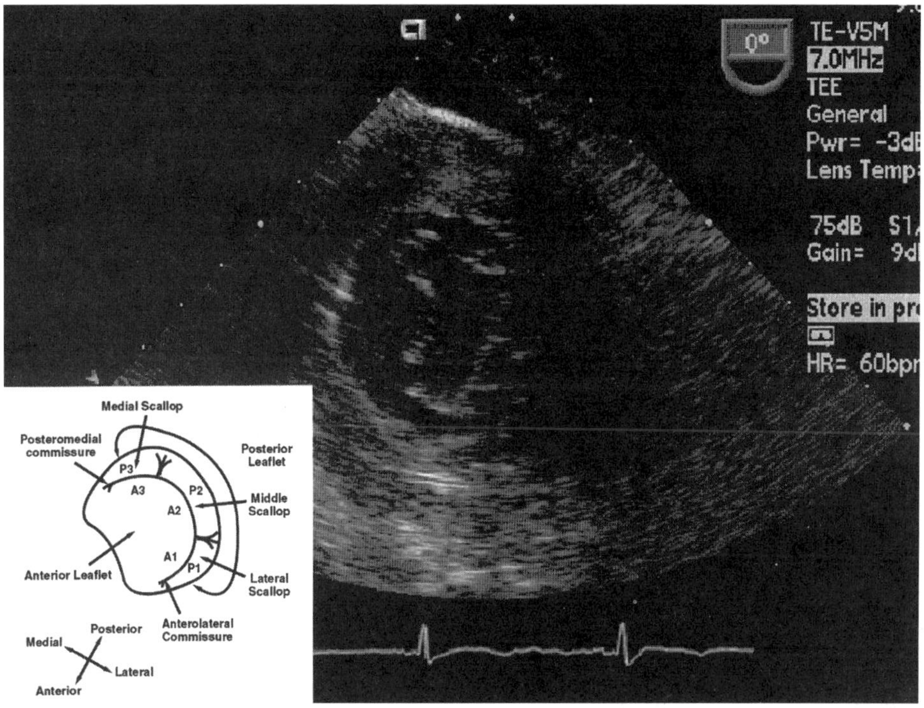

FIGURE 9-15. Short-axis view of the left ventricle and mitral valve.

in the center of the screen. The transducer angulation is increased to approximately 30° to 45°, with the probe being anteflexed and leftward flexed to align the imaging plane parallel to the annulus and perpendicular to the root axis. As illustrated in Fig. 9-17, all three coronary cusps are visualized, along with the left main and right coronary arteries. This is also an excellent view for visualizing the degree of stenosis (and planimetering the valve area).

The ME AV LAX view (Fig. 8-14I) is obtained by rotating the multiplane transducer angulation forward approximately 90° more in the range of 120° to 160°. The more anterior of the valve cusps is the right and the corresponding coronary artery may be easily visualized with CF Doppler. This view is used for measuring the size of the aortic annulus

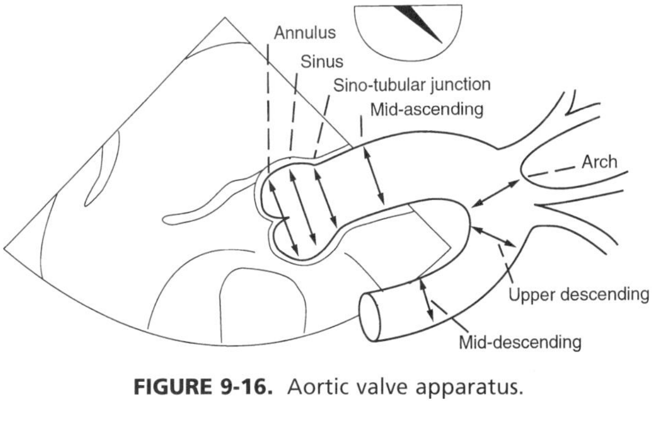

FIGURE 9-16. Aortic valve apparatus.

for purposes of sizing homograft size, size of a prosthetic valve annulus to be inserted, or for volumetric calculations involving the LVOT diameter at this point. Additionally, this view is useful for demonstrating the severity of aortic regurgitation (AR) into the LVOT. Use of color m-mode imaging permits better temporal resolution of the timing of flow in the LVOT, with regurgitation of the AV being visualized after the R wave on the electrocardiogram (ECG) (See Color Fig. 9-18, between pages 560 and 561).

To obtain the deep TG LAX view (Fig. 8-14K) of the AV, the probe transducer is rotated to a neutral position and advanced deep into the stomach with anteflexion. Leftward flexion may be necessary to place the LVOT and AV in the center of the screen. Due to the increased distance between the transducer and the AV, lower frequency transducer settings are often necessary to better visualize the valve. This image may be used in measuring the Doppler-derived velocity of flow across the LVOT or the AV. In addition, CF Doppler may demonstrate aortic regurgitant flow toward the transducer, which is not visualized in the other views when there is acoustic shadowing from annular calcification or a prosthetic valve in either the aortic or the mitral position. The TG LAX (Fig. 8-14J) view is developed from the TG mid-SAX view. The transducer angulation is rotated forward to approximately 90° to 120°, with the LVOT and AV appearing on the right of the screen. The AV and ascending aorta may be visualized in the lower right portion of the screen, depending on the depth settings. This is also

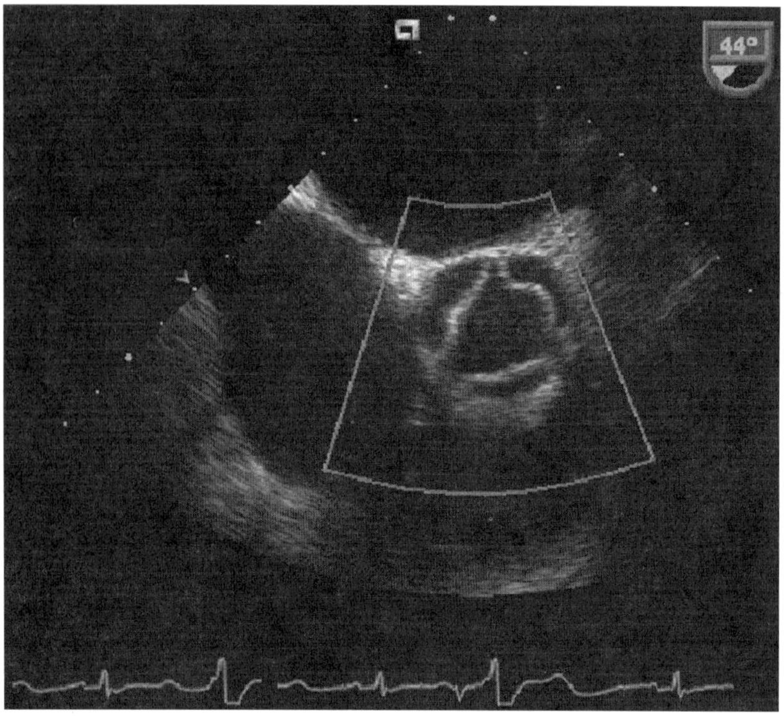

FIGURE 9-17. Midesophageal short axis image of the aortic valve demonstrating the three aortic valve cusps.

an excellent view for volumetric flow across the LVOT or AV as well as visualization of regurgitant AV flow.

Tricuspid valve: normal anatomy and echo doppler evaluation. The TV apparatus is similar in structure to the MV, being composed of valve leaflets, chordae, and papillary muscles. Due to the diminished muscle mass of the RV, it is not as structurally essential for RV function. It does maintain the integrity of blood flow through the RV. The three leaflets of the TV are the septal, anterior, and posterior leaflets. Structurally, the TV sits lower in the heart than the MV so there is a small but common wall between the RA and the LV. The examination of the TV begins in the ME four-chamber view (Fig. 8-14A). The probe is turned clockwise to the patient's right and the depth is adjusted so that the TV is in the center of the screen. The septal leaflet and posterior leaflets are visualized. As with the MV, the probe is slightly advanced and withdrawn to visualize the tricuspid apparatus. Rotating the transducer angulation forward toward 50° to 80° provides the RV inflow-outflow view with the anterior leaflet to the right and the posterior to the left. This is a useful view for CF Doppler imaging of tricuspid regurgitation (TR) of Doppler interrogation of the RV inflow. To obtain the TG views of the TV, the probe is advanced into the stomach and turned to the right with the RV in the center of the screen. By withdrawing the probe (slightly anteflexing) and rotating the transducer angulation toward 20°, a SAX view of the TV is visualized with the anterior leaflet to the left, the septal to the right, and the posterior leaflet in the near-field left of the screen. CF Doppler at this level permits identification of the origin of regurgitant jets.

Pulmonic valve. The PV lies superior, anterior, and to the left of the AV. The PV has three semilunar cusps (right, left, and anterior). The PV is best imaged using the ME RV inflow-outflow view (Fig. 8-14M). The PV is a trileaflet structure with the leaflets being thinner than the semilunar AV cusps. Given this and the far field location of the valve, lower frequency transducer settings provide the best visualization of the valve. Beginning with the ME AV SAX view (Fig. 8-14H), the PV is visualized directly adjacent to the right coronary cusp. To better visualize the PA, the probe is turned leftward, withdrawn slightly with a rotation of the multiplane angulation back toward 10°. Further withdrawing the probe demonstrates the bifurcation of the PA. Turning the probe to the left visualizes the proximal left PA, which is the usual site of persistent patent ductus arteriosus flow detected by CF Doppler. The right PA is visualized by turning the probe rightward and following it out to its branching arteries. In suspected pulmonary emboli, this view will often confirm their presence. The main PA and PV may also be seen from the UE aortic arch SAX view by turning the probe to the right (Fig. 8-14T). Rotating the transducer angulation to 90° permits the calculation of volumetric flow with a PW Doppler angle of interrogation nearly parallel to the PA flow.

Thoracic aorta. The thoracic aorta is in close proximity to the esophagus. This permits close inspection of the proximal ascending aorta and descending thoracic aorta with higher frequency transducer settings. As previously mentioned, the anatomic interposition of the trachea between the esophagus and the ascending aorta (distal to the right PA) make it extremely difficult, if not impossible, to image this portion of the aorta. The proximal aorta may be visualized using the ME AV LAX (Fig. 8-14I). The probe is withdrawn to examine the superior aspects of the proximal aorta proximal to the "blind spot." The outflow cannula insertion of implantable LV assist devices (LVADs) is best visualized in this imaging plane. As discussed previously, epiaortic standoff scanning with a sterile sleeve permits visualization of this anatomic locale. Occasionally, the more superior arch vessels may be visualized above the blind spot. By rotating the TEE transducer angulation to 0°, advancing and turning the probe to the left, the descending thoracic aorta is visualized in the descending aortic SAX view (Fig. 8-14Q). Keeping in mind that the position of the aorta, at the level of the diaphragm, is to the left and posterior to the esophagus (Fig. 9-19), the near-field image of the circular aorta represents the right anterior wall of the aorta. The rightward structures are therefore on the screen's left and the leftward on the right. By rotating the transducer angle toward 90°, the descending aortic LAX view is obtained. By returning the transducer angle to 0° rotation and withdrawing the probe, the proximal descending aortic arch is visualized in LAX and develops an oblong configuration. Further withdrawal may permit cross-sectional visualization of the great vessels of the head and neck. Rotating the transducer angulation toward 90°, from the UE aortic arch LAX view, permits visualization of the proximal origin of the left subclavian artery in the upper right screen and the PV and main PA in the lower left screen. Turning the probe rightward with the assistance of CF Doppler set for low-velocity aliasing permits visualization of the origin or the left common carotid artery and brachiocephalic artery with further rightward turning. At this level, the aorta is anterior to the esophagus, and therefore the posterior wall of the aortic arch is in the near-field image.

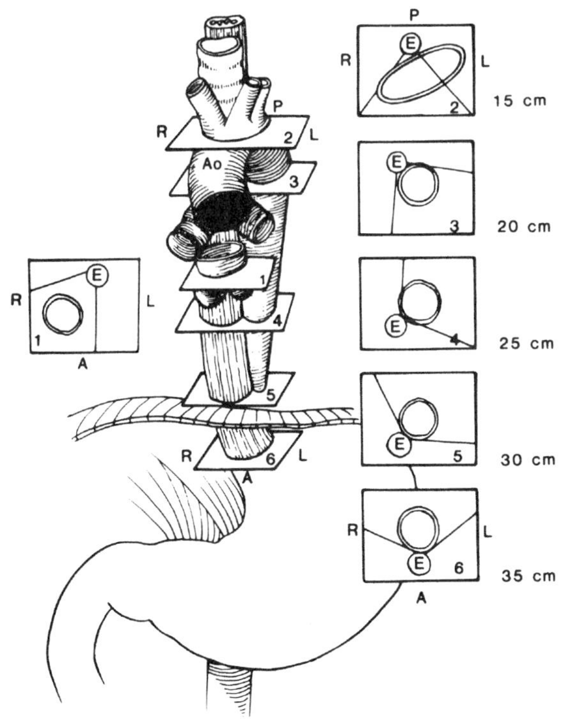

FIGURE 9-19. Relation of the esophagus and aorta at different levels of the esophagus.

CLINICAL APPLICATIONS

Monitoring

The monitoring indications for IOE include assessment of myocardial performance and hemodynamics, recognition of myocardial ischemia, and detection of unsuspected myocardial air. In addition to heart rhythm and rate, the major determinants of myocardial performance include preload, diastolic function, contractility, afterload, valvular function, and pericardial function. Although there are other methods of monitoring cardiac function intraoperatively, (Table 9-12), TEE provides a more direct physiologic method of assessing each of these parameters.

Preload

Intraoperatively, preload has been indirectly assessed using either the PA catheter (PAOP, PAEDP) or LA catheter (LA pressure [LAP]) for inferring LA and LV volume. As illus-

TABLE 9-12. TEE PROVIDES A MORE DIRECT PHYSIOLOGIC ASSESSMENT OF EACH OF THE DETERMINANTS OF CARDIAC FUNCTION

Determinant	PA catheter	TEE
Preload	Indirect pressures	Direct volume assessment
Diastolic function	Indirect PAOP	Inflow patterns
Afterload	SVR	Wall stress
Contractility	Cardiac output	Cardiac output elastance (ESPVR)
Valvular function	Indirect CV waves	Diagnostic and severity assessment
Pericardial function	Pressure tracing	Direct visualization inflow patterns

Note: PA, pulmonary artery; TEE, transesophageal echocardiography.

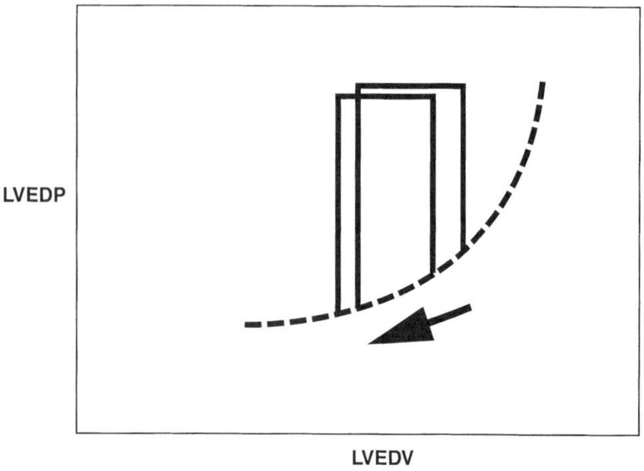

FIGURE 9-20. Physiologically, preload is not a pressure but a volume.

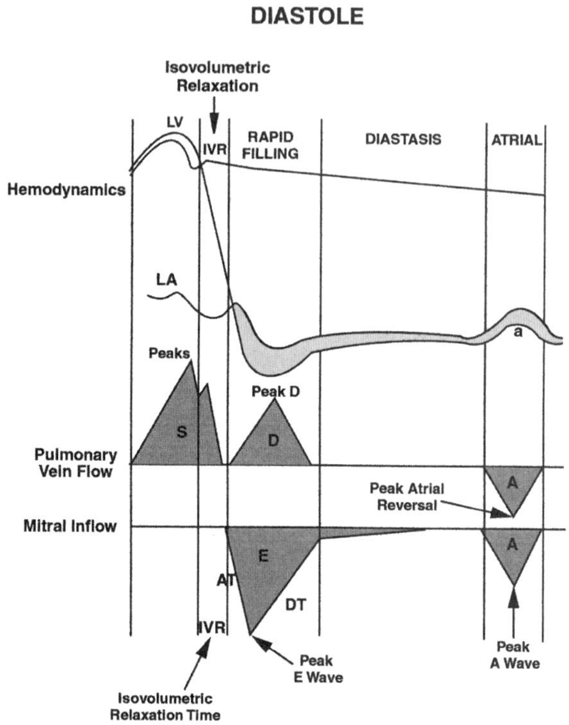

FIGURE 9-21. Diastole consists of four distinct phases. The relation of left atria and ventricular hemodynamic pressures are shown in relation to pulsed waved Doppler interrogation of the pulmonary veins and mitral inflow.

trated in Fig. 9-20, however, physiologically, preload is not a pressure but a volume. Depending on the compliance of the ventricular chamber, the preload may or may not accurately reflect the volume of the LV. Clements et al. (22) reported on 14 patients undergoing surgery for abdominal aortic aneurysms in which TEE, PA catheterization, and portable radionuclide measurements of end-diastolic volume (EDV) were simultaneously determined. There was a very close correlation between the TEE (end-diastolic diameter [EDD] and end-diastolic area[EDA]) and the accepted gold standard of radionuclide measurement of EDV. Interestingly, there was no correlation between PA catheter and the ultrasound or nuclear methods of preload assessment. Standard criteria for diagnosing hypovolemia include an EDD of less than 25 mm, systolic obliteration of the LV cavity, and an LV EDA of less than 55 cm^2.

Diastolic Function

In addition to the intravascular volume, the filling of the LV is determined by the intrinsic compliance and relaxation of the LV. Adequate filling of the LV during diastole is essential for normal systolic function. The determinants of normal diastolic function include not only the MV area but also the atrioventricular pressure gradient, ventricular relaxation and compliance, end-systolic volume (ESV), and the presence of atrial contraction. Diastole may be divided into four distinct phases (Fig. 9-21): (a) isovolumetric relaxation, (b rapid ventricular filling, (c) diastasis, and (d) atrial contraction. Upon opening of the MV after isovolumetric relaxation, there is a rush of blood, which has been accumulating in the LA during systole, into the LV. This early filling is referred to as the rapid filling phase, which is followed by a slower filling period (diastasis) and eventually the atrial contraction. Using PW Doppler, one can evaluate each of these phases. Evaluation of the LV diastolic function is best performed by measuring the mitral inflow velocity profile using PW Doppler at the level of the tips of the open MV leaflets. The early (E wave) and atrial (A wave) filling velocities are easily identified in the spectral envelope (Fig. 9-21). Normally, the atrial contraction contributes 15% to 20% of the LV preload before the onset of ventricular systole. Interrogation of the pulmonary veins with PW Doppler demonstrates reversal of flow during atrial contraction (PV_A wave), systolic (PV_S wave), and diastolic (PV_D wave) flow. Under normal circumstances, pulmonary vein flow is greater in systole than diastole (Fig. 9-21). Measurements that characterize the four phases of diastole are demonstrated in Table 9-13 and include (a) isovolumetric relaxation time or period between AV closure and MV opening, (b) peak E-wave and A-wave velocities, (c) E wave deceleration time (DT) from peak or (d) mean E- (TVI_E) or A- (TVI_A) wave velocities and (e) ratio of E- and A-wave velocities (E:A ratio), and (f) ratio of pulmonary (A_P) and mitral (A_M) A-wave duration. Recording the effects of volume loading or induced hypovolemia (nitrates or Valsalva maneuver) will also assist in distinguishing some patterns of diastolic dysfunction from one another. More recently, the use of Doppler tissue imaging ratio of the E-wave and A-wave mitral annular motion (E'_{MA}:A'_{MA}) has also been used to distinguish these patterns.

Diastolic dysfunction is defined as a condition in which filling of the LV is impeded, resulting in symptoms of low cardiac output, elevated LV filling pressures, or both. In the

TABLE 9-13. DISTINGUISHING THE PATTERNS OF DIASTOLIC DYSFUNCTION

Parameter	Normal Filling	Impaired Filling Stage I	Pseudonormal Filling Stage 2	Restrictive Filling Stages 3 & 4
E wave DT	160–240 msec	>240 msec	160–200 msec	<160 msec
IVRT	70–90 msec	>90 msec	<90 msec	<70 msec
E:A	1–2	<1	1–1.5	>1.5
A_M:A_P duration	$A_M \geq A_P$	$A_M > A_P$	$A_M < A_P$	$A_M \ll A_P$
PV_S:PV_D	$PV_S > PV_D$	$PV_S \gg PV_D$	$PV_S < PV_D$	$PV_S \ll PV_D$
$V_{E'MA}$:$V_{A'MA}$	$V_{E'MA} > V_{A'MA}$	$V_{E'MA} < V_{A'MA}$	$V_{E'MA} < V_{A'MA}$	$V_{E'MA} < V_{A'MA}$
Valsalva E:A	Decreased	Decreased	Reversal <1	Decreased
Volume loading A_M:A_P duration	—	$A_M < A_P$	$A_M \ll A_P$	$A_M <<< A_P$

intraoperative setting, diastolic dysfunction has heretofore been indirectly inferred by the correlation of increasing cardiac output with the addition of quantities of intravascular volume despite apparently normal or elevated PA catheter filling pressures. Echocardiographic techniques not only demonstrate that there may be diminished preload in the setting of elevated filling pressures but also permit the physiologic characterization of the diastolic dysfunction. There are four distinct physiologic stages of diastolic dysfunction (Fig. 9-22): (a) abnormal relaxation, (b) restrictive physiology (reversible), (c) a combined abnormal relaxation and restriction, and (d) irreversible restrictive physiology (23). Diastolic dysfunction may be detected either as a new abnormality (abnormal relaxation) or as a chronic progression from abnormal relaxation to a restrictive physiology (24).

Abnormal relaxation (*stage 1* diastolic dysfunction) is typically the initial pattern of diastolic dysfunction in a number of cardiac diseases including acute ischemia, LV hypertrophy, and hypertrophic cardiomyopathy. The criteria for its diagnosis are listed in Table 9-13 and include a prolonged E-wave deceleration time, an E:A ratio of less than 1.0, a $PV_S >> PV_D$ wave, and an A_M duration more than A_P duration. This pattern may be demonstrated intraoperatively with the onset of acute myocardial ischemia, utilization of inhalation anesthetics, and prolonged CPB.

The restrictive filling pattern (reversible) of diastolic dysfunction (*stage 3* physiology) must be clearly distinguished from the term restrictive cardiomyopathy. This pattern may occur in any cardiac disease process that results in a reduction of LV compliance and elevation of LAPs. Such disease processes would include advanced ischemic heart disease, uncompensated congestive failure, or restrictive cardiomyopathy. The diagnostic criteria (Table 9-13) include a D_T of less than 150 msec, $PV_S << PV_D$, A_M duration << A_P duration, and an E:A ratio of more than 1.5. The E:A ratio decreases with reduction of preload or positive pressure ventilation. With the administration of nitrates, diuretics, or positive pressure ventilation, stage 3 physiologic pattern of dysfunction reverts to stage 1 dysfunction.

Stage 2 diastolic dysfunction is a combined pattern of *abnormal relaxation* and *restrictive physiology* (Table 9-13). Such dysfunction occurs as the disease process associated with abnormal relaxation further deteriorates, causing increased LAPs. The increased LAP permits compensation for abnormal relaxation with a normalization of the mitral inflow E and A wave. This pattern, however, may be distinguished from the normal pattern by Doppler-derived indexes of elevated LAP including a $PV_S << PV_D$ wave, an increased PV_A velocity and an A_M duration << A_P duration. Stage 2 diastolic dysfunction is associated with end-stage cardiac disease. It has similar Doppler-derived indexes of diastolic dysfunction as those of stage 3; however, preload reduction does not revert to the pattern of pseudonormal

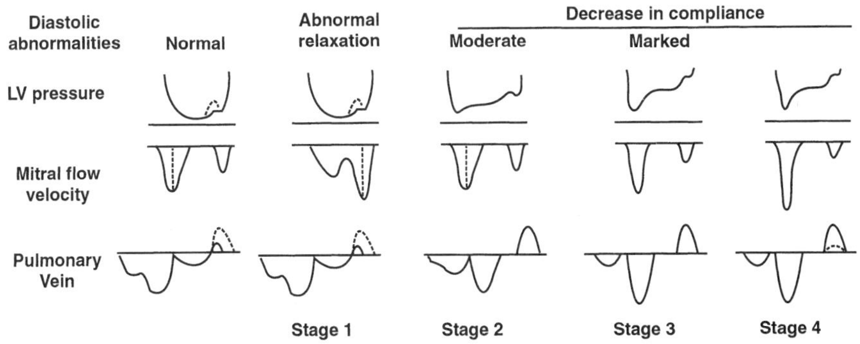

FIGURE 9-22. Patterns of diastolic dysfunction.

dysfunction with nitrate administration or the Valsalva maneuver.

Systolic Function

Assessment of systolic function is an essential feature of IOE and includes global LV and RV function, the hemodynamic assessment of Doppler-derived indexes of systolic function, and the detection of sudden changes in regional or segmental myocardial function. Visual estimations of global LV function have been employed since the initial experience with TEE in the intraoperative setting. Although controversy exists regarding the capability to "eye" acute and subtle changes in systolic performance, it is clear that detection of more substantial alterations in function lie within the capabilities of trained echocardiographers. The LV may be assessed using the ME four- or two-chamber views or the TG mid-SAX or LAX views (Fig. 8-14A, B, D, and E). The LV wall thickness is also best measured in this imaging plane with normal end-diastolic wall thickness less than 12 mm.

The percentage of 2D area change between end-diastole (measure at the ECG R-wave) and end-systole is estimated. Global LV function may be classified as normal (estimated ejection fraction [EF] of more than 50%), mild global LV dysfunction (estimated EF 30% to 50%), moderate global LV dysfunction (estimated EF more than 15% to 30%), and severe global LV dysfunction (estimated EF less than 15%).

The most frequently employed quantitative estimations of global LV are the fractional shortening, fractional area of change (FAC), EF, and cardiac output. The measurement of fractional shortening represents the percentage change in the LV diameter during systole as measured from the ME four- or two-chamber images. It is calculated by dividing the difference between the LVEDD (normally less than 55 mm) and the LV end-systolic diameter (LVESD) by the LVEDD:

$$\text{fractional shortening} = \text{LVEDD} - \text{LVESD/LVEDD}$$

A value greater than 30% is considered normal. Capturing a cine loop of the LV in the ME four-chamber view and tracing the end-systolic area (ESA) and EDA provides a means of assessing manually the FAC.

$$\text{FAC} = \text{EDA} - \text{ESA/EDA}$$

More recently, the ability to distinguish blood and tissue, using automated backscatter analysis, in these imaging planes has been incorporated into on-line measurements of the FAC. EF measurements represent the stroke volume as a percentage of the EDV.

$$\text{EF} = \text{EDV} - \text{ESV/EDV}$$

If there are no regional wall motional abnormalities, simple LV diameters, measured at the mid-PM level, may be used to estimate EF.

$$\text{EF} = \text{EDD}^2 - \text{ESD}^2/\text{EDD}^2$$

The volumes may be calculated using the modified Simpson method, whereby the length of the LV cavity and diameter of individual discs are used to calculate and summate the volume in each of a series of discs comprising the LV cavity. With the newer ultrasound platforms, these measurements may be determined on-line (using the automated backscatter technique described earlier) or off-line. The LVEDV and LVESV are determined automatically and the EF is calculated as in the formula expressed above. A measured EF of more than 50% is considered normal.

RV function similarly may be assessed by visual estimates of the RV size and EF (ME four-chamber or two-chamber RV inflow-outflow views) or calculating the RV FAC. Because the RV is a crescent-shaped chamber, simple formulas, such as the Simpson method used for the LV, are not as accurate. If the mid-cavity internal diastolic diameter of the RV is more than 35 mm, there is some degree of RV dysfunction. With RV dysfunction, there is a dilated tricuspid annulus with associated TR. A tricuspid annulus larger than 30 mm is dilated. If there is RV pressure overload, the LV septum is flattened, giving a D-shaped appearance in systole and diastole. The RV FAC is also a useful method of assessing global RV function. The RV FAC is the difference in the ESAs and EDAs of the RV in this view divided by the EDA and is normally more than 30%. In the absence of >1+ TR, this has been shown to correlate fairly well with the RV EF as measured by the RV EF thermodilution catheter (19).

Hemodynamic Assessment of Systolic Function

The two most commonly employed methods of assessing hemodynamic systolic function of the LV are (a) cardiac output determinations from volumetric flow calculations and (b) Doppler-derived indexes of contractility (LV dP/dt). It must be remembered that with the exception of calculating the end-systolic pressure volume elastance relation, all methods of contractility assessment are dependent on the LV loading conditions. Volume loading, systemic afterload reduction, or the presence of mitral regurgitation (MR) may enhance the overall appearance of LV systolic performance.

Volumetric Cardiac Output Calculation

Volumetric flow calculations are based on the principle that flow through a fixed orifice is equal to the product of cross-sectional area and the velocity time integral (or stroke-volume distance). If we think of the stroke volume as a cylinder, the cross-sectional area of the base is the orifice area and the cylinder height is the velocity time integral (VTI). Utilizing the TG midventricular LAX view, the PW cursor is placed parallel to the LVOT and AV. With PW interrogation at the level of the AV annulus where the diameter measurement for the area calculation is taken. All ultrasound platforms have calculation packages for determining the VTI by tracing the "modal" envelope or average outer intensity recording.

$$\text{stroke volume} = (\pi r^2_{AV}) \times (VTI_{AV})$$

or

$$\text{stroke volume} = d^2 \times 0.785 \times (VTI_{AV})$$
$$\text{cardiac output} = \text{stroke volume} \times \text{heart rate}$$

The pulmonic outflow, from the UE aortic arch SAX, may also be used for cardiac output determination. For all volumetric calculations, there are assumptions that must be met to ensure accuracy: (a) The interrogation angle must be <20°, (b) flow is nonturbulent with a homogenous flow profile, and (c) the orifice being interrogated has no valvular regurgitation.

Systolic Index of Contractility (dP/dt)

Using CW Doppler interrogation of a mitral regurgitant jet, the dP/dt may be determined (See Color Fig. 9-23, between pages 560 and 561). Because the systolic pressure difference between the LV and the LA is approximately 100 mm HG, the peak instantaneous velocity is expressed by the simplified Bernoulli equation (100 mm Hg = 4 V^2). Therefore the peak velocity squared = 25 or 5 m/second. If we know the time interval between the time at which the envelope velocity is 1 m/second (representing an LV-LA gradient of 4 V^2 or 4 mm Hg) and when the velocity is 3 m/second (representing an LV-LA pressure gradient of 4 V^2 or 4 × 3 × 3 = 36 mm Hg). We can calculate the dP/dt as follows: dP/dt = 36 mm Hg − 4 mm Hg / time interval. If the time interval is 0.45 seconds, the dP/dt = 32 mm Hg / 0.45 seconds = 800 mm Hg per second. A dP/dt of more than 800 mm Hg per second is considered normal (25). Similar calculations may be applied to the RV tricuspid regurgitant jet. Due to the smaller muscle mass of the RV, a dP/dt valve more than 250 mm Hg per second is considered to be indicative of normal RV contractility (19).

Afterload

Systolic wall stress may be calculated using a combination of ultrasound-determined measurements in combination with blood pressure measurements. The formula for wall stress represents the Laplace equation, which expresses the direct proportionality between stress and systolic blood pressure and the LVEDD and the inverse relation to the LV wall thickness. This is expressed in the equation

$$\text{wall stress} = 1.33 \times \text{systolic blood pressure} \times \text{LVEDD/4WTh/LVEDD}$$

Two simplifications of this formula are

$$\text{wall stress} = (P) \times (\text{LVEDD})/(\text{WTh})$$
$$\text{relative wall thickness} = 2 \times (P)\ (\text{WTh})/(\text{LVEDD})$$

where P equals systolic pressure and WTh equals wall thickness.

Wall stress calculations, although conceptually of interest, have not demonstrated a clinical usefulness to date.

Myocardial Ischemia

One of the first uses of IOE involved the detection of new or worsening segmental wall motion abnormalities that may be indicative of ischemia. IOE provides a sensitive method for detecting ischemia. Previous studies have demonstrated the sequence of events after a reduction of coronary blood flow to regions of the heart (26,27). Almost immediately, there is a reduction of active thickening of the myocardium followed by a reduction of regional compliance and diastolic relaxation. After 3 to 5 minutes, ECG evidence of ischemia may develop. It is only after prolonged myocardial ischemia that global dysfunction, detected by reductions in thermodilution cardiac output or elevated filling pressures, becomes apparent. Transient periods of ischemia, which are reversed, may not impact systolic function. However, there is clearly an increased stiffness of the LV resulting in higher filling pressures despite reduced LV volume. This diastolic dysfunction may persist for more than 48 hours. There are, however, limitations to the echocardiographic detection of ischemia. Segmental wall motion abnormalities may be related to sudden alterations in afterload, image foreshortening, or tethering to adjacent regions of abnormal myocardium. IOE provides a very sensitive indicator of acute ischemia, although one that may not be as specific as other monitors. Given the potential catastrophic consequences of not recognizing active ischemia, having a more sensitive indicator of regional ischemia is of value in an increasingly higher risk cardiac surgery population. As illustrated in Fig. 9-6A and B, the 16 segments of the LV may be evaluated for segmental wall motion and correlated with their corresponding coronary artery perfusion bed in five imaging views (ME two and four chamber, ME LAX, as well as the TG SAX (base, mid, and apex) and two chamber. The segmental wall motion is characterized by its thickening throughout systole and is graded as (a) normal, with more than 30% thickening, (b) mild hypokinesia, with 10% to 20% thickening, (c) severely hypokinetic, with less than 10% thickening, (d) akinetic, with no thickening, and (e) dyskinetic, with paradoxical systolic bulging.

Valvular Function

Using the PA catheter, valvular dysfunction is inferred by the presence of combined "*cv*" waves suggestive of MR or

TR. In contrast, using CF Doppler, IOE provides not only a direct method of assessing the presence of valve dysfunction but also a way of directly assessing its physiologic severity and mechanism. In addition, the 2D IOE may demonstrate pathologic features that may assist in the surgical decision-making process. Monitoring valve function intraoperatively usually involves evaluating the presence of AR while on bypass to determine the necessity of a LV vent to prevent overdistension.

Hemodynamic Assessment

In addition to volumetric methods of rapidly assessing changes in cardiac output, IOE enables the calculation of other indexes of myocardial performance including shunt fraction calculations, the hemodynamic assessment of the severity of valve dysfunction (discussed under Diagnostic Applications in valvular disease), and the noninvasive estimation of intracardiac pressures.

Shunt Flows and Ratio

In patients who have left-to-right shunts involving interatrial or interventricular septal defects, PW Doppler may be used to separately calculate right-sided and systemic stroke volume. Using the UE aortic SAX view, a PW Doppler interrogation cursor is placed (the exact site of determination PA diameter measurement) parallel to the main PA flow. Using the deep TG or TG longitudinal imaging views, PW Doppler of the LVOT is used to determine the systemic stroke volume, as discussed already. The ratio of the pulmonary flow (Q_p) to the systemic flow (Q_s) provides an index of the magnitude of the shunt severity and has been demonstrated to closely correlate with those measured invasively ($r = 0.92$) (31). A Q_p to Q_s ratio of more than 1.5 is considered to be clinically significant especially when associated with evidence of pulmonary hypertension, RV volume overload, or systemic hypoperfusion.

Intracardiac Pressure Estimation

The simplified Bernoulli equation states that the instantaneous pressure gradient between two chambers is related to the relation expressed as:

$$\text{gradient (mm Hg)} = 4 \times V^2 \text{ (m/second)} + \text{mean pressure (lower pressure chamber)}$$

Therefore the gradient between a higher pressured chamber and a lower (P1 − P2) = 4 V^2 (velocity of a regurgitant jet). Using this principle, a number of intracardiac pressures may be determined, as illustrated in Table 9-14.

Central Venous Pressure

The central venous pressure (CVP) may be estimated on the basis of respiratory variation of the inferior vena cava

TABLE 9-14. ESTIMATION OF INTRACARDIAC PRESSURES

Pressure Estimated	Required Measurement	Formula	Normal Valves (mm Hg)
Estimated CVP	Respiratory IVC collapse	≥40% = 5 mm Hg <40%, (nl RV) = 10 mm Hg 0% & RV Dysfx = 15 mm Hg	5–10
RVSP	Peak velocity$_{TR}$ CVP or measured	RVSP = $4(V_{TR})^2$ + CVP (no PS)	16–30
RV systolic (with VSD)	Systemic systolic BP Peak velocity$_{LV\text{-}RV}$	RVSP = SBP − $4(V_{LV\text{-}RV})^2$ (no LVOT obstruction)	With VSD usually >50
PASP	Peak velocity$_{TR}$ CVP* or measured	PASP = $4(V_{TR})^2$ + CVP (no PS)	16–30
PAD pressure	End-diastolic velocity$_{PR}$ CVP* or measured	PAEDP = $4(V_{PR\ ED})^2$ + CVP	0–8
PAM	AT to peak V_{PA}	PAM = (−0.45) AT + 79	10–16
RV dP/dt	TR spectral envelope $T_{TR(2\ m/sec)} - T_{TR(1\ m/sec)}$	RV dP = $4V^2$ TR(2 m/sec) − $4V^2$ TR(2 m/sec) RV dP/dt = dP/$T_{TR(2\ m/sec)}$ − T TR(1 m/sec)	>150 mm Hg/msec
LASP	Peak V_{MR} SBP	LASP = SBP − $4(V_{MR})^2$ (no LVOT gradient)	100–140
LA (PFO)	Velocity$_{PFO}$ CVP* or measured	LAP = $4(V_{PFO})^2$ + CVP	3–15
LV diastolic (LVEDP)	End-diastolic velocity$_{AR}$ DBP	LVEDP = DBP − $4(V_{AR})^2$	3–12
LV dP/dt	MR spectral envelope $T_{MR(2\ m/sec)} - T_{MR(1\ m/sec)}$	LV dP = $4V^2_{TR(2\ m/sec)} - 4V^2_{TR(2\ m/sec)}$ LV dP/dt = dP/$T_{MR(2\ m/sec)} - T_{MR(1\ m/sec)}$	>800 mm Hg/msec

Note: CVP, central venous pressure; IVC, inferior vena cava; RVSP, right ventricular systolic pressure; RV, right ventricle; VSD, ventricular septal defect; PASP, pulmonary artery systolic pressure; PAD, pulmonary artery diastolic; PAM, pulmonary artery mean; BP, blood pressure; AT, acceleration time; SBP, systolic blood pressure; V, velocity; LASP, left atrial systolic pressure; LVEOP, left ventricular end diastolic pressure; DBP, diastolic blood pressure.

or hepatic veins. If there is greater than a 40% in the inferior vena cava diameter with spontaneous inspiration or controlled expiration, then the CVP is approximately 5 mm Hg. If the reduction is less than 40 %, the CVP is estimated to be 10 mm Hg. If there is no respiratory variation in the inferior vena cava diameter in the presence of RV dysfunction, the CVP is 15 mm Hg or greater.

Right Ventricular and Pulmonic Valve Systolic Pressure

The RV systolic pressure (RVSP) or PA systolic pressure (PASP) is equal to the systolic gradient between the RA and RV plus the CVP. Consequently, if the peak TR velocity (V_{TR}) is 4.0 m/second and the CVP is 15 mm Hg, the RV or PASP is 4 (peak V_{TR})^2, therefore, RVSP or PASP is 4 (16 mm Hg) + 15 mm Hg = 79 mm Hg).

Pulmonary Artery Diastolic Pressure

The PA diastolic (PAD) pressure may be measured using the pulmonic regurgitant end-diastolic (PR ED) velocity. The end-diastolic gradient between the PA and RV is equal to $4 \times (\text{velocity}_{PR\ ED})^2 + \text{CVP}$. If the CVP is 10 mm Hg and the end-diastolic PR velocity is 1 m/second, then the PAD = 10 + 4 = 14 mm Hg.

$$\text{PA diastolic} = \text{CVP} + (\text{PA-RV gradient})$$
$$\text{PAD} = 4\,(V_{PR\ ED})^2 + \text{CVP}$$

RV Systolic Pressure in the Presence of Ventricular Septal Defect

In a patient with a ventricular septal defect (VSD), the RVSP is equal to the systemic/systolic blood pressure (SBP) minus the LV-RV gradient. The LV-RV gradient is estimated by the Bernoulli equation as equal to 4 (peak $V_{LV\text{-}RV}$). Therefore, if the systemic blood pressure is 140/65 and the peak VSD jet is 4 m/second then the RVSP is equal to 140 − (4 × 16) = 76 mm Hg.

$$\text{RVSP} = \text{systemic BP} - (\text{LV-RV gradient})$$
$$\text{LV-RV pressure gradient}$$
$$\text{gradient} = 4\,(\text{peak VSD jet velocity})^2$$
$$\text{systolic systemic BP} - (\text{LV-RV gradient})$$

Note: This equation assumes no LVOT obstruction or aortic stenosis.

LA Systolic Pressure

The LA pressure (LAP) (in systole, LASP) is equal to the systemic systolic BP minus the systolic gradient between the LV and the LA. If the systemic BP is 130 mm Hg and the peak MR velocity (V_{MR}) is 5 m/second, then the LAP = 130 mm Hg − (4 × 25 mm Hg) = 30 mm Hg.

$$\text{LASP} = \text{systolic BP} - (\text{LV-LA gradient})$$
$$\text{LASP} = \text{systolic BP} - 4\,(\text{peak MR velocity})^2$$

LV End-Diastolic Pressure

The LVEDP is equal to the diastolic BP (DBP) − (gradient between the aorta and LV). If the DBP = 80 mm Hg and the end-diastolic AR velocity ($V_{AR\ ED}$) = 4 m/second, then the LVEDP = 80 mm Hg − 4 (16 mm Hg) = 16 mm Hg

$$\text{LVEDP} = \text{diastolic BP} - 4\,(V_{AR\ ED})^2$$

DIAGNOSTIC APPLICATIONS

In addition to the development of techniques of myocardial protection during cardiac surgery, IOE has been one of the major advances in cardiac surgery during the last 15 years (28). It has permitted the surgical team to confirm their preoperative diagnosis and to screen for previously undetected cardiovascular abnormalities, and it has provided a safety net to ensure the optimal results for patients. In addition, it has hastened the development and understanding of newer surgical techniques including less invasive approaches to valve repair and surgical approaches to the management of end-stage heart failure. The major diagnostic applications of echocardiography involve its use in valvular heart surgery, congenital heart surgery, surgery for hypertrophic cardiomyopathy, myocardial revascularization, major vascular surgery, surgery for congestive heart failure, surgical treatment of pericardial disease, noncardiac surgery in patients with cardiac disease organ transplantation, and the perioperative evaluation of hemodynamic instability.

Valvular Disease

The physician involved in the IOE evaluation of valvular dysfunction should possess an understanding of the pathophysiology of the various etiologies of valvular disease and the associated anomalies. In addition to determining the severity of valvular dysfunction, it is necessary provide an assessment of the mechanism of the valvular lesion and the underlying pathologic process. To accomplish this, multiple views and methods of severity assessment are used so that the final diagnosis is based on multiple images or Doppler assessment modalities. Although the surgical team may be able to visualize anatomically the valvular abnormality, IOE provides a real-time assessment of the pathophysiology of valvular dysfunction.

Mitral Valve

Stenosis

Mitral stenosis most commonly results from long-standing rheumatic heart disease secondary to acute rheumatic fever. However, there are other potential causes of mitral stenosis including congenital, mitral annular calcification (extending into leaflets), parachute MV, obstructing masses (large atrial myxomas, thrombi), or endocarditis vegetations. Rarer causes of stenosis include valve abnormalities associated with inborn errors of metabolism, malignant carcinoid syndrome, systemic lupus, cardiac amyloid, and rheumatoid arthritis. The pathologic features of rheumatic valvular disease involving the MV include diffuse thickening, fibrosis, calcification of the valve leaflets, commissures, and subvalvular chordae. This results in thickened rigid valves, commissural fusion, and shortened fused chordae producing a fish-mouth–shaped valve with both valvular and subvalvular stenosis. In addition, rheumatic nodules are deposited in the myocardium (Aschoff bodies), which may produce underlying myocarditis. The mitral stenosis ultimately leads to elevated LAPs, PA hypertension, RV dysfunction, and TR (with or without rheumatic involvement). The chronic elevation of LAP may result in atrial enlargement, stagnant blood flow (detected as spontaneous contrast), and thrombus formation.

Methods for characterizing the severity of the valve stenosis are illustrated in Table 9-15 and include (a) 2D planimetry, (b) CW Doppler determination of mean valve gradient, and (c) calculation of the valve area (utilizing pressure half-time, deceleration time, or continuity equation), or (d) proximal isovelocity surface area (PISA). The mitral apparatus is evaluated first from the ME four-chamber image and may demonstrate the classic "hockey stick deformity" of the anterior MV leaflet and the restricted leaflet opening. The TG basal SAX view (Fig. 8-14F), which is aligned parallel to the valve annulus, may demonstrate the commissural fusion and restricted valve motion and opening. Capturing a digital image loop and freezing on the frame demonstrating maximal opening and electronically planimetering the valve area provides a reliable estimation of the true valve area (Fig. 9-24). There is a close correlation between valve area determined by planimetry and invasive catheterization using the Gorlin equation. Planimetry may underestimate the severity due to echogenic shielding from the presence of Ca^{2+} in the valve annulus and the subvalvular degree of flow obstruction. Doppler examination of the stenotic MV is performed by placing the interrogation cursor across the region of mitral blood flow, as directed by CF Doppler and using the CW mode due to the high-flow velocities and potential for aliasing. The resulting spectral envelope (See Color Fig. 9-25, between pages 560 and 561) demonstrates increased flow velocity across the valve upon opening, which corresponds to the increased valve gradient. It may also demonstrate a flattened E-to-F slope caused by the slower reduction in the gradient between the LA and LV caused

TABLE 9-15. MV STENOSIS SEVERITY ASSESSMENT

Left atrial size	LAE >45 mm AP diameter exclude LAA thrombi
Pulmonary artery pressure	$PASP = 4(V_{TR})^2 + CVP$*
	$PAM = (-0.45)\ AT + 79$
Planimeter valve area	Difficult with heavy Ca++, previous comissurotomy
Mean gradient	integrated area of $MV_{diastolic}$ spectral envelope
	With atrial fibrillation, average 5 consecutive diastoles
	Gradient α flow across MV and MVA, therefore severe MR produces larger than expected gradient
Continuity equation	$MVA = (D^2_{LVOT} \times 0.785)\ (TVI_{LVOT})/TVI_{MV}$
	No AR, LVOT obstruction, or MR
Deceleration time	$MVA = 759/DT$
	$PT_{1/2} = 0.29 \times DT$
	Altered by diastolic dysfunction
Pressure half-time	$MVA = 220/PT_{1/2}$
	Inaccurate with abnormal compliance (LA, LV), significant AR, or postvalvuloplasty (AR reduces $PT_{1/2}$ and overestimates valve area)
PISA	$MVA = 2\ \pi R^2 \times V_{Aliasing}/Peak\ V_{MS} \times \alpha°/180°$
	$V_{Aliasing}$ = aliasing velocity of color doppler
	R = radius from orifice to PISA interface
	Peak V_{MS} = peak CW diastolic Doppler velocity

Normal = 4–6 Cm²	Mild	Moderate	Severe
Planimetered Area	1.5–2.0 Cm²	1.0–1.5 cm²	≤0.9 Cm²
Mean $Gradient_{Diastolic}$	<6 mm Hg*	6–12 mm Hg*	>12 mm Hg*
Deceleration Time	<517 Msec	517–690 Msec	>759 Msec
Pressure Half-time	<150 Msec	150–200 Msec	>220 Msec

Note: Symptoms = gradient = MVA, if not, must explain (rest vs. exercise, other etiology). MV, mitral valve; PISA, proximal isovelocity surface area; PASP, pulmonary artery systolic pressure; PAM, pulmonary artery mean; CVP, central venous pressure; AT, acceleration time; LVOT, left ventricular outflow tract; DT, deceleration time.

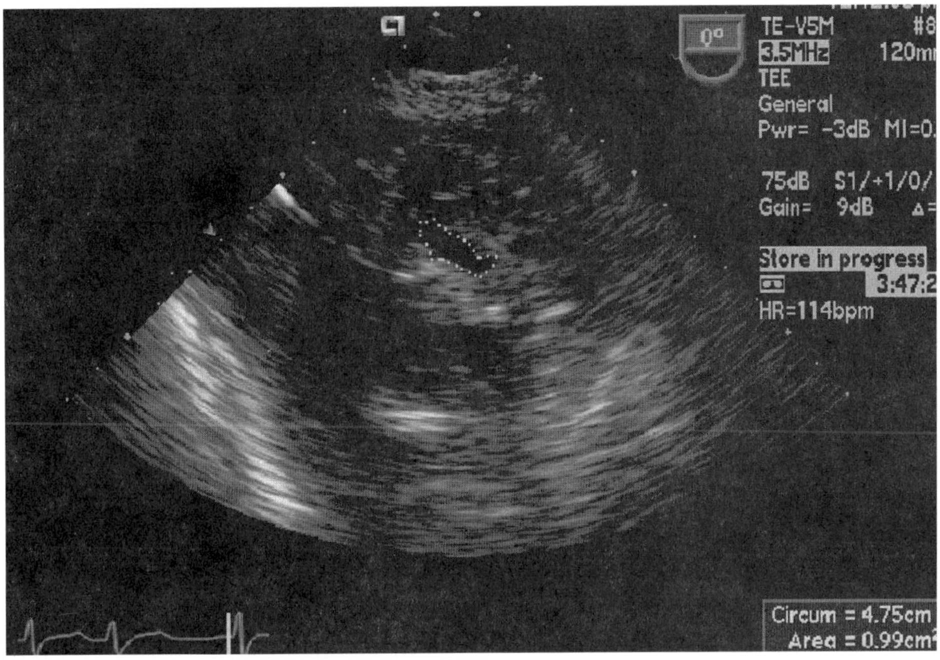

FIGURE 9-24. Planimetry of the mitral valve provides a reliable estimation of the true valve area.

by the restricted flow of valvular obstruction. This slowed gradient reduction is reflected in the calculation of the pressure half-time. The pressure half-time (PT½) is the time it takes for the initial peak instantaneous pressure gradient (4 × peak V^2) to drop by 50% (Fig. 9-26). It is measured by determining (a) the peak instantaneous gradient (using the simplified Bernoulli equation), where V is the initial peak instantaneous velocity and then (b) determining the time it requires for the gradient to drop by 50%. If the initial peak velocity is 2.5 m/second, then the corresponding gradient would be 25 mm Hg (4 V^2 or 4 × 2.52). The half-time pressure would be 12.5 mm Hg, which would equal 4 V^2 $PT_{1/2}$ (V^2 = 12.5/4 or V = 1.78 m/second.) The time it would take for the peak instantaneous velocity to decline to 1.78 m/second would be the $PT_{1/2}$. The MVA is calculated by the formula MVA = $K_{MV}/PT_{1/2}$, where the K_{MV} is equal to 220 based on relative diastolic properties of the LA and LV. Because severe mitral stenosis is classified as an MVA less than 1.0 cm^2, whenever $PT_{1/2}$ more than 220 milliseconds, there is severe mitral stenosis. A number of unique circumstances exist for this calculation, which may lead to miscalculation: (a) the presence of AR leads to a reduced $PT_{1/2}$ (more rapid equilibration of LA and LV pressures) and therefore leads to overestimation of MVA, (b) with aging, the compliance of the LV is diminished, and the LV diastolic pressure rises faster than in normal complaint ventricles, hence a shorter $PT_{1/2}$ with overestimation of MVA. The deceleration time, or time it takes the peak velocity to reach 0 m/second along the interpolated slope, may also be utilized to calculate the MVA. The relation is characterized by the formula MVA = 759 / DT. As illustrated in Fig. 9-27, $PT_{1/2}$ may be calculated from the DT ($PT_{1/2}$

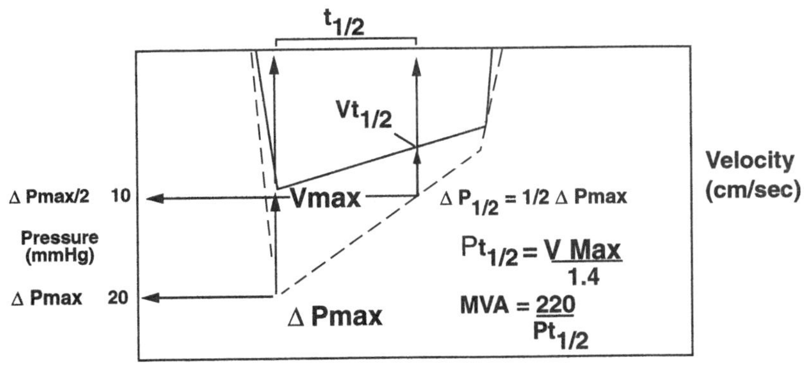

FIGURE 9-26. Calculation of mitral valve area using pressure half time method. The pressure half time ($PT_{1/2}$) represents the time it takes for the pressure gradient between the left atrium and left ventricle to decrease by 50%.

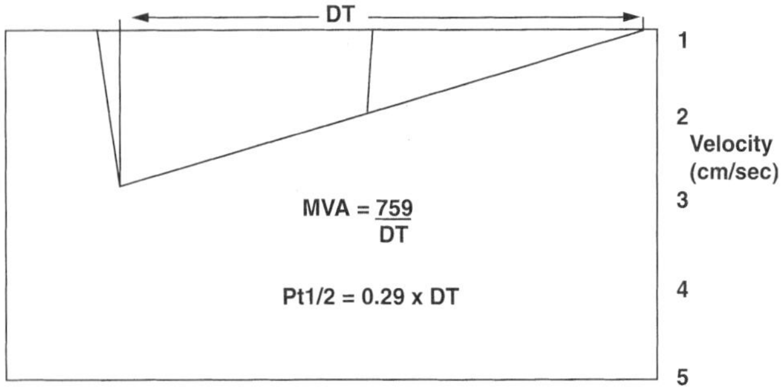

FIGURE 9-27. Mitral valve area may also be calculated using the deceleration time of the continuous wave interrogation of the mitral valve inflow.

= 0.29 × DT). Therefore, a DT of more than 760 milliseconds is also suggestive of severe stenosis. Another alternative for calculation of the MVA is by utilizing the *continuity equation.* The continuity states that the flow across one valve must equal the flow across another in the absence of regurgitation of either valve (28). Therefore,

$$\text{MV flow} = \text{LVOT flow}$$

therefore

$$MV_A \times TVI_{MV} = area_{LVOT} \times TVI_{LVOT}$$

therefore

$$MVA = (area_{LVOT}) \times (TVI_{LVOT})/TVI_{MV}$$

This technique involves obtaining the LVOT diameter (measured at the AV annulus), the PW Doppler VTI_{LVOT} and the CW Doppler VTI across the MV (29).

MVA may also be calculated using the proximal isovelocity surface area (PISA) method. Using the ME four-chamber view, CF Doppler interrogation of the MV stenotic jet is performed with the zero baseline shifted the upward to reduce the aliasing velocity away from the transducer. A digital looped is captured and the image is frozen in diastole to optimize the radius measurement of the first PISA interface zone. The atrial MV angle is then determined (30).

$$\text{MV flow rate} = \text{spherical area} \times \text{velocity}_{aliasing} \times (\text{angle}/180°) = 2\pi r^2 \times V_{aliasing} \times (\text{angle}/180°)$$

$$MVA = \text{flow rate/peak (CW Doppler)} V_{MS}$$

The TG two-chamber view is excellent for evaluating the severity of involvement of the subvalvular apparatus.

Mitral Regurgitation

Due to the reduced incidence of rheumatic MV disease in the United States and the increasing age of the patient population, MR has become the predominant valvular abnormality involving the MV. The more common causes of acute MR include myxomatous degeneration of the MV with associated chordal rupture, endocarditis, ischemic heart disease with PM rupture, and traumatic disruption of the MV apparatus. The chronic causes of MR include myxomatous degeneration of the MV, mitral annular calcification, rheumatic valve disease, endocarditis, global LV dysfunction, hypertrophic obstructive cardiomyopathy (HOCM), degenerative connective tissue disorders, and congenital abnormalities (cleft MV, parachute MV). Myxomatous degeneration of the MV results from the presence of excessive proteoglycans, which interfere with the production of normal elastin and collagen which is manifest as disorganized swirling of the collagen and elastic fibers. These changes make the support structures of the valve apparatus prone to disruption at the points of maximal stress where the primary chordae attach to the leaflet tips. The posterior leaflet is more commonly affected. MV prolapse is a common cause of MR and results from elongation of the chordal or PM structures. Some patients simply have a normal-size MV in a small heart and resulting mismatch.

Acute MR results in a sudden volume overload of the LV. Due to the increased preload, the LV may actually become hypercontractile (LV volume overload pattern) with much of the stroke volume proceeding into the more compliant LA during systole. However, in acute MR, both the LA and LV are not as compliant as in the chronic disease process, and patients rapidly develop pulmonary congestion, pulmonary hypertension, and eventually RV dysfunction with dilation and TR. In chronic MR, the LA has time to become more compliant, resulting in extremely large LA chamber sizes. Because the amount of regurgitant volume may be more than 50%, the forward stroke volume is diminished. Eventually the LV may fail with EDDs in excess of 70 mm. The patient may increasingly develop pulmonary hypertension and eventual right heart failure. During the IOE examination, it is important to determine the underlying pathologic process, the regurgitant mechanism, severity of MR, and the upstream impact of the MR. Mechanisms of MR include excessive leaflet motion (flail or prolapse), restricted leaflet motion (rheumatic disease, global LV dysfunction), and perforation. Methods of MR severity assessment (Table 9-16) include (a) spatial area mapping of the MR jet, (b) evaluation of the pulmonary venous flow pattern, (c) the volumetric calculation of the regurgitant volume or fraction, and (d) PISA determination of the regurgitant volume and orifice area (ROA) (30,32). Indirect methods of assessing the severity of MR include (a) LA size (more than 45 mm is severe), (b) peak *E* wave velocity (more than 1.5 m/second is severe), (c) denseness of the CW Doppler signal (denseness α severity), and (d) size of the LV at end-diastole, (LVEDD more than 70 mm is severe). *Spatial area mapping* is best accomplished utilizing the ME four- and two-chamber view of the MV using CF Doppler. Other imaging views such as the ME mitral commissural and LAX (Fig. 8-14C) may also provide important information regarding the size of the regurgitant jet. Spatial

TABLE 9-16. MITRAL VALVE REGURGITATION

Direct	
Regurgitant jet area	Severe >8 cm^2, Moderate MR (4–8 cm^2) Dependent on loading, eccentricity of jet, Coanda effect, PRF, gain settings, and depth
PW of pulmonary vein	Severe MR = Systolic Reversal of Flow Blunting of S wave indicates ↑ LAP only
Vena contracta width (narrowest Portion of MR jet)	if ≥0.5 cm^2 indicates severe MR
Volumetric regurgitant	Reg Fx = $Vol_{MR\ Reg}$/Stroke $Volume_{LVOT}$ Reg Fx = MV Flow − LVOT Flow/LVOT Flow × 100%
Fraction (Reg Fx)	$(A_{MV} \times TVI_{MV}) - (A_{LVOT} \times TVI_{LVOT})/(A_{LVOT} \times TVI_{LVOT})$ If ≥55% indicates severe
PISA	Flow Rate = $2\pi R^2 \times V_{Aliasing}$
Regurgitant orifice area (ROA)	ROA = Flow Rate/Peak V_{MR} ROA >0.40 cm^2 indicates severe MR
Regurgitant stroke volume (Reg SV)	ROA = Flow Rate/Peak V_{MR} Reg SV = $A_{ERO} \times TVI_{MR}$ Reg SV >60 cc indicates severe MR

Note:

$$\begin{aligned} \text{If } V_{Aliasing} &= \text{Color aliasing velocity} = 40 \text{ cm/sec (set)} \\ R &= \text{radius from orifice to PISA interface} \\ \text{Peak } V_{MR} &= 500 \text{ cm/sec (assuming } LV_{SP} - LA_{SP} = 100) \\ \text{Then ROA} &= 2\pi R^2 \times 40 \text{ cm/s}/500 \text{ cm/sec} \\ &= (6.28 R^2) \times 40 \text{ cm/sec}/500 \text{ cm/sec} = R^2\ 250/500 \\ &= R^2 \times \tfrac{1}{2} \end{aligned}$$

	Trivial MR <1+	Mild MR (1–2+)	Moderate MR (2–3)	Severe MR (3–4+)
MR jet area	0–0.5 cm^2	0.5–4 cm^2	4–8 cm^2	>8 cm^2
Vena contracta	0–0.1 cm	0.1–0.3 cm	>0.3–0.5 cm^2	>0.5 cm^2
Reg fraction	10% <	10%–24%	25–55%	>55%
Reg SV	<30 cc	30–44 cc	45–60 cc	>60 cc
ROA	<0.2 cm^2	0.20–0.29 cm^2	0.30–0.39 cm^2	0.4 cm^2
$R_{Aliasing}$ ($V_{Aliasing}$ = 40, V_{MR} = 5 m/sec)	<0.63	0.63–0.78	0.78–0.89 cm	>0.89 cm

Indirect	
CW spectral density	Density of spectral envelope
Mitral inflow velocity	E-wave velocity >1.5 m/sec suggests severe
LA & LV dimensions	LA >55 mm AP diameter or LVEDD >70 mm suggests severe
PA pressure	PASP = $4(V_{TR})^2$ + CVP*, PAM = (−0.45) AT + 79

area mapping closely correlates with the regurgitant severity determined at angiography. The absolute area of the regurgitant jet, (utilizing an aliasing velocity in the 40- to 50-m/second range) is highly predictive of the severity of MR. If the jet is eccentric, it may be directed into the LA wall giving the appearance of a smaller amount of MR. This is referred to as the *Coanda effect* and may lead to underestimation of MR (See Color Fig. 9-28, between pages 560 and 561). If the absolute jet area is more than 8 cm^2, there is severe regurgitation, whereas less than 4 cm^2 is considered mild. The measurement of percentage of the LA that the MR jet occupies is an inaccurate method due to the inability for IOE techniques to fully visualize the entire LA. Length of the jet is also an inaccurate method of determining the severity of MR due to variations in patient's LA sizes and compliances. Small but high velocity MR jet may penetrate further in the LA than a larger volume but lower velocity jet. The pulmonary veins may provide valuable information regarding the severity of MR (33). They may be interrogated by starting from the ME four-chamber image and turning the probe to the left and with drawing while visualizing with CF Doppler. Placing the cursor parallel to left upper PV flow into the LA at a PW depth of at least 2 cm into the pulmonary results in optimal spectral tracings. Normally most flow from the PV into the LA occurs during systolic. With increasing LAP, there is initial blunting of the S-wave velocity, followed by a systolic to diastolic ratio of less than 1 as the LAP increases further. As the systolic regurgitant jet increases, there is reversal of flow in the pulmonary veins during systole. It is important to understand that blunting of the systolic waves is more indicative of increased LAP than MR per se. Because increased LAP is associated with increasing MR, this association is usually consistent.

The mitral regurgitant fraction is expressed as the percentage of total stroke volume that regurgitates through the incompetent MV. To calculate the regurgitant fraction, one must determine the regurgitant volume and LVOT stroke volume, which requires time-velocity interval (TVI) of the mitral annular flow, the mitral annulus diameter, the aortic annulus diameter, and the TVI of the aortic annulus flow.

regurgitant fraction (%) =
regurgitant volume/aortic flow =
mitral flow − aortic flow/aortic flow

mitral flow = mitral stroke volume (cc) =
TVI_{MV} (cm) x CSA_{MV} (cm^2)

aortic flow = aortic stroke volume (cc) =
TVI_{AV} (cm) X CSA_{AV} (cm^2)

PISA may also be used to determine the severity of MR (See Color Fig. 9-29, between pages 560 and 561). As blood accelerates toward a regurgitant orifice, there are multiple concentric isovelocity hemispheres formed proximal to the regurgitant orifice. Based on the law of conservation of mass, all blood passing through these hemispheres must ultimately pass through the regurgitant orifice. Hence, the flow rate through any isovelocity hemisphere must equal the regurgitant flow rate at the valve. The regurgitant flow rate (Q) and the ROA may be determined using CF Doppler interrogation of the proximal flow convergent zone.

$$Q = 2\,\pi r^2 \times V_a$$

$$ROA = Q/\text{peak } V_{MR}$$

$$\text{regurgitant stroke volume} = ROA \times TVI_{MR}$$

Simplified PISA Method

There are two methods for simplifying PISA (30,34).

1. If we assume that the systolic pressure gradient between the LV and LA is 100 mm Hg (120 to 20 mm Hg), then we understand from the Bernoulli equation that the gradient 100 mm Hg equals 4 peak V^2; and therefore peak V equals 5 m/second.
   (a) aliasing velocity = 40 cm/second

   $$ROA = 2\,\pi r^2 \times V_a/V_P$$

   ROA =
   6.28 ×40 cm/second r^2 / 500 cm/second =
   251 r^2 / 500

   $$ROA = \tfrac{1}{2} r^2$$

   (b) aliasing velocity = 32 cm/second

Because any ROA of more than 0.40 cm^2 is severe MR, if VP is also assumed to be 500 cm/second, then the V_a must be 30 cm/second for the ROA to equal 0.4 cm^2.

$$V_a = 0.4\ cm^2 \times 500\ cm/second/6.28 \times r^2\ (1)$$

$$V_a = 200\ cm^3/second/6.28\ cm^2 = 32\ cm/second$$

Therefore, if the V_a is set at 30 cm/second and *r* is greater than 1 cm, the ROA is always more than 0.4 cm^2.

The antegrade velocity of the early E wave also provides a clue to the severity of MR. If this velocity exceeds 1.5 m/second, it suggests more severe regurgitant flow. It should be kept in mind that there are a number of factors that may affect the severity of MR; these include afterload, inotropic state, intravascular volume status, LA compliance, heart rate/rhythm, body temperature, and hemoglobin level. Each method of the MR severity assessment has its own disadvantages and inaccuracies. Consequently, care must be taken to always use multiple imaging planes for spatial area mapping and compare such results with the other methods of severity assessment. When the regurgitant severity is graded at 1 to 2+ or 2 to 3+, it is incumbent upon the intraoperative team to assess the severity by using all the methods of severity assessment in reaching a final decision. The question often arises regarding data that conflict with the preoperative echocardiographic assessment. Under such circumstances, attempts are made to duplicate the patient's "hemodynamic clinical state" before administration of the anesthetic and hemodynamic optimization. If an incongruity persists with the preoperative clinical evaluation results, alternative explanations for the patient's clinical course should be vigorously pursued during the comprehensive IOE examination.

Aortic Valve

Aortic stenosis

Obstruction to flow across the AV may result from a number of different etiologies including congenital malformations, rheumatic fusion of the cusps, and degeneration of normal or congenitally bicuspid valves. Under the age of 70, a congenitally bicuspid AV is the most common etiology, whereas over the age of 70, calcific degeneration of a TV is the most common. The mechanisms of aortic stenosis include fibrosis and/or calcification of the normal or congenitally abnormal AV cusp with a resulting lack of normal excursion during systole. Systolic doming of the AV occurs in more advanced grades of stenosis in addition to a decrease in the maximal aortic cusp separation (Fig. 9-30). Methods of AS severity assessment include (a) 2D planimetry of the AV, (b) measurement of the maximal cusp separation using M mode, (c) mean AV gradient, (d) AV area calculation by the continuity equation, and (e) the "dimensionless index" or ratio of the TVI_{LVOT} and TVI_{AV} (Table 9-17). Using the ME AV SAX view (with close-in focus of the AV cross section), a digital loop may be stored and frozen in systole at maximal AV leaflet excursion to planimeter the valve area. An AV area less than 1.0 cm^2 is considered severe stenosis. In addition, *m* mode of the ME AV LAX view, which is parallel to the plane of the AV annulus, demonstrates systolic excursion of the right and left or noncoronary cusps. If this excursion is more than 10 mm, severe AS is unlikely. CW interrogation of the AV, using either the TG LAX or deep TG LAX (Figs. 8-14J and 8-14K), results in a spectral envelope of the LV outflow. The peak instanta-

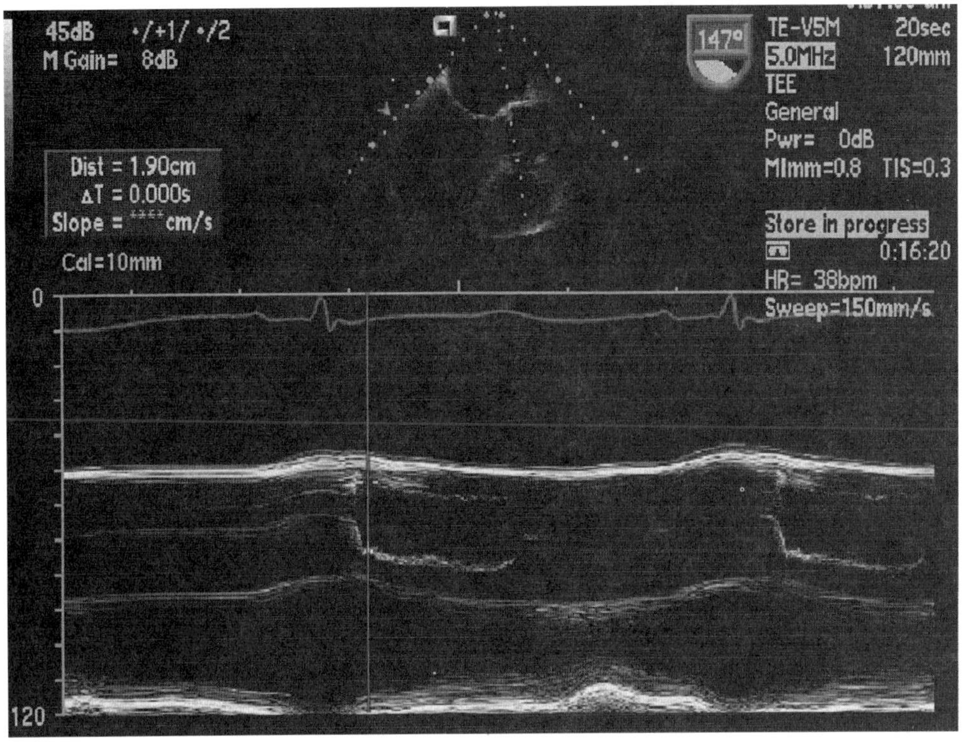

FIGURE 9-30. M-mode interrogation of the aortic valve demonstrating reduced maximum aortic cusp separation (MACS).

TABLE 9-17. AORTIC VALVE STENOSIS SEVERITY ASSESSMENT

Maximal cusp separation[a] (M-mode or 2D equivalent)	If < 10 mm, suggests restricted valve motion
Planimeter valve area[a]	Difficult with heavy Ca^{2+} <0.75 cm^2 indicates severe AS
Peak velocity[a]	Peak instantaneous velocity by CW >4.5 m/sec indicates severe AS
Mean gradient[a]	Integrated area of $AV_{Systolic}$ spectral envelope >50 mm HG, (with nl. CO and no AR), indicates severe AS Dependent on cardiac output (if reduced, dobutamine may assist) Even with AR, gradient >50 mm Hg suggestive of significant AS May underestimate gradient, cannot overestimate (except anemia, LVOT obstruction small aortic root)
TVI_{LVOT}/TVI_{AV} ratio	<0.25 indicates severe AS Avoids inaccuracies of LVOT measurement with Ca^{2+} annulus
Continuity equation	AV Area = $(D^2_{LVOT} \times 0.785)\ (TVI_{LVOT})/TVI_{AV}$ No AR, LVOT obstruction, or MR

Normal = 3 − 4 cm^2	Mild AS	Moderate AS	Severe AS
Planimetered area	2.0–1.5	1.5–0.75 cm^2	≤0.75 cm^2
Mean $gradient_{Diastolic}$	<20[a]	30–50[a]	>50 mmHg[a]
V peak	2.5<	2.5–4.5 msec	4.5 m/sec
TVI_{LVOT}/TVI_{AV}	<150 msec	150–200 msec	<0.25

Note: Clinical symptoms = AV area, which the gradient may or may not reflect. If gradient <30 mm Hg, AV area <1.3 with poor LVC function, dobutamine may clarify. LVOT, left ventricular outflow tract.

[a] Cardiac output or flow dependent.

neous gradient or mean AV gradient may be estimated by using the Bernoulli equation estimate of peak instantaneous gradient ($4V^2$) or by integrating the area of the CW systolic Doppler spectral profile. Using the continuity equation, the AV area (at the level of the orifice) may be calculated in a manner similar to that for the MV.

AV flow equals LVOT flow; therefore, $area_{AV}$ times TVI_{AV} equals $LVOT_A$ times TVI_{LVOT}; therefore, AVA equals ($LVOT_{area}$) × (VTI_{LVOT}) divided by VTI_{AV}.

Assumptions in using the continuity equation include that (a) the AV orifice is circular, (b) the angle of ζ is 0, (c) flow across the AV is laminar, and (d) there is no AR or MR. The correlation between AV area calculated by the continuity equation and that derived from the Gorlin formula at the time of cardiac catheterization demonstrates a close correlation ($r = 0.92$). It should be kept in mind that the peak instantaneous gradient determined by Doppler is different from the peak gradient derived at the time of cardiac catheterization. The latter is a nonphysiologic term obtained from subtracting the peak aortic pressure from the peak LV systolic pressure. Gradients obtained across the AV are dependent not only on the AV area, but the flow across the AV. Consequently, in patients with severe LV dysfunction and low cardiac output, the AV gradient may grossly underestimate the severity of stenosis. If there is shielding of the annulus due to severe calcification, the LVOT diameter measurement may be inaccurate. Resulting in a significant AV area error. In these circumstances, a dimensionless index ratio of the LVOT TVI and AV TVI may be used. A ratio less than 0.25 indicates severe AS.

Aortic Regurgitation

The etiology of AR may be classified according to four different mechanisms: (a) cusp abnormalities (congenitally bicuspid valve, bacterial endocarditis, rheumatic disease, rheumatoid disease), (b) aortic root distortion (associated with aortitis of ankylosing spondylitis, rheumatoid disease), (c) loss of commissural support (aortic dissection), and (d) aortic root dilation (syphilitic aortitis, Marfan syndrome, or Ehlers-Danlos syndrome). Cusp abnormalities from endocarditis may result in perforation of the AV cusp. Bicuspid AV most commonly involves fusion of the left and right coronary cusps. Frequently, this is associated with prolapse of the fused cusp with a posteriorly directed regurgitant jet. In myxomatous disease involving the AV, the redundant AV cusp may prolapse, resulting in a regurgitant jet directed away from the prolapsing cusp. With dilation of the aortic root, as seen in aortic inflammation, the cusp coaptation along the commissures is incomplete, resulting in AR. With dissection of the aorta, the architectural orientation of the AV orifice may be distorted with resulting regurgitation.

As illustrated in Table 9-18, AR severity may be assessed by five methods including (a) the size of the regurgitant jet or regurgitant orifice by CF Doppler, (b) determination of the pressure half-time or deceleration slope of the regurgitant jet by CW Doppler, (c) volumetric calculation of regurgitant volume or fraction, (d) reversal of diastolic flow in the descending aorta, and (e) calculation of the regurgitant orifice area using PISA (36). It should be kept in mind that the size of the regurgitant jet is dependent on a number of factors including aortoventricular pressure gradient, LV compliance, the Coanda effect (jet eccentricity along a tissue plane), and the AV lesion. Consequently, grading of regurgitation severity based on the depth or size of the regurgitant jet is the least accurate of the methods. From the longitudinal 2D view of the AV, CF interrogation will demonstrate a diastolic regurgitant jet. The diameter of this regurgitant jet in comparison to the diameter of the AV orifice or the LVOT can be used as a rough estimate of severity of regurgitation. If this value is more than 60%, the AR is considered severe. CW Doppler interrogation of the regurgitant jet demonstrates an initial peak gradient followed by a gradual deceleration toward the baseline (Fig. 9-31). The pressure half-time of this diastolic flow profile may be obtained and is equal to the time for the pressure gradient between the aorta and LV to drop by 50%. A pressure half-time of less than 250 milliseconds infers severe AR. The deceleration slope of the regurgitant jet is steeper in more severe AR because of the rapid gradient decay between the aorta and LV. A slope of greater than 3 m/second is consistent with severe AR. Utilizing PW Doppler interrogation of the descending thoracic aorta, the demonstration of holodiastolic reversal of flow is indicative of more severe AR. The regurgitant volume (Reg Vol) and fraction (Reg Fx) may be calculated using CW Doppler determination of transaortic and transmitral flow:

$$\text{Reg Vol} = \text{aortic flow} - \text{mitral flow} = (A_{Ao} \times VTI_{Ao}) - (A_{MV} \times VTI_{MV})$$

$$\text{Reg Fx} = \text{Reg Vol/aortic flow}$$

A regurgitant fraction of more than 40% to 50% implies more severe AR. PISA may also be used to quantify AR. Similar to the PISA technique described for MR, the radius of the proximal flow convergence aliasing sphere on the aortic side of the AV is measured. Regurgitant flow rate and orifice area may be calculated by the following relation, where V_{AR} is the peak velocity of AR jet:

$$\text{flow rate} = 2\pi r^2 \times V_{aliasing}$$

$$\text{ROA} = \text{flow rate/peak } V_{AR}$$

An ROA of AR of more than 0.3 cm^2 is indicative of severe AR. Indirect methods that suggest severe AR include an LVEDD of more than 75 mm, premature closure of the MV or diastolic MR, a dense CW AR spectral envelope, and a restrictive filling pattern by PW Doppler interrogation of the MV inflow.

Each of the techniques for evaluating the severity of AR

TABLE 9-18. AORTIC VALVE REGURGITATION SEVERITY ASSESSMENT

Direct	
$Area_{AR\ Jet}$: A_{LVOT}	Annular $Area_{AR\ Jet}/A_{LVOT}$ >60% indicates severe AR
$Diameter_{AR\ Jet}$: $Diameter_{LVOT}$	$D_{AR\ Jet}$: D_{LVOT} Eccentric jets may confound >60% indicates severe AR
AR CW pressure half-time	Time for Ao–LV pressure gradient to decrease 50% Reduced with greater AR PT1/2 <250 msec indicates severe AR
AR CW deceleration slope	Steeper slope with increasing AR Slope >3 m/sec^2 indicates severe AR
CW spectral envelope density	Increased with increasing AR
Diastolic retrograde flow	PW Doppler descending thoracic aorta
Descending thoracic aorta (Retro $Flow_{Desc\ Th\ Ao}$)	Holodiastolic or TVI >3 cm indicates severe
Regurgitant $volume_{AV}$ (RegV)	Reg V_{AV} = $Flow_{LVOT}$ − $Flow_{MV}$ $RegV_{AV} = (D^2_{LVOT} \times 0.785)\ TVI_{LVOT} - (D^2_{MV} \times 0.785)\ TVI_{MV}$ Cannot have MR >60 cc indicates severe AR
AV Reg $fraction_{AV}$	Reg $Fx_{AV} = RegV_{AV}/SV_{LVOT}$
PISA	Flow Rate = $2\pi R^2 \times V_{Aliasing}$
Regurgitant orifice area (ROA)	ROA = Flow Rate/Peak V_{AR} ROA >0.30 cm^2 indicates severe

	Trivial <1+)	Mild (1–2+)	Moderate (2–3)	Severe (3–4+)
AR Area Ratio	<10%	10–30%	30–60%	>60%
AR Diameter Ratio	<10%	10–30%	30–60%	>60%
AR Reg Vol	<30 cc	30–44 cc	45–60 cc	>60 cc
AR Reg Fraction	10%<	10–30%	30–55%	>55%
Retro $Flow_{Desc\ Th\ Ao}$	none	early diastolic	into mid diastole	holodiastolic
AR ROA	<0.1 cm^2	0.10–0.20 cm^2	0.2–0.3 cm^2	>0.3 cm^2
CW Signal	faint+	++	+++	++++dense
INDIRECT				
Color M-mode	Premature MV closure or diastolic MR or AV opening Diastolic Opening of AV			
Mitral inflow	Restrictive filling pattern (acute)			
LV dimensions	LVEDD >75 mm suggests severe			

Note: MV, mitral valve; LVOT, left ventricular outflow tract.

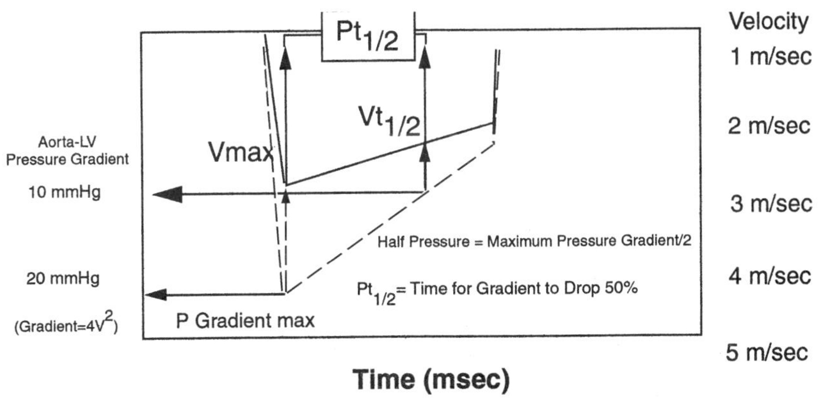

FIGURE 9-31. Pressure half-time ($Pt_{1/2}$) for severity of aortic regurgitation. Time for maximum aorta-LV gradient to decrease 50%.

has its own assumptions and inherent inaccuracies. Consequently, multiple techniques of assessing AR severity will result in a more accurate characterization of the hemodynamic pathophysiology.

Tricuspid Valve

Stenosis

Obstruction to blood flow into the RV results from either acquired (e.g., inflammatory disease, tumors, vegetations, or thrombi) or congenital deformities of the TV. Acquired TV stenosis is seen most frequently in patients with rheumatic heart disease but may occur in association with endocardial fibroelastosis, endomyocardial fibrosis, or malignant carcinoid. TV stenosis is characterized echocardiographically by thickened deformed TV leaflets, restriction of the diastolic leaflet motion, and an overall reduction in the orifice size. TS may be suspected in the presence of leaflet doming and the presence of turbulent flow across the TV during diastole. Using CW Doppler interrogation of the TV, gradients across the valve may be determined as for the MV. TV area may also be calculated by Doppler using the continuity equation or the pressure half-time method using the formula ($TVA = 190 / PT_{1/2}$). Due to differences in the diastolic properties of the RA and RV, the constant 190 is used for TVA calculation.

Tricuspid Regurgitation

Normal closure of the TV depends on the integrity of the TV complex. When there is dilation of the annulus or there is restriction of normal leaflet closure, regurgitation occurs. Most commonly TR occurs in the setting of RV dilation associated with an increase in annular diameter. TR may be classified as either acquired or congenital. Acquired causes include RV dysfunction, rheumatic valvular disease, myxomatous degeneration of the TV, endocarditis, carcinoid syndrome, or trauma. Congenital disorders involving the TV include the Epstein anomaly and incomplete cusp or chordal development that prevent normal closure. The diagnosis of TR is based on CF Doppler interrogation of the TV in the ME four- and two-chamber views of the RV. In the setting of tachycardia, color M mode may be used to distinguish retrograde systolic flow from the normal antegrade diastolic flow. CW Doppler interrogation of the tricuspid regurgitant jet may demonstrate peak velocities up to 5 m/second (depending on the right atrioventricular gradient). In the setting of pulmonary hypertension, this gradient is markedly increased. Assessment of the severity of TR is based on the relative jet size of the CF Doppler. PW Doppler interrogation of hepatic vein may demonstrate systolic reversal of flow which is indicative of severe TR.

Pulmonic Valve Dysfunction

Pulmonic Valve Stenosis

Obstruction to flow across the PV is either congenital or acquired. Congenital stenosis is more common and may either be bicuspid, unicuspid, tricuspid, or atretic. Commissural unicuspid PS is the most common form of congenital stenosis. Stenotic valves are characterized by systolic doming and varying degrees of cusp thickening and restriction. Acquired pulmonic stenosis (PS) is most commonly secondary to carcinoid disease but may also be associated with rheumatic heart disease or infective endocarditis. Valvular PS may also occur in association with complex congenital anomalies such as tetralogy of Fallot, double-outlet RV, complete atrial ventricular canal, or univentricular. IOE evaluation of PS uses the ME RV inflow-outflow (Fig. 8-14M), ME AV SAX (Fig. 8-14H), or UE aortic-arch SAX view (Fig. 8-14T). Systolic doming of the stenotic leaflets and abnormal systolic leaflet motion may be demonstrated. CF Doppler may demonstrate turbulent systolic flow in addition to the restricted leaflet motion. CW Doppler interrogation of the stenotic pulmonary valve demonstrates an increase in flow velocity.

Pulmonary Regurgitation

Causes of pulmonary regurgitation (PR) are congenital (bicuspid or quadricuspid) or acquired (secondary pulmonary hypertension), which is most commonly secondary to MV disease, LV dysfunction, or congenital defects resulting in increased PA flow. Other acquired causes include endocarditis, trauma, syphilis, carcinoid, and pulmonary valve prolapse. The IOE diagnosis of PR is best achieved using CF Doppler in the views discussed previously where a diastolic regurgitant jet may be demonstrated. Color M mode of the RV outflow tract may confirm PR in the setting of tachycardia.

Valvular Heart Surgery

The purposes of the IOE in patients undergoing valvular heart surgery are (a) to confirm the preoperative diagnosis, (b) to refine the pathoanatomy and mechanism of the valvular disorder, (c) to assess the secondary pathophysiology, (d) to evaluate the results of the valve repair or replacement surgery, and (e) to assess the postsurgical cardiac function.

Mitral Valve Surgery

Mitral Valve Repair

In the 1970s, the concept of valve repair was revolutionized when Carpentier et al. (39) introduced a physiologic classification detailing the anatomic changes in patients with MR. This provided the foundation of our current understanding of mechanisms of MR. Both Carpentier, in France, and Duran, in Spain, developed MV repair techniques to manage patients with rheumatic mitral disease (40,41). These procedures caught the attention of surgeons in the United States who foresaw potential benefits for an older patient population with MR as a result of myxomatous degeneration and ischemia (42). Over the course of the 20th century,

MV repair procedures have gone from surgical suggestion to surgical reality in more than 2,000 MV repair procedures performed annually in the United States alone (43). In comparison to MV replacement, repair offers the advantages of less perioperative morbidity and mortality, preservation of the mitral tensor apparatus with maintenance of ventricular function, freedom from need for anticoagulation, long-term durability, and freedom from reoperation (35). However, the surgical valve repair technique is more technically demanding. The development of improved myocardial protection during CPB and the technological advances of IOE have enhanced the development of repair techniques. Both TEE and EPE provide "real-time" information to the surgical team regarding the underlying valve structure and mechanism dysfunction as well as the pathologic process. Importantly, it serves as a safety net insuring the adequacy of repair. IOE has the added advantage of facilitating feedback to reduce the time of education for surgeons incorporating valve repair into their practice.

The IOE assessment of patients undergoing MV repair is separated into the pre-CPB and post-CPB assessment. The purpose of the pre-CPB study is to refine the preoperative diagnosis with regard to (a) dysfunction severity, (b) specific location and mechanism of the pathoanatomy, (c) underlying RV and LV function, and (d) physiologic sequelae secondary to the primary valve abnormality (including LA thrombi, pulmonary hypertension, PV or TV dysfunction, and hepatic venous congestion.) The post-CPB study assesses the success of the repair procedure, ventricular function, and the associated complications (44). In MV repair, IOE is used to characterize the mechanism and severity of valve dysfunction through a segment by segment analysis of the MV pathoanatomy. The use of IOE to systematically guide the mitral repair procedure was first reported by Stewart et al. (45) in 1992. In this study, 286 patients were prospectively studied with either monoplane TEE (235) or EPE echocardiography (45) with an overall accuracy of diagnosis of the mechanism and pathology of MR in 85% of patients. This accuracy varied according to the mechanism and etiology (from 94% for anterior or posterior leaflet flail or prolapse to 38% for patients with two or more mechanisms of regurgitation). Lambert et al. (46) confirmed these results. In their prospective study involving 13 patients, the mechanism of regurgitation and location of pathology was identified by this systematic echocardiographic examination in 12 patients (92%) and 96% of MV segments compared to a detailed surgical inspection of the valve. Lambert's study did not identify patients with bileaflet prolapse, ischemic MR, more than one surgically identifiable regurgitant mechanism, solitary leaflet perforation, or cleft MVs. Both studies confirm the importance of understanding the anatomy of the MV and the necessity for a comprehensive and systematic approach in evaluating MV during valve repair procedures.

This IOE assessment includes a comprehensive assessment of the pathoanatomy MV apparatus as well as the segmental evaluation leaflet anatomy and motion. As first suggested by Carpentier, segmental leaflet motion may be classified as either excessive, restricted or normal (Fig. 9-32). As illustrated in Table 9-19, examples of segmental mitral abnormalities with excessive leaflet motion include MV prolapse or flail (usually secondary to myxomatous degeneration). Restricted segmental valve motion is usually associated with rheumatic valve disease, whereas examples of mitral pathology with normal leaflet motion include valve endocarditis with associated vegetations or perforation. Although MV repair may be successfully performed in patients with restricted leaflet motion, it is far more successful in patients with either excessive or normal leaflet motion. Utilizing the commonly employed valve repair techniques (Table 9-20), the highest rates of successful repair (98%) occur in patients with myxomatous disease of the posterior

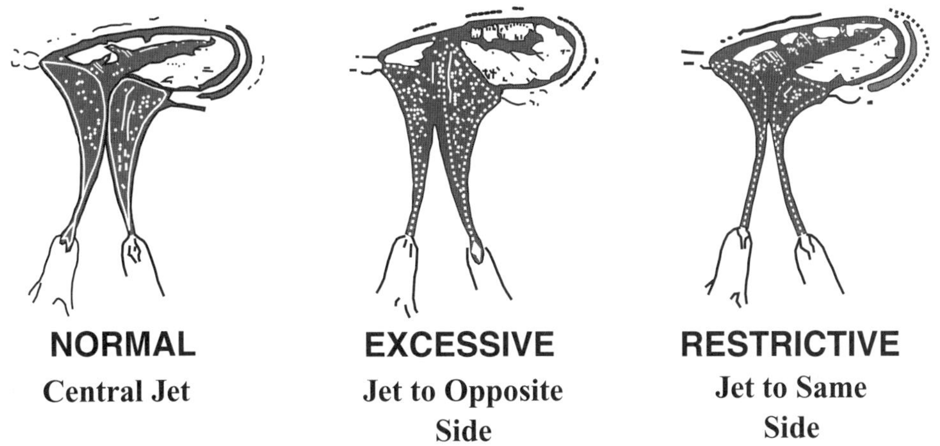

FIGURE 9-32. Mechanisms of mitral valve regurgitation classified by leaflet motion. (Adapted from Ref. 35.)

TABLE 9-19. MECHANISMS OF MITRAL REGURGITATION: SEGMENTAL LEAFLET MOTION

Excessive segmental motion
- Prolapse
- Flail
- Ruptured papillary muscle

Restricted
- Rheumatic restriction
- Dilated left ventricle
- Inflammatory

Normal leaflet motion
- Endocarditis (perforation)

TABLE 9-20. MITRAL VALVE REPAIR TECHNIQUES

Quadrilateral resection posterior leaflet
Anterior leaflet resection
Chordal transfer
Alferi repair (suture between central anterior mitral valve leaflet & posterior mitral valve leaflet)
Ring annuloplasty
Chordal shortening
Artificial (Gortex) chordae
Papillary muscle reattachment
Annular calcium resection
Commissural closure (suture)
Pericardial patch (for perforation)
Annular slide (elevation)

MV leaflet (flail or prolapsing segment)(45). This is followed by patients with MR secondary to LV enlargement (85%), bileaflet prolapse (83%), anterior leaflet myxomatous disease (61%), and restricted leaflet motion secondary to rheumatic disease (20% to 36%, depending on the number of involved leaflets)(45).

As previously discussed (see Guidelines for Comprehensive Examination), the jet in patients with MR may be used to guide the surgeon's repair of the valve. The anatomic localization of the regurgitant jet is accomplished by using all of the MV views (ME four and two chamber, ME mitral commissural, ME LAX, and TG SAX), as illustrated in Fig. 9-11. Particular attention is focused on the origin and subsequent direction of the MR jet. Each part of the MV tensor apparatus is evaluated for its anatomic integrity. Every segment of the MV leaflet is also evaluated for dysfunction and its mechanism. In patients with flail MV segments (valve tip comes above the coaptation plane), the regurgitant jet is directed opposite the segment of origin. Flail posterior MV segments characteristically have an origin from the line of coaptation and an anteriorly directed jet. The leaflet tips of prolapsing segments do not come above the line of coaptation unless the chordae are extremely redundant. Regurgitant MR jets in such valves originate along the line of coaptation and are directed either centrally or proceed opposite the involved segment (depending on the leaflet tip chordal laxity). MR associated with global LV dysfunction is usually central in direction due to restriction of both the anterior MV leaflet and posterior MV leaflet. This may or may not be associated with posterior annular dilation. Patient's with MR associated with rheumatic disease usually have restricted leaflet motion with the regurgitant jet directed toward the involved segments due to an override of the opposing valve leaflet segment. Perforated MV leaflets characteristically have an origin within the leaflet tissue, as visualized in the TG basal SAX view of the MV (Fig. 8-14F). Once identified in the TG SAX view, the transducer angle is rotated forward to demonstrate the jet origin and direction in the TG LAX view. The origin may also be similarly identified in the ME views.

The lowest successful repair rates occur in patients with severe bileaflet restriction secondary to rheumatic disease (20%). Similar to results involving balloon valvuloplasty, the likelihood of successful repair in patients with rheumatic disease is associated with the severity of four distinct features of the underlying pathoanatomy including (a) the degree of involvement of the subvalvular apparatus, (b) leaflet thickness, (c) the degree of restricted leaflet motion, and (d) the severity of leaflet calcification (Table 9-21) (31). In patients with either predominant MR or mitral stenosis, it is important to discuss all IOE findings related to MV anatomy and function with the surgeon to optimally assist in developing the valve repair procedure.

The post-CPB IOE focuses on identifying complications of MV repair and the patient's hemodynamic function. Complications of MV repair include (a) incomplete repair, (b) systolic anterior motion (SAM) of the mitral leaflets with LVOT obstruction (with or without associated MR), (c) mitral stenosis, (d) interruption of coronary circulation,

TABLE 9-21. ECHOCARDIOGRAPHIC INDEX OF REPARABILITY BASED ON MITRAL VALVE MORPHOLOGY

A. Grade	Mobility	Leaflet Thickening
1	Tips restricted	Normal 4–5 m
2	Base to midnormal	Midnormal
3	Base normal	Throughout leaflet
4	No movement	Marked throughout <8–10 mm
B. Grade	**Subvalvular**	**Calcification**
1	Minimal below leaflet	Area
2	1/3 of chordae	Scattered areas on leaflet margins
3	2/3 of chordae	Brightness to midportion of leaflets
4	All	Majority of leaflet tissue

Note: Score of <8 indicates repair more probable.

(e) avulsion of the posterior mitral annulus (secondary to debridement of annular calcification), and (f) trauma to the noncoronary cusp of the AV. The success rate for mitral repair is dependent on the underlying pathoanatomy. Currently, in patients with myxomatous disease, second pump runs are required in less than 3% to 5% of patients (35). Returning to CPB for further repair has not been associated with an increase in perioperative morbidity (47). In this circumstance, IOE provides crucial information regarding the mechanisms for the failed repair. Returning to CPB for further repair may be necessary in circumstances of incomplete repair or pathologic SAM. LVOT obstruction after MV repair is secondary to SAM of the coapted mitral leaflets. LVOT obstruction has been associated with an elongated anterior MV leaflet and a small ventricular cavity (with associated reduction in the diameter of the LVOT) in addition to precipitating factors including hypovolemia, excessive afterload reduction (vasodilators or anesthetic agents), and hyperdynamic ventricular function (increased sympathetic tone or inotropic agents). In these situations, the surgeon may elect to raise the posterior annulus superiorly using an annular "slide" procedure thereby moving the mitral coaptation point further from the interventricular septum and increasing the systolic diameter of the LVOT. In some circumstances, further attempts at valve repair are unsuccessful and valve replacement is necessary.

Mitral Valve Replacement

In MV replacement, the post-CPB echocardiographic evaluation focuses on the integrity of the valve, presence of perivalvular regurgitation, underlying LV function, and potential for valve strut interference with LVOT blood flow. Because of the left-sided systolic pressures, small spaces between the valvular sewing ring and mitral annulus may result in small, but high velocity, perivalvular regurgitation. Such high velocity has a propensity to cause hemolysis and requires further evaluation or repair of the sewing ring leak. It is imperative that regurgitant jets associated with valve replacement be localized either as originating from the sewing ring or as perivalvular. Localization and quantification of the regurgitant jet associated with prosthetic valves is one of the most difficult challenges in IOE due to the artifacts associated with an echo-dense valve ring or mechanical leaflets. Use of multiple imaging views and/or EPE technique is often necessary to achieve a confident conclusion. Helpful clues in this dilemma include the almost universal presence of small regurgitant jets with bioprosthetic valves and the characteristic regurgitant patterns of the various mechanical valves. In addition, the gentle application of manual pressure posteriorly by the surgeon on the sewing ring may obliterate some perivalvular leaks, confirming the diagnosis. There is an increased incidence of perivalvular regurgitation in the setting of severe mitral annular calcification and in valve reoperations due to the artifacts caused by an echo-dense valve ring and/or leaflets. In patients receiving a bileaflet (St. Jude, Carbomedics) or a tilting disc, it is important to visualize an appropriate range of motion of the individual leaflets or disc.

Due to the disruption of the mitral tensor apparatus, MV replacement is associated with reduced ventricular function. This is especially prevalent in those circumstances in which the surgeon was not able to maintain the continuity of the mitral tensor apparatus. In addition, the propensity for disruption of the posterior LV or annulus is increased in such circumstances. Such disruption is preceded by identifiable intramyocardial areas of turbulence permitting the echocardiographer to alert the surgeon before a catastrophic myocardial rupture.

With the implantation of higher profile valves in the mitral position, the valve struts may protrude into the LVOT if not appropriately aligned. Although some prosthetic valve models permit an in situ rotation of the valve, significant obstruction to LVOT flow may require reimplantation of the prosthetic valve.

Tricuspid Valve Repair or Replacement

Except in cases of TV stenosis (e.g., carcinoid valve disease) or TV endocarditis, dysfunction of the TV requiring surgical repair or replacement is usually secondary to RV dysfunction. RV dysfunction, resulting in significant TR, is most commonly associated with severe pulmonary hypertension (severe LV dysfunction, mitral stenosis, or MR). It may also be associated with intrinsic RV dysfunction (right coronary artery ischemia) or RV volume overload (left-to-right shunting). Such regurgitant dysfunction is usually associated with dilation of the RV (restricting the tricuspid apparatus and complete leaflet coaptation) and annular dilation. If there is associated hepatic congestion or more than moderate regurgitation, the TV is usually repaired using a ring valvuloplasty. Endocarditis of the TV may be associated with leaflet perforation or vegetations that interfere with complete coaptation. Repair of such valves is usually successful using a pericardial patch to repair the perforated leaflet or resection of the vegetation with or without a valvuloplasty ring. Replacement of the TV more frequently results from either stenosis or destruction of the valve leaflets from endocarditis. The echocardiographic evaluation after replacement is centered on evaluating the integrity of the valve ring seating, significant perivalvular regurgitation, and mechanical prosthetic leaflet motion.

Aortic Valve Surgery

Surgery involving the AV has undergone dramatic advances in recent years. Included among these have been the development of AV repair techniques, use of cadaveric homografts, further refinement of valve sparring techniques, pulmonary autograft placement (Ross procedure), stentless valves, and reimplantation of the native AV in the proximal ascending aorta. Although each of these procedures has unique echocardiographic requirements, there are common features to the examination that are similar to those previously described for MV repair. The purpose of the pre-CPB IOE study in AV repair is to determine (a) the severity of the valve dysfunction in addition its underlying mechanism and pathoanatomy, (b) the size of the aortic annulus and assess the ascending aorta for post–stenotic dilation, (c) the underlying LV function, (d) the presence of segmental wall motion abnormalities, indicative of associated coronary artery disease, (e) secondary valvular or ventricular dysfunction, and (f) an appropriate cannulation and perfusion strategy. The common features of the post-CPB IOE study for all AV surgery includes (a) evaluation of AV competence, (b) determination of the mechanism of any valve dysfunction, (c) evaluation of global and regional dysfunction, and (d) screening for potential complications, most commonly associated with coronary artery surgical anatomy.

Aortic Valve Repair or Replacement

Using various techniques, repair of dysfunctional AVs is an option in some centers and has been met with a high rate of success in the setting of regurgitation associated with a perforated valve leaflet or a congenitally bicuspid AV (48). AV endocarditis is usually associated with underlying valve pathology resulting in regurgitation or turbulent systolic flow secondary to stenosis. Perforation of the AV leaflet may be repaired utilizing a pericardial patch. A bicuspid AV most commonly involves fusion of the left and right coronary cusps with associated prolapse of the fused cusp beneath the plane of aortic coaptation. Consequently, the resulting regurgitant jet is directed posteriorly toward the anterior MV leaflet. Although repair may be successfully accomplished in the setting of AS, it is more challenging due to increased leaflet thickening and calcification. In comparison to AVs that are regurgitant, it is, however, associated with an increased incidence of subsequent valve replacement. In addition to the previously mentioned features, the post-CPB study is focused on the success of the valve repair (or mechanism of persistent dysfunction), the underlying ventricular function, secondary valve dysfunction, and detection of new regional wall motion abnormalities indicating either surgical interference with coronary flow or air embolism associate with open cardiac procedures. In those circumstances in which valve repair or one of the other AV techniques is not applicable, AV replacement is necessary. The critical issues of the pre-CPB include the sizing of the aortic annulus (under physiologic conditions) and determining the presence of secondary valve dysfunction (MR in the setting of severe AR and ventricular dilatation). In the setting of AS, there may be poststenotic dilation of the ascending aorta, which may require conduit replacement.

Aortic Homograft Implantation

Implantation of cadaveric AV homografts has grown in popularity given the initial reports of long-term outcome. Echocardiographic issues that must be addressed for the success of this procedure include (a) accurate pre-CPB sizing of the aortic annulus (to permit thawing of the appropriate size of homograft before implantation, (b) post-CPB assessment of AV competence, (c) evaluation of potential surgical trauma to the MV function, and (d) determination of healthy coronary by either direct coronary CF visualization or indirectly by assessment of segmental wall function (49).

Aortic Valve Resuspension

As previously discussed, aneurysmal dilation of the proximal ascending aorta frequently results in dilation of the AV annulus and distortion of the normal valve alignment for coaptation. To successfully achieve correction of this anatomic problem, the AV is either resuspended after implantation of the aortic conduit or replaced with a prosthetic valve. In addition, the coronary artery ostia are reimplanted into the conduit. To ensure the success of this procedure, the echocardiographic study must evaluate the post-CPB competence of the resuspended valve in addition to assessing indicators of successful reimplantation of the coronary arteries. Occasionally the proximal left main or right coronary artery is kinked due to the higher reimplantation location and requires coronary bypass grafting of the involved coronary artery.

Pulmonary Autograft (Ross Procedure)

The Ross procedure involves the implantation of the native pulmonary valve into the aortic position. Although the long-term viability of this procedure has been called into question (due to the development of AR or pulmonary homograft stenosis), this procedure is common in some centers. The critical issues that must be addressed in this procedure include (a) the patency of the septal perforator (which may be interrupted during pulmonary autograft harvest), (b) competency of the AV after implantation, (c) evaluation of the segmental function in coronary perfusion beds, which may indicate surgical disruption of coronary flow, and (d) evaluation of the competency and systolic gradient of the pulmonary valve homograft (50,51).

David Procedure

In patients with Marfan syndrome, some centers have advocated the prophylactic reimplantation of the AV in the ascending aorta in the early phase of aortic root dilation as a way of circumventing the complications of aortic dissection and AR associated with this syndrome. The surgery involves removal of the native AV and resuspension in the proximal ascending aorta. Critical features of this procedure that must be assessed include the competency of the AV and coronary perfusion after AV resuspension (52).

Intraoperative Evaluation of Prosthetic Valves

In 1960, Starr and Harken implanted the first prosthetic intracardiac valve (53). This operation launched 39 years of growth in the area of implanting prosthetic valves. These valves have provided patient benefits including improved survival and quality of life. But the implantation of these valves is palliative, not curative, and all valves have problems associated with them. To understand prosthetic valve dysfunction, it is necessary to be familiar with the various types of valve prostheses and their flow characteristics, which are illustrated in Table 9-22A–C.

The role of IOE in patients with prosthetic valves is to determine a baseline function during the initial operation and to detect perioperative valve dysfunction. The IOE of all the prosthetic valves can be limited by acoustic shadowing and reverberations by the echo-dense areas of the valves. As with other IOE studies, evaluation of a prosthetic valve begins with a review of the patient's chart to identify the type and size of the valve, length of implantation, past gradients, and problems associated with the valve. It may also be important to review the surgeon's report, looking for problems in seating the valve or severe annular calcification.

The types of prosthetic valves fall into three categories: caged-ball valves, discs, and bioprosthetic valves. In each category, there are many types of valves. The *caged-ball valves* are extremely durable, with some lasting more than 20 years. The classic example is the Starr-Edward valve. This valve is formed by a circular sewing ring attached to two metallic, U-shaped arches. This apparatus forms the cage and a Silastic ball is placed inside this cage. The ball moves to the apex of the cage (opening) when blood flows through the valve and returns to the base of the cage (closure) to prevent regurgitation. Blood flow through the valve is asymmetrical around the edges of the ball. Therefore, when measuring Doppler gradients across this valve, the CW Doppler should be measured around the periphery of the ball, where the flow velocities are the highest. The area behind the ball during blood flow is relatively stagnant, which may lead to thrombus formation. Despite required adequate anticoagulation, there is a continuing risk of thromboembolic events. There is also a low incidence of acute thrombotic occlusion, mechanical sticking, or encasement. Implantation of the valve may be limited due to the high cage profile. In the aortic position, the cage may reach up to the sinuses of Valsalva and in the mitral position, the cage may interfere with the LVOT and the intraventricular septum. In the mitral position, the larger valves function well, but the smaller valves are associated with unacceptable transvalvular gradients. The same is true for small caged-ball valves in the aortic position; in addition, there is a high incidence of hemolysis of these valves.

The *tilting-disc valves* are represented by many types including the Bjork-Shiley and Medtronics-Hall valves. These valves have a circular disc attached to a sewing ring via an eccentric strut mechanism. The back pressure on the largest portion of the disc causes closure of the valve; thus, to ensure closure, the strut system must be designed so that the opening arc of the disc must be less than 90° from the sewing ring. This design leads to a complex flow around the valve. The flow is laminar through the valve sewing ring. As the blood flow opens the tilting disc, it is directed laterally through a major and minor orifice. Thus, the sewing ring is not the limitation to blood flow through the valve, but it is the complex flow through the two orifices. These valves have functioned quite well, particularly when the larger sized prostheses are used. When this valve is fully open, there is an area of stagnation behind the valve, due to the less than 90° opening. This area of stagnation can lead to thrombus formation. Thus, complications of this valve type include acute thrombotic occlusion and thromboembolism despite adequate anticoagulation. Major valve design improvements have centered on improvement of the opening arc, thus decreasing the area of stagnation. Valve dysfunction can also occur from fibrous ingrowth (pannus formation) from the sewing ring interfering with either the strut mechanism or the disc function. This at times can lead to either obstruction of flow (the disc is restricted from opening) or regurgitation of flow (the disc is restricted from

TABLE 9-22. INTRAOPERATIVE ASSESSMENT OF PROSTHETIC VALVES

A. DOPPLER HEMODYNAMIC PROFILE OF NORMAL AORTIC VALVE PROSTHESES

Prosthesis	Number	V_{Peak}	$P_{Mean\ Gradient}$	TVI_{LVOT}/TVI_{Ao}
Heterograft	214	2.4	13.3	0.44
Ball-Cage	160	3.2	23.0	0.32
Bjork-Shiley	141	2.5	13.9	0.40
St. Jude Medical	44	2.5	14.4	0.41
Homograft	30	1.9	7.7	0.56
Medtronic-Hall	20	2.4	13.6	0.39
Total	609	2.6	15.8	0.40

B. DOPPLER HEMODYNAMIC PROFILE OF NORMAL MV PROSTHESES

Prosthesis	Number	V_{Peak}	$P_{Mean\ Gradient}$	Effective Area
Heterograft	150	1.6	4.1	2.3
Ball-Cage	161	1.8	4.9	2.4
Bjork-Shiley	79	1.7	4.1	2.6
St. Jude Medical	66	1.6	4.0	3.0

C. INTRAOPERATIVE ASSESSMENT OF PROSTHETIC VALVES

Valve	Aortic position (mean gradient) mm Hg	Mitral position (mean gradient) mm Hg
Heterograft	13.3 ± 6.1	4.1 ± 1.5
Ball Cage	22.8 ± 8.6	4.9 ± 1.8
Bjork Shiley	13.7 ± 7.0	4.1 ± 1.6
St. Jude	15.1 ± 7.3	4.0 ± 1.8
Homograft	7.8 ± 2.7	None
Hall Metronics	15.1 ± 5.2	None
CarboMedics	5.8–19.4	3.3–7

Note: V, velocity; P, pressure; LVOT, left ventricular outflow test.

closing). Clinically, patients develop congestive heart failure and flash pulmonary edema when this occurs.

The St. Jude valve is an example of a *low-profile bileaflet mechanical valve.* This valve consists of two semicircular discs (leaflets) attached to a sewing ring by a midline hinge mechanism. This configuration leads to two large lateral semicircular openings and a smaller midline rectangular opening. The hinge mechanism allows the leaflet opening to more than 80°, unlike the single disc valves that open from 55° to 70°, allowing the effective orifice of the valve to more closely approximate the area of the sewing ring. This mechanism allows more symmetrical and unobstructed flow along the axis of the valve inlet. The St. Jude design has two major advantages: There is a large unobstructed flow area through the valve, and there is a markedly decreased area of stagnation. The disadvantage of the wide open excursion of this valve is that it allows for significant regurgitant backflow. This backflow swings the leaflets through their long closing arc, and it is during this time that valvular regurgitation occurs. On color-mapping Doppler, this regurgitant flow is seen at the periphery (between the disc and the sewing ring) and centrally (between the disc leaflets). The normal regurgitation pattern is viewed as a small central jet and two or more small peripheral jets directed toward the central jet.

Because of the smaller area of stagnation, the St. Jude valve is thought to have a lower incidence of thromboembolism than the previously discussed mechanical valves. Anticoagulation of patients with St. Jude valves is still required. Valve dysfunction can occur either from pannus formation or from thrombi forming at the hinge mechanism. Generally, this causes the valve leaflets to stick in a partially open position, causing acute regurgitation. Due to the narrow sewing ring of the St. Jude valve, an improperly placed suture in the sewing ring can cause the valve leaflet to stick, causing the patient to develop acute congestive heart failure. Currently, due to the St. Jude valve's excellent hemodynamic profile, durability, and low thrombogenicity, it is one of the most commonly implanted mechanical valves.

The Carbomedics *bileaflet prosthetic heart valve* is another low-profile mechanical valve. This valve differs from the St. Jude valve in that it has an inner ring composed of pyrolitic carbon, rather than pyrolitic-covered graphite. The reported advantage of this valve is that the differences in the inner ring allow for more washing jets, thus reducing the risk of thromboembolism. In addition, the leaflet excursion is different so that even if the valve is implanted at an angle, the leaflets will close properly. Lastly, in some models, the inner ring can be rotated within the sewing ring at the time of implantation to optimize leaflet orientation. Just as in the newer models of the St. Jude valves, the pressure gradients produced by this valve are very similar to those of the St. Jude valve. With CF Doppler, there are four washing jets, one on either side of each pivotal point, one jet was commonly more prominent than the other three. This is similar to the St. Jude valve IOE findings. Overall, the characteristics from a surgical and echocardiographic standpoint are very similar.

There are two types of *stented porcine bioprostheses* currently used: the Hancock and the Carpentier-Edwards. Both types of valves, although different in design, are similar in echocardiographic appearance and thus will be considered together in this discussion. These valves are constructed using a preserved porcine AV attached to a mount (stented) and this apparatus is attached to a sewing ring. Before the valve leaflets are mounted, they are treated in glutaraldehyde, which acts as a tanning agent and reduces their antigenicity. These preserved leaflets are nonviable, unlike the homograft valves, and are thus stiffer. The porcine bioprostheses have been used in all valvular positions and their main advantages are low thrombogenicity (no anticoagulation is necessary) and their central blood flow. Because the porcine valves are stiff and the size of the porcine valve is limited by the size of the pig; placement of these valves in a previous large valve orifice can lead to significant obstruction to flow. Approximately 10% of these valves will have some degree of regurgitation. Since their widespread use over time, several problems have arisen. One is durability and the other is longevity. Both of these problems are more prominent with implantation in young people and placement in the MV position, rather than the aortic site. Mitral porcine failure is common after 5 years and very few valves last for 10 years. The dysfunction is usually associated with progressive leaflet thickening and calcification, followed by leaflet fracturing, tearing, and stenosis. A more active immune response to the foreign porcine valve is the postulated mechanism of higher failure in the younger porcine valve recipient. The higher incidence of failure in the mitral position is thought to be due to a greater "back pressure" between the LV and LA in systole, compared to the aorta and LV in diastole. The risk of endocarditis continues throughout the implanted life of the valve.

There are also *stentless porcine prosthetic valves* (Toronto SPV valve), which are similar to the stented bioprosthetic valve except for the lack of the mechanical framework. The reported advantages of this valve are increased effective orifice areas with peak pressure gradients similar to those obtained with the aortic homograft. The disadvantage of this valve is the greater technical demands placed on the surgeon. The echocardiographic findings are similar to those of an aortic homograft.

The *bovine pericardial valves* are very similar to the porcine valves except that the three leaflets are fashioned from bovine pericardium. The rest of the valve, including the sewing ring and leaflet support structure, are very similar to the porcine apparatus. Initially, the most commonly used valve of this type was the Ionescu-Shiley valve. Today, the Baxter-Carpentier-Edwards pericardial valve is the only one approved for use. The pericardial valves offer several advantages over the porcine valves. These advantages include unlimited sizes and the ability to make modifications in valve design due to the total artificial nature of the valve and the leaflets. The most common cause of failure with this valve is due to abrasion of the pericardial leaflets with the support frame and calcification of the pericardial leaflets, leading to valvular regurgitation. In the case of abrasion, the regurgitation is due to sudden perforation. The calcification also leads to progressive thickening and an increasing transvalvular gradient.

Evaluation of Gradients Across the Prosthetic Valve

These measurements (Table 9-22B) are important to determine whether a prosthetic valve is becoming stenotic. All prosthetic valves have some degree of intrinsic stenosis associated with them. The normal prosthetic gradient depends on the type of prosthetic valve, the size of the prosthetic valve, the location of the implanted valve, and the ventricular function. In the aortic position as valve size increases, the gradient decreases except for the caged-ball valve. In the mitral position, for all the valves, as the size increases the gradient decreases. The phenomenon of pressure recovery states that the conservation of energy requires that the pressure of fluid decrease as the velocity increases. As velocity increases, pressure decreases and the contrary to this principle. The orifice of a prosthetic valve is the narrowest point across the outflow tract. This area will have the highest velocity and the lowest pressure. As measurements are made further away from the valve, the velocity decreases and the pressure increases. This is pressure recovery. Baumgartner et al. demonstrated that *in vitro* the CW Doppler measurement of the St. Jude valve compared to catheter pullback measurements varied depending on where the Doppler measurements were taken (54). Thus, the mean gradient obtained by CW Doppler may not be the spatial mean gradient, and care must be taken when comparing St. Jude prostheses to other prostheses using CW Doppler.

Hypertrophic Cardiomyopathy

Hypertrophic obstructive cardiomyopathy (HOCM) is a rare progressive cardiac abnormality associated with dynamic systolic LVOT obstruction and diastolic dysfunction. In patients who remain symptomatic despite medical therapy, transaortic septal myectomy or percutaneous septal myectomy (selected higher risk patients) have been used in their surgical management. Without interfering with the surgical procedure, IOE is able to characterize the anatomic features and severity of hemodynamic obstruction, determine the presence of coexisting MR, evaluate diastolic dysfunction, and immediately demonstrate the surgical results of the myectomy. The surgical myectomy involves the removal of portions of the abnormal septum beneath the right coronary cusp. Two parallel incisions of the septum are made, which are approximately 1 cm in depth, up to 2 cm in width, and at a length that extends the incision to the bases of the PMs and directed by the intraoperative presurgical (See Color Fig. 9-33, between pages 560 and 561). The anatomic and functional substrates of LVOT obstruction include (a) a diminished LVOT diameter associated with SAM of the MV, (b) an increased velocity of LVOT blood flow, and (c) anterior displacement of the PMs (55,56). An LVOT diameter of less than 20 mm is associated with LVOT obstruction in up to 66% of patients (56,57). The severity of the LVOT obstruction has also been associated with the presence of leaflet SAM-septal contact and the length of the leaflet SAM-septal contact (57). Patients with HOCM may have a septal thickness ranging from 15 mm to more than 30 mm.

TABLE 9-23. ATTRIBUTES OF IOE THAT ENABLE ASSESSMENT OF SURGERY FOR HOCM

1. Ability of characterize HOCM anatomy
    - Septal thickness
    - MV septum relation
    - Left atrial enlargement
2. Accuracy
    - Gradient measurement
    - Anatomic measurement
        - Septal thickness
        - Distance AV to SAM-special contact
        - Length SAM-septal contact
3. MV evaluation
    - Redundancy of leaflets
    - SAM of MV leaflets
    - Associated MR
    - Intrinsic MV disease
    - Anterior papillary muscle displacement
4. Ability of characterize diastolic dysfunction
    - Abnormal relaxation
    - Pseudonormal pattern
    - Restriction
5. Lack of interference with surgery
    - (unless epicardial echo necessary)
4. Ability to evaluate immediate response to surgery
    - Complications
        - Persistent significant gradient
        - Ventricular septal defect
        - Coronary artery–ventricular communication
    - Response to isuprel provocation

Note: IOE, intraoperative echocardiography; HOCM, hypertrophic obstructive cardiomyopathy; MV, mitral valve; SAM, systolic anterior motion.

The role of IOE in the surgical management of patients with hypertrophic obstructive cardiomyopathy is organized into the pre-CPB and post-CPB assessment (Table 9-23 and 9-24A and B). The prepump study focuses on determining (a) the diastolic thickness of the septum, (b) the distance of the SAM-septal contact from the base of the right coronary cusp, (c) the severity of the LVOT obstructive gradient, and (d) the mechanism and severity of MR. In patients with HOCM, systolic contraction is followed by SAM of the MV, LVOT obstruction and MR (which is characteristically posterior in direction). As the coapted mitral leaflets move anteriorly during systole, they will frequently contact the septum and eventually create a echo-

TABLE 9-24. PRESURGICAL ASSESSMENT AND IOE EVALUATION OF HOCM

A. Assessment of HOCM
  1. 2D Examination of chambers
     Regional wall motion abnormalities
     LV wall thickness
       Septum
       Lateral wall
     LA size
     RV function
  2. 2D assessment of LVOT obstruction
     Diameter of LVOT
     Systolic anterior motion of MV
       SAM-septal contact
       Distance AV RCC to SAM-septal contact point
       Length of SAM-septal contact
     Intrinsic mitral disease
  3. Color Doppler assessment
     Systolic turbulence in LVOT
     MR
       Anterior, central, or posterior jet
  4. Pulse and continuous-wave Doppler
     Localize point of peak gradient
     Maximal instantaneous and mean gradient
     LV inflow characterization of diastolic function
       Normal, abnormal relaxation, pseudonormal, or restriction
     Pulmonary vein flow characterization
       Severity of MR
       Distinguish normal from pseudonormal pattern
  5. Routine comprehensive examination
     All valves and chambers, aorta

B. IOE evaluation of HOCM
  1. 2D assessment of LVOT obstruction
     Residual septal thickness
     Systolic anterior motion of the MV
     SAM-septal contact
     LV function
     RV function
     Intrinsic MV disease
  2. Color Doppler assessment
     Turbulent systolic flow in LVOT
     MR associated with SAM
     Ventricular septal defect
     Coronary-ventricular cavity blood flow
  3. Pulse and continuous-wave Doppler
     Maximal instantaneous and mean gradient
       Before and following provocation with isuprel
  4. Characterization of diastolic function
     Normal, abnormal relaxation, pseudonormal, or restriction
     Pulmonary vein flow
       Severity of MR
       Distinguish normal from pseudonormal pattern
  5. Routine comprehensive examination
     All valves and chambers, aorta

Note: IOE, intraoperative echocardiogram; HOCM, hypertrophic obstructive cardiomyopathy; LV, left ventricle; LA, left atrium; RV, right ventricle; LVOT, LV outflow tract; MV, mitral valve; SAM, systolic anterior motion; AV, aortic valve; MR, mitral regurgitation.

TABLE 9-25. INDICATIONS FOR EPICARDIAL IOE IN SURGERY FOR HOCM

1. Inability to insert TEE probe
2. Contraindications for TEE
3. Suboptimal Doppler interrogation angle LVOT gradient
4. Inconsistent 2D measurements
   Septal thickness
   AV to SAM-septal contact
   Length of SAM-septal contact

Note: IOE, intraoperative echocardiogram; HOCM, hypertrophic obstructive cardiomyopathy; TEE, transesophageal echocardiography; LVOT, left ventricular outflow tract; AV, aortic valve; SAM, systolic anterior motion.

genic fibrotic patch. To safely guide the surgical myectomy, the true septal diameter must be measured during diastole. The ME four-chamber, ME LAX, and TG basal SAX views permit measurement of the diastolic septal thickness (at the point of SAM-septal contact), the length of SAM-septal contact, and the distance from the right coronary cusp to the highest SAM-septal contact. If there is any significant variance in the septal thickness, it is essential that an EPE study be performed (Table 9-25). If the thickness measurement overestimates the true diastolic septal dimension, the surgeon may inadvertently create a VSD during the myectomy. We have used an epicardial probe held by the surgeon on the septum (through the open aortic root), to measure the septal thickness during the surgical procedure. This provides additional assurance that at least 5 mm of septum remains and that a VSD is unlikely to develop postoperatively. The LVOT systolic gradient is best measured using either the TG LAX or deep TG LAX views. Using color Doppler as a guide, the CW cursor is placed parallel to LVOT blood flow. The resulting spectral characteristic of obstruction (Fig. 9-34) is a late-peaking "dagger-shaped" spectral envelope. Provocative measures such as the Valsalva maneuver, pharmacologic afterload reduction, or Isuprel may increase a borderline gradient. It is possible to confuse the spectral envelope of MR with that of LVOT obstruction. As illustrated in Table 9-26, there are specific distin-

TABLE 9-26. DISTINGUISHING THE LVOT AND MITRAL REGURGITANT SPECTRAL ENVELOPE IN PATIENTS WITH HOCM

	LVOT Spectral Envelope	Mitral Regurgitation Spectral Envelope
Onset	AV opening	Initiation of LV systole
Duration	LV ejection	Holosystolic
Peak velocity	<4.5 m/sec	>4.5 m/sec
Contour	Dagger shaped	Symmetrical
Peak velocity timing	Delayed	Early systole

Note: LVOT, left ventricular outflow tract; AV, aortic valve; LV, left ventricular; HOCM, hypertrophic obstructive cardiomyopathy.

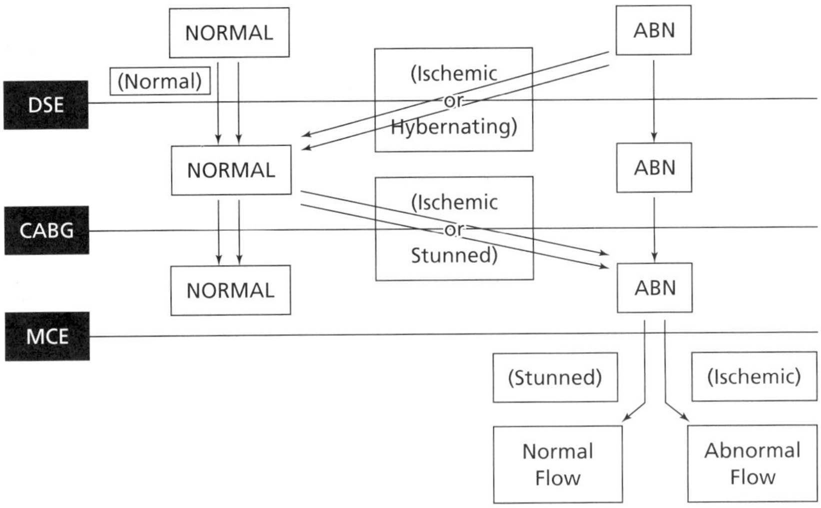

FIGURE 9-34. Myocardial function.

guishing characteristics that must be followed to prevent such misinterpretation. In MR, the peak velocity occurs earlier and is greater (usually more than 4.5 m/second) than that seen with LVOT obstruction. The mechanism of MR in HOCM involves the distortion of the plane of coaptation produced by SAM of the coapted leaflets (57). The results in an opening of the leaflets with a relative anterior override of the posterior leaflet. Therefore, the characteristic jet is posteriorly directed. If the jet is direct anteriorly or centrally, other possible mechanisms of MR should be investigated.

Diastolic dysfunction of the LV is commonly present in patients with HOCM and may include all four physiologic patterns. Although pharmacologic intervention, including lusitropic or chronotropic drugs, may assist in the management of diastolic dysfunction, the abnormalities commonly persist after correction of the systolic LVOT obstruction. It is important to recognize the implications for the perioperative management of these patients.

The postbypass study determines the success of the septal myectomy and evaluates for any potential complications (Table 9-27) or persistent diastolic dysfunction. The views that were used to perform the CW Doppler prebypass should provide the optimal interrogation post-CPB. A medically unresponsive persistent gradient or provocative peak instantaneous gradient of more than 36 mm Hg peak should be evaluated for further surgical myectomy (58). If the septal thickness or depth of the incision toward the apex will not permit further tissue removal, consideration is given to replacing the MV. In addition to significant persistence of the LVOT obstruction, the most significant complications of septal myectomy include an iatrogenic VSD, PM laceration, and a coronary-ventriculo fistula resulting from incision across a left anterior descending septal perforator. A septal thickness of less than 3 to 5 mm at the point of septal myectomy must be followed closely in the perioperative period to ensure that a VSD does not ensue. Color *m* mode may be used to distinguish a small VSD from the small coronary ventricular fistula.

TABLE 9-27. IOE ASSESSMENT OF COMPLICATIONS OF SURGERY FOR HOCM

1. Ventricular septal defect
2. Residual LVOT gradient
3. Persistent mitral valve SAM
4. Mitral regurgitation
5. Coronary artery ventricular fistula
6. Diastolic dysfunction

Note: IOE, intraoperative echocardiography; HOCM, hypertrophic obstructive cardiomyopathy; LVOT, left ventricular outflow tract; SAM, systolic anterior motion.

Recently interventional cardiologists have used the *percutaneous septal ablation* for the management of LVOT obstruction secondary to HOCM (59). This is accomplished through the catheter-directed infusion of a sclerosing concentration of alcohol into the first septal perforator of the left anterior descending coronary artery. As anesthesiologists become increasingly involved in the more complex catheterization laboratory interventions on higher risk patients, it will become more important for us to provide comprehensive management of these patients. In many circumstances, the patients are intubated and undergo simultaneous TEE evaluation of the procedure. The degree of obstruction is often reduced at the time of the procedure. Complications of such procedures include extensive septal infarction associated with the sclerosing agent being infused into a larger collateralized vessel or back-leakage into the left anterior descending circulation.

Higher Risk Myocardial Revascularization

Great strides have been made during the last 30 years of surgical revascularization of the myocardium. With the

TABLE 9-28.

82 consecutive patients
Cleveland Clinic severity score >4
Primary coronary bypass surgery
No planned valve or vascular surgery
No contraindications to intraoperative echocardiography transesophageal or epivascular
Documentation anesthetic/hemodynamic and surgical management plan
Staged blinding
 Pre-CPB, pre-CPB separation, post-CPB, post–chest closure
Reveal echo findings
Document management plans altered by intraoperative echocardiography findings

Note: CPB, cardiopulmonary bypass.

aging population, the increasing incidence of associated diseases, and the increasing numbers of cardiac reoperations, newer strategies for the surgical and anesthetic/hemodynamic management must be developed if we are to continue to maintain the low incidence of morbidity and mortality associated with this procedure. IOE has demonstrated its effectiveness in guiding the intraoperative decision-making process and potentially improving patient outcome (28). In a study by the authors, 82 consecutive high-risk patients undergoing coronary artery bypass surgery were studied in a four-stage protocol to determine the efficacy of IOE in management planning (Table 9-28). Alterations in major surgical and anesthetic/hemodynamic management initiated by IOE findings were documented in addition to perioperative morbidity and mortality. Major changes in the surgical management are illustrated in Table 9-29. Two patients required urgent CPB due to detection of a new irreversible regional wall motion abnormality (left main reoperation) in one patient and another with a previously undetected LV pseudoaneurysm. Twelve patients received unplanned coronary grafts on the basis of regional wall motion abnormalities in areas supplied by coronary arteries with less than or equal to 40% stenotic "luminal irregularities" and new regional wall motion abnormalities postbypass or after chest closure. These patients underwent unplanned valve surgery because of undiagnosed or underdiagnosed valve disease. Anesthetic hemodynamic management alterations were precipitated by IOE in 37 patients (Table 9-30) with global LV or RV dysfunction and 35 patients with new or worsening regional wall motion abnormalities. Fifteen patients with diastolic dysfunction had volume administered in the setting of elevated filling pressures on the basis of IOE findings. In these patients, 12 (80%) had a pattern of abnormal relaxation, 2 (13%) had a pseudonormal pattern, and 1 patient (7%) had reversible restrictive filling. When these results were collated, it was discovered that IOE initiated at least one major surgical management alteration in 33% of patients (27) and at least one major anesthetic/hemodynamic change in 51% of patients (42) (Table 9-31A). Comparing this consecutive high-risk study population with a similar group of patients with no IOE (Table 9-31B) demonstrated a decreased incidence of perioperative death (1.2% versus 3.8%), myocardial infarction (1.2% versus 3.5%), and central nervous system morbidity (1.2% versus 3.8%) in those patients receiving IOE. Although these patients had undergone preoperative assessment by the referring cardiologists, the IOE provided a final diagnostic screening for the unsuspected findings and altered the hemodynamic or surgical management as a consequence. It should be understood that the deployment of IOE in this study was not passive monitoring, but one in which comprehensive diagnostic studies were performed at four stages during the operation. Although this study may provide some insight into the impact IOE would potentially have if routinely utilized in this patient population, it is dependent on a number of factors. Included among these are (a) quality of the IOE, (b) correct interpretation of the IOE, (c) correct surgical or hemodynamic assessment, (d) development of an appropriate management plan, and (e) its skillful implementation. It was concluded that when all of the isolated diagnostic and monitoring ap-

TABLE 9-29. MAJOR SURGICAL MANAGEMENT ALTERATIONS PRECIPITATED BY INTRAOPERATIVE ECHOCARDIOGRAPHY

	Pre-CPB	Pre-CPB Separation	Post-CPB Separation	Post–chest Closure	Total of Patients
CABG Without CPB	3	—	—	—	3
Axillary Cannulation	6	—	—	—	6
Circulatory Arrest	1	—	—	—	1
Mitral Valve Repair	3	—	—	—	3
Aortic Valve Replacement	2	—	—	—	2
Pulmonic Valve Replacement	1	—	—	—	1
LV Rupture	1	—	—	—	1
Aortic Dissection	1	—	—	—	1
Chest Reopened	—	—	—	2	2
Rush To Bypass	2	—	—	—	2
Return To Bypass	—	—	3	1	4

Note: CPB, cardiopulmonary bypass; CABG, coronary artery bypass graft; LV, left ventricle.

TABLE 9-30. MAJOR ANESTHETIC/HEMODYNAMIC MANAGEMENT ALTERATIONS PRECIPITATED BY INTRAOPERATIVE ECHOCARDIOGRAPHY

	Pre-CPB	Pre-CPB Separation	Post-CPB Separation	Post–chest Closure	No. of Patients
Global Dysfx	6	25	37	37	37
RWMA	8	18	8	1	35
RV Dysfx	2	12	15	15	15
DIAST Dysfx	13	5	12	15	15
Un-DX Valve DZ	13	3	2	3	16
Under-DX Valve	15	0	0	0	16

Note: CPB, cardiopulmonary bypass.

plications of IOE are routinely and systematically performed, it may significantly impact the decision-making process in the intraoperative care of high-risk patients undergoing primary isolated coronary artery bypass surgery and may contribute to their optimal care.

As we enter into a new era of surgical revascularization, the key issues that impact the outcome of patients undergoing coronary artery surgery include (a) detection of complications associated with ischemic heart disease, (b) prevention of stroke, (c) prediction of myocardial viability after graft placement and long-term outcome, (d) myocardial protection, (e) detection of previously undiagnosed cardiac disease, (f) need for mechanical support (IABP, LVAD, biventricular assist device [BiVAD]), and (g) end-organ perfusion (kidneys, central nervous system, and so on). Complications associated with ischemic heart disease are more frequent in the higher risk population. After myocardial infarction, cardiogenic shock (cardiac index less than 2.1 L/m^2) occurs in approximately 8% of patients with a mortality of 80%. In a large multicenter retrospective analysis, it was found that the cause of shock in this patient population was largely due to LV failure but included acute ventricular septal or free-wall rupture, PM rupture, MR secondary to ischemic dysfunction, RV infarction, LV thrombus, tamponade, and LVOT obstruction. Each of these complications are readily detected using IOE. It is capable of not only diagnosing the presence of each of these complications but also assessing the success of subsequent therapeutic interventions.

TABLE 9-31. HIGH-RISK CORONARY ARTERY SURGERY IOE VERSUS NO IOE

A.	Study Group With IOE	Severity Score >4 No IOE
No. of patients	82	397
Age	68.4	64.8
Severity score	6.1	5.9
Hospital deaths	1 (1.2%)	18 (3.8%)
Preoperative myocardial infarct	1 (1.2%)	14 (3.5%)
Hospital CNS morbidity	1 (1.2%)	18 (3.8%)

B.	Major Management Alterations	% Patients
Anesthetic/hemodynamic	51	
Surgical	33	
Anesthetic/hemodynamic/surgical	64	

Note: IOE, intraoperative-echocardiography; CNS, central nervous system.

Kachouchus et al. clearly demonstrated that in a higher risk population of patients undergoing cardiac surgical procedures, IOE (including EPE and TEE) was capable of detecting significant atheroma, which were missed by manual palpation. Using aggressive management strategies (altering arterial and cardioplegia administration sights, replacing severely disease aorta, altering aortic cross-clamp technique), they demonstrated a significant improvement in patient outcome. Konstadt et al. (60) demonstrated that TEE may serve as a screen for EPE. Significant atheroma visualized in either the proximal ascending or descending aorta increases the likelihood of finding atheromatous disease in the "blind" portion of the ascending aorta accessible to EPE (61). Blauth et al. (62) demonstrated up to a 30% incidence of cognitive deficiencies in patients after the utilization of CPB. Using TEE, EPE, and intracranial Doppler may significantly diminish these cognitive disorders after cardiac surgery employing CPB.

Accurate prediction of myocardial viability after revascularization is important in the higher risk patient for three reasons: (a) It is a predictor of long-term outcome, (b) additional time on CPB required for unnecessary coronary grafting, and (c) postbypass ventricular function. In a study of 318 patients undergoing revascularization with severe LV dysfunction, Afridi et al. (63) demonstrated that the presence of contractile reserve by dobutamine stress testing was a reliable predictor of survivability after surgical revascularization. Dynamic imaging with stress echocardiography has been evaluated as a method to distinguish viable from nonviable myocardium. It is well recognized that regional LV dysfunction is often reversible and exists in territories of viable myocardium (63–66). Indeed, it is widely recognized that reversible segmental wall motion abnormalities caused by transient myocardial ischemia are the hallmark of atherosclerotic coronary artery disease. During the past decade, stress echocardiography has emerged as a safe and sensitive method for the detection of coronary artery disease and it has been used to provide data for risk stratification during the perioperative period (67–69).

The response of regional LV function to dobutamine is useful to characterize myocardium. In the therapeutic dose range (5 to 20 μg/kg/minute), cardiac output is augmented by an increase in ventricular contractility, heart rate, and stroke volume, and a β_2-mediated decrease in systemic vascular resistance. Contractility increases at higher doses (20 to 40 μg/kg/minute). Normal resting wall motion and the development of hyperdynamic function with increasing doses of dobutamine are hallmarks of normally perfused myocardium. The development of new wall motion abnormalities or the worsening of baseline systolic dysfunction with escalating doses of dobutamine increases myocardial ischemia. Contractile reserve, on the other hand, is consistent with viability and characterized by baseline wall motion abnormalities that improve with low-dose dobutamine (70–72). When such a low-dose augmentation of function is followed by progressive systolic dysfunction with higher doses (biphasic response), the accuracy of predicting postoperative cardiac morbidity or changes in regional function after revascularization is enhanced even greater (63). Regional segments that remain akinetic (or dyskinetic) despite dobutamine infusion are nonviable. Dobutamine stress echocardiography has a high sensitivity (85%) and specificity (88%) when compared to angiography in patients with recent myocardial infarction (73). A review of data from several studies revealed overall sensitivity and specificity of the test for detecting ischemic heart disease to be 82% and 86%, respectively (73). Stress echocardiography has been shown to be an efficient method for identifying patients undergoing major vascular surgery who are at high or low risk of perioperative cardiac events. In addition, intraoperative application of stress echocardiography enables the extent of myocardial salvage and viability during coronary revascularization surgery to be determined and therefore used to more reasonably direct therapeutic intervention. Recently Aronson and colleagues (74) demonstrated that functional changes after low-dose dobutamine before coronary artery bypass graft predicted functional changes post–coronary artery bypass graft when complete revascularization was achieved (74). Four hundred twenty segments in 30 patients were prospectively evaluated during elective coronary artery bypass graft for regional wall motion changes at four stages, including baseline (post induction of general anesthesia, before CPB) and after low-dose dobutamine (also before CPB), after separation from CPB (early), and 1 hour after administration of protamine (late). It was observed early ($p < .0001$) and late ($p < .0001$) functional changes for all regional myocardial wall motion scores.

Because there is increasing pressure to minimize cost and delays for preoperative patient evaluation, intraoperative stress echocardiography may be particularly well suited for use in patients who have known coronary artery disease or who are at high risk of postoperative cardiac morbidity (Fig. 9-35). An intraoperative paradigm that demonstrates postoperative outcome benefits and thereby enables more efficient utilization and allocation of otherwise scarce resources (e.g., intensive care unit beds) would improve quality of care and reduce cost.

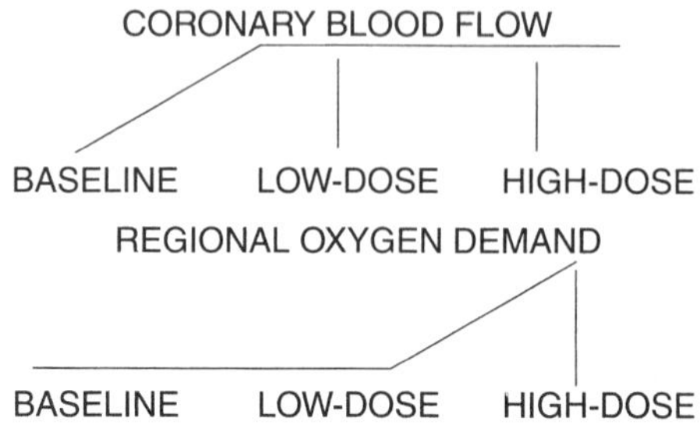

FIGURE 9-35. Low-dose and high-dose dobutamine effect on coronary blood flow and regional oxygen demand.

Understanding the relationship between ventricular function and coronary blood flow during coronary bypass surgery represents another limitation to provocative stress testing with echocardiography and has been limited by the inability to directly assess myocardial perfusion (See Color Fig. 9-36, between pages 560 and 561). Thallium scintigraphy, for example, is predicted on characterization of cell-membrane function of extract patterns of thallium with washout kinetics (14) and is not practical during surgery. Thallium imaging uptake is normal in healthy and stunned myocardial tissue, and decreased uptake is expected at rest in hibernating and infracted tissue with redistribution of thallium at 4 hours in ischemic myocardial tissue after initial decreased uptake. Thallium (and other nuclear pharmaceuticals) perfusion imaging does not, however, provide a functional correlation to flow conditions, is time-consuming, and cannot be used to assess flow intraoperatively.

The goals of intraoperative assessment of bypass surgery include the ability to assess graft patency and anastomotic sites and to identify that the correct stenoses are selected with adequate perfusion established and that a relationship between flow and function is understood before therapeutic intervention is initiated.

Previous techniques employed to understand coronary blood flow have included anatomic and hydraulic methods (measuring graft flow, probing anastomosis), as well as physiologic methods (intraoperative velocity measurements linked with assessment of coronary reserve). These techniques are not routinely used today largely because they all have limitations. Recently, intraoperative MCE has been used to assess myocardial perfusion after myocardial revascularization (74–77). MCE is a technique used to assess the integrity of the coronary microcirculation. The visualization of microbubbles by this technique assesses flow through vessels with a less than 100-μg diameter and provides evidence for microvascular integrity, which is a marker for viability.

Intraoperative stress-contrast echocardiography holds promise as a technique that may enable the identification of viable myocardium and differentiate ischemic dysfunction from nonischemic dysfunction, and this greatly enhances our therapeutic rationalization when treating low-output syndromes. Despite this important question, no studies have yet addressed the question of whether the identification and revascularization of dysfunctional but viable myocardium improves patient outcomes. Barill et al. (89) reported that patients with viable myocardium treated medically had less recovery of LV systolic function than those who were revascularized. Voci et al. (90) have shown that microvascular revascularization improves functional outcome. Unfortunately, many techniques to assess revascularization only provide anatomic evidence of vessel patency rather than microvascular flow into the tissue at risk.

In patients with acute myocardial infarction and occlusion of the infarct-related artery, the presence of collateral flow by MCE correlated with improvement in regional wall motion a month after successful coronary angioplasty (78). A subsequent study showed that in patients with documented patency of the infarct-related artery after recent myocardial infarction, there was a strong correlation between evidence of an intact microcirculation and subsequent improvement in regional wall motion. During acute myocardial infarction, patients with evidence of reflow by MCE in the myocardial area at risk after reperfusion therapy had greater improvement in global and regional LV function on follow-up than patients with no reflow (92). With respect to chronic ischemia, perfusion by MCE correlated with improvement in regional wall motion and global LV function after revascularization in a population of patients with previous myocardial infarction and reduced LV EF (93). The method and rationalization for performing intraoperative stress-contrast echocardiography has been reported and is briefly described later. The response of regional LV function to the β-adrenergic receptor agonist dobutamine is useful to characterize myocardial reserve capacity (79,80). Low-dose dobutamine infusion is expected to increase regional myocardial blood flow and contractility without causing myocardial ischemia, unlike high-dose dobutamine, which would be expected to increase oxygen nutrient delivery mismatch in areas at risk.

Normal resting wall motion and the development of hyperdynamic function with increasing doses of dobutamine are hallmarks of normally perfused myocardium (81,82). The development of new wall motion abnormalities or the worsening of baseline systolic dysfunction with escalating doses of dobutamine indicates myocardial ischemia. Contractile reserve, on the other hand, is consistent with viability and characterized by baseline regional wall motion abnormalities that improve with low-dose dobutamine. Anticipated low-dose augmentation of function would be followed by progressive systolic dysfunction if higher doses of dobutamine were used (a biphasic response) (83). The accuracy of predicting changes in regional systolic function after low-dose dobutamine in chronic coronary artery disease should optimally predict function after revascularization. LV segments that remain akinetic or dyskinetic despite dobutamine infusion are nonviable and likely reflect scar. We often only infuse low-dose dobutamine to augment baseline coronary blood flow and assess the changes in regional myocardial function reserved to be used as a gold standard to predict myocardial flow function after revascularization.

The patient's regional function should be evaluated with intraoperative TEE imaging in the TG SAX (basal, mid, and apical) view, ME four-chamber and ME two-chamber view, and TG two-chamber view using a multiple transducer. If contrast is used, images should be recorded during and after the contrast injection. Regions of interest can be marked on the 2D echocardiogram by using internal calipers to outline the segments. In the LV SAX view, the left coronary artery territory will extend from the anterior septum to the posterolateral wall. The anterior septum and anterior wall will typically be the left anterior descending territory while the lateral and posterior walls will be the circumflex artery territory. The right coronary territory will include the inferior wall and inferior septum. Further, the addition of intravenous perfusion contrast distinguishes stunned, hibernating, and dead myocardium, which directs the surgeon where time on CPB may be most efficiently used.

The infusion of potassium-rich cardioplegia solution has been instrumental in reducing the morbidity and mortality associated with open heart surgery. Optimal myocardial protection during CPB is predicated on adequate homogenous distribution of cardioplegia solution to all myocardial segments. Traditionally, the efficacy of cardioplegia perfusion has been assessed by quiescence of electrical activity on the ECG, a decrease in myocardial temperature, and direct visualization. Recently, contrast ultrasonography has been used to indicate the adequacy of cardioplegia distribution within the myocardium during cardiac surgery (84–86).

Monitoring cardioplegia delivery with contrast ultrasound is a direct, real-time, intraoperative technique that enables the surgeon and anesthesiologist to assess the adequacy of cardioplegia distribution to all myocardial segments. Zaroff et al. (87) retrospectively investigated the relationship between immediate outcome after cardiac surgery, preoperative LV EF, and homogeneous delivery of cardioplegia with intraoperative contrast echocardiography in 21 patients undergoing coronary artery bypass graft surgery. They found that low EF alone did not predict low-output failure after CPB while the combination of inadequate intraoperative myocardial protection (as indicated by nonhomogeneous delivery of cardioplegia to myocardial regions at risk) and low EF always predicted the need for exogenous support to separate from CPB.

Although critical, coronary artery stenosis may impair antegrade delivery of cardioplegia solutions through the aortic root and thereby contribute to perioperative ischemia and infarction, it has been shown with intraoperative contrast ultrasonography that retrograde infusion of cardioplegia provides myocardial distribution to areas subserved by the left anterior descending and left circumflex coronary arteries even in the presence of complete stenosis of these vessels (88). Furthermore, retrograde perfusion of cardioplegia in humans has been reported to provide information regarding transmural distribution of cardioplegia with the ratio of endocardial to epicardial flow 1.46 ± 0.27 and 1.39 ± 0.33 in the LV free-wall and interventricular septum, respectively (89).

In general, retrograde delivery of cardioplegia for myocardial protection is an approach fostered by coronary venous and arterial anatomy. Its efficacy is highly predicated on individual coronary venous drainage patterns that vary greatly. Winkelman et al. (90) have shown that retrograde-delivered cardioplegia through a balloon-tip coronary sinus catheter is not distributed equally to the RV and interventricular septum. They use intraoperative contrast echocardiography and on-line video densitometric analysis to demonstrate that RV free-wall opacification was significantly less (peak pixel intensity 48 + 9) compared to the posterior septum (peak pixel intensity 89 + 12) or anterior septum (peak pixel intensity 107 + 10), after retrograde-delivered cardioplegia.

In a related study by Allen et al. (91), it was confirmed that retrograde cardioplegia provided poor ventricular myocardial perfusion when assessed by contrast echocardiography and coronary ostial drainage. The poor perfusion was unable to meet the myocardial demands of the RV as assessed by oxygen extraction during retrograde perfusion. Villanueva et al. (92) in an experimental protocol used radio-labeled isotropes and MCE to evaluate microvascular flow and nutrient delivery during retrograde and antegrade delivery of cardioplegia. They concluded that microvascular and nutrient flow rates were lower during retrograde delivery due to microvascular differences between coronary arterial and venous systems. Myocardial cooling was however equally efficient with either delivery techniques, suggesting that the clinical benefits of retrograde delivery was primarily cooling and substrate replenishment was better achieved (at similar flow rates and temperatures) with antegrade delivery. Their data, however, presumed healthy coronary artery anatomy and did not consider the influence of collateralization. In patients with ischemic heart disease, predicting the distribution of cardioplegia and understanding its contribution to myocardial protection in each individual patient is difficult without direct assessment during delivery.

Quintilio et al. (93) used intraoperative MCE to determine the myocardial distribution of cardioplegia during combined antegrade and retrograde delivery. They showed that overall myocardial opacification was greater after retrograde delivery in patients with three-vessel disease undergoing elective coronary artery bypass graft surgery. However, collateral circulation was the most important determinate for adequacy of myocardial cardioplegia delivery. If adequate collaterals were present, than retrograde delivery offered no advantage for distribution of cardioplegia to regions at risk. On the other hand, they did show that aortic root delivery may not provide adequate myocardial protection in the subset of patients without evidence of significant collateral circulation. In a related study, we employed intraoperative MCE during coronary artery bypass graft surgery to determine the contribution of collateral blood flow for regional myocardial cardioplegia distribution when delivered antegrade and retrograde (94). The role of the preoperative ECG and coronary angiogram for determining the distribution of cardioplegia in 15 patients (all with total occlusion of their right coronary artery) was also evaluated and compared to direct assessment with intraoperative MCE. Coronary angiograms were evaluated and compared to direct assessment with intraoperative MCE. In that study, coronary angiograms were evaluated for native epicardial anatomy and evidence of collateral coronary circulation supplying the RV, LV apex, and interventricular septum. Evaluation of the preoperative ECG were also performed and prediction of regional distribution of cardioplegia was compared to delivery of cardioplegia determined with myocardial contrast echocardiography using Albunex. Eighty-seven out of 90 (97%) segments were analyzed for cardioplegia distribution at the time of CPB during delivery of cardioplegia. It was demonstrated that the preoperative angiogram and ECG poorly predicted regions at risk for incomplete cardioplegia distribution. Antegrade delivery of cardioplegia was distributed to the RV in 31% of patients despite 100% occlusion of the right coronary artery, whereas retrograde delivery of cardioplegia to the RV only occurred 20% of the time. It was concluded that in the presence of 100% occlusion of the right coronary artery, retrograde cardioplegia delivery is not often observed and antegrade delivery of cardioplegia to the RV is not expected unless coronary collateral circulation is well developed. Furthermore, compared to intraoperative contrast echocardiography, the preoperative angiogram and ECG were not predictive of coronary collateral circulation and therefore not predictive of cardioplegia distribution to the RV.

Currently there are a number of myocardial protection strategies available including (a) intermittent antegrade and retrograde paralysis, (b) simultaneous intermittent antegrade and retrograde paralysis, (c) direct administration of paralysis via manual coronary ostial cannulation, and (d) intermittent antegrade and continuous retrograde. Use of ultrasound contrast agents may help guide the surgical team in the optimal method of myocardial protection for the individual patient.

Ultrasound technology has also been used to visualize renal perfusion utilizing intravenous contrast. The potential exists for clinical application in determining quantitative perfusion indexes of the renal cortex and medulla. In addition, the use of intracranial Doppler provides the surgeon with an effective means of quantifying cerebral blood flow, detecting embolic phenomena, and potentially using retrograde cerebral perfusion to reverse catastrophic embolization.

CONGENITAL HEART DISEASE

IOE has become an essential part of the management of children and adults undergoing surgical repair of congenital cardiac defects. Initially, EPE was the only method available to perform imaging in younger children. In 1989, the first report (95) of using a miniaturized single-plane adult TEE probe in a 7-year-old child demonstrated the advantages of TEE. Compared to EPE, TEE does not interfere with or delay the surgical procedure, does not increase the risk of arrhythmias and infection, and can be performed continuously, as well as in the postoperative period. However, the use of a single-plane TEE probe failed to identify anterior structures, especially the RV outflow tract. Several companies have succeeded in developing pediatric-size, multiplane TEE probes that are currently in clinical use in very young children. Compared to the adult probes, a pediatric multiplane TEE probe has a gastroscope diameter of 7 mm, a tip of 9 by 8 mm, and a frequency of 5 to 7.5 MHz.

The training of physicians in pediatric TEE has the two main goals of achieving technical skills of imaging and interpretation ability. The current recommendations are the performance of 300 studies for basic training, 400 for advanced, and 750 for independent practice, with at least 50% of these cases in patients younger than 1 year old (96). A recent study demonstrated that patient outcome is affected beneficially when pediatric intraoperative TEE is performed by physicians who meet the training guidelines and whose sole responsibility is the performance of echocardiography (97). Significantly, more children had adequate TEE studies, more residual defects were detected, and managed by return to bypass.

Several reports have demonstrated the precautions that should be taken when performing TEE in children. Due to a higher risk of loose teeth, coagulopathy with cyanotic heart disease, and vertebral abnormalities, caution in the insertion and advancing of the TEE probe should be taken. In addition, the relative size of the probe to the smaller infant may cause vascular occlusion, airway obstruction, accidental extubation, or endobronchial advancement of the endotracheal tube (98). However, a recent prospective study reported no significant changes in ventilation variables, in 22 infants, 2 to 5 kg, undergoing TEE during cardiac surgery (99).

The basic echocardiographic examination in children with congenital cardiac defects identifies the cardiac situs, the anatomic structures, and the communications (100). The cardiac situs is identified by the axis of the heart and the relation of the great vessels to the vertebral column.

Venous Connections

To identify the superior vena cava and inferior vena cava connection to the RA, both the longitudinal and transverse views are needed. It is also essential to document the size of the coronary sinus at the base of the LA, to rule out the presence of a LSVC. A normal coronary sinus should be less than 30% of the LA size. The presence of a LSVC will change the plans for percutaneous as well surgical cannulation for CPB. The pulmonary venous drainage should be identified bilaterally, especially in the presence of an atrial septal defect.

Anatomic Structures

The atrioventricular and ventriculoarterial connections have to be documented to reach an adequate diagnosis. Thus, the different structures are identified using specific landmarks on TEE. To identify the atrial anatomy, the appendages of the RA and LA can be examined for differences in appearance. The RA is best seen in the ME bicaval view, as a short, blunt structure with a broad junction to the RA and a rudimentary Eustachian valve at the mouth of the inferior vena cava. The LAA is seen in the ME two chamber view as a long, crenelated structure with a narrow junction to the LAA and the possible presence of a membrane dividing the LA (cor triatriatum).

The ventricles also have distinctive morphologic appearances. The RV has a triangular cavity with a trabecular, endocardial surface, and a moderator band. The RV is always attached to the more broad, trileaflet, apically positioned TV with three PMs and septal chordae. The thicker LV has an ellipsoid cavity, with a smooth endocardial surface and two PMs. The LV is always attached to the bileaflet, basally inserted MV.

The great vessels can be identified by their position and branching. The PA is anterior and leftward with a short main pulmonary artery dividing into two branches. The aorta is posterior and rightward, with a longer ascending aorta, and coronary arteries originating at the sinuses.

Cardiac Crux

The interatrial septum is best seen in two views to avoid the misleading appearance of a drop-off as a defect. The interatrial septum may have a defect in the area of the fossa ovalis (secundum atrial septal defect), the more basal area of the atrioventricular valves (primum atrial septal defect), or the more inferior (sinus venosus atrial septal defect) with abnormalities in pulmonary venous drainage.

The interventricular septum may also have a defect in the muscular, perimembranous, or subarterial areas and must be examined in more than one view to correctly identify defects.

Doppler examination is an essential component of a complete pediatric TEE study. Using CF Doppler, PW Doppler, and CW Doppler, information about shunt amount and direction, degree of obstruction, and vascular resistance can be obtained (101,102). Using Doppler interpretation, several methods were identified and validated by cardiac catheterization results to calculate pulmonary-to-systemic shunt flow through a VSD. One such method uses the flow through the PA and the aorta and the continuity equation:

$$Q_p/Q_s = \text{area PA} \times \text{VTI/area Ao} \times \text{VTI}$$

In addition, the degree of pulmonary hypertension can be identified using Doppler examination of the pressure gradient between the LV and RV through a VSD and the systemic arterial pressure or using the jet of TR and the RA pressure (103).

The benefits of TEE in children with congenital heart disease are to improve accuracy of diagnosis, use as an intraoperative monitor, and identification of residual defects after a repair.

Intraoperative TEE is essential to confirm the preoperative diagnosis and the planned surgical procedure. In 8.5% of patients, TEE either added important information or significantly changed the surgical approach in children with a cardiac defect. In fact, the use of TEE in very small infants had an equal accuracy to cardiac catheterization with a significant decrease in morbidity and mortality, compared with children with similar diagnoses (104).

Intraoperatively, TEE is a viable monitor of cardiac function and ventricular filling that will help in the management of fluids and inotropic support. In a study of seven patients with transposition of the great arteries after an atrial switch who were undergoing PA banding to train the LV to become the systemic ventricle, TEE was a valuable tool to guide the degree of tightening of the PA band (104). These patients had no intracardiac shunts, so the pulse oximeter had a limited ability to direct the surgical procedure.

After surgical repair of congenital cardiac defects, patients with residual lesions identified by TEE had a longer hospital stay, a worse postoperative functional status, and a higher mortality compared to patients with no residual defects (105). In those patients whose residual lesions were immediately identified by TEE and managed in the same surgical encounter, the outcome as well as the cost of care was significantly improved (106).

Major Vascular (Aortic) Surgery

IOE is an important addition to the intraoperative management of patients with vascular disease involving the aorta including aneurysmal dilation, aortic dissection, traumatic aortic disruption, and pseudoaneurysm formation. Nondissecting thoracic aortic aneurysms may be either fusiform or sacular. Fusiform aneurysms may involve the proximal ascending aorta and coronary sinuses (such as occurs in Marfan's syndrome) or the aortic arch and descending aorta. With aneurysmal dilation, the velocity of blood flow diminishes and may become stagnant to the point of mural thrombus formation. In some circumstances, there may be a contained rupture of the aorta, commonly associated with trauma, penetrating ulcers, mycotic aneurysms, or aortic dissection. In these circumstances, it is important to identify the intima of the aorta using higher frequency imaging to distinguish the ruptured pseudoaneurysm from intramural hematoma formation.

Aortic Dissections and Intramural Hematoma

The diagnostic criteria for dissecting aortic aneurysms are grounded on the demonstration of an intimal flap and differential flows in the true and false lumen using CF Doppler imaging (See Color Fig. 9-36 between pages 560 and 561.) (107). Because of the management decisions that must be made, it is important to determine the location and extent of the aortic dissection, in addition to the presence of associated complications (including AR, cardiac tamponade, obstruction of cerebral blood flow, and coronary obstruction, which may result in regional myocardial dysfunction) (108). According to the Stanford classification, type A dissections are surgical emergencies and involve the proximal ascending aorta, whereas the type B dissections originate distal to the left subclavian aorta and are generally managed medically. It is important to distinguish an intimal flap from reverberation artifacts or normal AV suspension, which may mimic aortic dissections (Table 9-32). The intimal flap is generally

TABLE 9-32. AORTIC DISSECTION DIFFERENTIATION

Artifact
Intimal flap demonstrated in multiple imaging planes
Differential flow demonstrated in true and false lumen
Does not cross anatomic plane
Entry and exit site flow
Aortic aneurysm with thrombus
Intima central to thrombus
Normal venous structure
Venous contrast opacification
No entrance/exit site flow
No undulating flap identified
Intramural hematoma
Intima central identified
No entrance/exit site flow
May be associated with ulcerated plaque
Wall thickness (intima-adventitia) >7 mm

an undulating structure with demonstrable differential flow, which does not cross the plane of the intimal flap. Compared to other diagnostic imaging modalities, TEE offers a higher sensitivity (99% versus 88% by angiography and 83% by computed tomography scan) and a similar specificity (109). Not included in the standard classifications of the dissection (Stanford and DeBakey) are those dissections associated with retrograde passage of a catheter into the wall of the descending thoracic aorta. This type of aortic dissection usually does not progress more proximally due to the opposing direction of blood flow. Aortic plaques or ulcers are thought to represent precursors of true aortic dissection. CF Doppler may assist in identifying the extent of the ulceration.

Intramural Hematomas

Rupture of the blood vessels within the wall of the aorta may produce intramural hematoma formation. Intramural hematomas are commonly associated with chest trauma and may progress to aortic dissection formation in up to 30% of patients. Features that characterize the intramural hematoma include the absence of an intimal flap, presence of crescentic or circular mural thickening (5 to 7 cm) with identification of the intima adjacent to the lumen (110).

Intraoperative Assessment of Diastolic Dysfunction and Pericardial Disease

In addition to the patterns of diastolic dysfunction previously discussed, it is clinically important that constrictive pericarditis be distinguished from restrictive disease. In the former, the clinical approach is surgical pericardectomy or pericardial stripping, whereas irreversible end-stage restrictive physiology carries a more ominous clinical scenario treated by orthotopic heart transplantation and more recently developed surgical approaches to congestive heart failure. In constrictive pericarditis, the heart is encased in a fibrotic and often calcified peal (See Color Fig. 9-37, between pages 560 and 561), as frequently demonstrated by 2D echocardiography. Consequently, during respiration, the intrathoracic pressures are not transmitted to the ventricular cavities, resulting in extreme variations of blood flow into the heart (111,112). Consequently, despite similar Doppler indexes at rest, there is profound respiratory variation (Table 9-33).

TABLE 9-33. DISTINGUISHING CONSTRICTIVE PERICARDITIS FROM RESTRICTIVE CARDIOMYOPATHY

	Constrictive Pericarditis	Restrictive Cardiomyopathy
Calcified pericardium	Yes	No
Thickened pericardium	Yes	No
Septal bounce	Yes	No
Mitral valve inflow >30% "e" wave respiratory variation	Yes	No
Left atrium enlargement	+ +	+ + + +

TABLE 9-34. ECHOCARDIOGRAPHIC FINDINGS IN CARDIAC TAMPONADE

Echo free space throughout cardiac cycle
Swinging motion of heart in pericardial cavity
Early diastolic collapse of right ventricle
Diastolic inversion of right atrium
Abnormal (bouncing) septal motion
Interior vena cava congestion
  <10% respiratory variation by diameter
Mitral and tricuspid inflow
  >30 respiratory variation
  prolongs (left ventricular) isovolumetric relaxation time

In the setting of cardiac tamponade, there is impedance to diastolic flow due to compression of the more compliant right-sided chambers with the consequent echocardiographic findings (Table 9-34). Tamponade can also involve compression of the thicker LV, as may occur in post–cardiotomy tamponade. Although these features of tamponade are readily identified, they are not always present in the setting of posterior collections of blood or thrombus, (113) as occasionally occurs after cardiac surgery. In these circumstances, utilization of PW Doppler interrogation of blood flow at the tips of the tricuspid or mitral leaflets may identify exaggerated respiratory variation of peak *e*-wave velocities (more than 30%) and should be taken in the context of the patient's clinical circumstance.

Surgical Management of Congestive Heart Failure

Every year an additional 80,000 patients are diagnosed as having end-stage congestive heart failure, which would benefit from some form of surgical intervention (24). Despite newer pharmacologic approaches to this clinical dilemma, there is a growing population of patients who would benefit from orthotopic heart transplantation. Unfortunately, due to the availability of suitable donor hearts, more than 30% of potential orthotopic heart transplant recipients die every year. Consequently, the surgical approaches to end-stage congestive heart failure are rapidly expanding out of necessity. Included among these advances are mechanical LVADs and BiVADs, ventricular remodeling procedures in conjunction with revascularization and mitral valvuloplasty (Dor procedure, partial ventriculectomy), and more recently procedures intended to reduce ventricular dilation (external or internal splinting). These surgical procedures have unique issues that must be addressed to ensure their success (Table 9-35). The most important determinants of success

TABLE 9-35.

Surgical Procedure	Critical IOE Issues	Pre-CPB	Post-CPB
LVAD implantation	RV function Sequelae of CHF MR, pulmonary HTN Diastolic dysfunction Mural thrombi (LA,LV) Potential R → L shunt Potential Ao → LV circuit Cannulation perfusion LVAD cannula Inflow/outflow Position & function LVAD function LV volume Valve competence Complications of CPB	Global RV Fx, RV FAC MR (grade, mechanism) LAA or LV mural thrombi PW of MV inflow pulmonary vein contrast CFD, contrast with valsalva CFD of AV	Global RV Fx, RV FAC PW of MV & pulmonary vein CFD of AV TEE & EPE Apical inflow position CW, CFD Aortic outflow Air embolism Hypovolemia, flow <15 m/sec Regurgitant LVAD flow 2D Ascending & descending aorta
Bi-VAD, ECMO	(As above) Cannula positioning LA, PA, LV, Ao LA thrombus formation	(As above)	(As above)
Dor procedure remodeling LV	RV function	Global RV Fx, RV FAC, TR	(As above)
CABG MV Repair	LV function and scar Sequelae of CHF MR, pulmonary HTN Diastolic dysfunction Mural thrombi Potential R → L shunt Embolic source (LA, LV) Cannulation-perfusion Strategy Myocardial viability MR severity & mechanism	RWMA, scar MR (severity & mechanism) PWD MW & pulmonary vein Contrast CFD, contrast & valsalva EPE Resting RWMA Low-dose dobutamine stress	
Revascularization	Myocardial viability	Resting RWM Low-dose dobutamine stress Mitral valve function	(As above)
MV repair	Mitral regurgitation	MR severity & mechanism Pathoanatomy, annulus size	(As above)
External & internal splinting	Size LV, systolic, LV/RV Fx, MR, diastolic Fx Position of mechanical splints	As above, LV dimensions, LV & RV dimensions, ejection-fraction MR mechanism/severity, Mitral inflow, pulmonary Vein CW	(As above)

Note: IOE, intraoperative echocardiography; CPB, cardiopulmonary bypass; LVAD, left ventricular assist device; Bi-VAD, Bi-ventricular assist device; LV, left ventricle; CABG, coronary artery bypass graft; MV, mitral valve; RV, right ventricle; Fx, fraction; LA, left atrium.

of each of these procedures are RV function, concomitant valvular disease, and overall function of the other organ systems. In each of these procedures, the pre-CPB IOE focuses on (a) evaluating the underlying RV function, severity of TR, and the potential for BiVAD support, (b) baseline assessment of LV function, (c) evaluating potential sequelae of end-stage dilated cardiomyopathies (LV/LAA mural thrombi, MR, diastolic dysfunction), (d) potential right-to left-shunting, which may contribute to hypoxemia, (e) the presence of AR, which may increase forward-flow demands post-CPB, and (f) development of a CPB strategy. Common features of the post-CPB IOE study are centered on (a) RV function and presence of TR, (b) evaluation of potential consequences of CPB (micro air embolism, complications of cannulation, and (c) the issues uniquely associated with individual surgical approaches to congestive heart failure (Table 9-35). After separation from CPB, it is important to establish a comprehensive baseline study for future comparison. Given the importance of RV function in the overall success of the procedure, an objective measurement of RV function (RV FAC, TR severity, RVEDD, RV dP/dt, TV annulus measurement) is a priority. In the event of deteriorating RV function (due to respiratory insufficiency), this will permit comparison. In LVAD implantation, the potential for right-to-left shunting and AR is increased due to the reduction of left-sided pressures with LV mechanical assist. As LVAD pump flow is initiated, the potential for micro air embolism exists. IOE is used to gauge aortic and outflow cannula venting to reduce this potential. With angulation of the LVAD inflow cannula, there may be obstruction to LVAD inflow, which may be detected by turbulent flow detected by CF Doppler and CW Doppler velocity of more than 1.5 m/second (Fig. 9-38; also see right panel in color between pages 560 and 561). In the event of LVAD inflow prosthetic valve regurgitation, retrograde flow during LVAD pumping will be noted by either CF Doppler or CW Doppler.

The newer remodeling procedures (e.g., Dor and Jentile) involve (a) resection of the ischemic endocardial scar and endocardial patch, (b) revascularization of viable areas, and (c) MV repair if necessary. In addition to those general IOE concerns previously discussed, the pre-CPB study centers around determining those viable regions of myocardium that would respond to viable. Viability assessment may be accomplished with IOE low-dose dobutamine stress testing. Due to severe global dysfunction with a dilated LV, there is frequently significant secondary MR. The MR jet is typically central (due to symmetrical restriction of the tensor apparatus to the anterior MV leaflet and posterior MV leaflet), requiring an annuloplasty ring. An Alferi repair technique may also be used, which involves suturing the A2 and P2 segments of the anterior MV leaflet and posterior MV leaflet, resulting in a double-barreled MV orifice. A baseline area of the MV is measured by planimetry (usually more than 2.5 cm^2) in addition to CW Doppler determination of the mean transvalvular gradient.

External splinting with a constraining jacket or internal splinting is designed to reduce wall stress and myocardial demands by reducing the wall tension related to the internal LV diameter. Both procedures require similar IOE evaluation of those issues previously addressed. In addition, assessing the impact of such splinting on systolic and diastolic function are necessary. This may be accomplished by determination of global EF using volumetric calculations, global estimation of function, and PW interrogation of mitral inflow and pulmonary veins. 3D IOE has also been used to demonstrate the impact of such procedures on wall stress and overall LV performance. Given the expanding patient population of candidates for these procedures, this will become an expanding area for both research and clinical responsibilities shouldered by the cardiovascular anesthesiologist.

Organ Transplantation

Although the use of IOE in organ transplantation is not an absolute indication, its availability, on a moments notice, is required to evaluate problems encountered during these procedures. In addition to its use as an intraoperative monitor, each of the transplant procedures has specific diagnostic indications.

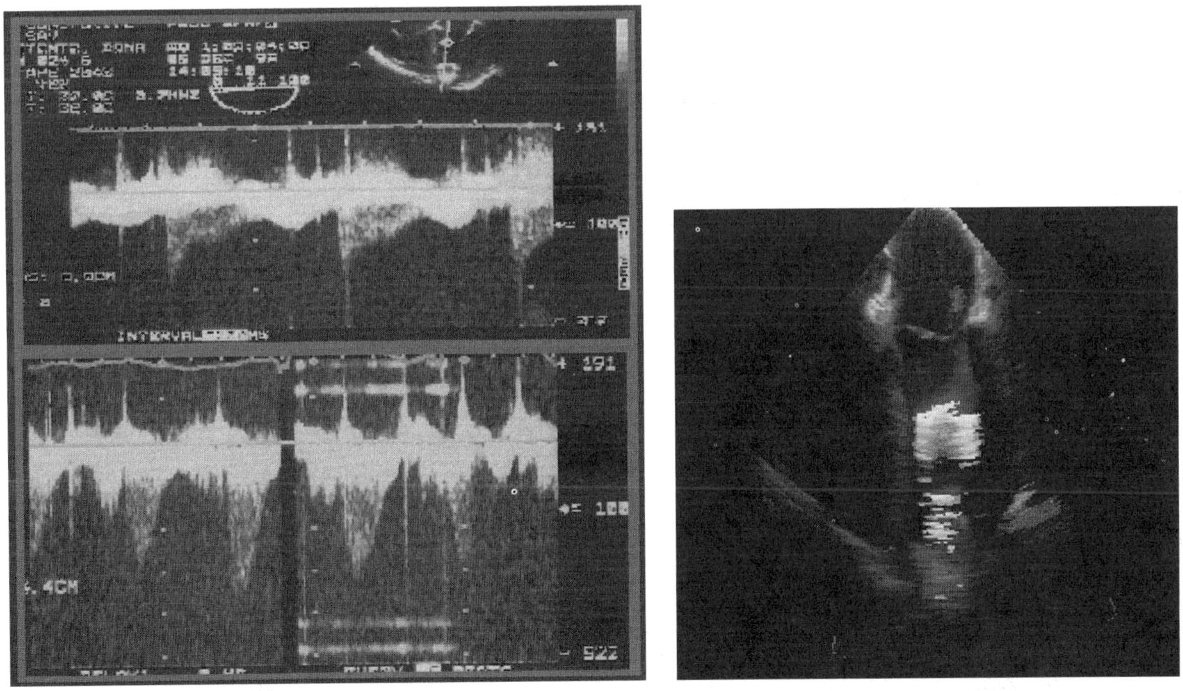

FIGURE 9-38. Left ventricular assist device cannula obstruction. Continuous wave doppler. Normal < 2.2 m/s; Obstructed > 3 m/s. (See right panel of figure in Color Figure 9-38, between pages 560 and 561.)

Heart Transplantation

The issues that must be addressed by IOE to ensure the success of heart transplant procedures include (a) RV function, (b) LV function, (c) vascular anastomoses, (d) potential shunting, which may lead to hypoxemia, (e) presence of embolic material (thrombi or intracardiac air), (f) unanticipated valve dysfunction, (g) status of ventricular support devices before explantation, and (h) evaluation of arterial cannulation and cross-clamp sites. One of the most important determinants of success of the transplant procedure is the function of the RV. IOE not only may characterize the degrees of RV dysfunction but also permits the determination of the underlying etiology (LV dysfunction, pulmonary hypertension, right coronary artery ischemia, TV dysfunction). With the growing number of patients awaiting cardiac transplantation, hearts that previously may not have been considered acceptable are being used increasingly. Consequently, there may be transient degrees of myocardial dysfunction, which require valve repair procedures or coronary grafting at the time of transplantation. Evaluation of the vascular anastomoses is required in circumstances of hemodynamic or respiratory instability. Any CW velocities that are more than 1.5 m/second or CF Doppler detection of turbulent flow should be evaluated thoroughly to exclude vascular obstruction (114).

Lung Transplantation

Lung transplantation is one of the most challenging anesthetics that anesthesiologists perform. These challenges include (a) preexisting cardiorespiratory disease, (b) the impact of one-lung ventilation on RV function and LV filling, (c) risk of embolism (air or thrombi), (d) potential for CPB, (e) reperfusion injury to the pulmonary vasculature, and (f) possible complications related to the vascular anastomoses. Due to the presence of pulmonary hypertension in many lung transplantation patients, commonly employed methods of assessing ventricular pressures are highly inaccurate. Consequently, IOE permits a more accurate method of preload assessment. Before removal of the lung, cross-clamping of the PA while imaging the RV permits the determination of the necessity for using CPB (115). Should the RV dilate and have a marked reduction in systolic function despite pharmacologic intervention, CPB should probably be employed. Additionally, IOE has proved useful in diagnosing unsuspected LVOT obstruction, pulmonary venous obstruction, and posttransplant RV dysfunction. In patients with posttransplant pulmonary edema, the differential diagnosis includes LV dysfunction, obstruction of pulmonary venous flow (secondary to stenosis of the venous anastomosis or compression of the veins from pulmonary hyperinflation), and reperfusion injury. Interrogation of the surgical venous anastomosis with PW or color Doppler may identify high-velocity flow (more than 1.5 m/second) or turbulence indicative of anastomotic stenosis that would require closer surgical inspection (116).

FUTURE CONSIDERATIONS

Perioperative echocardiography applications continue to evolve as new developments are introduced (Table 9-36). Currently the use of high-frequency 2D TEE transducers with CF and spectral Doppler are established modalities. The intraoperative application of dobutamine stress echocardiography has recently been introduced to establish myocardial function reserve and thus help guide revascularization strategies and validate adequacy of repair after coronary bypass surgery. Among the new emerging technologies introduced with potential application in the operating room with TEE, 3D imaging and perfusion echocardiography with harmonic imaging are at the forefront (Table 9-37). The use of intravascular echocardiography transducer technology is also evolving; however, only high-frequency (12 to 20 MHz) transducer technology is currently available.

Looking down the road of developing technologies, advances in real-time 3D reconstruction of 2D images will likely become reality, which will have immediate clinical applicability in valve repair and ventricular remodeling procedures as the technology becomes more timely. The use of smaller and smaller transducers (nasal-esophageal) and ultrasound systems (handheld) will enable perioperative echocardiography to be easily portable to the postanesthesia care unit, intensive care unit, and emergency code situations in the workplace. Advances in power-Doppler harmonic imaging with PW inversion will greatly enhance quantitative perfusion assessment efforts (Table 9-37). Finally, the use of ultrasound to deliver therapeutics has been introduced. By delivering specific radio frequency signals that

TABLE 9-36. ECHOCARDIOGRAPHY MODALITIES

Established	Emerging	Developing
2D	3D (reconstruction)	3D (real time)
Fundamental Imaging Doppler	Harmonic	Doppler harmonic-pulse Inversion
Transesophageal echocardiography	Intravascular	NEE
Stress	Myocardial contrast echocardiography	Tissue characterization

TABLE 9-37. PERFUSION ECHOCARDIOGRAPHY

Fundamental Imaging	Harmonic Imaging	Power Doppler Imaging
Frequency-dependent resolution	Better resolution	Decrease resolution
Artifact	No artifact (motion)	Motion artifact
Limited bandwidth	Increase bandwidth	Decrease bandwidth
Black & white resolution problem	Black & white resolution less problematic	No problem with black & white resolution
Semiquantitative	Semiquantaitative	Visually quantitative

disrupt ultrasound imaging agents, encapsulated drugs can be delivered to specific sites in the body, thereby avoiding systemic toxicity from large doses.

The future of ultrasound with specific application in the perioperative environment continues to be an exciting and growing area. Emerging and developing technologies will place new demands on our need to understand how to use them while enabling us to understand more about the physiology, anatomy, and viability of our patients' myocardial function.

CONCLUSIONS

IOE provides the anesthesiologist with a technology that permits a more definitive quality of patient care. As a result, the anesthesiologist has become more involved in the perioperative decision-making process. It has enhanced the overall stature of the discipline through an increased visibility in the clinical care of our patients, as well as involvement in interdisciplinary research and cooperative participation in multidisciplinary education. Although these advantages have done much to further the discipline of cardiovascular anesthesia, it presents all of us with daily challenges. These include the additional responsibility of becoming competent echocardiographers and understanding the surgical management decisions, which are established on the pivotal information IOE provides. Most critical to our discipline, however, is the recognition of the potential that this engaging technology has to reduce the intraoperative vigilance given to our patients. Only when we, as a discipline, are able to consistently address these challenges will IOE become an established responsibility for the cardiovascular anesthesiologist.

REFERENCES

1. Savage RM, Cosgrove DM. A systematic approach to the evaluation of the mitral valve during surgical repair: the evolution of a discipline into the 21st century. *Anesth Analg* 1999;88:1197.
2. Thys D. *Newsletter of the Society of Cardiovascular Anesthesiologists* 1999;June.
3. Side CD, Gosling RG. Nonsurgical assessment of cardiac function. *Nature* 1971;232:335.
4. Johnson ML, Holmes JH, Spangler RD, et al. Usefulness of echocardiography in patients undergoing mitral valve surgery. *J Thorac Cardiovasc Surg* 1972;64:922.
5. Frazin L, Talano. Esophageal echocardiography. *Circulation* 1976;54:102.
6. Hisanaga K, Hisanaga A, Nagata K. et al. Transesophageal cross-sectional echocardiography. *Am Heart J* 1980;100:605.
7. Kremer P, Roizen MT, Gutman J, et al. Cardiac monitoring by transesophageal 2D echocardiography during abdominal aortic aneurysmectomy. *Circulation* 1982;66:11.
8. Topol EJ, Weiss JL, Guzman PA, et al. Immediate improvement of dysfunctional myocardial segments after coronary revascularization: detection by intraoperative transesophageal echocardiography. *J Am Coll Cardiol* 1984;4:1123.
9. Erb JM, Shanewise JS, Michaelsen LG, et al. Changes in intraoperative regional wall motion assessment using contrast echocardiography during cardiac surgery. 1999;88SCA102.
10. Thys D, Abel M, Bollen B, et al. Practice guidelines for perioperative transesophageal echocardiography. *Anesthesiology* 1996;84:986.
11. Weinger MB, Herndon OW, Gaba DM, et al. The effect of electronic record keeping and transesophageal echocardiography on task distribution, workload, and vigilance during cardiac anesthesia. *Anesthesiology* 1997;87:144.
12. Khandheria BK, Seward JB, Tajik AJ. Transesophageal echocardiography. *Mayo Clin Proc* 1994;69:856.
13. Daniel WG, Erbel R, Kasper W, et al. Safety of transesophageal echocardiography. A multicenter survey of 10,419 examinations. *Circulation* 1991;83:817.
14. Rafferty T, La Mantia KR, Davis E. Quality assurance for intraoperative transesophageal echocardiography monitoring: a report of 846 procedures. *Anesth Analg* 1993;76:228.
15. Pearlman AS, Gardin JM, Martin RP, et al. Guidelines for physician training in transesophageal echocardiography: recommendations of the American Society of Echocardiography. *J Am Soc Echocardiogr* 1992;5:187.
16. Savage RM, Licina MG, Koch CG, et al. Educational program for intraoperative transesophageal echocardiography. *Anesth Analg* 1995;81:399.
17. Stewart WJ. Intraoperative echocardiography. In: Skorton D, ed. *Cardiac imaging: principles and practice.* Philadelphia: WB Saunders, 1996:566.
18. Shanewise JS, Cheung AT, Aronson S, et al. ASE/SCA guidelines for performing a comprehensive intraoperative multiplane transesophageal echocardiographic examination: recommendations of the American Society of Echocardiography Council on Intraoperative Echocardiography Board and the Society of Cardiovascular Anesthesiologists Task Force for Certification in Perioperative Transesophageal Echocardiography. *J Am Soc Echocardiogr* 1999;12:894.
19. Savage RM, McCarthy PM, Stewart WJ, et al. Intraoperative transesophageal echocardiography (TEE) predicts right ventricular failure following implantation of the left ventricular assist

device (Heartmate) as a prolonged bridge to transplant. *Anesth Analg* 1993.

20. Carpentier AF, Lessana A, Relland J, et al. The "Physio-Ring": an advanced concept in mitral valve annuloplasty. *Ann Thorac Surg* 1995;60:1177.
21. Kumar N, Kumea M, Duran C. A revised terminology for describing surgical findings of the mitral valve. *J Heart Valve Dis* 1995;4:70.
22. Clements FM, Harpole DH, Quill T, et al. Estimation of left-ventricular volume and ejection fraction by two-dimensional transesophageal echocardiography: comparison of short axis imaging and simultaneously radionuclide angiography. *Br J Anesth* 1990;64:331.
23. Appleton CP, Hatle LK. The natural history of left ventricular filling abnormalities: assessment by two-dimensional and Doppler echocardiography. *Echocardiography* 1992;9:43.
24. Oh JK, Seward JB, Tajik AJ. Assessment of diastolic function. In: *The echo manual.* Lippincott–Raven Publishers, 1999:45.
25. Isada LR, Stewart WJ, Torelli J, et al. Morbidity and mortality is not affected by a second pump run for initially unsuccessful mitral valve repair. *J Am Soc Echocardiogr* 1992;5:318.
26. Savage RM, Guth B, White F, et al. Correlation of regional myocardial blood flow and function with myocardial infarct size during acute ischemia in the conscious pig. *Circulation* 1981;64: 284.
27. Guth B, Savage RM, White FC, et al. Determining ischemic wall dysfunction: comparison of sonomicrometry and M-mode electrocardiography. *Am Heart J* 1984;March.
28. Savage RM, Lytle BW, Aronson S, et al. Intraoperative echo is indicated in high risk coronary artery bypass surgery. *Ann Thorac Surg* 1997;64:368.
29. Nakatani S, Masuyama T, Kodama K, et al. Value and limitation of Doppler echocardiography in the quantification of stenotic mitral valve area: comparison of the pressure half-time and continuity equation method. *Circulation* 1988;77:78.
30. Oh JK, Seward JB, Tajik AJ. Assessment of valvular heart disease. In: *The echo manual.* Lippincott–Raven Publishers, 1999: 103.
31. Marwick TH, Torelli J, Obarski T, et al. Assessment of the mitral valve splitability score by transthoracic and transesophageal echocardiography. *Am J Cardiol* 1991;68:1106.
32. Pu M, Vandervoort PM, Griffin BP, et al. Quantification of mitral regurgitation by the proximal convergence method using transesophageal echocardiography. Clinical validation of a geometric correction for proximal flow constraint. *Circulation* 1995;92:2169.
33. Klein AL, Stewart WJ, Bartlett L, et al. Effects of mitral regurgitation on pulmonary venous flow and left atrial pressure: an intraoperative transesophageal echocardiographic study. *J Am Coll Cardiol* 1992;20:1345.
34. Thomas JD. How leaky is that mitral valve? Simplified Doppler methods to measure regurgitant orifice area. *Circulation* 1997; 95:548.
35. Cosgrove DM, Stewart WL. Mitral valvuloplasty. *Curr Prob Cardiol* 1989;14:359.
36. Sutton DC, Kluger R, Ahmed SU, et al. Flow reversal in the descending aorta: a guide to intraoperative assessment of aortic regurgitation with transesophageal echocardiography. *J Thorac Cardiovasc Surg* 1994;108:576.
37. Brunton L. Preliminary note on the possibility of treating mitral stenosis by surgical methods. *Lancet* 1902;1:352.
38. Lillehei CW, Gott VL, DeWall RA, et al. Surgical correction of pure mitral insufficiency by annuloplasty under direct vision. 1957;2:446.
39. Carpentier A, Deloche A, Dauptain J, et al. A new reconstructive operation for correction of mitral and tricuspid insufficiency. *J Thorac Cardiovasc Surg* 1971;61:1.
40. Duran CG, Pomar JL, Revuelta JM, et al. Conservative operation for mitral insufficiency. Critical analysis supported by postoperative hemodynamic studies in 72 patients. *J Thorac Cardiovasc Surg* 1980;79:326.
41. Kumar N, Kumea M, Duran C. A revised terminology for describing surgical findings of the mitral valve. *J Heart Valve Dis* 1995;4:70.
42. McGoon DC, et al. Repair of mitral insufficiency due to ruptured chordae tendineae. *J Thorac Cardiovasc Surg* 1969;8:289.
43. *Society of Thoracic Surgeons Clinical Database* 1999 Feb 12.
44. Stewart WJ, Salcedo EE, Cosgrove DM. The value of echocardiography in mitral valve repair. *Cleve Clin J Med* 1991;58:177.
45. Stewart WI, Currie PJ, Salcedo EE, et al. Evaluation of mitral leaflet motion by echocardiography and jet direction by Doppler color flow mapping to determine the mechanisms of mitral regurgitation. *J Am Coll Cardiol* 1992;20:1353.
46. Lambert AS, Miller JP, Merrick SH, et al. Improved evaluation of the location and mechanism of mitral valve regurgitation with a systematic transesophageal echocardiography examination. *Anesth Analg* 1999:12:974.
47. Isada LR, Stewart WJ, Torelli J, et al. Morbidity and mortality is not affected by a second pump run for initially unsuccessful mitral valve repair. *J Am Soc Echocardiogr* 1992;5:318(abst).
48. Cosgrove DM, Rosenkranz ER, Hendren WG, et al. Valvuloplasty for aortic insufficiency. *J Thorac Cardiovasc Surg* 1991; 102:571.
49. Stewart WJ, Gillam L, Morehead AJ, et al. Impact of intraoperative echocardiography on homograft aortic valve surgery. *J Am Coll Cardiol* 1993;21:17a(abst).
50. al-Halees Z, Kumar N, Gallo R, et al. Pulmonary autograft for aortic valve replacement in rheumatic disease: a caveat. *Ann Thorac Surg* 1995;60:S172.
51. Rubay JE, Raphael D, Sluysmans T, et al. Aortic valve replacement with allograft/autograft: subcoronary versus intraluminal cylinder or root. *Ann Thorac Surg* 1995;60:S78.
52. David TE. Aortic valve repair in patients with Marfan syndrome and ascending aorta aneurysms due to degenerative disease. *J Cardiac Surg* 1994;9:182.
53. Starr A, Edwards ML. Mitral replacement: clinical experience with a ball valve prosthesis. *Ann Surg* 1961;154:726.
54. Baumgartner H, Kahn S, Der-Robertis M, et al. Discrepancies between Doppler and catheter gradients in aortic prosthetic valves *in vitro:* a manifestation of localized gradients and pressure recovery. *Circulation* 1990;82:1467.
55. Wigle ED, Adelman AG, Silver MD. Pathophysiologic considerations in muscular subaortic stenosis. In: Wolstenholme GEW, O'Conner M, eds. *Hypertrophic obstructive cardiomyopathy. CIBA Foundation Study.* London: J & A Churchill, 1971: 63.
56. Levine RA. Echocardiographic assessment of the cardiomyopathies. In: Weyman AE, ed. *Principles and practice of echocardiography,* 2nd ed. Philadelphia: Lea & Febiger, 1994.
57. Pollick C, Rakowski H, Wigle ED. Muscular subaortic stenosis; the quantitative relationship between systolic anterior motion and the pressure gradient. *Circulation* 1984;69:43.
58. Herrick B, Lytle BW, Rosencranz ER, et al. Myectomy for HOCM: early and late results. *Ann Thorac Surg* 1995:110:195.
59. Nagueh SH, Lakkis NM, He ZX, et al. Role of myocardial contrast echocardiography during nonsurgical septal reduction therapy for hypertrophic obstructive cardiomyopathy. *J Am Coll Cardiol* 1998:32:225.
60. Konstadt SN, Reich DL, Quintana C, et al. The ascending aorta: how much does transesophageal echocardiography see? *Anesth Analg* 1994;78:240.

61. Davila-Roman VG, Phillips KJ, Daily BB, et al. Intraoperative transesophageal echocardiography and epiaortic ultrasound for assessment of atherosclerosis of the thoracic aorta. *J Am Coll Cardiol* 1996;28:942.
62. Blauth C, Cosgrove DM, Webb BW. Atheroembolism from the ascending aorta: an emerging problem in cardiac surgery. *J Thorac Cardiovasc Surg* 1992:103:1104.
63. Afridi I, Grayburn PA, Panza JA, et al. Myocardial viability during dobutamine echocardiography predicts survival in patients with coronary artery disease and severe left ventricular systolic dysfunction. *J Am Coll Cardiol* 1998;32:921.
64. Davila-Roman VG, Waggoner AD, Sicard GA, et al. Dobutamine stress echocardiography predicts surgical outcome in patients with an aortic aneurysm and peripheral vascular disease. *J Am Coll Cardiol* 1993;21:957.
65. Langan EM III, Youkey JR, Franklin DP, et al. Dobutamine stress echocardiography for cardiac risk assessment before aortic surgery. *J Vasc Surg* 1993;18:905.
66. Poldermans D, Fioretti PM, Foster T, et al. Dobutamineatropine stress echocardiography for assessment of perioperative and late cardiac risk in patients undergoing major vascular surgery. *Eur J Vasc Surg* 1994;8:286.
67. Madu EC, Ahmar W, Arthur J, et al. Clinical utility of digital dobutamine stress echocardiography in the noninvasive evaluation of coronary artery disease. *Arch Intern Med* 1994;154:1065.
68. Afridi I, Kleiman NS, Raizer AK, et al. Dobutamine echocardiography in myocardial hibernation: optimal dose and accuracy in predicting recovery of ventricular function after coronary angioplasty. *Circulation* 1995;91:663.
69. Smart SC, Sawada S, Ryan T, et al. Low-dose dobutamine echocardiography detects reversible dysfunction after thrombolytic therapy of acute myocardial infarction. *Circulation* 1993;88: 405.
70. Senior R, Lahiri A. Enhanced detection of myocardial ischemia by stress dobutamine echocardiography utilizing the "biphasic" response of wall thickening during low and high dose dobutamine infusion. *J Am Coll Cardiol* 1995;26:26.
71. Berthe C, Pierard LA, Hiernaux M, et al. Predicting the extent and location of coronary artery disease in acute myocardial infarction by echocardiography during dobutamine infusion. *Am J Cardiol* 1986;58:1167.
72. Eichelberger JP, Schqarz KQ, Black ER, et al. Predictive value of dobutamine echocardiography just before noncardiac vascular surgery. *Am J Cardiol* 1993;72:602.
73. Kiat H, Maddahi J, Yang LD, et al. Late reversibility of thallium-201 myocardial tomographic defects: an acute marker of myocardial viability. *Circulation* 1987;76:IV.
74. Aronson S, Lee BK, Wiencek JG, et al. Assessment of myocardial perfusion during CABG surgery with two dimensional transesophageal contrast echocardiography. *Anesthesiology* 1991; 75(3):433.
75. Villanueva FS, Spotnitz WD, Jayaweera AR, et al. Online intraoperative quantitation of regional myocardial perfusion during coronary artery bypass graft operations with myocardial contrast two-dimensional echocardiography. *J Thorac Cardiovasc Surg* 1992;104(6):1524.
76. Spotnitz WD, Keller MW, Watson DD, et al. Success of internal mammary bypass grafting can be assessed intraoperatively using myocardial contrast echocardiography. *J Am Coll Card* 1998;12(1):196.
77. Aronson S, Savage R, Fernandez A, et al. Assessing myocardial perfusion with Albunex during coronary artery bypass surgery: technical considerations and safety of aortic root injections. *J Cardiothor Vasc Anesth* 1996;10(6):713.
78. Barilla F, Gheorghiade M, Alam M, et al. Low-dose dobutamine in patients with acute myocardial infarction identifies viable but not contractile myocardium and predicts the magnitude of improvement in wall motion abnormalities in response to coronary revascularization. *Am Heart J* 1991;122(6):1522.
79. Voci P, Bilotta F, Caretta Q, et al. Low dose dobutamine echocardiography predicts the early response of dysfunctional myocardial segments to coronary artery bypass grafting. *Am Heart J* 1995;129:521.
80. Sabia PJ, Power ER, Ragosta M, et al. An association between collateral blood flow and myocardial viability in patients with recent myocardial infarction. *N Engl J Med* 1992;327(26):1825.
81. Ito H, Tomooka T, Sakai N, et al. Lack of myocardial perfusion immediately after successful thrombolysis. A predictor of poor recovery of left ventricular function in anterior myocardial infarction. *Circulation* 1992;85(5):699.
82. Iliceto S, Galiuto L, Marchese A, et al. Analysis of microvascular integrity, contractile reserve, and myocardial viability after acute myocardial infarction by dobutamine echocardiography and myocardial contrast echocardiography. *Am J Cardiol* 1996; 77(7):441.
83. Afridi I, Kleiman NS, Raizner AK, et al. Dobutamine echocardiography in myocardial hibernation: optimal dose and accuracy in predicting recovery of ventricular function after coronary angioplasty. *Circulation* 1995;91(3):663.
84. Marcovitz PA, Armstrong WF. Dobutamine stress echocardiography: diagnostic utility. *Herz* 1991;16(5):372.
85. Villanueva FS, Kaul S, Glasheen WP, et al. Intraoperative assessment of the distribution of retrograde cardioplegia using myocardial contrast echocardiography. *Surg Forum* 1990;12:252.
86. Voci P, Bilotta F, Caretta Q, et al. Mechanisms of incomplete cardioplegia distribution during coronary artery surgery. An intraoperative transesophageal contrast echocardiography study. *Anesthesiology* 1993;79(5):904.
87. Zaroff J, Aronson S, Lee BK, et al. The relationship between immediate outcome after cardiac surgery, homogeneous cardioplegia delivery, and ejection fraction. *Chest* 1994;106(1):38.
88. Aronson S, Lee BK, Zaroff JG, et al. Myocardial distribution of cardioplegic solution after retrograde delivery in patients undergoing cardiac surgical procedures. *J Thorac Cardiovasc Surg* 1993;105(5):214.
89. Aronson S, Lee BK, Liddicoat JR, et al. Assessment of retrograde cardioplegia distribution using contrast echocardiography. *Ann Thorac Surg* 1991;52(4):810.
90. Winkelmann J, Aronson S, Young CJ, et al. Retrograde-delivered cardioplegia is not equally distributed to the right ventricle free wall and septum. *J Cardiothorac Vasc Anesth* 1995;9(2):135.
91. Allen BS, Winkelmann JW, Hanafy H, et al. Retrograde cardioplegia does not adequately perfuse the right ventricle. *J Thorac Cardiovasc Surg* 1995;109(6):1116.
92. Villanueva FS, Spotnitz WD, Glasheen WP, et al. New insights into the physiology of retrograde cardioplegia delivery. *Am J Physiol* 1995;268:H1555.
93. Quintilio C, Voci P, Bilotta F, et al. Risk factors of incomplete cardioplegic solution during coronary artery grafting. *J Thorac Cardiovasc Surg* 1995;109(3):439.
94. Aronson S, Jacobsohn E, Savage R, et al. The influence of collateral flow on the antegrade and retrograde distribution of cardioplegia in patients with an occluded right coronary artery. *Anesthesiology* 1998;89:1099.
95. Cyran SE, Kimball TR, Meyer RA, et al. Efficacy of intraoperative transesophageal echocardiography in children with congenital heart disease. *Am J Cardiol* 1989;63:594.
96. Fyfe DA, Ritter SB, Snider AR, et al. Guidelines for transesophageal echocardiography in children. *J Am Soc Echocardiogr* 1992; 5:640.
97. Stevenson JG. Adherence to physician training guidelines for pediatric transesophageal echocardiography affects the outcome

of patients undergoing repair of congenital cardiac defects. *J Am Soc Echocardiogr* 1999;12:165.
98. Zestos MM, Chehade M, Mossad EB. A transesophageal echocardiography probe causes airway obstruction in an older child. *J Cardiothorac Vasc Anesth* 1998;12:65.
99. Andropoulos DB, Ayres NA, Stayer SA, et al. The effect of transesophageal echocardiography on ventilation in small infants undergoing cardiac surgery. *Anesth Analg* 2000;90:47.
100. Russell IA, Miller-Hance WC, Silverman NH. Intraoperative transesophageal echocardiography for pediatric patients with congenital heart disease. *Anesth Analg* 1998;87:1058.
101. Sabry AF, Reller MD, Silberbach M, et al. Comparison of four Doppler echocardiographic methods for calculating pulmonary-to-systemic shunt flow ratios in patients with ventricular septal defect. *Am J Cardiol* 1995;75:611.
102. Stevenson JG. Comparison of several noninvasive methods for estimation of pulmonary artery pressure. *J Am Soc Echocardiogr* 1989;2:157.
103. Huhta JC, Glasow P, Murphy DJ, et al. Surgery without catheterization for congenital heart defects: management of 100 patients. *J Am Coll Cardiol* 1987;9:823.
104. Mossad EB, Murphy D, Siker D, et al. Transesophageal echocardiography in the management of children for pulmonary artery banding procedures. *Anesthesiology* 1995;83:A491.
105. Ungerleider RM, Kisslo JA, Greeley WJ, et al. Intraoperative echocardiography during congenital heart operations: experience from 1,000 cases. *Ann Thorac Surg* 1995;60:S539.
106. Ramamoorthy C, Lynn AM, Stevenson JG. Pro: transesophageal echocardiography should be routinely used during pediatric open cardiac surgery. *J Cardiothorac Vasc Anesth* 1999;13:629.
107. San Roman JA, Vilacosta L, Castillo LA, et al. Role of transesophageal echocardiography in the assessment of patients with composite aortic grafts for therapy in acute aortic dissection. *Am J Cardiol* 1994;73:519.
108. Simon P, Owen AN, Havel M, et al. Transesophageal echocardiography in the emergency surgical management of patients with aortic dissection. *J Thorac Cardiovasc Surg* 1992;103:1113.
109. Cigarroa JE, Isselbacher EM, DeSanctis RW, et al. Diagnostic imaging in the evaluation of suspected aortic dissection. *N Engl J Med* 1993;328:35.
110. Keren A., Kim CB, Hu BS, et al. Accuracy of biplane and multiplane esophageal echocardiography and transesophageal echocardiography. *J Am Coll Cardiol* 1996;28:627.
111. Hatle LK, Appelton CP, Popp RL, et al. Differentiation of constrictive pericarditis and restrictive cardiomyopathy by Doppler echocardiography. *Circulation* 1989;79:357.
112. Klodas E, Nishimura R, Appleton C, et al. Doppler evaluation of patients with constrictive pericarditis: use of tricuspid regurgitation velocity curves to determine enhanced ventricular interaction. *J Am Coll Cardiol* 1996:28:652.
113. Armstrong WF, Schilt BF, Helper DJ, et al. Diastolic collapse of the right ventricle with cardiac tamponade: an echocardiographic study. *Circulation* 1982;65:1491.
114. Suriana RJ. Transesophageal echocardiography during transplantation. *J Cardiothorac Vasc Anesth* 1998;12:686.
115. Licina M, Savage RM, Brown M. TEE should be utilized during anesthesia for patients undergoing lung transplantation. *Anesthesiology* 1994;81:3.
116. Reich DL, Resnick A, Shore-Lesserson L, et al. Doppler assessment of right ventricular function. *Anesthesiology* 1992;77:A10.
117. Hausman D, Daniel WE, Mugge A, et al. Imaging of pulmonary artery and vein anastomosis by transesophageal echocardiography after lung transplantation. *Circulation* 1992;86:11251.

10

CARDIOVASCULAR PHARMACOLOGY OF ANESTHETICS

MICHAEL P. EATON
PETER L. BAILEY

The practice of cardiac anesthesia has evolved considerably. Early techniques, employing predominantly high concentrations of halothane, presented significant challenges. Surgical and anesthetic morbidity and mortality rates were high. Lowenstein (1) and Stanley (2) introduced the practice of administering large doses of opioids as primary or sole anesthetics. Morphine, 0.5 to 3.0 mg/kg, administered intravenously, did not alter or sometimes improved the cardiovascular status of patients with significant valvular disease. Problems with incomplete amnesia, histamine release, prolonged postoperative respiratory depression, increased blood volume requirements secondary to marked vasodilation, hypotension, and hypertension diminished the popularity of morphine as a sole anesthetic (3–6).

Large doses of fentanyl did not produce many of the unwanted adverse hemodynamic effects associated with large doses of morphine. High-dose fentanyl (75 to 150 μg/kg), and subsequently sufentanil (15 to 30 μg/kg), administered as the primary anesthetic, was a mainstay of cardiac anesthetic techniques throughout the 1980s. Although numerous supplements (e.g., benzodiazepines, potent inhaled anesthetics) were frequently coadministered, only modest doses of these other agents were required to ensure amnesia and cardiovascular stability with high-dose opioid anesthetic regimens.

The popularity of high-dose opioid anesthesia for patients undergoing cardiac surgery has greatly diminished. The reasons for this are several. High doses of opioids as sole or primary anesthetics are not consistently reliable. There is a lack of evidence substantiating any significant outcome benefit associated with the use of large doses of opioids (7,8). Importantly, "fast-track" success can be impeded by large doses of opioids (see later discussion) (9,10).

The concept of a "cardiac" anesthetic has become more, not less, obscure over time (11). There is a lack of compelling evidence that one anesthetic, or combination of anesthetics, is superior or preferred. Nevertheless, anesthesiologists remain concerned with the impact that any drug or drug combination can have on the hemodynamic determinants of myocardial oxygen supply and demand and cardiovascular performance in a host of cardiac conditions. In addition, other factors, including concomitant medical conditions and the medications patients are receiving or have recently discontinued, can significantly alter the pharmacodynamic profile of anesthetics. Advances in the methods of administering intravenous agents have also influenced cardiac anesthetic practices (see Pharmacokinetics). Administering intravenous agents by giving appropriate loading doses and maintaining therapeutic drug concentrations via continuous infusion can be advantageous compared with single or even multiple bolus techniques (Table 10-1). Possible benefits of continuous infusion of intravenous drugs in anesthesia are more stable blood and effect site drug concentrations, better hemodynamic control, reduced drug wastage, reduced awareness, and more predictable emergence from anesthesia. The balanced anesthetic approach, often using continuous intravenous infusions of multiple anesthetic and vasoactive agents, combined with modest doses of inhaled agents, allows for optimal perioperative hemodynamic control in the patient undergoing cardiac surgery.

TABLE 10-1. POTENTIAL ADVANTAGES OF CONTINUOUS INFUSIONS OVER INTERMITTENT BOLUSES OF INTRAVENOUS DRUGS IN ANESTHESIA

Decreased total dose
Greater hemodynamic stability
Decreased side effects (e.g., rigidity)
Decreased need for intraoperative supplementation
More rapid recovery of consciousness
Less respiratory depression and need for antagonists
Less pain in the immediate postoperative period
Decreased discharge time
Decreased potential for patient awareness

M. P. Eaton and P. L. Bailey: Department of Anesthesiology, University of Rochester and Strong Memorial Hospital, Rochester, New York 14642

STRESS REDUCTION AND OUTCOME

There was considerable interest in the past in the pharmacologic modification of hormonal and metabolic indices of the stress response to surgical trauma (11–13). The term "stress response" has been used extensively to describe the physiologic and pathophysiologic processes that occur when patients encounter a significant insult (14,15). The main components of the neuroendocrine stress response are the corticotropin-releasing hormone brain centers (e.g., paraventricular hypothalamic nucleus) and the locus-ceruleus-norepinephrine/autonomic nervous system (13). Hormonal and metabolic responses to surgery can be extreme and may contribute to operative mortality (16).

Increases in metabolism and substrate mobilization are part of the stress response. Although such responses are undoubtedly important, at times they can be deleterious, especially when very ill patients undergo major procedures. Increases in plasma catecholamine concentrations may increase cardiac risk, and increases in protein catabolism may delay recovery. Some evidence suggests that anesthetic techniques or agents that minimize this stress response might reduce morbidity and mortality in a variety of circumstances (16–18). Others suggest that the anesthetic technique has no an impact on outcome (7). This may relate in part to the fact that anesthesia-induced reductions in metabolic responses to surgery are usually short lived (19–21). Strong interest continues in the investigation of certain stress responses, such as the systemic inflammatory response to cardiopulmonary bypass (CPB) (see Part III of this book).

FAST-TRACK APPROACHES

Cost containment efforts, as well as a recognition of the potential for harm and adverse events associated with mandatory periods of controlled mechanical ventilation, sedation, and intensive care, have led to the widespread endorsement of fast-track approaches to the care of patients undergoing cardiac surgery and anesthesia. "Fast track" and "early extubation" are terms intended to describe a clinical pathway or process of patient care that is broad in concept, multidisciplinary, and not limited to expeditious tracheal extubation. Successful fast-track programs incorporate virtually all aspects of patient care. Key principles to fast-track care of the cardiac patient are meticulous and expeditious surgical and anesthetic management and a comprehensive systems approach beginning with preoperative patient education and continuing through the postoperative period. All involved health care personnel need to participate in order to optimize fast-track care success.

There is consensus that the medical and economic implications of fast-track care are significant. Morbidity and mortality are not increased, and medical costs are decreased (22).

TABLE 10-2. PATIENT-RELATED FACTORS MOST COMMONLY ASSOCIATED WITH FAST-TRACK FAILURE

Preoperative
Emergency procedure
Recent myocardial infarction
Elderly patient
Complex surgery (reoperation, combination cases, circulatory arrest)
Intraoperative
Hemorrhage
Need for significant pharmacological support
Intraaortic balloon pump
Cardiopulmonary bypass time >2 hr
Postoperative
Excessive sedation and/or muscle relaxation
Coagulopathy, hemorrhage
Hemodynamic instability
Myocardial infarct
Renal insufficiency
Cerebrovascular accident, encephalopathy
Arrhythmias, atrial fibrillation

Studies continue to address how to predict which patients should be fast-track candidates. It appears that common sense rules: patients who are likely to fail fast-track care pathways include the very elderly, the very ill, and those who require complex operations (Table 10-2). The most likely factors to result in delayed tracheal extubation include increased age, female gender, need for intraaortic balloon counterpulsation and inotropes, hemorrhage, and arrhythmia (23). Nevertheless, prediction of fast-track pathway appropriateness and success remains imperfect. No doubt that other factors, such as emergency operation or reoperation, also impede fast-track success. However, it is usually feasible to employ fast-track–compatible anesthetic techniques for most patients undergoing cardiac anesthesia and to allow for fast tracking should patients meet criteria. Depending on the patient population, 50% to 75% of cardiac surgical patients should be able to undergo tracheal extubation within the first 10 hours after surgery. The incidence of tracheal reintubation with fast-track management ranges from 1 to 7% (24).

Potential risks associated with fast-track approaches can be controlled (22,25). Although tracheal extubation can be associated with myocardial ischemia, early extubation (4 to 10 hours postoperatively) may actually lead to reductions in overall sympathoadrenal stress. It is possible to extubate cardiac surgical patients at the end of surgery in the operating room, and patients undergoing beating heart surgery may be particularly suited to such an approach. However, several factors mitigate against extubating most cardiac surgical patients in the operating room when CPB is employed. It is advisable to first ensure adequate thermoregulation, hemostasis, and cardiovascular function.

PHARMACOKINETICS

Tremendous advances have been made in clinical pharmacology and especially in the field of pharmacokinetics. These advances have played an integral part in the evolution of cardiac anesthesia and have allowed safer and more precise anesthetic techniques to be developed. Briefly, these advances have highlighted the usefulness of the concept of the "context-sensitive half-time" and the irrelevance of the terminal half-life.

Half-life, perhaps the most familiar and widely used concept in pharmacokinetics, is the parameter employed to describe the rate at which a drug concentration declines. The clinical relevance of terminal elimination half-life is particularly obscure in anesthesia. In addition, with modern multicompartmental drug models there are as many half-lives to consider as there are compartments. Although the terminal half-life from multicompartmental models has traditionally been the pharmacokinetic parameter relied on for predictions regarding the duration of drug effect, it can be grossly misleading. Distribution volumes and clearances can be similarly confusing to apply clinically. This confusion relates to the complex way in which these multiple pharmacokinetic parameters interact. A drug whose pharmacokinetics is described by a three-compartment model, for example, has three half-lives, three clearances, and four distribution volumes (the steady-state distribution volume is the sum of the three compartment volumes). The interactions among these parameters are virtually impossible to predict without the aid of computers (26). The terminal elimination half-life has minimal impact on the overall decline in drug concentration within the range of clinical significance, because most of the concentration decrease is accounted for by other components of the model.

The primary shortcoming of half-lives in pharmacology is that they fail to account for the important influence of distribution processes on drug disposition. The term "distribution processes" refers to the net transfer of drug between the central compartment and the peripheral compartments. Depending on the size of the peripheral compartment and the rate at which drug transfer occurs, distribution into or out of peripheral compartments can have a major impact on the profile of drug concentration versus time.

Recently introduced computer simulation techniques predict the time necessary to achieve a 50% decrease in drug concentration after termination of a variable-length continuous infusion to a steady-state drug level. Using concepts developed by Shafer and Varvel, these simulations are an attempt to provide context-sensitive half-times ($CST_{1/2}$) as proposed by Hughes et al. (27). In this case the "context" is the duration of a continuous infusion. The $CST_{1/2}$ has also been referred to as the 50% decrement time (Fig. 10-1). Such simulations are intended to provide more clinically relevant meaning to pharmacokinetic parameters. The shapes and relationships of these curves vary depending on the percentage decrease in concentration required. For some

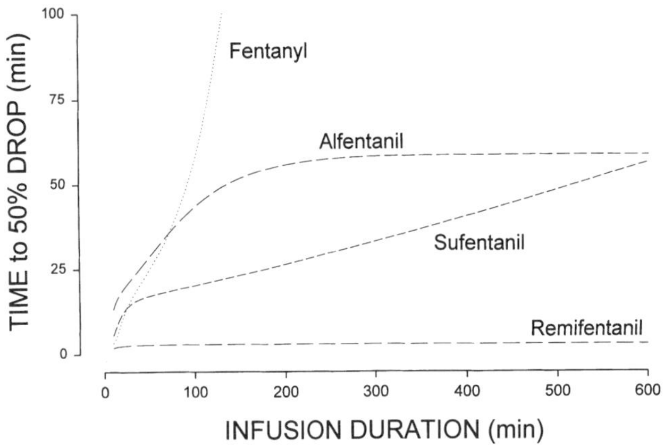

FIGURE 10-1. A graphical representation of the context-sensitive half-times for some of the fentanyl congeners. A simulation of the time required for a 50% decrease in plasma concentration after termination of continuous infusions of varying duration is depicted. (Reprinted with permission from Egan TD, Lemmens HJ, Fiset P, et al. The pharmacokinetics of the new short-acting opioid remifentanil (GI87084B) in healthy adult male volunteers [see comments]. *Anesthesiology* 1993;79:881.)

anesthetic techniques, a 50% decrease in concentration is not sufficient to permit spontaneous ventilation at the end of the operation (e.g., high-dose opioid anesthesia for cardiac surgery). In such cases, the 80% decrement time (or some other percentage) may be more clinically useful (28). Notably, the time-versus-drug concentration curves can differ in shape and slope depending on the targeted percentage decline that is simulated.

PHARMACODYNAMICS

Key to understanding the cardiovascular pharmacodynamics of drugs in anesthetic practice is knowing the impact of individual agents on myocardial contractility, preload, afterload, and heart rate. These important determinants of myocardial oxygen demand and cardiac performance are integral to understanding the goals of a cardiac anesthetic. Evaluations of the impact of anesthesia on myocardial ischemia and infarction, arrhythmias, the distribution of coronary artery blood flow, and baroreceptor function can further delineate how drugs can alter cardiovascular function (Fig. 10-2). Can a particular drug worsen perfusion of a myocardial area at risk for extension of infarction? What heart rate is optimal to minimize myocardial oxygen demand but maintain adequate diastolic blood pressure? Can an anesthetic alter coronary artery tone and redistribute blood flow in potentially deleterious ways? Although not always readily discernible clinically, is it preferable to preserve or blunt baroreceptor-mediated changes in heart rate? The astute clinician is aware of how these considerations, although often subtle, at times contribute to good clinical outcomes. Understanding how each anesthetic agent, alone

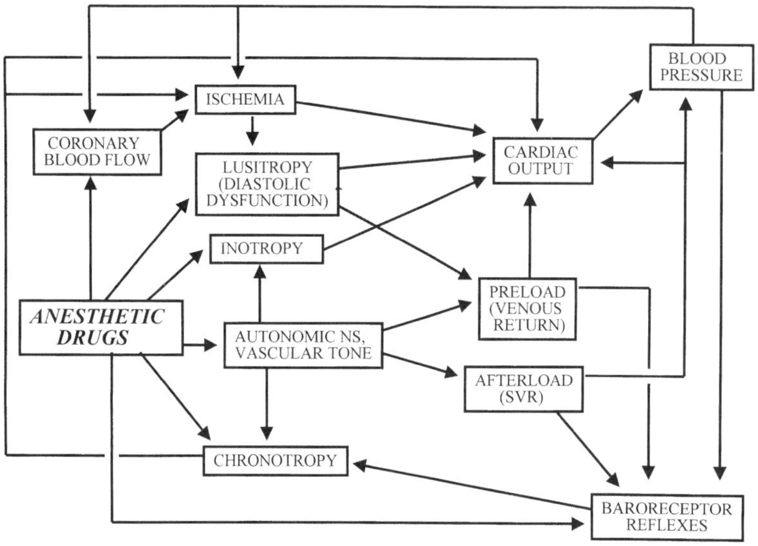

FIGURE 10-2. A schematic representation of the inter-related factors and mechanisms underlying the cardiovascular pharmacodynamic effects of anesthetic drugs. Many effects are directly mediated, but some are either directly or indirectly mediated. Compensatory effects may be advantageous (e.g., hypotension-induced tachycardia can help support cardiac output) or disadvantageous (e.g., hypotension-induced tachycardia can exacerbate ischemia).

and in combination with the other agents administered, affects cardiovascular function forms the pharmacologic basis of cardiac anesthesia.

ANESTHETIC AGENT CARDIOVASCULAR PHARMACODYNAMICS

Opioids

The utility of opioids in cardiac anesthesia goes beyond providing potent analgesia: they help promote hemodynamic stability both in the presence and in the absence of noxious stimuli. The direct cardiac actions of opioids, and in particular the effects on myocardial contractile mechanisms, are significantly less than those of many other intravenous and inhalation anesthetics. Most evidence indicates that fentanyl produces little or no change in myocardial contractility and that opioids have myocardial depression-sparing actions when combined with a potent inhaled agent (2,29).

Miller et al. (30) compared high doses of fentanyl, sufentanil, or alfentanil during anesthetic induction in patients who were scheduled for coronary artery surgery and had been premedicated with lorazepam. Anesthetic induction with fentanyl was associated with the least change in myocardial performance. Although sufentanil did not produce hemodynamic instability, it did cause some myocardial depression. Mild to no depression of cardiac index and pump function has been reported by others after use of sufentanil in humans (31,32).

Some authors have found that alfentanil causes decreases in heart rate, blood pressure, and cardiac index similar to those caused by fentanyl (32,33). Others report that alfentanil produces the least desirable hemodynamic profile (more hypotension as well as myocardial ischemia), compared with fentanyl and sufentanil, in patients undergoing coronary artery bypass grafting (CABG) (30,34,35). Remifentanil produces hemodynamic effects in dogs that include decreases in dp/dt and cardiac output, as well as in heart rate and blood pressure (36).

Maintaining preload can be integral to promoting hemodynamic stability and maintaining adequate cardiac function. During the course of an anesthetic induction, doses of opioids, such as 5 to 15 μg/kg of fentanyl or 0.5 to 1.5 μg/kg of sufentanil, usually produce minimal changes in preload. Some opioids, most notably morphine and meperidine, can cause decreases in preload through specific mechanisms such as histamine release. The modern opioids used in anesthetic practice—fentanyl, sufentanil, alfentanil, and remifentanil—do not cause histamine release.

Opioids may result in decreases in preload through venodilation in several conditions or circumstances. Most typically these are when a patient is volume depleted, is dependent on high intrinsic sympathetic tone, or requires high doses of exogenous catecholamines. Poorly compensated patients with very low ejection fractions may also be at risk. The mechanism whereby opioids can depress preload is through direct central nervous system sympatholytic and vagotonic actions (37). The widespread association between opioid receptors, endogenous opiates, and cardiovascular and autonomic regulatory areas within the central nervous system explains many opioid-induced cardiovascular pharmacodynamic actions (38).

Opioids also may have some direct vascular actions. Vasodilation after morphine may be caused by a direct effect of morphine on vascular smooth muscle (39). Sufentanil can directly relax vascular smooth muscle. Vascular studies evaluating alfentanil, fentanyl, and sufentanil in the dog demonstrated similar direct peripheral vessel smooth muscle relaxation (40). The administration of opioids does not usually decrease afterload or systemic vascular resistance (SVR) significantly.

The state of myocardial contractility can alter the apparent effects of opioids on afterload (41). Patients with good left ventricular (LV) function become hypertensive more frequently than patients with poor LV function during fentanyl anesthesia for coronary artery surgery. Patients with limited myocardial reserve cannot always maintain cardiac output in the face of an increased SVR. Blood pressure may not increase and can at times decrease in patients with poor LV function.

The predominant and usual effect of opioids on heart rate is to produce bradycardia due to stimulation of the central vagal nucleus (42). Asystole may follow opioid-induced bradycardia (43,44). Severe bradycardia and asystole can appear before or during laryngoscopy and intubation. Periods of asystole, lasting 10 to 20 seconds, may resolve on their own, or they may respond to atropine 0.4 to 0.8 mg IV, epinephrine 5 to 20 μg IV, or a precordial thump.

Compared with isoflurane, fentanyl anesthesia allows better preservation of myocardial function in a ventricular region subjected to experimental ischemia (45). During myocardial ischemia in dogs, fentanyl, compared with halothane, also allowed better functional compensation in nonischemic LV walls (46). On the other hand, functional recovery of the stunned myocardium was greater in dogs that were anesthetized with halothane, compared with fentanyl (47). Opioids were not found to protect against ischemia in animal models by some investigators (48,49).

Most recently it has been suggested that opioids can mimic ischemic preconditioning (IPC). IPC in the heart underlies the phenomenon whereby myocardial infarcts preceded by bouts of ischemia are smaller than infarcts not preceded by ischemia. Schultz and coworkers (50) demonstrated that opioid receptor stimulation results in a reduction in infarct size similar to that produced by ischemic preconditioning. The IPC effects of sufentanil are variable. It appears that IPC may be δ-opioid receptor mediated. Further studies are required to produce a better understanding of IPC (51).

Among the opioids, alfentanil is associated with more myocardial ischemia (as indicated by reversal of myocardial lactate extraction to production and worsening ventricular diastolic compliance) than fentanyl or sufentanil in patients having coronary artery surgery (30). Interestingly, hemodynamic conditions do not reliably indicate ischemia. Kleinman et al. (52) reported that hemodynamic changes were most often absent during ischemia in patients anesthetized with either fentanyl or halothane. Data from a prospective, randomized comparison of sufentanil versus enflurane, isoflurane, and halothane for coronary artery surgery revealed no difference in new intraoperative ischemia, incidence of postoperative myocardial infarction, or death (7). One report suggested that maintenance of intense analgesia into the postoperative period with sufentanil can reduce myocardial ischemia after coronary artery surgery (17).

Opioids appear to have no significant effect on coronary vasomotion or myocardial metabolism, do not produce steal phenomena, and do not diminish the ability of large coronary arteries or coronary arterioles to respond to vasoactive agents (53). In the dog, although coronary blood flow and myocardial oxygen consumption are reduced by fentanyl, the delivery of oxygen remains commensurate with demands of the heart. Regional blood flow distribution is not altered, and myocardial tissue perfusion is not compromised (54). Direct intracoronary fentanyl has no effect on LV mechanoenergetics in the dog (55).

Potent opioids applied in anesthesia usually produce little depression of great vessel and atrial baroreceptors (2,32). Opioids may depress arterial baroreflex control of the heart rate induced by hypotension or hypertension (56), but other reports suggest that this reflex is preserved under opioid anesthesia (57). Infants, after receiving 10 μg/kg of fentanyl, do demonstrate significant depression of baroreflex responses (58). This is significant because of the relationship between heart rate and cardiac output, especially in infants.

Benzodiazepines

Benzodiazepines exert their general effects by occupying benzodiazepine receptors, which modulate γ-aminobutyric acid (GABA), the major inhibitory neurotransmitter in the brain. This degree of modulation has a built-in limitation, which explains the significant degree of safety with benzodiazepines. Different benzodiazepine effects also reflect plasma and effect site concentrations; benzodiazepine receptor occupancies lower than 20% may be sufficient to produce the anxiolysis. Sedation is observed with 30% to 50% receptor occupancy, and unconsciousness requires 60% or more receptor occupancy (59). The hemodynamic effects of midazolam and diazepam also are dose dependent and related to effect site concentration. However, there is a plateau to the plasma drug concentration–cardiovascular effect relationship. The modest hemodynamic actions of the benzodiazepines, combined with their potent anxiolytic and amnestic properties, make them very useful anesthetic agents. In combination with opioids, they are a potent and complete anesthetic.

The hemodynamic effects of benzodiazepines have been widely studied (Table 10-3) (60,61). Benzodiazepines alone produce mild to modest hemodynamic effects (62). Diazepam and midazolam exert a direct myocardial depressant effect (63). Negative inotropic effects of benzodiazepines have also been reported in isolated organ preparations, although debate exists (64). In laboratory animals, both midazolam and diazepam produce dose-related decreases in maximum dP/dt (65,66). *In vivo* human studies of benzodiazepine effects, which also reflect central and local reflex

TABLE 10-3. HEMODYNAMIC CHANGES AFTER INDUCTION OF ANESTHESIA WITH VARIOUS AGENTS (%)

Parameter	Etomidate	Ketamine	Midazolam	Propofol	Thiopental
HR	−5 to +10	0 to 59	−14 to +12	−10 to +10	0 to +36
MABP	0 to 17	0 to +40	−12 to −26	−10 to −40	−18 to + 8
SVR	−10 to +14	0 to +33	0 to −20	−15 to −25	0 to +19
PAP	−9 to +8	+ 44 to +47	Unchanged	0 to −10	Unchanged
PVR	−18 to +6	0 to +33	Unchanged	0 to −10	Unchanged
PAOP	Unchanged	Unchanged	0 to −25	Unchanged	Unchanged
RAP	Unchanged	+ 15 to +33	Unchanged	0 to −10	0 to +33
CI	−20 to +14	0 to +42	0 to −25	−10 to −30	0 to −24
SV	0 to −20	0 to −21	0 to −18	−10 to −25	−12 to −35
LVSWI	0 to −33	0 to +27	−28 to −42	−10 to −20	0 to −26
dP/dt	0 to −18	Unchanged	0 to −12	Decreased	−18 to −28
References	98–100,233,234	235–238	76,239–242	80,90,243–250	240,251–254

Note: CI, cardiac index; dP/dt, pressure change over unit time; HR, heart rate; LVSWI, left ventricular stroke work index; MABP, mean arterial blood pressure; PAP, peak airway pressure; PAOP, pulmonary artery occlusion pressure; PVR, peripheral vascular resistance; RAP, right atrial pressure; SV, stroke volume, SVR, systemic vascular resistance.

compensatory changes after drug administration, do not indicate that these negative inotropic actions are problematic or very significant. Decreases in LV stroke work index and stroke index can occur due to decreases in myocardial contractility (67).

Ventricular filling pressures can decrease after induction of anesthesia with benzodiazepines. Studies of a wide variety of doses and patient populations indicate that midazolam may lower filling pressures more than diazepam and that patients with high filling pressures are more likely to experience decreases (60). These changes can be well tolerated in patients with coronary artery disease, resulting in a decrease in LV end-diastolic and arterial pressures but preserved coronary blood flow and cardiac index (68). Decreases in filling pressures may be exaggerated in the presence of hypovolemia (65,66). The mechanism whereby benzodiazepines decrease preload is not entirely clear, but it has been associated with reduced levels of circulating catecholamines, suggesting central sympatholysis (69,70).

The predominant hemodynamic change produced by benzodiazepines is a modest (0% to 20%) reduction in arterial blood pressure. This is often caused by a decrease in SVR that is similar in magnitude. Midazolam causes a somewhat greater decrease in arterial blood pressure than other benzodiazepines, but the hypotensive effect usually remains modest. The mechanism whereby benzodiazepines produce vasodilatation may include not only direct central autonomic nervous system effects but perhaps actions at postganglionic sites that control vasoreactivity (68,71). Midazolam may also produce vasodilation through endothelium-dependent (nitric oxide–releasing) and endothelium-independent (voltage-gated Ca^{2+} channel inhibiting) mechanisms (72).

Heart rate changes after benzodiazepine administration are variable, with modest (10% to 20%) decreases or increases occurring (60,73,74). However, after anesthetic induction with only a benzodiazepine and a muscle relaxant, tracheal intubation elicits significant increases in heart rate and other cardiovascular variables. Adjuvants, most commonly opioids, are required for hemodynamic stability to be maintained in the presence of noxious stimuli.

The hemodynamic stability and profile associated with benzodiazepines make them suitable agents for induction of anesthesia in the absence of noxious stimuli. In describing a purported "nitroglycerin-like" effect, Cote et al. found that diazepam (0.1 mg/kg) produced reductions in LV end-diastolic and systemic perfusion pressure but preserved coronary blood flow and cardiac index (68). Diazepam has been reported to cause significant increases in coronary artery blood flow in patients with coronary artery disease (75). Benzodiazepines also decrease total myocardial oxygen consumption (68,75), as well as some of the indices of myocardial oxygen consumption, such as the heart rate–systolic blood pressure product. Decreases in coronary blood flow that do occur after midazolam are matched with equal decreases in oxygen consumption (76).

Midazolam and presumably other benzodiazepines suppress arterial baroreflex control of the heart rate in humans (77). These effects can be reversed with flumazenil. The peripheral vascular resistance limb of the baroreflex system is not affected by benzodiazepines (78), perhaps explaining how benzodiazepines maintain hemodynamic stability (79).

Propofol

The cardiovascular actions of propofol have been well studied (Table 10-3) (80). More often than not, propofol has been demonstrated to be a direct myocardial depressant in animals and humans (81–83). Systolic shortening can be impaired by propofol, especially at high doses (250 μg/kg/minute) in either ischemic or nonischemic myocardial segments (84). Others suggest that propofol exerts a more profound negative inotropic effect in compromised than in normal myocardium. Studies of the effects of propofol using end-systolic pressure-volume relations in humans have demonstrated that propofol-induced depression of myocardial contractility is reversible with dobutamine and that the depressant effects are more pronounced and longer lasting than with equivalent doses of thiopental (85). More recently, with a relatively new technique (preload-adjusted maximal power), Schmidt et al. (86) suggested that sedative concentrations of propofol (0.65 to 2.6 μg/mL) produce significant vasodilation and hemodynamic disturbances but not direct negative inotropic effects.

It is clear that propofol causes vasodilation and, not infrequently, hypotension. It appears that both venous and arterial beds are affected, and the systemic circulation is affected more than the pulmonary circulation (87,88). Venodilation and reductions in LV preload as well as dose-related arterial vasodilation and decreases in afterload have been demonstrated to be important hemodynamic features of propofol (86). Propofol produces dose-dependent vascular smooth muscle relaxation in part via modulation of calcium influx through voltage-independent calcium channels (89).

Clinical studies report a range of heart rate effects associated with propofol (81,90). These effects may have multiple mechanisms, including modulation of the autonomic nervous system, resetting of the baroreflex, and negative dromotropic actions, mediated by muscarinic acetylcholine receptors (91,92). The negative chronotropic actions of propofol have been demonstrated to be dose dependent and mediated in part by M_2-acetylcholine receptor activation. Therefore, baroreflex-mediated tachycardia may be limited with propofol, with potentially beneficial effects on myocardial oxygen consumption (82).

Propofol does not seem to adversely affect myocardial oxygen supply and demand. Nakaigawa et al. (82) found that propofol, in the dog, produced progressive decreases in coronary blood flow that were matched by equal decreases in myocardial oxygen consumption, with no adverse effects on the coronary circulation.

Barbiturates

Barbiturates produce significant cardiovascular actions (Table 10-3). Cardiac contractility is decreased by barbiturates, through mechanisms involving calcium transport and its interaction with myofibrils (93,94). Barbiturate-induced cardiac depression may be endothelium dependent, suggesting the involvement of nitric oxide pathways (95). The dose-dependent negative inotropic actions of barbiturates are greater than those produced by benzodiazepines, etomidate, or ketamine (96) but probably not as great as the depression that can be produced by potent inhaled anesthetics.

In the absence of noxious stimulation, barbiturates decrease sympathetic tone, increase venous capacitance, and reduce preload. These effects are thought to be caused largely by medullary vasomotor center depression. These effects are greater in patients who are volume depleted or are dependent on a high degree of sympathetic tone, and they occasionally are exacerbated by associated histamine release.

Afterload is not as affected as preload by barbiturates, and it frequently remains unchanged, or modestly reduced, in the absence of noxious stimuli. Transient decreases in sympathetic outflow can lead to reductions in SVR. Sodium thiopental alone cannot prevent significant hemodynamic responses to noxious stimulation.

Heart rate typically increases after barbiturate administration, with even greater increases occurring after noxious stimulation. If the barbiturates possess any negative chronotropic actions, they are overridden by baroreceptor-mediated reflex increases in heart rate stimulated by vasodilation. Baroreceptor function does not appear to be significantly depressed by barbiturates.

Barbiturates can indirectly exacerbate myocardial ischemia through the effects delineated. The combination of decreased preload and tachycardia can create imbalances in oxygen supply and demand, especially if hypotension is significant.

Etomidate

Etomidate, 0.1 to 0.3 mg/kg, produces the fewest hemodynamic changes among the sedative-hypnotics (97–100) (Table 10-3). The inotropic effects of etomidate are slight; the drug itself has mild positive inotropic actions *in vitro* (101), but propylene glycol, the solvent that is used for the preparation of etomidate, may produce a slight negative inotropic effect. Dose-dependent decreases in sympathetic tone, venous return, preload, and cardiac contractility can occur with etomidate but are typically less than those associated with thiopental (102). Arterial blood pressure usually remains stable, and desirable myocardial oxygen supply and demand ratios are also better preserved than with other intravenous induction agents.

Ketamine

Ketamine is unique in its ability to produce generalized cardiovascular stimulation (103) (Table 10-3). Most notably, intravenous induction doses (e.g., 1 to 2 mg/kg) of ketamine result in increases in heart rate, cardiac output, pulmonary and systemic blood pressures, pulmonary vascular resistance (PVR), and SVR. Effects on pulmonary arterial pressure may be greater than on systemic arterial pressure. Increases in myocardial oxygen consumption occur and are usually met with proportional increases in coronary artery blood flow (104). These effects are not necessarily dose related, and repeat doses, or combining ketamine with other drugs, can result in opposite changes, with predominant hemodynamic depression instead of stimulation (105).

The mechanisms of action that determine the unique pharmacodynamic profile of ketamine are incompletely understood and probably complex. Direct inotropic actions may be dual and opposite (106). Cardiovascular stimulation probably results from central nervous system-mediated effects and sympathoneural and systemic release of norepinephrine (107,108). Ketamine also produces direct positive inotropic actions secondary to increased myocardial calcium influx. Functional impairment of the sarcoplasmic reticulum can occur with high concentrations of ketamine (109). The general stimulatory actions of ketamine make the drug less than ideal for routine use in cardiac anesthesia. However, in very poor-risk or hemodynamically unstable patients, induction of anesthesia with ketamine may be preferred (110–112).

α_2-Agonists

Clonidine and dexmedetomidine are agonists at α_2-adrenergic receptors. These drugs produce general inhibition of central sympathetic outflow and also have sedative and analgesic properties. Considerable interest has been generated in the use of these drugs because of the potentially beneficial effects they might have on myocardial oxygen supply-demand matching (113,114). Clonidine reduces anesthetic requirements and helps blunt hemodynamic responses to laryngoscopy and surgery. Its ability to decrease perioperative ischemia is unclear, and associated decreases in episodes of hypertension and tachycardia may also be associated with an increased incidence of hypotension and bradycardia. There may a need for more pharmacologic interventions to counter the hemodynamic effects of dexmedetomidine (115).

Dexmedetomidine, recently approved for sedation in intensive care units, is more selective for α_2- versus α_1-adrenergic receptors and is available as an intravenous agent. It has been shown to provide stable sedation and analgesia in patients after cardiac surgery, without significant respiratory depression (116). Its clinical utility remains to be completely explored and defined.

Inhaled Anesthetics

Currently used inhalation anesthetics are the gas, nitrous oxide (N_2O); the halogenated alkane, halothane; and the halogenated ethers, enflurane, isoflurane, sevoflurane, and desflurane. These agents share certain features, and other characteristics differ among classes of agents or among individual anesthetics.

All the inhalation anesthetics produce dose-related negative inotropic effects. N_2O has been demonstrated to depress various measures of LV contractile function (117), although to a lesser extent than potent inhaled agents do. Stimulation of the sympathetic nervous system by N_2O compensates, at least in part, for its negative inotropic effect.

Halothane and enflurane depress ventricular performance to similar degrees in animal and human studies (118). Isoflurane inhibits contractile function to a lesser degree than halothane and enflurane do (119). Sevoflurane and desflurane also produce negative inotropic effects, which are indistinguishable from those of isoflurane at equianesthetic concentrations (120,121). Rapid increases in desflurane concentration can stimulate the sympathetic nervous system and may temporarily mask its direct negative inotropic actions (122). The negative inotropic effects of inhalation agents can be greater in patients with poor baseline cardiac function (29,123–125). The negative inotropic effects of the potent inhaled agents appear to be mediated by alterations in intracellular calcium transport.

The effects of inhaled anesthetics on diastolic function are less well understood. Although all the inhalation agents produce a dose-related decrease in early diastolic relaxation, this appears to be caused by the negative inotropic effects of the drugs, rather than direct negative lusitropic effects. Indeed, the volatile anesthetics can improve diastolic function. These effects may be caused by a beneficial decrease in preload rather than improved lusitropy *per se*. Nevertheless, the improvement in diastolic function probably contributes to the ability of patients with poor ventricular function to tolerate anesthesia with potent inhaled agents despite their negative inotropic effects.

All the volatile agents are capable of producing vasodilation and afterload reduction through direct relaxant effects on arterial smooth muscle (126). The effect of the potent inhaled anesthetics on SVR in the intact organism is modified by intrinsic vasoregulatory mechanisms and the effects of these agents thereon (Fig. 10-2). For example, inhaled agents also directly cause decreases in preganglionic and postganglionic sympathetic activity (127), and they may decrease norepinephrine release from sympathetic postganglionic nerves (128). In studies in intact animals and humans, SVR is decreased in a dose-dependent fashion by isoflurane, enflurane, sevoflurane, and desflurane (129). Halothane has minimal direct effects on SVR (130).

As noted earlier, the inhalation anesthetics have effects on ventricular diastolic function that influence ventricular filling and preload regardless of venous capacitance and return. Atrial pressures can be increased secondary to inotropic and lusitropic effects. N_2O increases central venous pressure through increases in both venous tone and PVR, and possibly through a decrease in LV contractile function (131). Inhaled potent anesthetics can reduce preload through direct (vascular smooth muscle) and indirect (sympathetic nervous system) effects (130).

The chronotropic effects of inhaled agents may be directly or indirectly mediated (Fig. 10-2). The latter are most notably mediated through the baroreceptor reflex and central autonomic activity. The inhalation anesthetics have direct inhibitory effects on sinoatrial node activity, which would decrease heart rate in the absence of other compensatory mechanisms. Parasympathetic activity is also attenuated, as demonstrated by anesthetic-induced inhibition of the bradycardic response to hypertension (127,132). Halothane tends not to alter heart rate, because it inhibits the baroreceptor reflex (133). Enflurane also inhibits baroreceptor mechanisms, but to a lesser degree than halothane, resulting in variable increases in heart rate. Desflurane and isoflurane have little depressant effect on baroreceptor function, and these agents can be associated with significant positive chronotropic effects (122,134,135). Rapid increases in the inhaled concentrations of desflurane, and to a lesser extent those of isoflurane, may cause marked increases in heart rate due to sympathetic nervous system activation (122). The greater positive chronotropic potency of desflurane may be a result of the greater ease and rapidity with which rapid changes in plasma drug concentration can be achieved because of the poor solubility of desflurane. Sevoflurane, in contrast, has minimal effects on heart rate (136). N_2O increases heart rate through stimulation of the sympathetic nervous system (137).

The ability of halothane to sensitize the heart to the arrhythmogenic effects of epinephrine is well known (138). The other potent inhaled agents produce much less sensitization, but all of them have been demonstrated to possess some arrhythmogenic tendencies (139). In certain animal models of ventricular arrhythmias, such as those generated by disturbances in coronary flow, the potent inhaled agents can demonstrate some antiarrhythmic properties as well (140,141). Halothane, enflurane, and isoflurane have been shown to increase the electrocardiographic QT interval (142), theoretically increasing the risk of torsades de pointes.

Isolating the effects of inhalational anesthetics on coronary artery tone and blood flow in humans is difficult. The effects of surgery, concomitant medications, autonomic activity, and limitations in the ability to measure coronary flow all complicate such investigations. Halothane decreases myocardial oxygen demand (MVO_2) in accordance with its negative inotropic action; this drop in MVO_2 may be associated with an appropriate decrease in coronary flow (143,144). Volatile agents also appear to decrease neutrophil and platelet adherence to coronary endothelium after ischemia-reperfusion (145) and may even decrease platelet thrombus generation in the coronary circulation (146).

A report by Reiz et al. in 1983 (147) described apparent isoflurane-induced ischemia in patients with coronary artery disease. It was argued that isoflurane could cause myocardial ischemia by a "steal" mechanism. Steal results when one artery (artery x) has exhausted its vasodilatory reserve through autoregulation because of a flow-limiting lesion upstream and ischemia downstream. This usually occurs when stenosis becomes critical (more than 70%). It makes the flow in artery x entirely dependent on supply pressure. Drug-induced vasodilation in another artery (artery y), one that still has some vasodilatory reserve, increases flow and decreases pressure in that artery. If both arteries (x and y) are supplied by the same upstream artery, dilation of artery y can decrease pressure in the entire arterial bed and divert blood away from artery x, producing the so-called steal phenomenon. This phenomenon can produce or exacerbate ischemia. If artery x is a collateral that feeds an ischemic area, steal-prone anatomy may exist.

It was recognized early in the debate on the risk of myocardial ischemia associated with isoflurane that ischemia in anesthetized patients was more likely to be caused by tachycardia and/or hypotension than steal (148,149). Indeed, in a study of 955 patients undergoing CABG surgery, Slogoff et al. (150) failed to find an increased incidence of ischemia in patients who received isoflurane, compared with enflurane, halothane, or sufentanil. This finding did not change even when only patients with steal-prone anatomy were considered. Other studies have confirmed that isoflurane does not increase global or regional coronary artery blood flow or increase lactate production (151); nor does it increase the incidence of myocardial ischemia compared with a sufentanil-based anesthesia (152). The presence of steal-prone anatomy did not alter these findings (153). In summary, isoflurane is a weak coronary artery vasodilator. Although it may impair coronary autoregulation to some degree, there remains no clinical evidence that its use in patients with coronary artery disease and/or steal-prone coronary anatomy is likely to produce ischemia in the absence of other hemodynamic or vascular aberrations.

Desflurane produces changes in coronary artery flow similar to those of isoflurane (154). Sevoflurane appears to have weaker effects on coronary tone than isoflurane does (155). Neither desflurane nor sevoflurane has been implicated as causing or exacerbating the coronary artery steal phenomenon. N_2O has no direct effects on the coronary vasculature (156). Although there is some evidence that N_2O adversely affects myocardial oxygen supply and demand ratios, recent echocardiographic studies reveal no evidence of N_2O-induced ischemia (157).

Past concerns over the risk of coronary steal associated with isoflurane have perhaps overshadowed the fact that the potent inhaled agents can have significant protective effects in ischemic myocardium. The cardioprotective effects and mechanisms of action of the potent inhaled agents and their potential to ameliorate ischemia-reperfusion injury have been reviewed (158). The protective properties result from several mechanisms, including energy level preservation during ischemia, alteration of intracellular calcium concentrations, inhibition of free radicals, and interaction with potassium adenosine triphosphate (ATP) channels.

As early as 1976, it was documented that halothane decreases ischemia from reversible coronary occlusion in the dog (159). Potent inhaled agents have been demonstrated to also reduce infarct size after coronary ligation (160,161) and to improve diastolic mechanics during regional ischemia (162). These agents can also improve functional recovery and decrease reperfusion injury after global myocardial ischemia (163–165). These effects seem similar to those of ischemic preconditioning (166), and they may be mediated by adenosine receptor modulation.

Muscle Relaxants

Neuromuscular blocking agents (NMBs) produce their intended effects by mimicking acetylcholine at the motor end plate of skeletal muscle. Binding of drug to acetylcholine receptors at this site either produces prolonged depolarization of the muscle fiber (as with succinylcholine) or competitively prevents binding of acetylcholine to the receptors, preventing muscle depolarization (as with nondepolarizing agents). The structural resemblance between NMBs and acetylcholine explains many of the common adverse effects associated with these drugs. Because they mimic acetylcholine at sites other than the motor end plate, primarily in the autonomic nervous system, many NMBs can produce unwanted side effects.

Important cardiovascular effects mediated by muscarinic stimulation are primarily related to parasympathetic cardiac actions. Stimulation of parasympathetic vagal fibers primarily causes inhibition of sinus node function and decreased conduction in the atrioventricular node, resulting in decreased heart rate. Muscarinic receptors are also involved in negative feedback loops in the sympathetic nervous system, such that blockade of these receptors augments sympathetically mediated increases in cardiovascular tone.

Succinylcholine stimulates muscarinic receptors and can precipitate arrhythmias, including sinus bradycardia, junctional arrhythmias, and, rarely, significant ventricular arrhythmias.

Pancuronium, *d*-tubocurarine, and, to a lesser extent, rapacuronium, rocuronium, and metocurine produce increases in heart rate due to muscarinic blockade (167) (Table 10-4). Pancuronium also produces a non–receptor-mediated increase in the sympathetic response to a given stimulus by inhibiting catecholamine reuptake by adrenergic nerves (168). Nicotinic receptors mediate transmission in ganglia of both branches of the autonomic nervous system. Succinylcholine stimulates and *d*-tubocurarine and metocurine block ganglionic nicotinic receptors. Nonspecific binding to ganglionic receptors by muscle relaxants has different effects depending on the prior sympathetic/parasympathetic balance in the patient. For example, succinylcholine may be expected to produce tachycardia in a patient premedicated with an anticholinergic agent, but it would more likely produce bradycardia in a patient who has been taking β-blockers.

Histamine may be released from mast cells by immunologic mechanisms or directly by simple chemical displacement. It is the latter mechanism that is responsible for the rise in plasma histamine concentration seen after administration of certain muscle relaxants. A four- to nine-fold rise in plasma histamine produces vasodilation through actions mediated at histamine H_1 and H_2 receptors. Concomitant increases in heart rate can result from baroreceptor mechanisms. Although stimulation of myocardial H_2 receptors produces positive inotropic actions, this effect requires significantly higher histamine concentrations than those typically produced by muscle relaxants. Histamine release is seen primarily with the benzylisoquinolinium class of muscle relaxants, particularly *d*-tubocurarine, and to a lesser extent metocurine, atracurium, and mivacurium. High doses of the steroid relaxant rapacuronium may also release histamine. Histamine release may be minimized with slow or incremental administration of any of these agents. The hemodynamic consequences associated with histamine release can be attenuated by pretreatment with H_1 and H_2 blockers (169) or nonsteroidal antiinflammatory drugs (170).

TABLE 10-4. MUSCLE RELAXANT CHARACTERISTICS OF KEY INTEREST IN CARDIAC ANESTHESIA

Drug	Autonomic Ganglia	Cardiac Muscarinic	Histamine Release	Heart Rate	MAP	ED95 (mg/kg)	Clinical Duration[a]
Succinylcholine	⇑	⇑	⇑	⇑—⇓	⇑—⇓	0.3	5–10
Benzylisoquinilines							
D-tubocurarine	⇓⇓		⇑⇑⇑	—⇑	⇓	0.5	60–100
Metocurine	⇓		⇑⇑	—	⇓	0.28	60–120
Doxacurium				—	—	0.025	90–150
Atracurium			⇑⇑	—	—⇓	0.25	30–45
Mivacurium			⇑⇑	—	—⇓	0.08	15–20
Cisatracurium				—	—	0.05	40–75
Steroids							
Pancuronium		⇓⇓		⇑	⇑	0.06	60–120
Vecuronium				—	—	0.05	45–60
Pipecuronium				—	—	0.05	80–120
Rocuronium		— or ⇓		—⇑	—⇑	0.3	35–75
Rapacuronium		⇓⇓	— or ⇑	⇑	⇑	0.65	12–22

Note: ED_{95}, effective paralyzing dose in 95% of patients; MAP, mean arterial pressure.
[a] Time in minutes from intubating dose to 25% twitch recovery.

Pancuronium bromide has been used frequently for muscle relaxation during cardiac anesthesia and has been reported to provide superior hemodynamics compared with vecuronium (171) or with metocurine or metocurine-pancuronium combinations. The vagolytic actions of pancuronium tend to attenuate bradycardias and support blood pressure (172). However, others have cautioned against using pancuronium because of associated increases in heart rate and the potential to exacerbate myocardial ischemia (173). Shorten et al. (174) reported detecting no myocardial ischemia as assessed by transesophageal echocardiography after bolus injections of pancuronium in patients undergoing CABG surgery, even though increases in heart rate, blood pressure, and cardiac output occurred. Many factors alter the impact of pancuronium and other muscle relaxants on hemodynamics, including, as previously mentioned, the dose, timing, and rate of drug administration. Premedication, intravascular volume, LV function, and presence of other drugs with autonomic nervous system actions can also influence the hemodynamic consequences of NMBs (171). For example, β-adrenergic blockade often attenuates or eliminates significant pancuronium-induced tachycardias (175,176).

Vecuronium can potentiate decreases in heart rate and cardiac index after fentanyl (177), although alone it has minimal cardiovascular side effects. Combinations of vecuronium and opioids can produce negative chronotropic and inotropic effects, resulting in decreases in heart rate, cardiac output, and blood pressure and increases in the need for vasopressor support (173,178). Stimuli enhancing vagal tone may also predispose patients to bradycardia after vecuronium (179). This is probably the result of an absence of positive chronotropic effects (compared with pancuronium) rather than any direct or indirect negative inotropic effects.

O'Connor et al. (180) found that, compared with vecuronium (0.15 mg/kg), pancuronium (0.15 mg/kg) produced tachycardia more often in patients undergoing coronary artery surgery (32% versus 7%). However, pancuronium-induced tachycardia was easily and rapidly treated and caused no differences in ischemia or perioperative myocardial infarction. Some investigators have found more stable hemodynamics with vecuronium, and still others no significant differences in the frequency of intraoperative ischemic events, with pancuronium and vecuronium (176). Consideration of the effects of pancuronium and vecuronium should take into account the fact that many studies, unlike contemporary practice, evaluated the impact of NMBs in combination with high-dose opioid anesthesia.

Metocurine (0.5 mg/kg) alone has also been reported to produce less hemodynamic fluctuation than pancuronium, although high doses (more than 0.3 mg/kg) may cause hypotension. Combining metocurine and pancuronium has several advantages, including increased speed of onset and less tachycardia and hypotension.

Doxacurium, a very potent and long acting NMB, appears devoid of cardiovascular effects and produces little to no histamine release. Doxacurium causes no circulatory changes during sufentanil-midazolam anesthesia effects (181). Murray et al. (182) observed small decreases in blood pressure and heart rate in healthy patients receiving doxacurium during balanced anesthesia with fentanyl (210 μg/kg).

Pipecuronium, in doses as high as three times the effective dose in 95% of patients (ED_{95}), has also been found to be devoid of circulatory actions in patients undergoing CABG surgery under midazolam-fentanyl anesthesia (183). Starr et al. (184) reported that neither pipecuronium nor vecuronium produced significant hemodynamic changes in CABG surgery patients receiving sufentanil anesthesia.

Mivacurium chloride produces modest decreases in blood pressure when larger doses (e.g., two times ED_{95}) are injected rapidly (less than 30 seconds) (185,186). This response probably results from histamine release. Few significant circulatory changes were associated with mivacurium (0.15 to 0.25 mg/kg over 60 seconds) in patients undergoing CABG surgery and receiving sufentanil-midazolam anesthesia (187). The changes were modest and were limited to decreases in heart rate and increases in stroke volume.

Atracurium releases histamine in proportion to dose and speed of injection. Hemodynamic changes, predominantly increases in heart rate and decreases in blood pressure, can be minimized by administering small doses slowly.

Rocuronium is usually associated with a lack of hemodynamic side effects, although occasionally increases in heart rate have been reported. *Cis*-atracurium, even with large doses, does not have cardiovascular effects and does not release histamine.

Rapacuronium, a new short-acting steroid NMB, produces mild elevations of heart rate and mild decreases in blood pressure that are dose related and of short duration. Large doses may release histamine (188).

ANESTHETIC TECHNIQUES

Synergism Among Anesthetic Agents

No one agent produces the "best" cardiac anesthetic. Anesthesia with a single agent requires a dose that produces excessive hemodynamic depression. For example, the concentrations of propofol or isoflurane required to eliminate movement after skin incision frequently produce undesirable hypotension before such stimulation. At least two if not many more drugs are required to provide complete, stable anesthesia (189,190). Anesthesiologists, as clinical pharmacologists, practice polypharmacy every day in an attempt to optimally tailor anesthetic techniques, taking advantage of drug interactions and minimizing adverse effects.

The pharmacodynamic synergism between opioids and sedative-hypnotics such as propofol is profound. Therefore, when these drugs are combined, the amounts administered should be significantly reduced. For example, the optimal plasma level of propofol is estimated to be approximately 30% less when it is combined with remifentanil (191). Benzodiazepines also potentiate the effects of opioids and decrease opioid requirements for loss of consciousness, often in a synergistic fashion (192,193).

Combinations of benzodiazepines and opioids, although occasionally preserving ventricular function, can cause significant and sometimes profound decreases in blood pressure, cardiac index, heart rate, and SVR (194). Sudden dramatic hypotension has been reported when midazolam and sufentanil are combined (195). This drug regimen may be particularly hazardous in patients with poor LV function. Some investigators have found that administration of intravenous lorazepam after tracheal intubation during high-dose fentanyl anesthesia results in fewer hemodynamic changes than other benzodiazepines (196). The slow onset of action of lorazepam may contribute to an apparent reduction of associated adverse hemodynamic effects. Fluid loading may attenuate decreases in blood pressure, ventricular filling, and cardiac output that occur when benzodiazepines are combined with opioids.

Barbiturates, droperidol, ketamine, etomidate, and propofol have all been combined with opioids for patients undergoing cardiac surgery. Both thiopental and propofol can be employed safely in combination with opioids. However, either drug can potentiate or produce hypotension if too large a dose is administered. Attempts to ensure amnesia by combining barbiturates with opioids can significantly compromise hemodynamic stability (197). It is recommended that induction doses of barbiturate administered concomitantly with opioids be reduced by more than 50%.

Several clinical studies of cardiac anesthesia with propofol and opioids have reported favorable outcomes (10,83,198–201). Propofol-fentanyl (83) and propofol-sufentanil (202) anesthesia for CABG surgery may provide acceptable conditions, but the mean arterial pressure (MAP) can decrease to levels that might jeopardize coronary perfusion, especially during the induction of anesthesia. When a propofol infusion is followed by opioid administration, MAP and heart rate can decrease by as much as 35% and 16%, respectively. These changes may be associated with similar decreases in SVR and cardiac index. Comparisons of propofol-opioid anesthesia with potent inhaled agent-opioid anesthesia demonstrate that induction doses, but not infusions, of propofol produce greater degrees of hypotension (202,203).

Other anesthetic induction agents, such as etomidate and ketamine, may be combined in low doses with opioids with little loss of cardiovascular stability. In patients scheduled for CABG, Haessler et al. found that etomidate (0.25 mg/kg) plus fentanyl (6 μg/kg) resulted in less hypotension after induction and intubation than did propofol (1 mg/kg) plus fentanyl (6 μg/kg) (204). Combinations of etomidate and opioids reduce blood pressure, cardiac index, SVR, and heart rate 5% to 20%, and dosing with such drug combinations should still be done cautiously (205). The stimulatory properties of ketamine can be attenuated by concomitant administration of other agents, including α- and/or β-adrenergic blocking agents, calcium entry blockers, benzodiazepines, and opioids.

Deterioration of cardiac function with N_2O-opioid combinations may be a result of increases in afterload (SVR and PVR increases) (29,206), increases in coronary vascular resistance resulting in impaired coronary blood flow, lower inspired oxygen concentration associated with the use of N_2O, or direct myocardial depression (207). Myocardial dysfunction with N_2O may not be evident with routine monitoring (i.e., blood pressure) because of the elevated SVR (208). Segmental wall motion abnormalities in areas of marginal myocardial perfusion can be demonstrated in animals when N_2O and opioids are combined (208). However, in clinical studies of patients with ischemic cardiac disease, the addition of N_2O to fentanyl or sufentanil was reported not to be associated with any new ST-segment changes or segmental wall motion abnormalities (209).

Potent inhalation agents are frequently combined in low doses (one-third to one-half of the minimum alveolar concentration) with opioids to ensure amnesia and promote immobility and hemodynamic stability. Their ability to produce cardiovascular depression in a dose-dependent manner often allows titration toward these goals (202,210). Low concentrations of potent inhalation agents in combination with opioids are usually well tolerated in patients with normal or compromised ventricular function, although perhaps less so with halothane (210).

In general, clinical trials of opioids supplemented with newer potent inhaled agents for cardiac surgery demonstrate well preserved cardiac output and minimal decreases in MAP (200,201,211). The hemodynamic effects of combining opioids with modest doses of these inhalation agents are usually additive and do not resemble the exaggerated effect on hemodynamics that have been described with some intravenous agents such as the benzodiazepines. In addition, the added advantage of being able to remove potent inhaled anesthetics results in greater flexibility and perhaps safety.

Myocardial ischemia may not, however, always be ameliorated by approaches that combine opioids with potent inhaled agents, despite apparent "good" hemodynamic control. For example, the addition of halothane to a sufentanil anesthetic to control increases in arterial blood pressure may produce hemodynamic alterations (decreased blood pressure and cardiac output) that exacerbate regional myocardial hypoperfusion and increase lactate production.

Other pharmacologic agents known to inhibit contractility, such as β-adrenergic antagonists and calcium channel blockers, can also potentiate the negative inotropic actions of the inhaled anesthetics (212). Such negative effects can be reversed with commonly used positive inotropic agents, such as β-adrenergic agonists (213), phosphodiesterase III inhibitors (212), and calcium.

ANESTHETIC MANAGEMENT

As discussed earlier, a balanced approach—one that incorporates drugs from several different classes of agents—allows the most control and flexibility in anesthesia. "Balanced anesthesia" uses a combination of agents and techniques (e.g., premedication, regional anesthesia, general anesthesia with multiple agents) to produce the different components of anesthesia that are required (i.e., analgesia, amnesia, muscle relaxation, and abolition of autonomic reflexes with maintenance of physiologic homeostasis). In modern practice, balanced anesthesia is widely applied. The use of a variety of anesthetic agents (opioids, sedative-hypnotics, benzodiazepines, potent inhaled anesthetics, and muscle relaxants) and cardiovascular drugs (e.g., β-adrenergic blockers, vasodilators, inotropes) allows clinicians numerous options. Consideration of time to onset of action and peak effect as the basis for the timing of drug administration allows for proper preemptive administration before known noxious stimuli and control of the potentially significant hemodynamic responses they can elicit. For example, tracheal intubation, skin incision, sternal splitting, aortic manipulation, and cannulation are typical stimuli that can elicit hypertensive and tachycardic responses if not properly anticipated (214).

It is well accepted that β-adrenergic blockade medication should be maintained preoperatively (196,215,216). Indeed, most medications should be continued, with the exception of monoamine oxidase inhibitors. Calcium entry blockers do not provide the same degree of protection against intraoperative ischemia that β-adrenergic blockers do (217). Evaluation of the status of stomach contents and the possibility of reflux or regurgitation should be made and appropriate steps taken.

Before the practice of admitting elective cardiac surgery patients to the hospital only on the day of their operation was instituted, patients were heavily premedicated before being taken to the operating room. The goals of premedication were to reduce anxiety and fear, enhance amnesia, and provide analgesia, especially if potentially painful procedures were to be performed before the induction of anesthesia. It was common to administer intramuscular morphine and scopolamine or oral lorazepam or diazepam. Current emphasis on same-day admission of cardiac surgery patients reduces the opportunity and time available for anesthesiologists to interview and reassure patients before their operation. Effective preoperative evaluation can reduce preoperative anxiety as well as pharmacologic premedication can. Time pressures and concerns about interference with fast-tracking have also led to reductions in pharmacologic premedication. As a result, many cardiac patients are at risk for increased anxiety and potential related problems.

It is currently common practice to give modest doses of intravenous midazolam with or without an opioid immediately before placing invasive monitors and entering the operating room. It is well known that such drug combinations can result in hypoxemia (218,219). Although evidence is scant, anxiety may contribute to hemodynamic decompensation or ischemia. Preoperatively, oxygen should most likely be given to sedated patients, although there is only a weak association proven between preoperative hypoxemia and ischemia (220).

Premedication with morphine/scopolamine, compared with lorazepam, may result in more stable hemodynamics during anesthetic induction with fentanyl (194). α_2-Agonists such as clonidine have attributes that suggest utility as premedication (113), but care must be taken to avoid hypotension and bradycardia, particularly in patients taking other sympatholytic medications.

Anesthetic induction can be achieved by combining a loading dose of an opioid, such as fentanyl (5 to 15 μg/kg) or sufentanil (0.5 to 2 μg/kg) with a reduced dose of sedative-hypnotic, such as thiopental (0.5 to 2 mg/kg) or propofol (0.5 to 1 mg/kg), and a muscle relaxant. Etomidate (0.1 to 0.3 mg/kg) or ketamine (0.25 to 2.0 mg/kg) should be considered as potentially safer alternatives to barbiturates or propofol in severely compromised patients.

Although it is important to allow 4 to 5 minutes for full onset of effect after administration of fentanyl or sufentanil, opioid-induced rigidity and neuroexcitation can occur. Vocal chord closure usually occurs with rigidity, and it prevents ventilation by bag and mask, even with a patent upper airway (221). Only administration of a muscle relaxant will alleviate this problem. Therefore, before a significant dose of an opioid is administered, the possibility of a difficult airway should be assessed. In the absence of a difficult airway, completion of anesthetic induction of the cardiac patient should proceed expeditiously after administration of the previously mentioned doses of opioid and sedative-hypnotic. Once the patient loses consciousness (e.g., loss of response to command), muscle relaxation should be immediately achieved to avoid delays in establishing the ability to ventilate the patient and secure the airway. Otherwise, opioid-induced rigidity can be associated with numerous undesirable adverse effects (Table 10-5).

Maintenance of anesthesia can be achieved with a balance of several agents: N_2O, low concentrations of potent inhalation agents, and intermittent boluses or continuous infusions of benzodiazepines, sedative-hypnotics, and opioids (Table 10-6). Simple intravenous agent infusion schemes, such as those reported by Hall et al. employing a modified Wagner method (222), demonstrate that targeted drug plasma concentrations can be maintained throughout surgery (223). For example, a priming solution of fentanyl, 2.4 μg/kg/minute for 20 minutes in combination with a

TABLE 10-5. POTENTIAL PROBLEMS ASSOCIATED WITH OPIOID-INDUCED RIGIDITY

Hemodynamic
- Increases in central venous pressure, peak airway pressure, peripheral vascular resistance

Respiratory
- Decreases in compliance, functional reserve capacity, ventilation
- Vocal cord closure
- Hypercarbia
- Hypoxemia

Miscellaneous
- Increased oxygen consumption
- Increased intracranial pressure
- Occluded or dislodged intravenous lines

simultaneously started and maintained infusion of 0.3 μg/kg/minute, produced plasma concentrations between 20 and 27 ng/mL and effectively eliminated the need for supplements. Continuous infusions of fentanyl for cardiac surgery range from 0.1 to 1.0 μg/kg/minute up to or continuing through CPB.

Sufentanil, 0.5 to 2.0 μg/kg, administered several minutes before completion of induction of anesthesia, effectively prevents significant hemodynamic responses to laryngoscopy and intubation. In a multicenter report of computer-assisted continuous infusion (CACI) techniques for patients undergoing coronary artery surgery, modest induction doses (0.4 ± 0.2 μg/kg) and total maintenance doses (2.4 ± 0.8 μg/kg) of sufentanil were used in combination with propofol (1.5 ± 1 mg/kg for induction; 32 ± 12 mg/kg total) (224). Sufentanil requirements tripled when midazolam was employed instead of propofol.

Various mathematical models and calculations have been used to predict, establish, and maintain the desired plasma concentration of a drug, but their objective is the same: to achieve a desired plasma and effect site drug concentration and to maintain that state by replacing drug removed by redistribution and metabolism (222,225,226). More recent investigations offer better but more complex regimens (227) or computer-assisted delivery methods (228). The necessity or the presumed benefits of invoking complicated pharmacokinetic equations have been questioned as unduly cumbersome and complicated (229). Titration, based on a dose-response relation with limited attention to pharmacokinetic equations or concern about ideal plasma levels, may be equally effective. No outcome benefits are attributable to "tight" control of plasma drug concentrations. In addition, tremendous variability exists among patients in the drug doses and plasma concentrations required for anesthesia. Nevertheless, CACI systems that deliver drugs based on population-based pharmacokinetic data and target plasma or effect site concentrations can be accurate (230).

The choice of muscle relaxants for cardiac surgery is made with consideration of the hemodynamic side effects noted previously, as well as consideration of the duration of action and need for relaxation. Historically, pancuronium has been popular for relaxation with a high-dose opioid anesthetic, its vagolytic effects being used to offset the decrease in heart rate seen with fentanyl and its analogs. Pancuronium's long duration of action was considered desirable for patients who were mechanically ventilated for many hours postoperatively. The recent popularity of fast-tracking may decrease the utility of pancuronium for cardiac surgery. In addition, it is now recognized that continuous and/or profound neuromuscular blockade in cardiac surgery is not necessary. Although numerous factors can contribute to the problem of patient awareness under anesthesia (Table 10-7), patient immobility due to neuromuscular blockade is a primary and often avoidable cause. It is the patient who *cannot* move, and not the patient who can move, who experiences awareness. With the availability of the Bispectral Index monitor to monitor hypnosis (BIS, Aspect Medical, Nattic, MA), and the continuous delivery of intravenous and inhaled agents (including during CPB), an adequate depth of anesthesia can be maintained and patient movement avoided without the use of much, if any, neuromuscular blockade. Recent evaluations of fast-track patients indicated a low incidence of awareness (less than 1%), which

TABLE 10-6. APPROXIMATE OPIOID LOADING (BOLUS) DOSES, MAINTENANCE INFUSION RATES, AND ADDITIONAL MAINTENANCE DOSES FOR BALANCED CARDIAC ANESTHESIA

Drug	Loading Dose (μg/kg)	Maintenance Infusion Rate	Additional Boluses
Alfentanil	25–100	0.5–2 μg/kg/min	5–10 g/kg
Sufentanil	0.25–2	0.5–1.5 μg/kg/hr	2.5–10 μg
Fentanyl	4–20	2–10 μg/kg/hr	25–100 μg
Remifentanil	1–2	0.1–1.0 μg/kg/min	0.1–1.0 μg/kg

TABLE 10-7. FACTORS CONTRIBUTING TO AWARENESS IN CARDIAC ANESTHESIA

Inadequate anesthetic technique
- Inadequate premedication
- Ultra-short-acting intravenous induction agent
- Intermittent anesthetic administration
- Excessive or unnecessary neuromuscular blockade

Difficult and/or prolonged intubation
Equipment failure
American Society of Anesthesiologists physical status IV or V
Morbid obesity
Inexperience of the anesthesiologist
Pharmacologic autonomic blockade

was attributed in part to the use of continuous intravenous infusions of anesthetics (231).

Anesthetic techniques should allow patients to rapidly emerge in the immediate postoperative period if desired. Fentanyl, more so than sufentanil, carries the risk of postoperative narcosis as greater and multiple doses are administered intraoperatively. Sufentanil, in a total dose of 1 μg/kg/hour or less, should rarely impair the return of spontaneous ventilation within 1 to 2 hours postoperatively. The context-sensitive half-times for propofol, midazolam, sufentanil, and remifentanil make these drugs suitable for sedation and analgesia in the patient who is a fast-track candidate (27,232). Infusions of remifentanil or propofol (or both) can be used to achieve needed sedation and/or analgesia, and they provide the most flexibility if very rapid recovery is desired.

REFERENCES

1. Lowenstein E, Hallowell P, Levine FH, et al. Cardiovascular response to large doses of intravenous morphine in man. *N Engl J Med* 1969;281:1389.
2. Stanley TH, Webster LR. Anesthetic requirements and cardiovascular effects of fentanyl-oxygen and fentanyl-diazepam-oxygen anesthesia in man. *Anesth Analg* 1978;57:411.
3. Lowenstein E. Morphine "anesthesia": a perspective. *Anesthesiology* 1971;35:563.
4. Bedford RF, Wollman H. Postoperative respiratory effects of morphine and halothane anesthesia: a study in patients undergoing cardiac surgery. *Anesthesiology* 1975;43:1.
5. Stanley TH, Lathrop GD. Urinary excretion of morphine during and after valvular and coronary-artery surgery. *Anesthesiology* 1977;46:166.
6. Arens JF, Benbow BP, Ochsner JL, et al. Morphine anesthesia for aortocoronary bypass procedures. *Anesth Analg* 1972;51:901.
7. Slogoff S, Keats AS. Randomized trial of primary anesthetic agents on outcome of coronary artery bypass operations. *Anesthesiology* 1989;70:179.
8. Tuman KJ, McCarthy RJ, Spiess BD, et al. Does choice of anesthetic agent significantly affect outcome after coronary artery surgery? *Anesthesiology* 1989;70:189.
9. Mora CT, Dudek C, Torjman MC, et al. The effects of anesthetic technique on the hemodynamic response and recovery profile in coronary revascularization patients [see comments]. *Anesth Analg* 1995;81:900.
10. Bell J, Sartain J, Wilkinson GA, et al. Propofol and fentanyl anaesthesia for patients with low cardiac output state undergoing cardiac surgery: comparison with high-dose fentanyl anaesthesia. *Br J Anaesth* 1994;73:162.
11. Reves JG, Sladen RN, Newman MF. Cardiac anesthetic: is it unique? [Editorial; comment]. *Anesth Analg* 1995;81:895.
12. Weissman C. The metabolic response to stress: an overview and update. *Anesthesiology* 1990;73:308.
13. Chrousos GP, Gold PW. The concepts of stress and stress system disorders: overview of physical. and behavioral homeostasis [Published erratum appears in *JAMA* 1992 Jul 8;268(2):200]. *JAMA* 1992;267:1244.
14. Pick CG, Paul D, Pasternak GW. Nalbuphine, a mixed kappa 1 and kappa 3 analgesic in mice. *J Pharmacol Exp Ther* 1992; 262:1044.
15. Oyama T, Wakayama S. The endocrine responses to general anesthesia. *Int Anesthesiol Clin* 1988;26:176.
16. Cherny NJ, Chang V, Frager G, et al. Opioid pharmacotherapy in the management of cancer pain: a survey of strategies used by pain physicians for the selection of analgesic drugs and routes of administration. *Cancer* 1995;76:1283.
17. Mangano DT, Siliciano D, Hollenberg M, et al. Postoperative myocardial ischemia: therapeutic trials using intensive analgesia following surgery. The Study of Perioperative Ischemia (SPI) Research Group [see comments]. *Anesthesiology* 1992;76:342.
18. Yeager MP, Glass DD, Neff RK, et al. Epidural anesthesia and analgesia in high-risk surgical patients. *Anesthesiology* 1987;66: 729.
19. Cooper GM, Paterson JL, Ward ID, et al. Fentanyl and the metabolic response to gastric surgery. *Anaesthesia* 1981;36:667.
20. Sebel PS, Bovill JG, Schellekens AP, et al. Hormonal responses to high-dose fentanyl anaesthesia: a study in patients undergoing cardiac surgery. *Br J Anaesth* 1981;53:941.
21. Walsh ES, Paterson JL, O'Riordan JB, et al. Effect of high-dose fentanyl anaesthesia on the metabolic and endocrine response to cardiac surgery. *Br J Anaesth* 1981;53:1155.
22. Cheng DC. Fast track cardiac surgery pathways: early extubation, process of care, and cost containment [Editorial; comment]. *Anesthesiology* 1998;88:1429.
23. Wong DT, Cheng DC, Kustra R, et al. Risk factors of delayed extubation, prolonged length of stay in the intensive care unit, and mortality in patients undergoing coronary artery bypass graft with fast-track cardiac anesthesia: a new cardiac risk score [see comments]. *Anesthesiology* 1999;91:936.
24. London MJ, Shroyer AL, Grover FL. Fast tracking into the new millennium: an evolving paradigm [Editorial; comment]. *Anesthesiology* 1999;91:911.
25. Berry PD, Thomas SD, Mahon SP, et al. Myocardial ischaemia after coronary artery bypass grafting: early vs late extubation [Published errata appear in *Br J Anaesth* 1998 Apr;80(4):572 and 1998 Jul;81(1):111]. *Br J Anaesth* 1998;80:20.
26. Lemmens HJ, Egan TD, Fiset P, et al. Pharmacokinetic/dynamic assessment in drug development: application to the investigational opioid mirfentanil. *Anesth Analg* 1995;80:1206.
27. Hughes MA, Glass PS, Jacobs JR. Context-sensitive half-time in multicompartment pharmacokinetic models for intravenous anesthetic drugs [see comments]. *Anesthesiology* 1992;76:334.
28. Youngs EJ, Shafer SL. Pharmacokinetic parameters relevant to recovery from opioids [Published erratum appears in *Anesthesiology* 1995 Jan;82(1):326]. *Anesthesiology* 1994;81:833.
29. Lunn JK, Stanley TH, Eisele J, et al. High dose fentanyl anesthesia for coronary artery surgery: plasma fentanyl concentrations and influence of nitrous oxide on cardiovascular responses. *Anesth Analg* 1979;58:390.
30. Miller DR, Wellwood M, Teasdale SJ, et al. Effects of anesthetic induction on myocardial function and metabolism: a comparison of fentanyl, sufentanil and alfentanil. *Can J Anaesth* 1988; 35:219.
31. Mathews HM, Furness G, Carson IW, et al. Comparison of sufentanil-oxygen and fentanyl-oxygen anaesthesia for coronary artery bypass grafting. *Br J Anaesth* 1988;60:530.
32. Sebel PS, Bovil JG. Cardiovascular effects of sufentanil anesthesia. *Anesth Analg* 1982;61:115.
33. Ausems ME, Hug CC Jr, de Lange S. Variable rate infusion of alfentanil as a supplement to nitrous oxide anesthesia for general surgery. *Anesth Analg* 1983;62:982.
34. Rucquoi M, Camu F. Cardiovascular responses to large doses of alfentanil and fentanyl. *Br J Anaesth* 1983;55[Suppl 2]:223S.
35. Lemmens HJ, Bovill JG, Burm AG, et al. Alfentanil infusion in the elderly: prolonged computer-assisted infusion of alfentanil in the elderly surgical patient. *Anaesthesia* 1988;43:850.
36. James MK, Vuong A, Grizzle MK, et al. Hemodynamic effects of GI 87084B, an ultra-short acting mu-opioid analgesic, in anesthetized dogs. *J Pharmacol Exp Ther* 1992;263:84.

37. Flacke JW, Davis LJ, Flacke WE, et al. Effects of fentanyl and diazepam in dogs deprived of autonomic tone. *Anesth Analg* 1985;64:1053.
38. Parratt JR, Sitsapesan R. Stereospecific antiarrhythmic effect of opioid receptor antagonists in myocardial ischaemia. *Br J Pharmacol* 1986;87:621.
39. Lowenstein E, Whiting RB, Bittar DA, et al. Local and neurally mediated effects of morphine on skeletal muscle vascular resistance. *J Pharmacol Exp Ther* 1972;180:359.
40. White DA, Reitan JA, Kien ND, et al. Decrease in vascular resistance in the isolated canine hindlimb after graded doses of alfentanil, fentanyl, and sufentanil. *Anesth Analg* 1990;71:29.
41. Wynands JE, Townsend GE, Wong P, et al. Blood pressure response and plasma fentanyl concentrations during high- and very high-dose fentanyl anesthesia for coronary artery surgery. *Anesth Analg* 1983;62:661.
42. Reitan JA, Stengert KB, Wymore ML, et al. Central vagal control of fentanyl-induced bradycardia during halothane anesthesia. *Anesth Analg* 1978;57:31.
43. Starr NJ, Sethna DH, Estafanous FG. Bradycardia and asystole following the rapid administration of sufentanil with vecuronium. *Anesthesiology* 1986;64:521.
44. Egan TD, Brock-Utne JG. Asystole after anesthesia induction with a fentanyl, propofol, and succinylcholine sequence. *Anesth Analg* 1991;73:818.
45. Chinzei M, Morita S, Chinzei T, et al. Effects of isoflurane and fentanyl on ischemic myocardium in dogs: assessment by end-systolic measurements. *J Cardiothorac Vasc Anesth* 1991;5:243.
46. Kim YD, Danchek M, Myers AK, et al. Anaesthetic modification of regional myocardial functional adjustments during myocardial ischaemia: halothane vs fentanyl. *Br J Anaesth* 1992;68: 286.
47. White JL, Myers AK, Analouei A, et al. Functional recovery of stunned myocardium is greater with halothane than fentanyl anaesthesia in dogs. *Br J Anaesth* 1994;73:214.
48. MacLeod BA, Augereau P, Walker MJ. Effects of halothane anesthesia compared with fentanyl anesthesia and no anesthesia during coronary ligation in rats. *Anesthesiology* 1983;58:44.
49. Davis RF, DeBoer LW, Maroko PR. Thoracic epidural anesthesia reduces myocardial infarct size after coronary artery occlusion in dogs. *Anesth Analg* 1986;65:711.
50. Schultz JE, Hsu AK, Gross GJ. Morphine mimics the cardioprotective effect of ischemic preconditioning via a glibenclamide-sensitive mechanism in the rat heart. *Circ Res* 1996;78:1100.
51. Lee HT. Mechanisms of ischemic preconditioning and clinical implications for multiorgan ischemic-reperfusion injury. *J Cardiothorac Vasc Anesth* 1999;13:78.
52. Kleinman B, Henkin RE, Glisson SN, et al. Qualitative evaluation of coronary flow during anesthetic induction using thallium-201 perfusion scans. *Anesthesiology* 1986;64:157.
53. Blaise GA, Witzeling TM, Sill JC, et al. Fentanyl is devoid of major effects on coronary vasoreactivity and myocardial metabolism in experimental animals. *Anesthesiology* 1990;72:535.
54. Hirsch LJ, Rooney MW, Mathru M, et al. Effects of fentanyl on coronary blood flow distribution and myocardial oxygen consumption in the dog. *J Cardiothorac Vasc Anesth* 1993;7:50.
55. Kohno K, Takaki M, Ishioka K, et al. Effects of intracoronary fentanyl on left ventricular mechanoenergetics in the excised cross-circulated canine heart [Revised publication]. *Anesthesiology* 1997;87:658.
56. Kotrly KJ, Ebert TJ, Vucins EJ, et al. Baroreceptor reflex control of heart rate during morphine sulfate, diazepam, N_2O/O_2 anesthesia in humans. *Anesthesiology* 1984;61:558.
57. Zimpfer M, Kotai E, Mayer N, et al. [Effect of morphine on circulatory control in acute progressive hemorrhage]. *Anaesthesist* 1983;32:259.
58. Murat I, Levron JC, Berg A, et al. Effects of fentanyl on baroreceptor reflex control of heart rate in newborn infants. *Anesthesiology* 1988;68:717.
59. Osei-Gyimah P, Archer S, Gillan MG, et al. Some 14 beta-substituted analogues of *N*-(cyclopropylmethyl)normorphine. *J Med Chem* 1981;24:212.
60. Rao S, Sherbaniuk RW, Prasad K, et al. Cardiopulmonary effects of diazepam. *Clin Pharmacol Ther* 1973;14:182.
61. Forster A, Gardaz JP, Suter PM, et al. I.V. midazolam as an induction agent for anaesthesia: a study in volunteers. *Br J Anaesth* 1980;52:907.
62. Gutstein HB, Rubie EA, Mansour A, et al. Opioid effects on mitogen-activated protein kinase signaling cascades [see comments]. *Anesthesiology* 1997;87:1118.
63. Nakae Y, Kanaya N, Namiki A. The direct effects of diazepam and midazolam on myocardial depression in cultured rat ventricular myocytes. *Anesth Analg* 1997;85:729.
64. Reves JG, Kissin I, Fournier S. Negative inotropic effects of midazolam [Letter]. *Anesthesiology* 1984;60:517.
65. Adams P, Gelman S, Reves JG, et al. Midazolam pharmacodynamics and pharmacokinetics during acute hypovolemia. *Anesthesiology* 1985;63:140.
66. Jones DJ, Stehling LC, Zauder HL. Cardiovascular responses to diazepam and midazolam maleate in the dog. *Anesthesiology* 1979;51:430.
67. Reves JG, Samuelson PN, Lewis S. Midazolam maleate induction in patients with ischaemic heart disease: haemodynamic observations. *Can Anaesth Soc J* 1979;26:402.
68. Cote P, Gueret P, Bourassa MG. Systemic and coronary hemodynamic effects of diazepam in patients with normal and diseased coronary arteries. *Circulation* 1974;50:1210.
69. Hoar PF, Nelson NT, Mangano DT, et al. Adrenergic response to morphine-diazepam anesthesia for myocardial revascularization. *Anesth Analg* 1981;60:406.
70. Melsom M, Andreassen P, Melsom H, et al. Diazepam in acute myocardial infarction: clinical effects and effects on catecholamines, free fatty acids, and cortisol. *Br Heart J* 1976;38:804.
71. Abel RM, Staroscik RN, Reis RL. The effects of diazepam (Valium) on left ventricular function and systemic vascular resistance. *J Pharmacol Exp Ther* 1970;173:364.
72. Chang KS, Feng MG, Davis RF. Midazolam produces vasodilation by mixed endothelium-dependent and -independent mechanisms. *Anesth Analg* 1994;78:710.
73. D'Amelio G, Dalla VS, Stritoni P, et al. Acute cardiovascular effects of diazepam in patients with mitral valve disease. *Eur J Clin Pharmacol* 1973;6:61.
74. McCammon RL, Hilgenberg JC, Stoelting RK. Hemodynamic effects of diazepam and diazepam-nitrous oxide in patients with coronary artery disease. *Anesth Analg* 1980;59:438.
75. Ikram H, Rubin AP, Jewkes RF. Effect of diazepam on myocardial blood flow of patients with and without coronary artery disease. *Br Heart J* 1973;35:626.
76. Marty J, Nitenberg A, Blanchet F, et al. Effects of midazolam on the coronary circulation in patients with coronary artery disease. *Anesthesiology* 1986;64:206.
77. Marty J, Gauzit R, Lefevre P, et al. Effects of diazepam and midazolam on baroreflex control of heart rate and on sympathetic activity in humans. *Anesth Analg* 1986;65:113.
78. Sakamoto M, Yasumoto M, Ohsumi H, et al. Effects of midazolam and flumazenil on carotid sinus baroreflex control of circulation in rabbits. *Br J Anaesth* 1994;73:384.
79. Dickenson AH. Spinal cord pharmacology of pain [Review; 71 refs]. *Br J Anaesth* 1995;75:193.
80. Coates DP, Monk CR, Prys-Roberts C, et al. Hemodynamic effects of infusions of the emulsion formulation of propofol

during nitrous oxide anesthesia in humans. *Anesth Analg* 1987; 66:64.

81. Brussel T, Theissen JL, Vigfusson G, et al. Hemodynamic and cardiodynamic effects of propofol and etomidate: negative inotropic properties of propofol. *Anesth Analg* 1989;69:35.
82. Nakaigawa Y, Akazawa S, Shimizu R, et al. Effects of graded infusion rates of propofol on cardiovascular haemodynamics, coronary circulation and myocardial metabolism in dogs. *Br J Anaesth* 1995;75:616.
83. Lepage JY, Pinaud ML, Helias JH, et al. Left ventricular function during propofol and fentanyl anesthesia in patients with coronary artery disease: assessment with a radionuclide approach. *Anesth Analg* 1988;67:949.
84. Coetzee A, Fourie P, Coetzee J, et al. Effect of various propofol plasma concentrations on regional myocardial contractility and left ventricular afterload. *Anesth Analg* 1989;69:473.
85. Mulier JP, Wouters PF, Van Aken H, et al. Cardiodynamic effects of propofol in comparison with thiopental: assessment with a transesophageal echocardiographic approach [see comments]. *Anesth Analg* 1991;72:28.
86. Schmidt C, Roosens C, Struys M, et al. Contractility in humans after coronary artery surgery. *Anesthesiology* 1999;91:58.
87. Rouby JJ, Leger P, Andreev A, et al. [Peripheral vascular effects of propofol]. *Ann Fr Anesth Reanim* 1989;8[Suppl]:R15.
88. Boer F, Ros P, Bovill JG, et al. Effect of propofol on peripheral vascular resistance during cardiopulmonary bypass [see comments]. *Br J Anaesth* 1990;65:184.
89. Samain E, Bouillier H, Marty J, et al. The effect of propofol on angiotensin II-induced Ca(2+) mobilization in aortic smooth muscle cells from normotensive and hypertensive rats. *Anesth Analg* 2000;90:546.
90. Vermeyen KM, Erpels FA, Janssen LA, et al. Propofol-fentanyl anaesthesia for coronary bypass surgery in patients with good left ventricular function. *Br J Anaesth* 1987;59:1115.
91. Samain E, Marty J, Gauzit R, et al. Effects of propofol on baroreflex control of heart rate and on plasma noradrenaline levels. *Eur J Anaesthesiol* 1989;6:321.
92. Cullen PM, Turtle M, Prys-Roberts C, et al. Effect of propofol anesthesia on baroreflex activity in humans. *Anesth Analg* 1987; 66:1115.
93. Frankl WS, Poole-Wilson PA. Effects of thiopental on tension development, action potential, and exchange of calcium and potassium in rabbit ventricular myocardium. *J Cardiovasc Pharmacol* 1981;3:554.
94. Lehot JJ, Boulieu R, Foussadier A, et al. Comparison of the pharmacokinetics of methohexital during cardiac surgery with cardiopulmonary bypass and vascular surgery. *J Cardiothorac Vasc Anesth* 1993;7:30.
95. Bettens KM, De Hert SG, Sys SU, et al. Role of the endocardial endothelium in the negative inotropic effects of thiopental. *Anesthesiology* 1996;85:1100.
96. Gelissen HP, Epema AH, Henning RH, et al. Inotropic effects of propofol, thiopental, midazolam, etomidate, and ketamine on isolated human atrial muscle. *Anesthesiology* 1996;84:397.
97. Patschke D, Bruckner JB, Eberlein HJ, et al. Effects of althesin, etomidate and fentanyl on haemodynamics and myocardial oxygen consumption in man. *Can Anaesth Soc J* 1977;24:57.
98. Gooding JM, Corssen G. Effect of etomidate on the cardiovascular system. *Anesth Analg* 1977;56:717.
99. Colvin MP, Savege TM, Newland PE, et al. Cardiorespiratory changes following induction of anaesthesia with etomidate in patients with cardiac disease. *Br J Anaesth* 1979;51:551.
100. Gooding JM, Weng JT, Smith RA, et al. Cardiovascular and pulmonary responses following etomidate induction of anesthesia in patients with demonstrated cardiac disease. *Anesth Analg* 1979;58:40.
101. Riou B, Lecarpentier Y, Chemla D, et al. *In vitro* effects of etomidate on intrinsic myocardial contractility in the rat. *Anesthesiology* 1990;72:330.
102. Kissin I, Motomura S, Aultman DF, et al. Inotropic and anesthetic potencies of etomidate and thiopental in dogs. *Anesth Analg* 1983;62:961.
103. Jackson AP, Dhadphale PR, Callaghan ML, et al. Haemodynamic studies during induction of anaesthesia for open-heart surgery using diazepam and ketamine. *Br J Anaesth* 1978;50: 375.
104. Balfors E, Haggmark S, Nyhman H, et al. Droperidol inhibits the effects of intravenous ketamine on central hemodynamics and myocardial oxygen consumption in patients with generalized atherosclerotic disease. *Anesth Analg* 1983;62:193.
105. Savege TM, Colvin MP, Weaver EJ, et al. A comparison of some cardiorespiratory effects of althesin and ketamine when used for induction of anaesthesia in patients with cardiac disease. *Br J Anaesth* 1976;48:1071.
106. Riou B, Lecarpentier Y, Viars P. Inotropic effect of ketamine on rat cardiac papillary muscle. *Anesthesiology* 1989;71:116.
107. Zsigmond EK, Kelsch RC, Kothary SP. Rise in plasma free-norepinephrine during anesthetic induction with ketamine. *Behav Neuropsychiatry* 1974;6:81.
108. Traber DL, Wilson RD, Priano LL. The effect of alpha-adrenergic blockade on the cardiopulmonary response to ketamine. *Anesth Analg* 1971;50:737.
109. Riou B, Viars P, Lecarpentier Y. Effects of ketamine on the cardiac papillary muscle of normal hamsters and those with cardiomyopathy. *Anesthesiology* 1990;73:910.
110. Nettles DC, Herrin TJ, Mullen JG. Ketamine induction in poor-risk patients. *Anesth Analg* 1973;52:59.
111. Waxman K, Shoemaker WC, Lippmann M. Cardiovascular effects of anesthetic induction with ketamine. *Anesth Analg* 1980; 59:355.
112. Corssen G, Reves JG, Carter JR. Neuroleptanesthesia, dissociative anesthesia, and hemorrhage. *Int Anesthesiol Clin* 1974;12: 145.
113. Flacke JW, Bloor BC, Flacke WE, et al. Reduced narcotic requirement by clonidine with improved hemodynamic and adrenergic stability in patients undergoing coronary bypass surgery. *Anesthesiology* 1987;67:11.
114. Ghignone M, Quintin L, Duke PC, et al. Effects of clonidine on narcotic requirements and hemodynamic response during induction of fentanyl anesthesia and endotracheal intubation. *Anesthesiology* 1986;64:36.
115. Talke P, Li J, Jain U, et al. Effects of perioperative dexmedetomidine infusion in patients undergoing vascular surgery: The Study of Perioperative Ischemia Research Group. *Anesthesiology* 1995;82:620.
116. Venn RM, Bradshaw CJ, Spencer R, et al. Preliminary UK experience of dexmedetomidine, a novel agent for postoperative sedation in the intensive care unit. *Anaesthesia* 1999;54:1136.
117. Pagel PS, Kampine JP, Schmeling WT, et al. Effects of nitrous oxide on myocardial contractility as evaluated by the preload recruitable stroke work relationship in chronically instrumented dogs. *Anesthesiology* 1990;73:1148.
118. Van Trigt P, Christian CC, Fagraeus L, et al. The mechanism of halothane-induced myocardial depression: altered diastolic mechanics versus impaired contractility. *J Thorac Cardiovasc Surg* 1983;85:832.
119. Graves CL, McDermott RW, Bidwai A. Cardiovascular effects of isoflurane in surgical patients. *Anesthesiology* 1974;41:486.
120. Eger EI. New inhaled anesthetics. *Anesthesiology* 1994;80:906.
121. Bernard JM, Wouters PF, Doursout MF, et al. Effects of sevoflurane and isoflurane on cardiac and coronary dynamics in chronically instrumented dogs. *Anesthesiology* 1990;72:659.

122. Weiskopf RB, Moore MA, Eger EI, et al. Rapid increase in desflurane concentration is associated with greater transient cardiovascular stimulation than with rapid increase in isoflurane concentration in humans. *Anesthesiology* 1994;80:1035.
123. Kemmotsu O, Hashimoto Y, Shimosato S. Inotropic effects of isoflurane on mechanics of contraction in isolated cat papillary muscles from normal and failing hearts. *Anesthesiology* 1973;39:470.
124. Kemmotsu O, Hashimoto Y, Shimosato S. The effects of fluroxene and enflurane on contractile performance of isolated papillary muscles from failing hearts. *Anesthesiology* 1974;40:252.
125. Vivien B, Hanouz JL, Gueugniaud PY, et al. Myocardial effects of halothane and isoflurane in hamsters with hypertrophic cardiomyopathy. *Anesthesiology* 1997;87:1406.
126. Sprague DH, Yang JC, Ngai SH. Effects of isoflurane and halothane on contractility and the cyclic 3′, 5′-adenosine monophosphate system in the rat aorta. *Anesthesiology* 1974;40:162.
127. Seagard JL, Hopp FA, Donegan JH, et al. Halothane and the carotid sinus reflex: evidence for multiple sites of action. *Anesthesiology* 1982;57:191.
128. Rorie DK, Tyce GM, Mackenzie RA. Evidence that halothane inhibits norepinephrine release from sympathetic nerve endings in dog saphenous vein by stimulation of presynaptic inhibitory muscarinic receptors. *Anesth Analg* 1984;63:1059.
129. Lerman J, Oyston JP, Gallagher TM, et al. The minimum alveolar concentration (MAC) and hemodynamic effects of halothane, isoflurane, and sevoflurane in newborn swine. *Anesthesiology* 1990;73:717.
130. Pagel PS, Kampine JP, Schmeling WT, et al. Alteration of left ventricular diastolic function by desflurane, isoflurane, and halothane in the chronically instrumented dog with autonomic nervous system blockade. *Anesthesiology* 1991;74:1103.
131. Eisele JH, Smith NT. Cardiovascular effects of 40 percent nitrous oxide in man. *Anesth Analg* 1972;51:956.
132. Seagard JL, Elegbe EO, Hopp FA, et al. Effects of isoflurane on the baroreceptor reflex. *Anesthesiology* 1983;59:511.
133. Bagshaw RJ, Cox RH. Baroreceptor control of systemic haemodynamic at incremental halothane levels in the dog. *Acta Anaesthesiol Scand* 1981;25:416.
134. Weiskopf RB, Cahalan MK, Ionescu P, et al. Cardiovascular actions of desflurane with and without nitrous oxide during spontaneous ventilation in humans. *Anesth Analg* 1991;73:165.
135. Stevens WC, Cromwell TH, Halsey MJ, et al. The cardiovascular effects of a new inhalation anesthetic, Forane, in human volunteers at constant arterial carbon dioxide tension. *Anesthesiology* 1971;35:8.
136. Ebert TJ, Harkin CP, Muzi M. Cardiovascular responses to sevoflurane: a review. *Anesth Analg* 1995;81:S11.
137. Kawamura R, Stanley TH, English JB, et al. Cardiovascular responses to nitrous oxide exposure for two hours in man. *Anesth Analg* 1980;59:93.
138. Johnston RR, Eger EI II, Wilson C. A comparative interaction of epinephrine with enflurane, isoflurane, and halothane in man. *Anesth Analg* 1976;55:709.
139. Turner LA, Bosnjak ZJ, Kampine JP. Actions of halothane on the electrical activity of Purkinje fibers derived from normal and infarcted canine hearts. *Anesthesiology* 1987;67:619.
140. Jang TL, MacLeod BA, Walker MJ. Effects of halogenated hydrocarbon anesthetics on responses to ligation of a coronary artery in chronically prepared rats. *Anesthesiology* 1983;59:309.
141. Kroll DA, Knight PR. Antifibrillatory effects of volatile anesthetics in acute occlusion/reperfusion arrhythmias. *Anesthesiology* 1984;61:657.
142. Schmeling WT, Warltier DC, McDonald DJ, et al. Prolongation of the QT interval by enflurane, isoflurane, and halothane in humans. *Anesth Analg* 1991;72:137.
143. Reiz S, Balfors E, Gustavsson B, et al. Effects of halothane on coronary haemodynamics and myocardial metabolism in patients with ischaemic heart disease and heart failure. *Acta Anaesthesiol Scand* 1982;26:133.
144. Hilfiker O, Larsen R, Sonntag H. Myocardial blood flow and oxygen consumption during halothane-nitrous oxide anaesthesia for coronary revascularization. *Br J Anaesth* 1983;55:927.
145. Kowalski C, Zahler S, Becker BF, et al. Halothane, isoflurane, and sevoflurane reduce postischemic adhesion of neutrophils in the coronary system. *Anesthesiology* 1997;86:188.
146. Bertha BG, Folts JD, Nugent M, et al. Halothane, but not isoflurane or enflurane, protects against spontaneous and epinephrine-exacerbated acute thrombus formation in stenosed dog coronary arteries. *Anesthesiology* 1989;71:96.
147. Reiz S, Balfors E, Sorensen MB, et al. Isoflurane: a powerful coronary vasodilator in patients with coronary artery disease. *Anesthesiology* 1983;59:91.
148. Moffitt EA, Barker RA, Glenn JJ, et al. Myocardial metabolism and hemodynamic responses with isoflurane anesthesia for coronary arterial surgery. *Anesth Analg* 1986;65:53.
149. Sahlman L, Milocco I, Appelgren L, et al. Control of intraoperative hypertension with isoflurane in patients with coronary artery disease: effects on regional myocardial blood flow and metabolism. *Anesth Analg* 1989;68:105.
150. Slogoff S, Keats AS, Dear WE, et al. Steal-prone coronary anatomy and myocardial ischemia associated with four primary anesthetic agents in humans. *Anesth Analg* 1991;72:22.
151. O'Young J, Mastrocostopoulos G, Hilgenberg A, et al. Myocardial circulatory and metabolic effects of isoflurane and sufentanil during coronary artery surgery. *Anesthesiology* 1987;66:653.
152. Leung JM, Goehner P, O'Kelly BF, et al. Isoflurane anesthesia and myocardial ischemia: comparative risk versus sufentanil anesthesia in patients undergoing coronary artery bypass graft surgery. The SPI (Study of Perioperative Ischemia) Research Group. *Anesthesiology* 1991;74:838.
153. Leung JM, Hollenberg M, O'Kelly BF, et al. Effects of steal-prone anatomy on intraoperative myocardial ischemia: The SPI Research Group. *J Am Coll Cardiol* 1992;20:1205.
154. Merin RG, Bernard JM, Doursout MF, et al. Comparison of the effects of isoflurane and desflurane on cardiovascular dynamics and regional blood flow in the chronically instrumented dog. *Anesthesiology* 1991;74:568.
155. Tomiyasu S, Hara T, Hasuo H, et al. Comparative analysis of systemic and coronary hemodynamics during sevoflu. *J Cardiovasc Pharmacol* 1999;33:741.
156. Stowe DF, Marijic J, Bosnjak ZJ, et al. Direct comparative effects of halothane, enflurane, and isoflurane on oxygen supply and demand in isolated hearts. *Anesthesiology* 1991;74:1087.
157. Kozmary SV, Lampe GH, Benefiel D, et al. No finding of increased myocardial ischemia during or after carotid endarterectomy under anesthesia with nitrous oxide. *Anesth Analg* 1990;71:591.
158. Ross S, Foex P. Protective effects of anaesthetics in reversible and irreversible ischaemia-reperfusion injury. *Br J Anaesth* 1999;82:622.
159. Bland JH, Lowenstein E. Halothane-induced decrease in experimental myocardial ischemia in the non-failing canine heart. *Anesthesiology* 1976;45:287.
160. Davis RF, DeBoer LW, Rude RE, et al. The effect of halothane anesthesia on myocardial necrosis, hemodynamic performance, and regional myocardial blood flow in dogs following coronary artery occlusion. *Anesthesiology* 1983;59:402.
161. Kersten JR, Schmeling TJ, Pagel PS, et al. Isoflurane mimics ischemic preconditioning via activation of K(ATP) channels: reduction of myocardial infarct size with an acute memory phase. *Anesthesiology* 1997;87:361.

162. Pagel PS, Kampine JP, Schmeling WT, et al. Influence of volatile anesthetics on myocardial contractility *in vivo*: desflurane versus isoflurane. *Anesthesiology* 1991;74:900.
163. Freedman BM, Hamm DP, Everson CT, et al. Enflurane enhances postischemic functional recovery in the isolated rat heart. *Anesthesiology* 1985;62:29.
164. Schlack W, Preckel B, Stunneck D, et al. Effects of halothane, enflurane, isoflurane, sevoflurane and desflurane on myocardial reperfusion injury in the isolated rat heart. *Br J Anaesth* 1998; 81:913.
165. Mattheussen M, Rusy BF, Van Aken H, et al. Recovery of function and adenosine triphosphate metabolism following myocardial ischemia induced in the presence of volatile anesthetics [see comments]. *Anesth Analg* 1993;76:69.
166. Cope DK, Impastato WK, Cohen MV, et al. Volatile anesthetics protect the ischemic rabbit myocardium from infarction. *Anesthesiology* 1997;86:699.
167. Muir AW, Houston J, Marshall RJ, et al. A comparison of the neuromuscular blocking and autonomic effects of two new short-acting muscle relaxants with those of succinylcholine in the anesthetized cat and pig. *Anesthesiology* 1989;70:533.
168. Domenech JS, Garcia RC, Sastain JM, et al. Pancuronium bromide: an indirect sympathomimetic agent. *Br J Anaesth* 1976; 48:1143.
169. Hosking MP, Lennon RL, Gronert GA. Combined H_1 and H_2 receptor blockade attenuates the cardiovascular effects of high-dose atracurium for rapid sequence endotracheal intubation. *Anesth Analg* 1988;67:1089.
170. Hatano Y, Arai T, Noda J, et al. Contribution of prostacyclin to *d*-tubocurarine-induced hypotension in humans. *Anesthesiology* 1990;72:28.
171. Gravlee GP, Ramsey FM, Roy RC, et al. Rapid administration of a narcotic and neuromuscular blocker: a hemodynamic comparison of fentanyl, sufentanil, pancuronium, and vecuronium. *Anesth Analg* 1988;67:39.
172. Cote D, Martin R, Tetrault JP. Haemodynamic interactions of muscle relaxants and sufentanil in coronary artery surgery. *Can J Anaesth* 1991;38:324.
173. Paulissian R, Mahdi M, Joseph NJ, et al. Hemodynamic responses to pancuronium and vecuronium during high-dose fentanyl anesthesia for coronary artery bypass grafting [see comments]. *J Cardiothorac Vasc Anesth* 1991;5:120.
174. Shorten GD, Sieber T, Maslow AD, et al. Left ventricular regional wall motion and haemodynamic changes following bolus administration of pipecuronium or pancuronium to adult patients undergoing coronary artery bypass grafting. *Can J Anaesth* 1995;42:695.
175. Thomson IR, MacAdams CL, Hudson RJ, et al. Drug interactions with sufentanil: hemodynamic effects of premedication and muscle relaxants. *Anesthesiology* 1992;76:922.
176. Waldmann CS, Wark KJ, Sebel PS, et al. Hemodynamic effects of atracurium, vecuronium and pancuronium during sufentanil anesthesia for coronary artery bypass. *Acta Anaesthesiol Scand* 1986;30:351.
177. Inoue K, el Banayosy A, Stolarski L, et al. Vecuronium induced bradycardia following induction of anaesthesia with etomidate or thiopentone, with or without fentanyl. *Br J Anaesth* 1988; 60:10.
178. Heinonen J, Salmenpera M, Suomivuori M. Contribution of muscle relaxant to the haemodynamic course of high-dose fentanyl anaesthesia: a comparison of pancuronium, vecuronium and atracurium. *Can Anaesth Soc J* 1986;33:597.
179. Cozanitis DA, Lindgren L, Rosenberg PH. Bradycardia in patients receiving atracurium or vecuronium in conditions of low vagal stimulation. *Anaesthesia* 1989;44:303.
180. O'Connor JP, Ramsay JG, Wynands JE, et al. The incidence of myocardial ischemia during anesthesia for coronary artery bypass surgery in patients receiving pancuronium or vecuronium. *Anesthesiology* 1989;70:230.
181. Stoops CM, Curtis CA, Kovach DA, et al. Hemodynamic effects of doxacurium chloride in patients receiving oxygen sufentanil anesthesia for coronary artery bypass grafting or valve replacement. *Anesthesiology* 1988;69:365.
182. Murray DJ, Mehta MP, Choi WW, et al. The neuromuscular blocking and cardiovascular effects of doxacurium chloride in patients receiving nitrous oxide narcotic anesthesia. *Anesthesiology* 1988;69:472.
183. Tassonyi E, Neidhart P, Pittet JF, et al. Cardiovascular effects of pipecuronium and pancuronium in patients undergoing coronary artery bypass grafting. *Anesthesiology* 1988;69:793.
184. Starr NJ, Kraenzler EJ, Wong D, et al. Comparison of cardiovascular effects of pipecuronium versus vecuronium in patients receiving sufentanil anesthesia for myocardial revascularization. *J Cardiothorac Vasc Anesth* 1991;5:116.
185. Savarese JJ, Ali HH, Basta SJ, et al. The cardiovascular effects of mivacurium chloride (BW B1090U) in patients receiving nitrous oxide-opiate-barbiturate anesthesia. *Anesthesiology* 1989; 70:386.
186. Choi WW, Mehta MP, Murray DJ, et al. Neuromuscular and cardiovascular effects of mivacurium chloride in surgical patients receiving nitrous oxide-narcotic or nitrous oxide-isoflurane anaesthesia [see comments]. *Can J Anaesth* 1989;36:641.
187. Stoops CM, Curtis CA, Kovach DA, et al. Hemodynamic effects of mivacurium chloride administered to patients during oxygen-sufentanil anesthesia for coronary artery bypass grafting or valve replacement. *Anesth Analg* 1989;68:333.
188. Levy JH, Pitts M, Thanopoulos A, et al. The effects of rapacuronium on histamine release and hemodynamics in adult patients undergoing general anesthesia. *Anesth Analg* 1999;89:290.
189. Stanski DR, Shafer SL. Quantifying anesthetic drug interaction: implications for drug dosing [Editorial; comment]. *Anesthesiology* 1995;83:1.
190. Zbinden AM, Maggiorini M, Petersen-Felix S, et al. Anesthetic depth defined using multiple noxious stimuli during isoflurane/oxygen anesthesia: I. Motor reactions [see comments]. *Anesthesiology* 1994;80:253.
191. Vuyk J, Mertens MJ, Olofsen E, et al. Propofol anesthesia and rational opioid selection: determination of optimal EC50-EC95 propofol-opioid concentrations that assure adequate anesthesia and a rapid return of consciousness. *Anesthesiology* 1997;87: 1549.
192. Tverskoy M, Fleyshman G, Ezry J, et al. Midazolam-morphine sedative interaction in patients. *Anesth Analg* 1989;68:282.
193. Kissin I, Brown PT, Bradley EL Jr, et al. Diazepam-morphine hypnotic synergism in rats. *Anesthesiology* 1989;70:689.
194. Thomson IR, Bergstrom RG, Rosenbloom M, et al. Premedication and high-dose fentanyl anesthesia for myocardial revascularization: a comparison of lorazepam versus morphine-scopolamine. *Anesthesiology* 1988;68:194.
195. Spiess BD, Sathoff RH, el Ganzouri AR, et al. High-dose sufentanil: four cases of sudden hypotension on induction. *Anesth Analg* 1986;65:703.
196. Heikkila H, Jalonen J, Laaksonen V, et al. Lorazepam and high-dose fentanyl anaesthesia: effects on haemodynamics and oxygen transportation in patients undergoing coronary revascularization. *Acta Anaesthesiol Scand* 1984;28:357.
197. Pomane C, Paulin M, Lena P, et al. [Comparison of the hemodynamic effects of midazolam-fentanyl and thiopental-fentanyl combinations in the induction of general anesthesia]. *Ann Fr Anesth Reanim* 1983;2:75.
198. Roekaerts PM, Gerrits HJ, Timmerman BE, et al. Continuous

infusions of alfentanil and propofol for coronary artery surgery. *J Cardiothorac Vasc Anesth* 1995;9:362.
199. Gordon PC, Morrell DF, Pamm JD. Total intravenous anesthesia using propofol and alfentanil for coronary artery bypass surgery. *J Cardiothorac Vasc Anesth* 1994;8:284.
200. Phillips AS, McMurray TJ, Mirakhur RK, et al. Propofol-fentanyl anesthesia: a comparison with isoflurane-fentanyl anesthesia in coronary artery bypass grafting and valve replacement surgery. *J Cardiothorac Vasc Anesth* 1994;8:289.
201. Sorbara C, Pittarello D, Rizzoli G, et al. Propofol-fentanyl versus isoflurane-fentanyl anesthesia for coronary artery bypass grafting: effect on myocardial contractility and peripheral hemodynamics [see comments]. *J Cardiothorac Vasc Anesth* 1995;9:18.
202. Hall RI, Murphy JT, Moffitt EA, et al. A comparison of the myocardial metabolic and haemodynamic changes produced by propofol-sufentanil and enflurane-sufentanil anaesthesia for patients having coronary artery bypass graft surgery. *Can J Anaesth* 1991;38:996.
203. Underwood SM, Davies SW, Feneck RO, et al. Anaesthesia for myocardial revascularisation: a comparison of fentanyl/propofol with fentanyl/enflurane. *Anaesthesia* 1992;47:939.
204. Haessler R, Madler C, Klasing S, et al. Propofol/fentanyl versus etomidate/fentanyl for the induction of anesthesia in patients with aortic insufficiency and coronary artery disease. *J Cardiothorac Vasc Anesth* 1992;6:173.
205. Spiss CK, Coraim F, Haider W, et al. Haemodynamic effects of fentanyl or alfentanil as adjuvants to etomidate for induction of anaesthesia in cardiac patients. *Acta Anaesthesiol Scand* 1984;28:554.
206. Wong KC, Martin WE, Hornbein TF, et al. The cardiovascular effects of morphine sulfate with oxygen and with nitrous oxide in man. *Anesthesiology* 1973;38:542.
207. Stowe DF, Monroe SM, Marijic J, et al. Effects of nitrous oxide on contractile function and metabolism of the isolated heart. *Anesthesiology* 1990;73:1220.
208. Philbin DM, Foex P, Drummond G, et al. Postsystolic shortening of canine left ventricle supplied by a stenotic coronary artery when nitrous oxide is added in the presence of narcotics. *Anesthesiology* 1985;62:166.
209. Cahalan MK, Prakash O, Rulf EN, et al. Addition of nitrous oxide to fentanyl anesthesia does not induce myocardial ischemia in patients with ischemic heart disease. *Anesthesiology* 1987;67:925.
210. Heikkila H, Jalonen J, Arola M, et al. Low-dose enflurane as adjunct to high-dose fentanyl in patients undergoing coronary artery surgery: stable hemodynamics and maintained myocardial oxygen balance. *Anesth Analg* 1987;66:111.
211. Ramsay JG, DeLima LG, Wynands JE, et al. Pure opioid versus opioid-volatile anesthesia for coronary artery bypass graft surgery: a prospective, randomized, double-blind study. *Anesth Analg* 1994;78:867.
212. Makela VH, Kapur PA. Amrinone and verapamil-propranolol induced cardiac depression during isoflurane anesthesia in dogs. *Anesthesiology* 1987;66:792.
213. Pagel PS, Hettrick DA, Warltier DC. Left ventricular mechanical consequences of dihydropyridine calcium channel modulation in conscious and anesthetized chronically instrumented dogs. *Anesthesiology* 1994;81:190.
214. Philbin DM, Rosow CE, Schneider RC, et al. Fentanyl and sufentanil anesthesia revisited: how much is enough? [see comments]. *Anesthesiology* 1990;73:5.
215. Stanley TH, de Lange S, Boscoe MJ, et al. The influence of chronic preoperative propranolol therapy on cardiovascular dynamics and narcotic requirements during operation in patients with coronary artery disease. *Can Anaesth Soc J* 1982;29:319.
216. Miller RR, Olson HG, Amsterdam EA, et al. Propranolol-withdrawal rebound phenomenon: exacerbation of coronary events after abrupt cessation of antianginal therapy. *N Engl J Med* 1975;293:416.
217. Chung F, Houston PL, Cheng DC, et al. Calcium channel blockade does not offer adequate protection from perioperative myocardial ischemia. *Anesthesiology* 1988;69:343.
218. Saccomanno PM, Kavanagh BP, Cheng DC, et al. Comparison of lorazepam alone vs lorazepam, morphine, and perphenazine for cardiac premedication. *Can J Anaesth* 1997;44:146.
219. Bailey PL, Pace NL, Ashburn MA, et al. Frequent hypoxemia and apnea after sedation with midazolam and fentanyl. *Anesthesiology* 1990;73:826.
220. Keyl C, Lemberger P, Rodig G, et al. Hypoxaemia and myocardial ischaemia on the night before coronary bypass surgery [Published erratum appears in *Br J Anaesth* 1994 Dec (6):872]. *Br J Anaesth* 1994;73:157.
221. Bennett JA, Abrams JT, Van Riper DF, et al. Difficult or impossible ventilation after sufentanil-induced anesthesia is caused primarily by vocal cord closure [see comments]. *Anesthesiology* 1997;87:1070.
222. Wagner JG. A safe method for rapidly achieving plasma concentration plateaus. *Clin Pharmacol Ther* 1974;16:691.
223. Hall RI, Molderhauer CC, Hug CC Jr. Fentanyl plasma concentrations maintained by a simple infusion scheme in patients undergoing cardiac surgery. *Anesth Analg* 1993;76:957.
224. Jain U, Body SC, Bellows W, et al. Multicenter study of target-controlled infusion of propofol-sufentanil or sufentanil-midazolam for coronary artery bypass graft surgery: Multicenter Study of Perioperative Ischemia (McSPI) Research Group [see comments]. *Anesthesiology* 1996;85:522.
225. Schwilden H. A general method for calculating the dosage scheme in linear pharmacokinetics. *Eur J Clin Pharmacol* 1981;20:379.
226. Rigg JR, Wong TY. A method for achieving rapidly steady-state blood concentrations of I.V. drugs. *Br J Anaesth* 1981;53:1247.
227. Maitre PO, Shafer SL. A simple pocket calculator approach to predict anesthetic drug concentrations from pharmacokinetic data [see comments]. *Anesthesiology* 1990;73:332.
228. Alvis JM, Reves JG, Govier AV, et al. Computer-assisted continuous infusions of fentanyl during cardiac anesthesia: comparison with a manual method. *Anesthesiology* 1985;63:41.
229. Waud BE, Waud DR. Dose-response curves and pharmacokinetics. *Anesthesiology* 1986;65:355.
230. Glass PS, Jacobs JR, Smith LR, et al. Pharmacokinetic model-driven infusion of fentanyl: assessment of accuracy. *Anesthesiology* 1990;73:1082.
231. Dowd NP, Cheng DC, Karski JM, et al. Intraoperative awareness in fast-track cardiac anesthesia. *Anesthesiology* 1998;89:1068.
232. Egan TD, Lemmens HJ, Fiset P, et al. The pharmacokinetics of the new short-acting opioid remifentanil (GI87084B) in healthy adult male volunteers [see comments]. *Anesthesiology* 1993;79:881.
233. Criado A, Maseda J, Navarro E, et al. Induction of anaesthesia with etomidate: haemodynamic study of 36 patients. *Br J Anaesth* 1980;52:803.
234. Lindeburg T, Spotoft H, Bredgaard SM, et al. Cardiovascular effects of etomidate used for induction and in combination with fentanyl-pancuronium for maintenance of anaesthesia in patients with valvular heart disease. *Acta Anaesthesiol Scand* 1982;26:205.
235. Virtue RW, Alanis JM, Mori M, et al. An anesthetic agent: 2-orthochlorophenyl, 2-methylamino cyclohexanone HCl (CI-581). *Anesthesiology* 1967;28:823.

236. Cote P, Noble J, Bourassa MG. Systemic vasodilatation following diazepam after combined sympathetic and parasympathetic blockade in patients with coronary heart disease. *Cathet Cardiovasc Diagn* 1976;2:369.
237. Tweed WA, Minuck M, Mymin D. Circulatory responses to ketamine anesthesia. *Anesthesiology* 1972;37:613.
238. Tweed WA, Mymin D. Myocardial force-velocity relations during ketamine anesthesia at constant heart rate. *Anesthesiology* 1974;41:49.
239. Samuelson PN, Reves JG, Kouchoukos NT, et al. Hemodynamic responses to anesthetic induction with midazolam or diazepam in patients with ischemic heart disease. *Anesth Analg* 1981;60:802.
240. Nauta J, Stanley TH, de Lange S, et al. Anaesthetic induction with alfentanil: comparison with thiopental, midazolam, and etomidate. *Can Anaesth Soc J* 1983;30:53.
241. Schmucker P, van Ackern K, Franke N, et al. [Effect of the intravenous administration of lormetazepam on hemodynamics and arterial blood gases in patients with coronary heart disease]. *Anaesthesist* 1982;31:557.
242. Lebowitz PW, Cote ME, Daniels AL, et al. Comparative renal effects of midazolam and thiopental in humans. *Anesthesiology* 1983;59:381.
243. Larsen R, Rathgeber J, Bagdahn A, et al. Effects of propofol on cardiovascular dynamics and coronary blood flow in geriatric patients: a comparison with etomidate. *Anaesthesia* 1988; 43[Suppl]:25.
244. Aun C, Major E. The cardiorespiratory effects of ICI 35 868 in patients with valvular heart disease. *Anaesthesia* 1984;39:1096.
245. Grounds RM, Twigley AJ, Carli F, et al. The haemodynamic effects of intravenous induction: comparison of the effects of thiopentone and propofol. *Anaesthesia* 1985;40:735.
246. Al Khudhairi D, Gordon G, Morgan M, et al. Acute cardiovascular changes following disoprofol: effects in heavily sedated patients with coronary artery disease. *Anaesthesia* 1982;37:1007.
247. Patrick MR, Blair IJ, Feneck RO, et al. A comparison of the haemodynamic effects of propofol ("Diprivan") and thiopentone in patients with coronary artery disease. *Postgrad Med J* 1985;61[Suppl 3]:23.
248. Stephan H, Sonntag H, Schenk HD, et al. Effects of propofol on cardiovascular dynamics, myocardial blood flow and myocardial metabolism in patients with coronary artery disease. *Br J Anaesth* 1986;58:969.
249. Coates DP, Prys-Roberts C, Spelina KR, et al. Propofol ("Diprivan") by intravenous infusion with nitrous oxide: dose requirements and haemodynamic effects. *Postgrad Med J* 1985; 61[Suppl 3]:76.
250. Van Aken H, Meinshausen E, Prien T, et al. The influence of fentanyl and tracheal intubation on the hemodynamic effects of anesthesia induction with propofol/N_2O in humans. *Anesthesiology* 1988;68:157.
251. Seltzer JL, Gerson JI, Allen FB. Comparison of the cardiovascular effects of bolus v. incremental administration of thiopentone. *Br J Anaesth* 1980;52:527.
252. White PF. Comparative evaluation of intravenous agents for rapid sequence induction—thiopental, ketamine, and midazolam. *Anesthesiology* 1982;57:279.
253. Reiz S, Balfors E, Friedman A, et al. Effects of thiopentone on cardiac performance, coronary hemodynamics and myocardial oxygen consumption in chronic ischemic heart disease. *Acta Anaesthesiol Scand* 1981;25:103.
254. Tarnow J, Hess W, Klein W. Etomidate, alfathesin and thiopentone as induction agents for coronary artery surgery. *Can Anaesth Soc J* 1980;27:338.

PART III

CARDIOPULMONARY BYPASS

11

THE COAGULATION SYSTEM AND CARDIAC SURGERY

THOMAS F. SLAUGHTER

Despite recent strides made in improving the safety of cardiac surgery, perioperative complications related to bleeding and thrombosis remain a significant problem. Each year as many as 5% to 25% of patients experience serious bleeding after cardiac surgery; 2% to 3% of these patients require reoperation to control bleeding (1). In the past decade, major advances have been made in understanding the mechanisms underlying normal hemostatic control. In addition, increasing awareness of transfusion-acquired infections has generated renewed interest in pharmacologic approaches to limit postoperative hemorrhage. This chapter reviews the current understanding of the hemostatic process, the pathophysiologic effects of cardiopulmonary bypass (CPB) on coagulation, methods of monitoring coagulation during CPB, and pharmacologic approaches to limit hemorrhage after cardiac surgery.

PHYSIOLOGY OF HEMOSTASIS

Plasma-Mediated Hemostasis

In a concise summation, the coagulation cascade may be described as an amplification system designed to convert prothrombin to thrombin (2). Trace plasma proteins, activated on exposure to damaged tissue or foreign surfaces, initiate a series of reactions culminating in the conversion of prothrombin to thrombin. Thrombin then converts soluble fibrinogen into an insoluble fibrin clot. Thrombin is the key regulatory step in the hemostatic process; it results not only in fibrin formation but also in platelet activation and fibrinolysis. Coagulation factors circulate as inactive zymogen precursors until they are complexed with active proteases, cofactors, and in some cases calcium and platelet phospholipids (3,4). For ease of discussion, the coagulation cascade is traditionally split into extrinsic and intrinsic systems (Fig. 11-1). These two pathways may be viewed as the switches that turn on the prothrombin-activating system.

T. F. Slaughter: Department of Anesthesiology, Duke University Medical Center, Durham, North Carolina 27710

The extrinsic pathway of coagulation has only recently been recognized as the most important pathway to formation of thrombin *in vivo*. Activation of the extrinsic pathway requires exposure of circulating plasma factor VIIa to the membrane-bound tissue factor protein (5). An abundance of tissue factor is located in the subendothelium surrounding the vasculature; however, under normal circumstances tissue factor does not contact the blood. After damage to the vascular endothelium, tissue factor protein is exposed to plasma, leading to formation of a phospholipid-bound complex with factors VIIa and X. This tissue factor–factor VIIa complex activates not only factor X but also factor IX of the intrinsic pathway (6).

Initiation of the intrinsic pathway of coagulation occurs on exposure of Hageman factor, factor XII, to a negatively charged foreign surface (7). In the presence of high-molecular-weight kininogen and kallikrein, factor XIIa converts factor XI to factor XIa. In addition to activating the intrinsic pathway, factor XIIa plays a role in initiating fibrinolysis, kinin, and complement pathways. Factor XIa may be generated by the activity of either factor XIIa or thrombin itself (8). Factor XIa goes on to complex with factor IX to generate factor IXa. The major importance of the intrinsic pathway *in vivo* would appear to be as an amplification system for increased thrombin generation after initiation of the extrinsic pathway of coagulation (8).

Both platelet and platelet microvesicle membranes play an important role in propagation of the extrinsic and intrinsic pathways by acting as assembly sites for zymogen-cofactor complexes (2). These membrane-bound complexes accelerate enzymatic reaction rates to increase production of coagulation factors. Factor IXa forms the "tenase" complex with a cofactor, factor VIIIa, on the platelet phospholipid membrane, thereby accelerating the activation of factor X. The prothrombinase complex, comprising factors Xa, Va, and calcium, amplifies the conversion of prothrombin to thrombin. Platelet activation leads to conformational changes in the platelet membrane that optimize assembly of the prothrombinase complex. Although they participate in platelet-bound complexes, coagulation factors (Xa, Va, VIIa, IXa) are shielded from inactivation by intrinsic antico-

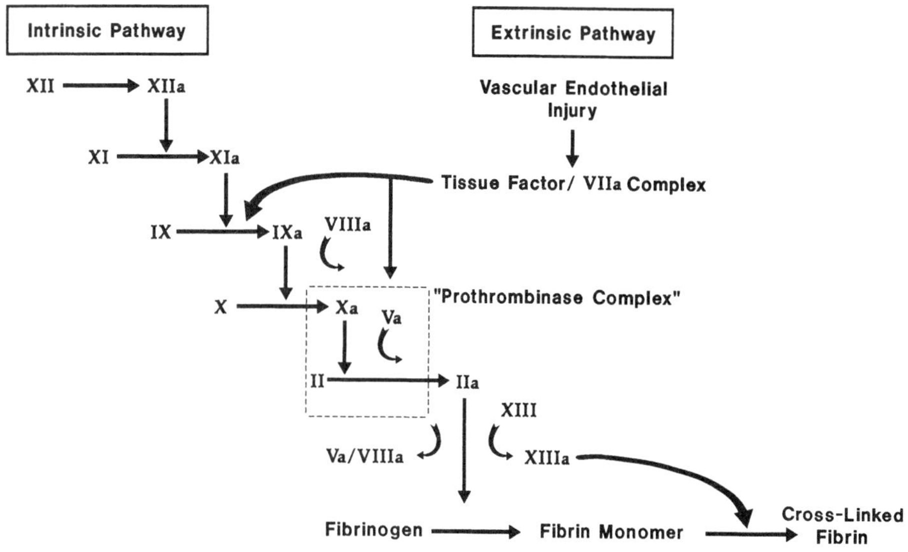

FIGURE 11-1. A summation of the extrinsic and intrinsic pathways of hemostasis.

agulant proteins circulating in plasma, such as antithrombin III (AT III) and activated protein C (9). Thrombin activates the essential cofactors V and VIII that function in the tenase and prothrombinase complexes. This feedback loop plays a major role in accelerating prothrombin activation (2).

The final pathway, common to both chains of the coagulation cascade, concludes with the proteolytic action of thrombin on fibrinogen to produce a stable hemostatic plug. Thrombin cleaves fibrinopeptides A and B from the fibrinogen molecule, producing fibrin monomers that spontaneously polymerize into long strands (10). These strands are cross-linked with covalent bonds by the action of factor XIIIa to produce an insoluble fibrin clot.

Platelet Adhesion and Aggregation

Platelets play a central role in the activation of prothrombin and the propagation of the hemostatic plug (11). Under normal physiologic conditions platelets do not adhere to the vascular endothelium; however, vascular damage results in the exposure of subendothelial matrix proteins (i.e., collagen, von Willebrand factor [vWF], fibronectin) that are capable of inducing platelet adhesion (12). vWF forms a bridge linking subendothelial proteins with a glycoprotein receptor on the platelet surface, glycoprotein Ib/IX (GP Ib/IX) (13). Platelet adhesion to the endothelium leads to platelet activation and initiates several nearly simultaneous platelet responses, including release of storage granule contents, production of prostaglandin endoperoxides, and expression of active glycoprotein receptors on the platelet surface.

The redistribution of membrane phospholipids that occurs with platelet activation proves essential to the interaction between plasma proteins of the coagulation pathway and the platelet membrane. As the platelet exterior assumes a "spiny" appearance, conformational changes occur in surface glycoproteins and phospholipids. The surface glycoprotein IIb/IIIa complex (GP IIb/IIIa) becomes "activated" to bind fibrinogen, which acts as a bridge to promote aggregation of adjacent platelets (14). In addition, anionic phospholipids exposed during structural changes in the platelet surface act as binding sites for factor Va and other proteins involved in formation of the coagulation activation complexes.

Fibrinolysis

The fibrinolytic system represents a carefully balanced group of profibrinolytic and antifibrinolytic enzymes that maintain vascular patency by dissolving fibrin (Fig. 11-2). Under normal physiologic conditions, the fibrinolytic system is not activated until thrombin converts fibrinogen to fibrin. The principal mediator of fibrinolysis is plasmin, a

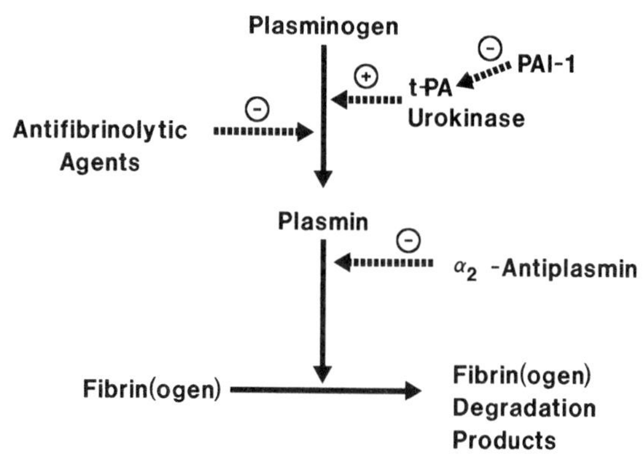

FIGURE 11-2. The principal mediators of fibrinolysis *in vivo*. Dashed lines demonstrate sites of action for promoters and inhibitors of fibrinolysis.

proteolytic enzyme that digests fibrin (15). Plasmin circulates as an inactive precursor, plasminogen. Contact activators intrinsic to the circulation, such as FXIIa or plasma kallikrein, activate plasminogen on contact with a foreign surface (16). In addition, tissue plasminogen activator (tPA) and urokinase are enzymes generated extrinsic to the blood that are capable of activating plasminogen. Fibrinolysis is normally activated concurrently with the coagulation cascade. Thrombin accelerates plasmin formation by triggering release of tPA from vascular endothelium and by producing fibrin (17). Fibrin accelerates the conversion of plasminogen to plasmin by plasminogen activators and acts to localize fibrinolysis to sites of active clot formation (18). Plasmin, and fibrin degradation products generated during fibrinolysis, manifest multiple anticoagulant activities, including degradation of the cofactors Va and VIIIa and interference with fibrin polymerization and platelet aggregation.

PATHOPHYSIOLOGIC HEMOSTATIC EFFECTS OF CARDIOPULMONARY BYPASS

Plasma Proteins

Numerous investigations have demonstrated a decline in circulating concentrations of coagulation factor proteins during CPB (19). Both bubble and membrane oxygenators denature plasma proteins; denaturation associated with air-fluid interfaces may partially explain the increases in postoperative bleeding associated with increased salvage of blood from the operative field (20). Protein denaturation becomes more pronounced with time, and it is particularly problematic with the bubble oxygenator (21). Hemodilution due to CPB pump priming volume accounts for much of the plasma protein decline; however, for unknown reasons factor V decreases to a greater extent than other plasma proteins during CPB (22). Interaction with the artificial surfaces of the CPB circuit undoubtedly accounts for some depletion of plasma proteins. Fibrinogen is rapidly adsorbed to the synthetic surface of the perfusion circuit during extracorporeal circulation (23).

Platelets

Initiation of CPB results in a rapid decline in both platelet number and function (24). Hemodilution accounts for the major reduction in platelets; however, platelets have been demonstrated to adhere to extracorporeal synthetic surfaces (25). At the outset of CPB, fibrinogen and other plasma proteins adhere to the artificial surfaces of the extracorporeal circuit, thereby providing a substrate for platelet adhesion (26). Membrane oxygenators, with a larger surface area, tend to generate greater degrees of thrombocytopenia at the outset of CPB. However, platelet counts seldom decrease below 100,000/mL during CPB (19). Alterations in platelet number clearly do not account for the majority of hemostatic abnormalities occurring after CPB.

Regardless of whether bubble or membrane oxygenators are used, several minutes after initiation of CPB the bleeding time becomes prolonged (27). Prolongation of the bleeding time correlates with the duration of CPB, and it is independent of platelet count. Elevated plasma concentrations of platelet-specific proteins (i.e., platelet factor 4 (PF4) and β-thromboglobulin) are indicative of platelet activation and release of alpha granule contents. Release of alpha granule contents has been further substantiated by electron microscopy and, more recently, by flow cytometry (28). Increasing numbers of platelets are progressively activated during CPB, with one study describing 29% of circulating platelets as being in an activated state during CPB (29).

Evidence exists for mechanical damage to the platelet membrane during extracorporeal circulation. Shear stress, turbulence, and adherence to synthetic surfaces may result in loss of platelet membrane glycoprotein receptors. In addition, plasmin generated during CPB may cleave glycoproteins from the platelet membrane, potentially interfering with subsequent platelet adhesion and aggregation (30). Several investigations have demonstrated reductions in platelet membrane glycoproteins Ib and IIb/IIIa after CPB (31,32). However, these findings have been contested, and their physiologic significance for postoperative bleeding remains unclear (33).

Fibrinolysis

The success of antifibrinolytic drugs in limiting hemorrhage after CPB has generated increasing interest in the role of fibrinolysis in post-CPB hemorrhage. Fibrin degradation products frequently attain measurable concentrations during CPB (34). Investigators have demonstrated increasing concentrations of both tPA antigen and activity during CPB (35,36). The presence of circulating D-dimer during CPB suggests that cross-linked fibrin has undergone fibrinolytic degradation (37). Systemic fibrinolysis appears to be short-lived, with a return of plasma tPA concentrations to baseline within a few hours after completion of CPB. Although the source of plasminogen activator is probably the vascular endothelium, mechanisms regulating the release of tPA during CPB are unknown. Proposed mechanisms for initiation of the fibrinolytic state include release of plasminogen activators from pericardial and periosteal surfaces, factor XIIa-mediated activation of plasminogen, and thrombin-mediated release of tPA from the vascular endothelium (19).

MANAGEMENT OF ANTICOAGULATION DURING CARDIOPULMONARY BYPASS

Heparin Anticoagulation

The intensity of thrombogenic stimuli occurring during surgery and CPB necessitate a level of anticoagulation exceeding that in other medical settings. An activated coagulation

TABLE 11-1. COMMON MECHANISMS OF EXCESSIVE BLEEDING AFTER CARDIOPULMONARY BYPASS

Preexisting acquired or congenital bleeding disorder
Inadequate surgical hemostasis
Qualitative disorders of platelet function
Fibrinolysis
Inadequate reversal of heparin
Hypothermia

time (ACT) in excess of 400 seconds is generally accepted as the minimal degree of anticoagulation necessary before institution of CPB (38). The major risk associated with lesser degrees of anticoagulation is not that the CPB circuit will occlude but rather that a consumptive coagulopathy will ensue, resulting in increased postoperative hemorrhage (Table 11-1).

Almost 80 years after its discovery (39), heparin remains the only widely available pharmacologic agent for anticoagulation during CPB. The heparin molecule is composed of long sulfated mucopolysaccharide chains belonging to the glycosaminoglycan family. The basic structure of heparin consists of alternating uronic acid and glucosamine saccharide subunits (40). Heparin preparations are derived primarily from partial purification of bovine lung or porcine intestinal mucosa. The end product is structurally heterogeneous, with molecular weights ranging from 3,000 to 35,000 Da. Heparins of different molecular weights possess differing abilities to inhibit thrombin and other serine proteases.

Heparin functions as a catalyst rather than as a direct inhibitor of coagulation. Heparin binds with antithrombin (AT III), resulting in a conformational change that accelerates subsequent binding with target serine proteases (41). The heparin–AT III complex irreversibly binds and inactivates thrombin as well as factors IXa, Xa, XIa, and XIIa (42). After inactivation of a serine protease, heparin is released from the complex to catalyze additional inhibitory reactions.

Protocols for anticoagulation before CPB vary somewhat from one medical center to another. At our institution, porcine heparin, 300 units/kg, is administered by central venous catheter before CPB is initiated. An additional 5,000 units of heparin is included in the CPB pump priming volume. The ACT is determined 5 minutes after injection of heparin to ensure that intravascular administration occurred. The ACT is determined every 30 minutes during CPB and more frequently during rewarming. Additional heparin is administered as necessary to maintain the ACT in excess of 400 seconds.

Rarely, a patient is encountered in whom the ACT fails to increase after heparin administration. Patients receiving heparin preoperatively (43) and those with ongoing thrombotic disorders are more likely to experience such "heparin resistance" (44). Several mechanisms have been proposed to explain this phenomenon. Interpatient anticoagulant responses to identical doses of heparin vary widely (45,46); in many cases resistance may be merely an extreme manifestation of the normal variable response to heparin. Preexisting deficiencies in AT III, as might be acquired during prolonged heparin infusions, limit the ability of heparin to produce adequate anticoagulation. The release of platelet stores of PF4, a potent inhibitor of heparin, has been proposed as an explanation for heparin resistance in the setting of ongoing thrombosis.

Several approaches are available for the management of heparin resistance. Initially, technical errors of administration must be ruled out. Blood should be aspirated before and after injection of heparin. Administration of hepa·in from a different manufacturing lot may prove more effective at producing anticoagulation. In most cases, administration of additional heparin will produce an ACT in excess of 400 seconds. Administration of fresh-frozen plasma as a means of repleting AT III has been described as a method to overcome heparin resistance in extreme cases (47). Heat-sterilized or transgenic AT III concentrates may provide a safer and more specific therapeutic approach to these patients (48).

Heparin Neutralization

Perhaps the greatest advantage in using heparin as an anticoagulant is the ability to antagonize its effect with protamine. Protamine is a small cationic protein derived from salmon sperm. The mechanism of heparin inhibition is simply that of a stoichiometric acid-base reaction. Heparin is a highly anionic molecule that readily complexes with the cationic protamine, milligram for milligram. For this reason, protamine is typically administered in a dose of 1 mg for each 100 units of heparin present. Heparin inhibition is complicated by the unpredictable rate of heparin uptake and metabolism after intravascular administration. Bull et al. (45) demonstrated a large variability in heparin sensitivity and elimination half-life among patients. This observation necessitates monitoring of heparin effect as opposed to reliance on a fixed dosing protocol. Using the ACT, heparin dose-response curves may be constructed to better estimate heparin and protamine requirements during surgery (Fig. 11-3). Alternatively, heparin concentration may be monitored by automated protamine titration assays (e.g., Hepcon Heparin Management System, Medtronic Blood Systems, Parker, CO).

Numerous adverse effects have been attributed to protamine, including interference with hemostasis, anaphylactoid reactions, and a pulmonary vasoconstrictive response. Evidence for a physiologically significant anticoagulant effect from protamine is scant and is derived primarily from *in vitro* investigations. It has been suggested that protamine contributes to thrombocytopenia and inhibits platelet ag-

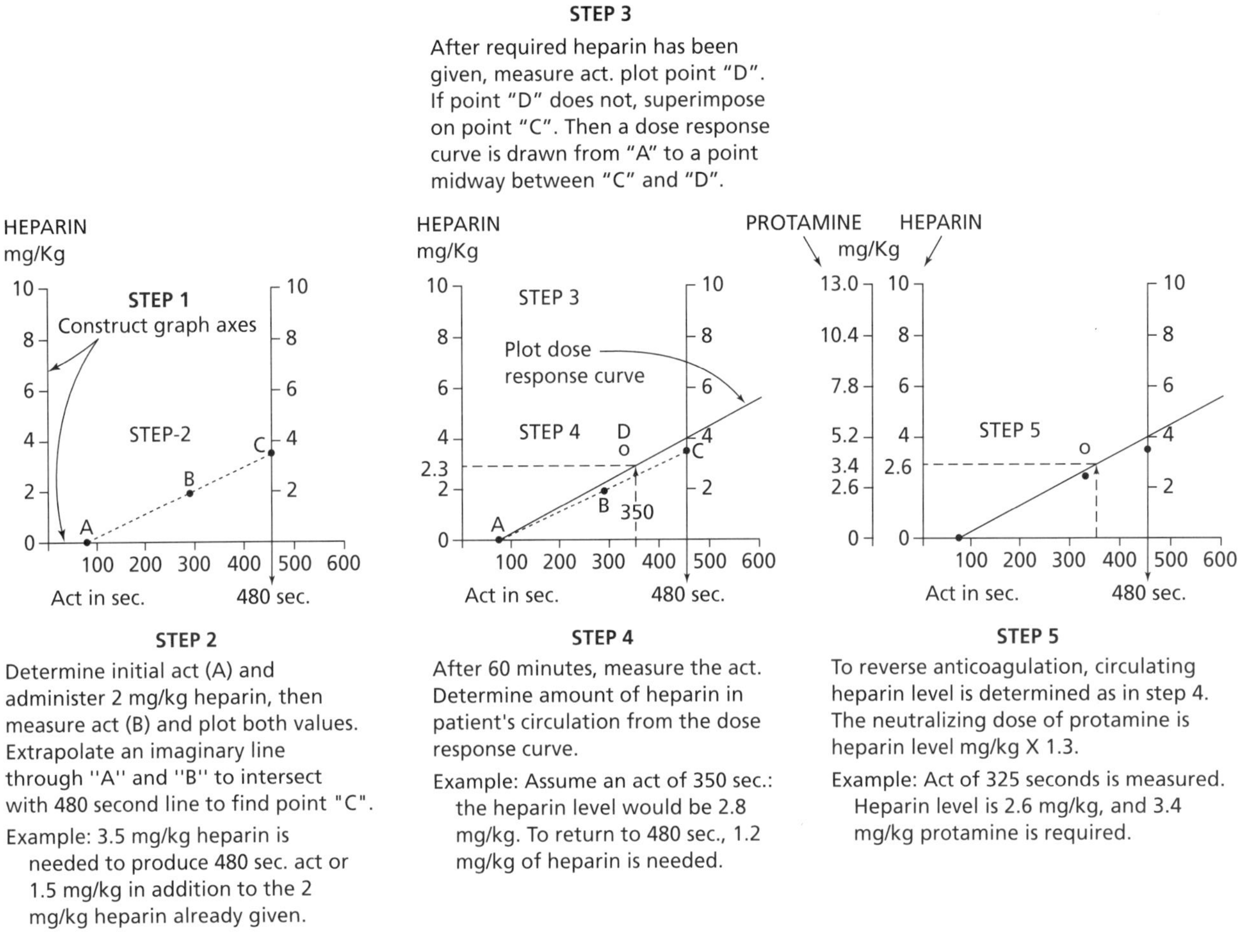

FIGURE 11-3. Bull's method for the construction of heparin dose-response curves. Heparin dose is more properly reported in units per kilogram. One milligram of heparin is roughly equal to 100 units. ACT, activated coagulation time. (From Bull BS, Huse WM, Brauer FS, et al. Heparin therapy during extracorporeal circulation: II. The use of a dose-response curve to individualize heparin and protamine dosage. *J Thorac Cardiovasc Surg* 1975;69:685, with permission.)

gregation (49,50). Again, the *in vivo* significance of these findings remains uncertain.

Adverse hemodynamic responses to protamine appear to be a more prevalent and identifiable complication. Systemic hypotension often accompanies the administration of protamine (51,52). The mechanism appears to be related primarily to systemic vasodilation rather than impaired myocardial contractility (53). Histamine release has been implicated as the likely mediator (54). However, vascular endothelial release of nitric oxide may play a contributory role (55). Slowing the administration rate of protamine appears to be an effective means of reducing the frequency of adverse hemodynamic responses.

Several risk factors have been implicated in protamine-mediated anaphylactoid reactions, including fish allergy, a history of vasectomy, and prior exposure to protamine (i.e., protamine-containing insulin) (56). Regardless of whether any of these conditions actually increases the probability of an anaphylactoid reaction to protamine, the risk to any individual patient appears quite low (57,58).

A third reaction seen after administration of protamine is severe pulmonary vasoconstriction. This complication is manifested by systemic hypotension and increased pulmonary artery pressure, occasionally leading to right ventricular failure (59). Complement-mediated release of prostaglandin endoperoxides has been implicated in the mechanism underlying this reaction (60,61). Treatment is largely empirical. Vasodilating inotropes may be required for management of pulmonary hypertension and ventricular failure. Administration of additional heparin has been suggested as a means of reducing the size of heparin-protamine complexes and thereby alleviating the symptoms (62). Inhaled nitric oxide proved efficacious in a single report (63).

The patient with a history of a prior protamine reaction presents a therapeutic dilemma. Protamine is the only widely available pharmacologic agent for reversal of heparin.

Protamine may be withheld at the conclusion of CPB. As might be expected, the blood loss associated with this approach is considerable (64). Preoperative administration of a cyclooxygenase inhibitor may attenuate the hemodynamic response to protamine (65). A more practical approach may be the slow infusion of protamine after successful administration of a test dose (56). Viable alternatives to protamine, heparinase and PF4, are currently undergoing clinical trials and may in the near future provide a safer alternative to protamine for reversal of heparin anticoagulation (66,67).

MONITORING ANTICOAGULATION DURING CARDIOPULMONARY BYPASS

The high degree of patient-to-patient variability in both pharmacokinetic and pharmacodynamic response to heparin necessitates some form of intraoperative coagulation monitoring to ensure that adequate anticoagulation has been achieved before initiation of CPB. Traditional laboratory tests for heparin response, such as the activated partial thromboplastin time (aPTT) and thrombin time, are extremely sensitive to low doses of heparin and therefore of little use during CPB (68). Several monitors with limited applicability outside the operative setting have proved useful for monitoring anticoagulation at heparin concentrations achieved during CPB.

Activated Coagulation Time

The ACT was initially described by Hattersly in 1966 as a modification of the whole blood clotting time (69). As a measure of the intrinsic pathway of coagulation, the ACT is prolonged in the presence of heparin. Since Hattersly's description, instrument automation has greatly simplified ACT determination in patient care settings. Although ACT detection methodology differs somewhat among manufacturers, the principle remains the same. Whole blood from the patient is directly added to a glass vial containing either celite or kaolin—contact activators. One popular automated method for ACT determination (Hemochron, International Technidyne, Edison, NJ) incorporates a magnet into the ACT sample vial. As the vial containing a blood sample and contact activator is rotated continuously within the instrument, the magnet maintains contact with a proximity detection switch. Clot formation entraps the magnet. As the sample vial continues to rotate, the magnet is pulled away from the proximity detection switch, triggering an end to the assay. Another variation of the ACT (ACTII, Medtronic) exploits a plumb bob–flag assembly that is repeatedly raised and lowered through the sample of whole blood and contact activator. As clot formation occurs, descent of the flag through the blood slows, triggering an optical detector that ends the assay.

The normal range for the ACT, as determined in a healthy cohort, is 107 ± 13 seconds (69). Heparin administration results in prolongation of the ACT. Measurements greater than 600 seconds exceed the linear dose-response range for the test. The coefficient of variation for the ACT has been estimated to be less than 10% (70). The ACT is relatively insensitive to platelet abnormalities; however, hypothermia and hemodilution prolong the measurement (71). After neutralization of heparin with protamine, the ACT should return to within 10% of the preoperative baseline value. Although the ACT is well suited to monitoring anticoagulation during CPB, this measurement is relatively insensitive to low heparin concentrations. Therefore, return of the ACT to baseline does not ensure that heparin is entirely neutralized (72). Low concentrations of circulating heparin may be detected by measuring the plasma heparin concentration.

Heparin Concentration

The direct stoichiometric inactivation of heparin by protamine provides a method for estimating the circulating heparin concentration (73). As increasing concentrations of protamine are added to samples of heparin-containing blood, the time required to form a fibrin clot decreases. As the concentration of protamine exceeds that of heparin, the time to clot formation increases owing to the *in vitro* anticoagulant effects of protamine. These measurements have been automated in the Hepcon Heparin Management System (Medtronic). Assuming that the heparin-protamine titration curve remains constant during a given surgery, these instruments theoretically allow maintenance of a desired heparin concentration throughout the intraoperative period. However, these assays are not functional measures of heparin activity. Protamine titration assays do not verify anticoagulation but merely indicate that a given concentration of heparin is present in the blood sample. In contrast to the ACT, protamine titration tests are relatively resistant to interference from hypothermia and hemodilution. Maintenance of stable heparin concentrations during CPB may reduce thrombin activity and potentially improve postoperative hemostasis (74,75). The greatest benefit of heparin titration assays may be in diagnosis of unneutralized heparin after CPB and in estimation of the protamine dose necessary to neutralize remaining heparin.

Viscoelastic Measures of Coagulation

Viscoelastic measures of coagulation have undergone a resurgence in popularity associated with their applications in monitoring perioperative hemostasis. The thromboelastograph (TEG) (Haemoscope, Morton Grove, IL), the viscoelastic monitor in most widespread use, was initially introduced by Hartert in 1948 as a qualitative measure of clot formation (76). The unique feature of the TEG is its ability to measure overall hemostatic response, from initial acti-

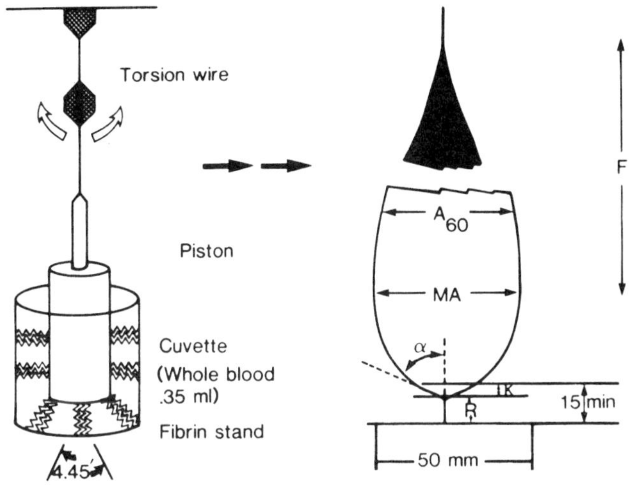

FIGURE 11-4. Structural components of the thromboelastograph (TEG) and normal measured parameters. R, reaction time, 7.5 to 15 minutes; K, 3 to 7 minutes; alpha angle, 40 to 60 degrees; MA, maximum amplitude, 40 to 60 mm; A_{60}, amplitude after 60 minutes; A_{60}/MA, whole blood clot lysis index greater than 0.85; F, whole blood clot lysis time greater than 300 minutes. (From Tuman KJ, Spiess BD, McCarthy RJ, et al. Effects of progressive blood loss on coagulation as measured by thromboelastography. *Anesth Analg* 1987;66:856, with permission.)

vation of coagulation to clot formation, retraction, and eventual lysis. The TEG is operated by placing 0.35 mL of whole blood into a disposable cuvette. The cuvette is placed into the TEG, where it is continuously rotated and maintained at a temperature of 37°C. A metal piston, suspended by a torsion wire attached to an electronic recording device, is lowered into the spinning cuvette (Fig. 11-4). As clot formation occurs, fibrin strands form between the cuvette and the piston, transferring rotational motion of the cuvette to the torsion wire and recording device (77).

Although TEG-derived variables do not correlate directly with other, more specific laboratory-based measures of coagulation, information derived from the TEG can identify abnormalities in clot formation and lysis (77). The reaction time (R; normal range, 7.5 to 15 minutes) is a measure of time to initial clot formation. The R value is comparable to the whole blood clotting time and may be accelerated by adding a contact activator to the sample cuvette. Prolongation of the R value would be consistent with a deficiency in one or more plasma coagulation factors. The maximum amplitude (MA; normal range, 50 to 60 mm) provides a measure of clot strength and may be decreased by qualitative or quantitative platelet dysfunction or by hypofibrinogenemia. Both the alpha angle and the clot formation time (K) provide measures of the rate of clot growth. Any factors that slow the kinetic rate of clot formation would prolong these variables.

Preliminary data suggest that the TEG may be useful in differentiating postoperative hemorrhage related to a coagulopathy from that resulting from a surgically correctable cause (78). The TEG has proved particularly adept in the diagnosis of fibrinolysis during liver transplantation (79). In addition, it is possible to perform titration tests using antifibrinolytic agents while assessing therapeutic effect with the TEG (80). Principally because of the limited specificity of findings associated with thromboelastography, viscoelastic measurements of hemostasis have failed to gain popularity outside the operative setting. Recent advances in computerized data analysis may improve issues of quality assurance and lead to wider acceptance of viscoelastic monitoring of hemostasis.

Platelet Function Monitors

Although platelet dysfunction has long been recognized as a major component of coagulopathies after CPB, simple point-of-care monitors to detect these disorders have not, until recently, been available. Preliminary investigations with these instruments suggest potential to detect platelet dysfunction in the perioperative setting and to modify postoperative hemorrhage by directing therapeutic interventions. HemoSTATUS (Medtronic), the first commercially available point-of-care platelet function test, exploits platelet activating factor (PAF) as an agonist to accelerate platelet-mediated clot formation. Using the Heparin Management System (Medtronic) as a monitoring platform, the HemoSTATUS performs kaolin ACT measurements in the presence and absence of PAF. A clot ratio reflecting the effect of PAF on kaolin ACT formation for a particular patient is compared with a manufacturer-provided "maximal clot ratio" derived from healthy volunteers. In the presence of intrinsic platelet dysfunction, additional PAF would be required to achieve kaolin ACT results comparable to those of healthy control subjects. This PAF "insensitivity" is reflected in the clot ratio, allowing identification of patient samples with reduced platelet function. In preliminary investigations, platelet dysfunction detected by the HemoSTATUS test correlated with postoperative mediastinal drainage (81). However, other investigators have failed to corroborate these results, suggesting the need for further investigation (82,83).

A particularly novel approach to monitoring platelet function is manifested in the PFA-100 (Platelet Function Analyzer, Dade Behring International, Miami, FL) (84). The PFA-100 measures the time required for a sample of whole blood to occlude an aperture within a collagen/adenosine diphosphate or collagen/epinephrine membrane. Test conditions are optimized to measure platelet plug formation under physiologic high-shear conditions, and both platelet adherence and aggregation must be optimal to obtain a normal "closure time." Clinical trials with the PFA-100 remain in progress, but preliminary investigations have demonstrated the sensitivity and specificity of this instrument to detect both congenital and acquired disorders of platelet function (85).

PHARMACOLOGIC HEMOSTATIC AGENTS IN THE MANAGEMENT OF POSTOPERATIVE HEMORRHAGE

Desmopressin

Desmopressin acetate [1-desamino-8-D-arginine vasopressin, or DDAVP] is a synthetic analog of the antidiuretic hormone vasopressin. Structural modifications provide increased potency and duration but less pressor effect than the parent compound (86). Since the 1970s, DDAVP has been recognized as an effective therapy for mild hemophilia and some forms of von Willebrand disease. Beneficial hemostatic effects also have been reported after DDAVP administration in patients with uremia and in those requiring extensive spinal surgery (87,88). The proposed mechanism for these hemostatic effects is release of factor VIII and vWF from the vascular endothelium (89).

Investigations focusing on the ability of DDAVP to limit bleeding after cardiac surgery have yielded conflicting results. In a double-blind, randomized, prospective study of 72 patients undergoing surgery for valve replacement, repeat coronary artery bypass graft (CABG) surgery, or atrial septal defect repair, DDAVP (0.3 g/kg administered after protamine neutralization of heparin) significantly reduced blood loss (90). Initial enthusiasm for DDAVP has been dampened by the failure of follow-up investigations to demonstrate any benefits from DDAVP administration in either adults or children (91–93). Some authors suggest that DDAVP may have a role in a subpopulation of patients who are at particularly high risk for postoperative hemorrhage; however, evidence currently available does not support widespread administration of DDAVP as a prophylactic measure to limit bleeding after cardiac surgery.

Antifibrinolytics

Two synthetic antifibrinolytic drugs, ϵ-aminocaproic acid (EACA) and tranexamic acid, have been widely administered for control of bleeding associated with CPB (94). Both agents are lysine analogs; they bond with the lysine binding site of plasminogen, thereby impeding interactions between plasminogen and fibrin (Fig. 11-5) (95). In the absence of fibrin binding, conversion of plasminogen to plasmin by plasminogen activators is no longer a kinetically favored reaction (96). Fibrinolytic activity is reduced, and the fibrin clot is "protected" from degradation.

Both EACA and tranexamic acid may be administered by either the intravenous or the oral route. Elimination is by renal excretion, with a plasma half-life of 1.5 hours (97). As a perioperative hemostatic agent, EACA is typically administered intravenously in a loading dose of 100 to 150 mg/kg, followed by a continuous infusion of 10 to 15 mg/kg/hour. Tranexamic acid is considered to be approximately ten-fold more potent than EACA, and it is typically administered as a 10 to 15 mg/kg loading dose, followed by an infusion of 1–1.5 mg/kg/hour (94). Administration of antifibrinolytic agents is absolutely contraindicated in the management of patients with either disseminated intravascular coagulation or upper urinary tract bleeding, owing to the associated risk for thrombosis.

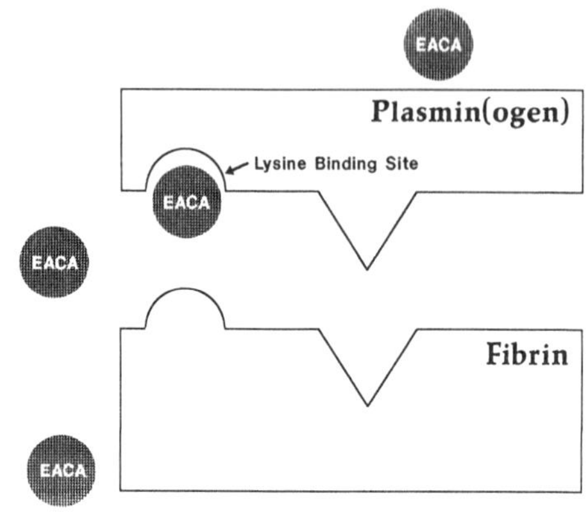

FIGURE 11-5. Mechanism of action of synthetic antifibrinolytic drugs. These drugs interact with lysine binding sites of plasmin and plasminogen, thereby interfering with the ability of these fibrinolytic components to bind fibrin. EACA, ϵ-aminocaproic acid.

Both EACA and tranexamic acid have proved efficacious in reducing bleeding after CPB. EACA has been in clinical use as a hemostatic agent since the mid-1960s (98); however, the full hemostatic potential of the synthetic antifibrinolytics was recognized only with the advent of increased doses and prophylactic administration before CPB. Randomized prospective trials generally have demonstrated 30% to 40% reductions in blood loss, compared with a control group that did not receive antifibrinolytics before CPB (99–102). Concerns have been raised regarding the potential for the synthetic antifibrinolytic drugs to induce thrombotic complications. The lack of significant drug-related morbidity in clinical trials to date suggests that this risk, in the setting of cardiac surgery, is low; however, the sample size of clinical trials to date has been limited.

Aprotinin

During the past decade, aprotinin has emerged as the most promising pharmacologic agent for control of perioperative hemorrhage associated with cardiac surgery. Initially described in the 1930s, aprotinin has long been a popular serine protease inhibitor for *in vitro* laboratory investigations. In fact, aprotinin's potential as a hemostatic agent was first noted during clinical trials attempting to limit cell activation and pulmonary injury associated with CPB (103).

Initial dosing regimens for aprotinin were based on pharmacokinetic modeling and estimates of the aprotinin concentration necessary for *in vitro* plasmin and kallikrein inhibition (104). With an initial elimination half-life of less than 1 hour, aprotinin must be administered by constant infusion to maintain stable plasma concentrations. The standard "high-dose" regimen consists of a loading dose of 2×10^6 KIU (280 mg) administered over 20 minutes, followed by a constant infusion of 5×10^5 KIU (70 mg) per hour. In addition, 2×10^6 KIU (280 mg) is added to the CPB pump priming volume to adjust for hemodilution (103). Administration of a loading dose of aprotinin should always be preceded by a 1-mL test dose to assess the risk for subsequent anaphylactoid reactions.

Numerous investigations have demonstrated the efficacy of aprotinin in reducing blood loss associated with cardiac surgery. A summary of five randomized, double-blind, placebo-controlled trials in Europe demonstrated consistent 40% to 50% reductions in blood loss for primary CABG surgery (103). Aprotinin also has been demonstrated to reduce postoperative bleeding in patients undergoing repeat CABG surgery (105,106), in patients with bacterial endocarditis (107), and those taking aspirin (108).

Despite considerable investigative efforts, the primary mechanism by which aprotinin reduces perioperative hemorrhage remains unclear. Aprotinin has been isolated from tissues of many species, including humans (109); however, the normal physiologic role for this protein is unknown. Although aprotinin clearly inhibits plasmin activity, the significance for *in vivo* fibrinolysis is unclear (110,111). Several studies have suggested that aprotinin "protects" platelets during CPB. Reductions in fibrinolytic activity may reduce proteolytic degradation of platelet surface receptors. Preliminary data indicate that aprotinin does indeed preserve platelet GP Ib receptors, which are essential to platelet adhesion and the primary hemostatic response, during CPB (112).

Several drug interactions of note have been reported with aprotinin. As might be expected, aprotinin inhibits the action of both fibrinolytic drugs and angiotensin-converting enzyme inhibitors (113,114). In addition, aprotinin-mediated inhibition of the intrinsic pathway of coagulation results in artifactual elevation of several screening tests of coagulation, including the celite ACT (103,115). Some authors have suggested increasing the minimally acceptable celite ACT to 750 seconds during aprotinin administration; however, a more prudent course of action would appear to be avoidance of celite ACT monitoring in this setting. The kaolin ACT has demonstrated greater resistance to aprotinin interference (116). Kaolin binds aprotinin in solution, thereby reducing the free drug concentration in plasma. Measurement of heparin concentration, as determined by heparin/protamine titration, is unaffected by aprotinin and offers an alternative method for ensuring adequate anticoagulation during CPB.

The major risk associated with aprotinin administration appears to be that of anaphylactoid reactions (117). Aprotinin is derived from a bovine source, increasing the potential for allergic reactions. In the absence of prior exposure, the incidence of anaphylactoid reactions appears to be extremely low. However, aprotinin reexposure occurring within 6 months may carry a risk for anaphylactoid reaction as high as 4.5%. After 6 months the incidence of anaphylactoid reaction decreases to 1.5% (118). Dietrich et al. (118) suggested several interventions to minimize the risk of anaphylactoid reactions associated with aprotinin reexposure. First, aprotinin reexposure should be avoided for a period of 6 months, if possible. Second, an aprotinin test dose should always be administered before treatment. Third, H_1/H_2 histamine blocking drugs should be administered to patients requiring aprotinin reexposure. And finally, aprotinin administration should be delayed until the surgical team has completed preparations for immediate institution of CPB.

Questions regarding the potential for antifibrinolytic drugs to promote thrombosis have been a recurring concern. It would seem logical that reductions in intrinsic fibrinolytic activity might shift the hemostatic balance toward a prothrombotic state. The fact that patients receiving antifibrinolytic therapy experience reduced postoperative bleeding appears to support this concern. However, to date there have been few reports of thrombotic complications associated with antifibrinolytic therapy in the setting of cardiac surgery. Clearly, the risk for thrombosis, if present, must be low. There is some evidence to suggest that aprotinin may be a safer antifibrinolytic choice in this regard. In contrast to the synthetic antifibrinolytics, high-dose aprotinin therapy has been demonstrated to reduce thrombin and fibrin generation associated with cardiac surgery (116). Suppression of fibrinolytic activity in the absence of concomitant reductions in fibrin generation suggests the possibility that the synthetic antifibrinolytics, EACA and tranexamic acid, may actually increase the potential for thrombosis (119). The recently completed International Multicenter Aprotinin Graft Patency Experience (IMAGE) trial directly assessed coronary patency by angiography in almost 800 patients randomized to receive either high-dose aprotinin or a placebo before CABG surgery (120). Although an overall increase in saphenous vein graft occlusion was detected initially in patients receiving aprotinin (15.4% versus 10.9%; $p = .03$), adjustment of the data to account for coexisting risks for graft occlusion reduced the relative risk of graft occlusion associated with aprotinin from 1.7 to only 1.05. No trials directly assessing vein graft patency are available for the synthetic antifibrinolytics. Patients undergoing cardiac surgery with CPB experience multiple adverse effects to the hemostatic system--quantitative and qualitative platelet dysfunction, hemodilution, hypothermia, heparin rebound. The occurrence of a prolonged "anticoagulated" state in these patients may limit any risk posed by inhibition of intrinsic fibrinolysis.

COMMON PERIOPERATIVE HEMOSTATIC DISORDERS AND THEIR MANAGEMENT

Heparin-Associated Thrombocytopenia and Thrombosis

Heparin-associated thrombocytopenia and thrombosis (HATT) is a life-threatening complication that occurs unpredictably in a subpopulation of patients exposed to heparin. The disorder is characterized by progressive thrombocytopenia that most often occurs within 7 days after heparin exposure, although patients with prior heparin exposure may develop symptoms within 1 to 2 days (121). HATT occurs independently of dose or site of heparin administration. In fact, HATT has been described after exposure to heparin-coated vascular catheters (122).

Laboratory investigations have long suggested an immunologic mechanism as the basis for heparin-associated thrombocytopenia (123). Only recently, Amiral et al. (124) demonstrated that a complex of heparin and PF4 represents the primary antigenic target in HATT. In contrast to other forms of drug-induced thrombocytopenia, heparin-associated thrombocytopenia results in activation of platelets before clearance from the circulation. Evidence supports a model in which heparin–immunoglobulin G immune complexes bind to Fc receptors on the platelet surface, triggering platelet activation and aggregation (125,126).

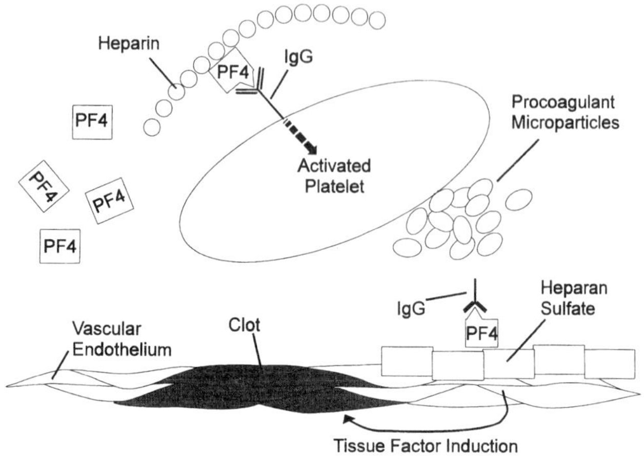

FIGURE 11-6. Heparin-associated thrombocytopenia: proposed thrombotic mechanisms. Immune complexes comprising antibodies directed against heparin/platelet factor (PF4) complexes bind to and activate platelets through FcRII receptors. Procoagulant microparticles released from activated platelets provide additional binding sites to promote generation of activated coagulation factors. Immune complexes also bind heparin or heparin-like molecules of the vascular endothelial surface, resulting in localized expression of tissue factor. (From Slaughter TF, Greenberg CS. Heparin-associated thrombocytopenia and thrombosis. *Anesthesiology* 1997;87:667, with permission.)

Thromboses have been reported in as many as 10% of patients with heparin-associated thrombocytopenia (127). The mechanism for thrombosis remains unclear; however, endothelial binding sites for heparin have been described (128), and immunoglobulin G from the serum of patients with HATT has been demonstrated to bind endothelial cells (129). A recently proposed model (Fig. 11-6) suggests that antibodies directed against heparin/PF4 complexes bind to and activate platelets by way of platelet FcγRII receptors (130). Heparin/PF4 complexes may also bind the vascular endothelium to induce tissue factor expression and thereby promote vascular thrombosis (131). Vascular injury appears to increase the incidence of thrombosis in the setting of heparin-associated thrombocytopenia. Retrospective analysis suggests that patients who undergo surgery in the presence of heparin-associated thrombocytopenia have an increased mortality rate (132).

Several approaches are available for the management of HATT in a patient presenting for cardiac surgery (133). Clearly, all heparin exposure must be eliminated. Elective surgery should be postponed until a time at which the patient's platelets no longer aggregate *in vitro* in response to heparin. A single clinical exposure to heparin in the absence of heparin-induced platelet aggregation appears to pose minimal risk. Concurrent administration of aspirin may further decrease the incidence of thrombotic complications (134). Low-molecular-weight heparins cross-react with heparin-associated antibodies in more than 90% of cases and are therefore not generally useful as substitute therapy for patients with HATT. However, danaparoid has proved efficacious as an alternative anticoagulant (135). This heparinoid, composed of a mixture of polysulfated glycosaminoglycans, fails to induce platelet aggregation in 90% of samples from patients with HATT (136), and it has been safely administered to achieve anticoagulation for CPB (137). Additional alternatives include ancrod, a venom derivative from the Malayan pit viper, and specific thrombin inhibitors (138). The major limitations to ancrod administration include the prolonged preoperative preparatory time required to achieve an adequate state of anticoagulation and the inability to rapidly reverse anticoagulation. Blood losses reported after ancrod administration for CPB are high, requiring substantial exposure to blood products postoperatively. As specific thrombin inhibitors such as hirudin and argatroban become more widely available, they may offer safer alternatives for anticoagulation during CPB in the patient with HATT. However, at present, thrombin inhibitors have limitations similar to those of ancrod and danaparoid. Lack of specific reversal agents and limited monitoring capabilities frequently result in excessive blood loss in the perioperative setting.

Von Willebrand Disease

Von Willebrand disease is the most common of the inheritable bleeding disorders, with a prevalence of 1% of the population (139). This disorder is characterized by quantitative and/or qualitative defects of the vWF protein. vWF, synthesized by the vascular endothelium and megakaryocytes, plays an essential role in platelet adhesion under conditions of high shear (140). In addition, vWF acts as a carrier protein for factor VIII, providing protection from plasma proteases.

In order to optimize management of the patient with von Willebrand disease, the patient's disease must be subtyped on the basis of agarose gel electrophoresis (141). Type I von Willebrand disease, present in the majority of patients, is characterized by a quantitative deficiency in vWF. This subtype of disease is frequently amenable to treatment with desmopressin acetate (DDAVP). Infusion of DDAVP generates increased plasma concentrations of both vWF and factor VIII (142). Administration in a dose of 0.3 mg/kg produces maximal plasma concentrations of vWF within 30 to 90 minutes (143). Rapid infusion may lead to systemic hypotension, and tachyphylaxis frequently accompanies repetitive dosing. Type II von Willebrand disease is characterized by a qualitative defect in vWF and is usually unresponsive to DDAVP administration. In fact, DDAVP may prove detrimental, leading to thrombocytopenia (144). Type III disease is characterized by a homozygous or doubly heterozygous genetic defect that results in near-total or total absence of vWF. DDAVP is usually ineffective in this subtype of von Willebrand disease.

Treatment for both type II and type III von Willebrand disease has traditionally relied on vWF replacement by administration of cryoprecipitate. Exposure to this homologous blood product and the risks of viral transmission make this a less than ideal option. Recent advancements in the manufacture of factor VIII concentrates have resulted in preservation of vWF through the manufacturing process (145). Humate-P (Armour Pharmaceutical, Kankakee, IL) is a third-generation pasteurized factor VIII concentrate with high concentrations of both vWF and high-molecular-weight vWF multimers. This product offers a safer and more specific replacement for vWF and has been successfully administered for the management of von Willebrand disease after cardiac surgery (146).

Emergency Coronary Artery Bypass Graft Surgery after Thrombolytic Therapy

Administration of intravenous thrombolytic therapy in the early management of acute myocardial infarction has become an increasingly widespread practice. Thrombolytic therapy fails to achieve reperfusion in as many as 20% of vessels, necessitating, in some cases, CABG surgery in the setting of a systemic fibrinolytic state (147). Thrombolytic therapy alone is an infrequent cause of bleeding; however, in the setting of a major surgical procedure, postoperative hemorrhage becomes a much greater concern. CABG surgery performed immediately after thrombolytic therapy is associated with significant increases in blood loss (148,149). In a group of patients requiring CABG surgery within 6 hours after receiving intravenous tPA, Kereiakes et al. (147) described an 8% incidence of surgical reexploration for postoperative bleeding.

Unfortunately, the pharmacologic goal of localizing fibrinolytic activity to sites of vascular occlusion has not been achieved. Each of the thrombolytic agents currently used generates plasmin by accelerating the activation of plasminogen. In addition to degrading fibrin at the site of clot formation, plasmin exerts nonspecific proteolytic effects throughout the hemostatic system. Degradation of fibrinogen is the most frequently observed laboratory finding associated with thrombolytic therapy (150). Degradation fragments of fibrin and fibrinogen subsequently interfere with the process of fibrin polymerization (151). Plasmin degrades the cofactors Va and VIIIa, which are essential to thrombin formation (152). Also, plasmin has been demonstrated *in vitro* to degrade platelet membrane glycoproteins GP Ib and GP IIb/IIIa.

No single approach to the management of hemorrhage after thrombolytic therapy and CABG surgery is likely to be uniformly successful. Both interventions are associated with the development of a coagulopathy of multifactorial etiologies. Bleeding is not associated with the dose of thrombolytic agent, nor is it possible to predict the degree of hemorrhage based on currently available laboratory tests. The simplest approach is to delay surgery after thrombolytic therapy. Patients undergoing CABG surgery within 12 hours of streptokinase administration experience significantly greater blood loss than those patients whose surgery is postponed (153). Cryoprecipitate, containing high concentrations of both fibrinogen and factor VIII, has been suggested as the treatment of choice for bleeding after thrombolytic therapy. Platelet concentrates contain intracellular stores of factor V as well as both factors V and VIII in the plasma diluent (154). Because of the frequency with which qualitative platelet defects occur postoperatively (155), platelet concentrates may offer a better therapeutic option than fresh-frozen plasma in this setting. Use of antifibrinolytic agents, aprotinin in particular, may prove to be an effective prophylactic approach to limit bleeding after thrombolytic therapy and cardiac surgery.

REFERENCES

1. Bick RL. Hemostasis defects associated with cardiac surgery, prosthetic devices, and other extracorporeal circuits. *Semin Thromb Hemost* 1985;11:249.
2. Furie B, Furie BC. Molecular and cellular biology of blood coagulation. *N Engl J Med* 1992;326:800.
3. Davie EW, Ratnoff OD. Waterfall sequence for intrinsic blood clotting. *Science* 1964;145:1310.
4. Macfarlane RG. An enzyme cascade in the blood clotting mechanism and its function as a biochemical amplifier. *Nature* 1964; 202:498.
5. Rao LV, Rapaport SI. Activation of factor VII bound to tissue factor: a key early step in the tissue factor pathway of blood coagulation. *Proc Natl Acad Sci USA* 1988;85:6687.

6. Osterud B, Rapaport SI. Activation of factor IX by the reaction product of tissue factor and factor VII: additional pathway for initiating blood coagulation. *Proc Natl Acad Sci USA* 1977;74:5260.
7. Griffin JH. The role of surface in the surface-dependent activation of Hageman factor (blood coagulation factor XII). *Proc Natl Acad Sci USA* 1978;75:1998.
8. Gailani D, Broze GJ. Factor XI activation in a revised model of blood coagulation. *Science* 1991;253:909.
9. Marciniak E. Factor Xa inactivation by antithrombin III: evidence for biological stabilization of factor Xa by factor V-phospholipid complex. *Br J Haematol* 1973;24:391.
10. Ferry JD. The mechanism of polymerization of fibrin. *Proc Natl Acad Sci USA* 1952;38:566.
11. Weiss H. Platelet physiology and abnormalities of platelet function: parts 1 and 2. *N Engl J Med* 1975;293:531, 580.
12. Tranzer JP, Baumgartner HR. Filling gaps in the vascular endothelium with blood platelets. *Nature* 1967;216:1126.
13. Kroll MH, Harris TS, Moake JL, et al. Von Willebrand factor binding to platelet GpIb initiates signals for platelet activation. *J Clin Invest* 1991;88:1568.
14. Bennett JS, Vilaire G. Exposure of platelet fibrinogen receptors by ADP and epinephrine. *J Clin Invest* 1979;64:1393.
15. Vassalli JD, Sappino AP, Belin D. The plasminogen activator/plasmin system. *J Clin Invest* 1991;88:1067.
16. Ogston D, Ogston CM, Ratnoff OD, et al. Studies on a complex mechanism for the activation of plasminogen by kaolin and chloroform: the participation of Hageman factor and additional cofactors. *J Clin Invest* 1969;48:1786.
17. Levin EG, Marzec U, Anderson J, et al. Thrombin stimulates tissue plasminogen activator release from cultured human endothelial cells. *J Clin Invest* 1984;74:1988.
18. Ranby M. Studies on the kinetics of plasminogen activation by tissue plasminogen activator. *Biochim Biophys Acta* 1982;704:461.
19. Woodman RC, Harker LA. Bleeding complications associated with cardiopulmonary bypass. *Blood* 1990;76:1680.
20. Lee WH, Krumhaar D, Fonkalsrud EW, et al. Denaturation of plasma proteins as a cause of morbidity and death after intracardiac operations. *Surgery* 1961;50:29.
21. Pruitt KM, Stroud RM, Scott JW. Blood damage in the heart-lung machine. *Proc Soc Exp Biol Med* 1971;137:741.
22. Harker LA, Malpass TW, Branson HE, et al. Mechanisms of abnormal bleeding in patients undergoing cardiopulmonary bypass: acquired transient platelet dysfunction associated with selected alpha granule release. *Blood* 1980;56:824.
23. Mason RG. The interaction of blood hemostatic elements with artificial surfaces. *Prog Hemost Thromb* 1972;1:141.
24. Addonizio VP. Platelet function in cardiopulmonary bypass and artificial organs. *Hematol Oncol Clin North Am* 1990;4:145.
25. Hope AF, Heyns A duP, Lotter MG, et al. Kinetics and sites of sequestration of indium[111]-labeled human platelets during cardiopulmonary bypass. *J Thorac Cardiovasc Surg* 1981;81:880.
26. Musial J, Niewiarowski S, Hershock D, et al. Loss of fibrinogen receptors from the platelet surface during simulated extracorporeal circulation. *J Lab Clin Med* 1985;105:514.
27. Edmunds LH Jr, Ellison N, Colman RW, et al. Platelet function during cardiac operation: comparison of membrane and bubble oxygenators. *J Thorac Cardiovasc Surg* 1982;83:805.
28. Zilla P, Fasol R, Groscurth P, et al. Blood platelets in cardiopulmonary bypass operations. *J Thorac Cardiovasc Surg* 1989;97:379.
29. Rinder CS, Bohnert J, Rinder HM, et al. Platelet activation and aggregation during cardiopulmonary bypass. *Anesthesiology* 1991;75:388.
30. Adelman B, Michelson AD, Loscalzo J, et al. Plasmin effect on platelet glycoprotein Ib-von Willebrand factor interactions. *Blood* 1985;65:32.
31. Wenger RK, Lukasiewicz H, Mikuta BS, et al. Loss of platelet fibrinogen receptors during clinical cardiopulmonary bypass. *J Thorac Cardiovasc Surg* 1989;97:235.
32. George JN, Picket EB, Saucerman S, et al. Platelet surface glycoproteins: studies on resting and activated platelets and platelet microparticles in normal subjects and observations in patients during adult respiratory distress syndrome and cardiac surgery. *J Clin Invest* 1986;78:40.
33. Kestin AS, Valeri CR, Khuri SF, et al. The platelet function defect of cardiopulmonary bypass. *Blood* 1993;82:107.
34. Spiess BD. The contribution of fibrinolysis to postbypass bleeding. *J Cardiothorac Anesth* 1991;5:13.
35. Stibbe J, Kluft C, Brommer EJP, et al. Enhanced fibrinolytic activity during cardiopulmonary bypass in open-heart surgery in man is caused by extrinsic (tissue-type) plasminogen activator. *Eur J Clin Invest* 1984;14:375.
36. Tanaka K, Takao M, Yada I, et al. Alterations in coagulation and fibrinolysis associated with cardiopulmonary bypass during open heart surgery. *J Cardiothorac Anesth* 1989;3:181.
37. Gram J, Janetzko T, Jespersen J, et al. Enhanced effective fibrinolysis following the neutralization of heparin in open heart surgery increases the risk of post-surgical bleeding. *Thromb Haemost* 1990;63:241.
38. Young JA, Kisker CT, Doty DB. Adequate anticoagulation during cardiopulmonary bypass determined by activated clotting time and the appearance of fibrin monomer. *Ann Thorac Surg* 1978;26:231.
39. McClean J. The thromboplastic action of cephalin. *Am J Physiol* 1916;41:250.
40. Warkentin TE, Kelton JG. Heparin and platelets. *Hematol Oncol Clin North Am* 1990;4:243.
41. Villanueva GB, Danishefsky I. Evidence for a heparin-induced conformational change in antithrombin III. *Biochem Biophys Res Commun* 1977;74:803.
42. Damus PS, Hicks M, Rosenberg RD. Anticoagulant action of heparin. *Nature* 1973;246:355.
43. Anderson EF. Heparin resistance prior to cardiopulmonary bypass. *Anesthesiology* 1986;64:504.
44. Collen D, Schetz J, DeCock F, et al. Metabolism of antithrombin III (heparin cofactor) in man: effect of venous thrombosis and of heparin administration. Eur *J Clin Invest* 1977;7:27.
45. Bull BS, Korpman RA, Huse WM, et al. Heparin therapy during extracorporeal circulation: 1. Problems inherent in existing heparin protocols. *J Thorac Cardiovasc Surg* 1975;69:674.
46. Bull BS. Heparin anticoagulation. *Ann Thorac Surg* 1980;30:204.
47. Sabbagh AH, Chung GKT, Shuttleworth P, et al. Fresh frozen plasma: a solution to heparin resistance during cardiopulmonary bypass. *Ann Thorac Surg* 1984;37:466.
48. Hoffman DL. Purification and large-scale preparation of antithrombin III. *Am J Med* 1989;87[Suppl 3B]:23S.
49. Jacques LB. Protamine-antagonist to heparin. *Can Med Assoc J* 1973;108:1291.
50. Anderson MN, Mendelow M, Alfano G. Experimental studies of heparin-protamine activity with special reference to protamine inhibition of clotting. *Surgery* 1959;46:1050.
51. Goldman BS, Joison J, Austen WG. Cardiovascular effects of protamine sulfate. *Ann Thorac Surg* 1969;7:459.
52. Gourin A, Streisand RL, Greineder JK, et al. Protamine sulfate administration and the cardiovascular system. *J Thorac Cardiovasc Surg* 1971;62:193.
53. Taylor RL, Little WC, Freeman GL, et al. Comparison of the cardiovascular effects of intravenous and intraaortic protamine

in the conscious and anesthetized dog. *Ann Thorac Surg* 1986; 42:22.

54. Levy JH, Faraj BA, Zaidan JR, et al. Effects of protamine on histamine release from human lung. *Agents Actions* 1989;28:70.
55. Akata T, Yoshitake J, Nakashima M, et al. Effects of protamine on vascular smooth muscle of rabbit mesenteric artery. *Anesthesiology* 1991;75:833.
56. Horrow JC. Protamine allergy. *J Cardiothorac Anesth* 1988;2: 225.
57. Levy JH, Schwieger IA, Zaidan JR, et al. Evaluation of patients at risk for protamine reactions. *J Thorac Cardiovasc Surg* 1989; 98:200.
58. Weiss ME, Nyhan D, Peng Z, et al. Association of protamine IgE and IgG antibodies with life-threatening reactions to intravenous protamine. *N Engl J Med* 1989;320:886.
59. Lowenstein E, Johnston WE, Lappas DG, et al. Catastrophic pulmonary vasoconstriction associated with protamine reversal of heparin. *Anesthesiology* 1983;59:470.
60. Rent R, Ertel N, Eisenstein R, et al. Complement activation by interaction of polyanions and polycations: I. Heparin-protamine induced consumption of complement. *J Immunol* 1975; 114:120.
61. Colman RW. Humoral mediators of catastrophic reactions associated with protamine neutralization. *Anesthesiology* 1987;66: 595.
62. Lock R, Hessel EA. Probable reversal of protamine reactions by heparin administration. *J Cardiothorac Vasc Anesth* 1990;4:604.
63. Ralley FE. The use of nitric oxide for managing catastrophic pulmonary vasoconstriction arising from protamine administration. *Anesth Analg* 1999;88:505.
64. Castaneda AR. Must heparin be neutralized following open-heart operations? *J Thorac Cardiovasc Surg* 1966;52:716.
65. Hobbhahn J, Conzen PF, Zenker B, et al. Beneficial effect of cyclooxygenase inhibition on adverse hemodynamic responses after protamine. *Anesth Analg* 1988;67: 253.
66. Michelsen LG, Kikura M, Levy JH, et al. Heparinase I (Neutralase) reversal of systemic anticoagulation. *Anesthesiology* 1996; 85:339.
67. Dehmer GJ, Fisher M, Tate DA, et al. Reversal of heparin anticoagulation by recombinant platelet factor 4 in humans. *Circulation* 1995;91:2188.
68. Colman RW, Oxley L, Giannusa P. Statistical comparison of the automated activated partial thromboplastin time and the clotting time in the regulation of heparin therapy. *Am J Clin Pathol* 1970;53:904.
69. Hattersly PC. Activated coagulation time of whole blood. *JAMA* 1966;196:436.
70. Gravlee GP, Case LD, Angert KC, et al. Variability of the activated coagulation time. *Anesth Analg* 1988;67:469.
71. Ammar T, Fisher CF, Sarier K, et al. The effects of thrombocytopenia on the activated coagulation time. *Anesth Analg* 1996; 83:1185.
72. Culliford AT, Gitel SN, Starr N, et al. Lack of correlation between activated clotting time and plasma heparin during cardiopulmonary bypass. *Ann Surg* 1981;193:105.
73. Perkins HA, Osborn JJ, Hurt R, et al. Neutralization of heparin *in vivo* with protamine: a simple method of estimating the required dose. *J Lab Clin Med* 1956;48:223.
74. Despotis GJ, Joist JH, Hogue CW Jr, et al. More effective suppression of hemostatic system activation in patients undergoing cardiac surgery by heparin dosing based on heparin blood concentrations rather than ACT. *Thromb Haemost* 1996;76: 902.
75. Despotis GJ, Joist JH, Hogue CW Jr, et al. The impact of heparin concentration and activated clotting time monitoring on blood conservation: a prospective, randomized evaluation in patients undergoing cardiac operation. *J Thorac Cardiovasc Surg* 1995;110:46.
76. Hartert H. Blutgerinnungstudien mit der Thrombelastographie, einem neuen Untersuchungsverfahren. *Klin Wochenschr* 1948;26:577.
77. Tuman KJ, Spiess BD, McCarthy RJ, et al. Comparison of viscoelastic measures of coagulation after cardiopulmonary bypass. *Anesth Analg* 1989;69:69.
78. Spiess BD, Tuman KJ, McCarthy RJ, et al. Thromboelastography as an indicator of post-cardiopulmonary bypass coagulopathies. *J Clin Monit* 1987;3:25.
79. Kang YG, Martin DJ, Marquez J, et al. Intraoperative changes in blood coagulation and thromboelastographic monitoring in liver transplantation. *Anesth Analg* 1985;64:888.
80. Kang Y, Lewis JH, Navalgund A, et al. Epsilon-aminocaproic acid for treatment of fibrinolysis during liver transplantation. *Anesthesiology* 1987;66:766.
81. Despotis GJ, Levine V, Filos KS, et al. Evaluation of a new point-of-care test that measures PAF-mediated acceleration of coagulation in cardiac surgical patients. *Anesthesiology* 1996;85: 1311.
82. Ereth MH, Nuttall GA, Klindworth JT, et al. Does the platelet-activated clotting test (HemoSTATUS) predict blood loss and platelet dysfunction associated with cardiopulmonary bypass? *Anesth Analg* 1997;85:259.
83. Ereth MH, Nuttall GA, Santrach PJ, et al. The relation between the platelet-activated clotting test (HemoSTATUS) and blood loss after cardiopulmonary bypass. *Anesthesiology* 1998;88:962.
84. Mammen EF, Comp PC, Gosselin R, et al. PFA-100 system: a new method for assessment of platelet dysfunction. *Semin Thromb Hemost* 1998;24:195.
85. Fressinaud E, Veyradier A, Truchaud F, et al. Screening for von Willebrand disease with a new analyzer using high shear stress: a study of 60 cases. *Blood* 1998;91:1325.
86. Shiffrin JS, Glass DD. DDAVP administration for postbypass bleeding. *J Cardiothorac Anesth* 1991;5:285.
87. Mannucci PM, Remuzzi G, Pusineri F, et al. Deamino-8-D-arginine vasopressin shortens the bleeding time in uremia. *N Engl J Med* 1983;308:8.
88. Kobrinsky NL, Letts RM, Patel LR, et al. 1-Deamino-8-D-arginine vasopressin (desmopressin) decreases operative blood loss in patients having Harrington rod spinal fusion surgery. *Ann Intern Med* 1987;107:446.
89. Mannucci PM. Desmopressin: a nontransfusional form of treatment for congenital and acquired bleeding disorders. *Blood* 1988;72:1449.
90. Salzman EW, Weinstein MJ, Weintraub RM, et al. Treatment with desmopressin acetate to reduce blood loss after cardiac surgery. *N Engl J Med* 1986;314:1402.
91. Hackman T, Gascoyne RD, Naiman SC, et al. A trial of desmopressin (1-deamino-8-D-arginine vasopressin) to reduce blood loss in uncomplicated cardiac surgery. *N Engl J Med* 1989;321: 1437.
92. Seear MD, Wadsworth LD, Rogers PC, et al. The effect of desmopressin acetate (DDAVP) on postoperative blood loss after cardiac operations in children. *J Thorac Cardiovasc Surg* 1989;98:217.
93. Brown MR, Swygert TH, Whitten CW, et al. Desmopressin acetate following cardiopulmonary bypass: evaluation of coagulation parameters. *J Cardiothorac Anesth* 1989;3:726.
94. Slaughter TF, Greenberg CS. Antifibrinolytic drugs and perioperative hemostasis. *Am J Hematol* 1997;56:32.
95. Hardy JF, Desroches J. Natural and synthetic antifibrinolytics in cardiac surgery. *Can J Anaesth* 1992;39:353.
96. Alkjaersig N, Fletcher AP, Sherry S. The mechanism of clot dissolution by plasmin. *J Clin Invest* 1959;38:1086.

97. Verstraete M. Clinical application of inhibitors of fibrinolysis. *Drugs* 1985;29:236.
98. Marin HM. Hemostatic mechanism in extracorporeal circulation. *Arch Surg* 1964;88:988.
99. Vander Salm TJ, Ansell JE, Okike ON, et al. The role of epsilon-aminocaproic acid in reducing bleeding after cardiac operation: a double-blind randomized study. *J Thorac Cardiovasc Surg* 1988;95:538.
100. DelRossi AJ, Cernaianu AC, Botros S, et al. Prophylactic treatment of postperfusion bleeding using EACA. *Chest* 1989;96:27.
101. Horrow JC, Hlavacek J, Strong D, et al. Prophylactic tranexamic acid decreases bleeding after cardiac operations. *J Thorac Cardiovasc Surg* 1990;99:70.
102. Munoz JJ, Birkmeyer NJO, Birkmeyer JD, et al. Is ϵ-aminocaproic acid as effective as aprotinin in reducing bleeding with cardiac surgery: a meta-analysis. *Circulation* 1999;99:81.
103. Royston D. High-dose aprotinin therapy: a review of the first five years' experience. *J Cardiothorac Anesth* 1992;6:76.
104. Van Oeveren W, Jansen NJG, Bidstrup BP, et al. Effects of aprotinin on haemostatic mechanisms during cardiopulmonary bypass. *Ann Thorac Surg* 1987;44:640.
105. Royston D, Bidstrup BP, Taylor KM, et al. Effect of aprotinin on the need for blood transfusion after repeat open heart surgery. *Lancet* 1987;2:1289.
106. Bidstrup BP, Royston D, Sapsford RN, et al. Reduction in blood loss and blood use after cardiopulmonary bypass with high dose aprotinin (Trasylol). *J Thorac Cardiovasc Surg* 1989;97:364.
107. Royston D. The serine antiprotease aprotinin (Trasylol): a novel approach to reducing postoperative bleeding. *Blood Coag Fibrinol* 1990;1:55.
108. Bidstrup BP, Royston D, McGuiness C, et al. Aprotinin in aspirin treated patients. *Perfusion* 1990;5:77.
109. Fioretti E, Binotti I, Barra D, et al. Heterogeneity of the basic pancreatic inhibitor (Kunitz) in various bovine organs. *Eur J Biochem* 1983;130:13.
110. Dietrich W, Spannagl M, Jochum M, et al. Influence of high-dose aprotinin treatment on blood loss and coagulation patterns in patients undergoing myocardial revascularization. *Anesthesiology* 1990;73:1119.
111. Clozel JP, Banken L, Roux S. Aprotinin: an antidote for recombinant tissue-type plasminogen activator (rt-PA) active *in vivo*. *J Am Coll Cardiol* 1990;16:507.
112. Van Oeveren W, Harder MP, Roozendaal KJ, et al. Aprotinin protects platelets against the initial effect of cardiopulmonary bypass. *J Thorac Cardiovasc Surg* 1990;99:788.
113. Wiman B. On the reaction of plasmin or plasmin-streptokinase complex with aprotinin or alpha 2 antiplasmin. *Thromb Res* 1980;17:143.
114. Overlack A, Stumpe KO, Kuhnert M, et al. Evidence for participation of kinins in the antihypertensive effect of converting enzyme inhibition. *Klin Wochenschr* 1981;59:69.
115. Royston D, Bidstrup BP, Sapsford RN, et al. Reduced blood loss after open heart surgery with aprotinin is associated with an increase in the activated clotting time (ACT). *J Cardiothorac Anesth* 1989;3:80.
116. Dietrich W, Dilthey G, Spannagl M, et al. Influence of high-dose aprotinin on anticoagulation, heparin requirement, and celite- and kaolin-activated clotting time in heparin pretreated patients undergoing open-heart surgery: a double-blind, placebo-controlled study. *Anesthesiology* 1995;83:679.
117. Dobkowski WB, Murkin JM. A risk-benefit assessment of aprotinin in cardiac surgical procedures. *Drug Saf* 1998;18:21.
118. Dietrich W, Spath P, Ebell A, et al. Prevalence of anaphylactic reactions to aprotinin: analysis of two hundred forty-eight reexposures to aprotinin in heart operations. *J Thorac Cardiovasc Surg* 1997;113:194.
119. Slaughter TF, Faghih F, Greenberg CS, et al. The effects of ϵ-aminocaproic acid on fibrinolysis and thrombin generation during cardiac surgery. *Anesth Analg* 1997;85:1221.
120. Alderman EL, Levy JH, Rich JB, et al. Analyses of coronary graft patency after aprotinin use: results from the International Multicenter Aprotinin Graft Patency Experience (IMAGE) trial. *J Thorac Cardiovasc Surg* 1998;116:716.
121. Warkentin TE, Kelton JG. Heparin-induced thrombocytopenia. *Annu Rev Med* 1989;40:31.
122. Laster J, Silver DS. Heparin-coated catheters and heparin-induced thrombocytopenia. *J Vasc Surg* 1988;7:667.
123. Rhodes GR, Dixon RH, Silver D. Heparin-induced thrombocytopenia with thrombotic and hemorrhagic manifestations. *Surg Gynecol Obstet* 1973;136:409.
124. Amiral J, Bridey F, Dreyfus M, et al. Platelet factor 4 complexed to heparin is the target for antibodies generated in heparin-induced thrombocytopenia. *Thromb Haemost* 1992;68:95.
125. Kelton JG, Sheridan D, Santos A, et al. Heparin-induced thrombocytopenia: laboratory studies. *Blood* 1988;72:925.
126. Chong BH, Ismail F. The mechanism of heparin-induced platelet aggregation. *Eur J Haematol* 1989;43:245.
127. Kelton JG. Heparin-induced thrombocytopenia. *Haemostasis* 1986;16:173.
128. Barzu T, Van Rijn JLML, Petitou M, et al. Endothelial binding sites for heparin. *Biochem J* 1986;238:847.
129. Cines DB, Tomaski A, Tannenbaum S. Immune endothelial-cell injury in heparin-associated thrombocytopenia. *N Engl J Med* 1987;316:581.
130. Warkentin TE, Hayward CPM, Boshkov LK, et al. Sera from patients with heparin-induced thrombocytopenia generate platelet-derived microparticles with procoagulant activity: an explanation for the thrombotic complications of heparin-induced thrombocytopenia. *Blood* 1994;11:3691.
131. Visentin GP, Ford SE, Scott JP, et al. Antibodies from patients with heparin-induced thrombocytopenia/thrombosis are specific for platelet factor 4 complexed with heparin or bound to endothelial cells. *J Clin Invest* 1994;93:81.
132. Walls JT, Curtis JJ, Silver D, et al. Heparin-induced thrombocytopenia in open heart surgical patients: sequelae of late recognition. *Ann Thorac Surg* 1992;53:787.
133. Slaughter TF, Greenberg CS. Heparin-associated thrombocytopenia and thrombosis: implications for perioperative management. *Anesthesiology* 1997;87:667.
134. Makhoul RG, McCann RL, Austin EH, et al. Management of patients with heparin-associated thrombocytopenia and thrombosis requiring cardiac surgery. *Ann Thorac Surg* 1987;43:617.
135. Ortel TL, Gockerman JP, Califf RM, et al. Parenteral anticoagulation with the heparinoid lomoparan (Org 10172) in patients with heparin induced thrombocytopenia and thrombosis. *Thromb Haemost* 1992;67:292.
136. Makhoul RG, Greenberg CS, McCann RL. Heparin-associated thrombocytopenia and thrombosis: a serious clinical problem and potential solution. *J Vasc Surg* 1986;4:522.
137. Doherty DC, Ortel TL, DeBruijn N, et al. "Heparin-free" cardiopulmonary bypass: first reported use of heparinoid (Org 10172) to provide anticoagulation for cardiopulmonary bypass. *Anesthesiology* 1990;73:562.
138. Zulys VJ, Teasdale SJ, Michel ER, et al. Ancrod (Arvin) as an alternative to heparin anticoagulation for cardiopulmonary bypass. *Anesthesiology* 1989;71:870.
139. Rodeghiero F, Castaman G, Dini E. Epidemiological investigation of the prevalence of von Willebrand's disease. *Blood* 1987;69:454.
140. Sadler JE. Von Willebrand factor. *J Biol Chem* 1991;266:22777.

141. Hoyer LW, Rizza CR, Tuddenham EGD, et al. Von Willebrand factor multimer patterns in von Willebrand's disease. *Br J Haematol* 1983;55:493.
142. Mannucci PM. Desmopressin (DDAVP) for treatment of disorders of hemostasis. *Prog Hemost Thromb* 1986;8:19.
143. Kohler M, Harris A. Pharmacokinetics and haematological effects of desmopressin. *Eur J Clin Pharmacol* 1988;35:281.
144. Holmberg L, Nilsson IM, Borge L, et al. Platelet aggregation induced by 1-desamino-8-D-arginine vasopressin (DDAVP) in type IIB von Willebrand's disease. *N Engl J Med* 1983;309:816.
145. Fricke WA, Yu MW. Characterization of von Willebrand factor in factor VIII concentrates. *Am J Hematol* 1989;31:41.
146. Slaughter TF, Mody EA, Oldham HN, et al. Management of a patient with type IIC von Willebrand's disease during coronary artery bypass graft surgery. *Anesthesiology* 1993;78:195.
147. Kereiakes DJ, Topol EJ, George BS, et al. Emergency coronary artery bypass surgery preserves global and regional left ventricular function after intravenous tissue plasminogen activator therapy for acute myocardial infarction. *J Am Coll Cardiol* 1988; 11:899.
148. Kay P, Ahmad A, Floten S, et al. Emergency coronary artery bypass surgery after intracoronary thrombolysis for evolving myocardial infarction. *Br Heart J* 1985;53:260.
149. Skinner JR, Phillips SJ, Zeff RH, et al. Immediate coronary bypass following failed streptokinase infusion in evolving myocardial infarction. *J Thorac Cardiovasc Surg* 1984;87:567.
150. Sane DC, Califf RM, Topol EJ, et al. Bleeding during thrombolytic therapy for acute myocardial infarction: mechanisms and management. *Ann Intern Med* 1989;111:1010.
151. Marder VJ, Shulman NR. High molecular weight derivatives of human fibrinogen produced by plasmin: II. Mechanisms of their anticoagulant activity. *J Biol Chem* 1969;244:2120.
152. Omar MN, Mann KG. Inactivation of factor Va by plasmin. *J Biol Chem* 1987;262:9750.
153. Lee KF, Mandell J, Rankin JS, et al. Immediate versus delayed coronary grafting after streptokinase treatment. *J Thorac Cardiovasc Surg* 1988;95:216.
154. Simon TL, Henderson R. Coagulation factor activity in platelet concentrates. *Transfusion* 1979;19:186.
155. Campbell FW. The contribution of platelet dysfunction to postbypass bleeding. *J Cardiothorac Anesth* 1991;5[Suppl 1]:8.

Cardiac Anesthesia: Principles and Clinical Practice, Second Edition, edited by Fawzy G. Estafanous, Paul G. Barash, and J.G. Reves. Lippincott Williams & Wilkins, Philadelphia © 2001.

12

CARDIOPULMONARY BYPASS EQUIPMENT

EUGENE A. HESSEL, II

The management of the patient undergoing cardiopulmonary bypass (CPB) is one of the defining characteristics of cardiac anesthesia. It is this author's perception that the involvement and knowledge of new trainees and graduates in cardiothoracic surgery in CPB has diminished. Therefore, there is an opportunity, need, and role to be played by anesthesiologists in the conduct of clinical CPB. This demands that the cardiac anesthesiologist have a thorough knowledge of the basic physiology, principles, and practical application and management of CPB. This chapter attempts to provide some of this essential information.

There is abundant evidence that anesthesiologists are becoming increasingly involved in the study of CPB. This is evident by the recent publication of two textbooks on CPB edited principally by anesthesiologists (1,2), the appearance of many articles related to CPB in surgical and anesthesia journals in which anesthesiologists were principal investigators, the multidisciplinary annual course on CPB sponsored by the Society of Cardiovascular Anesthesiologists, and the workshops and papers presented at the annual meeting of the Society of Cardiovascular Anesthesiologists.

The conduct of CPB is obviously a team effort including the cardiac surgeon, perfusionist, and scrub nurse, but it is an endeavor in which anesthesiologists may provide leadership. In the operating room the anesthesiologist is in a unique position: he or she is the only one who can observe the entire circuit and what is going on in the surgical field. In addition, the anesthesiologist has more time than other team members to think about and observe the conduct of CPB; the surgeons and scrub nurse are concentrating on performing the surgical procedure, while the perfusionist is concentrating on running the heart-lung machine. Further, the anesthesiologist has a thorough knowledge about the patient (including the results of baseline intraoperative transesophageal echocardiographic [TEE] examination), what confounding conditions the patient may have, what the surgeon is planning to do, what has transpired with the case before CPB, what problems the surgeon is encountering, and what can be anticipated in the near future. Based on these data, the anesthesiologist is in a position to think, monitor, troubleshoot, and make recommendations concerning the conduct of CPB, including cannulation techniques, flow rates, arterial pressure (and how to treat), temperature and hematocrit management, venting, and so on, especially if changes or problems develop. In addition, the anesthesiologist can provide leadership in establishing and maintaining the institution's Cardiopulmonary Bypass Service, addressing such issues as development of written protocols for conduct of CPB and management of emergencies, employment of safety and monitoring devices, credentialing and continuing medical education (for all those who participate in CPB), quality assessment and improvement, and adverse event monitoring, investigation, and prevention. Fostering a periodic multidisciplinary conference to review these issues can be helpful.

Even in the short period since the first edition of this book was published, there have been significant changes that have affected the practice of CPB. These include emphasis on cost containment and minimally invasive cardiac surgery (including off-bypass procedures that still demand preparedness for CPB, often in awkward conditions), virtual replacement of bubble oxygenators with microporous hollow-fiber membrane oxygenators, use of augmented venous return, the frequent use of heparin-coated or -bonded circuits (HBCs), more frequent conduct of CPB at normothermic or "tepid" (32° to 35°C) temperature, the avoidance of excessive rewarming temperatures (higher than 37° to 38°C), the near-ubiquitous prophylactic use of some type of antifibrinolytics, better appreciation of the mechanisms involved in the systemic inflammatory response to CPB and of the incidence and cause of overt and subtle neurologic and neuropsychometric abnormalities (with particular appreciation of the significance of the atherosclerotic aorta), and the frequent use of perioperative TEE in conjunction with cardiac surgery and CPB. As a consequence CPB has become safer, partly because of improved equipment, monitoring, education, and credentialing of perfusionists.

This chapter, in addition to covering the technical details of the CPB circuit, emphasizes potential complications and

E. A. Hessel, II: Department of Anesthesiology, University of Kentucky College of Medicine, Lexington, Kentucky 40536

those options in the conduct of CPB that may benefit from the input of an anesthesiologist or may affect how the anesthesiologists cares for and monitors the patient. Because bubble oxygenators have virtually disappeared from the clinical practice of CPB in North America and Europe, we have opted to limit most references to these devices. To supplement this chapter, the interested reader is encouraged to consult recent textbooks on CPB (1–5), the journal *Perfusion* published by Edward Arnold (London), and other contemporary anesthesiology and surgical journals.

HISTORICAL PERSPECTIVE*

The birth of total CPB for cardiac surgery occurred on May 6, 1953, when Dr. John Gibbon, for the first time, successfully repaired an atrial septal defect with the aid of total CPB using a heart-lung machine of his design. This represented the culmination of work that had germinated while he was a surgical resident at the Massachusetts General Hospital in 1931. Dr. Gibbon's success was preceded by other pioneering work. Dr. Clarence Dennis first attempted to repair an atrial septal defect with total CPB on April 5, 1951, but the patient died. On September 2, 1952, Dr. John Lewis first performed intracardiac surgery under direct vision (repair of atrial septal defect) by employing inflow (venous) occlusion and circulatory arrest during surface-induced hypothermia. On October 21, 1952, Dr. F.D. Dodrill successfully corrected pulmonary stenois using right heart bypass. After his initial case Gibbon achieved little further success, and his contribution was met with skepticism. It was left to C. Walton Lillehei of the University of Minnesota to demonstrate the potential offered by extracorporeal circulation for the surgical treatment of cardiac disease; he introduced the use of cross-circulation, in which the patient's parent served as the extracorporeal pump oxygenator. On April 20, 1954, he used this method to perform the first successful repair of a ventricular septal defect. During the next year, he performed 45 repairs of various congenital heart defects using parental cross-circulation, with 66% patient survival and no loss of donors. Although this experience demonstrated the potential for CPB, it was obviously not a long-term solution to the problem. Finally, Dr. John Kirklin at the Mayo Clinic, using a modified Gibbon heart-lung machine, demonstrated in a series of eight patients from March to May, 1955, that the heart-lung machine was a viable tool for cardiac surgery. By October of that year, he had operated on 38 patients with 16 survivors. Many small steps have been taken since that time to bring us to our present state of practice, including disposable bubble oxygenators, nonblood priming, pulsatile bypass, centrifugal pumps, membrane oxygenators, microfiltration, and cardiopulmonary perfusionists (6,7).

GENERAL SURVEY OF THE CIRCUIT

The primary function of CPB is to divert blood away from the heart (both right and left sides, and hence usually the lungs as well) and return it to the systemic arterial system. Therefore, the CPB equipment must replace the function of both the lungs, for gas exchange, and the heart, to provide energy to ensure circulation of blood. Typically, blood is drained by gravity via cannulas in the superior and inferior venae cavae (SVC and IVC, respectively) and/or the right atrium to the heart-lung machine, where it passes through the artificial lung (usually a membrane "oxygenator"); it is then pumped, usually with a roller or centrifugal pump, back into the systemic arterial system via an arterial cannula, which usually is placed in the ascending aorta. With a membrane oxygenator, the pump is usually placed proximal to the oxygenator (Fig. 12-1).

Because of the need to offset the cooling that occurs during the extracorporeal passage of blood, as well as the frequent desire to intentionally cool and then rewarm the patient, a heat exchanger is included in the extracorporeal circuit. It is often part of the oxygenator and is usually placed just before gas exchange. The separate bypass of the right and left sides of the heart, by returning right pump (venous) blood to the pulmonary artery and keeping the

A,B

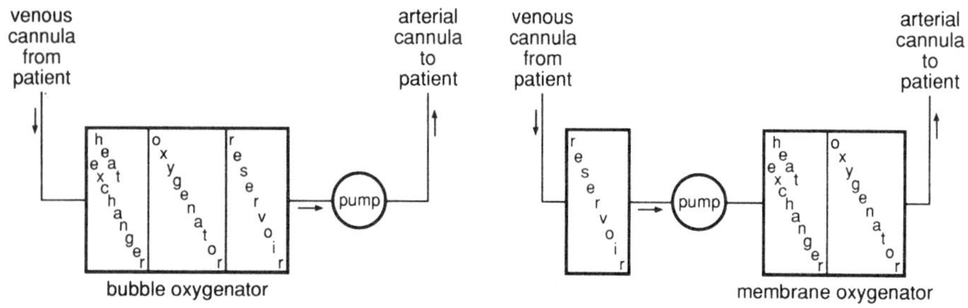

FIGURE 12-1. Usual pattern of cardiopulmonary bypass circuits with bubble **(A)** and membrane **(B)** oxygenators. The bubble oxygenators usually include an integral heat exchanger (venous) and reservoir (postoxygenator-defoamer), whereas the membrane oxygenators usually incorporate an integral heat exchanger. (Modified from Hensley FA Jr, Martin DE, eds. *The practice of cardiac anesthesia.* Boston: Little, Brown, 1990:585, with permission.)

* Please see Chapter 1 for more details.

patient's own lungs in the circuit to negate the need for an artificial lung, was used in the early days of cardiac surgery. However, the procedure is now primarily relegated to circulatory assistance (i.e., as a combined right and left ventricular assist device), although it is being reexplored for use in cardiac surgery (8,9). Peripheral cannulation, using the femoral or other veins and arteries, is occasionally employed for cardiac surgery when central cannulation is not technically possible, for initiating bypass before the chest is opened, especially for "reentry" (reoperation) (10), for emergency resuscitation, for aortic surgery, and for extracorporeal membrane oxygenation, but it is being used more commonly today to facilitate minimal access (minimally invasive) surgery. Left heart bypass or proximal descending aorta bypass (with "venous cannulation" of the left atrium, left ventricle, or proximal aorta) and distal infusion into the distal aorta or femoral artery, incorporating only an extracorporeal pump (commonly a centrifugal pump with minimal anticoagulation) is often used for aortic surgery.

In addition to the major venous and arterial connections and the oxygenator, heat exchanger, and pump, the heart-lung machine has many other components when used for cardiac surgery (Fig. 12-2). An adjustable clamp guards the main venous drainage line, and a separate clamp is used on the arterial line whenever CPB is not being performed, so as to prevent backflow out of the arterial cannula. The venous reservoir serves as a buffer for fluctuations in venous return and as a source of fluid for rapid transfusion. It usually is placed proximal to the membrane oxygenator (before the pump). Various fluids, including blood and crystalloids, and drugs may be added to this reservoir. Several suction devices and systems, usually using one or more of the roller pumps, may aspirate blood and air from the open heart chambers (hence the term, "cardiotomy suction"), the surgical field,* the aortic root (during aortic cross-clamping as a left ventricular vent, and after unclamping as an air vent), and the left heart vent. This blood is then passed into the cardiotomy reservoir, from which it is returned to the venous reservoir. A cardioplegia delivery and/or coronary perfusion system is another component that typically would use another one of the roller pumps for administering blood or cardioplegia solution into the coronary arteries, aortic root, or coronary sinus. This circuit may include a separate heat exchanger and reservoir, and sometimes a recirculation line from the surgical field, which is used when cardioplegia fluid is not being administered into the heart. A source of oxygen and air, with or without carbon dioxide, with appropriate flow meters and blenders, supplies gas to the oxygenator, usually through an anesthetic gas vaporizer. Although at times hot water and cold water are supplied from wall outlets to a temperature blender and regulator for adjustment of water temperature in the heat exchanger, more commonly a dedicated stand-alone water heater-cooler is used for this purpose. A number of filters (macrofilters or microfilters) are often included in various sites (e.g., cardiotomy reservoir, venous reservoir, oxygenator, and arterial line). Blood sampling ports (before and after the oxygenator); pressure monitoring sites (on the cardioplegia-coronary perfusion delivery line, on the arterial line—after the arterial pump but before the arterial filter, and sometimes also before the membrane oxygenator); in-line blood gas monitors (arterial and/or venous); and temperature monitoring sites (water inflow and outflow for major heat exchanger, venous and arterial blood—i.e, before and after heat exchanger, cardioplegia fluid, and water bath) are also included. Whenever a centrifugal pump is used, a flow meter must be included in the arterial outflow line.

Various other safety devices and monitors are frequently present. These include a bubble trap on the arterial line, which usually incorporates a microfilter and a bubble purge line passing (through a one-way valve) back to the cardiotomy reservoir, as well as a bypass line that goes around the arterial microfilter in case the latter becomes obstructed. Other safety devices are a bubble detector on the arterial line and a low-level alarm on the venous reservoir. A hemoconcentrator is sometimes attached between the arterial line and the venous or cardiotomy reservoir.

CANNULATION AND TUBING

Venous Cannulation and Drainage

Principles of Venous Drainage

Venous drainage is usually accomplished by siphonage or so-called gravity drainage. (However, recently there has been a renewed interest in applying suction to venous lines, a technique that had been discarded early in the history of CPB [see Augmented Venous Return]). Gravity drainage places two constraints on successful venous drainage: first, the venous reservoir must be below the level of the patient, and second, the lines must be full of blood or fluid, or else an air lock will occur to disrupt the siphon. The amount of venous drainage is determined by the pressure in the central veins, the difference between the height of the patient and the top of the blood level in the venous reservoir (gravity negative pressure equals this height differential in centimeters of water), and the resistance in the venous cannulas, venous line, and connectors (as well as the venous clamp, if one is used). The central venous pressure is influenced by intravascular volume and venous compliance, which is influenced by medications, sympathetic tone, and anesthesia. Excessive drainage (i.e., at a faster rate than that

* It is now more common to use a "cell washer/concentrator" or autotransfusion device suction to remove extracardiac blood and cardioplegia, thereby allowing the red blood cells to be washed and concentrated, and the debris and excessive crystalloid to be discarded, before returning them to the extracorporeal circuit.

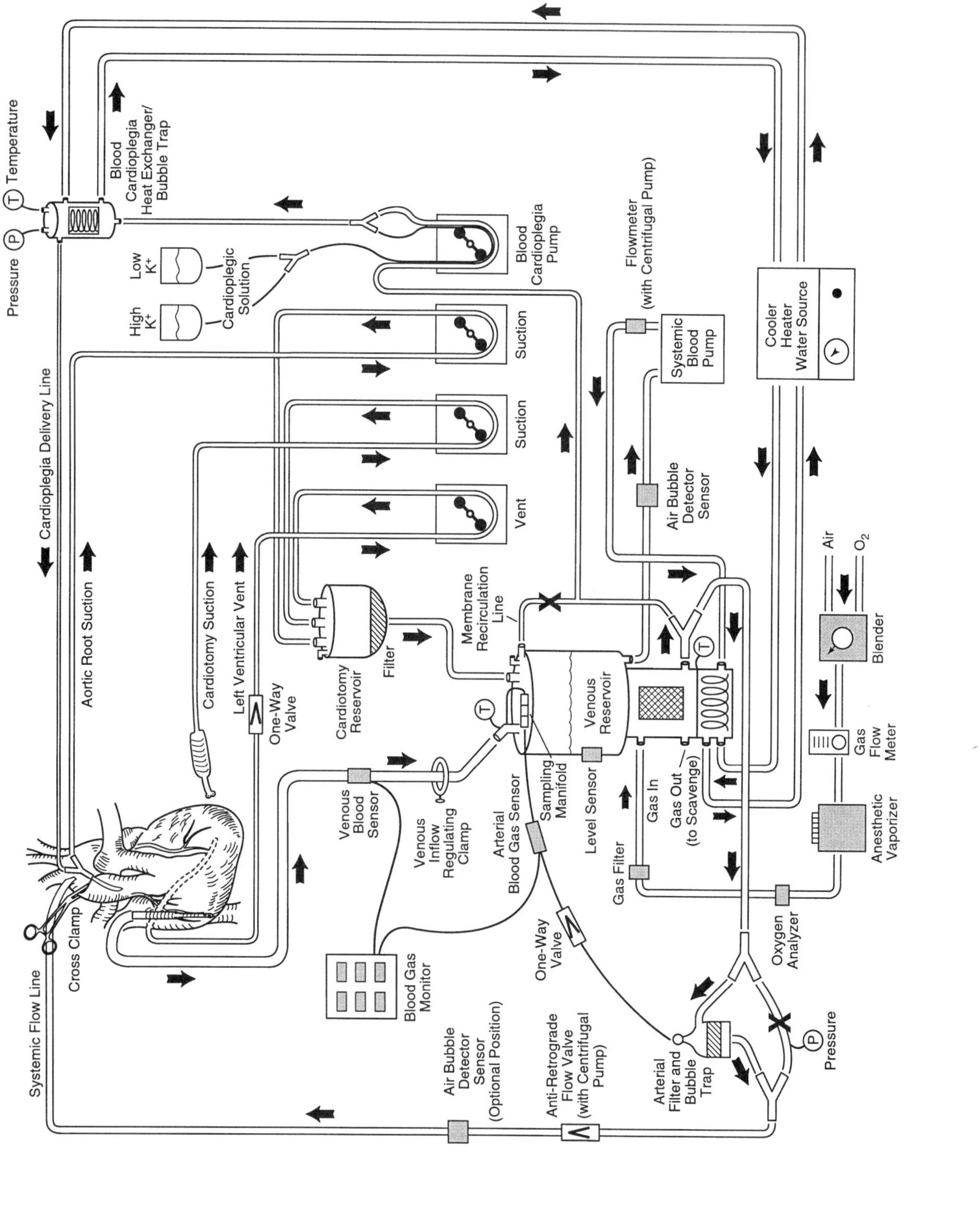
Pressure
Temperature
Blood Cardioplegia Heat Exchanger/ Bubble Trap
High K+
Low K+
Cardioplegic Solution
Blood Cardioplegia Pump
Suction
Suction
Vent
Flowmeter (with Centrifugal Pump)
Systemic Blood Pump
Cooler Heater Water Source
Air Bubble Detector Sensor
Air
O2
Blender
Gas Flow Meter
Anesthetic Vaporizer
Cardioplegia Delivery Line
Aortic Root Suction
Cardiotomy Suction
Left Ventricular Vent
One-Way Valve
Cardiotomy Reservoir
Filter
Membrane Recirculation Line
Venous Reservoir
Sampling Manifold
Level Sensor
Gas In
Gas Out (to Scavenge)
Gas Filter
Oxygen Analyzer
Venous Blood Sensor
Venous Inflow Regulating Clamp
Arterial Blood Gas Sensor
One-Way Valve
Blood Gas Monitor
Cross Clamp
Systemic Flow Line
Air Bubble Detector Sensor (Optional Position)
Anti-Retrograde Flow Valve (with Centrifugal Pump)
Arterial Filter and Bubble Trap
Pressure

of blood returning to the central veins) may result from an excessive negative pressure caused by gravity; this situation may cause the compliant vein or atrial walls to collapse around the ends of the venous cannulas (known as "chattering" or "fluttering") and may cause reduction of venous drainage. This condition can be ameliorated by partially occluding the clamp on the venous line, which paradoxically may increase venous drainage. Obviously, the ultimate limit of venous flow is the amount of blood returning from the body to the great veins.

Types and Sizes of Cannulas

Venous cannulas are either single or two-stage (cavoatrial) (Fig. 12-3). The latter type has a wider portion with holes designed to sit in the right atrium and a narrower tip designed to rest in the IVC. A single cannula may be placed in the right atrium, or separate cannulas may be positioned in each vena cava (see Connection to the Patient). Cannulas are usually made of a flexible plastic. Some are wire-reinforced to reduce the risk of kinking. They may be straight or right-angled. Some of the latter are constructed of hard plastic or metal for an optimal ratio of inner to outer diameter. The venous cannulas are typically the narrowest component and therefore represent a limiting factor for venous drainage. By knowing the flow characteristics of the particular catheter, which are available from the manufacturer, and the required flow (about one third of the total flow from the SVC and two thirds of that from IVC), one can select the appropriate-size venous cannula for a patient. For a 1.8-m^2 patient (total flow, 5.4; SVC flow, 1.8; IVC flow, 3.6 L/minute) at a siphon (gravity) gradient of 40 cm H_2O (about 30 mm Hg), this would require at leasst an SVC cannula of 30F, a 34F IVC cannula, or a 38F single catheter in the atrium. These requirements are easily met by various 36F to 51F cavoatrial cannulas.

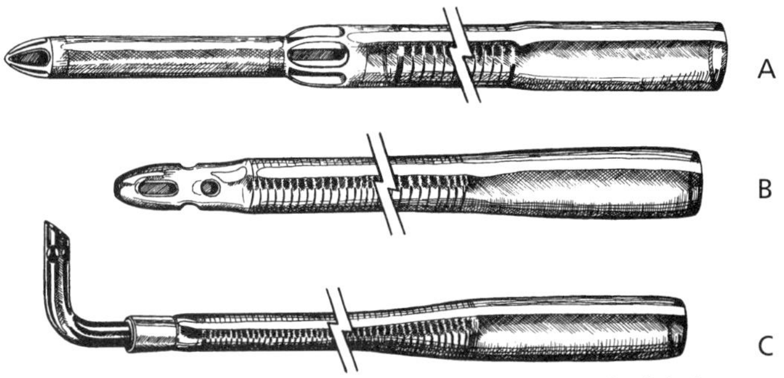

FIGURE 12-3. Venous cannulas. **(A)** Two-stage cannula. **(B)** Plastic cannula for atrial or caval cannulation. **(C)** Cannula with right-angled tip usually constructed of metal (because the thin wall offers superior inner- to outer-diameter dimensions); it is often used for pediatric cases and may be inserted directly into cavae near caval-right atrial junctions. (From Gravlee GP, Davis RF, Kurusz M, eds. *Cardiopulmonary bypass: principles and practice,* 2nd ed. Philadelphia: Lippincott, Williams & Wilkins, 2000, with permission.)

Connection to the Patient

Usually the venous connection for CPB is accomplished by inserting cannulas into the right atrium. Three basic approaches are used (Fig. 12-4): bicaval (separate cannulas

FIGURE 12-2. Detailed schematic diagram of a typical cardiopulmonary bypass circuit employing a membrane oxygenator that includes a heat exchanger sitting beneath an integral hard-shell venous reservoir *(lower center)* and an external cardiotomy reservoir. Venous cannulation is accomplished with the use of a cavoatrial cannula, and arterial cannulation is in the ascending aorta. Systemic venous blood flows by gravity into the venous reservoir (which sits on top of the membrane oxygenator in this figure). Cardiotomy suction and vent lines pass through roller pumps and then into the cardiotomy reservoir, from which the blood drains into the venous reservoir (sometimes the cardiotomy reservoir is physically incorporated into the venous reservoir). Venous blood is then pumped out of the venous reservoir by the systemic blood pump (centrifugal or roller), through the systemic heat exchanger and membrane oxygenator (combined), and then back to the patient (usually through an arterial filter and bubble trap). Other components depicted include the cardioplegia delivery system *(on the right)*, which in this case is a one-pass system that mixes blood (from out of the membrane oxygenator) with cardioplegia solution before passing it through a heat exchanger and bubble trap; a cooler-heater water source that supplies water to the systemic and cardioplegia heat exchangers; and the gas source with air-oxygen blender and anesthetic vaporizer for the membrane oxygenator.

The air bubble detector may be placed on the line between the venous reservoir and systemic pump, between the pump and membrane oxygenator inlet, between the oxygenator outlet and arterial filter (not shown), or on the line after the arterial filter *(optional position on drawing)*. One-way valves prevent retrograde flow (some circuits with a centrifugal pump also incorporate a one-way valve after the pump and within the systemic flow line). Other safety devices include (1) an oxygen analyzer placed between the anesthetic vaporizer (if used) and the oxygenator gas inlet and (2) a reservoir level sensor attached to the housing of the hard-shell venous reservoir *(on the left)*. Arrows indicate direction of flow. Bold Xs depict placement of tubing clamps. P and T denote pressure and temperature sensors, respectively. Hemoconcentrator (described in text) is not shown. (From Gravlee GP, Davis RF, Kurusz M, ed. *Cardiopulmonary bypass: principles and practice,* 2nd ed. Philadelphia: Lippincott, Williams & Wilkins, 2000, with permission.)

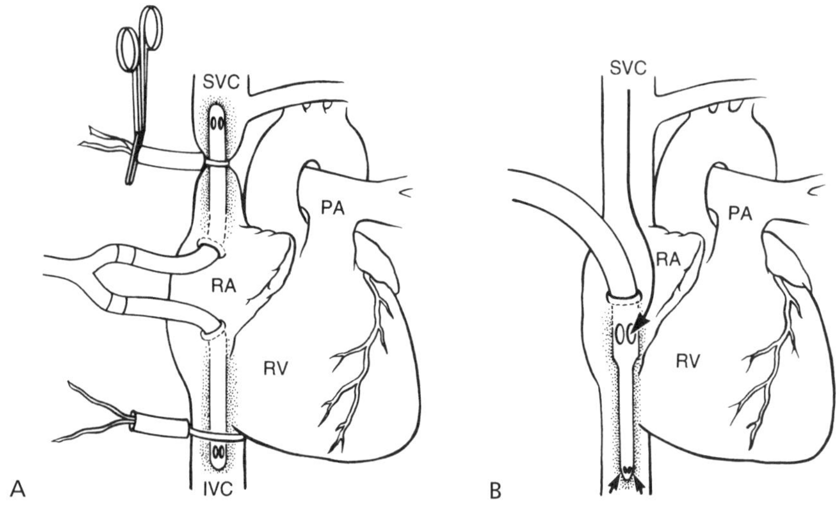

FIGURE 12-4. Methods of venous cannulation. **(A)** Separate cannulation of superior vena cava (SVC) and inferior vena cava (IVC). Loops are placed around the cavae and venous cannulas and passed through tubing to act as tourniquets or snares. The tourniquet on the SVC has been tightened to divert all of the SVC flow into the SVC cannulas and to prevent communication with the right atrium (RA). **(B)** Single cannulation of RA with a "two-stage" cannula. This is typically inserted through the right atrial appendage. Note that the narrower tip of the cannula is in the IVC and drains this vein. The wider portion, with additional holes, resides in the RA, where it receives blood from the coronary sinus and SVC. SVC blood must drain via the RA.

inserted into the SVC and IVC), single atrial, and cavoatrial (two-stage). The last type has a wider proximal section, with holes, that lies within the right atrium and a narrower extension, with end and side holes, that extends into the IVC (Fig. 12-3). When bicaval cannulas are used, tapes are frequently placed around the cavae and passed through small tubes so they may be cinched down as tourniquets or snares around the cannula, thereby forcing all of the venous return to pass into the extracorporeal circuit; this prevents any systemic venous blood from entering the right heart and any air (if the right side of the heart is opened) from entering the venous lines. This procedure is sometimes imprecisely referred to as "caval occlusion."

Arom et al. (11) and Bennett et al. (12) compared the efficiency of the various approaches for venous drainage (Table 12-1). *Bicaval cannulation with caval occlusion* is required whenever the right side of the heart is going to be entered. This system may provide best caval decompression *if properly positioned.* However, caval cannulas cause greater interference with venous flow (and hence with cardiac output) when the patient is not on CPB (i.e., after cannulation but before CPB and after CPB, but before decannulation). When the caval tapes are tightened, no decompression of the right heart (atrium and ventricle) is provided. If the right ventricle is not able to eject, then coronary sinus blood returning to the right atrium must be removed by opening or venting the right heart or releasing the caval tourniquets. This situation would be aggravated by a persistent left superior vena cava (PLSVC) (see later discussion). When the aorta is cross-clamped, coronary sinus flow is much reduced. However, the problem of right heart decompression recurs whenever antegrade cardioplegia or direct coronary perfusion is administered.

Bicaval cannulation without caval tourniquets is often preferred for mitral valve surgery because the necessary retraction often distorts the cavoatrial junctions, interfering with venous drainage if only a single atrial cannula is used (see later discussion). Right heart decompression is much better than when caval tourniquets are used but may not be as good as with atrial cannulation.

Single atrial cannulation has the advantage of being simpler, faster, and less traumatic with one less incision, and it provides fairly good drainage of both the cavae and the right heart. It interferes least with caval return when off bypass. However, the quality of its drainage of the cavae and right heart is very sensitive to positioning, especially with distortion of the heart (e.g., in the so-called circumflex position, when the heart is lifted to make anastomosis to posterior branches of the coronary arteries). The *cavoatrial cannula* has many of the advantages of a simple right atrial cannula but may provide superior drainage of the right side of the heart, especially in the circumflex position (perhaps by providing some stability to the position of the atrial holes) (12). Although drainage of the IVC remains good with cavoatrial cannulation in the circumflex position, drainage of the SVC is often compromised, and SVC (not right atrial) pressure should be carefully monitored at this time. Proper location of the atrial holes is critical to optimal drainage by this cannula (11), and adequate decompression of the right heart (and myocardial temperature) must be monitored and appropriate adjustments made when needed.

Some controversy has surrounded the effect of the type of venous cannulation on adequacy of myocardial protection during aortic cross-clamping using cardioplegic arrest. The concern is that, with atrial cannulation alone, relatively warm (about 25° to 30°C) blood returning from the body may bathe the right heart and interfere with myocardial protection (15). Bennett et al. (13) studied the effects of venous drainage on myocardial preservation in a dog model and compared cavoatrial cannulation with biatrial cannulation with or without caval tourniquets. They observed greatest myocardial cooling, slowest rewarming (between cardi-

TABLE 12-1. COMPARISON OF VENOUS CANNULATION METHODS

Parameter	Bicaval: With Tourniquet	Bicaval: Without Tourniquet	Single: Atrial	Single: Cavoatrial
Atrial incisions	2[a]	2[a]	1	1
Speed of cannualtion	Slowest	Slow	Fast	Fast
Technical difficulty	Most difficult	Difficult	Easy	Moderately easy
Right heart exclusion	Complete	Incomplete	No	No
Coronary sinus return	Excluded	Partial	Included	Included
Right heart decompression	None	Fair	Good	Best
Right Heart decompression with heart lifted up	Bad	Bad	Bad	Good
Caval drainage	Best	About as good	Good (less good for IVC)	Good (less good for SVC)
Caval drainage with heart lifted up	Good	Good	Bad	IVC OK; SVC bad
Adequate venous drainage for all types of surgery	Yes	Yes	No	No
Potential rewarming of heart by systemic venous return	No	Yes	Yes	Yes
Myocardial preservation	Best	Good	Suboptimal	Controversial[b]

Note: IVC, inferior vena cava; SVC, superior vena cava.
[a] Some surgeons place both catheters through a single atriotomy.
[b] See reference 13.
Source: Data from references 4, 11–14, and others.

oplegic dosages), and least evidence of myocardial ischemia with cavoatrial cannulation, which they attributed to superior decompression of the right side of the heart. The fact that most surgeons employ a cavoatrial cannula for coronary artery bypass graft surgery with apparently good results corroborates these observations (16).

Taylor and Effler (17) and Kirklin and Barratt-Boyes (18) reviewed the surgical technique of venous cannulation. Single atrial cannulas are usually inserted through the right atrial appendage after a pursestring suture is made. Bicaval cannulas are usually placed through separate incisions, although some surgeons place both through a single incision in the atrial appendage. The SVC cannula is usually passed through the right atrial appendage. The IVC cannula is usually passed through a pursestring suture placed in the posterior inferior portion of the lateral wall of the right atrium near the IVC and avoiding the right coronary artery. The cavoatrial junctions may be dangerously thin. Some surgeons place pursestrings directly in the SVC and IVC, but this could cause narrowing when they are closed (19).

At times, venous cannulation is accomplished *peripherally,* usually via the femoral or iliac vein. This is used for emergency closed cardiopulmonary assist, for support of particularly ill patients before induction of anesthesia, for prevention or management of bleeding complications during sternotomy for reoperations (10), and for certain types of aortic and thoracic surgery. The key to adequate flow rates with peripheral cannulation is using a cannula that is as large as possible and advancing the catheter into the right atrium (guided by TEE if available) if possible. Specially designed commercially manufactured long, ultrathin nonkinkable (wire-reinforced) catheters are available for this purpose. Insertion may be facilitated by use of an internal stylet and guidewire. Flow through these catheters may be improved by the use of augmented venous return (see later discussion). Alternatively, percutaneous venous catheters intended for percutaneous CPB may be used. A 29F and 33F bicaval femoral venous cannula is available commercially that allows drainage of the SVC and IVC while isolating the right atrium by snaring the SVC and IVC around the cannula (20). Others (21,22) have used the right internal jugular vein by cutdown or percutaneously for peripheral venous cannulation of the heart.

Persistent Left Superior Vena Cava

A PLSVC is present in 0.3% to 0.5% of the general population but in about 2% to 10% of patients with congenital heart disease. It usually drains into the coronary sinus and thence into the right atrium, but in about 10% of cases it drains into the left atrium (23–25). The presence of a PLSVC should be suspected when the (left) innominate vein is small or absent and when a large coronary sinus or the PLSVC itself is seen on baseline TEE (26,27). (Other causes of a large coronary sinus include right-sided venous hypertension, tricuspid regurgitation, and stenosis of the ostium of the coronary sinus). Its presence is confirmed by injecting agitated saline echo contrast medium into the left internal jugular vein or left arm vein and noting passage of contrast into the coronary sinus by TEE.

The presence of a PLSVC poses a number of problems during cardiac surgery. It may confuse and complicate passage of a pulmonary artery catheter or and interfere with administration of retrograde cardioplegia (28). The latter problem is difficult because the coronary sinus is usually quite large in this circumstance, so that the balloon on the retrograde catheter does not seal and cardioplegia solution leaks into the right atrium. Furthermore, the cardioplegia solution may run off into the PLSVC; and finally, the cardioplegia solution will be diluted with systemic venous blood draining down the PLSVC. Patients with this anomaly may also be more prone to atrial trachycardia, and they may have other congenital cardiac abnormalities. The presence of a PLSVC also poses obvious problems if the right side of the heart is to be entered, or with right heart decompression and adequacy of venous return if bicaval cannulation is used, because of the flow of the additional systemic venous blood into the right atrium.

If the right heart is not going to be opened and a single simple or two-staged venous cannula is employed for venous drainage *and* retrograde cardioplegia is not used, the presence of a PLSVC poses no problems. If the right heart needs to be entered, several options are available. If an adequate-sized innominate vein is present (true in about 30% of cases), the PLSVC can simply be occluded during CPB. (However, one must be wary of the rare associated anomaly of atresia of the coronary sinus, in which case the PLSVC provides the main outlet for cardiac venous drainage and it occlusion could injure the myocardium [29]. This condition should be suspected if the coronary sinus in not enlarged, and by failure of echocontrast material injected into the left arm or PLSVC from entering the right atrium via the coronary sinus during TEE.) Another obvious circumstance in which the left SVC cannot be occluded despite the presence of an adequate-sized innominate vein is when there is associated absence of the right SVC (true in about 20% of cases).

If the innominate vein is absent (true in about 40% of cases) or small (about 33% of cases), occlusion of the PLSVC can cause serous venous hypertension and potentially cerebral injury or ischemia and should not be done without documenting acceptable venous pressure in the left jugular system cephalad to the occlusion. Otherwise, some other arrangement must be made to provide drainage of the PLSVC. Use of cardiotomy suction in the coronary sinus ostium may be adequate, but cannulation, usually via a cannula passed retrograde into the PLSVC through the ostium of the coronary sinus, is preferred, with a caval tape (tourniquet) placed around the PLSVC. Alternatively, a cuffed caval cannula or endotracheal tube may be used (30). A caval cannula could be placed directly into the PLSVC through a pursestring suture placed externally. Finally, in small infants, induction of deep hypothermia with perfusion cooling using a single venous cannula followed by circulatory arrest obviates the need for extra cannulation of the PLSVC. Management of retrograde cardioplegia in the presence of a PLSVC is discussed later.

Augmented Venous Return

Early in the history of CPB, suction pumps (roller or finger) were used for venous drainage; however, because they were difficult to control, they were discarded in favor of the simpler and more effective gravity siphon described previously. More recently, there has been a renewed interest in the use of suction to overcome the resistance of longer and/or narrower venous cannulas used during limited access (transthoracic) or peripheral venous access (e.g., jugular or femoral vein) (31). With these narrower and longer venous cannulas, gravity siphon may not provide adequate flow for full bypass even with maximal table (patient) height above the heart-lung machine. However, use of narrower and shorter venous lines does reduce pump prime volume.

At least three systems to "augment" venous return have been described. One places a *roller pump* in the venous line between the venous cannula and the venous reservoir. This carries a high risk of generating excessive negative pressure and collapsing the right atrium or great veins around the cannula tip and requires constant attention and adjustment of the roller pump rate. A second method substitutes a *kinetic (centrifugal) pump* for the roller pump in the venous line and is referred to as *kinetic-assisted venous drainage, or KAVD)* (32). The third method involves applying a regulated vacuum to a closed, hard-shell venous reservoir (see later discussion) that is attached to the venous line (*vacuum-assisted venous drainage, or VAVD*) (33). This system is relatively simple and does not require regulation of a second pump. When a pump (roller or centrifugal) is used to generate the suction, some advocate placing a shunt around the pump with the use of two Y-connectors. When a centrifugal pump is used, the shunt is cross-clamped but can be opened in case massive air deprimes and inactivates the pump. When a roller is used, the shunt is only partially occluded to prevent generation of excessive negative pressures. With all three systems, an arterial pump (centrifugal or roller) then pumps blood out of the venous reservoir through the oxygenator and to the patient. This constitutes a second pump in the aforementioned pump-assisted methods.

Use of these systems require careful regulation of the degree of negative pressure applied to the venous line. This is best accomplished by monitoring the pressure in the venous line about 10 cm before the inlet to the venous pump head (if using a roller or kinetic pump) or within the hard-shell reservoir (if using a VAVD system). The negative pressure (vacuum) measured at this site should not exceed -60 to -100 mm Hg. It is also desirable to keep an eye on the right atrium directly or via TEE.

When the vacuum-assisted system is used, the amount of vacuum applied should be controlled with a vacuum regulator that can be adjusted and that displays low levels of suction in 10 mm Hg increments. Vacuum should never be applied when there is no forward blood flow through the oxygenator (to prevent air from being pulled across the membrane into the blood path), and the reservoir should be open to the atmosphere when vacuum is not being applied (to prevent overpressuring of the venous reservoir with reduction of venous return and risk of retrograde or antegrade air embolization). The venous reservoir should also have a low positive and a high negative pressure relief valve (about +15 mm Hg and −150 mm Hg, respectively).

Usually, adequate venous drainage is achieved with speeds of 1,000 to 1,200 rpm of the kinetic pump or application of 20 to 60 mm Hg vacuum to the venous reservoir.

When a vacuum-assisted system is used with a closed reservoir, the amount of vacuum within the reservoir is influenced not only by the amount of vacuum applied to the system but also the relative flow of blood and air into the reservoir (from the venous line and from cardiotomy suckers and vents) and the flow of blood out of the reservoir (by the arterial pump).

There are a number of potential problems and risks associated with the use of augmented venous return systems. Excessive negative pressure may cause microcavitation (microair bubbles) and generation of systemic gaseous microembolization and or hemolysis (red blood cells are more easily damaged by negative than by positive pressure [34]); collapse of right atrial, tricuspid valve, or venous structures around the cannula tip resulting in impaired venous return and chattering in the venous line; and possible damage to cardiovascular structures. Application of additional negative pressure (beyond gravity) increases the risk and amount of gross air aspiration from holes in walls of the right atrium or great veins, through a patent foramen ovale if the left heart is open or through any intravenous lines or introducers that may be in place (these should be closed or connecting lines placed in infusion pumps during augmented venous return). The aspirated air could cause an air lock or "deprime" and defunctionalize a kinetic pump, or it could fill the venous reservoir and contribute to systemic air embolization. If vacuum is applied to the closed reservoir system during a no-flow state, there is the theoretic risk of pulling air across the membrane oxygenator into the blood path, with subsequent systemic air embolism. If the venous reservoir is not open to the atmosphere when vacuum is not being applied, or when KVAD is in use, the venous reservoir could become overpressurized, with reduction of venous return and risk of retrograde (through cardiac vents or cardioplegia line) or antegrade (systemic arterial line) air embolization. When a pump is being used to augment venous return, there is the potential for imbalance of flow between the venous (inflow) and arterial (outflow) pumps, resulting in a change in intravascular volume in the patient or a risk of systemic air embolism, so the perfusionist must be even more attentive.

Complications Associated with Achieving Venous Drainage

Complications include atrial arrhythmias, tears and bleeding of the atrium, air embolization (especially if atrial pressure is low; systemic embolization is possible if there are potential right-to-left shunts), tears of the venae cavae (IVC is particularly prone to this), and malposition of the tips (or atrial portion of the cavoatrial catheter), including insertion of the tips into the azygos, innominate, or hepatic veins, or across an atrial septal defect into the left heart. Placement of the low atrial pursestring for cannulation of the IVC requires retraction of the heart, which may have adverse hemodynamic consequences and sometimes is deferred until CPB is instituted with a single cannula. Placing tapes around the cavae may result in lacerations of the cavae themselves or branches thereof, or, when encircling the SVC, may cause lacerations of the right pulmonary artery. Once the venous cannulas are in place, they may interfere with venous return and cardiac output until CPB is initiated. Placing venous cannulas may displace central venous or pulmonary artery catheters (35). Caval tapes may occlude these monitor lines, and conversely their presence may prevent tight caval occlusion by the tapes (with the risk of air entering venous line when the right atrium is open). Further, these monitor lines may become caught in atrial pursestrings, causing malfunction and preventing their removal (36). Finally the cava may become obstructed when pursestrings placed for direct cannulation are closed after catheter removal (19).

Causes of Low Venous Return

Reduced venous drainage may result from reduced venous pressure, inadequate height of the patient above the reservoir, malposition of the venous cannulas (sometimes due to manipulation of heart), or obstruction or excessive resistance of the lines and cannulas. Inadequate venous pressure may be caused by venodilation with drugs (e.g., nitroglycerin, inhalational anesthetics) or hypovolemia. Obstruction may be caused by kinks, clamps, air lock, or insertion of a pulmonary artery balloon catheter into a cannula (37), or the cannulas may be too small.

Arterial Cannulation

Cannulas

Many different types of cannulas are available (Fig. 12-5), and they are made of various materials. Some, designed for insertion into the ascending aorta, have right-angled tips; some are tapered, and some have flanges to aid in fixation and prevent introduction of a too-great length into the aorta. The arterial cannula is usually the narrowest part of the extracorporeal circuit. High flow through narrow can-

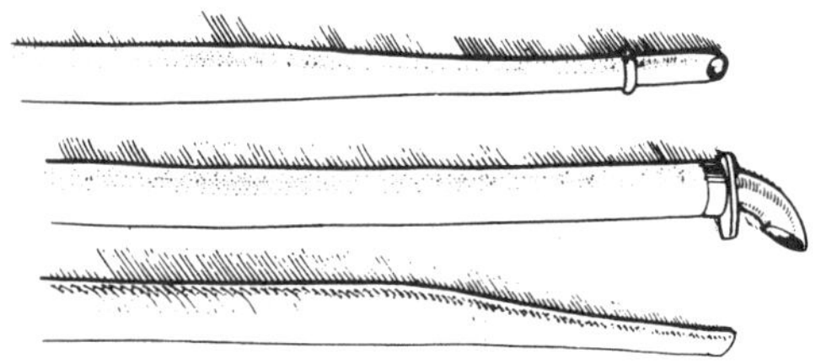

FIGURE 12-5. Arterial cannulas. The top figure depicts a plastic cannula with a flange near the tip to prevent inserting it too far and to help with fixation. The middle cannula has a right-angled tip, usually constructed of metal because the thin wall offers a superior ratio of inner to outer diameter, and a fixation flange. The lower cannula has a tapered tip. (Modified from Hensley FA Jr, Martin DE, eds. *The practice of cardiac anesthesia.* Boston: Little, Brown, 1990:219, with permission.)

nulas may lead to high-pressure gradients, high velocity of flow (jets), turbulence, and cavitation with undesirable consequences (see later discussion). The key characteristic of an arterial cannula is its performance index (pressure gradient versus external diameter at any given flow) (38). The narrowest portion of the catheter that enters the aorta should be as short as is compatible with safety, and thereafter the cannula size should enlarge to minimize the gradient. Long catheters with a uniformly narrow diameter are undesirable. Metal or hard plastic tips provide the best ratio of inner to outer diameter.

Pressure gradients greater than 100 mm Hg are associated with excessive hemolysis and protein denaturation (39). Therefore, a cannula should be selected that provides adequate flow (e.g., 3 L/minute/m^2) with a pressure gradient of no more than 100 mm Hg based on gradient-flow data provided by the manufacturer or bench tests conducted by the practice group using fluids with a viscosity similar to that of blood with a hematocrit of 20% to 30%.

The jets produced by small cannulas may damage the aortic wall and dislodge atheroemboli, cause dissections and disturbing flow into nearby vessels (see later discussion of the Coanda effect). Muehrcke et al. (40) described a new aortic cannula (Soft-Flow: Sarns 3M Health Care, Ann Arbor, MI) that features a closed tip with an internal cone and side holes; it is designed to reduce exit forces and velocities, thereby reducing these adverse jet effects.

Connection to the Patient

In the early days of CPB, arterial inflow was accomplished via the subclavian or femoral artery, but currently it is usually accomplished via a cannula inserted into the ascending aorta (16). The advantages of this approach over the femoral approach (Table 12-2) include ease and safety and the fact that it does not require an additional incision. The surgical technique for aortic cannulation has been reviewed in detail by many others (17,18,41). The site for cannulation is selected based on the type of cannula to be used, the operation planned (how much of the ascending aorta must be available), and the quality of the aortic wall (42).

Atherosclerosis of the Ascending Aorta

Atherosclerosis with or without calcification frequently involves the ascending aorta and poses problems regarding arterial cannulation as well as application of clamps and vascular grafts. The review by Beique et al. (43) is highly recommended. Dislodgment of atheromatous debris, either by direct mechanical disruption or from the "sandblasting" effect of the jet coming out of the arterial cannula, is thought to be a major cause of perioperative stroke (44,45). Atherosclerosis is also considered to be a risk factor for perioperative aortic dissection (46) and postoperative renal dysfunc-

TABLE 12-2. ARTERIAL CANNULATION

Parameter	Ascending Aorta or Arch	Femoral or Illiac
Accessibility	Easy	Difficult
Additional incision	No	Yes
Cannula size	Usually unlimited	Limited
Obstruct ascending aorta	Possible	No
Risk of malperfusion of arch vessels	Yes	No
Perfusion direction	Antegrade	Retrograde
Leg ischemia	No	Possible
Aortic dissection incidence	0.01%–0.09%	0.2%–1.3%
Leg wound and artery complications	0	~ 4%
Indications	Most cases	When aortic cannulation is not feasible or desirable; peripheral cannulation under local anesthesia; bleeding complications during reentry
Contraindications	Ascending aortic aneurysms; diseased ascending aorta	When aortic cannulation is feasible; occlusive disease of vessels; extensive atheroma (especially mobile) in arch and/or descending aorta

Source: Data from reference 14 and others; see text for details.

tion (47). Traditionally, surgeons have relied on palpation to detect these changes and select sites for cannulation, cross-clamping, and other procedures, and the sensitivity of this technique is improved by briefly reducing the systemic arterial pressure to 40 to 50 mm Hg with venous inflow occlusion (42) or administration of vasodilators. Palpation should continue to be a component of evaluation of the aorta (48), but it is less sensitive and less accurate than epivascular ultrasonic scanning (43,49,50). TEE, which is more convenient, is also not as sensitive as epiaortic scanning because of limited views of the ascending aorta (49,50,51). However, some believe that TEE can be used as a screening method to determine which patients need epiaortic scanning (52). If no significant atherosclerosis is detected in the ascending, transverse, or proximal descending aorta, then these authors contend that epiaortic imaging is not necessary (52); others disagree (49,53). Epiaortic imaging and TEE should be considered complementary (49). Beique et al. (43) suggest using epiaortic scanning in all patients who have a history of transient ischemic attack, stroke, severe peripheral vascular disease, palpable calcification in the ascending aorta, calcified aortic knob on chest radiograph, age older than 60 years, or TEE findings of moderate aortic atherosclerosis. Others advocate epiaortic scanning of the ascending aorta in all patients older than 50 years of age (54). If atherosclerosis is detected, then sites for insertion of cannulas, grafts, and application of vascular clamps are modified (55). If extensive atherosclerosis precludes arterial cannulation in the ascending aorta, then the femoral route is considered (see later discussion). However, in this case, the transverse and descending aorta should be evaluated by TEE to rule out extensive atheromata that might be embolized into the brain or elsewhere with retrograde flow from a femoral cannula. If such is the case, then axillary-subclavian cannulation should be considered (see later discussion). If there is extensive atheroma in the ascending or transverse aorta, some have suggested using a long arterial cannula that is inserted in the ascending aorta and threaded around into the proximal descending aorta to reduce the sandblasting effect (56). Others have advocated performing an endarterectomy under deep hypothermic circulatory arrest if severely protruding or mobile atheromata are detected (57), but this procedure has been associated with higher rates of stroke (35% versus 12%) and mortality (19% versus 12%) than when endarterectomy was not performed (58). If the ascending aorta is totally calcified and rigid (so-called porcelain aorta), then entirely different strategies for cannulation and surgery must be employed (59). These include no clamping of the ascending aorta, femoral or axillary-subclavian arterial cannulation, and in selected cases graft replacement or endarterectomy of the ascending aorta during deep hypothermic circulatory arrest (54,60), although this may be a high-risk procedure (61). When there was no intraluminal debris, Liddicoat et al. (62) employed an intraluminal balloon (Heartport Endoaortic Clamp, Heartport, Redwood City, CA) inserted through a pursestring suture in an atherosclerotic free portion of aortic arch to occlude the aorta; others have used a Foley catheter (63). Studies using historical controls suggest improved neurologic outcome with echocardiographic-based modification of surgical techniques in handling the ascending aorta (55,64).

If possible, the intrapericardial aorta is chosen for arterial cannulation because it is usually stronger. Many surgeons insert two concentric pursestring sutures into the aortic wall, but not to full thickness. Most avoid using a partial excluding clamp, except in children, to minimize clamp trauma. Optimal arterial blood pressure (mean arterial pressure about 80 to 100, systolic about 100 to 120 mm Hg) is important: if it is too high, there is greater chance of tears, dissection, blood loss, and blood spray; if too low, the aorta tends to collapse, it is harder to make an incision and insert the cannula, and there is greater risk of damaging the back wall. If a right-angled tip is used, it is often initially directed toward the heart and then rotated 180° to confirm intraluminal placement. Some back-bleeding is allowed to eliminate air and atheromatous material and to further confirm intraluminal placement; the placement is additionally confirmed by noting a pulsatile pressure in the arterial line pressure monitor on the heart-lung machine that is at least as high as the that shown on the radial artery monitor. Proper position of the tip of the cannula is critical (see later discussion). Most surgeons insert the cannula only 1 to 2 cm into the aorta and direct it toward the middle of the transverse arch to avoid entering the arch vessels. As mentioned previously, others advocate threading a long cannula into the proximal descending aorta to reduce velocity and turbulence in the aortic arch and thereby reduce the sandblasting effect and emboli (56).

Complications of Ascending Aorta Cannulation

Complications include difficulty introducing the cannula (because of interference by adventitia or plaques, a too-small incision, fibrosis of wall, or low arterial pressure), intramural placement, dislodgment of atheroemboli, air embolism from the cannula, injury to the back wall of the aorta, persistent bleeding around the cannula (or after its removal), malposition of the tip (retrograde and even across the aortic valve, against the wall, or into the arch vessels), abnormal cerebral perfusion, obstruction of aorta (in infants), aortic dissection, and high line pressure (65,66). *High line pressure* may be a clue to malposition of the tip (against the wall, into an arch vessel), cannula occlusion by an aortic cross-clamp, aortic dissection, a kink anywhere in the arterial inflow system (including a line clamp still left on), or a too-small cannula. Inadvertent *cannulation of the arch vessels* may cause irreversible cerebral injury and reduced systemic perfusion (67–70). Suggestive evidence of cannulation of aortic arch vessels includes high arterial line pressure; high pressure in a radial artery if supplied by the cannulated vessel (or low pressure if not supplied by the cannulated vessel); unilateral blanching of the face when CPB is first instituted with a clear prime (68) or asymmetric cooling of the neck during perfusion cooling (70); and unilateral hyperemia, edema, petechiae, and dilated pupil or pupils. Before CPB, palpation of the carotids may reveal asymmetric pulsation (reduced on the cannulated side), and the opposite may be observed during pulsatile bypass (increased pulsation on cannulated side) (70). Before CPB, the radial artery line may reveal sudden dampening if the cannula is inserted into the arch vessel supplying the monitored radial artery (71).

It has been suggested that the Coanda effect (in which the jet stream adheres to boundary wall and therefore produces a lower pressure along the opposite wall), which has been shown experimentally to be associated with carotid hypoperfusion (72), may account for some cerebral dysfunction after CPB with aortic cannulation. Salerno et al. (73) detected major electroencephalogram (EEG) abnormalities caused by malposition of a cannula in 3 of 84 patients undergoing arch perfusion, possibly on the basis of the Coanda effect.

Aortic dissection ("antegrade") associated with ascending aortic cannulation has reportedly occurred in 0.01% to 0.09% of cases (Table 12-3) (41,46,66,74,75); it is more common in patients with abnormal aortic roots. Aortic dissection may manifest as a blue discoloration of the aortic root (differential diagnosis is subadventitial hematoma) and with bleeding from needle holes or cannulation sites in the aortic root. Other clues include a sudden decrease in venous return and arterial pressure, excessive loss of perfusate, increased arterial line pressure, and evidence of decreased organ perfusion (e.g., oliguria, dilated pupil or pupils, EEG changes, myocardial ischemia). TEE may be useful in establishing the diagnosis (76). Gott et al. (74) and Still et al. (75) have discussed this complication and its management in detail. The aortic cannula should be promptly transferred to a location distal to the dissection (usually femoral, but occasionally into the distal arch). Meanwhile, arterial pressure and pulse pressure should be kept to a minimum by administration of vasodilator and β-adrenergic blocking agents. Deep hypothermia (less than 20°C) is then induced, the aorta is opened, and the extent of injury is evaluated and repaired either by direct closure, use of a patch, or replacement of ascending aorta with a tubular graft. Occasionally, small injuries can be repaired off bypass by closed plication (74). The survival rate of patients whose dissections were recognized and treated in the operating room has ranged from 66% to 85%; when dissection was not recognized until postoperatively, survival has been only 50% or less (Table 12-3). Late bleeding and infected or noninfected false aneurysms are late complications of aortic cannulation.

Cannulation of the Femoral or Iliac Artery

Cannulation of the femoral or iliac artery (exposed via a retroperitoneal suprainguinal approach) is indicated when there is an aneurysm of the ascending aorta or when the aorta is otherwise unsatisfactory for cannulation (due to thinning or severe atherosclerosis). It is also indicated when

TABLE 12-3. ASCENDING AORTIC DISSECTION COMPLICATING CARDIAC SURGERY

Author (Reference No.)	Murphy et al. (46)	Gott et al. (74)	Still et al. (75)	All
Year published	1983	1990	1992	—
Institution	Emory	Emory	MGH	—
Years covered	1971–1981	1982–1988	1982–1990	1971–1990
Total cases	6,943	11,145	14,877	32,965
Dissections (incidence %)	24 (0.35)	27 (0.24)	24 (0.16)	75 (0.23)
Site of origin				
Aortic cannulation (incidence %)	4 (0.06)	10 (0.09)	10 (0.07)	24 (0.07)
Partial occlusion clamp	8	3	7	18
Aortic cross clamp	1	4	8	13
Proximal SV anastamosis	4	2	1	7
Cardioplegia cannula	2	5	—	7
Vent site	—	1	—	1
Aortotomy	2	—	—	2
Unknown or other	3	2	1	6
When recognized				
OR	15	27	20	62
Postoperative	9	—	4	13
Mortality (%)				
If recognized in OR	33	15	20	—
If recognized postoperatively	78	—	50	0

Note: SV, saphenous vein; OR, operating room.

no space is available owing to multiple procedures involving the ascending aorta, for peripheral cannulation under local anesthesia in unstable patients, prophylactically during reoperations (10) or if bleeding complications occur during reentry, or when dissection complicates cannulation of the ascending aorta. Femoral cannulation is also used during limited-access cardiac surgery. Femoral cannulation requires a second incision and limits the size of cannula that may be used. The latter may cause the adverse consequences of a jet and high-pressure gradients to be more likely. Lees et al. (77) found no difference in the distribution of blood flow and vascular resistance between retrograde (femoral artery infusion) and antegrade (aortic root infusion) flow in monkeys.

Femoral cannulation is associated with many complications (10,73,78). These include trauma to the cannulated vessel, including tears, dissection, late stenosis or thrombosis, bleeding, lymph fistula, and infection. Because the retrograde perfusion cannula may completely occlude the blood supply to the cannulated limb, ischemic complications (acidosis, compartment syndrome, muscle necrosis, neuropathy) may develop if cannulation exceeds 3 to 6 hours (79,81), and reperfusion of the limb may be associated with acidosis or acute pulmonary hypertension. Therefore the femoral ischemic time should be monitored. The risk of femoral ischemia may be minimized by perfusing the distal limb with a separate cannula "Y-ed" off of the arterial line (80), or by suturing a side graft onto the femoral artery into which the arterial cannula is inserted (82). This latter technique may also reduce the risk of arterial injury and retrograde dissection. If the limb is perfused by these methods and the ipsilateral femoral vein is also cannulated, then an additional venous cannula is sometimes placed in the distal femoral vein to prevent venous congestion. If limb ischemia does occur, Beyersdorft et al. (83) have described a method of controlled limb reperfusion to improve outcome.

Femoral perfusion may lead to cerebral and coronary atheroembolism if there is extensive atheroma in the distal arch or descending aorta; ideally this should be assessed by TEE before the femoral route is selected. If severe atherosclerosis is present, an alternate route (e.g, subclavian-axillary) should be used if possible (see earlier discussion). Femoral perfusion may also aggravate preexisting aortic dissections, and an alternative site for cannulation (see discussion) is recommended by some authors (84).

The most serious complication of femoral cannulation is retrograde arterial dissection, which may lead to retroperitoneal hemorrhage or retrograde extension all the way to the aortic root and has been associated with a mortality rate of about 50%. The incidence appears to be between 0.2% and 1.3% (85–89), although higher and lower rates have been reported. A rate of 0.75% was reported recently with the Port Access System (Heartport), although the rate may be lower more recently with improved technology, techniques, and patient screening and selection (90).

Retrograde arterial dissection is thought to be caused by either direct (cannula) or indirect (jet) trauma, and it is thought to be more likely to occur in the presence of atherosclerosis or cystic medial necrosis and in patients older than 40 years of age (78).

Retrograde aortic dissection may manifest like antegrade aortic dissection (already described), but it may be more difficult to recognize if it does not extend into the ascending aorta, in which case it may be signaled only by a sudden decrease in venous return and arterial pressure, excessive loss of perfusate, increased arterial line pressure in the extracorporeal circuit, and oliguria. In this situation, TEE is extremely helpful (76).

Because of the nature of the dissection and the flap, discontinuation of retrograde perfusion and resumption of antegrade flow (via a cannula in the ascending aorta or by normal cardiac function) may resolve the problem. This may permit management that is different from that for antegrade dissections. If the dissection occurs early in the procedure, success can be achieved by simply discontinuing CPB (and hence retrograde femoral perfusion) immediately and restoring intravascular volume (which can be facilitated by attaching the arterial line to the venous cannula and infusing from the pump), and then aborting the planned operation and doing nothing to the ascending aorta, even when it is affected by the dissection (86). If the dissection occurs later, when it is not possible or desirable to discontinue CPB, retrograde perfusion should be immediately discontinued, and the arterial cannula should be introduced into the true lumen in the ascending aorta (often through the false lumen); CPB is resumed with antegrade perfusion, and the planned operation may be completed *without* repair of the dissection itself or of the ascending aorta (87). Others recommend graft replacement of the ascending aorta (85).

A pre-CPB test infusion with the arterial pump through the arterial line (regardless of the location of the arterial cannula) that indicates increased line pressure may warn of possible dissection and may avoid extensive dissection.

Other Sites for Arterial Cannulation

Use of the *axillary-subclavian artery* instead of the femoral artery when ascending aortic cannulation is not feasible or is undesirable is being increasingly advocated (91–93). Advantages of the axillary artery over the femoral artery include that it is less likely to be involved by atherosclerosis, it has good collateral flow and therefore ischemic complications are less likely, and that, because it provides antegrade flow, it is less likely to cause cerebral atheroembolization. Its use has also been advocated for establishing deep hypothermia before repair of type I aortic dissections, because it is less likely to result in malperfusion and further expansion of the dissection, as may occur with femoral perfusion (84,94). Use of the right artery is favored by some (84) and the left by others (94). The axillary artery is approached through a subclavicular incision, although the intrathoracic subclavian artery may be cannulated if a left thoracotomy has been used. Of course, the contralateral radial or brachial artery (usually the left) must be used for intraarterial pressure monitoring. However, some surgeons suture a graft onto the side of the axillary artery for cannulation (93), in which case the ipsilateral radial or brachial artery pressure may still be monitored. Brachial plexus injury and axillary artery thrombosis are reported complications (91).

Antegrade aortic perfusion can be also accomplished by cannulating through the *left ventricular apex* and passing the cannula across the aortic valve into the aortic root (95). Coselli and Crawford (96) described retrograde perfusion through a *graft sewn onto the abdominal aorta* when distal occlusive disease prevented femoral cannulation and ascending aortic cannulation was not feasible. Cannulation of the *supraceliac aorta* (approached via an extension of the median incision into the abdomen) has been described in infants (97).

Tubing and Connectors

Minimization of blood trauma, prime volume, and resistance to flow, as well as avoidance of leaks (the outward flow of blood or aspiration of air), are considerations in the selection of tubing and connectors. To minimize blood trauma, one should strive to have smooth, nonwettable inside walls made of nontoxic materials and to avoid velocities greater than 100 cm/second and a Reynolds number higher than a critical value (1,000 to 2,000).* One also wishes to minimize the gradient necessary to propel the blood along the tubing. Selection of wide tubing aids in achieving these objectives. On the other hand, larger tubing is associated with greater priming volume. Keeping the tubing as short as possible reduces prime volume, pressure gradient (resistance to flow), and blood trauma. Desirable tubing characteristics include transparency, resilience (reexpansion after compression), flexibility, kink resistance, hardness (resistance to collapse), toughness (resistance to cracking and rupture), inertness, smooth and nonwettable inner surface, tolerance of heat sterilization, and blood compatibility. Medical grade polyvinyl chloride (PVC) (e.g., Tygon) seems to meet these standards. Silicone or latex rubber tubing is sometimes used in roller pumps. New formulations of PVC are being developed for use in roller pumps to minimize spallation (see later discussion).

It is desirable to use disposable, hard plastic connectors (e.g., polycarbonate) with smooth, nonwettable, hemocompatible inner surfaces that make smooth junctions with plastic tubing to minimize turbulence. Smooth curves rather than sharp-angled bends also minimize turbulence.

Connections must be tight enough to prevent the leakage of blood when exposed to positive pressures (up to 500 mm Hg beyond the arterial pump) and the aspiration of air (on the venous side before the arterial pump). The friction of fluted connectors with an outer diameter larger than the inner diameter of the plastic tubing or cannula into which the connector is inserted may provide sufficient tightness; otherwise, plastic bands should be applied tightly around all such connections. For convenience and safety, most tubing and connectors are prepackaged and disposable. Heparin bonding is discussed in a later section.

* In general, turbulence occurs when disrupting forces (inertial) overcome the retaining forces (viscous). This relation is expressed by the Reynolds number (density × velocity × diameter ÷ viscosity). Empirically, turbulence has been found to occur in blood when this number exceeds 1,000 to 2,000, although its occurrence is also influenced by curvature, smoothness, and inlet conditions.

PUMPS

Types of Pumps

Two types of pumps are currently used: roller pumps and centrifugal pumps (Fig. 12-6 and Table 12-4).

Roller Pumps

Roller pumps (Fig. 12-6A) have been the most commonly used pumps in CPB for the past 40 years. They consist of a length of tubing located inside a curved raceway at the perimeter of the travel of rollers (usually two) mounted on the ends of rotating arms (usually 180° apart), arranged so that one roller is compressing the tubing at all times. Flow of blood is induced by compression of the tubing, which pushes the blood ahead of the moving roller. Flow rate depends on the size of the tubing, the length of the track, and the rotation rate of the rollers. For a given pump, tubing type, and tubing size, flow is proportional to pump speed (revolutions per minute). *In vitro* calibration curves must be constructed and checked periodically. This is done by measuring the output of the pump over a measured period of time at various pump settings in a mock circulation, preferably using blood. Silastic rubber, latex rubber, and PVC (e.g., Tygon) tubing have been used in the raceway, with the last type favored by many because it is an integral part of the circuit, is durable, and is associated with acceptable rates of hemolysis (98). It does become stiff during hypothermia and is subject to release of particulate material (spallation). Latex rubber is associated with greater hemolysis; Silastic rubber has less hemolysis when the pump is completely occlusive (98) and is said to resist fracture over long periods (99). Spallation refers to the release of microparticles of plastic from the inner walls of tubing due to compression by roller pumps. Silicone releases more particles than PVC does (99); new formulations of PVC that release even fewer particles are being developed.

The degree of compression of the tubing by the rollers

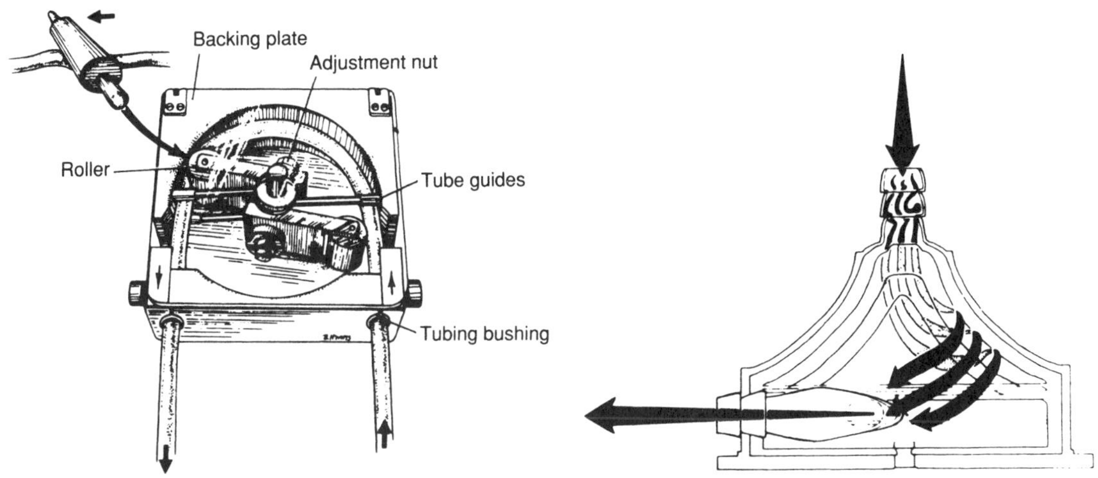

FIGURE 12-6. Arterial pumps. **(A)** Roller pump. **(B)** Centrifugal pump. (**A,** from Reed CC, Stafford TB. *Cardiopulmonary bypass,* 2nd ed. Houston, TX: Medical Press, 1985:377, with permission. **B,** from Lake CL, ed. *Pediatric cardiac anesthesia.* Norwalk, CT: Appleton & Lange, 1988:162, with permission.)

(occlusiveness) can be adjusted and appears to be critical. Excessive compression aggravates hemolysis and tubing wear; too little occlusion may also aggravate hemolysis but, more importantly, compromises forward output. Although there is some disagreement, most authors believe that the least hemolysis occurs when compression is adjusted to be barely nonocclusive (98). This is accomplished by holding the outflow line vertically so that the top of the fluid (blood or asanguineous) is about 60 to 100 cm (24 to 39 inches) above the pump and then gradually decreasing the occlusiveness until the fluid level falls at a rate of 1 cm in 5 to 60 seconds (98,100–102). The tighter setting ensures more accurate forward flow, makes the roller pump relatively insensitive to afterload, and may not be associated with more hemolysis.

Complications associated with roller pumps include malocclusion (with the consequences noted previously), miscalibration, miscalculation (including setting the wrong tube size into the pump controller [103]), fracture of the pump tubing, "runaway" (104) or loss of power, spallation

TABLE 12-4. ROLLER VERSUS CENTRIFUGAL PUMP

Parameter	Roller Pump	Centrifugal Pump
Principle characteristics	Nearly occlusive	Nonocclusive
	Afterload independent	Afterload dependent
Favorable features	Low prime volume	Portable and can function in any position
	Less expensive	Will not develop excessive positive or negative pressure
	Reliable forward flow	Adapts to venous return
	Can produce fair pulsatile flow	Superior for left- or right-sided heart bypass
		Good for long-term bypass (ECMO, VAD)
		Will not pump massive amounts of air (but can pass up to 50 ml)
Unfavorable features	Can develop excessive positive (rupture arterial line) and negative (cavitation, hemolysis) pressure	Large prime volume
	Spallation	Expensive
	Tube rupture	Requires flow meter
	Can pump massive amounts of air	Backward flow out of aorta if low revolutions per minute or turned off unless line is clamped or one-way valve is employed
	Must adjust occlusion	Cannot produce much pulsatile flow
	Requires close monitoring	
Conflicting data	Hemolysis and systemic inflammatory response	

(99,105), and pumping of large amounts of air. If the *outflow* becomes occluded, pressure in the line progressively rises until the tubing or connections break. This can be avoided by use of a pressure-regulated shunt between the outflow and inflow lines of the roller pump (Better Header [102]) or by servoregulation of the pump-to-arterial line pressure so that the pump is turned off when excessive pressures are detected. If *inflow* becomes limited, the roller pumps develop high negative pressures, producing cavitation (microbubbles).

Centrifugal Pumps

Centrifugal pumps (Fig. 12-6B) consist of a vaned impeller or a nest of smooth plastic cones that sit inside a plastic housing (106). The impeller or cones are magnetically coupled with an electric motor. When rotated rapidly, they generate a pressure differential that causes the movement of blood. Unlike roller pumps, they are totally nonocclusive and afterload dependent, which has both favorable and unfavorable consequences. Flow is not determined by rotational rate alone; therefore, a *flow meter* must be incorporated in the arterial outflow line to quantitate pump flow. Furthermore, when the arterial cannula is connected to the patient's arterial system and the pump is not running fast enough or is turned off, blood will flow backward through the pump and out of the patient *unless* the arterial line is clamped. This can cause exsanguination of the patient or aspiration of air into the arterial line (e.g., from around the pursestring). Therefore, *whenever the centrifugal pump is not running the arterial line must be clamped.* Incorporation of a check valve on the arterial line may minimize this problem (107). On the other hand, if the arterial line becomes occluded, these pumps do not generate excessive pressure (maximum only about 700 to 900 mm Hg) and do not rupture the arterial line. Likewise, they do not generate as much negative pressure (maximum only about −400 to −500 mm Hg), and hence not as much cavitation and microemboli production as does a roller pump, if inflow becomes occluded. A reputed advantage of centrifugal pumps over roller pumps is less risk of passage of massive air emboli into the arterial line. This is because the pumps become "deprimed" and stop pumping if more than 30 to 50 mL of air is introduced into the circuit (*however, they will pass smaller but potentially lethal quantities of air* and can generate microbubbles).

Roller versus Centrifugal Pumps

In *in vitro* studies, Moen et al. (108) noted less hemolysis and reduction in complement lytic inhibitors with centrifugal pumps but no differences in complement, coagulation, granulocyte activation, platelet activation, or endotoxin release. Hoerr et al. (109) observed less hemolysis and loss of clottable fibrinogen with centrifugal pumps compared with roller pumps. Tamari et al. (110) analyzed the effects of pressure and flow on the hemolysis caused by centrifugal versus roller pumps and found the former to be superior only when the ratio of pressure difference to flow is less than 0.25 mm Hg/mL/minute. In small clinical studies, Wheeldon et al. (111) found better preservation of platelet numbers, decreased complement activation, and reduced microbubble transmission, while Drissen et al. (112) noted less fall in the white blood cell count with centrifugal than with roller pumping. On the other hand, Wahba et al. (113) observed no difference in levels of free hemoglobin, lactate dehydrogenase, or bilirubin, or in activation of platelet surface receptors glycoprotein IIb, IIIa, and GMP140 between patients perfused with centrifugal versus roller pumps. And Ashraf et al. (114) observed no difference in release of serum S100β (a marker for cerebral injury) among patients exposed to either type pump. In other randomized clinical studies, Baufreton et al. (115) and Ashraf et al. (116) observed evidence of *greater* systemic inflammatory response with the use of *centrifugal* versus roller pumps. They speculated that this could be related to the completely nonpulsatile nature of perfusion with a centrifugal pump, compared with the slight pulsatility delivered by roller pumps (117).

In a prospective randomized study of 1,000 patients, published only in abstract form, Klein et al. (118) observed less bleeding and transfusion, shorter ventilator and intensive care unit stays, and fewer complications with centrifugal versus roller pumping. Other smaller, published studies have *not* observed differences in clinical outcome (111–113).

Centrifugal pumps are probably superior for use as temporary extracorporeal assist devices (119), for left heart bypass (120,121), and for generating pump-augmented venous return (see earlier discussion). Some believe that they require less anticoagulation (120). On the other hand, roller pumps are simpler, cheaper (especially the disposables), have a lower prime volume and are easier to prime (de-air), produce a predictable output that is independent of afterload, produce a slight pulsatile outflow, and can be modified to generate greater degrees of pulsatile flow.

Pulsatile Bypass

The complex issues surrounding pulsatile bypass have been reviewed elsewhere (122–126). Benefits are attributed to (a) the transmission of more energy to the microcirculation, which reduces critical capillary closing pressure, improves lymph flow, and improves tissue perfusion and cellular metabolism, and (b) reduction of adverse neuroendocrine responses (mainly vasoconstrictive) to nonpulsatile flow emanating from the baroreceptors, the kidneys, and probably the endothelium (e.g., regulation of nitric oxide release). Therefore, pulsatile bypass may result in increased oxygen consumption; reduced acidosis, improved cerebral, coronary, and renal perfusion; and reduced morbidity and mortality.

The *generation of pulsatile flow* and, more importantly, its transfer into the patient are complex. Several methods have been described, including an extracorporeal balloon (Pulsatile Assist Device: Datascope Corp, Paramus, NJ) and ventricular-type or hydraulic pumps (e.g., Keele pump, Polystan pulsatile pump: Polystan A/S, Copenhagen), but only modified roller pumps (e.g., Sarns: Ann Arbor, MI [127], Stockert: Cobe Stockert Inc., Lakewood, CO [128]), centrifugal pumps (e.g., Sarns [112]), and intraaortic balloon pumps (129) are used clinically at this time. Wright (130,131) compared the hydraulic power output of various pulsatile pumps; he found that the ventricular pumps (which have not found acceptance in clinical bypass) are more powerful and that a popular modified roller pulsatile pump (Stockert) was only able to produce, at most, about 12% (and usually only about 5%) of the pulsatile power of the human heart. Computer-controlled variable pulsatility may be advantageous (132).

Transfer of this pulsatile energy into the patient is influenced by factors within the extracorporeal circuit (such as passage through membrane oxygenators, arterial line filters, the arterial line [and its compliance], and the arterial cannula); patient factors (age, compliance of the vascular tree, systemic vascular resistance, anesthetic state, carotid sinus responsiveness [133]); physiologic autoregulation (130, 131,134); and the complex issue of impedance matching, without which pulsatile energy is either wasted or may even be damaging (124). Optimal transfer of pulsatile energy requires short, wide arterial cannulas (greater than 24F or 6.5 mm or, according to one author [135], greater than 11.6 mm!) and the use of a second (pulsatile) pump distal to the membrane oxygenator (which increases the complexity of the circuit) or a single pump system beyond the membrane oxygenator (if a gravity-perfused membrane oxygenator [e.g., Capiox-E, Terumo Corporation, Tokyo, Japan] is employed). However, only a modest amount of dampening has been reported with pulsatile bypass through some hollow-fiber membrane oxygenators, although control of the pulsatile output of the pump is critical to limit the generation of microbubbles (136).

A long-standing controversy exists concerning the importance of pulsatility during CPB (126,137,138). Hornick and Taylor (126) have nicely reviewed the evidence favoring pulsatile bypass and identified certain groups of patients in whom it may be more important (e.g., those with poor cardiac reserve, hypertension, vascular occlusive disease, renal or hepatic insufficiency; during deep hypothermia; after circulatory arrest). Mangano et al. (138) summarized some of the conflicting experimental data from more than 25 studies (see Table 30-3 of their review). For example, in two different prospective randomized studies comparing pulsatile (Stockert roller pump) with nonpulsatile CPB in patients undergoing coronary artery surgery, Minami et al. (139) observed lower mean arterial pressure, lower total peripheral resistance, and lower levels of epinephrine and norepinephrine with pulsatile perfusion, whereas Alston et al. (140,141) observed no difference in peripheral vascular resistance nor systemic oxygen uptake. Some of the conflicting data relate to failure to quantitatively define the degree of pulsatility produced in terms of pulsatile pressure and flow (including pulse pressure, shape, and size; ejection time; stroke volume; and dP/dt) within the aorta despite the availability of quantitative measures (e.g., the energy equivalent pressure [142] and the pulsatility index and pulse power index [143]). In addition, there is lack of agreement about what is the optimal form of pulsatility (144). Other factors that may influence the outcome of various experimental studies include species studied, patient group (e.g., low versus high risk), age, flow rate, pressures and temperatures employed during CPB, duration of CPB, type of anesthesia, and means of assessing organ effects (145). Some confusion may relate to the fact that even "nonpulsatile" roller pumps produce some pulsatility (117).

Despite many favorable laboratory studies, the demonstration of improved clinical outcome with pulsatile CPB has been limited. Shaw et al. (146), Henze et al. (147) and Murkin et al. (148) found no difference in neurologic or cognitive outcome; this confirms recent clinical (149) and animal studies (144,145), which have found no difference in cerebral metabolism or blood flow between pulsatile and nonpulsatile CBP. (This is in distinction to Mutch et al. [132], who reported increased jugular venous oxygen during rewarming when computer-controlled pulsation was used in pigs.) Ohri et al. (150) observed no difference in incidence of intraabdominal complications and Badner et al. (151) found no difference in perioperative renal function or dysfunction. Louagie et al. (152) could detect no differences in numerous hemodynamic, fluid balance, organ function, and clinical outcome variables in a prospective randomized study of 100 elective coronary artery surgery patients when they compared pulsatile with nonpulsatile perfusion. On the other hand, both Taylor et al. (153) and Murkin et al. (154), in studies involving more than 150 patients in each group, observed lower rates of mortality and of myocardial infarction or low cardiac output in patients undergoing coronary artery and other cardiac procedures when pulsatile versus nonpulsatile perfusion was used.

On the negative side, pulsatile CPB is more expensive and more complicated, requires the use of larger arterial cannulas, and is associated with higher nozzle velocities out the arterial cannula and hence greater theoretic risk of adverse effects including hemolysis, platelet injury, and vascular trauma (135). With the concern that aortic atheroembolism may be a major cause of neurologic morbidity associated with CPB, arterial cannula jet effects are worrisome. If pulsation is carried out through a membrane oxygenator, there is risk of generation of gaseous microbubbles and damage to the membrane oxygenator (136).

Wright (124) concluded his analysis of pulsatile CPB on a pessimistic note: "Modern cardiopulmonary bypass systems incorporate so many pulse damping devices and impedance mismatches that the pulsatile power delivered to the aorta by modified roller pumps is probably insignificant. Conversely, pulsatile flow that resembled the output of the normal left ventricle would probably result in blood cell trauma and even mechanical damage to the extracorporeal circuit . . . . It is difficult to see how this dilemma is going to be resolved."

OXYGENATORS

Although numerous types of oxygenators have been used in the past (including heterologous biologic lungs, vertical screens, and disk oxygenators), currently only two varieties are in use—the bubble oxygenator and the membrane oxygenator (155)—and bubble oxygenators are rapidly disappearing from use in most parts of the world (Fig. 12-7).

Bubble Oxygenators

Bubble oxygenators (Fig. 12-7A) were among the earliest types of oxygenators used for CPB; they are simple and are the least expensive type. They include three components—an oxygenation chamber, a defoaming chamber, and a reservoir—although most now also include an integral heat exchanger within the inflow or oxygenator chamber. Oxygen is passed through a dispersion plate at the site of venous inflow, which results in the formation of bubbles. Gas exchange occurs through the walls of the bubbles and is determined by the number and size of bubbles. The number of bubbles is determined by gas flow rate and bubble size, and the size is influenced by the size of holes in the dispersion plate. Smaller bubbles result in a larger surface area and better oxygen exchange, but they also limit carbon dioxide exchange and may be harder to remove; therefore, a compromise is made by the manufacturer. Oxygenation is usually superior to carbon dioxide removal. Arterial partial pressure of carbon dioxide (P_{CO_2}) is controlled by gas flow (i.e., ratio of gas flow to blood flow), which is kept at a minimal acceptable level to minimize blood trauma and gaseous microemboli production. Only pure oxygen should be used, because inclusion of inert gases (e.g., nitrogen) increases the risk of difficult-to-reabsorb gaseous microemboli. Hence, the arterial partial pressure of oxygen (P_{O_2}) tends to be high and difficult to control independent of P_{CO_2}.

Next the blood (foam) passes through a defoamer consisting of plastic sponges coated with silicone A antifoam, which lowers surface tension and causes the bubbles to dissi-

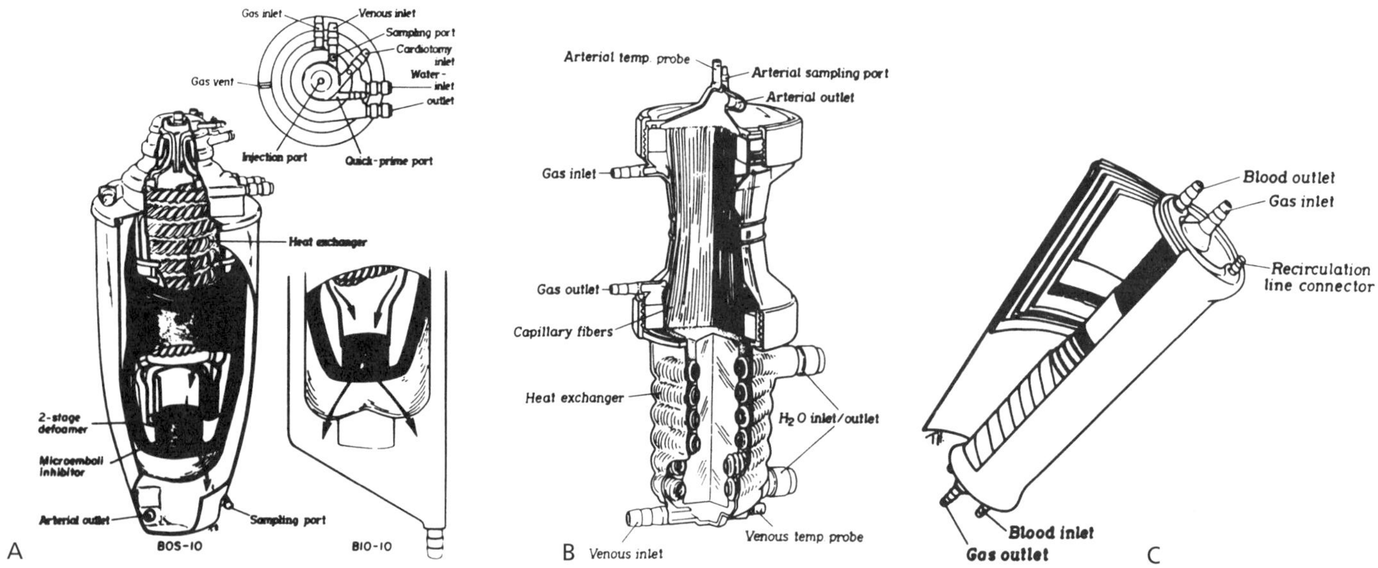

FIGURE 12-7. Oxygenators. **(A)** A typical bubble oxygenator (Bentley BOS 10). Venous blood enters the top, where it is mixed with bubbles of oxygen and passes over an integral heat exchanger. It then passes through defoaming and debubbling stages and collects in the reservoir at the bottom. **(B)** A capillary microporous membrane oxygenator (Bentley BOS CM 50). Venous blood enters the bottom; it passes over the heat exchanger tubes and then into the oxygenating column, where it passes around the multiple capillary tubes (through which the fresh gas—oxygen and air—passes) and out the top as oxygenated blood. **(C)** A true silicone membrane (sheet) oxygenator (Avecor). An envelope that consists of a silicone rubber membrane enclosing a nylon screen separator is wound in spiral fashion around a core. Blood passes within the envelope, and the fresh gas passes on the outside of the envelope in a countercurrent fashion. (Blood enters the bottom and exits out the top; fresh gas passes in the opposite direction.) (**A** through **C**, from Reed CC, Stafford TB. *Cardiopulmonary bypass,* 2nd ed. Houston, TX: Medical Press, 1985:293,441,448, with permission.)

pate. The defoamer must have the capacity to cope with the maximal rated flow of the oxygenator. Some gas exchange also occurs in the defoamer. The liquefied blood then collects in the reservoir in which further debubbling occurs. The reservoir also serves as the "atrium" for the arterial pump, as a buffer to modulate fluctuations in venous drainage, and as an emergency reserve in case of complete loss of venous return (providing time to slow or turn off the arterial pump before air embolism can occur). Maintenance of a large volume in this reservoir favors bubble removal and safety but increases the prime volume. Blood moves through a bubble oxygenator by being passively driven by the oxygen flowing into it. Oxygen flow must be initiated before the oxygenator is primed; otherwise fluid and/or blood may back-leak through the dispersion plate and interfere with bubble formation.

Bubble oxygenators are efficient and less expensive than membrane oxygenators, but they cause more gaseous and particulate microemboli and blood trauma and they preclude independent control of arterial oxygen and carbon dioxide.

Membrane Oxygenators

Membrane oxygenators imitate the natural lung by interspersing a thin membrane between the gas and blood phases. This eliminates gaseous microemboli formation and minimizes blood trauma. Most membranes are made of either solid silicone rubber or microporous (0.3 to 0.8 μm) polypropylene. The microporous membranes are not considered true membranes, but the pores quickly become filled with plasma and proteins, which serve as a very efficient "membrane." The true silicone membrane is typically arranged as a coiled sheet (Fig. 12-7C), whereas the microporous polymers are usually made into hollow-fiber capillaries arranged in vertical bundles (Fig. 12-7B). Either the gas or the blood passes through the capillary tubes, and the other on the outside, depending on the manufacturer's design. The limitation to gas exchange is not primarily diffusion through the membrane but rather diffusion through the thin film of blood (approximately 100 μm), which requires some turbulence within the blood film to succeed. Because of the relatively high resistance to blood flow through most membrane oxygenators, venous blood must be pumped through them. Arterial P_{CO_2} is controlled by gas flow, and P_{O_2} is controlled by the fraction of inspired oxygen (F_{IO_2}) through the use of an air-oxygen blender (which is safe because the nitrogen cannot form bubbles in the blood). More precise independent control of blood gases is possible with membrane oxygenators compared with bubble oxygenators. De-airing during priming is somewhat more difficult than with bubble oxygenators, but preflushing with carbon dioxide facilitates this procedure. Microporous membranes are not optimal for extended periods (i.e., days) of oxygenation because of protein leakage, which degrades membrane function; therefore, only true silicone membrane oxygenators (e.g., ECMO Oxygenator, Avecor Cardiovascular, Plymouth, MN) (Fig. 12-7C) are recommended for extracorporeal membrane oxygenation.

Because membrane oxygenators are inherently safer, produce less particulate and gaseous microemboli (156), exhibit superior hemocompatibility, and allow superior blood gas control (157), they have largely replaced bubble oxygenators for clinical CPB (155,158,159). Nevertheless, it has been difficult to demonstrate improved clinical outcome with membrane oxygenators, especially for CPB of less than 2 hours' duration (160,161), although in a retrospective study of 1,078 patients Utley et al. (162) found by one-way analysis of variance that use of a bubble (versus the membrane) oxygenator was associated with increased rates of death, stroke, and leg wound complications.

Autologous Oxygenation

Interest in an old form of oxygenation, use of the patient's own lungs, was renewed by a report of improved pulmonary function and lower levels of interleukin-6 when the patient's own lungs were used, compared with conventional oxygenator use (9). This approach requires a more complex cannulation and extracorporeal circuit perfusion management (right atrium to pulmonary artery with a pulmonary pump and left atrium to aorta with a systemic pump), but it merits further investigation (see also Sweeney and Frazier [8]).

Circuit Configuration

The type of oxygenator does influence the configuration of the extracorporeal circuit (Fig. 12-1), and often the oxygenator includes other components of the circuit (163). The heat exchanger is usually an integral part of the oxygenator and commonly is situated just proximal to the gas-exchanging section (or sometimes within the bubble chamber of the bubble oxygenator). Bubble oxygenators are positioned before the pump and include an arterial reservoir, which is located distal to the oxygenating column and defoaming area and before the arterial pump for which it serves as an atrium. No additional venous reservoir is included in this circuit, because the venous return empties directly into the oxygenating column of the oxygenator (as does the cardiotomy reservoir). Membrane oxygenators are usually positioned distal to the pump, because the resistance in most membrane oxygenators requires that blood be pumped through them. A venous reservoir receives the venous return (as well as the drainage from the cardiotomy reservoir) and serves as the atrium for the arterial pump, which pumps the blood through the oxygenator and into the patient. Some low-resistance membrane oxygenators may be adequately perfused by gravity drainage of venous blood and therefore are positioned like a bubble oxygenator. For pulsatile bypass with a membrane oxygenator circuit, often a second (pulsatile) pump is placed distal to the membrane oxygenator to avoid the dampening that would occur if it were placed before the membrane oxygenator. This requires inclusion of a second ("arterial") reservoir and a bypass line to handle the excessive flow of the first ("venous") pump, which must run slightly faster than the arterial pump. If there is no arterial reservoir between the membrane oxygenator and the arterial pump, there is risk of drawing bubbles of gas across the membrane and into the bypass circuit. Some membrane oxygenators permit pulsatile pumping through them and do not require a second pump; however, control of the pulsatile output of the pump is critical to limit generation of gaseous microbubbles, and these systems do reduce the amount of transmitted hydraulic power (136).

Often, to gain maximum benefit from the membrane oxygenator (elimination of blood-gas interface), collapsible reservoirs are used in these circuits (see Venous/Arterial and Cardiotomy Reservoirs and Suction).

Oxygenators Require a Gas Supply System

Oxygenators require at least a source of oxygen (but usually also air [only with membrane oxygenators] and sometimes carbon dioxide), flow regulators, and flow meters. When oxygen and air are used, a blender is needed. An oxygen analyzer should be incorporated in the circuit—after the blender, if one is used—as should a microfilter and a moisture trap. An anesthetic vaporizer is usually incorporated in the gas supply line to the oxygenator. Because volatile anesthetic liquids may be destructive to the plastic components of extracorporeal circuits, one must consider the location of these vaporizers and use extreme care when filling them with anesthetic liquid so as not to "contaminate" any plastic component, including tubing. Gravlee et al. (164) called attention to the risk of hypoxemia during CPB caused by leaks in the gas supply system at various sites, and they described and advocated a low-pressure leak test. Obstruction (165) or disconnection of the oxygen supply line also causes hypoxemia during CPB.

Oxygenator Malfunction

Oxygenator malfunction requiring changing of the oxygenator during CPB has been reported to occur in 0.02% to 0.26% of cases (166–171). The most common cause is development of abnormal pressure gradients across the blood path (in membrane oxygenators), although the cause of this phenomenon is unresolved (171). Other problems include leaks and deteriorating gas-exchanging performance. Svenmaker et al. (168) found a wide variability in "oxygenator incident rate" among different types of membrane oxygenators. Wahba et al. (170) observed one-tenth the rate of development of abnormal pressure gradients with heparin-coated compared with uncoated membrane oxygenators.

VENOUS/ARTERIAL AND CARDIOTOMY RESERVOIRS AND SUCTION

Venous/Arterial Reservoir

A reservoir is placed immediately before the arterial pump to serve as its "holding tank" or "atrium" and to act as a buffer for fluctuations and imbalances between venous return and arterial flow. It also serves as a high-capacitance (i.e., low-pressure) receiving chamber for venous return and therefore facilitates gravity drainage of venous blood. In addition, it functions as a place to store excessive blood from the venae cavae when the heart and lungs are exsanguinated. Additional venous blood may become available from the patient when CPB is initiated and systemic venous pressure is reduced to low levels. As much as 1 to 3 L of blood may need to be translocated from the patient to the extracorporeal circuit when full CPB is initiated, especially in a patient who has been in congestive heart failure. The reservoir may also serve as a gross bubble trap for air that enters the venous line; as the site where blood, fluids, or drugs may be added and into which the cardiotomy reservoir empties (see later discussion); and as a ready source of blood for transfusion into the patient. It may also be used as a site to apply vacuum for VAVD (see earlier discussion). One of its most important functions, however, is to provide time for the perfusionist to act if venous drainage is sharply reduced or stopped, in order to avoid pumping the system dry and risking systemic air embolism. The reaction time is determined by the volume of blood in the reservoir and the flow rate. At a flow of 4.3 L/minute (2.4 L/minute/m^2 in a 1.8-m^2 subject), a reservoir volume of 500 mL allows 7 seconds, and a volume of 1 L allows 14 seconds. Another problem with running a low level in a hard-shell venous reservoir (see later discussion) is that this may result in greater formation of microemboli (172).

With membrane oxygenators, the reservoir is the first component of the extracorporeal circuit; it directly receives the venous drainage as well as the cardiotomy drainage. Blood then passes through the arterial pump and proceeds through the membrane oxygenator. If the reservoir is of the hard-shell type, it may be physically attached to and part of the oxygenator housing. Reservoirs may be rigid (hard) plastic canisters ("open" types) or soft, collapsible plastic bags ("closed" types). The rigid canisters facilitate measurements of volume and handling of venous air, often have a larger capacity, are easier to prime, permit application of suction for VAVD, and may be less expensive. Some hard-shell venous reservoirs incorporate macrofilters and microfilters and can also serve as cardiotomy reservoirs and to directly receive vented blood (see discussion). The soft bags eliminate the blood-gas interface and reduce the risk of pumping massive air emboli because they collapse when empty and prevent air from entering the arterial pump.

Schonberger et al. (173) observed more blood activation, blood loss, and blood administration with the use of hard-shell versus collapsible venous reservoirs, which they attributed to additional exposure to filters and blood-air interface. Another limitation of hard-shell reservoirs is that their defoaming elements are coated with silicone compounds (antifoam) which may cause systemic microembolization (174).

Cardiotomy Reservoir and Field Suction

During cardiac surgery it is necessary to aspirate variable but often large amounts of blood from the cardiac chambers and surgical field. The aspiration prevents distention of the cardiac chambers and air embolization and provides adequate exposure of the surgical field. It is not practical to discard the blood, and most of it is returned to the heart-lung machine via the cardiotomy reservoir.

The cardiotomy reservoir receives blood that has been aspirated from the heart or pericardium, or out of various vents (see later discussion). It usually includes a defoaming chamber containing a sponge impregnated with a substance that lowers surface tension, a storage chamber, and filters (macrofilters and microfilters; see later discussion). Blood is returned, usually by gravity, to the venous arterial reservoir, either intermittently or continuously. When a hard-shell (rigid) venous reservoir is used in conjunction with a membrane oxygenator, usually this reservoir serves as a combined or integrated venous and cardiotomy reservoir, although the blood path of the cardiotomy section usually includes more extensive defoaming and microfiltration before this blood joins the venous return blood in the common reservoir section.

Suction is usually and most conveniently and simply generated by the use of a roller pump. The disadvantage of this system is that if the sucker tip becomes occluded a high degree of negative pressure is developed, causing hemolysis of red blood cells. It also requires constant adjustment of the speed of the roller pump by the perfusionist and coordination with the surgeon. Alternatively, suction can be generated by connecting the cardiotomy reservoir to a vacuum suction (e.g., "wall suction"). This method avoids development of excessive negative pressure, but it requires a closed cardiotomy reservoir and increases the risk of developing positive pressure in the cardiotomy reservoir and therefore the risk of systemic air embolization.

The cardiotomy suction and reservoir have been found to be a major source of hemolysis, particulate and gaseous microemboli (see later discussion), fat globule formation, cellular aggregation, platelet injury and loss, and activation of coagulation and fibrinolysis (174–178). A major contributor to these adverse effects is the amount of air aspirated along with the blood. This adds gaseous microemboli to the blood that are particularly hard to dissipate because they contain mainly nitrogen, a gas that is quite insoluble. In addition, the air-blood mixture causes turbulence and high shear stresses that injure both red blood cells and platelets. Pearson et al. (179) analyzed the ability of various commercial cardiotomy reservoirs to remove bubbles from aspirated blood and described desirable features: directly injecting blood into the defoamer and avoiding turbulence at inlet (which may generate microemboli), ensuring that all blood passes through the defoamer, avoiding the free fall of blood into the reservoir (which causes splashing and microemboli), and incorporating a micropore filter. Storing the blood in the cardiotomy reservoir for as long as possible, rather than letting it flow continuously into the main circuit, reduces the number of microemboli, as does reducing the ratio of air in the aspirated blood.

Edmunds et al. (175) found that the fall in platelet count was directly proportional to the amount of cardiotomy suction, expressed either as the total amount (liters per case) or as a fraction of total extracorporeal flow during CPB. de Jong et al. (180), in a canine study, observed progressively greater reduction in platelet number and function and a prolongation of bleeding time as increasing amounts of air were aspirated along with blood during cardiotomy suction. Boonstra et al. (181) conducted a prospective study of patients undergoing coronary artery bypass grafting with a membrane oxygenator. They noted less release of β-thromboglobulin and less postoperative bleeding when they used an automatically controlled cardiotomy suction device that prevented aspiration of air with the blood, compared with conventional ("uncontrolled") suction. Wright and Sanderson (176) also documented the adverse effects of coaspiration of air on platelet count and formation of microaggregates (manifested by a rise in screen filtration pressure). The cardiotomy suction also appears to be a principal source of hemolysis during CPB. This has been attributed to blood contact with the pericardium, excessive negative pressure (182,183), and, most importantly, coaspiration of air (176,180). Wright and Sanderson noted less hemolysis when a vacuum suction pump was used, rather than a roller pump (176).

The amount of cardiotomy suction that is necessary is influenced by the type of surgery; it is greater with surgery for valvular and congenital heart disease, especially if the patient is cyanotic (175), than with coronary artery surgery. The amount of blood damage can be minimized by avoiding or minimizing coaspiration of air (i.e., the sucker tip should be kept below the blood level and the field should not be sucked dry), by not allowing the blood to remain in the pericardium for long periods, by using the slowest flow rates and largest suction tips possible, and by avoiding generation of high degrees of negative pressure (i.e., not occluding the sucker tip and using controlled vacuum suction rather than a roller pump). This last method, however, is somewhat more complicated and requires a closed system, increasing the risk of developing positive pressure in the cardiotomy reservoir and thereby the risk of systemic air embolism.

An alternative method of handling blood and fluid in the surgical field is the use of centrifugal cell washers (e.g., Haemonetics Cell Saver: Maemonetics Corp., Braintree,

MA). These washers aspirate the blood with a controlled vacuum; the red cells are automatically washed with saline and separated from the fluid by centrifugation, and the washed red blood cells may then be returned to the extracorporeal circuit. The advantages of this method are that it removes undesirable materials (e.g., microaggregates, fat, gross air, tissue debris, potassium, bioactivators); hemoconcentrates (raises the hematocrit of the fluid); and may improve biocompatiability. The disadvantages are the slow turnaround time and the loss of plasma proteins, coagulation factors, platelets, and other desirable substances that are in the blood. Many teams use both cell washer suction and cardiotomy suction, choosing one or the other depending on the type of fluid (e.g., predominantly cardioplegic solution or ice melt versus predominantly blood) and the location (e.g., pleural versus intracardiac); however, cost considerations have reduced the routine use of cell washers.

HEAT EXCHANGERS

Heat exchangers are designed to add or remove heat from the blood and hence to control body temperature. During its flow in the extracorporeal circuit, the blood cools and therefore heat must be added to avoid patient cooling. In addition, the patient's temperature is often deliberately lowered during the case and then needs to be restored to normothermia before CPB is discontinued. Although in the past separate heat exchangers were used in extracorporeal circuits, currently they are invariably included as an integral part of the disposable oxygenators. They are usually located proximal to the gas-exchanging section of the circuit to minimize the risk of releasing microbubbles of gas from the blood, which might occur if the blood is warmed after being saturated with gas at a colder temperature. The warming gradient (the difference between the temperature of inflowing warming water and that of inflowing blood) should be kept at less than 5° to 10°C, and the water temperature should not be allowed to exceed 40°C to further minimize release of microbubbles of gas (184) and damage to blood elements; and some recommend restricting water temperature to below 37° to 38°C to reduce the risk of cerebral injury. Excessive cooling gradients could theoretically also cause gas emboli formation when the cooled oxygenated blood enters the warmer patient, but this may be of limited clinical significance (184). An additional risk of heat exchangers is leakage of water into the blood path, which might be manifested by an appearance of hemolysis. A source of hot and cold water, a regulator/blender, and temperature sensors are supplemental requirements of heat exchangers. Although the hospital water supply may provide such a source, more commonly a dedicated freestanding water heater-cooler is used. Malfunctions of these heater-coolers are among the more common incidents during CPB (169).

Separate heat exchangers are needed for administration of cardioplegia fluid and/or blood for coronary perfusion. In the former case, the simplest system is to use bags of precooled (i.e., in a refrigerator or ice bucket) cardioplegia solution. Alternatively, the cardioplegia fluid is circulated through coils of plastic tubing, which are placed in an ice bath or a warm-water bath, or through a dedicated separate heat exchanger.

MICROEMBOLIZATION, FILTERS, AND BUBBLE TRAPS

Gross and Microembolic Material

Gross and microembolic materials are always present during CPB (177,185). They are subclassified as gas, biologic, and nonbiologic substances. Gaseous emboli may be gross or microscopic—the latter, referred to as gaseous microemboli, may consist predominantly of air (i.e., 80% nitrogen) or of oxygen. The sources of gaseous emboli include the oxygenator, cardiotomy reservoir, roller pump, heat exchanger, prime solution and any fluid added to the circuit, the circuit itself (inadequate de-airing), and the heart. Taylor et al. (186) identified sampling of blood and administration of drugs into the bottom of a soft-shell venous reservoir as a major source of microemboli during CPB. Bubble oxygenators were a major source of gaseous microemboli, whereas membrane oxygenators produce little or none (155,156,177,187). Warming of cold fluid or blood causes a release of gas, which is more likely to occur if the fluid is fully saturated (e.g., high PaO_2). This may occur when cold fluids are added to the extracorporeal circuit, when hypothermia is induced (cold perfusate is warmed inside warmer body), or during warming (warming of cold blood in the heat exchanger) (184). Cardiotomy suction is a major source of gaseous microemboli, and factors influencing this effect were discussed previously. Cavitation describes the creation of microbubbles when a fluid is exposed to sudden negative pressure. This is said to occur when blood exits at high velocity out of an arterial cannula and in the tubing behind the moving rollers of a roller pump, especially if set occlusively, and even with centrifugal pumps. Microbubbles as well as gross air may be entrained around venous and vent cannulas if the pursestrings are not tight or excessive suction is applied. Any time the left heart (or aortic root) is opened, air enters and, unless it is completely removed, embolizes systemically.

Biologic particulate emboli include fat, fibrin, clots, microaggregates of red blood cells, platelets and white blood cells, calcium, atherosclerotic material, bone, and tissue. Microaggregation may be precipitated by exposure of blood to pleural and pericardial surfaces or to foreign surfaces of the extracorporeal circuit—in particular to the blood-gas interfaces in cardiotomy suctions (178,188). Release of various substances from platelets and activation of the complement cascade also contribute to microaggregation. Donor blood may be an important source of biologic particles (188).

Nonbiologic particulate emboli may come from the surgical field via the cardiotomy suction and can include fibers, talc, thread, and dust, or they may come from the circuit, consisting of fibers, antifoam, plastic chips, and tubing particles (spallation) (105,188).

Emboli have been detected experimentally and/or clinically by examination of tissues at autopsy, fluorescein angiography (156), measurement of screen filtration pressure, use of an electronic particle size analyzer (188), and examination and weighing of microfilters. The most commonly used clinical methods are ultrasound detectors on the arterial line* (189), transcranial Doppler (190–193), and TEE (184).

It is generally accepted that microemboli can be responsible for injury to many systemic organs (188,194), and many believe that microemboli are responsible for much of the neurologic dysfunction that can be detected after CPB (186). Although this belief seems reasonable, it has not been proven (185,195). Several canine studies that have demonstrated cerebral vascular obstruction, decreased cerebral blood flow, decreased oxygen and glucose metabolism, and release of enzymes into the cerebrospinal fluid during CPB—and their amelioration by micropore arterial filtration—are among the most convincing evidence supporting this hypothesis (196–198).

Reduction of Microembolization

Many strategies have been suggested to reduce the hazards of microembolization (Table 12-5), but the most obvious is the use of micropore filters (199–201).† Two types of micropore filters are available. The depth filter consists of packed fibers or porous foam. The predominant example of this type is the Swank Dacron wool filter. It has no defined pore size, presents a tortuous large wetted surface, and filters by impaction and absorption. The screen filters are usually made of woven polymer thread, which has a defined pore size and filters by interception, although the smallest pored screen filters (0.2 to 5.0 μm) are made out of membranes. Screen filters vary in pore size, material used (principally polyester and nylon), and configuration. They block not only particulate emboli but also gross and microscopic air emboli, the latter because the pores are filled with liquid maintained by surface-active forces (excessive pressure could overcome this, the so-called bubble point pressure).

TABLE 12-5. PROCEDURES AND PRACTICES THAT HAVE BEEN PROPOSED TO REDUCE AMOUNT OF MICROEMBOLIZATION

Membrane oxygenator (vs. bubble)
Centrifugal pump (vs. roller)
Micropore filter below cardiotomy reservoir ($\leq$40 μm)
Arterial line micropore filter ($\leq$40 μm)
Vent arterial filter continuously to cardiotomy reservoir
Microfiltration of blood added to circuit
If using bubble oxygenator
Maintain high reservoir volume
Use lowest gas-to-blood flow ratio possible
Regarding cardiotomy suction
Use as little as possible
Aspirate as little air as possible
Use lowest flow possible
Regarding cardiotomy reservoir
Should have an integral micropore filter
Maintain high reservoir volume
Retain blood in reservoir as long as possible
If using roller pump
Set barely nonocclusive
Use polyvinyl chloride vs. silicone rubber
During priming
Flush with carbon dioxide before prime
Prime with warmed fluids
Use prebypass micropore filter (5 μm)
Prolonged recirculation with tapping of components
Keep temperature gradients during warming and cooling to less than 8°–10°C
Use largest arterial cannula possible
Adequate anticoagulation
Keep pursestring sutures around cannula as tight as possible
Minimal acceptable suction on vents
Vigorous de-airing at end of any procedure, if left side of heart has been opened
Avoid use of nitrous oxide during or after cardiopulmonary bypass

Several studies have compared the performance of various micropore filters designed for cardiotomy (202,203) or arterial lines (179,197,204–206), and most have found the Dacron wool (depth) filter to be the most effective. Gourlay et al. (204,205) in an *in vitro* study of 13 commercially available arterial line filters, found that they all had similar pressure drops (24 to 34 mm Hg at 5 L/minute flow) but exhibited varying degrees of hemolysis and platelet loss and of handling gross and microscopic air; these variations did not appear to be related to pore size or type of material, except that the Dacron wool (Swank) filter was best at removal of both microscopic and gross air. For other filters there was no parallel between their effectiveness in handling gross versus microscopic air. However, all were vastly superior to the use of no filter in regard to interdiction of microemboli. Other authors have expressed concern that the Dacron wool filter might cause significantly more hemo-

* For an interesting debate on the validity of the ultrasonic bubble counter, see the correspondence between Wright and Furnes and Pearson et al. in *Perfusion*, volume 1 (1986), pages 216–219, and the review by Butler and Kurusz (185).

† The potential for bias, in the two, otherwise excellent review articles by Berman and Marin (199) and Marshall (200), must be recognized since these authors were employed by a manufacturer (Pall Biomedical Corporation) of screen-type filters.

lysis and thrombocytopenia and might develop channeling and saturation breakthrough (199). Gourlay et al. (205) did not note excessive hemolysis, and Ware et al. (203) determined that although platelet counts were lower after use of Dacron wool cardiotomy filters, the number of functional platelets was the same (i.e., the screen filter allowed more dysfunctional platelets to pass). Some concern has also been expressed regarding screen filters made of nylon, which may activate complement (199,200).

Micropore filters may be used in several locations in the extracorporeal circuits. A survey conducted in 1993 found their frequency of use in the various locations to be as follows: arterial line, 92%; cardiotomy reservoir, 89%; gas line to oxygenator, 83%; blood product administration sets, 80%; prebypass (i.e., after priming but before connecting to patient), 78%; and cardioplegia delivery system, 46% (207).

Most commercial cardiotomy reservoirs now contain an integrated micropore filter. Because cardiotomy suction is a major source of microemboli, and because a micropore filter is more effective if it is placed in the cardiotomy reservoir line (rather than in the arterial line) (179), this would appear to be a reasonable practice. With the demonstrated presence of various types of foreign particulate matter in the disposables used for extracorporeal circuits, it also seems reasonable to use a prebypass filter during priming. The need for micropore filters on the cardioplegia delivery system has been questioned on the basis of recent experimental studies (208).

Arterial Micropore Filtration

The need for and benefits of arterial micropore filtration are still debated (201). *In vitro* studies (179,197,204,205) have documented that micropore arterial filtration does reduce the number of microemboli measured by ultrasound, and clinical studies have confirmed this finding (187,190,191). Muraoka et al. (209) noted fewer abnormal computed tomographic scans when a 20-μm filter was used, but just as many abnormal scans when a 40-μm filter was used, compared with no filter during CPB in children with a bubble oxygenator. However, Blauth et al. (156) observed no reduction in microembolic retinal ischemia when a 40-μm arterial filter (Ultipore, Pall Biomedical Corporation, New York, NY) was used in a bubble oxygenator circuit, and Henriksen et al. (210) observed only a modest reduction in the cerebral hyperemic response to bypass (which they attribute to microembolization) with the use of arterial micropore filtration.

Several authors, using historical controls, have reported a reduced incidence of neurologic damage with use of micropore filters (211–214); however, Garvey et al. (215) found statistically insignificantly less incidence of impairment of function on a psychometric test with one arterial micropore filter (Pall 40 μm) and statistically insignificantly greater incidence of impairment with another filter (Bentley 25 μm), compared with historical controls. Three prospective controlled studies have failed to detect differences in neurologic outcome with or without the use of micropore filters (216–218), and another observed no difference in performance on a sophisticated neuropsychometric test with the use of arterial micropore filtration (195). Ohri et al. (150) observed no difference in incidence of intraabdominal complications with the use of arterial microfiltration. The most persuasive study demonstrating clinical benefits from the use of arterial microfiltration was the prospective, double-blinded and randomized study of Pugsley et al. (219), which compared 50 patients in each of two groups with or without use of a 40-μm screen filter (EC Plus, Pall) in the arterial line. Although there were no focal neurologic changes in either group, the incidence of "soft neurologic deficits" was lower (16% versus 38%; $p < .05$) in the filtered group, and the incidence of neurologic deficits in two or more neuropsychometric tests (of a battery of ten) at 8 weeks after operation was lower (8% versus 27%; $p < .03$) in the filtered group. They also found a correlation between the number of microemboli ("HITS") during transcranial Doppler monitoring of the middle cerebral artery and the incidence of neuropsychometric deficits (9% if less than 200 HITS, 23% to 31% if 200 to 1,000 HITS, and 43% if more than 1,000 HITS), as did Sylivris et al. (220). However it is important to note that a bubble oxygenator was used in the Pugsley study. When membrane oxygentators are used, the embolic load is much less than when bubble oxygenators are used, and in fact is comparable to the load seen with a bubble oxygenator and micropore filter, so arterial line microfiltration may be less critical (201). Other observations that may suggest limits to the benefits of arterial line microfiltration are that the times of greatest microembolic load are during arterial cannulation (220–222), application and release of aortic clamps (221,222), and initiation of cardiac ejection after open heart procedures (223) and that surgically induced emboli (compared with perfusion-induced emboli) are more likely to lead to postoperative morbidity (224). These non–perfusion-related sources of microemboli are not likely to be interdicted by arterial line filtration. Further, Brooker et al. (178), in a canine study, found that cardiotomy suction was the major source of cerebral emboli and that these emboli were not prevented by use of arterial line filtration. Also, Taylor et al. (186) noted that an arterial line microfilter (32 μm) did not prevent the passage of microemboli (presumably gaseous microemboli) introduced by perfusionist interventions.

There are other limitations of arterial line microfilters: they add to the cost, may obstruct, are harder to de-air (and therefore may be a source of gaseous microemboli), may generate microemboli, cause hemolysis and platelet loss, and cause complement activation.

However, the wide experience and available studies on these filters suggest that there are few adverse effects from

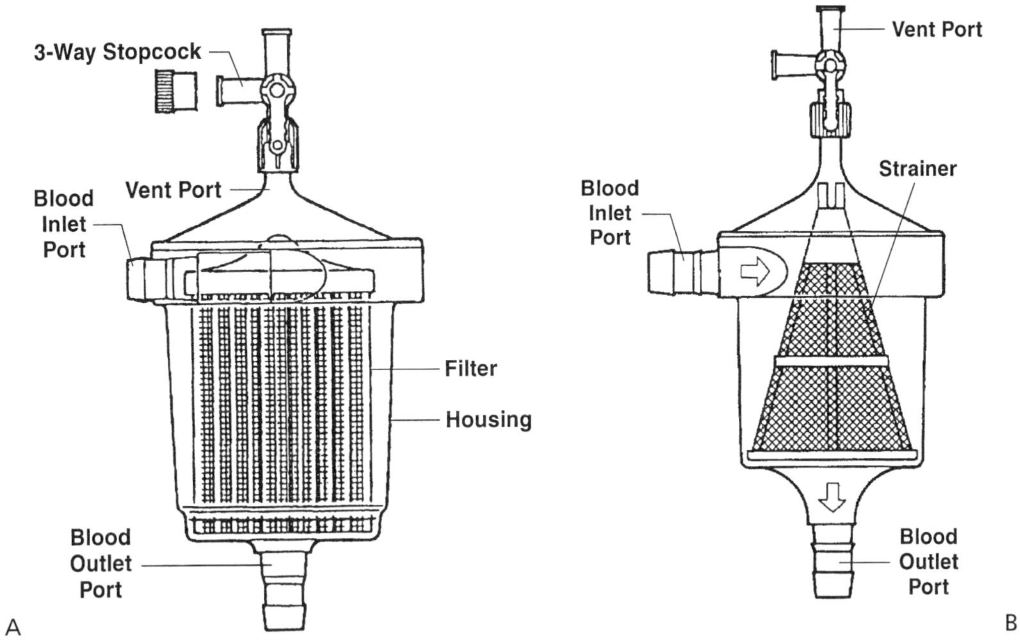

FIGURE 12-8. Arterial line filters and bubble traps. **(A)** A conventional adult arterial line microfilter and bubble trap. Blood enters tangentially at the top **(left)**, which encourages any possibly entrained bubbles to rise to the top, where they are vented out through a continuous purge line connecting the three-way stopcock to the cardiotomy or venous reservoir. Blood then passes through a screen microfilter (20 to 40 μm size), which also serves as a barrier to the passage of gaseous microemboli and out the bottom. **(B)** An arterial line bubble trap. The design and flow dynamics are similar to those of the arterial filter, but blood only passes through a coarse screen strainer (approximately 170 μm pore size). (From Gravlee GP, Davis RF, Kurusz M, eds. *Cardiopulmonary bypass: principles and practice,* 2nd ed. Philadelphia: Lippincott, Williams & Wilkins, 2000, with permission.)

their use. Micropore arterial filters (Fig. 12-8) are excellent gross bubble traps, and on this basis alone their routine use can probably be justified. However, if they are used for that purpose, they must (unless they are self-venting) have a continuously open purge line (including a one-way valve) that goes from the filter to the cardiotomy reservoir, to allow escape of trapped air, and a bypass safety line that goes around the filter and is usually clamped but can be opened in case the filter clogs.

Leukocyte-Depleting Filters

The use of leukocyte-depleting filters is receiving much attention. Activation of leukocytes is thought to be a major contributor to the inflammatory response to CPB and post-ischemic injury. Active removal of leukocytes and platelets with a separate cell separator throughout CPB seems to have beneficial clinical effects (225,226). However, the benefits of use of leukocyte-depleting filters are less clear. Animal studies have been encouraging (e.g., Lazar et al. [227]), but most clinical studies have failed to document significant leukocyte depletion or clinical benefits (e.g., Hurst et al. [228], Baksaas et al. [229]). Gu et al. (230) described significant leukocyte depletion (but without clinical benefits) from leukofiltration of part of the systemic venous drainage. On the other hand, Suzuki et al. (231) noted reduced cardiac enzyme levels when a leukocyte removal filter was used in the blood cardioplegia delivery circuit. Gu et al. (232) observed improved postoperative oxygenation with leukocyte filtration of residual pump blood, and Gott et al. (233) reported reduced length of stay and cost savings with aggressive use of multiple leukocyte filters (arterial line, cardioplegia line, autotransfused blood, and all blood product administration lines). However, this benefit was noted only in low-risk patients and despite the fact that no difference was observed in morbidity or mortality! Further research is required to define the role, if any, of leukocyte filtration during CPB (230).

CARDIOPLEGIA DELIVERY SYSTEMS

To provide a quiet surgical field and/or access to the aortic root for aortic valve surgery, the aorta is cross-clamped. This deprives the heart of its blood supply. In the past the resulting myocardial ischemia was ameliorated by topical hypothermia (with cold saline or ice slush or a coolant flow pad that was placed around the heart) or by continuous direct coronary perfusion. The latter technique has virtually been replaced by the administration of cardioplegia solutions. These solutions contain potassium and may be asanguineous or mixed with blood; they may be administered at very cold (4°C), "tepid" (28° to 35°C), or normothermia (35° to 37°C) temperatures. They may be administered either *antegrade* (i.e., into the aortic root, coronary ostia, or the proximal end of bypass grafts that have been sewn onto coronary arteries) or *retrograde* (i.e., into the coronary sinus). If cold cardioplegia is administered, it is often supplemented with topical hypothermia. The simplest cardioplegia system is an ice-cold bag of crystalloid cardioplegia solution placed under external pressure (150 to 300 mm Hg) often managed by the anesthesiologist. The bag is connected to a weighing scale to monitor volume administered. Care must be taken to avoid infusing air. However, most groups deliver cardioplegia from the heart-lung machine managed by the perfusionist.

Two general types of delivery systems are employed: recirculating and nonrecirculating (234). Both systems include a pump (usually roller), a heat exchanger (which may simply be a coil of plastic tubing in a water bath or a formal metal heat exchanger), a bubble trap, and a site for monitoring line pressure and temperature of the fluid going to the patient. With the *recirculating system,* the cardiplegia fluid (asanguineous crystalloid or mixed with oxygenated pump blood) is stored in a reservoir bag. One line goes from this bag through the pump and heat exchanger and to the surgical field and a switching device, where it may be directed either into the cardioplegia cannula (antegrade or retrograde) or to return back to the reservoir bag for recirculation. The *nonrecirculating system* lacks the recirculation line. When the nonrecirculating system is used to administer blood cardioplegia, often this is accomplished by running two lines of different caliber through a single roller pump. One line is connected to a source of oxygenated blood and the other to concentrated crystalloid cardioplegia. Based on the relative size of the tubing in the pump head, a ratio of blood and crystalloid (typically 4:1) is mixed and joined in a single tube before passing through the heat exchanger and to the patient. There are also commercially available dedicated, self-contained cardioplegia consoles that permit mixing of blood and crystalloid in variable ratios.

Antegrade Cardioplegia

Antegrade cardioplegia is usually administered through a cannula placed in the aortic root proximal to the aortic cross-clamp (and the arterial inflow cannula). These cannulas are often Y-shaped, with one end connected to the source of cardioplegia solution and the other to suction for venting the left ventricle out the aortic root when antegrade cardioplegia is not being administered. Some of these cannulas possess a third lumen for measuring aortic root pressure during cardioplegia administration. This is desirable because the size of the cardioplegia cannula is usually small (12 to 18 gauge) so that a considerable gradient exists between the cardioplegia line pressure and the aortic root; yet it is important to maintain an adequate but not excessive pressure (60 to 100 mm Hg) in the aortic root during cardioplegia administration to ensure adequate perfusion of the myocardium, especially in the presence of coronary artery disease. In the absence of a perfusion monitoring port, surgeons often palpate the aortic root to assess the pressure. It is also important to watch for left ventricular distention during administration of antegrade cardioplegia. In the presence of significant aortic regurgitation or when the aorta root must be opened for aortic valve or intraventricular surgery, antegrade cardioplegia must be given by inserting (sometimes handheld) cannulas directly into the coronary artery orifices through the aortotomy. These cannulas come in various sizes and should fit snugly in the coronary ostia to avoid significant back-leak. Care must be taken not to injure the coronary artery or to insert the catheter in too far (thereby failing to perfuse critical branches). This is more likely with perfusion of the left main coronary artery in the presence of left dominance, because the left main is shorter in this circumstance.

Retrograde Cardioplegia

Retrograde cardioplegia is administered into the coronary sinus (235). Frequency of use varies among surgical teams. It may be particularly desirable in the presence of severe proximal coronary artery disease that may impair antegrade distribution, when aortic regurgitation negates antegrade administration, while the aortic root is open (as for aortic valve surgery), and in repeat coronary operations (to limit or wash out atheroemboli from vein grafts). Many groups use both antegrade and retrograde methods in the same patient (236). Special cannulas are designed for administering retrograde cardioplegia. All have an extra port near the tip for monitoring coronary sinus pressure and a cuff or balloon to prevent back-leakage. Some cuffs require manual inflation, and some autoinflate with infusion of the cardioplegic solution. The cannula may be inserted blindly through an atrial pursestring, which may be aided by intraatrial palpation with a finger passed through a separate atrial pursestring or by the use of TEE (237). It is often easier to insert the retrograde cardioplegia cannula before the atrial cannulas are inserted and CPB has begun, but the patient may not tolerate this in terms of hemodynamics or rhythm. When the cannula is inserted during CPB, there may be problems with air entrainment and subsequent air lock. Special care must be taken not to insert the cannula too far into the coronary sinus (which would prevent the perfusion of proximal tributaries and hence adequate delivery to the right ventricle). Clements et al. (238) reviewed the anatomy and variability of the cardiac venous system, which helps explain some of the limitations associated with retrograde cardioplegia. The same cardioplegic delivery systems are employed as for antegrade cardioplegia. Coronary sinus pressure should be monitored during infusion, and pressures lower than 30 mm Hg or higher than 40 to 50 mm Hg should be avoided (239). Optimal flow is probably between 200 and 400 mL/minute (240). In the presence of a PLSVC, retrograde coronary sinus cardioplegia may still be administered by intermittent occlusion of the left SVC with a tourniquet and application of external finger pressure at the junction of the IVC and right atrium to occlude the coronary sinus ostium during administration of cardioplegia (28). Rupture, perforation, and hematoma have been observed during retrograde coronary sinus cardioplegia, usually during insertion or manipulation of the catheter (239). Although retrograde delivery may provide superior cardioplegia distributions to the left ventricle in the presence of coronary artery disease, it may provide less optimal protection of the right ventricle (236,238).

When first inducing cardioplegia, one should watch for prompt cooling and electrical arrest of the heart. Often this effect is slower with retrograde than antegrade administration. When cooling or arrest is delayed with antegrade administration, one should consider inadequate flow or pressure, aortic regurgitation, incomplete occlusion by the aortic cross-clamp, malposition of the cannula, or error in temperature or composition of the cardioplegia solution. When induction is slower than expected with retrograde delivery, one should consider, in addition, malposition of the cannula (too deep, too shallow, or not in the coronary sinus), leak around the cuff (especially if the coronary sinus is large), a PLSVC, or a coronary sinus-left atrial fenestration.

VENTING OF THE HEART

The right side of the heart is normally drained or vented by the venous cannulas. The relative efficiencies of various types of venous lines in venting the right heart has been studied by Arom et al. (11) and Bennett et al. (12,13) and was summarized earlier (see Venous Cannulation and Drainage and Table 12-1). When bicaval cannulation with caval tourniquets is used, venting of the right heart is not provided, and if the right ventricle is not able to eject, the right heart must be vented by a cannula, by cardiotomy suction, or by opening it to drain into the pericardial sac. The rest of this discussion pertains to venting of the left ventricle.

Purpose

The purpose of left ventricular venting is to prevent distention of the ventricle, reduce myocardial rewarming, prevent ejection of air, facilitate surgical exposure (e.g., when working on aortic valve), and facilitate recovery of the ventricle from a period of ischemia. Preventing distention of the left ventricle is desirable to prevent mechanical damage to the muscle from excessive stretching; to improve myocardial preservation by decreasing myocardial oxygen demand (wall tension decreased as a result of decreased radius of ventricle); to facilitate subendocardial perfusion (subendocardial perfusion pressure equals aortic pressure minus left ventricular pressure); and to prevent pulmonary venous hypertension, with possible pulmonary injury or edema, and pulmonary artery hypertension with right ventricular dysfunction.

Sources of Blood Returning to the Left Heart

The normal sources of blood returning to the left side of the heart during CPB include blood returning to the right heart that gets past the systemic venous cannulas and passes through the pulmonary circulation, bronchial veins, and thebesian veins. Abnormal sources include a PLSVC (see previous discussion), patent ductus arteriosus (PDA), or systemic-to-pulmonary artery shunt (e.g., Blalock-Taussig, Waterston); atrial septal defect; ventricular septal defect; anomalous systemic venous drainage into the left side of the heart; and aortic regurgitation. Even if it is not present preoperatively, *aortic regurgitation* commonly occurs when cold cardioplegia is administered into the aortic root and from distortion of the aortic root with other surgical manipulations. Even hemodynamically mild aortic regurgitation (e.g., 1 L/minute) becomes catastrophic when the heart fibrillates during CPB (yielding continuous aortic regurgitation without the ability of the left ventricle to empty itself). The *bronchial blood flow* to the periphery of lung normally drains with the pulmonary veins. On CPB, this drainage averages about 140 ± 182 mL/minute (241) and the amount is influenced by the mean arterial pressure (which is one rationale for maintaining low perfusion pressures during CPB). Patients with chronic lung infections or inflammatory lung disease (e.g., bronchiectasis) and those with cyanotic congenital heart disease have exaggerated bronchial blood flow. Coronary sinus flow into the right side of the heart should greatly diminish with aortic cross-clamping, except for noncoronary collateral flow (average, 48 ± 74 mL/minute [241]), when antegrade cardioplegia is administered, and in the presence of a PLSVC. Most coronary sinus blood should be removed if the venous cannulas are working properly (unless bicaval cannulas with caval tourniquets are employed). When excessive return of blood in the left side of the heart is encountered, improper function or placement of the venous cannulas, a PLSVC, a PDA, or aortic regurgitation should be suspected. Unsuspected PDA has been discovered in about 1 of every 3,500 coronary artery bypass operations (242) and in 1 of 1,750 adults undergoing echocardiography for other reasons (243). PDA may be detected during baseline intraoperative TEE (244).

Monitoring for Left Ventricular Distention

Monitoring for left ventricular distention is multimodal and includes inspection and palpation, observation of pulmonary artery or left atrial pressure, and TEE. *Inspection and palpation of the heart* is the most common and simplest method, but it requires the constant attention of the surgical team, which often is directing its attention elsewhere. Furthermore, moderate distention of the left ventricle may not be easy to detect because of its posterior location, often covered by blood, fluid, or ice, and because its thick walls make it difficult to assess. One advantage of a *pulmonary artery catheter* is that it can provide an indication of left atrial hypertension that accompanies left heart distention. It may be somewhat late in rising if the cause of left heart distention is aortic regurgitation, and it is rendered invalid by a pulmonary artery vent (see later discussion). The pulmonary artery pressure may become falsely elevated if the tip of the pulmonary artery catheter becomes wedged against a wall or if the pulmonary artery catheter is caught in an aortic cross-clamp or SVC tourniquet; therefore, a high reading should be confirmed by palpation of the pulmonary artery or left ventricle. If a *left atrial line* is placed early in the course of CPB, it can provide an early warning of left heart distention; however, these lines are rarely used currently. TEE is a helpful monitor of left heart distention during CPB. The transgastric short-axis view is optimal but can be obscured if a sponge or pad is placed behind the left ventricle (to aid exposure or to protect the phrenic nerve from ice and the heart from warming), in which case the transatrial views may still be used.

Particular attention should be paid to looking for evidence of left heart distention when CPB is first instituted,

TABLE 12-6. METHODS OF VENTING THE LEFT VENTRICLE

Method	Advantages	Disadvantages
Ascending aortic (cardioplegia cannula)	Simple; no additional cannula Also vents air when aorta unclamped and when LV starts to eject Can be used to monitor aortic root infusion pressure	Works only when aorta is cross-clamped Does not work during administration of antegrade cardioplegia Can cause air to be aspirated into the aortic root
Indirect LV (via stab wound in RSPV, through LA and MV)	Handles all sources of blood causing LV distention Best for aortic regurgitation Provides optimal decompression of LV Avoids problems of direct LV vent	Somewhat difficult exposure of insertion site May be difficult to thread cannula into LV and position correctly Risk of bleeding and tears at insertion site in RSPV Potential for air entry into left heart Potential problem if mechanical prosthesis in MV Potential embolism if tumor or clots in LA or LV
Direct LV (through stab wound in apex)	Direct and simple Avoids going across prosthetic MV Handles all sources of blood causing LV distention	Positioning may be a problem—tip becomes easily obstructed by LV wall or MV apparatus Risk of damage to LV and injury to coronary arteries and collaterals (myocardial ischemia) May be difficult to control bleeding from stab wound Late LV aneurysm Potential embolism if clots in LV Potential for air entry into the left heart
Direct LA (via LA appendage, roof of LA, or RSPV)	Relatively simple Avoids going across the MV	Does not handle AR Potential embolism if clots in LA Potential for air entry into the left heart
Pulmonary artery	Simple Less risk of admitting air into the left heart	Does not handle AR. Renders use of PA pressure as a monitor of LV distention invalid Risk of damage and bleeding from pulmonary artery

Note: AR, aortic regurgitation; LA, left atrium; LV, left ventricle; MV, mitral valve; PA, pulmonary artery; RSPV, right superior pulmonary vein.

if the heart fibrillates, when the aorta is cross-clamped, whenever antegrade cardioplegia is administered, and when the aortic cross-clamp is released (the left ventricle is usually asystolic and hence unable to empty itself of any blood returning to it).

Indications for Venting of the Left Heart

Venting of the left heart is indicated whenever the left ventricle is unable to handle the amount of blood returning to it. There is considerable debate about the need to vent the left heart during cardiac surgery, especially in the era of cold cardioplegia, and during coronary artery surgery (16,245–248). Excellent results have been reported without venting in aortic (249) and coronary artery surgery (250). On the other hand, experimental studies suggest that optimal myocardial recovery after an ischemic insult is best provided by full CPB and venting of the left ventricle (251). Otherwise, myocardial oxygen demand may be considerable, even though the left ventricular diastolic pressure is low and the heart is not ejecting (251). Left ventricular venting during reperfusion may be warranted in hearts with limited reserve and in those that have been incompletely revascularized or have sustained a particularly severe ischemic insult. Olinger and Bonchek (252) found better left ventricular performance immediately after coronary artery surgery when a vent was used.

Methods of Venting the Left Ventricle

Methods of venting the heart are summarized in Table 12-6 and described in Fig. 12-9. During coronary artery surgery, either no venting or *venting out the cardioplegia cannula** in the aortic root (253) is the most common practice (Fig. 12-9A). One of the limits of aortic root venting is that it cannot function while cardioplegia is being administered, and if there is any aortic regurgitation or excessive blood return to the left heart it may be necessary to intermittently interrupt the administration of cardioplegia and suck on the vent with or without external compression of the left ventricle. When direct venting of the left ventricle is desired, it is most commonly accomplished by *inserting a catheter through a pursestring placed in the junction of the right superior pulmonary vein and the left atrium* and advancing the catheter across the mitral valve into the left ventricle (Fig. 12-9B). Today, vents are rarely placed directly through the *apex of the left ventricle* (Fig. 12-9C). This approach has been largely abandoned owing to risk of hemorrhage and myocardial

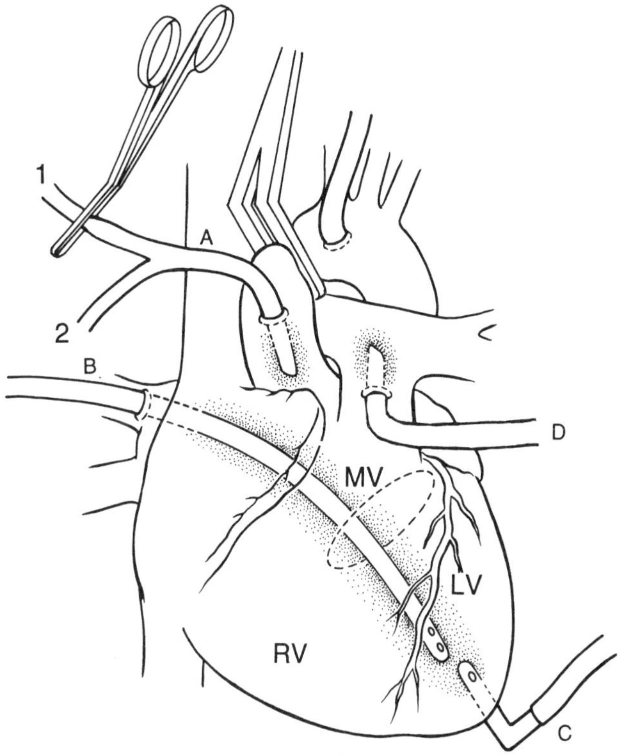

FIGURE 12-9. Sites for venting the left ventricle. *(A)* Aortic root cannula; one limb of Y *(1)* is connected to the cardioplegia administration system; other limb *(2)* is connected to suction for venting of the left heart. *(B)* Cannula is inserted at junction of right superior pulmonary vein and left atrium and threaded through left atrium and mitral valve into the left ventricle. *(C)* The cannula is inserted directly into apex of left ventricle. *(D)* The cannula is inserted into the pulmonary artery. (Modified from Bensley FA Jr, Martin DE, eds. *The practice of cardiac anesthesia.* Boston: Little, Brown, 1990:637, with permission.)

injury. Some surgeons insert vents *into the left atrium only.* Others vent via the *pulmonary artery* (Fig. 12-9D) (246,254), thereby minimizing some of the risks of direct left heart venting, but the results are variable. Pulmonary artery venting may not prevent left ventricular distention in the presence of aortic regurgitation if the mitral valve is competent (255).

These vents are then attached to a suction device (roller pump or regulated wall suction), and the blood is returned to the cardiotomy reservoir. When the tip of the vent is in the ventricle, the degree of suction must be constantly adjusted to avoid excessive suction (with resultant collapse and trauma to the ventricle and risk of air aspiration) or inadequate suction (with overdistention). For this reason, some teams employ gravity (siphon) drainage instead of suction. This technique requires that the drainage reservoir be located well below the patient; it may not provide adequate drainage if large volumes of blood are returning to the left side of the heart, and it will not work when the left heart is open because air interrupts the siphon effect. Some split

* Special cardioplegia cannulas are available with a Y-arm, which may be connected to suction when cardioplegia is not being administered through the main arm of the cannula. Other antegrade cardioplegia cannulas have a third lumen, which permits monitoring of aortic root pressure while cardioplegia is being administered.

the line coming from the ventricular vent so that either gravity or suction drainage can be used. Another method of applying suction to these vents is to connect them via a Y-connector to the systemic venous line (256,257). This provides automatic gravity (siphon) or venturi suction of about 18 to 35 mm Hg without generating excessive suction or need for extra pumps, but it does increase the risk of getting air into the venous lines.

Complications of Left Heart Venting

Complications include introduction of air into the left heart and subsequent systemic air embolism. This is most likely to occur at the time of insertion or removal if the left heart volume is low. To minimize this risk, the heart is usually allowed to fill before insertion, and the vents are often removed while the insertion site is covered with fluid. Excessive suction is another source of air. This air may be sucked in from around pursestring sutures in the left atrium or aorta or retrograde out of open coronary arteries during coronary artery surgery (258). Even pulmonary artery vents may suck air into the left heart and pulmonary veins (personal observation by the author, using TEE). Finally, erroneous function of the suction apparatus (positive pressure in reservoir, misdirection of tubing into roller pump head, reversal of roller pump) may cause air to be pumped into the ventricle. Use of a one-way valve in the left ventricular vent line is advocated by some to prevent this complication, although a valve inserted backwards will prevent adequate venting as well. Most surgeons test the function of the vent line (to enssure that it aspirates fluid) before attaching it to the heart. Other risks are bleeding and damage to the heart, including late left ventricular aneurysms (259).

Significant blood return through a left heart vent (from aortic regurgitation or bronchial blood flow) reduces the amount of systemic tissue perfusion and should be compensated for by increasing the arterial pump flow rate by an equivalent amount.

Aortic Root Air Venting

Any time the left side of the heart is entered, even simply by placing a catheter in a chamber, air may collect in the heart and, if not removed, will embolize. Right heart air may pass into the left heart via septal defects or even through the lungs. In addition to vigorous attempts at removal of all air before the left heart is closed, the use of left heart vents, and repeated aspirations of left-sided chambers, venting of the highest point of the aorta is considered the "final safety valve" against systemic air embolism (260). Brenner et al. (261) analyzed the physical principles relevant to efficiency of aortic root air vents and studied various systems in an *in vitro* model. They found that a freely bleeding stab wound containing a nonconstricted fenestrated 10F plastic catheter connected to suction was most efficient (97%). A freely bleeding stab wound was almost as efficient (91%), but insertion of a catheter, not connected to suction, into the stab wound decreased its efficiency to 79%. Freely bleeding needles and catheter vents not connected to suction were very inefficient (20% to 36%), but efficiency was improved (to about 90%) by the application of suction. Marco and Barner (260) demonstrated that larger vent needle area and a greater flow out of the vent (suction) are associated with greater efficiency. There are obvious limits to this approach, including loss of forward flow and hemolysis. Gundry (262) advocated infusing blood into the left ventricular vent (using the blood in the cardioplegic circuit) to facilitate de-airing out of the aortic root before unclamping of the aorta. Verification of the need for and effectiveness of various de-airing techniques can be accomplished by use of TEE.

HEMOCONCENTRATORS (HEMOFILTRATION, ULTRAFILTRATION)

Hemofiltration

Hemoconcentrators contain semipermeable membranes (typically hollow fibers) that permit passage of water and electrolytes out of the blood. They are used *in lieu* of diuretics to remove excessive fluid or electrolytes (e.g, potassium) and to raise the hematocrit. They may also exert beneficial effects by removal of inflammatory mediators (263). They can be connected to the extracorporeal circuit in several different configurations. Blood may be drawn from the venous line, the arterial or venous reservoir, or the arterial line (sometimes from the air purge vent of the micropore filter), and filtered blood may be returned to the venous line or to the cardiotomy or venous reservoir. Except when blood is taken from a high-pressure port (e.g., arterial line), a pump must be used to drive blood through the device, and one may be used to control flow even if blood comes from the arterial line. Pressure is generated within the blood channels by resistance to flow through the capillaries or by a partially occluding clamp downstream. Suction may or may not be applied to the air side of the membrane to facilitate filtration. Fluid removal can be as great as 180 mL/minute (at a 500 mL/minute flow) (264). Various types of membranes are used. Molecules with molecular weights up to 20,000 Da are removed. Despotis et al. (265) found that hemofiltration did not remove an appreciable amount of low-molecular-weight heparin and in fact concentrated the heparin and resulted in an increase in heparin activity. This effect could vary with differing types of hemofilters, and therefore the adequacy of heparinizaton should be monitored. Hematocrit should not be raised until the start of rewarming. The hemofilter can be used after CPB to concentrate the pump blood before it is given back to the patient. Advantages of using hemofilters compared with centrifugal cell washers (e.g., Cell Saver) is that they conserve platelets, albumin (colloid osmotic pressure), and coagulation factors (264), and they may be cheaper.

Potential adverse consequences (besides cost) are additional entrance into the circuit, potential for complement activation, retention of free hemoglobin and proteolytic enzymes (e.g., polymorphonuclear elastase), loss of heparin, and excessive rise in hematocrit. However, no adverse effects were encountered by Boldt et al. (264). They compared six different hemofiltration devices with the Cell Saver and identified some significant differences. Compared with diuretics, hemofiltrators are more easily controlled and do not cause excessive potassium losses (266).

Modified Ultrafiltration

The term "modified ultrafiltration" (MUF) refers to a practice of withdrawing blood out of the patient (usually from the arterial cannula) *after weaning from bypass,* passing it through a hemofilter, and pumping it back into the patient via the venous cannulas. It is mainly used in pediatric cases. It has been shown to be effective in reducing total body water; raising hematocrit; removing inflammatory mediators; reducing bleeding; improving hemodynamics, ventricular function, and cerebral and pulmonary recovery; and reducing postoperative morbidity and convalescence (267,268). In a survey conducted in 1996, about 44% of pediatric cardiac surgery programs in North America used MUF (269). About 41% used it on all pediatric cases, while 45% based its use on the patient's weight (about one half of these chose a weight of less than 10 or 15 kg). In most centers, the arteriovenous MUF configuration is used. (Venovenous MUF is also used [268] and carries less risk of air cavitation and hemodynamic instability, but it may be associated with recirculation of filtered blood and does not deliver oxygenated blood to the pulmonary vasculature.) Many groups use the blood cardioplegia system as the MUF circuit, removing the crystalloid cardioplegia tubing from the cardioplegia roller head, flushing the cardioplegia solution out with CPB circuit blood, and inserting a primed hemoconcentrator distal to the blood cardioplegia pump and proximal to the blood cardioplegia system (270). The advantage of using this system is that it includes a roller pump, bubble trap, heat exchanger, and line pressure monitor and is already connected to the arterial line. It does carry the risk of accidental infusion of cardioplegia if not adequately flushed. Other methods of setting up MUF circuits have been described (269,271–273).

In the aforementioned survey (269), technical complications were encountered by 84% of the centers and included air cavitation, patient cooling, circuit disruption, unintended infusion of cardioplegia solution, clotted circuit, and transient exsanguination. Because blood is typically aspirated from the arterial cannula by the MUF pump, air cavitation and air aspiration (from around the arterial cannulation site or through the membrane oxygenator) may occur if excessive negative pressure develops. Because of the risk of air entering the arterial circuit, antegrade flow should not be permitted once MUF has begun. For this reason, the arterial pump flow rate (which may be used to add volume from the pump oxygenator to the MUF circuit) should never exceed the MUF pump flow rate. Strategies to reduce air entry and cavitation in the arterial line (caused by developing negative pressure) include extravigilant monitoring of the arterial line pressure (sometimes by the use of an additional perfusionist), use of pressure servoregulation to stop the MUF pump if negative pressure develops in the arterial line, bypass of the arterial line filter, and having the surgeon maintain optimal aortic cannula position. Other safety measures include use of a bubble trap and bubble detector, inversion of the hemoconcentrator (so that blood enters the top), and monitoring of the pressure in the MUF return line beyond the MUF pump (with or without positive pressure servoregulation of the MUF pump).

PRIMING

Adult extracorporeal circuits have priming volumes of about 1,500 to 2,000 mL (e.g., about 25 mL/kg in a 70-kg patient or approximately 35% of the patient's blood volume). In the early days, whole blood was used to prime the pump, and the conversion to use of asanguineous primes is considered a major reason for the reduced morbidity associated with CPB. The use of asanguineous prime results in a reduction in the hematocrit that has both favorable and unfavorable features. As in other clinical situations, the safe lower limit—not to mention the optimal hematocrit during CPB—is debated and unknown. Many advocate hematocrit values of 20% to 25% for moderate (25° to 32°C) hypothermia. (Viscosity remains approximately stable when the hematocrit, expressed in percent, equals the temperature expressed in degrees Celsius.) Mixed venous oxygen concentration has been advocated as a useful clue to the adequacy of hematocrit (in conjunction with pump flow) (274–276). Higher flows and/or hematocrit are required during rewarming. If the prime volume is 1,750 mL, for a 70-kg subject, the baseline hematocrit must be at least 27% to maintain a hematocrit of 20%; for a 50-kg subject, the critical baseline hematocrit is 30%. These calculations discount any added crystalloid cardioplegia solution, which would cause further hemodilution.

To minimize to effect of asanguineous primes, effort is being directed to reducing the prime volume: use of smaller and shorter venous lines (facilitated by bringing the heart-lung machine closer to the operating table and raising the level of the venous reservoir, which in turn is made possible by the use of augmented venous return, discussed earlier) is one approach. Tolerating lower levels in the venous reservoir is another approach (but with the hazards discussed previous, which perhaps can be minimized by the use of collapsible venous reservoirs and low-level and bubble sensors that turn off the arterial pump). Others practice displacing much of the prime with the patient's venous blood when CPB is first instituted, discarding the asanguineous blood before commencing arterial infusion (so-called autologous priming techniques). This requires careful monitoring of the patient's hemodynamic status when beginning CPB.

As substitutes for blood prime, most groups use various balanced electrolyte solutions (e.g., lactated Ringer's solution, Normosol-A, Plasma-Lyte). There is little scientifically valid evidence favoring one over another. The absence of calcium has raised concern, whereas, if calcium is present, most groups add heparin to any units of banked blood that are added to the prime to reduce the risk of clot formation (1,000 units of heparin per 1 unit of packed red blood cells; 2,000 units of heparin per 1 unit of whole blood). Many groups add heparin to the prime (typically 2,500 units per 1,000 mL of prime) in any case, to minimize the risk of thrombosis if patient anticoagulation is imperfect. Many also add mannitol to the prime (12.5 to 50 g) to ensure brisk diuresis and to minimize the risk of renal injury during CPB. Although there are theoretic rationales for this practice, there are no valid studies proving its benefit or effectiveness. Controversy exists regarding the need for colloids (277). Use of colloids clearly better maintains colloid osmotic pressure during CPB (it falls by about 50% if no colloid is used) and is associated with less fluid loss into the patient during CPB. At issue is whether the addition of colloids influences outcome. Current evidence suggests that they do no harm but that their use does not improve clinical outcome (278). McKnight et al. (279) found no influence of prime composition on postoperative nitrogen balance. Kongsgaard et al. (280) found that use of dextran 70 did not influence the changes in plasma protease systems, whereas Bosner et al. (281) reported that the use of polygeline reduced complement activation. Controversy also surrounds the use of glucose solutions in the prime. McKnight et al. (282) noted that the presence of glucose and/or lactate in the prime resulted in very high levels of these substances, which may have adverse consequences. Many now recommend avoiding glucose because of possible adverse neurologic effects (283), but others have expressed skepticism (284).

SPECIAL TOPICS

Unusual Cannulations

Most CPB procedures are conducted with the heart approached through a median sternotomy, which provides excellent exposure for venous and arterial cannulation. Approaching the heart through a right or left thoracotomy or through a limited sternotomy (limited to the upper or lower portion), or initiating CPB before or without ever exposing the heart, presents special cannulation problems. These alternative approaches may be used to avoid sternotomy because of prior sternotomy, especially if complicated by prior infection or aneurysms of the ascending aorta or right ventricle, and to avoid patent coronary grafts that might pass beneath the sternum (e.g., right internal mammary artery to left coronary circulation); for focused access to specific coronary arteries (e.g., right coronary artery or circumflex [285]); for surgery involving the descending aorta; and when one wishes to support the heart on CPB before entering the chest (e.g., severe cardiac failure or problems anticipated or encountered during attempted reentry [10]). These alternative approaches are also being used for minimal-access (minimally invasive) cardiac surgery (see later discussion).

Cannulation through Right Thoracotomy

This approach poses little problem with venous (atrial) cannulation but provides poor access to the ascending aorta and no access to the left ventricle. Peters et al. (20) evaluated various options for bicaval cannulation during minimal-access right thoracotomies. Aortic cannulation and cross-clamping can be difficult, as is de-airing the left ventricle. Arterial cannulation may be more conveniently accomplished using the femoral or axillary artery (see earlier discussion). Femoral-femoral bypass with deep hypothermia has been advocated by others (286). Placing external defibrillator pads on the left chest (front and back over the heart) may facilitate defibrillation if needed.

Cannulation through Left Thoracotomy

One can conduct partial or complete left heart bypass and partial or complete heart-lung bypass through the left chest.

Left Heart Bypass

Left heart bypass (i.e., left atrium to aorta without oxygenator) relies on the right side of the patient's heart to pump blood through the lungs to the left heart and on the lungs to provide gas exchange. Blood is usually removed from the left heart with a large venous cannula placed directly into the left atrium (via the atrial appendage or the left upper pulmonary vein at its junction with the left atrium). This carries a risk of systemic air embolism if one is not careful during insertion and removal of this cannula (the left heart should be well filled and ventilation should be interrupted during these procedures). Also, if excessive suction is applied to the venous line, especially if the atrial pursestring is not secure, air can be entrained into the left heart and into the venous cannula (and subsequently pumped into the systemic arterial system). Another problem is that improper positioning or movement of the tip of the left atrial cannula can impair drainage of the left heart and flow into the left heart bypass circuit. Another way of draining blood from the left heart is by placing a cannula into the apex of the left ventricle. This method may provide excellent flow of blood into the left heart bypass circuit, but it adds the risks of injury to the left ventricle, bleeding, and late aneurysm formation. Arterial return may be into the descending aorta or femoral artery (usually the left, since patient is in the right lateral decubitus position). The extracorporeal circuit typically consists only of tubing and a centrifugal pump and does not include a reservoir, heat exchanger, or bubble trap. This minimizes the need for heparinization but precludes the ability to add or sequester fluid, adjust temperature, or prevent systemic air embolization. The anesthesiologist must be prepared to administer intravascular volume expanders as needed through other sites of vascular access. Some have advocated including a heat exchanger in the circuit to restore normothermia (287).

Partial Left Heart Bypass

Partial left heart bypass is used to facilitate surgery on the descending thoracic aorta. The patient's left ventricle supplies blood to the aorta proximal to the clamps, and the left heart bypass circuit supplies blood to the body distal to the clamps. Typically about two-thirds normal basal cardiac output (i.e., two thirds of 2.4 L/minute/m^2, or 1.6 L/minute/m^2) is pumped to the lower body, and the remainder is pumped by the left ventricle to the upper body. Arterial pressure should be measured in the proximal (right radial or brachial) artery and the distal aorta (right femoral artery) to assess adequacy of flow to each part of the body, and the central venous pressure and pulmonary artery diastolic or occlusion pressure should be monitored to assess filling of the two ventricles. Use of TEE is particularly helpful in assessing filling and function of the left heart and left atrial cannula placement and function. If arterial pressure is too high proximally and too low distally, more blood should be pumped by the left heart bypass. Conversely, if arterial pressure is too low proximally and too high distally, less blood should be pumped by the left heart bypass. If both pressures are low, blood volume, and possibly a vasoconstrictor, may need to be added. If both pressures are high, more anesthesia and possibly a vasodilator should be added (see Table 5 on Hemodynamic Management During Femoral-Femoral Bypass in O'Connor and Rothenberg's review [288] for a more extensive outline). Although left heart bypass should eliminate the need for an oxygenator during descending thoracic aortic surgery (leading to less heparinization and cost), some critically ill or traumatized patients have such severe pulmonary shunting and hypoxemia that inclusion of an oxygenator would be beneficial.

Full Left Heart Bypass

Full left heart bypass may be employed for left-sided coronary artery surgery using the cannulation techniques described previously, by draining all of the pulmonary venous return out of the left atrium, leaving no blood for the left ventricle to eject. If the heart fibrillates, blood can still passively pass through the right heart and lungs, but often an elevated central venous pressure is required.

Partial Cardiopulmonary Bypass

The technique of partial CPB (i.e., systemic veins to aorta with oxygenator) is also used to facilitate descending aortic surgery. The major issue is how to obtain systemic venous drainage. Several options are available, including drainage through the pulmonary artery (with the tip left in the main pulmonary artery or threaded retrograde into the right ventricle [289]), through the right ventricular outflow tract, directly into the right atrium through the right atrial appendage, or via the femoral vein. The problem with the last method is achieving adequate venous drainage through long, small catheters; this is usually solved by the use of thin-walled cannulas threaded up into the right atrium (proper positioning facilitated by TEE), with or without use of augmented venous return (see earlier discussion). Direct cannulation of the right atrium is quite different, with risk of compression of the heart, tearing of the atrium, and bleeding. Cannulation of the pulmonary artery is somewhat easier. The extracorporeal circuit resembles that previously described for full CPB. In addition to the pump or pumps, it includes a reservoir, oxygenator, heat exchanger, and bubble trap. The left ventricle is still the source of blood supply to the upper part of the body and the heart, and the patient's own lungs are providing gas exchange for that blood. Therefore, the principles of relative flows to lower and upper parts of the body, described for left heart bypass, apply here. Furthermore, the adequacy of gas exchange of blood going to the upper body must be assessed separately (via the radial or brachial artery) from that coming out of the extracorporeal oxygenator and going to the lower body.

Full Cardiopulmonary Bypass

With full CPB, the only difference from what has just been discussed is that virtually all of the systemic venous return must be drained from the right heart, which accentuates the demand on venous cannulation and drainage. All systemic flow and gas exchange is supplied by the heart-lung machine. Ascending aortic cross-clamping and administration of antegrade cardioplegia can be problematic. Sasaguri et al. (290) have described a special double-lumen balloon catheter (Model 10F-60, Ideas for Medicine, Inc, St. Petersburg, FL) that is inserted through the left ventricular apex into the ascending aorta with TEE guidance for occlusion of the ascending aorta and administration of cardioplegia during thoracic aortic surgery via a left thoracotomy.

Femoral Vein to Femoral Artery Bypass

Femoral vein to femoral artery bypass is used to initiate bypass outside the operating room (as for supportive angioplasty [291] or circulatory assistance) or in the operating room for hemodynamically deteriorating patients or during reoperations—especially if bleeding is encountered during reentry (10); for aortic surgery; during some pulmonary surgeries (e.g., lung transplantation, upper airway reconstruction); and to induce (e.g., for neurosurgery) or treat accidental hypothermia. The principles of femoral cannulation for venous drainage and arterial return have been reviewed in earlier sections.

Femoral vein to femoral artery bypass requires inclusion of an oxygenator, but heparin requirements may be reduced by employing an HBC (292). When the technique is used to augment oxygenation, one must recognize the effect of femoral flow rate (expressed as a percentage of total body flow) on how far proximally in the aorta the oxygenated blood extends (293). When it is used to unload the left ventricle and reduce myocardial oxygen demand, near-full bypass may be required. When it is used for descending thoracic aortic surgery, the flow permitted through the lungs, which supplies the heart and upper portion of body, and that removed for pumping to the lower portion of the body must be carefully balanced (see earlier discussion).

Cannulation for Minimally Invasive (Limited-Access) Surgery

Minimally invasive cardiac surgery includes that done off-bypass (including MID-CAB and OP-CAB) and that done on bypass but via smaller incisions (e.g., partial sternotomy, small anterior thoracic incisions). The former avoid the needs and complications of CPB, but the latter complicates cannulation for CPB (31,294). Some of the cannulation options have just been discussed. In some cases, central cannulation of the aorta and atrium or systemic veins is accomplished with the use of smaller cannulas placed through the operative incision or through separate smaller incisions in the chest wall. The use of smaller arterial lines increases the risk of complications from high-velocity jets and affects pressure gradients. The use of the Soft-Flow arterial cannula tip may minimize some of these potential hazards (40). The problems of achieving adequate venous drainage with smaller venous cannulas are overcome by use of augmented venous return (see earlier discussion). Use of wire-reinforced cannulas, special angled venous cannulas, and flattened-contour venous cannulas, discussed previously, also contributes to solving cannulation problems through small chest incisions. An alternative approach is the use of peripheral (jugular or femoral vein and subclavian or femoral artery) cannulation, which have been discussed earlier.

The most sophisticated and complex system for providing peripheral cannulation–based CPB for minimal-access cardiac surgery (coronary and valve procedures) is the commercial Port Access System (Heartport) (90,295). This system permits total CPB, proximal aortic occlusion, and antegrade and retrograde cardioplegia administration. It features a transcutaneously placed (internal jugular vein) coronary sinus catheter (for administering retrograde cardioplegia, and which includes a balloon inflation port and a pressure monitoring port); a pulmonary artery drainage cannula (also introduced via an internal jugular puncture); a venous drainage cannula that is threaded into the right atrium from the femoral vein; and a femoral arterial perfusion cannula through which another multiorifice catheter is passed retrograde into the ascending aorta. This last catheter includes an inflatable balloon designed to occlude the ascending aorta *in lieu* of an aortic cross-clamp ("endoaortic clamp"), as well as a lumen through which antegrade cardioplegia is delivered out the tip and another lumen for monitoring pressure in the proximal aorta during cardioplegia delivery. Successful application of this technique requires special training and unique cooperation among the cardiac surgeon, anesthesiologist, and perfusionist. Fluoroscopy and TEE are essential additional monitoring and imaging techniques. Port Access surgery is associated with many potential complications, including perforation of cardiac structures, retrograde aortic dissection, incomplete de-airing, systemic air embolism, and malposition of the endoaortic clamp. The clamp can prolapse through the aortic valve into the left ventricle or move distally, occluding arch vessels with subsequent cerebral ischemia. Monitoring methods (in addition to TEE and fluoroscopy) that have been advocated to ensure proper positioning and to detect this complication include monitoring of pressure in both radial arteries, transcranial Doppler, cerebral oximetry (near-infrared spectroscopy), and EEG (296).

Retained intracardiac air and subsequent systemic air embolization is a risk with all minimal-access surgery because of limited access to the cardiac structures for de-airing and because the left ventricular apex can not be reached for needle aspiration. Many advocate flooding the operative field with carbon dioxide (5 to 10 L/minute). This gas is heavier than air and therefore displaces the latter from the field; because it is more readily dissolved in the blood, the adverse consequences of carbon dioxide gas embolization are less. Despite these potential complications, the outcome with use of the Port Access System in many cases have been acceptable (90).

Retrograde and Antegrade Cerebral Perfusion

During surgery involving aortic arch, as well as during some surgery on the ascending aorta (e.g., porcelain aorta, dissections) and on the descending aorta, the flow to the cerebral vessels is interrupted. Commonly, this is managed with the use of deep hypothermic circulation arrest. Although the safe time limit of this technique is not known, it is probably finite. Two techniques are used to minimize this limitation: selective (antegrade) cerebral perfusion (SCP or "cerebroplegia") and retrograde cerebral perfusion (RCP).

Selective Cerebral Perfusion

Selective cerebral perfusion is an old technique that requires one or more pumps (typically roller), a heat exchanger, and cannulation of at least some of the cerebral vessels. The latter are typically cannulated from within the aortic lumen. Higami et al. (297) have designed special two-lumen catheters featuring a ribbed balloon for intraluminal occlusion and a port for measuring perfusion pressure (SP Stud, Fuji Systems, Tokyo, Japan). They insert a 14F catheter into the innominate artery and a 12F catheter into the left carotid and left subclavian arteries. A single roller pump perfuses all three vessels at a flow of 300 to 350 mL/m^2/minute to maintain a perfusion pressure of 30 mm Hg using oxygenated blood at 16° to 18°C. Others have advocated flows of 10 mL/kg/minute (298,299) or total flows of 100 to 600 mL/minute (300), 250 to 350 mL/minute (301,302), or 500 to 1,000 mL/minute (303) at lower temperatures: 6° to 12°C (301,302) or 10°C (300). Some have used retrograde coronary sinus cannulas with inflatable balloons for intraluminal cannulation; others insert special cannulas with right-angled tips directly into the cerebral vessels through pursestring suture lines with proximal cross-clamping of the vessel (301,302). Some have cannulated both subclavian arteries through infraclavicular incisions (299), while others have solely relied on perfusion through a graft sewn onto the right axillary artery (used initially for total CPB) and during circulatory arrest have perfused the brain via the right carotid and vertebral arteries after clamping of the innominate and left carotid arteries (93). This method also permits monitoring of the cerebral perfusion pressure via the right radial artery line. Others perfuse only the right innominate and left carotid arteries (298,302). Griepp (300) described a method of sewing an 18-mm graft onto an island of the superior wall of the aortic arch that includes the orifices of the innominate, left carotid, and left subclavian arteries; this is then perfused with the main arterial cannula. If a pressure port is not contained within the perfusion cannula but the innominate artery is being infused, one can use the right radial artery to monitor cerebral perfusion pressure, which is maintained at 40 to 70 mm Hg (298,300); others simply monitor line pressure (302). Tanaka et al. (304), based on a canine study conducted at 25°C, recommended a minimal flow of 50% of normal (normal flow, about 10 mL/minute/kg) and a carotid arterial pressure of at least 30 mm Hg. Some have advocated monitoring jugular venous saturation, cerebral oximetry (near-infrared spectroscopy), or transcranial Doppler (303) to assess adequacy of cerebral oxygenation and flow during selective cerebral perfusion. Problems associated with this technique include extra complexity, risk of cerebral air or atheromatous embolization, cerebral edema or other injury from excessive perfusion, and unproven benefit (303).

Retrograde Cerebral Perfusion

Retrograde cerebral perfusion (RCP) was first introduced in 1980 by Mills and Ochsner for treatment of massive air embolism, and Lemole and colleagues described the use of intermittent RCP during aortic surgery in 1982, but Ueda and associates first introduced *continuous RCP* as an adjunct to deep hypothermic circulatory arrest during *aortic surgery* in 1990 (305). Although it has been used clinically by many groups with apparently good results (306–313), many questions remain concerning technical details of how it should be performed and monitored and about its benefits and risks (305,314–316). It is usually performed by perfusing cold oxygenated blood into an SVC cannula (either previously placed as part of bicaval venous cannulation or specifically placed for RCP) while a tourniquet snugs the SVC around the cannula. Often a line is "Y-ed" off of the arterial line and "Y-ed" into the SVC venous cannula line, and with appropriate clamping the systemic arterial pump supplies the RCP. Alternatively, a second pump is used to provide RCP when simultaneous systemic perfusion is required (some have advocated simultaneous retrograde perfusion of the IVC as well). Blood perfusate temperatures are commonly 10°C but have ranged from 8° to 18°C; flow rates commonly are between 250 and 400 mL/minute but have been as high as 1,600 mL/minute (317). Based on a canine study in which the IVC and azygous vein were occluded, Usui et al. (318) found the optimal jugular venous pressure to be 25 mm Hg (lower pressure reduces cerebral flow and higher pressure causes cerebral edema), and most groups follow these guidelines. Jugular venous pressure is most commonly assumed to equal to that measured in the SVC or the SVC cannula. However, because valves are present in the internal jugular veins near the junction with the subclavian veins in 80% to 90% of humans and are competent in about 10% to 20% (319), pressure in the SVC or the SVC cannula may significantly overestimate the jugular venous pressure and lead to underperfusion (317). This suggests the need to measure pressure in the jugular vein cephalad to these valves (with a separate monitor catheter) or to insert the RCP cannula into the jugular vein beyond the valves. Okamoto et al. (319) described a technique in which a guidewire is threaded through a small right atriotomy retrograde through a 7F catheter previously placed in the right internal jugular vein and then a tapered-tip 24F to 26F venous cannula is passed retrograde into the internal jugular vein. Alternatively, a coronary sinus perfusion cannula can be advanced retrograde from the right atrium into the right internal jugular vein (320). The balloon is then inflated to ensure retrograde cerebral perfusion, and the distal pressure port is used to monitor jugular venous pressure.

Ganzel et al. (317) used multimodal neurophysiologic monitoring (EEG, transcranial Doppler, and near-infrared spectroscopy ["cerebral oximeter"]) to monitor the adequacy of RCP flow and venous pressure (as measured in the SVC). They found that the average pressure in the SVC necessary to demonstrate retrograde cerebral flow by transcranial Doppler during RCP was 40 mm Hg (range, 30 to 49 mm Hg) and that the average flow required to *prevent* the rapid decline in cerebral oximetric saturation (less than 1% per minute) was 1.2 L/minute (range, 0.9 to 1.64 L/minute). These are much higher values than recommended by most groups and may relate to the pressure discrepancies caused by jugular venous valves, mentioned earlier, and to diversion of perfusate away from the brain. Despite these high pressures and flows, these authors noted no adverse neurologic consequences; however, the duration of RCP was quite short (average, 26 minutes; range, 22 to 30 minutes).

No consistent practice dictates the management of the azygous vein and IVC (316). The azygous vein, if left open during RCP, may provide another route for cerebral perfusion (via epidural veins), especially when the jugular valves are competent (321), or a site for runoff of retrograde perfused blood away from the head, depending on whether the IVC is occluded (forcing azygous blood into the brain) or is left open (allowing diversion of SVC perfusate away from the brain via the azygous drainage into the IVC). In studies of a chronic porcine model, Juvonen et al. (322) noted higher cerebral blood flow and superior removal of cerebral arterial particulate emboli (250 to 750 μm) when the IVC was occluded during RCP but observed more histologic damage and poorer neurologic recovery after 90 minutes of RCP with IVC occlusion, compared with no occlusion (323). They hypothesized that these effects were caused by cerebral edema from the increased RCP. Others have advocated inflating cuffs around the arms to 60 mm Hg to prevent diversion of retrograde flow into the extremities (317), but the merits and hazards of this approach have not been established.

The pressure in the internal jugular vein (in distinction to the SVC) should be monitored (although many groups do not do so). Little further monitoring is done by most groups, but the potential benefits of multimodal monitoring (EEG, transcranial Doppler, and cerebral oximetry using near-infrared spectroscopy), as suggested by Ganzel et al. (317), are appealing.

The proposed rationales for RCP include washout of cerebral air and particulate emboli (the latter are thought to be a major cause of neurologic injury after aortic arch surgery) (322,324); reduced cerebral rewarming during circulatory arrest; and provision of oxygen and metabolic substrates to reduce ischemic injury (316). Several concerns persist: is the brain really being perfused? (315); does it cause harm? (323); and does it improve outcome during deep hypothermic circulatory arrest? (see Cosselli [305] versus Griepp [314]). Several authors have reviewed the data, which indicate only limited cerebral perfusion during RCP (315,316,325). In humans Lin et al. (308) measured cortical flows equal to only 10% of the control value. Ganzel et al. (317) and Higami et al. (297) noted that in humans RCP only slows but does not prevent the decline in cerebral oxygen saturation during circulatory arrest, and Cheung et al. (326) observed the same to be true of the decay in amplitude of somatosensory evoked potentials. This suggests a time limitation to the benefits of RCP, as supported by a review of the initial clinical results in Japan (poorer outcomes after 60 minutes) (307). However for intermediate durations, animal studies have shown improved outcome with RCP, compared with deep hypothermic circulatory arrest alone, at 60 minutes (327) and 90 minutes (323), and the same has been suggested (but using historical controls) in human studies (310,311,317). Further, some remarkably good clinical results have been reported with circulatory arrest periods exceeding 90 to 120 minutes (308,313). Animal studies (which avoid some of the problems encountered clinically) (323,328) and one clinical study (297) have shown the superiority of selective cerebral perfusion over RCP: the former is able to maintain normal cerebral metabolic activity and to prevent the fall in cerebral oxygenation.

Heparin-Coated or -Bonded Circuits

Heparin can be attached to the blood interface surface of all components of the extracorporeal circuit to render them more biocompatible with the objectives of reducing or eliminating the need for systemic heparinization and reducing the activation of other components of the blood (besides coagulation), including platelets, kalikrien, complement, fibrinolytic systems, and leukocytes, and hence reducing the systemic inflammatory response to CPB. Two proprietary commercial methods of hepain coating are commonly employed (329). One is referred to as *covalent bonding*; it first deposits a polyethylenimine polymer *spacer* onto the plastic surface, to which heparin fragments are covalently bonded (Carmeda Bioactive Surface, Medtronic Inc, Minneapolis, MN). This is also referred to as end-point attachment or "universal surface." The second method is *ionic bonding:* heparin is first bound (ionically) to a quaternary ammonium carrier (alkylbenzyl dimethyl-ammonium chloride), and this complex then binds to the plastic surfaces (Duraflow II, Baxter Healthcare Corporation, Bentley Laboratories, Irvine, CA). This is also referred to as a "universal coating." The covalent-bonded surface (Carmeda) is more expensive but leaches off less heparin; may expose more of the heparin molecule; and may provide superior results. Numerous laboratory and clinical studies have documented that use of HBC is associated with decreased platelet activation, thrombin generation, complement activation, cytokine production (tumor necrosis factor-α, interleukin-6, interleukin-8), and endothelial leukocyte activation, including release of neutrophil granular proteases (lactoferrin) (329–333), although the reduced leukocyte activation may require concomitant reduction in heparin dose (334). However, the clinical relevance and safety of its use is debated (e.g., see

Shore-Lesserson [331] versus Woolff and Mythen [335]). The clinical results are probably influenced by patient population, heparin dosing protocol, surface coating used (although there have been no direct comparative studies), duration of CPB, details of conduct of CPB (e.g., use of cardiotomy suction), and other intangibles (e.g., type of pump used, postoperative autotransfusion of chest drainage). Most studies have found reduced bleeding and transfusion requirements associated with use of HBC *only* if reduced heparin dosing (100 to 150 units/kg; activated clotting time [ACT], 180 to 250 seconds) is employed (336,337), and the safety of such practice has been questioned (338—342). Aldea et al. (222) documented that, with the use of HBC, low-heparin protocols (ACT greater than 250 seconds; average initial dose, 114 ± 29 units/kg) are not associated with increased thrombin generation, cerebral microemboli (by transcranial Doppler), neurologic events, or neuropsychometric test score deterioration, compared with full heparinization protocol (ACT greater than 450 seconds). However, cardiotomy suckers were used sparingly if at all, and cannulas were removed promptly after termination of CPB.

Mahoney (343) performed a metaanalyses of 12 acceptable studies published between 1992 and 1996 and concluded that HBC improved clinical outcome and was associated with a theoretic cost savings (although the added cost of the HBC was not taken into account). He also concluded that covalently bonded circuits provided a greater magnitude of clinical benefits than did ionically bonded circuits. However, several recent clinical studies with HBC using full-dose heparinization have detected no clinical benefit in low-risk patients (344) and no benefit (233,333) or only modest benefit (332,345) in certain subgroups of high-risk patients. Aldea et al. (222,336) reported studies suggesting that the combined use of HBC and low systemic heparinization protocols provides complementary and additive clinical benefits.

The use of HBC has not eliminated the need for systemic heparinization for CPB, but it may permit safe lower heparin dosing in patients who are at particular risk with heparinization, and it has permitted the elimination of systemic heparinization for left heart bypass (extracorporeal circuits that exclude a reservoir and oxygenator).

Other surface modification methods are being introduced, but their clinical relevance is yet to be established (346,347).

Pediatric Circuits

Pediatric CPB places extreme demands on the extracorporeal circuit (348–351). Every effort must be directed at reducing the extracorporeal prime volume (e.g., use of tubing as narrow and short as possible). Because of complex anatomy, cannulation may be complex. Bicaval venous cannulation is invariably required, and one must always consider the possibility of a PLSVC. Cannulas with maximal inner- to outer-diameter ratios are extremely important, and so right-angled metal cannulas for caval cannulation are favored. Nevertheless, interference with native caval return when not on CPB is more likely, so the time between caval cannulation and CPB must be kept to a minimum. Likewise, interference with left ventricular outflow by the arterial cannula is more likely, as is the risk of inadvertent cannulation of the great vessels and jet effects (due to small-bore cannulas). It is also more likely for the stiff cannula to distort the anatomy of the patient's veins and arteries. Because of lower prime volumes, roller pumps are more commonly used than centrifugal pumps. Because of the large volume of the extracorporeal circuit compared with the blood volume of the patient, composition of the priming solution is more critical. Hemoconcentration and MUF are commonly employed.

Computerized Control

Computerized control of CPB has been described (352,353) and used clinically (354), but aside from automated data collection (see later discussion) it has not yet become accepted in general clinical practice.

MONITORING

Overall monitoring of the patient during CPB is covered in Chapter 14. This section concentrates on monitors of the function of the heart-lung machine and its interface with the patient (355).

In-line Blood Gas Monitors

Noninvasive flowthrough devices are available to measure blood gases and other electrolytes and hemoglobin/hematocrit in the arterial and venous lines (355). The arterial monitor provides continuous assessment of arterial oxygenation (like a pulse oximeter) and permits more rapid and precise control of blood gases (157,356). Venous oximetry permits rapid assessment of the balance of oxygen supply and demand (274–276,357). Rubsamen (358), a medicolegal scholar, asserted that in-line blood gas monitoring is a standard of care that is essential from the standpoint of both patient safety and prevention of devastating malpractice suits. However, there appears to be little scientific data documenting that this approach is superior to (more safe than) the visual monitoring of arterial and venous lines combined with periodic blood gas sampling, nor that its use does prevent malpractice suits. Further, currently available devices are imperfect and may provide misleading information (359); a determination of "adequate" mixed venous oxygen saturation may give a false sense of security (360). Finally, economic considerations cannot be ignored.

Another approach to more timely monitoring of blood

gases and various electrolytes is the use of automated operating room analyzers (361,362), but the perfusion team or other individuals in the operating room must accept responsibility for quality control and recognize their limitations (361). One must also beware that blood drawn from the sampling port of some oxygenators can give misleading information (363). Stammers (355) has summarized the clinical evaluation studies of varous in-line and off-line blood gas and electrolyte monitoring devices.

Arterial Line Pressure

The pressure in the arterial line, after the pump but before the arterial line filter, should be monitored continuously to detect obstruction in the arterial line, malposition of the arterial cannula, arterial dissection, or obstruction of the filter. This pressure must be interpreted in the context of the expected pressure drop across the arterial cannula at the indicated flow rate and the patient's monitored intraarterial pressure (364). It is also a useful guide to proper initial arterial cannulation and as a monitor of central arterial pressure in the early postbypass period, when radial artery pressure may be misleading. It is desirable to include an audible alarm in this pressure monitoring system to alert the team if pressures are excessive. Some also connect the arterial line pressure monitoring system to the arterial pump (servocontrolled) to turn off the pump when excessive pressures develop.

Arterial Line Flow Meter

An arterial line flow meter is essential if a centrifugal pump is being used, and it is a helpful adjunct to confirm proper occlusiveness and calibration when a roller pump is used. Akers et al. (365) compared four different extracorporeal blood flow meters and the influence of changing hematocrit. The differences they observed were small and did not appear to be clinically significant.

Oxygen Concentration of the Gas Entering the Oxygenator

Just as monitoring oxygen concentration in the gas delivered to a patient during anesthesia is part of standard basic monitoring, an oxygen analyzer should be placed in the gas supply line to the oxygenator. This is essential if oxygen is being diluted with another gas, and the analyzer should be placed "downstream" to the blender (166). Monitoring the *flow* of gas into the oxygenator is also desirable. Kirson and Goldman (365b) described a comprehensive system for monitoring the delivery of ventilating gas to the oxygenator.

Expired Gas Monitoring

Monitoring the concentrations of oxygen, carbon dioxide, and anesthetic vapors exiting the oxygenator ensures that oxygen is passing through the oxygenator and provides clues to metabolic activity and depth of anesthesia (365b), but it may not correlate with arterial carbon dioxide when a membrane oxygenator is used (366).

Pressure Gradient across Membrane Oxygenator

Some manufacturers recommend monitoring the pressure gradient across membrane oxygenators. Development of excessive pressure gradients has been reported to be the most common problem encountered with membrane oxygenators and may be an early indicator of possible oxygenator failure (167,168,170,171). If the gradient is not being monitored but a centrifugal arterial pump is being used, a high pressure gradient through the membrane should be suspected when the flow rate is low for the pump speed setting and the arterial line pressure.

Temperature Monitoring

Monitoring the temperature of the water entering the heat exchangers is helpful to ensure adequate cooling, avoid excessive heating, and avoid potentially hazardous cooling and warming gradients (184). Knowledge of the temperature of the venous blood draining from the patient provides a clue to adequacy of cooling when inducing hypothermia and of rewarming when restoring normothermia. With increased interest in the possible role of cerebral hyperthermia as a contributor to cerebral dysfunction after CPB, monitoring of the temperature of the blood (arterial) being delivered to the patient from the extracorporeal circuit is considered by many to be essential for the safe conduct of CPB.

Low-Level Sensor and Alarms and Bubble Detector

A low-level sensor with alarms on the arterial or venous reservoir and a bubble detector on the arterial line are additional desirable safety devices. Whether they should be connected to the pump controller to automatically turn off the pump is the subject of debate (faster response time versus risk of false alarms). Furthermore, some reservoirs and oxygenators in current use preclude the application of low-level alarms, emphasizing the essential role of a vigilant perfusionist.

Echocardiography

Epiaortic echocardiography and TEE can be extremely helpful in the conduct of CPB. Previously their role in evaluating the aorta in regard to arterial cannulation was described. TEE is very accurate in detecting atherosclerosis in the descending aorta which might influence the use of femoral artery inflow. It can also detect clots or tumors in the left atrium, left atrial appendage, or left ventricle, as well as in the right-sided chambers, which could influence venous cannulation and left-sided venting. Detection of a patent foramen ovale (two-dimensional images, color flow Doppler, and agitated saline echocontrast study) may anticipate a source of venous air if the left side of the heart is to be opened, and detection of a PDA may explain excessive return of blood to the left heart during CPB (244). Evaluation of the degree of aortic regurgitation (367) and the presence of a dilated coronary sinus (26) affect the administration of antegrade and retrograde cardioplegia. The detection of clues to the presence of a PLSVC (see earlier discussion) has obvious impact on venous cannulation and administration of retrograde cardioplegia (27). TEE can facilitate the positioning of peripherally introduced systemic venous cannulas, long arterial cannulas introduced into ascending aorta, retrograde coronary sinus cannulas (238), and left-sided venting cannulas; this is particularly helpful when the surgeon cannot directly inspect or palpate the heart due to limited access or adhesions. Use of TEE is essential for placement of various cannulas during Port Access (Heartport) surgery (295), and it is helpful for the proper placement and assessment of proper function of intraaortic balloon pumps, especially when placed antegrade through the ascending aorta, and for the proper placement of endovascular aortic occluders (63). During CPB, TEE helps assess the degree of left ventricular distention and decompression and helps with the differential diagnosis of ascending aortic hematoma and the diagnosis of aortic dissection. This is particularly important during femoral artery perfusion. With femoral perfusion during surgery for aortic dissection, TEE may be useful in detecting malperfusion (369). During partial left heart bypass (femoral vein to artery and left atrial to distal aorta or femoral artery) it is helpful in guiding the balance of flow between the upper and lower body and blood volume regulation. Finally, TEE is useful in detecting intracardiac air and assessing adequacy of de-airing after cardiac surgery (370,371).

Automated Data Collection Systems

Automatic data collection systems are available to assist with the preoperative calculations and to process and store data during CPB, which should free the perfusionist to attend to more important tasks (372). Whether this will indeed improve outcome remains to be demonstrated (356,373).

COMPLICATIONS SAFETY, RISK MANAGEMENT, AND RISK CONTAINMENT

Throughout, this chapter has emphasized various complications associated with CPB and the roles of specific monitors on the heart-lung machine to detect and reduce adverse events. Others have reviewed issues in perfusion safety (100,374–379). Four surveys conducted between 1972 and 1986 found a life-threatening incident rate of 0.4% to 1% and a permanent injury or death rate attributed to such accidents of about 1 in 1,000 to 1,400 cases (Table 12-7) (376). Principal types of incidents were inadequate oxygenation, electrical failure, gas embolization, clotting, line separation, blood leaks, mechanical failure, and failure of the blender-flow meter; principal causes of permanent injury or death were gas embolism, an inadequate oxygenator, and clotting. Other reported incidents that may not have been directly related to the CPB equipment *per se* included hypoperfusion, coagulopathy, protamine reaction, drug errors, and transfusion-related complications. Like most other adverse incidents in anesthesia, most of these were estimated to be caused by human error and only 20% by device failure (377–379).

TABLE 12-7. INCIDENCE OF CRITICAL INCIDENTS DURING PERFUSION

Type Of Critical Incident	Incidence (per 1,000)	Permanent Injury or Mortality (%)
Gas embolism	1.2	25
Electrical failure	0.9	1
Oxygenator failure	0.6	7
Mechanical failure	0.2	4
Reversed left ventricular vent	0.05	—

Source: Summary of data from four studies between 1972 and 1987 as presented by Kurusz and Wheeldon (377–379).

Jenkins et al. (169) have presented a contemporary survey from Australia and New Zealand. They observed a higher rate of incidents (2.9%) but lower rate of serious injury or death (1 in 2,500) than in previous surveys. A list of those incidents is summarized in Table 12-8. More recently, Mejak et al. (379b) published a survey from the United States covering the years 1996–1998 and reported an incident rate of 0.7% and a serious injury or death rate of 1 in 1,453.

Gross and Massive Air Embolism

Gross and massive air embolism is one of the most common serious adverse events associated with CPB (380–382) (see Tables 12-7 and 12-8), but it is largely preventable. Kurusz et al. (383) thoroughly reviewed the incidence, pathophysiology, consequences, sources and mechanisms, treatment, and prevention of macro air embolism during CPB. Air may enter the patient's arterial system from the arterial inflow line, from intracardiac vents, or from cardioplegia lines. Principal causes include pumping air out of a dry or almost empty reservoir (vortexing), disconnection, leaks, oxygenator break or line occlusion before the arterial pump (with air entrainment or cavitation), incomplete de-airing of the

TABLE 12-8. PERFUSION INCIDENTS RELATED TO CANNULATION AND EQUIPMENT

Type of Perfusion Incident	Incidence (per 1,000)	Serious Injury or Death (% of Incidents)
Heater-cooler require changing	3.0	—
Air	3.3	1.1
Air in circuit not reaching patient	(2.0)	
Embolism	(1.3)	
Massive air embolism	(0.07)	(50)
Hospital power failure	1.8	—
Cannula displacement	1.6	7.1
Oxygenator require replacement	1.3	—
Other oxygenator problems	0.9	—
Gas supply failure	0.9	—
Aortic or femoral dissection	0.8	14.3
Tubing rupture or disconnect	0.6	—
Arterial pump electrical or mechanical failure	0.4	—
Other pump electrical or mechanical failure	0.5	—
Arterial line filter failure	0.3	—
Tubing rupture or disconnect	0.6	—
Heparin resistance	2.1	2.6
Inadequate anticoagulation	0.3	
Clotting in circuit	0.3	
Drug incident	1.6	—
Severe hypoperfusion/ hypotension	1.1	6.9
Unplanned circulatory arrest to deal with problem with heart-lung machine	0.2	—
Protamine-induced clotting of circuit after bypass	1.4	—
Urgent circuit resetup after disposal	2.9	13.0

Source: Modified from Jenkins OF, Morris R, Simpson JM. Australasian perfusion incident survey. *Perfusion* 1997;12:289.

circuit before CPB, reversal of arterial and venous lines, reversal of arterial pump head, backflow into the arterial cannula (air may be aspirated into the arterial line from around the pursestring suture if there is backflow while the arterial pump is off and if the arterial line is not occluded, as when using a centrifugal pump [107]), occlusion of the exhaust port of membrane oxygenators (forcing air bubbles into the blood), development of positive pressure in the cardiotomy reservoir (which may force air back through the arterial filter bleed line or through left ventricular or aortic root vents), injection of air into the aortic root from the cardioplegia delivery system, ejection of air from the heart, or introduction of air at the time of cannulation or decannulation of the aorta or left heart. Air entrainment during the latter procedures may be aggravated by low arterial or left heart pressures and filling. The deflation phase of an intraaortic balloon pump may aspirate air through an open aorta. Air may be entrained into the heart by the patient's own inspiratory effort (inadequate muscle relaxation) when the left heart is open or by injudicious mechanical ventilation when the pressures in the heart cavities fall precipitously with expiration. If there are septal defects (including patent foramen ovale), right-sided air may get into the left heart.

Pumping air out of the reservoir is principally caused by inattention on the part of the perfusionist but can be aggravated by a sudden decline in venous return or a runaway pump. Ejection of air from the left ventricle occurs whenever air gets into the left heart and is allowed to eject before adequate de-airing. Insertion of lines and vents into the left heart, deep suction into the pulmonary arteries, reverse flow of air through a left-sided vent (due to reversal of pump head or development of positive pressure in the cardiotomy reservoir), and septal defects all may permit air to enter the left heart. Kurusz and Weldon (378) reported that 44% of 458 episodes of gas embolization came from the arterial line, and half of these cases were attributed to inattention on the part of the perfusionist. Nine percent were attributed to reversed left ventricular vent line, 10% to unexpected resumption of heartbeat, 5% to pressurized cardiotomy reservoir, and 5% to unnoticed rotation of the arterial pumphead.

Vigilance is the key to prevention. Other helpful components are protection of the venous lines by the surgical team and communication to the perfusionist when venous return is likely to be compromised (e.g., when lifting the heart); maintenance of a safe volume of blood in the reservoir; use of collapsible venous reservoirs, centrifugal pumps, arterial line filters, or bubble traps with a continuously open air-purge line guarded by a one-way valve; placement of one-way valves in left heart vent lines; checking the flow direction in vent lines on the table before connection; and use of low-level alarms and bubble detectors, which may or may not be connected to automatic shutoff devices connected to the arterial pump. The survey reported by Jenkins et al. (169) noted a significant reduction in the incidence (0.007%) and rate of adverse outcomes (0.003%) from massive air embolism compared with earlier surveys. The survey by Mejak et al. (379b) noted an incidence of 0.003% and a rate of adverse outcomes of 0.002%.

If a massive air embolism occurs, suggested management is summarized in Table 12-9 (381,382,384,385). Clearly, no controlled studies are available to prove the benefit of any of these components. In one retrospective review, 61% of 64 patients treated with retrograde perfusion were without apparent neurologic injury (382), but such treatment should not inordinately delay resumption of antegrade perfusion. Induced hypothermia with 100% oxygen should favor absorption of nitrogen emboli and improve cerebral tolerance to ischemia. There is little proof that barbiturates given after an ischemic insult are beneficial, and they could cause harm by depressing postbypass perfusion and cardiac

TABLE 12-9. SUGGESTED MANAGEMENT OF MASSIVE SYSTEMIC AIR EMBOLISM DURING CARDIOPULMONARY BYPASS

1. Stop arterial pump immediately, and clamp both venous and arterial lines.
2. Place patient in steep Trendelenburg position.
3. Remove aortic cannula and vent air out.
4. De-air arterial line and cannula.
5. Insert arterial cannula into SVC cannula (if one is present and after excluding all air); otherwise into the SVC through a stab wound. Snare SVC cannula (if present; otherwise clamp SVC between cannula and the right atrium and initiate retrograde SVC perfusion.)
   a. Flow rate 1–2 L/min/70 kg
   b. Perfusate temperature 20°–24°C
   c. For 1–3 min or until no more froth is seen to egress from the aorta
   d. Anesthesiologists should temporarily compress the carotids during the later phase of retrograde perfusion (to purge air from vertebral system)
6. Resume antegrade hypothermic (20°–22°C), pulsatile (if available) perfusion for about 45 min at higher-than-usual pressure (high flow, vasoconstrictors, intermittent clamping of descending aorta for 2–3 min).
7. Express coronary air.
8. Consider retrograde IVC perfusion.
9. Consider giving the following:
   a. Methylprednisone 30 mg/kg
   b. Mannitol 25 g
   c. Barbiturates (pentobarbital 10 mg/kg or thiopental 16 mg/kg)
   d. Low-molecular-weight dextran
10. Wean from bypass after cauteous rewarming to about 36°C; avoid inflow temperature higher than 37°C.
11. Maintain on 100% O_2 for at least 6 hr postoperatively; avoid body temperature higher than 37°C.
12. Initiate hyperbaric oxygen therapy, if available and patient's condition permits (3 ATA × 30 min; 2 ATA × 90 min)

Note: ATA, atmospheres absolute; IVC, inferior vena cava; SVC, superior vena cava.
Source: Modified from references 381, 382, 384, and 385.

output and delaying ability to assess neurologic status. Prompt initiation of hyperbaric oxygen therapy is advocated by some (385,386), with impressive outcomes if initiated within 3 hours and occasional successes even at 30 hours (387); however, the logistic issues may be daunting, although not insurmountable.

Other Malfunctions and Catastrophes during Cardiopulmonary Bypass

The cardiac surgical team (surgeon, anesthesiologist, and perfusionist) must be aware of the potential complications during CPB (see Table 12-8) in order to prevent, recognize, and manage them if they should occur (169,266,378, 384,388). Many of these problems are discussed earlier in this chapter and elsewhere in this book.

1. Problems associated with venous cannulation and venous return
   a. Bleeding, arrhythmias, injury to cardiovascular structures, malposition, air embolism
   b. Low venous return
   c. High venous pressure and failure to decompress right heart
   d. Reversal of arterial and venous lines
   e. Inadvertent decannulation
   f. Air lock
2. Problems associated with arterial cannulation and inflow
   a. Bleeding, air, and atheroembolism
   b. Malposition, carotid malperfusion
   c. Dissection
   d. High pressure in arterial line; line rupture
   e. Reversal of arterial and venous lines
   f. Retrograde flow when pump is off due to lack of occlusiveness (may lead to hypovolemia and air aspiration—and subsequent air embolism if CPB is resumed)
   g. Inadvertent decannulation
3. Problems associated with venting
   a. Bleeding, air embolization, injury to cardiac structures
   b. Reverse flow (infusion of air into left heart)
   c. Inadequate decompression of left heart
4. Massive air embolism (see earlier discussion)
5. Malfunction of arterial pump
   a. Electrical failure
   b. Runaway pump due to malfunction of control system (can lead to systemic air embolism [104]). The pump must be turned off (occasionally the power source may need to be disconnected) and an alternative pump used; meanwhile, hand cranking is required.
   c. Loss of the RPM indicator light
   d. Loss of flow meter indicator
   e. Pump creep (pump continues to move even when flow rate control knob has been turned to zero; it may need to turn off). This can cause excessive transfusion into the patient or air embolization.
   f. Occlusion malfunction (roller pump): if too tight, it may cause excessive tubing wear, hemolysis, spallation, and a "frozen" pump; if too loose, it may cause hemolysis and inadequate (uncalibrated, afterload-sensitive) forward flow
   g. Reverse flow (due to misplacement of line in pump head or switching error)
   h. Rupture of pump head tubing
6. Oxygenator failure or malfunction (166,378,389,390)
   a. Hypercapnia
   b. Hypoxemia
      (1) Failure of oxygen supply (leaks, obstruction, nonconnection, blender failure) (165)

(2) Oxygenator failure (obstructed disperser plate, excessive reservoir volume)
(3) Low venous oxygen content (inadequate perfusion rate, inadequate hematocrit, inadequate anesthesia, hyperthermia [malignant hyperthermia])

c. Gas embolization (obstruction of gas outlet or vent)
d. Excessive pressure gradient through blood path (167,168,170,171)

7. Electrical failure (e.g., loss of electrical power to operating room or electrical outlets, electrical disconnection, tripping of circuit breaker or fuse). Troianos (391) has reviewed the catastrophic problem of total electrical failure during CPB. Such failure can lead to loss of all room lighting, loss of monitoring and controls, and loss of monitors on the heart-lung machine (e.g., RPM indicator, line pressure indicator, timers), as well as loss of the arterial pump (forward flow) and field suction pumps. Loss of the latter may result in flooding of the surgical field and a reduced amount of blood returning to the heart-lung machine, and hence contribute to the risk of air embolism. Troianos (391) outlined a logical approach to deal with electrical failure and essential preparations to minimize the negative impact of such an event. Emergency lighting and hand cranking of the arterial and suction pumps must be available and initiated.
8. Clotting in machine (due to inadequate heparinization, inadvertent administration of protamine, administration of unheparinized fresh-frozen plasma into the reservoir, or use of cardiotomy suction after heparin reversal with protamine [169]). This is a critical problem if there is urgent need to return to CPB (see later discussion) and suggests the need to limit return of field suction blood to the heart-lung machine once protamine administration has begun (or to retain such blood in a separate reservoir).
9. Water leak
10. Disconnection of line and connector, loose connection (leading to blood leakage if on positive side of pump or air entrainment if on negative side of pump), or rupture
11. Hemolysis. Potential sources of hemolysis include cardiotomy suction, bubble oxygenator, roller pump, micropore arterial filter, small arterial cannulas, water leak into the circuit, chemical contamination, and transfusion reactions (34,98,392–394). Hemolysis is further discussed in the sections on specific components of the circuit. Lamon et al. (395) suggested that extracorporeal circuits do not directly damage red blood cells but do so indirectly via the immunologic consequences of bypass.
12. Hypotension. The differential diagnosis must include monitor error, artifactually low radial artery pressure, dissection, malposition of arterial cannulas, low arterial inflow (calibration error, nonocclusive roller pump), and low systemic vascular resistance (drop in hematocrit, anesthetic and vasoactive drug administration).
13. Need to urgently return to CPB after disposal of the circuit (169) or after the circuit has become clotted (see item 8 above). This suggests that one should delay dismantling the circuit until the case is over.

Risk Containment (100,169,374,375,377–379)

In Table 12-10 are listed some of the safety devices and procedures employed during CPB. Accidents are caused principally by human error, although device failures account for some. A risk containment program therefore should include the following:

TABLE 12-10. SAFETY DEVICES AND PROCEDURES

	Percent Used	
Device Or Procedure	Australasian Survey[a]	Other Surveys
Low blood level alarm	100	60–80,[b] 70[d]
with pump cutoff	83	34[d]
High arterial line pressure alarm	84	94[d]
with pump cutoff	75	35[d]
Macrobubble detector	78	42–80[b], 88[d]
with pump cutoff	62	63[d]
Arterial line filter	82	44–97,[b] 99[d]
Prebypass filter	75	78,[c] 81[d]
Oxygen supply filter	81	83,[c]7 95[d]
In-line venous oxygen saturation	76	75[d]
In-line arterial oxygen saturation	12	13[d]
Oxygenator gas supply oxygen analyzer	43	53[d]
One-way valve in intracardiac vent lines	18	73[b]
Electrical power backup	92	
Batteries in heart-lung machine	(29)	85[d]
Alternative dedicated power supply	(36)	
Generator	(28)	
Backup arterial pump head	80	
Backup heater-cooler	97	
Backup oxygen supply	88	91[d]
Emergency lighting	62	91[d]
Prebypass check list	80	74–77,[b] 95[d]
Prebypass ACT	74	96–99[b]
ACT during bypass	83	
Check flow direction in cardiac vents on-the-table	16	
Keep log of perfusion incidents	46	
Keep log of device failures	52	
Have written protocols	49	75[b]

Note: ACT, activated clotting time.
[a] Jenkins, O.F., et al. (169) "Percent of respondents always using."
[b] Kurusz, M (376) (results of various surveys 1991–1996).
[c] Silvay, G., et al. (207).
[d] Mejak BL, et al (379b).

1. Adequate education, practice, experience, training, and certification (and recertification) (396) of all members of the team (and proper accreditation of training centers). A formal system of continuing education that emphasizes safety, practical techniques, and new techniques is essential. The well-trained, vigilant human is the key to risk containment.
2. Development of written protocols for all routine and emergency situations (e.g., Policy and Procedure Manual). Emergency protocols and contingency plans should be periodically reviewed and practiced by all team members.
3. Use of checklists
4. Checking of backup equipment and supplies
5. Employment (and activation) of safety equipment and alarms (see Table 12-10 and the section on monitoring above)
6. Appropriate preventive maintenance program (and documentation)
7. Evaluation of the capabilities of all power supplies (capacity of outlets—beware of overloading, especially with heater-coolers)
8. Appropriate replacement of old equipment
9. Thorough familiarity with and testing of new equipment or components added
10. Avoidance of distraction of any team member during the procedure
11. Team communication. The three key members of the team (surgeon, anesthesiologist, and perfusionist) must keep in constant communication with one another. In particular, they must mention any activity in which they engage that may affect the work of the other two. Commands must be clear and must be positively (verbally) acknowledged. *The role of the anesthesiologist* during bypass is often underemphasized or underused. The anesthesiologist should be responsible for management of ventilation and anesthetic agents and can assist with heparin and protamine administration and their monitoring. The anesthesiologist should provide an "extra set of eyes" for vigilance (e.g., kinked lines, clamps, air bubbles). Being able to observe both the operative field and the heart-lung machine, the anesthesiologist can help keep both the surgeon and the perfusionist apprised of activities that may affect the other. The anesthesiologist should assist with monitoring, troubleshooting, and recognition and management of problems. Obviously, the drugs that the anesthesiologist administers (anesthetics, muscle relaxants, vasoactive agents) have important effects on the conduct of CPB, and the other two team members must be kept informed of their administration.
12. Automatic control or regulation of CPB. This is being explored and has the potential of reducing the workload on the perfusionist and improving patient safety (352,353,372,373).
13. Keeping a log of all perfusion incidents and device failures. Systematically review all incidents with the entire team to analyze contributing factors and implement preventive strategies.
14. Implementing a program of continuous quality assurance and improvement (397)
15. Formal training of other team members to take over running the heart-lung machine in the event that the perfusionist becomes incapacitated and a second perfusionist is not available (along with the development of written policies covering this eventuality)

ACKNOWLEDGMENT

The author greatfully acknowledges the art work of Norman P. Pregent CCP and Steve Scheunke for Figures 12-2, 12-3, and 12-8.

REFERENCES*

1. Gravlee GP, Davis RF, Kurusz M, et al. *Cardiopulmonary bypass: principles and practice.* 2nd Ed. Baltimore: Williams & Wilkins, 2000.
2. Mora CT, ed. *Cardiopulmonary bypass: principles and techniques of extracorporeal circulation.* New York: Springer-Verlag, 1995.
3. Kay PH, ed. *Techniques in extracorporeal circulation,* 3rd ed. Oxford: Butterworth-Heinemann, 1992.
4. Casthely PA, Bregman D, eds. *Cardiopulmonary bypass: physiology, related complications, and pharmacology.* Mount Kisco, NY: Futura Publishing, 1991.
5. Taylor KM, ed. *Cardiopulmonary bypass: principles and management.* Baltimore: Williams & Wilkins, 1986.
6. Utley JR. Early development of cardiopulmonary bypass. *Perfusion* 1986;1:1.
7. Westaby S, Bosher C. *Landmarks in cardiac surgery.* Oxford: Isis Medical Media, 1997.
8. Sweeney MS, Frazier OH. Device-supported myocardial revascularization: safe help for sick hearts. *Ann Thorac Surg* 1992; 54:1065.
9. Tassani P, Richter JA, Barankay A, et al. Is the patient's own lung a superior oxygenator regarding pulmonary and inflammatory parameters after CABG? [Abstract]. *Anesth Analg* 1999;88: SCA96.
10. Merin O, Silberman S, Brauner R, et al. Femoro-femoral bypass for repeat open-heart surgery. *Perfusion* 1998;13:455.
11. Arom KV, Ellestad C, Grover FL, et al. Objective evaluation of the efficacy of various venous cannulas. *J Thorac Cardiovasc Surg* 1981;81:464.
12. Bennett EV Jr, Fewel JG, Ybarra J, et al. Comparison of flow differences among venous cannulas. *Ann Thorac Surg* 1983;36: 59.

* The interested reader is alerted to the existence of a Cardiopulmonary Bypass Bibliography, edited by J.R. Utley, H.D. Johnson, and M.S. Morgan, covering the years 1967 through 1988. It was published in 1989 by the Cardiothoracic Research and Education Foundation (P.O. Box 8100, Spartanburg, SC 29305.)

13. Bennett EV Jr, Fewel JG, Grover FL, et al. Myocardial preservation: effect of venous drainage. *Ann Thorac Surg* 1983;36:132.
14. Lake CL. Controversies in the management of cardiopulmonary bypass. *Cardiothoracic and Vascular Anesthesia Updates* 1990;1: 1.
15. Rosenfeldt FL, Watson DA. Interference with local myocardial cooling by heat gain during aortic cross-clamping. *Ann Thorac Surg* 1979;27:13.
16. Miller DW, Ivey TD, Bailey WW, et al. The practice of coronary artery bypass surgery in 1980. *J Thorac Cardiovasc Surg* 1981;81:423.
17. Taylor PC, Effler DB. Management of cannulation for cardiopulmonary bypass in patients with adult-acquired heart disease. *Surg Clin North Am* 1975;55:1205.
18. Kirklin JW, Barrett-Boyes BE. *Cardiac surgery,* 2nd ed. New York: John Wiley & Sons, 1993;Chapter 2.
19. Ambesh SP, Singh SK, Dubey DK, et al. Inadvertent closure of the superior vena cava after decannulation: a potentially catastrophic complication after termination of bypass [Letter]. *J Cardiothorac Vasc Anesth* 1998; 12:723.
20. Peters WS, Stevens JH, Smith JA, et al. Minimally invasive right heart operations: techniques for bicaval occlusion and cardioplegia. *Ann Thorac Surg* 1997;64:1843.
21. Westaby S. Extrathoracic cannulation for urgent cardiopulmonary bypass in cardiac tamponade: use of internal jugular vein. *J Cardiovasc Surg* 1988;29:103.
22. Flege JB Jr, Wolf RK. Venous drainage to the heart-lung machine via the internal jugular vein. *Ann Thorac Surg* 1997;63: 861.
23. Winter FS. Persistent left superior vena cava: survey of world literature and report of thirty additional cases. *Angiology* 1954; 5:90.
24. Choudhry AK, Conacher ID, Hilton CJ, et al. Persistent left superior vena cava. *J Cardiothorac Anesth* 1989;3:616.
25. Horrow JC, Lingaraju N. Unexpected persistent left superior vena cava: diagnostic clues during monitoring. *J Cardiothorac Anesth* 1989;3:611.
26. Hasel R, Barash PG. Dilated coronary sinus on pre-bypass echocardiography. *J Cardiothorac Vasc Anesth* 1996;10:430.
27. Garduno C, Chew S, Forbess J, et al. Persistent left superior vena cava and partial anomalous pulmonary venous connection: incidental diagnosis by transesophageal echocardiography during coronary artery bypass surgery. *J Am Soc Echocardiogr* 1999; 12:682.
28. Shahian DM. Retrograde coronary sinus cardioplegia in the presence of persistent left superior vena cava. *Ann Thorac Surg* 1992;54:1214.
29. Yokota M, Kyoku I, Kitano M, et al. Atresia of the coronary sinus orifice: fatal outcome after intraoperative division of the drainage left superior vena cava. *J Thorac Cardiovasc Surg* 1989; 98:30.
30. Harris AM, Shawkat S, Bailey JS. The use of an endotracheal tube for cannulation of left superior vena cava via coronary sinus for repair of a sinus venosus atrial septal defect. *Br Heart J* 1987; 58:676.
31. Toomasian JM. Cardiopulmonary bypass for less invasive procedures. *Perfusion* 1999;14:279.
32. Toomasian JM, McCarthy JP. Total extrathoracic cardiopulmonary support with kinetic assisted venous drainage: experience in 50 patients. *Perfusion* 1998;13:137.
33. Taketani S, Sawa Y, Massai T, et al. A novel technique for cardiopulmonary bypass using vacuum system for venous drainage with pressure relief valve: an experimental study. *Artif Organs* 1998;22:337.
34. Indeglia RA, Shea MA, Varco RE, et al. Mechanical and biologic considerations in erythrocyte damage. *Surgery* 1967;114:126.
35. Ratnaraj J, Manohar G. Pulmonary artery catheter displacement during cannulation for CPB [Letter]. *J Cardiothorac Vasc Anesth* 1991;5:648.
36. Troianos CA. Transesophageal echocardiographic diagnosis of pulmonary artery catheter entrapment and coiling. *Anesthesioloy* 1993;79:602.
37. Herrema IH, Winsser LJA. Flow directed pulmonary artery catheter obstructs venous drainage cannula of cardiopulmonary bypass machine [Letter]. *Anaesthesia* 1988;43:799.
38. Brodman R, Siegel H, Lesser M, et al. A comparison of flow gradients across disposable arterial perfusion cannulas. *Ann Thorac Surg* 1985;39:225.
39. Galletti PM, Brecher GA. *Heart-lung bypass.* New York: Grune & Stratton, 1962.
40. Muehrcke DD, Cornhill JF, Thomas JD, et al. Flow characteristics of aortic cannulae. *J Card Surg* 1995;10:514.
41. Taylor PC, Groves LK, Loop FD, et al. Cannulation of the ascending aorta for cardiopulmonary bypass. *J Thorac Cardiovasc Surg* 1976;71:255.
42. Mills NL, Everson CT. Atherosclerosis of the ascending aorta and coronary artery bypass: pathology, clinical correlates, and operative management. *J Thorac Cardiovasc Surg* 1991;102:546.
43. Beique FA, Joffe D, Tousignant G, et al. Echocardiographic-based assessment and management of atherosclerotic disease of the thoracic aorta. *J Cardiothorac Vasc Anesth* 1998;12:206.
44. Blauth CI, Cosgrove DM, Webb BW, et al. Atheroembolism from the ascending aorta. *J Thorac Cardiovasc Surg* 1992;103: 1104.
45. Barbut D, Grassineau D, Lis E, et al. Posterior distribution of infarcts in strokes related to cardiac operation. *Ann Thorac Surg* 1998;65:1656.
46. Murphy DA, Craver JM, Jones EL, et al. Recognition and management of ascending aortic dissection complicating cardiac surgical operations. *J Thorac Cardiovasc Surg* 1983;85:247.
47. Davila-Roman VG, Kouchoukos NT, Schechtman KB, et al. Atherosclerosis of the ascending aorta is a predictor of renal dysfunction after cardiac operations. *J Thorac Cardiovasc Surg* 1999;117:111.
48. Bar-El Y, Goor DA. Clamping of the atherosclerotic ascending aorta during coronary artery bypass operations: its cost in strokes. *J Thorac Cardiovasc Surg* 1992;104:469.
49. Davila-Roman V, Phillips K, Davila R, et al. Intraoperative transesophageal echocardiography and epiaortic ultrasound for assessment of atherosclerosis of the thoracic aorta. *J Am Coll Cardiol* 1996;28:942.
50. Sylivris S, Calafiore P, Matalanis G, et al. The intraoperative assessment of ascending aortic atheroma: epiaortic imaging is superior to both transesophageal and direct palpation. *J Cardiothorac Vasc Anesth* 1997;11:704.
51. Konstadt SN, Reich DL, Quintana C, et al. The ascending aorta: how much does transesophageal echocardiography see? *Anesth Analg* 1994;78:240.
52. Konstadt SN, Reich DL, Kahn R, et al. Transesophageal echocardiography can be used to screen for ascending aortic atherosclerosis. *Anesth Analg* 1995;81:225.
53. Guzzetta NA, Lee E, Sadel SM, et al. Does the degree of atheromatous disease in the descending aorta correlate with atheromatous disease in the ascending aorta? [Abstract]. *Anesth Analg* 1995;80:SCA 95.
54. Rokkos CF, Kouchoukos NT. Surgical management of the severely atherosclerotic ascending aorta during cardiac operations. *Semin Thorac Cardiovasc Surg* 1998;10:240.
55. Wareing TH, Davila-Roman VG, Barzilai B, et al. Management of the severely atherosclerotic ascending aorta during cardiac operations: a strategy for detection and treatment. *J Thorac Cardiovasc Surg* 1992;103:453.

56. Grossi EA, Kanchuger MS, Schwartz DS, et al. Effect of cannula length on aortic arch flow: protection of the atheromatous aortic arch. *Ann Thorac Surg* 1995;59:710.
57. Ribakov GH, Katz ES, Galloway AC, et al. Surgical implications of transesophageal echocardiography to grade the atheromatous aortic arch. *Ann Thorac Surg* 1992;53:758.
58. Stern A, Tunick PA, Culliford AT, et al. Aortic arch endarterectomy increases the risk of stroke during heart surgery in patients with protruding aortic arch atheromas [Abstract 1024]. *Circulation* 1997;96:I-185.
59. Byrne JG, Aranki SF, Cohn LH. Aortic valve operations under deep hypothermic circulatory arrest for the porcelain aorta: "no-touch" technique. *Ann Thorac Surg* 1998;65:1313.
60. Svensson LG, Sun J, Cruz HA, et al. Endarterectomy for calcified porcelain aorta associated with aortic valve stenosis. *Ann Thorac Surg* 1996;61:149.
61. King RC, Kanithanon RC, Shockley KS, et al. Replacing the atherosclerotic ascending aorta is a high-risk procedure. *Ann Thorac Surg* 1998;66:396.
62. Liddicoat JR, Doty JR, Stuart RS. Management of the atherosclerotic ascending aorta with endoaortic occlusion. *Ann Thorac Surg* 1998;65:1133.
63. Paul D, Hartman GS. Foley balloon occlusion of the atheromatous ascending aorta: the role of transesophageal echocardiography. *J Cardiothorac Vasc Anesth* 1998;12:61.
64. Duda AM, Letwin LB, Sutter FP, et al. Does routine use of aortic ultrasonography decrease the stroke rate in coronary artery bypass surgery? *J Vasc Surg* 1995;21:98.
65. Magner JB. Complications of aortic cannulation for open-heart surgery. *Thorax* 1971;26:172.
66. Salama FD, Blesovsky A. Complications of cannulation of the ascending aorta for open heart surgery. *Thorax* 1970;25:604.
67. Krous HF, Mansfield PB, Sauvage LR. Carotid artery hyperperfusion during open-heart surgery. *J Thorac Cardiovasc Surg* 1973;66:118.
68. Dalal FY, Patel KD. Another sign of inadvertent carotid cannulation [Letter]. *Anesthesiology* 1981;55:487.
69. Ross WT Jr, Lake CL, Wassons HA. Cardiopulmonary bypass complicated by inadvertent carotid cannulation. *Anesthesiology* 1981;54:85.
70. Watson BG. Unilateral cold neck. *Anaesthesia* 1983;38:659.
71. McLeskey CH, Cheney FW. A correctable complication of cardiopulmonary bypass. *Anesthesiology* 1982;56:214.
72. Magilligan DJ Jr, Eastland MW, Lell WA, et al. Decreased carotid flow with ascending aortic cannulation. *Circulation* 1972;45[Suppl 1]:I-130.
73. Salerno TA, Lince DP, White DN, et al. Arch versus femoral artery perfusion during cardiopulmonary bypass. *J Thorac Cardiovasc Surg* 1978;78:681.
74. Gott JP, Cohen CL, Jones EL. Management of ascending aortic dissections and aneurysms early and late following cardiac operations. *J Card Surg* 1990;5:2.
75. Still RJ, Hilgenberg AD, Akins CW, et al. Intraoperative aortic dissection. *Ann Thorac Surg* 1992;53:374.
76. Troianos CA, Savino JS, Weiss RL. Transesophageal echocardiographic diagnosis of aortic dissection during cardiac surgery. *Anesthesiology* 1991;75:149.
77. Lees MH, Herr RH, Hill JD, et al. Distribution of systemic blood flow of the rhesus monkey during cardiopulmonary bypass. *J Thorac Cardiovasc Surg* 1971;61:570.
78. McAlpine WA, Selman MW, Kawakami T. Routine use of aortic cannulation in open heart operations. *Am J Surg* 1967; 114:831.
79. Herman BE, Wallace HW, Gadboys HL, et al. Anterior crural syndrome as a complication of cardiopulmonary bypass. *J Thorac Cardiovasc Surg* 1966;52:755.
80. Hendrickson SC, Glower DD. A method for perfusion of the leg during cardiopulmonary bypass via femoral cannulation. *Ann Thorac Surg* 1998;65:1807.
81. Gates JD, Bichell DP, Rizzu RJ, et al. Thigh ischemia complicating femoral vessel cannulation for cardiopulmonary bypass. *Ann Thorac Surg* 1996;61:730.
82. Van derSalm TJ. Prevention of lower extremity ischemia during cardiopulmonary bypass via femoral cannulation. *Ann Thorac Surg* 1997;63:251.
83. Beyersdorf F, Mitrev Z, Ihnken K, et al. Controlled limb reperfusion in patients having cardiac operations. *J Thorac Cardiovasc Surg* 1996;111:873.
84. Svensson LG. Autopsies in acute Type A aortic dissection: surgical implications [Editorial comment]. *Circulation* 1998;98:II-302.
85. Bilgutay AM, Garamella JJ, Danyluk M, et al. Retrograde aortic dissection occurring during cardiopulmonary bypass. *JAMA* 1976;236:465.
86. Benedict JS, Buhl TL, Henney RP. Acute aortic dissection during cardiopulmonary bypass. *Arch Surg* 1974;108:810.
87. Carey JS, Skow JR, Scott C. Retrograde aortic dissection during cardiopulmonary bypass: "nonoperative" management. *Ann Thorac Surg* 1977;24:44.
88. Kay JH, Dykstra FC, Tsuji HK. Retrograde ilioaortic dissection: a complication of common femoral artery perfusion during open heart surgery. *Am J Surg* 1966;111:464.
89. Matar AF, Ross DN. Traumatic arterial dissection in open-heart surgery. *Thorax* 1967;22:82.
90. Galloway AC, Shemin RJ, Glower DD. et al. First report of the Port Access International Registry. *Ann Thorac Surg* 1999; 67:51.
91. Sabik JF, Lytle BW, McCarthy PM, et al. Axillary artery: an alternative site of arterial cannulation for patients with extensive and peripheral vascular disease. *J Thorac Cardiovasc Surg* 1995; 109:885.
92. Bichell DP, Balaguer JM, Aranki SF, et al. Axilloaxillary cardiopulmonary bypass: a practical alternative to femorofemoral bypass. *Ann Thorac Surg* 1997;64:702.
93. Baribeau YR, Westerbrook BM, Charlesworth DC, et al. Arterial inflow via an axillary artery graft for the severely atherosclerotic aorta. *Ann Thorac Surg* 1998;66:33.
94. Neri E, Massetti M, Capannini G, et al. Axillary artery cannulation in type A aortic dissection operations. *J Thorac Cardiovasc Surg* 1999;118:324.
95. Golding LAR. New cannulation technique for the severely calcified ascending aorta. *J Thorac Cardiovasc Surg* 1985;90: 626.
96. Coselli JS, Crawford ES. Femoral artery perfusion for cardiopulmonary bypass in patients with aortoiliac artery obstruction. *Ann Thorac Surg* 1987;43:437.
97. Mishima A, Asano M, Yonamoto S, et al. Cannulation of the supraceliac aorta for perfusion in small infants. *Ann Thorac Surg* 1999,67:874.
98. Bernstein EF, Gleason LR. Factors influencing hemolysis with roller pumps. *Surgery* 1967;61:432.
99. Uretzky G, Landsburg G, Cohn D, et al. Analysis of microembolic particles originating in extracorporeal circuits. *Perfusion* 1987;2:9.
100. Reed CC, Kurusz M, Lawrence AE. *Safety techniques in perfusion.* Stafford, TX: Quali-Med, 1988.
101. Stammers AH. Extracorporeal devices and related technologies. In: Kaplan JA, ed. *Cardiac anesthesia,* 4th ed. Philadelphia: WB Saunders Co, 1999:1018.
102. Mongero LB, Beck JR, Orr TR, et al. Clinical evaluation of setting pump occlusion by the dynamic method: effect on flow. *Perfusion* 1998;13:360.

103. Tempe DK, Khana SK. Accidental hyperperfusion during cardiopulmonary bypass: suggested safety features. *Ann Thorac Surg* 1998;65:306.
104. Kurusz M, Shaffer CW, Christman EW. Runaway pump head. *J Thorac Cardiovasc Surg* 1979;77:792.
105. Kurusz M, Christman EW, Williams EH, et al. Roller pump induced tubing wear: another argument in favor of arterial line filtration. *J Extracorp Technol* 1980;12:49.
106. Leschinsky BM, Zimin NK. Centrifugal blood pumps—a brief analysis: development of new designs. *Perfusion* 1991;6:115.
107. Kolff J, McClurken JB, Alpern JB. Beware centrifugal pumps: not a one-way street, but a dangerous siphon! *Perfusion* 1990; 5:225.
108. Moen O, Fosse E, Broten J, et al. Difference in blood activation related to roller/centrifugal pumps and heparin coated/uncoated surfaces in a cardiopulmonary bypass model circuit. *Perfusion* 1996;11:113.
109. Hoerr HR, Kraemer MF, Williams JL, et al. *In vitro* comparison of the blood handling by the constrained vortex and twin roller blood pumps. *J Extracorp Technol* 1987;19:316.
110. Tamari Y, Lee-Sensiba K, Leonard EF, et al. The effects of pressure and flow on hemolysis caused by Bio-Medicus centrifugal pumps and roller pumps: guidelines for choosing a blood pump. *J Thorac Cardiovasc Surg* 1993;106:997.
111. Wheeldon DR, Bethune DW, Gill RD. Vortex pumping for routine cardiac surgery: a comparative study. *Perfusion* 1990;5: 135.
112. Driessen JJ, Fransen G, Rondelez L, et al. Comparison of the standard roller pump and a pulsatile centrifugal pump for extracorporeal circulation during routine coronary artery bypass grafting. *Perfusion* 1991;6:303.
113. Wahba A, Philip A, Bauer MF, et al. The blood saving potential of vortex versus roller pump with and without aprotinin. *Perfusion* 1995;10:333.
114. Ashraf S, Bhattacharya K, Zachanias S, et al. Serum S100B release after coronary artery bypass grafting: roller versus centrifugal pump. *Ann Thorac Surg* 1998;66:1958.
115. Baufreton C, Intractor L, Jansen PGM, et al. Inflammatory response to cardiopulmonary bypass using roller or centrifugal pumps. *Ann Thorac Surg* 1999;67:972.
116. Ashraf S, Butler J, Tian Y, et al. Inflammatory mediators in adults undergoing cardiopulmonary bypass comparison of centrifugal and roller pump. *Ann Thorac Surg* 1998;65:480.
117. James SD, Peters J, Maresca L, et al. The roller pump does produce pulsatile flow. *J Extracorp Technol* 1987;19:376.
118. Klein M, Dauben HP, Boeken W, et al. The benefits of centrifugal pumping during open heart surgery [Abstract]. In: Utley JR, ed. *Pathophysiology and Techniques of Cardiopulmonary Bypass.* Spartanburg, SC: Cardiothoracic Research and Education Foundation, 1995:229.
119. Odom NJ, Richens D, Glenville BE, et al. Successful use of mechanical assist device for right ventricular failure after orthotopic heart transplantation. *J Heart Lung Transplant* 1990; 9:652.
120. Everts P, Schonberger JPAM, Steenbrink J, et al. Partial left heart bypass with centrifugal pump and limited anticoagulation during the resection of coarctation of the aorta. *Perfusion* 1991; 6:285.
121. Walls JT, Crutis JJ, Boley T. Sarns centrifugal pump for repair of thoracic aortic injury: case reports. *J Trauma* 1989;29:1283.
122. Hickey PR, Buckley MJ, Philbin DM. Pulsatile and non pulsatile cardiopulmonary bypass: review of a counterproductive controversy. *Ann Thorac Surg* 1983;36:720.
123. Wright G. Hemodynamic analysis could resolve the pulsatile blood flow controversy [Current review]. *Ann Thorac Surg* 1994;58:1199.
124. Wright G. Mechanical simulation of cardiac function by means of pulsatile blood pumps. *J Cardiothorac Vasc Anesth* 1997;11: 299.
125. Munoz HR, Sacco CM. Cardiac mechanical energy and effects on the arterial tree. *J Cardiothorac Vasc Anesth* 1997;11:289.
126. Hornick P, Taylor K. Pulsatile and non pulsatile perfusion: the continuing controversy. *J Cardiothorac Vasc Anesth* 1997;11: 310.
127. Adams S, Fleming J, Gourley T, et al. Clinical experience with the Sarns pulsatile pump during open-heart surgery. *Perfusion* 1986;1:53.
128. Taylor KM, Bain WH, Maxted KJ, et al. Comparative studies of pulsatile and nonpulsatile bypass: I. Pulsatile system employed and its hematologic effects. *J Thorac Cardiovasc Surg* 1978;75:569.
129. Pappas G, Winter SD, Kopriva CJ, et al. Improvement of myocardial and other vital organ functions and metabolism with a simple method of pulsatile flow (IABP) during clinical cardiopulmonary bypass. *Surgery* 1975;77:34.
130. Wright G. The hydraulic power outputs of pulsatile and nonpulsatile cardiopulmonary bypass pumps. *Perfusion* 1988;3:251.
131. Wright G. Factors affecting the pulsatile hydraulic power output of the Stockert roller pump. *Perfusion* 1989;4:187.
132. Mutch WAC, Lefevre GR, Thiessen DR, et al. Computer-controlled cardiopulmonary bypass increases jugular venous oxygen saturation during rewarming. *Ann Thorac Surg* 1998;65:59.
133. Minami K, Vyska K, Korfer K. Role of the carotid sinus in response of integrated venous system to pulsatile and nonpulsatile perfusion. *J Thorac Cardiovasc Surg* 1992;104:1639.
134. Taylor KM. The hemodynamics of cardiopulmonary bypass. *Semin Thorac Cardiovasc Surg* 1990;2:300.
135. Rees W, Schiessler A, Schulz F, et al. Pulsatile extra-corporeal circulation: fluid-mechanic considerations. *Perfusion* 1993;8: 459.
136. Gourlay T, Taylor KM. Pulsatile flow and membrane oxygenators. *Perfusion* 1994;9:189.
137. Shevde K vs. Finlayson DC. Pro and con: pulsatile flow is preferable to non-pulsatile flow during cardiopulmonary bypass. *J Cardiothorac Anesth* 1987;2:165.
138. Mangano CM, Hill L, Cartwright CR, et al. Cardiopulmonary bypass and the anesthesiologist: nonpulsatile versus pulatile perfusion. In: Kaplan JA, ed. *Cardiac anesthesia,* 4th ed. Philadelphia: WB Saunders Co, 1999;1065.
139. Minami K, Korner MM, Vyska K, et al. Effects of pulsatile perfusion on plasma catecholamine levels and hemodynamics during and after cardiac operations with cardiopulmonary bypass. *J Thorac Cardiovasc Surg* 1990;99:82.
140. Alston RP, Singh M, McLaren AD. Systemic oxygen uptake during hypothermic cardiopulmonary bypass: effects of flow rate, flow character and arterial pH. *J Thorac Cardiovasc Surg* 1989;98:757.
141. Alston RP, Murray L, McLaren AD. Changes in hemodynamic variables during hypothermic cardiopulmonary bypass: effect of flow rate, flow character and arterial pH. *J Thorac Cardiovasc Surg* 1990;100:134.
142. Shepard RA, Simpson MS, Sharp JF. Energy equivalent pressure. *Arch Surg* 1966;93:730.
143. Grossi EA, Connolly MW, Drieger KH, et al. Quantification of pulsatile flow during cardiopulmonary bypass to permit direct comparison of the effectiveness of various types of "pulsatile" and "nonpulsatile" flow. *Surgery* 1985;98:547.
144. Hindman BJ, Dexter F, Ryu K, et al. Pulsatile versus non pulsatile cardiopulmonary bypass. *Anesthesiology* 1995;82:241.
145. Cook JJ, Orszulak TA, Daly RC. The effects of pulsatile cardiopulmonary bypass on cerebral and renal blood flow in dogs. *J Cardiothorac Vasc Anesth* 1997;11:420.
146. Shaw PJ, Bates D, Cartlige NEF. Analysis of factors predispos-

ing to neurological injury in patients undergoing coronary bypass operations. *Q J Med* 1989;72:633.

147. Henze T, Stephen H, Sonntag H. Cerebral dysfunction following extracorporeal circulation for aorta coronary bypass surgery: no difference in neuropsychological outcomes after pulsatile versus non pulsatile flow. *Thorac Cardiovasc Surg* 1990;38:65.
148. Murkin JM, Martzke JS, Buchan AM, et al. A randomized study of the influence of perfusion technique and pH management strategy in 316 patients undergoing coronary artery bypass surgery: II. Neurological and cognitive outcomes. *J Thorac Cardiovasc Surg* 1995;110:349.
149. Chow G, Roberts IG, Harris D, et al. Stockert roller pump generated pulsatile flow: cerebral metabolic changes in adult cardiopulmonary bypass. *Perfusion* 1997;12:113.
150. Ohri SK, Desai JB, Gaer JAR, et al. Intra-abdominal complications after cardiopulmonary bypass. *Ann Thorac Surg* 1991;52:826.
151. Badner NH, Murkin JM, Lok P. Differences in pH management and pulsatile/nonpulsatile perfusion during cardiopulmonary bypass do not influence renal function. *Anesth Analg* 1992;75:696.
152. Louagie YA, Gonzalez M, Collard E, et al. Does flow character of cardiopulmonary bypass make a difference? *J Thorac Cardiovasc Surg* 1992;104:1628.
153. Taylor KM, Bain WH, Davidson KG, et al. Comparative clinical study of pulsatile and non-pulsatile perfusion in 350 consecutive patients. *Thorax* 1982;37:324.
154. Murkin JM, Martzke JS, Buchan AM, et al. A randomized study of the influence of perfusion technique and pH management in 316 patients undergoing coronary artery bypass surgery: I. Mortality and cardiovascular morbidity. *J Thorac Cardiovasc Surg* 1995:110:340.
155. Pearson DT. Gas exchange: bubble and membrane oxygenators. *Semin Thorac Cardiovasc Surg* 1990;2:313.
156. Blauth CI, Smith PL, Arnold JV, et al. Influence of oxygenator type on the prevalence and extent of micro-emboli retinal ischemia during cardiopulmonary bypass. *J Thorac Cardiovasc Surg* 1990;99:61.
157. Pearson DT. Blood gas control during cardiopulmonary bypass. *Perfusion* 1988;3:113.
158. Masters RG vs. Bethune DW. Pro and con: bubble oxygenators are outdated and no longer appropriate for cardiopulmonary bypass. *J Cardiothorac Anesth* 1989;3:235.
159. Peirce EC. Membrane oxygenation. In: Taylor KM, ed. *Cardiopulmonary bypass: principles and management.* Baltimore: Williams & Wilkins, 1986:177.
160. Clark RE, Beauchamp RA, Magrath, RA, et al. Comparison of bubble and membrane oxygenators with short and long term perfusions. *J Thorac Cardiovasc Surg* 1979;78:655.
161. Hessel EA II, Johnson DD, Ivey TD, et al. Membrane versus bubble oxygenator for cardiac operations. *J Thorac Cardiovasc Surg* 1980;80:111.
162. Utley JR, Leyland SA, Johnson HD, et al. Correlation of preoperative factors, severity of disease, type of oxygenator and perfusion times with mortality and morbidity of coronary bypass. *Perfusion* 1991;6:15.
163. Kirson LE, Laurnen ME, Tornbene MA. Position of oxygenators in the bypass circuit [Letter]. *J Cardiothorac Anesth* 1989;3:817.
164. Gravlee GP, Wong AA, Charles DJ. Hypoxemia during cardiopulmonary bypass from leaks in the gas supply system [Letter]. *Anesth Analg* 1985;64:649.
165. Robblee JA, Crosby E, Keon WJ. Hypoxemia after intraluminal oxygen line obstruction during cardiopulmonary bypass. *Ann Thorac Surg* 1989;48:575.
166. Kurusz M, Conti VR, Arens JF. Oxygenator failure [Letter]. *Ann Thorac Surg* 1990;49:511.
167. Blomback M, Kronlund P, Aberg B, et al. Pathologic fibrin formation and cold-induced clotting of membrane oxygenators during cardiopulmonary bypass. *J Cardiothorac Vasc Anesth* 1995;9:34.
168. Svenmarker S, Haggmark S, Jansson E, et al. The relative safety of an oxygenator. *Perfusion* 1997;12:289.
169. Jenkins OF, Morris R, Simpson JM. Australasian perfusion incident survey. *Perfusion* 1997;12:279.
170. Wahba A, Philipp A, Behr R, et al. Heparin-coated equipment reduces the risk of oxygenator failure. *Ann Thorac Surg* 1998;65:1310.
171. Fisher AR. The incidence and cause of emergency oxygenator changeovers. *Perfusion* 1999;14:207.
172. Mitchell SJ, Wilcox T, McDougal C, et al. Emboli generation by the Medtronic Maxima hardshell adult venous reservoir in cardiopulmonary bypass circuits: a preliminary report. *Perfusion* 1996;11:145.
173. Schonberger JPAM, Everts PAM, Hoffman JJ. Systemic blood activation with open and closed venous reservoirs. *Ann Thorac Surg* 1995;59:1549.
174. Orenstein JM, Sato N, Arron B, et al. Microemboli observed in deaths following cardiopulmonary bypass surgery: silicone antifoam agents and polyvinyl chloride tubing as source of emboli. *Hum Pathol* 1982;13:1082.
175. Edmunds LH Jr, Saxena NH, Hillyer P, et al. Relationship between platelet count and cardiotomy suction return. *Ann Thorac Surg* 1978;25:306.
176. Wright G, Sanderson JM. Cellular aggregation and trauma in cardiotomy suction systems. *Thorax* 1979;34:621.
177. Pearson DT. Micro-emboli: gaseous and particulate. In: Taylor KM, ed. *Cardiopulmonary bypass: principles and management.* Baltimore: Williams & Wilkins, 1986:313.
178. Brooker RF, Brown WR, Moody DM, et al. Cardiotomy suction: a major source of brain lipid emboli during cardiopulmonary bypass. *Ann Thorac Surg* 1998;65:1651.
179. Pearson DT, Watson BG, Waterhouse PS. An ultrasonic analysis of the comparative efficiency of various cardiotomy reservoirs and micropore blood filters. *Thorax* 1978;33:352.
180. de Jong JCF, ten Duis HJ, Sibinga CT. Hematologic aspects of cardiotomy suction in cardiac operations. *J Thorac Cardiovasc Surg* 1980;79:227.
181. Boonstra PW, van Imhoff GW, Eysman L, et al. Reduced platelet activation and improved hemostasis after controlled cardiotomy suction during clinical membrane oxygenator perfusions. *J Thorac Cardiovasc Surg* 1985;89:900.
182. Hirose T, Burman SD, O'Connor RA. Reduction of perfusion hemolysis by use of atraumatic low pressure suction. *J Thorac Cardiovasc Surg* 1964;47:242.
183. Wielgorski JR, Cross DE, Nwadike EVD. The effects of subatmospheric pressure on the hemolysis of blood. *J Biomech* 1975;8:321.
184. Geissler HJ, Allen JS, Mehlhorn U, et al. Cooling gradients and formation of gaseous microemboli with cardiopulmonary bypass: an echocardiographic study. *Ann Thorac Surg* 1997;64:100.
185. Butler BD, Kurusz M. Gaseous microemboli: a review. *Perfusion* 1990;5:81.
186. Taylor RL, Borger MA, Weisel RD, et al. Cerebral microemboli during cardiopulmonary bypass: increased emboli during perfusionist interventions. *Ann Thorac Surg* 1999;68:89.
187. Griffin S, Pugsley W, Treasure T. Microembolism during cardiopulmonary bypass: a comparison of bubble oxygenator with arterial line filter and membrane oxygenator alone. *Perfusion* 1991;6:99.

188. Liu J-F, Su Z-F, Ding W-X. Quantitation of particle microemboli during cardiopulmonary bypass: experimental and clinical studies. *Ann Thorac Surg* 1992;54:1196.
189. Wright G, Furness A, Haigh S. Integral pulse frequency modulated ultrasound for the detection and quantification of gas microbubbles in flowing blood. *Perfusion* 1987;2:131.
190. Padayachee TS, Parsons S, Theobold R, et al. The effect of arterial filtration on reduction of gaseous microemboli in the middle cerebral artery during cardiopulmonary bypass. *Ann Thorac Surg* 1988;45:647.
191. Pugsley WD. The use of Doppler ultrasound in the assessment of microemboli during cardiac surgery. *Perfusion* 1989;4:115.
192. van der Linden J, Casimir-Ahn H. When do cerebral emboli appear during open heart operations? A transcranial Doppler study. *Ann Thorac Surg* 1991;51:237.
193. Ringelstein EB, Droste DW, Babikian VL, et al. Consensus on microembolus detection by TCD. *Stroke* 1998;29:725.
194. Allardyce DB, Yoshida SH, Ashmore PG. The importance of microembolism in the pathogenesis of organ dysfunction caused by prolonged use of the pump oxygenator. *J Thorac Cardiovasc Surg* 1966;52:706.
195. Nussmeier NA, Fish KJ. Neuropsychologic dysfunction after cardiopulmonary bypass: a comparison of two institutions. *J Cardiothorac Vasc Anesth* 1991;5:584.
196. Brennan RW, Patterson RH Jr, Kessler J. Cerebral blood flow and metabolism during cardiopulmonary bypass: evidence of microembolic encephalopathy. *Neurology* 1971;21:665.
197. Patterson RH Jr, Wasser JS, Porro RS. The effect of various filters on microembolic cerebrovascular blockade following cardiopulmonary bypass. *Ann Thorac Surg* 1974;17:464.
198. Taylor KM, Devlin BJ, Mittra SM, et al. Assessment of cerebral damage during open heart surgery: a new experimental model. *Scand J Thorac Cardiovasc Surg* 1980;14:197.
199. Berman L, Marin F. Micropore filtration during cardiopulmonary bypass. In: Taylor KM, ed. *Cardiopulmonary bypass: principles and management.* Baltimore: Williams & Wilkins, 1986: 355.
200. Marshall L. Filtration in cardiopulmonary bypass: past, present and future. *Perfusion* 1988;3:135.
201. Joffe D, Silvay G. The use of microfilters in cardiopulmonary bypass. *J Cardiothorac Vasc Anesth* 1994;8:685.
202. Solis RT, Horak J. Evaluation of a new cardiotomy blood filter. *Ann Thorac Surg* 1979;28:487.
203. Ware JA, Scott MA, Horak JK, et al. Platelet aggregation during and after cardiopulmonary bypass: effect of two different cardiotomy filters. *Ann Thorac Surg* 1982;34:204.
204. Gourlay T, Gibbons TG, Fleming J, et al. Evaluation of a range of arterial line filters: part I. *Perfusion* 1987;2:297.
205. Gourlay T, Gibbons M, Taylor KM. Evaluation of a range of arterial line filters: part II. *Perfusion* 1988;3:29.
206. Gourlay T. The role of arterial line filters in perfusion safety. *Perfusion* 1988;3:195.
207. Silvay G, Ammar T, Reich DL, et al. Cardiopulmonary bypass for adult patients: a survey of equipment and techniques. *J Cardiothorac Vasc Anesth* 1995;9:420.
208. Munsch C, Rosenfeldt F, Chang V. Absence of particle-induced coronary vasoconstriction during cardioplegic infusion: is it desirable to use a microfilter in the infusion line? *J Thorac Cardiovasc Surg* 1991;101:473.
209. Muraoka R, Yokota M, Aoshima M, et al. Subclinical changes in brain morphology following cardiac operations as reflected by computed tomographic scans of the brain. *J Thorac Cardiovasc Surg* 1981;81:364.
210. Henriksen L, Hjelms E. Cerebral blood flow during cardiopulmonary bypass in man: effect of arterial filtration. *Thorax* 1986; 41:386.
211. Aberg T, Kihlgren M. Cerebral protection during open heart surgery. *Thorax* 1977;32:525.
212. Branthwaite MA. Prevention of neurological damage during open-heart surgery. *Thorax* 1975;30:258.
213. Hill JD, Osborn JJ, Swank RL, et al. Experience using a new Dacron wool filter during extracorporeal circulation. *Arch Surg* 1970;101:649.
214. Skagseth E, Froysaker T, Refsum SB. Disposable filter for microemboli in cardiopulmonary bypass. *J Cardiovasc Surg* 1974; 15:318.
215. Garvey JW, Willner A, Wolpowitz A, et al. The effect of arterial filtration during open heart surgery on cerebral function. *Circulation* 1983;64[Suppl 2]:2.
216. Aris A, Solanes H, Camara ML, et al. Arterial line filtration during cardiopulmonary bypass. *J Thorac Cardiovasc Surg* 1986; 91:526.
217. Loop F. Cleveland Clinic Foundation, Cleveland, OH. Personal communication, 1971.
218. Mossing KA. Post cardiotomy delirium and microfiltration [Master of Arts Dissertation]. University of Washington, 1975.
219. Pugsley W, Klinger L, Paschalie C, et al. The impact of microemboli during cardiopulmonary bypass on neurological functioning. *Stroke* 1994;25:1393.
220. Sylivris S, Levi C, Matalanis G, et al. Pattern and significance of cerebral microemboli during coronary artery bypass grafting. *Ann Thorac Surg* 1998;66:1674.
221. Grocott HP, Croughwell ND, Amory DW, et al. Cerebral emboli and serum S-100-B during cardiac operation. *Ann Thorac Surg* 1998;65:1645.
222. Aldea GS, O'Gara P, Shapira OM, et al. Effects of anticoagulation protocol on outcome in patients undergoing CABG with heparin-bonded cardiopulmonary bypass circuits. *Ann Thorac Surg* 1998;65:425.
223. Milsom FP, Mitchell SJ. A dual-vent left heart de-airing technique markedly reduces carotid artery microemboli. *Ann Thorac Surg* 1998;66:785.
224. Clark RE, Brillman J, Davis DA, et al. Microemboli during coronary artery bypass grafting: genesis and effect on outcome. *J Thorac Cardiovasc Surg* 1995;109:249.
225. Morioka K, Muraoka R, Chiba Y, et al. Leukocyte and platelet depletion with a blood separator: effects on lung injury after cardiac surgery with cardiopulmonay bypass. *J Thorac Cardiovasc Surg* 1996;111:45.
226. Chiba Y, Morioka K, Muraoka R, et al. Effect of depletion of leukocytes and platelets on cardiac dysfunction after cardiopulmonary bypass. *Ann Thorac Surg* 1998;65:107.
227. Lazar HL, Zhang X, Hamasaki T, et al. Role of leukocyte depletion during cardiopulmonary bypass and cardioplegic arrest. *Ann Thorac Surg* 1995;60:1745.
228. Hurst T, Johnson D, Cujec B, et al. Depletion of activated neutrophils by a filter during cardiac valve surgery. *Can J Anaesth* 1997;44:131.
229. Baksaas ST, Videm V, Mollnes TE, et al. Leukocyte filtration during cardiopulmonary bypass hardly changed leukocyte counts and did not influence myeloperoxidase, complement, cytokinin or platelets. *Perfusion* 1998;13:429.
230. Gu YJ, deVries AJ, Voa P, et al. Leukocyte depletion during cardiac operations: a new approach through the venous bypass circuit. *Ann Thorac Surg* 1999;67:604.
231. Suzuki I, Ogoshi N, Chiba M, et al. Clinical evaluation of a leukocyte-depleting blood cardioplegia filter (BCIB) for elective open-heart surgery. *Perfusion* 1998;13:205.
232. Gu YJ, deVries AJ, Boonstra PW, et al. Leukocyte depletion results in improved lung function and reduced inflammatory response after cardiac surgery. *J Thorac Cardiovasc Surg* 1996; 112:494.
233. Gott JP, Cooper WA, Schmidt FE, et al. Modifying risk for

extracorporeal circulation: trial of four anti-inflammatory strategies. *Ann Thorac Surg* 1998;66:747.
234. Stammers AH. Advances in myocardial protection: the role of mechanical devices in providing cardioprotective strategies. *Int Anesthesiol Clin* 1996;34:61.
235. Chitwood WR Jr. Retrograde cardioplegia: current methods. *Ann Thorac Surg* 1992;53:352.
236. Honkonen EL, Kaukinen L, Pehkoneu EJ, et al. Myocardial cooling and right ventricular function in patients with right coronary artery disease: antegrade vs. retrograde cardioplegia. *Acta Anaesthesiol Scand* 1997;41:287.
237. Aldea GS, Connelly G, Fonger JD, et al. Directed atraumatic coronary sinus cannulation for retrograde cardioplegia administration. *Ann Thorac Surg* 1992;54:789.
238. Clements F, Wright SJ, deBruijn N. Coronary sinus catheterization made easy for port-access minimally invasive cardiac surgery. *J Cardiothorac Vasc Anesth* 1998;12:96.
239. Panos AL, Ali IS, Birnbaum PL, et al. Coronary sinus injuries during retrograde continuous normothermic blood cardioplegia. *Ann Thorac Surg* 1992;54:1132.
240. Ikonomidis JS, Yau IM, Weisel RD,. et al. Optimal flow rates for retrograde warm cardioplegia. *J Thorac Cardiovasc Surg.* 1994;107:510.
241. Baile EM, Ling IT, Heyworth JR, et al. Bronchopulmonary anastomotic and noncoronary collateral blood flow in humans during cardiopulmonary bypass. *Chest* 1985;87:749.
242. Killen DA, Piehler JM, Borkon AM, et al. Occult patent ductus arteriosus encountered during coronary artery bypass procedures [Letter]. *J Thorac Cardiovasc Surg* 1994;108:588.
243. Tunick PA, Kronzon I. Diagnoses of patent ductus arteriosus by serendipity in the adult. *J Am Soc Echocardiogr* 1988;1:446.
244. Amir IM, Maranets I, Barash P. Transesophageal echocardiography of the distal aortic arch. *J Cardiothorac Vasc Anesth* 1998; 12:599.
245. Arom KV, Vinas JF, Fewel JE, et al. Is the left ventricular vent necessary during cardiopulmonary bypass? *Ann Thorac Surg* 1977;24:566.
246. Burton NA, Graeber GM, Zajtchuk R. An alternate method of ventricular venting—the pulmonary artery sump. *Chest* 1984; 85:814.
247. Breyer RN, Meredith JW, Mills SA, et al. Is a left ventricular vent necessary for coronary artery bypass procedures performed with cardioplegia arrest? *J Thorac Cardiovasc Surg* 1983;86:338.
248. Buckberg GD. The importance of venting the left ventricle [Editorial]. *Ann Thorac Surg* 1975;20:488.
249. Najafi H, Javid H, Golding MD, et al. Aortic valve replacement without left heart decompression. *Ann Thorac Surg* 1976;21: 131.
250. Salerno TA, Charrette EJP. Elimination of venting in coronary artery surgery. *Ann Thorac Surg* 1979;27:340.
251. Kanter KR, Schaff HV, Gott VL. Reduced oxygen consumption with effective left ventricular venting during postischemic reperfusion. *Circulation* 1982;66[Suppl 1]:1.
252. Olinger GM, Bonchek LI. Ventricular venting during coronary revascularization: assessment of benefit by intraoperative ventricular function curves. *Ann Thorac Surg* 1978;26:525.
253. Salomon NW, Copeland JG. Single catheter technique for cardioplegia and venting during coronary artery bypass grafting. *Ann Thorac Surg* 1980;29:88.
254. Little AG, Lin CY, Wernley JA, et al. Use of the pulmonary artery for left ventricular venting during cardiac operations. *J Thorac Cardiovasc Surg* 1984;87:532.
255. Roach GW, Bellow WH. Left ventricular distention during pulmonary artery venting in a patient undergoing coronary artery bypass surgery. *Anesthesiology* 1992;76:655.
256. Casha AR. A simple method of aortic root venting for CABG [Letter]. *Ann Thorac Surg* 1998;66:608.
257. Victor S, Kobeer M. Venting and de-airing without a roller pump [Letter]. *Ann Thorac Surg* 1993;55:807.
258. Robicsek F, Duncan GD. Retrograde air embolization in coronary operations. *J Thorac Cardiovasc Surg* 1987;94:110.
259. Weesner KM, Byrum C, Rosenthal A. Left ventricular aneurysms associated with intraoperative venting of the cardiac apex in children. *Am Heart J* 1981;101:622.
260. Marco JD, Barner HB. Aortic venting: comparison of vent effectiveness. *J Thorac Cardiovasc Surg* 1977;73:287.
261. Brenner WI, Wallsh E, Spencer FC. Aortic vent efficiency: a quantitative evaluation. *J Thorac Cardiovasc Surg* 1971;61:258.
262. Gundry SR. Facile left ventricular de-airing by administration of cardioplegia into the left ventricular vent. *Ann Thorac Surg* 1998;66:2117.
263. Journois D, Israel-Biet E, Pouard P, et al. High volume, zero-balance hemofiltration to reduce delayed inflammatory response to cardiopulmonary bypass in children. *Anesthesiology* 1996;85: 965.
264. Boldt J, Zickmann B, Fedderson B, et al. Six different hemofiltration devices for blood conservation in cardiac surgery. *Ann Thorac Surg* 1991;51:747.
265. Despotis GJ, Levine V, Filosk S, et al. Hemofiltration during cardiopulmonary bypass: effect on anti-Xa and anti-IIa heparin activity. *Anesth Analg* 1997;84:479.
266. High KM, Williams DR, Kurusz M. Cardiopulmonary bypass circuits and design. In: Hensley FA Jr, Martin DE, eds. *A practical approach to cardiac anesthesia,* 2nd ed. Boston: Little, Brown, 1995:465.
267. Bando K, Turreutine MW, Vijay P, et al. The effect of modified ultrafiltration in high-risk patients undergoing operations for congenital heart disease. *Ann Thorac Surg* 1999;66:821.
268. Hennein HA, Kiziltepe U, Barst S, et al. Veno venous modified ultrafiltration after cardiopulmonary bypass in children: a prospective randomized study. *J Thorac Cardiovasc Surg* 1999;117: 496.
269. Darling E, Nanry K, Shearer I, et al. Techniques of paediatric modified ultrafiltration. *Perfusion* 1998;13:93.
270. Groom RC, Aki BF, Albus RA, et al. Alternative method of ultrafiltration after cardiopulmonary bypass. *Ann Thorac Surg* 1994;58:573.
271. Sutton RG. Renal considerations, dialysis, and ultrafiltration during cardiopulmonary bypass. *Intern Anesth Clin* 1996;34: 165.
272. Naik S, Elliott M. Ultrafiltration. In: Jonas RA, Elliott MJ. *Cardiopulmonary bypass in neonates, infants and young children.* Boston: Butterworth Henemann, 1994:158.
273. Portela FA, Densado A, Sanchez A, et al. A simple technique to perform combined ultrafiltration. *Ann Thorac Surg* 1999;67: 859.
274. Baraka A, Barody M, Harous S, et al. Continuous venous oximetry during cardiopulmonary bypass: influence of temperature changes, perfusion flow and hematocrit level. *J Cardiothorac Anesth* 1990;4:35.
275. Swan H, Sanchez M, Tyndall M, et al. Quality control of perfusion: monitoring venous blood oxygen tension to prevent hypoxic acidosis. *J Thorac Cardiovasc Surg* 1990;99:868.
276. Willford DC, Hill EP, Moores WY. Theoretical analysis of oxygen transport during hypothermia. *J Clin Monit* 1986;2:30.
277. London MJ vs. D'Ambra MN, Philbin DM. Pro and con: colloids should be added to the pump prime. *J Cardiothorac Anesth* 1990;4:401.
278. Marelli D, Paul A, Samson R, et al. Does the addition of albumen to the prime solution in cardiopulmonary bypass affect clinical outcome? *J Thorac Cardiovasc Surg* 1989;98:751.

279. McKnight CK, Elliott MJ, Holden MP, et al. The cardiopulmonary bypass pump priming fluid and nitrogen balance after open heart surgery in adults. *Perfusion* 1986;1:47.
280. Kongsgaard UE, Smith-Erichsenn L, Geiran O, et al. Changes in the plasma protease systems during open-heart surgery with dextran vs. Ringer's acetate as priming solution. *Scand J Cardiovasc Surg* 1989;23:253.
281. Bosner RS, Dave JR, Davies ET, et al. Reduction of complement activation during bypass by prime manipulation. *Ann Thorac Surg* 1990;49:279.
282. McKnight CK, Elliott MJ, Pearson DT, et al. The effect of four different crystalloid bypass pump priming fluids upon the metabolic response to cardiac operations. *J Thorac Cardiovasc Surg* 1985;90:97.
283. Lanier WL. Glucose management during cardiopulmonary bypass: cardiovascular and neurologic implications. *Anesth Analg* 1991;72:423.
284. Metz S, Keats AS. Benefits of a glucose containing priming solution for cardiopulmonary bypass. *Anesth Analg* 1991;72:428.
285. Uppal R, Mills NL, Wechsler AS, et al. 1993 Update: left thoracotomy for reoperative coronary artery bypass procedures. *Ann Thorac Surg* 1993;55:1575.
286. Cohn LH. Update of right thoracotomy, femoro-femoral bypass, and deep hypothermia for re-replacement of mitral valve. *Ann Thorac Surg* 1997;64:578.
287. Ireland KW, Follette DM, Iguidbashian J, et al. Use of a heat exchanger to prevent hypothermia during thoracic and thoracoabdominal aneurysm repairs. *Ann Thorac Surg* 1993;55:534.
288. O'Connor CJ, Rothenberg DM. Anesthetic considerations for descending thoracic aortic surgery: part II. *J Cardiothorac Vasc Anesth* 1995;9:734.
289. Westaby S, Katsumata T. Proximal aortic perfusion for complex arch and descending aortic disease. *J Thorac Cardiovasc Surg* 1998;115:162.
290. Sasaguri S, Fukuda T, Yamamoto T, et al. Transapical aortic occlusion for cardioplegic delivery during reconstruction of thoracoabdominal aortic aneurysm with deep hypothermic circulatory arrest. *J Thorac Cardiovasc Surg* 1999;117:186.
291. Hedlund KD, Dattilo R. Supportive angioplasty [Letter]. *Perfusion* 1990;5:297.
292. von Segesser LK, Weiss BM, Garcia E, et al. Clinical application of heparin-coated perfusion equipment with special emphasis on patients refusing homologous transfusions. *Perfusion* 1991; 6:227.
293. Hanson EL, Lehr JL, Stetz CW, et al. Retrograde aortic perfusion by partial cardiopulmonary bypass: effect of mixing on measured arterial oxygen tension. *Arch Surg* 1975;110:86.
294. Taylor KM, ed. 1997 Hammersmith Perfusion Workshop: Perfusion techniques for minimally invasive cardiac surgery. *Perfusion* 1998;13:225.
295. Siegel LC, StGoar FG, Stevens JH, et al. Monitoring considerations for Port-Access cardiac surgery. *Circulation* 1997;96:562.
296. Grocott HP, Smith MS, Glower DD, et al. Endovascular aortic balloon clamp malposition during minimally invasive cardiac surgery: detection by transcranial Doppler monitoring. *Anesthesiology* 1998;88:1396.
297. Higami T, Kozawa S, Asada T, et al. Retrograde cerebral perfusion versus selective cerebral perfusion as evaluated by cerebral oxygen saturation during aortic arch reconstruction. *Ann Thorac Surg* 1999;67:1091.
298. Kazui T, Kimura N, Yamada O, et al. Surgical outcome of aortic arch aneurysms using selective cerebral perfusion. *Ann Thorac Surg* 1994;57:904.
299. Ohmi M, Tabayashi K, Hata M, et al. Brain damage after aortic arch repair using selective cerebral perfusion. *Ann Thorac Surg* 1998;66:1250.
300. Griepp RB. Strategies for cerebral protection during aortic aneurysm surgery. In: Kawashima Y, Takamoto S, eds. *Brain protection in aortic surgery.* New York: Elsevier Science BV, 1997: 127.
301. Bachet J, Guilmet D, Goudot B, et al. Cold cerebroplegia: a new technique of cerebral protection during operations on the transverse aortic arch. *J Thorac Cardiovasc Surg* 1991;102:85.
302. Bachet J, Guilmet D, Banfi C, et al. Surgery of aortic arch aneurysm with cold blood antegrade cerebroplegia. In: Kawashima Y, Tokamoto S, eds. *Brain protection in aortic surgery.* New York: Elsevier Science BV, 1997:139.
303. Alamanni F, Agrifoglio M, Pompilio G, et al. Aortic arch surgery: pros and cons of selective cerebral perfusion. A multivariable analysis for cerebral injury during hypothermic circulatory arrest. *J Cardiovasc Surg* 1995;36:31.
304. Tanaka H, Kazui T, Sato H, et al. Experimental study on the optimal flow rate and pressure for selective cerebral perfusion. *Ann Thorac Surg* 1995;59:651.
305. Coselli JS. Retrograde cerebral perfusion is an effective means of neural support during deep hypothermic circulatory arrest. *Ann Thorac Surg* 1997;64:908.
306. Lytle BW, McCarthy PM, Meaneu KM, et al. Systemic hypothermia and circulatory arrest combined with arterial perfusion of the superior vena cava. *J Thorac Cardiovasc Surg* 1995;109: 738.
307. Usui A, Abe T, Murase M. Early clinical results of retrograde cerebral perfusion for aortic arch operations in Japan. *Ann Thorac Surg* 1996;62:94.
308. Lin PJ, Chang GH, Tan PPC, et al. Prolonged circulatory arrest in moderate hypothermia with retrograde cerebral perfusion: Is brain ischemic? *Circulation* 1996;95[Suppl II]:II-166.
309. Raskin SA, Fuselier VW, Reeves-Viets JL, et al. Deep hypothermic circulatory arrest with and without retrograde cerebral perfusion. *Intern Anesth Clin* 1996;34:177.
310. Coselli JS, LeMaire SA. Experience with retrograde cerebral perfusion during proximal aortic surgery in 290 patients. *J Card Surg* 1997;12:322.
311. Safi HJ, Letson GV, Illiopoulous DC, et al. Impact of retrograde cerebral perfusion on ascending aorta and arch aneurysm repair. *Ann Thorac Surg* 1997;63:1601.
312. Moshkovitz Y, David TE, Caleb M, et al. Circulatory arrest under moderate systemic hypothermia and cold retrograde cerebral perfusion. *Ann Thorac Surg* 1998;66:1179.
313. Okita Y, Takamota S, Ando M, et al. Mortality and cerebral outcome in patients who underwent aortic arch operations using deep hypothermic circulatory arrest with retrograde cerebral perfusion: no relation of early death, stroke, delirium to the duration of circulatory arrest. *J Thorac Cardiovasc Surg* 1998; 115:129.
314. Griepp RP, Juvoneu T, Griepp EB, et al. Is retrograde cerebral perfusion an effective means of neural support during deep hypothermic circulatory arrest? *Ann Thorac Surg* 1997;64:913.
315. Murkin JM. Retrograde cerebral perfusion: is the brain really being perfused? [Editorial]. *J Cardiothorac Vasc Anesth* 1998; 12:249.
316. Wong CH, Bonser RS. Retrograde cerebral perfusion: clinical and experimental aspects. *Perfusion* 1999;14:247.
317. Ganzel BL, Edmonds HL Jr, Pank JR, et al. Neurophysiologic monitoring to assure delivery of retrograde cerebral perfusion. *J Thorac Cardiovasc Surg* 1997;113:748.
318. Usui K, Oohara K, Liu T-L, et al. Determination of optimal retrograde cerebral perfusion conditions. *J Thorac Cardiovasc Surg* 1994;107:300.
319. Okamoto H, Sato K, Matsuura A, et al. Selective jugular cannu-

lation for safer retrograde cerebral perfusion. *Ann Thorac Surg* 1993;55:538.

320. McLoughlin TM Jr, Carter WR Jr, King CD. Continuous retrograde cerebral perfusion as an adjunct to brain protection during deep hypothermic systemic circulatory arrest. *J Cardiothorac Vasc Anesth* 1995;9:205.
321. DeBrux J-L, Subayi J-B, Pegis J-D, et al. Retrograde cerebral perfusion: anatomic study of the distribution of blood to the brain. *Ann Thorac Surg* 1995;60:1294.
322. Juvonen T, Weisz DJ, Wolfe D, et al. Can retrograde perfusion mitigate cerebral injury after particulate embolization? A study in a chronic porcine model. *J Thorac Cardiovac Surg* 1998;115: 1142.
323. Juvonen T, Zhang N, Wolfe D, et al. Retrograde cerebral perfusion enhances cerebral protection during prolonged hypothermic circulatory arrest: a study in a chronic porcine model. *Ann Thorac Surg* 1998;66:38.
324. Kouchoukos NT. Adjuncts to reduce the incidence of embolic brain injury during operations on the aortic arch. *Ann Thorac Surg* 1994;57:243.
325. Katz MG, Khazin V, Steinmetz A, et al. Distribution of cerebral flow using retrograde versus antegrade cerebral perfusion. *Ann Thorac Surg* 1999;97:1065.
326. Cheung AT, Bavaria JE, Weiss SJ, et al. Neurophysiologic effects of retrograde cerebral perfusion used for aortic reconstruction. *J Cardiothorac Vasc Anesth* 1998;12:252.
327. Safi HT, Illiopoulos DC, Gopinath SP, et al. Retrograde cerebral perfusion during profound hypothermia and circulatory arrest in pigs. *Ann Thorac Surg* 1995;59:1107.
328. Ye J, Ryner LN, Kozlowski P, et al. Retrograde cerebral perfusion results in flow distribution abnormalities and neuronal damage. *Circulation* 1998;98:II-313.
329. Gravlee GP. Heparin-coated cardiopulmonary bypass circuits. *J Cardiothorac Vasc Anesth* 1994;8:213.
330. Miller BE, Levy JH. Inflammatory response to cardiopulmonary bypass. *J Cardiothorac Vasc Anesth* 1997;11:355.
331. Shore-Lesserson L. Pro: heparin-bonded circuits represents a desirable option for cardiopulmonary bypass. *J Cardiothorac Vasc Anesth* 1998;12:705.
332. Ranucci M, Mozzucco A, Pessotto R, et al. Heparin-coated circuits for high-risk patients: a multi-center prospective randomized trial. *Ann Thorac Surg* 1999;67:994.
333. Videm V, Mollnes TE, Fosse E. et al. Heparin-coated cardiopulmonary bypass equipment: I. Biocompatability markers and development of complications in a high risk population. *J Thorac Cardiovasc Surg* 1999;117:794.
334. Ovrum E, Mollnes TE, Fosse E, et al. High and low heparin dose with heparin-coated cardiopulmonary bypass: activation of complement and granulocytes. *Ann Thorac Surg* 1995;60: 1755.
335. Woolf RL, Mythen MG. Con: heparin-bonded cardiopulmonary bypass circuits do not represent a desirable and cost-effective advance in cardiopulmonary bypass technology. *J Cardiothorac Vasc Anesth* 1998;12:710.
336. Aldea GS, Doursounian M, O'Gara P, et al. Heparin-bonded circuits with a reduced anticoagulation protocol in primary CABG: a prospective randomized study. *Ann Thorac Surg* 1996; 62:410.
337. VonSegesser LK, Weiss BM, Dasic M, et al. Risk and benefit of low systemic heparinization during open heart operations. *Ann Thorac Surg* 1994;58:391.
338. Cheung AT, Levin SK, Weiss SJ, et al. Intracardiac thrombosis: a risk of incomplete anticoagulation for cardiac operations. *Ann Thorac Surg* 1994;58:541.
339. Edmunds LH Jr. Surface-bound heparin: panacea or peril [Editorial]. *Ann Thorac Surg* 1994;58:285.
340. Muehrcke DD, McCarthy PM, Stewart RW, et al. Complications of extracorporeal life support systems using heparin-bound surfaces: the risk of intracardiac clot formation. *J Thorac Cardiovasc Surg* 1995;110:843.
341. Bannan S, Danby A, Cowan D, et al. Low heparinization with heparin-bonded bypass circuits: is it a safe strategy? *Ann Thorac Surg* 1997;63:663.
342. Kuitunen AH, Heikkila LJ, Salmenpera MT. Cardio-pulmonary bypass with heparin-coated circuits and reduced systemic heparinization. *Ann Thorac Surg* 1997;63:438.
343. Mahoney CB. Heparin-bonded circuits: clinical outcome and costs. *Perfusion* 1998;13:1892.
344. Wildevuur CRH, Jansen DGM, Bezemer PD, et al. Clinical evaluation of Duraflo II heparin treated extrcorporeal circuits. *Eur J Cardiothorac Surg* 1997;11:616.
345. McCarthy PM, Yared J-PP, Foster RC, et al. A prospective randomized trial of Duraflow II heparin-coated circuits in cardiac reoperations. *Ann Thorac Surg* 1999;67:1268.
346. Gu YJ, Boonstra PW, Rijnsburger AA, et al. Cardiopulmonary bypass circuit treated with surface-modifying additives: a clinical evaluation of blood compatibility. *Ann Thorac Surg* 1998;65: 1343.
347. Rubens FS, Labow RS, Lavalee GR, et al. Hematologic evaluation of cardiopulmonary bypass circuits prepared with a novel block copolymer. *Ann Thorac Surg* 1999;67:689.
348. Jonas RA, Elliott MJ. *Cardiopulmonary bypass in neonates, infants and young children.* Boston: Butterworth-Heinemann, 1994.
349. Groom RC, Aki BF, Albus R, et al. Pediatric cardiopulmonary bypass: A review of current practice. *Intern Anesth Clin* 1996; 34;141.
350. Davies LK. Cardiopulmonary bypass in infants and children: how is it different [Review article]. *J Cardiothorac Vasc Anesth* 1999;13:330.
351. Elliott MJ. Recent advances in pediatric cardiopulmonary bypass. *Perfusion* 1999;14:337.
352. Wada J, Hino T, Kaisuka H, et al. Automatic regulation of the cardiopulmonary bypass. *Perfusion* 1986;1:117.
353. Wabeke E, Mook PH, et al. An automatically regulated low prime heart-lung machine for infants: a rabbit model. *Perfusion* 1987;2:109.
354. Beppu T, Imai Y, Fukui Y. A computerized control system for cardiopulmonary bypass. *J Thorac Cardiovasc Surg* 1995;109: 428.
355. Stammers AH. Monitoring controversies during cardiopulmonary bypass: how far have we come? *Perfusion* 1998;13:35.
356. Justison GA, Parsons S. Improved quality control utilizing continuous blood gas monitoring and computerized perfusion systems. In: *Proceedings of the 27th International Conference of the American Society of Extracorporeal Technology,* 1989:83.
357. Philbin DM, Inada E, Sims N, et al. Oxygen consumption and on-line blood gas determinations during rewarming on cardiopulmonary bypass. *Perfusion* 1987;2:127.
358. Rubsamen DS. Continuous blood gas monitoring during cardiopulmonary bypass: how soon will it be the standard of care? [Editorial]. *J Cardiothorac Anesth* 1990;4:1.
359. Mark JB, Fitzgerald D, Fenton T, et al. Continuous arterial and venous blood gas monitoring during cardiopulmonary bypass. *J Thorac Cardiovasc Surg* 1991;102:431.
360. McDaniel LB, Zwischenberger JM, Vertrees RA, et al. Mixed venous oxygen saturation during cardiopulmonary bypass poorly predicts regional venous saturation. *Anesth Analg* 1994; 80:466.
361. Bashein G, Greydanus WK, Kenny MA. Evaluation of a blood gas and chemistry monitor for use during surgery. *Anesthesiology* 1989;70:123.

362. Nicolson SC, Jobes DR, Steven JM, et al. Evaluation of a user-operative patient-site blood gas and chemistry monitor in children undergoing cardiac surgery. *J Cardiothorac Anesth* 1989; 3:741.
363. Kent AP, Tarr JT, Fox MA. Where to sample during cardiopulmonary bypass [Letter]. *J Cardiothorac Anesth* 1989;3:136.
364. Delius RF, Montoya JP, Merz SJ, et al. A new method for describing the performance of cardiac surgery cannulas. *Ann Thorac Surg* 1992;33:278.
365. Akers T, Bolen G, Gonez J, et al. *In vitro* comparison of ECC blood flow measurement techniques. Proceedings, 28th International Conference. *J ExtraCorp Technol* 1990;17.
365b. Kirson LE, Goldman JM. A system for monitoring the delivery of ventilating gas to the oxygenator during cardiopulmonary bypass. *J Cardiothorac Vasc Anesth* 1994;8:51.
366. O'Leary MJ, MacDonnell SP, Ferguson CN. Oxygenator exhaust capnography as an index of arterial carbon dioxide during cardiopulmonary bypass using a membrane oxygenator. *Br J Anaesth* 1999;82:843.
367. Moisa RB, et al. Aortic regurgitation in coronary artery bypass grafting: implication for cardioplegia administration. *Ann Thorac Surg* 1995;60:665.
369. Yamada E, Matsumura M, Kimura S. et al. Usefulness of transesophageal echocardiography in detecting changes in flow dynamics responsible for malperfusion phenomena observed during surgery of aortic dissection. *Am J Cardiol* 1997;79:1149.
370. Orihashi K, Matsuura Y, Hamanaka Y, et al. Retained intracardiac air in open heart operations examined by transesophageal echocardiography. *Ann Thorac Surg* 1993;55:1467.
371. Tingleff J, Joyce FS, Pettersson G. Intraoperative echocardiographic study of air embolism during cardiac operations. *Ann Thorac Surg* 1995;60:673.
372. Berg E, Knudsen N. Automatic data collection for cardiopulmonary bypass. *Perfusion* 1988;3:263.
373. Gourlay T. Computers in perfusion practice. *Perfusion* 1987;2: 79.
374. Taylor KM, ed. Proceedings of 1996 Hammersmith Perfusion Workshop: safety, standards and education. *Perfusion* 1997;12: 217.
375. Palanzo DA. Perfusion safety: past present and future. *J Cardiothorac Vasc Anesth* 1997;11:383.
376. Kurusz M. Lessons from perfusion surveys. *Perfusion* 1997;12: 221.
377. Kurusz M, Wheeldon DR. Perfusion safety. *Perfusion* 1988;3: 97.
378. Kurusz M, Wheeldon DR. Risk containment during cardiopulmonary bypass. *Semin Thorac Cardiovasc Surg* 1990;2:400.
379. Wheeldon DR. Safety during cardiopulmonary bypass. In: Taylor KM, ed. *Cardiopulmonary bypass: principles and management.* Baltimore: Williams & Wilkins, 1986:398.
379b. Mejak BL, Stammers A, Rauch E, et al. A retrospective study on perfusion incidents and safety devices. *Perfusion* 2000;15: 51.
380. Mills NL, Ochsner JL. Massive air embolism during cardiopulmonary bypass: causes, prevention, and management. *J Thorac Cardiovasc Surg* 1980;80:708.
381. Bayindir O, Paker T, Akpinar B, et al. Case conference: a 58-year-old man had a massive air embolism during cardiopulmonary bypass. *J Cardiothorac Vasc Anesth* 1991;5:627.
382. Mills NL, Morris JM. Air embolism associated with cardiopulmonary bypass. In: Waldahausen JA, Orringer MB. *Complications in cardiothoracic surgery.* St. Louis: Mosby-Year Book, 1991:60.
383. Kurusz M, Butler BD, Katz J, et al. Air embolism during cardiopulmonary bypass. *Perfusion* 1995;10:361.
384. Larach DR. Anesthetic management during cardiopulmonary bypass. In: Hensley FA, Martin DE, eds. *A practical approach to cardiac anesthesia,* 2nd ed. Boston: Little, Brown, 1995:Chapter 6.
385. Kols A, Ammar R, Weisz G, et al. Hyperbaric oxygenation for arterial air embolism during cardiopulmonary bypass. *Ann Thorac Surg* 1993;55:401.
386. Ziser A, Adir Y, Lavon H, et al. Hyperbaric oxygen therapy for massive arterial air embolism during cardiac operations. *J Thorac Cardiovasc Surg* 1999;117:818.
387. Armon C, Deschamps C, Adkinson C, et al. Hyperbaric treatment of cerebral air embolism sustained during an open heart surgical procedure. *Mayo Clin Proc* 1991;66:565.
388. Pae WE, Williams DR, Troncellitti EK, et al. Prevention of complications during cardiopulmonary bypass. In: Waldhausen JA, Orringer MB. *Complications in cardiothoracic surgery.* St. Louis: Mosby-Year Book, 1991:39.
389. Peirce EC. Are oxygenators (airplanes, oil spills, pesticides) safe? *Ann Thorac Surg* 1989;48:467.
390. Peirce EC II. Oxygenator failure [Response to letter]. *Ann Thorac Surg* 1990;49:112.
391. Troianos CA. Complete electrical failure during cardiopulmonary bypass. *Anesthesiology* 1995;82:298.
392. Hirayama T, Yamaguchi H, Allers M, et al. Evaluation of red cell damage during cardiopulmonary bypass. *Scand J Thorac Cardiovasc Surg* 1985;19:263.
393. Larson DF, Mayall B, Anderson RM. Hemolysis due to chemical contamination of clinical perfusion apparatus. *Ann Thorac Surg* 1977;23:374.
394. Martin R, McKentry S, Thisdale Y, et al. Hemolysis during cardiopulmonary bypass. *J Cardiothorac Anesth* 1989;3:737.
395. Lamon EW, Bethard A, Powell TJ Jr, et al. Hemolysis after cardiopulmonary bypass [Letter]. *J Thorac Cardiovasc Surg* 1990;99:751.
396. Fosburg RG, Anderson RD, Nolan SP, et al. Invited letter concerning: certification of perfusionists. *J Thorac Cardiovasc Surg* 1990;100:455.
397. Pedersen T, Kaargen AL, Benze S. An approach toward total quality assurance in cardiopulmonary bypass: which data to register and how to assess perfusion quality. *Perfusion* 1996;11:39-44.

13

MYOCARDIAL PRESERVATION

ELIOT R. ROSENKRANZ

During the first one-half century of cardiac surgery using cardiopulmonary bypass, numerous technical advances have allowed the repair of diseased cardiac valves, bypassing of obstructed coronary arteries, the replacement of diseased great vessels, and the extensive reconstruction of congenital cardiac malformations. Early on in this continuum of development, surgeons recognized the occurrence of early myocardial dysfunction after cardiac surgery, despite the technical success of the procedure. Taber et al.,(1) Najafi et al.,(2) and others noted histologic evidence of myocardial necrosis on postmortem examination of such patients, suggesting an injury induced by perioperative ischemia. Such injury was most prevalent in the subendocardium due presumably to its greater metabolic requirements and its jeopardized blood supply in patients with coronary artery disease (3–5). As such, attention was directed in the laboratory and in the clinic to the avoidance of perioperative ischemic injury by better myocardial protection.

Although in recent years, myocardial protection is often considered synonymous with cardioplegia, the avoidance of perioperative myocardial injury is truly multifactorial. Preexisting systemic and myocardial disease, pre–cardiopulmonary bypass hemodynamic stability during anesthetic induction and maintenance, the success and adequacy of the surgical procedure, the separation from cardiopulmonary bypass, and the hemodynamic stability in the early postoperative period all play pivotal roles, along with chemical cardioplegic (or noncardioplegic) techniques used for intraoperative protection of the heart muscle to avoid myocardial injury. This problem is all the more evident in the current era of cardiac surgery, in which we are increasingly operating on higher risk patients and exploring alternative approaches for exposure to the heart and even performing coronary revascularization on the beating heart. Older patients with less systemic organ reserve and often more advanced cardiac disease are an increasing percentage of those undergoing surgery in most practices. The percentage of reoperative coronary revascularization surgery, valvular procedures, and congenital operations continues to increase in all centers.

Although percutaneous transluminal coronary angioplasty has reduced the incidence of simple coronary artery bypass surgeries in low-risk patients, it has increased the frequency of emergency revascularization for acute coronary occlusion, which demands particular attention perioperatively in terms of myocardial protection. Aggressive treatment of acute myocardial infarction by thrombolysis, catheter manipulation, and surgery requires specialized attention to the appropriate management of the acutely ischemic and reperfused myocardium (6). The increasing emphasis on complex reconstruction of congenital heart disorders in newborns and children presents the challenge of protecting the immature myocardium with the complicating influences of chronic hypoxia and myocardial hypertrophy. Finally, heart transplantation is increasingly being applied clinically, pressing the need for improved methods of myocardial preservation to extend donor availability and prevent ischemic and reperfusion injury during the implantation process.

To meet the challenges outlined, the surgeon and operating room team must understand and address the pathophysiology of myocardial ischemia and reperfusion and be conceptually and practically able to apply this understanding to the clinical practice of cardiac surgery and cardiac anesthesia. As so simply stated by Wechsler and associates (7) in a recent review, "adaptation of techniques that allow reaction to rapidly changing intraoperative and perioperative events is only possible when the cardiac surgeon is a skilled physiologist with as great an understanding of injury mechanisms as of protective techniques." Therefore, to meet this goal, this chapter discusses current approaches to perioperative myocardial protection, along with a review of the pathophysiology of ischemia and reperfusion as it applies to the varied environments (e.g., adult coronary disease, the immature heart, and acute myocardial infarction) within which cardiac surgery is performed today. This chapter develops a historical perspective of the development of myocardial protection and cardioplegic techniques, along with alternatives available for current clinical practice. Preoperative factors that influence the risk of and complicate

E. R. Rosenkranz: Department of Surgery, State University of New York at Buffalo; Department of Cardiothoracic Surgery, The Children's Hospital of Buffalo, Buffalo, New York 14222

the avoidance of perioperative myocardial damage are described, as well as postoperative factors that may cause or exacerbate the perioperative injury. Finally, current clinical strategies for myocardial protection for elective, emergency, and redo adult cardiac surgery, as well as pediatric and transplant surgery are detailed.

PATHOPHYSIOLOGY OF MYOCARDIAL INJURY, ISCHEMIA, AND REPERFUSION

An in-depth analysis of the pathophysiology of myocardial ischemia and reperfusion is beyond the scope of this chapter and can be found in recent reviews in the literature (8–14). Instead, we present the concepts pertinent to the development of myocardial protection strategies for varying clinical applications.

Much like myocardial protection, myocardial injury is a multifactorial event. Even in the absence of frank myocardial ischemia, injury to the heart muscle can occur if metabolic demands outweigh the available metabolic supply (e.g., oxygen, glucose, and fatty acids). Although inadequate blood perfusion (e.g., ischemia) is the most common insult, perioperative myocardial injury can occur due to ventricular distention, which impairs subendocardial perfusion and increases myocardial oxygen requirements due to increased wall tension (law of Laplace). Tachycardia, hypotension, or hypertension play important roles in altering the adequacy of the supply of myocardial metabolic requirements.

The concept developed by Buckberg, Hoffman, and colleagues (4,15–17) of myocardial supply-demand balance expressed as the ratio of diastolic pressure time index (DPTI) divided by the time-tension index (TTI) (18) is a useful way to conceptualize these situations clinically (Fig. 13-1). Although more sophisticated parameters of the interrelationship of contractile state, mechanical work, and metabolic demands recently developed (pressure-volume area–MV_{O_2} relationships, end-systolic stress-strain relationships)(19–21) may more accurately describe the complex functional and metabolic changes imposed by ischemia physiologically, the current state of clinical practice prevents routine monitoring of these parameters in the operating room or intensive care unit settings.

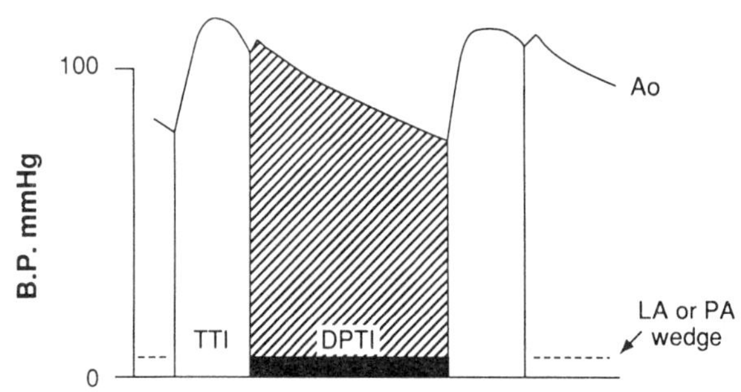

FIGURE 13-1. Relationship between myocardial oxygen supply (*DPTI,* diastolic pressure time index) and myocardial oxygen demands (*TTI,* tension time index) during the cardiac cycle. Left atrial or pulmonary artery wedge pressure tracings and aortic blood pressure tracings can be used to estimate these indexes clinically. (From Buckberg GD. Recent progress in myocardial protection during cardiac operations. In: McGoon DC, ed. *Cardiac surgery,* 2nd ed. Philadelphia: FA Davis Co, 1987:291, with permission.)

Transmural blood supply of the healthy heart is not uniform during the cardiac cycle, the left ventricular subendocardium being principally perfused during diastole. When subendocardial blood vessels are maximally dilated in response to increased metabolic needs (or decreased supply), subendocardial blood flow is determined by diastolic coronary driving pressure (aortic diastolic blood pressure minus the left ventricular end-diastolic pressure)(4,16). Buckberg et al. and colleagues (4,15) described the area below the aortic diastolic and left atrial pressure tracing (Fig. 13-1) (i.e., DPTI) as a way to estimate the potential subendocardial blood flow and oxygen supply. The area between the left ventricular systolic pressure tracing (Fig. 13-1) (i.e., TTI) provides an estimate of left ventricular subendocardial oxygen requirements (18). The influence of ventricular distension, tachycardia, hypotension, and hypertension on myocardial muscle function can be expressed by how they alter the ratio of DPTI to TTI.

Ventricular distention increases left ventricular end-diastolic pressure, reducing the DPTI and therefore the driving pressure for subendocardial blood flow. Tachycardia disproportionately reduces the diastolic portion of the cardiac cycle, thereby reducing the DPTI. Hypertension increases the area under the left ventricular systolic pressure trace, in disproportion to any increase in the aortic diastolic pressure. This results in an increase in the TTI and therefore a fall in the ratio between DPTI and TTI. Conversely, hypotension may decrease both TTI and DPTI, but the impact on coronary perfusion of a maximally vasodilated bed is greater particularly when compromised by coronary stenoses. Ventricular hypertrophy can compromise subendocardial blood flow by increasing coronary resistance, and chronic hypoxemia (e.g., cyanosis) will decrease oxygen content and therefore subendocardial oxygen supply (DPTI $\times$ O_2 content) (22,23).

Once a supply-demand imbalance exists, a complex cascade of events occurs determined by the degree of the supply inadequacy (hypoxia versus anoxia versus ischemia), the duration of ischemia, and the events that follow (e.g., reperfusion). Furthermore, inadequate coronary blood supply will not only fail to meet the supply of metabolites but also allow the accumulation of potentially toxic metabolic waste products such as lactate, hydrogen ion, fatty acids, and oxygen radicals, as well as the development of an oxidation reduction potential imbalance resulting in an alteration or cessation of enzyme activity. Similarly, reperfusion may allow the resumption of arrested metabolic production but may also wash out nutrient metabolites that diffuse into the interstitium of the heart muscle cells during the period of ischemia. These events are summarized in the next section.

Ischemia

Regional myocardial ischemia secondary to coronary occlusion is frequently a heterogenous event in the portion of the heart fed by the involved artery. There are islands of severely impaired cells destined for myocardial necrosis intermingled with mildly injured cells that will rapidly recover once blood flow is restored (11,24,25). Global myocardial ischemia induced by aortic cross-clamping also causes heterogeneous injury in that the left ventricular subendocardium is more vulnerable to irreversible injury than the epicardial layer. Subendocardial injury without transmural necrosis may manifest itself with transient left ventricular dysfunction ("stunning") that resolves with mild inotropic support and time (26). This may, however, result in significant left ventricular dysfunction in patients with preexisting areas of old myocardial infarction and scar or acute transmural ischemia.

Within the first few seconds after the onset of ischemia, contractile function of the heart deteriorates with associated changes in cardiac rhythm (27). This occurs before any significant decline in myocardial tissue adenosine 5′-triphosphate (ATP) level, which has lead to speculation that the initial decline in contractile function is related to a loss of calcium-mediated coupling of ATP hydrolysis within the contractile apparatus of the myocyte (28,29). Residual contractile activity after the onset of ischemia rapidly depletes ATP stores despite anaerobic metabolism. Due to oxygen depletion, mitochondrial control of substrate utilization is altered due to changes in the balance of the oxidation-reduction potential and hydrogen ion accumulation. Beta-oxidation of fatty acids ceases, resulting in a depletion of acetyl-coenzyme A (acetyl-CoA) availability for subsequent oxidative phosphorylation and the accumulation of fatty acids that are toxic to cellular and organelle membrane function (30–34). Anaerobic glycolysis is simultaneously stimulated with utilization of cell glycogen stores for ATP production (34,35). Energy production by anaerobic glycolysis is inadequate however to sustain myocardial contractile function because it is energetically less efficient than aerobic metabolism of free fatty acids or glucose. Furthermore, nicotinamide adenine dinucleotide (NADH), a byproduct of anaerobic glycolysis accumulates in the cytoplasm of the myocyte, resulting in feedback inhibition of glycolytic enzymes. Under aerobic conditions, NADH is oxidized inside the mitochondria regenerating NAD and promoting continued glucose utilization. Pyruvate, an end product of glycolysis is further metabolized to lactate in an attempt to oxidize NADH anaerobically but results in regional tissue acidosis and further shutdown of cellular metabolic activity (34,36).

The net result of the loss of cellular energy generation mechanisms is the inability to maintain ATP-dependent ion gradients. Energy-dependent calcium sequestration by the sarcoplasmic reticulum is halted, further impairing any residual coupling of ATP hydrolysis and muscle contraction. Mitochondrial function terminates in a loss of the connection between oxygen consumption and ATP generation (respiratory control) and a loss of membrane-bound components of the electron transport chain (37–39). From the accumulation of end products of fatty acid metabolism and water and the failure to generate energy for cell repair, membrane integrity is lost, leading to a leakage of intracellular proteins (enzyme release), metabolites (adenine nucleotides), and eventual tissue necrosis due to cell death. On a tissue level, the leakage of adenine nucleotides and adenosine causes coronary vasodilation.

By the end of 15 to 20 minutes of normothermic ischemia, total diastolic arrest occurs due to cell-membrane depolarization. This may progress to myocardial contracture formation, which presents the most significant morphologic change noted histologically (40,41). Contraction bands, myofibrillar disarray, and distorted Z bands are visible, along with a spherical shape of the mitochondria. Further organelle changes include vacuolization of the sarcoplasmic reticulum and the mitochondria and release of lysosomal enzymes from lysozyme granules, resulting in further tissue self-destruction (42).

As mentioned already, the ischemic process is heterogenous. Areas of viable cells are found adjacent to and/or mixed with irreversibly injured cells. Histologically, it can be difficult (if not impossible) to distinguish irreversible injury from reversible injury. The classical studies of Jennings et al. (25) describe specific histopathologic criteria that they felt represented irreversible injury after ischemia. They felt that such injury would be widespread after 45 minutes of normothermic ischemia; however, these criteria and the reversibility of the duration of ischemia has been questioned (43). The recent evidence for the "stunned" myocardium helps explain the lack of early return of myocardial function due to the time-related processes of substrate and adenine nucleotide replenishment and cell repair. Therefore, a complete pathophysiologic understanding of the impact of ischemia must consider not only its duration but also the conditions under which ischemia occurs (e.g., temperature, hemodynamic status and loading conditions, and degree of collateral blood flow), which can be manipulated clinically to prolong the safety period of ischemia. Furthermore, the events occurring after ischemia (reperfusion) have been extensively studied, particularly how they impact on early and late metabolic functional recovery.

Reperfusion Injury

Restoration of blood flow to the ischemic myocardium should be expected to reactivate ATP generation for the repair of ischemic injury and the return of myocardial pump function. It has long been recognized that this simplistic view does not hold true clinically or experimentally (11,12, 25). Depending on the duration and conditions of ischemia, unmodified blood reperfusion may not fully restore healthy histopathology, metabolism, and mechanical function of the heart. It had been debated whether these observed changes represent a new injury induced by the process of reperfusion or reveal an injury induced by ischemia that would become manifest with more time. This argument, which is more than semantic, is incompletely resolved (14, 43). The conditions of reperfusion (e.g., temperature, pressure, hemodynamics), as well as the composition of the reperfusate (e.g., pH, calcium content, oxygen) have an important impact on the degree of reperfusion damage seen histopathologically, metabolically, and functionally (44,45).

Unmodified Reperfusion

After very brief episodes of ischemia (5 minutes), reperfusion of the ischemic myocardium results in restoration of ventricular function that is mildly depressed from normal ("stunned"). Murry and colleagues (46) noted that if one then exposes the reperfused heart to a more prolonged period of ischemia, the heart is preconditioned in that restoration of function and prevention of necrosis occurs in contrast to the heart exposed only to a period of prolonged ischemia without the preconditioning period of brief ischemia. The pathophysiology of the preconditioning phenomenon is incompletely understood but appears to be initiated by chemicals released by ischemic tissues (adenosine, bradykinin), which via cell-membrane receptors, initiate a series of intracellular signals that result in inducing the preconditioned state.

Restoration of blood flow to the ischemic heart even after a longer time of ischemia (15 to 20 minutes) results in more significant and prolonged dysfunction. Reperfusion ventricular arrhythmias are common and may be accompanied by impaired ventricular pump function. After brief periods of ischemia, the histologic appearance after reperfusion may be fairly normal with only subtle changes including myocyte and organelle edema and focal calcium deposition. With time, the heart recovers functionally and histopathologically and may have only small areas of subendocardial scar (13,26).

After longer periods of ischemia, blood reperfusion results in more significant histologic changes with evidence of mitochondrial damage, disarray of the contractile apparatus, and organelle and/or cell disruption. Functionally, this is paralleled by significant muscle dysfunction. Metabolically, the determinant of the extent of dysfunction and the likelihood of recovery is the preservation of mitochondrial function. Three mitochondrial processes are fundamentally involved: (a) oxidative phosphorylation and ATP generation, (b) calcium regulation, and (c) generation of oxygen radicals.

Oxidative Phosphorylation and ATP Generation

Ischemia promptly halts mitochondrial oxidative phosphorylation and therefore ATP production. Upon reperfusion, oxidative metabolism is restored, but tissue ATP levels do not return to within the normal range either because of uncoupling of oxidative metabolism and high-energy bond formation (respiration) or because adequate precursor for ATP generation (adenine nucleotide) is not available despite the mitochondrial production of high-energy bonds. Oxidation may continue with energy expended to sequester calcium and expel hydrogen ion without significant recovery of subsequent mechanical function. In contrast, loss of adenine nucleotide is generally transient, being replenished by de novo and salvage resynthesis pathways

Calcium Regulation

An important hallmark of the reperfusion-damaged heart is uncontrolled, excessive calcium uptake in the cytosol and mitochondria of myocytes, resulting in cellular and organelle dysfunction (8,14,24). Histologically, this is manifested as contraction bands and deposition of calcium phosphate crystals in the mitochondrial matrix. Calcium enters the myocytes by energy-dependent mitochondrial membrane pumps that expel intramitochondrial hydrogen ion. Excessive mitochondrial calcium accumulation damages the respiratory chain and results in a failure of ATP production (47,48). Experimentally, this process can be halted by agents that poison energy-generation processes in the mitochondria (10) (clinically impractical), preventing calcium passage in slow calcium channels (49,50) or by reducing (but not eliminating) the calcium content of the initial reperfusate solution following ischemia (44,50) (see Modified Reperfusion).

Generation of Oxygen Radicals

Upon reoxygenation of the ischemic myocardium, oxygen-derived radicals (superoxide anion, hydroxyl anion, and hydrogen peroxide) are rapidly generated (51–53). These cytotoxic agents are normally byproducts of cellular metabolism and are scavenged and deactivated enzymatically (superoxide dismutase, catalase, and peroxidase) (54,55) and by antioxidant receptors (glutathione, vitamin E, hemoglobin, and so on). During reperfusion, oxygen-derived radical production is markedly increased while the normal endogenous mechanisms of radical scavenging are decreased. Glucose depletion prevents activity of the pentose phosphate shunt that regenerates the reduced form of glutathione. Mitochondrial and cellular membrane damage allow enzyme leakage into the tissue interstitium, resulting in depletion of superoxide dismutase and catalase. The net result is extensive mitochondrial membrane damage and the failure of ATP generation and all mitochondrial functions (51, 53,56).

REPERFUSION MODIFICATION

In developing a clinical strategy for the intraoperative management of myocardial ischemia and reperfusion, it has become evident that attention to the pathophysiology of these states is mandatory. Ischemic damage can be avoided by providing the ischemic heart with substrates to optimize anaerobic metabolism between cardioplegia infusions and enhance aerobic metabolism during reinfusion. With this concept in mind, the cardioplegic and reperfusate solutions must be formulated to prevent the previously outlined events associated with reperfusion of the ischemic myocardium. Therefore, the ideal reperfusate solution should enhance aerobic metabolism to allow cellular repair and energy replenishment but minimize oxygen-derived radical generation by providing antioxidants and oxygen-derived radical scavenging compounds. Intracellular acidosis should be buffered to enhance enzymatic activity and substrates should be provided to take advantage of aerobic and anaerobic metabolic pathways. To minimize mitochondrial injury, calcium sequestration must be avoided by either reducing calcium delivery or preventing its entry into the cell. Tissue edema must be avoided to prevent unfavorable changes in ventricular compliance, and finally energy requirements must be minimized during early reperfusion to allow maximal organ recovery before separation from bypass (57). The remainder of this chapter describes several approaches to achieve these goals.

MYOCARDIAL PROTECTION

As mentioned previously, myocardial protection is a multifactorial problem that extends well beyond the scope of cardioplegic delivery techniques alone. Factors occurring before the operation including the patients age, disease, and degree of illness set the environment in which myocardial ischemia and reperfusion is to occur. Events occurring in the operating room including anesthetic induction in preparation for cardiopulmonary bypass, as well as the process of separation from cardiopulmonary bypass and stabilization thereafter, will also have direct impact on the patients tolerance of the perioperative period of myocardial ischemia. The success of the surgical procedure (e.g., adequacy of revascularization, relief of pressure, and/or volume loads, relief of intracardiac shunts) will also impact the demands placed on the heart at the conclusion of the operative procedure. It is therefore important that the surgeon and the anesthesiologist consider these problems in conjunction with the planning of the surgical procedure when laying out the operative strategy.

PREOPERATIVE FACTORS

It is evident from recent laboratory and clinical investigation that important developmental and metabolic differences exist between pediatric and adult patients exposed to intraoperative ischemia (58–60). Similarly, adult patients with coronary artery disease versus those with valvular heart disease and hypertrophy differ in their tolerance to intraoperative ischemia (61–63). Finally, the patient's preoperative hemodynamic stability, particularly the presence of acute ischemia or infarction, will influence his or her tolerance of intraoperative events. These patient characteristics will be reviewed in reference to the development of surgical strategies to avoid perioperative injury. Although certain patient groups may come to surgery with anticipated risk factors because of the nature of their disease (64), a myocardial protection regimen should also provide the physiologic redundancy to cope with unanticipated episodes or metabolic stress such as arrhythmias and hypotension.

Adult Patients: Ischemic/Coronary Artery Disease

As reviewed already, the subendocardium of the healthy heart is more vulnerable to ischemic injury. It has further been shown experimentally in animals and in humans that the myocardium distal to significant coronary stenoses has a lower level of ATP in the subendocardium and develops ischemic contracture more rapidly than tissues supplied by unobstructed coronary arteries (65–67). This situation is exacerbated by physiologic stress (such as tachycardia, hypertension, and ventricular distention). Acute ischemia either due to critical coronary lesions or induced by acute occlusion during catheterization or percutaneous transluminal coronary angioplasty results in sudden metabolic and physiologic dysfunction in the ischemic region (see previous descriptions), which is extended or intensified by subsequent episodes of ischemia in the operating room. Prolonged regional or global myocardial dysfunction is well recognized in such situations and may severely compromise postoperative hemodynamics and survival. In a similar sense, patients with preexisting impairment of regional or global ventricular function due to earlier ischemia or scar formation will have less functional reserve and therefore lesser tolerance to even limited intraoperative stress. Patients with significant distal coronary obstructions not accessible to bypass grafting will not be completely revascularized and may not be adequately protected, due to inadequate distribution of cardioplegic solution beyond these stenoses (68). Similarly, patients with patent bypass grafts undergoing a second revascularization are not as adequately protected by standard cardioplegic administration techniques and may therefore be at greater risk for intraoperative ischemia and infarction. It is then of the utmost importance that a myocardial protection regimen be designed to address these factors, which can be anticipated preoperatively. These strategies may require modification of the anesthetic induction (including preoperative use of an intraaortic balloon pump) and conduct of cardiopulmonary bypass. Alterations of cardioplegic solution components and of its infusion may also be indicated.

Valvular Heart Disease

Acquired or congenital stenosis or insufficiency of the atrioventricular or semilunar valves causes metabolic and physiologic adaptations that affect myocardial ischemia tolerance. The metabolic consequences of ventricular hypertrophy included more rapid subendocardial ATP depletion and subsequent contracture development in experimental models when the heart was exposed to even brief periods of ischemia (61–63). Similar transmural ATP gradients were also identified in humans with left ventricular hypertrophy due to valvar aortic stenosis (69). This is particularly important in reference to the observations reported by Cooley et al. and Katz et al. of the "stone" heart occurring after intraoperative ischemia followed by reperfusion (40,70). This occurred almost exclusively in hypertrophic hearts. Of particular note was the observation by Peyton and colleagues (71) that baseline subendocardial ATP depletion in the hypertrophic heart could be repleted and the tolerance to ischemia (contracture formation) be returned to normal by preischemic perfusion of the heart with a normothermic substrate solution (see warm induction strategy). This implies, and subsequent studies confirm, that this preischemic state is remediable by appropriate modification of the myocardial protection strategy.

In pediatric patients, a similar problem is seen particularly in the right ventricle with tetralogy of Fallot. Del Nido et al. (72) have demonstrated significant depletion of both ATP and creatine phosphate in subendocardial right ventricular biopsies. Therefore, similar attention to reperfusate modification may be necessary in these patients with hypertrophied myocardium.

Aortic insufficiency presents more subtle metabolic myocardial dysfunction that becomes more important only when more advanced disease exists. Global left ventricular dilation secondary to chronic volume overload increases wall tension and therefore basal oxygen requirements and may create preoperative energy depletion (73). More commonly, aortic insufficiency complicates the intraoperative conduct of cardioplegic induction and avoidance of ventricular distention before aortic clamping (see further in this chapter).

Chronic mitral valve disease elevates pulmonary artery pressure with secondary right ventricular dysfunction. Perioperative protection of the right ventricle is often less successful due to right ventricular hypertrophy. Postoperative right ventricular dysfunction, therefore, may significantly complicate an otherwise adequate mitral valve operation.

Pediatric Patients

The overall subject of protection of the immature heart is presently receiving careful reevaluation in several laboratories. Although generally more tolerant to comparable periods of unprotected myocardial ischemia than the adult heart, the immature heart may in fact be injured by cardioplegic techniques that are used routinely in adults (59). Furthermore, the cardiac lesions requiring repair with associated hypertrophy or cyanosis present unique metabolic adaptations and requirements during periods of surgical ischemia. Some of these unique requirements are reviewed more fully in later sections.

PERIOPERATIVE FACTORS

The details of anesthetic management of cardiac surgical patients are fully described in other chapters of this book. This discussion will limit itself to particular events in the operating room that may directly impact myocardial perfusion and metabolism, and therefore tolerance to intraoperative ischemia.

Despite the advances in intraoperative monitoring including ST segment T-wave analysis by computer, flotation catheters, transesophageal echo to monitor wall motion, and more, a sound appreciation for the physiologic balance of myocardial energy supply and demand must be kept in mind. Anesthetic agents, tachycardia, hypovolemia, and left ventricular dysfunction may cause hypotension, decrease myocardial perfusion, and cause regional or global myocardial ischemia. Similarly, hypertension, pain, or tachycardia may all increase myocardial oxygen demands at a time when supply is limited by coronary stenoses. Inadequate ventilation resulting in hypoxemia, hypercarbia, and acidosis alter oxygen supply, myocardial contractility, and pulmonary vascular resistance. These factors acutely affect cardiac output and myocardial blood supply. These are particularly dangerous events in pediatric patients with more reactive pulmonary vascular beds.

During cannulation for cardiopulmonary bypass, the surgical team must be advised of hypotension or arrhythmias induced by direct cardiac manipulation. More urgent cannulation by the transthoracic or femoral routes with prompt ventricular decompression may avoid ischemia induced by hemodynamic compromise during preparations for bypass. Similarly, the anesthesiologist plays a critical role in managing patients undergoing coronary revascularization via new minimally invasive approaches (see discussion later in this chapter) performed on the beating heart. To improve exposure to bypass target sites, pharmacologic agents may be employed to slow the heart rate, and various strategies to position and immobilize are often employed that may alter the hemodynamic stability of the patient while the anastomoses are being performed.

PHARMACOLOGIC CARDIOPLEGIC MYOCARDIAL PROTECTION

Historical Overview

The issues related to preservation of myocardial function, structure, and metabolism have evoked significant debate and laboratory and clinical investigation since the earliest days of cardiac surgery. Several reviews of the literature describe in detail the development of the many approaches surgeons have employed for intraoperative myocardial protection (74–76). This section highlights pertinent events to put our current concepts in historical perspective.

Although most cardiac surgeons today employ hypothermic chemical cardioplegia, others still successfully employ different approaches with satisfactory results including procedures performed without the aid of cardiopulmonary bypass. It is advantageous for the surgeon and anesthesiologist to understand these alternatives because a single standard approach may not always be suitable or successful and the surgical team must be flexible enough to employ alternative strategies when the intraoperative conditions dictate such changes.

With the introduction of cardiopulmonary bypass in the early 1950s, surgical repair of cardiac defects became technically possible. However, even in the empty heart, ongoing contraction and the risk of air embolus during normothermic perfusion made all but the simplest intracardiac lesions impractical for repair. Similarly, the need for precise anastomoses during coronary artery bypass graft (CABG) surgery made cardiac standstill in a bloodless field a necessity until recent methods of off-pump bypass were developed. The relationship between sodium and potassium concentration and heart rate was reported by Ringer in 1883 (77) and the direct effect of potassium ion on myocardial contraction was reported by Hooker in 1929 (78). Melrose applied these observations and developed the first methods of induced chemical cardioplegia using high concentrations of potassium citrate (79). Although initially promising, several instances of fatal postoperative myocardial failure were reported with this solution and these early cardioplegic solutions fell into disfavor. Subsequent reexamination of these solutions revealed that the problem was excessive osmolality due to the high-concentration potassium citrate (80). Today's cardioplegic solutions of very similar composition are quite effective when potassium concentration and osmolality are more physiologic. However, before the reintroduction of chemical cardioplegia in the early 1970s, other strategies in myocardial protection were employed.

Hypothermia was introduced to reduce myocardial metabolic requirements and to prolong the "safe period" of elective myocardial ischemia. Topical hypothermia was popularized by Shumway et al. in 1960 (81) and allowed safe periods of aortic cross-clamping for up to 30 to 60 minutes (82,83). Systemic hypothermia with intermittent aortic occlusion was subsequently introduced to improve myocardial cooling, allow a reduction of systemic flow on cardiopulmonary bypass, and therefore reduce coronary collateral blood flow. Ventricular fibrillation during aortic occlusion provided better surgical conditions as well. This technique, often augmented by topical hypothermia, was widely used and remains a technique employed clinically by some today (84).

In the early 1970s, Bretschneider et al., Kirsch et al., and colleagues (85–87) reintroduced clinical cardioplegia using a low-sodium solution that appeared safe and provided more satisfactory surgical conditions for safer periods of aortic cross-clamping. Similar results were reported by Hearse et al. and Gay et al. (88,89), who reintroduced potassium chloride as the arresting ion. A multitude of cold crystalloid solutions have since gained clinical popularity.

Despite these improvements, myocardial recovery was not always complete. Histologic evaluation revealed significant changes in the myocardial structure after blood reperfusion (reperfusion injury; see previous discussion) and Hearse et al. described the associated influence of calcium and oxygen on tissue damage after blood reperfusion (10,90). To address this pathophysiologically, Buckberg systematically identified the components of oxygenated blood that impacted on reperfusion damage and developed a modified blood reperfusate to avoid such damage, which was reported in the literature in 1978 (91,92). Describing cardioplegia as the first phase of reperfusion of the ischemic heart, Buckberg and associates subsequently introduced blood as a vehicle for cardioplegic solutions and further refined these solutions to address the specific requirements of the energy-depleted heart, the acutely ischemic heart, and the premature heart. Such solutions and strategies of administration have found widespread clinical acceptance.

MYOCARDIAL PROTECTION STRATEGIES

Design of Cardioplegic Solutions

Buckberg (93) identified four specific prerequisites in the design of a cardioplegic solution that can be generalized to the design of an overall myocardial protection strategy. First, the solution or strategy must be demonstrated to be safe in experimental models and proven in carefully controlled clinical settings. Second, the solution must be delivered to all regions of the myocardium and the overall strategy must consider the protection of all regions of the heart. Third, the continued maintenance of myocardial preservation must be ensured by periodic replenishment of the cardioplegic solution, and fourth, flexibility of the protection technique must be available to allow adaptation to varying clinical situations. Specific metabolic principles must be addressed in the design of a protection strategy, because these are unavoidable factors that determine myocardial ischemic tolerance.

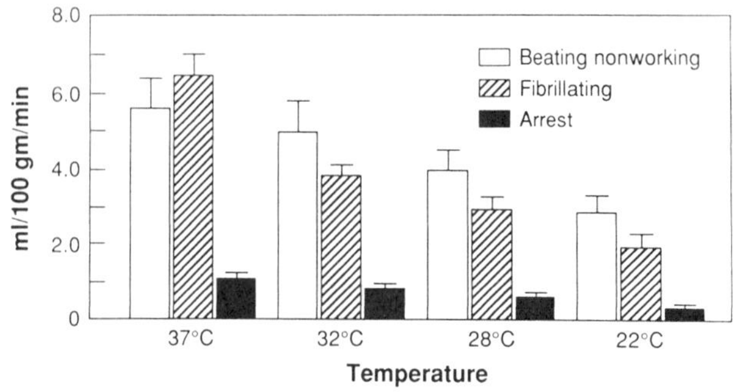

FIGURE 13-2. Changes in myocardial oxygen consumption in mL/100 g/minute relative to myocardial work condition and myocardial temperature. Myocardial oxygen consumption decreases linearly as temperature is reduced. At any specific myocardial temperature, inducing myocardial arrest markedly decreases oxygen consumption. (From Buckberg GD. Recent progress in myocardial protection during cardiac operations. In: McGoon DC, ed. *Cardiac surgery,* 2nd ed. Philadelphia: FA Davis Co, 1987:291, with permission.)

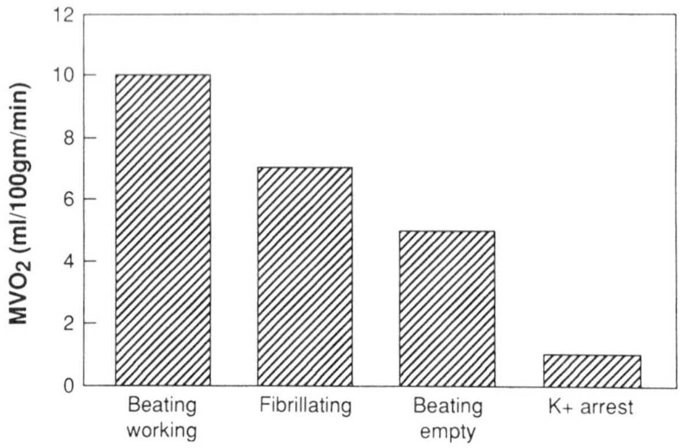

FIGURE 13-3. Myocardial oxygen consumption (MVo_2, mL/100 g/minute) relative to the work status of the heart at normothermia. Note that the oxygen consumption of the fibrillating heart is 75% that of the beating working heart. The nonworking heart on cardiopulmonary bypass (beating empty) consumes approximately 50% of the amount of oxygen as the working heart. Potassium arrest reduces oxygen consumption to approximately 10% of the working heart.

Temperature

The most consistent component of myocardial protection strategies until the more recent introduction of warm cardioplegia (see later section) has been myocardial cooling or hypothermia. The direct correlation between lowering heart temperature and lowering oxygen requirements of the heart is well recognized (Fig. 13-2). Perfusion hypothermia by moderately cooling the cardiopulmonary bypass perfusate to 24°C to 28°C and further cooling the cardioplegia temperature to between 4°C to 10°C is the most popular approach used clinically today. Myocardial cooling jackets may add further protection, particularly during longer periods of aorta cross-clamping as well as in situations in which distribution of cardioplegia beyond coronary stenoses is in doubt (94).

Electromechanical Work

The direct association between cardiac work (loading conditions) and myocardial oxygen and substrate requirement has also been well-documented experimentally and clinically (18,95). In the working state, myocardial oxygen consumption is approximately 10 to 14 mL of oxygen per 100 g of myocardium per minute and increases as the workload (i.e., afterload, cardiac output, and so on) increases (Fig. 13-3). By inducing cardiopulmonary bypass and allowing the heart to beat without ejection at 37°C (i.e., the beating empty state), myocardial oxygen consumption is reduced by approximately 50% and coronary blood flow distribution remains normal except in the hypertrophic or pediatric heart in which subendocardial underperfusion may occur due to changes in the subendocardial coronary vascular resistance (96,97). Although the induction of ventricular fibrillation can provide more satisfactory operating conditions than the beating empty heart (quite heart, avoidance of air embolus, coronary perfusion), it is at the cost of a significantly elevated oxygen requirement. Furthermore, subendocardial coronary resistance is elevated during ventricular fibrillation, increasing the risk of subendocardial ischemia. Hypothermia will decrease the heart's oxygen requirement and improve its tolerance to ventricular fibrillation (Fig. 13-2) (95).

Diastolic arrest results in a major reduction in myocardial oxygen consumption to approximately 1 mL/100 g/minute at 37°C. Pharmacologic arrest with potassium overcomes the limitations of ischemic arrest while providing maximal reduction of oxygen requirements at a given temperature. By avoiding continued electromechanical activity after aortic occlusion, ATP stores are used only to maintain cell integrity and are not wasted by unnecessary work. Oxygen requirements during pharmacologic arrest can be further reduced by hypothermia (0.3 mL/100 g/minute), which prolongs the period of safe ischemia and minimizes the degree of tissue injury.

pH Concentration

It is a physicochemical property of water that the neutrality point rises to a more alkalotic pH level as water is cooled (98,99). Similarly, animals that vary their body temperature to that of the environment (poikilotherms) also vary their blood pH concentration according to the temperature of the ambient environment (100,101). In clinical cardiopulmonary bypass, maintaining a pH level of 7.40 without correction for temperature may make the heart "inappropriately" acidotic, and this has been shown to decrease myocardial performance (102,103). By inducing relative alkalosis at the time of cooling, "appropriate" pH level is ensured during hypothermia, maintaining optimal myocardial enzyme function. In addition, anaerobic metabolism during aortic occlusion induces tissue acidosis, which can be more adequately buffered by adjusting the pH level of the cardioplegia solution (see section on methods of buffering).

Metabolic Substrate, Cofactors, and Additives

Anaerobic utilization of glucose by glycolysis is the main source of myocardial ATP generation during ischemia. Free fatty acids cannot be used during ischemia because of the cessation of normal oxidative metabolism via the Krebs cycle (Fig. 13-4). Although amino acids, primarily glutamate, aspartate, and other branched chained amino acids, normally represent approximately 5% of myocardial energy substrates, laboratory and clinical studies have shown an increase in anaerobic amino acid metabolism and ATP generation during ischemia and during the period after reperfusion (104–117). Using the Krebs cycle enzymatic pathways, glutamate and aspartate can be deaminated anaerobically to the Krebs cycle intermediates (α-ketoglutarate and succinate) and yield ATP by the mechanism of substrate level phosphorylation in the absence of oxygen while altering the intracellular oxidation-reduction potential, which helps sustain anaerobic glucose metabolism (Fig. 13-4) (106,107, 109–111). By supplying exogenous amino acid before and during aortic occlusion, ischemic damage can be avoided and possibly reversed (113–115). Several other metabolic substrates have been tested experimentally, including the Krebs cycle intermediates, carnitine, and others with variable results (118).

Tolerance to myocardial ischemia during aortic occlusion can also be enhanced by providing periodic replenishments of oxygen. Many methods have been investigated including simple intermittent aortic occlusion and reperfusion, which unfortunately results in reperfusion injury as described previously (92). Oxygenating the cardioplegic solution is an effective means of delivering oxygen, and we have preferred oxygenation of a modified blood solution as the cardioplegic vehicle (45,57,91–93,119). Other components of blood also provide additional salutary effects including the phosphate buffering system, endogenous glucose and amino acids, and oxygen-derived radical scavengers. Oxygenation of nonhemoglobin-containing solutions (crystalloid cardioplegia) by directly dissolving oxygen in solution has also been effective in improving myocardial function, compared to nonoxygenated solutions (120–123).

Oxygen-derived free-radical generation during reperfusion of the ischemic heart has been discussed previously in this chapter as a source of intracellular tissue damage. By reducing their generation from white blood cells (filtration) or by enhancing their rapid consumption by endogenous enzymes (superoxide dismutase, catalase), the toxic effects of these substances can be limited by inclusion of oxygen-derived radical scavengers in cardioplegic and reperfusate solutions. Such agents under investigation include superoxide dismutase, catalase, mannitol, allopurinol, coenzyme Q_{10}, deferoxamine mesylate, and several other agents (52, 54,55,124–127).

Although ATP depletion can be minimized by hypothermia, by reducing electromechanical work and by providing substrates for ATP generation, the regeneration of high-energy phosphates also requires an intact oxidative phosphorylation capacity and a source of ATP precursors needed for ATP resynthesis (adenine nucleotides) (128). Adenine nucleotides that result from ATP utilization are freely diffusible from the myocardial cell and are lost in the coronary venous blood. These building blocks for ATP generation can be resynthesized de novo, but this is a relatively slow process. Adenine nucleotides can also be restored by the

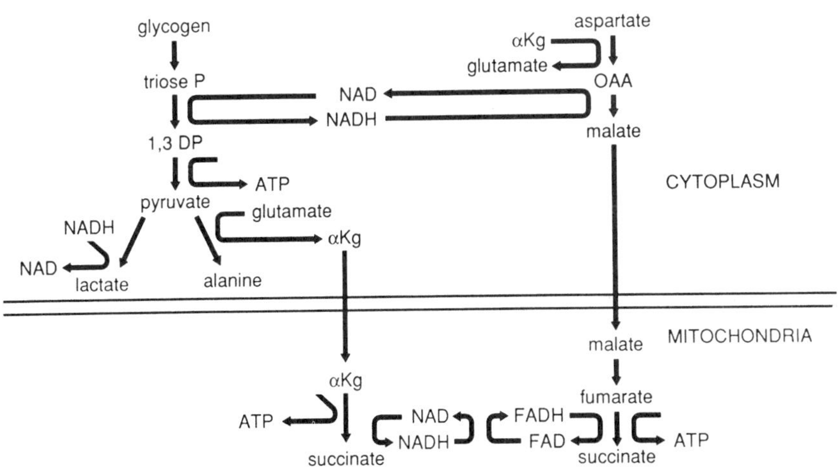

FIGURE 13-4. Myocardial anaerobic metabolism. On the left is the glycolytic pathway, whereby endogenous glycogen or exogenously supplied glucose is metabolized to pyruvate yielding two moles of adenosine 5′-triphosphate (ADP) for each mole of glucose consumed. Pyruvate can be further metabolized to lactate during anaerobic conditions. Alternatively, pyruvate can be transaminated with glutamate, yielding α-ketoglutarate, which can enter the mitochondria and yield an additional mole of ATP anaerobically. On the right is the pathway for anaerobic amino acid metabolism, whereby aspartate can be deaminated with α-ketoglutarate, yielding malate, which can enter the mitochondria and yield an additional mole of ATP in the absence of oxygen. Note that these pathways also regenerate nicotinamide adenine dinucleotide, which helps sustain continued anaerobic glycolysis.

so-called salvage pathway by inhibiting catabolic enzymes (129–131) or by supplying the heart with exogenous replacement of adenine nucleotide precursor lost by catabolism (adenosine, 5-aminoimidazole-4-carboxamide riboside, ribose, and so on) (132–137). Although a certain basal level of adenine nucleotide must be available to replenish ATP, adequate restoration of regional and global myocardial function can be achieved without complete restoration of ATP as long as oxidative phosphorylation capacity has been preserved (128,138).

The significant alterations of myocardial cell volume and ion gradients that occur with ischemia must be avoided or reversed to allow prompt restoration of cellular function after reperfusion of the heart with blood. Loss of cell volume regulation can be avoided by maintaining basal cell metabolism (provide substrates, avoid ATP depletion) and by drawing water from cells with osmotic agents (mannitol, glucose, albumin) included in the cardioplegic solution (44, 139–141).

Calcium regulation, as discussed previously, is significantly deranged during ischemia and reperfusion and can be managed by reducing calcium concentration by calcium chelation agents during the early stages of reperfusion (44, 142) or by inhibiting calcium uptake by blocking calcium channels pharmacologically (143). By maintaining basal metabolic integrity, one can also minimize the loss of intracellular calcium regulation. Normal calcium sequestration and release will allow restoration of normal intracellular calcium distribution and availability after the period of ischemia.

Intracellular acid-base buffering to provide an appropriate tissue pH level and counteract ischemic acidosis is an important determinant of myocardial function, as just reviewed. Endogenous buffers are found in blood-based solutions (e.g., phosphate buffer, histidine buffer, hemoglobin, and others) and may be substituted or augmented by diffusible buffers such as bicarbonate or tromethamine (44,144, 145) added to the cardioplegic solution.

The growing list of components included in current cardioplegic solutions in many respects reflects our growing understanding of the pathophysiology of myocardial ischemia and reperfusion. The ideal solution is as yet undetermined and it is unlikely that a single solution will be universally applicable to all patients and in all clinical conditions.

MYOCARDIAL PROTECTION TECHNIQUES

As discussed previously, the cardiac surgeon and the anesthesiologist must be familiar with alternative methods of myocardial protection to allow flexibility when standard techniques are either ineffective or not applicable to a specific clinical circumstance. The next section will summarize several techniques that are still of utility in specific circumstances. The growing application of off-pump coronary revascularization may obviate the need for noncardioplegic techniques for isolated coronary bypass surgery.

Noncardioplegic Techniques

Systemic Hypothermia with Ventricular Fibrillation

Systemic hypothermia with induced fibrillation of the heart was introduced as a method of myocardial preservation in the earliest years of cardiac surgery and provided suitable conditions to allow intracardiac repairs. Although this method has largely been replaced by chemical cardioplegic arrest, this technique continues to be used by some with satisfactory results (146–148). In the past, this technique was a useful alternative to cardioplegic arrest when aortic clamping was not possible or dangerous (e.g., with a heavily plaqued or calcified aorta) or when patent internal mammary grafts could not be temporarily occluded and therefore prevent adequate regional administration of cardioplegia by antegrade or retrograde techniques. Today, off-pump procedures provide a better alternative.

Method

After cannulation, cardiopulmonary bypass is initiated with systemic cooling to 25°C to 28°C. The pericardial well is then perfused with 4°C lactated Ringer's solution to further augment myocardial cooling. The mean aortic blood pressure is maintained at 80 to 100 mm Hg to ensure adequate subendocardial blood flow. If spontaneous fibrillation does not occur with hypothermia alone, ventricular fibrillation is induced electrically. Ventricular distention is avoided by the routine use of a transatrial left ventricular vent and the aorta is left unclamped unless the procedure (aortic valve replacement) or conditions (aortic insufficiency with subsequent ventricular distention) dictate aortic occlusion. In centers experienced with this technique, a perioperative myocardial infarction rate of 1.8% and a perioperative mortality rate of 0.4% have been reported for elective operations (145,147,148).

Ischemic Arrest with Hypothermia

Ischemic arrest was the method of choice for many years before chemical cardioplegic arrest became accepted and has served as a point of comparison during the development of cardioplegic strategies (44,92). In contrast to fibrillatory arrest, ischemic arrest requires aortic clamping. It is tempting to speculate that intermittent ischemic arrest induces myocardial preconditioning, which is the reason this technique has been clinically successful.

Methods

For intermittent ischemic arrest, the aorta is cross-clamped and the surgical repair carried out. The aorta is unclamped every 15 to 20 minutes allowing brief periods (3 to 5 minutes) of reperfusion of the ischemic myocardium. After aortic unclamping, the heart is defibrillated, if necessary, during the period of brief reperfusion. The aorta is again clamped and the procedure continued. In cases in which the aortic root is opened, direct coronary ostial perfusion is required to reperfuse the heart.

Prolonged ischemic arrest with topical cooling was popularized by Shumway (81–84). Cardiopulmonary bypass with mild hypothermic or normothermic perfusion is established, the heart vented, and 2 to 3 L of 4°C saline poured into the pericardial well to rapidly decrease intramyocardial temperature to 15°C to 20°C. The aorta is left clamped throughout the procedure while continuous irrigation of the heart with cold saline is used to maintain myocardial hypothermia. This technique was found to be safe for periods of up to approximately 1 hour of aortic occlusion and superior in its safety to an equivalent period of hypothermic fibrillatory arrest.

Continuous Coronary Perfusion

This method of myocardial protection provided continuous blood perfusion of the beating nonworking heart, completely avoiding ischemia. Perfusion is carried out either by aortic root infusion or by direct coronary ostial intubation and perfusion with blood from the pump oxygenator. This technique may be a good alternative if cardiac manipulation results in hemodynamic instability during attempted off-pump surgery. This technique is considered unsafe, however, for open heart repairs due to the risk of air embolism. More recently, continuous retrograde coronary sinus perfusion has been employed with aortic cross-clamping to allow open heart operations such as valve repairs or replacements.

Chemical Cardioplegic Techniques

Since the reintroduction of chemical cardioplegic techniques, surgeons have largely adopted these methods in preference to noncardioplegic strategies, although off-pump and noncardioplegic on-pump modalities have growing acceptance for CABG surgery. A large list of cardioplegic solutions with various components and methods of administration have been promoted often with quite comparable results. This section will present our view on the requirements of a chemical cardioplegic solution and clinical strategy and describe the general alternatives to meet these principles.

Cardioplegic Principles

Buckberg and colleagues (45,57) have identified six physiologic requirements in the design of a cardioplegic solution. These requirements are principles that serve as useful criteria by which one can compare various cardioplegic techniques and compare their clinical results.

Immediate Arrest

By chemically inducing diastolic arrest and terminating electromechanical work, the heart's energy requirements will be immediately lowered to that required to sustain basal cell metabolism and integrity during the period of ischemia.

Hypothermia

Hypothermia reduces the heart's metabolic rate and energy requirements. Therefore, cooling the cardioplegic solution to 8°C to 10°C will promptly cool the myocardium and reduce oxygen needs to a minimum. Recently, the concepts of warm or "tepid" cardioplegic arrest and cardiopulmonary bypass have been introduced to avoid the systemic effects of hypothermia (149). Although hypothermia remains a fundamental principle of chemical cardioplegic strategies, normothermic cardioplegic induction (150), reperfusion, or continuous warm cardioplegic infusion (149) have promising results.

Provide Substrate

Energy utilization continues, although at a reduced rate, during the period of cardioplegic arrest; therefore, metabolic substrate must be provided to meet these demands and avoid significant tissue depletion of energy stores that will be needed to renew electromechanical work. Glucose is a major source of energy for sustained anaerobic and aerobic glycolysis. Free fatty acid utilization ceases with anaerobic conditions and remains depressed during the early phases of reperfusion (117,151). Anaerobic and aerobic metabolism of amino acids is enhanced in the ischemic heart and can provide the heart with an important source of energy during the period of ischemia (104–118).

Maintain Appropriate pH

The issue of adjusting the cellular pH level, particularly during hypothermia to a more alkalotic pH level has been discussed previously. Many types of buffers are available and may be suitable for inclusion in the cardioplegic solution to correct intracellular acidosis and adjust pH level to the appropriate range for temperature.

Avoidance of Cellular Reperfusion Damage

Reperfusion damage is principally manifested by cellular membrane disruption and intracellular or organelle calcium deposition, as was described in detail previously. The mediators of such damage include calcium ion in the reperfusate, oxygen radicals generated after reintroduction of oxygen in the ischemic heart, and failure of energy-dependent cell-membrane pumps that normally regulate cell homeostasis. Cardioplegic solution can avoid excessive calcium deposition by reducing calcium content in the solution by chelation or preventing its entry with calcium channel blockers, as discussed previously. Oxygen radical damage can be reduced by including inhibitors of the enzymes that generate oxygen radicals, enzymes that enhance their catabolism, substrates that bind oxygen radicals (e.g., mannitol, and deferoxamine mesylate) or by reducing the oxygen tension of the reperfusate solution.

Avoidance of Edema

Myocardial edema occurs because of compromised cell-membrane integrity and inactivity of membrane-bound ATP-dependent pumps that maintain cell volume. Raising the cardioplegic solution osmolality with mannitol, glucose, or albumin provides an osmotic gradient favoring water withdrawal from the cell. Perfusing the heart with a lower blood pressure (e.g., 50 mm Hg), particularly during the early phases of reperfusion and before reinitiation of myocardial contraction, also combats the development of cell edema.

Cardioplegic Delivery

Cardioplegic solution in adequate amounts must be distributed to all segments and layers of the myocardium to provide adequate myocardial protection. Several factors play important roles in determining regional cardioplegic delivery. The most obvious problem is coronary artery obstruction that prevents antegrade infusion of cardioplegic solution via the native coronary circulation. Similarly, aortic valve insufficiency may prevent adequate filling of the aortic root and therefore compromise adequate antegrade cardioplegic administration. If the aortic root is open, as, for example, during aortic valve replacement, then direct cannulation of the coronary ostia is required for antegrade cardioplegic delivery. During mitral valve surgery, retraction of the atrium often distorts the aortic root, resulting in aortic valve incompetence, which prevents adequate antegrade cardioplegic delivery without intermittent removal of the retraction apparatus.

The hypertrophic heart presents additional problems with cardioplegic delivery to the subendocardium due to increased coronary vascular resistance (95,97). In cases of reoperative coronary revascularization, patent internal mammary grafts may prevent cardioplegic distribution in the region of this graft.

Although substantial collateral vessels may exist in patients with coronary artery disease, these vessels may not adequately supply cardioplegic solution to protect the myocardial tissue distal to significant coronary obstructions (152,153). Regions distal to the coronary stenoses receive inadequate amounts of cardioplegic solution with antegrade cardioplegic infusion alone.

Several strategies during coronary revascularization surgery have been developed to ensure better cardioplegic delivery. Vessels serving the most ischemic, but still viable, areas of the left ventricle may be grafted first and cardioplegic solution infused down the vein graft. This method does not, however, provide cardioplegic protection before construction of the graft during the initial induction of cardioplegic arrest and cannot be used to protect the region that will be revascularized by an in situ internal thoracic or gastroepiploic artery graft (119).

Many of the limitations of antegrade cardioplegic delivery can be overcome by the use of retrograde delivery of cardioplegia via the coronary venous system introduced into the coronary sinus or right atrium (154). The delivery of blood in a retrograde manner via the coronary sinus was first reported in 1956 by Lillehei for repair of calcific aortic stenosis (155). Laboratory investigations reported by Partington and coworkers have shown that retrograde coronary sinus infusion of blood cardioplegia provided better coronary blood flow, better myocardial cooling, and an appropriate ratio of endocardial to epicardial blood flow distribution (1.4:1), compared to that seen with control antegrade technique when there were no coronary stenoses (156–158). When significant proximal coronary artery stenoses were present, antegrade cardioplegic delivery provided less than 10% of control antegrade cardioplegic volume with a preferential flow distribution of the solution to the epicardium. In contrast, retrograde cardioplegic infusion alone provided approximately 60% of control antegrade cardioplegic volume with a normal distribution of cardioplegic solution to the endocardium and the epicardium (1.2:1).

The right ventricle however may not be as adequately protected by retrograde cardioplegia alone (156–159). This is thought to be due to direct drainage of coronary sinus perfusion into the right ventricular cavity by the thebesian system in the right ventricle. To address this issue, Buckberg and colleagues developed combined antegrade and retrograde cardioplegia, delivered sequentially or simultaneously (154,160–163), which ensures more prompt initial arrest of the heart and better distribution of cardioplegic solution. During reoperative coronary revascularization surgery, particularly in patients with patent internal thoracic artery or gastroepiploic artery grafts, retrograde infusion during internal thoracic or gastroepiploic graft occlusion provides cardioplegic distribution to the bed distal to the patent graft while antegrade infusion provides protection for the more proximal segments.

To address the problems of maintaining myocardial cooling and arrest and counteracting the problems of cardioplegic solution washout by noncoronary collateral blood flow, most surgeons administer periodic reinfusions of cardioplegic solution after the initial dose given to induce diastolic arrest (maintenance cardioplegic infusion). The frequency and duration of these multidose infusions depends on whether one uses nonoxygenated crystalloid or an oxygenated blood or crystalloid solution (57). With nonoxygenated crystalloid solutions, myocardial protection is principally conveyed by rapid arrest and cooling because nonoxygenated solutions carry little, if any, oxygen for the ischemic myocardium to use. Therefore, rapid infusion is desirable to ensure immediate arrest and cooling. When oxygen delivery is desired, infusion for a fixed time is necessary to allow uptake of the oxygen by the ischemic myocardium. As demonstrated experimentally, it takes approximately 2 minutes of infusion of blood cardioplegic solution until the oxygen uptake by the heart returns to approximately that of the basal requirement of the myocardium for a specific temperature (44,92,150). Therefore, maintenance blood cardioplegic reinfusions of 2-minute duration delivered every 20 minutes are generally used clinically.

Continuous blood cardioplegia, delivered in antegrade or retrograde fashion can completely avoid myocardial ischemia. When continuous crystalloid infusion is used, rewarming is avoided due to the continuous infusion of the cooled solution. Continuous cardioplegia infusion during CABG can impair visualization during the anastomosis, which can be remedied by brief, intermittent interruption of the cardioplegia infusion or by brief occlusion of the coronary artery by snares or intraluminal occluder devices.

CARDIOPLEGIC SOLUTION DEVELOPMENT AND ADMINISTRATION

Crystalloid Cardioplegia

The earliest clinical cardioplegic solutions used were crystalloid solutions, based on Ringer's solution (77). Melrose and colleagues (79) added high concentrations of potassium citrate (approximately 250 mEq of potassium per liter) to their cardioplegic solution, which was subsequently found to be toxic to the myocardium due to severe hyperosmolality (80). Subsequent refinement led to a reduction of the potassium concentration to an amount that provided sustained diastolic arrest without residual myocardial depression.

A principal division in solution design is into the intracellular versus extracellular types of solutions, which is based on the relative content of sodium and potassium in the solution and therefore the means of inducing myocardial arrest. Intracellular solutions have a low sodium content and a moderate potassium content, much like one would find in the cell cytoplasm. Diastolic arrest is induced with these solutions by rapid extracellular sodium depletion causing a loss in the transmembrane sodium gradient and a resultant loss in membrane potential. The two most commonly used low-sodium intracellular-type solutions are Bretschneider's solution (86), used mainly in Europe, and Roe's solution (164), used more commonly in the United States (Table 13-1). Bretschneider's solution contains little additional potassium, whereas Roe's solution contains 20 mEq of potassium per liter. Both solutions are buffered, Bretschneider's with histidine, (which adds a significant osmolar load) and Roe's solution with tromethamine. Both solutions have a small amount of supplemental magnesium, but no calcium.

TABLE 13-1. CRYSTALLOID CARDIOPLEGIA SOLUTIONS: INTRACELLULAR TYPES

Component	Bretschneider's Solution No. 3	Roe's Solution
Na (mEq/L)[a]	12	27
K (mEq/L)	10	20
Ca (mEq/L)	0	0
Mg (mEq/L)	4	3
pH (buffer)	7.4 (histidine)	7.6 (tham[b])
Osm (mOsm)	320	347
Substrates		Glucose 278 mm
Other	Procaine 0.2% Mannitol 239 mm/L	

Note: Na, sodium; K, potassium; Ca, calcium; Mg, magnesium; Osm, osmolality.
[a] Delivered concentration into aorta or coronary sinus.
[b] Tromethamine 0.3 m.

Extracellular solutions are based on saline, and diastolic arrest is induced by hyperkalemia resulting in depolarization of the cell membrane. Extracellular-type solutions are composed of sodium and chloride concentrations that are similar to that of plasma with exogenous potassium added to induce and maintain diastolic arrest of the heart. A large variety of solutions have been described and similarly employed clinically with comparable results. By far, the most widely used solution is St. Thomas's no. 2 solution available commercially as Plegisol (Abbot Laboratories, North Chicago, IL). This solution, developed by Hearse and Braimbridge (88,165) has a sodium content similar to that of plasma (110 mEq/L) and a moderate amount of supplemental potassium (16 mEq/L) (Table 13-2). The importance of magnesium concentration in crystalloid solutions has been emphasized by laboratory studies (166,167). It is hypothesized that the inclusion of magnesium improves myocardial function because of its important role as a cofactor in several myocardial enzyme systems. Several types of crystalloid cardioplegic solutions have been reported, including a solution popularized at the National Institutes of Heath that also contained procaine hydrochloride. None of these solutions has gained as wide a clinical following as that of St. Thomas, however.

Oxygenated cardioplegic solutions have been popularized to provide oxygen during reperfusion, which has resulted in improved postischemic ventricular function, compared to identical crystalloid solutions without oxygenation. Oxygen extraction and uptake by the heart during cardioplegic infusion, as well as better ATP retention after aortic unclamping, is found with oxygenated solutions. The methods of oxygenation have varied but usually involve equilibra-

TABLE 13-2. CRYSTALLOID CARDIOPLEGIA SOLUTIONS: EXTRACELLULAR TYPES

Component Clinic	St. Thomas's I	St. Thomas's II	Tyer's	Cleveland
Na (mEq/L)[a]	144	110	138	147
K (mEq/L)	20	16	25	20
Ca (mEq/L)	4.8	2.4	1	4.5
Mg (mEq/L)	32	32	3	32
pH (buffer) (bicarbonate)	5.5 (none)	7.8 (bicarbonate)	7.8 (bicarbonate)	7.8
Osm (mOsm)	285	324	275	285
Substrate	None	±oxygen	None	Oxygen
Other	Procaine (1 mEq)	None	Acetate (27 mm) Gluconate (23 mm)	Procaine (1 mEq)

Note: Na, sodium; K, potassium; Ca, calcium; Mg, magnesium; Osm, osmolality.
[a] Delivered concentration into aorta or coronary sinus.

tion of the crystalloid solution with oxygen bubbled into the cardioplegic reservoir bag after its preparation.

Crystalloid Cardioplegia Delivery Methods

When using a nonoxygenated crystalloid solution, the primary modalities for avoiding ischemic damage during aortic clamping are providing prompt arrest and immediate cooling, both steps aimed at immediate reduction of myocardial energy requirements. With oxygenated crystalloid solutions, aerobic energy regeneration may be possible during cardioplegic induction and maintenance infusions. This may help prevent further ischemia during aortic occlusion and avoid subsequent reperfusion damage at the conclusion of the period of myocardial ischemia. Therefore, the duration of cardioplegia infusion may be important to allow the time-dependent transfer of oxygen from solution to the myocardial cells.

In many centers, crystalloid cardioplegia delivery is regulated by the anesthesiologist. Initial myocardial arrest is achieved by antegrade infusion of cold (4°C to 10°C) crystalloid solution administered rapidly at high pressure into the aortic root. Cooling is achieved by circulating the pressurized solution through an ice bath and cooling coil connected to the aortic root cardioplegia delivery cannula. Bag pressure is generally raised to approximately 300 mm Hg and 1 to 2 L of cardioplegic solution is delivered rapidly for 1 to 2 minutes after aortic occlusion to induce prompt arrest.

Cardioplegia may be delivered as a set volume of cardioplegic solution (irrespective of the time of infusion) or over a set time (irrespective of the total volume). Experimental evidence suggests that a minimum volume of cardioplegic solution of approximately 2 mL per gram of heart weight (approximately 500 mL in an average adult) over a period not less than 30 seconds provides adequate myocardial protection in healthy hearts with crystalloid solutions (168). Volumes and durations beyond those parameters are of unclear benefit.

The cardioplegic solution is most commonly delivered antegradely into the aortic root and then the remaining half delivered retrogradely via the coronary sinus cannula. The use of retrograde delivery enhances cardioplegic distribution beyond the areas of coronary stenoses and may be of significant benefit in washout of atheromatous debris embolized into the distal coronary bed during reoperative coronary revascularizations. Direct coronary ostial antegrade infusion is employed in cases of severe aortic insufficiency or other valve operations where the aortic root is opened.

Multidose reinfusions of crystalloid cardioplegia may be based on a preset time interval (e.g., 15 to 30 minutes), by a measured rise in the myocardial temperature, or by evidence of resumption of electromechanical activity. Maintenance doses of crystalloid solution can be administered antegradely into the aortic root, down the newly constructed distal grafts, or in a combined fashion by both antegrade aortic root and retrograde coronary sinus infusions.

Systemic rewarming is initiated 15 to 30 minutes before the anticipated time of aortic unclamping, and subsequent modified reperfusions are not generally used. Technical modifications may be required during mitral valve procedures due to the retraction-induced aortic valve incompetence compromising the ability to delivery aortic root infusions. In this setting, retrograde infusion alone may be an option during the period of mitral valve retraction. Similarly, when antegrade delivery via the coronary ostia is not practical (e.g., Bentall operation), retrograde infusions may be satisfactory.

Blood Cardioplegia

Historically, it has been interesting to note that Melrose in his initial work on cardioplegic myocardial protection suggested that the ideal means of allowing correction of intracardiac lesions would be to develop a method to stop and restart the heart while maintaining coronary blood flow, thereby avoiding myocardial injury (79). This led to Melrose's initial series of experimental studies using coronary blood as the vehicle for cardioplegic solution delivery. Similarly, Bretschneider also proposed the inclusion of blood in cardioplegic solutions due to his concerns that asanguineous solutions would not provide the heart with an adequate energy replenishment by anaerobic means alone (86). The reintroduction and subsequent clinical use of blood cardioplegia occurred with the studies of Follette and Buckberg in 1978 (92), who reported the first laboratory and clinical evidence for an advantage of blood as the vehicle for potassium cardioplegia compared to continuous coronary perfusion or intermittent ischemia. Subsequent reports by several groups including randomized clinical trials increased the clinical interest in this method of myocardial protection (169–177).

Buckberg's concept for using blood cardioplegia was borne from his elegant series of studies in the late 1970s aimed at understanding the process of reperfusion injury in the ischemic heart and developing methods to prevent this otherwise inevitable consequence of blood reperfusion (166). Buckberg and colleagues used a model of 1 hour of ischemic arrest with topical hypothermia and tested the hypothesis that by adjustment of the blood reperfusate composition and methods of its administration, reperfusion damage could largely be avoided. The first modification was a reduction of the ionic calcium concentration to 1.0 mEq/L in the reperfusate by chelating ionic calcium with citrate-phosphate dextrose solution added to the reperfusate blood (44,142). A minimum level of calcium must be present in the reperfusion solution to avoid injury to the cell membranes, which depend on calcium for their integrity (178).

The next series of studies investigated the benefits of buffering the reperfusate solution to counteract intracellular acidosis induced by anaerobic metabolism during the period of ischemia. A reperfusion solution pH level of 7.6 to 7.8 was found to result in superior postreperfusion myocardial function than solutions that were kept at a pH level of 7.4 (44). The alkalotic pH level of this solution, when used as a cold cardioplegic solution, also provided the appropriate physiologic rise in pH of an aqueous solution, based on the change in the neutrality point of water during cooling.

The next series of studies employed the earlier observations on basal oxygen requirements of the heart according to its state of function and workload. To minimize oxygen requirement, potassium was included in the reperfusate solution to maintain myocardial arrest and to reduce myocardial oxygen requirements. This resulted in better postreperfusion myocardial function and metabolic recovery than seen in hearts allowed to continue to fibrillate during the period of reperfusion (44). In hearts fibrillating at 37°C, the oxygen requirements are nearly equivalent to those of the working heart (Fig. 13-3). The basal oxygen requirements could also only be met by including oxygen in the reperfusate solution.

It was noted histologically that myocardial edema, occurring during the period of ischemia due to the cessation of energy-dependent cell volume regulation mechanisms, was worsened by unmodified blood reperfusion. Reduction of the reperfusate pressure to approximately 50 mm Hg minimizes the hydraulic forces that otherwise encouraged reperfusion edema. Moderately raising the reperfusate osmolality to approximately 350 mOsmol with potassium, mannitol, or glucose also encouraged the osmotic dehydration of the edematous ischemic cellular tissue. These methods improved postreperfusion myocardial contractility and diastolic compliance (44,140).

Finally, warming the reperfusate temperature was evaluated to test the hypothesis that normothermia would enhance the resumption of myocardial aerobic metabolism and therefore increase the rate of metabolic activity and cellular repair before the time of aortic unclamping and resumption of myocardial work. By infusing the reperfusate at 37°C while maintaining myocardial arrest, maximum oxygen consumption, ATP regeneration, and subsequent postischemic recovery was achieved.

The combination of the reperfusate solution modifications (e.g., calcium reduction, oxygenation, increased osmolality, buffering, and warm temperature) resulted in near-complete recovery of myocardial function. The efficacy of the combination of these modifications was superior to that of any individual modification when tested alone (Fig. 13-5). It is important to note that like confirmatory evidence of the validity of these principles of blood reperfusate modification, comparable results have been achieved experimentally and clinically by others employing the identical components suggested by Buckberg as well as by similarly designed solutions that achieve the same goals of reperfusate modification using different components (119).

By extension of these benefits of reperfusate modification

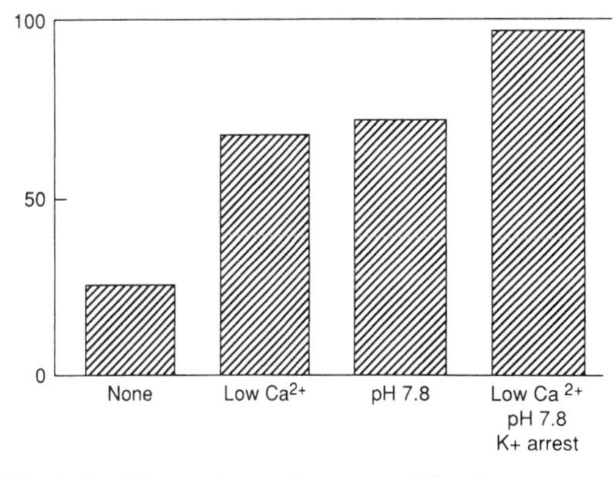

FIGURE 13-5. Effects of reperfusate modification on myocardial functional recovery after ischemic injury. Note the cumulative improvement in functional recovery by the combination of reperfusate modifications.

to the process of induction and maintenance of myocardial arrest, routine use of blood cardioplegia was instituted in the late 1970s by several groups in the United States and have since been widely used clinically around the world. In human investigation, oxygen extraction and ATP and creatine phosphate replenishment have clearly been demonstrated during infusions of blood cardioplegia (169). Several studies have shown improved early myocardial metabolic and functional recovery with less ischemic damage using blood cardioplegic protection compared to using crystalloid cardioplegic techniques in patients with coronary artery disease (172–175,177). Other studies have been equivocal, particularly when these techniques were used in patients with normal preoperative myocardial function.

Patients with unstable angina or those requiring emergency revascularization often have myocardial ATP depletion and require modifications of the cardioplegia solution composition and administration. In the energy-depleted heart, induction of cardioplegic arrest at 37°C for 5 minutes (warm cardioplegic induction) restores depleted myocardial energy stores and enhances oxidative metabolism. This period of warm cardioplegic induction is followed by a subsequent period of aortic clamping using cold blood cardioplegic protective techniques. We found that the injured heart consumed oxygen in excess of basal requirements, particularly when blood cardioplegia was given at 37°C and that this persisted for approximately 10 minutes, although the large majority of the excess oxygen consumption occurred during the first 5 minutes of cardioplegic induction. The increased oxygen consumption with warm induction was paralleled metabolically by greater recovery of tissue creatine phosphate and less residual anaerobic metabolism (lactate production), both suggesting more intact oxidative phosphorylation. Functionally, there was a significant return of left ventricular function measured by Sarnoff curves (150) (Fig. 13-6).

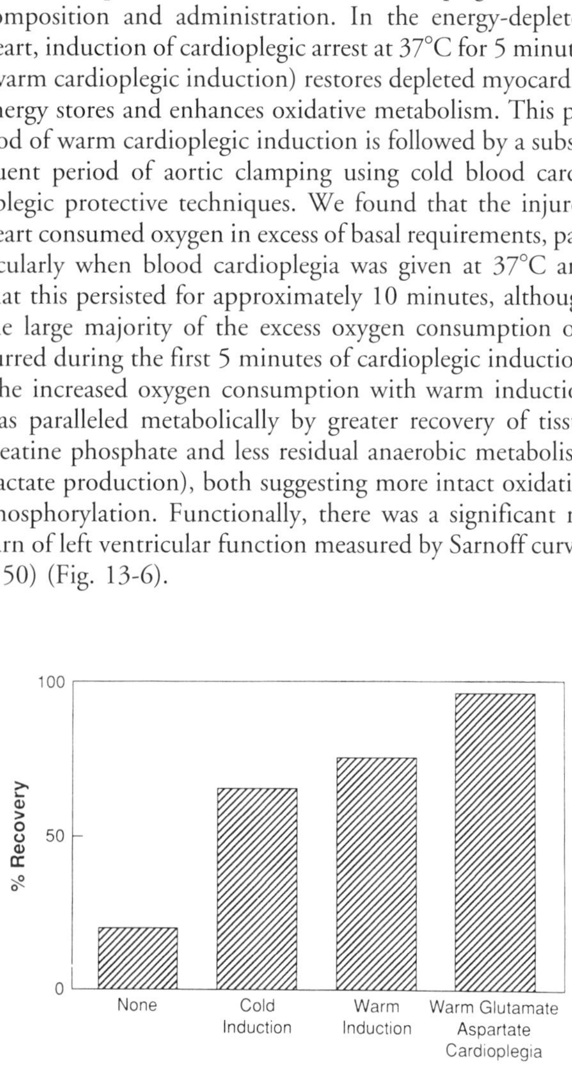

FIGURE 13-6. Effects of cardioplegic induction temperature and amino acid enrichment on postischemic recovery in energy-depleted hearts. Note the near-complete functional recovery achieved by the combination of warm (37°C) cardioplegic induction temperature and amino acid enrichment of the blood cardioplegia solution.

Subsequent modifications included amino acid supplementation (glutamic acid, aspartic acid) of blood cardioplegia as a means of enhancing metabolic and functional recovery of the energy-depleted heart, using substrate-level phosphorylation. By enriching blood cardioplegia with glutamic acid and aspartic acid, particularly when combined with warm cardioplegic induction, near-complete metabolic and functional recovery could be achieved reliably in the experimentally injured heart destined otherwise to lethal, low cardiac output state when reperfused in an unmodified fashion (114,115) (Fig. 13-6). These same solutions were then employed clinically in studies at several centers, with results demonstrating a lower perioperative mortality rate, a significant reduction in perioperative myocardial injury, and a better recovery of left ventricular function with less dependence on inotropic drug and intraaortic balloon support due to a lower incidence of low cardiac output state (179,180). Amino acid uptake is enhanced in the postischemic human heart after aortic unclamping in patients with ischemic coronary artery disease. Furthermore, this preferential consumption of amino acids persisted for several hours after intraoperative ischemia and directly correlated with myocardial oxygen consumption, suggesting a direct link between myocardial amino acid uptake, postischemic energy metabolism, and oxidative phosphorylation (117).

Blood Cardioplegia Delivery Principles

The practical aspects of blood cardioplegic delivery have been significantly improved by the commercial availability of several cardioplegia delivery systems that mix crystalloid and blood components in specifically determined proportions at a controllable temperature via a disposable heat exchanger. Several systems are available to readily allow antegrade blood cardioplegia solution delivery via the aortic root, via bypass grafts, or directly into the coronary ostia, combined with retrograde coronary sinus infusion (Fig. 13-7).

Several important principles concerning the delivery of blood cardioplegia bear emphasis to ensure consistent results (57,93,119). The solution composition must adhere to the principles of reperfusate modifications previously discussed (e.g., hypercalcemia, alkalosis, hyperosmolar, and substrate enriched). The solution also must be administered over a set time frame, not by a set volume, to ensure adequate delivery and uptake of oxygen during the periods of cardioplegic induction, maintenance, and reperfusion. Antegrade infusion pressure must be controlled to avoid myocardial edema (particularly during reperfusion), and retrograde infusion pressure monitoring must be employed to avoid coronary sinus injury. Adequate cardioplegic delivery must be ensured by combined antegrade and retrograde infusion methods (181). Finally, a warm reperfusate with modified blood cardioplegia enriched with amino acids prevents reperfusion damage and may reverse ischemic/reperfusion

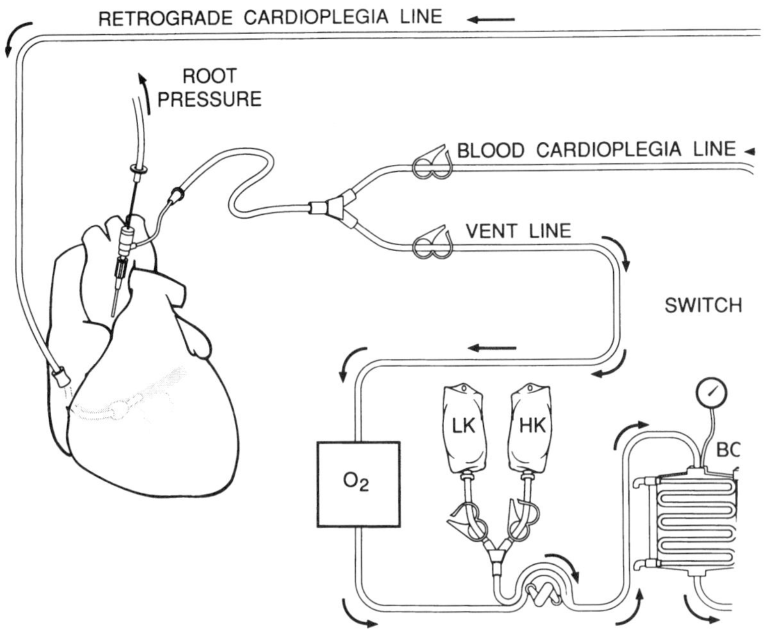

FIGURE 13-7. Blood cardioplegia delivery circuit. Two reservoir bags of crystalloid solution, a high potassium (*HK*) induction solution and a low potassium (*LK*) maintenance solution selectively mix with blood from the pump oxygenator (O_2) via a roller head. The temperature of the blood cardioplegia solution is regulated by a heat exchanger (*BCD*) and is delivered either antegrade into the aortic root (*blood cardioplegia line*) or retrograde via a transatrially placed cannula into the coronary sinus (*retrograde cardioplegia line*). Delivery into the aortic root or coronary sinus is controlled by the perfusionist (*switch*).

damage that had occurred during the preceding period of aortic occlusion.

Blood Cardioplegic Solution Preparation and Delivery

Three crystalloid solutions containing the cardioplegic additives (Tables 13-3 and 13-4) are prepared under sterile techniques in the pharmacy or may be purchased commercially. The solutions used for induction of cardioplegic arrest at cold temperature (cold induction) and for the maintenance of cardioplegic arrest (maintenance infusion) differ only in the amount of potassium chloride that they contain (Table 13-3). When delivered in a blood to crystalloid solution ratio of 4 : 1, they provide a blood cardioplegia composition, as listed in Table 13-3.

A third solution (reperfusate) containing the amino acids glutamic acid (13 μm) and aspartic acid (13 μm) is used for warm reperfusion or for induction of cardioplegic arrest at normothermic temperature (warm induction) (Table 13-4). This solution also varies from the cold induction and maintenance solutions in that it has more citrate-phosphate dextrose to further lower ionic calcium, less tromethamine to appropriately adjust the pH level for a warmer temperature, more dextrose to raise the osmolality, and a lower potassium concentration to allow prompt resumption of sinus rhythm after aortic unclamping.

The prepared solutions are delivered by the cardiopulmonary bypass machine through a single roller head on the heart-lung machine, resulting in a 4 : 1 blood to crystalloid mixture. Others have used a more concentrated solution to minimize the amount of crystalloid delivered. The temperature is regulated by circulation of warm or cold water from

TABLE 13-3. BLOOD CARDIOPLEGIA SOLUTIONS

Component	Cold Induction	Maintenance Infusion
Na (mEq/L)[a]	118	118
K (mEq/L)	18	11
Ca (mEq/L)	0.3–0.5	0.3–0.5
Mg (mEq/L)	1.6	1.6
pH (buffer)	7.6–7.8 (tham)[b]	7.6–7.8 (tham)[b]
Osm (mOsm)	320–340	320–340
Substrates	Glucose, oxygen	Glucose, oxygen

[a] Delivered concentration based on 4:1 blood:crystalloid mixture. Will vary slightly according to patient's electrolytes.
[b] Tromethamine 0.3 m.

TABLE 13-4. BLOOD CARDIOPLEGIA SOLUTIONS SUBSTRATE ENRICHED

Component	Warm Induction	Warm Reperfusate
Na (mEq/L)[a]	122	120
K (mEq/L)	25	9
Ca (mEq/L)	0.15–0.25	0.15–0.25
Mg (mEq/L)	1.6	1.6
pH (buffer)	7.5–7.6 (tham)[b]	7.5–7.6 (tham)[b]
Osm (mOsm)	340–360	340–360
Substrates	Glucose, oxygen Glutamate, aspartate	Glucose, oxygen Glutamate, aspartate

[a] Delivered concentration based on 4:1 blood:crystalloid mixture. Will vary slightly according to patients electrolytes.
[b] Tromethamine 0.3 m.

the heater-cooler system through a disposable heat exchanger (Fig. 13-7). A disposable regulator switch on the heart-lung machine or the operating room table to alternately or simultaneously delivers antegrade and retrograde cardioplegia. The circuit is completed by connection to a pump suction that allows venting of the aortic root between antegrade cardioplegic infusions or decompression of the aortic root during retrograde infusions.

Clinical Protocols

Primary Coronary Revascularization or Valvular Surgery

Cardiopulmonary bypass is established normothermically or with mild to moderate systemic hypothermia. Aortic root and transatrial coronary sinus cardioplegic delivery cannulas are positioned with pressure monitoring lines used to transduce cardioplegic infusion delivery pressures. After aortic cross-clamping, cold blood cardioplegic arrest is induced (induction solution) by antegrade infusion delivered at 60 to 80 mm Hg for 2 minutes. The infusate temperature averages 10°C to 11°C when delivered into the aortic root or the coronary sinus. Retrograde infusion is then started while venting the aortic root in coronary revascularization cases. The pressure of retrograde infusion is maintained at or below 50 mm Hg and the entire infusion period is continued for 1.5 to 2 minutes. Antegrade infusion technique is modified when the aortic valve is insufficient, substituting direct coronary ostial infusion for aortic root infusion followed by retrograde infusion, as previously described. By ensuring adequate cardioplegic distribution beyond critical coronary stenoses with retrograde coronary sinus administration of the cardioplegic solution, the surgeon can then construct coronary bypass grafts based on the technical ease or preference, as opposed to placing the first graft to the most critical coronary lesion. In most instances, aortic valve excision, annulus sizing, and initial steps of intracardiac repairs can be carried out during retrograde infusion periods. In mitral valve procedures, antegrade infusion is completed before retraction of the left atrium to avoid aortic root distortion and secondary valve insufficiency. Retrograde infusion can easily be performed while the retractors are being inserted.

Cardioplegic arrest is maintained by multidose antegrade and retrograde cold blood cardioplegic reinfusions of the maintenance solution (Table 13-3). These are delivered every 15 to 20 minutes or after each distal graft anastomosis is complete. Infusions of cardioplegic solution down bypass grafts can be accomplished directly into the reversed saphenous vein grafts via a multilimb infusion head or via the aortic root by sequential construction of distal and then proximal graft anastomoses. Antegrade and retrograde infusions are maintained for 1 and 1.5 minutes, respectively (total reinfusion period of 2 of 3 minutes).

Fifteen to 20 minutes before aortic unclamping, systemic rewarming is started and the warm blood cardioplegia reperfusate is prepared, circulated, and warmed through the cardioplegic delivery system. The warm reperfusate is administered antegradely and then retrogradely each for 1 and 1.5 minutes, respectively (total infusion of 2 to 3 minutes), and the infusion pressure is maintained at 50 mm Hg to prevent myocardial edema. The aorta is then unclamped and the procedure completed.

Reoperative Procedures. Reoperative coronary revascularization requires additional attention to the method of blood cardioplegic administration. Old patent bypass grafts often contain friable atheromatous debris and may embolize into the native coronary bed during the period of dissection. For this reason, cardiac and great vessel dissection is minimized, allowing suitable placement of cannulas for cardiopulmonary bypass and administration of cardioplegic solution. In addition, several centers are employing off-pump or minimally invasive approaches if limited revascularization is required.

After establishing cardiopulmonary bypass, patent internal thoracic artery grafts are temporarily occluded and antegrade cold blood cardioplegic induction is carried out via the aortic root, as described for primary cases. Retrograde cardioplegic infusion then proceeds as detailed previously for primary procedures. Old vein bypass grafts, if patent, are ligated and excised during the period of retrograde cardioplegic infusion to decrease the likelihood of distal atheromatous embolization. Subsequent cardiac dissection and placement of new grafts is then carried out. Antegrade and retrograde maintenance blood cardioplegic infusions proceed as described for primary operations, being repeated at 20-minute intervals. Systemic rewarming, warm blood cardioplegic reperfusate preparation, and infusion are carried out as previously described and the aorta is then unclamped. Simultaneously, the internal thoracic artery clamp is removed and flow is restored through this conduit. Construction of proximal and distal anastomoses during a single period of aortic cross-clamping is again advised to reduce the incidence of atheroembolism.

Reoperative valve surgery procedures in general do not require significant alteration in their protection techniques compared to those described for primary procedures. Using a slightly lower systemic temperature on bypass may improve surgical exposure by allowing a decrease in systemic flow rates on the heart-lung machine and therefore reducing the noncoronary collateral blood return to the heart.

"Energy-Depleted" Hearts

As described earlier, patients with cardiogenic shock, unstable angina, or acute or extending myocardial infarction present far greater challenges in preventing intraoperative ischemia and reperfusion damage. Preventing intraoperative damage begins with the preoperative stabilization of the patient, including the early use of the intraaortic balloon pump, providing pharmacologic support within inotropic and vasodilator drugs, and intubation and mechanical ventilation in the appropriate circumstances.

Cardiopulmonary bypass is established and a left atrial vent is used to ensure ventricular decompression and reduce myocardial rewarming from noncoronary collateral blood returning to the left atrium. Blood cardioplegic arrest is induced at a warm temperature (37°C) with amino acid–enriched blood cardioplegia solution (Table 13-4) containing 25 mEq of potassium chloride to ensure prompt normothermic arrest during this period of warm cardioplegic induction. Warm cardioplegic infusion is carried out for 5 minutes (2.5 minutes antegrade, 2.5 minutes retrograde). This is followed by 2 to 3 minutes of cold (10°C to 11°C) blood cardioplegic infusion to reduce myocardial temperature and metabolic rate for the remainder of the period of aortic cross-clamping. Maintenance reinfusions and the warm blood cardioplegic reperfusion are administered as previously described. Patients in low cardiac output states from acute valvular lesions (severe aortic or mitral regurgitation) will also benefit from warm cardioplegic induction therapy although conduct of the procedure need not deviate significantly from the surgeon's usual routine.

Clinical Results of Blood Versus Crystalloid Cardioplegic Protection

As described previously, several clinical studies in the literature report superior perioperative myocardial protection in patients receiving blood cardioplegia, as opposed to crystalloid cardioplegia. This is most notable in patients undergoing urgent coronary revascularization for unstable angina, myocardial infarction or low cardiac output state, and cardiogenic shock (176,177,179,180). Loop and colleagues (182) reported their results of primary and reoperative coronary vascularization, valve procedures, and combined coronary revascularization and valve operations looking at both perioperative morbidity and mortality rates. This study clearly documented a reduction in morbidity in patients receiving blood cardioplegia compared to a matched control group given crystalloid cardioplegia. A further improvement was seen in patients receiving antegrade and retrograde cardioplegia delivery compared to those receiving only antegrade blood cardioplegic protection.

SPECIAL CIRCUMSTANCES

Pediatric Patients

As noted already, the immature heart appears to be more tolerant to equivalent periods of unprotected normothermic ischemia than the adult heart (58,60). Recent evidence suggests that this may be due to a more avid and prolonged capacity for anaerobic metabolism of glucose by glycolysis, more efficient use of amino acids, and Krebs cycle intermediates for prolonged anaerobic metabolism during the period of aortic occlusion and an endogenous state of myocardial preconditioning (183–185).

The requirements for intraoperative cardioplegic myocardial protection of the immature heart are less well identified and understood than those currently recognized for the mature heart. Cold St. Thomas's crystalloid cardioplegia is a popular method for clinical myocardial protection, although modified blood cardioplegic techniques have gained acceptance. We and others use a blood cardioplegic protocol essentially identical to that described in the preceding section for adult patients undergoing repair of congenital heart lesions (186,187). Cardioplegia volume is limited to 30 mL/kg for the cardioplegic induction dose, 15 to 20 mL/kg for maintenance reinfusions, and 20 mL/kg for warm reperfusion. The time intervals for infusion are the same as those outlined for adult patients. Retrograde delivery of cardioplegia via the coronary sinus is employed selectively for cases in which aortic root reconstruction is required such as with the arterial switch operation and the Ross operation (186). Other groups report satisfactory results with single dose, dilute blood cardioplegic protection (188,189). The different requirements for cyanotic versus acyanotic children are as yet unidentified, although laboratory evidence suggests that important differences may exist (190). Pediatric myocardial protection remains an area of active but incomplete investigation.

Heart Transplantation

Myocardial protection of the heart for orthotopic transplantation had until recently been focused on long-term (more than 24 hours) storage and preservation. Recent efforts have also focused on evaluating the physiologic and metabolic changes that occur in the heart of the brain-dead donor and how best to prevent further ischemic and reperfusion damage during the phase of allograft reimplantation.

The brain-dead donor has a massive release of circulating catecholamines, resulting in an eventual decline in myocardial function. This is due to a depletion of myocardial ATP and creatine phosphate (191), which experimentally can be reversed by initially inducing arrest with a normothermic perfusate (i.e., warm induction). Hann and colleagues (192) showed that including glutamic acid in the reperfusate solution further improved graft functional recovery. Clinically, Hardesty and colleagues (193) reported a significant benefit of using blood cardioplegia during graft implantation.

Warm Cardioplegia/Warm Cardiopulmonary Bypass

Although hypothermia has been a fundamental tool and hallmark of myocardial protection, Salerno and colleagues (149,194–196) from Toronto reintroduced the concept of normothermic cardiac surgery to avoid the systemic metabolic disadvantages of hypothermia and minimize perioperative myocardial ischemia. Their technique involves the use of continuous retrograde warm blood cardioplegia to eliminate periods of intraoperative ischemia and maintain continued aerobic metabolism in the potassium-arrested heart. Their results showed that postischemic myocardial function was superior in patients undergoing warm heart surgery with continuous retrograde warm blood cardioplegia, compared to a similar group of patients receiving cold blood cardioplegia with systemic hypothermia. Furthermore, patients maintained at normothermia (33°C to 34°C) had a shorter period on cardiopulmonary bypass (no need for cooling and rewarming time) and required less fluid replacement in the early postoperative period. To facilitate visualization of coronary artery anastomoses, Salerno and others (194,196) use periodic interruptions of cardioplegic administration, which has not proven to be detrimental.

Less-Invasive and Off-Pump Heart Surgery

In an effort to reduce the trauma and expense of heart surgery, several groups have introduced less-invasive techniques for performing heart surgery that have altered the types and methods of surgical exposure, whereas others have explored performing coronary bypass operations without the use of cardiopulmonary bypass. Although these approaches are early in their development and long-term results are not available, there is growing enthusiasm for these new techniques. The traditional methods of myocardial protection and the role played by the anesthesiologist in myocardial protection are also under rapid transition as these techniques mature and develop.

Less-invasive cardiac surgery is often referred to as minimally invasive surgery, which is in many ways a misnomer. The fundamental change in these procedures is the size of the surgical incision and the method of exposure of the heart. These techniques still use cardiopulmonary bypass and periods of aortic cross-clamping with some variations of the myocardial protection techniques. In contrast, off-pump surgery, which is limited to coronary revascularization surgery, has the noted advantage of not using cardiopulmonary bypass or aortic cross-clamping, and as such, it does not employ the methods of myocardial protection discussed in this chapter. Despite areas of overlap, for the purpose of this chapter, these less-invasive approaches to cardiac surgery will be discussed separately, because from the perspective of myocardial protection, substantial differences exist.

Minimally Invasive Procedures

The main innovation of minimally invasive heart surgery is a reduction in the size and location of the surgical incision. Advocates of these approaches have proposed that by avoiding full median sternotomy, postoperative pain and morbidity will be reduced, thereby reducing the length of hospitalization and convalescence. Several approaches have been introduced, which can be categorized as those using modified incisions in the thorax versus those employing principally endoscopic exposure to the heart.

The modified thoracic incisions have included partial sternotomy (197), parasternal incisions (198), and more traditional methods of anterior thoracotomy (199). Depending on the type of incision, transthoracic, percutaneous, or a combination of these, cannulation techniques for cardiopulmonary bypass have been employed. Similarly, modified aortic occlusion techniques have been described, ranging from using the fairly standard application of the cross-clamp through the thoracic incision to placing the clamp through an additional incision to endovascular aortic occlusion with a percutaneously positioned balloon catheter in the ascending aorta. Cardioplegia delivery methods have also been modified. Depending on the incision chosen, fairly traditional insertion of aortic root and coronary sinus cannulas can often be employed. Alternative routes such as antegrade delivery via the endoaortic occlusion balloon and retrograde delivery via a coronary sinus cannula placed percutaneously via the jugular vein have also been employed.

The endoscopic approach has largely employed the HeartPort System (HeartPort, Inc., Redwood City, CA), which requires percutaneous cannulation for cardiopulmonary bypass, endoaortic aortic catheter occlusion, and cardioplegia delivery and access to the heart via multiple thoracoscopic ports. Early experience with this approach has been reported for performing mitral valve repairs or replacements, closure of atrial septal defects, and coronary bypass operations (200).

Off-Pump Operations

Coronary bypass graft operations have been performed on the beating heart without the use of cardiopulmonary bypass since Kolosov reported his initial experience in 1967 (201). Several groups continued to use this technique for selected situations, but it was largely ignored until 1985 when Benetti (202) and Buffolo (203) reintroduced this approach and reported remarkable success. Two general approaches have been employed for off-pump CABG. Isolated revascularization of the left anterior descending coronary artery with the left internal thoracic artery via a limited left anterior thoracotomy that have been referred to as minimally invasive coronary bypass, left anterior small thoracotomy (204), and less invasive clinical approach (LISA) (205) procedures by differing authors. This approach enjoys both the advantage of being less invasive than traditional CABG, like angioplasty and stenting, and the advantage of the documented long-term patency of the surgically placed LIMA graft. However, it has limited application in situations of multivessel revascularization. For this reason, off-pump, multivessel CABG via a traditional median sternotomy incision has been promoted. Access to the inferior (posterior descending artery) and lateral (circumflex) surfaces of the heart were difficult until several stabilizing apparatuses were developed, along with methods of distracting the heart vertically out of the mediastinum (205).

All of these approaches require a period of coronary artery occlusion with snares or insertion of an intraluminal stent that allows limited distal flow to control bleeding from the anastomosis site of the target vessel. As such, periods of unprotected myocardial ischemia and subsequent reperfusion are a part of this surgical approach. Due to concerns about the safety of these periods of regional myocardial ischemia, several groups have investigated a process of preconditioning the heart to improve its tolerance to the subsequent period of ischemia. Preconditioning is the phenomenon described by Murry (46) in which a brief (i.e., 5-minute) interval of myocardial ischemia followed by reperfusion improves the heart's tolerance to a subsequent, more prolonged period of sustained ischemia, as would be required for performing a coronary bypass graft anastomosis. The pathophysiology of the preconditioning phenomenon is incompletely understood but appears to be initiated by chemicals released by ischemic tissues (adenosine, bradykinin) which via cell membrane receptors, initiate a series of intracellular signals that result in inducing the preconditioned state. The clinical application of ischemic preconditioning or pharmacologic preconditioning are both under active investigation and may represent important adjuncts to off-pump coronary bypass surgery.

POSTOPERATIVE FACTORS

Although we often focus our attention on the period of myocardial ischemia during aortic cross-clamping as the sole determinant of the outcome of the surgical procedure, myocardial protection truly extends beyond this period into the postoperative phase as well. The phases of separation from cardiopulmonary bypass, reestablishing a stable hemodynamic state, and the gradual emergence from anesthetic agents represent periods in which myocardial damage can also occur.

The processes of systemic rewarming and aortic unclamping elicit significant fluctuations in sympathetic tone (206). This is manifested by an increase in heart rate, fever, changes in systemic vascular resistance, and a rise in the circulating levels of catecholamines. These physiologic effects on the heart and systemic vascular bed result in a decrease in oxygen supply and an increase in oxygen demands precisely at a time the myocardium is vulnerable to ischemic damage despite having undergone a satisfactory technical operation. After cardioplegic arrest, the heart is frequently more compliant than before the period of cardioplegic arrest and therefore may be functioning at a significantly greater left ventricular end-diastolic volume. This in turn will increase wall tension and myocardial oxygen requirements unless the heart is properly unloaded. The native coronary arteries and the bypass conduits may become subject to vasomotor disturbances due to changes in endogenous stimuli as well as due to the acute withdrawal of exogenous pharmacologic agents such as β-blockers and calcium channel blockers. Significant vasospasm may compromise myocardial perfusion in the early period after aortic unclamping. Metabolically, the recovering postischemic myocardium has elevated oxygen requirements that are needed to replenish depleted ATP stores, reestablish intracellular ion gradients, and allow the resumption of electromechanical work. Adequate ventilation and control of tracheobronchial secretions must precede separation from cardiopulmonary bypass to ensure adequate oxygenation and to avoid respiratory acidosis.

A major factor in causing early postoperative myocardial dysfunction is ventricular distention while weaning from cardiopulmonary bypass. If ventricular distention occurs, immediate reinstitution of cardiopulmonary bypass will allow assessment of the cause of ventricular dysfunction while minimizing metabolic demands. The immediate institution of high-dose inotropic drug support should be avoided until other options have been considered, due to evidence that significantly elevated oxygen demands induced by these agents may actually delay recovery of the postischemic heart. To maintain cardiac output, an adequate level of preload should be provided, without significantly increasing wall tension, and afterload reduction with pharmacologic or mechanical means (intraaortic balloon) should be considered. Adequate mean arterial blood pressure must also be maintained however, to ensure adequate coronary arterial and bypass graft perfusion. Tachycardia due to pain, inotropic drugs, fever, or arrhythmia should be controlled to ensure an adequate period for diastolic coronary perfusion during each cardiac cycle. All attempts to maximize this complex physiologic balance should be made before transition from cardiopulmonary bypass. Finally, excessive bleeding should also be promptly corrected before separation from bypass to prevent intravascular volume changes.

COMPLICATIONS OF MYOCARDIAL PROTECTION

The most common and potentially fatal complication of intraoperative myocardial protection is the failure to adequately protect the heart, resulting in significant postoperative ventricular dysfunction at the conclusion of the procedure. By careful preoperative planning of the procedure, stable induction and maintenance of anesthesia, meticulous attention to the requirements for and administration of intraoperative cardioplegic technique, and gentle separation from cardiopulmonary bypass, the surgeon can limit inadequate postoperative results to situations in which the patient's anatomy or the severity of the disease prevents complete surgical correction of the underlying problem.

Postoperative right ventricular dysfunction is a more complex issue and remains a clinical challenge (207–209). The right ventricle physiologically is less tolerant to sudden increases in pressure-work than the left ventricle. Therefore, poor postoperative right ventricular function most frequently is a manifestation of inadequate left ventricular function and therefore a pressure-loaded right ventricle. Uniform cardioplegic solution distribution may be difficult to achieve in the right ventricle for several reasons. Although major left ventricular coronary artery stenoses are generally bypassed during coronary artery revascularization, acute marginal branches are rarely bypassed, therefore potentially limiting the antegrade delivery of cardioplegic solution beyond stenoses in these vessels. Retrograde coronary sinus distribution of cardioplegic solution to the right ventricle is less uniform than that in the left ventricle, and this is particularly notable in the right ventricular subendocardium (156). Finally, rewarming of the right ventricular free wall during the period of aortic cross-clamping is a significant problem due to exposure to the ambient room temperature (210). This may be avoided by topical cooling solutions or the use of a cooling jacket.

Mechanical injuries induced by cardioplegic delivery are infrequent. A particularly serious lesion is coronary ostial stenosis related to ischemic injury of the ostial endothelium by the incorrect use of ostial cannulas. This can be avoided by the use of soft-tipped cannulas and/or by allowing a small degree of leak around the cannula by gentle contact with the ostial lumen. Increased reliance on retrograde delivery may also reduce the incidence of this complication. Finally, coronary sinus injury, a potentially lethal complication of retrograde cardioplegic delivery, can all but be eliminated by careful palpation during the insertion of the cannula or by insertion under direct vision in situations in which transatrial technique meets with resistance during insertion. Constant control of the infusion pressure at or below 50 mm Hg should also prevent sinus perforation or iatrogenic edema formation.

CONCLUSIONS

Of the many advances developed in the first half century of cardiac surgery, improved intraoperative myocardial protection has had the greatest impact on improving the conditions under which repairs are performed and the tolerance of the patient's heart to undergo these often lengthy and complex procedures. These major advances have largely been made possible by careful investigation into the basic science of myocardial ischemia and reperfusion. The application of these scientific discoveries to the clinical arena has been directly responsible for our ability to reduce perioperative morbidity and mortality rates in a patient population presenting with increasingly greater risk factors and with an increasing need for reoperative surgery. Unlocking the mechanisms of myocardial preconditioning so that it can be induced pharmacologically promises to open new avenues for reducing the risk of myocardial injury during surgery.

The continued quest for improved surgical results increases the demand for a concerted team approach of the surgeon and anesthesiologist in minimizing all factors that contribute to myocardial damage during the time of anesthetic induction, the surgical procedure, and the period of separation from cardiopulmonary bypass. By exercising a practical understanding of cardiac physiology and metabolism to varying perioperative risk factors and events, we can achieve consistent and improving results. As the challenges of patient care continue to increase, the requirement for perfect myocardial protection becomes more significant.

REFERENCES

1. Taber RE, Norales AR, Fine G. Myocardial necrosis and the postoperative low cardiac output syndrome. *Ann Thorac Surg* 1967;4:12.
2. Najafi H, Henson D, Dye WS, et al. Left ventricular hemorrhagic necrosis. *Ann Thorac Surg* 1969;7:550.
3. Buckberg GD. Left ventricular subendocardial necrosis. *Ann Thorac Surg* 1977;24:379.
4. Buckberg GD, Fixler DW, Archie JP, et al. Experimental subendocardial ischemia in dogs with normal coronary arteries. *Circ Res* 1972;30:67.
5. Buckberg GD, Towers B, Paglia D, et al. Subendocardial ischemia after cardiopulmonary bypass. *J Thorac Cardiovasc Surg* 1972;64:669.
6. Allen BS, Buckberg GD, Schwaiger M, et al. Studies of controlled reperfusion after ischemia. XVI: consistent early recovery of regional wall motion following surgical revascularization after eight hours of acute coronary occlusion. *J Thorac Cardiovasc Surg* (Suppl) 1986;92[Suppl]:686.
7. Wechsler AS, Abd-El fattah AS, Murphy CE, et al. Myocardial protection. *J Cardiac Surg* 1986;1:271.
8. Nayler WG, Elz JS. Reperfusion injury: laboratory artifact or clinical dilemma. *Circulation* 1986;74:215.
9. Jennings RB, Reimer KA, Steenbergen C. Myocardial ischemia revisited: the osmolar load, membrane damage, and reperfusion. *J Mol Cell Cardiol* 1986;18:769.
10. Hearse DJ, Humphrey SM, Bullock GR. The oxygen paradox and the calcium paradox: two facets of the same problem? *J Mol Cell Cardiol* 1978;10:641.
11. Hearse DJ. The pathophysiology of myocardial ischemia. In: Roberts AJ, ed. *Myocardial protection is cardiac surgery.* New York: Marcel Dekker Inc, 1987:7.
12. Kloner RA, Przyklenk K, Lange R, et al. Reperfusion pathophysiology. In: Roberts AJ, ed. *Myocardial protection in cardiac surgery.* New York: Marcel Dekker Inc, 1987:29.
13. Bolli R. Mechanism of myocardial "stunning." *Circulation* 1990;82:723.
14. Opie LH. Reperfusion injury and its pharmacologic modification. *Circulation* 1989;80:1049.
15. Brazier J, Cooper N, Buckberg GD. The adequacy of subendocardial oxygen delivery: the interaction of determinants of flow, arterial oxygen content and myocardial oxygen need. *Circulation* 1974;49:968.
16. Buckberg GD, Ross G. The effects of isoprenaline on coronary

blood flow, its distribution and myocardial performance. *Cardiovasc Res* 1973;7:429.
17. Hoffman JIE, Buckberg GD. Transmural variation in myocardial perfusion. In: Yu PN, Goodwin JF, eds. *Progress in cardiology*. Philadelphia: Lea & Febiger, 1976:38.
18. Sarnoff SJ, Braunwald E, Welch GD. Hemodynamic determinants of oxygen consumption of the heart with special reference to the tension time index. *Am J Physiol* 1958;192:148.
19. Suga H. Total mechanical energy of a ventricle model and cardiac oxygen consumption. *Am J Physiol* 1979;236:H498.
20. Furukawa S, Bavaria JE, Kreiner G, et al. Relationship between total mechanical energy and oxygen consumption in the stunned myocardium. *Ann Thorac Surg* 1990;49:543.
21. Burkhoff D. Myocardial energetics and the postischemic heart. *Ann Thorac Surg* 1990;49:525.
22. Brazier JR, Buckberg GD. Effects of tachycardia on the adequacy of subendocardial oxygen delivery in aortic stenosis. *Am Heart J* 1975;90:222.
23. Buckberg GD, Fixler DE, Archie JP, et al. Variable effects of heart rate on phasic and regional left ventricular muscle blood flow in anesthetized dogs. *Cardiovasc Res* 1975;9:1.
24. Jennings RB, Reimer KA. Factors involved in salvaging ischemic myocardium. Effects of reperfusion of arterial blood. *Circulation* 1983;68[Part 2]:I25.
25. Jennings RB, Ganote CE. Structural changes in myocardium during acute ischemia. *Circ Res* 1974:34/35[Suppl 3]:156.
26. Braunwald E, Kloner RA. The stunned myocardium: prolonged, postischemic ventricular dysfunction. *Circulation* 1982; 66:1146.
27. Katz AM. Effects of ischemia on the contractile process of heart muscle. *Am J Cardiol* 1973;32:456.
28. Hearse DJ. Oxygen deprivation and early contractile failure: reassessment of the possible role of ATP. *Am J Cardiol* 1979; 44:1115.
29. Gudbjarnason S, Mathea P, Ravens KG. Functional compartmentation of ATP and creatine phosphate in heart muscle. *J Mol Cell Cardiol* 1970;1:325.
30. Neely JR, Morgan HE. Relationship between carbohydrate and lipid metabolism and the energy balance of heart muscle. *Ann Rev Physiol* 1974;36:413.
31. Evans JR. Cellular transport of long-chain fatty acids. *Can J Biochem* 1964:42:955.
32. Liedtke AJ, Nellis S, Neely JR. Effects of excess free fatty acids on mechanical and metabolic function in normal and ischemic myocardium in swine. *Circ Res* 1978;43:652.
33. Mjos OD, Vik-Mo H. Influence of free fatty acids on myocardial oxygen consumption and ischemic injury. *Am J Cardiol* 1981;48:361.
34. Opie LH. Effects of regional ischemia on metabolism of glucose and fatty acids. Relative rates of aerobic and anaerobic energy production during myocardial infarction and comparison with effects of anoxia. *Circ Res* 1976;38[Suppl 1]:52.
35. Dobson JG, Moyer SE. Mechanisms of activation of cardiac glycogen phosphorylase in ischemia and anoxia. *Circ Res* 1973; 33:412.
36. Rovetto MJ, Lamberton WF, Neely JR. Mechanisms of glycolytic inhibition in ischemic rat hearts. *Circ Res* 1975;47:742.
37. Kane JJ, Murphy ML, Bissett JK, et al. Mitochondrial function, oxygen extraction, epicardial ST segment changes and tritiated digoxin distribution after reperfusion of ischemic myocardium. *Am J Cardiol* 1975;36:218.
38. Lochner A, Opie LH, Owen P, et al. Oxidative phosphorylation in infarcting baboon and dog myocardium: effects of mitochondrial isolation and incubation media. *J Mol Cell Cardiol* 1975; 7:203.
39. Jennings RB, Herdson PB, Sommers HM. Structural and functional abnormalities in mitochondria isolated from ischemic dog myocardium. *Lab Invest* 1969;20:548.
40. Cooley DA, Reul GJ, Wukasch DC. Ischemic contracture of the heart, "stone heart." *Am J Cardiol* 1972;29:575.
41. Hearse DJ, Garlick PB, Humphrey SM. Ischemic contracture of the myocardium: mechanism and precaution. *Am J Cardiol* 1977;39:986.
42. Ricciutti MA. Lysosomes and myocardial cellular injury. *Am J Cardiol* 1972;30:498.
43. Buckberg GD. Studies of controlled reperfusion after ischemia: I. When is cardiac muscle damaged irreversibly? *J Thorac Cardiovasc Surg* 1986;92:483.
44. Follette DM, Fey K, Buckberg GD, et al. Reducing postischemic damage by temporary modification of reperfusate calcium, potassium, pH and osmolarity. *J Thorac Cardiovasc Surg* 1981; 82:221.
45. Rosenkranz ER, Buckberg GD. Myocardial protection during surgical coronary reperfusion. *J Am Coll Cardiol* 1983;1:1235.
46. Murry C, Jennings R, Reimer K. Preconditioning with ischemia: a delay of lethal cell injury in ischemic myocardium. *Circulation* 1986;74:1124.
47. Jennings RB, Shen AC. Calcium in experimental myocardial ischemia. In: Bajusz E, Rona G, eds. *Recent advances in studies on cardiac structure and metabolism.* Baltimore, MD: University Park Press, 1972:639.
48. Jennings RB, Ganote C. Mitochondrial structure and function in acute myocardial ischemic injury. Circ Res 1976;38[Suppl I]:80.
49. Nayler WG, Ferrari R, Williams A. Protective effect of pretreatment with verapamil, nifedipine and propranolol on mitochondrial function in the ischemic and reperfused myocardium. *Am J Cardiol* 1980;46:242.
50. Fitzpatrick DB, Karmazyn M. Comparative effects of calcium channel blocking agents and varying extracellular calcium concentration on hypoxia/reoxygenation and ischemia/reperfusion cardiac injury. *J Pharmacol Exp Ther* 1984;228:761.
51. Guarnieri C, Flamigni F, Calderen CM. Role of oxygen in the cellular damage induced by reoxygenation of the hypoxic heart. *J Mol Cell Cardiol* 1980;12:797.
52. Menasché P, Piwnica A. Free radicals and myocardial protection: a surgical viewpoint. *Ann Thorac Surg* 1989;47:939.
53. Hammond B, Hess ML. The oxygen free radical system: potential mediator of myocardial injury. *J Am Coll Cardiol* 1986;6: 215.
54. Shlafer M, Kane PF, Kirsh M. Superoxide dismutase plus catalase enhances the efficacy of hypothermic cardioplegia to perfect the globally ischemic, reperfused heart. *J Thorac Cardiovasc Surg* 1982;83:830.
55. Menasché P, Grousset C, Gaudmel Y, et al. A comparison study of free radical scavengers in cardioplegic solutions. Improved protection with peroxidase. *J Thorac Cardiovasc Surg* 1986;92: 264.
56. Kako KJ. Free radical effects on membrane protein in myocardial ischemia/reperfusion injury. *J Mol Cell Cardiol* 1987;19: 209.
57. Buckberg GD. Strategies and logic of cardioplegic delivery to prevent, avoid and reverse ischemic and reperfusion damage. *J Thorac Cardiovasc Surg* 1987;93:127.
58. Murashoita T, Kempsford Rd, Hearse DJ. Age-dependent changes in tolerance of the rabbit heart to ischemia. *Eur J Cardiothorac Surg* 1990;4:492.
59. Baker JE, Boerboom LE, Olinger GN. Age-related changes in the ability of hypothermia and cardioplegia to protect ischemic rabbit myocardium. *J Thorac Cardiovasc Surg* 1988;96:717.
60. Bove E, Stammers A. Recovery of left-ventricular function after hypothermic global ischemia. Age-related differences in the iso-

lated working rabbit heart. *J Thorac Cardiovasc Surg* 1986;91:115.
61. Bladergroen MR, Takei H, Christopher TD, et al. Accelerated transmural gradients of energy compound metabolism resulting from left ventricular hypertrophy. *J Thorac Cardiovasc Surg* 1990;100:506.
62. Attarian DE, Jones RN, Cumé WD, et al. Characteristics of chronic left ventricular hypertrophy induced by subcoronary valvular aortic stenosis. II. Response to ischemia. *J Thorac Cardiovasc Surg* 1981;81:389.
63. Vincent RW, Buckberg GD, Hoffman JIE. Left-ventricular subendocardial ischemia in severe valvular and supravalvular aortic stenosis. *Circulation* 1974;49:326.
64. Higgins TL, Estafanous FG, Loop FD, et al. Evaluation of operative risk in patients undergoing coronary artery bypass grafting. *Anesth Analg* 1991;72:S107.
65. Jones RN, Peyton RB, Sabina RL, et al. Transmural gradients in high-energy phosphate content in patients with coronary artery disease. *Ann Thorac Surg* 1981;32:546.
66. Allison TB, Ramey CA, Hollsinger JW. Transmural gradient of left ventricular tissue metabolites after circumflex coronary artery ligation in dogs. *J Mol Cell Cardiol* 1977;9:837.
67. Lowe JE, Cummings RG, Adams DH, et al. Evidence that ischemic cell death begins in the subendocardium independent of variations in collateral flow or wall tension. *Circulation* 1983;68:190.
68. Becker H, Vinten-Johansen J, Buckberg GD, et al. Critical importance of ensuring cardioplegic delivery with coronary stenoses. *J Thorac Cardiovasc Surg* 1981;81:407.
69. Peyton RB, Jones RN, Attarian D, et al. Depressed high-energy phosphate content in hypertrophied ventricles in animal and man. The biologic basis for increased sensitivity to ischemic injury. *Ann Surg* 1982;196:278.
70. Katz AM, Tada M. The "stone heart": a challenge to the biochemist. *Am J Cardiol* 1972;29:578.
71. Peyton RB, Van Trigt P, Pellom GS, et al. Improved tolerance to ischemia in hypertrophied myocardium by preischemic enhancement of adenosine triphosphate. *J Thorac Cardiovasc Surg* 1982;84:11.
72. Del Nido PJ, Mickle DAG, Wilson GJ, et al. Inadequate myocardial protection with old cardioplegic arrest during repair of tetralogy of Fallot. *J Thorac Cardiovasc Surg* 1988;95:223.
73. Papadimitriou JM, Hopkins BE, Taylor RR. Regression of left ventricular dilation and hypertrophy after removal of volume overload. *Circ Res.* 1974;35:127.
74. Gay WA. The evolution of intraoperative myocardial protection. In: Roberts AJ, ed. *Myocardial protection in cardiac surgery.* New York: Marcel Dekker Inc, 1987:1.
75. Gay WA. Potassium-induced cardioplegia: evaluation and present status. *Ann Thorac Surg* 1989;48:441.
76. Kirklin JW, Conti VR, Blackstone EH. Prevention of myocardial damage during cardiac operation. *N Engl J Med* 1979;301:135.
77. Ringer S. A further contribution regarding the influence of different constituents of the blood on the contraction of the heart. *J Physiol* 1883;4:29.
78. Hooker DR. On recovery of the heart in electric shock. *Am J Physiol* 1929;91:305.
79. Melrose DG, Dreyer B, Bentall HH, et al. Elective cardiac arrest. *Lancet* 1955;2:21.
80. Tyers GFO, Todd GJ, Niebauer IM, et al. The mechanism of myocardial damage following potassium citrate (Melrose) cardioplegia. *Surgery* 1975;78:45.
81. Shumway NE, Lower RR. Topical cardiac hypothermia for extended periods of anoxic cardiac arrest. *Surg Forum* 1960;10:563.
82. Griepp RB, Stinson EB, Shumway NE. Profound local hypothermia for myocardial protection during open-heart surgery. *J Thorac Cardiovasc Surg* 1973;66:731.
83. Pupello DF, Blank RH, Connor RG, et al. Fifty-two consecutive aortic valve replacements employing local deep hypothermia. *Ann Thorac Surg* 1976;21:508.
84. Griepp RB, Stinson EB, Oyer PE, et al. The superiority of aortic cross-clamping with profound local hypothermia for myocardial protection during aorta-coronary bypass grafting. *J Thorac Cardiovasc Surg* 1975;70:995.
85. Reidmeister JC, Heberer G, Bretschneider HJ. Induced cardiac arrest by sodium and calcium depletion and application of procaine. *Int Surg* 1967;47:535.
86. Bretschneider H, Hubner G, Knoll D, et al. Myocardial resistance and tolerance to ischemia: physiological and biochemical basis. *J Cardiovasc Surg* 1975;16:241.
87. Kirsch U, Rodewald G, Kalmar P. Induced ischemic arrest: clinical experience with cardioplegia in open heart surgery. *J Thorac Cardiovasc Surg* 1972;63:121.
88. Hearse DJ, Stewart DA, Braimbridge MV. Cellular protection during myocardial ischemia: the development and characterization of a procedure for the induction of reversible ischemic arrest. *Circulation* 1976;54:193.
89. Gay WA, Ebert PA. Functional, metabolic and morphologic effects of potassium-induced cardioplegia. *Surgery* 1973;74:284.
90. Hearse DJ, Humphrey SM, Nayler WG, et al. Ultrastructural damage associated with reoxygenation of the aerobic myocardium. *J Mol Cell Cardiol* 1975;7:315.
91. Follette D, Fey K, Mulder D, et al. Prolonged safe aortic clamping by combined membrane stabilization, multidose cardioplegia and appropriate pH reperfusion. *J Thorac Cardiovasc Surg* 1977;74:682.
92. Follette DM, Mulder DG, Maloney JV, et al. Advantages of blood cardioplegia over continuous coronary perfusion and intermittent ischemia. *J Thorac Cardiovasc Surg* 1978;76:604.
93. Buckberg GD. Recent progress in myocardial protection during cardiac operations. In: McGoon DC, ed. *Cardiac surgery,* 2nd ed. Philadelphia: FA Davis Co, 1987:291.
94. Daily PO, Kinney TB. Optimizing myocardial hypothermia: I. Cooling jacket modification and clinical results. *Ann Thorac Surg* 1991;51:284.
95. Buckberg GD, Brazier JR, Nelson RL, et al. Studies of the effects of hypothermia on regional myocardial blood flow and metabolism during cardiopulmonary bypass. I. The adequately perfused beating, fibrillating and arrested heart. *J Thorac Cardiovasc Surg* 1977;73:87.
96. Hottenrott C, Towers B, Kurkji H, et al. The hazard of ventricular fibrillation in hypertrophied hearts during cardiopulmonary bypass. *J Thorac Cardiovasc Surg* 1973;66:742.
97. Steed D, Follette D, Foglia R, et al. Unavoidable subendocardial underperfusion during bypass especially in infants. *Circulation* 1977;55/56[Suppl 3]:248.
98. Rahn H. Body temperature and acid-base regulation. *Pharmacologie* 1974;15:87.
99. Swan H. The hydroxyl-hydrogen ion concentration ratio during hypothermia. *Surg Gynecol Obstet* 1982;155:897.
100. Howell BJ, Baumgartner FW, Bondi K, et al. Acid-base balance in cold-blooded vertebrates as a function of body temperature. *Am J Physiol* 1970;218:600.
101. Goodrich CA. Acid-base balance in ectothermic and liberating marmots. *Am J Physiol* 1973;224:1185.
102. Streisand RL, Gourin A, Stuckey JH. Respiratory and metabolic alkalosis and myocardial contractility. *J Thorac Cardiovasc Surg* 1971;62:431.
103. Becker H, Vinten-Johansen J, Buckberg GD, et al. Myocardial

damage caused by keeping pH 7.40 during systemic deep hypothermia. *J Thorac Cardiovasc Surg* 1981;82:810.

104. Mudge GH, Mills RM, Taegtmeyer HJ, et al. Alterations of myocardial amino acid metabolism in chronic ischemic heart disease. *J Clin Invest* 1976;58:1185.
105. Galis L, Benmoyal E. Endogenous alanine, glutamate aspartate and glutamine in the perfused guinea pig heart: effect of substrates and cardioactive agents. *Can J Biochem* 1973;51:11.
106. Davis EJ, Bremmer J. Studies with isolated surviving rat hearts: independence of free amino acids and citric-acid cycle intermediates. *Eur J Biochem* 1973;38:86.
107. Sanborn T, Gavin W, Berkowitz S, et al. Augmented conversion of aspartate and glutamate to succinate during anoxia in rabbit hearts. *Am J Physiol* 1979;237:H535.
108. Burns AH, Reddy WJ. Amino acid stimulation of oxygen and substrate utilization by cardiac myocytes. *Am J Physiol* 1978; 235:E461.
109. Penny DG, Cascarano J. Anaerobic rabbit heart: effects of glucose and tricarboxylic acid cycle intermediates on metabolism and physiological performance. *Biochem J* 1970;118:221.
110. Rau EE, Shine KT, Gervais A, et al. Enhanced mechanical recovery of anoxic and ischemic myocardium by amino acid perfusion. *Am J Physiol* 1979;236:H873.
111. Safer B. The metabolic significance of the malate aspartate cycle in the heart. *Circ Res* 1975;51:521.
112. Thomassen AR, Nielsen TT, Bagger JP, et al. Myocardial exchange of glutamate, alanine and citrate in controls and patients with coronary artery disease. *Clin Sci* 1983;64:33.
113. Lazar HL, Buckberg GD, Manganaro AM, et al. Reversal of ischemic damage with amino acid substrate enhancement during reperfusion. *Surgery* 1980;88:702.
114. Rosenkranz ER, Okamoto F, Buckberg GD, et al. The safety of prolonged aortic clamping with blood cardioplegia. II. Glutamate enrichment in energy-depleted hearts. *J Thorac Cardiovasc Surg* 1984;88:402.
115. Rosenkranz ER, Okamoto F, Buckberg GD, et al. Safety of prolong aortic clamping with blood cardioplegia. III. Aspartate enrichment of glutamate blood cardioplegia in energy depleted hearts after ischemic and reperfusion injury. *J Thorac Cardiovasc Surg* 1986;91:428.
116. Schwalb H, Izhar U, Yaroslavsky E, et al. The effect of amino acids on the ischemic heart. Improvement of oxygenated crystalloid cardioplegic solution by an enriched branched chain amino acid formulation. *J Thorac Cardiovasc Surg* 1989;98:551.
117. Svedjeholm R, Ekroth R, Joachinisson P, et al. Myocardial uptake of amino acids and other substrates in relation to myocardial oxygen consumption four hours after cardiac operations. *J Thorac Cardiovasc Surg* 1991;101:688.
118. Sako EY, Kingsley-Hickman PB, From AHL, et al. Substrate effects in the post-ischemic myocardium. *J Surg Res* 1988;44: 430.
119. Buckberg GD. A proposed "solution" to the cardioplegia controversy. *J Thorac Cardiovasc Surg* 1979;77:803.
120. Bodenhammer R, DeBoer LWV, Geffin GA, et al. Enhanced myocardial protection during ischemic arrest. Oxygenation of a crystalloid cardioplegic solution. *J Thorac Cardiovasc Surg* 1983;85:769.
121. Ledinghorn SJM, Braimbridge MV, Hearse DJ. Improved myocardial protection by oxygenation of the St. Thomas' Hospital cardioplegic solutions. Studies in the rat. *J Thorac Cardiovasc Surg* 1988;95:103.
122. Digerness SB, Vanini V, Wideman FE. In vitro comparison of oxygen availability from asanguineous and sanguineous cardioplegic media. *Circulation* 1981;64:80.
123. Coetzee A, Roussouw G, Fourie P, et al. Preservation of myocardial function and biochemistry after blood and oxygenated crystalloid cardioplegia during cardiac arrest. *Ann Thorac Surg* 1990; 50:230.
124. Myers CL, Weiss SJ, Kirsh MM, et al. Effects of supplementary hypothermic crystalloid cardioplegic solution with catalase, superoxide dismutase, allopurinol, or deferoxamine on functional recovery of globally ischemic and reperfused isolated hearts. *J Thorac Cardiovasc Surg* 1986;91:281.
125. Moorhouse PC, Grootveld M, Holliwell B, et al. Allopurinol and oxypurinol are hydroxyl radical scavengers. *FEBS Lett* 1987; 213:23.
126. Ferreira R, Burgos M, Lleusy S, et al. Reduction of reperfusion injury with mannitol cardioplegia. *Ann Thorac Surg* 1989;48: 77.
127. Ferreira R, Burgos M, Milei J, et al. Effect of supplementing cardioplegic solution with deferoxamine on reperfused human myocardium. *J Thorac Cardiovasc Surg* 1990;100:708.
128. Rosenkranz ER, Okamoto F, Buckberg GD, et al. Studies of controlled reperfusion after ischemia. II. Biochemical studies: failure of tissue adenosine triphosphate levels to predict recovery of contractile function after controlled reperfusion. *J Thorac Cardiovasc Surg* 1986;92:488.
129. Reimer KA, Hill MJ, Jennings RB. Prolonged depletion of ATP and the adenine nucleotide pool due to delayed resynthesis of the adenine nucleotide following reversible myocardial ischemic injury in dogs. *J Mol Cell Cardiol* 1981;13:229.
130. Zimmer HG, Trendelenburg C, Kammermeier H, et al. De novo synthesis of myocardial adenine nucleotides in the rat. Acceleration during recovery from oxygen deficiency. *Circ Res* 1973;32:635.
131. Reibel DK, Rovetto MJ. Myocardial adenosine salvage rates and restoration of ATP content following ischemia. *Am J Physiol* 1979;237:H247.
132. Rosenkranz ER, Okamoto F, Vinten-Johansen J, et al. Improved adenosine-triphosphate recovery in energy-depleted hearts treated in 5-amino-4-imidazole carboxamide riboside (AICAR). *Surg Forum* 1983;34:330.
133. Swain JL, Hines JJ, Sabina RL, et al. Accelerated repletion of ATP and GTP pools in post-ischemic canine myocardium using a precursor or pure de novo synthesis. *Circ Res* 1982;51:102.
134. DeWitt DF, Jochiem KE, Behrendt DM. Nucleotide degradation and functional impairment during cardioplegia. Amelioration by inosine. *Circulation* 1983;67:171.
135. Humphrey SM, Selye RN. Improved functional recovery of ischemic myocardium by suppression of adenosine metabolism. *J Thorac Cardiovasc Surg* 1982;84:16.
136. Pasque MK, Spray TK, Pellum GL, et al. Ribose-enhanced myocardial recovery following ischemia in the isolated working rat heart. *J Thorac Cardiovasc Surg* 1982;83:390.
137. Bolling S, Bies L, Gallagher K, et al. Enhanced myocardial protection with adenosine. *Ann Thorac Surg* 1989;47:809.
138. Feinstein MB. Effects of experimental congestive heart failure, ouabain and asphyxia on the high-energy phosphate and creatine content of the guinea pig heart. *Circ Res* 1962;10:333.
139. Leaf A. Cell swelling, a factor in ischemic tissue injury. *Circulation* 1973;48:455.
140. Foglia RP, Steed DL, Follette DM, et al. Iatrogenic myocardial edema with potassium cardioplegia. *J Thorac Cardiovasc Surg* 1979;78:217.
141. Powell WJ, DiBona DR, Flores J, et al. Effects of hyperosmotic mannitol in reducing ischemic cells swelling and minimizing myocardial necrosis. *Circulation* 1976;53:45.
142. Follette D, Fey K, Livesay J, et al. The beneficial effects of citrate reperfusion of ischemic heart on cardiopulmonary bypass. *Surg Forum* 1976;27:244.
143. deJong JW. Cardioplegia and calcium antagonist. A Review. *Ann Thorac Surg* 1986;42:593.

144. Furness FN. In vitro and in vivo effects of amino buffers. *Ann NY Acad Sci* 1961;92:333.
145. Holmdahl MH, Nahas GG. Volume of distribution of C14 labeled tris (hydroxymethyl) amino methane. *Am J Physiol* 1962; 202:1101.
146. Akins CW. Noncardioplegic myocardial preservation for coronary revascularization. *J Thorac Cardiovasc Surg* 1984;88:174.
147. Akins CW. Early and late results following emergency isolated myocardial revascularization during hypothermic fibrillatory arrest. *Ann Thorac Surgery* 1987;43:131.
148. Akins CW. Fibrillatory arrest. In: Roberts AJ, ed. *Myocardial protection in cardiac surgery.* New York: Marcel Dekker Inc, 1987:221.
149. Lichtenstein SV, Ashe KA, El Dalati H, et al. Warm heart surgery. *J Thorac Cardiovasc Surg* 1991;101:269.
150. Rosenkranz ER, Vinten-Johansen J, Buckberg GD, et al. Benefits of normothermic induction of blood cardioplegia in energy-depleted hearts with maintenance of arrest by multidose cold blood cardioplegic infusions. *J Thorac Cardiovasc Surg* 1982; 84:667.
151. Teoh KH, Mickel DAG, Weisel RD, et al. Decreased postoperative myocardial fatty acid oxidation. *J Surg Res* 1988;44:36.
152. Becker H, Vinten-Johansen J, Buckberg GD, et al. Critical importance of ensuring cardioplegic delivery with coronary stenoses. *J Thorac Cardiovasc Surg* 1981;81:507.
153. Grondin CM, Helias J, Vouhe PR, et al. Influence of critical coronary stenosis on myocardial protection through cold potassium cardioplegia. *J Thorac Cardiovasc Surgery* 1981;82:608.
154. Buckberg GD. Antegrade cardioplegia, retrograde cardioplegia, or both? *Am Thorac Surg* 1988;45:589.
155. Lillehei CW, Deverall RA, Gott VL, et al. A direct vision correction of calcific aortic stenosis by means of a pump oxygenator and retrograde coronary sinus perfusion. *Dis Chest* 1956;30: 123.
156. Partington MT, Acar C, Buckberg GD, et al. Studies of retrograde cardioplegia. I. Advantages of antegrade/retrograde cardioplegia to optimize distribution in jeopardized myocardium. *J Thorac Cardiovasc Surg* 1989;97:613.
157. Partington MT, Acar C, Buckberg GD, et al. Studies of retrograde cardioplegia. II. Nutritional blood flow distribution in normal and jeopardized myocardium. *J Thorac Cardiovasc Surg* 1989;97:613.
158. Partington MT, Acar C, Buckberg GD, et al. Studies of retrograde cardioplegia. III. Capillary blood flow distribution to myocardium supplied by open and occluded arteries. *J Thorac Cardiovasc Surg* 1989;97:605.
159. Stirling MC, McClanahan TB, Schott RJ, et al. Distribution of cardioplegic solution infused antegradely and retrogradely in normal canine hearts. *J Thorac Cardiovasc Surg* 1989;98:1066.
160. Buckberg GD, Beyersdorf F, Allen BS, et al. Integrated myocardial management: background and initial application. *J Cardiac Surg* 1995;10:68.
161. Shirai T, Rao V, Weisel RD, et al. Antegrade and retrograde cardioplegia: alternate of simultaneous? *J Thorac Cardiovasc Surg* 1996;112:787.
162. Drinkwater DC, Laks H, Buckberg GD. A new simplified method of optimizing cardioplegic delivery without right heart isolation. Antegrade/retrograde blood cardioplegia. *J Thorac Cardiovasc Surg* 1990;100:56.
163. Buckberg GD. Antegrade/retrograde blood cardioplegia to ensure cardioplegic distribution: operative techniques and objectives. *J Cardiac Surg* 1989;4:216.
164. Roe BB, Hutchinson JC, Fishman NH, et al. Myocardial protection with cold, ischemic, potassium-induced cardioplegia. *J Thorac Cardiovasc Surg* 1977;73:366.
165. Ledingham SJM, Braimbridge MV, Hearse DJ. The St. Thomas' Hospital cardioplegic solution. A comparison of the efficacy of two formulations. *J Thorac Cardiovasc Surg* 1987; 93:240.
166. Hearse DJ, Steward DA, Braimbridge MV. Myocardial protection during ischemic cardiac arrest. The importance of magnesium in cardioplegic infusates. *J Thorac Cardiovasc Surg* 1978; 75:877.
167. Reynolds TR, Geffin GA, Titus JS, et al. Myocardial preservation related to magnesium content of hyperkalemic cardioplegic solution of 8 C. *Ann Thorac Surg* 1989;47:907.
168. Takahashi A, Chambers DJ, Braimbridge MV, et al. Optimal myocardial protection during crystalloid cardioplegia. Interrelationship between volume and duration of infusion. *J Thorac Cardiovasc Surg* 1988;96:730.
169. Cunningham JN, Adams PX, Knopp EA, et al. Preservation of ATP, ultrastructural, and ventricular function after aortic cross-clamping and reperfusion. Clinical use of blood potassium cardioplegia. *J Thorac Cardiovasc Surg* 1979;78:708.
170. Laks H, Barner HB, Kaiser G. Cold blood cardioplegia. *J Thorac Cardiovasc Surg* 1979;77:319.
171. Engelman RM, Rousou JH, Dobbs W, et al. The superiority of blood cardioplegia in myocardial preservation. *Circulation* 1980;62:I62.
172. Roberts AJ, Moran JM, Sanders JH, et al. Clinical evaluation of the relative effectiveness of multidose crystalloid cardioplegia and cold blood cardioplegia in coronary artery bypass graft surgery: a non-randomized matched-pair analysis. *Ann Thorac Surg* 1982;33:421.
173. Shapira N, Kirsh M, Jochiem K, et al. Comparison of the effect of blood cardioplegia to crystalloid cardioplegia on myocardial contractility in man. *J Thorac Cardiovasc Surg* 1980;80:647.
174. Singh EK, Farrugia R, Teplitz C, et al. Electrolyte versus blood cardioplegia: randomized clinical and myocardial ultrastructural study. *Ann Thorac Surg* 1982;33:218.
175. Feindel CM, Tait GA, Wilson GJ, et al. Multidose blood versus crystalloid cardioplegia. Comparison by a quantitative assessment of irreversible myocardial injury. *J Thorac Cardiovasc Surg* 1984;87:585.
176. Christakis GT, Fremes SE, Weisel RD, et al. Reducing the risk of urgent revascularization for unstable angina: a randomized clinical trial. *J Vasc Surg* 1986;3:764.
177. Fremes SE, Christakis GT, Weisel RD, et al. A clinical trial of blood and crystalloid cardioplegia. *J Thorac Cardiovasc Surg* 1984;88:726.
178. Langer GA. Control of calcium movement in the myocardium. *Eur Heart J* 1983;2:3.
179. Rosenkranz ER, Buckberg GD, Laks H, et al. Warm induction of cardioplegia with glutamate-enriched blood in coronary patients with cardiogenic shock who are dependent on inotropic drugs and intra-aortic balloon support. Initial experience and operative strategy. *J Thorac Cardiovasc Surg* 1983;86:507.
180. Allen BS, Rosenkranz ER, Buckberg GD, et al. Studies on prolonged acute regional ischemia. VI: Myocardial infarction with left ventricular power failure. A medical/surgical emergency requiring urgent revascularization with maximal protection of remote muscle. *J Thorac Cardiovasc Surg* 1989;98:691.
181. Buckberg GD. Antegrade-retrograde blood cardioplegia to ensure cardioplegic distribution: operative techniques and objectives. *J Cardiac Surg* 1989;4:216.
182. Loop FD, Higgins TL, Panda R, et al. Improved effectiveness of myocardial protection with blood cardioplegia and coronary sinus perfusion. *J Thorac Cardiovasc Surg* 1992;104:608.
183. Jarmarkani JM, Nagatomo T, Nakazawa M, et al. Effects of hypoxia on myocardial high-energy phosphates in neonatal mammalian heart. *Am J Physiol* 1978;235:H475.
184. Julia PL, Kofsky ER, Buckberg GD, et al. Studies of myocardial

protection in the immature heart. I. Enhanced tolerance of immature versus adult myocardium to global ischemia with reference to metabolic differences. *J Thorac Cardiovasc Surg* 1990;100:879.

185. Julia PL, Young H, Buckberg GD, et al. Studies of myocardial protection in the immature heart. II. Evidence for importance of amino acid metabolism in tolerance to ischemia. *J Thorac Cardiovasc Surg* 1990;100:888.
186. Drinkwater DC, Cushen CF, Laks H, et al. The use of combined antegrade-retrograde infusion of blood cardioplegia solution in pediatric patients undergoing heart operations. *J Thorac Cardiovasc Surg* 1992;104:1349.
187. Williams WG, Rebeyka IM, Tibshiran RJ, et al. Warm induction blood cardioplegia in the infant. A technique to avoid rapid cooling myocardial contracture. *J Thorac Cardiovasc Surg* 1990;100:896.
188. De Leon SY, Idriss FS, Ilbawi MN, et al. Comparison of single versus multidose blood cardioplegia in arterial switch procedures. *Ann Thorac Surg* 1988;45:548.
189. Iannettoni MD, Bove EL. Myocardial preservation in the newborn. In: Kron IL, Mavroudis C, eds. *State-of-the-art reviews. Innovations in congenital heart surgery.* Philadelphia: Hanley and Belfus, 1989:809.
190. Fujiwara T, Kurtts T, Anderson W, et al. Myocardial protection in cyanotic neonatal lambs. *J Thorac Cardiovasc Surg* 1988;96:700.
191. Tixier DB, Matheis GF, Buckberg GD, et al. Donor hearts with impaired hemodynamics: benefits of warm substrate enriched blood cardioplegia induction during harvesting. *J Thorac Cardiovasc Surg* 1991;102:207.
192. Haan CK, Lazar HL, Rivers S, et al. Improved myocardial preservation during cold storage using substrate enhancement. *Ann Thorac Surg* 1990;50:80.
193. Hardesty RL, Griffith PB, Deeb GM, et al. Improved cardiac function using cardioplegia during procurement and transplantation. *Transplant Proc* 1983;15:1253.
194. Lichtenstein SV, Fremes SE, Abel JQ, et al. Technical aspects of warm heart surgery. *J Cardiac Surg* 1991;6:278.
195. Salerno TA, Houck JP, Barrozo CAM, et al. Retrograde continuous warm blood cardioplegia: a new concept in myocardial protection. *Ann Thorac Surg* 1991;51:245.
196. Christakis GT, Koch JP, Deemar KA, et al. A randomized study of the systemic effects of warm heart surgery. *Ann Thorac Surg* 1992;54:449.
197. Doty DB, DiRusso GB, Doty JR. Full-spectrum cardiac surgery through a minimal incision: mini-sternotomy (lower-half) technique. *Ann Thorac Surg* 1998;65:573.
198. Cosgrove DM, Sabik JF, Navia JL. Minimally invasive valve operations. *Ann Thorac Surg* 1998;65:1525.
199. Calafiore AM, Angelini GD, Bergsland J, et al. Minimally invasive coronary artery bypass grafting. *Ann Thorac Surg* 1997;62:1545.
200. Gulielmos V, Dangel M, Solowjowa N, et al. Clinical experiences with minimally invasive mitral using a simplified Port Access technique. *Eur J Cardiothorac Surg* 1998;14:141.
201. Kolessov VI. Mammary artery-coronary artery anastomosis as a method of treatment for angina pectoris. *J Thorac Cardiovasc Surg* 1967;54:535.
202. Benetti FJ, Naselli G, Wood M. Direct coronary artery surgery with saphenous vein bypass without either cardiopulmonary bypass or cardiac arrest. *J Cardiovasc Surg* 1985;26:217.
203. Buffolo E, Andrade JCS, Succi JC. Direct myocardial revascularization without cardiopulmonary bypass. *J Thorac Cardiovasc Surg* 1985;33:26.
204. Calafiore AM, Vitolla G, Mazzei V, et al. The last operation: techniques and results before and after the stabilization era. *Ann Thorac Surg* 1998;66:998.
205. Bergsland J, Hasnain S, Lajos TZ, et al. Elimination of cardiopulmonary bypass: a prime goal of reoperative coronary bypass surgery. *Eur J Cardiothorac Surg* 1998;14:59.
206. Mangano DT. Myocardial ischemia following surgery: preliminary findings. *J Cardiac Surg* 1990;5:288.
207. Christakis GT, Weisel RD, Mickle DAG. Right ventricular function and metabolism. *Circulation* 1990;80:IV332.
208. Hines R. Management of acute right ventricular failure. *J Cardiac Surg* 1990;5:285.
209. Mullen JC, Weisel RD, Fremes SE, et al. Right ventricular function: a comparison between blood and crystalloid cardioplegia. *Ann Thorac Surg* 1987;43:17.
210. Boldt J, Kling D, Dapper F, et al. Myocardial temperature during cardiac operations: influence on right ventricular function. *J Thorac Cardiovasc Surg* 1990;100:562.

Cardiac Anesthesia: Principles and Clinical Practice, Second Edition, edited by Fawzy G. Estafanous, Paul G. Barash, and J.G. Reves. Lippincott Williams & Wilkins, Philadelphia © 2001.

14

PATHOPHYSIOLOGY AND MANAGEMENT OF CARDIOPULMONARY BYPASS

SUGANTHA GANAPATHY
JOHN M. MURKIN

Since its initial clinical introduction by Gibbon in 1953 (1), cardiopulmonary bypass (CPB) has found increasing use as a circulatory support modality in a wide variety of clinical situations. In addition to widespread application during cardiac surgery, CPB is being used in conjunction with hypothermia and circulatory arrest during certain cerebrovascular neurosurgical procedures (2), and to provide circulatory support during coronary angioplasty (3), as well as for certain resuscitative procedures, such as after accidental hypothermia (4) and cardiac arrest following bupivacaine cardiac toxicity (4a).

The following chapter considers circulatory pathophysiology during CPB and examines the functioning of specific organ systems during CPB, to understand the utility as well as the limitations and potential sequelae of the clinical use of CPB.

CIRCULATORY PATHOPHYSIOLOGY

Venous Return

CPB procedures employ either a single two-stage venous cannula or two single-stage venous cannulas to drain venous blood from the right atrium and venae cavae into the pump-oxygenator, with oxygenated blood being returned via an aortic cannula into the ascending aorta. In emergency situations in which atrial and aortic cannulation cannot be rapidly secured or in which sternotomy is not required for the surgical procedure, arterial and venous access is obtained most commonly by cannulation of the great femoral vessels. Rarely, massive bleeding during chest opening in patients with previous chest surgery or after trauma may require use of blood from the wound suction directed to the venous reservoir.

Perfusion flow rates during CPB are controlled by varying the speed of the roller pump head, but the rate of venous return to the oxygenator dictates the upper limit of perfusion flows. Because the atria and venae cavae are highly compliant structures, they are readily collapsible and may invaginate with the application of negative pressure unless specific techniques are used (see later discussion). This may result in a diminution or loss of blood returning to the oxygenator. Venous return to the pump is therefore most commonly by gravity. The difference between the height of the atrial cannulas and the meniscus of the venous reservoir of the pump provides the pressure differential necessary for the return of blood.

Obstruction to venous return because of kinking of the atrial cannulas or compression of the venae cavae can significantly decrease venous return and necessitate a reduction in perfusion flow rates. In addition, distal venous hypertension may result. Elevated venous pressures within the superior vena cava (SVC) may be produced by dislocation of the heart, particularly in the presence of a single two-stage atrial cannula.

Whereas bicaval cannulation using two single-stage venous cannulas drains the SVC and inferior vena cava (IVC) separately, use of a single two-stage atrial cannula is being increasingly favored (Fig. 14-1A). It affords greater surgical exposure of the heart, and it eliminates one atriotomy site. With a two-stage cannula, the IVC is drained by an orifice at the tip of the cannula while blood returning via the SVC is drained through more proximal holes in the segment of cannula located within the atrium. One potential disadvantage is that with elevation or rotation of the heart, although IVC drainage is generally unimpeded, flow from the SVC may be significantly restricted—leading to cerebral venous hypertension (Fig. 14-1B). Unless specifically monitored, this obstruction may go undetected because right atrial pressures may remain below or within the normal range. Unrecognized cerebral venous hypertension may produce signifi-

S. Ganapathy: Department of Anesthesia, University of Western Ontario, London, Ontario, N6A 5A5 Canada; and Department of Anesthesia, London Health Sciences Center, London, Ontario, N6A 5A5 Canada

J. M. Murkin: Department of Anesthesia, University of Western Ontario, London, Ontario, N6A 5A5 Canada; and Department of Cardiac Anesthesiology, London Health Sciences Center, London, Ontario, N6A 5A5 Canada

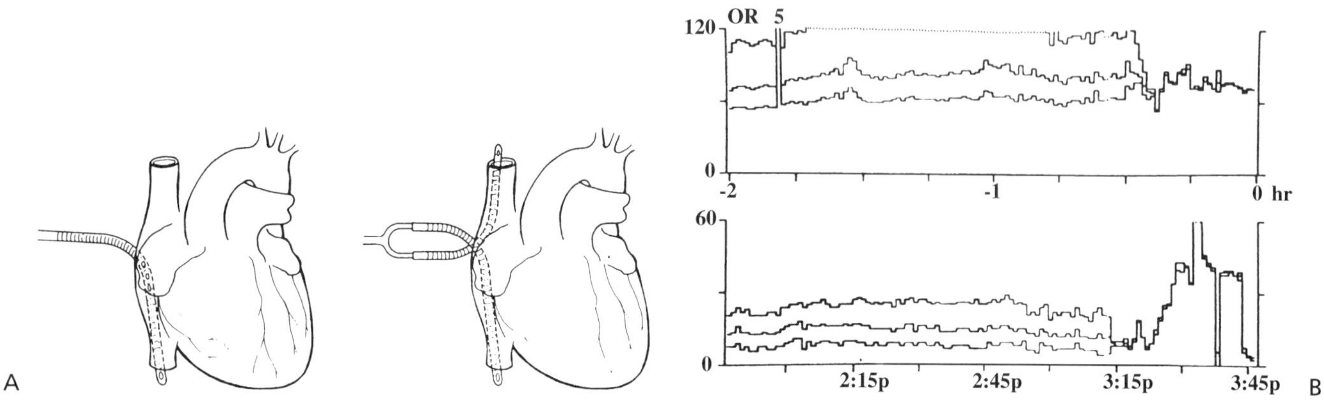

FIGURE 14-1. A: Two-stage venous cannula **(left)** draining the inferior vena cava (IVC) and right atrium. Only one atriotomy site is required, but only indirect drainage of the superior vena cava (SVC). Two single-stage venous cannulas **(right)** draining IVC and SVC directly. **B: (top)** Systolic, mean, and diastolic arterial pressures before and immediately after onset of cardiopulmonary bypass (CPB). **(Bottom)** Pulmonary artery pressures before CPB, and proximal SVC pressure after onset of CPB. Using a single two-stage venous cannula, venous return to oxygenator was decreased and SVC pressures approached systemic values with dislocation of the heart. After repositioning the venous cannula, SVC pressures were immediately reduced, avoiding prolonged compromise of the cerebral circulation. (JVP, jugular venous pressure.)

cant impairment of cerebral perfusion due to the resulting reduction in cerebral perfusion pressure while cerebral venous hypertension *per se* may produce cerebral edema. Transcranial Doppler assessment of cerebral blood flow (CBF) during such dislocation of the heart has demonstrated significant decreases in cerebral flow consequent to elevated SVC pressures (Fig. 14-1B) (5). Monitoring SVC pressure via a proximally placed central venous pressure catheter, or the sheath introducer of a pulmonary artery catheter, may help identify such obstruction to cerebral venous drainage. Alternately, the pulmonary artery catheter should be withdrawn so that the proximal opening (central venous pressure port) is in the SVC and the transducer is set to measure central venous pressure.

Use of vacuum-assisted venous drainage was introduced by McCusker et al. in 1992. They were able to maintain high-flow femoro-femoral bypass using small cannulas (17 French on the arterial side and 21 French for the venous side) and a centrifugal pump on the venous side to facilitate venous return (6). The venous cannula is positioned in the right atrium with the aid of transesophageal echocardiography (TEE). Toomasian et al. have been able to maintain adequate support of circulation via a femoral cannula using a similar kinetic-assisted venous drainage with a 40% increase in venous drainage in patients undergoing port-access surgery or redo thoracotomies requiring circulatory support (7). Recently, the innominate vein has been used instead of the femoral vein to insert the venous cannula in the right atrium using TEE to guide tip placement (8).

Small volumes of air within the venous line will not interfere with venous return, but venous air lock with complete prevention of blood return to the pump can result if

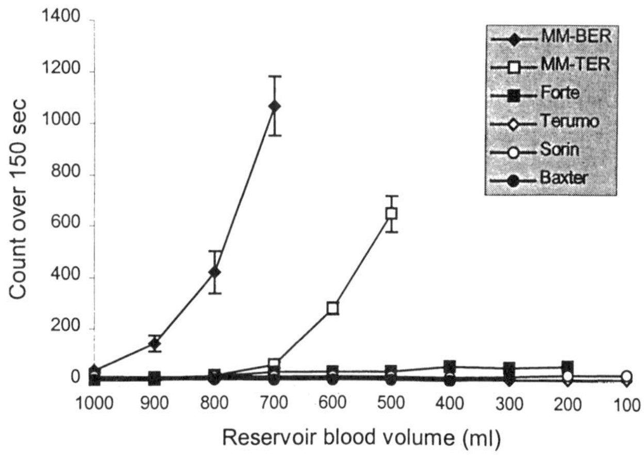

FIGURE 14-2. Investigation of gaseous emboli generation by venous reservoirs comparing emboli generation by the Medtronic Maxima (top and bottom entry versions); the Medtronic Forte; the Sorin Monolyth; the Baxter Bentley HSR-4000; and the Terumo Capiox SX. Salvaged clinical circuits with an appropriate blood receptacle were employed to stimulate the patient. The prime, restored with date expired suspended red cells, was circulated at 3.5 L/minute^{-1}. Reservoir blood volume was lowered in 100-mL decrements from a starting volume of 1,000 mL. At each new volume, emboli counts over 150 seconds were made immediately downstream of the reservoir. A total of eight such runs in two separate circuits were completed for each reservoir. The mean emboli counts averaged over all runs for each reservoir are shown. Note that the manufacturers recommended minimum volume for the Maxima reservoirs was 300 mL. (From Mitchell SJ, Willcox T, Gorman DF. Bubble generation and venous air filtration by hardshell venous reservoirs: a comparative study. *Perfusion* 1997; 12:325, with permission.)

the volume of air within the line is excessive (more than 50 to 100 mL). There is also evidence that air introduced into the venous side of the CPB circuit can transit the oxygenator and be delivered into the arterial circulation (9–13) (Fig. 14-2). Using transcranial Doppler, Taylor et al. demonstrated increased numbers of cerebral microemboli during CPB associated with perfusionist interventions (blood sampling and drug administration) versus surgical instrumentation of the aorta and all other times, despite usage of 32 μ arterial line filter (13). Air emboli have also been demonstrated with certain venous reservoirs at minimal volume levels where there was entrainment of air into the upwardly directed fountain of venous inflow blood. This entrainment was totally abolished by flushing the field with carbon dioxide (10). Similar situations can arise when pump flow is increased with inadequate venous return. Wilcox et al. have documented a 10-fold increase in arterial gas emboli after entrainment of large volumes of venous air during vacuum-assisted venous drainage, compared to gravity-assisted venous drainage (9). Thus, vacuum-assisted venous drainage devices should not be used to drain trapped air from the venous system. Correct priming of all lines within the CPB circuit, as well as the prevention or prompt correction of air entrainment occurring during CPB, can minimize such eventualities. New devices with a pressure-relief valve to assist with venous drainage are under development (14).

Arterial Cannulation

Unless the ascending aorta has dissected, is aneurysmal or thin-walled, or contains extensive atherosclerotic plaque, cannulation of the ascending aorta is the preferred site for the return of oxygenated blood to the patient. The arterial cannula used for return of oxygenated blood produces directional flow because of the curved tip of the cannula. When inserted into the ascending aorta, if care is not taken to ensure correct orientation of the tip of the cannula, preferential perfusion of the innominate or left carotid arteries may occur with resultant unilateral cerebral hyperperfusion (15,16). Although reports of this complication are quite rare, when unrecognized it has most commonly resulted in extensive cerebral damage and severe neurologic injury or death (15). Yet when recognized early, it can be readily corrected without clinical sequelae (16). A high index of suspicion is therefore necessary to avoid this potential catastrophe.

Of the patients in whom miscannulation has been reported, commonly there has been some associated abnormality of the great vessels of the aortic arch that predisposes to miscannulation. With initiation of CPB in such situations, either hypertension or hypotension may be observed depending on whether the radial artery being pressure monitored is ipsilateral or contralateral to the miscannulated vessels (15). Because of the pattern of inhomogeneous perfusion, a "harlequin facies" with a demarcation of hemispheric pallor and ipsilateral plethora may result. Facial swelling, ipsilateral conjunctival edema, rhinorrhea, and otorrhea have all been reported after unilateral cerebral hyperperfusion but are all late signs and result after prolonged cerebral hyperperfusion (15). Noticeable alteration in the temperature of the ipsilateral head and neck, as well as the identification of ipsilateral carotid pulsations during pulsatile perfusion, have been reported as early signs of unilateral hyperperfusion and resulted in early correction of aortic miscannulation with successful recovery of the patient (16). Clearly, a high index of suspicion, particularly in the presence of known abnormalities of the heart and great vessels, is necessary to avoid such complications.

The most important determinant of perioperative stroke after cardiac surgery and CPB is increasingly recognized as the extent of ascending aortic atherosclerosis (17). This correlates strongly with age, insulin-dependent diabetes mellitus, peripheral vascular disease, and history of cerebrovascular accident (18,19). In one study of more than 200 patients dying after cardiac surgery, atheroemboli were demonstrated at autopsy in 37% of patients with severe aortic atherosclerotic disease (19). These investigators found a direct correlation between age, presence of peripheral vascular disease, and severe atherosclerosis of the ascending aorta and cerebral atheroemboli, at autopsy. Atherosclerosis of the ascending aorta is present in 20% to 38% of cardiac surgical patients aged 50 or older, with the percentage increasing with age, and is an independent risk factor for cerebrovascular accidents (20,21). Stump et al. demonstrated that older patients have increased emboli during coronary artery bypass (CAB) graft surgery (22). The risks of embolic complications and stroke from the severely atherosclerotic ascending aorta have been well documented (23–25). In one study, 23% of patients with severe aortic atherosclerotic disease suffered perioperative cerebrovascular complications (25). Plaque fracture and cerebral embolization during aortic instrumentation are felt to be a primary mechanism of such perioperative strokes (26).

Epiaortic Scanning

Routine intraoperative echocardiographic studies of the aorta using TEE have been recommended before cannulation (27); however, the ability of TEE to reliably detect all ascending aortic and arch lesions has been questioned (28, 29). As shown in Fig. 14-3, this is due to the air-tissue interface from the overlying lung and right main bronchus preventing TEE visualization of potential lesions in the mid ascending and upper ascending aorta and the aortic arch, sites where cannulation and clamping generally occur. In the distal ascending aorta, Katz et al. showed that in all five patients in whom severe atherosclerotic plaque was found on direct epiaortic scanning, these lesions were missed on biplanar TEE examination (30). A more recent study comparing TEE with epiaortic scanning has confirmed these

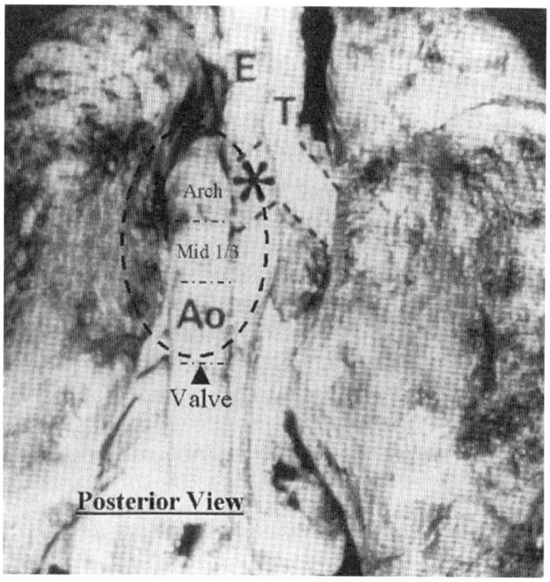

FIGURE 14-3. Anatomic specimen seen from the posterior aspect, showing the relationship of the esophagus (*E*), trachea (*T*), and the thoracic aorta (*Ao*). The asterisk marks the crossing of the esophagus and the left main bronchus. Note that the distal ascending aorta and proximal aortic arch (*Arch, Mid 1/3*) are anterior to the lower trachea and right main bronchus. (From Konstadt SN, Reich DL, Quintana C, et al. The ascending aorta: how much does transesophageal echocardiography see? *Anesth Analg* 1994;78:240, with permission.)

results and concluded that TEE is an insensitive technique for such evaluations and is of little value in guiding surgical manipulations such as aortic cross-clamping, in contrast to the high sensitivity of epiaortic scanning (29). Although there have been few prospective studies of epiaortic scanning, it has been recently shown in a prospective randomized study that both surgical selection of cannulation and clamp sites and consequent cerebral embolization are reduced by epiaortic scanning (31,32).

Identifying severe aortic disease has important clinical implications because surgical technique, including assessment of stroke risk, selection of sites for aortic cannulation, and techniques for anastomosing proximal ends of coronary grafts, all may be altered to minimize the risk of producing cerebral emboli and neurologic injury. An example of severe ascending aortic disease seen on epiaortic ultrasonic scanning in the operating room is shown in Fig. 14-4. These images from Wareing and colleagues illustrate the high likelihood of fracturing plaque and having it embolize to the brain or other organs during cannulation or cross-clamping (33). It is easy to imagine how embolic debris from just such atherosclerotic plaque within the aorta can be a primary cause of stroke or of more subtle neurocognitive dysfunction that occurs after CAB surgery.

Cardiac Venting

Although most venous return to the right ventricle occurs via the venae cavae, a variable amount is also delivered by the coronary sinus. Venous blood from the bronchial and thebesian systems is drained into the left ventricle and in the presence of extensive lung disease, can result in relatively large volumes of blood being returned to the left ventricle (34). The potential for ventricular distention is most pronounced when vena caval ties are used, minimizing drainage of blood directly from the right atrium and promoting passage of blood through the pulmonary circulation and into

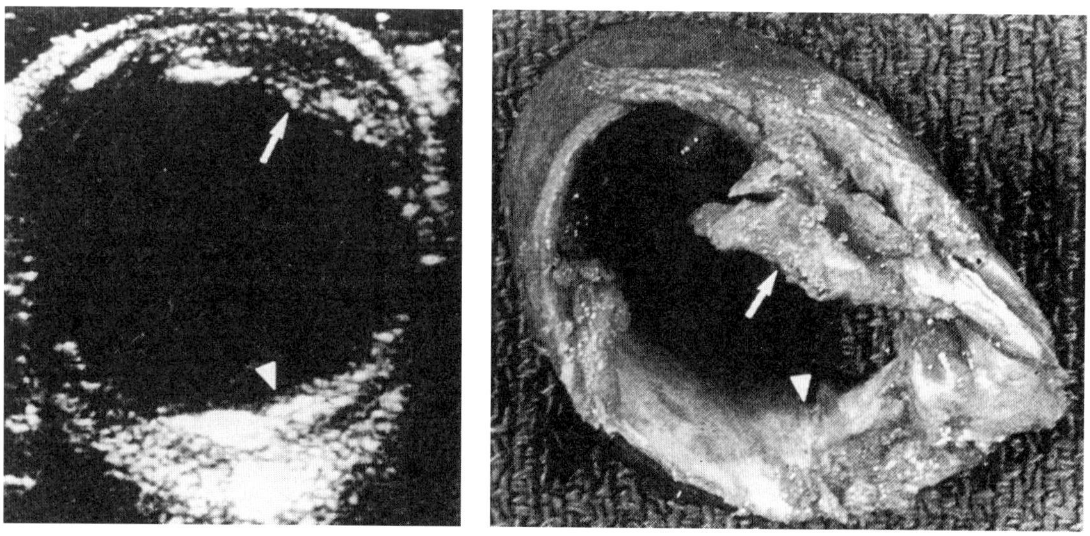

FIGURE 14-4. Transverse ultrasonic image of the ascending aorta and the corresponding segment of the aorta in a patient with severe atherosclerosis. Note the calcification (*triangle*) and the projection of atheroma (*arrow*) into the lumen. (From Wareing TH. Management of the severely atherosclerotic ascending aorta during cardiac operations. *J Thorac Cardiovasc Surg* 1992;103:453, with permission.)

the left ventricle (34). This can distend the left ventricle, increasing myocardial oxygen consumption (35,36). As a result, venting of the left side of the heart is commonly practiced to avoid ventricular distention and the potential for the development of subendocardial ischemia (35). In addition, venting facilitates exposure during coronary artery surgery by minimizing back-bleeding through enhanced emptying of the distal segment of the coronary artery.

The left ventricular vent cannula can be inserted through the right superior pulmonary vein, passing through the left atrium and into the left ventricle. Alternatively, the ascending aorta proximal to the arterial cross-clamp is an increasingly common site of vent insertion (35). If suction is used to enhance drainage of blood through the vent, there is the possibility of air being entrained through the vent site and being drawn into the left ventricle. Unless this air is carefully eliminated before commencement of ventricular ejection, it can be a source of emboli released into the arterial circulation. In most centers, therefore, when ventricular venting is required, gravity drainage is used for ventricular evacuation. The observation of air in the vent line should indicate the possibility of air being entrained into the left ventricle and thus prompt some corrective action. Milsom et al. have reported significantly reduced cerebral embolization after valve operations with dual left ventricular and aortic root vent de-airing technique (Fig. 14-5) (37).

In percutaneous cardiopulmonary support, transaortic catheter venting has been recommended as an adjunctive technique for left ventricular unloading (38,39). Vent insertion into a main pulmonary artery has also been used, and it is claimed to be relatively easy to perform (36). This technique withdraws blood from the left side of the heart via the pulmonary vasculature in addition to returning right side of the heart spillover and scavenging bronchial flow. This may also avoid introducing air into the left ventricle.

The left atrial appendage and the body of the left atrium are alternative sites for venting of the heart (35). If venting is not employed, continuous observation for ventricular distention—with or without use of left atrial or pulmonary artery pressure monitoring—should be used to avoid the development of myocardial dysfunction or pulmonary congestion secondary to pressure-related complications.

Perfusion Flow Rates

The adequacy of perfusion flow rates can basically be considered as reflecting the balance between the oxygen requirements of tissues and oxygen delivery by the circulation, although a number of organs have autoregulatory mechanisms to independently regulate blood supply according to regional tissue oxygen requirements (40,41). Tolerance to ischemia thus differs among various tissues and organs in the body. However, the unique circumstances of CPB with nonpulsatile perfusion, hypothermia, hemodilution, and differing pH management strategies—all variously influencing metabolic demand and tissue oxygen supply—must be considered in assessing the appropriateness of any given perfusion flow rate. Vital organ perfusion, cardiac protection, and improved operative field exposure are additional factors to consider in determining perfusion rates.

In healthy resting individuals, systemic oxygen consumption ($\dot{V}O_2$) averages 250 mL·minute^{-1} or 150 mL·minute^{-1}·m^{-2}, and adequacy of tissue oxygen supply is generally reflected in mixed venous oxygen saturations ($S\bar{v}O_2$) averaging 75% (42). During anesthesia in paralyzed, normothermic adult patients, $\dot{V}O_2$ averages 100 to 120 mL ·minute^{-1}·m^{-2} and $S\bar{v}O_2$ averages 70% (43). During hypothermic nonpulsatile CPB without neuromuscular blockade, VO2 averages 90 mL·minute^{-1}·m^{-2} while $S\bar{v}O_2$ is approximately 70% (44). Profound neuromuscular blockade

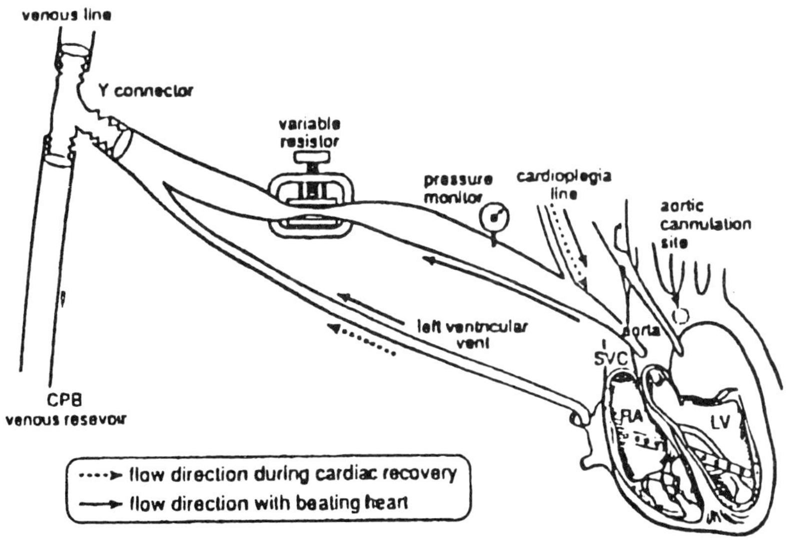

FIGURE 14-5. Schematic layout of the dual-vent de-airing apparatus (see text for details). (CPB, cardiopulmonary bypass; LV, left ventricle; RA, right atrium; SVC, superior vena cava.) (From Milsom FP. A dual-vent left heart de-airing technique markedly reduces carotid artery microemboli. *Ann Thorac Surg* 1998;66:785, with permission.)

during hypothermic CPB at 27°C significantly decreases V_{O_2} to about 45 mL·minute^{-1}·m^{-2}(44–46), demonstrating the importance of resting muscle tone on V_{O_2} during hypothermia (44). This decreased V_{O_2} is approximately one half the normothermic values, in accordance with the effect of temperature on the rate of reactions (van't Hoff's law). After more uniform cooling, the decrease in systemic oxygen consumption during a 10°C reduction in body temperature (Q_{10}) ranges between 2.71 and 2.8 (47).

In addition to temperature and anesthesia, several other factors are important in determining V_{O_2}. Resting muscle tone makes a significant contribution to V_{O_2}, particularly during hypothermia, with which profound neuromuscular blockade can significantly decrease V_{O_2} by up to 30% (44). In animals, it has been observed that pH management during hypothermia may also play a significant role in determining V_{O_2}. During hypothermic (28°C) nonpulsatile CPB in dogs, pH-stat pH management has been shown to result in V_{O_2} approximately 20% higher than predicted, and greater than with alpha-stat management, presumably as a result of the metabolic effect of elevated levels of circulating catecholamines resulting from the increased Pa_{CO_2} (48). To date, this has not been confirmed with any clinical studies.

Based on the aforementioned considerations, it is possible to derive guidelines for optimal perfusion flow rates during both hypothermic and normothermic CPB.

At 37°C and a hemoglobin (Hb) concentration of 8g·dL^{-1}, arterial oxygen content (Ca_{O_2}) would be approximately (1.34 × 8 × 1.0) 10.7 mL·dL^{-1} or 107 mL·L^{-1}. To maintain a normal $S\bar{v}_{O_2}$ level of 75%, with a V_{O_2} level of 80 mL·minute^{-1}·m^{-2}, an indexed perfusion flow rate (pulsatility index [PI]) of 3.0 L·minute^{-1}·m^{-2} would be required. A lower PI value could be tolerated by raising the Hb level or by allowing $S\bar{v}_{O_2}$ to decrease, but the latter risks a tissue oxygen debt and the development of systemic acidosis. Using similar parameters but during hypothermic CPB at 28°C, the hypothermia-induced lowering of V_{O_2} to 45 mL·minute^{-1}·m^{-2} indicates that a PI of 1.5 L·minute^{-1}·m^{-2} should be well tolerated from the standpoint of systemic oxygen delivery.

During profoundly hypothermic nonpulsatile CPB, Fox et al. varied PI between 0.25 and 2.0 L·minute^{-1}·m^{-2} (49). At 20°C and an average hematocrit level of 22%, they observed progressive decreases in V_{O_2} below PI of 1.8 and decreasing mixed venous P_{O_2} and oxygen saturation at a PI of less than 1.2. They concluded that a PI of 1.2 L·minute^{-1}·m^{-2} is adequate despite evidence of limited reserves. Rebeyka et al. studied cerebral cortical metabolism in dogs and somatosensory evoked potentials in patients during low-flow hypothermic CPB (50). Cerebral lactate levels increased significantly at flow rates of less than 0.5 L·minute^{-1}·m^{-2}, and complete depletion of cerebral adenosine triphosphate was observed at flow rates of 0.25 L·minute^{-1}·m^{-2}. Preservation of somatosensory evoked potential was seen until flow rates were reduced to 0.25 L·minute^{-1}·m^{-2}. They concluded that in the absence of cerebrovascular disease, the threshold for incurring functional cerebral injury during hypothermic nonpulsatile CPB is less than 1.0 L·minute^{-1}·m^{-2}. This is consistent with the studies of Fox et al. in which they demonstrated in monkeys that with decreases in PI to 0.5 L·minute^{-1}·m^{-2}, CBF and cerebral metabolism are maintained by preferential diversion of blood flow from the rest of the body (49).

In patients during nonpulsatile CPB using moderate hypothermia, Govier et al. demonstrated that CBF is independent of PIs between 1.0 and 2.0 L·minute^{-1}·m^{-2} (51). Murkin et al. demonstrated that over a similar range of PI values, both CBF and cerebral metabolic rate for oxygen are unchanged (52). In a study employing a hypothermic CPB model, Schwartz et al. demonstrated that changes in mean arterial pressure (MAP) below the apparent cerebral autoregulatory range were shown to influence CBF directly (53). Conversely, profound reductions in pump flow rate produced no significant effects on CBF, provided that MAP was preserved. Other studies, both clinical and experimental, have suggested such effects, but generally either the variables in these studies were altered over a fairly limited range or flow rate and perfusion pressure interacted and were not kept as totally independent variables. The data of Schwartz et al. effectively confirmed the primacy of perfusion pressure over flow rates.

There is thus significant evidence that during hypothermic CPB, moderate flow reductions with a PI of between 1.2 and 1.5 L·minute^{-1}·m^{-1} can be safely employed. Because oxygen saturation is not influenced by temperature, in-line Sv_{O_2} measurement using commercially available oximeters represents a readily available technique for the continuous evaluation of the adequacy of matching systemic oxygen supply to demand under any given flow parameters.

Arterial Pressure During CPB

Since the initial report by Stockard et al. in which a perfusion pressure less than 50 mm Hg was incriminated in the incidence of neurologic dysfunction after CPB (54), the influence of hypotension during CPB on postoperative neurologic dysfunction has been debated (55,56). A recent clinical outcome trial in 248 coronary bypass patients was able to show significant outcome differences by using a cumulative end point comprised of mortality rate (1.6% versus 4.0%), stroke rate (2.4% versus 7.2%), and cardiovascular complications (2.4% versus 4.8%) in a group in whom MAP was maintained at 80 to 100 mm Hg versus one in which systemic pressure averaged 50 to 60 mm Hg (57). This study has not yet been independently confirmed, however.

As noted previously, it should also be recognized that during CPB, cerebral venous hypertension with resultant decreases in cerebral perfusion pressure may result, independent of maintenance of even high MAPs, particularly when using a single two-stage venous cannula. Manipulation of the heart to access posterior coronary vessels may occlude venous return from the SVC, resulting in an elevation of jugular pressures, decreases in cerebral perfusion pressure, and significant decreases in CBF, independent of MAP (5). It is noteworthy that this potential was initially identified more than 35 years ago by Paton et al., who suggested employing electroencephalographic (EEG) monitoring to identify just such cerebral venous obstruction (58).

Murkin et al., Rogers et al., and others have shown that CBF is not affected by changes in pump flow rates within 2.2 L/m^2/minute to 1.0 L/m^2/minute (52,59). The larger, physiologic question of whether the limits of cerebral autoregulation are extended during moderate hypothermic CPB, as several clinical studies have suggested (51,60), remains unclear. Cerebral autoregulation is lost at extremes of hypotension. Further, there is evidence from the meticulous work of Newman et al. that during nonpulsatile CPB, cerebral autoregulation exhibits a small pressure dependence such that a 20 mm Hg increase in MAP results in approximately a 10% increase in CBF (61). Studies from this group have also shown that hypotension (MAP less than 50 mm Hg) and rapid rewarming during CPB contributed significantly to postoperative cognitive dysfunction in the elderly patient who underwent CAB surgery (62).

While Henriksen et al. (63) reported hyperemic CBF during hypothermic CPB that was directly related to arterial pressure, falling significantly with pressures less than 55 mm Hg, Govier et al. (51) observed much lower CBF that was independent of MAP down to 30 mm Hg. These observations were subsequently reconciled by Murkin et al., who demonstrated the pivotal role of pH management in influencing CBF (60). They showed that alpha-stat pH management preserves cerebral autoregulation and cerebral flow-metabolism coupling, whereas pH-stat management produces pressure-passive CBF and uncouples the normal relationship between CBF and cerebral metabolic rate for O_2. Prough et al. further demonstrated the influence that changes in $Paco_2$, according to alpha-stat or pH-stat management during hypothermic CPB, exerted on CBF (64). They confirmed the preservation of cerebral autoregulation with alpha-stat and demonstrated loss of autoregulation with pH-stat pH management. The apparently conflicting observations of CBF during hypothermic CPB by Govier et al. and Henriksen et al. were thus reconciled as being due to the use of differing pH management strategies, alpha-stat and pH-stat, respectively, in the two studies (51,63). These observations have again been confirmed more recently (65).

Although it should be recognized that in all these investigations, patients with untreated hypertension, diabetes mellitus, or overt cerebrovascular disease were excluded from study, case reports of patients with significant carotid or vertebral artery stenoses have demonstrated similar preservation of CBF with alpha-stat pH management (66). The apparent loss of cerebral autoregulation during hypothermic CPB in diabetic patients, as demonstrated by Croughwell et al. (67), raises concern however, it may be a further manifestation of a diabetic autonomic neuropathy, and it implies that these patients may be at increased risk for postoperative neurologic dysfunction independent of the risks associated with hyperglycemia *per se* (68).

During normothermic CPB in patients, Cook et al. have documented increased CBF secondary to hemodilution and decreased cerebrovascular resistance with apparently appropriate coupling of cerebral oxygen demand and delivery (69). Similarly Philipott et al. have documented an 85% increase in CBF from baseline, proportional to the degree of hemodilution, during normothermic CPB with a PI of more than $2.1 \cdot \text{minute}^{-1} \cdot \text{m}^{-2}$ and perfusion pressures of 50 to 70 mm Hg (70). This hyperemia gave rise to modest increases in intracranial pressure. In animals maintained at lower perfusion pressures during normothermic CPB, decreased CBF with increased oxygen extraction was observed. Postoperatively, a paradoxical cerebral hyperperfusion with increased CBF and reduced cerebral metabolic rate for O_2 was noted after such cerebral hypoperfusion (70).

Clinically, these data suggest that when flow reductions are required during CPB, efforts must be made to maintain cerebral perfusion pressure to preserve CBF. Similarly, even when hypotension is accompanied by high pump flow rates—such as sometimes occurs during normothermic CPB—adequacy of cerebral perfusion cannot be assumed. By default, maintaining pressures at the normal lower limit of cerebral autoregulation—50 mm Hg—or higher, appears judicious.

Hemodilution

During the initial clinical introduction of CPB, the perfusion circuit was primed with donor blood (1). Within a few years, reports of pulmonary congestion and problems associated with postoperative hypervolemia appeared, implicating the use of hemic prime and raising concerns about this practice (71). Subsequently, the use of a blood-free prime was reported in the early 1960s (72,73), and as further experience was gained, hemodilution has become standard practice during adult cardiac surgery.

The volume of an average CPB circuit incorporating a membrane oxygenator, heat exchanger, arterial line filter, and venous return and arterial inflow lines ranges between 1,800 mL and 2,300 mL. Depending on the Hb concentration and the circulating blood volume of the patient, the pump circuit is primed with either a crystalloid solution or blood.

Given that the blood volume in an adult is approximately 7% of body weight, an estimate of the circulating blood volume can be made to calculate the effective Hb concentration after hemodilution during institution of CPB. This can be approximated by considering the increased effective circulating blood volume resulting from the incorporation of the pump circuit as follows:

$$\{[7\% \times \text{body wt(kg)}]/[7\% \times \text{body wt(kg)} + \text{pump vol}]\} \times \text{Hb} = \text{effective Hb} \quad [14\text{-}1]$$

For example, in a 70-kg adult with a Hb concentration of 15 g/dL, calculated blood volume would be (7% × 70 = 4.9) 4.9 L, and given a 2.2-L CPB circuit volume, the resultant Hb concentration would be approximately (5/7 × 15 = 10.7) 10.7 g/dL. Alternatively, if Hb concentration was 12 g/dL, the resultant Hb concentration would be approximately 8.5 g/dL. As determined previously, as long as an adequate pump flow can be maintained, transfusion should not be necessary.

To determine the maximal allowable degree of hemodilution, the necessity for an increased oxygen carrying capacity should be analyzed in a similar fashion as described earlier. The importance of minimizing Vo_2 by ensuring an adequate level of neuromuscular blockade (44) and of minimizing increases in Vo_2 associated with shivering secondary to inadequate core rewarming are of fundamental importance if unnecessary transfusion is to be avoided.

Cook et al. have determined the minimum hematocrit level supporting cerebral oxygenation during normothermic CPB in dogs. They note that the critical hematocrit at which metabolism becomes delivery dependent is between 9% ± 2% and 14% during normothermic CPB (74). Paradoxically, Liam et al. found that a hematocrit level of more than 18% was needed to maintain systemic oxygen delivery and consumption during normothermic CPB (75). This implies that the critical hematocrit value for the whole body may be higher than that required for the brain, due to cerebral compensation via autoregulation.

Fluid Management: Crystalloid Versus Colloid

Several studies have investigated the efficacy of various types of priming fluids for the CPB circuit in relation to the total volume of perioperative fluids required and examined differences in organ system functioning after CPB.

Byrick et al. evaluated colloid osmotic pressure and postoperative extravascular lung water accumulation in two groups of patients in whom the CPB circuit had been primed with either 2,000 mL of lactated Ringer's solution (RL) or with 400 mL of plasma and 1,600 mL of RL (76). Although colloid osmotic pressure was significantly lower in the group who received RL during CPB, this difference between groups disappeared postoperatively, and colloid osmotic pressure remained significantly lower than control in both groups. Postoperatively, they were unable to demonstrate any difference between groups with respect to extravascular lung water, with the greatest accumulations in both groups appearing on the second postoperative day.

Hollowell et al. examined the practice of administering either 75 g albumin or RL to the pump circuit during CPB (77). They were unable to demonstrate any significant difference in clinical course or blood usage between groups. Although the RL group demonstrated a positive postoperative fluid balance that was 1,000 mL more than that in the albumin-treated group, the RL group had a tendency for a lower incidence of abnormal indexes of renal function postoperatively, leading the authors to conclude that administration of albumin does not positively influence the outcome of patients undergoing CPB.

When the effects of hypothermia, hemodilution, and CPB were examined separately by Utley et al. in dogs, they demonstrated that hemodilution with RL to a hematocrit level of 25% produced increased water content in tissue and that normothermic nonpulsatile CPB decreased blood flow to the outer cortex of the kidney and the subendocardium while hemodilution increased it (78). Hypothermia to 25°C, or CPB, decreased renal free-water clearance but did not alter glomerular filtration rate. Overall, they demonstrated that hemodilution counters the adverse effects of hypothermia and pump-oxygenation on blood flow, oxygen delivery, and renal function, but that hemodilution produces an increased water content of gastrointestinal (GI) organs and the myocardium.

The metabolic responses to CPB after usage of either dextrose, RL, dextrose and RL, or plasmolyte for pump primes were assessed with regard to glucose, lactate, and pyruvate concentrations, as well as insulin, glucagon, and cortisol levels in patients during and after hypothermic CPB (79). The inclusion of glucose-containing solutions was demonstrated to produce dramatic increases in blood glucose concentrations during CPB, with no differences in glucagon or cortisol levels, although insulin levels were highest in the groups receiving glucose-containing primes. When the use of a hypertonic saline hydroxyethyl starch solution (2,400 mOsmol/L) was compared with standard hydroxyethyl starch for volume replacement after acute hemodilution, a significantly lower fluid balance and higher cardiac index was found in the hypertonic group (80).

The use of glucose-containing fluids during CPB has been advocated by some because of an apparent decrease in postoperative fluid balance in comparison to RL treated patients (81). Also, these authors did not observe any difference in neurologic complications in patients managed with glucose-containing fluids (81). This study has been criticized for downplaying the potential neurologic risks of hyperglycemia however (82), particularly because neurologic functioning was assessed retrospectively. Retrospective surveys are notoriously insensitive for the detection of neurologic abnormalities (83), and there is a growing and persuasive body of literature demonstrating the potential for enhanced neurologic injury during hyperglycemia with either focal or global cerebral ischemia (84–86).

There appear to be several different mechanisms by which hyperglycemia can give rise to increased neuronal injury in the presence of ischemia. Formation of advanced glycosylation end products decreases microvascular endothelial and smooth-muscle relaxation with resulting microcirculatory disturbances (87). Anaerobic glycolysis produces intracellular acidosis, with subsequent free radical generation also impairing smooth-muscle relaxation, again leading to microvascular dysregulation (88). Decreased glutamine transport associated with decreased cerebral plasma volume results in endothelial cell swelling and microvascular plugging (89). In addition, in patients presenting with ischemic strokes, hemorrhagic transformation of ischemic infarcts has been strongly correlated with elevated blood glucose concentrations (90). Further, anaerobic glycolysis has been shown to enhance energy-dependent DNA fragmentation during delayed neuronal death (apoptosis) (91). Interestingly, at least one study has been able to demonstrate an improvement in postoperative cognitive performance in normoglycemic versus hyperglycemic CAB patients (92). This study demonstrated improved central nervous system outcome related to intraoperative glucose management and avoidance of hyperglycemia, consistent with the experimental evidence cited earlier.

Neurologic injury alone is not the only detriment to hyperglycemia during cardiovascular surgery, however. There is also evidence that hyperglycemia impairs white blood cell function and leads to a greater incidence of wound infection. In a prospective study of 26 diabetic patients randomized to aggressive insulin infusion or standard therapy, continuous insulin infusion and tight glucose control during surgery significantly improved white blood cell function in diabetic patients, leading the authors to speculate that this "may increase resistance to infection after surgery"(93). Interestingly, in a prospective study of 2,467 diabetic open heart surgery patients, continuous insulin infusion induced a significant reduction in perioperative blood glucose levels (less than 200 mg/dL), which led to a significant reduction in the incidence of sternal wound infection to 0.8% versus 2.0% in patients in whom hyperglycemia was documented (94).

A strong correlation between preoperative hyperglycemia and postoperative renal failure has also been made. In a prospective observational, multicenter study of 2,222 patients undergoing elective CAB surgery, preoperative serum glucose level of more than 16.6 mmol/L was associated with the highest relative risk (RR) being 3.7, versus age 80 to 95 years (RR = 3.5), elevated serum creatinine level of 124 to 177 μmol/L (RR = 2.3), previous CAB surgery (RR = 1.8), and even preoperative congestive heart failure (RR = 1.8) (95). Even mortality has been correlated with elevated blood glucose levels after cardiac surgery. In a single-center observational study of 1,157 CAB patients more than 75 years of age, one significant predictor of postoperative mortality included postoperative a plasma glucose level of more than 300 mg/dL (96).

Currently, it appears as though there is no particular benefit to be derived from the routine use of other than crystalloid-based fluids for routine fluid management during CPB, but hyperglycemia, which can be precipitated or aggravated by the administration of glucose-containing fluids during CPB, should be avoided (82,97).

Tissue Perfusion

The adequacy of tissue perfusion during CPB can be monitored by direct and indirect means. Clinical assessment of tissue perfusion such as capillary refill and tissue coloration are useful but nonspecific indicators during normothermia, but they become ambiguous during hypothermia. Continuous in-line monitoring of $S\bar{v}O_2$ using an infrared analyzer, combined with intermittent blood gas analysis or continuous in-line fluorometric analysis of arterial pH, PO_2 and PCO_2 gives useful and quantifiable indication of the adequacy of tissue perfusion (98). Mixed venous oxygen saturation correlates inversely with VO_2 and directly with perfusion rates (44). Overall tissue oxygen delivery can be estimated using $S\bar{v}O_2$, which should normally be more than 70%. Inadequate perfusion results in venous desaturation, and $S\bar{v}O_2$ of less than 60% should be corrected by either increasing perfusion flow rates, decreasing metabolic demand (e.g., by the administration of muscle relaxants), or by red blood cell transfusion or administration of synthetic oxygen carriers.

Urinary output as a measure of adequacy of overall perfusion is generally an unreliable indicator during CPB. Urinary volume is influenced by several factors, including the degree of hypothermia, pulsatility, use of diuretics, and use of mannitol in the prime solution. Also, narcotics such as fentanyl can induce increased levels of antidiuretic hormone, resulting in lower urine output (99). Venous hypertension as produced by partial obstruction of the IVC cannula can result in oliguria. This can be manifested as a combination of poor venous return and low urinary volumes and may require repositioning of the IVC cannula.

PULSATILE PERFUSION

In most centers, nonpulsatile perfusion remains the most common mode of perfusion used during CPB. This is partly because the nature of the apparatus required to produce pulsatile flow was relatively cumbersome, and in part because there has been no clear consensus on the relative merits of pulsatile perfusion.

Pulsatile Perfusion Techniques

Until the advent of the variable-speed roller pump, commercially available devices for the production of a pulsatile waveform during CPB had included the use of a separate intraaortic balloon pump (100) or involved the interposition of specially constructed sections of tubing into the arterial line for use with in-line pulsators. The pulsatile assist device used by Bregman et al. incorporated a balloon through which arterial blood was pumped, surrounded by a rigid external jacket connected by a pneumatic line to an intraaortic balloon pump console (101,102). Although Bregman et al. reported increased urinary output and increased coronary graft blood flow when using this device during CPB (102), others were unable to duplicate these results and reported evidence of increased blood trauma (103). The Tamari-Kaplitt pulsator represents another older type of device also producing pulsations by phasic external compression of the arterial line. Rather than using an interposed section of balloon, as in the pulsatile assist device, arterial blood is pumped through a dilated section of arterial tubing, which is similarly surrounded by a noncompliant jacket and connected to an external pneumatic device (104). With both of these devices, however, concerns have been expressed about hemolysis and the potential development of gaseous microemboli resulting from cavitation of blood during the negative-pressure phase of pulsation when the compressed section of arterial tubing is reexpanding (103, 105).

An alternate approach to the production of pulsatile flow during CPB is the use of a variable-speed roller pump, as reported by Jacobs et al. and Taylor et al (106,107). This type of device has been commercially available as the pulsatile flow controller, and clinical outcome studies have now been reported based on its use (108,109). This device regulates the speed of the roller pump heads, producing a cyclical increase and decrease in the instantaneous flow velocity of blood pumped into the aorta. Advantages inherent in this approach include the avoidance of separate cannulation sites, as is required with the intraaortic balloon pump, and the elimination of the need for the interposition of a separate segment of tubing into the arterial line, preserving the structural integrity of the arterial line.

Unlike in-line pulsators, oxygenator design becomes an important consideration with use of the pulsatile flow controller. With the exception of certain gravity-feed oxygenators such as the Capiox-E (TerumoR), most other oxygenators require that blood be pumped through them and are thus placed distal to the roller pump head. In contrast, because of its placement proximal to the roller pump head, use of a gravity-feed oxygenator may permit the oscillations produced by the roller pump head to be transmitted into the arterial tree. This configuration of the CPB circuit also permits maximal undamped transmission of the pulsatile waveform produced by the pulsatile flow controller.

Depending on their compliance characteristics, pump-through–type oxygenators may exert a significant degree of pressure/flow modulation, producing a variable degree of damping of the arterial flow characteristics. When Gourley et al. used a pulsatile flow controller to examine pulsatile flow characteristics with use of different oxygenator types, they demonstrated that in comparison to a bubble oxygenator, flat-sheet membrane oxygenators resulted in a highly significant degree of pressure/flow modulation, with virtually complete loss of pulsatile flow (110). Hollow-fiber membrane oxygenators, however, whether employing a blood-inside or blood-outside the fiber design, produced a characteristic pulsatile waveform (Fig. 14-6) and are thus preferable for use during pulsatile perfusion (110).

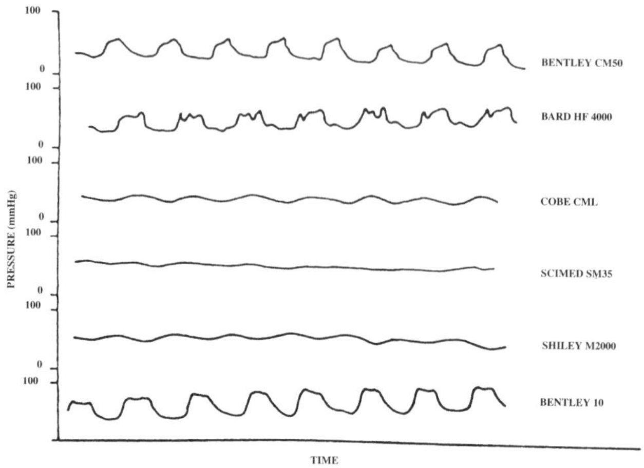

FIGURE 14-6. The efficacy of various membrane oxygenators to transmit a pulsatile waveform when roller pump is proximal to oxygenator. Flat-plate membrane oxygenators (Shiley M@000, Scimed SM35, Cobe CML) produce maximal damping of pulse, whereas hollow-fiber membrane oxygenators all transmit pulsatile pressure equally effectively whether they are blood-inside or blood-outside design. (From Gourlay T, Gibbons M, Taylor KM. Pulsatile flow compatibility of a group of membrane oxygenators. *Perfusion* 1987;2:115, with permission.)

Indexes of Pulsatility

When the results of pulsatile perfusion are being interpreted, critical analysis of the perfusion characteristics that were produced during CPB becomes an important consideration. In the extensive review by Hickey et al. (111), as well as in the editorials and commentaries by Wright et al. and Grossi et al. (112,113), it has been recognized that the designation "pulsatile perfusion" represents an inherently polymorphous continuum. These authors have identified that many of the diverse and apparently contradictory results that have been reported after use of pulsatile perfusion have resulted from the employment of pulsatile techniques having varying degrees of efficacy. Some types of pulsatile flow are more effective than nonpulsatile flow in preserving tissue function while others are not. The inconsistency in results reported after comparisons of pulsatile and nonpulsatile perfusion is thus partly attributable to a lack of agreement in the definition and hence the achievement of pulsatile perfusion (112). Analysis of many of the studies in which pulsatile perfusion was evaluated has highlighted the lack of any consistent definition, or in some cases lack even of a functional description, of the type of pulsatile waveform produced (111).

Wright et al. (112) have emphasized that the one type of pulsatile flow that is by definition physiologic is that produced in the aorta by the healthy left ventricle. They advocate the use of harmonic analysis to describe the frequency, amplitude, and phase characteristics of the output from various pulsatile pumps in order to form a basis for comparisons of their efficacy in reproducing a physiologic waveform. This approach is important for evaluation in an experimental model but remains difficult to achieve in clinical conditions.

Grossi et al. (113,114) analyzed the output produced during pulsatile perfusion by various combinations of rate and pulse shape in a perfusion model and categorized them according to the PI after Gosling et al. (115) This unitless measure is based on a harmonic analysis of the pulsatile waveform produced and reflects the relative "sharpness" of a given waveform with respect to its mean flow, independent of frequency. The pulse-power index (PPI) was formulated as the PI not normalized for frequency (115). When differing combinations of rate and various pulsatile waveforms were characterized according to PI and PPI and evaluated with respect to their ability to decrease serum lactate production in dogs during normothermic CPB, all combinations produced significant decreases in PI and PPI as compared to prebypass control measures. The authors concluded that it is very difficult to reproduce the stroke volume characteristics of blood that is normally ejected through the aortic annulus during a small portion of the cardiac cycle, by mechanically pumping blood through the commonly used sizes of aortic cannulas. This simple fact is unquestionably of profound importance in the pursuit of "physiologically relevant" pulsatile flow.

Rather than discounting systems that do not completely mimic the characteristics of pulsatile perfusion as produced by ventricular ejection, however, a systematic evaluation of various pulsatile pumps used for CPB and assessing various indexes of end-organ function, coupled with a description of the characteristics of the waveform produced, would allow the selection of the most clinically appropriate method of perfusion during CPB. Grossi et al. did observe that there was a high correlation between the PI measured through the arterial inflow cannula and that in the descending aorta (113). The fidelity of pulse characteristics recorded in the radial artery in comparison to those present within the cerebral circulation is presently unclear. Overall, it was demonstrated that a minimum rate of 80 beats/minutes and a pulse shape with the stroke volume delivered over the shortest portion of the pulse period were most effective in decreasing lactate production, as compared with nonpulsatile roller pump perfusion. The duration of pump flow in this system occurred within 50% of each pump cycle.

Organ Blood Flow

Despite the extensive clinical experience that has been gained over the past three decades demonstrating the relative safety of nonpulsatile perfusion during CPB, there is evidence that pulsatile perfusion during CPB may be better able to preserve the function of certain organ systems. Pulsatile flow contains more energy (power × time), which can be transmitted distally to perform work such as tissue perfusion and the promotion of metabolic exchange, and which encourages the movement of tissue fluids and the promotion of the flow of lymph (116).

Of the positive results that have been reported to accrue from pulsatile perfusion, decreases in systemic vascular resistance (117), increases in urinary output (117), decreased renin release (118,119), and lower levels of stress hormones (118) are among the most consistent. As is discussed later, improved organ perfusion has also been reported for the kidneys, liver, and brain with use of pulsatile CPB.

Metabolic indexes implying more homogeneous perfusion, including a lower systemic vascular resistance (117, 120–123), lower systemic lactate production (114), higher systemic oxygen consumption (122), and shorter times for rewarming (123), have been demonstrated after use of pulsatile perfusion. Whether these parameters reflect a "mechanical" effect of pulsatile perfusion to promote formation and flow of lymph fluid, as has been demonstrated in isolated tissue (116), or alternatively, whether the greater energy associated with pulsatile perfusion better maintains "critical opening pressures" necessary for capillary perfusion is still unresolved.

Most measures of renal function during CPB have demonstrated improved indexes with pulsatile perfusion, compared with nonpulsatile perfusion. In dogs, nonpulsatile perfusion of one kidney resulted in decreased urine output and sodium excretion from both kidneys (124). A significant increase in urine output has also been demonstrated during pulsatile CPB as compared with nonpulsatile CPB in monkeys (125). Although several studies have reported increased urine output in patients managed with pulsatile perfusion during CPB (103,106,117,123), Badner et al. were unable to distinguish any differences in urine output or sodium excretion among patients randomized to pulsatile or nonpulsatile CPB (126). In this latter study, however, pulsatile perfusion was only maintained during the hypothermic phase of CPB and thus accounted for only about one half the total duration of CPB. In addition, only patients with normal preoperative renal function were evaluated; thus, the role of pulsatile perfusion in patients with impaired renal function remains unclear.

A redistribution of blood flow from outer cortical layers to the deeper juxtamedullary cortex, accompanied by increased renin secretion, was demonstrated after 1 and 2 hours of nonpulsatile perfusion in dogs (127). Another study was unable to demonstrate any difference in the distribution of renal blood flow upon conversion from nonpulsatile to pulsatile perfusion, however, possibly due to the much shorter duration of nonpulsatile perfusion, only about 10 minutes (128).

Hepatic blood flow has also been investigated during pulsatile and nonpulsatile CPB. Using indocyanine green (ICG) clearance as an indirect means of assessing hepatic blood flow, Howie et al. demonstrated a significant difference in hepatic blood flow in patients depending on whether pulsatile or nonpulsatile CPB was employed (129). Based on ICG clearance, they determined that there was no change in hepatic plasma flow from control in the pulsatile CPB group while there was a significant decrease in the nonpulsatile group. Pulsatile or nonpulsatile perfusion does not appear to influence metabolism of thiopental during CPB, however (130).

The influence of perfusion characteristics on cerebral physiology have also been studied. Early studies identified decreases in cerebral metabolism (131) and reductions in cortical CBF and progressive increases in cerebrovascular resistance with increasing durations of nonpulsatile CPB (132). Microscopic examinations of cerebral and conjunctival capillary beds after pulsatile and nonpulsatile perfusion using an isolated dog head model demonstrated increased red blood cell sludging, capillary closure, and venous distention with nonpulsatile as compared to pulsatile perfusion (133). Sanderson et al. demonstrated histologic changes indicative of ischemia and areas of cerebral capillary closure after nonpulsatile but not after pulsatile CPB in dogs (134). When this same group examined cerebral histology postoperatively in dogs after pulsatile or nonpulsatile CPB, they observed focal ischemic lesions in brains of both groups but evidence of additional diffuse cerebral nerve cell damage only in the nonpulsatile group (135). Although most studies have shown either no abnormalities or a decreased incidence of histologic abnormalities after pulsatile CPB, not all studies of pulsatile and nonpulsatile CPB have demonstrated improvements in brain histology after pulsatile perfusion. Laursen et al. reported increased brain edema and apparent evidence of increased blood-brain barrier permeability after 3 hours of normothermic pulsatile CPB, as compared to nonpulsatile CPB (136).

CBF during normothermic CPB was assessed by Tranmer et al. in the presence and absence of middle cerebral artery ligation, during either pulsatile or nonpulsatile CPB (137). In ischemic hemispheres, pulsatile perfusion increased CBF by 55% while in the nonischemic brain CBF increased by 19% (137). Consistent with these observations, Murkin et al. demonstrated that in patients during hypothermic CPB, institution of pulsatile perfusion significantly increased CBF by 15% in comparison to nonpulsatile perfusion (138).

During core cooling for deep hypothermic circulatory arrest in dogs, pulsatile perfusion significantly decreased cerebral lactate production compared with nonpulsatile CPB (139). During deep hypothermia in dogs, low-flow CPB has been shown to maintain brain tissue pH and Pco_2 more optimally than circulatory arrest, with pulsatile CPB able to restore these measures toward control more rapidly than nonpulsatile CPB (140). Overall, it would appear that organ perfusion is better maintained with pulsatile as compared with nonpulsatile perfusion during CPB. Whether this influences postoperative outcome, however, remains an open question.

There have been discouragingly few clinical outcome studies assessing the impact of pulsatile compared to nonpulsatile CPB. Most of the clinical studies reported to date have looked at intermediary, process-related variables such as urine output, vascular resistance, and hormone profiles. This is not surprising, given the much greater number of subjects that must be examined to achieve sufficient power to detect a significant difference in outcome. Given the presence of the very large number of uncontrolled and potentially confounding clinical variables such as myocardial function, postoperative complications, hemodynamic perturbations, concomitant disease, and surgical technique, randomization of several hundred patients is required.

In what still constitutes the largest prospective clinical comparison of pulsatile and nonpulsatile CPB reported to date, Taylor et al. demonstrated a significantly lower total mortality rate (4.6% versus 10.3%) and a lower incidence of inotropic drug and circulatory assist device usage in 350 patients using pulsatile as compared to nonpulsatile CPB, without significant differences in hemolysis, postoperative bleeding, or blood transfusion requirements (109). Murkin and colleagues randomized 316 patients undergoing closed chamber coronary bypass surgery to either pulsatile or nonpulsatile perfusion and demonstrated significant decreases in overall in-hospital mortality rate (0.6% versus 5.8%), myocardial infarction rate (0.7% versus 6%), and overall complication rates (8% versus 16%), in patients randomized to receive pulsatile perfusion (108).

Given the aforementioned, why is the use of pulsatile perfusion during CPB essentially unchanged over the past two decades? Although there are obviously many reasons, ranging from the apparent dichotomy of results after pulsatile CPB to the reluctant acceptance of the surgical team of the pulsations of the arterial cannula, the most likely reason remains a degree of clinical inertia "nonpulsatile CPB has served us well enough." Newer developments using beating heart surgery for coronary revascularization without the use of CPB may well render these issues increasingly irrelevant.

HYPOTHERMIA

Metabolic Rate

The metabolic activity of various organ systems includes a series of biochemical reactions, the nature of which is determined by the complex interactions of a variety of biochemical, hormonal, neuronal, and metabolic influences—all of which summate to influence the degree to which a particular biochemical reaction occurs. The rate of that reaction is also determined in part by the thermal energy, or temperature, of the tissues. According to van't Hoff's law, the rate of a chemical reaction is directly dependent on the temperature at which it occurs. Regardless of whether a reaction takes place in a test tube or in a biological system, a similar temperature dependency of rate is evident. There is an exponential relationship between temperature and metabolic rate that can be described by an Arrhenius equation, in which the natural logarithm (ln) of the metabolic rate is inversely related to temperature (T) by the rate constant ($-k$):

$$\ln \text{metabolic rate} = -k \cdot 1/T \qquad [14\text{-}2]$$

The influence of temperature on the metabolic activity of an organ system can be characterized by a ratio, the temperature coefficient, referred to as Q_{10}. The Q_{10} for a given system is determined as the quotient of the metabolic rate of the tissue measured at two temperatures separated by 10°C. By convention, the metabolic rate at the lower temperature forms the divisor, thus the resulting index is greater than unity. The larger the value of Q_{10}, the more profound the decrease in metabolic rate for a given reduction in temperature. The inverse of the Q_{10} represents the metabolic activity at the lower temperature expressed as a portion of the metabolic activity at the higher temperature; simply put, a Q_{10} of 2 implies that cooling by 10°C decreases metabolic activity by one half. The metabolic rates for various mammalian organ systems, including the brain, have been measured both *in vitro* and *in vivo,* and temperature dependency has been demonstrated.

Temperature exerts an influence on metabolic activity that is exponential rather than linear. Change in the rate of activity, rather than change in the amount of activity, is represented by Q_{10}. Therefore, an apparently greater degree of metabolic suppression occurs with initial decreases in temperature from normothermia, than that which occurs during hypothermia (141). For whole-body oxygen consumption in patients during nonpulsatile CPB, values of Q_{10} range from 1.9 to 2.6, depending on whether a period of normothermic CPB perfusion precedes cooling (46).

For the brain, this relationship becomes more complex. Over the range from 37°C to 27°C, Q_{10} is approximately 2.2 as measured *in vitro* (142), in dogs (143), and in surgical patients during nonpulsatile CPB (52). Over the range from 28°C to 18°C, however, Q_{10} has been calculated as being much greater, at approximately 5.0 (144). In an elegant review of this topic, John D. Michenfelder has cogently argued that this substantial increase in Q_{10} occurs because there is a loss of EEG activity between 18°C and 22°C that produces a disproportionate decrease in cerebral metabolic rate over this range (145). If EEG activity is suppressed by thiopental administration, the absolute metabolic activity of the brain is proportionately lower than in the presence of a similar degree of hypothermia, during which EEG activity is occurring, and Q_{10} is decreased and approaches 2.2 over the entire range from 37°C to 18°C.

This is considerably important in the clinical management of patients undergoing CPB, particularly if circulatory arrest or low flows are employed. It implies that in the presence of EEG activity, the tolerable duration of ischemia for the brain at 27°C is doubled and is further increased five-fold at 18°C. If barbiturate suppression of EEG is to be employed for cerebral protection in patients at risk for cerebral ischemia during CPB (146), however, it would be predicted to be of most benefit during normothermia and would have decreased efficacy when the cerebral metabolic rate for O_2 is lowered either by hypothermia or when cerebral activity and metabolic rate are decreased by other anesthetic agents (147). In fact, this is consistent with what has been demonstrated clinically to date. Nussmeier et al. have reported decreases in persistent neurologic deficits after thiopental-induced EEG suppression during CPB at 34°C for open chamber cardiac surgery (148) while Zaiden et al. were unable to demonstrate a benefit using a similar thiopental administration protocol during CPB at 28°C for coronary bypass procedures (149). More recently, Roach et al. have been unable to show central nervous system benefits from administration of propofol to induce burst suppression during hypothermic CPB in patients undergoing valvular surgery (150).

Viscosity

Not only does hypothermia produce a decrease in the metabolic rate for various organ systems, as discussed earlier, but hypothermia can also affect tissue perfusion characteristics resulting from changes in blood rheology due to an increase in blood viscosity.

The viscosity of a fluid is a measure of its resistance to flow or "thickness." For whole blood at rest, fibrinogen and erythrocytes produce a three-dimensional matrix wherein red blood cells are interconnected by negatively charged fibrinogen molecules producing aggregation and rouleaux formation (151). Yield stress is a measure of the force that must be applied to disrupt red blood cell aggregates when blood is stationary, and shear rate or velocity gradient is a measure of the rate at which fluid particles separate from one another. Yield stress is responsible for a significant portion of the peripheral resistance when flow is low and is not affected by anticoagulants (152).

Fluids for which viscosity is constant and thus independent of shear rate are considered newtonian liquids. Whole blood is a non-newtonian fluid because it exhibits an anomalous viscosity such that viscosity increases at low shear rates, and in small-caliber vessels, the apparent viscosity at all shear rates is less than that found in larger vessels (153). This is due to axial streaming of red blood cells in small arterioles in which a boundary layer of plasma is in contact with the vessel walls, resulting in an effective viscosity in 20 μm arterioles that is two thirds that measured in a viscometer. If whole blood is defibrinogenated or washed, red blood cells are suspended in saline, a more characteristically newtonian fluid behavior is observed (154).

Independent of fibrinogen concentrations, the viscosity of whole blood is also influenced by hematocrit level and temperature (155). There is an exponential increase in viscosity with increases in hematocrit, such that viscosity increases nearly 70% for an increase in hematocrit from 40% to 60% while viscosity decreases by 30% with a reduction in hematocrit from 40% to 20%. The effect of a change in temperature is an inverse change in viscosity, so a decrease in temperature from 37°C to 27°C increases viscosity by 30%. The net result is that at 22°C and a hematocrit of 20%, viscosity is virtually identical over a range of shear rates to that at 37°C and a hematocrit of 40%. At 27°C and a hematocrit of 20%, viscosity is slightly less over a wide range of shear rates to that measured at 37°C with a hematocrit of 40% (155). As such, hemodilution is essential during procedures employing hypothermia, and the increased yield stress that must be overcome to restore capillary circulation during profound hypothermia and circulatory arrest may contribute to some of the decrease in CBF that has been reported after total circulatory arrest (156).

pH Management

Among numerous other physiologic effects, hypothermia increases the solubility of oxygen and carbon dioxide in the blood such that for a given content of each, the measured tensions are proportionately reduced. In the case of CO_2, this leads to a corresponding rise in pH and what is perceived as "respiratory alkalosis."

Two main types of acid-base management may be followed during hypothermic CPB: pH-stat, whereby a pH value of 7.4 and Pco_2 value of 40 mm Hg are maintained when these values are corrected for the patients core temperature, and alpha-stat, in which the non–temperature-corrected pH is kept at 7.4 and the Pco_2 at 40 mm Hg (measured at 37°C), so the temperature-corrected pH value varies inversely with body temperature. Given an average 10°C reduction in body temperature during hypothermic CPB, these two approaches result in a difference in pH of approximately 0.16 pH units and in Pco_2 of 15 mm Hg.

Until the mid 1980s, the pH-stat approach was the most commonly employed. The reasons for the popularity of this approach are multiple but are primarily based on an underlying concern about cerebral ischemia during CPB and the possibility that pH-stat might prevent it. Several clinical series from the early 1960s describe focal brain lesions in patients dying after open heart surgery using hypothermic CPB (157,158). With the demonstration of the powerful cerebral vasodilatory properties of CO_2 (159) and the increased concern about the effects of hypothermia in reducing CBF, many cardiac centers began to add CO_2 (approximating pH-stat) during hypothermic CPB.

Due to the inherently greater Pco_2, the pH-stat approach increases CBF and was felt to offset the hypothermia-induced left shift of the oxyhemoglobin dissociation curve, thus potentially increasing oxygen availability at the tissue level. Beyond these considerations was the belief that a temperature-corrected pH value of 7.4 was "normal" and therefore that pH-stat was more physiologic.

It is now apparent that pH-stat is not physiologic in humans; the pH level of arterialized blood is rather governed in accordance with alpha-stat, containing a heterogeneity of pH values depending on the temperature of the tissues being perfused. In intact humans, thermal gradients exist between the tissues at the core and those of the periphery; at a skin temperature of 27°C, arterialized blood perfusing the extremities will fall from a core value pH value of 7.4 and Pco_2 of 40 mm Hg at 37°C to a pH value of 7.56 and Pco_2 of 25 mm Hg (Fig. 14-7) (160). This observation has also been confirmed in patients undergoing hypothermic CPB (161).

To preserve the functional charge ratios of intracellular enzymes and intermediary metabolites, optimal intracellular pH is determined by the neutral pH of water (pNH_20), water being the primary source of intracellular hydrogen ion (H^+) (162,163). Because the dissociation of water is proportionally decreased with falling temperature, intracellular pH rises during hypothermia. To eliminate acid metabolites and CO_2, a constant H^+ gradient of 0.6 to 0.8 pH units is required across the cell membrane, so at all temperatures, blood pH is more alkaline (163). The key buffering mechanism anchoring intracellular pH to pNH_20, and changing its dissociation constant (pK) with tempera-

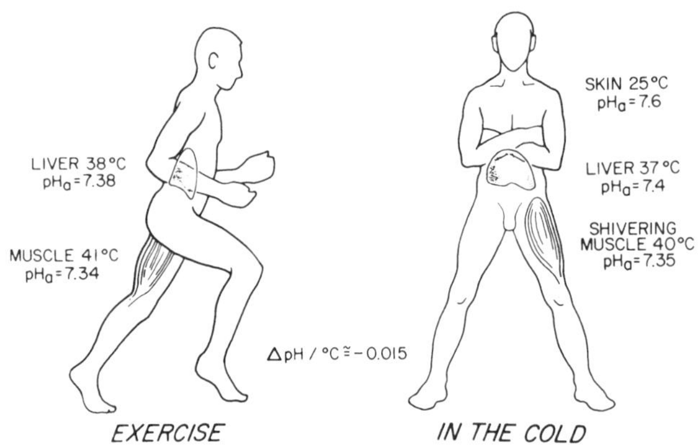

FIGURE 14-7. In intact humans, various thermal gradients exist, depending on the degree of metabolic activity of that tissue. In this closed system, pH regulation is governed in accordance with alpha-stat theory, such that tissue pHa and $Paco_2$ represent a heterogeneous range of values determined by the local temperature. (From White FN. A comparative physiological approach to hypothermia. *J Thorac Cardiovasc Surg* 1981;82:821, with permission.)

ture parallel to pNH_20, was identified by Reeves as a protein buffer, the imidazole group of the amino acid histidine (164).

The degree of buffer dissociation is expressed by "alpha," where alpha refers to the percentage of the imidazole portion of histidine that has dissociated and lost a proton. Alpha-stat acid-base management implies the maintenance of a constant alpha (i.e., a constant charge ratio relative to pNH_20 of this key metabolic buffer over all ranges of temperatures). Constancy of alpha at all temperatures preserves the optimal transmembrane H^+ gradient and intracellular electrochemical neutrality, which facilitates many aspects of metabolic activity including the egress of metabolic byproducts. Alpha-stat acid-base management, by keeping total CO_2 content constant and allowing Pco_2 to vary with temperature, maintains alpha constant (163).

Another rationale for the use of pH-stat is to counter the leftward shift of the oxyhemoglobin dissociation curve engendered by hypothermia (165). This shift is increased by alkalosis and can potentially reduce tissue oxygenation because the increased affinity of Hb for oxygen may impair oxygen unloading at the tissue level. The left shift may be partially offset by lowering pH through the addition of CO_2 (i.e., pH-stat). However, a 10°C reduction in blood temperature increases the dissolved oxygen fraction 25%, reduces total systemic oxygen consumption by more than 60%, and reduces the cerebral metabolic rate for oxygen by more than 70% (60), so adequate tissue oxygen delivery becomes significantly less dependent on oxyhemoglobin kinetics. When this hypothesis was clinically tested during moderately hypothermic CPB, no significant difference was found in the position of the oxyhemoglobin dissociation curve between alpha-stat and pH-stat management, the oxyhemoglobin curve being 50% saturated (p50) at approximately 12 mm Hg with either approach (166).

CO_2 is a potent cerebral vasodilator and will directly increase CBF. This response is maintained during hypothermia, profoundly influencing CBF and having the potential to disrupt cerebral autoregulation (60,64). Murkin et al. demonstrated that alpha-stat maintains cerebral autoregulation and flow/metabolism coupling, enabling the brain to adjust CBF in response to metabolic demands and maintaining CBF over a wide range of perfusion pressures (60). In contrast, pH-stat overrides cerebral autoregulation (64), produces a pressure passive CBF and disrupts flow/metabolism coupling (60), and theoretically has the potential to produce an intracerebral "steal"(167). When specifically sought for, however, evidence of intracerebral steal has not been demonstrated even in patients with cerebrovascular disease managed with pH-stat during hypothermic CPB (168).

CO_2-induced cerebral vasodilation can also reduce perfusion pressure, jeopardizing areas of the brain dependent on flow through critically stenosed vessels (165). In addition, because cerebral emboli are felt to account for a significant portion of neurologic deficits after CPB (19,22,27), unnecessary elevations of CBF have the potential to directly increase delivery of emboli into the cerebral circulation.

Studies in intact dogs during hypothermic CPB have demonstrated significantly better subendocardial blood flow, contractility, and metabolism (169,170), and elevated fibrillation thresholds (171), using alpha-stat versus pH-stat. In one of the few dissenting studies, isolated rat hearts were used, and although a statistically significant difference was not found, it also demonstrated a slight decrease in myocardial efficiency at the lower pH (172). Additionally, in the context of organ transplantation, the optimum perfusate pH for hypothermic organ preservation has been demonstrated to be consistent with the alpha-stat concept (173). Also of potential importance during CPB is the influence of alpha-stat on red blood cell tonicity. Alpha-stat prevents the "chloride shift," with its attendant increase in red blood cell fragility, which accompanies pH-stat and may therefore lessen hemolysis during CPB (174).

With the exception of certain species, in whom pH-stat appears to be operative during hibernation (perhaps because intracellular acidosis serves certain adaptive functions (175), a pH value of 7.4 and Pco_2 of 40 mm Hg can be seen as merely points in a continuum of physiologic acid-base values, appropriate only at 37°C, rather than representing fixed biological end points (163).

Whether these considerations apply during the special circumstances of deep hypothermic circulatory arrest is unclear. During deep hypothermic circulatory arrest in infants, additional factors may be at work. In a prospective study in infants undergoing surgical repair of congenital heart defects using deep hypothermic circulatory arrest, use of pH-stat strategy was associated with lower postoperative morbidity rates, shorter time to first EEG activity, and numerically fewer seizures (though not statistically significantly less), compared with those infants managed using alpha-stat (176). It appears then that in contrast to continuous perfusion during moderate hypothermic or normothermic CPB, reperfusion injury rather than cerebral embolization *per se,* may be a greater factor in postoperative injury during deep hypothermic circulatory arrest. There is no similar data in adults undergoing deep hypothermic circulatory arrest, where appropriate pH management would still appear to be alpha-stat.

NORMOTHERMIC CARDIOPULMONARY BYPASS

The demonstration of apparently improved myocardial performance after normothermic CPB has prompted several outcome studies to assess the efficacy of this approach, with particular focus now centered on CNS outcomes. In a prospective study of 1,732 patients undergoing CAB surgery and randomized to normothermic or hypothermic CPB, a decreased incidence of low-output syndrome and lower cardiac isoenzyme fractions in the warm group was not associated with any difference in stroke rates in comparison to hypothermic CPB group, 1.6% versus 1.5%, respectively (177). In contrast, a study by Martin et al. of 1,001 patients similarly randomized to warm or cold CPB again demonstrated marginally better myocardial protection with warm CPB but found a significantly higher rate of stroke in the warm group compared with the hypothermic CPB group, 3.1% versus 1.0%, respectively (178). Although reasons for this striking difference in stroke rate using two ostensibly similar techniques at different centers are not apparent, it does appear as though the group reported by Martin et al. were at higher risk, because there were more diabetics (25% versus 5.5%, respectively), and more of their patients had undergone prior CAB surgery (14.5% versus prior vascular surgery 8%, respectively) than in the other trial. Additionally, patients rewarmed during normothermia in the Martin et al. group appear much more likely to have had estimated brain temperatures at or exceeding 37°C (179).

While many clinicians have observed cerebral hyperthermia during rewarming after hypothermic CPB, and some have speculated about a potential link between this and postbypass impairment (180,181), until now this phenomenon has been poorly documented. In attempting to quantify clinical practice with respect to the extent of cerebral hyperthermia, a 1995 survey by Nathan et al. provided some important indicators regarding standards of practice (182). In 24 of 28 centers responding to their survey, some attempt was made to monitor cerebral temperature, i.e., either nasopharyngeal or esophageal temperatures. When it is recognized that in the context of cardiac surgery and CPB, esophageal temperature—representing as it does a heterogeneous measure that is variably influenced by core body temperature as well as blood temperature from the aortic inflow cannula and iced slush or fluid within the pericardium—is not reliably representative of temperatures of any specific organ system (183), this is concerning. Seen from this perspective, only about 50% of cardiac centers routinely monitor a site, e.g., nasopharynx, that provides even a moderately reliable index of brain temperature. Furthermore, Nathan et al. reported that even in those centers monitoring nasopharyngeal temperature, brain temperatures routinely exceed 38°C. Transient cerebral hyperthermia is thus the rule rather than the exception for many patients undergoing moderate hypothermic CPB.

It is known that the vulnerability of the normothermic brain to focal ischemic insult demonstrates a surprising variability in the presence of small gradations in temperature (184). Small increases in brain temperature (e.g., 39°C) have been shown to profoundly enhance the susceptibility of the brain to focal ischemic insult and result in ischemic lesions of much greater extent in comparison to controls at 37°C (185). Active rewarming during CPB to bladder temperatures of more than or equal to 37°C may result in nasopharyngeal temperatures of 38°C to 39°C and thus produce significantly greater likelihood of exacerbation of focal neurological injury (186).

Physiologic studies assessing cerebral oxygenation during normothermic or hypothermic CPB have been described. Using continuous jugular oximetry, a higher incidence and extent of cerebral venous oxygen desaturation was found in patients undergoing normothermic CPB, in comparison to those undergoing hypothermic CPB (187). Whether this potential cerebral stress is etiologic in producing overt stroke in a high-risk subset of patients, e.g., diabetics, or whether other more subtle technical differences account for the differing stroke rates after normothermic CPB remains unclear. One study by Newman et al. assessing the effects of MAP and rate of rewarming on the incidence of cognitive dysfunction after cardiac surgery was able to demonstrate a differential susceptibility to rapid rewarming and hypotension in older patients (62).

ORGAN FUNCTION

Various perturbations inherent in the use of CPB include systemic heparinization, extensive exposure of blood to the foreign surfaces presented by tubing, oxygenator, and cardiotomy suction, as well as the potential development of splanchnic ischemia during CPB, production of an acute dilutional anemia, changes in perfusion pressure and flow characteristics, exclusion of the pulmonary circulation, potential employment of moderate or profound degrees of hypothermia, release of cytokines, perturbation in levels of nitric oxide, and activation of various blood element cascades. All have been implicated as factors in the development of the systemic inflammatory response syndrome (188). These perturbations interact to varying degrees to influence the functioning of different organ systems. Gut-induced translocation of endotoxin initiates production of cytokines and complement, as well as activation of neutrophils. Endotoxemia *per se* can cause lactic acidosis, low systemic vascular resistance, and depressed ventricular function. This has been extensively reviewed by Hall et al. and others (189,190). Activation of platelets and leukocytes has also been demonstrated during CPB (191).

Endotoxin

Endotoxins are biologically active substances derived from the breakdown of cell walls of Gram-negative bacteria. In a study of 12 patients undergoing CAB surgery, endotoxin levels and leukocyte activation, as measured by neutrophil generation of oxygen-derived free radicals, were demonstrated to increase significantly during CPB after the aortic cross-clamp was released (192). It was concluded that during CPB, circulating blood is contaminated with endotoxin and that neutrophils become primed for generation of oxygen-derived free radicals and thus may be instrumental in postoperative end-organ dysfunction. Methylprednisolone (30 mg/kg) has been demonstrated to cause a significant decrease in complement activation during CPB; however, it was also observed that endotoxin concentrations were significantly higher in the steroid-treated group during bypass, possibly reflecting decreased clearance of systemic endotoxins. There was no difference in clinical outcome after the first postoperative week in either group, however (193).

It is unclear whether the measured endotoxins are generated by the patient during CPB—possibly by translocation from the GI tract—or alternatively, whether they are introduced during the manufacturing process, because even sterile water may also contain large amounts of endotoxins. No causative relationship between endotoxin levels during CPB and postoperative morbidity has yet been identified (194). The clinical significance of circulating endotoxin levels found in association with CPB remains unknown.

White Blood Cells, Cytokines, and Complement

CPB and the activation of the inflammatory pathways have effects on the circulating blood components, either via direct damage or through activation of secondary mechanisms. Activation of platelets and neutrophils by CPB is thought to play a key role in the production of injury to the endothelium (191). Neutrophils contain various enzymes and cytotoxic substances that when released, result in many of the systemic manifestations of the inflammatory response to CPB. In addition to neutrophil activation, other granulocytes, T and B lymphocytes, and monocytes are involved. Monocytes are critically important, because they produce and release cytokines, in particular tumor necrosis factor-α (TNF-α) and interleukins. Increased levels of circulating TNF-α have been shown in patients undergoing normothermic CPB and are implicated in the vasodilation frequently seen in these patients (195). Cytokines have important actions to regulate the margination and adherence of neutrophils to the endothelial surface and subsequent transendothelial migration. The vascular endothelium, platelets, and neutrophils all have either constitutively present or mediator-stimulated adhesion molecules that initiate and regulate these events.

The first stage in the process of adhesion involves margination of neutrophils. Normally, leukocytes travel with red blood cells in the center of the postcapillary venule at speeds of approximately 1,000 mm/second. The expression of adhesion molecules (selectins) on either the neutrophil (L selectin) or endothelial cell (E selectin) results in the neutrophil "rolling" along the endothelial surface at slower speeds (about 30 mm/second) (see Fig. 14-8) (196). Both E selectin and L selectin can be up-regulated by TNF-α, IL-1, and endotoxin (197,198). Integrins, a different set of adhesion molecules, mediate the ultimate sticking of the neutrophil to the endothelial wall. The integrins CD11a/18 and CD11b/18 are expressed by neutrophils on exposure to chemotactic stimuli. CD11a/18 is expressed at relatively constant levels, whereas CD11b/18 expression can be increased 300% to 400% within seconds. Immunoglobulin adhesion molecules on the endothelium, in particular intercellular adhesion molecule-1 (ICAM-1), are ligands for these integrins and are induced by cytokine stimulation. There is evidence that adherence by CD11b/18 primes the neutrophil to degranulate (199) and to produce the respiratory burst (200). These mechanisms are an essential part of the host defense against invading microbes, but when stimulated inappropriately—as occurs during CPB—unwanted

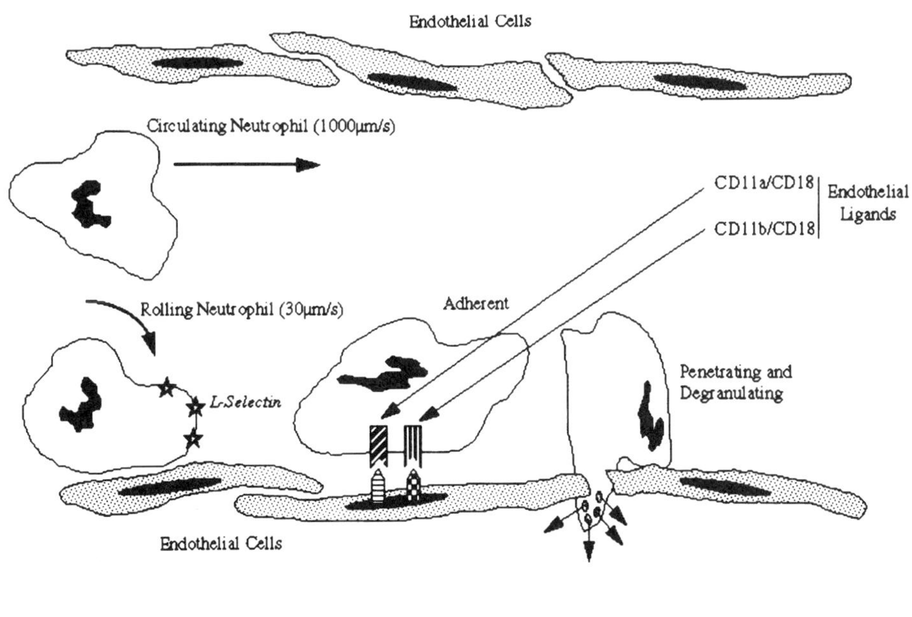

FIGURE 14-8. Processes thought to be involved in primary and secondary adhesion of neutrophils. (From Elliott MJ, Finn AHR. Interaction between neutrophils and endothelium. *Ann Thorac Surg* 1993;56:1503, with permission.)

tissue injury may result from the release of proteolytic enzymes, e.g., elastase, and the generation of oxygen-derived free radicals.

Cytokine rises associated with CPB include TNF-α, IL-1β, IL-2, IL-6, IL-8, and IL-10. Some investigators could not demonstrate any evidence of endotoxemia and demonstrated an antiinflammatory, rather than a proinflammatory cytokine response, in a small number of patients during CPB. Menasche et al. measured levels of IL-1 receptor antagonist (IL-1RA), soluble ICAM-1 (sICAM-1), and elastase as markers of cytokine production, cytokine–up-regulated endothelial ligands for neutrophil adhesion molecules, and degranulation secondary to adhesion of neutrophils to endothelial cells, respectively (201). IL-1RA levels peaked 4 hours after bypass, and sICAM peaked 24 hours after bypass. All three were higher in a normothermic versus a hypothermic CPB group. Other investigators have not been able to demonstrate significant differences in cytokine production between hypothermic and normothermic CPB (202,203). Normothermic CPB has also been documented to induce a fast increase in CD11b/18 expression, similar to hypothermic CPB (204). Neutrophil sequestration by the lung during pulmonary reperfusion may maintain and perseverate CD11b/18 expression. Release of IL-8 by neutrophils could lead to positive feedback inducing further neutrophil recruitment and endothelial injury (205,206).

The role of cytokines in cardiac surgery has been extensively reviewed by a number of authors (189,190,206,207). The proinflammatory cytokines (IL-1β, IL-6, IL-8, and TNF-α) increase within 10 minutes after induction of anesthesia with high-dose fentanyl and continues until initiation of CPB (190). This proinflammatory response is subject to tight physiologic control, as within 2 hours after initiation of CPB, there is increased release of antiinflammatory cytokines such as IL-10, TNF-1SR and TNF-2SR (soluble receptor), and IL-1RA (receptor antagonist), which persist in the immediate postoperative period. Such increases in antiinflammatory cytokines do not occur during *in vitro* CPB, suggesting this is an *in vivo* physiologic response (190). Ischemia reperfusion injury may play a major role in cytokine balance. Wan et al. have noted that the levels of proinflammatory cytokines such as TNF-α, IL-6, and IL-8 correlate with the duration of cardiac ischemia and hypothesize that ischemic myocardium may be the major source of these three cytokines, whereas IL-10 levels correlate with the duration of CPB and seem to be primarily derived from liver (208–210).

A number of interventions have been shown to influence cytokine production, including high-dose aprotinin (211, 212), use of heparin-coated CPB circuits (213,214), normothermic cardioplegia (215), pulsatile perfusion (216), leukocyte filtration (217,218), administration of methylprednisolone (219,220), milrinone (221), ketamine (222), TNF-SR (223), and sodium nitroprusside (224). Whether any of these interventions results in lower end-organ morbidity rates, however, is currently unclear.

Kallikrein, Bradykinin, and Serine Protease Inhibitors

Activation of kallikrein and complement also occur during routine CPB (225). Kallikrein plays a seminal role in the incitement and amplification of the inflammatory response (Fig. 14-9). The foreign surface of the CPB circuit activates trace amounts of bound factor XII that in the presence of prekallikrein and surface-bound high-molecular-weight kininogen result in kallikrein production. Kallikrein greatly accelerates factor XII activation, and a positive feedback loop thus amplifies the intrinsic coagulation cascade. The potent action of kallikrein to liberate bradykinin from high-molecular-weight kininogen is an important reaction in relation to the whole-body inflammatory response to CPB. Bradykinin enhances vascular permeability, produces hypotension, contracts smooth muscle, causes pain, and releases tissue-type plasminogen activator. Increases in vascular permeability can result in both diffuse and specific organ edema. Kallikrein also converts plasminogen to plasmin, activates the complement system, liberates renin from prorennin, and primes neutrophils for chemotactic activity. Activation of both the kallikrein-kinin system and the complement cascade has been shown in patients undergoing cardiac surgery with CPB (225).

Many of the various inflammatory cascades in the body are enzyme-mediated, involving serine proteases. Serine protease inhibitors have specificity for enzymes with trypsin-like tertiary structures in the vicinity of the active site and are thus capable of competitive inhibition of certain enzymes within various inflammatory cascades, in a concentration-dependent manner. The dissociation constant (K*d*) is a measure of the affinity of the inhibitor for a specific enzyme, wherein the lower the K*d*, the greater the degree of inhibition. In clinically relevant concentrations, the nonspecific serine antiprotease, aprotinin, has a low K*d*, and thus significant inhibitory activity against factors XIIa, IXa, leukocyte elastase and protease, trypsin, kallikrein, and other enzymes while not influencing the enzymatic activity of other proteases including angiotensin converting enzyme, lysozyme, and liver esterases (226).

Because kallikrein plays a seminal role in the incitement and amplification of the inflammatory response and is intimately linked to bradykinin activation (227), kallikrein inactivation by aprotinin may ameliorate some of the inflammatory consequences of CPB. In a study of patients undergoing CPB, low-dose aprotinin administration was found to have a similar antiinflammatory effect to methylprednisolone in blunting release of systemic TNF-α and neutrophil integrins CD11b/18 up-regulation in comparison to untreated controls (228). Additionally, in patients after major vascular surgery, activation of neutrophils, mani-

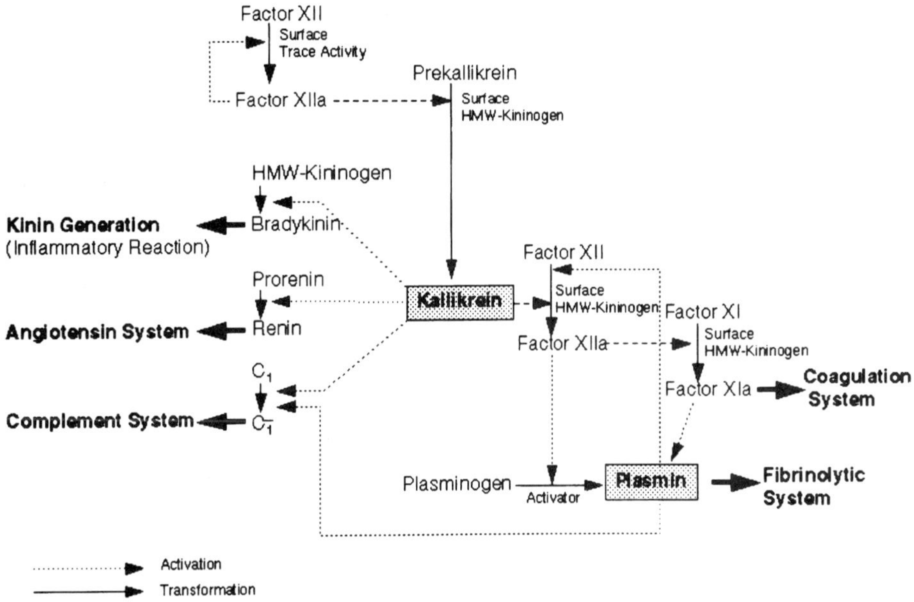

FIGURE 14-9. Role of kallikrein and plasmin as mediators in the coagulation, fibrinolytic, kinin, angiotensin, and complement systems. (From Verstraete M. Clinical application of inhibitors of fibrinolysis. *Drugs* 1985;29:236, with permission.)

festing as increased superoxide production and impaired chemotaxis, has been shown to be significantly suppressed by aprotinin administration (229). In CPB patients, aprotinin has also been shown to suppress the rise of the inflammatory mediator and leukocyte activator IL-6 during CPB in comparison to a control group (230).

It has been demonstrated that cerebral edema is an accompaniment of routine cardiac surgery with both hypothermic and normothermic CPB in adults (231,232). Bradykinin has been shown to be intimately linked to cerebral edema formation and in an animal model was accompanied by progressive loss of adenosine triphosphate and a corresponding rise in lactate. In this ischemic brain model, aprotinin administration was found to significantly decrease the extent of cerebral edema formation and to result in lower lactate and greater adenosine triphosphate preservation than control animals (233). Subsequently, Aoki and colleagues examined the use of aprotinin in hypothermic circulatory arrest in a piglet model undergoing 60 minutes of hypothermic circulatory arrest at 15°C (234). Aprotinin was shown to enhance recovery of cerebral adenosine triphosphate and pH and demonstrated better preservation of endothelium-mediated vasoreactivity. In other ischemic models including heart preservation, aprotinin treatment was shown to be highly effective in suppressing lysosomal enzyme release and maintaining myocardial adenosine diphosphate and adenosine monophosphate levels (235). In a multicenter clinical trial in patients receiving a second CAB surgery, Levy et al. confirmed the efficacy of aprotinin therapy to decrease blood loss and transfusion requirements and demonstrated a significant reduction in the incidence of stroke in the aprotinin group (236). This data suggest that some of the antiinflammatory properties of aprotinin, particularly its inhibition of bradykinin, may be of clinical significance in decreasing central nervous system sequelae of CPB. A related compound, nafamostat mesilate, a synthetic antiprotease with a similar pharmacologic profile to that of aprotinin, has been shown in a rabbit model of head injury to significantly decrease cerebral vasospasm after subarachnoid hemorrhage (237). In a clinical trial of patients presenting with subarachnoid hemorrhage, lower incidences of cerebral vasospasm and better clinical outcomes were seen in those treated with nafamostat in comparison to those receiving historical controls (238).

Brain

In one of the largest prospective surveys of postoperative central nervous system sequelae after CAB surgery to date, Roach and colleagues reported outcomes from 2,108 CAB patients from 24 U.S. cardiac centers in 1996 (239). They found that adverse cerebral outcomes occurred in 129 patients (6.1%), of which half (66 patients) were characterized as type I outcomes including 55 nonfatal strokes, 8 cerebral deaths, and 3 instances of stupor or transient ischemic attacks. Type II outcomes including deterioration of intellectual function or seizures occurred in 63 patients. Patients with such adverse neurologic events also had a ten-fold (21% versus 2%) increase in mortality rate, as opposed to those without a neurologic event. Additionally, these patients required prolonged hospitalization (25 days versus 10 days) and a significantly higher transfer rate to chronic care facilities (47% versus 8%). These authors concluded that adverse cerebral outcomes after CAB surgery are relatively common and serious and are associated with substantial increases in mortality rate, length of hospitalization, and use of intermediate and chronic care facilities.

It is apparent that the incidence of neuropsychologic dysfunction after CPB is much greater than had been formerly been appreciated. Prospective studies by Shaw et al. (240, 241), as well as by Carella et al. (242), Murkin et al. (243), and Smith et al. (244), have demonstrated incidences of postoperative neuropsychological dysfunction ranging from 48% to more than 60%. When compared to control groups undergoing major surgery without CPB, the incidence of neuropsychologic dysfunction was significantly greater in patients in whom CPB was employed (243,244). Although the etiology of this dysfunction is unclear, it is becoming increasingly apparent the cerebral microemboli and macroemboli are occurring in most patients undergoing CPB (245). Although open chamber procedures are considered to be associated with a greater number of macroparticulate emboli delivered into the cerebral circulation (246), contradictory observations have been made regarding the relative impact of the duration of CPB versus open chamber valvular surgery, or closed chamber CAB operations, on the incidence of postoperative neurologic dysfunction and stroke (247). It has now been demonstrated that insufflation of carbon dioxide into the surgical field during valvular operations can significantly decrease the amount of residual air, as assessed by TEE when compared with conventional deairing techniques (248). Whether this influences central nervous system outcomes, however, has not yet been rigorously assessed.

Lipid microembolization during CPB is common and can be detected in the brain as lipid deposits producing small capillary and arterial dilations distributed diffusely throughout the cerebral microvasculature roughly in proportion to regional CBF (Fig. 14-10) (249). Brooker et al. have documented that use of cardiotomy suction to scavenge and return shed blood to the venous reservoir is associated with increased numbers of histologically detected cerebral emboli (250). Reduced small capillary and arterial dilation density has been observed in animals after use of cell saver to wash salvaged blood before return during CPB. Similarly, Stump et al. have noted reduced numbers of lipid microemboli when the quantity of blood returned via cardiotomy sucker was reduced via administration of the antiprotease aprotinin (251).

Others have demonstrated that arterial line filters, with the attendant reduction in cerebral microemboli, were associated with significant improvements in performance on postoperative neuropsychometric testing (252). Blauth et al. have demonstrated the relationship between usage of different oxygenator types, arterial line filtration, and reductions in retinal microemboli (253) while Padayachee et al. have used transcranial Doppler techniques to demonstrate a similar reduction in delivery of emboli into the middle cerebral artery (254). As demonstrated by Moody and colleagues in postmortem histologic specimens, instrumentation of the ascending aorta is associated with cerebral capillary inclusions that may represent gaseous or fat emboli generated during aortic instrumentation (248).

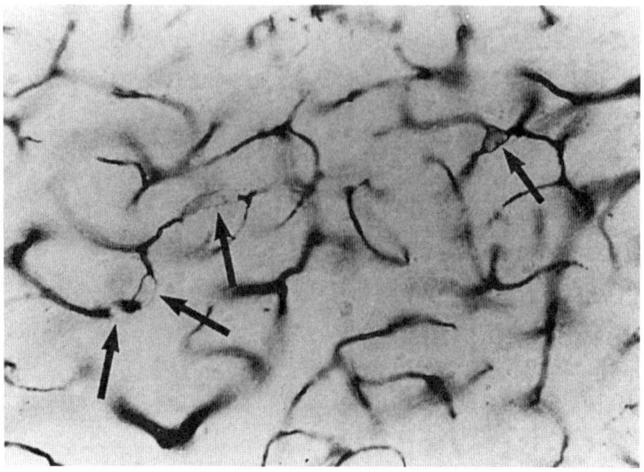

FIGURE 14-10. Microemboli (or small capillary and arteriolar dilations (SCADs) in arterioles of human brain 1 day after cardiopulmonary bypass. The afferent microvessels are black. The SCADs are dilated clear areas (*arrows*): The largest one here measures 25 μm in diameter. It is believed these represent the "footprints" of emboli that were almost completely removed by the reagents employed in this histochemical staining method. (Alkaline phosphatase-stained 100-μm thick celloidin section; ×300 before 50% reduction.) (From Moody DM, Bell A, Phil D, et al. Brain microemboli during cardiac surgery or aortography. *Ann Neurol* 1990; 28:477, with permission.)

It has been demonstrated that pH management can markedly influence neuropsychologic outcome after prolonged CPB (more than 90 minutes). In 316 patients undergoing CAB surgery and randomized to either alpha-stat or pH-stat management, Murkin and colleagues were able to show significantly lower incidences of neuropsychologic dysfunction 2 months postoperatively in patients managed with alpha-stat in whom CPB durations exceeded 90 minutes, in comparison with those in whom pH-stat management was employed (27% versus 44%) (Fig. 14-11) (243). Thus, it appears that despite impressive decreases in generation of cerebral emboli with membrane oxygenators and the inclusion of arterial line filters, prolonged exposure to CPB (more than 90 minutes) results in a "threshold" effect, after which the benefits of proportional decreases in CBF (and thus cerebral emboli) produced by alpha-stat become manifest and result in decreased neuropsychologic impairment. Similar results favoring alpha-stat were also demonstrated by Patel et al., in their study of 250 CAB patients (65).

Future efforts aimed at decreasing the neurologic morbidity associated with CPB may involve different cannulation strategies (e.g., femoral artery or carotid compression during aortic cannulation), usage of epiaortic scanning before surgical instrumentation to detect otherwise unrecognized aortic atherosclerosis, routine employment of micro-

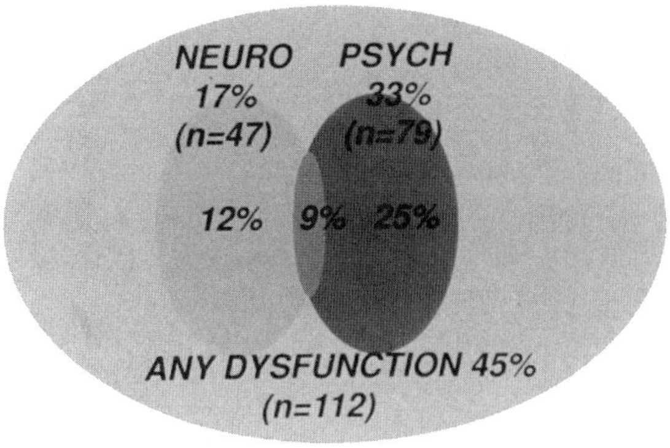

FIGURE 14-11. Assessment of cognitive dysfunction at 2 months after coronary bypass surgery in 249 patients, where *Neuro* indicates patients with a significant decrease in neurologic score, *Psych* indicates patients having a significant decrease in cognitive test scores, and *Any Dysfunction* refers to patients having significant decreases in either Neuro or Psych scores. (From Murkin JM, Martzke JS, Buchan AM, et al. A randomized study of the influence of perfusion technique and pH management strategy in 316 patients undergoing coronary artery bypass surgery. *J Thorac Cardiovasc Surg* 1995;110:349, with permission.)

pore arterial line filters, routine intraoperative monitoring using Doppler-based emboli detectors over carotid or middle carotid artery, or administration of pharmacologic/anesthetic regimens designed to be either primarily cerebroprotective (255) or indirectly cerebroprotective by decreasing CBF by reducing the cerebral metabolic rate of O_2 (thus decreasing the proportion of emboli delivered into the cerebral circulation, though this latter approach has only been shown as successful in one of three clinical trials to date) (148–150).

Lungs

Alterations in pulmonary function after CPB can result from changes in chest wall mechanics (256), hypothermia-induced phrenic nerve dysfunction (257,258), increases in extravascular lung water,(76) differing perfusion characteristics during CPB (259,260), mode of pulmonary ventilation and oxygenation during CPB (261,262), and selection of oxygenator type (263). Macherini et al. have documented elimination of diaphragmatic paralysis with warm CPB and attribute previous instances of phrenic nerve dysfunction to the effect of hypothermia and topical cooling (264).

The influence of CPB on pulmonary gas exchange was examined by Rea et al., who demonstrated that with use of a bubble oxygenator, functional residual capacity and tidal volume decreased between 15% and 25% at 48 hours postoperatively while venous admixture increased by 50%, although in inverse proportion to the magnitude of the preoperative value (265). Byrick et al. reported that pulmonary vascular resistance and extravascular lung water were significantly decreased after use of a membrane as compared to a bubble oxygenator (263). Some of these ultrastructural alterations in lung tissue appear to result from endothelial cell damage as a result of capillary leukocyte deposition (266).

There is some evidence from animal studies that static inflation of lungs using 50% to 100% oxygen at 5 cm H_2O inflation pressure results in better preservation of pulmonary lactate/pyruvate ratio and normal levels of high-energy phosphates (262), as well as less evidence of ultrastructural damage (261), in comparison to passive lung deflation during CPB.

The employment of nonpulsatile perfusion for lung perfusion has been shown to produce thickening of alveolar walls and increases in pulmonary vascular resistance, although pulmonary gas exchange was not affected significantly (259). MAP and body surface area have been found to exert influences that are either directly or inversely related, respectively, to the magnitude of postoperative alveolar-arterial oxygen tension gradients (259). Ostensibly, increased MAP acts to produce increased pulmonary capillary hydrostatic pressure, and patients with smaller body surface areas have relatively greater exposure to inflammatory mediators that are generated during CPB (267), such as complement C3a and C5a (268) and activated neutrophils and leukocytes (269,270). Increased leukocyte elastase during hypothermic or normothermic CPB has been shown to correlate with extent of postoperative intrapulmonary shunt and respiratory index (271).

Liver

Decreased hepatic perfusion has been reported in patients and in animal experiments during CPB. Koizumi et al. studied the effect of normothermic and hypothermic CPB on hepatic arterial blood flow, portal venous blood flow, hepatic oxygen delivery, and hepatic oxygen consumption in beagles (272). They found no change in hepatic blood flow with normothermic CPB with low-dose fentanyl. Large doses of fentanyl (50 μg/kg) and hypothermic CPB were associated with reduced hepatic blood flow, portal venous blood flow, and impaired hepatic delivery of oxygen. Koizumi also noted that the hepatic oxygen consumption was periodically well maintained by spontaneous rises in the oxygen-uptake ratio, despite the decrease in hepatic oxygen delivery (272). Wakiyama et al. noted that increased portal endothelin-1 level is associated with hepatocellular damage resulting in abnormal liver enzymes and serum ammonia after hypothermic CPB in rabbits (273). A high incidence (11.4%) of hyperamylasemia was reported in children after CPB by Torre Rodriguez et al., noting that episodes of shock and systemic ischemia appeared to be etiologic in its pathogenesis (274).

Gut

It is apparent that in a low but still significant number of patients, postoperative GI tract morbidity is a significant complication. In a review of 4,473 patients undergoing cardiac surgery with CPB, an overall incidence of GI complications of 0.78% was recorded (275). Such complications included GI bleeding (45%), intestinal infarction (37%), and acute pancreatitis (18%). Associated mortality rate was high, with 63% of such patients dying. These deaths accounted for 11.5% of overall mortality rates in this series. Data from this study indicated the relative risk of GI complications to be 1:249 when the heart was not opened versus 1:66 when it was. This rose to an astonishingly high 1:5 after cardiac transplantation. The authors concluded that acute surgical intervention for GI complications was potentially lifesaving, whereas inappropriate conservative therapy was poorly tolerated (275).

In another series of 6,452 patients undergoing CPB, an incidence of GI tract complications of 0.94% was noted (276). GI bleeding, ischemic bowel, pancreatitis, and bowel obstruction were again the most common entities, and they resulted in a 59% mortality rate. Advanced age, valvular surgery, and prolonged pump time were significant risk factors for GI morbidity. In a series of 1,686 patients, another group reported an incidence of GI complications of 1.6% associated with use of CPB, in whom an overall mortality rate of 36% occurred (277). Prolonged CPB and valvular surgery were again significantly correlated with abdominal complication rates.

Initiation of CPB results in a moderate increase in intestinal microvascular permeability to protein and an increase in intestinal tissue water. The increase in tissue water is not due to increased capillary pressure (278). Haisjackl et al. measured hepatic (splanchnic) blood flow, splanchnic oxygen transport and consumption, splanchnic lactate uptake, and gastric mucosal pH in adults during normothermic nonpulsatile CPB (279). They concluded that normothermic CPB is not associated with deterioration in global intestinal oxygen delivery and attributed the increase in plasma lactate, decreased gastric mucosal pH, and increased extraction of indocyanine green to the systemic inflammatory response to CPB.

Mrozek et al. have used continuous gastric tonometry to evaluate splanchnic perfusion (280). The critical period was 4 to 12 hours after CPB when cardiac output decreases while the oxygen consumption increases, resulting in anaerobic metabolism and accumulation of lactate. It is during this period that they noted the lowest (although noncritical) gastric mucosal pH. O'Dwyer et al. compared the effects of increasing pump flow to infusion of phenylephrine to restore aortic pressure on visceral organ, brain, and muscle perfusion during CPB in swine (281). Infusion of phenylephrine significantly reduced splanchnic blood flow, thus suggesting it may exacerbate ongoing hypoperfusion of splanchnic organs, despite restoration of perfusion pressure. Given the almost ubiquitous administration of phenylephrine during CPB, the clinical significance of this observation is currently unclear.

Using laser Doppler flow measurements and gastric tonometry, Ohri et al. found that nonpulsatile CPB resulted in a 60% reduction in gastric mucosal blood flow, which persisted during CPB and for 4 hours into recovery (202). They noted gastric hyperemia on termination of CPB in all groups. Gastric hypoperfusion and related GI tract disturbances may have clinical implications, particularly during "fast-track" management of patients after CPB.

These studies demonstrate a low but relatively constant incidence of GI complications related to CPB and show that advancing age, prolonged CPB, open chamber procedures, and immunosuppressive therapies all contribute to the risk of GI complications. The implications of the detection of circulating endotoxin, whether as an indicator of an alteration in GI mucosal integrity or as an epiphenomenon resulting from a manufacturing artifact, remain unclear.

Renal

As with GI complications, the incidence of renal failure after CPB remains a low but clinically significant factor influencing morbidity and overall outcome. In a review of 1,686 patients undergoing CPB-related procedures, the incidence of acute renal failure was 0.9% (282). Valvular surgery, CPB duration, and development of postoperative infection were main factors contributing to acute renal failure.

In high-risk children undergoing cardiac surgical procedures, a much higher incidence of acute renal failure (9% of 156 patients) has been reported and resulted in an overall mortality rate of 58% in one series (283). Another survey of 441 pediatric cardiac patients reported a 4% incidence of acute renal failure, which was associated with a 72% mortality rate (284). In most of the cases reported in both studies, acute renal failure was either present preoperatively or subsequently developed as a component of multisystem failure.

In a study of 775 adults undergoing CPB, Zanardo et al. noted that postoperative renal dysfunction (creatinine level of 1.5 to 2.5 mg/dL) occurred in 11.4% of patients (285). Renal failure (creatinine level of more than 2.5 mg/dL) occurred in 3.7%. Both were found to be independent predictors of mortality (9.5% with renal dysfunction and 44.4% with acute renal failure). Use of intraaortic balloon pump, deep hypothermic circulatory arrest, low output syndrome, advanced age, emergency surgery, and low urine output during CPB were all independent risk factors for postoperative renal failure, although exposure to CPB *per se* appeared to be a relatively less important risk. In a retrospective study examining post-CPB renal failure in 2,262 children, Picca et al. noted the incidence of acute renal failure to be 2.7% (286). High inotropic use, systemic hypotension, and elevated central venous pressure were shown to be risk factors.

In a prospective, observational, multicenter study of 2,222 patients, Mangano et al. noted an incidence of postoperative renal dysfunction of 7.7%, with 1.4% of patients having oliguric renal failure requiring dialysis (95). Patients with renal failure or dysfunction had higher in-hospital mortality rates (63% and 19% versus 0.9%), a more prolonged stay in the intensive care unit (14.9 days and 6.5 days versus 3.1 days), and a more prolonged hospital stay overall (28.8 days and 18.2 days versus 10.6 days), compared to patients who had neither form of renal complication. CPB lasting 3 or more hours was an independent risk factor for development of renal dysfunction.

A number of pharmacologic interventions have been studied for potential efficacy in reducing the incidence of postoperative renal dysfunction. In a study of 142 children undergoing CPB, no superiority of prophylactic administration of low-dose dopamine versus dobutamine could be determined with regard to urine output, creatinine levels, or diuretic requirement (287). Unfortunately, whether either agent was beneficial was not adequately addressed. In a small study of 17 CAB patients with renal impairment, Lema et al. compared low-dose dopamine infusion versus elevation of perfusion pressure with phenylephrine for effects on intraoperative and postoperative renal function (288). They found clinically relevant differences showing an apparent effect of dopamine to decrease renal vasoconstriction, but only during surgery before CPB.

In a randomized, prospective study of 40 pediatric patients undergoing CPB, prophylactic mannitol 0.5 $g \cdot kg^{-1}$ was shown to decrease plasma creatinine concentrations and urinary albumin excretion rates, compared with an untreated control group (289). Fisher et al. have similarly noted an improvement in perioperative renal function when mannitol was added to the pump prime, which extended into the perioperative period in adult patients who received higher doses of 20 or 30 g (290).

There is also some indication of efficacy for the intraoperative administration of calcium channel antagonists during CPB. Continuous infusion of diltiazem at 2 $\mu g/kg/$ minute during surgery has been shown to prevent decreases in glomerular function secondary to CPB (291). Others have documented similar benefits with infusions of felodipine and nifedipine (292,293). Improved renal function has also been seen after CPB following use of prostaglandin E_1 (294) and infusion of human atrial natriuretic peptide (295).

Significant reductions in renal cortical blood flow occur during nonpulsatile flow (296). Pulsatile perfusion during CPB has been investigated both in animals and in patients to determine whether any potential benefits are demonstrable with respect to postoperative renal function. In dogs, some potential benefits of pulsatile perfusion were apparent at flow rates of 80 and 100 $mL \cdot kg^{-1} \cdot minute^{-1}$, but at higher or lower rates, no difference was apparent in terms of hemodynamics, renal circulation, or renal metabolism (297). Badner et al. were unable to demonstrate any beneficial effect of pulsatile perfusion and differing pH management during CPB on postoperative renal function in a group of 156 patients with normal preoperative renal function (126). In 12 patients with impaired renal function, defined as creatinine clearance below 30 $mL. \cdot minute^{-1}$, serum creatinine and creatinine clearance were better preserved at 7 days in a group in whom pulsatile perfusion was employed, in contrast to a nonpulsatile perfusion group (298). Perfusion pressure rather than pump flow has been shown to correlate with urinary output during CPB (299) while no influence of perfusion temperatures between hypothermic or normothermic CPB has been shown (300).

Increased renal glucose reabsorption during CPB, with resultant greatly increased blood levels, may play a major role in the hyperglycemia seen during normothermic CPB. Without careful management during CPB, serum glucose concentrations will often become elevated far above the normal range, even in nondiabetic patients. Surprisingly small amounts of intraoperative glucose, on the order of 100 g (about 2 L dextrose)—particularly if administered during CPB—have been shown to produce significant hyperglycemia with average peak serum glucose values in the range of 31 mmol/L (438 mg/dL) (301). This effect is multifactorial and reflects acute glucose intolerance in the form of insulin suppression, stress hormone–induced gluconeogenesis, and impaired glucose excretion as a consequence of enhanced renal tubular resorption (301,302).

REFERENCES

1. Gibbon JH. Application of a mechanical heart and lung apparatus to cardiac surgery. *Minn Med* 1954;37:171.
2. Cameron DE, Reitz BA, Carson BS, et al. Separation of craniopagus Siamese twins using cardiopulmonary bypass and hypothermic circulatory arrest. *J Thorac Cardiovasc Surg* 1989;98: 961.
3. Lincoff AM, Popma JJ, Ellis SG, et al. Percutaneous support devices for high risk or complicated coronary angioplasty. *J Am Coll Cardiol* 1991;17:770.
4. Field J, Shearman FA, Martin AW. Effect of temperature on oxygen consumption of brain tissue. *J Neurophysiol* 1944;7:117.

4a. Long WB, Rosenblum S, Grady IP. Successful resuscitation of bupivacaine-induced cardiac arrest using cardiopulmonary bypass. *Anesth Analg* 1989;69:403.

5. Aavramides EJ, Murkin JM. The effect of surgical dislocation of the heart on cerebral blood flow in the presence of a single, two-stage venous cannula during cardiopulmonary bypass. *Can J Anesth* 1996;43:A36.
6. McCusker K, Hoffman D, Maldarelli W, et al. High flow femoro-femoral bypass utilizing small cannulae and a centrifugal pump on the venous side. *Perfusion* 1992;7:295.
7. Toomasian JM, McCarthy JP. Total extrathoracic cardiopulmonary support with kinetic assisted venous drainage: experience in 50 patients. *Perfusion* 1998;13:137.
8. Zlotnick AY, Gilfeather MS, Adams DH, et al. Innominate vein cannulation for venous drainage in minimally invasive aortic valve replacement. *Ann Thorac Surg* 1999;67:864.
9. Wilcox TW, Mitchell SJ, Gorman DF. Entrained venous air during cardiopulmonary bypass: a source of arterial emboli exacerbated by vacuum assisted venous drainage. *Ann Thorac Surg* 1999;68:1459.

10. Mitchell SJ, Willcox T, Gorman DF. Bubble generation and venous air filtration by hardshell venous reservoirs: a comparative study. *Perfusion* 1997;12:325.
11. Mitchell SJ, Willcox T, McDougal C, et al. Emboli generation by the Medtronic Maxima hard-shell adult venous reservoir in cardiopulmonary bypass circuits: a preliminary report. *Perfusion* 1996;11:145.
12. Pearson DT, Holden MP, Poslad SJ, et al. A clinical evaluation of the performance characteristics of one membrane and five bubble oxygenators: gas transfer and gaseous microemboli production. *Perfusion* 1986;1:15.
13. Taylor RL, Borger MA, Weisel RD, et al. Cerebral microemboli during cardiopulmonary bypass: increased emboli during perfusionist interventions. *Ann Thorac Surg* 1999;68:89.
14. Taketani S, Sawa Y, Masai T, et al. A novel technique for cardiopulmonary bypass using vacuum system for venous drainage with pressure relief valve: an experimental study. *Artif Organs* 1998,22:337.
15. Ross WT, Lake CL, Wellons HA. Cardiopulmonary bypass complicated by inadvertent carotid cannulation. *Anaesthesiology* 1981;54:85.
16. Watson BG. Unilateral cold neck. A new sign of misplacement of the aortic cannula during cardiopulmonary bypass. *Anaesthesia* 1983;38:659.
17. Hartman GS, Yao FSF, Bruefach M III, et al. Severity of aortic atheromatous disease diagnosed by transesophageal echocardiography predicts stroke and other outcomes associated with coronary artery surgery: a prospective study. *Anesth Analg* 1996; 83:701.
18. Tuman KJ, McCarthy RJ, Najafi H, et al. Differential effects of advanced age on neurologic and cardiac risks of coronary artery operations. *J Thorac Cardiovasc Surg* 1992;104:1510.
19. Blauth CI, Cosgrove DM, Webb BW, et al. Atheroembolism from the ascending aorta. *J Thorac Cardiovasc Surg* 1992;103: 1104.
20. Davila-Roman VG, Barzilai B, Wareing TH, et al. Atherosclerosis of the ascending aorta. *Stroke* 1994;25:2010.
21. Tobler HG, Edwards JE. Frequency and location of atherosclerotic plaques in the ascending aorta. *J Thorac Cardiovasc Surg* 1988;96:304.
22. Stump DA, Tegeler CH, Newman SP, et al. Older patients have more emboli during coronary artery bypass graft surgery. *Anesthesiology* 1992;77:A52.
23. Culliford AT, Colvin SB, Rohrer K, et al. The atherosclerotic ascending aorta and transverse arch: a new technique to prevent cerebral injury during bypass: experience with 13 patients. *Ann Thorac Surg* 1986:41:27.
24. Marschall K, Kanchuger M, Kessler K, et al. Superiority of transesophageal echocardiography in detecting aortic arch atheromatous disease: identification of patients at increased risk of stroke during cardiac surgery. *J Cardiothorac Vasc Anesth* 1994; 8:5.
25. Hosoda Y, Watanabe M, Hirooka Y, et al. Significance of atherosclerotic changes of the ascending aorta during coronary bypass surgery with intraoperative detection by echocardiography. *J Cardiovasc Surg* 1991;32:301.
26. Hogue CW Jr, Barzilai B, Davila-Roman VG. Stroke reduction: diagnosis and management of the atherosclerotic aorta during cardiac surgery. *J Thorac Cardiovasc Anesth* 1999;3:17.
27. Seward JB, Khandheria BK, Tajik J. Wide-field transesophageal echocardiographic tomography: Feasibility Study. *Mayo Clin Proc* 1990;65:31.
28. Konstadt SN, Reich DL, Quintana C, et al. The ascending aorta: how much does transesophageal echocardiography see? *Anesth Analg* 1994;78:240.
29. Sylviris S, Calafiore P, Matalanis G, et al. The intraoperative assessment of ascending aortic atheroma: epiaortic imaging is superior to both transesophageal echocardiography and direct palpation. *J Cardiothorac Vasc Anesth* 1997;11:704.
30. Katz ES, Tunick PA, Rusinek H, et al. Protroding aortic atheromas predict stroke in elderly patients undergoing cardiopulmonary bypass: experience with intraoperative transesophageal echocardiography. *J Am Coll Cardiol* 1992;20:70.
31. Menkis AH, St-Amand MA, Murkin JM, et al. Epiaortic scanning can influence surgical management during cardiac surgery. *Ann Thorac Surg* 1997;64:919.
32. Murkin JM, Menkis AH, Downey D, et al. Epiaortic scanning decreases cerebral emboli during aortic cannulation and application of partial occlusion clamp. *Ann Thorac Surg* 1999;68:1461.
33. Wareing TH, Davila-Roman VG, Barzilai B, et al. Management of the severely atherosclerotic ascending aorta during cardiac operations. *J Thorac Cardiovasc Surg* 1992;103:453.
34. Arom KV, Vinas JF, Fewel JE, et al. Is a left ventricular vent necessary during cardiopulmonary bypass? *Ann Thorac Surg* 1977;24:566.
35. Miller DW, Hessel EA, Winterscheid LC, et al. Current practice of coronary artery bypass surgery. *J Thorac Cardiovasc Surg* 1977;73:75.
36. Little AG, Lin CY, Wernly JA, et al. Use of the pulmonary artery for left ventricular venting during cardiac operations. *J Thorac Cardiovasc Surg* 1984;87:532.
37. Milsom FP, Mitchell SJ. A dual-vent left heart deairing technique markedly reduces carotid artery microemboli. *Ann Thorac Surg* 1998;66:785.
38. Shibuya M, Kitamura M, Kurihara H, et al. Significant left ventricular unloading with transaortic catheter venting during venoarterial bypass. *Artif Organs* 1997;21:789.
39. Morishita A, Kitamura M, Shibuya M, et al. Effectiveness of transaortic venting from a failing left ventricle during venoarterial bypass. *ASAIO* 1999;45:69.
40. Nunn JF. Oxygen. In: *Applied respiratory physiology,* 3rd ed. London: Butterworth-Heineman, 1987:375.
41. Swan H. The importance of acid-base management for cardiac and cerebral preservation during open heart operations. *Surg Gynecol Obstet* 1984;158:391.
42. Snyder JV, Carroll GC. Tissue oxygenation: a physiological approach to a clinical problem. *Curr Probl Surg* 1982;19:650.
43. Fiaccadori E, Vezzani A, Coffrini E, et al. Cell metabolism in patients undergoing major valvular heart surgery: relationship with intra and postoperative hemodynamics, oxygen transport, and oxygen utilization patterns. *Crit Care Med* 1989;17:1286.
44. Irish CL, Murkin JM, Cleland A, et al. Neuromuscular blockade significantly decreases systemic oxygen consumption during hypothermic cardiopulmonary bypass. *J Cardiothorac Vasc Anesth* 1991;5:132.
45. Hickey RF, Hoar PF. Whole-body oxygen consumption during low-flow hypothermic cardiopulmonary bypass. *J Thorac Cardiovasc Surg* 1983;86:903.
46. Harris EA, Seelye ER, Squire AW. Oxygen consumption during cardiopulmonary bypass with moderate hypothermia in man. *Br J Anaesth* 1971;43:1113.
47. Kent B, Peirce EC. Oxygen consumption during cardiopulmonary bypass in the uniformly cooled dog. *J Appl Physiol* 37:917, 1974.
48. Willford DC, Moores WY, Ji S, et al. Importance of acid-base strategy in reducing myocardial and whole body oxygen consumption during perfusion hypothermia. *J Thorac Cardiovasc Surg* 1990;100:699.
49. Fox LS, Blackstone EH, Kirklin JW, et al. Relationship of brain blood flow and oxygen consumption to perfusion flow rate dur-

ing profoundly hypothermic cardiopulmonary bypass. *J Thorac Cardiovasc Surg* 1984;87:658.

50. Rebeyka IM, Coles JG, Wilson GJ, et al. The effect of low-flow cardiopulmonary bypass on cerebral function: an experimental and clinical study. *Ann Thorac Surg* 1987;43:391.
51. Govier AV, Reves JG, McKay RD, et al. Factors and their influence on regional cerebral blood flow during nonpulsatile cardiopulmonary bypass. *Ann Thorac Surg* 1984;38:592.
52. Murkin JM, Farrar JK, Cleland CP, et al. The influence of perfusion flow rates on cerebral blood flow and oxygen consumption during hypothermic cardiopulmonary bypass. *Anesthesiology* 1987;67:A9.
53. Schwartz AE, Sandhu AA, Kaplon RJ, et al. Cerebral blood flow is determined by arterial pressure and not cardiopulmonary bypass flow rate. *Ann Thorac Surg* 1995;60:165.
54. Stockard JJ, Bickford RG, Schauble JF. Pressure-dependent cerebral ischemia during cardiopulmonary bypass. *Neurology* 1973;25:521.
55. Ellis RJ, Wisniewski A, Potts R, et al. Reduction of flow rate and arterial pressure at moderate hypothermia does not result in cerebral dysfunction. *J Thorac Cardiovasc Surg* 1980;79:173.
56. Kolkka R, Hilberman M. Neurologic dysfunction following cardiac operation with low-flow, low-pressure cardiopulmonary bypass. *J Thorac Cardiovasc Surg* 1980;79:432.
57. Gold JP, Charlson ME, Williams-Russo P, et al. Improvement of outcomes after coronary artery bypass. A randomized trial comparing intraoperative high versus low mean arterial pressure. *J Thorac Cardiovasc Surg* 1995;110:1302.
58. Paton B, Pearcy WC, Swan H. The importance of the electroencephalogram during cardiac surgery with particular reference to superior vena caval obstruction. *Surg Gynecol Obstet* 1960;111:197.
59. Rogers AT, Prough DS, Roy RC, et al. Cerebrovascular and cerebral metabolic effects of alterations in perfusion flow rate during hypothermic cardiopulmonary bypass in man. *J Thorac Cardiovasc Surg* 1992;103:363.
60. Murkin JM, Farrar JK, Tweed WA, et al. Cerebral autoregulation and flow/metabolism coupling during cardiopulmonary bypass: the influence of $Paco_2$. *Anesth Analg* 1987;66:825.
61. Newman MF, Croughwell ND, Blumenthal JA, et al. Effect of aging on cerebral autoregulation during cardiopulmonary bypass. Association with postoperative cognitive dysfunction. *Circulation* 1994;90(5, Part 2):II243.
62. Newman MF, Kramer D, Croughwell ND, et al. Differential effects of mean arterial pressure and rewarming on cognitive dysfunction after cardiac surgery. *Anesth Analg* 1995;81:236.
63. Henriksen L, Hjelms E, Lindeburgh T. Brain hyperperfusion during cardiac operations. *J Thorac Cardiovasc Surg* 1983;86:202.
64. Prough DS, Stump DA, Roy RC, et al. Response of cerebral blood flow to changes in carbon dioxide tension during hypothermic cardiopulmonary bypass. *Anesth Analg* 1986;64:576.
65. Patel RL, Turtle MR, Chambers DJ, et al. Alpha-stat acid-base regulation during cardiopulmonary bypass improves neuropsychologic outcome in patients undergoing coronary artery bypass grafting. *J Thorac Cardiovasc Surg* 1996;111:1267.
66. Brusino FG, Reves JG, Prough DS, et al. Cerebral blood flow during cardiopulmonary bypass in a patient with occlusive cerebrovascular disease. *J Cardiothorac Anesth* 1989;3:87.
67. Croughwell N, Lyth M, Quill T, et al. Diabetic patients have abnormal cerebral autoregulation during cardiopulmonary bypass. *Circulation* 1990;82:IV407.
68. Lanier WL. Glucose management during cardiopulmonary bypass: cardiovascular and neurologic implications. *Anesth Analg* 1991;72:423.
69. Cook DJ, Oliver WC Jr, Orszulak TA, et al. Cardiopulmonary bypass temperature, hematocrit, and cerebral oxygen delivery in humans. *Ann Thorac Surg* 1995;60:1671.
70. Philipott JM, Eskew TD, Sun YS, et al. A paradox of cerebral hyperperfusion in the face of cerebral hypotension: the effect of perfusion pressure on cerebral blood flow and metabolism during normothermic cardiopulmonary bypass. *J Surg Res* 1998;77:141.
71. Gadboys HL, Slonim R, Litwak RS. Homologous blood syndrome. *Ann Surg* 1962;156:793.
72. Zuhdi N, McCollough B, Carey J, et al. Double-helical reservoir heart-lung machine. *Arch Surg* 1961;82:166.
73. De Wall RA, Lillehei RC, Sellers RD. Haemodilution perfusions for open heart surgery. *N Engl J Med* 1962;266:1078.
74. Cook DJ, Orszulak TA, Daly RC, et al. Minimum hematocrit for normothermic cardiopulmonary bypass in dogs. *Circulation* 1997;96[Suppl 9]:II200.
75. Liam BL, Plochl W, Cook DJ, et al. Hemodilution and whole body oxygen balance during normothermic cardiopulmonary bypass in dogs. *J Thorac Cardiovasc Surg* 1998;115:1203.
76. Byrick RJ, Kay JC, Noble WH. Extravascular lung water accumulation in patients following coronary artery surgery. *Can Anaesth Soc J* 1977;24:332.
77. Hollowell P, Bland JH, Dalton BC, et al. The effect of hemodilution with albumin or Ringer's lactate on water balance and blood use in open-heart surgery. *Ann Thorac Surg* 1978;25:22.
78. Utley JR, Wachtel C, Cain RB, et al. Effects of hypothermia, hemodilution, and pump oxygenation on organ water content, blood flow and oxygen delivery, and renal function. *Ann Thorac Surg* 1981;31:121.
79. McKnight CK, Elliott MJ, Pearson DT, et al. The effects of four different crystalloid bypass pump-priming fluids upon the metabolic response to cardiac operation. *J Thorac Cardiovasc Surg* 1985;90:97.
80. Boldt J, Kling D, Weidler B, et al. Acute preoperative hemodilution in cardiac surgery: volume replacement with a hypertonic saline-hydroxyethyl starch solution. *J Cardiothorac Vasc Anesth* 1991;5:23.
81. Metz S, Keats AS. Benefits of a glucose-containing priming solution for cardiopulmonary bypass. *Anesth Analg* 1991;72:428.
82. Lanier WL. Glucose management during cardiopulmonary bypass: cardiovascular and neurologic implications. *Anesth Analg* 1991;72:423.
83. Sotaniemi KA. Cerebral outcome after extracorporeal circulation. Comparison between prospective and retrospective evaluations. *Arch Neurol* 1983;40:75.
84. Longstreth WT Jr, Inui TS. High blood glucose level on hospital admission and poor neurologic recovery after cardiac arrest. *Ann Neurol* 1984;15:59.
85. Pulsinelli WA, Waldman S, Rawlinson D, et al. Moderate hyperglycemia augments ischemic brain damage: a neuropathologic study in the rat. *Neurology* 1982;32:1239.
86. Woo E, Chan YW, Yu Yl, et al. Admission glucose level in relation to mortality and morbidity outcome in 252 stroke patients. *Stroke* 1988;19:185.
87. Li PA, Siesjo BK. Role of hyperglycaemia-related acidosis in ischaemic brain damage. *Acta Physiol Scand* 1997;161:567.
88. Davies MG, Hagen PO. Alterations in venous endothelial cell and smooth muscle cell relaxation induced by high glucose concentrations can be prevented by aminoguanidine. *J Surg Res* 1996;63:474.
89. Kawai N, Stummer W, Ennis SR, et al. Blood-brain barrier glutamine transport during normoglycemic and hyperglycemic focal cerebral ischemia. *J Cereb Blood Flow Metab* 1999;19:79.

90. Broderick JP, Hagen T, Brott T, et al. Hyperglycemia and hemorrhagic transformation of cerebral infarcts. *Stroke* 1995;26: 484.
91. Niwa M, Hara A, Iwai T, et al. Prevention of ischemia-induced hippocampal neuronal damage by 2-deoxy-D-glucose in gerbils. *Life Sci* 1999;64:PL193.
92. Griffin S, Klinger L, Newman S, et al. The effect of substrate load and blood glucose management on cerebral dysfunction following cardiopulmonary bypass. *Vasc Surg* 1992;21:656.
93. Rassias AJ, Marrin CAS, Arruda J, et al. Insulin infusion improves neutrophil function in diabetic cardiac surgery patients. *Anesth Analg* 1999;88:1011.
94. Furnary AP, Zerr KJ, Grunkemeier GL, et al. Continuous intravenous insulin infusion reduces the incidence of deep sternal wound infection in diabetic patients after cardiac surgical procedures. *Ann Thorac Surg* 1999;67:352.
95. Mangano CM, Diamondstone LS, Ramsay JG, et al. Renal dysfunction after myocardial revascularization: risk factors, adverse outcomes, and hospital resource utilization. *Ann Intern Med* 1998;128:194.
96. Rady MY, Ryan T, Starr NJ. Perioperative determinants of morbidity and mortality in elderly patients undergoing cardiac surgery. *Crit Care Med* 1998;26:225.
97. Murkin JM. Intraoperative tight glucose control improves outcome in cardiovascular surgery—pro. *J Cardiothorac Vasc Anesth* 2000;14:475.
98. Bashein G, Greydanus WK, Kenny MA. Evaluation of a blood gas and chemistry monitor for use during surgery. *Anesthesiology* 1989;70:123.
99. Hynynen M, Lehtinen AM, Salmenpera M, et al. Continuous infusion of fentanyl or altentanil for coronary artery surgery. Effect on plasma cortisol concentration, beta-endorphin immunoreactivity and arginine vasopressin. *Br J Anaesth* 1986;58: 1260.
100. Grover FL, Fewel JG, Vinas J, et al. Effects of aortic balloon pumping during cardiopulmonary bypass on myocardial perfusion, metabolism, and contractility. *Chest* 1979;75:37.
101. Bregman D, Bailin M, Bowman FO, et al. A pulsatile assist device (PAD) for use during cardiopulmonary bypass. *Ann Thorac Surg* 1977;24:574.
102. Bregman D, Bowman FO, Parodi EN, et al. An improved method of myocardial protection with pulsation during cardiopulmonary bypass. *Circulation* 1977;56:157.
103. Zumbro GL, Shearer G, Fishback ME, et al. A prospective evaluation of the pulsatile assist device. *Ann Thorac Surg* 1979; 28:269.
104. Kaplitt MJ, Tamari Y, Frantz SL, et al. Clinical experience with tamari-kaplitt pulsator. *NY State J Med* 1978;78:1090.
105. Wise EA, Mandl JP, Zaayer WE. Gaseous emboli generation by a pulsatile assist device. *J Extracorp Tech* 1978;10:93.
106. Jacobs LA, Klopp EH, Seamore W, et al. Improved organ function during cardiac bypass with a roller pump modified to deliver pulsatile flow. *J Thorac Cardiovasc Surg* 1969;58:703.
107. Taylor KM, Bain WH, Maxted KJ, et al. Comparative studies of pulsatile and nonpulsatile flow during cardiopulmonary bypass. *J Thorac Cardiovasc Surg* 1978;75:569.
108. Murkin JM, Martzke JS, Buchan AM, et al. A randomized study of perfusion technique and pH management strategy in 316 patients undergoing coronary artery bypass surgery: I. Mortality and cardiovascular morbidity. *J Thorac Cardiovasc Surg* 1995; 110:340.
109. Taylor KM, Bain WH, Davidson KG, et al. Comparative clinical study of pulsatile and nonpulsatile perfusion in 350 consecutive patients. *Thorax* 1982;37:324.
110. Gourlay T, Gibbons M, Taylor KM. Pulsatile flow compatibility of a group on membrane oxygenators. *Perfusion* 1987;2: 115.
111. Hickey PR, Buckley MT, Philbin DM. Pulsatile and nonpulsatile cardiopulmonary bypass: review of a counterproductive controversy. *Ann Thorac Surg* 1983;36:720.
112. Wright G, Furness A. What is pulsatile flow? *Ann Thorac Surg* 1985;39:401.
113. Grossi EA, Baumann FG. Pulsatile flow. *Ann Thorac Surg* 1985; 40:638.
114. Grossi EA, Connolly MW, Krieger KH, et al. Quantification of pulsatile flow during cardiopulmonary bypass to permit direct comparison of the effectiveness of various types of "pulsatile" and "nonpulsatile" flow. *Surgery* 1985;98:547.
115. Gosling RG, King DH, Woodcock JP. Blood-velocity waveforms in the evaluation of atheromatous changes. In: Roberts C, ed. *Blood flow measurement.* Baltimore: Williams & Wilkins, 1972:33.
116. Parsons RJ, McMaster PD. The effect of the pulse upon the formation and flow of lymph. *J Exp Med* 1938;68:353.
117. Nakamura K, Koga Y, Sekiya R, et al. The effects of pulsatile and nonpulsatile cardiopulmonary bypass on renal blood flow and function. *Jpn J Surg* 1989;19:334.
118. Canivet JL, Larbuisson R, Damas P, et al. Plasma renin activity and urine B2-microglobulin during and after cardiopulmonary bypass: pulsatile vs nonpulsatile perfusion. *Eur Heart J* 1990; 11:1079.
119. Kaul TK, Swaminathan R, Chatrath RR, et al. Vasoactive pressure hormones during and after cardiopulmonary bypass. *Int J Artif Organs* 1990;13:292.
120. Minami K, Korner MM, Vyska K, et al. Effects of pulsatile perfusion on plasma catecholamine levels and hemodynamics during and after cardiac operations with cardiopulmonary bypass. *J Thorac Cardiovasc Surg* 1990;99:82.
121. Taylor KM, Bain WH, Russell M, et al. Peripheral vascular resistance and angiotensin II levels during pulsatile and nonpulsatile cardiopulmonary bypass. *Thorax* 1979;34:594.
122. Dunn J, Kirsh MM, Harness J, et al. Hemodynamic, metabolic, and hematologic effects of pulsatile cardiopulmonary bypass. *J Thorac Cardiovasc Surg* 1974;68:138.
123. Williams GD, Seifen AB, Lawson NW, et al. Pulsatile perfusion versus conventional high-flow nonpulsatile perfusion for rapid core cooling and rewarming of infants for circulatory arrest in cardiac operation. *J Thorac Cardiovasc Surg* 1979;78:667.
124. Many M, Soroff HS, Birtwell WC, et al. The physiologic role of pulsatile and nonpulsatile blood flow. *Arch Surg* 1968;97: 917.
125. Boucher JK, Rudy LW, Edmunds LH. Organ blood flow during pulsatile cardiopulmonary bypass. *J Appl Physiol* 1974;36:86.
126. Badner NA, Murkin JM, Lok P. Differences in pH management and pulsatile/nonpulsatile perfusion during CPB do not influence renal function. *Anesth Analg* 1992;75:696.
127. Goodman TA, Gerard DF, Bernstein EF, et al. The effects of pulseless perfusion on the distribution of renal cortical blood flow and on renin release. *Surgery* 1976;80:31.
128. Sink JD, Chitwood WR, Hill RC, et al. Comparison of nonpulsatile and pulsatile extracorporeal circulation on renal cortical blood flow. *Ann Thorac Surg* 1980;29:57.
129. Howie MB, Mortimer W, Rathburn S, et al. Does pulsatile flow maintain liver blood flow during CPR? *Anesthesiology* 1986; 65:A52.
130. Hynynen M, Olkkola KT, Naveri E, et al. Thiopentone pharmacokinetics during cardiopulmonary bypass with a nonpulsatile or pulsatile flow. *Acta Anaesth Scand* 1989;33:554.
131. Creech O, Bresler E, Halley M, et al. Cerebral blood flow during extracorporeal circulation. *Surg Forum* 1957;8:510.

132. Lees MH, Herr RH, Hill JD, et al. Distribution of systemic blood flow of the rhesus monkey during cardiopulmonary bypass. *J Thorac Cardiovasc Surg* 1971;61:570.
133. Matsumoto T, Wolferth CC, Perlman MH. Effects of pulsatile and nonpulsatile perfusion upon cerebral and conjunctival microcirculation. *Am Surg* 1971;37:61.
134. Sanderson JM, Wright G, Sims FW. Brain damage in dogs immediately following pulsatile and nonpulsatile blood flows in extracorporeal circulation. *Thorax* 1972;27:275.
135. Wright G, Sanderson JM. Brain damage and mortality in dogs following pulsatile and nonpulsatile blood flows in extracorporeal circulation. *Thorax* 1972;27:738.
136. Laursen H, Bodker A, Andersen K, et al. Brain oedema and blood-brain barrier permeability in pulsatile and nonpulsatile cardiopulmonary bypass. *Scan J Thorac Cardiovasc Surg* 1986; 20:161.
137. Tranmer BI, Gross CE, Kindt GW, et al. Pulsatile versus nonpulsatile blood flow in the treatment of acute cerebral ischemia. *Neurosurgery* 1986;19:724.
138. Murkin JM, Farrar K. The influence of pulsatile vs nonpulsatile cardiopulmonary bypass on cerebral blood flow and cerebral metabolism. *Anesthesiology* 1989;71:A41.
139. Mori A, Sono J, Nakashima M, et al. Application of pulsatile cardiopulmonary bypass for profound hypothermia in cardiac surgery. *Jpn Circ J* 1981;45:315.
140. Watanabe T, Orita H, Kobayashi M, et al. Brain tissue pH, oxygen tension, and carbon dioxide tension in profoundly hypothermic cardiopulmonary bypass. *J Thorac Cardiovasc Surg* 1989;97:396.
141. Busto R, Dietrich WD, Globus MY, et al. Small differences in intraischemic brain temperature critically determine the extent of ischemic neuronal injury. *J Cereb Blood Flow Metab* 1987; 7:729.
142. Field J, Shearman FA, Martin AW. Effect of temperature on oxygen consumption of brain tissue. *J Neurophysiol* 1944;7:117.
143. Michenfelder JD, Theye RA. Hypothermia: effect of canine brain and whole-body metabolism. *Anesthesiology* 1968;29: 1107.
144. Steen PA, Newberg L, Milde JH, et al. Hypothermia and barbiturates: individual and combined effects on canine cerebral oxygen consumption. *Anesthesiology* 1983;58:527.
145. Michenfelder JD. The hypothermic brain. In: *Anesthesia and the brain.* New York: Churchill Livingstone, 1988:23.
146. Michenfelder JD. A valid demonstration of barbiturate-induced brain protection in man—at last. *Anesthesiology* 1085;64:140.
147. Woodcock TE, Murkin JM, Farrar JK, et al. Pharmacologic EEG suppression during cardiopulmonary bypass: cerebral hemodynamic and metabolic effects of thiopental or isoflurane during hypothermia and normothermia. *Anesthesiology* 1987; 67:218.
148. Nussmeier NA, Arlund C, Slogoff S. Neuropsychiatric complications after cardiopulmonary bypass: cerebral protection by a barbiturate. *Anesthesiology* 1986;64:165.
149. Zaidan JR, Dlochany A, Martin WM, et al. Effect of thiopental on neurologic outcome following coronary artery bypass grafting. *Anesthesiology* 1991;74:406.
150. Roach GW, Newman MF, Murkin JM, et al. Ineffectiveness of burst suppression therapy in mitigating perioperative cerebrovascular dsyfunction. *Anesthesiology* 1999;90:1255.
151. Gordon RJ, Ravin MB. Rheology and anesthesiology. *Anesth Analg* 1978;57:252.
152. Greenbaum R. The blood and transfusion fluids in shock. In: Freeman J, ed. *Physiological and practical aspects of shock.* Boston, MA: Little, Brown and Company, 1969:775.
153. Hill DW. Properties of liquids, gases and vapours. In: *Physics applied to anaesthesia.* London: Butterworth-Heineman, 1980: 170.
154. Replogle RL, Meiselman HJ, Merrill EW. Clinical implications of blood rheology studies. *Circulation* 1967;36:148.
155. Rand PW, Lacombe E, Hunt HE, et al. Viscosity of normal human blood under normothermic and hypothermic conditions. *J Appl Physiol* 1964;19:117.
156. Greeley WJ, Ungerleider RM, Smith LR, et al. The effects of deep hypothermic cardiopulmonary bypass and total circulatory arrest on cerebral blood flow in infants and children. *J Thorac Cardiovasc Surg* 1989;97:737.
157. Brierly JB. Neuropathological findings in patients dying after heart surgery. *Thorax* 1963;18:291.
158. Egerton N, Egerton SW, Kay JH. Neurological changes following profound hypothermia. *Ann Surg* 1963;157:366.
159. Payne SW, Theye RA, Kirklin JW. Effect of carbon dioxide on rate of brain cooling during induction of hypothermia by direct cooling. *J Surg Res* 1963;3:54.
160. Rahn H. Body temperature and acid-base regulation. *Pneumonologie* 1974;151:87.
161. Blayo MC, Lecompte Y, Pocidalo JJ. Control of acid-base status during hypothermia in man. *Respir Physiol* 1980;42:287.
162. Hazel JR, Carlick WS, Sellner PA. The effects of assay temperature upon the pH optima of enzymes from poikilotherms: a test of the imidazole alphastat hypothesis. *J Comp Physiol* 1978; 123:97.
163. Rahn H, Reeves RB, Howell BJ. Hydrogen ion regulation, temperature, and evolution. *Am Rev Respir Dis* 1975;112:165.
164. Reeves RB. An imidazole alphastat hypothesis for vertebrate acid-base regulation: tissue carbon dioxide content and body temperature in bull frogs. *Respir Physiol* 1972;14:219.
165. Astrup P, Engel S, Severinghaus, et al. The influence of temperature and pH on the dissociation curve of oxyhemoglobin of human blood. *Scand J Clin Lab Invest* 1965;17:512.
166. Baraka AS, Baroody MA, Haroun ST, et al. Effects of alphastat versus pH stat strategy on oxyhemoglobin dissociation and whole-body oxygen consumption during hypothermic cardiopulmonary bypass. *Anesth Analg* 1992;74:32.
167. Boysen G, Ladegaard-Pederson JH, Henriksen H, et al. The effects of PaCO2 on regional cerebral blood flow and internal carotid pressure during carotid clamping. *Anesthesiology* 1971; 35:286.
168. Gravlee GP, Roy RC, Stump DA, et al. Regional cerebrovascular reactivity to carbon dioxide during cardiopulmonary bypass in patients with cerebrovascular disease. *J Thorac Cardiovasc Surg* 1990;99:1022.
169. McConnell DH, White F, Nelson RL, et al. Importance of alkalosis in maintenance of "ideal" blood pH during hypothermia. *Surg Forum* 1975;26:263.
170. Becker H, Vinten-Johansen J, Buckberg GD, et al. Myocardial damage caused by keeping pH 7.40 during systemic deep hypothermia. *J Thorac Cardiovasc Surg* 1981;82:810.
171. Swain JA, White FN, Peters RM. The effect of pH on the hypothermic ventricular fibrillation threshold. *J Thorac Cardiovasc Surg* 1984;87:445.
172. Sinet M, Muffat-Joly M, Bendaace T, et al. Maintaining blood pH at 7.4 during hyupothermia has no significant effect on work of the isolated rat heart. *Anesthesiology* 1985;62:582.
173. Carter JN, White FN, Collins GM, et al. Studies of the ideal [H +] for perfusional preservation. *Transplantation* 1980;30: 409.
174. Reeves RB. Temperature-induced changes in blood acid-base status. Donnan rC1 and red cell volume. *J Appl Physiol* 1976; 40:762.

175. Wilson TL. Theoretical analysis of the effects of two pH regulation patterns on the temperature sensitivities of biological systems in nonhomeothermic animals. *Arch Biochem Biophys* 1977; 182:409.
176. Du Plessis AJ, Jonas RA, Wypij D, et al. Perioperative effects of alpha-stat versus pH-stat strategies for deep hypothermic cardiopulmonary arrest bypass in infants. *J Thorac Cardiovasc Surg* 1997;114:991.
177. The Warm Heart Investigators. Randomised trial of normothermic versus hypothermic coronary bypass surgery. *Lancet* 1994; 343:559.
178. Martin TD, Craver JM, Gott JP, et al. Prospective, randomized trial of retrograde warm blood cardioplegia: myocardial benefit and neurologic threat. *Ann Thorac Surg* 1994;57:298.
179. Guyton RA, Mellitt RJ, Weintraub WS. A critical assessment of neurological risk during warm heart surgery. *J Cardiac Surg* 1995;10:488.
180. Murkin JM. Hypothermic cardiopulmonary bypass—time for a more temperate approach? *Can J Anaesth* 1995;42:663.
181. Drummond JC. Brain protection during anesthesia: a reader's guide. *Anesthesiology* 1993;79:877.
182. Nathan HJ, Lavallee G. The management of temperature during hypothermic cardiopulmonary bypass: I—Canadian survey. *Can J Anaesth* 1995;42:669.
183. Muravchick S. Deep body thermometry during general anesthesia. *Anesthesiology* 1983;58:271.
184. Busto R, Dietrich WD, Globus MY-T, et al. The importance of brain temperature in cerebral injury. *Stroke* 1989;20:1113.
185. Chopp M, Knight R, Tidwell CD, et al. The metabolic effects of mild hypothermia on global cerebral ischemia and recirculation in the cat: comparison of normothermia to hyperthermia. *J Cereb Blood Flow Metab* 1989;9:141.
186. Taylor KM. Central nervous system effects of cardiopulmonary bypass. *Ann Thorac Surg* 1998;66[Suppl 5]:S20.
187. Cook DJ, Oliver WC, Orszulak TA, et al. A prospective, randomized comparison of cerebral venous oxygen saturation during normothermic and hypothermic cardiopulmonary bypass. *J Thorac Cardiovasc Surg* 1994;107:1020.
188. Westaby S. Organ dysfunction after cardiopulmonary bypass. A systemic inflammatory reaction initiated by the extracorporeal circuit. *Int Care Med* 1987;13:89.
189. Hall RI, Smith MS, Rocker G. The systemic inflammatory response to cardiopulmonary bypass: pathophysiological, therapeutic, and pharmacological considerations. *Anesth Analg* 1997; 85:766.
190. McBride WT, Armstrong MA, Crockard AD, et al. Cytokine balance and immunosuppressive changes in cardiac surgery: contrasting response between patients and isolated CPB circuits. *Br J Anaesth* 1995;75:724.
191. Colman RW. Platelet and neutrophil activation in cardiopulmonary bypass. *Ann Thorac Surg* 1990;49:32.
192. Kharzami A, Anderson LW, Baek L, et al. Endotoxemia and enhanced generation of oxygen radicals by neutrophils from patients undergoing cardiopulmonary bypass. *J Thorac Cardiovasc Surg* 1989;98:381.
193. Anderson LW, Baek L, Thomsen BS, et al. Effect of methylprednisolone on endotoxemia and complement activation during cardiac surgery. *J Cardiothorac Anesth* 1989;3:544.
194. Nilsson L, Kulander L, Nystrom SO, et al. Endotoxins in cardiopulmonary bypass. *J Thorac Cardiovasc Surg* 1990;100:777.
195. Frering B, Philip I, Dehoux M, et al. Circulating cytokines in patients undergoing normothermic cardiopulmonary bypass. *J Cardiovasc Surg* 1994;108:636.
196. Elliott MJ, Finn AHR. Interaction between neutrophils and endothelium. *Ann Thorac Surg* 1993;56:1503.
197. Bevilacqua M, Poberr J, Mendrick D, et al. Identification of an inducible endothelial-leukocyte adhesion molecule. *Proc Natl Acad Sci USA* 1987;84:9238.
198. Smith CW, Kishimoto TK, Abbassi O, et al. Chemotactic factors regulate lectin adhesion molecule 1 (LECAM-1)-dependent neutrophil adhesion to cytokine-stimulated endothelial cells in vitro. *J Clin Invest* 1991;87:609.
199. Richter J, Ng Sikorski J, Olsson I, et al. Tumor necrosis factor-induced degranulation in adherent human neutrophils is dependent on CDllb/CD18-integrin-triggered oscillations of cytosolic free Ca^{2+}. *Proc Natl Acad Sci USA* 1990;87:9472.
200. Shappell SB, Toman C, Anderson DC, et al. Mac-1 (CD1lb/CD18) mediates adherence-dependent hydrogen peroxide production by human and canine neutrophils. *J Immunol* 1990; 144:2702.
201. Menasche P, Peynet J, Lariviere J, et al. Does normothermia during cardiopulmonary bypass increase neutrophil-endothelium interactions? *Circulation* 1994;90(Nov, Part 2):II275.
202. Ohri SK, Bowles CW, Mathie RT, et al. Effect of cardiopulmonary bypass perfusion protocols on gut tissue oxygenation and blood flow. *Ann Thorac Surg* 1997;64:163.
203. Quigley RL, Caplan MS, Perkins JA, et al. Cardiopulmonary bypass with adequate flow and perfusion pressure prevents endotoxemia and pathologic cytokine production. *Perfusion* 1995; 10:27.
204. Paugam C, Chollet-Martin S, Dehoux M, et al. Neutrophil expression of CD11b/CD18/CD18 and IL-8 secretion during normothermic cardiopulmonary bypass. *J Cardiothorac Vasc Anesth* 1997;11:575.
205. John AE, Galea J, Francis SE, et al. Interleukin-8 mRNA expression in circulating leucocytes during cardiopulmonary bypass. *Perfusion* 1998;13:409.
206. Boyle EM Jr, Pohlman TH, Johnson MC, et al. Endothelial cell injury in cardiovascular surgery: the systemic inflammatory response. *Ann Thorac Surg* 1997;63:277.
207. Menasche P. The inflammatory response to cardiopulmonary bypass and its impact on postoperative myocardial function. *Curr Op Cardiol* 1995;10:597.
208. Wan S, LeClerc JL, Vincent JL. Cytokine responses to cardiopulmonary bypass: lessons learned from cardiac transplantation. *Ann Thorac Surg* 1997;63:269.
209. Liebold A, Keyl C, Birnbaum D. The heart produces but the lungs consume proinflammatory cytokines following cardiopulmonary bypass. *Eur J Cardiothorac Surg* 1999;15:340.
210. Wan S, LeClere JL, Schmartz D, et al. Hepatic release of interleukin-10 during cardiopulmonary bypass in steroid pretreated patients. *Am Heart J* 1997;133:335.
211. Hill GE, Diego RP, Stammers AH, et al. Aprotinin enhances the endogenous release of interleukin-10 after cardiac operations. *Ann Thorac Surg* 1998;65:66.
212. Ashraf S, Tian Y, Cowan D, et al. "Low dose" aprotinin modifies hemostasis but not proinflammatory cytokine release. *Ann Thorac Surg* 1997;63:68.
213. Parolari A, Alamanni F, Gherli T, et al. "High dose" aprotinin and heparin-coated circuits: clinical efficacy and inflammatory response. *Cardiovasc Surg* 1999;7:117.
214. Schreurs HH, Wijers MJ, Gu YJ, et al. Heparin-coated bypass circuits: effects on inflammatory response in pediatric cardiac patients. *Ann Thorac Surg* 1998;66:166.
215. Wan S, Yim AP, Arifi AA, et al. Can cardioplegia management influence cytokine responses during clinical cardiopulmonary bypass? *Ann Thorac Cardiovasc Surg* 1999;5:81.
216. Orime Y, Shiono M, Hata H, et al. Cytokine and endothelial damage in pulsatile and nonpulsatile cardiopulmonary bypass. *Artif Organs* 1999;23:508.
217. Hurst T, Johnson D, Cujec B, et al. Depletion of activated

neutrophils by a filter during cardiac valve surgery. *Can J Anaesth* 1997;44:131.

218. Baksaas ST, Videm V, Mollners TE, et al. Leucocyte filtration during cardiopulmonary bypass hardly changed leucocyte counts and did not influence myeloperoxidase, complement, cytokines or platelets. *Perfusion* 1998;13:429.
219. Tassani P, Richter JA, Barankay A, et al. Does high-dose methylprednisolone in aprotinin-treated patients attenuate the systemic inflammatory response during coronary artery bypass grafting procedures? *J Cardiothorac Vasc Anesth* 1999;13:165.
220. Kawamura T, Inada K, Nara N, et al. Influence of methylprednisolone on cytokine balance during cardiac surgery. *Crit Care Med* 1999;27:545.
221. Mollhoff T, Loick HM, Van Aken H, et al. Milrinone modulates endotoxemia, systemic inflammation, and subsequent acute phase response after cardiopulmonary bypass. *Anesthesiology* 1999;90:72.
222. Roytblat L, Talmor D, Rachinsky M, et al. Ketamine attenuates the interleukin-6 response after cardiopulmonary bypass. *Anesth Analg* 1998;87:266.
223. Carney DE, Lutz CJ, Picone AL, et al. Soluble tumor necrosis factor receptor prevents post-pump syndrome. *J Surg Res* 1999; 83:113.
224. Massoudy P, Zahler S, Barankay A, et al. Sodium nitroprusside during coronary artery bypass grafting: evidence for an antiinflammatory action. *Ann Thorac Surg* 1999;67:1059.
225. Kongsgaard UE, Smith-Erichsen N, Geiran O, et al. Different activation patterns in the plasma kallikrein-kinin and complement systems during coronary bypass surgery. *Acta Anaesth Scand* 1989;33;343.
226. Fritz H, Wunder G. Biochemistry and applications of aprotinin, the kallikrein inhibitor from bovine organs. *Arzneim-Forschl Drug Res* 1983;33:479.
227. Verstaete M. Clinical application of inhibitors of fibrinolysis. *Drugs* 1985;29:236.
228. Hill GE, Alonso A, Spurzem JR, et al. Aprotinin and methylprednisolone equally blunt cardiopulmonary bypass-induced inflammation in humans. *J Thorac Cardiovasc Surg* 1995;110: 1658.
229. Lord RA, Roath OS, Thompson JE, et al. Effect of aprotinin on neutrophil function after major vascular surgery. *Br J Surg* 1992;79;517.
230. Whitten CW, Latson TH, Allison PM, et al. Does aprotinin inhibit cardiopulmonary bypass-induced inflammation? *Anesthesiology* 1992:77:A266.
231. Harris DNF, Bailey SM, Smith PLC, et al. Brain swelling in the first hour after coronary artery bypass surgery. *Lancet* 1993; 342:586.
232. Harris DN, Oatridge A, Dob D, et al. Cerebral swelling after normothermic cardiopulmonary bypass. *Anesthesiology* 1998;88: 340.
233. Karniya T, Katayarna Y, Kashiwagi F, et al. The role of bradykinin in mediating ischemic brain edema in rats. *Stroke* 1993;24: 571.
234. Aoki M, Jonas RA, Nomura F, et al. Effects of aprotinin on acute recovery of cerebral metabolism in piglets after hypothermic circulatory arrest. *Ann Thorac Surg* 1994;58:146.
235. Sultan I, Sunamori M, Suzuki A. Heart preservation: analysis of cardioprotective infusate characteristics. Membrane stabilization, calcium antagonism, and protease inhibition on myocardial viability: a biochemical, ultrastructural, functional study. *J Heart Lung Transplant* 1992;11:607.
236. Levy JH, Pifarre R, Schaff HV, et al. A multicenter, double-blind, placebo-controlled trail of aprotinin for reducing blood loss and the requirement for donor-blood transfusion in patients undergoing repeat coronary artery bypass grafting. *Circulation* 1995;92:2236.
237. Yanamoto H, Kikuchi H, Okamoto S, et al. Preventive effect of synthetic serine protease inhibitor, FUT-175, administered in the acute stage after subarachnoid hemorrhage. *Neurosurgery* 1992;30:351.
238. Yanamoto H, Kikuchi H, Sato M, et al. Therapeutic trial of cerebral vasospasm with the serine protease inhibitor, FUT-175, administered in the acute stage after subarachnoid hemorrhage. *Neurosurgery* 1992;330:358.
239. Roach GW, Kanchuger M, Mora Mangano C, et al. Adverse cerebral outcomes after coronary bypass surgery. *N Engl J Med* 1996;335:1857.
240. Shaw PJ, Bates D, Cartlidge NE, et al. Early intellectual dysfunction following coronary bypass surgery. *J Med* 1986;58:59.
241. Shaw PJ, Bates D, Cartlidge NE, et al. Neurologic and neuropsychological morbidity following major surgery: comparison of coronary artery bypass and peripheral vascular surgery. *Stroke* 1987;18:700.
242. Carella F, Travaini G, Contri P, et al. Cerebral complications of coronary bypass surgery. A prospective study. *Acta Neurol Scand* 1988;77:158.
243. Murkin JM, Martzke JS, Buchan AM, et al. A randomized study of the influence of perfusion technique and pH management strategy in 316 patients undergoing coronary artery bypass surgery. II Neurologic and cognitive outcomes. *J Thorac Cardiovasc Surg* 1995;110:349.
244. Smith P, Treasure T, Newman S, et al. Cerebral consequences of cardiopulmonary bypass. *Lancet* 1986;2:823.
245. Blauth C, Arnold J, Kohner EM, et al. Retinal microembolism during cardiopulmonary bypass demonstrated by fluorescein angiography. *Lancet* 1986;2:827.
246. Slogoff S, Girgis KA, Keats AS. Etiologic factors in neuropsychiatric complications associated with cardiopulmonary bypass. *Anesth Analg* 1982;61:903.
247. Murkin JM. Neurological dysfunction after CAB or valvular surgery: is the medium the miscreant? *Anesth Analg* 1993;76: 213.
248. Webb WR, Harrison LH, Helmcke FR, et al. Carbon dioxide field flooding minimizes residual intracardiac air after open heart operations. *Ann Thorac Surg* 1997;64:1489.
249. Moody DM, Bell A, Phil D, et al. Brain microemboli during cardiac surgery or aortography. *Ann Neurol* 1990;28:477.
250. Brooker RF, Brown WR, Moody DM, et al. Cardiotomy suction: a major source of brain lipid emboli during cardiopulmonary bypass. *Ann Thorac Surg* 1998;65:1651.
251. Stump DA, Jones TJ, Hammon JW, et al. Does aprotinin use influence the volume of shed blood and the number of microemboli during CPB? *Ann Thorac Surg* 1999;68:1460.
252. Pugsley W, Klinger L, Paschalis C. Microemboli and cerebral impairment during cardiac surgery. *Vasc Surg* 1990;34.
253. Blauth CI, Smith PL, Arnold JV, et al. Influence of oxygenator type on the prevalence and extent of microembolic retinal ischemia during cardiopulmonary bypass. *J Thorac Cardiovasc Surg* 1990;99:61.
254. Padayachee TS, Parsons S, Theobold R, et al. The detection of microemboli in the middle cerebral artery during cardiopulmonary bypass: a transcranial Doppler ultrasound investigation using membrane and bubble oxygenators. *Ann Thorac Surg* 1987;44:298.
255. Roach GW. Pro: prevention of neurologic dysfunction associated with cardiac surgery requires pharmacologic brain protection. *J Cardiothorac Vasc Anesth* 1997;11:793.
256. Zin WA, Caldeira MP, Cardoso WV, et al. Expiratory mechanics before and after uncomplicated heart surgery. *Chest* 1989; 95:21.

257. Wilcox P, Baile EM, Hards J, et al. Phrenic nerve function and its relationship to atelectasis after coronary artery bypass surgery. *Chest* 1988;93:693.
258. Olopade CO, Staats BA. Time course of recovery from frostbitten phrenics after coronary artery bypass graft surgery. *Chest* 1991;99:1112.
259. Clarke CP, Kahn DR, Dufek JH, et al. The effects of nonpulsatile blood flow on canine lungs. *Ann Thorac Surg* 1968;6:450.
260. Hewson JR. Perfusion characteristics during cardiopulmonary bypass and subsequent changes in alveolar-arterial oxygen tension gradients. *Anesth Analg* 1978;57:298.
261. Weedon RJ, Coalson JJ, Greenfield LJ. Effects of oxygen and ventilation on pulmonary mechanics and ultrastructure during cardiopulmonary bypass. *Am J Surg* 1970;120:584.
262. Hewson JR, Shaw M. Continuous airway pressure with oxygen minimizes the metabolic lesion of "pump lung." *Can Anaesth Soc J* 1983;30:37.
263. Byrick RJ, Noble WH. Postperfusion lung syndrome. *J Thorac Cardiovasc Surg* 1978;76:685.
264. Maccherini M, Davoli G, Sani G, et al. Warm heart surgery eliminates diaphragmatic paralysis. *J Cardiac Surg* 1995;10:257.
265. Rae HH, Harris EA, Seelye ER, et al. The effects of cardiopulmonary bypass upon pulmonary gas exchange. *J Thorac Cardiovasc Surg* 1978;75:104.
266. Ratliff NE, Young WG, Hackel DB, et al. Pulmonary injury secondary to extracorporeal circulation. *J Thorac Cardiovasc Surg* 1973;65:425.
267. Royston D, Fleming JS, Desai JB, et al. Increased peroxide product generation associated with open heart surgery; evidence for free radical generation. *J Thorac Cardiovasc Surg* 1986;91:759.
268. Kirklin JW, Westaby S, Blackstone EH, et al. Complement and the damaging effects of cardiopulmonary bypass. *J Thorac Cardiovasc Surg* 1983;86:845.
269. Kharzami A, Anderson LW, Baek L, et al. Endotoxemia and enhanced generation of oxygen radicals by neutrophils from patients undergoing cardiopulmonary bypass. *J Thorac Cardiovasc Surg* 1989;98:381.
270. Paugam C, Chollet-Martin S, Dehoux M, et al. Neutrophil expression of CD11b/CD18/CD18 and IL-8 secretion during normothermic cardiopulmonary bypass. *J Cardiothorac Vasc Anesth* 1997;11:575.
271. Tonz M, Mihaljevic T, von Segesser LK, et al. Acute lung injury during cardiopulmonary bypass. Are the neutrophils responsible? *Chest* 1995;108:1551.
272. Koizumi M, Matsumoto N, Ueda K. Influences of cardiopulmonary bypass and fentanyl anesthesia on hepatic circulation and oxygen metabolism in beagles. *Anesth Analg* 1998;86:1177.
273. Wakiyama H, Yamashita C, Okada M, et al. Increased portal endothelin-1 level is associated with the liver function after cardiopulmonary bypass in rabbits: influence of hypothermia on the damage. *Kobe J Med Sci* 1997;43:245.
274. Torre Rodriguez I, Lopez-Herce Cid J, Vazquez Gonzalez P, et al. Hyperamylasemia after cardiac surgery in children. *Ann Esp Pediatr* 1997;46:156.
275. Huddy SP, Joyce WP, Pepper JR. Gastrointestinal complications in 4,473 patients who underwent cardiopulmonary bypass surgery. *Br J Surg* 1991;78:293.
276. Leitman IM, Paull DE, Barie PS, et al. Intra-abdominal complications of cardiopulmonary bypass operations. *Surg Gynecol Obstet* 1987;165:251.
277. Heikkinen LO, Ala-Kulju KV. Abdominal complications following cardiopulmonary bypass in open-heart surgery. *Scand J Thorac Cardiovasc Surg* 1987;21:1.
278. Cox CS, Allen SJ, Brennan M. Analysis of intestinal microvascular permeability associated with cardiopulmonary bypass. *J Surg Res* 1999;83:19.
279. Haisjackl M, Birnbaum J, Redlin M, et al. A Splanchnic oxygen transport and lactate metabolism during normothermic cardiopulmonary bypass in humans. *Anesth Analg* 1998;86:22.
280. Mrozek R, Wos S, Bachowski R, et al. Gastric tonometry as a method of visceral oxygenation monitoring in patients undergoing coronary revascularization. *Eur J Cardiothorac Surg* 1997;11:1158.
281. O'Dwyer C, Woodson LC, Conroy BP, et al. Regional perfusion abnormalities with phenylephrine during normothermic bypass. *Ann Thorac Surg* 1997;63:728.
282. Heikkinen L, Harjula A, Merikallio E. Acute renal failure related to open heart surgery. *Ann Chir Gynaecol* 1985;74:203.
283. Gomez-Campadera FJ, Maroto-Alvaro E, Galinanes M, et al. Acute renal failure associated with cardiac surgery. *Child Nephrol Urol* 1988-89;9:138.
284. Baxter P, Rigby ML, Jones OD, et al. Acute renal failure following cardiopulmonary bypass in children: results of treatment. *Int J Cardiol* 1985;7:235.
285. Zanardo G, Michielon P, Pacagnella A, et al. Acute renal failure in the patient undergoing cardiac operation, prevalence, mortality rate, and main risk factors. *J Cardiothorac Surg* 1994;107:1489.
286. Picca S, Principato F, Mazzera E, et al. Risks of acute renal failure after cardiopulmonary bypass surgery in children: a retrospective 10 year case control study. *Nephrol Dial Transplant* 1995;10:630.
287. Wenstone R, Campbell JM, Booker PD, et al. Renal function after cardiopulmonary bypass in children: comparison of dopamine with dobutamine. *Br J Anaesth* 1991;67:591.
288. Lema G, Urzua J, Jalil R, et al. Renal protection in patients undergoing cardiopulmonary bypass with preoperative abnormal renal function. *Anesth Analg* 1998;86:3.
289. Rigden SP, Dillon MJ, Kind PR, et al. The beneficial effect of mannitol on postoperative renal function in children undergoing cardiopulmonary bypass surgery. *Clin Nephrol* 1984;211:48.
290. Fisher AR, Jones P, Barlow P, et al. The influence of mannitol on renal function during and after open heart surgery. *Perfusion* 1998;13:181.
291. Zanardo G, Michielon P, Rosi P, et al. Effects of continuous diltiazem infusion on renal function during cardiac surgery. *J Cardiothorac Vasc Anesth* 1993;7:711.
292. Andersson LG, Jeppsson A, Bratteby LE, et al. Renal function during cardiopulmonary bypass: influence of the calcium entry blocker felodipine. *Anesth Analg* 1996;83:34.
293. Bertolissi M, Antonucci F, Monte A, et al. Effects on renal function of a continuous infusion of nifedipine during cardiopulmonary bypass. *J Cardiothorac Vasc Anesth* 1996;10:238.
294. Abe K, Sakakibara T, Yoshiya I. The effect of prostaglandin E1 on renal function after cardiac surgery involving cardiopulmonary bypass. *Prostoglandins Leukotrienes Essent Fatty Acids* 1993;49:627.
295. Sezai A, Shiono M, Orime Y, et al. Effectiveness of low dose continuous infusion of alpha hANP from the start of cardiopulmonary bypass. *Kyobu Geka* 1999;52:384.
296. Toda K, Tatsumi E, Taenaka Y, et al. Impact of systemic depulsation on tissue perfusion and sympathetic nerve activity. *Ann Thorac Surg* 1996;62:1737.
297. Nakamura K, Koga Y, Ishii K, et al. The effects of pulsatile and nonpulsatile cardiopulmonary bypass on renal blood flow and function. *Jpn J Surg* 1989;19:334.

298. Matsuda H, Hirose H, Nakano S, et al. Results of open heart surgery in patients with impaired renal function as creatinine clearance below 20 mL/min. The effects of pulsatile perfusion. *J Cardiovasc Surg* 1986;27:595.
299. Andersson LG, Bratteby LE, Ekroth R, et al. Renal function during cardiopulmonary bypass: influence of pump flow and systemic blood pressure. *Eur J Cardiothorac Surg* 1994;8:597.
300. Regragui IA, Izzat MB, Birdi I, et al. Cardiopulmonary bypass perfusion temperature does not influence perioperative renal function. *Ann Thorac Surg* 1995;60:160.
301. Werb MR, Zinman B, Teasdale SJ, et al. Hormonal and metabolic responses during coronary artery bypass surgery: role of infused glucose. *J Clin Endocrinol Metab* 1989;69:1010.
302. Braden H, Cheema-Dhadli S, Mazer CD, et al. Hyperglycemia during normothermic cardiopulmonary bypass: the role of the kidney. *Ann Thorac Surg* 1998;65:1588.

15

TERMINATION OF CARDIOPULMONARY BYPASS AND POSTBYPASS HEMODYNAMIC MANAGEMENT

GERARD McCLOSKEY

The termination of cardiopulmonary bypass (CPB) and post-CPB management presents a challenging task to the anesthesiologist. Often the myocardium is compromised by acute dysfunction from the residual effects of cardioplegia, iatrogenic ischemia, and hyperkalemia superimposed on chronic deterioration in ventricular performance. Vasomotor instability at a time when the myocardium may be sensitive to minor changes in the preload is superimposed on dynamic changes in fluid requirements. Anticoagulation must be reversed, anesthesia and muscle relaxation requirements must be addressed, and the patient must be prepared for transport while being continuously monitored. Smooth execution of all these tasks takes experience, good clinical judgment, and a knowledge base that can deal with a number of complex and serious problems that may arise very quickly.

Communication between anesthesiologist, surgeon, perfusionist, and nurses is critical. Supervision of weaning from CPB varies from institution to institution, but it is appropriate for the anesthesiologist to be primarily responsible for establishing optimal hemodynamics and ventilatory patterns, choosing pharmacologic therapies, and managing fluid replacement. The surgeon has a number of other complex responsibilities including early evaluation of the surgical procedure, hemostasis, and closure of the wound. An orderly routine with defined responsibilities should be established.

As the anesthesiologist prepares for termination of CPB, it is useful to have a checklist (Table 15-1) to serve as a starting point for clinical actions. The use of this checklist assumes that physiologic parameters during bypass have been monitored and attended to. Obviously, this protocol must also account for individual patient difference and variation. The components of Table 15-1 are considered individually.

G. McCloskey: Department of Anesthesiology, Yale University School of Medicine; Cardiothoracic Intensive Care Unit, Yale-New Haven Hospital, New Haven, Connecticut 06510

ANALYSIS AND CORRELATION OF ELECTROLYTE, ACID-BASE, AND OXYGEN TRANSPORT STATUS

The metabolic status is evaluated primarily through analysis of arterial and mixed venous blood gas samples. Often mixed venous oxygen saturation and arterial and mixed venous blood gases are continuously monitored during CPB. Acid-base status should be optimized, with particular attention paid to metabolic acidosis. Respiratory acidosis is easily managed by the perfusionist altering oxygenator gas flow rates and can aid in the correction of pH level. Acidosis of either type not only acts as a direct myocardial depressant (1,2) but also can cause an elevation in pulmonary vascular resistance (PVR) leading to a progressive decrement in right ventricular function (3). The presence of metabolic acidosis is usually a consequence of inadequate tissue perfusion resulting from inadequate perfusion flow, a low hemoglobin level, inadequate arterial oxygenation, or increased oxygen consumption. Less common causes of metabolic acidosis include diabetic ketoacidosis and renal failure. If necessary, sodium bicarbonate can be administered to correct the metabolic component of an acidosis, but treatment of the primary cause is more desirable.

The serum potassium level should be maintained well above 4.0 mEq/L to reduce the incidence of arrhythmia or conduction problems. Depending on the type and amount of myocardial protective solution, corrective measures may be required to reduce elevated potassium levels. Often elevated potassium levels recede quickly to acceptable levels toward the end of CPB due to an increased osmotic diuresis seen during this period. If, however, the urine output is judged inadequate, corrective measures would include the administration of a loop diuretic (typically furosemide) to

TABLE 15-1. CHECKLIST FOR SEPARATION FROM CARDIOPULMONARY BYPASS

1. Analysis and correction of electrolyte, acid-base, and oxygen transport status
2. Reestablishment of adequate pulmonary ventilation
3. Evaluation of circulation
   - Reliability and function of monitors
   - Cardiac rate and rhythm
   - Anticipated state of ventricular performance and possible need for pharmacologic and/or mechanical support
   - State of the peripheral and pulmonary circulation
   - Evaluation of reservoir volume
4. Temperature
5. Anesthetic state
6. Elapsed time since removal of aortic cross-clamp; possible need for continued cardiopulmonary bypass and/or reperfusion

facilitate the removal of excess potassium in the urine. There is a notion that patients treated with high doses of ϵ-aminocaproic acid in the perioperative period to reduce blood loss often have elevated serum potassium levels toward the end of the CPB period. These elevations may be quite impressive, often reaching 6 to 7 mEq/L. Possible renal mechanisms have been recently proposed to explain this clinical observation (S. Garwood, *written communication, Nov. 1999*). Clearly, at these levels, the hyperkalemia will result in impaired myocardial cell hyperpolarization, which will result in reduced myocardial contractility, deranged conduction system function, and elevated pacemaker thresholds. In these more urgent clinical situations, administration of intravenous regular insulin may be required to translocate the potassium to the interior of the cells, thereby lowering serum potassium concentrations temporarily (4). The administration of insulin in this instance may also help serve a second purpose, treating the commonly seen hyperglycemia associated with the administration of glucose containing cardioplegic solutions (5) and the elevated catecholamines of CPB. Elevated glucose levels may be damaging to the central nervous system (6–8). Thus, insulin administration may be warranted even in the nondiabetic patient.

The routine administration of calcium is controversial. Although some evidence exists that elevated serum calcium levels may aggravate reperfusion injury (10–13), it is important that serum calcium levels be adequate. Ionized calcium levels should be monitored and corrected if they are low (9). The importance of magnesium has been increasingly recognized. The serum level of magnesium is often low following termination of bypass and has been associated with an increased incidence of ventricular arrhythmias and impaired contractile function (14–19). Many practitioners advocate routine treatment for hypomagnesemia in the immediate post-CPB period.

The hematocrit level must be adequate to provide oxygen-carrying capacity. Although there is no magic number for hematocrit at the termination of bypass, logic dictates that a low hematocrit level is better tolerated in a healthy individual with good preoperative ventricular function than in a physiologically compromised patient with a chronically failing or hypertrophic myocardium (20–22). In general, a hematocrit level of 20% or more is thought to be appropriate for the termination of bypass (23). The complications of blood administration are well known (24), and blood conservation is always prudent. Hematocrit level can be increased while on CPB in two ways. In patients who are judged to be low in overall volume toward the end of CPB, the level of hematocrit can be increased by adding packed cells to the bypass reservoir. If, however, the patient's volume is adequate or even high, the level of hematocrit can be improved by using ultrafiltration techniques to hemoconcentrate the blood as it passes through the extracorporeal circuit. This latter technique is particularly useful when dealing with patients with coexisting renal impairment and poor urine output.

The clinician, faced with the decision to transfuse or withhold red blood cells in the post-CPB period should consider, in addition to the patient's overall cardiovascular reserve, the amount and availability of sequestered or salvaged blood and the rate of ongoing diuresis. In this manner, the experienced clinician can extrapolate to an estimated appropriate "intensive care unit arrival" hematocrit level.

REESTABLISH ADEQUATE VENTILATION

Until weaning from CPB is initiated and ventricular ejection (pulsatile arterial waveform) is seen, ventilation is not required. However, ventilation is usually started before actual separation from CPB for several reasons. Careful manual ventilation allows the clinician to assess the compliance of the lungs and detect bronchospasm or reduced lung compliance, allowing for early detection and treatment while still oxygenating on CPB. In addition, in patients in whom the left internal mammary artery has been used as a graft for coronary revascularization, careful gradual reexpansion of the deflated left lung allows the surgeon to assess the position of the pedicle and reposition it if necessary to allow complete lung excursion.

Early gentle ventilation is also used to assist in the elimination of intravascular air (pulmonary veins). Lastly, during this critical period, the team's attention may be diverted to other clinical problems, which may result in a lack of ventilation. It is essential that the anesthesiologist develop a protocol that will avoid such lapses in ventilation. Use of a mnemonic is suggested (Table 15-2). Care must be taken with the first few reinflation breaths to ensure patency of the airway, acceptable pulmonary compliance, and proper position of the internal mammary graft. As the lungs are reexpanded, they must be observed for signs of atelectasis.

TABLE 15-2. FIVE *P*'s of PUMP SEPARATION

Premature separation: rewarming, reperfusion time
Pulmonary preparation: reexpansion, ventilation, monitoring
P waves: rate, rhythm and pacing
Preload: titrate, avoid overdistention
Power assist: inotropes, mechanical assistance

Source: From Gravlee GP. Management of cardiopulmonary bypass. In: Barash PG, Deutch S, Tinker J, eds. *The American Society of Anesthesiologists annual refresher course lectures.* Philadelphia: JB Lippincott, 1992:106, with permission.

The pleural cavities are suctioned so that no blood or fluid is trapped in the partially open hemithorax and to allow complete lung expansion. The time of initial ventilation may be performed with the aortic cross-clamp in position to assist in left ventricular de-airing. Often ventilation is continued while the operating room table is tilted head down and occasionally side to side (25). Sustained positive pressure may facilitate removal of air from the pulmonary veins and left ventricle. These traditional ventilation and positioning maneuvers may reduce the risk of embolic neurologic sequelae, but none is totally effective in eliminating intracranial air (26).

EVALUATION OF THE CIRCULATION

Monitors

Hemodynamic monitoring is pivotal to the decisions made while separating a patient from CPB (Fig. 15-1). Before separation, the zero balance and calibration of all transducers should be checked and all placed at the appropriate anatomic level (midatrium). Blood pressure data obtained via the radial artery catheter may indicate pressures considerably below those measured simultaneously in the brachial artery, femoral artery, or aorta at this point (Fig. 15-2) (27). Stern et al. have postulated that vasodilation in the forearm and redistribution of flow around the wrist at least partially explain this phenomenon (28). Pauca et al. have also implicated vasodilation in the hand (29). These phenomena together may temporarily create a situation analogous to that of an arteriovenous fistula. Consequently, before initiating a therapeutic plan based on low blood pressure measured in the radial artery, it is advisable to place a needle into the aorta and measure aortic pressure.

Once weaning has been completed, measuring aortic pressure via a three-way stopcock connected to the aortic cannula becomes convenient and equally effective. If the latter option is selected, the aortic infusion tubing from the oxygenator circuit should be clamped just proximal to the cannula reading when reading the aortic pressure to prevent exaggeration of aortic systolic pressure from resonance artifact (28,29). Usually, this phenomenon of low radial artery pressure is transient. Radial artery pressure usually equilibrates rapidly with that measured in the central aorta. If this does not occur in hemodynamically unstable patients, a femoral artery catheter becomes necessary to accurately monitor central arterial pressure in the postbypass period.

Many anesthesiologists rely heavily on the data received from the pulmonary artery catheter during weaning from CPB. The pulmonary artery catheter provides pressure and flow data that can be obtained in no other way with a single device. Modifications of the standard thermodilution pulmonary artery catheter also can provide continuous cardiac output, continuous mixed venous oxygen saturation, right ventricular ejection fraction, and right ventricular end-diastolic volume (30,31). It is common practice to establish the relationship between pulmonary capillary wedge pressure and pulmonary artery diastolic pressure or pulmonary artery mean pressure before CPB and thereby have a continuous estimation of left-sided filling pressure. This practice is useful and often allows continuous fine-tuning of left ventricular preload during weaning and after bypass. However, if the PVR changes significantly, this technique will lead to incorrect estimations (32). Many clinicians avoid inflation of the pulmonary artery catheter balloon after CPB, particularly while still anticoagulated, fearing the possibility of pulmonary artery rupture. If the catheter has been left in place in the pulmonary artery during CPB, the anesthesiologist must confirm that the tip of the catheter has not migrated distally during CPB. The pulmonary artery waveform must be seen to change from the low, flat pattern seen on complete bypass to the familiar systolic/diastolic pattern typical of the pulmonary artery as the patient separates from CPB and pulmonary blood flow increases. The absence of pulsatile pulmonary artery flow in the presence of detectable left ventricular ejection strongly suggests that the pulmonary artery catheter has migrated to a "wedged" position.

Even pulmonary capillary wedge pressure can yield poor estimations of left ventricular end-diastolic pressure (LVEDP) at the end of CPB (33,34). The purpose of estimating LVEDP is to assess left ventricular end-diastolic volume (LVEDV), which is the closest clinical correlate of left ventricular preload (35). The relationship between LVEDP and LVEDV may change significantly, depending on left ventricular diastolic compliance (36,37). Transesophageal echocardiography (TEE) provides the most clinically accurate assessment of LVEDV, although it is seldom critical to successful weaning from CPB (38–40). However, TEE has been used successfully to detect patients having difficulty weaning from CPB, to monitor cardiac function as therapy was instituted and finally to guide CPB termination after normalizing echocardiographic parameters of left ventricular fractional area change, regional wall motion abnormalities, and left ventricular end-diastolic volume. If the clinical situation warrants a more accurate determination of left atrial pressure, consideration should be given to the placement of a left atrial catheter.

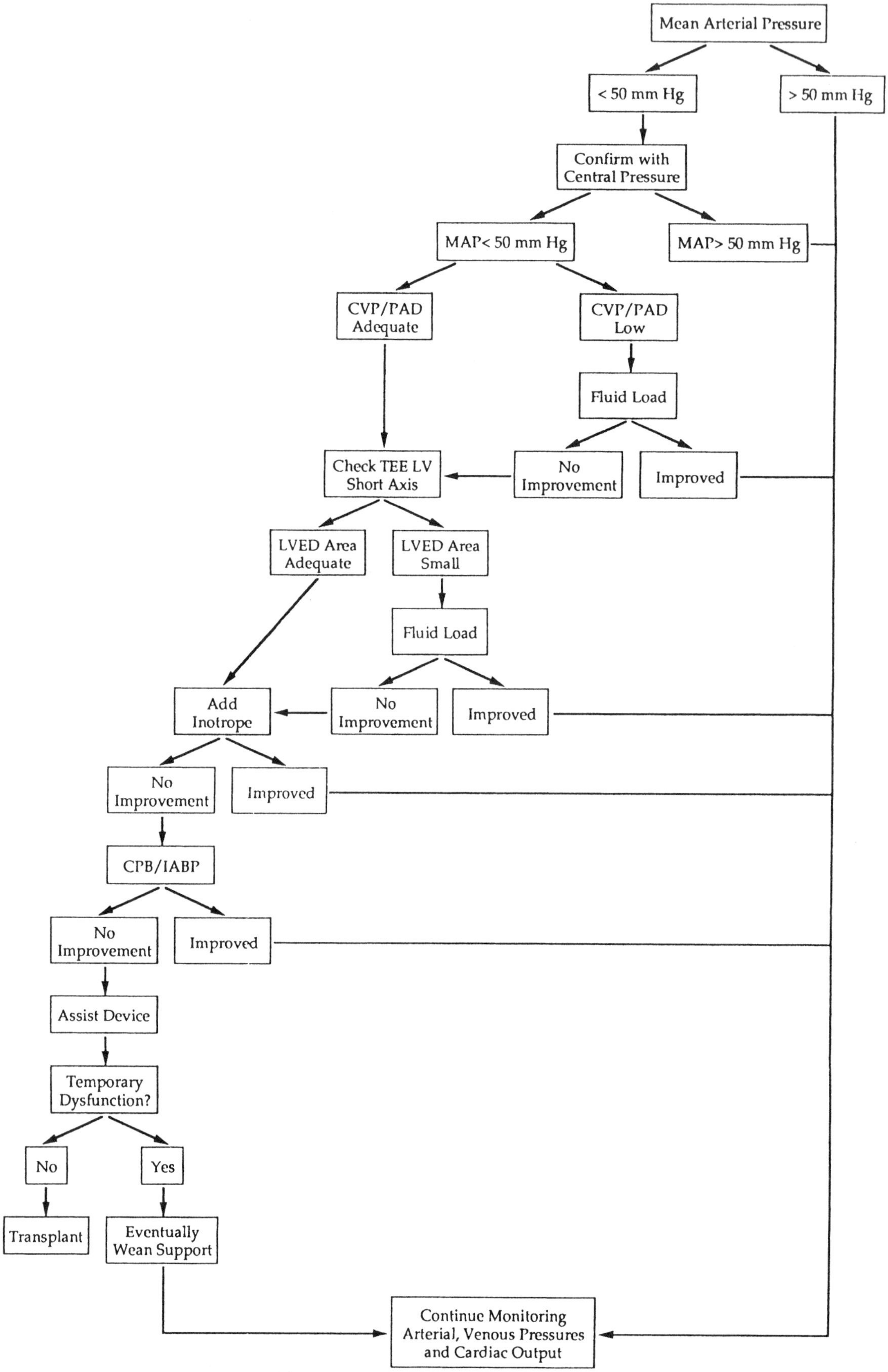
Mean Arterial Pressure
< 50 mm Hg
> 50 mm Hg
Confirm with Central Pressure
MAP< 50 mm Hg
MAP> 50 mm Hg
CVP/PAD Adequate
CVP/PAD Low
Fluid Load
No Improvement
Improved
Check TEE LV Short Axis
LVED Area Adequate
LVED Area Small
Fluid Load
Add Inotrope
No Improvement
Improved
No Improvement
Improved
CPB/IABP
No Improvement
Improved
Assist Device
Temporary Dysfunction?
No
Yes
Transplant
Eventually Wean Support
Continue Monitoring Arterial, Venous Pressures and Cardiac Output

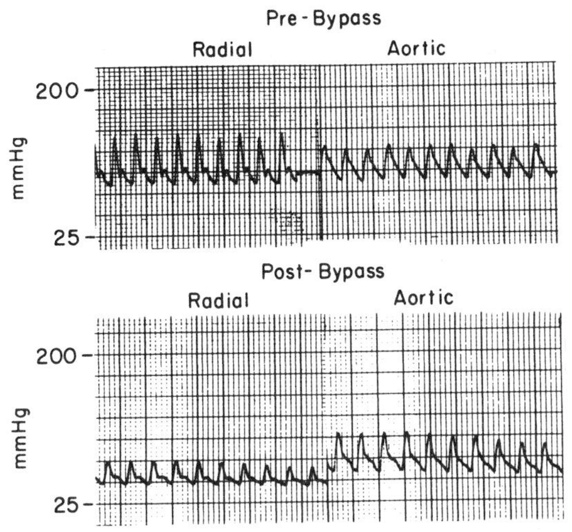

FIGURE 15-2. Arterial pressure tracings from the radial artery and aorta. The normal (prebypass) relationship shows the radial artery pressure higher than the central aorta pressure. After bypass, this relationship is reversed in this patient, allowing erroneous diagnosis of postbypass hypotension. (From Stern DH, Gerson JI, Allen FB, et al. Can we trust the direct radial artery pressure immediately following cardiopulmonary bypass? *Anesthesiology* 1985;62:558, with permission.)

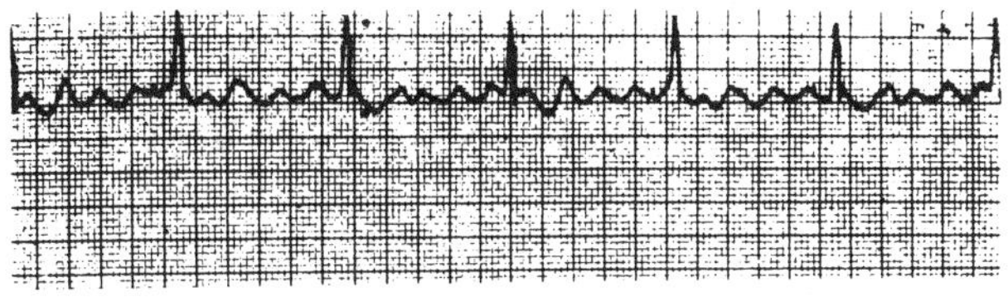

FIGURE 15-3. Electrocardiogram of a patient in normal sinus rhythm while on bypass. The roller head of the bypass apparatus has produced a static charge artifact that could easily be mistaken for atrial flutter. (From Griffin RM, Kaplan JA. ECG lead systems. In: Thys D, Kaplan JA, eds. *The ECG in anesthesia and critical care.* New York: Churchill Livingstone, 1987:29, with permission.)

Rate and Rhythm

Before cessation of CPB, the native cardiac rhythm should be analyzed. Because of the relationship of surface electrodes to the heart with an open chest, the presence of pericardial fluid, and the possible electrostatic disturbance from the CPB apparatus, the amplitude of the P waves and QRS complexes may be diminished and the isoelectric segments obscured by artifacts, preventing appropriate rhythm interpretation (Fig. 15-3). These artifacts may also interfere with electrocardiogram diagnosis of ischemia. Hard copy of the rhythm strips of all available leads (commonly I, II, III, aVR, aVL, aVF, and V_5) is often useful when there is difficulty analyzing the presence of P waves, regularity of rhythm, width of ventricular complexes, and so forth. Many patients experience rhythm disturbances and conduction abnormalities during weaning from bypass (41,42). Fortunately, most of the abnormalities are amenable to treatment. Bradycardia, heart block, and asystole represent the most common problems (43). Sinus or junctional bradycardia can be treated effectively by atrial pacing. Heart blocks and asystole can be managed with atrioventricular sequential pacing (44). Many rate, rhythm, and conduction abnormalities resolve within the first half hour after CPB separation, at which time pacing can be discontinued. Electrical pacing then appears to be more useful during the weaning process than the use of agents such as atropine or isoproterenol, which may be associated with both undesirable side effects and difficulty in achieving a specific heart rate (45). Even in patients with preserved sinus mechanism after CPB, a significant number will exhibit significant atrioventricular delay. This delay, although moderate in severity, always is associated with a decrement in cardiac output (compared to baseline) and responds well to atrioventricular sequential pacing at a smaller atrioventricular delay. The magnitude of the benefit appears to be largest in those patients with poor preoperative left ventricular function (46). Atrioventricular dissociation poses specific clinical problems. When present, the synchrony between the atria and ventricles varies cyclically over periods of several beats, leading to substantial fluctuations in arterial pressure. This pattern is easily recognized when right atrial pressure (central venous pressure [CVP]) is monitored. The periods of lower arterial pressure are accompanied by periods of higher CVP with prominent *v* waves. This can be treated by faster asynchronous atrioventricular sequential pacing (to exceed the atrial rate), by the use of temporary DDD pacing or by attempting to slow the atrial rate pharmacologically with β-blockers (47).

Tachyarrhythmias are more difficult to manage. Patients who require high doses of inotropic drugs for weaning from bypass mat develop tachyarrhythmias as drug dosages increase (discussed later under Therapy). Small doses of either a β-blocker or calcium channel blocker may be administered with good effect in the presence of many of these arrhythmias. Both sinus tachycardia and ventricular arrhythmias may indicate myocardial ischemia, so a search for an etiology

FIGURE 15-1. Algorithm for weaning from cardiopulmonary bypass in a patient with hypotension (MAP less than 50 mm Hg). Note the use of transesophageal echocardiography to guide therapy. (MAP, mean arterial pressure; CVP, central venous pressure; PAD, pulmonary artery diastolic pressure; TEE, transesophageal echocardiography; LV, left ventricle; LVED, left ventricular end-diastolic; CPB, cardiopulmonary bypass; IABP, intraaortic balloon pump.)

should be undertaken (45,47,48). This search might include automated or visual multilead ST-segment analysis, wall motion disturbance seen in the surgical field, or by TEE analysis. Tachycardia may also be precipitated by inadequate anesthesia and central hyperthermia from excessive rewarming.

Although most patients benefit from the atrial contribution to ventricular filling seen with the reestablishment of sinus rhythm, there are some patients with chronic atrial fibrillation or severe atrial enlargement (e.g., chronic mitral valve pathology) in whom atrial systole may provide little or no hemodynamic advantage over ventricular pacing. However, other patients with a history of chronic atrial fibrillation demonstrate a higher cardiac output and lower filling pressures during actual or "simulated" sinus rhythm than during single-chamber ventricular pacing (49). It is therefore advisable to attempt electrical cardioversion and atrioventricular sequential pacing in such patients. Even if atrial fibrillation remits for only several hours, this brief period of rhythm stability may assist the patient through the difficult period immediately following CPB.

Sinus rhythm is particularly important to patients with left ventricular hypertrophy or any other problem such as acute ischemia that may render the left ventricle noncompliant. Atrial "kick" may contribute 20% to 40% of the stroke volume in these situations, so every effort should be made to establish a sinus rhythm (50–52).

Anticipated Ventricular Performance and the Need for Pharmacologic or Mechanical Support

Although one cannot predict precisely how the heart will function upon resuming its work after CPB, a number of historical and perioperative factors may help predict myocardial performance. Compromised preoperative ventricular function (defined as an ejection fraction of less than 0.40), preoperative wall motion abnormalities in the distribution of one or more of the three major coronary arteries, and the magnitude of rise in LVEDP following contrast dye injection for left ventriculogram serve as predictors of the need for inotropic drugs after CPB (53). Intraoperatively, the use of TEE before bypass provides a first-hand look at preoperative anatomy, chamber size, and wall motion (38–40). This technique allows a subjective assessment of global ventricular function, regional wall motion abnormalities, and ejection fraction (54). The anesthesiologist may use TEE to determine ventricular function after induction and throughout the procedure as preload, afterload, and contractility are manipulated or modified (55–57). Most often, if the patient had poor left ventricular function before the procedure, one can expect poor ventricular performance during weaning form CPB. Furthermore, the pre-CPB response to anesthetics may serve as a post-CPB predictor of function. If the blood pressure and cardiac output decrease precipitously with administration of small doses of anesthetic agents (in the absence of hypovolemia), then it is possible that high basal sympathetic tone was present and that the heart required endogenous sympathetic support preoperatively. The patient may then require exogenously administered catecholamine support after CPB. Low cardiac outputs before CPB also seem to predict the need for inotropic support following CPB unless the low output resulted from deliberate hypovolemia, from anesthetic-induced myocardial depression by inhalation agents that are no longer present, or from bradycardia related to short-acting β-blocking drugs.

The quality of myocardial protection is important to the preservation of myocardial function after CPB. A good rapport with the surgeon and astute observation of the surgical field during the procedure are useful in assessing the situation at the end of CPB. Although the surgeon may not be eager to critically judge the quality of his or her work at this point, not all coronary revascularizations or valve repairs are of equal quality. The surgeon's opinion of the quality of the revascularization or surgical repair of a valve may be a valuable predictor of myocardial function. Sometimes a request for prophylactic inotropic therapy after a procedure that appeared straightforward may be the first clue that the surgeon is not pleased with the quality of revascularization, repair, or myocardial preservation.

The total time of aortic cross-clamping and the total time of CPB are valuable factors that predict how the heart will perform postoperatively. Cross-clamping times of 120 minutes or longer are associated with a significant risk of irreversible cell damage (58). The shorter the cross-clamp time the better, although the importance of this factor is mitigated to some degree by efficient myocardial preservation techniques. There is evidence for a direct relationship between cross-clamp times and adverse outcomes (53,58,59). If the cross-clamp time was excessive, one should consider the possibility of prolonging reperfusion time to facilitate recovery from global ischemic ventricular dysfunction ("myocardial stunning") (60). Extending reperfusion time or going back on bypass after a troubled postbypass course has been shown to result in improved ventricular function over time (61, 62).

The clinical appearance of the heart at the end of CPB can give insight into post-CPB performance. Although visual examination of the heart from the anesthesiologist's position at the head of the table usually only provides a view of the anterior wall of the right ventricle and a small portion of the left ventricle, this information is still very useful. Are the contractions of the right ventricle as forceful as they were before bypass? Are they as vigorous as they should be? Does the heart seem to be contracting symmetrically? Although these observations are usually helpful, occasionally a heart looks quite vigorous while empty and perfused by the pump-oxygenator, only to fail upon resumption of a normal workload at separation from CPB. The astute anesthesiologist must be alert for the harbingers of acute ventricular dysfunction during removal of the left ventricular vent.

The surgeon often requests that the heart be filled to avoid air entry into the left side of the heart. During this maneuver, partial separation from CPB occurs. If left ventricular ejection is brisk, as evidenced on the arterial waveform, and relatively low pressure is seen on the CVP or pulmonary artery trace, weaning will usually proceed without hemodynamic deterioration. Conversely, if the pulmonary artery diastolic pressure reaches 15 to 20 mm Hg with little or no detectable left ventricular ejection, the patient may need considerable pharmacologic or mechanical support to provide an adequate cardiac output.

In most patients, it seems wise to discontinue volatile anesthetic agents for at least 10 minutes before separation from bypass. If necessary, anesthesia can be supplemented at this time by intravenous agents that have less negative inotropic effects. Even a small dose of a volatile agent can cause significant myocardial depression at this sensitive stage (63,64).

State of the Peripheral and Pulmonary Circulation

The tone of the circulation during bypass can be extremely variable. The use of vasodilators or vasoconstrictors during the bypass period can give an indication of the state of the vasculature immediately preceding weaning. It is useful to do a quick calculation of systemic vascular resistance (SVR) before termination from bypass. The standard formula for calculation of SVR can be used. The pump flow rate is the cardiac output, and CVP is equal to atmospheric pressure (CVP = 0). Before the patient is weaned from bypass, this calculated SVR can be brought into a reasonable range by vasoactive drugs.

The pulmonary vasculature should also be considered, particularly if there was prebypass pulmonary hypertension or right ventricular dysfunction. Acute increases of PVR can be devastating to a right ventricle not exposed to elevated PVR on a chronic basis. Although one cannot measure PVR while the patient is on bypass, every effort should be made to keep pulmonary vasoconstriction as low as possible. Use of nitroglycerin or other pulmonary artery vasodilators may be indicated, as well as careful attention to acidosis and adequacy of ventilation and oxygenation (3,65). Although nitroglycerin and to a lesser extent nitroprusside are the most commonly used drugs to reduce PVR acutely after CPB, their use is often limited by the arterial hypotension that often ensues. In patients with elevated PVR and subsequent poor left ventricular filling despite adequate right ventricular preload after CPB, 15 minutes of inhaled nitric oxide (20 parts per million) reduced PVR and improved left ventricular filling without reducing mean arterial pressure (66).

Evaluation of Reservoir Volume

Consultation with the perfusionist will help determine whether additional circulating blood volume will be needed to successfully separate from CPB. This will depend to some degree on the anticipated level of preload required for separation, which will be lower in patients with good ventricular function. As noted previously, filling the heart for removal of the left ventricular vent allows one to predict the preload necessary for separation as well as the need for inotropic or mechanical support. The presence of a vigorous ejection at a low filling pressure also suggests that intravascular volume augmentation before discontinuation of CPB is required. If additional fluid volume is needed, the hematocrit should be an important consideration. One should not reflexively add crystalloid if this will result in a hematocrit level below 20%, particularly when ischemic ventricular dysfunction is anticipated and when ventricular hypertrophy is present.

TEMPERATURE

Systemic hypothermia is widely used during bypass; therefore, the patient must be rewarmed, and a rewarming end point at which it is considered safe to terminate CPB must be established. Practices vary as to the appropriate gauge of adequate rewarming. Depending on the level of cooling and the point at which the surgeon requests initiation of rewarming, complete rewarming may prolong bypass time, which carries inherent risks. Alternatively, incomplete rewarming sets the stage for exaggerated hypothermic "afterdrop," which results from gradual equilibration of the warm central circulation with peripheral tissues that have remained hypothermic (67–69). Some practitioners choose to accept a moderate degree of afterdrop, reserving the completion of rewarming for the postoperative period. This approach leads to a more vasoconstricted patient in the early period after CPB (68,70). Successful use of this technique requires maintaining adequate anesthesia and muscle relaxation until the patient is fully rewarmed, because striking increases in systemic oxygen consumption will otherwise result from muscle activity as the patient attempts to rewarm himself or herself (70). The physiology of rewarming by heating the bloodstream is dependent on tissue blood flow relationships and is analogous to the uptake and distribution of inhalation anesthetics. The vessel-rich group warms most quickly, the muscle group next, and the fat group last. By the same analogy, the duration of rewarming (similar to the length of time to awaken after inhalation anesthesia) depends on the depth and duration of hypothermia (like the depth and duration of anesthesia). Because the body rewarms from the central circulation, temperature measurements that reflect perfusion by the vessel-rich group (e.g., pulmonary artery catheter, esophageal, and nasopharyngeal measurements) will not adequately reflect rewarming in muscle and fat (67,70). Temperatures measured in the rectum and skin rise more slowly but better indicate the global adequacy of systemic rewarming (69,72). Another convenient and accurate measure of core temperature can also be made in the urinary bladder with a catheter-mounted thermistor. If afterdrop becomes severe enough that it appears to increase postoperative bleeding or risk ventricular arrhythmias, then the duration of rewarming during CPB should be increased.

ANESTHETIC STATE

Because of the potential for hemodynamic instability during and shortly after weaning from CPB, it makes sense to avoid additional anesthetic administration during that period. Supplemental intravenous anesthetics such as opiates, benzodiazepines, and muscle relaxants are best given during rewarming. Even drugs with supposedly benign hemodynamic effects (e.g., fentanyl) can induce hypotension unless given quite cautiously after CPB (73). The lack of hemodynamic effect from a particular drug or drug dose before CPB does not necessarily predict the same response after CPB. In most patients, inhalation anesthetics should be discontinued in anticipation of separation from CPB, because their tendency to depress the heart or decrease SVR is generally undesirable at this time. Despite a lack of objective evidence of harm (74,75), because of its ability to increase the volume of closed gas spaces and the risk of intravascular air after CPB, many practitioners avoid nitrous oxide after CPB.

TIME SINCE CROSS-CLAMP REMOVAL

In a well-intended effort to minimize the total duration of CPB, surgeons and anesthesiologists alike may push to separate the patient from CPB before the heart has had adequate time to recover from the ischemic period during aortic cross-clamping. Even if the cross-clamp was removed before the aortic anastomosis of an aortocoronary vein graft was constructed, the conditions of CPB and the state of the native coronary circulation may limit myocardial recovery during that period (76). The optimal reperfusion time between aortic declamping and separation from CPB cannot be easily specified, because it will vary with the patient's cardiac pathology, the perfusion conditions during CPB, and most important, the quality of myocardial preservation. Clinical observation suggests that even under relatively low-risk conditions, at least 10 to 15 minutes should elapse after removal of the aortic cross-clamp before attempting separation from CPB.

The ideal perfusion pressure during the reperfusion period is unknown. Experimental evidence in animal models strongly suggests that myocardial injury and edema are reduced by avoiding myocardial perfusion pressures of more than 60 mm Hg for the first 10 to 15 minutes after reperfusion (77). Thereafter, sustaining coronary perfusion pressures above 70 mm Hg for the last 5 to 10 minutes of CPB improves outcome (78,79).

HEART FAILURE

Pathophysiology

The etiology of heart failure in the post-CPB period is often multifactorial. It can be related to ischemia incurred from inadequate myocardial protection during the aortic cross-clamp period (53,58), from residual cardioplegic effects (46, 60,61), or from the underlying chronic myocardial dysfunction (10,53). Important also are any acute myocardial insults immediately preceding surgery. Perhaps the myocardium was ischemic at that time or there was a recent infarction. It is useful to try to assess the degree to which postbypass myocardial dysfunction is chronic or acute, because differences in pathophysiology may affect treatment.

Chronic congestive heart failure (CHF) from ischemia, cardiomyopathies, or valvular heart disease results in mechanisms of compensation that involve the myocardium as well as autonomic neurohormonal systems (80). Muscle mass increases, thereby reducing wall stress (Laplace relationship) in the presence of the volume and pressure overload that often accompanies CHF. Thus cardiac hypertrophy does not increase "normal" myocardium. Hypertrophic myocardium exhibits reduced capillary and mitochondrial density, limiting both oxygen delivery and utilization while energy demands increase (81). These conditions reduce the ability of the coronary circulation to deliver substrate for energy production. Although this reduction may not cause ischemia at rest, there may be little reserve for increased energy demands. Systolic contraction abnormalities will result from reduced cyclic adenosine monophosphate (cAMP) levels and a slowing of myosin adenosine triphosphatase activity (81). Further, the action potential is slowed because lack of energy substrate impairs the biochemical pumps necessary for intracellular calcium sequestration. Both systolic contraction and diastolic relaxation are impaired in CHF, because both processes require energy, and energy delivery and utilization are impaired.

Autonomic and endocrine mechanisms attempt to compensate for the low cardiac output state that results from chronic CHF. Sodium overload may be created by increased levels of aldosterone secreted by the adrenal cortex. This sodium excess expands intravascular volume and increases preload to a noncompliant ventricle in an effort to increase cardiac output via the Frank-Starling relationship (81). Increased basal sympathetic tone increases myocardial norepinephrine levels and increases contractility temporarily. This increased sympathetic tone also increase epinephrine secretion from the adrenal medulla, which increases both preload and contractility. A higher level of circulating catecholamines and a secondary activation of angiotensin II and III increase SVR in an effort to support blood pressure. This combination of sodium retention and its concomitant fluid retention, along with increased sympathetic tone and elevated SVR, are the hallmarks of compensated CHF.

These mechanisms, while compensating for decreased

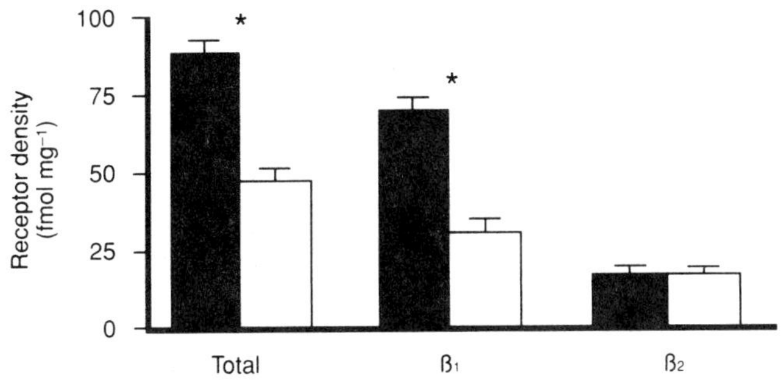

FIGURE 15-4. Alterations in β-receptor populations in failing and nonfailing myocardium. Note the overall decline in β-receptor population in the failing myocardium. However, the β_2-receptors are preserved. Therefore, the relative contribution of these receptors' subtypes is actually increased. β_1- and β_2-receptor densities in ventricular myocardial membranes prepared from nonfailing (■ n = 27) and failing (□ n = 28) human hearts. * = P < 0.05. (From Bristow MR, Port JD, Hershberger RE, et al. The beta-adrenergic receptor–adenylate cyclase complex as a target for therapeutic intervention in heart failure. *Eur Heart J* 1989; 10(B):45, with permission.)

cardiac output, may be detrimental to overall cardiac function. Endogenous myocardial stores of norepinephrine are depleted, due to the chronic stimulation (83). β-Receptor density is reduced by increased serum catecholamines (see Chapter 2). This down-regulation occurs primarily with the β_1-receptors (84). The normal β_1:β_2-receptor ratio of 80:20 decreases in chronic heart failure to approximately 60:40 (Fig. 15-4). The degree to which these phenomena occur relates directly to the degree of ventricular dysfunction. In addition to diminishing receptor density, there is evidence that existing receptors may function abnormally (85). In the healthy heart, stimulation of a β_1-receptor initiates a series of events that increases intracellular cAMP levels, which are important for the release of intracellular calcium stores to initiate contraction. β_1-Receptors in the failing heart do not increase cAMP levels to the same extent (85).

In addition to causing peripheral vasoconstriction, α-receptor stimulation increases myocardial contractility. This increased contractility is not mediated by increased intracellular cAMP levels (86). Vago has found that myocardial α-receptor down-regulation does not occur and that receptor density is not reduced in chronic CHF (87). This supports the assertion that norepinephrine, with its strong stimulation of α-receptors (88), may be beneficial in treating patients with CHF. Smith has demonstrated that the effect of α-adrenergic agonists on the peripheral circulation diminishes in patients with chronic CHF and that higher doses of α-agonists are needed to achieve comparable increases in SVR (89).

The problems of acute ventricular dysfunction caused by CPB are superimposed on whatever chronic abnormalities exist. Myocardium that has been ischemic and possibly damaged presents the greatest challenge. Myocardium that is not perfused and becomes ischemia can show a range of responses from "stunned myocardium"(60, 61) to frankly necrotic muscle tissue—in other words, from fully reversible to totally irreversible injury.

Stunned myocardium is defined as muscle that functions abnormally after being subjected to ischemia (60). This reversible abnormality affects both systolic and diastolic function and may last from hours to days. The mechanisms generating stunned myocardium are completely understood and appear to involve several processes, including a reduction in high-energy phosphate levels (90), generation of superoxide radicals (61), intracellular calcium overload (12), and abnormalities in the microcirculation (probably from cellular edema and capillary compression) (91, 92). The function of this reversibly injured myocardium will improve with inotropes during the recovery period and will return to normal if the proper conditions of oxygen supply and demand are maintained (60). The myocardium is still at risk for irreversible injury. Therefore, appropriate clinical management may influence outcome.

TABLE 15-3. MOST COMMON CAUSES OF RIGHT VENTRICULAR FAILURE AFTER CARDIOPULMONARY BYPASS

Component of biventricular failure
Right coronary artery ischemia or embolism
Increased pulmonary vascular resistance
Tricuspid valvular insufficiency
Localized cardiac tamponade

Although most patients who experience difficulty separating from CPB do so because of left ventricular failure, some patients experience isolated right ventricular dysfunction. Table 15-3 lists the most common causes of post-CPB right ventricular failure. The pathophysiology of increased PVR and tricuspid insufficiency is discussed in Chapter 20, Valvular Heart Disease. The pathophysiology of the other causes of right ventricular failure is similar to that of left ventricular failure.

Therapy

Pharmacologic support is the first line of treatment for the failing myocardium. The final common pathway for most inotropic drugs is the increase in available intracellular calcium for use in the contractile mechanism (64,82,86). Myocardial muscle contains two contractile proteins, actin and myosin. These are under the regulatory control of two other proteins, troponin and tropomyosin. The myocardium develops contractile force by forming cross-bridges between the actin and myosin filaments. In the absence of calcium, the inhibitory protein tropomyosin prevents the interaction between actin and myosin. Depolarization of the cell membrane allows calcium to enter the cell via slow channels during the plateau phase of the action potential. This small amount of extracellular calcium then triggers a large release from the intracellular stores in the sarcoplasmic reticulum. This causes an abrupt rise in calcium available to initiate contraction. Administration of exogenous calcium increases the calcium gradient across the cell membrane, which facilitates transmembrane calcium transport, thereby potentially exerting an inotropic effect. Relaxation is also an energy-dependent process that occurs as calcium is sequestered by the sarcoplasmic reticulum or transported outside the cell.

Myocardial cAMP is produced by the membrane-bound enzyme adenylate cyclase, which is partly under the control of membrane receptors exposed to the extracellular environment. When these receptors are activated, cAMP is produced and activates a protein kinase that modifies the slow channels and allows calcium ions to traverse the slow channels and increase the intracellular calcium concentration. Stimulation of cardia β-adrenergic receptors increases contractility by this mechanism of increasing intracellular levels of cAMP. Phosphodiesterase inhibitors such as milrinone and amrinone exert their inotropic effect by slowing the degradation of cAMP, thus allowing intracellular levels to remain higher longer. The pharmacology of circulatory drugs is discussed in detail in Chapter 3. Anesthesiologists and cardiac surgeons, like clinicians in most other specialties, tend to select a familiar drug for use in particular situations in which they are faced with several options. The most popular first-line drugs for inotropic support after CPB appear to be epinephrine, dobutamine, and dopamine.

Catecholamines

Our institution favors epinephrine for the purpose of post-CPB inotropic support because it is the single drug most likely to simultaneously elevate the blood pressure and cardiac output without causing tachycardia (93). Doses in the range of 0.01 to 0.05 μg/kg/minute are usually effective. This relative predictability makes epinephrine an attractive inotrope for situations in which the frequent measurement of cardiac output is not possible. Tachycardia from catecholamine inotropes can occur after CPB. Patients often require temporary pacing for bradycardia or atrioventricular block at the time of separation from CPB. However, the cardiac conduction system may resume function to unmask the tachycardiac effects of the catecholamine. Although epinephrine clearly can cause tachycardia, this is more likely to occur with moderately inotropic doses of dopamine and dobutamine (5 to 10 μg/kg/minute) (Fig. 15-5) (93).

Dobutamine also increases blood pressure less reliably

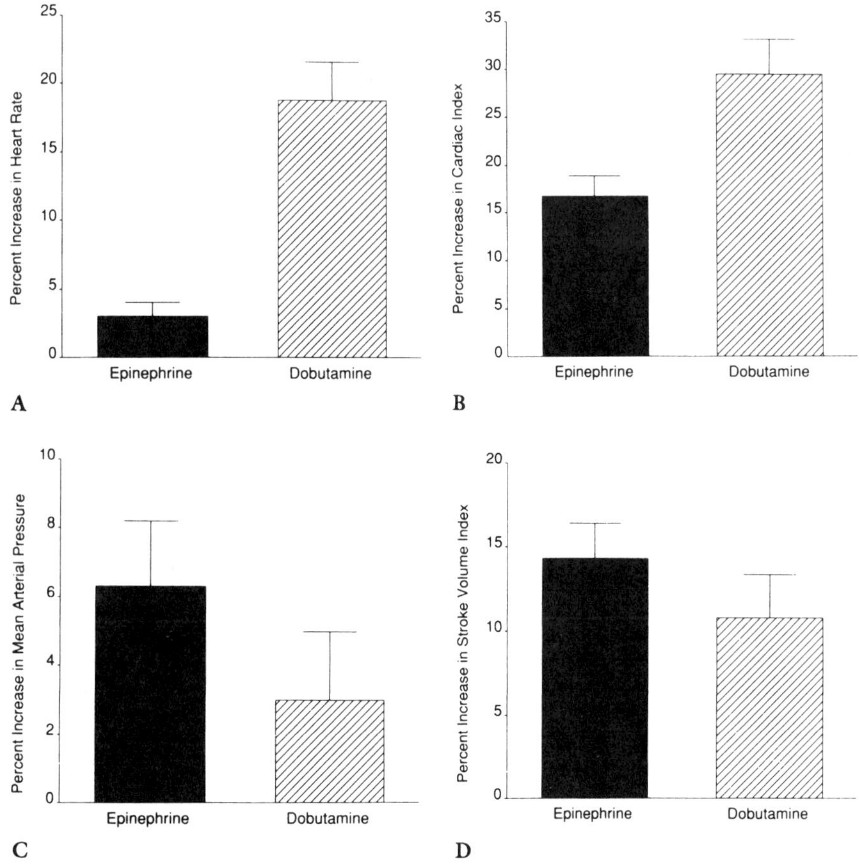

FIGURE 15-5. Hemodynamic responses to dobutamine or epinephrine in postoperative cardiac surgical patients. Note the marked increase in heart rate and cardiac index seen with dobutamine compared to epinephrine. Epinephrine produced a smaller increase in cardiac index but was more effective at increasing arterial pressure. (From Butterworth JF, Prielipp RC, Royster RL, et al. Dobutamine increases heart rate more than epinephrine in patients recovering from aortocoronary bypass surgery. *J Cardiothorac Vasc Anesth* 1992;6:535, with permission.)

than epinephrine or dopamine. Low doses (0.01 to 0.03 μg/kg/minute) of epinephrine may also decrease SVR and blood pressure, apparently because of predominantly nonselective β-adrenergic effects at that dosing level. Clinical experience suggests that when dobutamine and dopamine are used at higher doses for severely depressed hearts, the inotropic effects are more likely to plateau than with epinephrine (93,94). Increase in blood pressure achieved by dopamine doses of more than 10 μg/kg/minute probably result primarily from an α-mediated effect(94,95); therefore, blood pressure might increase at the expense of cardiac output. A similar phenomenon occurs at high doses of epinephrine, but the specific dose level at which this occurs is less well-defined for epinephrine than for dopamine. Despite a lack of efficacy at blood pressure elevation, dobutamine does have one advantage. Some evidence supports the popularity of dobutamine because of its beneficial effects on collateral coronary blood flow in the presence of ischemia, particularly in comparison to dopamine (96,97).

Vasoconstrictors

Vasoconstrictors such as phenylephrine (100 μg intravenously) may be useful either by themselves or in combination with one of the inotropes mentioned previously when low SVR and hypotension coexist either during weaning from CPB or thereafter (89). Elevation of perfusion pressure during the final minutes of CPB would theoretically benefit the heart by increasing coronary blood flow in a beating, nonworking heart. This might enhance myocardial recovery or facilitate washout of small amounts of air that often reach the coronary circulation during coronary revascularization procedures (98). On the other hand, higher coronary perfusion pressures enhance myocardial edema formation during reperfusion from ischemia. Some have chosen to balance these two considerations by avoiding vasopressors for the first 5 to 10 minutes following release of the aortic cross-clamp, then judiciously raising the mean arterial pressure to 70 to 80 mm Hg for the final 5 to 10 minutes preceding separation from bypass. If α_1-agonists are used to raise the blood pressure after CPB, one must be aware of the possibility that SVR may be elevated excessively with this therapy. The most obvious result of this condition is hypertension, but the afterload sensitivity of the left ventricle (and the right ventricle) after CPB makes it possible for arterial pressures to remain low or in the normal range in the face of dangerous elevations in SVR or PVR. Therefore, a potential pitfall in using α_1-agonists after CPB is the resultant rise in SVR, which may provide an adequate arterial pressure at the expense of increased myocardial wall tension, increased oxygen consumption, and declining cardiac output and oxygen delivery. This therapy can lead to progressive myocardial ischemia, metabolic acidosis, and eventually hemodynamic deterioration.

A novel approach to the problem of hypotension and decreased SVR following CPB has been reported. Recently, the use of vasopressin as a continuous infusion has been shown effective in increasing mean arterial pressure after CPB in patients requiring norepinephrine to maintain adequate blood pressure. An infusion rate of 0.1 U/minute increased blood mean arterial pressure and SVR significantly in all patients studied (99).

Drug Combinations

Various combinations of inotropes, vasoconstrictors, and vasodilators are commonly used after CPB. An inotrope-vasoconstrictor combination makes sense when preload is adequate and SVR and cardiac output are both low. It should be remembered that hemodilution is a significant cause of decreased SVR (100). Consequently, the "normal" range of SVR should probably be adjusted downward during and shortly after CPB. This range should be readjusted as hematocrit rises during red blood cell transfusion after CPB. Often, the need for a vasoconstrictor decreases or disappears during reinfusion of washed red blood cells after CPB. Some clinicians choose norepinephrine alone when an inotrope-vasoconstrictor combination appears indicated. This approach offers the simplicity of a single drug, but sacrifices the flexibility of an inotrope-vasoconstrictor combination. Hemodynamics are dynamic after CPB. Therefore, increased flexibility is often an asset. A vasoconstrictor may be needed to support coronary perfusion pressure and SVR while nitroglycerin is used to prevent or treat myocardial ischemia. Vasoconstrictors are also commonly needed to support blood pressure when "inodilator" phosphodiesterase inhibitors are used (101).

Combinations of inotropes and vasodilators are commonly used when the inotrope has mixed α- and β-adrenergic activity. The vasodilator offsets the α-adrenergic–mediated afterload increase caused by such agents as dopamine, epinephrine, and norepinephrine (102). Commonly used vasodilators include sodium nitroprusside and nitroglycerin. Nitroprusside more reliably reduces SVR while nitroglycerin tends to dilate coronary arteries and systemic veins more than the arterioles (103). The combination of norepinephrine and phentolamine (a nonselective α-adrenergic blocker) is used in some centers as first-line therapy for cardiovascular support after CPB. This combination offers the advantage of norepinephrine's potent β-adrenergic inotropic effect while phentolamine is titrated to offset the α-adrenergic vasoconstricting effect.

Phosphodiesterase III Inhibitors

Phosphodiesterase III inhibitors such as amrinone and milrinone have played a major role in the pharmacologic circulatory support following CPB. These agents can be used alone or in combination with another inotrope, a vasopressor, or both (101,104). They are sometimes referred to as "inodilators" because they induce both vasodilation and increased myocardial contractility. A loading dose is required, which is ideally accomplished with the support of CPB, because arterial pressure sometimes decreases (104). Typical loading doses for separation from CPB are 1.5 mg/kg for amrinone and 50 μg/kg for milrinone. If done during CPB, adjustments in perfusion flow and in vasomotor tone can be accomplished readily to create a hemodynamically stable state before imposing a mechanical workload on the heart (105). Often a vasoconstrictor is needed to counteract the vasodilating effect. Using a pure α-adrenergic agonist such as phenylephrine holds some appeal, particularly in view of the gradual rise in SVR that occurs after CPB to which one can easily adapt by titrating the α-agonist. Phosphodiesterase inhibitors synergistically enhance β-adrenergic agonists by slowing the metabolic degradation of the cAMP created by the β-adrenergic agonist. After administration of the loading dose of phosphodiesterase inhibitor, a constant infusion may be started to maintain a stable plasma level. Infusion rates of 0.5 μg/kg/minute for milrinone and 2 to 10 μg/kg/minute for amrinone are commonly used. However, for temporary, transient support required at the time of CPB termination, alternative single dose methods have been described (106,107). The efficacy of phosphodiesterase inhibitors in allowing patients with severely depressed cardiac function to separate from CPB has been well described (104).

Bolus Drugs

Vasoactive drugs probably are most often administered by continuous infusion after CPB, but drugs in this category can be administered as a bolus, either to assist in separation from bypass or to achieve rapid hemodynamic response. Most drugs administered as an infusion can also be given safely as a bolus, but some vasoactive drugs commonly given as a bolus are seldom given as continuous infusions. Calcium chloride and ephedrine are examples of the latter category. Long a mainstay of separation from CPB, calcium chloride (or gluconate) has recently seen less use because of evidence that it attenuates the inotropic response to epinephrine and its detrimental effect on reperfusion injury (108,109). Its popularity may have derived from its predictable ability to elevate blood pressure while seldom inducing hypertension, even in large doses. Drop et al. (109) showed that the hemodynamic response to calcium depends upon the level of ionized calcium at the time of administration. An inotropic response is possible only if the ionized calcium level is subnormal, but the increase in blood pressure seen after administration of intravenous calcium results primarily from an increase in SVR when ionized calcium levels are within the normal range or elevated (9). Additionally, administration of calcium has been shown to cause a impairment of ventricular relaxation and worsening of diastolic dysfunction (110). Because ionized calcium levels are easily obtained, it now appears that calcium administration is not an ideal choice if ionized calcium levels are within the normal range or high. The clinician is cautioned that calcium chloride and calcium gluconate are not equivalent. In addition to providing different amounts of ionized calcium, the gluconate form requires hepatic metabolism. A mixed adrenergic agonist such as ephedrine can also be used as a bolus in this setting with the likely production of an increase in SVR, cardiac output, and heart rate (111). Its best use is in situations in which it is likely that the heart and peripheral circulation will sustain themselves if brief hemodynamic support is given at separation from CPB.

Cardiac Assist Devices

If pharmacologic support is unsuccessful, cardiac assist devices such as the intraaortic balloon pump, venoarterial assist device, ventricular assist device, or total artificial heart may be considered. Theoretically, a reduction in the workload and the subsequent decompression of the failing ventricle will reduce wall tension, reduce oxygen consumption, and allow for myocardial recovery and improved ventricular function. The intraaortic balloon pump is used in situations of low cardiac output syndrome because of its beneficial effects on myocardial energy balance. The inflation of an appropriately sized and positioned balloon in the central aorta, carefully timed to coincide with aortic valve closure, will result in an increased early diastolic pressure, improved coronary perfusion pressure, and improved coronary blood flow. In addition, sudden deflation of the balloon, just before left ventricular ejection, results in a lower arterial pressure at the time of ejection. Consequently, afterload and left ventricular wall tension are decreased and oxygen consumption is reduced.

Animal studies of long-term ventricular support models indicate that improved coronary perfusion pressure, not ventricular decompression, was responsible for preserved left ventricular systolic function and improved response to catecholamine exposure (dobutamine). Interestingly, left ventricular diastolic function worsened in all cases over time regardless of perfusion pressure or degree of left ventricular decompression (112). There have been a number of techniques developed for the mechanical assistance of a failing heart after CPB. Many of these entail the temporary use of external pumps to reduce or eliminate the workload of the struggling heart. These techniques are referred to as "cardiopulmonary support" devices to differentiate them from standard bypass apparatus (CPB) and more specialized extracorporeal membrane oxygenation systems. Temporary cardiopulmonary support assistance is appropriate if the myocardial dysfunction is judged to be amenable to treatment or is otherwise likely to be transient (113). Recovery of significant cardiac function after "resting" a stunned myocardium is a typical scenario. Other indications for the use of a temporary external device would entail emergency "bridging" to either transplant or the implantation of a more permanent internal device. There is no doubt that such inexpensive, temporary external devices work in these situations. In a review of 129 post-CPB cardiac failure patients placed on a centrifugal pump device, fully 56% were later successfully weaned from the device and 21% were later discharged from the hospital (114). These results are typical of a single chamber assist for cardiac failure following CPB (114–117). In many studies of mechanical support following bypass, more than half of the patients die during or after the support. Both weaning rates and survival-to-discharge rates may be higher in those patients treated with biventricular assistance. Kitamura et al. have reported very similar weaning and discharge rates for patients treated with single ventricle assist: 50% of all venoarterial bypass patients were successfully weaned and 26.7% were discharged. Eighty-seven percent of left ventricular assist patients were weaned, but only 37.5% were discharged. Contrast these survival rates with those of the patients treated with both right and left ventricular assist devices. Seventy-six percent were successfully weaned and 57% survived to discharge from the hospital (116). The authors conclude that early application of the devices to patients in need and the application of a biventricular device improve outcome and survival.

Although there is no doubt that ventricular assist devices improve outcome in patients who cannot be separated from bypass, there are other less invasive and less expensive measures that can be used in select individuals. Simple methods such as insertion of an intraaortic balloon pump or delayed sternal closure may be all that is necessary to permit termination of CPB. In a review of 60 patients with postbypass low cardiac output syndrome, delayed sternal closure allowed for resolution of the low cardiac output state in 75% of the patients. The remaining 25% required either intraaortic balloon pump or left ventricular assist device support. The overall patient survival rate of 47% was typical for post-CPB cardiac failure (118).

Patients who require more than transient cardiovascular support and for whom transplantation is not likely to occur promptly may require a more permanent form of mechanical assistance. Semipermanent devices exist—and more are in development—that can maintain adequate circulation for weeks, months, and potentially years (119–121). Totally implantable biventricular devices weighing less than 6 kg have been developed (122). Others are completely internalized and require no physical connection with the external environment for electrical or control functions (123).

HYPERTENSION

Although hypertension seldom occurs during or immediately after weaning from CPB, it may occur before the patient leaves the operating room. Vasodilators may be needed to control the blood pressure. Systolic blood pressure exceeding 150 mm Hg or mean arterial pressures of more than 100 mm Hg shortly after CPB are undesirable because hypertension may disrupt fresh aortic suture lines or cannulation sites, causing severe hemorrhage or aortic dissection. The anesthesiologist should consider the causes of hypertension—inadequate anesthesia, hypoxia, and hypercarbia—before assuming that vasodilation or β-adrenergic blockade constitute the best initial approach. If the blood pressure or heart rate increase in response to surgical stimulation such as sternal wire placement or transfer of the patient to the intensive care unit, strong consideration should be given to the need for additional anesthesia. Often a short-acting vasodilator will also be needed. Nitroglycerin or nitroprusside are often selected because they are easily titrated and their effects rapidly remit upon discontinuation. Esmolol is the β-adrenergic blocker of choice in these patients for similar reasons. The short duration of action and titratability are important because of the hemodynamic liability of postoperative cardiac surgical patients. More recently, fenoldopam, a dopamine-1 receptor agonist has been proposed as a safe and effective alternative to sodium nitroprusside for the treatment of post-CPB hypertension (124). Although clinical experience in the cardiac surgical arena is scant, fenoldopam appears to have the advantage over nitroprusside in its ability to lower blood pressure while maintaining renal blood flow and glomerular filtration rate in healthy kidneys and in those acutely impaired by contrast-induced dysfunction (125,126).

Later in the postoperative course, longer acting vasodilating agents can be used to control persistent hypertension. labetalol, hydralazine, and chlorpromazine have been used in this situation. However, their relatively long half-lives limit their usefulness in the dynamic post-CPB setting. Chlorpromazine, although effective, is particularly dangerous to the unwary anesthesiologist. Supplied in ampules containing 25 mg, the drug must be diluted and administered carefully in 1-mg increments until the desired effect is reached. Its combined sedative and α-receptor blocking properties, combined with its long duration of action, make treatment of an inadvertent overdose difficult.

PROTAMINE REACTIONS

One of the more dramatic complications of separation from CPB can occur during reversal of heparin-induced anticoagulation with protamine. An otherwise uncomplicated cardiac surgical case can be transformed into a true medical emergency with the administration of protamine. However, heparin must be reversed in the immediate post-CPB period to allow adequate assessment of surgical homeostasis. Failure of adequate and prompt heparin reversal with protamine can result in hemodynamic instability and increased utilization of blood and blood products.

Protamine reactions are not rare. The reported incidence is typically less than 2% (127). A higher apparent clinical incidence probably reflects differing practice patterns, different patient populations, and a lack of a uniform definition of what constitutes a protamine reaction. Most commonly, administration of protamine to human patients results in transient arterial hypotension (128). This reaction is associated with an increase in plasma histamine levels and results in a decrease in blood pressure without alteration in cardiac output or right- and left-sided filling pressures (129). Therapy is limited to administration of additional intravascular volume and/or a change in patient position.

A second and more serious type of reaction to protamine is an anaphylactoid response to the drug. This response may be mediated by immunoglobulins, which react with protamine as an antigen. If the immunoglobulin is of the IgE variety, a true anaphylactoid response can occur. Vasoactive mediators liberated from degranulated mast cells result in hypotension, increased vascular permeability, and cardiovascular collapse. Skin tests have demonstrated protamine-reacting immunoglobulins in humans, including some who have suffered a protamine reaction (129,130). However, these skin tests are dangerous, lack sensitivity and specificity (131), and cannot be used reliably shortly after a protamine reaction (132). In addition, some anaphylactoid reactions can occur without immunoglobulin-mediated alterations in vascular reactivity. These reactions are probably mediated by the complement system or by direst pharmacologic triggers (133). Although the are complex enzyme-linked immunoelectrophoretic techniques (135) and radioallergosorbent assays (136) to detect antiprotamine antibodies, the presence of antibodies is not a reliable predictor of protamine sensitivity (127,136,137). Treatment of a suspected protamine allergic response is supportive. Additional fluid administration and the Trendelenburg position may need to be supplemented with an infusion of epinephrine to support blood pressure and limit the reaction. Administration of steroids has been advocated.

The most serious type of protamine reaction is that associated with catastrophic pulmonary vasoconstriction. Unlike the common hypotensive response associated with a decreased SVR or the anaphylactoid type characterized by a sudden decrease in filling pressures, this response is associated with sudden, dramatic increases in PVR and acute dysfunction of the right side of the heart (138). This particular cardiovascular response to protamine is easily reproduced in the laboratory in both sheep and dog models (139–141). The vasoconstriction is associated with transient thrombocytopenia, leukopenia, and hypoxia. Although the exact mechanism is controversial, it is probably produced by complement activation and/or release of vasoconstricting cyclooxygenase products of arachidonic acid, thromboxane (Fig. 15-6). High levels of complement C5a, thromboxane A_2, and its more stable metabolite, thromboxane B, are found in both animal models and in human subjects (141–143). The receptors for thromboxane can be blocked in animal models, which effectively prevents the pulmonary vasoconstrictive consequences of protamine exposure (141, 144). However, these receptor blockers also interfere with platelet function and are too long-acting for clinical use in humans in their present form (145). Catastrophic pulmonary vasoconstriction can be so hemodynamically devastating that reheparinization and a return to CPB may be indicated. After institution of supportive catecholamine infusions, pulmonary vascular dilators, and possibly intraaortic balloon pump placement, a second separation from CPB should be attempted. Strong consideration should be given to omit reversal of anticoagulation.

Protamine administration is not without risk. The risk can be minimized by administration of the drug slowly and in dilute form. The incidence of hypotensive reactions associated with protamine increases with increased rate of deliv-

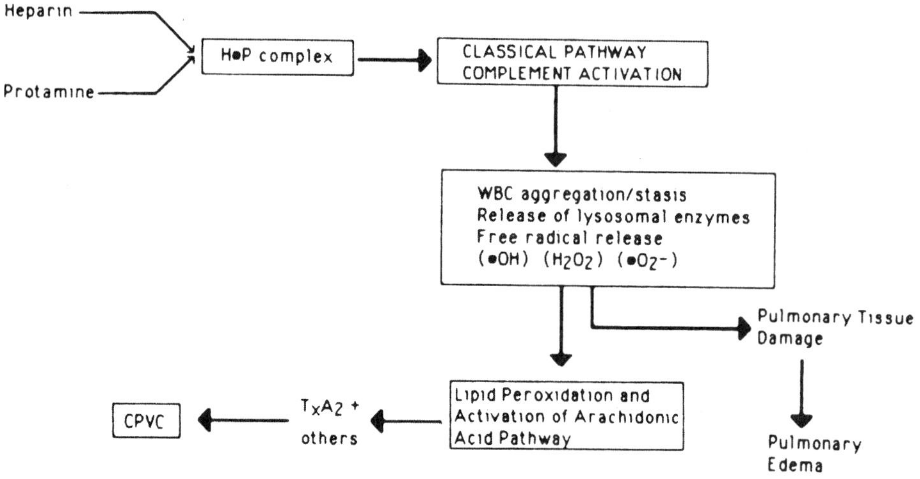

FIGURE 15-6. One theory of the etiology of the catastrophic pulmonary vasoconstriction reaction to protamine. (From Horrow JC. Protamine allergy. *J Cardiothorac Anesth* 1988; 2:225, with permission.)

ery (141,146,147). Dilution may confer even more of a safety margin (148). On the other hand, administration of protamine into the left side of the heart or into the arterial system appears to be of no additional benefit and should be avoided (149,150).

REFERENCES

1. Cingolani HE, Faulkner SL, Mattiazzi AR, et al. Depression of human myocardial contractility with "respiratory" and metabolic acidosis. *Surgery* 1975;77:427.
2. Cingolani HE, Mattiazzi AR, Blesa ES, et al. Contractility in isolated mammalian heart muscle after acid base changes. *Circ Res* 1970;26:269.
3. Fullerton DA, Kirson LE, Cyr JA, et al. The influence of respiratory acid-base status on adult pulmonary vascular resistance before and after cardiopulmonary bypass. *Chest* 1993;103:1091.
4. Frazier HS. Life threatening electrolyte abnormalities. In: May HL, ed. *Emergency medicine.* New York: John Wiley and Sons, 1984:222.
5. Lehot JJ, Piriz H, Villard J, et al. Glucose homeostasis: comparison between hypothermic and normothermic cardiopulmonary bypass. *Chest* 1992:102:106.
6. D'Alecy LG, Lundy ER, Barton KJ. Dextrose-containing intravenous fluid impairs outcome and increases death after eight minutes of cardiac arrest and resuscitation in dogs. *Surgery* 1986; 100:505.
7. Longstreth WT, Invi TS. High blood glucose level on hospital admission and poor neurological outcome after cardiac arrests. *Ann Neurol* 1984;15:59.
8. Pulsinelli WA. Increased damage after ischemic stroke in patients with hyperglycemia with or without established diabetes mellitus. *Am J Med* 1983;74:540.
9. Shapira N, Scharf HV, White RD, et al. Hemodynamic effects of calcium chloride injection following cardiopulmonary bypass: response to bolus injection and continuous infusion. *Ann Thorac Surg* 1984;37:133.
10. Reimer KA, Jennings RB, Tatum AH. Pathobiology of acute myocardial ischemia: metabolic, functional and ultrastructural studies. *Am J Cardiol* 1983;52:72A.
11. Opie LH, Coetzee WA. Are calcium ions involved in the genesis of early ischemic ventricular arrhythmias? In: Hearse DJ, Manning AS, Janse MJ, eds. *Life threatening arrhythmia's during ischemia and infarction.* New York: Raven Press, 1987:63.
12. Kusuoka H, Proterfield JK, Weisman HF, et al. Pathophysiology and pathogenesis of stunned myocardium: depressed Ga +2 activation of contraction as a consequence of reperfusion-induced cellular calcium overload in ferret hearts. *J Clin Invest* 1987;79:950.
13. Kitakaze M, Weisman HF, Marban E. Contractile dysfunction and ATP depletion after transient calcium overload in perfused ferret hearts. *Circulation* 1988;77:685.
14. Burch GE, Giles TE. The importance of magnesium deficiency in cardiovascular disease. *Am Heart J* 1977;95:649.
15. Iseri LT, Freed J, Bures AR. Magnesium deficiency and cardiac disorders. *Am J Med* 1975;58:837.
16. Turlapy PD, Altura BM. Magnesium deficiency produces spasms of coronary arteries: relationship to etiology of sudden death and ischemic heart disease. *Sconce* 1980;208:198.
17. Scheinmen MM, Sullivan RW, Hyatt KH. Magnesium metabolism in patients undergoing cardiopulmonary bypass. *Circulation* 1969;39:235.
18. Chernow B, Smith J, Rainey TG, et al. Hypomagnesemia: implications for critical care specialists. *Crit Care Med* 1982;10: 193.
19. England MR, Gordon G, Salem M, et al. Magnesium administration and dysrhythmia after cardiac surgery: a placebo-controlled double-blind, randomized trial. *JAMA* 1992;17:2395.
20. Folk FS, Bailey CP, Hirose T. Open-heart surgery without blood transfusion. *J Natl Med Assoc* 1969;61:213.
21. Ott DA, Cooley DA. Cardiovascular surgery in Jehovah's Witnesses. *JAMA* 1977;238:736.
22. Niinikosi J, Laaksonen V, Meretoja O. Oxygen transport to tissue under normovolemic moderate and extreme hemodilution during coronary bypass operation. *Ann Thorac Surg* 1981; 31:1354.
23. Tyson GS, Sladen RN, Spainhour V, et al. Blood conservation in cardiac surgery. Preliminary results with an institutional commitment. *Ann Surg* 1989;209:736.
24. Kolins J, Kolins MB. Informed consent, risk, and blood transfusion. *J Thorac Cardiovasc Surg* 1990;100:88.
25. Butler BD, Laine GA, Seiman BC, et al. Effect of Trendelenbuerg position on the distribution of arterial air emboli in dogs. *Ann Thorac Surg* 1988;45:198.
26. Oka Y, Moriwaki KM, Hong Y, et al. Detection of air emboli in the left heart by M-mode transesophageal echocardiography following cardiopulmonary bypass. *Anesthesiology* 1985;63:109.
27. Mohr R, Lavee J, Goor DA. Inaccuracy of radial artery pressure measurement after cardiac operations. *J Thorac Cardiovasc Surg* 1987;94:286.
28. Stern DH, Gerson JI, Allen FB, et al. Can we trust the direct radial artery pressure immediately following cardiopulmonary bypass? *Anesthesiology* 1980;62:364.
29. Pauca AL, Meredith JW. Possibility of A-V shunting upon cardiopulmonary bypass discontinuation. *Anesthesiology* 1987;67: 91.
30. Yelderman M, Quinn MD, McKown RC, et al. Continuous thermodilution cardiac output measurement in sheep. *J Thorac Cardiovasc Surg* 1992;104:315.
31. Yelderman M, Ramsay MA, Quinn MD, et al. Continuous thermodilution cardiac output measurement in intensive care patients. *J Cardiothorac Vasc Anesth* 1992;6:270.
32. Douglas PS, Edmunds LH, Sutton MS, et al. Unreliability of hemodynamic indexes of left ventricular size during cardiac surgery. *Ann Thorac Surg* 1987;44:31.
33. Hansen RM, Viquerat CE, Matthay R, et al. Poor correlation between pulmonary arterial wedge pressure and left ventricular end-diastolic volume after coronary artery bypass graft surgery. *Anesthesiology* 1986;64:764.
34. Ellis RJ, Mangano DT, Van Dyke DC. Relationship of wedge pressure to end-diastolic volume in patients undergoing myocardial revascularization. *J Thorac Cardiovasc Surg* 1979;78:605.
35. Braunwald E. Regulation of the circulation. *N Engl J Med* 1974; 290:1124.
36. Braunwald E. Contraction of the normal heart. In: Braunwald E, ed. *Heart disease.* Philadelphia: WB Saunders, 1992.
37. Grossman W, McLaurin LP. Diastolic properties of the left ventricle. *Ann Intern Med* 1976;84:316.
38. Leung JM, O'Kelly B, Browner WS, et al. Prognostic importance of post-bypass regional wall-motion abnormalities in patients undergoing coronary artery bypass surgery. *Anesthesiology* 1989;70:19.
39. Van Daele MERM, Sutherland GR, Mitchell MM, et al. Do changes in pulmonary capillary wedge pressure adequately reflect myocardial ischemia during anesthesia? A correlative preoperative hemodynamic, electrocardiographic, and transesophageal echocardiographic study. *Circulation* 1990;81:865.
40. Smith JS, Cahalan MK, Benefiel DJ, et al. Intraoperative detection of myocardial ischemia in high-risk patients: electrocardiog-

raphy versus two-dimensional transesophageal echocardiography. *Circulation* 1985;72:1015.
41. Montero JA, Anguita M, Concha M, et al. Pacing requirements after orthotopic heart transplantation: incidence and related factors. *J Heart Lung Transplant* 1992;11:799.
42. Thormann J, Schwarz F. Long-term observation of cardiac arrhythmia's urine and after cardiac surgery. *Scan J Thorac Cardiovasc Surg* 1976;10:149.
43. Magilligan DJ, Vij D, Peper W, et al. Failure of standard cardioplegic techniques to protect the conducting system. *Ann Thorac Surg* 1985;39:403.
44. Latson TW, Lappas DG. Use of a pacing catheter to control heart rate in a patient with aortic insufficiency and coronary artery disease. *Anesthesiology* 1985;63:712.
45. Dennis SC, Coetzee WA, deJong JW, et al. Effects of coronary flow, pacing rate, isoprenaline and diltiazem on ischemic ventricular arrhythmia's in guinea pig hearts. *J Pharmacol Exp Ther* 1989;248:372.
46. Broka SM, Ducart AR, Collard EL, et al. Hemodynamic benefit of optimizing atrioventricular delay after cardiopulmonary bypass. *J Cardiothorac Vasc Anesth* 1997;11(6):723.
47. Elsherif N, Scherlag BJ, Lazzara R. Electrode catheter recording during malignant ventricular arrhythmia following experimental acute myocardial ischemia: evidence for re-entry due to conduction delay and block in ischemic myocardium. *Circulation* 1975;51:1003.
48. Donovan KD, Dobb GJ, Lee K-Y. Hemodynamic benefit of maintaining atrioventricular syndrome during cardiac pacing in critically ill patients. *Crit Care Med* 1991;19:320.
49. Wiggers CJ, Katz LN. The contours of ventricular volume curves under different conditions. *Am J Physiol* 1965;209:1601.
50. Gesell RA. Auricular systole and its relation to ventricular output. *Am J Physiol* 1911;29:32.
51. Stauffer J-C, Gaash WH. Recognition and treatment of left ventricular diastolic dysfunction. *Prog Cardiovasc Dis* 1990;32:319.
52. Royster RL, Butterworth JF, Prough DS, et al. Perioperative and intraoperative predictors of inotropic support and long-term outcome in patients having coronary artery bypass grafting. *Anesth Analg* 1991;72:729.
53. Smith MD, MacPhail B, Harrison MR, et al. Value and limitations of transesophageal echocardiography in determination of left ventricular volumes and ejection fraction. *J Am Coll Cardiol* 1992;19:1213.
54. Harpole DH, Rankin JS, Wofle WG, et al. Effects of standard mitral valve replacement on left ventricular function. *Ann Thorac Surg* 1989;209:356.
55. Dormehl IC, Hugo N, van Gelder AL, et al. Left ventricular volume and function changes during beta-blockade and accompanying atrial pacing. *Am J Physiol Imaging* 1991;4:151.
56. Harpole DH, Clements FM, Quill T, et al. Right and left ventricular performance during and after abdominal aortic aneurysm repair. *Ann Surg* 1989;209:356.
57. Cooley DA, Reul GJ, Wwukasch DC. Ischemic myocardial contracture ("stone heart"): a complication of cardiac surgery. *Isr J Med Sci* 1975;11:203.
58. Townes BD, Bashein G, Hornbein TF, et al. Neurobehavioral outcomes in cardiac operations: a prospective controlled study. *J Thorac Cardiovasc Surg* 1989;98:774.
59. Braunwald E, Kloner RA, The stunned myocardium: prolonged post-ischemic ventricular dysfunction. *Circulation* 1982;66:1146.
60. Bolli R. Mechanism of myocardial "stunning." *Circulation* 1990;82:723.
61. Bolli R. Oxygen-derived free radicals and post-ischemic myocardial dysfunctions ("stunned myocardium"). *J Am Coll Cardiol* 1988;12:239.
62. Marijic J, Bosnjak ZJ, Stowe DF, et al. Effects and interaction of verapamil and volatile anesthetics on the isolated perfused guinea pig heart. *Anesthesiology* 1988;69:914.
63. Rusy BF, Komai H. Anesthetic depression of myocardial contractility: a review of possible mechanisms. *Anesthesiology* 1987;67:745.
64. D'Ambra MN, Laraia PJ, Philbin DM, et al. Prostaglandin E: a new therapy for refractory right heart failure and pulmonary hypertension after mitral valve replacement. *J Thorac Cardiovasc Surg* 1985;89:567.
65. Argenziano M, Choudhri AF, Moazami N, et al. Randomized, double-blind trial of inhaled nitric oxide in LVAD recipients with pulmonary hypertension. *Ann Thorac Surg* 1998;66(5):1862.
66. Davis FJ, Paraimelzhagan KN, Harris EA. Thermal balance during cardiopulmonary bypass with moderate hypothermia in man. *Br J Anaesth* 1977;49:1127.
67. Sladen RN. Temperature and ventilation after hypothermic cardiopulmonary bypass. *Anesth Analg* 1985;64:816.
68. Stupfel M, Severinghaus JW. Internal body temperature gradients during anesthesia and hypothermia and effect of vagotomy. *J Appl Physiol* 1956;9:380.
69. Zwischenberger JB, Mirsh MM, Dechert RE, et al. Suppression of shivering decreases oxygen consumption and improves hemodynamic stability during postoperative rewarming. *Ann Thorac Surg* 1987;43:428.
70. Bone ME, Feneck RO. Bladder temperature as an estimate of body temperature during cardiopulmonary bypass. *Anaesthesia* 1988;43:181.
71. Horrow JC, Rosenberg H. Does urinary temperature reflect core temperature during cardiac surgery? *Anesthesiology* 1988;69:986.
72. Bovill JG, Sebel PS, Stanley TH. Opioid analgesics in anesthesia: with special reference to their use in cardiovascular anesthesia. *Anesthesiology* 1987;61:731.
73. Wells DG, Podalakin W, Mohr M, et al. Nitrous oxide and cerebral spinal fluid markers of ischemia following cardiopulmonary bypass. *Anaesth Intensive Care* 1987;15:431.
74. Adams HA, Kling D, Boldt J, et al. Effects of nitrous oxide on endocrine stress response and hemodynamic parameters during coronary artery surgery. *Thorac Cardiovasc Surg* 1990;38:73.
75. Schaff HV, Ciardullo RC, Flaherty JT, et al. Development of regional myocardial ischemia distal to critical coronary stenosis during cardiopulmonary bypass: comparison of the fibrillating vs the beating nonworking states. *Surgery* 1978;83:57.
76. Slogoff S, Reul GJ, Keats AS, et al. Role of perfusion pressure and flow in major organ dysfunction after cardiopulmonary bypass. *Ann Thorac Surg* 1990;50:911.
77. Leonov Y, Sterz F, Safarr P, et al. Hypertension with hemodilution prevents multifocal cerebral hypoperfusion after cardiac arrest in dogs. *Stroke* 1992;23:453.
78. Steers F, Leonov Y, Safar P, et al. Hypertension with or without hemodilution after cardiac arrest in dogs. *Stroke* 1990;21:1178.
79. Katz AM. The myocardium in congestive heart failure. *Am J Cardiol* 1989;63:12A.
80. Krowski W. Compensatory and adaptive mechanisms in congestive heart failure. *J Cardiovasc Pharmacol* 1989;14:55.
81. Royster RL. Intraoperative administration of inotropes in cardiac surgery patients. *J Cardiothorac Anesth* 1990;70:125.
82. Rutenberg HL, Sponn JF. Alterations of cardiac sympathetic neurotransmitter activity in congestive heart failure. *Am J Cardiol* 1973;32:472.
83. Bristow MR, Ginsberg R, Umans U, et al. β_1 and β_2-adrenergic

receptor subpopulations in normal and failing human ventricular myocardium: coupling of both receptor subtypes to muscle contraction and selective β_1 receptor down regulation in heart failure. *Circ Res* 1986;59:297.
84. Brodde OE, Schuler S, Kretsch R, et al. Regional distribution of beta-adrenoceptors in the human heart: coexistence of functional $beta_1$- and $beta_2$-adrenoceptors in both atria and ventricles in severe congestive cardiomyopathy. *J Cardiovasc Pharmacol* 1986;8:1235.
85. Beveridge MJ, Irvine RF. Inositol triphosphate: a novel second messenger in cellular transudation. *Nature* 1984;312:315.
86. Vago T. Identification of alpha-adrenergic receptors on sarcolemma from normal subjects and patients with idiopathic dilated cardiomyopathy: characteristics and linkage to GTP-binding protein. *Circ Res* 1989;64:474.
87. Ruffolo RR, Messick K. Inotropic selectively of dobutamine enantiomers in pithed rats. *J Pharmacol Exp Ther* 1985;235:344.
88. Smith C. Alpha-adrenergic agonist drugs: left ventricular function and emergence from cardiopulmonary bypass. *J Cardiothorac Anesth* 1990;4:681.
89. Reimer KA, Hill ML, Jennings RB. Prolonged depletion of ATP and of the adenine nucleotide pool due to delayed resynthesis of adenine nucleotides following reversible myocardial ischemic injury in dogs. *Mol Cell Cardiol* 1981;13:229.
90. Kloner RA, Ganote CE, Jennings RB. The "no-reflow" phenomenon after temporary coronary occlusion in the dog. *J Clin Invest* 1974;54:1496.
91. Kloner RA, Rude RE, Carlson N, et al. Ultrastructural evidence of microvascular damage and myocardial cell injury after coronary artery occlusion: which comes first? *Circulation* 1974;62:945.
92. Butterworth JF, Prielipp RC, Royster RL, et al. Dobutamine increases heart rate more than epinephrine in patients recovering from aortocoronary bypass surgery. *J Cardiothorac Vasc Anesth* 1992;6:535.
93. Szerlip HM. Renal-dose dopamine: fact and fiction. *Ann Intern Med* 1991;115:153.
94. Brown L. Pharmacological responses to dopamine isolated guinea pig cardiovascular tissues: mechanisms of action. *Arch Int Pharmacodyn Ther* 1990;308:47.
95. Muller HS, Evans R, Ayres SM. Effect of dopamine on hemodynamics and myocardial metabolism in shock following acute myocardial infarction in man. *Circulation* 1978;57:361.
96. Maekawa K, Liang CS, Hood WB Jr.. Comparison of dobutamine and dopamine in acute myocardial infarction. *Circulation* 1983;67:750.
97. Robicsek P, Duncan GD. Retrograde air embolization in coronary operations. *J Thorac Cardiovasc Surg* 1987;94:110.
98. Argenziano M, Choudhri AF, Oz MC, et al. A prospective randomized trial of arginine vasopressin in the treatment of vasodilatory shock after left ventricular assist device placement. *Circulation* 1997;96[Suppl 9]:286.
99. Rand PW, Lacombe E, Hunt HE, et al. Viscosity of normal human blood under normothermic and hypothermic conditions. *J Appl Physiol* 1964;19:117.
100. Goenen M. Historical perspectives and update of amrinone. *J Cardiovasc Anesth* 1989;3:15.
101. Dell'Italia LJ, Starling MR, Blumhardt R, et al. Comparative effects of volume loading, dobutamine, and nitroprusside in patients with predominant right ventricular infarction. *Circulation* 1985;72:1327.
102. Abrams J. Mechanism of action of nitrates. In: Abrams J, Pepine CJ, Thadani V, eds. *Medical therapy of ischemic heart disease: nitrates, beta-blockers and calcium antagonists.* Boston, MA: Little, Brown and Company, 1992:79.
103. Rutman HI, LeJemtel TH, Sonnenblick EH. Newer cardiotonic agents: implications for patients with heart failure and ischemic heart disease. *J Cardiothorac Anesth* 1987;1:59.
104. Baim DS. Effect of phosphodiesterase inhibition on myocardial oxygen consumption and coronary blood flow. *Am J Cardiol* 1989;63:23.
105. Kikura M, Levy JH, Bailey JM, et al. A bolus dose of 1.5 mg/kg amrinone effectively improves low cardiac output state following separation from cardiopulmonary bypass in cardiac surgical patients. *Acta Anaesth Scand,* 1998;42(7):825.
106. Kikura M, Levy JH, Michelsen LG, et al. The effect of milrinone on hemodynamics and left ventricular function after emergence from cardiopulmonary bypass. *Anesth Analg* 1997;85(1):16.
107. Royster RL, Butterworth JF, Prielipp RC, et al. A randomized blinded placebo-controlled evaluation of calcium chloride and epinephrine for inotropic support after emergence from cardiopulmonary bypass. *Anesth Analg* 1992;74:3.
108. Zaloga GP, Strickland RA, Butterworth JF, et al. Calcium attenuates epinephrine's beta-adrenergic effects in postoperative heart surgery patients. *Circulation* 1990;81:196.
109. Drop LJ, Scheidegger D. Plasma ionized calcium concentration: important determinant of the hemodynamic response to calcium infusion. *J Thorac Cardiovasc Surg* 1980;795:425.
110. DeHert SG, Ten Broecke PW, DeMulder PA, et al. Effects of calcium on left ventricular function early after cardiopulmonary bypass. *J Cardiothorac Vasc Anesth* 1997;11(7):864.
111. Weiner N. Norepinephrine, epinephrine and the sympathomimetic amines. In: Gillman AG, Goodman LS, Rall TW, et al., eds. *The pharmacologic basis of therapeutics.* New York: Macmillan, 1985:145.
112. Komeda M, DeAnda A Jr, Glasson JR, et al. Complete unloading alone may not adequately protect the left ventricle. *Ann Thorac Surg* 1997;64(5):1250.
113. von Segesser LK. Cardiopulmonary support and extracorporeal membrane oxygenation for cardiac assist. *Ann Thorac Surg* 1999;68(2):627.
114. Noon GP, Ball JW Jr, Short HD. Bio-Medicus centrifugal ventricular support for postcardiotomy cardiac failure: a review of 129 cases. *Ann Thorac Surg* 1996;61(1):291.
115. Orime Y, Shiono M, Hata H, et al. Clinical experiences of percutaneous cardiopulmonary support: its effectiveness and limit. *Artif Organs* 1998;22(6):498.
116. Kitamura M, Aomi S, Hachida M, et al. Current strategy of temporary circulatory support for severe cardiac failure after operation. *Ann Thorac Surg* 1999;68(2):662.
117. Koyanagi H, Kitamura M, Aomi S, et al. Mechanical circulatory support for severe heart failure after operation. *Artif Organs* 1998;22(1):82.
118. Freeman RK, Daily PO, Dembitsky WP, et al. The treatment of low cardiac output syndrome following cardiopulmonary bypass using delayed sternal closure. *Am Surg* 1997;63(10):882.
119. Scheld HH, Hammel D, Schmid C, et al. Beating heart implantation of a wearable NOVACOR left-ventricular assist device. *Thorac Cardiovasc Surg* 1996;44(2):62.
120. Hendry PJ, Masters RG, Ibrahim M, et al. In vivo evaluation of an intrathoracic ventricular assist device. *ASAJO J* 1999;45(3):123.
121. Tector AJ, Kress DC, Downey FX, et al. Transition from cardiopulmonary bypass to the HeartMate left ventricular assist device. *Ann Thorac Surg* 1998;65(3):643.
122. von Segesser LK, Tkebuchava T, Lesosek B, et al. Biventricular assist using a portable driver in combination with implanted devices: preliminary experience. *Artif Organs* 1997;21(1):72.
123. Musivand T, Hendry PJ, Masters RG, et al. A remotely controlled and powered artificial heart pump. *Artif Organs* 1996;20(12):1314.

124. Gombotz H, Plaza J, Mahla E, et al. DA-1 receptor stimulation by fenoldopam in the treatment of postcardiac surgical hypertension. *Acta Anaesth Scand* 1998;42(7):834.
125. Mathur VS, Swan SK, Lambrecht LJ, et al. The effects of fenoldopam, a selective dopamine receptor agonist, on systemic and renal hemodynamics in normotensive subjects. *Crit Care Med* 1999;27(9):1832.
126. Bakris GL, Lass NA, Glock D. Renal hemodynamics in radiocontrast medium-induced renal dysfunction: a role for dopamine-1 receptors. *Kidney Int* 1999;56(1):206.
127. Levy JH, Zaidan JR, Faraj B. Prospective evaluation of risk of protamine reactions in patients with NPH insulin-dependent diabetes. *Anesth Analg* 1986;65:739.
128. O'Reilly RA. Anticoagulant, antithrombotic, and thrombotic drugs. In: Gillman AG, Goodman LS, Rall TW, et al., eds. *The pharmacologic basis of therapeutics.* New York: Macmillan, 1985: 1344.
129. Michaels IA, Barash PG. Hemodynamic changes during protamine administration. *Anesth Analg* 1983;62:831.
130. Samuael T, Kolk A. Auto-antigenicity of human protamines. In: Leopow IH, Croizer R, eds. *Vasectomy: immunologic and pathophysiologic effects in animals and man.* San Diego, CA: Academic Press, 1979;203.
131. Fisher MM. Intradermal testing in the diagnosis of acute anaphylaxis during anesthesia: results of five years' experience. *Anaesth Intensive Care* 1979;58.
132. Dockhorn RJ. Diagnostic tests for allergic disease. In: Korenblat PE, Weber HJ, eds. *Allergy: theory and practice.* Philadelphia: Grune & Stratton, 1984:57.
133. Levy JH. *Anaphylactic reactions in anesthesia and intensive care.* Boston, MA: Butterworth-Heineman, 1986:39.
134. Levy JH. A laboratory test to detect antibodies to protamine. *Anesthesiology* 1987;67:281.
135. Oggel JD, Bukstein DA. Radioallergosorbent test. In: Bukstein DA, Strunk KG, eds. *Manual of clinical problems in asthma, allergy and related disorders.* Boston, MA: Little, Brown and Company, 1984:29.
136. Samuel T, Kolk AHJ, Rumpke P, et al. Autoimmunity to sperm antigens in vasectomized men. *Clin Exp Immunol* 1975;21:65.
137. Kurtz AB, Gray RS, Markand S. Circulating IgG antibody to protamine in patients treated with protamine-insulin. *Diabetalogia* 1983;25:322.
138. Lowenstein E, Johnston WE, Lappas DG. Catastrophic pulmonary vasoconstriction associated with protamine reversal of heparin. *Anesthesiology* 1983;59:470.
139. Radegran K, Taylor GA, Olson P. Mode of action of protamine in regard to its circulatory and respiratory side effects. *Eur Surg Res* 1971;3:139.
140. Jastrzebski J, Hilgard P, Sykes MK. Pulmonary vasoconstriction produced by protamine and protamine-heparin complex in the isolated cat lung perfused with blood or dextran. *Cardiovasc Res* 1975;9:691.
141. Morel DR, Mo Costabella PM, Pittet JF. Adverse cardiopulmonary effects and increased plasma thromboxane concentrations following the neutralization of heparin with protamine in awake sheep are infusion dependent. *Anesthesiology* 1990;73:415.
142. McIntyre RW, Fezzani P, Knopes KD. Pulmonary hypertension and prostaglandin after protamine. *Am J Cardiol* 1986;58:857.
143. Morel DR, Zapol WM, Thomas SJ, et al. C5a and thromboxane generation associated with pulmonary vaso- and broncho-constriction during protamine reversal of heparin. *Anesthesiology* 1987;66:597.
144. Montalescot G, Lowenstein E, Ogletree M, et al. Thromboxane receptor blockade prevents protamine-induced pulmonary hypertension in awake sheep. *Circulation* 1990;82:1765.
145. Lowenstein E, Zapol WM. Protamine reactions, explosive mediator release, and pulmonary vasoconstriction. *Anesthesiology* 1990;73:373.
146. Shapira N, Schaff HV, Piehler JM, et al. Cardiovascular effects of protamine sulfate in man. *J Thorac Cardiovasc Surg* 1982; 84:505.
147. Frater RWM, Oka Y, Hong Y, et al. Protamine-induced circulatory changes. *J Thorac Cardiovasc Surg* 1984;87:687.
148. Castley PA, Goodman K, Fyman PH, et al. Hemodynamic changes after the administration of protamine. *Anesth Analg* 1986;65:78.
149. Alaoui A. Administration of protamine through the left atrium. *J Thorac Cardiovasc Surg* 1985;90:153.
150. Horrow JC. Protamine allergy. *J Cardiothorac Anesth* 1988;2: 225.

Cardiac Anesthesia: Principles and Clinical Practice, Second Edition, edited by Fawzy G. Estafanous, Paul G. Barash, and J.G. Reves. Lippincott Williams & Wilkins, Philadelphia © 2001.

16

BRAIN INJURY AND BRAIN PROTECTION

PAULA M. BOKESCH

Neurologic complications—be they stroke, seizures, or even insidious neurobehavioral dysfunction—are devastating when associated with successful cardiac surgery. Very little progress has been made toward reducing neurologic injury from cardiopulmonary bypass (CPB) despite arterial filters, advances in monitoring, acid-base management, improvement in bypass technology, meticulous placement of the aortic cross-clamp, and methods to decrease the embolic load. Recent findings during a large prospective, multicenter blinded study by Roach et al. (1) showed that present practice is still associated with a 50% incidence of neurologic injury persisting at 2 months after surgery. The social and economic impact of unemployment and the requirement for long-term institutional care may be enormous.

Since the development of open heart surgery in the early 1950s, brain injury has been recognized as a complication of CPB (Table 16-1) (2). Although most likely the current methods of CPB are inflicting subtle degrees of brain injury in all patients, patients at the extremes of age are known to be at increased risk for manifestation of neurologic complications. Elderly patients who undergo cardiac surgery are more likely to develop complications, including stroke, encephalopathy, and neuropsychologic dysfunction, because of either coexisting atherosclerosis and hypertension, a genetic predisposition to cerebrovascular injury, or a higher incidence of diabetes and previous neurologic injury (3–5). Patients aged 75 years or older who undergo coronary revascularization are nine times more likely to experience a postoperative adverse neurologic event than are patients younger than 65 years of age (4). Even though the operative mortality after CPB has steadily declined since its inception, the incidence of death caused by neurologic complications has increased from 7.2% to 19.6% (6). Besides stroke, numerous studies have documented a significant incidence of neuropsychologic dysfunction, agitation and delirium, depression, and diminished intellectual functions. Depending on the type and time of neurologic testing and the accuracy of outcome measurements, the reported incidence of neurologic complications ranges from 19% to 80% (1,7–10). Neurologic and developmental abnormalities occur in 30% of infants and children who undergo cardiac surgery (11). Seizures, developmental delays, and lower intelligence are some of the possible consequences of CPB in infants and children, particularly in those subjected to deep hypothermic circulatory arrest (DHCA) (12,13).

This chapter reviews the pathophysiology of brain injury after CPB, methods to investigate cerebral injury, and interventions to reduce damage.

P. M. Bokesch: Department of Cardiothoracic Anesthesiology, The Cleveland Clinic Foundation, Cleveland, Ohio 44195

CAUSES OF BRAIN INJURY FROM CARDIOPULMONARY BYPASS

The risk of neurologic injury from cardiac surgery differs according to the support technique used. Although CPB alone can injure the brain, the addition of DHCA, which is the cessation of all blood flow, has the highest risk for global neurologic ischemia. The etiology of brain injury after open heart surgery is multifactorial; damage results from intraoperative microemboli and macroemboli, abnormal cerebral perfusion, reperfusion injury, and inflammatory and neurohumoral responses, as well as premorbid disease and postoperative events (Fig. 16-1). Focal stroke, reported to occur in 0.8% to 5.2% of patients, is usually attributed to macroembolic causes (10). Transient postoperative neurologic dysfunction is thought to be induced by inadequate cerebral perfusion or microembolism. Microemboli during cardiac surgery consist of atheromatous debris, fat, air, and fibrin-platelet complexes (14–17). Stroke is an obvious complication, easy to document and to follow. However, transient neurologic dysfunction, memory impairment, diminished intelligence, depression, and other forms of subtle neuropsychologic abnormalities are difficult to diagnose, document, or quantitate and even more difficult to duplicate in animal models.

It is unlikely that *all* neurologic changes are caused by emboli, particularly microemboli. CPB is an abnormal circulatory state, and neurons are particularly vulnerable to perturbations in blood flow, blood pressure, and oxygen delivery. CPB provides ample opportunities for neurons to

TABLE 16-1. PATIENTS AT RISK FOR BRAIN INJURY FROM CPB

Age >75 yr or <1 mo
Previous neurologic injury
Genetic predisposition: APOEε4 allele
Diabetes mellitus
Hypertension
Peripheral vascular disease
Three-vessel coronary artery disease

be stressed, particularly in patients with advanced age, a previous neurologic injury, or specific genetic markers that place them at increased risk. Whether the cause is hypoperfusion, emboli, reperfusion injury, or inflammation, the end result is the same: neuronal hypoxia and/or ischemia. Regardless of the cause of the insult, what follows is a cascade of cellular events ending in either the destruction of neurons or their survival (Fig. 16-2). Ischemic neurologic morbidity and mortality result from both rapid and delayed neuronal death and chronic impairment of cerebral metabolism. Cells denied blood flow and oxygen delivery quickly lose their ability to maintain the energy-requiring sodium and potassium pumps and die rapidly, whereas cells in the adjacent penumbra region may be damaged by the consequences of excitotoxicity.

Pathways of Brain Injury—Excitotoxicity

Glutamate is the principal excitatory neurotransmitter in the brain, released by 90% of neurons during excitation. Through interactions with membrane receptors, glutamate is responsible for numerous neurologic functions, including cognition, memory, sensation, synaptogenesis, development, and plasticity. It is now known that under pathologic conditions such as stroke, seizures, traumatic brain injury, perinatal hypoxia, and some neurodegenerative disorders (e.g., Alzheimer's disease, amyotrophic lateral sclerosis, dementia), excessive release of glutamate and concomitant activation of its receptors leads to neuronal injury and death (18,19). Olney coined the term "excitotoxicity" to describe this condition whereby a variety of pathologic processes share a common final pathway for neuronal injury as a result of either excessive release or inadequate removal of the excitatory neurotransmitters (20).

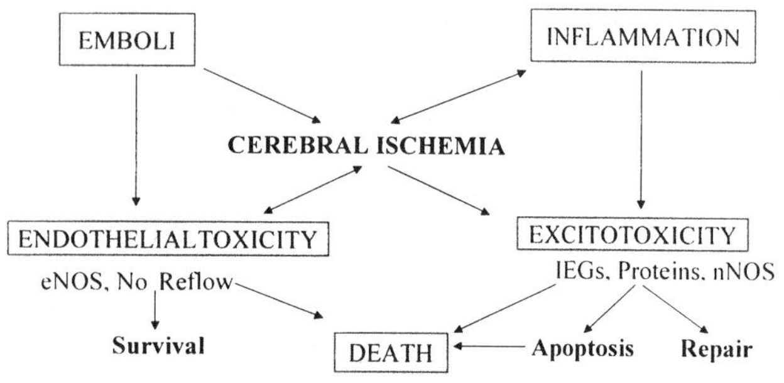

FIGURE 16-1. Sources of neuronal injury from cardiopulmonary bypass. IEGs, immediate-early genes; nNOS, neuronal nitric oxide synthase; eNOS, endothelial nitric oxide synthase.

In response to a stimulus-induced depolarization, glutamate is released from the presynaptic membrane and binds to receptors on the postsynaptic membrane, the most notable being the *N*-methyl D-aspartate (NMDA) receptor (Fig. 16-2). The agonist-operated NMDA receptor is coupled directly to membrane ion channels. In contrast to most ion channels, the NMDA receptor is both a ligand and a voltage-gated channel. Opening of the channel requires both binding of the neurotransmitter glutamate and depolarization of the membrane (21). With activation of the receptor, the cation channel undergoes a conformational change that permits calcium and sodium ions to enter the neuron (22, 23). Excessive activation of these receptors results in prolonged influx of calcium into the cell (24). Stimulation of the NMDA receptor is one means of directly increasing intracellular calcium. Glutamate-mediated α-amino-3-hydroxy-5-methyl-4-isoxazole propionic acid (AMPA) receptor depolarization indirectly activates voltage-dependent calcium channels to increase intracellular calcium (25). Additional sources of intracellular calcium include the release of calcium stores from mitochondria and uncoupling of calcium from other intracellular organelles (26).

The excessive cytosolic Ca^{2+} initiates a cascade of biochemical events. Calcium is a second messenger in neurons and plays an important role in the regulation of many enzymatic pathways (27). Increased intracellular calcium activates certain isoforms of protein kinase C, phospholipase A_2 and C, Ca^{2+}/calmodulin-dependent protein kinase, nitric oxide synthase (NOS), and a number of proteases and endonucleases which, if not properly regulated, can produce considerable cellular damage (28,29). Calcium signals are also propagated to the nucleus, where they promote profound changes in gene expression crucial for proper neuronal function (30). Within the nucleus, increased intracellular calcium rapidly (within minutes) results in transcription of the messenger ribonucleic acids (mRNAs) for the early response genes known as immediate-early genes (IEGs). The translated protein products of the IEGs act as transcriptional regulators initiating a sequence of biochemical events leading to long-term adaptive changes in neurons. IEGs modulate transcription of numerous other genes, including p53, bcl-2, tyrosine hydroxylase, neuronal NOS (nNOS), and opiate peptides, to name a few (35–37). Whereas some of these genes are associated with programmed cell death, or apoptosis, others are neuroprotective and enhance neuronal survival, repair, and recovery (35–37) (Fig. 16-2).

Glutamate-mediated excitotoxic injury to neurons from CPB with circulatory arrest has been confirmed in animal models. CPB with circulatory arrest significantly increases

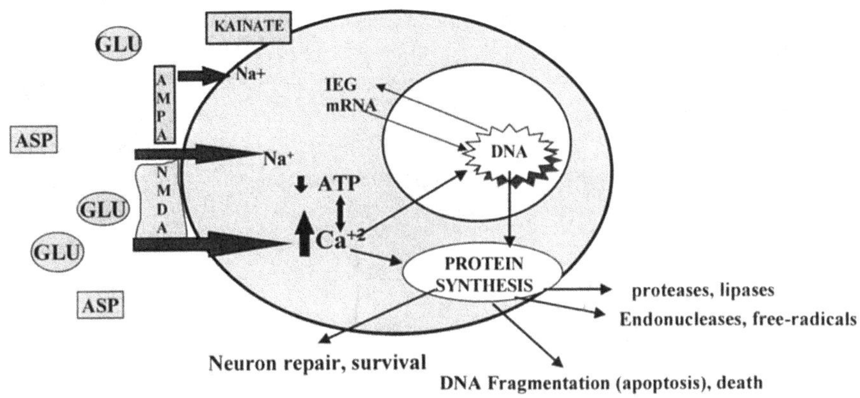

FIGURE 16-2. Molecular pathways of hypoxia/ischemia-induced neuronal injury. The excitatory neurotransmitters, glutamate (GLU) and aspartate (ASP), are released with excitation, after which they diffuse across the synaptic cleft and bind to receptors (*N*-methyl D-aspartate [NMDA], α-amino-3-hydroxy-5-methyl-4-isoxazole propionic acid [AMPA], Kainate) on the postsynaptic neuron. Increased intracellular calcium (Ca+) activates a cascade of cellular reactions, including the transcription of immediate-early genes (IEGs) that promote the synthesis of numerous proteins leading to either cell survival or cell death.

the release of glutamate and other excitatory neurotransmitters in the brain (38). Both CPB and DHCA alter IEG transcription and translation in the brain that may result in neuronal death (39). The pattern of brain damage follows closely the distribution of NMDA receptors in the hippocampal formation, basal ganglia, and cerebellum, the brain regions that are the most vulnerable to injury from CPB and DHCA (40). The hippocampal formation is the area of the brain important to memory and learning. Damage to the hippocampus from CPB is reflected in neuropsychologic tests as impaired memory and difficulty with learning new information.

The neonatal brain is hypersensitive to the toxic effects of the excitatory amino acids. Clinical investigations have demonstrated that the concentrations of the excitatory amino acids, glutamate and aspartate, in the cerebrospinal fluid are higher after asphyxia in neonates than in infants and older children (41). The NMDA receptors are hyperactive during brain development, and NMDA-mediated toxicity is 60 times greater in 7-day old rats than in adults (42).

Inflammation

During CPB, tissue trauma, ischemia-reperfusion injury, temperature changes, protamine, and the release of endotoxin from the gut induce a complex inflammatory response including complement activation, cytokine release, expression of adhesion molecules, leukocyte activation, and release of multiple factors leading to tissue injury, increased microvascular permeability, and organ dysfunction. Numerous studies have documented that CPB induces a systemic inflammatory response (43–45). The inflammatory response begins as soon as the patient's blood makes contact with air or with the synthetic nonendothelial cell surfaces of the CPB circuit. Complement is immediately activated via the alternative pathway leading to the cleavage of C3 and C5 (46). Blood flow to the brain, gut, and kidneys declines significantly with the onset of CPB (47). In addition, emboli—both gaseous and particulate during CPB—further diminish perfusion in the microcirculation. Diminished perfusion activates neutrophils and endothelial cells within the vasculature, promoting the inflammatory response. Reestablishing "normal" circulation after CPB maintains the inflammatory response. In something of a paradox, reperfusion injury may be defined as the conversion of reversible cell injury to irreversible cell injury on perfusion of a previously ischemic area, reintroducing oxygen (48–50). The temporary interruption of cerebral blood flow produces a transient hyperemic response followed by a gradual decline in cerebral blood flow called the no-reflow phenomenon (51). Neutrophil adherence to the vascular endothelium is the initial step of the postischemic microvascular dysfunction that occurs in the no-reflow phenomenon (48). Neutrophil adherence is followed by the release of toxic substances causing edema and perivascular swelling, creating more perfusion abnormalities of the microvasculature (50).

Although the inflammatory response to CPB has been extensively studied in other organs, there have been only a few reports investigating cerebral inflammatory processes. It is not feasible, in most cases, to obtain cerebrospinal fluid samples or brain tissue from patients after CPB. However, by simultaneously measuring both jugular bulb and arterial blood samples, the serum markers of inflammation can be localized to the brain. Nandate et al. (52) reported increases in juguloarterial gradients of interleukin-8 (IL-8) after CPB that were significantly larger with normothermic compared to hypothermic CPB. The inflammatory response may be responsible for the marked cerebral swelling that is visible on magnetic resonance images taken immediately after CPB (53).

Nitric Oxide

Experiments suggest that nitric oxide (NO) may be involved with ischemia-induced brain damage. NO is synthesized from L-arginine by the enzyme NOS. Although it is produced in only 1% to 2% of neurons (via nNOS) in the brain, NO is a gas and, like carbon dioxide and oxygen, passes freely across membranes (54). In the brain, NO is also produced by the vascular endothelium (via endothelial NOS, or eNOS), astrocytes, and neutrophils (inducible-NOS or iNOS) (55,56). Unlike the NO produced by neurons, NO production by the vascular endothelium is cerebroprotective during hypoxia (57). The *in vivo* effects of endothelial NO include vasodilatation, decreased platelet aggregation, and down-regulation of the NMDA receptors (58,59). However, NO production in the parenchyma of the hypoxic brain may be injurious rather than protective (60). Acute hypoxia leads to increased production of neuronal NO that becomes neurotoxic by reacting with other free radicals, paralyzing the glycolytic pathway and adenosine triphosphate production and inhibiting the mitochondrial electron transport chain (60). Neuronal NO production is linked to activation of glutamate and the excitatory amino acid receptors, including the NMDA receptors. As a result of glutamate-mediated increases in intracellular Ca^{2+}, more nNOS is expressed (61). Cerebral ischemia increases both the expression of the genes encoding nNOS and the synthesis of neuronal NO (62–64). Although the results of early investigations have been controversial, abnormally high concentrations of NO in the brain have been associated with neurotoxicity in animal models of brain ischemia. However, whether NO is destructive or protective depends on the stage of evolution of the ischemic process and the cellular source of NO (i.e., blood vessel or neuron). Therefore, in some studies the severity of neuronal loss was reduced by the prior administration of inhibitors of NOS, whereas in other studies there was no benefit (65).

BRAIN PROTECTION

Unlike a stroke, CPB is a scheduled event permitting protective interventions and preemptive therapy. Historically, hypothermia has been used to diminish brain injury. Technologic advances introduced over the past 20 years include membrane oxygenators (replacing bubble oxygenators), arterial filters, pulsatile perfusion, heparin-bonded circuits, retrograde perfusion of the brain, and improved cannulation techniques. Not all of these techniques have proved successful in reducing brain injury, however. Presently, the strategy is to use pharmacologic approaches that selectively attenuate the mediators of brain injury (Fig. 16-3). In the future, protective strategies will shift again to molecular therapeutics (once available) that modulate gene expression to enhance neuronal repair and survival and inhibit apoptosis. Whatever the choice of therapy, it will be most effective if applied preemptively before the onset of CPB.

Hypothermia

Hypothermia is the mainstay of cerebral protection during CPB. Bigelow et al. (66) demonstrated in 1950 that cardiac surgery could be successfully performed on dogs using deep hypothermia. The neuroprotective effects of hypothermia were initially attributed to metabolic suppression and decreased brain energy demands. But even modest decreases (2°C) in brain temperature attenuate neuronal damage in vulnerable neurons within the hippocampus and striatum, even though high-energy phosphate depletion and lactate accumulation are not affected (67). In addition, the degree of neuropathology does not correlate with the magnitude of metabolic suppression, casting further doubt on inhibition of the cerebral metabolic rate for oxygen ($CMRO_2$) as the sole mechanism of hypothermia's protection (68). As pointed out by Michenfelder and others, the brain's utilization of oxygen can be divided into that associated with support of electrophysiologic activity (about 60%) and that associated with maintenance of membrane and organelle homeostasis (40%) (69). Even with an anesthetic-induced isoelectric electroencephalogram (EEG), the brain will suffer very quickly at normothermia in the event of severe reduction of substrate delivery. Therefore, reduction of $CMRO_2$ or burst suppression is probably not the only mechanism of brain protection by hypothermia.

Another mechanism by which even small variations in brain temperature exert a protective effect is by reduction in ischemia-induced glutamate release and attenuation of the excitotoxic cascade. Using *in vivo* microdialysis techniques, Busto et al. (70) measured extracellular glutamate in rat brains subjected to 20 minutes of ischemia. In animals whose intraischemic brain temperature was maintained at

Technology	Pharmacology	Molecular
⇓	⇓	⇓
Hypothermia (< 35°C)	Monoclonal Abs (C3a, C5a, cytokines, lectins, ICAMS)	↓Apoptosis genes
Arterial Filters‾	Inhalational anesthetics	Anti-sense
Membrane Oxygenators	Corticosteroids	Proteases↑↓
Placement of Ao Xclamp	Ketamine, Magnesium	↑Repair genes
α- or pH stat	Other NMDA antagonists (aptiganel, lamotrigine)	
↓ CPB time	Vasodilators	
↓ or avoid DHCA		

FIGURE 16-3. Protective strategies to decrease brain injury from cardiopulmonary bypass. ICAMS, intercellular adhesion molecules.

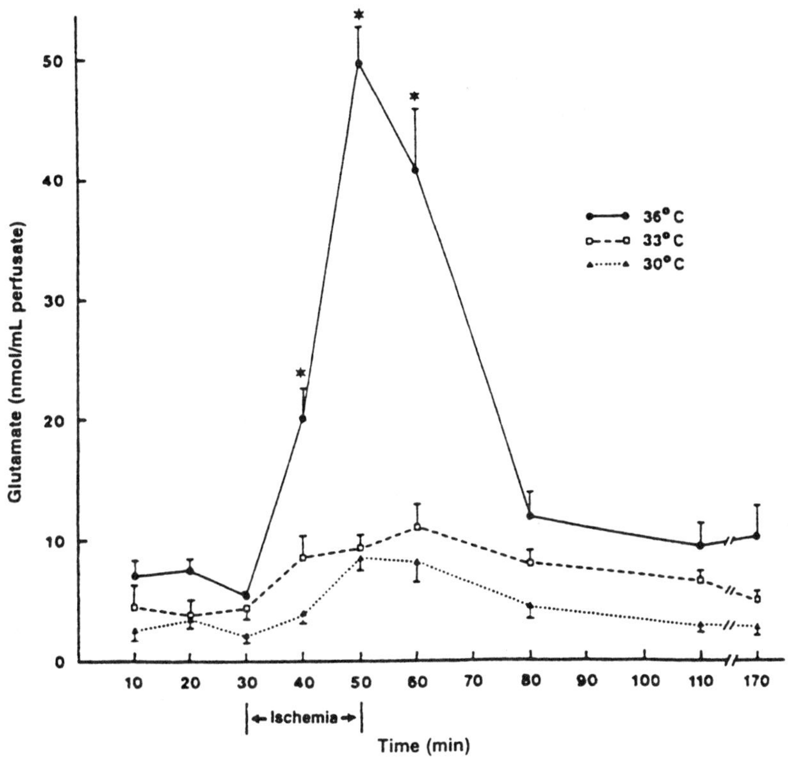

FIGURE 16-4. Changes in cerebral microdialysis perfusate concentrations of glutamate (nmol/mL) in animals whose intraischemic brain temperature was maintained at 36°C (n = 10), 33°C (n = 4), or 30°C (n = 8). The data are presented as mean ± SEM. Statistical significance was assessed by two-way analysis of variance. In the animals whose intra-ischemic brain temperature was maintained at 36°C, there was a massive increase in extracellular glutamate (*, $p < .01$). No significant changes were found in those animals whose intraischemic brain temperature was maintained at 30° or 33°C. (From Busto R, Globus M, Bietrich WD, et al. Effect of mild hypothermia on ischemia-induced release of neurotransmitters and free fatty acids in rat brain. *Stroke* 1989;20:904, with permission.)

36°C, a massive increase in extracellular glutamate was demonstrated (Fig. 16-4). No significant changes in extracellular glutamate were observed in animals with brain temperature maintained at 33° or 30°C. Illievich et al. (71) reported similar reductions in ischemia-induced glutamate release at 32°C in a rabbit model using microdialysis in the brain. Other beneficial effects of hypothermia at the molecular level may involve increasing intracellular pH and attenuating calcium-mediated injury by preserving Ca^{2+}/calmodulin-dependent protein kinase and other enzymes needed for normal calcium homeostasis. Bickler et al. (72) documented in brain slices that reducing the temperature to 28°C caused a 57% reduction in the rate of intracellular calcium accumulation during ischemia.

Although hypothermia has significant protective effects on the brain, it has also been fraught with systemic complications. Disturbances in coagulation, choreoathetosis, infection, arrhythmias, and exacerbation of the inflammatory response (during rewarming) are some of the adverse effects attributed to hypothermia (73,74). Overzealous rewarming during CPB with cerebral temperatures exceeding 37°C may also produce neuropsychologic dysfunction (75–77). Nevertheless, hypothermia (35°C or less) increases the tolerance of ischemia in the brain during CPB and circulatory arrest and is still used in most practices.

In clinical practice, brain temperature is best monitored with a nasopharyngeal, tympanic, or jugular bulb thermistor. Care must be taken in placing any of these probes. The nasopharyngeal probe is frequently advanced too far into the mouth or even into the esophagus. The tympanic probe can perforate the tympanic membrane if pushed in too far. The use of bladder, rectal, esophageal, or skin thermometers is unacceptable for monitoring brain temperature.

Managing Emboli

Another effort to protect the brain during cardiac surgery has been to decrease the delivery of emboli. The use of arterial filters on the pump and meticulous placement of the aortic cross-clamp by the surgeon decrease considerably the number of macroemboli entering the brain. Although macroembolic events from the release of aortic plaque are most certainly related to stroke, it is not clear that the more subtle neuropsychologic disturbances can be attributed to microembolism. If the latter were true, then techniques that decrease cerebral blood flow, and hence the embolic load, should improve neurologic outcome. Drugs such as propofol that decrease cerebral blood flow also reduce the number of cerebral microemboli received during surgery. However, propofol does not improve neurologic outcome (1). Similarly, the use of alpha-stat pH management (temperature-uncorrected pH and arterial carbon dioxide tension [Pa_{CO_2}], with no CO_2 added to the CPB circuit) reduces cerebral blood flow and embolic load (78). Although this technique has been practiced in adults for the past 10 years, it may not be desirable to decrease cerebral blood flow in patients with preexisting neurologic injury who may have limited cerebral perfusion reserves (79). The use of pH-stat management (temperature-corrected pH and Pa_{CO_2}, with CO_2 added to the CPB circuit), which increases cerebral blood flow, increases the rate of brain cooling and decreases the rate of oxygen depletion during DHCA (80). Hypercapnea during rewarming from hypothermic CPB also increases cerebral blood flow and prevents jugular bulb desaturation (81). Therefore, increased cerebral blood flow has been demonstrated to be beneficial in certain patients despite the theoretically negative effects of increased delivery of microemboli to the brain.

Anesthetics

The question of whether anesthetics are neuroprotective in intact animals is controversial. The magnitude of neuroprotection has varied depending on the animal model, the severity of ischemia, and the choice of anesthetic. Illievich et al. (82) showed that volatile and intravenous anesthetics did not reduce extracellular accumulation of glutamate in the brain during global ischemia. Other animal models indicate that both inhalational anesthetics and lidocaine reduce hypoxia-induced glutamate release at clinically relevant concentrations (83,84). Isoflurane, in comparison with a nitrous oxide/fentanyl anesthetic, significantly attenuated ischemia-induced glutamate release in the rat hippocampus, and the effects of isoflurane were comparable to those of mild hypothermia (34°C) (85).

Metabolic suppression alone does not provide neuroprotection during cardiac surgery. For example, induced EEG-burst suppression with propofol during cardiac valve replacement did not significantly reduce the incidence or severity of neurologic or neuropsychologic dysfunction (1). Anesthetics that reduce $CMRO_2$ do not provide equivalent protection from ischemia (86). Although clinical trials have demonstrated that the neuropsychologic complications of intracardiac operations can be lessened by barbiturate (thiopental) administration, patients had significant cardiac instability and required prolonged postoperative intubation and time in the intensive care unit for recovery (87). Besides reducing $CMRO_2$, barbiturates also reduce glutamate release and calcium influx, block sodium channels, and inhibit free radical formation (88). Thiopental administration before DHCA failed to preserve energy stores in neurons and was detrimental to the recovery of neurons after CPB and DHCA (89). Even though barbiturates have proved beneficial in cases of acute head injury, they may be harmful in the setting of CPB/DHCA.

Because of their cardiovascular stability, large doses of opiates are frequently used for cardiac surgery. Although high-dose opiate "anesthesia" and postoperative analgesia can markedly attenuate the hormonal and cardiovascular stress responses to CPB and DHCA (90), there is no evidence that opiates diminish glutamate-mediated excitotoxicity mechanisms in the brain. Unlike volatile anesthetics, fentanyl is not protective against ischemic injury to hippocampal neurons when used in concentrations comparable to those produced in clinical practice (91). Neither does fentanyl attenuate ischemia-induced excitatory neurotransmitter release in the hippocampus (85).

Vasodilators

Inadequate tissue perfusion during CPB results from local intravascular coagulation (fibrin formation), vasoconstriction, and cellular plugging of the microcirculation by neutrophils, platelets, and possibly air microemboli. Although early reperfusion can salvage tissue, reperfusion also increases mortality by increasing the inflammatory response. Therefore, a logical approach to preventing reperfusion injury in the first place is to enhance perfusion of the microcirculation during CPB by vasodilatation. Phenoxybenzamine, 1 mg/kg, is being used at some centers to achieve this purpose in infants (92). Phenoxybenzamine is a noncompetitive α-adrenergic blocker that has a long half-life (18 hours) and facilitates high pump flows on bypass, even at low temperatures (93). Unlike other α-adrenergic blockers, phenoxybenzamine does not cause cardiac stimulation. The effects of phenoxybenzamine persist in the postbypass period, providing excellent afterload reduction and organ perfusion (93). Phenoxybenzamine is not the drug of choice for the adult cardiac surgery patient on the fast track.

Corticosteroids

Corticosteroids have been used during cardiac surgery since the 1960s. Although they have been used for more than 40 years, and the intention behind their administration has changed during this time, the mechanism of steroid intervention is still incompletely understood or defined. Neither is there agreement on the doses of steroids or the timing of their administration. For that matter, not all steroids are alike. Steroids differ considerably in their antiinflammatory potency and mineralocorticoid (sodium-retaining) effects.

Initially steroids were given for their hemodynamic effects, namely vasodilation with increased venous capacitance as a therapy for low cardiac output syndrome after CPB. In the late 1960s, steroids were reported to exert an ill-defined "membrane stability" effect on lysosomal membranes (94). In a large series of patients reported by Dietzman et al. in 1975 (95), steroid administration before the onset of CPB was shown to cause significantly less vasoconstriction and improved perfusion flows that translated into decreased intensive care unit length of stay. Later, Engelman et al. (96) reported that steroids inhibit phospholipase activation and improve myocardial preservation.

With the introduction of molecular biology techniques, the antiinflammatory mechanisms of steroids have been better described. Although the effect of steroids on complement activation is controversial (97–99), they clearly inhibit the expression of the proinflammatory cytokines, tumor necrosis factor-α (TNF-α), IL-1B, IL-6, and IL-8 (100,101). Furthermore, steroids enhance the production of the anti-inflammatory cytokine IL-10 (102). Therefore, the inflammatory reaction to CPB should be reduced with steroids and postoperative recovery should be improved, but outcome studies have not shown this to be true.

The downside of steroid pretreatment for cardiac surgery includes increased expense, increased endotoxin release during CPB, glucose intolerance, increased infection and wound dehiscence, and possibly increased intubation time (99,102,103). Also, the vasodilatory effects of steroids may be undesirable in some patients (100). The hippocampus is rich in corticosteroid receptors. Corticosteroids easily cross cell membranes to bind to the glucocorticoid receptor in the cytoplasm, which then translocates to the nucleus, where it activates or inhibits gene transcription. Exposure to high concentrations of circulating steroids may increase the loss of hippocampal neurons that have endured transient ischemia. The mechanism of cell death is thought to involve inhibition of glucose transport and, subsequently, failure to sequester calcium mobilized by the excitatory neurotransmitters (104).

Inflammatory Modulators

The sequential manner of the inflammatory response that results in the "inflammatory cascade" provides multiple opportunities for therapeutic interventions to selectively interrupt the events and enhance or eliminate specific mediators. Many of the mediators require transcription and translation for their release, and these processes frequently take several hours. Furthermore, CPB is a planned event, providing an ideal model in which to study preemptive treatments. Current concepts of intervention focus on methods of inhibiting complement activation and attenuating the cytokine response. Animal studies have shown improved outcome after inhibition of the cytokine response (105). The clinical relevance of complement activation is uncertain. Several studies have related postoperative morbidity to complement activation, whereas other groups have found no correlation between complement activation and outcome.

The appearance of increased serum concentrations of IL-6 after CPB is a consistent marker for activation of the inflammatory cascade and a predictor of subsequent organ dysfunction and death. Serum IL-6 concentrations are highest in patients with complications after CPB and correlate with the duration of CPB and ventricular dysfunction (106). Opioids and regional anesthesia have little effect on IL-6 concentrations (107,108). Adding ketamine to opioid-based anesthesia, however, attenuates the IL-6 response after CPB and inhibits TNF-α–mediated reduction of cardiac intracellular cyclic adenosine monophosphate (cAMP) and contractility (106,109).

Several companies are developing mediators of complement activation with recombinant complement protein inhibitors and monoclonal antibodies to specific complement fragments (110,111). These compounds will specifically target the extrinsic pathway of complement activation, leaving the intrinsic Ab/Ag pathway intact. Similar therapeutic maneuvers have been directed at suppressing neutrophil adhesion to the endothelial cells and synthesis of cytokines (112). Protease inhibitors (aprotinin) have been shown to reduce serum concentrations of proinflammatory cytokines released during cardiac surgery, but without any improvement in patient outcome (113). Proteases terminate the effects of many inflammatory mediators, so protease inhibitors will enhance some inflammatory pathways and diminish others.

Heparin-coated CPB circuits have been suggested as a method to reduce the inflammatory response. Heparin bonding on the artificial surface can reduce thrombus formation, decrease complement activation via the alternative pathway, reduce platelet adhesion, and inhibit the release of the inflammatory cytokines (114). However, it is still unclear whether these effects can lead to improved clinical outcome. Also, various coating techniques used in the design of the CPB circuits may have a major impact on activation of complement and heparin doses.

Future Therapeutics

There is growing enthusiasm for an alternative therapeutic approach directed at improving the intrinsic ability of neurons to withstand ischemia and inflammation. Initial attempts with barbiturates were unsuccessful because the massive doses required to benefit the brain were harmful to the heart and had numerous other undesirable side effects. Similarly, calcium channel blockers create cardiovascular instability and excessive bleeding in the setting of heart disease and CPB (115). The NMDA antagonist, remacemide, has been tried in patients undergoing coronary artery surgery with CPB. Although the patients had better cognitive outcomes, they reported more frequent side effects (dizziness, drowsiness, and ataxia) than control patients did (117). Both ketamine and magnesium noncompetitively block the NMDA-receptor complex and are available for clinical use (Fig. 16-5). More specific NMDA-receptor antagonists are in clinical trials in patients with stroke and traumatic brain injury, but they have not been tried in patients before CPB. NMDA receptors are located only in the brain and spinal cord, and that gives their antagonists the advantage of not directly affecting the cardiovascular system. Several animal studies have reported improved neurologic outcome with the use of novel NMDA antagonists during CPB and DHCA when given preemptively (106,116).

Blocking NMDA receptors alone will not completely prevent the increase in intracellular calcium, because calcium entry is from multiple sources besides those mediated by glutamate. The survival of neurons depends on inhibit-

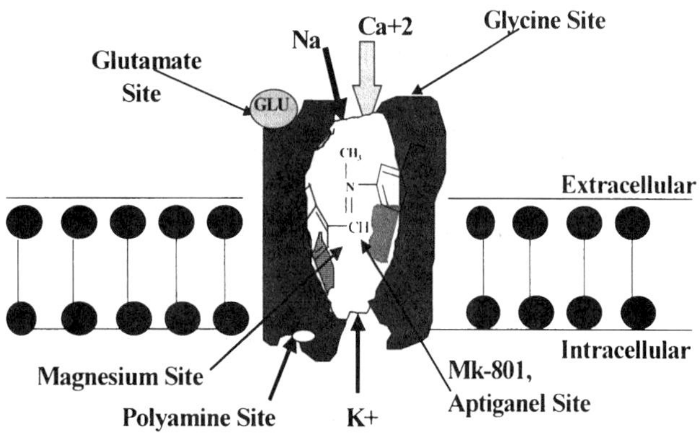

FIGURE 16-5. The *N*-methyl D-aspartate (NMDA) receptor. With excitation, glutamate binds to the NMDA receptor, causing the channel to open, permitting sodium and calcium ions to enter into the neuroplasm. Glycine is a coagonist at the NMDA receptor. Noncompetitive NMDA antagonist sites are shown for magnesium, MK-801, and aptiganel.

ing, or at least attenuating, the cascade of events triggered by increased calcium that lead to death and preserving those that protect or repair the neuron. Although understanding of the molecular mechanisms of ischemic brain injury has advanced considerably in recent years, several important questions need to be resolved. It has not yet been sorted out which processes are detrimental and which are beneficial. Once the genes and gene products are identified, specific therapies can be designed to facilitate the pathways that lead to neuronal repair and survival and to inhibit those leading to death. Until then, "cocktails" that combine therapies attacking specific components (e.g., complement activation, inflammation, reperfusion injury, vasoconstriction, free radicals) are needed (Fig. 16-3).

We have been taught that the adult mammalian brain lacks the mechanisms needed to replenish neurons and reestablish neuronal networks after acute injury. Some recent work suggests that adult brains have a much greater potential for producing new neurons and repairing damaged regions than previously thought (118). In 1913 the Spanish neuroscientist Dr. S.R. yCajal responded to the brain's lack of regenerative ability by stating "It is for the science of the future to change, if possible, this harsh decree. Inspired with high ideals, it must work to impede or modulate the gradual decay of the neurons, to overcome the almost invincible rigidity of their connections, and to reestablish normal nerve paths when disease has severed centers that were intimately associated" (119). At the beginning of the new millennium, we will achieve this goal.

REFERENCES

1. Roach GW, Newman MF, Murkin JM, et al., for The Multicenter Study of Perioperative Ischemia (McSPI) Research Group. Ineffectiveness of burst suppression therapy in mitigating perioperative cerebrovascular dysfunction. *Anesthesiology* 1999;90:1255.
2. Lillehei CW. Historical development of cardiopulmonary bypass. In: Gravlee GP, Davis RF, Utley JR. *Cardiopulmonary bypass: principles and practice.* Baltimore: Williams & Wilkins, 1993:1.
3. McKhann GM, Goldsborough MA, Borowicz MS, et al. Predictors of stroke in coronary artery bypass patients. *Ann Thorac Surg* 1997;63:516.
4. Tuman KJ, McCarthy RJ, Najafi H, et al. Differential effects of advanced age on neurologic and cardiac risks of coronary artery operations. *J Thorac Cardiovasc Surg* 1992;104:1510.
5. Tardiff BE, Newman MF, Saunders AM, et al. Preliminary report of a genetic basis for cognitive decline after cardiac operations. *Ann Thorac Surg* 1997;64:715.
6. Ravi G, Murkin JM. Neuropsychologic dysfunction after cardiac surgery: what is the problem? *J Cardiothorac Vasc Anesth* 1996;10:91.
7. Elsass P, Henriksen L. Acute cerebral dysfunction after open-heart surgery: a reaction-time study. *Scand J Thorac Cardiovasc Surg* 1984;18:161.
8. Shaw PJ, Bates D, Cartlidge NF, et al. Neurologic and neuropsychological morbidity following major surgery: comparison of coronary artery bypass and peripheral vascular surgery. *Stroke* 1987;18:700.
9. Hammeke TA, Hastings JE. Neuropsychologic alterations after cardiac operation. *J Thorac Cardiovasc Surg* 1988;96:326.
10. Roach GW, Kanchuger M, Mangano CM, et al. Adverse cerebral outcomes after coronary bypass surgery: Multicenter Study of Perioperative Ischemia Research Group and the Ischemia Research and Education Foundation Investigators. *N Engl J Med* 1996;335:1857.
11. Pua HL, Bissonnette B. Cerebral physiology in paediatric cardiopulmonary bypass. *Can J Anesth* 1998;45:960.
12. Newburger JW, Jonas RA, Wernovsky G, et al. A comparison of the perioperative neurologic effects of hypothermic circulatory arrest versus low-flow cardiopulmonary bypass in infant heart surgery. *N Engl J Med* 1993;329:1057.
13. Glauser TA, Rorke LB, Weinberg PM, et al. Acquired neuropathologic lesions associated with the hypoplastic left heart syndrome. *Pediatrics* 1990;85;991.
14. Blauth CI, Arnold JV, Schulenberg WE, et al. Cerebral microembolism during cardiopulmonary bypass. *J Thorac Cardiovasc Surg* 1988;95:668.
15. Brooker RF, Brown WR, Moody DM, et al. Cardiotomy suction: a major source of brain lipid emboli during cardiopulmonary bypass. *Ann Thorac Surg* 1998;65:1651.
16. Reasoner DK, Hindman BJ, Dexter F, et al. Doxycycline reduces early neurologic impairment after cerebral arterial air embolism in the rabbit. *Anesthesiology* 1997;87:569.
17. Blauth CI, Cosgrove DM, Webb BW, et al. Atheroembolism from the ascending aorta: an emerging problem in cardiac surgery. *J Thorac Cardiovasc Surg* 1992;103:1104.
18. Lipton SA, Rosenberg PA. Excitatory amino acids as a final common pathway for neurologic disorders. *N Engl J Med* 1994;330:613.
19. Meldrum B, Garthwaite J. Excitatory amino acid neurotoxicity and neurodegenerative disease. *Trends Pharmacol Sci* 1990;11:379.
20. Rothman SM, Olney JW. Glutamate and the pathophysiology of hypoxic-ischemic brain damage. *Ann Neurol* 1986;19:105.
21. Choi DW. Calcium-mediated neurotoxicity: relationship to specific channel types and role in ischemic damage. *Trends Neurosci* 1988;11:465.

22. Orrenius S, Ankarcrona M, Nicotera P. Mechanisms of calcium-related cell death. *Adv Neurol* 1996;71:137.
23. MacDermott AB, Mayer ML, Westbrook GL, et al. NMDA-receptor activation increases cytoplasmic calcium concentration in cultured spinal cord neurones. *Nature* 1986;321:519.
24. Choi DW. Ionic dependence of glutamate neurotoxicity. *J Neurosci* 1987;7:369.
25. Greenamyre JT, Porter HP. Anatomy and physiology of glutamate in the CNS. *Neurology* 1994;44:S7.
26. Choi DW. Glutamate neurotoxicity and diseases of the nervous system. *Neuron* 1988:1:623.
27. Siesjo BK, Bengtsson F. Calcium fluxes, calcium antagonists, and calcium-related pathology in brain ischemia, hypoglycemia, and spreading depression: a unifying hypothesis. *J Cereb Blood Flow Metab* 1989;9:127.
28. Dawson TM, Dawson VL, Snyder SH. A novel neuronal messenger molecule in the brain: the free radical, nitric oxide. *Ann Neurol* 1992;32:297.
29. Chan PH, Fishman RA. Free fatty acids, oxygen free radicals, and membrane alterations in brain ischemia and injury. In: Plum F, Pulsinelli W, eds. *Cerebrovascular diseases.* New York: Raven Press, 1985:161.
30. Ghosh A, Greenberg ME. Calcium signaling in neurons: molecular mechanisms and cellular consequences. *Science* 1995;268: 239.
31. Bullitt E. Expression of *c-fos*-like protein as a marker for neuronal activity following noxious stimulation in the rat. *J Comp Neurol* 1990;296:517.
32. Sheng M, Greenberg ME. The regulation and function of *c-fos* and other immediate-early genes in the nervous system. *Neuron* 1990;4:477.
33. Ikeda J, Nakajima T, Gerfen C, et al. *In situ* hybridization analysis of c-fos and prodynorphin mRNA levels and distribution in gerbil hippocampus after transient ischemia. *Stroke* 1990; 21:1.
34. Bading H, Ginty DD, Greenberg ME. Regulation of gene expression in hippocampal neurons by distinct calcium pathways. *Science* 1993;260:181.
35. Benveniste H. The excitotoxin hypothesis in relation to cerebral ischemia. *Cerebrovasc Brain Metab Rev* 1991;3:213.
36. Sonnenberg JL, MacGregor-Leon PF, Curran T, et al. Dynamic alterations occur in the levels and composition of transcription factor AP-1 complexes after seizure. *Neuron* 1989;3:359.
37. Smeyne RJ, Vendrell M, Hayward M, et al. Continuous *c-fos* expression precedes programmed cell death *in vivo. Nature* 1993;363:166.
38. Conroy BP, Lin CY, Jenkins LW, et al. Hypothermic modulation of cerebral ischemic injury during cardiopulmonary bypass in pigs. *Anesthesiology* 1998;88:390.
39. Bokesch PM, Marchand J, Seirafi PA, et al. Immediate-early gene expression in ovine brain after cardiopulmonary bypass and hypothermic circulatory arrest. *Anesthesiology* 1996;85: 1439.
40. Bokesch PM, Halpin D, Ranger W, et al. Immediate-early gene expression in ovine brain after hypothermic circulatory arrest: effects of the noncompetitive NMDA antagonist, aptiganel Hcl (Cerestat). *Ann Thorac Surg* 1998;64:1082.
41. Hagberg H. Hypoxic-ischemic damage in the neonatal brain: excitatory amino acids. *Dev Pharmacol Ther* 1992;18:139.
42. McDonald JW, Johnston MV. Physiological and pathophysiological roles of excitatory amino acids during central nervous system development. *Brain Res Rev* 1990;15:41.
43. Hall RI, Smith MS, Rocker G. The systemic inflammatory response to cardiopulmonary bypass: pathophysiological, therapeutic, and pharmacological considerations. *Anesth Analg* 1997; 85:766.
44. Wan S, LeClerc JL, Vincent JL. Inflammatory response to cardiopulmonary bypass. *Chest* 1997;112:676.
45. Khabar KSA, ElBarbary MA, Khouqeer F, et al. Circulating endotoxin and cytokines after cardiopulmonary bypass: differential correlation with duration of bypass and systemic inflammatory response/multiple organ dysfunction syndromes. *Clin Immunol Immunopathol* 1997;85:97.
46. Chenoweth DE, Cooper SW, Hugli TE, et al. Complement activation during cardiopulmonary bypass: evidence for generation of C3a and C5a anaphylatoxins. *N Engl J Med* 1981;304: 497.
47. Lazenby WD, Wilson K, Zelano JA, et al. Effects of temperature and flow rate on regional blood flow and metabolism during cardiopulmonary bypass. *Ann Thorac Surg* 1992;53:957.
48. Ames A, Wright RL, Kowada M, et al. Cerebral ischemia II: the no-reflow phenomenon. *Am J Pathol* 1968;52:437.
49. Smith DS, Levy W, Maris M, et al. Reperfusion hyperoxia in brain after circulatory arrest in humans. *Anesthesiology* 1990;73: 12.
50. Del Zoppo GJ, Schmid-Schoenbein GW, Mori E, et al. Polymorphonuclear leukocytes occlude capillaries following middle cerebral artery occlusion and reperfusion in baboons. *Stroke* 1991;22:1276.
51. Rogers MC, Kirsch JR. Current concepts in brain resuscitation. *JAMA* 1989;261:3143.
52. Nandate K, Vuylsteke A, Crosbie AE, et al. Cerebrovascular cytokine responses during coronary artery bypass surgery: specific production of interleukin-8 and its attenuation by hypothermic cardiopulmonary bypass. *Anesth Analg* 1999;89:823.
53. Harris DNF, Oatridge A, Dob D, et al. Cerebral swelling after normothermic cardiopulmonary bypass. *Anesthesiology* 1998;88: 340.
54. Garthwaite J. Nitric oxide signalling in the nervous system. *Neurosciences* 1993;5:171.
55. Moncada C, Palmer RMJ, Higgs EA. Nitric oxide: physiology, pathophysiology, and pharmacology. *Pharmacol Rev* 1991;43: 109.
56. Bredt DS, Hwang PM, Snyder SH. Localization of nitric oxide synthase indicating a neural role for nitric oxide. *Nature* 1990: 347:768.
57. Choi DW. Calcium: still center-stage in hypoxic-ischemic neuronal death. *Trends Neurosci* 1995;18:58.
58. Meldrum BS. Cellular and molecular mechanisms of ischemic brain damage: the role of nitric oxide in ischemic damage. *Adv Neurol* 1996;71:355.
59. Lipton SA, Wang YF. NO-related species can protect from focal cerebral ischemia/reperfusion. In: Krieglstein J, ed. *Pharmacology of cerebral ischemia.* Stuttgart, Germany: Medpharm Scientific Publishers 1996:186.
60. Garthwaite J, Garthwaite G, Palmer RM, et al. NMDA receptor activation induces nitric oxide synthesis from arginine in rat brain slices. *Eur J Pharmacol* 1989;172:413.
61. Beckman JS, Koppenol WH: Nitric oxide, superoxide, and peroxynitrite: the good, the bad, and the ugly. *Am J Physiol* 1996; 271:C1424.
62. Garthwaite J. Glutamate, nitric oxide and cell-cell signalling in the nervous system. *Trends Neurosci* 1991;14:60.
63. Nishikawa T, Kirsch JR, Koeshler RC, et al. Nitric oxide synthase inhibition reduces caudate injury following transient focal ischemia in cats. *Stroke* 1994;25:877.
64. Zhang ZG, Chopp M, Gatam S, et al. Upregulation of neuronal nitric oxide synthase and mRNA, and selective sparing of nitric oxide synthase-containing neurons after focal cerebral ischemia in rat. *Brain Res* 1994;654:85.
65. Litt L, Espanol MT, Hasegawa K, et al. NOS inhibitors decrease

hypoxia-induced ATP reductions in respiring cerebrocortical slices. *Anesthesiology* 1999;90:1392.
66. Bigelow WG, Callaghan JC, Hopps JA. General hypothermia for experimental intracardiac surgery. *Ann Surg* 1950;132:531.
67. Busto R, Dietrich WD, Globus MYT, et al. Small differences in intra-ischemic brain temperature critically determine the extent of ischemic neuronal injury. *J Cereb Blood Flow Metab* 1987;7:729.
68. Todd MM, Warner DS. A comfortable hypothesis reevaluated: cerebral metabolic depression and brain protection during ischemia. *Anesthesiology* 1992;76:161.
69. Michenfelder JD, Milde JH. The relationship among canine brain temperature, metabolism, and function during hypothermia. *Anesthesiology* 1991;75:130.
70. Busto R, Globus M, Bietrich WD, et al. Effect of mild hypothermia on ischemia-induced release of neurotransmitters and free fatty acids in rat brain. *Stroke* 1989;20:904.
71. Illievich UM, Zornow MH, Choi KT, et al. Effects of hypothermic metabolic suppression on hippocampal glutamate concentrations after transient global cerebral ischemia. *Anesth Analg* 1994;78:905.
72. Bickler PE, Buck LT, Feiner JR. Volatile and intravenous anesthetics decrease glutamate release from cortical brain slices during anoxia. *Anesthesiology* 1995;83:1233.
73. Almond CH, Jones JC, Snyder HM, et al. Cooling gradients and brain damage with deep hypothermia. *J Thorac Cardiovasc Surg* 1964;48:890.
74. Mora CT, Henson WB, Weintraub WS, et al. The effect of temperature management during cardiopulmonary bypass on neurological and neuropsychological outcomes in coronary revascularization patients. *J Thorac Cardiovasc Surg* 1996;112:514.
75. Murkin J. Hypothermic cardiopulmonary bypass: time for a more temperate approach. *Can J Anesth* 1995;42:663.
76. Cook DJ, Orszulak TA, Daly RC, et al. Cerebral hyperthermia during cardiopulmonary bypass in adults. *J Thorac Cardiovasc Surg* 1996;111:663.
77. Mangano CM. Optimal temperature management during cardiopulmonary bypass: warm, cold, or tepid? *Semin Cardiothorac Vasc Anesth* 1998:2:293.
78. Patel RL, Turtle MR, Chambers DJ, et al. Alpha-stat acid-base regulation during cardiopulmonary bypass improves neuropsychologic outcome in patients undergoing coronary artery bypass grafting. *J Thorac Cardiovasc Surg* 1996;111:1267.
79. Hindman BJ. Choice of α-stat or pH-stat management and neurologic outcomes after cardiac surgery. *Anesthesiology* 1998;89:5.
80. Kurth CD, O'Rourke MM, O'Hara IB. Comparison of pH-stat and alpha-stat cardiopulmonary bypass on cerebral oxygenation and blood flow in relation to hypothermic circulatory arrest in piglets. *Anesthesiology* 1998;89:110.
81. Haenel F, von Knobelsdorff G, Werner C, et al. Hypercapnia prevents jugular bulb desaturation during rewarming from hypothermic cardiopulmonary bypass. *Anesthesiology* 1998;89:19.
82. Illievich UM, Zornnow MH, Choi KT, et al. Effects of hypothermia or anesthetics on hippocampal glutamate and glycine concentrations after repeated transient global cerebral ischemia. *Anesthesiology* 1994;80:177.
83. Miura Y, Grocott HP, Bart RD, et al. Differential effects of anesthetic agents on outcome from near-complete but not incomplete global ischemia in the rat. *Anesthesiology* 1998;89:391.
84. Terada H, Ohta S, Nishikawa, et al. The effect of intravenous or subarachnoid lidocaine on glutamate accumulation during transient forebrain ischemia in rats. *Anesth Analg* 1999;89:957.
85. Patel PM, Drummond JC, Cole DJ. Isoflurane reduces ischemia-induced glutamate release in rats subjected to forebrain ischemia. *Anesthesiology* 1995;82:996.
86. Drummond JC. Brain protection during anesthesia: a reader's guide. *Anesthesiology* 1993;79:877.
87. Nussmeier NA, Arlund C, Slogoff S. Neuropsychiatric complications after cardiopulmonary bypass: cerebral protection by a barbiturate. *Anesthesiology* 1986;64:165.
88. Kirsch JR, Traystman RJ, Hurn PD. Anesthetics and cerebroprotection: experimental aspects. *Int Anesthesiol Clin* 1996;34:73.
89. Siegman MG, Anderson RV, Balaban RS, et al. Barbiturates impair cerebral metabolism during hypothermic circulatory arrest. *Ann Thorac Surg* 1992;54:1131.
90. Anand KJS, Hickey PR. Halothane-morphine compared with high-dose sufentanil for anesthesia and postoperative analgesia in neonatal cardiac surgery. *N Engl J Med* 1992;326:1.
91. Charchaflieh J, Cottrell JE, Kass IS. The effect of fentanyl on electrophysiologic recovery of CA1 pyramidal cells from anoxia in the rat hippocampal slice. *Anesth Analg* 1998;87:68.
92. Tweddell JS, Hoffman GM, Fedderly RT, et al. Phenoxybenzamine improves systemic oxygen delivery after the Norwood procedure. *Ann Thorac Surg* 1999;67:161.
93. Nickerson M, Collier B. Drugs inhibiting adrenergic nerves and structures innervated by them. In: Goodman LS, Gilman A, eds. *The pharmacological basis of therapeutics,* 5th ed. New York: MacMillan, 1975:533.
94. Replogle RL, Gazzania AB, Gross RE. Use of corticosteroids during cardiopulmonary bypass: possible lysosome stabilization. *Circulation* 1966;33[Suppl I]:I-86.
95. Dietzman RH, Lunseth JB, Goott B, et al. The use of methylprednisolone during cardiopulmonary bypass: a review of 427 cases. *J Thorac Cardiovasc Surg* 1975;69:870.
96. Engelman RM, Rousou JA, Flack JE, et al. Influence of steroids on complement and cytokine generation after cardiopulmonary bypass. *Ann Thorac Surg* 1995;60:801.
97. Andersen LW, Baek L, Thomsen BS, et al. Effect of methylprednisolone on complement-mediated neutrophil activation during cardiopulmonary bypass. *Surgery* 1986;100:134.
98. Jansen NJG, van Oeveren W, Gu YJ, et al. Endotoxin release and tumor necrosis factor formation during cardiopulmonary bypass. *Ann Thorac Surg* 1992; 54:744.
99. Andersen LW, Baek L, Thomsen BS, et al. Effect of methylprednisolone on endotoxemia and complement activation during cardiac surgery. *J Cardiothorac Anesth* 1989;3:544.
100. Kawamura T, Inada K, Okada H, et al. Methylprednisolone inhibits increase of interleukin 8 and 6 during open heart surgery. *Can J Anaesth* 1995; 42:399.
101. Teoh KHT, Bradley CA, Gauldie J, et al. Steroid inhibition of cytokine-mediated vasodilation after warm heart surgery. *Circulation* 1995;92[Suppl II]:II-347.
102. Tabardel Y, Duchateau J, Schmatz D, et al. Corticosteroids increase blood interleukin 10 levels during cardiopulmonary bypass in men. *Surgery* 1996; 119:76.
103. Gurwitz JH, Bohn RL, Glynn RJ, et al. Glucocorticoids and the risk for initiation of hypoglycaemic therapy. *Arch Intern Med* 1994;154:97.
104. Sapolsky R, Pulsinelli W. Glucocorticoids potentiate ischemic injury to neurons: therapeutic implications. *Science* 1985;229:1397.
105. Giroir BP. Mediator of septic shock, new approaches for interrupting the endogenous inflammatory cascade. *Crit Care Med* 1993;21:780.
106. Roytblat L, Roy-Shapira A, Greenberg L, et al. Ketamine and IL-6 response after CPB. *Anesth Analg* 1998;87:266.

107. Moore CM, Desborough JP, Powell H, et al. Effects of extradural anaesthesia on IL-6 and acute phase response to surgery. *Br J Anaesth* 1994;72:272.
108. Taylor NM, Lacoumenta S, Hall GM. Fentanyl and the interleukin-6 response to surgery. *Anaesthesia* 1997;52:112.
109. Hill GE, Anderson JL, Lyden ER. Ketamine inhibits the proinflammatory cytokine-induced reduction of cardiac intracellular cAMP accumulation. *Anesth Analg* 1998;87:1015.
110. Bokesch PM, Bansal R, Parent JB, et al. Anti-human properdin monoclonal antibodies block the alternative pathway in a model of cardiopulmonary bypass. *Anesthesiology* 1999;91:A121.
111. Park KW, Tofukuji M, Dai HB, et al. Attenuation of endothelium-dependent relaxation of pig microvessels following cardiopulmonary bypass is mediated by C5a. *Anesth Analg* 1998;86: SCA4.
112. Clark WM, Madden KP, Rothlein R, et al. Reduction of central nervous system ischemic injury in rabbits using leukocyte adhesion antibody treatment. *Stroke* 1991;22:877.
113. Aoki M. Jonas RA, Nomura F, et al. Anti-CD 18 attenuates deleterious effects of cardiopulmonary bypass and hypothermic circulatory arrest in piglets. *J Card Surg* 1995;10:407.
114. Wan S, LeClerc JL, Vincent JL. Inflammatory response to cardiopulmonary bypass. *Chest* 1997;112:676.
115. Legault C, Furberg CD, Wagenknecht LY, et al. Nimodipine neuroprotection in cardiac valve replacement: report of an early terminated trial. *Stroke* 1996:27:593.
116. Bokesch PM, Kapural M, Drummond-Webb J, et al. Neuroprotective, anesthetic and cardiovascular effects of the NMDA antagonist, CNS 5161A, in isoflurane-anesthetized lambs. *Anesthesiology* 2000;93:202.
117. Arrowsmith JE, Harrison MJG, Newman SP, et al. Neuroprotection of the brain during cardiopulmonary bypass: a randomized trial of remacemide during coronary artery bypass in 171 patients. *Stroke* 1998;29:2357.
118. Lowenstein DH, Parent JM. Brain, heal thyself. *Science* 1999; 283:1126.
119. yCajal SR, May RT, eds. *Degeneration and regeneration of the nervous system,* vol II. New York: Hafner, 1959.

Cardiac Anesthesia: Principles and Clinical Practice, Second Edition, edited by Fawzy G. Estafanous, Paul G. Barash, and J.G. Reves. Lippincott Williams & Wilkins, Philadelphia © 2001.

PART

IV

INTENSIVE CARE MEDICINE

17

ADULT INTENSIVE CARE AND COMPLICATIONS

THOMAS L. HIGGINS
JEAN-PIERRE YARED

INTRODUCTION

The profile of the cardiac surgical patient continues to change, affecting the need for and intensity of postoperative management. Widespread adoption of "fast-track" management has resulted in very short postoperative length of stay and reduced intubation time for the majority (1–3). On the other hand, surgery is now accomplished on patients not previously considered ideal operative candidates. An increasing number of patients are older than 75 years of age, reoperation candidates, or affected by severe left ventricular dysfunction or concurrent medical illnesses (4). Patients undergoing simultaneous coronary artery bypass grafting (CABG) plus valve replacement or repair, carotid surgery, arrhythmia surgery, insertion of ventricular assist devices (VADs), or cardiomyoplasty represent a growing percentage of the total cardiac cases.

Although postoperative care of low-risk cardiac surgical patients may now resemble a recovery room model, high-risk patients require increasing postoperative involvement of anesthesiologists, cardiologists, and critical care specialists (5,6). The presence of full-time intensive care unit (ICU) staff physicians improves outcome in intensive care (7,8), pointing to a continued and growing involvement of intensive care specialists. This chapter highlights the usual course and potential pitfalls of the postoperative period and discusses the sometimes conflicting goals in the early management of the patient recovering from cardiac surgery. Because the total scope of postoperative management of these patients involves knowledge covered elsewhere in this book, this chapter concentrates on the following areas of importance:

Recovery from anesthesia with control of the stress response

Respiratory management and weaning from mechanical ventilation

Monitoring for adverse events that can be prevented or ameliorated with ICU care

Intervention for expected and unexpected events such as shivering, return to the operating room (OR) for control of bleeding, and respiratory failure.

Delivery of the Patient to the Intensive Care Unit

Smooth postoperative management begins with uneventful transport from the OR to the ICU or postsurgical recovery area. Transport of a critically ill patient is associated with acute physiologic changes and the potential for mishap (9). During this period, the intense monitoring of the OR may be momentarily relaxed while attention is focused on physically moving the patient and the associated infusion pumps, ventilation equipment, and monitors. Ideally, the ICU should be in close proximity to the cardiac OR to minimize transport time and distance.

Common problems encountered during transport include sudden hypotension as a result of fluid shifts or vasodilatation and extreme hypertension precipitating afterload increase and augmenting the risk for serious bleeding. Wide swings in blood pressure can be minimized with adequate volume loading of the patient and continuing adequate anesthesia during transport. Care must be taken to ensure that intravenous medications do not become disconnected or the doses inadvertently altered. Particular attention must be directed to all tubes connected to the patient, including endotracheal tubes, chest tubes, Foley bladder catheters, and vascular cannulas.

Information Transfer

A thorough understanding of each patient's anatomy and physiology is essential, and this information must be conveyed from the OR team to the ICU team. Although there is a generally accepted range of appropriate cardiac filling pressures, the OR team has the unique advantage of having

T. L. Higgins: Departments of Medicine and Anesthesiology, Tufts University School of Medicine, Boston, Massachusetts 02111; Adult Critical Care Service, Baystate Medical Center, Springfield, Massachusetts 01199

J. P. Yared: Department of Cardiac Anesthesia, The Cleveland Clinic Foundation, Cleveland, Ohio 44195

seen the patient's heart while the chest was open, perhaps with concurrent intraoperative transesophageal echocardiography. This experience allows a much better understanding of a given patient's optimal filling pressures in the early postbypass period. Basic information such as the timing of antibiotics, response to anesthetics, and trends in hematocrit and blood glucose should also be transferred. Important operative information gleaned from the surgical and anesthesia staff and residents should be documented in designated locations on the bedside flow sheets or clinical information system screen. Table 17-1 contains a checklist that may be used by the anesthesia team before leaving the OR and a summary of information to be communicated to the ICU team.

TABLE 17-1. CHECKLIST FOR TRANSFER OF OPEN HEART SURGICAL PATIENTS FROM THE OPERATING ROOM (OR) TO THE INTENSIVE CARE UNIT (ICU) OR POSTANESTHESIA CARE UNIT (PACU)

On leaving the OR
Connect transport monitor (continuous ECG and arterial pressure)
Turn on oxygen tank
Disconnect patient from anesthesia ventilator
Ventilate with self-inflating "Ambu"-type bag
Bring all records and blood products
Have ready in ICU
Ventilator set to V_T, 10 cc/kg; rate, 8 breaths/min, FiO_2, 0.60; PEEP, 2–5 cm
Bedside monitor for ECG, CVP, arterial-line, and, if used, PA or LA pressure
Infusion pumps for inotropes, vasopressors, and vasodilators
Defibrillator, resuscitation cart, surgical "bleeder" tray
On arrival in ICU
Connect ECG, pressure monitors, and pulse oximeter
Connect on ventilator
Auscultate breath sounds and observe chest excursion
Zero pressure transducers, and correlate with cuff pressure
Determine cardiac output
Check function of IABP and/or assist devices
Communicate to ICU physician and nursing staff
Patient's name, age, gender, and brief history
Exact nature of surgical repair
Completeness of revascularization
CPB/circulatory arrest times
Complications encountered
Optimal filling pressures as determined in OR
Current drug infusions and titration plans
Pacemaker and antiarrhythmic information
Anesthetics given and plans for awakening
Fluids and blood products given; urine output
Hemostasis and heparin reversal
Last hematocrit, potassium, and antibiotic dose
Availability of blood products and surgical salvage
Before leaving ICU
Ensure hemodynamic stability
Ensure adequate oxygenation and ventilation
Check drainage from and function of chest tubes
Place blood products in refrigerator
Complete ICU orders including postoperative chest radiography, ECG, and laboratory work

Note: CPB, cardiac pulmonary bypass; CVP, central venous pressure; ECG, electrocardiography, FiO_2, fraction of inspired oxygen; IABP, intraaortic balloon pump; LA, left atrium; PA, pulmonary artery; PEEP, positive end-expiratory pressure; V_T, tidal volume.

RESPIRATORY MANAGEMENT

Surgery and anesthesia together produce a number of respiratory system changes, including decreases of up to 40% in vital capacity, total lung capacity, inspiratory capacity, and functional residual capacity. These changes occur immediately but require up to several weeks to return to baseline (10). Cardiopulmonary bypass (CPB) creates a systemic inflammatory response with alterations in pulmonary vascular permeability proportionate to the length of bypass (11). Better oxygenation and lower shunt fraction can be achieved by keeping the lungs inflated at 5 cm H_2O continuous positive airway pressure (CPAP) and 0.21 fraction of inspired oxygen (FiO_2), compared with collapsing the lungs during CPB (12). Atelectasis occurs in up to 90% of patients, whether or not prophylactic positive end-expiratory pressure (PEEP) is used (13), and this atelectasis results in increased work of breathing. In addition, direct trauma to the lungs or pleura may occur during surgical retraction or insertion of chest tubes. Pain and splinting cause the patient to limit lung expansion and limit the ability to cough and clear secretions. Adequate pain relief is therefore an important ICU consideration. Respiratory management goals and possible interventions are outlined in Table 17-2.

Routine Support

On arrival in the ICU, the patient's chest is auscultated to ensure proper positioning of the endotracheal tube, and mechanical ventilation is reinitiated. Patients with normal lungs and those recovering from high-dose opioid/relaxant anesthesia normally receive an initial tidal volume (V_T) of 8 to 10 cc/kg, a respiratory rate of 8 to 10 breaths/minute, an inspired oxygen percentage of 60%, and 5 cm H_2O of PEEP. Other settings may be indicated by experience in the OR. Patients maintained on short-acting agents and whose neuromuscular blockade has been reversed may progress directly to CPAP and pressure support as long as a respiratory rate of at least 6 beats/minute and a V_T greater than 5 cc/kg can be supported.

The use of PEEP may not provide any benefits. Increased levels of PEEP decrease cardiac output, unless volume loading is used to maintain transmural filling pressures (14). The effects of PEEP are most marked in the presence of abnormal right ventricular function, particularly if the right coronary artery is compromised (15). PEEP neither protects against the development of adult respiratory distress syndrome (16) nor reduces the amount of mediastinal bleeding (17). In the event of difficulty with oxygenation, pressure-controlled inverse-ratio ventilation may be more clinically

TABLE 17-2. RESPIRATORY MANAGEMENT AFTER CARDIOPULMONARY BYPASS

Management	Immediate	Later
Goals	Complete O_2 saturation of hemoglobin Normocarbia Minimization of ventilation's hemodynamic effects	Extubation with adequate reserve Restoration of FRC
Assessment	ABGs Cardiac output and filling pressures CXR	VT, rate on CPAP (f/Vt) Vital capacity and MIP ABGs, CXR, fluid balance Chest tube output
Interventions	Changes in rate and VT Positive end-expiratory pressure Limited opiates Reversal of muscle relaxants Sedation and neuromuscular blockade if necessary Pressure control ventilation to limit PIPs	Control of secretions Upright position Incentive spirometry Ambulation

Note: ABGs, arterial blood gases; CXR, chest radiography; CPAP, continuous positive airway pressure; FRC, functional residual capacity; F/VT, ratio of frequency to tidal volume; MIP, maximal inspiratory pressure; PIP, peak inspiratory pressures; VT, tidal volume.

useful than high levels of PEEP (18), as long as hemodynamics are monitored for potential compromise. In patients with airflow obstruction, occult positive end-expiratory pressure (auto-PEEP) (19) may occur and cause hypotension and low cardiac output. Auto-PEEP can be detected by respiratory waveform monitoring or by monitoring pressures with the ventilator's expiratory port held closed at the end of exhalation. Auto-PEEP is minimized by using bronchodilators and/or lengthening the expiratory time to allow full exhalation to occur.

A portable chest radiograph can be used to confirm chest tube, endotracheal tube, and line placement and to rule out pneumothorax or significant atelectasis. A baseline arterial blood gas determination, drawn 30 minutes after the initiation of ventilation, is helpful in calibrating O_2 saturation and end-tidal CO_2 monitors, which may then be followed for further ventilator changes. Hemodynamic measurements may be determined with the patient connected to the ventilator, because hypervolemic and normovolemic patients do not experience dramatic hemodynamic changes when mechanical ventilation is interrupted (20). Pulmonary pressures may be altered by ventilation pressures in hypovolemic patients, but the advantage of more accurate readings is often outweighed by the disadvantage of the persistent hypoxemia that can result when unstable patients are removed from the ventilator for monitoring or even for suctioning.

When To Wean and Extubate

Factors that enter into the timing of extubation of the post-CPB patient include metabolism and elimination of opioids, anesthetic agents, and neuromuscular blocking agents; the degree of hypothermia and rewarming; the hemodynamic status of the patient; and the need to maintain an airway in an unstable patient who may need to return to the OR for tamponade or control of bleeding. Figure 17-1 contains an algorithm for early postoperative respiratory management that addresses the most common considerations. Overnight mechanical ventilation, long the accepted practice for the cardiac surgical patient, has been supplanted by early extubation protocols (2,3,21,22). Shorter-acting intravenous and inhaled anesthetics now make it possible to provide a nearly stress-free anesthesia without the need for prolonged postoperative ventilation. The presence of an endotracheal tube impairs cough efficiency, and positive airway pressure decreases preload to both ventricles, increases right-sided afterload, and decreases cardiac output. Because prophylactic ventilation does not affect the level of intrapulmonary shunt (23) and is uncomfortable and stressful for the nonsedated patient, the endotracheal tube should be removed as soon as criteria for extubation are met (Table 17-3). Documented advantages of early endotracheal extubation after cardiac surgery include improved left ventricular performance, decreased ICU length of stay, diminished requirement for postoperative medication, lessened cardiopulmonary morbidity, improved patient comfort, and lower costs (2,22,24). The stress of endotracheal extubation is modest compared with that of intubation (25).

Initiation of ventilator weaning can begin when the patient has begun to awaken, is hemodynamically stable with minimal chest tube drainage and adequate urine output, and can maintain a reasonable spontaneous VT and respiratory rate, indicating sufficient reversal of both narcotics and neuromuscular blocking agents. Often these conditions are met shortly after ICU arrival. Although various respiratory parameters and scoring systems (26–29) have been proposed to predict successful extubation, none is infallible, and they may unnecessarily delay extubation if used too rigidly. In the otherwise stable patient, the ability to maintain arterial pH greater than 7.35 while decreasing the rate of intermittent mandatory ventilation (IMV) to a CPAP of 5 cm H_2O is a convenient and easily applied test for ability to sustain spontaneous respiration. The ratio of respiratory rate to tidal volume (f/VT) quantifies the degree of rapid shallow breathing as a marker of work of breathing and readiness for extubation (30); values greater than 100 on

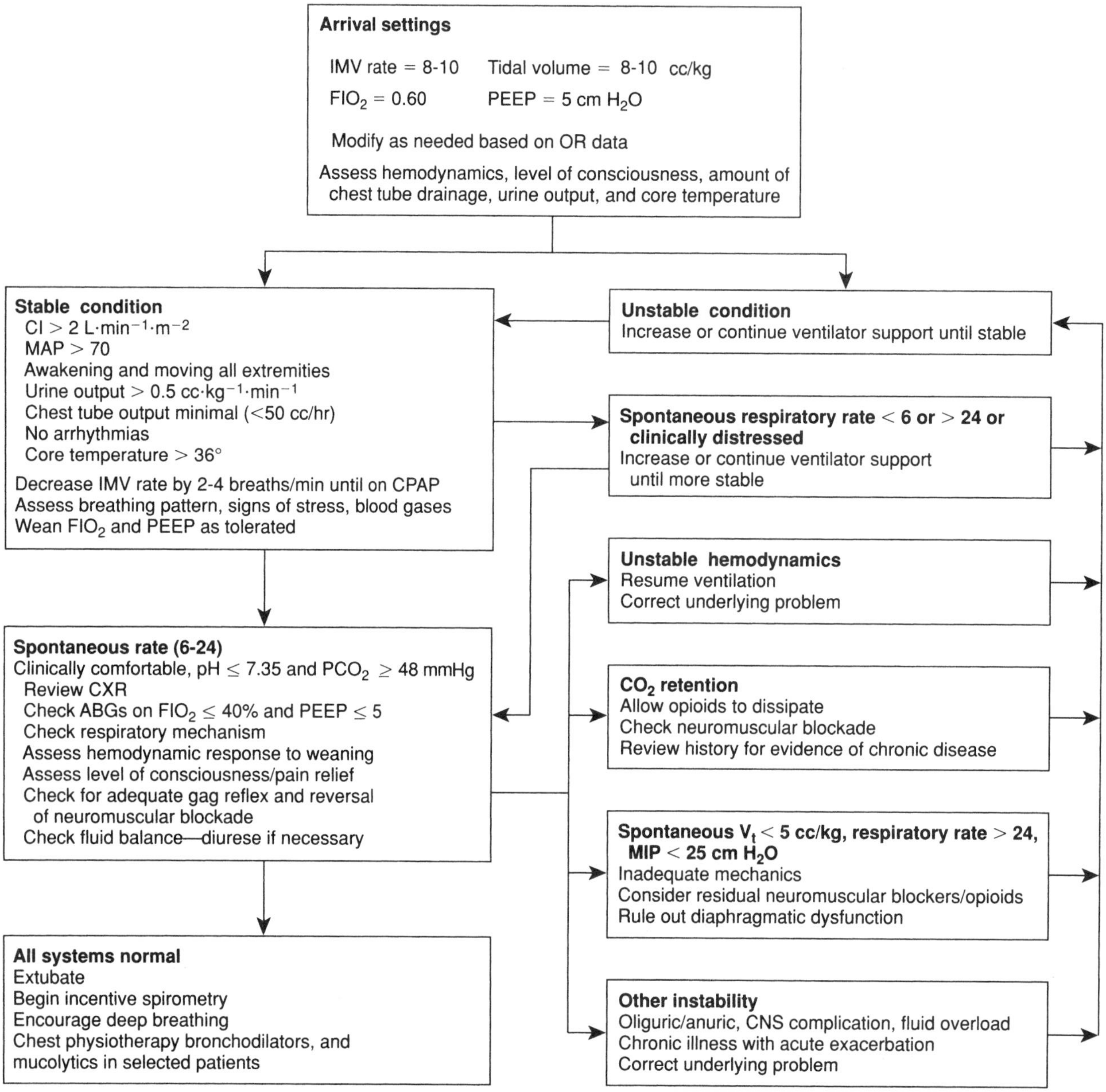

FIGURE 17-1. Early postoperative management. The initial settings are based on clinical experience and result in mild hyperventilation while the patient is cold. Weaning should occur only when the patient is stable from a hemodynamic, respiratory, neurologic, renal, and metabolic standpoint. A good test of readiness for extubation is the ability to maintain a pH greater than or equal to 7.35. Laboratory and radiographic findings should be reviewed and the patient's neurologic integrity ensured before extubation. IMV, intermittent mandatory ventilation; Fio_2, fraction of inspiratory oxygen; PEEP, positive end-expiratory pressure; OR, operating room; CI, cardiac index; MAP, mean arterial pressure; CXR, chest radiography; MIP, maximum inspiratory pressure; ABGs, arterial blood gases; CNS, central nervous system; Vt, tidal volume; CPAP, continuous positive airway pressure.

CPAP generally are associated with respiratory failure and the need for reintubation.

Nonrespiratory factors such as poor urine output or presence of ongoing sepsis become increasingly important in determining readiness to extubate in complex cases (31). In a 1999 study, extubation failure was independently predicted by age greater than 65 years, inpatient hospitalization before surgery, arterial vascular disease, chronic obstructive pulmonary disease (COPD), pulmonary hypertension, severe left ventricular dysfunction, cardiac shock, hematocrit

TABLE 17-3. EXTUBATION CRITERIA

Neurologic	Awake and cooperative, able to cough and protect airway
	Neuromuscular blockade fully reversed
Cardiac	Stable; not on IABP, index >2.2 l $min^{-1} \cdot m^{-2}$
	MAP >70 mm Hg; no serious arrhythmias
Respiratory	Acceptable CXR, ABGs (pH ≥7.35) at PEEP 5, Fio_2 40, f/VT <100
	Optional: MIP < −25, VT >5 cc/kg, Vc >10 cc/kg
	Minimal secretions
Renal	Diuresing well; not markedly fluid overloaded
	Urine output >0.5 mL/kg per hour
Hematologic	Chest tube drainage <50 mL/hr
Temperature	Fully rewarmed

Note: ABGs, arterial blood gases; CXR, chest radiography; CPAP, continuous positive airway pressure; Fio_2, fraction of inspired oxygen; f/VT, ratio of frequency to tidal volume; IABP, intra-aortic balloon pump; MAP, mean arterial pressure; MIP, maximum inspiratory pressure; PEEP, positive end-expiratory pressure; Vc, vital capacity; VT = tidal volume.

34% or less, blood urea nitrogen 24 mg/dL or more, serum albumin 4.0 g/dL or less, oxygen delivery (Do_2) 320 mL/minute or less, reoperation, thoracic aortic procedures, transfusion of 10 or more units of blood products, and CPB time 120 minutes or longer (32).

Sudden changes in preload and afterload may occur during the transition from mechanical ventilation to spontaneous ventilation. They are most marked in patients who have undergone mitral valve surgery and in those with preoperative congestive heart failure. The ability to excrete fluid volumes administered perioperatively is compromised with cardiac and/or renal dysfunction. Success in the treatment of acute respiratory failure after cardiac surgery has been reported with the application of continuous arterial venous hemofiltration (CAVH) (33); however, in the patient with some renal function, furosemide and other diuretics may be equally efficacious in reducing the volume overload (34).

Sternotomy with internal thoracic artery (ITA) harvesting is accompanied by a greater impairment in pulmonary function tests than when saphenous vein grafts alone are used (35). Some of this impairment may be caused by the irritating presence of pleural chest tubes, and patients with pleural tubes *in situ* have reduced forced vital capacity and 1-second forced expiratory volume (FEV_1) and higher pain scores. Removal of both pleural and mediastinal chest tubes reduces discomfort and results in modest improvement in pulmonary function, normally of clinical importance only in the patient with baseline borderline pulmonary function (36).

After extubation, the patient must be encouraged to cough and breathe deeply to restore lung volume. Incentive spirometry, while routine, is sometimes ineffective at increasing diaphragmatic movement, particularly after the abdomen has been entered for gastroepiploic artery harvest, or in the presence of phrenic nerve dysfunction. Intermittent positive-pressure breathing (IPPB) treatments, although not routinely needed when the patient can perform incentive spirometry, can be useful in improving lung expansion in the patient with neurologic impairment or poor cooperation due to language difficulty (37). Useful adjuncts to maintaining lung expansion include early mobilization and use of the sitting position while in bed. Adequate analgesia is important and can be provided with intravenous opioids, ketorolac, patient-controlled analgesia (PCA), and regional techniques.

LONG-TERM VENTILATION

Prolonged mechanical ventilation (longer than 48 to 72 hours) is required in about 5% to 8% of patients after CABG (38,39); the corresponding figure for valve surgery patients is about the same. Patients with preexisting COPD have higher rates of pulmonary complications (12%), atrial fibrillation (27%), and death (7%) (40). The odds of requiring prolonged ventilation increase with preoperative presence of congestive heart failure, azotemia, valvular heart disease, advanced age, or diffuse vascular disease and with reoperation and emergency procedures. The rate of nosocomial infection for ventilated patients is approximately 1% per day for the first 30 days (41). Patients requiring long-term ventilation are prone to malnutrition, stress ulceration, and gastrointestinal bleeding, so early enteral feeding and gastric cytoprotection are appropriate. The use of sucralfate rather than histamine blockers has been shown to decrease the incidence of nosocomial pneumonia (42).

Factors limiting the removal of mechanical ventilatory support include sepsis, renal failure with fluid overload, marked neurologic dysfunction, and unstable hemodynamic status. Figure 17-2 outlines an approach to investigation and treatment of failure to wean after open heart surgery. Respiratory failure can be precipitated by high carbohydrate loads delivered during attempts to provide nutritional support. Acute left ventricular dysfunction may occur in patients with COPD during the shift from mechanical to spontaneous ventilation (43). Careful attention to fluid balance and aggressive diuresis or use of ultrafiltration ameliorates the abrupt rise in left ventricular filling pressure and allows weaning from ventilation to proceed. Although it is useful to compare the patient's current and preoperative body weights, catabolic states arising postoperatively, and especially during sepsis, reduce lean body weight. It is not usual to find patients "unweanable" until fluid removal reduces body weight to several kilograms below the preoperative value.

Patients with valvular disease have significantly higher respiratory system and lung elastances and resistances than those undergoing surgery for ischemic heart disease, but

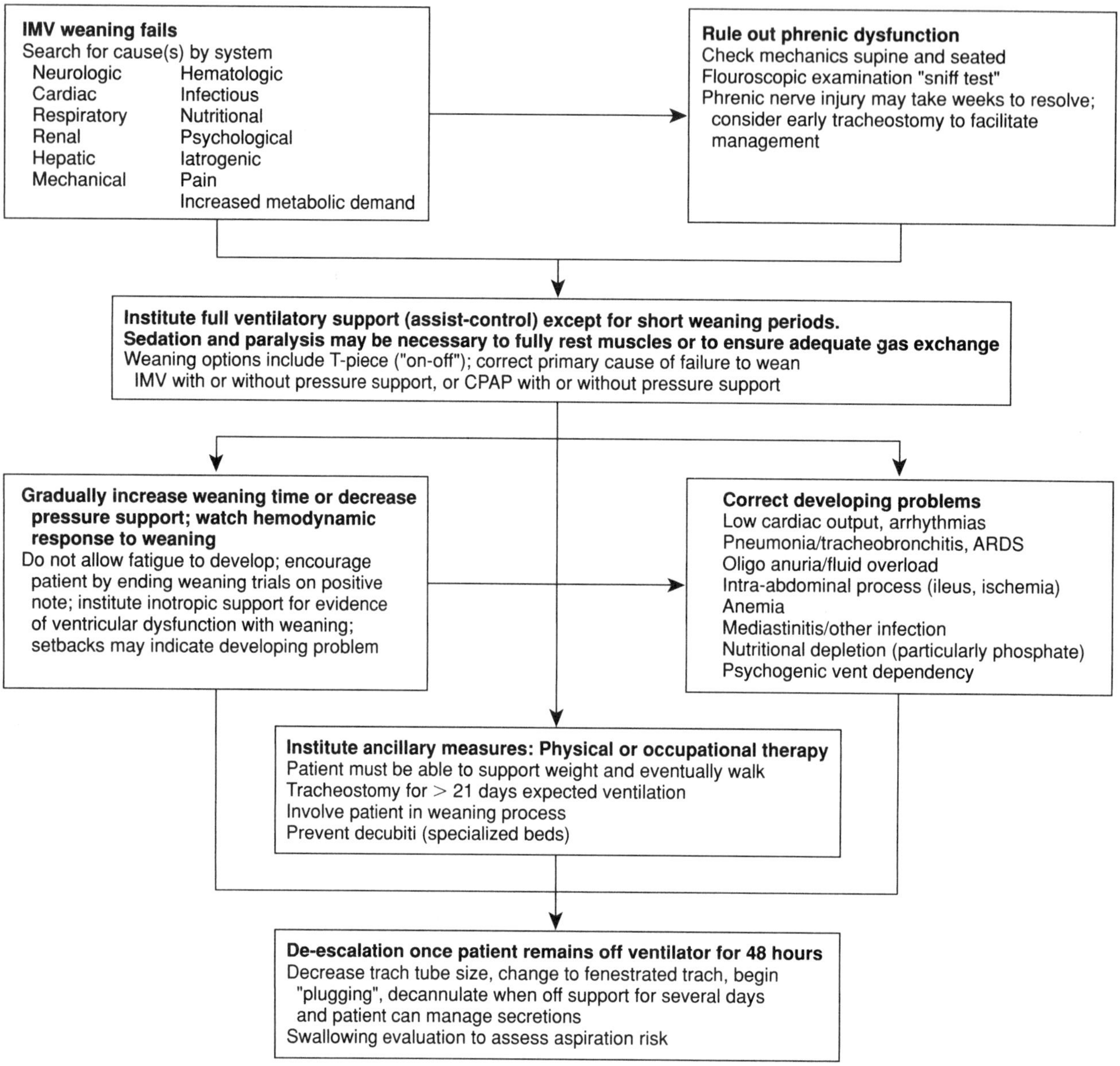

FIGURE 17-2. Long-term postoperative ventilatory management. Failure to tolerate intermittent mandatory ventilation (IMV) weaning is most often a result of inadequate cardiopulmonary reserve. While the search for causes of failure is conducted, the patient should be provided full ventilatory support, using the assist-control mode to minimize work of breathing. Short weaning periods may then be started as long as the patient is not showing signs of fatigue. Temporary phrenic nerve dysfunction is common and may be confirmed by fluoroscopic examination. Our preference for complicated weaning is to combine 5 cm H_2O of continuous positive airway pressure (CPAP) with sufficient pressure support to allow the patient to breathe at a respiratory rate of 24 breaths/minute or less for increasing periods. Once the patient is able to breathe for 8 continuous hours on CPAP with pressure support, the level of pressure support is gradually decreased. Full ventilatory support is maintained during the night shift to allow the patient full rest and adequate sleep. If the weaning period is expected to last longer than 21 days, a tracheostomy and a jejunostomy feeding tube should be considered. When the patient is able to sustain respiration for 24 hours without ventilatory support, the tracheostomy is changed from a size 6 or 8 to a size 4 Airlon (uncuffed) tube to allow plugging while retaining access for secretion control. Aspiration is sufficiently common after long-term intubation that all patients should have a swallowing evaluation by a speech therapist before nutrition by mouth is allowed. ARDS, adult respiratory distress syndrome.

with successful surgery and recovery these parameters decrease to values similar to those of patients undergoing surgery for coronary ischemia (44). The correlation of this finding is that valve surgery patients may exhibit diminished work of breathing and improved respiratory function after correction of the valvular pathology, but CABG patients are less likely to show dramatic improvement.

Patients receiving chronic amiodarone therapy are prone to have postoperative respiratory failure, longer intubation times, and longer ICU stays, even with only subclinical evidence of pulmonary amiodarone toxicity (45). Uncommonly, patients taking amiodarone develop life-threatening pulmonary complications, including adult respiratory distress syndrome, possibly related to increased effects of CPB time, high levels of oxygen, and infection on already-damaged lungs. Histologic lung examination of these patients demonstrates marked interstitial fibrosis with enlarged air spaces ("honeycomb" appearance), and hyperplasia of type II pneumocytes (46).

Diaphragmatic paralysis may complicate any thoracic procedure, but it is more common in patients undergoing reoperation, owing to the difficulty in identifying the phrenic nerve in fibrotic pericardial tissue. The incidence of diaphragmatic paralysis has not been well characterized; in our experience, permanent bilateral diaphragmatic paralysis occurs in fewer than 0.1% of patients after CPB, but temporary diaphragmatic weakness may occur in 4% or more. The diagnosis of diaphragmatic paralysis should be suspected whenever a patient fails to wean from mechanical ventilation; it should be documented by observing paradoxic movement of the diaphragm during inspiration and by comparing vital capacity and V_T in the supine and seated positions. Differences in supine and seated vital capacity of more than 10% to 15% should prompt fluoroscopic examination of the diaphragm ("sniff" test). Bilateral paralysis may be missed by this test, because comparison of left and right diaphragmatic excursion has lower specificity when both diaphragms are involved. Transient diaphragmatic paralysis may occur secondary to cold injury to the phrenic nerve (47). Less often, the phrenic nerve is injured or transected during dissection of the internal mammary arteries or during mobilization of the heart in patients undergoing reoperation.

Patients with respiratory failure and systemic inflammatory response syndrome (SIRS) can also develop critical illness polyneuropathy, the first sign of which may be failure to wean from the ventilator (48). Disuse atrophy (49) and steroid administration (50) may also contribute to diaphragmatic weakness. Other causes of apparent diaphragmatic weakness include noncompliant lung, muscle weakness and wasting, hypophosphatemia, and hypomagnesemia. Patients who are dependent on diaphragmatic breathing preoperatively (e.g., those with severe COPD) are most likely to manifest diaphragmatic weakness as postoperative ventilator dependency. Full recovery of diaphragmatic function may take from 4 months to more than 2 years; and partial recovery is apparent when the patient can assume the supine position without dyspnea (51). Important adjuncts to improving diaphragmatic strength include inspiratory muscle training (52), normalizing calcium and phosphate levels, and the use of dopamine (53) or aminophylline (54). Long-term management of diaphragmatic paralysis is facilitated by tracheostomy, which allows better secretion control and use of intermittent respiratory support.

Weaning a patient from long-term mechanical ventilation requires an individualized approach, with the goal of optimizing function in all body systems. Diuresis and inotropic support forestall respiratory failure from cardiovascular causes. Nutritional support and training of the inspiratory muscles avoids failure caused by respiratory muscle fatigue. Any underlying infection or metabolic disturbance must also be treated. It is important for the patient to become an active participant in the weaning process, which may require psychotherapy or psychopharmacology, because situational depression is common. The exact method of weaning ("on-off" T-piece, IMV, pressure support ventilation) is less important than developing a comprehensive plan that allows for the inevitable setbacks and complications. Daily screening of respiratory function reduces ventilation time, ICU length of stay, and costs (55). Other necessary care (e.g., physical therapy, diagnostic tests) can interfere with the weaning plan unless it is clearly communicated to the ICU nursing staff and consulting physicians. Respiratory muscle fatigue must be avoided by keeping the patient's respiratory rate well below 30 breaths/minute during weaning. Appropriate sedation reduces the patient's sensation of dyspnea and allows longer weaning periods. On particularly busy days, when other tests and procedures tire the patient, weaning may need to be postponed. If the patient is allowed to fatigue and become uncomfortable, psychologic resistance and preweaning anxiety may occur. It is therefore essential that each day's period of ventilatory weaning end with a sense of success rather than failure. Provision of a good night's sleep on full ventilatory support allows the patient to recover strength and readiness for the next day's work.

Tracheostomy should be considered for patients who will be ventilated for longer than 2 to 3 weeks (56). Percutaneous tracheostomy can be accomplished at the bedside, eliminating the need to transport the patient to the OR. At some point in the weaning process, the patient will be ready to breathe spontaneously for part of the day and require only intermittent mechanical support. Use of a fenestrated tracheostomy tube then permits "plugging" the tracheostomy, allowing the patient to communicate verbally during periods off the ventilator. The presence of active mediastinitis is a relative contraindication to tracheostomy, and these patients can be switched from oral to nasal intubation to improve comfort and tube support. Nasal intubation, however, increases the risk of nosocomial sinusitis (57).

After both short- and long-term ventilatory support, tracheal strictures and stenoses may develop. These may be apparent as inability to "plug" a fenestrated tracheostomy tube or as extubation failure resulting from increased work of breathing. Arytenoid dislocation is a rare complication of tracheal intubation, but it should be considered in the differential diagnosis of noisy inspiration and painful swallowing after extubation (58). Surgical treatment of this complication should happen early, before fibrosis occurs.

Swallowing dysfunction occurs commonly in patients with neurologic impairment and prolonged periods of ventilatory support (59). Because aspiration can snatch defeat from the jaws of weaning victory, a careful swallowing evaluation should precede any attempts to feed the patient. Patients with swallowing dysfunction should be referred to a speech pathologist for retraining in the use of pharyngeal muscles and staged reintroduction of food.

CARDIOVASCULAR SUPPORT

Cardiovascular support in the early postoperative period involves hemodynamic monitoring and intervention during the period of myocardial recovery from CPB. Four major goals can be identified during stabilization of the postoperative cardiac patient:

1. Maintenance of appropriate perfusion pressure
2. Delivery of adequate oxygen to the tissues
3. Balancing of oxygen supply versus demand
4. Maintenance of a stable cardiac rhythm

Perfusion Pressure

Adequate perfusion pressure is essential for proper cerebral and visceral function and to ensure perfusion through newly placed bypass grafts; therefore, a mean arterial pressure of more than 70 mm Hg is generally maintained. ITA grafts are more vulnerable to closure with decreased perfusion pressure. Elderly patients and patients with renal or cerebrovascular stenoses may require higher minimal perfusion pressures. In the absence of solid data on where mean pressure should be maintained, it is reasonable to aim for a level within 20 mm Hg of the resting preoperative mean values.

Postoperative hypotension can be precipitated by decreased preload, decreased systemic vascular resistance, or insufficient cardiac output. Increased preload can result from mannitol-induced diuresis, vasodilatation from mediator release after CPB, fluid compartmental shifts, or bleeding. Volume status is not always easily assessed, even when a pulmonary artery (Swan-Ganz) catheter is employed to measure intracardiac pressures. Left atrial catheters provide a constant indication of left-sided pressures while avoiding the necessity of frequent balloon inflation in the pulmonary artery. However, left atrial catheters introduce the risk of air embolization to the systemic circulation and have occasionally been associated with bleeding after their removal. Correlations between pressures and volumes are best made during direct observation at operation, bearing in mind that ventricular compliance may change during the first 4 to 5 hours after bypass (60). Observation of the response to fluid challenge is the best noninvasive measurement of optimal filling pressure for each individual patient. Transesophageal echocardiography (TEE) is increasingly used to determine optimal ventricular loading and in the diagnosis of cardiac tamponade or outflow obstruction occurring postoperatively.

Although maintenance of adequate perfusion pressure is important, the postoperative patient is also prone to develop significant arterial hypertension, with resulting increases in myocardial oxygen consumption and stress on suture lines. Diagnosis and treatment of hypertension often focuses on the role of the heart, although noncardiac factors such as resolution of hemodilution, pressor reflexes from the heart, and changes in serum catecholamine levels determine hemodynamics as well (61). In patients with normal or only mild left ventricular impairment and normal volume status, the major factor influencing postoperative arterial pressure variation is peripheral resistance, not alterations in cardiac output (62). For most patients, the clinical course is marked by a slow increase in mean arterial pressure as systemic vascular resistance increases, beginning after bypass and continuing through the first few postoperative hours.

Variations in vascular resistance, which are affected by the degree of hemodilution, also need to be considered in the treatment of early postoperative hypertension. Causes of postoperative hypertension include pain, hypoxia, hypercarbia, hypothermia with shivering, visceral distention, and inadequate sedation, particularly in the presence of residual neuromuscular blockade. CPB results in variable increases in circulating epinephrine and norepinephrine levels, which correlate with blood pressure changes and sympathetic overdrive. This concept is supported by the ability of a stellate ganglion block to abolish the hypertensive response (63).

Because postoperative hypertension is often related to an increased systemic vascular resistance, vasodilator therapy is effective and is indicated once adequate ventilation and sedation are assured. Nitroglycerin and nitroprusside are the most commonly used vasodilators, but other agents such as nicardipine (64), labetalol (65), hydralazine, and prazosin are alternatives. Sublingual nifedipine has also been used for emergency blood pressure control, but its use remains controversial (66). The vasodilating properties of propofol may also be useful in this setting (67). Nitroprusside is widely used because it can be precisely titrated in response to sudden changes. Long-term nitroprusside administration, particularly at high doses, may be accompanied by increased blood cyanide and thiocyanate levels in hepatic or renal failure, respectively. Arterial oxygen saturation may be reduced via an unknown mechanism, and there may be rebound vasoconstriction after discontinuation of the drug. An automated closed loop system for nitroprusside administration can achieve superior control of hypertension with less nursing effort and less chest tube drainage (68).

Intravenous labetalol usually lowers both heart rate and cardiac index, whereas sodium nitroprusside can cause significant increases in heart rate and cardiac index. When the cardiac output is borderline (less than 2.3 L/minute/m^2), sodium nitroprusside is probably the dilating agent of choice, but labetalol, which has α- and β-adrenergic blocking effects, is preferred when the circulation is hyperdynamic. Esmolol also effectively reduces blood pressure by depressing a hyperdynamic circulation, and its half-life is sufficiently short that any adverse effects may be reversed by stopping the infusion of the drug. Fenoldopam, a catecholamine with vasodilating properties, is effective for blood pressure control and also increases renal blood flow via a dopaminergic effect (69), but its routine use is presently limited by cost concerns.

Cardiac Output

The second hemodynamic goal is maintenance of sufficient cardiac output. Acute myocardial dysfunction occurs in almost all patients, reaching a nadir at 262 $\pm$ 116 minutes after CPB. Patients with persistent low-output syndrome have an increased frequency of cardiac death, as well as complications such as renal failure, respiratory failure, disseminated intravascular coagulation, gastrointestinal bleeding, and neurologic sequelae. Regional differences in blood flow can also occur even in the presence of an adequate overall cardiac output, so a normal whole-body cardiac index does not guarantee adequate perfusion of individual organs. Evidence suggests that multiorgan failure may be precipitated by a period of gut ischemia or hyperpermeability followed by translocation of gut bacteria and release of endotoxin and other vasoactive substances that then produce generalized inflammation and organ injury (70). Monitoring of gastric tonometry offers a potential approach to detecting and treating hypoperfusion (71) but has not achieved widespread use.

Clinical indicators such as capillary refill and pedal pulses are unreliable markers for adequate peripheral perfusion after cardiac surgery, although there is a correlation between cardiac index and toe-core temperature gradient (72). Without the technology to monitor regional organ perfusion, most clinicians aim for a whole-body cardiac index of at least 2.2 L/minute/m^2. Evidence of adequate global perfusion can also be obtained by monitoring mixed venous oxygenation and the generation of lactic acid. Even these markers may be misleading, particularly in the "washout" period after CPB, when elevated serum lactic acid may represent only improved perfusion and clearance of lactate. Some investigators suggest that supranormal values of cardiac index may be necessary, and that tissue oxygen debt, reflected by insufficient oxygen consumption, is a major determinant of morbidity and mortality (73). However, the outcome benefit of supranormal cardiac output has not been demonstrated and may not be achievable in any case in the cardiac surgical population.

The most common causes of low cardiac output in the early postoperative period are hypovolemia, myocardial dysfunction, and cardiac tamponade. In the absence of the need for specific component therapy, volume expansion can be achieved with electrolyte solutions, such as Ringer's lactate or normal saline. Plasma expanders such as hetastarch or albumin are more likely to remain intravascular but are more expensive. Although colloids may reduce total volume requirements initially with endothelial injury and capillary leak, they ultimately accumulate in the interstitial compartment, where they exert an osmotic gradient, further worsening "third-spacing" (74). Once sufficient filling pressures have been attained, increasing cardiac output requires use of inotropes, reduction of afterload, or a combination of the two. The selection and use of catecholamines and vasodilators is covered in Chapter 3. Phosphodiesterase inhibitors such as milrinone and amrinone are often effective in catecholamine-refractory shock (75) in the immediate postbypass period.

Refractory right-sided heart failure is a difficult problem that often occurs after prolonged periods of ischemic arrest, mitral valve replacement, or cardiac transplantation. Treatment success has been improved by separately treating the left and right circulations, using a left atrial catheter for drug infusion to the systemic circulation and a central venous or pulmonary artery catheter for the pulmonary circulation. Prostaglandin E_1, a potent pulmonary vasodilator, has the desirable effect of specifically dilating coronary, renal, and cutaneous circulations in addition to pulmonary vasodilating effects (76). Most patients treated with prostaglandin need high doses of norepinephrine, optimally delivered via a left arterial line, to compensate for systemic vasodilation. Since the advent of phosphodiesterase inhibitors, however, we have infrequently had to employ this approach.

About 5% of patients require mechanical cardiac support after CPB, primarily with an intraaortic balloon pump (IABP), but rarely (0.3%) with VADs (77). Indications for the use of the IABP include cardiogenic shock, failure to wean from CPB, and prophylactic perioperative support in the high-risk patient. Patients with mild reversible postcardiotomy ventricular failure are most likely to respond to the 10% to 15% improvement in cardiac output achievable with IABP alone. Complications of IABP use include severe leg ischemia (5%), infection (less than 1%), and hematomas requiring drainage (0.2%) (78). IABPs may be placed via a femoral artery cutdown or percutaneously. Because surgical placement with an arteriotomy requires surgical removal under anesthesia, these patients are often left intubated and sedated until the balloon is removed. With percutaneous IABP placement, stable patients may be extubated with the balloon in place, bearing in mind that they may not be able to sit up and cough effectively while the balloon is in place or for a period of 6 hours for groin compression after balloon removal.

Although the IABP can be used to augment mildly depressed cardiac function, the presence of severe dysfunction requires a true pump capable of replacing the function of the heart until recovery occurs. A number of left and right VADs are available and can be classified as pulsatile (HeartMate, Pierce-Donachy, Abiomed BVS 5000, Novacor) or nonpulsatile. Among the nonpulsatile devices, one of the most commonly used is the Biomedicus centrifugal pump. Generally, the VAD is used to achieve a cardiac index greater than 2.2 L/minute/m^2 for a minimum of 24 hours. Daily assessments are made for the return of ventricular contractility, which manifests as measurable cardiac ejection while the patient is receiving pump support. Weaning from the VAD is accomplished by decreasing pump flow while ascertaining by thermodilution or TEE that cardiac output is maintained without a significant increase in atrial pressure. If adequate systemic flows can be sustained with the device pumping at about 500 mL/minute, the VAD can usually be removed while inotropic support or IABP counterpulsation, or both, are maintained. Survival statistics with postcardiotomy mechanical support are gradually increasing; the reader is referred to a recent review (77).

Myocardial Oxygen Supply and Demand

Optimization of the balance between myocardial oxygen supply and demand is the third postoperative hemodynamic goal. Supply-side problems can be acute (early graft occlusion or coronary artery spasm) and subacute (ITA hypoperfusion syndrome, systemic hypotension). Demand can be increased by tachycardia, shivering, and agitation. An imbalance between supply and demand may manifest as electrocardiographic ST-segment changes, ventricular dyssynergy on echocardiographic examination, and increased left- or right-sided filling pressures, but it is often unrecognized clinically (79).

Coronary artery spasm occurs in about 1% of patients, more often in those with preoperative unstable angina and/or a right-dominant coronary circulation (80). Exogenous catecholamines, preoperative β-blocked or calcium channel blockade, hypomagnesemia, and hyperventilation have all been implicated as contributing to spasm. The manifestations of coronary artery spasm occurring after revascularization (with either saphenous vein or internal mammary conduits) range from asymptomatic electrocardiographic changes to total sudden hemodynamic collapse. If the chest is open or TEE is available, examination of the heart will reveal diffuse hypokinesis. Recognition of coronary artery spasm is important because standard measures such as catecholamine and volume administration and IABP counterpulsation cannot reverse hypotension during severe episodes of spasm. Large doses of intravenous or intracoronary nitroglycerin are sometimes helpful, but nifedipine and other calcium channel blockers also appear to be effective (81). Some clinicians believe that prophylactic postoperative calcium channel therapy is indicated for patients who were taking calcium channel blockers preoperatively, to minimize the chance of spasm.

A syndrome of acute perioperative ischemia caused by hypoperfusion through ITA bypass grafts has been described (82). ITA hypoperfusion typically occurs 30 to 40 minutes after discontinuation of CPB, but it may also occur early in the ICU. This condition, which may be confused with ITA or coronary artery spasm, results from inability of an ITA to supply its large area of distribution due to mismatch between the size of the ITA and the coronary artery it is intended to supply. When it occurs, hypoperfusion syndrome often requires a return to the OR for revision of the initial operation. Experimental evidence suggests that milrinone is a direct endothelium-independent vasodilator of the human ITA and therefore may be useful for treatment of ITA spasm (83).

Cardiac Rhythm

The final early hemodynamic goal is maintenance of a stable cardiac rhythm, optimally normal sinus rhythm at a rate of 70 to 100 beats/minute. Perioperative heart rates greater than 100 beats/minute are associated with ischemia and postoperative myocardial infarction (84); bradycardia may depress cardiac output. If pacing wires have been placed, not only is treatment of bradycardia facilitated but the pacing wires may be used as leads for electrocardiographic arrhythmia detection.

Arrhythmias are common postoperatively and may result from electrolyte imbalance, myocardial ischemia, acid-base abnormalities, and excess catecholamines. Supraventricular tachycardias associated with hemodynamic instability should be treated immediately with synchronous cardioversion at 50 to 150 joules. Adenosine has become the drug of choice for reentry supraventricular tachycardias. Adenosine is given in incremental doses beginning with 6 mg, preferably through a central line. Hypotension is a common side effect, but it resolves rapidly due to adenosine's short half-life. Overdrive pacing is also useful if the rapid atrial rate can be captured and then controlled.

Atrial fibrillation is a common postoperative arrhythmia even in the absence of preexisting atrial fibrillation (85). Prophylactic magnesium administration (178 mEq over the first 4 postoperative days) lessens the incidence and severity of atrial fibrillation after CABG (86). Rate control can be accomplished with β-adrenergic blockade, electrical cardioversion, diltiazem, or amiodarone (87).

First-line treatment of ventricular dysrhythmias continues to be immediate defibrillation in the event of hemodynamic instability and use of intravenous lidocaine—1 mg/

kg bolus followed by a continuous infusion of 2 mg/minute. Ibutilide, amiodarone, bretylium, procainamide, quinidine, and diphenylhydantoin are alternatives to consider. Torsades de pointes, a special form of ventricular tachycardia associated with a long QT interval, is commonly seen in patients with ongoing ischemia. Torsades may be precipitated or worsened by type 1a antiarrhythmic drugs, and first-line therapy of torsades in the post-CPB setting involves repletion of Mg^{2+} and control of heart rate and ischemia rather than use of antiarrhythmics.

Tamponade

Signs and symptoms of cardiac tamponade in the postoperative cardiac patient can differ markedly from those seen after chest trauma or as a complication of constrictive diseases of the pericardium. First, the pericardial sac is usually left open, thus altering the compliance of the cavity and preventing classic equalization of pressures. Isolated tamponade may occur, involving only the left or the right atrium. Secondly, in the presence of coexisting left ventricular dysfunction, pulsus paradoxus may be absent. Tamponade may be also caused by acute cardiac dilatation without hemopericardium or by a small clot strategically placed so that it compresses a vital structure and decreases venous return (88). The diagnosis of tamponade should always be suspected when hemodynamic status deteriorates and fails to respond to fluid challenge and pharmacologic manipulation. The cause of mediastinal tamponade after heart surgery is usually excessive postoperative bleeding with accumulated clot producing compression of one or more chambers of the heart. Although pericardiocentesis is lifesaving in nonsurgical tamponade, it is rarely useful in the postbypass patient because clot cannot be aspirated and the procedure risks disrupting newly placed grafts. Surface echocardiography can be frustrated by the presence of bandages, edema, and overexpansion of the lungs with positive-pressure ventilation. TEE can be helpful if the time course of deterioration is not rapid. With a high index of suspicion, the usual course is to transport the patient back to the OR, open the chest and evacuate clot, at which point hemodynamic improvement is usually dramatic. If immediate return to the OR is not possible, the lower end of the sternotomy incision can be opened in the ICU and clot evacuated manually or with a suction device.

Myocardial Infarction

Perioperative myocardial infarction is recognized by new electrocardiographic changes (new Q wave) and cardiac enzyme elevation (creatinine kinase MB fraction greater than 8%, aspartate aminotransferase concentration greater than 80 units/dL). Using these criteria, the rate of infarction is in the range of 3% to 6%. Although no combination of enzyme activity changes can completely discriminate patients with perioperative myocardial infarction from those without, experience suggests that elevated creatine kinase MB exhibits diagnostic association with the presence of histologically proven infarction (89). Troponin I is specific and sensitive in the diagnosis of acute myocardial infarction and can be used for specific confirmation, late presentation, and risk stratification (90). Reinfusion of shed mediastinal and chest tube drainage can complicate enzyme diagnosis of infarction, because autotransfusion results in elevation of creatinine kinase, aspartate aminotransferase, and lactic dehydrogenases (91). Myoglobin levels increase rapidly and peak at 3 hours after reperfusion in uncomplicated patients. However, the rise in myoglobin may continue for 24 hours and may exhibit a delayed peak in those with myocardial injury accelerated by reperfusion after ischemia (92).

Calcium in Resuscitation

The routine use of calcium to treat hypotension and low output after cardiac surgery has been called into question. Calcium inhibits the cardiotonic action of β-adrenergic agonists such as dobutamine, possibly by interfering with signal transduction (93). Administration of a calcium infusion has been shown to blunt dobutamine-induced increases in cardiac output by 30%, without altering the effects of phosphodiesterase inhibitors such as amrinone. In addition, hyperamylasemia, a marker of pancreatic cellular injury, is more common in patients receiving large doses of calcium chloride, raising the possibility that calcium administration can precipitate postoperative pancreatitis (94). Some clinicians have also implicated bolus administration of calcium in coronary spasm, although the data are inconclusive. Our practice is to treat symptomatic ionized hypocalcemia but otherwise to avoid routine calcium administration, at least until this therapeutic question has been more clearly settled.

RECOVERY FROM ANESTHESIA

A variety of anesthetic regimens are used for cardiac surgery patients; they involve low- to high-dose opioid administration and muscle relaxation supplemented as needed with inhaled anesthetic agents, benzodiazepines, or propofol. Depending on the drugs and dosages used, the effects of these agents may dissipate early in the ICU stay or be prolonged. Care must be taken to ensure that patients do not awaken while they are still neuromuscularly blocked. Renarcotization, manifested by elevated carbon dioxide tension (P_{CO_2}) and somnolence, may occur as a result of either mobilization of stored opioids from muscle or trapping of opioid in the stomach with subsequent reabsorption from the alkaline small intestine (95). Factors influencing opioid pharmacokinetics include age of the patient, use of β-blocking agents and other drugs, and the patient's habitual consumption of alcohol or other agents active in the central nervous system.

Usually the most marked increases in oxygen consumption and carbon dioxide production occur during the first 6 postoperative hours, simultaneously with maximum spontaneous rewarming. The risk of decompensation is highest during these first few hours of hypermetabolism, and it is in these same few hours that perioperative ischemic episodes are most common (96). Heart rate, hypertension, and hypermetabolic responses can be well controlled with sedative agents such as propofol (97).

TEMPERATURE CONTROL AND SHIVERING

Shivering commonly occurs after CPB, and it may increase oxygen consumption beyond what a depressed heart can adequately deliver, resulting in lactic acidosis. Patients who shiver may also develop acute respiratory acidosis as a result of the inability to increase spontaneous minute ventilation appropriately after a narcotic/relaxant anesthesia. Calculated minute ventilation may be normal or even excessive on admission to the ICU when the patient is hypothermic, but it may become deficient as rewarming occurs. Because respiratory alkalosis exacerbates hypokalemia and ventricular irritability, and respiratory acidosis can compromise catecholamine function, proper ventilatory management and control of shivering is essential. Shivering may be inhibited with radiant heat or meperidine. Although radiant heat takes slightly longer to affect shivering, it is more easily controlled, does not impose additional medication on the patient, and has a lower incidence of shivering recurrence

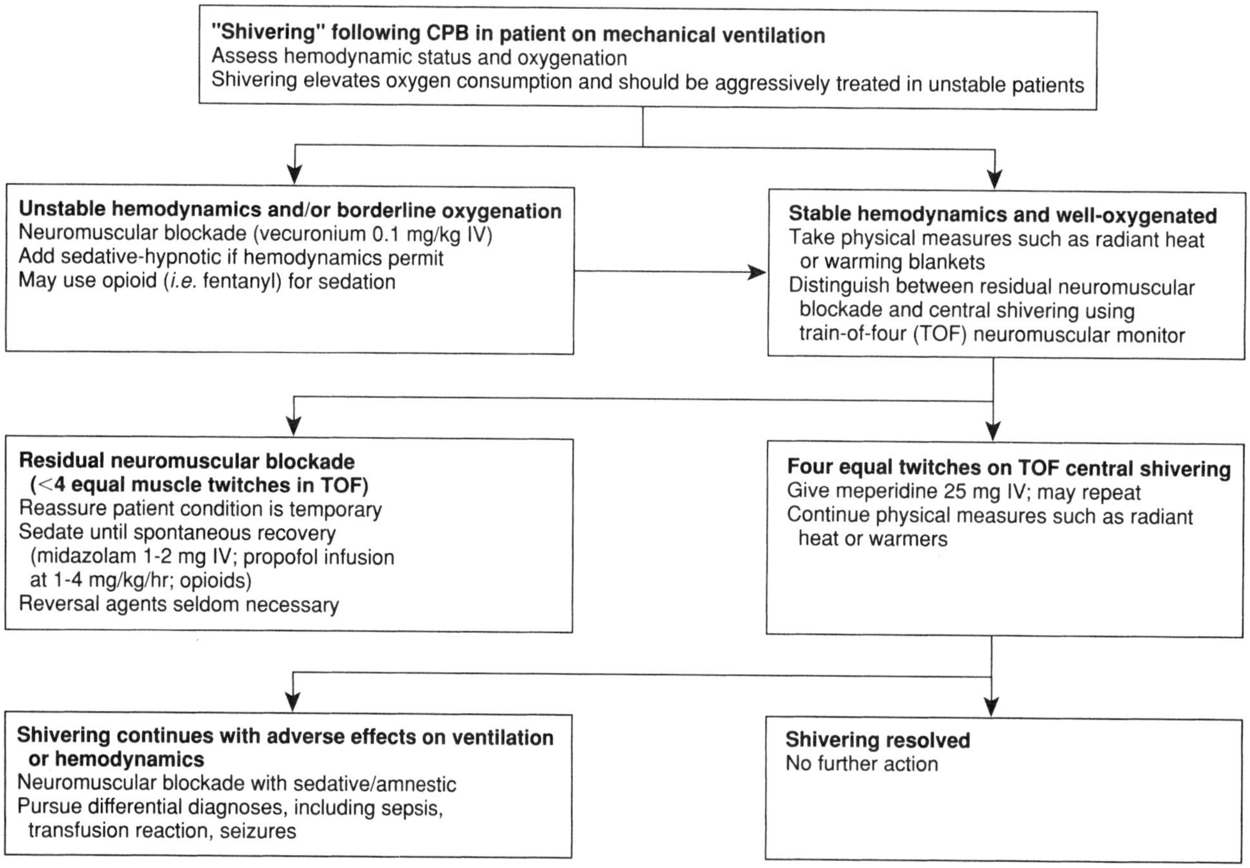

FIGURE 17-3. "Shivering" after cardiopulmonary bypass (CPB) in patients receiving mechanical ventilation. The period of hypermetabolism after CPB occurs within the first 4 hours after arrival at the intensive care unit. Although true shivering is common, it must be differentiated from the frequently seen partial neuromuscular blockade as the patient recovers from operative medications. Shivering in an unstable patient should be treated with neuromuscular blockade and a small dose of a sedative-hypnotic agent if the patient is awake and hemodynamics permit. Opioids such as fentanyl and sufentanil may be given by bolus or infusion with very little risk of hemodynamic compromise. Radiant heat and warming blankets are effective physical measures. If neuromuscular blockade has been ruled out and shivering persists, meperidine 25 to 50 mg IV often alleviates shivering. Should it be necessary to use a neuromuscular blocking agent for uncontrolled shivering, small doses (e.g., vecuronium 4 mg) suffice. Although residual neuromuscular blockade may be reversed, we prefer to keep the patient sedated while spontaneous recovery occurs.

than does meperidine (98). Small doses of a neuromuscular blocking agent such as pancuronium or vecuronium may be needed for intubated, ventilated patients whose shivering is severe or cannot be controlled by other methods. An algorithmic approach to shivering is displayed in Fig. 17-3. Dexamethasone has been shown to decrease the incidence of shivering independently from temperature, suggesting that shivering may be part of the febrile response that occurs after the release of cytokines during CPB (99).

RENAL CONSIDERATIONS

Oliguric or anuric renal failure occurs after 1% to 4% of open heart surgery procedures, and lesser degrees of renal dysfunction, marked by elevated serum creatinine, occur in 2% to 30% (100). Univariate predictors of serious acute renal failure include low cardiac output at the end of CPB, advanced age, preoperative cardiac failure, need for postoperative circulatory support, blood transfusions, and prolonged time on CPB (101). Despite aggressive ICU care and the availability of renal replacement therapy, the mortality rate is high, as much as 88% with the combination of renal and hepatic failure (102).

Prevention of renal failure is clearly desirable, although evidence for the efficacy of interventions is scant. Urine output must be monitored throughout the perioperative period. Dopamine has been shown to produce functional improvement in the setting of new-onset oliguria after CPB (103), but data are lacking to support prophylactic use. Post-CABG patients given dopamine are prone to develop hypokalemia and arrhythmias. An algorithm for management of perioperative oliguria is presented in Fig. 17-4.

When renal failure occurs, it usually follows one of three well-defined patterns (104) (Fig. 17-5). Abbreviated acute renal failure occurs after an isolated insult, results in a peak in serum creatinine around the fourth postevent day, and generally has a favorable prognosis if no other events occur. The second pattern initially resembles the first, except that the acute insult is accompanied by prolonged circulatory failure. This pattern runs a longer course, with recovery typically occurring in the second or third week after injury, in tandem with improvements in cardiac output. In the third pattern, recovery is complicated by a second insult such as sepsis, massive gastrointestinal bleeding, or myocardial infarction. Permanent failure may result from this pattern, and other coexisting organ failure is common. Because fluid overload with renal failure may precipitate respiratory and cardiac failure, there has been a trend toward early application of CAVH and related techniques to remove excess fluid (105). There is speculation that aggressive fluid removal may decrease tissue edema and intraabdominal pressure, thereby improving renal perfusion pressure and, consequently, renal function.

CENTRAL NERVOUS SYSTEM CONSIDERATIONS

Potential neurologic complications after open heart surgery include focal cerebral lesions resulting in gross sensory-motor abnormalities such as hemiparesis and aphasia, severe global encephalopathy, peripheral nerve injury, phrenic nerve injury, and neuropsychiatric changes. The reported incidence depends on how and where the study was conducted, with prospective studies identifying early postoperative neurologic changes in more than 60% of patients (106). Fortunately, most of these resolve by 6-month follow-up, and the residual findings are often of little functional importance. Major disability occurs in slightly more than 1% of patients and is almost always identified very early in the postoperative period (107). ICU care of these patients is usually concerned with maintaining reasonable perfusion pressure and ensuring continued protection of the airway, because aspiration is a major risk. Seizures, occasionally seen in association with focal neurologic deficits, can be controlled by usual measures such as intravenous benzodiazepine and phenytoin (Dilantin) or phosphenytoin. Physical therapy and occupational therapy should be initiated while the patient is still in the ICU.

An approach to the management of the patient who fails to awaken is outlined in Fig. 17-6. Sedatives, narcotics, and muscle relaxants should be withheld, and peripheral neuromuscular function should be assessed with the use of a nerve stimulator. Computed tomography or magnetic resonance imaging can rule out structural lesions or cerebral edema. Lumbar puncture is rarely helpful. Electroencephalography and evoked potentials are indicated to assess brain electrical activity and to rule out seizures only when other tests have not delivered a diagnosis. There is currently very little that can be done acutely once a major focal or global neurologic injury is identified; prevention of these injuries and early institution of rehabilitation are important. In the absence of cerebral hemorrhagic infarct and after the early postoperative phase, anticoagulation may be useful. The use of thrombolytics for postoperative stroke has not been well studied.

Transient postoperative delirium occurs in about 7% of patients, resolving spontaneously or with pharmacologic intervention in almost all patients by postoperative day 6 (108). Alcohol or benzodiazepine withdrawal should be considered in the differential diagnosis of delirium. Initial management of agitation consists of reassurance and orientation of the patient and control of pain with opioids. Agitation accompanied by disorientation may be worsened by benzodiazepines, which should be restricted to treatment of oriented but anxious patients or for prophylaxis of alcohol and benzodiazepine withdrawal. If the patient remains agitated and disoriented, haloperidol is often useful (109).

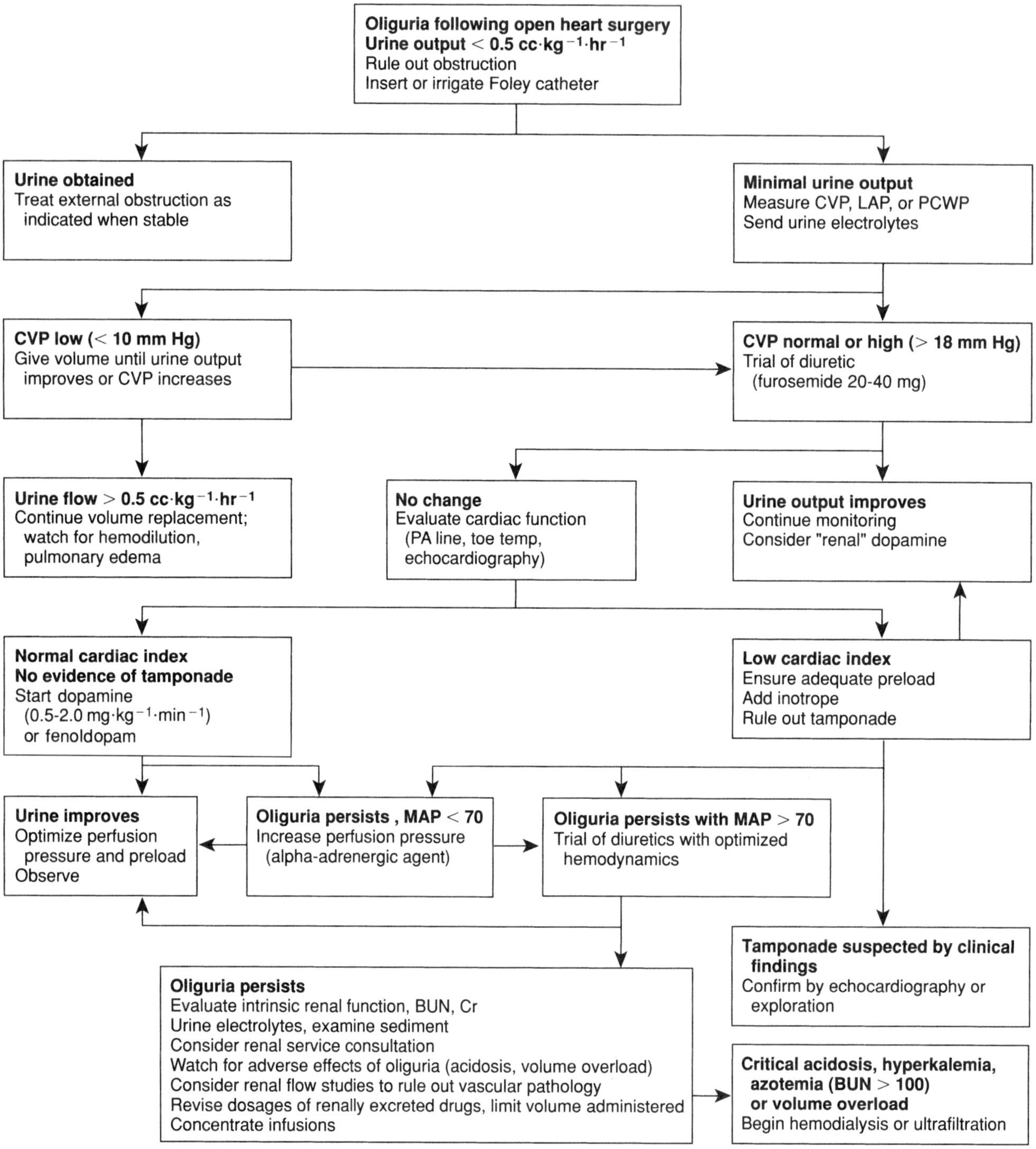

FIGURE 17-4. Oliguria after open heart surgery. Compromised renal function may occur as a result of a low-flow state or embolic occlusion of the renal arteries. Postrenal obstruction should be ruled out with passage or irrigation of the Foley catheter. A sonogram of the kidneys may also be helpful in delineating obstructive pathology. Adequacy of filling pressures and inotropic support should then be considered. Many times, response to diuretics occurs only when the mean arterial pressure is increased above the patient's baseline values. Low urine output may be a marker of a low cardiac output state, which can be documented by pulmonary artery catheterization or echocardiographic examination. Oliguria that persists after adequate blood flow and perfusion pressure are ensured requires an extensive workup, and consultation from a nephrologist can be very helpful. CVP, central venous pressure; LAP, left arterial pressure; PCWP, pulmonary capillary wedge pressure; PA, pulmonary artery; MAP, mean arterial pressure; BUN, blood urea nitrogen; Cr, creatinine.

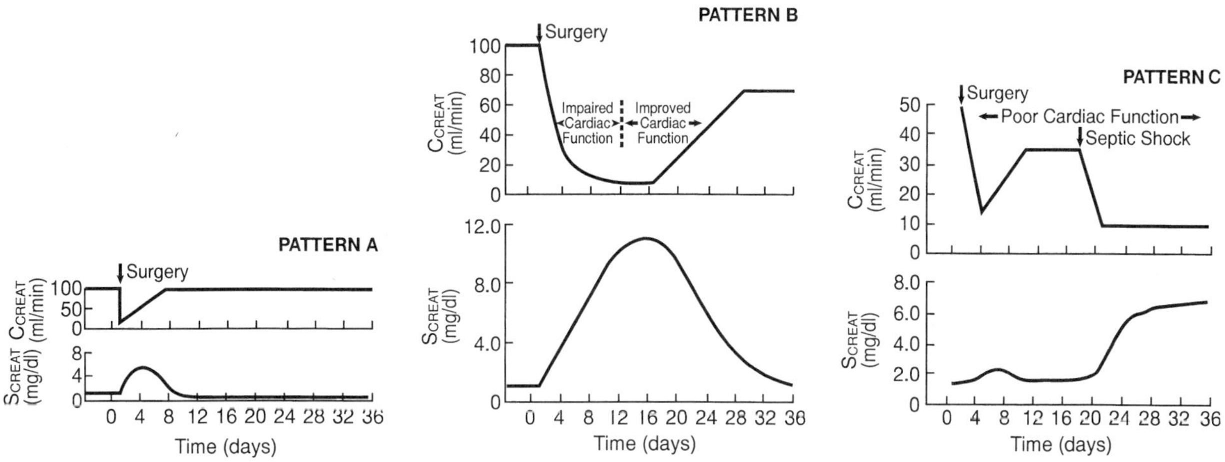

FIGURE 17-5. Three typical courses of acute renal failure after cardiac surgery are illustrated by creatinine clearance (^{c}CREAT) and serum level of creatinine (^{s}CREAT) in representative patients who did not undergo dialysis (38). The upper portion (pattern A) displays a step decrement that is followed immediately by a ramp increment in ^{c}CREAT typical of abbreviated acute renal failure. The middle portion (pattern B) displays an exponential decrement of ^{c}CREAT that is accompanied by a linear increase in ^{s}CREAT (days 1 to 12). Recovery, which follows improved cardiac performance from day 12, is manifested during days 16 through 30 by a ramp increment in ^{c}CREAT that is accompanied by a sigmoidal decline in ^{s}CREAT. In the lower portion (pattern C), successive ramp decrements in ^{c}CREAT (days 1 to 4 and 18 to 21) are accompanied by sigmoidal elevation of ^{s}CREAT. Recovery of ^{c}CREAT (ramp increment, days 4 to 7) is seen only after the first episode. A persistent low-cardiac-output state prevents recovery from the second insult. (From Meyers BD, Moran SM: hemodynamically mediated acute renal failure. *N Engl J Med* 1986;314:97, with permission.)

RETURN FOR BLEEDING

The cycle of systemic heparinization, hypothermia (if used), and protamine reversal is followed by persistent bleeding in a small but important subset of patients. Several aspects of the immediate management deserve emphasis.

Causes of postoperative bleeding include inadequate heparin neutralization, fibrinolysis, complement activation, quantitative or qualitative platelet defects, and less often, decreased levels of factors V, VIII, XIII, fibrinogen, and plasminogen. No single test of hemostasis is sufficient. Postoperative coagulation profiles may include an activated clotting time (ACT), prothrombin time (PT), an international normalized ratio (INR), partial thromboplastin time (PTT), platelet count, and fibrinogen level. Most of these values are abnormal immediately after CPB, even without excessive bleeding. D-dimer or fibrin split products may be ordered if there is suspicion of disseminated intravascular coagulation as the result of low cardiac output and hypoperfusion. One approach to postoperative bleeding is to determine the ACT, and, if it is elevated, administer protamine 50 mg IV, and then recheck the ACT. If bleeding persists and the ACT is normal, then a clotting profile should be drawn. At this point, platelet transfusion may be indicated even in the presence of a normal count, because function may be impaired. The use of desmopressin (110), ϵ-aminocaproic acid (111), and aprotinin (112) can be supported, although controversy persists (113).

The majority of patients still undergo cardiac surgery without need for exogenous transfusion. Red blood cell volume, followed by age, is the best determinant of blood use during myocardial revascularization (114). The mortality rate increases with hemoglobin values of less than 9.5 g/dL in patients with heart disease, and high-risk patients have improved outcome when transfused (115). Specific transfusion guidelines for cardiac surgical patients have been published (116).

The decision to reexplore a patient for postoperative bleeding must be individualized, with a bias toward earlier rather than later reexploration. Bleeding of more than 300 mL in the first hour, 250 mL in the second hour, or 150 mL/hour thereafter without signs of abatement are common indications for surgical exploration and have been correlated with surgically correctable bleeding (117). Exploration is also indicated if a large hemothorax or pericardial tamponade occurs. Wound complications are diminished with early exploration in patients whose blood loss exceeded 200 mL/hour for 4 hours (118).

INFECTIOUS COMPLICATIONS

Mediastinitis, sternal dehiscence, or both, are rare complications of coronary revascularization, with an incidence of about 1%, but a mortality rate of 13%. Predisposing factors

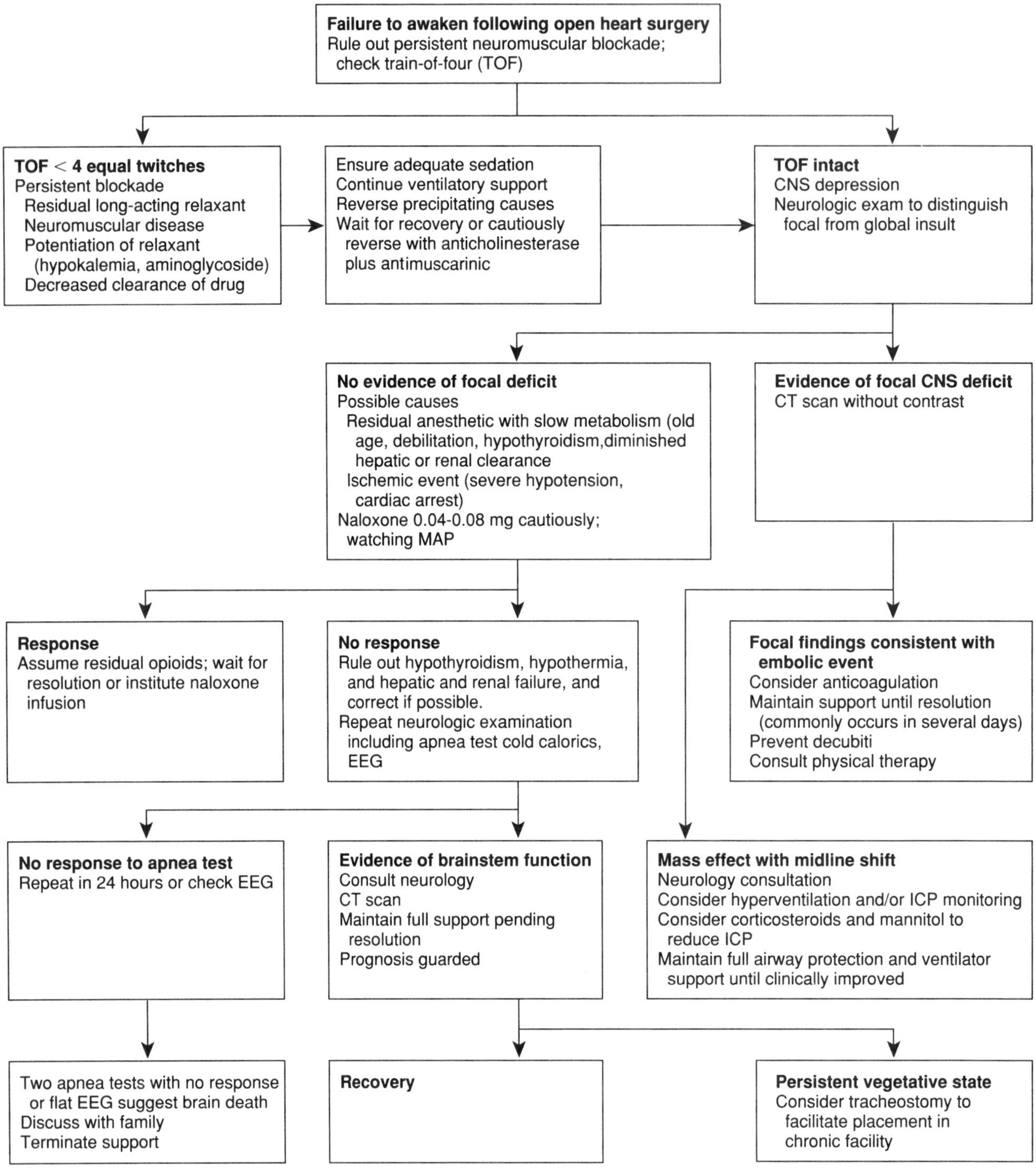

FIGURE 17-6. Failure to awaken after open heart surgery. Persistent neuromuscular blockade is surprisingly common and must be ruled out in any patient who does not awaken after open heart surgery. Once this has been ruled out, a careful neurologic examination should be made to search for evidence of a focal central nervous system deficit, which can further be evaluated with computed tomographic scanning. Many focal lesions are of embolic origin, and the prognosis for recovery is good. Persistent coma without evidence of a focal deficit is more worrisome. Aside from the situation in which barbiturate loading has been used for cerebral protection, it is unusual to see a patient fail to metabolize operative anesthetics by the end of 24 hours. If naloxone is used, it should be cautiously titrated in doses of 40 to 80 μg, watching for tachycardia and hypertension. Lack of response to a naloxone challenge requires further workup, and neurologic consultation is well advised at this point.

for wound complications after open heart surgery include diabetes, low cardiac output, use of bilateral internal mammary grafts, and reoperation for control of bleeding (119). Maintenance of blood glucose lower than 200 mg% in the perioperative period reduces the sternal wound infection rate from 2.4% to 1.5% (120). Mediastinal infection is often manifested as failure to wean, unexplained fever, and an unstable sternum. Confirmation of infection may be difficult, because radionuclide bone scans "light up" with normal healing. Surgical exploration and drainage of the wound may be necessary to obtain adequate material for culture. Polymicrobial isolates are associated with particularly poor outcome. Management of mediastinitis requires selective antibiotic therapy, debridement, irrigation, drainage, and reclosure. In cases of severe sternal necrosis, early debridement and plastic surgical reconstruction using omental and/or myocutaneous flaps are recommended.

Pneumonia, tracheobronchitis, line sepsis, and urinary tract infections are frequently seen in the ventilator-dependent long-term ICU patient. The organisms encountered are influenced by the type of antibiotic prophylaxis used and the portal of entry. Because typical perioperative antibiotic prophylaxis consists of an anti-staphylococcal penicillin or cephalosporin, nosocomial pneumonia is likely to occur with organisms such as *Pseudomonas, Klebsiella, Serratia, Acinetobacter,* or, rarely, methicillin-resistant staphylococcus aureus (MRSA). Treatment of the secondary infection may be followed by a tertiary infection with even more difficult organisms, such as *Candida, Torulopsis,* or other fungal species. Selective digestive decontamination was initially received with enthusiasm but controlled studies suggested lack of outcome benefit; the latest metaanalysis indicates utility in selected patients (121).

GASTROINTESTINAL COMPLICATIONS

Gastrointestinal complications requiring intervention occur in 1% to 3% of patients but are associated with substantial mortality (122). Postoperative ileus and upper gastrointestinal bleeding from ulceration are common. Pancreatitis, mesenteric ischemia, perforation, and bleeding elsewhere in the gastrointestinal tract are problems of the critically ill patient with developing multisystem failure. Mesenteric ischemia can occur as a result of low perfusion or embolic atheroma from large-vessel manipulation. The risk of gastrointestinal bleeding in the complicated postoperative case can be minimized with antacid therapy, histamine blockers, or barrier protection agents such as sucralfate. Enteral nutritional support also appears to protect the gastric mucosa (123).

If the gastroepiploic artery is used as a conduit for revascularization, it is wise to leave a gastric sump tube in place postoperatively and to monitor for postoperative ileus and pancreatitis. These precautions are not necessary when the inferior epigastric, which supplies the rectus sheath, is used as a conduit.

Jaundice occurs in approximately 20% of patients after CPB, often in association with replacement of multiple valves, higher transfusion requirements, longer times on CPB, or hepatic defects in the excretion of bilirubin (124). Jaundice plus renal failure carries a mortality rate as high as 88%.

Acute postoperative pancreatitis is uncommon but carries a poor prognosis, especially when it occurs in the setting of multisystem organ failure. Evidence of pancreatitis is found in 25% of autopsied patients dying after open heart surgery (125). Transient elevation of amylase may occur unrelated to pancreatic injury, so hyperamylasemia is less valuable as a diagnostic test than is a serum lipase assay.

RISK ASSESSMENT AND OUTCOME SCORING

Knowledge of the factors that place an individual patient at high risk is helpful for surveillance and intervention. Factors shown to increase mortality risk include emergency surgery, combined valve and coronary surgery, left main coronary artery occlusion greater than 90%, aneurysm and great vessel surgery, and any reoperation. Demographic and historical predictors include advanced age, female gender, low body weight, poor left ventricular function, congestive heart failure, diabetes, COPD, and diffuse vascular disease represented by peripheral or carotid occlusive disease (126–129). Stratification of risks is necessary to assess overall outcome, to examine the effects of ICU care, and to assist with triage and therapeutic decisions.

Systems designed for general ICU risk stratification do not necessarily apply to the cardiac surgical population. Variables scored by the APACHE-II study (130), for example (temperature, mean pressure, heart rate, respiratory rate, arterial pH, sodium, potassium, and hematocrit), are controlled by the OR team and therefore may not reflect the patient's physiologic reserve. Only chronic disease history and emergency surgery remain as measurable mortality risks. APACHE-III has been successfully applied to evaluate ICU length of stay and costs in cardiac surgical patients (131). Scoring systems for cardiac surgical patients can be used to assess risk either preoperatively (132) or at ICU admission (Table 17-4). Sequential use of a preoperative and ICU admission score helps isolate the OR and ICU components of care. These systems have utility in outcome assessment for administration, quality assurance, and research. Using the Cleveland Clinic Preoperative Score (Table 17-5), we have observed a steady increase in the number of high-risk patients (Fig. 17-7) but a declining risk-adjusted morbidity rate (Fig. 17-8). For more detailed information on risk stratification and outcome assessment in the adult cardiac surgical patient, the reader is referred to several recent articles (133–136).

TABLE 17-4. INTENSIVE CARE UNIT RISK STRATIFICATION SCORE

Variable	Value
Preoperative factors	
Small body size (BSA <1.72m^2)	1
Prior heart operation	
One	1
Two or more	2
History of operation or angioplasty for peripheral vascular disease	3
Age ≥70 yr	3
Preoperative creatinine ≥1.9 mg/dL	4
Preoperative albumin <3.5 mg/dL	5
Intraoperative factors	
CPB time ≥160 min	3
Use of IABP after CPB	7
ICU admission physiology	
A-a O_2 gradient ≥250 mm Hg	2
Heart rate ≥100 beats/min	3
Cardiac index <2.1 L/min^1/m^2	3
CVP ≥17 mm Hg	4
Arterial bicarbonate <21 mmol/L	4

Note: A-a, alveolar-arterial; BSA, body surface area; CPB, cardiopulmonary bypass; CVP, central venous pressure; IABP, intraaortic balloon pump; ICU, intensive care unit.

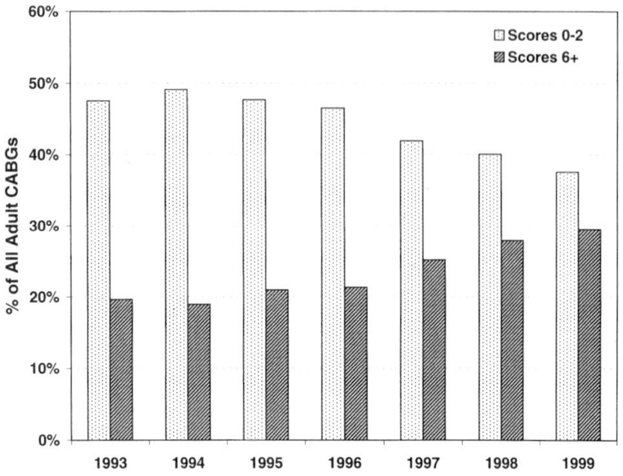

FIGURE 17-7. Change in risk profile over time.

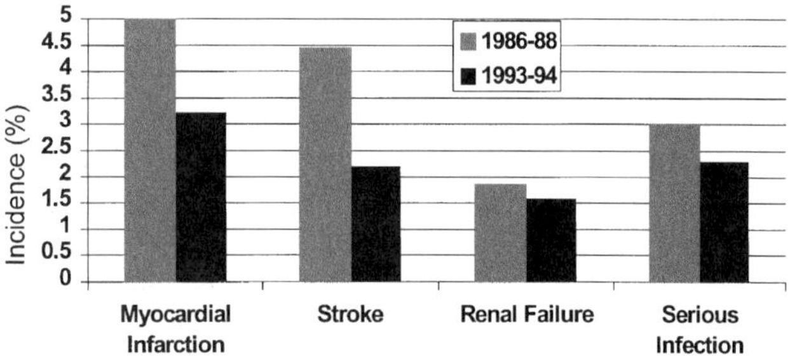

FIGURE 17-8. Changes in risk-adjusted morbidity after coronary after bypass grafting. (Data from Estafanous F, Loop FD, Higgins TL, et al. Increased risk and decreased morbidity of coronary artery bypass grafting between 1986 and 1994. *Ann Thorac Surg* 1998;65:383, with permission.)

TABLE 17-5. PREOPERATIVE SEVERITY SCORING SYSTEM FOR CARDIAC SURGERY

Preoperative Factors	Score
Emergency case	6
Serum creatinine (mg/dL)	
≥1.6 and ≤1.8	1
≥1.9	4
Severe LV dysfunction	3
Reoperation	3
Operative mitral valve insufficiency	3
Age ≥65 and ≤74 yr	1
Age ≥75 yr	2
Prior vascular surgery	2
Chronic obstructive pulmonary disease	2
Anemia (HCT ≤34%)	2
Operative aortic valve stenosis	1
Weight ≤65 kg	1
Diabetes, oral or insulin therapy	1
Cerebrovascular disease	1

Note: HCT, hematocrit; LV, left ventricular.
Source: Higgins TL, Estafanous FG, Loop FD, et al. Stratification of morbidity and mortality outcome by preoperative risk factors in coronary artery bypass patients. *JAMA* 1992;267:2344, with permission.

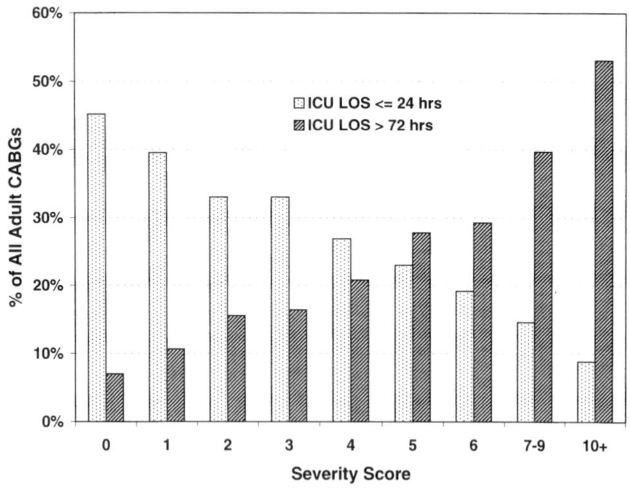

FIGURE 17-9. Intensive care unit length of stay (LOS) by severity score.

UTILIZATION OF THE INTENSIVE CARE UNIT

Admission and discharge criteria are necessary for patient care and to ensure equitable use of resources. For a dedicated cardiothoracic unit, the admission criteria are fairly straightforward, because patients undergoing cardiac surgery typically require postoperative monitoring and interventions. However, an increasing number of fast-track patients may be managed in recovery areas, thus avoiding occupancy of a full-service ICU bed (137). Length of stay is highly correlated with preoperative severity of illness (Fig. 17-9). Discharge criteria form the basis for triage decisions. Allowing patients to leave the ICU prematurely increases the rate of readmissions and can set the stage for catastrophic problems. On the other hand, keeping patients in the ICU unnecessarily increases costs and may force cancellation of other surgeries. Discharge criteria for the Cleveland Clinic Cardiothoracic ICU are listed in Table 17-6. Using these criteria as the basis for triage decisions, more than 40% of all CPB patients leave the unit on the first postoperative day. Early ICU discharge is possible for almost half of low-risk patients but falls off progressively with higher preoperative risk scores (Fig. 17-8).

QUALITY IMPROVEMENT IN THE INTENSIVE CARE UNIT

The goals of a quality improvement program are to monitor and evaluate the quality of patient care objectively and systematically, to identify opportunities to improve patient care, and to resolve problems as they are identified (138). The ICU quality improvement program is usually the responsibility of the medical director of the unit, in coordination with the directors of the surgical and anesthesia services and representatives from nursing and respiratory therapy.

The quality improvement plan at the Cleveland Clinic has four components: (a) quarterly analysis of a set of indicators collected routinely on every patient, using a risk-adjusted epidemiologic approach; (b) focused structure and process reviews conducted on a regular basis; (c) a problem log for events noted in the day-to day work of physicians, nurses, and allied health workers; and (d) *ad hoc* analysis of the impact of changes in patient management on outcome. A recent year's worth of quarterly reports is displayed in Table 17-7. Outcome indicators have been chosen to reflect important aspects of ICU care, particularly organ system failure and occurrence of preventable events such as self-extubation. The relative patient severity for each quarter is included, using a previously described scoring system. Indicators that exceed predetermined thresholds are first evaluated for the contribution of patient severity, to ensure that, for example, an increased mortality rate is not just a function of an increased number of seriously ill patients, based on preoperative severity scoring. This process involves

TABLE 17-6. CRITERIA FOR DISCHARGE FROM THE CARDIOVASCULAR INTENSIVE CARE UNIT

Neurologic and psychological
- Able to protect airway (adequate gag reflex or tracheostomized)
- Able to signal distress (verbal or using call button)
- If requiring psychotropic drugs or withdrawing from alcohol or other drugs, pharmacologic regimen should be stable for at least 24 hr

Cardiac
- Stable MAP $\geq$70 mm Hg without pressor support
- Adequate perfusion (CI $\geq$2.1; warm extremities; satisfactory urine output)
- No inotropic support other than "renal" dopamine ($\leq$3 μg/ kg^{-1}/min^{-1})
- Rhythm sinus <6 PACs/min or atrial fibrillation with controlled rate <120 beats/min
- Not pacer-dependent (unless suitable junctional-ventricular escape rate)

Respiratory
- Maintaining pH >7.35 and Pco_2 within 8 mm Hg of baseline value
- Oxygen saturation $\geq$92% on nasal cannula or simple mask (<50% Fio_2)
- Coughing well and clearing secretions; suctioned twice per shift or less
- No pneumothorax, large effusions, or marked fluid overload on chest radiography
- No subcutaneous emphysema that will interfere with respiratory status or vision

Renal
- Urine output at least 0.5 mL/kg^{-1}/hr
- Weight within 5 μg of preoperative value
- Creatinine less than 50% greater than preoperative value

Hematologic
- Hematocrit $\geq$26%
- Chest tube output <50 mL/hr
- No evidence of ongoing DIC
- Clotting parameters within normal unless deliberately anticoagulated

Infectious
- No evidence of acute pneumonia or sepsis
- Temperature $\leq$39.0°C
- WBC < 18,000/mm^3

Gastrointestinal
- Taking and holding clear liquids or on enteral/parenteral support
- No active gastrointestinal bleeding
- No ileus or bowel obstruction unless resolving
- No evidence of active cholecystitis or pancreatitis

Endocrine/metabolic
- Blood glucose adequately controlled
- Serum potassium $\geq$3.5 mEq

Exceptions
- Patients with "DNR" status written need not meet any other criteria
- Patients sent to floor on ventilator need not meet respiratory criteria
- Patients who will be discharged on chronic dobutamine therapy may go to floor on inotropes
- Inotropic support and more frequent suctioning acceptable on stepdown floor

Note: CI, cardiac index; DIC, disseminated intravascular coagulation; DNR, do not resuscitate; Fio_2, fraction of inspired oxygen; MAP, mean arterial pressure; PAC, premature atrial contraction; Pco_2, partial pressure of carbon dioxide; WBC, white blood cell count.

TABLE 17-7. CARDIOTHORACIC INTENSIVE CARE UNIT QUARTERLY REPORT (PERCENTAGES IN PARENTHESES)

Indicator	Year Quarter				Grand Total	1995 Level	Expected Range	
	1998 Q1	1998 Q2	1998 Q3	1998 Q4			Lower	Upper
No. cases	857	861	910	896	3524	3302		
No. CABG ± other procedures	538 (62.8)	531 (61.7)	555 (61.0)	551 (61.5)	2175 (61.7)	73.20%	70.3%	76.1%
Isolated CABGs	368 (42.9)	380 (44.1)	397 (43.6)	373 (41.6)	1518 (43.1)	56.9%	53.6%	60.2%
Average Severity Score (CABG plus others)	3.98	4.16	3.68	4.23	4.01	3.4	3.1	3.6
Mortality	24 (2.8)	31 (3.6)	16 (1.8)	30 (3.4)	101 (2.9)	3.2%	2.0%	4.4%
All CABG	7 (0.8)	16 (1.9)	10 (1.1)	13 (1.5)	46 (1.3)	2.1%	1.1%	3.0%
Isolated CABG	5 (0.6)	10 (1.2)	4 (0.4)	3 (0.2)	21 (0.6)	1.3%	0.5%	2.0%
Non-CABG	17 (1.9)	15 (1.7)	6 (0.7)	17 (1.9)	55 (1.6)	1.2%	0.4%	1.9%
Morbidity	102 (11.9)	111 (12.9)	99 (10.9)	85 (9.5)	397 (11.3)	12.0%	9.9%	12.2%
Cardiac	28 (3.3)	36 (4.2)	26 (2.9)	25 (2.8)	115 (3.3)	2.2%	1.2%	3.1%
Intubated ≥72 hr	77 (8.9)	76 (8.8)	64 (7.0)	64 (7.1)	281 (7.8)	9.2%	7.2%	11.1%
Renal failure	21 (2.5)	22 (2.6)	12 (1.3)	20 (2.2)	75 (2.1)	2.1%	1.1%	3.0%
Neurologic	17 (1.9)	25 (2.9)	28 (3.1)	18 (2.0)	88 (2.5)	2.6%	1.6%	3.7%
Serious infection	42 (4.9)	53 (6.2)	42 (4.6)	48 (5.4)	185 (5.3)	4.8%	3.4%	6.2%
Initial intubation time								
Average (hr)	18.1	25.9	18.8	22.6	21.3	30.2	23.3	37.1
Median (hr)	9.9	9.5	10.1	9.1	9.7	12.3		
Time ≤4 hr	53 (6.2)	66 (7.7)	64 (7.0)	69 (7.7)	252 (7.2)	2.4%	1.4%	3.4%
Time >4 and ≤8 hr	260 (30.3)	260 (28.6)	254 (27.9)	290 (32.4)	1064 (30.2)	17.5%	15.0%	20.1%
No. reintubated	79 (9.2)	64 (7.4)	77 (8.5)	65 (7.3)	285 (8.1)	8.0%	6.2%	9.8%
ICU LOS								
Average Total (hr)	79.2	76.8	69.7	71.4	74.2	84.8	72.8	96.7
Median Total (hr)	38.7	31.3	29.9	29.7	30.6	39.3		
Time ≤24 hr	218 (25.4)	213 (24.7)	250 (27.5)	259 (28.9)	940 (26.7)	28.9%	25.9%	31.9%
Time >72 hr	230 (26.8)	200 (23.2)	197 (21.6)	195 (21.8)	822 (23.3)	23.5%	20.7%	26.3%
No. cases with at least 1 readmission	74 (8.6)	89 (8.0)	65 (7.1)	49 (5.7)	257 (7.3)	8.2%	6.3%	9.9%
Atrial arrhythmia	166 (19.4)	139 (16.1)	143 (15.7)	142 (15.9)	590 (16.7)	17.9%	15.2%	20.3%
Ventricular arrhythmias	43 (5.0)	43 (4.9)	39 (4.3)	41 (4.6)	166 (4.7)	4.4%	3.1%	5.8%
Respiratory morbidity	53 (6.2)	60 (6.9)	67 (7.4)	76 (8.5)	256 (7.3)	7.2%	5.5%	8.9%
No. returned to OR for bleeding or tamponade	36 (4.2)	35 (4.1)	36 (3.9)	32 (3.6)	139 (3.9)	4.9%	3.5%	6.4%
MSOF	11 (1.3)	15 (1.7)	7 (0.8)	16 (1.8)	49 (1.4)	1.2%	0.5%	1.9%
Died without awakening	3 (0.4)	3 (0.4)	4 (0.4)	0 (0)	10 (0.3)	0.6%	0.1%	1.2%
Lip/Dental injury	1 (0.1)	1 (0.1)		1 (0.1)	3 (0.1)	0.3%	0.0%	0.7%
Transfusion therapy	2 (0.2)	0 (0)	0 (0)	– (0)	2 (0.1)	0.2%	0.0%	0.4%
Wound dehiscence	1 (0.1)	0 (0)	0 (0)	0 (0)	1 (0.0)	0.1%	0.0%	0.2%
Self-extubation	14 (1.6)	3 (0.4)	5 (0.6)	8 (0.9)	30 (0.9)	1.9%	1.1%	2.9%
Ulnar neuropathy	0 (0)	0 (0)	1 (0.1)	0 (0)	1 (0.1)	0.03%	0.0%	0.6%
Brachial plexus injury	0 (0)	3 (0.4)	0 (0)	0 (0)	3 (0.1)	0.03%	0.0%	0.2%

Note: CABG, coronary artery bypass grafting; ICU, intensive care unit; LOS, length of stay; MSOF, multiple system organ failure; OR, operating room.

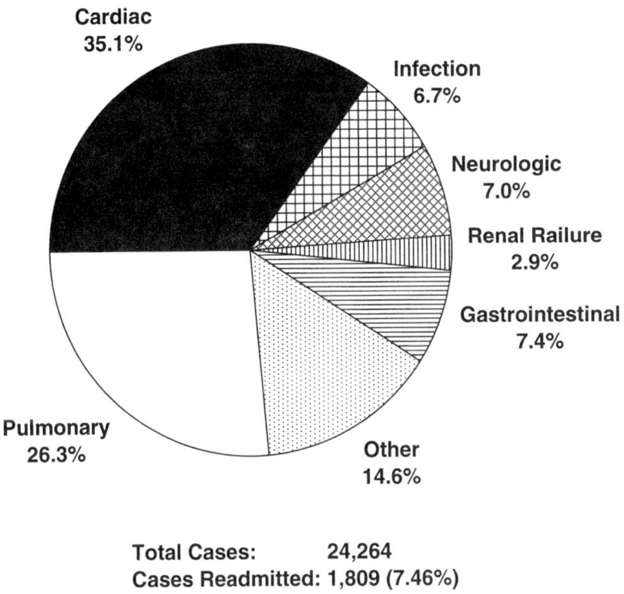

FIGURE 17-10. Primary reasons for readmission to the intensive care unit after cardiac surgery.

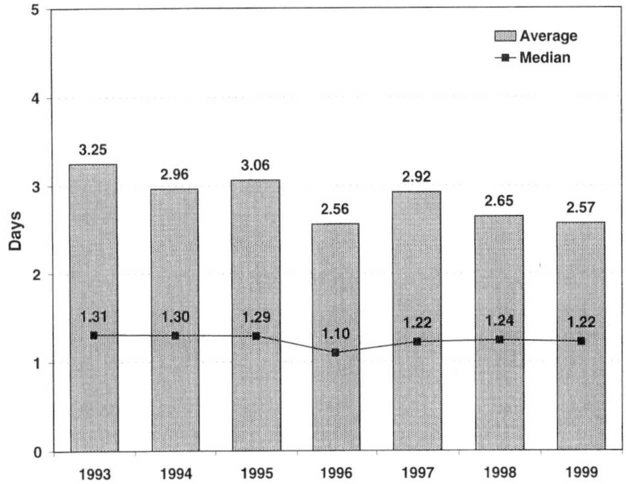

FIGURE 17-12. Initial intensive care unit length of stay after cardiac surgery.

calculating 95% confidence intervals around the expected occurrence of events at each severity level and then evaluating a given interval's data to determine whether the values fall within expected limits. Indicators that truly exceed thresholds are then subjected to focused review.

Focused reviews generally take the form of small-scale studies, examining a given outcome event, and determining why the incidence has increased. Several years ago, for example, a high incidence of readmissions triggered by respiratory events prompted the ICU team to closely follow high-risk patients after ICU discharge and intervene before they needed to return to the unit in respiratory distress. Readmission for respiratory reasons, once 46% of all readmissions, now account for only 27% (Fig. 17-10). Another focused review identified suction failure as a cause of recurrent pneumothoraces in patients with pleural chest tubes. Once a focused review has identified a problem and a solution, continued follow-up is necessary to document that the problem is truly solved. All quality assurance data is maintained in a file for regular review by the medical staff, hospital administration, and reviewing agencies such as the Joint Commission on Accreditation of Health Care Organizations.

Focused review can also be applied to existing processes in an effort to reduce the baseline (or historical) rate of complications. Examples include early extubation as part of a fast-track recovery process (Fig. 17-11) and reduction of ICU length of stay (Fig. 17-12) and reintubation rates.

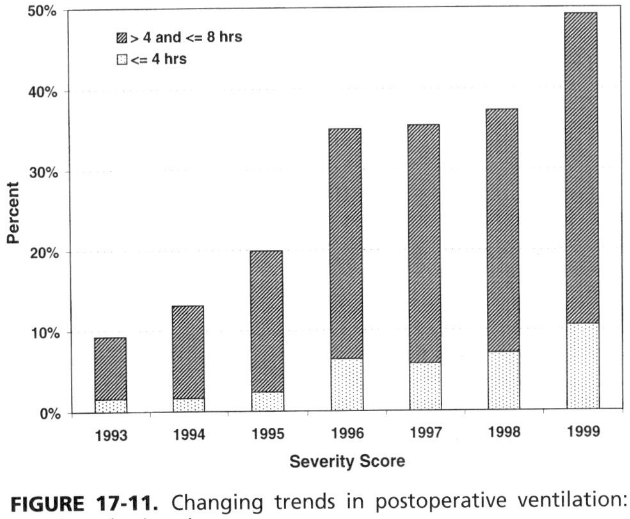

FIGURE 17-11. Changing trends in postoperative ventilation: initial intubation time.

PSYCHOSOCIAL SUPPORT OF THE PATIENT'S FAMILY

An often overlooked aspect of ICU responsibility is communication with the families of critically ill patients. Although most clinicians enthusiastically give updates on routine postoperative patients, there is a progressive reluctance to bear bad news to families of long-stay ICU patients who are doing poorly. Often this lack of communication results in family dissatisfaction, progressively difficult interactions, and potential lawsuits. Accurate transfer of information may be thwarted by a large number of family members or by differing viewpoints of multiple consultants. We try to identify one family member, usually the next of kin, as the family spokesperson and to funnel all communications through that person. The nurses also take an active role in updating the families if the physicians are not immediately available. The ICU Critical Care staff are available to answer questions from family members when the surgeon is in the OR or otherwise unavailable. Regular conferences are scheduled to outline the care plans for long-term patients who are monitored by multiple consulting services. Once a week, interdisciplinary ICU "long-term" rounds are conducted to share information among nursing, surgery, anesthesia, respiratory therapy, dietary, social service, occupational therapy, physical therapy, speech pathology, and the chaplain's office. Members of the bioethics consultation service are immediately available to assist with ethical concerns (139). We involve social services for every long-term patient to address issues of finances and housing arrangements for out-of-town families and to assist with arrangements for hospital discharge or transfer to another facility. Patients requiring extended weaning from mechanical ventilation are candidates for specialized subacute facilities, once acute medical issues have been treated. Visiting hours for the families of long-term patients are extremely liberal. Some family members can even be used to assist in ventilator weaning, feeding a patient, or helping with aspects of physical or occupational therapy. As long as the lines of communication are kept open, minor problems can be dealt with before they become a source of contention (140).

SUMMARY

Constant vigilance with attention to details is as important in the ICU as in the OR. Of necessity, this chapter has only touched on some issues relevant to postoperative management. Other chapters in this book contain greater detail on inotropic support for low-output states, therapy for cardiac rhythm disturbances, and management of specific complications.

The concept of risk identification and risk reduction can be applied to the postoperative cardiac patient. Statistically, certain patients are more likely to experience postoperative complications (130), and it is in this high-risk group that greater attention and interventions can be directed. By understanding the risk factors for catastrophic deterioration and undertaking preventive measures, outcome can be improved. Management of the cardiac surgery patient is becoming ever more complex with changes in demographics and extent of surgery. The clinician must thoroughly understand the effects of anesthesia and surgical therapy on the patient's physiology to appropriately care for the patient in the immediate postoperative period. Attention to the details of postoperative management helps avoid morbidity and mortality. Such an effort requires a team approach and constant communication among all those who are involved in the patient's immediate postoperative care.

REFERENCES

1. Higgins TL. Safety issues regarding early extubation after coronary artery bypass surgery. *J Cardiothorac Vasc Anesth* 1995;9:24.
2. Cheng DCH, Karski J, Peniston C, et al. Early tracheal extubation after coronary artery bypass graft surgery reduces costs and improves resource use. *Anesthesiology* 1996;85:1300.
3. Reyes A, Vega G, Blancas R, et al. Early vs conventional extubation after cardiac surgery with cardiopulmonary bypass. *Chest* 1997;112:193.
4. Estafanous FG, Loop FD, Higgins TL, et al. Increased risk and decreased morbidity of coronary artery bypass grafting between 1986 and 1994. *Ann Thorac Surg* 1998;65:383.
5. Lee A, Lum ME, O'Regan WJ, et al. Early postoperative emergencies requiring an intensive care team intervention: the role of ASA physical status and after-hours surgery. *Anesthesia* 1998;53:529.
6. Higgins TL, Yared J-P, Ryan T. Immediate postoperative care of cardiac surgical patients. *J Cardiothorac Vasc Anesth* 1996;10:643.
7. Reynolds HN, Haupt MT, Thill-Baharozian MC, et al. Impact of critical care physician staffing on patients with septic shock in a university hospital medical intensive care unit. *JAMA* 1988;260:3446.
8. Brown JJ, Sullivan G. Effect on ICU mortality of a full-time critical care specialist. *Chest* 1989;96:127.
9. Smith I, Fleming S, Cernaianu A. Mishaps during transport from the intensive care unit. *Crit Care Med* 1990;18:278.
10. Johnson D, Hurst T, Thomson D, et al. Respiratory function after cardiac surgery. *J Cardiothorac Vasc Anesth* 1996;10:571.
11. Hall RI, Smith MS, Rocker G. The systemic inflammatory response to cardiopulmonary bypass: pathophysiological, therapeutic and pharmacological considerations. *Anesth Analg* 1997;85:766.
12. Michalopoulos A, Anthi A, Rellos K, et al. Effects of positive end-expiratory pressure (PEEP) in cardiac surgery patients. *Respir Med* 1998;92:858.
13. Good JT Jr, Wolz JF, Anderson JT, et al. The routine use of positive end-expiratory pressure after open heart surgery. *Chest* 1979;76:397.
14. Guyton RA, Chiavarelli M, Padgett CA, et al. The influence of positive-end expiratory pressure on intrapericardial pressure and cardiac function after coronary artery bypass surgery. *J Cardiothorac Vasc Anesth* 1987;1:98.
15. Boldt J, Kling D, Bormann BV, et al. Influence of PEEP ventilation immediately after cardiopulmonary bypass on right ventricular function. *Chest* 1988;94:566.
16. Pepe PE, Hudson LD, Carrico CJ. Early application of positive end-expiratory pressure in patients at risk for the adult respiratory-distress syndrome. *N Engl J Med* 1984;311:281.
17. Zurick AM, Urzua J, Ghattas M, et al. Failure of positive end-expiratory pressure to decrease postoperative bleeding after cardiac surgery. *Ann Thorac Surg* 1982;34:608.
18. Abraham E, Yoshihara G. Cardiorespiratory effects of pressure controlled inverse ratio ventilation in severe respiratory failure. *Chest* 1989;96:1356.
19. Pepe PE, Marini JJ. Occult positive end-expiratory pressure in mechanically ventilated patients with airflow obstruction. *Am Rev Respir Dis* 1982;126:166.
20. Schwartz SZ, Shoemaker WC, Nolan-Avila LS. Effects of blood volume and discontinuance of ventilation on pulmonary vascular pressures and blood gases in patients with low levels of positive end-expiratory pressure. *Crit Care Med* 1987;15:671.
21. Higgins TL. Early endotracheal extubation is preferable to late

extubation in patients following coronary artery surgery. *J Cardiothorac Vasc Anesth* 1992;6:488.
22. Engelman RM, Rousou JA, Flack JE, et al. Fast-track recovery of the coronary bypass patient. *Ann Thorac Surg* 1994;58:1742.
23. Dantzker DR, Cowenhaven WM, Willoughby WJ, et al. Gas exchange alterations associated with weaning from mechanical ventilation following coronary artery bypass grafting. *Chest* 1982;82:674.
24. Gall SA, Olsen CO, Reves JG, et al. Beneficial effects of endotracheal extubation on ventricular performance. *J Thorac Cardovasc Surg* 1988;95:819.
25. Paulissian R, Salem MR, Joseph NJ, et al. Hemodynamic responses to endotracheal extubation after coronary artery bypass grafting. *Anesth Analg* 1991;73:10.
26. Michel L, McMichan JC, Marsh HM, et al. Measurement of ventilatory reserve as an indicator for early extubation after cardiac operation. *J Thorac Cardiovasc Surg* 1979;78:761.
27. Prakash O, Meij S, Borden BVD. Spontaneous ventilation test vs intermittent mandatory ventilation. *Chest* 1982;81:403.
28. Sahn SA, Lakshiminarayan S. Bedside criteria for discontinuation of mechanical ventilation. *Chest* 1973;63:1002.
29. Millbern SM, Downs JB, Jumper LC, et al. Evaluation of criteria for discontinuing mechanical ventilatory support. *Arch Surg* 1978;113:1441.
30. Chatila W, Jacob B, Guaglionone D, et al. The unassisted respiratory rate-tidal volume ratio accurately predicts weaning outcome. *Am J Med* 1996;101:61.
31. Higgins TL, Yared JF, Paranandi L, et al. Risk factors for respiratory complications after cardiac surgery. *Anesthesiology* 1991;75: 3A.
32. Rady MY, Ryan T. Perioperative predictors of extubation failure and the effect on clinical outcome after cardiac surgery. *Crit Care Med* 1999;27:340.
33. Coraim FJ, Coraim HP, Ebermann R, et al. Acute respiratory failure after cardiac surgery: clinical experience with the application of continuous arteriovenous hemofiltration. *Crit Care Med* 1986;14:714.
34. Sivak ED, Tita J, Meden G, et al. Effects of furosemide versus isolated ultrafiltration on extravascular lung water in oleic acid-induced pulmonary edema. *Crit Care Med* 1986;14:48.
35. Berrizbeitia LD, Tessler S, Jacobowitz IJ, et al. Effect of sternotomy and coronary bypass surgery on postoperative pulmonary mechanics. *Chest* 1989;96:873.
36. Higgins TL, Barrett C, Riden DJ, et al. Influence of pleural and mediastinal chest tubes on respiration following coronary artery bypass grafting (CABG). *Chest* 1989;96:237S.
37. Oikkomen M, Karjalainen K, Kachara V, et al. Comparison of incentive spirometry and intermittent positive pressure breathing after coronary artery bypass graft. *Chest* 1991;99:60.
38. Spivack SD, Shinozaki T, Albertini JJ, et al. Preoperative prediction of postoperative respiratory outcome: coronary artery bypass grafting. *Chest* 1996;109:1222.
39. Mahfood SS, Higgins TL, Loop FD. Management of complications related to perioperative care in cardiothoracic surgery. In: Waldhausen JA, Orringer MB, eds. *Management of complications related to coronary artery bypass surgery.* St. Louis: Mobsy–Year Book, 1991:265.
40. Samuels LE, Kaufman MS, Morris RJ, et al. Coronary artery bypass grafting in patients with COPD. *Chest* 1998;113:878.
41. Fagon J-Y, Chastre J, Domart Y, et al. Nosocomial pneumonia in patients receiving continuous mechanical ventilation: prospective analysis of 52 episodes with use of a protected specimen brush and quantitative culture techniques. *Am Rev Respir Dis* 1989;139:877.
42. Daschner K, Kappstein I, Engels I, et al. Stress ulcer prophylaxis and ventilation and ventilation pneumonia: prevention by antibacterial cytoprotective agents? *Infect Control Hosp Epidemiol* 1988;9:59.
43. Manthous CA, Zarich S. Myocardial ischemia during weaning from mechanical ventilation. *Semin Cardiothorac Vasc Anesth* 1998;2:78.
44. Zin WA, Caldeira MPR, Cardoso WV, et al. Expiratory mechanics before and after uncomplicated heart surgery. *Chest* 1989:1:21.
45. Tuzcu EM, Maloney JD, Sangani BH, et al. Cardiopulmonary effects of chronic amiodarone therapy in the early postoperative course of cardiac surgery patients. *Cleve Clin J Med* 1987;54: 491.
46. Nalos PC, Kass RM, Gang ES, et al. Life-threatening postoperative pulmonary complications in patients with previous amiodarone pulmonary toxicity undergoing cardiothoracic operations. *J Thorac Cardiovasc Surg* 1987;93:904.
47. Wilcox P, Baile EM, Hards J, et al. Phrenic nerve function and its relationship to atelectasis after coronary artery bypass surgery. *Chest* 1988;93:693.
48. Lorin S, Sivak M, Nierman DM. Critical illness polyneuropathy: what to look for in at-risk patients. Diagnosis requires a high index of suspicion. *J Crit Illness* 1998;13:608.
49. Ibebunjo C, Martyn JAJ. Fiber atrophy, but not changes in acetylcholine receptor expression, contributes to the muscle dysfunction after immobilization. *Crit Care Med* 1999;27:275.
50. Van Balkom RHH, Dekhuijzen R, Folgering HTM, et al. Effects of long-term low-dose methylprednisolone on rat diaphragm function and structure. *Muscle Nerve* 1997;20:983.
51. Abd AG, Braun NMT, Baskin MI, et al. Diaphragmatic dysfunction after open heart surgery: treatment with a rocking bed. *Ann Intern Med* 1989;111:881.
52. Weiner P, Zeidan F, Zamir D, et al. Prophylactic inspiratory muscle training in patients undergoing coronary artery bypass graft. *World J Surg* 1998;22:427.
53. Aubier M, Murciano D, Menu Y, et al. Dopamine effects on diaphragmatic strength during acute respiratory failure in chronic obstructive pulmonary disease. *Ann Intern Med* 1989; 110:17.
54. Aubier M, DeTroyer A, Sampson M, et al. Aminophylline improves diaphragmatic contractility. *N Engl J Med* 1981;305: 249.
55. Ely EW, Baker AM, Dunagan DP, et al. Effect on the duration of mechanical ventilation of identifying patients capable of breathing spontaneously. *N Engl J Med* 1996;335:1864.
56. American College of Chest Physicians. Consensus conference on artificial airways in patients receiving mechanical ventilation. *Chest* 1989;96:178.
57. American Thoracic Society. Hospital-acquired pneumonia in adults: diagnosis, assessment of severity, initial antimicrobial therapy, and preventative strategies. *Am J Respir Crit Care Med* 1995;153:1711.
58. Castella X, Gilabert J, Perez C. Arytenoid dislocation after tracheal intubation: an unusual cause of acute respiratory failure? *Anesthesiology* 1991;74:613.
59. Hogue CW, Lappas GD, Creswell LL, et al. Swallowing dysfunction after cardiac operation: associated adverse outcomes and risk factors including intraoperative transesophageal echocardiography. *J Thorac Cardiovasc Surg* 1995;110:517.
60. Breisblatt WM, Stein KL, Wolfe CJ, et al. Acute myocardial dysfunction and recovery: a common occurrence after coronary artery bypass. *J Am Coll Cardiol* 1990;15:1261.
61. Fouad FM, Estafanous FG, Bravo EL, et al. Possible role of cardioaortic reflexes in postcoronary bypass hypertension. *Am J Cardiol* 1979;44:866.
62. Estafanous FG, Urzua J, Yared JP, et al. Pattern of hemody-

namic alterations during coronary artery operations. *J Thorac Cardiovasc Surg* 1984;87:175.
63. Tarazi RC, Estafanous FG, Fouad FM. Unilateral stellate block in the treatment of hypertension after coronary bypass surgery: implications of a new therapeutic approach. *Am J Cardiol* 1978; 42:1013.
64. Van Wezel HB, Koolen JJ, Visser CA, et al. The efficacy of nicardipine and nitroprusside in preventing post-sternotomy hypertension. *J Cardiothorac Vasc Anesth* 1989;3:700.
65. Chauvin M, Deriaz H, Viars P. Continuous I.V. infusion of labetalol for postoperative hypertension. *Br J Anesth* 1987;59: 1250.
66. Grossman E, Messerli FH, Grodzicki T, et al. Should a moratorium be placed on sublingual nifedipine capsules given for hypertensive emergencies and pseudoemergencies? *JAMA* 1996; 276:1328.
67. Higgins TL, Tared J-P, Estafanous FG, et al. Propofol versus midazolam for intensive care unit sedation after coronary artery bypass grafting. *Crit Care Med* 1994;22:1415.
68. Bednarski P, Siclari F, Voigt A, et al. Use of a computerized closed-loop sodium nitroprusside titration system for antihypertensive treatment after open heart surgery. *Crit Care Med* 1990; 18:1061.
69. Post JB, Frishman WH. Fenoldopam: a new dopamine agonist for the treatment of hypertensive urgencies and emergencies. *J Clin Pharmacol* 1998;38:2.
70. Riddington DW, Venkatesh B, Boivin CM, et al. Intestinal permeability, gastric intramucosal pH and systemic endotoxemia in patients undergoing cardiopulmonary bypass. *JAMA* 1996;275:1007.
71. Landow L, Phillips DA, Heard SO, et al. Gastric tonometry and venous oximetry in cardiac surgery patients. *Crit Care Med* 1990;19:1226.
72. Bailey JM, Levy JH, Kopel MA, et al. Relationship between clinical evaluation of peripheral perfusion and global hemodynamics in adults after cardiac surgery. *Crit Care Med* 1990;18: 1353.
73. Shoemaker WC, Appel PL, Kram HB. Tissue oxygen debt as a determinant of lethal and nonlethal postoperative organ failure. *Crit Care Med* 1988;16:1117.
74. Cochrane Injuries Group Albumin Reviewers. Human albumin administration in critically ill patients: systematic review of randomized controlled trials. *BMJ* 1998;317:235.
75. Doolan LA, Jones EF, Kalman J, et al. A placebo-controlled trial verifying the efficacy of milrinone in weaning high-risk patients from cardiopulmonary bypass. *J Cardiothorac Vasc Anesth* 1997;11:37.
76. D'Ambra MN, LaRaia PJ, Phillbin DM, et al. Prostaglandin E: a new therapy for refractory right heart failure and pulmonary hypertension after mitral valve replacement. *J Thorac Cardiovasc Surg* 1985;89:567.
77. Smedira NG, Hlozek CC, McCarthy PM. Mechanical support after cardiac surgery. *Semin Cardiothorac Vasc Anesth* 1998;2: 66.
78. Golding LAR. Postcardiotomy mechanical support. *Semin Thorac Cardiovasc Surg* 1991;3:29.
79. Smith RC, Leung JM, Mangano DT. Postoperative myocardial ischemia in patients undergoing coronary artery bypass graft surgery. *Anesthesiology* 1991;74:464.
80. Kemmer JH, Kirse MM. Coronary artery spasm following coronary artery surgery. *Ann Thorac Surg* 1988;46:108.
81. Eide TR, Katz RI, Poppers PJ. The effect of sublingual nifedipine on coronary venous graft resistance immediately following cardiopulmonary bypass. *Anesth Analg* 1989;68:462.
82. Jones EL, Lattouf O, Weintraub WS. Catastrophic consequences of internal mammary artery hypoperfusion. *J Thorac Cardiovasc Surg* 1989;98:902.
83. Liu JJ, Doolan LA, Xie B, et al. Direct vasodilator effect of milrinone, an inotropic drug, on arterial coronary bypass grafts. *J Thorac Cardiovasc Surg* 1997;113:108.
84. Slogoff S, Keats AS. Does perioperative myocardial ischemia lead to postoperative myocardial infarction? *Anesthesiology* 1985; 62:107.
85. Mathew JP, Parks R, Savino JS, et al. Atrial fibrillation following coronary artery bypass graft surgery: predictors, outcomes and resource utilization. *JAMA* 1996;276:300.
86. Fanning WJ, Thomas CS, Roach A, et al. Prophylaxis of strial fibrillation with magnesium sulfate after coronary artery bypass grafting. *Ann Thorac Surg* 1991;52:529.
87. Clemo HF, Wood MA, Gilligan DM, et al. Intravenous amiodarone for acute heart rate control in the critically ill patient with atrial tachyarrhythmias. *Am J Cardiol* 1998;81:594.
88. Maggiano HJ, Higgins TL, Lobo W, et al. Superior vena cava syndrome after open heart surgery. *Cleve Clin J Med* 1992;59: 93.
89. VanLente F, Martin A, Ratliff NB, et al. The predictive value of serum enzyme for perioperative myocardial infarction after cardiac operations: an autopsy study. *J Thorac Cardiovasc Surg* 1989;98:704.
90. Kost GJ, Kirk JD, Omand K. A strategy for the use of cardiac injury markers (troponin I and T, creatine kinase, MB mass and isoforms, and myoglobin) in the diagnosis of acute myocardial infarction. *Arch Pathol Lab Med* 1998;122:245.
91. Wahl GW, Feins RH, Alfieres G, et al. Reinfusion of shed blood after coronary operation causes elevation of cardiac enzyme levels. *Ann Thorac Surg* 1992;53:625.
92. Kinoshita K, Tsuruhara Y, Tokunaga K. Delayed time to peak serum myoglobin level as an indicator of cardiac dysfunction following open heart surgery. *Chest* 1991;99:1398.
93. Butterworth JF, Zaloga GP, Prielipp RC, et al. Calcium inhibits the cardiac stimulating properties of dobutamine but not of amrinone. *Chest* 1992;101:174.
94. Fernandez-Del Castillo C, Harringer W, Warshaw AL, et al. Risk factors for pancreatic cellular injury after cardiopulmonary bypass. *N Engl J Med* 1991;325:382.
95. Caspi J, Klausner JM, Safadi T, et al. Delayed respiratory depression following fentanyl anesthesia for cardiac surgery. *Crit Care Med* 1988;16:238.
96. Knight AA, Hollenberg M, London MJ, et al. Perioperative myocardial ischemia: importance of the preoperative ischemic pattern. *Anesthesiology* 1988;68:681.
97. Plunkett JJ, Reeves JD, Ngo L, et al. Urine and plasma catecholamine and cortisol concentrations after myocardial revascularization. *Anesthesiology* 1997;86:785.
98. Saunders PR, Banish P, Kipton JM, et al. Localized regulated radiant heat vs. meperidine in the control of postanesthetic shivering. *Anesthesiology* 1989;71:A184.
99. Yared J-P, Staff NJ, Hoffman-Hogg L, et al. Dexamethasone decreases the incidence of shivering after cardiac surgery: a randomized, double-blind, placebo-controlled study. *Anesth Analg* 1998;87:795.
100. Hilberman M, Myers BD, Carrie BJ, et al. Acute renal failure following cardiac surgery. *J Thorac Cardiovasc Surg* 1979;77: 880.
101. Koning HM, Koning AJ, Leusink JA. Serious acute renal failure following open heart surgery. *J Thorac Cardiovasc Surg* 1985; 33:283.
102. Higgins TL, Blum JM, Lytle BW. Postoperative complications following coronary bypass grafting: implications of elevated bilirubin and elevated creatinine. *Abstracts of Society of Cardiovascular Anesthesiologists 1992 meeting.* Boston, MA; May 1992:326.

103. Davis RF, Lappas DG, Kirklin JK, et al. Acute oliguria after cardiopulmonary bypass: renal functional improvement with low-dose dopamine infusion. *Crit Care Med* 1982;10:852.
104. Myers BD, Moran SM. Hemodynamically mediated acute renal failure. *N Engl J Med* 1987;314:97.
105. Joy MS, Matzke GR, Armstrong DK, et al. A primer on continuous renal replacement therapy for critically ill patients. *Ann Pharmacother* 1998;32:362.
106. Shaw PJ, Bates D, Cartlidge NEF, et al. Neurological complications of coronary artery bypass graft surgery: six month follow-up study. *Br Med J* 1986;293:165.
107. Bojar RM, Najafi H, DeLaria GA, et al. Neurological complications of coronary revascularization. *Ann Thorac Surg* 1983;36: 427.
108. Calabrese JR, Skwerer RG, Gulledge AD, et al. Incidence of postoperative delirium following myocardial revascularization. *Cleve Clin J Med* 1987;54:29.
109. Tesar GE, Murray GB, Cassem NH. Use of high-dose intravenous haloperidol in the treatment of agitated cardiac patients. *J Clin Psychopharmacol* 1985;5:344.
110. Salzman EW, Weinstein MJ, Weintraub RM, et al. Treatment with desmopressin acetate to reduce blood loss after cardiac surgery: a double-blind randomized trial. *N Engl J Med* 1986; 314:1402.
111. DelRossi AJ, Carnaiann AC, Botros S, et al. Prophylactic treatment of postperfusion bleeding using EACA. *Chest* 1989;96: 27.
112. Royston D, Taylor KM, Bidstrup BP, et al. Effect of aprotinin on need for blood transfusion after repeat open-heart surgery. *Lancet* 1987;1289.
113. Westaby S. Aprotinin in perspective. *Ann Thorac Surg* 1993; 55:1033.
114. Cosgrove DM, Loop FD, Lytle BW, et al. Determinants of blood utilization during myocardial revascularization. *Ann Thorac Surg* 1985;40:380.
115. Hebert PC, Wells G, Tweeddale M, et al. Does transfusion practice affect mortality in critically ill patients? *Am J Respir Crit Care Med* 1997;155:1618.
116. Goodnough LT, Johnston MFM, Ramsey G, et al. Guidelines for transfusion support in patients undergoing coronary artery bypass grafting. *Ann Thorac Surg* 1990;50:675.
117. Michelson EL, Torosian M, Morganroth J, et al. Early recognition of surgically correctable causes of excessive mediastinal bleeding after coronary artery bypass graft surgery. *Am J Surg* 1980;139:313.
118. Talamonti MS, LoCirceo J, Hoyne WP, et al. Early re-exploration for excessive postoperative bleeding lowers wound complication rates in open heart surgery. *Am Surgeon* 1987:102.
119. Loop FD, Lytle BW, Cosgrove DM, et al. Sternal wound complications after isolated coronary artery bypass grafting: early andlate mortality, morbidity, and cost of care. *Ann Thorac Surg* 1990;49:179.
120. Zerr KJ, Furnary AP, Grunkemeier GL, et al. Glucose control lowers the risk of wound infection in diabetics after open heart operations. *Ann Thorac Surg* 1997;63:356.
121. D'Amico R, Pifferi S, Leonetti C, et al. Effectiveness of antibiotic prophylaxis in critically ill adult patients: systemic review of randomized controlled trials. *BMJ* 1998;316:1275.
122. Krasna MJ, Flanchbaum L, Trooskin ZS, et al: Gastrointestinal complications after cardiac surgery. *Surgery* 1988;104:733.
123. Ephgrave KS, Kleinman-Wexler RL, Adar CG. Enteral nutrients prevent stress ulceration and increase intragastric volume. *Crit Care Med* 1990;18:621.
124. Collins JD, Ferner R, Murray A, et al. Incidence and prognostic importance of jaundice after cardiopulmonary bypass surgery. *Lancet* 1983:1119.
125. Haas GS, Warshaw AL, Daggett WM, et al. Acute pancreatitis after cardiopulmonary bypass. *Am J Surg* 1985;149:508.
126. Barsonnet V, Dean D, Berstein AD. A method of uniform stratification of risk for evaluating the results of surgery in acquired adult heart disease. *Circulation* 1989;79:I3.
127. Hammermeister KE, Burchfiel C, Johnson R, et al. Identification of patients at greatest risk for developing major complications at cardiac surgery. *Circulation* 1990;82:IV380.
128. Higgins TL, Estafanous FG, Loop FD, et al. Stratification of morbidity and mortality outcome by preoperative risk factors in coronary artery bypass patients. *JAMA* 1992;267:2344.
129. Higgins TL, Estafanous FG, Loop FD, et al. ICU admission score for predicting morbidity and mortality risk after coronary artery bypass grafting. *Ann Thorac Surg* 1997;64:1050.
130. Knaus WA, Draper EA, Wagner DP, et al. APACHE II: a severity of disease classification system. *Crit Care Med* 1985; 13:818.
131. Becker RB, Zimmerman JE, Kanus WA, et al. The use of APACHE III to evaluate ICU length of stay, resource use and mortality after coronary artery surgery. *J Cardiovasc Surg* 1995; 36:1.
132. Tu JV, Jagial SB, Naylor CD. Multicenter validation of a risk index for mortality, intensive care unit stay, and overall hospital length of stay after cardiac surgery. *Circulation* 1995;91:677.
133. Higgins TL. Quantifying risk and assessing outcome in cardiac surgery. *J Cardiothorac Vasc Anesth* 1998;12:330.
134. Orr RK, Maini BS, Sottile FD, et al. A comparison of four severity-adjusted models to predict mortality after coronary artery bypass graft surgery. *Arch Surg* 1995;130:301.
135. Iezzoni LI, Ash AS, Shwartz M, et al. Predicting in-hospital deaths from coronary artery bypass graft surgery: do different severity measures give different predictions? *Med Care* 1998;36: 28.
136. Silber JH, Rosenbaum PR, Schwartz JS, et al. Evaluation of the complication rate as a measure of quality of care in coronary artery bypass graft surgery. *JAMA* 1995;274:317.
137. Chong JL, Pillai R, Fisher A, et al. Cardiac surgery: moving away from intensive care. *Br Heart J* 1992;68:430.
138. Shahian DM, Williamson WA, Svensson LG, et al. Applications of statistical quality control to cardiac surgery. *Ann Thorac Surg* 1996;62:1351.
139. Balgyga AP. Ethical issues in the postoperative intensive care unit. *Semin Cardiothorac Vasc Anesth* 1998;2:90.
140. Mosley KR, Wise MG. The family of the critically ill patient. *Problems in Critical Care* 1988;2:188.

18

PEDIATRIC INTENSIVE CARE

FRANK H. KERN
WILLIAM J. GREELEY
SCOTT R. SCHULMAN
IRA M. CHEIFETZ
JON N. MELIONES

The postoperative care of the pediatric patient who has undergone cardiothoracic surgery is an important part of the overall sequence of anesthetic and surgical management. The postoperative period should therefore begin by acquiring a full knowledge of the intraoperative course and developing a therapeutic plan based on management after cardiopulmonary bypass (CPB). Hemodynamic responses to specific pharmacologic interventions in the early post-CPB period and concerns raised during the operative period should be discussed. Difficulty in weaning the patient from CPB, unusually high doses of inotropic support, and poor systemic perfusion should alert the intensive care team to an abnormal postoperative convalescence. The significance of residual anatomic defects as a cause of an abnormal postoperative recovery cannot be overemphasized. Uncomplicated recovery, low postoperative morbidity, and long-term disease-free survival are predicated on an anatomically precise operative repair in the patient with congenital heart disease (1).

When the postoperative course is complicated by abnormal hemodynamics despite adequate preload, inotropy, and ventilatory support, we assume that it represents either a residual anatomic defect, new loading conditions incurred by the operative repair, or the effects of CPB. In the early postoperative period, we critically evaluate the surgical repair to detect the presence of residual or previously undiagnosed defects. Indwelling pressure monitors, arterial blood gas determinations, hematocrit, mixed venous saturation, and lactic acid monitoring are commonly used to assess the adequacy of oxygen delivery and to ascertain whether right ventricular (RV), left ventricular (LV), biventricular, or pulmonary artery (PA) hypertension is present. In patients with evidence for abnormal convalescence, transthoracic or transesophageal echocardiography (or both) is a valuable bedside diagnostic tool for evaluating the quality of the repair and elucidating the cause of reduced systemic perfusion in congenital heart disease patients. Echocardiography is extremely helpful in detecting RV dysfunction, LV dysfunction, residual intracardiac shunts, valvular stenosis or regurgitation, residual obstruction of the proximal great vessels, pulmonary venous abnormalities, pericardial effusion with cardiac tamponade, and hypovolemia.

If significant structural defects exist, early reoperation and repair are indicated. For instances in which reoperation is considered hazardous, interventional catheterization may be an effective alternative to surgery. Closure of residual ventricular septal defects (VSDs), dilation of PAs, and placement of PA or pulmonary vein stents have been effective alternatives to surgery in some centers (2).

If residual structural defects are absent, then pharmacologic and ventilatory manipulations are instituted to maximize myocardial contractility and offset the new loading conditions imposed on the heart by the corrective or palliative procedure. Clinicians caring for a postoperative congenital heart disease patient must constantly evaluate the patient's hemodynamics and must alter loading conditions to maximize cardiac output and systemic perfusion. In addition, the effects of hypothermic CPB and/or deep hypothermic circulatory arrest on postoperative organ function must be appreciated so that the clinician can anticipate potential physiologic problems from the extreme conditions associated with CPB and circulatory arrest.

Finally, communication among the anesthesiologists, surgeons, cardiologists, and critical care team is essential

F. H. Kern and S. R. Schulman: Departments of Anesthesiology and Pediatrics, Duke University Medical Center; and Duke Children's Hospital, Durham, North Carolina 27710

W. J. Greeley: Departments of Anesthesiology and Pediatrics, University of Pennsylvania; and Departments of Anesthesiology and Critical Care Medicine, Children's Hospital of Philadelphia, Philadelphia, Pennsylvania 19104

I. M. Cheifetz: Department of Pediatrics, Duke University Medical Center and Duke Children's Hospital, Durham, North Carolina 27710

J. N. Meliones: Division of Pediatric Critical Care Medicine, Duke University Medical Center, Durham, North Carolina 27710

to optimize postoperative care in these patients. This team approach minimizes diagnostic errors and promotes open and effective patient care.

This chapter presents a management approach to postoperative care of the congenital heart disease patient. It is divided into five sections: monitoring considerations, a general treatment approach to postoperative physiologic problems, anatomic and physiologic problems as they relate to specific repairs, cardiac dysrhythmias, and end-organ dysfunction (cerebral, pulmonary, renal, and hepatic).

MONITORING

Monitoring is a critical part of postoperative management for the congenital heart disease patient. Although different approaches have evolved at different centers, the general management strategy involves a combination of invasive and noninvasive monitors to assess the quality of the operative repair, myocardial function, and valvular function and to assist in the balancing of blood flow between the systemic and pulmonary circulation in patients with shunt physiology. All children who have undergone CPB require a continuous monitor of right-sided filling pressures. This may be accomplished through a percutaneously placed line through the internal jugular vein, external jugular vein, or subclavian vein with the catheter advanced to the superior vena cava (SVC)–right atrial junction, or by placing a catheter directly into the right atrial appendage at the time of surgery.

Right atrial or internal jugular catheters are used to assess preload, RV function, right-sided atrioventricular (AV) valve function, and dysrhythmias and to obtain measurements of mixed venous saturations in congenital heart disease patients. Intermittent or continuous sampling of high SVC oxygen saturation is an effective method of corroborating that the child's cardiac output is adequate. In the absence of an atrial-level left-to-right shunt and radiographic evidence that the right atrial catheter is not near the coronary sinus ostium, right atrial catheters can also be used. In many congenital cardiac lesions, atrial-level shunting is common and therefore right atrial blood samples contain an admixture of oxygenated blood from the left atrium, creating an artificially high saturation and inaccurate measurement. High SVC catheter sampling is a good surrogate for mixed venous oxygen saturations in patients with atrial-level shunting. In general, a mixed venous oxygen saturation of 70% or higher implies good cardiac output (3). In neonates and children with palliated repairs, such as after an arterial switch repair, stage I Norwood operation for hypoplastic left heart syndrome, or Fontan procedure, high SVC saturations of 55% or greater are quite acceptable.

In patients younger than 6 months of age, a 5-cm-long double-lumen catheter allows for reproducible placement of the distal tip of the catheter at the SVC–right atrial junction. Sampling from the proximal port provides reliable saturation measurements from the high SVC. With intracardiac lines, placement depends on the experience of the surgeon and on postoperative evaluation by chest radiography.

Acute increases in central venous pressure (CVP) associated with tachycardia and decreased systemic perfusion alert the physician to cardiac tamponade, reactive pulmonary vascular resistance (PVR), hemodynamically significant dysrhythmias, or moderate-to-severe tricuspid regurgitation. Less commonly, an acute pneumothorax or hemothorax may result in similar effects on CVP and hemodynamics. Chest auscultation, chest radiography, and echocardiography should be used to reach the correct diagnosis.

Left atrial catheters are used routinely in some centers and selectively in others. The left atrial catheter provides data on the function of the left-sided AV valve and the LV. Although these catheters have a low rate of complications, constant diligence must be employed to avoid air entrainment into the left-sided circulation (4). Because of the introduction of intraoperative echocardiography for congenital heart disease patients, continuous evaluation of left-sided pressures can be chosen more selectively (1,2,5). If echocardiography demonstrates good LV and left-sided AV valve function after weaning from CPB and if inotropic support is low, a left atrial line is less likely to contribute to postoperative management and teams in some centers will choose not to place one. The placement of a left atrial line is clearly helpful for children undergoing the modified Fontan operation or a cavopulmonary shunt. It is also valuable for young children who require a mitral valve replacement or repair, AV canal defects, or aortic valve surgery and in children with anticipated LV dysfunction in the postoperative period (e.g., after an arterial switch operation). In general, left atrial pressure monitoring is a valuable tool and may be particularly useful when unanticipated problems with cardiac output develop in the postoperative period.

PA catheters are individualized on the basis of the operative procedure performed and the presence of PA hypertension. PA catheters should be considered for children whose postoperative PA pressures are greater than one half to two thirds of the systemic pressure and in patients who are at risk for reactive PA hypertension during the postoperative period. Newborns and infants with preexisting large left-to-right shunts (truncus arteriosus, complete AV canal) and patients with flow obstruction at the pulmonary venous or mitral valve level (total pulmonary venous connection or severe mitral stenosis) are candidates for continuous monitoring of PA pressure. PA catheters may also be used in patients undergoing repair of tetralogy of Fallot to assess the postoperative gradient across the RV outflow tract reconstruction (4). A PA catheter is also an excellent source of mixed venous blood samples in the absence of residual shunts and can be used in conjunction with a right atrial or central venous catheter to obtain cardiac output measurements (6).

Pulse oximetry is a crucial monitor in the postoperative management of these patients. Acute decreases in oxygen saturation due to unplanned extubation, mucus plugging of the endotracheal tube, or failure of the mechanical ventilator are well-recognized reasons for continuous pulse oximetry monitoring in all intensive care unit (ICU) patients. In the congenital heart disease patient, however, elevations in PVR or RV dysfunction may manifest as right-to-left shunting at the atrial level (7–10); clinically this presents as an acute reduction in systemic oxygen saturation. Pulse oximetry is therefore an excellent monitor of acute changes in pulmonary vascular reactivity. Similarly, a rise in systemic saturation serves as an indicator of improved RV compliance, resulting in a reduced right-to-left pressure gradient at the atrial level and resolution of the atrial-level shunt.

In patients with single-ventricle physiology, the goal is to maintain unobstructed systemic blood flow and to regulate pulmonary blood flow in such a way that the ratio of pulmonary to systemic flow remains balanced (Qp : Qs = 1 : 1) (11). The most convenient means of ensuring a 1 : 1 ratio is to achieve and maintain a systemic oxygen saturation of approximately 75% to 80% and a high SVC saturation of approximately 60% (12–15). Acute changes in lung compliance, systemic vascular resistance (SVR), and myocardial function are common in the postoperative period (3,16). In single-ventricle physiology these changes significantly alter the distribution of blood flow between the systemic and pulmonary circulations or reduce total cardiac output (Qt). Pulse oximetry provides a continuous assessment of Qp : Qs and allows prompt recognition and early treatment of unbalanced blood flow (11).

Invasive arterial monitoring—radial, ulnar, umbilical, or femoral—is routinely used in the postoperative period. Arterial lines also provide rapid access to repeated measures of arterial blood gases, electrolytes, calcium, glucose, lactic acid, and hematocrit.

Arterial blood gas monitoring is important in ensuring effective gas exchange (oxygenation and ventilation) and adequate tissue perfusion through monitoring of total HCO_3^- and base deficits. However, after reparative or palliative operations for congenital heart disease, oxygenation and ventilation exert a significant influence on measured hemodynamics. This is especially true in neonates and infants with reactive pulmonary vascular beds. In this population, maintenance of alkalemia and an inspired oxygen concentration of 100% remains the most effective means of lowering PVR (17–22). Alkalemia is achieved by mild hyperventilation and adding $NaHCO_3$.

Ionized calcium levels should be frequently monitored in the early postoperative period in neonates and infants. The lack of a well-developed intracellular transport system for calcium makes the immature heart much more dependent on extracellular calcium levels for effective contractility (23–25). In addition, marked fluctuations in ionized calcium levels are associated with the transfusions of citrate- and albumin-containing blood products used for preload support in the early postoperative period (23). Failure to maintain normal or slightly elevated ionized calcium levels may result in significant alterations in hemodynamics. In the critical care setting there is a poor correlation between serum and ionized calcium levels (25).

Intermittent monitoring of lactic acid is another method of monitoring oxygen delivery to tissue. Lactic acid levels are high (6 to 10 nmol/L) after circulatory arrest and deep hypothermic CPB. With improved tissue perfusion, lactate levels decrease rapidly during the first several hours of ICU care (26). Persistently elevated or rising lactate levels are a foreboding sign that requires therapeutic interventions with systemic vasodilators, inotropic agents, and perhaps extracorporeal life support (extracorporeal membrane oxygenation, or ECMO).

Hourly assessment of hematocrit, once bleeding has resolved, is a method of evaluating extravasation of water into the extravascular space caused by endothelial cell injury from the exaggerated inflammatory state induced by CPB. Hemoconcentration despite colloid or crystalloid administration suggests an ongoing endothelial cell injury and inflammation. When the need for volume support lessens and the hematocrit level stabilizes or begins to fall, capillary leak is resolving. Extravascular fluid begins to mobilize back into the vascular space, urine output improves, and diuretics may be employed to hasten extravascular water elimination. In neonates and infants, extravascular water accumulation occurs to a much greater extent than is typically seen in adults (27,28). Attempts to modify this response with the use of modified ultrafiltration (MUF) in the immediate postbypass period and the use of high-dose steroids 6 to 12 hours before CPB has reduced the marked postoperative inflammatory response in neonates. The most important, yet least quantitative, assessment of cardiac function remains physical assessment. Warm distal extremities, brisk capillary refill, strong peripheral pulses, and a urine output of more than 1 mL/kg/hour remain critical bedside measures of an effective cardiac output. An abnormal clinical assessment despite normal filling pressure and arterial blood pressure is a harbinger of systemic hypoperfusion and increased SVR. Corroboration with lactic acid or mixed venous oxygen saturation values is helpful.

Echocardiography is a valuable tool for evaluating the patient with an abnormal postoperative convalescence. Echocardiography provides a detailed picture of the anatomic and functional characteristics of the postoperative heart. Unanticipated hemodynamic alterations, failure to wean from mechanical ventilation, inotrope dependence, poor systemic cardiac output, and low systemic saturations in the postoperative period are all indications for echocardiographic assessment. Because the morbidity and mortality of congenital cardiac surgery depend heavily on the structural integrity of the operative repair, the isolation of potentially life-threatening residual defects early in the postoperative period is essential. The liberal use of echocardiographic evaluation in patients with abnormal convalescence is now an essential part of postoperative monitoring.

Cardiac catheterization should be considered when echocardiography is not definitive or when additional information about ventricular pressures, vascular gradients, atrial gradients, pulmonary venous gradients, presence of aortopulmonary collaterals, or residual shunts is needed to "fine tune" or alter management. Interventional approaches such as dilation or stenting of PAs, veins, or coarctation sites or coiling of collateral vessels can be entertained or attempted in an effort to avoid additional surgical intervention requiring cardiopulmonary bypass (29–31).

PATIENT MANAGEMENT

This discussion provides a comprehensive approach to postoperative management of the reconstructed pediatric heart. Patient management is approached in two ways. The first topic discussed is functional abnormalities common to all neonates, infants, and children after undergoing reparative or palliative operations for congenital heart disease. Management strategies for PA hypertension, RV dysfunction, and LV dysfunction are discussed. With this as background, a second discussion focuses on the approach to specific congenital cardiac defects and types of operative repair. Because recognizing residual anatomic defects is a major part of the postoperative management of congenital heart disease patients, ICU physicians must understand the repair and be cognizant of potential structural defects that may persist or become apparent after reconstructive heart surgery. The type, extent, and tolerance of residual cardiac defects depend on the method of repair. They also depend on whether the operation results in a complete anatomic and physiologic correction that uses the patient's native tissue, an anatomic and physiologic repair requiring artificial material to provide normal blood flow patterns, or a palliative operation necessitated by missing or diminutive ventricular chambers.

In patients undergoing a complete operative reconstruction (e.g., patients receiving an anatomic and physiologic correction), residual defects are less common and occur at more obvious locations. Because blood flow patterns are normal, mild to moderate anatomic defects are more readily tolerated in the postoperative period. Patients who receive a physiologic reconstruction (e.g., children who are missing cardiac structures) require artificial material such as a conduit or a baffle to restore normal blood flow patterns. In this group of patients anatomic problems are more common because of the interposition of artificial material within the

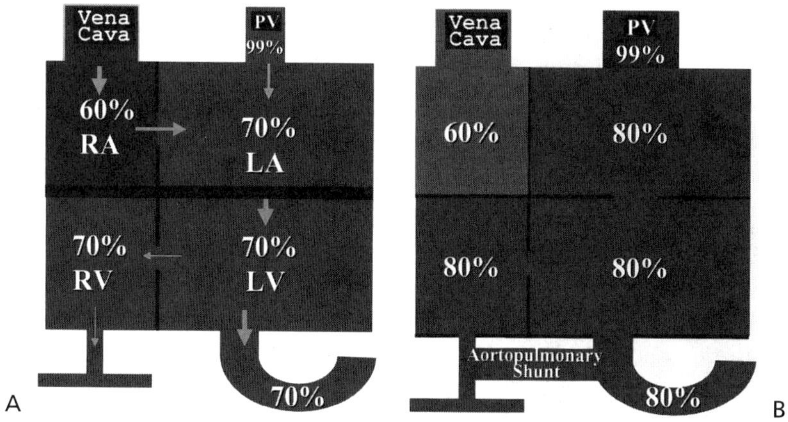

FIGURE 18-1. (A) Illustration of tricuspid atresia. In this lesion, blood enters the right atrium and is shunted right to left across an atrial septal defect (ASD) or patent foramen ovale (PFO) because of the absence of a patent tricuspid valve. A smaller volume of blood returns from the lungs through the pulmonary veins owing to a reduction in pulmonary blood flow. This small volume of blood mixes with desaturated blood from the body, resulting in blood with a low saturation (70% in this illustration). **(B)** The patient has undergone an aortopulmonary shunt procedure. Blood flows from the aorta through the shunt to the pulmonary arteries. If the volume of blood going to the body is equal to the amount of blood going to the lungs (Qp/Qs = 1), equal volumes of blood will return to the heart through the systemic veins and pulmonary veins. Assuming the cardiac output is normal, the saturation of blood returning from the body through the vena cava fSvo_2) will be 60%. And assuming there is no lung disease, so that the blood returning to the heart from the lungs is fully saturated (99%), then the mixed blood with in the left atrium and left ventricle will have a saturation of 80% (saturation of the systemic venous blood + saturation of the pulmonary venous blood divided by 2). The mixed blood with a saturation of 80% will be ejected by the left ventricle into the aorta and through the shunt into the pulmonary arterial circulation.

heart. Residual anatomic defects are somewhat less well tolerated in this group because of the abnormal loading conditions that existed in the prerepair period and because the conduit is usually positioned in a location that differs from the natural location of the great vessel it replaces. This situation reduces the efficiency of ventricular contractility. Long-term problems are more common in these patients due to conduit or baffle obstruction, aneurysms of the artificial material, valvular regurgitation, or supervalvar obstruction. Myocardial dysfunction from volume or pressure overload and the late development of atrial or ventricular rhythm disturbances are more common in patients receiving a physiologic reconstruction.

Patients requiring palliative reconstruction have only a single ventricle. Reconstruction is based first on having the single ventricle provide balanced blood flow to both the pulmonary and systemic circulations. A second procedure (or series of procedures) uses the single ventricle as a systemic ventricle. Pulmonary blood flow is provided by anastomosing systemic venous return directly to the PAs. Pulmonary blood flow is maintained by a passive gradient from the systemic veins through the lungs and into the left atrium. This procedure, known as the modified Fontan procedure, is now widely applied to a variety of anatomic variants of the single ventricle (32). Most patients undergo staged repairs. In infancy, palliative procedures are performed to either increase pulmonary blood flow, decrease pulmonary blood flow or establish systemic blood flow. If the physiologic problem is inadequate pulmonary blood flow, such as tricuspid atresia (Fig. 18-1), an aortopulmonary shunt is placed. If the physiologic problem is inadequate systemic blood flow, as in hypoplastic left heart syndrome, the main PA and diminutive ascending aorta are anastomosed to create a single neoaorta to provide systemic blood flow, and an aortopulmonary shunt is placed from the innominate artery or aorta to the PAs to provide pulmonary blood flow (Fig. 18-2A,B). In patients with complex single-ventricle anatomy in which a normal sized PA and aorta are present and are supplied by a single ventricle, the physiologic problem is excessive pulmonary blood flow and the treatment is a PA band to restrict or control pulmonary blood flow.

A second stage is planned at approximately 4 to 6 months to convert the physiology of all three infant palliative proce-

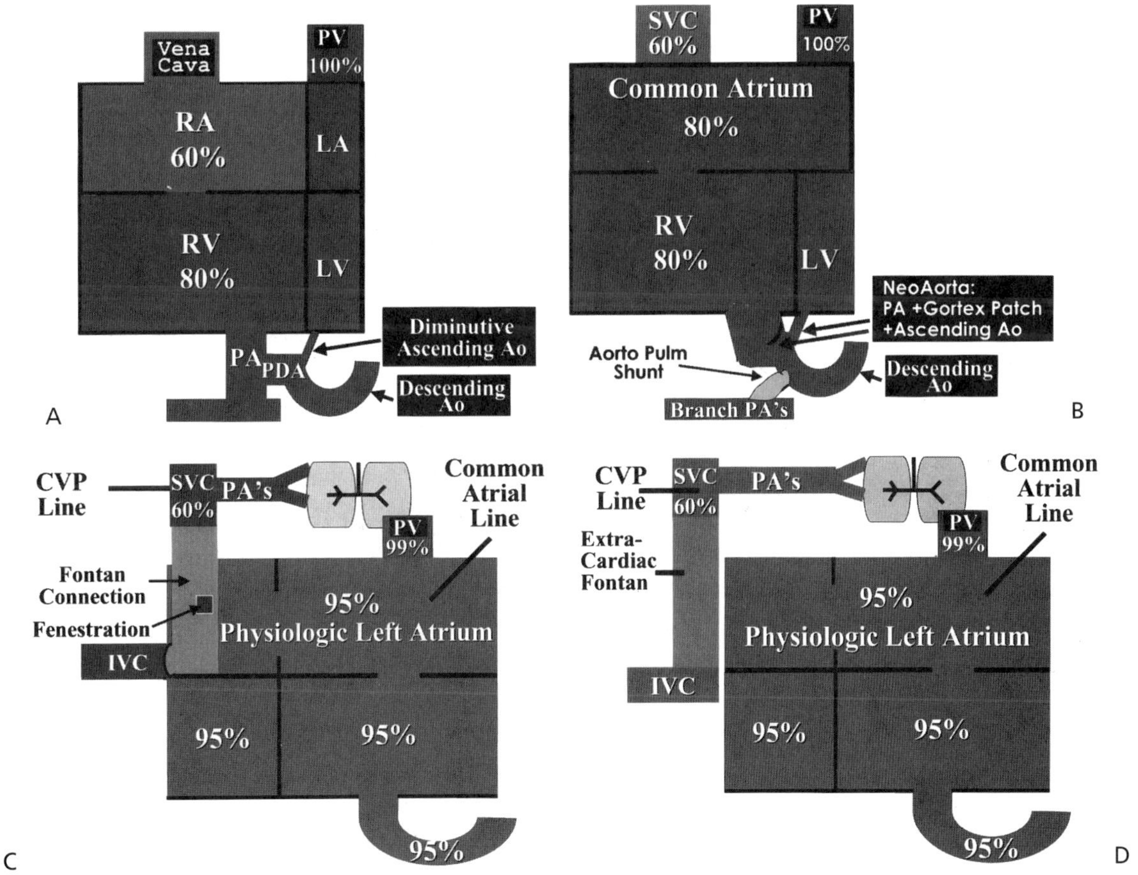

FIGURE 18-2. **(A)** through **(D)**. The anatomic correction and physiologic saturations expected in patients undergoing the bidirectional Glen operation, hemi-Fontan operation, Fontan operation, and extracardiac Fontan operation.

dures in either a bidirectional Glenn or a hemi-Fontan operation. In both procedures, a direct connection is created between the SVC and the branch PAs. In the bidirectional Glenn operation, the SVC is disarticulated from the right atrium and anastomosed to the branch PAs. In the hemi-Fontan procedure, a baffle is extended from the SVC to the right atrium and the SVC is connected to the branch PAs. The distal end of the atrial baffle is occluded with a dam so that blood flow from the SVC is channeled into the branch PAs (Fig. 18-2A,B).

MANAGEMENT APPROACH TO FUNCTIONAL ABNORMALITIES IN THE POSTOPERATIVE PERIOD

Pulmonary Artery Hypertension

All neonates are at risk for the development of PA hypertension owing to the *in utero* environment of high PA pressures and the muscularization of the pulmonary arterioles. In patients with congenital cardiac anomalies, the presence of cardiac defects with increased pulmonary blood flow and pressure increases the risk for postoperative pulmonary hypertension, because the vascular reactivity and muscularity of the pulmonary arterioles is maintained and progresses with persistent high flow and pressure. Congenital heart defects such as complete AV canal, large VSD, and truncus arteriosus are examples of high-flow lesions.

Another cause of elevated PVR is high venous pressure. An example is total anomalous pulmonary venous return (TAPVR). Patients with TAPVR presenting in the newborn period commonly have obstruction to pulmonary venous flow. Venous outlet obstruction results in high pulmonary vascular pressure, pulmonary edema, and hypoxemia, contributing to postoperative elevations in PVR.

Elevations in PVR increase RV afterload as well as RV end-diastolic and end-systolic pressure. As RV end-diastolic pressure increases, right atrial pressure increases and right-to-left shunting occurs at the atrial level if a persistent foramen ovale is present. This decreases pulmonary blood flow; oxygen saturation falls and oxygen delivery is reduced. As RV pressure increases, RV coronary perfusion is reduced, creating RV ischemia, decreased RV function, and a further reduction in cardiac output and oxygen delivery. Metabolic acidosis and hypoxemia further contribute to pulmonary vascular reactivity and contribute to a cyclic crisis resulting in RV failure and, ultimately, death.

Therapy for elevated PA pressures is aimed at lowering PVR and unloading the RV (Fig. 18-3). Reductions in PVR are accomplished by the use of inhaled medical gases (oxygen and nitric oxide [NO]), systemic alkalinization, ventilatory manipulations, and, if necessary, ECMO. Specifically, manipulating the pulmonary vascular bed in newborns and infants is a matter of regulating the arterial partial pressure of carbon dioxide ($PaCO_2$), pH, partial pressure of oxygen

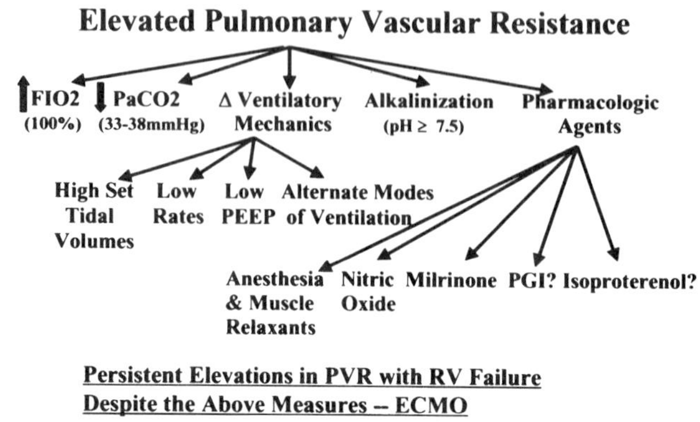

FIGURE 18-3. Decision-making algorithm for postoperative congenital heart disease patients with elevated pulmonary artery hypertension. Manipulations of the $PaCO_2$, pH, FIO_2, and ventilatory mechanics are the most crucial points. FIO_2, fraction of inspired oxygen; $PaCO_2$, partial pressure of arterial carbon dioxide; PEEP, positive end-expiratory pressure; PGE_1, prostaglandin E_1.

in the alveoli (PAO_2), partial pressure of arterial oxygen (PaO_2), and ventilatory mechanics (17,18,21,33,34). $PaCO_2$, $PACO_2$, and pH are potent mediators of PVR, especially in the newborn and the young infant (17).

Drummond and colleagues showed that reducing $PaCO_2$ and increasing pH to 7.6 produced a consistent and reproducible reduction in PVR in infants with PA hypertension (15). Manipulation of serum bicarbonate levels to achieve a pH between 7.5 and 7.6 while maintaining a $PaCO_2$ of 40 mm Hg has equal salutary effects on PVR (19–21). From a physiologic perspective, alkalinization with bicarbonate and mild hyperventilation ($PaCO_2$ of 35 mm Hg) reduces PVR while minimizing the negative impact of elevated mean airway pressure on cardiac preload. Elevations in mean airway pressure increase the intrathoracic pressure, reduce systemic venous return, and promote further reductions in cardiac output. High peak airway pressures may contribute to pulmonary barotrauma. Excessive ventilatory rates may result in an inadequate length of time for completing exhalation (premature termination of exhalation), resulting in gas trapping and intrinsic positive end-expiratory pressure (auto-PEEP), which would further contribute to high mean airway pressure. Finally, low $PaCO_2$ reduces cerebral blood flow, which may be problematic after circulatory arrest when cerebral autoregulation may be impaired, or after a bidirectional Glenn, hemi-Fontan, or Fontan procedure, when cerebral venous pressure may be high.

Both the arteriolar PaO_2 and the alveolar PAO_2 decrease PVR (21). In the circumstance of intracardiac shunts, changes in FIO_2 have little effect on the PaO_2. Therefore, by inference, a reduction in PVR induced by increasing the inspired oxygen concentration is probably a direct pulmonary vasodilatory effect of the alveolar rather than the arterial PO_2.

Work by Custer and Hales (18) showed that increased

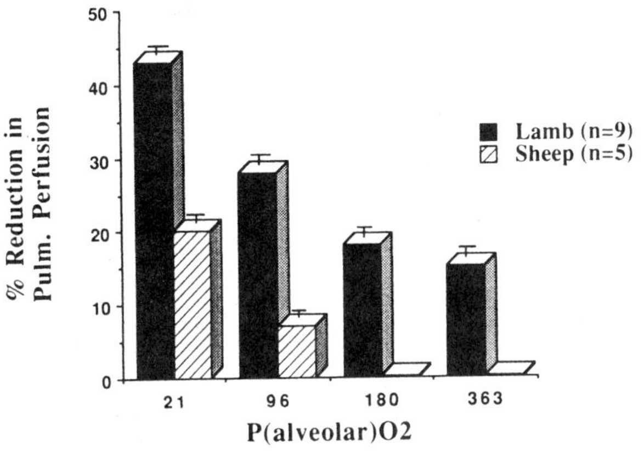

FIGURE 18-4. Oxygen is a more potent pulmonary vasodilator in neonatal than in adult animals. In this study, reductions in alveolar oxygen tension (Po_2) resulted in a much greater reduction in pulmonary blood flow in newborn lambs than in adult sheep.

Fio_2 is a more potent vasodilator in neonatal than in adult animals (Fig. 18-4). Increases in Fio_2 have shown similar dilatory effects on the pulmonary vascular bed of children with VSD in the cardiac catheterization laboratory (22). Ventilatory mechanics also play a major role in reducing PVR (35–37). Cardiorespiratory interactions are exaggerated in neonates and infants because peak and mean airway pressures are relatively high compared with RV and LV pressures. High mean airway pressures have a more dramatic impact on cardiac filling. For this reason, lower respiratory rates and shorter inspiratory times are preferred. In addition, newborns and infants have a closing volume below their functional residual capacity (FRC), so at the end of a normal breath some airway closure occurs (38). This process results in areas of lung that are perfused and yet underventilated (atelectatic). As these lung segments become increasingly hypoxemic, a secondary hypoxic vasoconstriction occurs (21). The net effect is an increase in PVR. Therefore, careful inflation of the lungs to maintain FRC and selectively reduce PVR is beneficial. In practice this is accomplished with relatively large set tidal volumes (measured at the ventilator) and low respiratory rates, which produce an exaggerated chest excursion during clinical observation in the early postoperative period. Usually tidal volumes of 10 to 15 mL/kg are required. When delivered tidal volumes are measured (at the endotracheal tube), they are usually in a more physiologic range of 7 to 10 mL/kg (39). Because most ventilators measure a set tidal volume, it is important to anticipate the need to set a higher than normal tidal volume on the ventilator.

A large array of modes of ventilation are available in current pediatric ventilators. In the immediate postoperative period, controlled ventilation is used. Continuous-flow and variable-flow patterns result in different pressures when assessed with a pneumotac placed at the airway. Continuous-flow patterns result in a square wave flow pattern, with higher peak inflation pressures and lower mean airway pressures for the same delivered tidal volume. In contrast, a decelerating flow pattern results in a higher mean airway pressure and lower peak pressure for a given delivered tidal volume. With a decelerating flow pattern, gas is distributed to the lung in the early portion of the breath. The net effect is decreased barotrauma owing to a lower peak or plateau pressure and better recruitment of atelectatic lung segments. Reductions in barotrauma and improvements in PAo_2 enhance management of PA hypertension. Modes such as pressure control, pressure-regulated volume control, and volume support generally provide a decelerating flow pattern (40).

The respiratory rate for newborns and infants is maintained at 15 to 20 breaths/minute. A reduced ventilatory rate provides a longer expiratory phase of ventilation. Because pulmonary blood flow occurs predominantly during the expiratory phase of the respiratory cycle, the ventilatory pattern should be adjusted to allow an adequate distribution of gas throughout the lung during inspiration and a more prolonged expiratory phase to promote blood flow through the lungs. In neonates, CPB results in a significant decrease in lung compliance. Decelerating flow patterns improve oxygenation without contributing to an increase in barotrauma (39,40). End-expiratory pressure must be applied cautiously in postoperative congenital heart disease patients. Low levels of PEEP (3 to 5 cm H_2O) prevent narrowing of the capillary and precapillary blood vessels, thereby reducing PVR (34). Higher levels of PEEP or excessive mean airway pressure results in alveolar overdistention and compression of the capillary network in the alveolar wall and interstitium. This situation causes elevated PVR and reduced pulmonary blood flow (16,40).

The final, and perhaps the least recognized, use of the mechanical ventilator is to assist in unloading the RV. During inspiration, intrathoracic pressure increases. Inspiration may therefore assist RV systole by creating an increased pressure gradient from the lung to the left atrium. This ventilatory assist is commonly seen in patients with PA hypertension or RV dysfunction. We typically see an augmentation of the arterial pressure trace during inspiration. The mechanical ventilator used to augment systemic blood flow is based on a concept similar to the thoracic pump mechanism used to explain blood flow during cardiopulmonary resuscitation (41). The inspiratory assist must be balanced by the potential negative effects of increased mean airway pressure on PVR (e.g., increased RV afterload). To maximize these cardiopulmonary interactions, high tidal volume with low respiratory rates should be employed. Inspiratory time should be limited to one to two cardiac cycles. A more prolonged inspiratory time reduces LV preload and minimizes cardiac output.

Nonconventional modes of ventilation include high-frequency oscillatory and high-frequency jet ventilation. High-frequency oscillatory ventilation utilizes an electrically powered piston diaphragm oscillator to rapidly alternate positive and negative pressure in the airway. Low tidal volumes of between 1 and 3 mL/kg are generated, and cycles range from 180 to 900 per minute (3 to 15 Hz). Oscillatory ventilation is active during both inspiration and expiration. Because expiration is active, CO_2 removal may be less efficient, particularly in patients with reactive airway disease. In neonatal and pediatric studies, high-frequency oscillatory ventilation was shown to reduce the incidence of chronic lung disease after treatment for infant respiratory distress syndrome and pediatric forms of adult respiratory distress syndrome (ARDS) (42). However, this mode of ventilation should be used with caution in patients with congenital cardiac abnormalities, because it requires a higher mean airway pressure than does conventional ventilation; with initiation of high-frequency oscillatory ventilation, the mean airway pressures required are commonly 5 to 10 mm Hg greater than for conventional modes of ventilation (42). The higher mean airway pressure increases intrathoracic pressure and significantly reduces LV preload.

High-frequency jet ventilation is another alternative method of ventilation for patients with RV failure. Because jet ventilation reduces mean airway pressure and PVR, it should be ideally suited for patients with RV dysfunction. In postoperative Fontan patients whose cardiac index is inversely related to PVR and mean airway pressure, jet ventilation significantly decreases mean airway pressure, reduces PVR, and increases cardiac index (Fig. 18-5) (43,44).

Patients with elevated PVR are also quite sensitive to hypovolemia. A patient with PA hypertension has an increased RV afterload. This may result in worsening RV

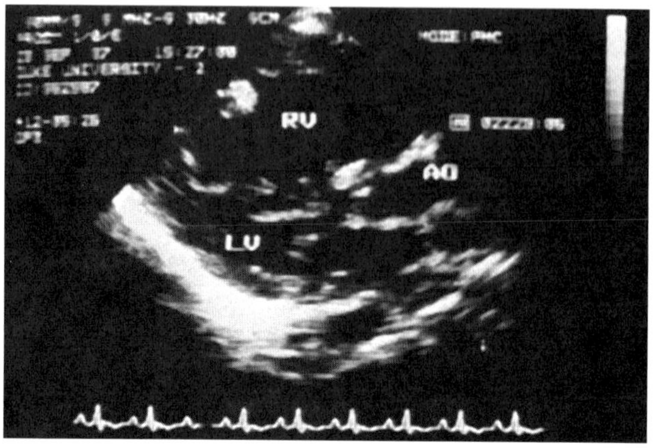

FIGURE 18-6. Echocardiogram demonstrating pulmonary artery hypertension, a dilated right ventricle, and shifting of the ventricular septum into the left ventricular chamber. The net result is decreased left ventricular filling and loss of effective contraction of the intraventricular septum.

function. The RV end-systolic volume increases, resulting in a volume-overloaded RV and a volume-underloaded LV (Fig. 18-6). LV stroke volume is dependent on left atrial preload, which requires a reduction in PVR to allow effective filling.

Newer agents aimed at lowering PVR through pharmacologic interventions have been introduced over the last decade. Perhaps the most successful agents have been inhaled NO and the phosphodiesterase type III inhibitors (45–47). NO is an endothelium-derived vasodilator that can be administered as an inhaled gas. Although nonselective, NO is rapidly inactivated by hemoglobin; therefore,

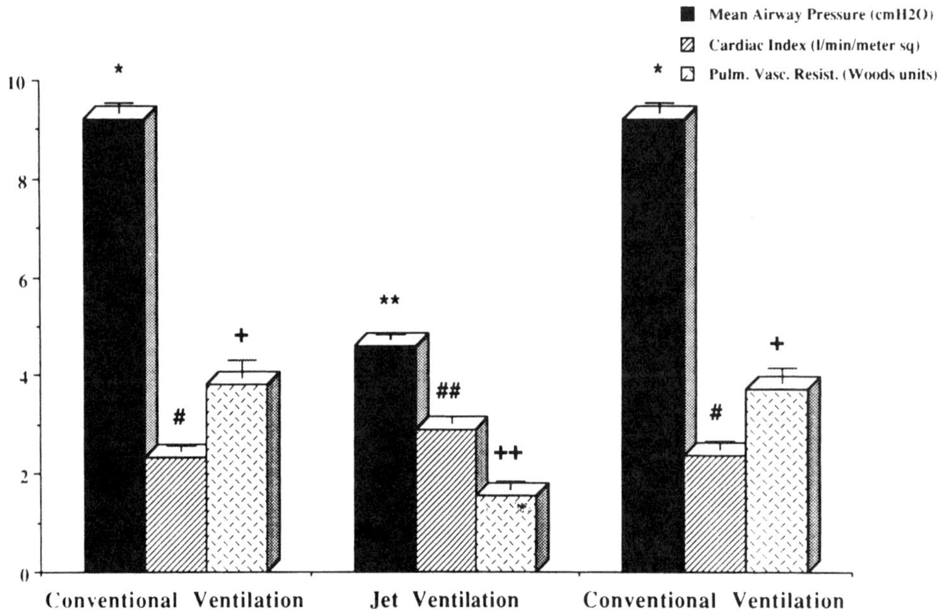

FIGURE 18-5. Jet ventilation provides equally effective ventilation and oxygenation at a lower mean airway pressure. In postoperative congenital heart disease patients, pulmonary vascular resistance is reduced and cardiac index is improved when patients are ventilated by jet rather than conventional methods.

when it is administered via inhalation, the systemic circulation is protected from its vasodilating properties. When used as an inhaled gas, it diffuses from the alveolus through the pulmonary vascular endothelium and enters the smooth muscle cells of the pulmonary vasculature. NO activates guanylate cyclase, which increases cyclic guanosine monophosphate (cGMP). cGMP decreases intracellular calcium levels, resulting in smooth muscle relaxation in the pulmonary vasculature. NO then diffuses into the blood, where it is rapidly deactivated by hemoglobin into nitrates, nitrites, and methemoglobin (45–47). The clinical action of inhaled NO is limited to the pulmonary vasculature because it is rapidly deactivated in blood; therefore it has limited systemic vascular side effects, which separates NO from other vasodilatory agents. Because NO is administered as an inhaled gas, it is effective only in ventilated regions of lung. In these regions, NO increases perfusion, decreases PVR, improves ventilation-perfusion matching, and improves oxygen delivery. In most cases low-dose NO (2 to 5 ppm) is effective. Clinical trials of inhaled NO in congenital cardiac patients with postoperative PA hypertension have been mixed. Consistent efficacy has been demonstrated in children with pulmonary venous hypertension due to mitral valve disease or TAPVR. In other congenital cardiac lesions the results have been inconsistent, with some patients responding to NO and others not. Patients with bidirectional Glenn or Fontan physiology and elevated PVR have benefited from NO with a reduction in PA pressure and measured gradient between the SVC and common atrium (physiologic left atrium) (47). In most studies, NO reduces PA pressure and PVR by approximately 20% in NO responders (48). Although beneficial, a 20% reduction may not be adequate in patients with significant RV dysfunction. Reductions in PA pressure from 35 to 28 mm Hg may be statistically but not clinically significant in these patients. Therefore, measures of mixed venous saturations (high SVC measures), systemic saturations, base deficits, and lactates should be used to demonstrate an improvement in cardiac output and oxygen delivery.

Phosphodiesterase type III inhibitors have also shown promise in reducing PVR. Milrinone is a mixed phosphodiesterase inhibitor in that it increases both cyclic adenosine monophosphate (cAMP) and cGMP. In clinical studies, milrinone reduced SVR by 38%, increased cardiac index by 30%, and reduced PVR by approximately 25% in neonates undergoing surgery for congenital cardiac conditions. Loading doses of 50 μg/kg and infusions of 0.5 μg/kg/minute are recommended (48). Amrinone, an older phosphodiesterase inhibitor, has less effect on cGMP, but it does reduce PVR and SVR and mildly increases RV contractility (48,51–53). Milrinone has become the preferred drug because of its shorter half-life, reduced systemic vasodilatory effect, and lack of a platelet inhibiting action (48).

Other agents include isoproterenol, prostaglandins E_1 (PGE_1), and prostacyclin (PGI_2). Isoproterenol, a β_1- and β_2-agonist, has mild PA vasodilating properties in the normal pulmonary circulation (54–56). Isoproterenol causes mild PVR reductions in adults after cardiac transplant surgery, but data are scant to support PVR reduction in infants and young children after cardiac surgery. In immature animals, compared with adult animals, the myocardium has been less responsive to isoproterenol (56). In addition, isoproterenol causes tachycardia and an increase in myocardial oxygen consumption (55). These effects may reduce coronary perfusion and result in relative myocardial ischemia. This may be especially problematic for the RV, which is being made to pump against a high PVR.

PGE_1 and PGI_2 both have a pulmonary vasodilating effect. The problem is that neither drug's effects are limited to the pulmonary circulation (57–59,61). Although PGE_1 has been used to treat pulmonary hypertensive crisis with varying degrees of success in newborns with persistent pulmonary hypertension, in our neonatal cardiac experience we have not been able to appreciate as consistent a pulmonary vasodilatory effect from this drug, although systemic vasodilatory effects are common. PGI_2 infusions have been used with some success in Europe. Bush et al. (58) reported the successful use of PGI_2 to prevent pulmonary hypertensive crisis in five patients with congenital heart defects (58). It also is being used with moderate success as a long-term treatment for elevated PVR in patients with primary pulmonary hypertension who are awaiting lung transplantation (60).

Because of the lack of specificity of intravenous vasodilator drugs on the pulmonary bed, newer pharmacologic methods of controlling PA hypertension and elevated PVR are being sought. The final approach to manipulating PVR has been to extend the anesthetic period through the first 24 to 48 hours of postoperative care (62–64). Narcotic-based anesthetic regimens prevent sympathetic-mediated increases in PVR (62–64). Continuous infusions of fentanyl or fentanyl plus midazolam may be particularly useful in patients who are prone to develop labile pulmonary hypertension.

Reactive pulmonary responses to endotracheal suction can be prevented by the prior administration of fentanyl (63,64). Because fentanyl does not block the effects of hypoxic pulmonary vasoconstriction, its effect probably results from the attenuated release of sympathomimetic mediators that produce a direct vasoconstrictive effect on PA smooth muscle. Continuous infusions of opioids such as fentanyl or sufentanil alone, or any opioid plus a benzodiazepine (midazolam), are considered beneficial in the postoperative treatment of infants prone to reactive pulmonary vascular responses after congenital heart surgery (63,64).

The addition of a neuromuscular blocking agent should be considered in patients with ventilatory dyssynchrony. Neuromuscular blockade allows for a more precise control of ventilation, pH, and $Pa{CO_2}$, thus optimizing therapy directed at reducing PVR. A schematic approach to PA hypertension management in neonates and infants is shown in Fig. 18-3.

Rebound pulmonary hypertension may be seen with NO withdrawal. In most cases this resolves within 60 minutes (49). However, on occasion, more prolonged and severe rebound has been reported. Approaches to this problem include slow weaning and maintenance of low levels of NO (approximately 1 ppm) for 12 to 24 hours before discontinuation of the drug, and the use of a substitute pulmonary vasodilator. Drugs such as PGI_2 or dipyridamole have been evaluated. Dipyridomole is particularly interesting because it is a selective inhibitor of the phosphodiesterase enzyme for cGMP (49,50). cGMP mediates vascular relaxation by decreasing intracellular calcium in vascular smooth muscle.

Right Ventricular Dysfunction

Primary RV dysfunction is a common finding after open heart surgery in neonates, infants, and children. Common causes of postoperative RV dysfunction in congenital heart disease patients are hypertrophied RV in tetralogy of Fallot, surgically induced RV dysfunction due to closing of a VSD through a right ventriculotomy, placement of transannular patches across the RV outflow tract (causing acute pulmonary regurgitation), and RV volume overload (stage one palliation of hypoplastic left heart syndrome) (65).

The diagnosis of RV dysfunction is suggested by high right-sided filling pressures, liver engorgement, hypotension, tachycardia, reduced cardiac output, and systemic venous desaturation (low mixed venous saturations). Reduced RV function leads to a decrease in systemic cardiac output because the LV can only pump the fraction of blood it receives from the RV. Low systemic arterial saturations may also occur as a result of right-to-left shunting across a persistent foramen ovale or atrial septal defect. If RV stroke volume is low, LV stroke volume will be low as well. A significant right-to-left shunt at the atrial level preserves cardiac output if LV function is normal, but at a reduced systemic arterial saturation. Atrial-level right-to-left shunting generally improves oxygen delivery by markedly increasing cardiac output while having a smaller effect on oxygen content.

The treatment of RV dysfunction consists of a paradigm aimed at improving oxygen delivery by increasing RV preload, direct and indirect augmentation of RV contractility through improving contractility and enhancing coronary perfusion, and reducing RV afterload (Fig. 18-7). Ventilatory strategies are used and are directed at reducing RV afterload and promoting LV filling. The RV is generally less responsive than the LV to inotropic support and therefore may require higher doses of inotropic agents. Epinephrine demonstrates the greatest improvement in RV contractility in animal models (66,67).

In contrast to the LV, the low-pressure RV receives a significant portion of its coronary filling during ventricular systole (68). In patients with RV dysfunction, maintaining a normal to slightly elevated systolic pressure maximizes coronary perfusion to the RV and augments contractility. RV coronary perfusion pressure can be significantly reduced with RV dysfunction (65). Under the low-pressure conditions of the RV, a significant portion of coronary blood flow occurs during ventricular systole. As RV pressure increases, the systolic component of coronary blood flow is reduced. Tachycardia reduces diastolic filling time, thereby compromising diastolic coronary perfusion. With further reductions in systemic blood pressure and elevations in RV end-diastolic pressure, RV coronary perfusion is further compromised, contractility is reduced, and significant RV failure ensues. Phenylephrine is a beneficial agent for rapidly increasing RV coronary blood flow by enhancing aortic blood pressure. Calcium also increases SVR and may be used intermittently to augment RV coronary perfusion. Epinephrine and dopamine increase systemic blood pressure and myocardial contractility, and these agents should be considered to maintain RV coronary blood flow (65,66,69). Drugs that decrease SVR and lower systemic blood pressure, such as nitroprusside, nicardipine, dobutamine, and phosphodiesterase inhibitors (amrinone or milrinone), should be used with caution if RV dysfunction exists, because of their tendency to decrease SVR and coronary blood flow to the RV. Epinephrine and dopamine enhance RV contractility directly by increasing myocardial excitation contraction coupling and indirectly by improving coronary perfusion pressure. If increases in inotropic support persist and frequent supplemental doses of calcium or phenylephrine are required after the early postoperative period, a critical evaluation for other structural and/or functional abnormalities should be aggressively pursued (69,70).

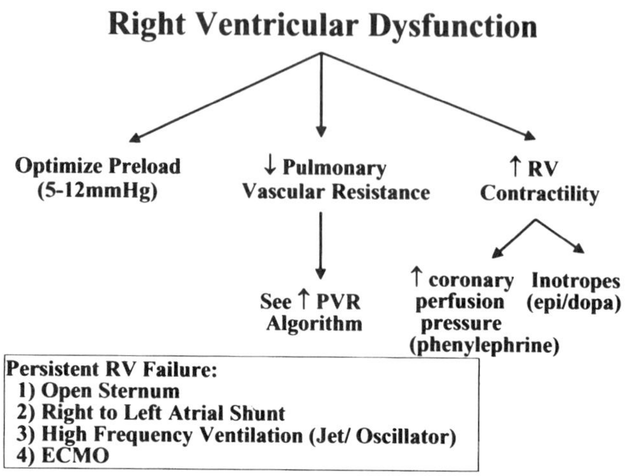

FIGURE 18-7. Decision-making algorithm for postoperative congenital cardiac patients with right ventricular dysfunction. Important concerns are preload augmentation, reducing pulmonary vascular resistance, and maintaining coronary perfusion. $Paco_2$, partial pressure of arterial carbon dioxide; Fio_2, fraction of inspired oxygen; ECMO, extracorporeal membrane oxygenation.

Preload should be maintained at a normal to slightly elevated level. Because RV contractility is reduced, it is important to maximize preload to the highest portion of the Starling curve (71). Excessive volume is not well tolerated owing to ventricular noncompliance (diastolic dysfunction) and tricuspid regurgitation resulting in a reduction in RV cardiac output. Generally, a CVP much above 12 to 14 mm Hg is poorly tolerated in neonates and young infants with RV dysfunction and leads to systemic venous hypertension, liver engorgement, and systemic capillary leak syndrome (endothelial cell dysfunction) (72).

Mechanical ventilation should be adjusted to assist RV function and minimize elevations in PVR. The RV is extremely sensitive to alterations in intrathoracic pressures. Venous return to the right side of the heart is passive and occurs as a result of pressure gradients between the systemic veins and the right atrium. As right atrial pressure increases, the gradient between the systemic veins and the right atrium falls and venous return is diminished, resulting in a reduction in RV preload and stroke volume. Positive-pressure ventilation, PEEP, and ventilatory strategies that increase mean airway pressure increase intrathoracic pressure and thereby reduce RV preload. In addition, high peak inspiratory pressure, particularly with a long inspiratory time, increases intrathoracic pressure and lowers the gradient between the aorta and RV. Therefore, during inspiration RV coronary perfusion may be compromised. This is particularly important in neonates because they require higher peak inspiratory pressures (30 mm Hg) relative to aortic pressures (65 mm Hg) compared with adults. Maintaining FRC is critical to RV afterload, because reductions in lung volume below FRC causes atelectasis and hypoxic pulmonary vasoconstriction, which increase PVR. If lung volumes exceed FRC, then alveolar overdistention occurs, contributing to increased resistance in the capillary and arteriolar vascular beds within the alveolus. This contributes to increased PVR and RV afterload.

If RV dysfunction persists or worsens because of elevations in PA pressure or if a low cardiac output state persists despite aggressive ventilatory and inotropic support, the sternum should be reopened (58). If mild ventricular distention has occurred and lung compliance is poor, eliminating the impedance imposed by the chest wall and allowing the RV to increase end-diastolic volume is an effective maneuver. If ventricular function and pulmonary blood flow improve after opening of the chest, a Silastic membrane can be sewn in place and covered with a povidone-iodine (Betadine) dressing.

An additional strategy in neonates, infants, and children with significant postoperative RV dysfunction is to allow right-to-left shunting at the atrial level. Typical patients who would benefit from this strategy include those undergoing neonatal repairs for tetralogy of Fallot, tetralogy with pulmonary atresia, and truncus arteriosus. In tetralogy of Fallot and tetralogy with pulmonary atresia, a hypertrophied noncompliant RV has undergone a ventriculotomy and may be further compromised by volume loading from a regurgitant pulmonary valve, induced by a transvalvular RV outflow tract patch. In truncus arteriosus, a noncompliant hypertrophied RV is compromised by exaggerated PA hypertension. Under these circumstances, allowing an atrial communication to remain open, with blood shunting in a right-to-left direction, preserves cardiac output and oxygen delivery to the systemic circulation. Although these patients may remain blue, their effective cardiac output is enhanced, systemic perfusion pressure is improved, and coronary perfusion to the RV is maintained. Over time, as RV pressure falls, right-to-left shunting decreases and systemic saturation improves. This same strategy of leaving an atrial communication to improve cardiac output has been extended to children with single-ventricle physiology.

Children with single ventricles and either reduced ventricular function or moderate elevations in PVR are high-risk candidates for a modified Fontan operation. By creating an atrial-level shunt, cardiac output can be augmented in this patient group. This modification is called the fenestrated Fontan procedure (Fig. 18-2C). This procedure is covered more completely in the discussion of palliative operations (73,74).

If RV dysfunction persists despite these maneuvers, consideration should be given to extracorporeal life support (ECMO). When ECMO is used for circulatory support, venoarterial cannulation is chosen. Venovenous bypass provides gas exchange but does not provide cardiac support. Venous and arterial access may be achieved through a large central artery and vein (usually the carotid and internal jugular) or by direct chest cannulation. Recovery from severe ventricular dysfunction is predicated on the concept that the myocardium sustained a transient injury and is capable of recovery with time ("stunned myocardium") (75–77) or that RV dysfunction is due to persistent increases in RV afterload from PA hypertension. ECMO is used to decrease ventricular wall tension, increase coronary perfusion pressure, and maintain systemic perfusion with oxygenated blood; ECMO's role in patients with myocardial injury or pulmonary hypertension is to provide adequate systemic oxygen transport and systemic perfusion while allowing the ventricles to "rest." Theoretically, ECMO provides adequate systemic and coronary oxygen transport while reducing myocardial oxygen demand. This favorable shift in the oxygen supply-to-demand ratio may allow the heart to recover from reversible myocardial failure.

The ECMO registry suggests that of all patients placed on ECMO for circulatory support, patients with tetralogy of Fallot or tetralogy-like physiology have the greatest likelihood of weaning from ECMO. This finding suggests that myocardial injury due to severe hypertrophy may result in an ischemic ventricle that, with prolonged rest, coronary reperfusion, and reduced RV afterload, may significantly recover function (78,79). An alternative approach is the use of a ventricular assist device. This approach is most beneficial when pulmonary function is adequate and PVR remains low. If significant lung disease exists and systemic oxygenation remains low conversion to ECMO may be indicated. The advantage to ventricular assist devices resides in the reduced need for anticoagulation. This is particularly valuable when coagulopathy is present and hemostasis has not been achieved.

Left Ventricular Dysfunction

The contractile state of the LV may be depressed after pediatric cardiac surgery. This results at least partly from the preoperative condition of the myocardium (myocardial hypertrophy, elevated end-diastolic pressure, systolic dysfunction); the response of the myocardium to the new loading conditions imposed by the operative repair (changes in afterload or preload); the effects of deep hypothermia, CPB, and/or circulatory arrest on myocardial compliance; and surgical problems such as ineffective myocardial protection, residual anatomic problems that interfere with LV function such as valvular regurgitation or stenosis, residual LV outflow obstruction, residual VSD, or mitral valve dysfunction (3,79–85). A further factor complicating LV function after cardiac surgery in newborns is the reduced myocardial reserve, the limited recruitable stroke work, and the reduced compliance characteristic of the immature neonatal heart.

The ultrastructure of the neonatal heart is characterized by a 50% reduction in the number of myofibrils, nonlinear or chaotic arrangement of the myofibrils, absence of the transverse tubular system, and an immature sarcoplasmic reticulum that has to store and release calcium (86–90). This condition effectively reduces the contractile mass of the heart and results in a ventricle with low compliance (88). Preload augmentation is effective at low filling pressures (1 to 12 mm Hg); however, when left-sided filling pressures exceed 10 to 12 mm Hg, further increases in LV stroke volume are minimal (91). As a consequence, neonates are more dependent on heart rate and, to a lesser extent, on preload to maintain cardiac output at higher filling rates (82,92).

The newborn LV is further handicapped by a reduced number of β-receptors and a resting level of circulating catecholamines that is much higher than typically seen in adults or older children. This limits contractile reserve and results in an LV with a high level of resting tone (88). Experiments in newborn lambs showed only a modest increase in preload-independent measures of contractility at dobutamine doses of 8 to 10 μg/kg/minute, whereas a moderately severe reduction in contractility was demonstrated with a 0.5-mg/kg dose of propranolol (93).

The diagnosis of LV dysfunction is made by clinical, radiographic, laboratory, invasive monitoring, and echocardiographic evaluation. Evidence of poor systemic perfusion includes tachycardia, hypotension, decreased pulses, delayed

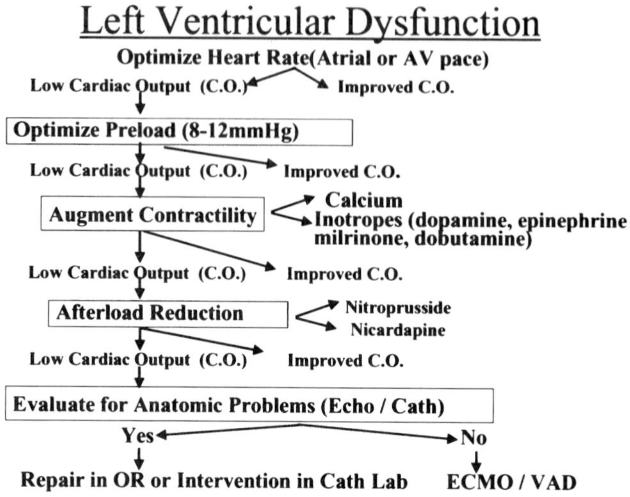

FIGURE 18-8. Decision-making algorithm for postoperative congenital cardiac patients with left ventricular dysfunction. A, atrial; AV, atrioventricular; OR, operating room; ECMO, extracorporeal membrane oxygenation; VAD, ventricular assist device.

capillary refill, and cool extremities. Radiographic findings are cardiomegaly and pulmonary edema. Abnormal laboratory values include persistent metabolic acidosis, low mixed venous saturations, high lactate concentration and high base deficit, decreased urine output, and rising creatine levels. Invasive pressure monitoring demonstrates elevated left atrial or capillary wedge pressures, and noninvasive echocardiographic provides evidence of decreased systolic function and increased end-diastolic volume.

LV dysfunction can be treated by optimizing heart rate and preload, then adding inotropic support, and finally reducing LV afterload (Fig. 18-8). Optimizing heart rate, however, reduces diastolic filling time. LV coronary blood flow occurs during diastole. Therefore, excessive tachycardia (greater than 180 to 190 beats/minute) may impair LV function. Pacing should be considered in neonates whose heart rates are less than 120 to 130 beats/minute. Usually atrial or AV sequential pacing is preferred to provide an atrial kick to improve LV filling. In patients with significant LV dysfunction, atrial contraction can augment cardiac output by up to 25% to 30%. Once the heart rate is optimized, preload should be optimized. Filling pressures in excess of 10 to 12 mm Hg are usually not beneficial unless LV compliance is severely impaired (left-sided obstructive lesion).

Once heart rate and preload have been optimized, increasing the inotropic state of the heart becomes paramount. Inotropic support is usually initiated with dopamine (5 to 10 μg/kg/minute). Dopamine has the unique property of binding to dopaminergic receptors in the renal and mesenteric beds and improving perfusion to the gut and the kidneys. Dopamine augments cardiac contractility by means of two mechanisms: a direct stimulation of β_1-receptors in the heart and inducement of norepinephrine release from sympathetic nerve endings (95). Several studies suggest that the effect of dopamine in children is age dependent. In young children after cardiac surgery, dopamine-induced increases in cardiac output correlate more with elevations in heart rate than with augmentation of stroke volume, whereas in young adults dopamine clearly increases stroke volume (94–98). Nonetheless, infants and neonates respond favorably to dopamine infusions, with increases in systemic blood pressure and improved peripheral and renal perfusion.

Although calcium supplementation has fallen into disfavor because of concerns about reperfusion injury, calcium administration remains important in augmenting cardiac contractility after pediatric cardiac surgery. In particular, the underdeveloped sarcoplasmic reticular system in neonatal myocardium makes the neonatal heart more dependent than the adult myocardium on extracellular calcium concentrations (23). Because intracellular calcium concentrations play a central role in myocardial contractility, normal or even elevated plasma levels of ionized calcium may be necessary to augment stroke volume (99). Additionally, fluctuations in ionized calcium levels occur commonly in the early postoperative period. These fluctuations most often result from the relatively large transfusions of citrate- and albumin-rich blood products, such as packed red blood cells, whole blood, fresh-frozen plasma, platelets, and cryoprecipitate, that are necessary to promote postoperative hemostasis and maintain an effective preload (24). Routine monitoring of ionized calcium levels and regular calcium supplementation during the first 24 hours of postoperative care are commonly employed. This approach is especially helpful in patients with diminished LV function. In patients with a slow sinus or junctional rate calcium must be administered cautiously, because marked slowing of AV conduction may occur.

Epinephrine is a potent α-, β_1-, and β_2-agent. In lower doses of 0.03 to 0.1 μg/kg/minute β effects predominate. Doses of 0.1 to 0.2 μg/kg/minute have a mixed α and β effect, and with doses greater than 0.2 μg/kg/minute α-mediated responses predominate. Epinephrine is useful in patients with significant LV dysfunction after cardiac repair who remain hypotensive or hypoperfused based on poor systemic perfusion, low mixed venous saturations, or rising serum lactate levels (100). It is effective in patients who do not respond to equivalent doses of dopamine or dobutamine and is particularly valuable in patients with mild to moderate degrees of hypotension and echocardiographic or electrocardiographic (ECG) evidence of regional ischemia.

Milrinone and amrinone are nonglycoside, noncatecholamine inotropic drugs. Their mechanism of action is the inhibition of phosphodiesterase type III enzyme. These agents prevent the breakdown of cAMP (amrinone) or of both cAMP and cGMP (milrinone), resulting in increased calcium transport. An increase in myocardial contractility and both systemic and PA vasodilation are produced (45, 48,51,101–103).

Clinical studies of the effects of amrinone and milrinone in pediatric patients have shown a considerable benefit, especially in patients whose myocardium is afterload-sensitive, such as those who have undergone arterial switch (45,48, 51). Pharmacokinetic studies suggest milrinone doses of 50 μg/kg load followed by an infusion of 0.5 μg/kg/minute. Amrinone loading doses in postoperative pediatric cardiac patients are 1.5 to 3 mg/kg, and infusion rates are 10 to 15 mg/kg/minute. Higher doses (3 to 4 mg/kg) have been associated with a profound systemic vasodilation in the postoperative pediatric cardiac patient. Because the onset of peripheral vasodilation precedes the increase in inotropy during the loading phase of amrinone, a significant reduction in afterload and hypotension may occur if loading occurs too quickly (102). This effect, coupled with the prolonged elimination half-life, necessitates caution when administering loading doses of phosphodiesterase type III inhibitors to children with borderline low blood pressures. In the postoperative period, we usually load over a 20- to 30-minute period.

Dobutamine is an effective, albeit weaker, inotropic agent in children. It has much less peripheral α-effect than dopamine does, and its β_2 effect predominates, yielding a mild peripheral vasodilation. Although dobutamine is reported to have fewer chronotropic effects than dopamine, in neonates it may cause significant tachyarrhythmias. This effect may relate to structural similarities between dobutamine and isoproterenol (104). In children who have undergone cardiac surgery, dobutamine increases cardiac output primarily through increases in heart rate. The efficacy of dobutamine seems to be reduced in immature animals (98). This finding is consistent with the previous discussion of reduced β-receptors and a higher level of circulating catecholamines in newborns (81,104). For these reasons, routine use of dobutamine after CPB in neonates is less effective, so selective use of dobutamine should be considered when LV afterload reductions are an important component of therapy or in older children.

Ventilation management in the postoperative congenital cardiac patient tends to use the ventilator to augment LV filling while minimizing mean airway pressure (105). Although experimental evidence supports the fact that increases in intrathoracic pressure reduce afterload to the LV, the reduction in LV preload secondary to increased intrathoracic pressure is usually the dominant pathophysiologic process (105). Mechanical assist devices in children include ECMO and ventricular assist devices. Intraaortic balloon pumps have had limited success in children because of the inability to inflate and deflate at rapid heart rates and because the inherent increased elasticity of the pediatric aorta tends to limit balloon pump augmentation. ECMO and ventricular assist devices have become the mainstay of mechanical ventricular support in children. Usually ECMO is preferred because of greater familiarity and a support staff with greater ECMO experience. In addition, many centers have rapid deployment capabilities with ECMO, allowing for earlier stability and better outcomes. Overall success rates are approximately 50% for ECMO in patients with LV dysfunction (105,106). These have improved over the last several years, probably as a result of increased experience and early implementation of ECMO. If LV function is impaired and both RV and pulmonary function are adequate, ventricular assist devices can be used as an alternative. Reduced heparin requirements and fewer hemorrhagic complications are the benefit, although perfusion services are usually required to run the device in most centers.

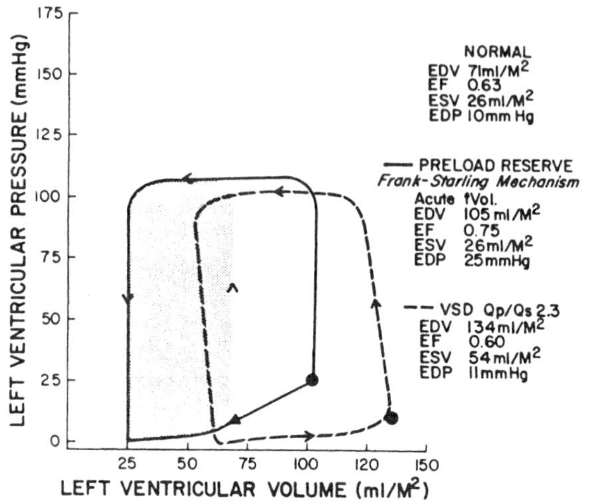

FIGURE 18-9. Pressure-volume relationship in a normal child showing normal preload reserve. This is compared with a child with chronic volume overload due to a large ventricular septal defect. EDV, end-diastolic volume; EF, ejection fraction; ESV, end-systolic volume; EDP, end-diastolic pressure. (From Graham TP Jr. Ventricular performance in congenital heart disease. *Circulation* 1991;84:2259, with permission.)

MANAGEMENT APPROACH TO SPECIFIC ANATOMIC REPAIRS

Complete Anatomic and Physiologic Repairs

The postoperative management of the patient with a complete anatomic and physiologic correction is simplified because blood flow patterns after surgical correction are normal; if an anatomic abnormality exists, its physiologic effect is more predictable and the location for the problem more obvious. Examples of complete anatomic repair include closure of a VSD, repair of tetralogy of Fallot, repair of AV canal defects, and arterial switch operation for transposition of the great arteries (TGA).

Postoperative Management of Ventricular Septal Defect

A VSD is a condition of chronic volume overload in which large increases in diastolic volume are tolerated with only minimal change in end-diastolic pressure (Fig. 18-9) (105, 108,109). The LV end-diastolic volume is usually twice normal, whereas the LV end-diastolic pressure and ejection fraction are unchanged (105). RV dilation also occurs with VSD, although it is usually less severe (108–110). The effects of a persistent VSD on LV and RV function depend on the length of time the ventricle has been exposed to the chronic volume-overload state (108). Large VSDs left unrepaired for 2 to 3 years or longer have a greater incidence of permanent ventricular dysfunction. These patients, along with neonates and infants with poorly compensated heart failure due to a large VSD, form a subset of patients at increased risk of postoperative ventricular dysfunction.

Most children who have undergone VSD closure convalesce normally. Patients are usually extubated shortly after surgery and, increasingly, in the operating room (111).

After VSD closure, patients infrequently require more than modest preload support and low-dose inotropy (e.g., 5 μg/kg/minute of dopamine). Postoperative problems, however, can be anticipated in patients with a residual VSD, neonates and infants with a large VSD and/or associated patent ductus arteriosus, repair after 2 to 3 years of age, postoperative complete heart block, and associated cardiac anomalies such as coarctation of the aorta, interrupted aortic arch, or mitral valve anomalies (108–110).

Residual septal defects are suggested by a low cardiac output and a residual holosystolic murmur. Bedside Doppler color flow echocardiography is usually diagnostic, although repeat cardiac catheterization may be necessary to better define the anatomic location of the defect before reoperation. Previously undiagnosed defects are usually found in the muscular septum. Residual defects around the patch are usually isolated to an area poorly visualized by the surgeon or near the conduction tissue (avoided to prevent heart block). Small defects of less than 4 mm have a high likelihood of closing on their own, and if the child is hemodynamically stable and convalescing well these defects usually do not require reoperation (112).

Neonates and infants with a large VSD and/or associated patent ductus arteriosus are susceptible to postoperative PA hypertensive crisis due to preexisting high pulmonary blood flow (80). After closure of the VSD, the RV must pump against increased PVR. It can no longer recruit the LV to assist in pumping against increased PVR. It must suddenly change from pumping against a volume load to supporting a pressure load. Similarly, the LV must pump a smaller volume load against SVR without the luxury of pumping any extra volume through the VSD and into the lower-pressure right-sided circulation. The LV may be at a further disadvantage if PA pressures are high and if the RV dilates and the septum shifts leftward. This situation significantly alters LV geometry and impairs LV ejection (Figs. 18-10

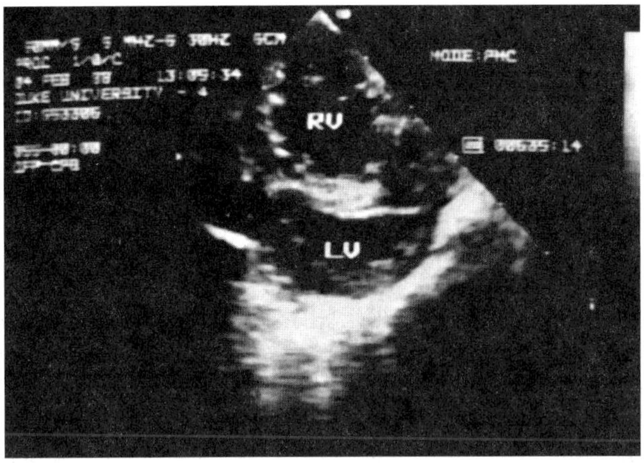

FIGURE 18-10. Echocardiogram demonstrating right ventricular dilation impinging on the left ventricle. This alters left ventricular filling, and, through alterations in left ventricular geometry, a secondary reduction in cardiac output occurs.

and 18-6) (113). Management is directed at reducing PVR and improving RV contractility. These maneuvers improve blood return to the LV, restore LV geometry, and improve cardiac output.

Patients undergoing repair at a late age and those with poor myocardial protection are similarly subject to RV and LV dysfunction. Elevations in PA pressures may also be a component of their disease; however, reactive PVR does not commonly occur with VSD outside the newborn and early infancy periods. PA pressures generally decrease to one third of the systemic values within 24 hours after surgery. Failure of the PA pressures to fall is very suggestive of a residual shunt, mitral regurgitation, or, less commonly, fixed changes associated with medial hypertrophy of the pulmonary arterioles.

Postoperative complete heart block is an uncommon finding today, owing to the precise anatomic knowledge concerning the location of the conduction tissue in different types of VSDs (114). Transient heart block, however, is not uncommon. Stretching of the conduction tissue at the time of surgery to more clearly visualize the defect, ion fluxes associated with cardioplegic solutions, and low-calcium–containing primes are other contributing factors. Temporary ventricular wires should be placed in all patients who experience periods of heart block in the operating room. In many institutions, atrial and ventricular wires are routinely placed after all operations involving closure of a VSD.

Associated cardiac anomalies such as left-sided obstructive lesions (interrupted aortic arch and coarctation) result in a pressure-overloaded dysfunctional LV. These patients frequently require much higher doses of inotropic infusions to improve LV contractility after repair.

Postoperative Management of Tetralogy of Fallot

Although the surgical approach to primary repair of tetralogy of Fallot has not changed significantly over the last decade, the timing of repair has changed. Evidence has accumulated that a considerable portion of the myocardial, pulmonary, and central nervous system damage attributable to "tetralogy of Fallot" is more specifically caused by prolonged exposure to abnormal blood flow patterns, hypoxemia, and cyanosis (115–118). Surgery involving multiple palliations and long-term medical management does not alleviate these problems, and a marked increase in long-term morbidity and mortality has been demonstrated (116, 119). Today there is a greater impetus to repair rather than palliate these defects in infancy (119).

The repair of tetralogy of Fallot includes a right ventriculotomy, patch closure of the VSD, resection of the infundibular stenosis, and patch augmentation of the RV outflow tract. In attempts to minimize RV dysfunction, closure of the VSD can be performed through the right atrium and the ventriculotomy kept to a minimum (120,121). In some cases, resection of subpulmonic muscle bundles is performed through the PA and no RV incision is required. The surgeon should evaluate the size of the pulmonary valve, and if it is too small the RV incision should be extended across the pulmonary valve annulus and onto the PA. Transannular patching creates postoperative pulmonary insufficiency, which may contribute a volume load to an already pressure-loaded RV (Fig. 18-11) (122). The need for a right ventricu-

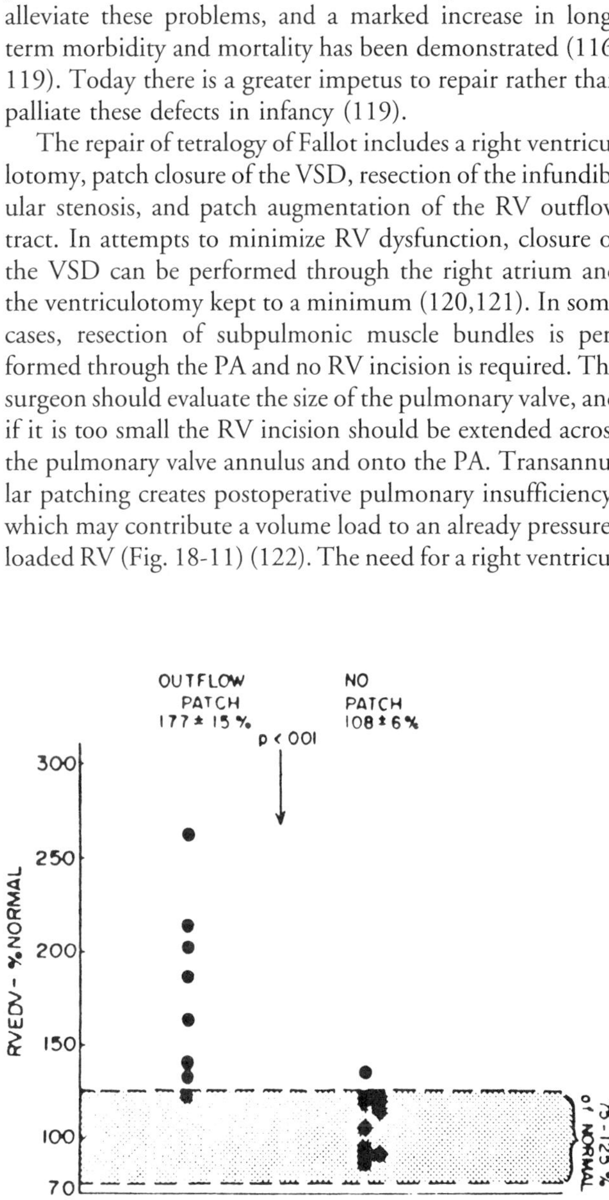

FIGURE 18-11. Right ventricular end-diastolic volume (RVEDV) is greater in postoperative tetralogy of Fallot patients receiving a transannular outflow patch, compared with patients whose pulmonary valve is preserved. (From Graham TP Jr, Cordell D, Atwood GF, et al. Right ventricular volume characteristics before and after palliative and reparative operation in tetralogy of Fallot. *Circulation* 1976;54:417, with permission.)

lotomy may also contribute to RV dysfunction in the postoperative period. These concerns are more pronounced when surgery is performed in early infancy.

Repair within the first few months of life is usually predicated on severe RV outflow obstruction, a small pulmonary valve orifice, and the presence of preoperative hypercyanotic spells. These patients commonly have a hypertrophied, noncompliant RV and frequently require a transannular patch. Postoperatively, RV systolic and mild diastolic dysfunction are is common. Higher right-sided filling pressures and lower pulmonary blood flow are seen. The LV receives less filling, resulting in reduced stroke volume, decreased cardiac output, and reflex tachycardia in an attempt to augment oxygen delivery.

Leaving the foramen ovale open or creating a small atrial septal defect at the time of surgery provides a right-to-left shunt at the atrial level. This shunt bypasses the noncompliant RV, preserving LV filling and systemic perfusion. The patient is somewhat hypoxemic, but this is well tolerated in the face of improved cardiac output and an overall improvement in oxygen delivery to tissue.

Persistently low cardiac output, despite an atrial-level shunt, suggests either a residual anatomic problem or severe ventricular dysfunction. Echocardiography and/or cardiac catheterization should be used to evaluate the repair for a residual VSD or inadequate relief of the RV outflow obstruction. If anatomic considerations persist, reoperation should be considered. If primary ventricular dysfunction exists, therapy should be directed toward RV or LV dysfunction, as previously discussed, and should include ECMO or use of a ventricular assist device.

Anatomic variants in coronary anatomy alter the surgical approach and may affect postoperative management in patients with tetralogy of Fallot. If the right coronary artery gives rise to the left anterior descending artery, the coronary artery courses directly across the RV outflow tract. A standard transannular enlargement is not feasible, because the right coronary would have to be transected. Under these circumstances the surgeon must decide either to place a conduit over the outflow tract or to resect as much infundibular tissue as possible and place a patch above and below the coronary artery (123,124). In the latter case, the narrowest part of the RV outflow tract is beneath the right coronary artery. In the postoperative period, ventricular distention and excessive preload may distend the RV, stretch the right coronary artery, and cause RV ischemia. Although ischemic changes are uncommon in pediatric cardiac surgery, this anatomic arrangement of the coronary arteries substantially increases the likelihood of ventricular ischemia. Careful observation for ischemic changes is essential. When the preload is augmented in the early postoperative period, the ECG should be watched closely for signs of ischemia. Volume supplementation should be given in small, frequent increments, and right-sided filling pressures should be maintained within a narrow range to avoid increases in ventricular end-diastolic and end-systolic dimension resulting in right coronary artery myocardial ischemia.

Postoperative Management of Atrioventricular Canal

AV canals behave physiologically as large VSDs. Their postoperative managements are similar, except that patients with AV canal are more prone to PA hypertension and valvular regurgitation in the postoperative period, owing respectively to the large left-to-right shunt imposed by the canal defect and abnormal valve tissue. AV canal defects are commonly found in patients with trisomy 21. This genetic defect is associated with small conducting airways and architecturally small PAs. Therefore, elevations in PVR may be caused by an underdeveloped pulmonary vascular tree as well. Reports of fixed PA hypertension have been documented in trisomy 21 patients with AV canal who are younger than 6 months of age (125).

Valvular regurgitation is not an uncommon finding after AV canal repair (126). Mild-to-moderate regurgitation is generally well tolerated and is managed in the postoperative period with systemic vasodilators. If concomitant ventricular dysfunction exists with AV valve regurgitation, low-dose dopamine, dobutamine, or milrinone may be added. If severe AV valve regurgitation exists, valve replacement may be necessary. Because the defect involves annular as well as valvular tissue, the artificial valve is difficult to seat and there is a greater risk of perivalvular leaks. Complete heart block, although generally uncommon, has an increased risk after valve replacement in AV canals, owing to a lack of normally developed annular tissue necessary for suturing the mechanical valve in place (127).

Postoperative Management of the Arterial Switch Operation for the Great Arteries

In TGA, the aorta arises from the RV and the PA arises from the LV. The arterial switch operation for TGA allows the LV to be the systemic ventricle. Theoretically, maintaining the LV as the systemic chamber improves ventricular longevity and reduces the incidence of systemic ventricular dysfunction.

The LV's cylindric shape and concentric contraction, and the location of the ventricular inlet and outlet at the base of the heart, allow the LV to function better as a pressure pump and account for improved long-term patient survival and reduced long-term morbidity after the arterial switch procedure. In contrast, atrial switch procedures that use the RV as the systemic pumping chamber have a 10% incidence of late systemic ventricular failure (128,129).

Improvements in coronary transfer techniques and myocardial preservation have reduced perioperative mortality for this operation to less than 3%, almost indistinguishable from atrial switch procedures. These results are more impressive in view of the late complications of atrial switch procedures, which include atrial dysrhythmias (50%), baffle stenosis (8% to 10%), and pulmonary venous obstruction and right (systemic) ventricular dysfunction (10%) (128, 129,131).

The arterial switch operation involves mobilization of the PA and dissection far out into the periphery. Marking sutures are placed in the predicted sites of the coronary artery anastomoses. The aorta and main PA are transected. The aorta is divided above the coronary arteries and aortic valves. The LeCompte maneuver (passage of the PA anterior to the aorta) is then performed. The coronary arteries are subsequently mobilized with 3 to 4 mm of surrounding aortic tissue and reimplanted into the "neoaorta." Previously harvested patches of pericardium are used to close the defects resulting from removal of the coronary arteries.

Although the arterial switch operation is preferred, two factors dictate the patient's ability to survive after an arterial switch operation: global function of the LV and focal ischemia (132,133). Global ventricular function addresses how well the LV is prepared to pump against a systemic pressure load after the arterial switch procedure. In patients who do not have a VSD (which allows both ventricles to see systemic pressure), the LV loses its ability to pump against systemic resistance 3 to 4 weeks after birth. In these patients, the LV must be "prepared." Preparation entails providing a pressure and volume load on the LV to allow it to pump against SVR. A PA band, which creates an LV pressure of 60% or more of systemic pressure, and a 4-mm aorta-to-pulmonary shunt are usually placed, to provide pressure and volume load on the LV respectively. These patients are frequently quite ill in the early postoperative period, but LV function recovers to the point of being able to pump against systemic afterload and tolerate an arterial switch within 5 to 7 days (130). Alternatively, use of a left ventricular assist device should be anticipated in the early postoperative period (134). In the postoperative period, the arterial switch patient exhibits global systolic and diastolic LV dysfunction occurring 6 to 12 hours after repair. The LV is typically dilated and poorly tolerant of volume loading.

The reason that LV function decreases in the early postoperative period is not entirely clear. On the basis of the timing of the peak reduction in cardiac output, one can speculate that myocardial, or perhaps coronary, edema might play a role. In the neonate, a small amount of coronary swelling might significantly narrow the coronary ostia and result in a transient period of reduced perfusion and myocardial dysfunction.

Another common anatomic problem that might contribute to LV dysfunction in the early postoperative period is LV outflow tract obstruction. This occurs in approximately 20% of patients with TGA (116,133). If unrecognized, excessive LV afterload may result in increased LV pressures and a reduced oxygen supply to the myocardium.

Inotropic support and afterload reduction are highly effective in maximizing cardiac output in the arterial switch patient. However, if inotropic support is excessive in the very early postoperative period and cardiac output and systemic perfusion remain marginal, early introduction of a ventricular assist device should be considered, because myocardial function predictably worsens in these patients. Nitroglycerin may be beneficial to reduce the incidence of coronary artery spasm in the early postoperative period.

Focal ischemia may be recognized in the postoperative period by ST-T wave changes. Kinking, twisting, or excessive tension placed on the coronary arteries and compression of the coronary arteries because the main PA crosses tightly over the aorta (due to inadequate dissection of the branch PAs in combination with the LeCompte maneuver) are causes of focal ischemic changes in these patients postoperatively. These changes are difficult to treat and may be poorly tolerated. Echocardiography is helpful in diagnosing abnormal coronary blood flow by demonstrating regional wall motion abnormalities and by visualizing decreased coronary flow at the coronary ostia.

Physiologic Repairs

A variety of complex congenital cardiac lesions allow for physiologic correction (i.e., return of normal blood flow patterns) but require an extracardiac conduit or an intracardiac baffle or tunnel to complete the repair. Conduits and baffles increase the likelihood of blood flow obstruction within the conduits and of extrinsic compression of the tracheobronchial tree or vascular structures from the conduit. Examples of physiologic corrections requiring conduits and baffles include (a) atrial switch for TGA (Mustard or Senning procedure), (b) the Rastelli repair for TGA with a VSD and LV outflow tract obstruction, (c) RV-to-PA conduits in patients with truncus arteriosus or various forms of pulmonary atresia, and (d) repair of the Taussig-Bing variety of double-outlet RV (double-outlet RV with a subpulmonic VSD), which requires an intracardiac baffle to connect the VSD with the PA. The intracardiac baffle creates TGA, which is then corrected by an arterial switch operation.

Postoperative Management of the Senning or Mustard Operation for the Great Arteries

Atrial repair of TGA is an example of a physiologic, rather than an anatomic, correction. Although indications for atrial-level repairs for transposition are much less common, patients with unusual coronary anatomy (e.g., coronary arteries with a prolonged intramural course) have a higher risk of coronary injury and death when the arterial switch operation is performed. Under these circumstances, atrial-level repairs may be preferred.

The Senning operation uses tissue from the right atrial wall and interatrial septum to fashion a conduit for the flow of deoxygenated (systemic venous) blood through the mitral valve and into the left (pulmonary) ventricle. The LV ejects this deoxygenated blood into the PA. The Mustard operation accomplishes the same physiologic correction, but it uses a pericardial or prosthetic baffle to redirect the flow of systemic venous blood.

The early postoperative course for both Mustard and Senning procedures is generally benign. Because the operation occurs in the atrium, ventricular function is usually well preserved. In patients with low cardiac output, the question of baffle obstruction versus inadequate intraoperative myocardial preservation should be entertained. Poor cardiac output after an atrial switch procedure and/or symptoms of SVC or inferior vena cava (IVC) obstruction are highly suggestive of a baffle obstruction. The most common location for baffle obstruction is where the SVC channel crosses the atrial septum. SVC obstruction occurs in approximately 8% to 10% of patients (129,131). If there is satisfactory collateral venous drainage and the obstruction is not severe, this is usually well tolerated. However, some patients develop full-blown SVC syndrome and need an emergency revision of the baffle. Reoperation is required in only about 1% of patients. The possibility of SVC obstruction should be entertained in patients with low cardiac output who develop progressive venous engorgement of the head and neck vessels. SVC syndrome can be diagnosed clinically, although angiography localizes the area of obstruction by pressure gradient. IVC obstruction is less common, but it should be considered in the diagnosis of patients with hepatomegaly, ascites, and protein-losing enteropathy.

Dysrhythmias are the most common complication after atrial correction of TGA. The incidence of dysrhythmia ranges from 20% to 60%, the higher number being more common with the Mustard repair (135). Although bradycardia is most commonly seen, supraventricular tachyarrhythmias are also observed. In the Mustard repair, the wide excision of atrial tissue and the long atrial suture line commonly damage the sinoatrial node or its blood supply. Temporary atrial and ventricular pacing wires should be routinely placed in these patients at the time of surgery because of the likelihood of postoperative atrial dysrhythmias.

Systemic (right) ventricular dysfunction occurs in patients with TGA who have undergone an atrial switch procedure. The RV is well suited to perform against a high afterload *in utero*. However, with the initiation of respiration at birth, PVR drops and the RV becomes a low-pressure ventricle. Several studies have questioned the long-term ability of the RV to function as the systemic pumping chamber (136). Despite being asymptomatic at rest, children who have undergone atrial rerouting procedures can have severe hemodynamic and electrophysiologic abnormalities during exercise (137). Late systemic ventricular dysfunction occurs in approximately 10% of patients after atrial switch repair.

Postoperative Management of Baffle and Extracardiac Conduit Repairs

The Rastelli procedure (an operation for TGA with a VSD and LV outflow tract obstruction) combines an intracardiac baffle or tunnel from the VSD to the aorta with an extracardiac conduit. The intracardiac baffle establishes continuity between the LV and the aorta. A large, nonrestrictive VSD is required to allow uninterrupted flow between the LV and the aorta. The VSD may need to be enlarged at the time of surgery. The extracardiac conduit establishes continuity between the RV and the PA.

Postoperatively, LV outflow tract obstruction can occur because of inadequate enlargement of the VSD or obstruction of the intracardiac tunnel, resulting in an acute pressure load on the LV. High left-sided filling pressures, low cardiac output, high inotropic requirements, and a distended, poorly contractile LV are typical postoperative findings. Bedside echocardiography and, frequently, cardiac catheterization are necessary to localize the area of LV obstruction (e.g., VSD, baffle). Postoperative management should maintain effective preload and avoid significant reductions in systemic afterload, the former to augment stroke volume and the latter to support coronary perfusion pressure, because these patients behave like those with severe left-sided obstructive lesions (138). Reoperation should be considered early if significant obstruction exists.

The extracardiac RV-to-PA conduit can also become obstructed. Although this is more commonly seen in late follow-up, early postoperative obstruction does occur. This condition is most commonly a result of extrinsic compression of the conduit by the sternum. The conduit can also drape across coronary vessels and, once the chest is closed, impinge on right coronary artery flow. Furthermore, the conduit can cause compression of the trachea or the right bronchus. Difficulty in weaning patients from mechanical ventilation, postoperative wheezing, and a chest radiograph demonstrating overinflation or areas of atelectasis mixed with segmental overinflation all suggest airway compression as a diagnostic possibility (139). Bronchoscopy should be considered in patients who have conduits and demonstrate these symptoms.

Heart block is an uncommon finding after Rastelli repair; however, if the VSD was surgically enlarged, the risk of transient or permanent heart block increases. All patients undergoing VSD enlargement should have temporary atrial and ventricular pacing wires placed during rewarming from CPB. Low pacing thresholds must be ensured in the operating room, because postoperative myocardial edema generally results in increasing pacing thresholds. In neonates and infants with heart-rate-dependent cardiac output, pacing wire failure resulting in a slow idioventricular rhythm that is poorly tolerated and it may become life-threatening in the infant with marginal cardiac output in the early postoperative period.

Palliations

In the early 1980s the preferred approach to the neonate with congenital heart disease (CHD) was palliation in infancy and repair later in childhood. Today the tendency is to repair congenital cardiac lesions as early as possible, preferably in the neonatal period. This important philosophic change in the operative management of the child with CHD stems from the recognition that (a) early repair is safe and feasible; (b) a considerable portion of the myocardial, pulmonary, and central nervous system damage attributable to CHD is more specifically caused by prolonged exposure to abnormal blood flow patterns, hypoxemia, and cyanosis; and (c) an increase in morbidity and mortality is associated with multiple palliations, multiple exposures to the risks of CPB, and long-term medical management of congenital cardiac patients (116–118,140–142). Therefore, the goal of early surgical intervention is to restore normal blood flow patterns where possible and to reduce long-term morbidity. Palliative surgery is reserved for cardiac lesions in which anatomic parts are missing, such as pulmonary atresia with intact septum (absent RV and PA), tricuspid atresia (absent RV and tricuspid valve), hypoplastic left heart syndrome (absent mitral valve and small LV), mitral atresia (absent LV), and univentricular heart (absent or minuscule RV or LV with other associated anomalies) (143). Underdeveloped or absent chambers and great vessels preclude reconstruction of a normal four-chambered heart and produce marked alterations in postoperative physiology. The postoperative management of patients receiving palliative operations is not intuitive. These patients remain the most difficult group to care for because their blood flow patterns are abnormal and the impact of preload augmentation, inotropic support, and afterload manipulations may redirect blood flow patterns rather than simply improving cardiac output and tissue oxygen delivery. Additionally, minor changes in PA pressure, PVR, AV valve function, and ventricular performance may significantly increase postoperative morbidity (143,144,152).

The ultimate goal of palliative surgery is to separate the pulmonary and systemic circulations and, in the case of a univentricular heart, to use the single ventricle as a systemic pumping chamber. The Fontan operation, initially described in 1971, and its modifications have been adapted to all forms of univentricular heart, including hypoplastic left heart syndrome (143,144). The modified Fontan operation provides pulmonary blood flow by anastomosing all of the systemic venous return (SVC and IVC) to the PAs without an interposed pumping chamber. Pulmonary blood flow therefore depends on maintaining a passive gradient from the systemic veins through the pulmonary vasculature and into the left atrium. This arrangement requires a low PVR and low-to-normal single-ventricular filling pressure. Because newborns have high PVR, they are not suitable candidates for a Fontan-type procedure. The goal in the newborn period is to establish permanent pulmonary blood flow (pulmonary atresia), establish systemic blood flow (hypoplastic left heart syndrome), or limit pulmonary blood flow (double outlet RV) and then achieve balanced blood flow between the pulmonary and systemic circulations until the PVR falls, rendering the child suitable for a modified Fontan procedure at 1 to 2 years of age or a cavopulmonary anastomosis at 4 to 12 months of age.

Postoperative Management of Newborn Palliations for Single Ventricles

A palliative procedure is performed in the newborn period to limit excessive pulmonary blood flow and provide balanced blood flow between the systemic and pulmonary circulations. Excessive pulmonary blood flow results in two problems that increase the risk of the Fontan procedure: (a) a large volume load on the single ventricle with development of a dilated cardiomyopathy and (b) persistent high pressure and high-flow pulmonary blood flow, which results in elevations in PVR. Therefore, palliation in the newborn period to balance pulmonary and systemic blood flow and minimize the volume load on the single ventricle is of critical importance. In patients with two great arteries emanating from a single ventricle, this may be accomplished by placing a restrictive band around the main PA. If the main PA is very small or atretic and pulmonary blood flow is primarily from the ductus arteriosus, pulmonary blood flow is maintained by placing a restrictive PA-to-aorta shunt and ligating the ductus arteriosus, thereby limiting pulmonary blood flow and reducing the volume load on the single ventricle. In more complex anatomy (e.g., hypoplastic left heart syndrome), the entire aorta must be reconstructed to establish systemic blood flow first, and then a shunt is placed from the aorta or, more commonly, from the innominate artery to provide restrictive pulmonary blood flow.

Regardless of the surgical technique, the physiologic goals are to minimize the volume load on the single ventricle by restricting excessive pulmonary blood flow and maintaining balanced flow between the pulmonary and systemic circulations (11,13). During the newborn period and early infancy, the univentricular heart has to pump blood to both the pulmonary and the systemic circulation. The direction of predominant blood flow depends on downstream resistance (i.e., the flow is determined by the PVR and the SVR). Ideally, balanced flow results in equal portions of cardiac output to the systemic and pulmonary vascular beds, resulting in a 1 : 1 shunt. If pulmonary resistance is low, then a greater proportion of the cardiac output is directed to the lungs, and the single ventricle is required to increase its cardiac output by increasing stroke volume and heart rate (13,145). The newborn's heart has a reduced capacity to increase stroke volume, especially when volume-loaded. When flow becomes unbalanced and a large left-to-right shunt provides a disproportionate amount of blood flow to the lungs, systemic hypoperfusion and metabolic acidosis result. Once low systemic perfusion is evident, therapy must be implemented to improve cardiac output, correct metabolic acidosis, and redistribute blood flow to the systemic circulation.

Postoperative management is based on balancing blood flow between the systemic and pulmonary circuits. A modification of the Fick equation can be used to approximate the systemic-to-pulmonary blood flow ratio (Qp:Qs). The Fick equations for systemic (Qs) and pulmonary blood flow (Qp) are

$$Qs = VO_2/[aO_2] - [mvO_2]$$
$$Qp = VO_2/[pvO_2] - [paO_2] \quad [18\text{-}1]$$

where VO_2 = oxygen consumption and $[aO_2]$, $[mvO_2]$, $[pvO_2]$, $[paO_2]$ = oxygen content of systemic arterial, mixed venous, pulmonary venous, and pulmonary arterial blood, respectively (51,116). From this equation, the ratio of pulmonary-to-systemic blood flow, Qp:Qs, can be estimated by substituting O_2 saturation for content (since we are interested in the ratio of the pulmonary and systemic flow, not the absolute flows). The equation simplifies to

$$Qp:Qs = (SO_2sa - SO_2mv)/(SO_2pv - SO_2pa) \quad [18\text{-}2]$$

where the SO_2 terms indicate oxygen saturations and sa equals systemic arterial.

A Qp:Qs ratio of 1:1 indicates no shunting or bidirectional shunting of equal magnitude. In the presence of complete mixing, such as occurs in patients with a single ventricle, aortic and PA saturations are equal (10). In these circumstances, the arterial O_2 saturation, in conjunction with mixed venous saturations sampled from the high SVC, can be used to approximate the Qp:Qs ratio. The only remaining assumption is that the pulmonary venous blood is fully saturated at 100%, in the absence of pulmonary disease; then the systemic arterial oxygen saturation can be calculated for a Qp:Qs of 1:1, or balanced pulmonary and systemic flow. If the chest radiograph demonstrates pulmonary edema or atelectasis, a pulmonary venous saturation of 95% rather than 100% should be considered. Substituting this information into the equation shows that a systemic arterial saturation of 80% yields a 1:1 shunt or balanced pulmonary-to-systemic flow if the mixed venous saturation is 60% (i.e., the cardiac output is near normal). If the mixed venous saturation is low (40%) and the arterial saturation is 80%, then Qp:Qs = 2:1. The patient has an increased Qp:Qs ratio and low cardiac output. Under these conditions, the patient's condition can be optimized by both balancing Qp:Qs and increasing inotropy to improve cardiac output. Therefore, arterial saturations of 80% imply either balanced pulmonary blood flow or low cardiac output with increased pulmonary blood flow. Arterial saturations of less than 80% are caused by either decreased pulmonary blood flow, low cardiac output with balanced pulmonary-to-systemic blood flow, or severe reduction in cardiac output with increased pulmonary-to-systemic blood flow. A reliable way of assessing shunt physiology in the postoperative period is by continuous monitoring of arterial saturation with pulse oximetry and monitoring of high SVC saturations (Fig. 18-12).

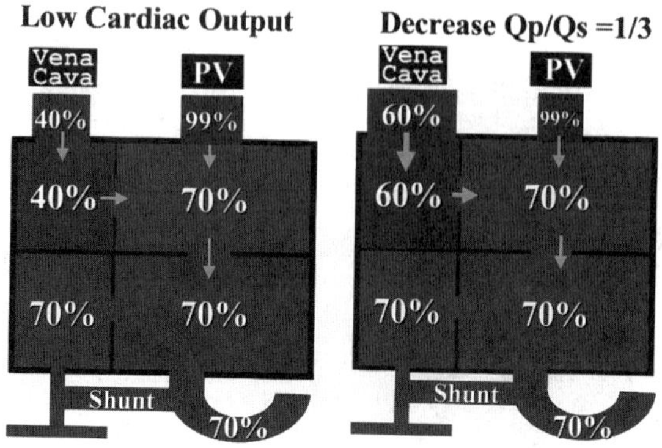

FIGURE 18-12. There are three causes of low systemic oxygen saturation values in stage I palliation (Norwood stage I) for hypoplastic left heart syndrome: low cardiac output, decreased pulmonary blood flow (low Qp), and lung disease with pulmonary venous desaturation. This figure depicts how low cardiac output and low Qp can manifest with similar clinical findings. Measuring the venous oxygen saturation (SvO_2) from the high superior vena cava (SVC) is an essential component to evaluating and correctly managing patients with low systemic saturations.

Inotropic agents are important for improving stroke volume in patients with a single ventricle, although they must be administered cautiously and maintained in a β-predominant range, since high levels of SVR may further increase pulmonary blood flow (145,146). A study completed in our laboratory demonstrated that dopamine, 10 μg/kg/minute, increases cardiac output without increasing Qp:Qs or altering coronary blood flow in newborn piglets with a 5-mm aortic-to-PA shunt. This finding suggests that cardiac output, and therefore systemic perfusion, can be enhanced in shunt-dependent patients with moderate doses of inotropic drugs. Work by Reddy, Hanley, and colleagues in a model of single-ventricle physiology demonstrated that epinephrine, 0.1 μg/kg/minute, improves cardiac output without changing the Qp:Qs ratio (145,146). In contrast, dobutamine increased Qp:Qs and actually decreased systemic cardiac output. Dobutamine is probably not the inotrope of choice in shunt-dependent physiology. Ventricular dysfunction in these patients is caused by shunt-dependent volume overload and reduced coronary blood flow resulting from shunt runoff. Although high systemic afterload may enhance shunt runoff, moderate doses of dopamine (10 μg/kg/minute) and epinephrine (0.1 μg/kg/minute) enhance cardiac output without affecting Qp:Qs ratio (145,146, 148).

Bicarbonate administration is another valuable adjunct to low cardiac output in shunt-dependent patients. Sodium bicarbonate corrects metabolic acidosis, providing an optimal pH for inotropic performance. Alkalinization with sodium bicarbonate decreases PVR without altering mean airway pressure.

Vasodilators such as nitroprusside or nicardipine reduce SVR and help decrease pulmonary blood flow. In combination with both ventilatory manipulations and bicarbonate administration, vasodilators should augment systemic perfusion. Vasodilators should be used cautiously, however, if systemic pressure is low. Volume support and inotropic agents should be optimized before a systemic vasodilator is administered. Phosphodiesterase type III agents (milrinone) are a useful alternative to sodium nitroprusside in terms of systemic vasodilation, and they have the added advantage of increasing contractility. Loading doses, however, may drop SVR and result in low systemic pressure. In contrast to nitroprusside, phosphodiesterase type III inhibitors have a long-lasting effect that cannot be rapidly reversed by stopping the infusion.

If PVR exceeds SVR, then inadequate pulmonary blood flow results and the child is severely hypoxemic. An FiO_2 of 100%, hyperventilation, alkalinization, and NO may be used to reduce PVR and improve pulmonary blood flow. Other therapeutic modalities, such as high-frequency jet ventilation, phosphodiesterase inhibitors, fentanyl, and muscle relaxant administration, should be considered as adjunctive therapy for reducing PVR. Persistent unresponsive hypoxemia may be caused by shunt dysfunction (clotting or kinking) and should be investigated. Urgent reoperation is indicated if shunt flow remains inadequate despite ventilatory maneuvers.

Phenoxybenzamine is currently being used at a handful of institutions during CPB. Phenoxybenzamine is a noncompetitive α-blocking agent. During CPB, pump flow rates are maintained at 200 mL/kg/min or more (high flow rates), and norepinephrine is used to maintain systemic blood pressure. After circulatory arrest, blood lactate levels are touted to be low and Qs (systemic cardiac output) elevated. Data supporting this methodology and its effect on oxygen delivery in the ICU have not been systematically evaluated, so these claims remain anecdotal, although institutions using this approach have reported low mortality rates after hypoplastic left heart surgery (149). ECMO for hypoplastic left heart syndrome can be effective. Complete occlusion of the systemic-to-pulmonary shunt does not allow for effective nutrient blood flow to the lungs, and pulmonary necrosis may ensue. ECMO should be run at high flows with pulmonary blood flow controlled medically. The overall survival for patients undergoing ECMO in hypoplastic left heart syndrome is low.

Postoperative Management of Fontan and Cavopulmonary Anastomosis Patients

If all of the systemic venous return (SVC and IVC) is directed to the PAs, the arrangement is termed a modified

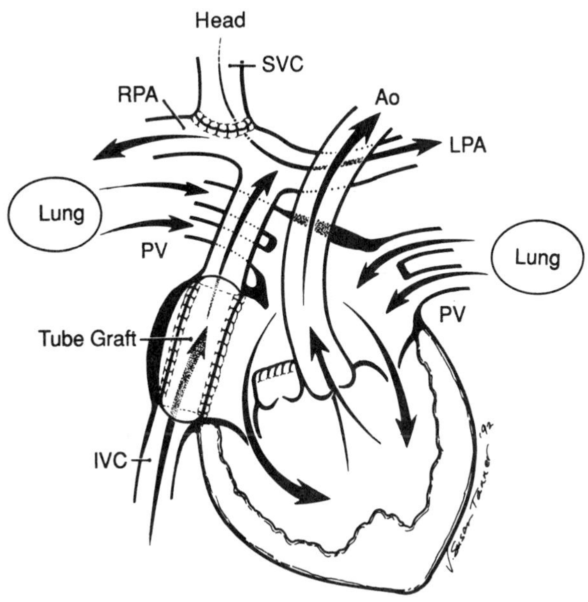

FIGURE 18-13. Blood flow patterns in the modified Fontan procedure. All inferior vena cava (IVC) blood is directed to the superior vena cava (SVC) through a tube graft. The SVC is directly anastomosed to the right and left pulmonary arteries. The functional right atrium is the tube graft. All surrounding atrial tissue is exposed to lower pressure and constitutes the physiologic left atrium. LPA, left pulmonary artery; Ao, aorta; RPA, right pulmonary artery; PV, pulmonary vein.

Fontan procedure. In the modified Fontan operation, the IVC blood is directed to the SVC by an intraatrial tube graft or baffle (Fig. 18-13) (147,150). This surgical arrangement allows all systemic venous return to enter the pulmonary circulation.

Cavopulmonary anastomoses are "partial Fontan procedures," that is, the SVC alone is anastomosed to the PAs, and IVC flow is allowed to mix with pulmonary venous return. A classic Glenn shunt is a cavopulmonary anastomosis that connects the SVC directly to the right PA and oversews the SVC–right atrial junction. The LPA is left separated from the right PA and SVC, and therefore systemic venous blood flow from the SVC is directed only to the right lung. A preferred form of cardiopulmonary anastomosis is the bidirectional Glenn anastomosis, which leaves the right and left PAs in continuity (Fig. 18-14). SVC blood flow is distributed to both the right and the left PA. IVC flow enters the physiologic left atrium, mixes with pulmonary venous blood, and enters the single ventricle.

The Patient Undergoing a Modified Fontan Procedure

In the modified Fontan procedure, cardiac output is limited by the ability of blood to passively flow from the systemic veins through the Fontan anastomosis into the PAs and through the pulmonary vasculature to the systemic ventricle. Blood return to the single ventricle depends on maintaining a pressure gradient from the SVC to the single ven-

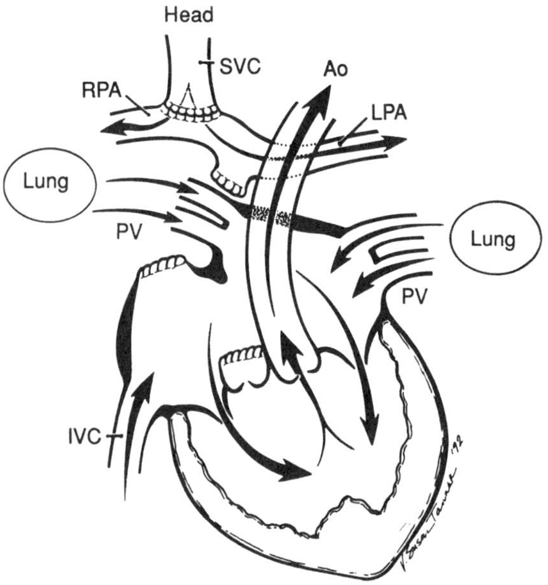

FIGURE 18-14. Blood flow patterns in the bidirectional cavopulmonary anastomosis (bidirectional Glenn procedure). In this procedure all the superior vena cava (SVC) blood flow is directed to the right and left pulmonary arteries (RPA and LPA, respectively). Inferior vena caval (IVC) flow enters the physiologic left atrium, mixes with pulmonary venous (PV) blood, and enters the single ventricle. After the bidirectional cavopulmonary anastomosis, the patient is moderately cyanotic but cardiac output is preserved because IVC blood enters directly into the single ventricle. Ao, aorta.

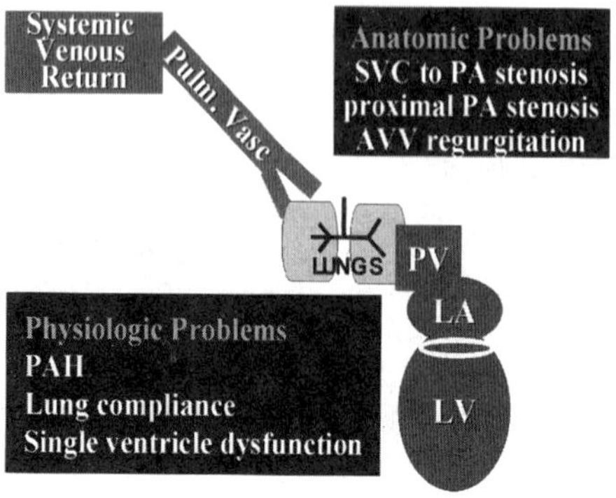

FIGURE 18-15. Diagrammatic illustration of causes for low cardiac output in the Fontan operation. Problems are divided into physiologic and anatomic causes. SVC, superior vena cava; PA, pulmonary artery; AVV, atrioventricular valve; PV, pulmonary veins; PAH, pulmonary artery hypertension.

tricle. Increased PVR, elevated PA pressures, distortion of the PAs, obstruction of the SVC-to-PA or IVC-to-SVC baffle, pulmonary venous obstruction, AV valve regurgitation, and systolic or diastolic ventricular dysfunction all limit blood return to the single ventricle (113,151). Clinically, these abnormalities are manifested as low cardiac output in the Fontan patient. Postoperatively in these patients, right atrial and left atrial pressure monitoring is necessary to identify the cause of low cardiac output.

In postoperative Fontan patients with good hemodynamic results, adequate systemic perfusion and age-appropriate blood pressures should be maintained with a maximal right atrial pressure of 15 mm Hg and a left atrial pressure of less than 10 mm Hg (147,150). If the right atrial pressure exceeds 15 mm Hg, the gradient between the right atrial and left atrial pressure is 10 mm Hg or less, and left atrial pressures are high (10 to 15 mm Hg), then ventricular dysfunction, AV valve regurgitation, or ventricular outflow obstruction (aortic valve stenosis or supravalvular stenosis) may exist. If CVP is high, the gradient between the SVC and left atrium is more than 10 mm Hg and left atrial pressure is low, then elevated PVR, baffle obstruction, or previously unrecognized obstruction of the pulmonary veins may be present. As previously mentioned, all of these problems are clinically manifested as low cardiac output (Fig. 18-15).

High Central Venous Pressure and Low Physiologic Left or Common Atrial Pressure. High CVP and low left atrial pressure in the postoperative Fontan patient have a physiologic or an anatomic origin. Anatomic problems include baffle obstruction, obstructed pulmonary veins, and PA distortion. Baffle obstruction is easily remedied, but it must be diagnosed early, before significant and irreversible consequences of abnormal hemodynamics occur.

Baffle obstruction is most reliably diagnosed by cardiac catheterization; transthoracic or transesophageal echocardiography may or may not allow adequate visualization or detect minor pressure gradients within the atrial baffle or the SVC-to-PA anastomoses. Mean pressure gradients as low as 3 to 4 mm Hg are significant and suggest an important stenosis in the right atrial-to-PA pathway. High right atrial pressure, low left atrial pressure, and a reduced systemic perfusion are clinically observed with baffle obstruction.

Pulmonary venous obstruction can occur after Fontan operation, especially in patients with complex venous anatomy (heterotaxy syndromes) and in patients with a small left atrium (hypoplastic left heart syndrome). In patients who do not receive a tube graft (Gore-Tex tube from the IVC to SVC), obstruction may develop because of pressure differences between the right and left atria. The higher right-sided pressures cause the intraatrial portion of the less rigid baffle to bow across the atrial septum. A simple tube graft such as the IVC-to-SVC intraatrial baffle minimizes the risk of pulmonary venous obstruction. If a left-sided SVC is present, it may be anastomosed directly to the left PA and the left-sided SVC–atrial junction may be oversewn. Abnormal pulmonary veins can occur in univentricular hearts and may be treated with balloon dilation and/or placement of small stents in the cardiac catheterization laboratory. Anatomic narrowing of pulmonary veins should be diagnosed preoperatively and treated before the Fontan procedure is performed, because pulmonary venous obstruction is poorly tolerated with Fontan physiology.

PA distortion is usually a result of previous shunt procedures. It can be treated by balloon dilation in the catheterization laboratory before surgery, or the PA may be reconstructed in the operating room at the time of the Fontan procedure.

Physiologic problems resulting in high CVP and low left atrial pressure are caused by elevations in PVR or PA pressure. Fontan patients have a very limited ability to compensate for these changes. Common treatable causes of increased PVR in the postoperative Fontan patient include hypoxia, hypercarbia, acidosis, excessive mean airway pressure, excessive PEEP, and extrapleural compression of the lung due to pleural effusion, hemothorax, or pneumothorax. In the absence of a clearly reversible cause of increased PVR, therapy is directed toward controlling pH, $Pa\text{CO}_2$, $Pa\text{O}_2$, and lung volumes through mechanical ventilation, high-frequency jet ventilation, systemic administration of bicarbonate, NO, and pulmonary vasodilators. Negative-pressure ventilation may also be beneficial because it decreases mean arterial pressure, thereby lowering the pressure gradient from the SVC to the single ventricle. Conventional ventilation in the early postoperative period uses a high set tidal volume (delivered tidal volume of 7 to 10 mL/kg) with relatively short inspiratory times to achieve $Pa\text{CO}_2$ values of approximately 35 mm Hg and to avoid the effects of high $Pa\text{CO}_2$ on PVR. Positive-pressure ventilation, which results in high mean airway pressures or uses high end-expiratory pressure, has a negative impact on pulmonary blood flow. In general, one must provide a short inspiratory phase and a prolonged expiratory phase with low mean airway pressure. Pulmonary blood flow predominates during exhalation, so an inspiratory-to-expiratory ratio of 1 : 3 or greater is preferred. PEEP may be used judiciously in Fontan patients to maintain FRC, as previously discussed. Excessive PEEP, however, is poorly tolerated in patients with Fontan physiology. Jet ventilation is an alternative mode of ventilation in patients with PA hypertension and Fontan physiology. Jet ventilation allows improved CO_2 removal at a lower mean airway pressure and therefore improves cardiac output and systemic oxygen delivery in Fontan physiology (43).

High Central Venous Pressure and High Left Atrial Pressure. There are three major causes of high CVP and high left atrial pressure in the postoperative Fontan patient: ventricular dysfunction (primarily diastolic dysfunction), AV valve regurgitation, and ventricular outflow tract obstruction.

The most troublesome consequence after Fontan operation is diastolic dysfunction of the systemic ventricle. Because many preoperative Fontan candidates have a volume-loaded, hypertrophied ventricle, elevated ventricular end-diastolic pressures are not uncommon after the operation (86,152–154). Inotropic agents that improve systolic function may actually worsen diastolic function by impairing ventricular relaxation. Vasodilators reduce ventricular volume and are beneficial in patients with diastolic dysfunction; however, in the postoperative Fontan patient, cardiac output is limited by the ability of blood to passively fill from the SVC to the single ventricle, and these patients may be highly sensitive to reductions in filling pressure. Drugs that promote ventricular relaxation or only minimally increase contractility and unload the heart, such as calcium channel blockers (nifedipine, nicardipine) or phosphodiesterase inhibitors (milrinone), may be helpful.

AV valve regurgitation may be caused either by a preexisting abnormal valve or by the chronic volume load on the single ventricle in the pre-Fontan period (85,151). In either case, AV valve regurgitation is poorly tolerated in the postoperative period because of the critical dependence of this physiology on ventricular filling. When valve replacement is combined with a Fontan operation, a higher than anticipated postoperative mortality rate has been observed (152). This may be related to the gradient that is present in an artificial valve and the consequent increase in left atrial pressure (152,153). Afterload reduction coupled with preload augmentation and mild increases in inotropy with milrinone, low-dose dopamine, low-dose epinephrine, or dobutamine may be helpful in these patients.

Ventricular outflow tract obstruction results in a pressure load on a previously volume-loaded heart. This worsens ventricular systolic and diastolic function, increasing the risk of a poor outcome after the Fontan procedure. Interventional cardiac catheterization and balloon dilation of supravalvular aortic stenosis is an important adjunctive therapy in preparing these patients for Fontan operation. Supravalvular aortic stenosis is common after a stage I hypoplastic left heart surgery repair (Norwood procedure)

All patients undergoing Fontan procedures have right atrial pressures that are higher than normal. Elevated right atrial pressures result in many objectionable complications (127,152). High systemic venous pressures result in diminished drainage through the thoracic duct and the release of atrial natriuretic factor, which may contribute to pleural effusions. IVC flow may also be impaired; when this condition is coupled with low cardiac output, systemic organ perfusion is significantly reduced. The net result is a diminished perfusion pressure for the abdominal viscera, hepatic and renal dysfunction, a significant accumulation of ascites fluid, and, less commonly, a protein-losing enteropathy. A poorly functioning Fontan repair with high CVP may result in severe, acute, and fatal hepatic failure due to high hepatic venous pressure and a diminution in effective hepatic blood flow.

Staging Operations in Single-Ventricle Patients. The Fontan procedure has been applied to an increasing number of patients who have risk factors that make them poor candidates for Fontan physiology. PA distortion, increased PVR, pulmonary hypertension, AV valve regurgitation, diminished ventricular performance, ventricular hypertrophy, complex cardiac anatomy (other than tricuspid atresia), and complex systemic or pulmonary venous connections increase the risk of a Fontan operation, from 1% to 10%, to 20% to 30% in some series (127,141,148,152). Although the optimal management of these patients is in evolution, it is clear that continued palliation with aorta-to-pulmonary shunts is a poor alternative. Ventricular function worsens with prolonged shunt physiology (84,155). Patients with tricuspid atresia have less ventricular dilation and hypertrophy after Fontan repair than do those who undergo a second aortopulmonary shunt procedure. In addition, the construction of a second palliative shunt has been shown to produce less favorable Fontan candidates because of greater distortion of the PA and chronic volume load on the single ventricle resulting in a dilated cardiomyopathy and elevation of PVR (84,150,155).

A fenestrated Fontan operation is the most common approach to a completed modified Fontan procedure performed today. Only in patients with tricuspid atresia and favorable physiology is a nonfenestrated Fontan the preferred approach. In the fenestrated Fontan arrangement, a 4-mm punch hole is placed in the tube graft connecting the IVC and SVC (117). The punch hole produces a right-to-left shunt, which allows approximately 20% of venous return to cross directly from the tube graft (physiologic right atrium) to the physiologic left atrium, thereby increasing cardiac output with minimal reductions in systemic saturation. This technique provides the added advantage of not requiring a second surgical procedure, because these small punch holes can be closed in the cardiac catheterization laboratory with the use of catheter-positioned atrial septal defect closure devices or, in many cases, they close on their own (Fig. 18-2C).

Staging operations, such as the bidirectional cavopulmonary anastomoses (bidirectional Glen procedure) or hemi-Fontan operation, are interim procedures performed in patients who require a Fontan procedure (143,156–159) (Fig. 18-16). The operation can be performed at an early age (4 to 8 months), allowing the patient to have a shorter period of exposure to shunt physiology and thereby decreasing the risk for development of a dilated cardiomyopathy. Hemi-Fontan and bidirectional Glen procedures are well tolerated, with low morbidity and mortality (156,157). The advantage of these procedures over the fenestrated Fontan procedure is that effective pulmonary blood flow is maintained while ventricular volume load is minimized and systemic oxygenation is improved (154,158,159). Additionally, cardiac output is not limited by high pressure or flow resistance across the pulmonary vascular bed. Cavopulmonary anastomoses or hemi-Fontan are modifications that allow IVC blood to enter the functional left atrium and the systemic ventricle without passing through the lungs. In the bilateral cavopulmonary anastomosis and hemi-Fontan, the entire IVC flow enters the physiologic left atrium, mixes with pulmonary venous blood, and enters the single ventricle. Cardiac output can be augmented because all the IVC return goes directly to the systemic ventricle and is pumped to the systemic circulation. The hemi-Fontan has the added advantage of being technically simple to convert to a complete Fontan procedure, because the SVC remains connected to the atrium and a partial tube graft is left in the atrium but closed off with a dam. On completion of the Fontan procedure the atrium is opened, the dam removed, and the atrial tube graft extended to the IVC. The bidirectional Glenn operation requires dissecting out the PAs and the right atrium. The main physiologic advantage of a bidirectional Glenn or hemi-Fontan over a fenestrated Fontan procedure is lower IVC pressure and a larger augmentation in cardiac output. In the fenestrated Fontan, higher IVC pressure results in reduced hepatic, renal, and mesenteric perfusion. The approximate 20% increase in cardiac output afforded by the fenestration may not be adequate in some patients. Careful evaluation of the repair and treatment of PA hypertension should be aggressively pursued.

Extracardiac Fontan procedures are also being applied to

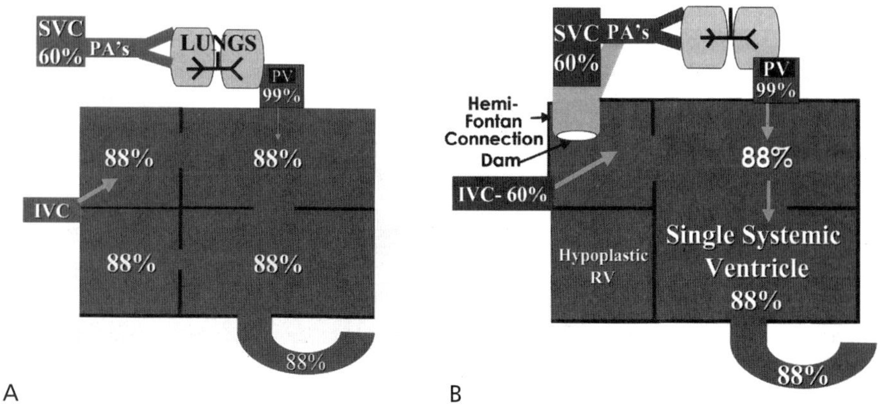

FIGURE 18-16. Diagrammatic illustration of the bidirectional Glenn **(A)** and the hemi-Fontan **(B)** procedures. In the bidirectional Glenn operation, the SVC is disarticulated from the right atrium. In contrast, the hemi-Fontan operation maintains continuity between the right atrium and the SVC, allowing the complete Fontan to procede with less dissection. SVC, superior vena cava; PV, pulmonary veins; IVC, inferior vena cava; PA, pulmonary arteries.

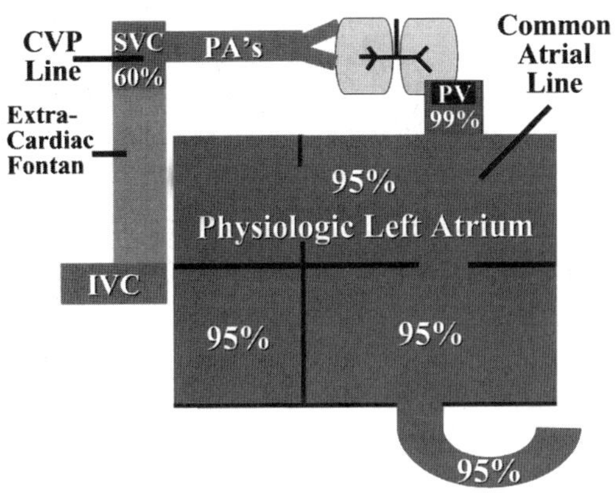

FIGURE 18-17. Diagrammatic representation of the extracardiac Fontan operation. In this procedure the conduit between the SVC and IVC is created outside of the heart, thus avoiding exposure of the native right atrial tissue to high pressures. The native atrium, after atrial septectomy, becomes the "physiologic" left atrium. Also depicted are the typical locations of monitoring lines in Fontan procedures. CVP, central venous pressure; SVC, superior vena cava; PV, pulmonary veins; IVC, inferior vena cava; PA, pulmonary arteries.

patients with abnormal atrial situs, abnormal pulmonary venous anatomy, or abnormal systemic venous drainage (Fig. 18-17). To complete a Fontan procedure in patients with these anatomic variants, a complex atrial baffle would be required. Complex baffles crossing the atrium have a higher likelihood of causing pulmonary venous obstruction. To minimize complications, an extracardiac conduit may be used to connect the SVC to the IVC. Extracardiac conduits can be fenestrated, although the fenestration tends to be less reliable because of atrial contraction and potential kinking. In addition, the extracardiac tube graft has no native atrial tissue, so it does not grow with the patient. The lack of atrial tissue exposed to high pressure and the absence of an atrial suture line may actually decrease the incidence of atrial fibrillation and flutter after the Fontan operation, and this is a potential benefit of the extracardiac conduit (Fig. 18-2D).

The postoperative management of these patients is similar to that for the completed Fontan patient. CVP and left atrial pressure are monitored and similarly maintained. Systemic saturations are lower because of the right-to-left atrial shunt and generally run between 80% and 90%. Lower systemic saturations are generally well tolerated because of an increase in oxygen delivery afforded by augmented cardiac output (right-to-left shunt) and because of red blood cell transfusion (increased oxygen-carrying capacity). Reduced pulmonary blood flow is usually better tolerated in the bidirectional Glenn or hemi-Fontan patients because cardiac output and oxygen delivery are maintained. In contrast to the Fontan patient, the patients undergoing a hemi-Fontan or bidirectional Glenn procedure who has reduced pulmonary blood flow due to anatomic obstruction or physiologic causes (elevated PVR or high single-ventricle end-diastolic pressure) presents with low saturations yet adequate systemic output. Therefore, in contrast to the situation with the completed Fontan or fenestrated Fontan, low systemic saturation values must to be carefully evaluated for anatomic or physiologic causes of reduced pulmonary blood flow. Other causes for very low saturations (50% to 60%) include venous collaterals and significant ventricular dysfunction. If saturations are very low, early cardiac catheterization is recommended, because extensive venous collaterals can be coil-occluded in the cardiac catheterization laboratory (152). If collaterals are not present, surgical options include conversion from a fenestrated Fontan to a bidirectional Glenn or hemi-Fontan operation or placement of an aorta-to-pulmonary shunt to improve pulmonary blood flow.

Complications after the Glenn procedure or the fenestrated Fontan are lower than those after the completed Fontan. The incidences of pleural effusions, ascites, atrial dysrhythmias, and renal, hepatic, and mesenteric perfusion problems are diminished. The bidirectional Glenn or hemi-Fontan is also a useful "bailout" operation. If the child does not tolerate Fontan physiology in the early postoperative period and there is no anatomically correctable problem, the patient can be returned to the operating room and converted to a cavopulmonary anastomosis.

Rhythm disturbances from the Fontan operation are common. It was originally thought that the absence of sinus rhythm was a risk factor for Fontan operation; however, more recent evidence suggests that sinus rhythm is not an absolute requirement for successful outcome after the Fontan procedure (160). Nevertheless, atrial pacing can improve cardiac output and systemic blood pressure, especially when junctional rhythm is present in the early postoperative period. Atrial pacing lowers left atrial pressure and provides an atrial kick, which supplements systemic stroke volume (159). More significant rhythm disturbances, such as atrial flutter and junctional ectopic tachycardia (JET), increase the risk of mortality in the early postoperative period. In a study by Balaji et al. (160), the presence of atrial tachydysrhythmias (atrial flutter, supraventricular atrial ectopic tachycardia, and JET) carried a very high mortality rate in the early postoperative period. When a total cavopulmonary connection, rather than an atriopulmonary connection, was used, atrial tachydysrhythmias were less common and were more easily controlled with antiarrhythmic therapy, overdrive pacing, or direct-current cardioversion (161). This finding suggests that a major contributor to postoperative dysrythmias in the Fontan patient is exposure of native atrial tissue to high pressure; this may favor a bidirectional Glenn approach over a hemi-Fontan.

Historically, a classic Fontan operation anastomoses the atrial appendage to the PA, thus exposing right atrial tissue to high pressures. This may explain the greater likelihood of atrial dysrythmias and why medical control is so difficult. In the lateral tunnel with a Gore-Tex tube graft, elevated right atrial pressure is confined to a small area of native atrial tissue as venous blood flow is channeled through the atrium. Atrial tissue is primarily exposed to left atrial pressures that are substantially lower (generally 5 to 8 mm Hg). The presence of AV valve regurgitation has also been suggested as an increased risk factor for postoperative dysrhythmias. This again suggests high atrial pressure as a principal factor (161).

RHYTHM DISTURBANCES IN THE POSTOPERATIVE PERIOD

The primary rhythm disturbances seen in the postoperative congenital heart disease patient are atrial or junctional in nature. Automatic tachycardias are more commonly seen in neonates and infants, whereas reentry tachycardias (atrial flutter, AV node reentry, accessory atrial pathway reentry tachycardia, and ventricular tachycardia) are more commonly seen after infancy. The preponderance of automatic tachydysrhythmias in infants reflects the conduction properties of the immature myocardium. In neonatal myocardium, calcium channel activity is high, and sodium channel activity is relatively low (162,163). The resting membrane potential of neonatal conduction tissue is higher than is typically seen in adult conduction tissue, and the action potential duration is shorter, with a more rapid repolarization phase (163).

Distinguishing atrial from junctional dysrhythmias in the postoperative period is complicated by the intrinsically rapid heart rate of infants and further complicated by the use of rate-enhancing inotropic agents. In neonates with rapid heart rates of 150 to 200 beats/minute, the P wave is typically buried in the T wave. Accurate diagnosis from a bedside monitor or 12-lead ECG is difficult. The two most effective means of bedside ECG analysis are an atrial or esophageal electrogram (164). An atrial electrogram is obtained by attaching two atrial pacing wires to the right and left arm leads of a standard ECG machine while maintaining normal leg lead recordings. This configuration provides maximal accentuation of the P wave. In the absence of atrial wires, an esophageal lead can be placed. A wire is placed in the mouth or nose and advanced to the midesophageal level. Because the midesophagus lies directly behind the left atrium, the presence or absence of P waves can be readily detected. Atrial pacing can also be instituted with an esophageal lead, which may be useful for overdrive pacing of a reentry tachycardia or in treating hemodynamically significant bradycardia in the postoperative period.

Reentry tachycardias include atrial flutter, AV node reentry, Wolff-Parkinson-White (and other forms of accessory pathways), and some forms of ventricular tachycardia. The most benign methods of treating reentrant tachycardias in the postoperative period are vagal maneuvers (e.g., placing ice on the head or face, gag reflex, placing a rectal thermometer) or overdrive pacing; these methods avoid the negative inotropic effects of antiarrhythmic drugs and the myocardial damage seen with repeated cardioversion (165). Adenosine and overdrive pacing have reported success rates of 75% to 95%. They are preferred techniques in the postoperative child with stable hemodynamics (166). Adenosine in doses of 100 μg/kg by rapid intravenous push is an effective treatment for reentrant supraventricular tachycardia (SVT). Experience with adenosine has shown it to be highly effective and well tolerated, even in infants with moderate hemodynamic instability. Several pacing techniques have been used to interrupt reentry tachycardias, including (a) brief bursts of pacing above the atrial rate (usually 200 to 250 beats/minute); (b) pacing above the SVT rate and, once a rapid atrial rate is captured, a gradual reduction in the pacing rate toward normal; and (c) introduction of a premature beat, which allows a sinus beat to occur during the refractory period of the reentry loop. If pacing is unsuccessful and the patient is hemodynamically stable, drug therapy with digoxin may be useful. In patients with unstable hemodynamics, synchronized cardioversion is the procedure of choice. In infants with significant myocardial dysfunction, verapamil may be contraindicated.

Perhaps the most common dysrhythmia in children older than 1 year of age is AV node or accessory pathway reentry tachycardia. In most cases a preoperative history of SVT can be elicited and should be investigated before surgery. An electrophysiologic study can diagnose the location of a bypass tract, which can then be treated medically or ablated in the electrophysiologic catheterization laboratory before corrective cardiac surgery. In the postoperative period AV node or accessory pathway SVT is treated with vagal maneuvers, overdrive pacing, synchronized cardioversion, or drug therapy with adenosine, digoxin, β-blockers, or occasionally verapamil. Adenosine and overdrive pacing have very high success rates in converting these forms of reentry tachycardia (135).

Atrial flutter is much more common in older children who have a preexisting pressure- or volume-loaded atrium before cardiac surgery. Flutter does occur in infants, however, and rates of up to 400 beats/minute have been observed. If AV conduction is 1:1 or 2:1, hemodynamic changes are severe, and synchronized cardioversion is the treatment of choice. If hemodynamic measures are stable, digoxin can slow AV conduction, and procainamide or sotalol can be added to prevent flutter. Atrial fibrillation is an uncommon arrhythmia in young children because of their very small atrial mass. Atrial fibrillation is treated with synchronized cardioversion or digoxin and procainamide. Overdrive pacing cannot be used because of the absence of organized atrial activity.

Of the automatic tachycardias, JET is the most common dysrhythmia, particularly after infant heart surgery. Heart rates usually vary between 120 and 170 beats/minute and are generally well tolerated. In some cases, however, JET can be rapid (180 to 280 beats/minute) and can result in significant reductions in cardiac output and systemic perfusion. The exact cause of JET is unknown; however, damage to junctional tissue from stretching of the AV node or from high catecholamine states, common to patients undergoing CPB, may increase the risk of postoperative JET. Fortunately, JET is a transient dysrhythmia that resolves in several hours to several days. Therefore, if hemodynamics can be temporarily supported, outcome can be improved and therapy can be withdrawn usually within 1 to 2 days.

Historically, postoperative JET carried a mortality rate of 50% (167). Diagnostic features of JET include a variable-rate tachycardia with a QRS pattern indistinguishable from the patient's normal sinus rhythm. Tachydysrhythmia with AV dissociation or a retrograde Wenckebach phenomenon is diagnostic of JET. In the absence of these signs, reentry tachycardias should be ruled out by esophageal or atrial electrogram, vagal maneuvers, adenosine therapy, aggressive overdrive pacing, and synchronized cardioversion. If these are unsuccessful, a working diagnosis of JET is made. Offending problems should be eliminated first, including aggressive treatment of fever and reduced inotropic support if possible. Fever therapy should include acetaminophen, nonsteroidal antiinflammatory agents, and steroids. This may lower the JET rate and improve systemic cardiac output. If the JET rate remains high, a safe and occasionally effective approach to lowering the JET rate is administration of digoxin. In patients with stable hemodynamics, digoxin is a safe first-line therapy (168,169). If digoxin is unsuccessful or hemodynamic status is deteriorating, intravenous amiodarone has been a very effective therapy for rapidly reducing the rate of JET and is becoming the treatment of choice. Intravenous amiodarone, however, it is a negative inotrope and causes vasodilation, both of which can result in significant hemodynamic changes. Amiodarone should be loaded slowly to decrease the likelihood of hypotension. An alternative and highly successful therapy for JET is induced hypothermia (168). In this technique, the patient is cooled to a rectal temperature of 34°C and given a muscle relaxant to eliminate shivering. Hypothermia slows the junctional rate, and the patient can be atrial-paced at slightly higher rates. The end result is a dramatic improvement in hemodynamics. Cold temperatures slow ion pumps and thereby reduce conduction rate. All conduction tissue is equally affected by hypothermia, so atrial pacing is an important adjunct therapy. Once the patient's hemodynamic status is controlled, rewarming trials are reinstituted on a 12- to 24-hour basis until the JET resolves.

Atrial ectopic tachycardia is much less common than JET. It is characterized by a stepwise increase and stepwise reduction in rate and a P-wave morphology that differs from sinus rhythm. As with JET, overdrive pacing and cardioversion are not useful. Drug therapy with digoxin slows the tachycardia but does not convert the rhythm to sinus. Procainamide and phenytoin (Dilantin) have been used successfully in atrial ectopic tachycardias in the postoperative period. Although β-blockers and the calcium channel blocker verapamil may be used, this should be done cautiously in infants because of the negative inotropic properties of these agents (170).

POSTOPERATIVE END-ORGAN DYSFUNCTION

Renal Effects

After CPB, the combined effects of hypothermia, nonpulsatile perfusion, and reduced mean arterial pressure cause release of angiotensin, renin, catecholamines, and antidiuretic hormones (171–175). These circulating hormones promote renal vasoconstriction and reduce renal blood flow. Yet despite the negative impact of CPB on renal function, studies have been unable to link low-flow, low-pressure, nonpulsatile perfusion with postoperative renal dysfunction. The factors that correlate most strongly with postoperative renal dysfunction are profound reduction in post-CPB cardiac output and preoperative renal dysfunction. Preoperative factors include primary renal disease, low cardiac output, and dye-related renal injury after cardiac catheterization (170, 172,173).

The incidence of acute renal failure after pediatric cardiac surgery is approximately 8%. This entity represents a heterogeneous group of insults whose final common pathway is oliguria and an elevated serum creatinine concentration. Diuretics have been the mainstay of promoting urine flow after pediatric CPB. Furosemide in doses of 1 to 2 mg/kg and/or ethacrynic acid 1 mg/kg every 4 to 6 hours induces a diuresis and reverses renal cortical ischemia associated with CPB in an animal model. After periods of total circulatory arrest (TCA), it is not unusual to observe a 24-hour period of oliguria that resolves over 12 to 24 hours. Furosemide infusions at 1 mg/hour provide an effective alternative to bolus diuretics and generally reduce the incidence of hypotension associated with larger intermittent doses of furosemide. Diuretics are generally effective only after patients have begun to diurese on their own.

One other factor in pediatric bypass is organ immaturity. Glomerular filtration rate and medullary concentrating ability are substantially reduced in pediatric patients. Therefore, prolonged periods of CPB may result in greater fluid retention than is typically seen in adult patients. The net result may be increased total body water and greater difficulty with postoperative weaning from ventilatory support.

Pulmonary Effects

Lung protection during CPB is a topic of ongoing investigation. Although cardioplegia protects the heart, there is no parallel chemical protection afforded to the airways during

CPB. Pulmonary dysfunction is common after CPB, yet its pathogenesis is poorly understood. In the broadest terms, lung injury is mediated in one of two ways: first, by an inflammatory response resulting largely from complement activation and endothelial cell injury, and second, by a mechanical effect culminating in atelectasis with resultant ventilation-perfusion mismatch, loss of lung volumes, and altered mechanics of breathing.

Laboratory data have demonstrated that exposure to hypothermic CPB is a primary cause of lung injury as opposed to circulatory arrest. Circulatory arrest, which limits the time the lung is exposed to bypass, seems to protect the lung and to minimize reductions in lung compliance and elevations in airway resistance (177,178). A study comparing ECMO and conventional ventilator therapy for persistent pulmonary hypertension of the newborn (PPHN) supported hypothermia as a primary mediator of lung injury (177,178). Neither conventional ventilator therapy nor the initiation of normothermic bypass (ECMO) increased the level of the circulating plasma vasoconstrictors (thromboxane or PGF_{2a}) in PPHN patients. In fact, vasoconstrictor concentrations fell as lung function improved in both therapies. Similarly, an increase in concentrations of thromboxane could not be detected across the pump oxygenator in children undergoing CPB (179). This suggests that the bypass circuit and oxygenator may not be as important as the effect of nonpulsatile cold perfusion or hypothermia in causing lung injury.

Pulmonary function after CPB is characterized by reduced static and dynamic compliance, reduced FRC, and an increased alveolar-arterial gradient (16,180,181). Atelectasis with increased capillary leakage due to hemodilution and hypothermic CPB are the most likely causes. Hemodilution reduces circulating plasma proteins, reduces intravascular oncotic pressure, and favors water extravasation into the extravascular space. Hypothermic CPB causes complement activation, release of cytokines, and leukocyte degranulation (176). Leukocytes and complement have a major role in promoting capillary-alveolar membrane injury (endothelial cell dysfunction) and microvascular dysfunction by means of platelet plugging and the release of mediators that increase PVR.

Neurologic Effects

A majority of neonatal and infant cardiac procedures are performed at temperature extremes of 15° to 20°C to significantly reduce tissue oxygen requirements and allow repairs to be performed under conditions of low-flow CPB or TCA. Hypothermia has been shown to decrease the cerebral metabolic rate for oxygen, decrease excitatory neurotransmitter release, retard calcium entry into the cell, and prevent ischemic injury. The length of "safe" circulatory arrest remains controversial. Clinical studies have not been able to consistently demonstrate a length of circulatory arrest that is safe. Periods of circulatory arrest in excess of 45 to 60 minutes have been suggested as potentially injurious (18). Therefore, most centers prefer to limit circulatory arrest times to this range if possible. However, survival and low morbidity depend on a repair with no residual defects, so that sacrificing a good technical repair to limit or avoid circulatory arrest may not be prudent. Attempts to reduce the risk of TCA include longer cooling times before initiation of TCA, intermittent perfusion periods during arrest, and the use of pH-stat blood gas management strategy during cooling. PH-stat management adds CO_2 to the blood during cooling and thereby increases cold cerebral blood flow to the brain. This has been particularly useful in patients with aortopulmonary collaterals, which tend to steal blood from the cerebral vasculature into the low resistance of the pulmonary vascular bed (182–185).

When possible, institutions are limiting the use of circulatory arrest and using deep hypothermic low-flow CPB as an alternative technique. Flow rates commonly employed are 50 mL/kg/minute, but evidence suggests that flow rates as low as 8 mL/kg/minute at 15°C may provide adequate cerebral perfusion (186,187). Studies of the neurologic outcome of low-flow CPB versus TCA has suggested a reduced incidence of clinical seizures in the low flow group (188). However, in later follow-up studies, TCA was not found to cause demonstrable long-term neurologic injury by school age (188).

Abnormalities of the microcirculation after TCA and increased capillary permeability after low-flow CPB (see Chapter 16) place the brain at increased risk of postoperative insults. If the brain cannot increase its metabolic rate (as occurs after TCA), events that increase metabolic demand (e.g., hyperthermia) or decrease substrate delivery (e.g., low cardiac output, hypoglycemia) may result in increasing neurologic injury. Hyperthermia occurs frequently after deep hypothermic CPB and is believed to result from hypothalamic dysfunction. Hypoglycemia is common in neonates and is also seen in older patients with low cardiac output and hepatic hypoperfusion.

Increased capillary permeability may result in cerebral edema. Evidence suggests that after TCA anterior fontanel pressure increases. This appears to be of limited significance in the immediate post-CPB period (189–192). However, if during the ICU period RV function worsens and right atrial pressures increases, cerebral edema may increase owing to increased hydrostatic forces. The end result is reduced intracranial compliance, elevations in intracranial pressure, and reduced cerebral perfusion pressure. These factors may be additive to any injury incurred during CPB and/or TCA. Patients who have received palliative procedures such as shunts or Fontan procedures would be at increased risk because of shunt runoff, collateral blood vessels, and high right-sided filling pressures, respectively (152,189).

SUMMARY

Optimal postoperative management of patients with congenital heart disease requires a sound knowledge of normal and pathologic cardiac and respiratory physiology, an understanding of the impact inotropic and ventilatory maneuvers have on postoperative hemodynamics, and a knowledge of acceptable and unacceptable organ dysfunction attributable to CPB and deep hypothermic circulatory arrest. Although postoperative intensive care is an important part of the management of these patients, it is the team-oriented approach of cardiologists, cardiac surgeons, anesthesiologists, critical care physicians, ICU nurses, operating room nurses, and perfusionists that is essential to a successful outcome. Expert surgical and anesthetic management should establish an initial therapeutic approach to postoperative care. The "intensivists" then begin managing these patients with a full knowledge of the intraoperative course and modify care as necessary to achieve a stable postoperative convalescence. Causes of an abnormal postoperative course depend on the congenital heart defect and the type of operative repair performed. However, alterations in anticipated postoperative convalescence should alert the critical care team to a possible structural problem. Structural problems must be aggressively treated, because residual anatomic defects are a major contributor to postoperative morbidity and mortality.

REFERENCES

1. Ungerleider RM, Greeley WJ, Sheikh KH, et al. Intraoperative echo with Doppler color flow imaging to predict outcome after repair of congenital cardiac defects. *Ann Surg* 1989;210:526.
2. Mullins CE. Pediatric and congenital therapeutic cardiac catheterization. *Circulation* 1989;79:1153.
3. Parr GVS, Blackstone EH, Kirklin JW. Cardiac performance and mortality early after intracardiac surgery in infants and young children. *Circulation* 1975;51:867.
4. Gold JP, Jonas RA, Lang P, et al. Transthoracic intracardiac monitoring lines in pediatric surgical patients: a ten-year experience. *Ann Thorac Surg* 1986;42:185.
5. Ungerleider RM, Greeley WJ, Sheikh KH, et al. Routine use of intraoperative epicardial echo and Doppler color flow imaging to guide and evaluate repair of congenital heart lesions: a prospective study. *J Thorac Cardiovasc Surg* 1990;100:297.
6. Lang P, Chipman CW, Siden H, et al. Early assessment of hemodynamic states after repair of tetralogy of Fallot: a comparison of 24 hour (intensive care unit) and 1 year postoperative data in 98 patients. *Am J Cardiol* 1982;50:795.
7. Moorthy SS, Haselby KA, Caldwell RL, et al. Transient right-left shunt during emergence from anesthesia demonstrated by color flow Doppler mapping. *Anesth Analg* 1989;68:20.
8. Moorthy SS, Dierdorf SF, Krishna G, et al. Transient hypoxemia from a transient right to left shunt in a child during emergence from anesthesia. *Anesthesiology* 1987;66:234.
9. Nundel D, Berman N, Talner N. Effects of acutely increasing systemic vascular resistance on arterial oxygen tension in tetralogy of Fallot. *Pediatrics* 1976;58:248.
10. McGoon DC, Mair DD. On the unmuddling of shunting, mixing and streaming. *J Thorac Cardiovasc Surg* 1990;100:77.
11. Norwood WI, Murphy JD. Hypoplastic left heart syndrome. In: Sabiston DC, Spencer FC, eds. *Surgery of the chest.* Philadelphia: WB Saunders Co, 1990:1493.
12. Hansen DD, Hickey PR. Anesthesia for hypoplastic left heart syndrome: use of high-dose fentanyl in 30 neonates. *Anesth Analg* 1986;65:127.
13. Nicolson SC, Jobes DR. Hypoplastic left heart syndrome. In: Lake CL, ed. *Pediatric cardiac anesthesia.* Norwalk, CT: Appleton & Lange, 1988:243.
14. Barnea O, Santamore WP, Rossi A, et al. Estimation of oxygen delivery in newborns with a univentricular circulation. *Circulation* 1998;98:1407.
15. Riordan CJ, Locher JP Jr, Santamore WP, et al. Monitoring systemic venous oxygen saturations in the hypoplastic left heart syndrome. *Ann Thorac Surg* 1997;63:835.
16. Jenkins J, Lynn A, Edmonds J, et al. Effects of mechanical ventilation on cardiopulmonary function in children after open heart surgery. *Crit Care Med* 1985;13:77.
17. Drummond WH, Gregory GA, Heyman MA, et al. The independent effects of hyperventilation, tolazoline, and dopamine in infants and persistent pulmonary hypertension. *J Pediatr* 1981;98:603.
18. Custer JR, Hales CA. Influence of alveolar oxygen on pulmonary vasoconstriction in newborn lambs vs sheep. *Am Rev Respir Dis* 1985;132:326.
19. Lyrene RK, Welch KA, Godoy G, et al. Alkalosis attenuates hypoxic pulmonary vasoconstriction in neonatal lambs. *Pediatr Res* 1985;19:1268.
20. Malik AB, Kidd SL. Independent effects of changes in H^+ and CO_2 concentrations on hypoxic pulmonary vasoconstriction. *J Appl Physiol* 1973;34:318.
21. Rudolph AM, Yuan S. Response of the pulmonary vasculature to hypoxia and H^+ ion concentration changes. *J Clin Invest* 1966;45:399.
22. Lock JE, Einjig S, Bass JL, et al. Pulmonary vascular response to oxygen and its influence on operative results in children with ventricular septal defects. *Pediatr Cardiol* 1982;3:41.
23. Jarmakani JM, Nakanishi T, George L, et al. Effect of extracellular calcium on myocardial mechanical function in neonatal rabbit. *Dev Pharmacol Ther* 1982;5:1.
24. Rebeyka IM, Yeh T Jr, Hanan SA, et al. Altered contractile response in neonatal myocardium to citrate-phosphate-dextrose infusion. *Circulation* 1990;82:IV-367.
25. Meliones JN, Moler FW, Custer JR, et al. Hemodynamic instability after the initiation of extracorporeal membrane oxygenation: role of ionized calcium. *Crit Care Med* 1991;19:1247.
26. Cheifetz IM, Kern FH, Schulman SR, et al. Serum lactates correlate with mortality after operations for complex congenital heart disease. *Ann Thorac Surg* 1997:64:735.
27. Haneda K, Sato S, Ischizawa E, et al. The importance of colloid osmotic pressure during open heart surgery in infants. *Tohoku J Exp Med* 1985;147:65.
28. Rosenthal SM, LaJohn LA. Effect of age on transvascular fluid movement. *Am J Physiol* 1975;228:134.
29. Rome JJ, Mayer JE, Castaneda AR, et al. Tetralogy of Fallot with pulmonary atresia: rehabilitation of diminutive pulmonary arteries. *Circulation* 1993;88:1691.
30. Kreutzer J, Perry SB, Jonas RA, et al. Tetralogy of Fallot with diminutive pulmonary arteries: preoperative pulmonary valve dilation and transcatheter rehabilitation of pulmonary arteries. *J Am Coll Cardiol* 1996;27:1741.
31. Kreutzer J, Lock JE, Jonas RA, et al. Transcatheter fenestration dilation and/or creation in postoperative Fontan patients. *Am J Cardiol* 1997;79:228.
32. Fontan F, Deville C, Quagebeur J, et al. Repair of tricuspid atresia in 100 patients. *J Thorac Cardiovasc Surg* 1983;85:647.

33. Deal CW, Warden JC, Monk I. Effect of hypothermia on lung compliance. *Thorax* 1970;25:105.
34. Hammon JW, Wolfe WG, Moran JF, et al. The effect of positive end-expiratory pressure on regional ventilation and perfusion in the normal and injured primate lung. *J Thorac Cardiovasc Surg* 1976;72:680.
35. Fagan DG. Shape changes in V-P loops for children's lungs related to growth. *Thorax* 1977;32:198.
36. Nelson NM. Neonatal pulmonary function. *Pediatr Clin North Am* 1966;13:769.
37. Zapletal A, Paul T, Samenek M. Pulmonary elasticity in children and adolescents. *J Appl Physiol* 1976;40:953.
38. Mansell A, Bryan AC. Airway closure in children. *J Appl Physiol* 1972;33:711.
39. Meliones JN, Wilson BW, Cheifetz IM, et al. Respiratory monitoring. In: Rogers MC, ed. *Textbook of pediatric intensive care.* Baltimore: Williams & Wilkins, 1996:331.
40. Cannon ML, Cornell J, Tripp DS, et al. Tidal volume measurements in infants should be obtained with a pneumotachometer located at the endotracheal tube. *Am J Resp Crit Care Med* 2000; 162:6.
41. Weisfeldt ML, Halpern HR. Cardiopulmonary resuscitation: beyond cardiac massage. *Circulation* 1986;74:443.
42. Toro-Figuero LO, Gutierrez J, Berens RJ, et al. Prospective, randomized comparison of high-frequency oscillatory ventilation and conventional mechanical ventilation in pediatric respiratory failure [see comments]. *Crit Care Med* 1994;22:1530.
43. Meliones JN, Bove EL, Dekeon MK, et al. High-frequency jet ventilation improves cardiac function after the Fontan procedure. *Circulation* 1991;84[Suppl III]:III-364.
44. Kocis KC, Meliones JN, Dekeon MK, et al. High-frequency jet ventilation for respiratory failure after congenital heart surgery. *Circulation* 1992;86[Suppl 5]:II-127.
45. Wessel DL, Triedman JK, Wernovsky G, et al. Pulmonary and systemic hemodynamics of amrinone in neonates following cardiopulmonary bypass. *Circulation* 1989;80[Suppl II]:II-488.
46. Zobel G, Gamillscheg A, Schwinger W, et al. Inhaled nitric oxide in infants and children after open heart surgery. *J Cardiovasc Surg* 1998;39:79.
47. Russell IA, Zwass MS, Fineman JR, et al. The effects of inhaled nitric oxide on postoperative pulmonary hypertension in infants and children undergoing surgical repair of congenital heart disease. *Anesth Analg* 1998;87:46.
48. Chang AC, Atz AM, Wernovsky G, et al. Milrinone: systemic and pulmonary hemodynamic effects in neonates after cardiac surgery. *Crit Care Med* 1995;23:1907.
49. Atz AM, Adatia I, Wessel DL. Rebound pulmonary hypertension after inhalation of nitric oxide. *Ann Thorac Surg* 1996;62: 1759.
50. Ivy DD, Ziegler JW, Kinsella JP, et al. Hemodynamic effects of dipyridamole and inhaled nitric oxide in pediatric patients with pulmonary hypertension. *Chest* 1996;114[Suppl 1]:17S.
51. Konstam MA, Cohen SR, Weiland DS, et al. Relative contribution of inotropic and vasodilator effects to amrinone-induced hemodynamic improvement in congestive heart failure. *Am J Cardiol* 1986;57:242.
52. Konstam MA, Cohen SR, Salem DN, et al. Effect of amrinone on right ventricular function: predominance of afterload reduction. *Circulation* 1986;74:359.
53. Molloy DW. Effects of noradrenaline and isoproterenol on cardiopulmonary function in a canine model of acute pulmonary hypertension. *Chest* 1985;88:432.
54. Parks IS, Michael LH, Driscoll DJ. Comparative responses of the developing canine myocardium to inotropic agents. *Am J Physiol* 1982;242:H13.
55. Schwartz DA, Grove FL, Horowitz LD. Effect of isoproterenol on regional myocardial perfusion and tissue oxygenation in acute myocardial infarction. *Am Heart J* 1979;97:339.
56. Drummond WH, Lock JE. Neonatal pulmonary vasodilator drugs. *Dev Pharmacol Ther* 1984;7:1.
57. Heymann MA, Hoffman JIE. Persistent pulmonary hypertension syndromes in the newborn. In: Weir EK, Reeves JT, eds. *Pulmonary hypertension.* New York: Futura, 1984.
58. Bush A, Busset C, Knight WB, et al. Modification of pulmonary hypertension secondary to congenital heart disease. *Am Rev Respir Dis* 1987;136:767.
59. Zall S, Milocco I, Rickstein S-E. Effects of adenosine on myocardial blood flow and metabolism after coronary artery bypass surgery. *Anesth Analg* 1991;73:689.
60. Girard C, Lehot JJ, Clerc J, et al. Inhaled nitric oxide (NO) in pulmonary hypertension following mitral valve replacement. *Anesthesiology* 1991;75:A984.
61. Higenbottam TW, Spiegelhalter D, Scott JP, et al. Prostacyclin (epoprostenol) and heart-lung transplantation as treatments for severe pulmonary hypertension. *Br Heart J* 1993;70:366.
62. Hickey PR, Hansen DD. Fentanyl and sufentanil-oxygen-pancuronium anesthesia for cardiac surgery in infants. *Anesth Analg* 1984;63:117.
63. Hickey PR, Hansen DD, Wessel DL, et al. Blunting of the stress responses in the pulmonary circulation of infants by fentanyl. *Anesth Analg* 1985;64:1137.
64. Anand KJS, Hansen DD, Hickey R. Hormonal-metabolic stress response in neonates undergoing cardiac surgery. *Anesthesiology* 1990;73:661.
65. Greeley WJ, Kern FH. Anesthesia for pediatric cardiac surgery. In: Otoyama EK, Davis PJ, eds. *Smith's anesthesia for infants and children,* 6th ed. St Louis: Mosby, 1996:475.
66. McGovern JJ, Craig DM, Bengur AR, et al. RV contractility and pulmonary vascular mechanics: effects of catecholamines in an immature animal model of RV injury. *Pediatr Res* 1996; 39:32A.
67. Perloff J. Development and regression of increased ventricular mass. *Am J Cardiol* 1982;50:605.
68. Friedman WF. The intrinsic properties of the developing heart. *Prog Cardiovasc Dis* 1972;15:87.
69. Berner M, Oberhansli I, Rouge JC, et al. Chronotropic and inotropic supports are both required to increase cardiac output early after corrective operations for tetralogy of Fallot. *J Thorac Cardiovasc Surg* 1989;97:297.
70. Hines R, Barash PG. Right ventricular failure. In: Kaplan JA, ed. *Cardiac anesthesia,* 2nd ed, vol 2. New York: Grune & Stratton, 1986:995.
71. Berne RM, Levy MN. Coronary circulation and cardiac metabolism. In: Berne RM, Levy MN, eds. *Cardiovascular physiology.* St Louis: Mosby, 1981:211.
72. Rudolph AM. Distribution and regulation of blood flow in the fetal and newborn lamb. *Circ Res* 1985;57:811.
73. Gentles TL, Mayer JE Jr, Gauvreau K, et al. Fontan operation in five hundred consecutive patients: factors influencing early and late outcome. *J Thorac Cardiovasc Surg* 1997;114:376.
74. Jacobs ML, Rychik J, Rome JJ, et al. Early reduction of the volume work of the single ventricle: the hemi-Fontan operation. *Ann Thorac Surg* 1996;62:456.
75. Pearl JM, Laks H, Drinkwater DC, et al. Repair of truncus arteriosus in infancy. *Ann Thorac Surg* 1991;52:780.
76. Eugene J, McClogan SJ, Moore-Jefferies EW, et al. Cardiac assist by extracorporeal membrane oxygenation with in-line left ventricular venting. *Trans Am Soc Artif Intern Organs* 1984;30: 98.
77. Klein MD, Shaheen KW, Whittlesey GC, et al. Extracorporeal membrane oxygenation for the circulatory support of children

after repair of congenital heart disease. *J Thorac Cardiovasc Surg* 1990;100:498.
78. Golding LAR. Postcardiotomy mechanical support. *Semin Thorac Cardiovasc Surg* 1991;3:29.
79. Meliones JN, Custer JR, Snedecor MS, et al. Extracorporeal life support for cardiac assist in pediatric patients. *Circulation* 1991;84:III-168.
80. Baylen B, Meyer RA, Korfhagen J, et al. Left ventricular performance in the critically ill premature infant with patent ductus arteriosus and pulmonary disease. *Circulation* 1977;55:182.
81. Berner M, Rouge JC, Friedli B. The hemodynamic effect of phentolamine and dobutamine after open-heart operations in children: influence of underlying heart defect. *Ann Thorac Surg* 1983;35:643.
82. Borow KM, Green LH, Castaneda AR, et al. Left ventricular function after repair of tetralogy of Fallot and its relationship to age at surgery. *Circulation* 1980;61:1150.
83. Downing SE, Talner NS, Gardner TH. Ventricular function in the newborn lamb. *Am J Physiol* 1965;208:931.
84. Graham TP, Franklin RCG, Wyse RKH, et al. Left ventricular wall stress and contractile function in childhood: normal values and comparison of Fontan repair versus palliation only in patients with tricuspid atresia. *Circulation* 1986;74:61.
85. Jarmakani JM, Graham TP, Canent RV. Left ventricular contractile state in children with successfully corrected ventricular septal defect. *Circulation* 1972;45,46[Suppl I]: F-102.
86. Nishioka K, Kamiya T, Ueda T, et al. Left ventricular volume characteristics in children with tricuspid atresia before and after surgery. *Am J Cardiol* 1981;47:1105.
87. Humpherys JE, Cummings P. Atrial and ventricular tropomysin and troponin-I in the developing bovine and human heart. *J Mol Cell Cardiol* 1984;16:643.
88. Legato MJ. Ultrastructural changes during normal growth in the dog and rat ventricular myofiber. In: Lieberman M, ed. *Developmental and physiological correlates of cardiac muscle.* New York: Raven Press, 1975:249.
89. Nasser R, Reedy MC, Anderson PAW. Developmental changes in the ultrastructure and sarcomer shortening of the isolated rabbit myocardium. *Circ Res* 1987;61:465.
90. Vetter R, Will H, Kuttner I, et al. Developmental changes of Ca+ + transport systems in chick heart. *Biomed Biochem Acta* 1986;45:S219.
91. Becker AE, Caruso G. Congenital heart disease: a morphologist's view on myocardial dysfunction. In: Losekoot G, Becker AE, Marcelleti C, et al, eds. *Paediatric cardiology.* Edinburgh: Churchill Livingstone, 1981.
92. Thornburg KL, Morton MJ. Filling and arterial pressure as determinants of RV stroke volume in the sheep fetus. *Am J Physiol* 1983;244:H656.
93. Kirkpatrick SE, Johnson GH, Assali NS. Frank-Starling as an important determinant of fetal cardiac output. *Am J Physiol* 1976;231:495.
94. Teitel DF, Sidi D, Chin T, et al. Developmental changes in myocardial contractile reserve in the lamb. *Pediatr Res* 1985; 19:948.
95. Goldberg LI. Cardiovascular and renal actions of dopamine: potential clinical applications. *Pharmacol Rev* 1972;24:1.
96. Stephenson LW, Edmunds LH, Raphaely R, et al. Effects of nitroprusside and dopamine on pulmonary artery vasculature in children after cardiac surgery. *Circulation* 1979;60[Suppl I]: I-104.
97. Lang P, Williams RG, Norwood WI. The hemodynamic effects of dopamine in infants after corrective cardiac surgery. *J Pediatr* 1980;96:630.
98. Driscoll DJ, Gillette PC, Fukushige J, et al. Comparison of the cardiovascular action of isoproterenol, dopamine and dobutamine in the neonatal and mature dog. *Pediatr Cardiol* 1980;1: 307.
99. Nakanishi T, Seguchi M, Takao A. Intracellular calcium concentrations in the newborn myocardium. *Circulation* 1987; 76[Suppl IV]: IV-455.
100. Bohn DJ, Poirer CS, Edmonds JF, et al. Efficacy of dopamine, dobutamine, and epinephrine during emergence from cardiopulmonary bypass in children. *Crit Care Med* 1980;8:367.
101. Hess W, Arnold B, Veit S. The hemodynamic effects of amrinone in patients with mitral stenosis and pulmonary hypertension. *Eur Heart J* 1986;7:800.
102. Bailey JM, Miller BE, Lu W, et al. The pharmacokinetics of milrinone in pediatric patients after cardiac surgery. *Anesthesiology* 1999;90:1012.
103. Lawless S, Burckart G, Diven W, et al. Amrinone pharmacokinetics in neonates and infants. *J Clin Pharmacol* 1988;28:283.
104. Robatham JL, Peters J, Takata M, et al. Cardiorespiratory interactions. In: Rogers MC, ed. *Textbook of pediatric critical care.* Baltimore: Williams & Wilkins 1996:369.
105. Bohn DJ, Piorier CS, Edmonds JF, et al. Hemodynamic effects of dobutamine after cardiopulmonary bypass in children. *Crit Care Med* 1980;8:367.
105. Duncan BW, Hraska V, Jonas RA, et al. Mechanical circulatory support in children with cardiac disease. *J Thorac Cardiovasc Surg* 117:529, 1999.
106. Borowski A, Korb H. Experience with uni- (LVAD) and biventricular (ECMO) circulatory support in postcardiotomy pediatric patients. *Int J Artif Organs* 1997;20:695.
107. Rankin JS, Olsen CO, Arentzen CE, et al. The effects of airway pressure on cardiac function in intact dogs and man. *Circulation* 1982;66:108.
108. Graham TP Jr. Ventricular performance in congenital heart disease. *Circulation* 1991;84:2259.
109. Cordell D, Graham TP, Atwood GJ, et al. Left heart volume characteristics following ventricular septal defect closure in infancy. *Circulation* 1976;54:294.
110. Graham TP Jr, Atwood GJ, Boucek RJ Jr, et al. Right ventricular volume characteristics in ventricular septal defect. *Circulation* 1976;54:800.
111. Heinle JS, Diaz LK, Fox LS. Early extubation after cardiac operations in neonates and young infants. *J Thorac Cardiovasc Surg* 1997;114:413.
112. Pacifico AD, Kirklin JW, Kirklin JK. Surgical treatment of ventricular septal defect. In: Sabiston DC Jr, Spencer FC, eds. *Surgery of the chest,* 6th ed. Philadelphia: WB Saunders Co, 1995.
113. Rychik J, Norwood WI, Chil AJ. Doppler color flow mapping assessment of residual shunt after closure of large ventricular septal defects. *Circulation* 1991;84[Suppl III]: III-153.
114. Meyer RA, Schwartz DC, Benzing G, et al. Ventricular septum in right ventricular volume overload. *Am J Cardiol* 1972;30: 349.
115. Dickinson DF, Wilkinson JL, Smith A, et al. Variations in the morphology of the ventricular septal defect and disposition of the atrioventricular conduction tissues in tetralogy of Fallot. *Thorac Cardiovasc Surg* 1982;30:243.
116. Castaneda AR, Mayer JE, Jonas RA, et al. The neonate with critical congenital heart disease: repair—a surgical challenge. *J Thorac Cardiovasc Surg* 1989;98:869.
117. Newberger JW, Silbert AR, Buckley LP, et al. Cognitive function and age at repair of transposition of the great arteries in children. *N Engl J Med* 1984;310:1495.
118. Rabinovitch M, Herrera-DeLeon V, Castaneda AR, et al. Growth and development of the pulmonary vascular bed in patients with tetralogy of Fallot with and without pulmonary atresia. *Circulation* 1981;64:1234.

119. Borow KM, Keane JF, Castaneda AR, et al. Systemic ventricular function in patients with tetralogy of Fallot, ventricular septal defect and transposition of the great arteries repaired during infancy. *Circulation* 1981;64:878.
120. Castaneda AR, Freed MD, Williams RG, et al. Repair of tetralogy of Fallot in infancy: early and late results. *J Thorac Cardiovasc Surg* 1977;74:372.
121. Brizard CP, Mas C, Sohn YS, et al. Transatrial-transpulmonary tetralogy of Fallot repair is effective in the presence of anomalous coronary arteries. *J Thorac Cardiovasc Surg* 1998;116:770.
122. Ilbawi MN, Idriss FS, DeLeon SY, et al. Factors that exaggerate the deleterious effects of pulmonary insufficiency on the right ventricle after tetralogy repair: surgical implications. *J Thorac Cardiovasc Surg* 1987;93:36.
123. Hurwitz RA, Smith W, King H, et al. Tetralogy of Fallot with abnormal coronary artery: 1967 to 1977. *J Thorac Cardiovasc Surg* 1980;80:129.
124. Humes RA, Driscoll DJ, Danielson GK, et al. Tetralogy of Fallot with anomalous origin of the left anterior descending coronary artery. *J Thorac Cardiovasc Surg* 1987;94:784.
125. Frescura C, Thiene G, Franceschini E, et al. Pulmonary vascular disease in infants with complete atrioventricular septal defect. *Int J Cardiol* 1987;15:91.
126. McGrath LB, Gonzales-Lavin L. Actuarial survival, freedom from reoperation and other events after repair of atrioventricular septal defects. *Thorac Cardiovasc Surg* 1987;94:582.
127. Kirklin JW, Barratt-Boyes BG. Cardiac surgery. In: Kirklin JW, Barratt-Boyes BG, eds. Cardiac Surgery. New York: Churchill Livingstone, 1993:863.
128. Castaneda AR, Trusler GA, Paul MH, et al. The early results of treatment of transposition in the current era. *J Thorac Cardiovasc Surg* 1988;95:14.
129. Trusler GA, Williams WG, Duncan KF, et al. Results with the Mustard operation in simple transposition of the great arteries. *Ann Surg* 1987;206.
130. Wernovsky G, Giglia TM, Jonas RA, et al. Course in the intensive care unit after "preparatory" pulmonary artery banding and aortopulmonary shunt placement for transposition of the great arteries with low left ventricular pressure. *Circulation* 1992; 86[Suppl 5]:II-133.
131. Helbing WA, Hansen B, Ottenkamp J, et al. Long-term results of atrial correction for transposition of the great arteries: comparison of Mustard and Senning operations. *J Thorac Cardiovasc Surg* 1994;108:363.
132. Tamisier D, Ouaknine R, Pouard P, et al. Neonatal arterial switch operation: coronary artery patterns and coronary events. *Eur J Cardiothorac Surg* 1997;11:810.
133. Blume ED, Altmann K, Mayer JE, et al. Evolution of risk factors influencing early mortality of the arterial switch operation. *J Am Coll Cardiol* 1999;33:1702.
134. Mee RB, Harada Y. Retraining of the left ventricle with a left ventricular assist device (Bio-Medicus) after the arterial switch operation [Letter]. *J Thorac Cardiovasc Surg* 1991;101:171.
135. Gillette PC, Kugler JD, Garson A Jr. Mechanisms of cardiac arrhythmias after the Mustard operation for transposition of the great arteries. *Am J Cardiol* 1980;45:1225.
136. Bender HW Jr, Stewart JR, Merrill WH, et al. Ten year experience with the Senning operation for transposition of the great arteries: physiologic results and late followup. *Ann Thorac Surg* 1989;47:218.
137. Parrish MD, Graham TP Jr, Bender HW, et al. Radionuclide evaluation of right and left ventricular function during exercise after repair of transposition of the great arteries. *Circulation* 1983;67:178.
138. Kreselis DA, Rocchin AP, Rosenthal A, et al. Hemodynamic determinants of exercise induced ST segment depression in children with valvular aortic stenosis. *Am J Cardiol* 1985;55:1133.
139. Dekeon MK, Meldrum M, Meliones JN, et al. Pulmonary functioning testing demonstrates airway obstruction secondary to cardiovascular abnormalities. *Proceedings of the Fifth Pediatric Critical Care Colloquium, Seattle, WA, January 30, 1992.*
140. Flanagan MF, Fuji AM, Colan SD, et al. Inhibitory effects of myocardial perfusion in pressure overload hypertrophy in immature lambs. *Pediatr Res* 1988;23:218A.
141. Wernovsky G, Hougen TJ, Walsh EP, et al. Mid-term results following the arterial switch operation for transposition of the great arteries with intact ventricular septum: clinical, hemodynamic, echocardiographic, and electrophysiologic data. *Circulation* 1988;77:1333.
142. Rabinovitch M, Herrera-DeLeon V, Castaneda AR, et al. Growth and development of the pulmonary vascular bed in patients with tetralogy of Fallot with and without pulmonary atresia. *Circulation* 1981;64:1234.
143. Bridges ND, Jonas RA, Mayer JE, et al. Bidirectional cavopulmonary anastomosis as interim palliation for high-risk Fontan candidates: early results. *Circulation* 1990;82[Suppl IV]:IV-170.
144. Pigott JD, Murphy JD, Barber G, et al. Palliative reconstructive surgery for hypoplastic left heart syndrome. *Ann Thorac Surg* 1988;45:122.
145. Reddy VM, Liddicoat JR, Fineman JR, et al. Fetal model of single ventricle physiology: hemodynamic effects of oxygen, nitric oxide, carbon dioxide, and hypoxia in the early postnatal period. *J Thorac Cardiovasc Surg* 1996;112:437.
146. Reddy VM, Liddicoat JR, McElhinney DB, et al. Hemodynamic effects of epinephrine, bicarbonate and calcium in the early postnatal period in a lamb model of single-ventricle physiology created in utero. *J Am Coll Cardiol* 1996;28:1877.
147. Mayer JE, Helgason H, Jonas RA, et al. Extending the limits of modified Fontan procedures. *J Thorac Cardiovasc Surg* 1986; 92:1021.
148. Shigeaki O, Mault JR, Lilly MK, et al. Effect of a systemic-pulmonary artery shunt on myocardial function and perfusion in a piglet model. *Surg Forum* 1991;42:200.
149. Li DM, Mullaly R, Ewer P, et al. Effects of vasodilators on rates of change of nasopharyngeal temperature and systemic vascular resistance during cardiopulmonary bypass in anaesthetized dogs. *Aust N Z J Surg* 1988;58:327.
150. Mayer JES. Risk factors for modified Fontan operations. In: Norwood WI, Jacobson ML, eds. *Pediatric cardiac surgery.* Boston: Butterworth-Heinemann, 1992:70.
151. Jonas RA, Castaneda AR. Modified Fontan procedure: atrial baffle and systemic venous to pulmonary artery anastomotic techniques. *J Cardiol Surg* 1988;3:91.
152. Gentles TL, Mayer JE Jr, Gauvreau K, et al. Fontan operation in five hundred consecutive patients: factors influencing early and late outcome *J Thorac Cardiovasc Surg* 1997;114:376.
153. Sanders SP, Wright GV, Keane JF, et al. Clinical and hemodynamic results of the Fontan operation for tricuspid atresia. *Am J Cardiol* 1982;49:1733.
154. Gewillig M, Lundstrom UR, Deanfield JE, et al. Impact of Fontan operation on left ventricular size and contractility in tricuspid atresia. *Circulation* 1990;81:118.
155. Mietus-Snyder M, Lang P, Mayer JE, et al. Childhood systemic-pulmonary shunts: subsequent suitability of Fontan operation. *Circulation* 1987;76:39.
156. Deleon SY, Idriss FS, Ilbawi MN, et al. The role of the Glenn shunt in patients undergoing the Fontan operation. *J Thorac Cardiovasc Surg* 1983;85:669.
157. Mazzera E, Corno A, Picardo S, et al. Bidirectional cavopulmo-

nary shunts: clinical applications as a staged or definitive palliation. *Ann Thorac Surg* 1989;47:415.
158. Forbess JM, Cook N, Serraf A, et al. An institutional experience with second- and third-stage palliative procedures for hypoplastic left heart syndrome: the impact of the bidirectional cavopulmonary shunt. *J Am Coll Cardiol* 1997;29:665.
159. deLaval MR, Kilner P, Gewillig M, et al. Total cavopulmonary connection: a logical alternative to atriopulmonary connection for complex Fontan operations. *J Thorac Cardiovasc Surg* 1988; 96:682.
160. Balaji S, Gewillig M, Bull C, et al. Arrythmias after the Fontan procedure: comparison of total cavopulmonary connection and atriopulmonary connection. *Circulation* 1991;84:III-162.
161. Alboliras ET, Porter CJ, Danielson GK, et al. Results of the modified Fontan operation for congenital heart lesions in patients without preoperative sinus rhythm. *J Am Coll Cardiol* 1985;6:228.
162. Bernard C. Establishment of ionic permeabilities of the myocardial membrane during embryonic development of the rat. In: Lieberman M, Sano T, ed. *Developmental and physiologic correlates of cardiac muscle.* New York: Raven Press, 1975:169.
163. Reder R, Danilo P Jr. Effects of tetrodotoxin on fetal canine cardiac Purkinje fibers. *Fed Proc* 1981;40:2618.
164. Waldo AL. Modes and methods of recording electrograms. In: Waldo AL, MacLean WAH, eds. *Diagnosis and treatment of cardiac arrhythmias following open heart surgery.* Mt. Kisco, NY: Futura, 1980:21.
165. Dahl CF, Ewy GA, Warne E, et al. Myocardial necrosis from direct current countershock. *Circulation* 1974;50:956.
166. Campbell RM, Dick M, Jenkins DM. Atrial overdrive pacing for conversion of atrial flutter in children. *Pediatrics* 1985;75: 730.
167. Garson A, Gillette PC. Junctional ectopic tachycardia in children: electrocardiographic, electrophysiologic and pharmacologic response. *J Am Coll Cardiol* 1979;44:298.
168. Bash SE, Shah JJ, Albers WH, et al. Hypothermia for the treatment of postsurgical greatly accelerated junctional ectopic tachycardia. *J Am Coll Cardiol* 1987;10:1095.
169. Grant JW, Serwer GA, Armstrong BA, et al. Junctional tachycardia in infants and children after open heart surgery for congenital heart disease. *Am J Cardiol* 1987;59:1216.
170. Gillette PC, Garson A, Hesslein A, et al. Effects of verapamil on superventricular tachycardia in children. *Am J Cardiol* 1981; 48:487.
171. German JC, Chalmers GS, Mukherjee D, et al. Comparison of nonpulsatile and pulsatile extracorporeal circulation on renal tissue perfusion. *Chest* 1972;61:65.
172. Gomez-Campdera FJ, Maroto-Alvaro E, Galinanes M, et al. Acute renal failure associated with cardiac surgery. *Child Nephrol Urol* 1988;9:138.
173. Goodman TA, Gerard DF, Bernstein EF, et al. The effects of pulseless perfusion on the distribution of renal cortical blood flow and renin. *Surgery* 1976;80:31.
174. Hilberman M, Derby GC, Spencer RJ, et al. Sequential pathophysiological changes characterizing the progression from renal dysfunction to acute renal failure following cardiac operation. *J Thorac Cardiovasc Surg* 1980;79:838.
175. Kron IL, Joob AW, Van Meter C. Acute renal failure in the cardiovascular surgical patient. *Ann Thorac Surg* 1985;39:590.
176. Howard RJ, Crain C, Franzini DA, et al. Effects of cardiopulmonary bypass on pulmonary leukostasis and complement activation. *Arch Surg* 1988;123:1496.
177. Bui KC, Hammerman C, Hirshl RB, et al. Plasma prostanoids in neonates with pulmonary hypertension treated with conventional therapy and with extracorporeal membrane oxygenation. *J Thorac Cardiovasc Surg* 1991;101:973.
178. Skaryak LA, Lodge AJ, Kirshbom PM, et al. Low-flow cardiopulmonary bypass produces greater pulmonary dysfunction than circulatory arrest. *Ann Thorac Surg* 1996;62:1284.
179. Greeley WJ, Bushman GA, Kong D, et al. Effects of cardiopulmonary bypass on ecosanoid metabolism during pediatric cardiovascular surgery. *J Thorac Cardiovasc Surg* 1988;95:842.
180. Zapol WM, Peterson MB, Wonders TR, et al. Plasma thromboxane and prostacyclin metabolites in sheep partial cardiopulmonary bypass. *Trans Am Soc Artif Intern Organs* 1980;26:556.
181. Zapletal A, Paul T, Samenek M. Pulmonary elasticity in children and adolescents. *J Appl Physiol* 1976;40:953.
182. Greeley WJ, Kern FH, Ungerleider RM, et al. The effect of hypothermic cardiopulmonary bypass and total circulatory arrest on cerebral metabolism in neonates, infants and children. *J Thorac Cardiovasc Surg* 1991;101:783.
183. Kern FH, Jonas RA, Mayer JE, et al. Temperature monitoring during infant CPB: does it predict efficient brain cooling? *Ann Thorac Surg* 1992;54:749.
184. Messmer BJ, Schallberger U, Galliker R, et al. Psychomotor and intellectual development after deep hypothermic circulatory arrest in early infancy. *J Thorac Cardiovasc Surg* 1976;72:494.
185. McConnell JR, Fleming WH, Chu WK, et al. Magnetic resonance imaging of the brain in infants and children before and after cardiac surgery. *Am J Dis Child* 1990;144:374.
186. Ferry PC. Neurologic sequelae of open-heart surgery in children. *Am J Dis Child* 1990;144:369.
187. Swain JA, McDonald TJ, Griffith PK, et al. Low flow hypothermic cardiopulmonary bypass protects the brain. *J Thorac Cardiovasc Surg* 1991;102:76.
188. Rappaport LA, Wypij D, Bellinger DC, et al. Relation of seizures after cardiac surgery in early infancy to neurodevelopmental outcome. Boston Circulatory Arrest Study Group. *Circulation* 1998;97:773.
189. Burrows FA, Hillier SC, McLeod ME, et al. Anterior fontanel pressure and visual evoked potentials in neonates and infants undergoing profound hypothermic circulatory arrest. *Anesthesiology* 1990;73:632.
190. Friesen RH, Thieme R. Changes in fontanel pressure during cardiopulmonary bypass and hypothermic arrest in infants. *Anesth Analg* 1987;66:94.
191. Stow PJ, Burrows FA, McLeod ME, et al. The effect of cardiopulmonary bypass and profound hypothermic circulatory arrest on anterior fontanelle pressure in infants. *Can J Anaesth* 1987; 34:450.
192. Glauser TA, Rorke LB, Weinberg PM, et al. Acquired neuropathologic lesions associated with the hypoplastic left heart syndrome. *Pediatrics* 1990;85:991.

Cardiac Anesthesia: Principles and Clinical Practice, Second Edition, edited by Fawzy G. Estafanous, Paul G. Barash, and J.G. Reves. Lippincott Williams & Wilkins, Philadelphia © 2001.

PART V

SPECIAL CONSIDERATIONS

19

ANESTHESIA FOR CORONARY ARTERY BYPASS SURGERY

RICHARD J. BONDY
J. EARL WYNANDS
B. HUGH DORMAN
J. G. REVES

Surgeons have been attempting to revascularize the myocardium in patients with coronary artery disease (CAD) for well over half a century. Advances in perioperative anesthetic management have contributed significantly to the care and outcome of these high-risk patients. This chapter summarizes the principles of anesthesia for coronary artery bypass (CABG) surgery. A brief review of the pertinent history and epidemiology of myocardial revascularization and the perioperative risks promotes a better understanding of current anesthetic practices.

HISTORICAL AND PATHOPHYSIOLOGIC PERSPECTIVES

Physicians in the 18th century recognized the association between CAD and angina pectoris. Fothergill (1712–1780), a prominent physician of his time, described the postmortem findings on one of his patients with angina: "The two coronary arteries from their origins to many of their ramifications upon the heart were become one piece of bone" (1). The pathophysiology of ischemic heart disease is well known now and involves atherosclerosis of the coronary arteries that impairs oxygen delivery to the myocardium. When oxygen delivery is unable to meet myocardial demand, myocardial ischemia occurs (Fig. 19-1) (2). Total obstruction of coronary arteries leads to myocardial infarction. Under normal conditions coronary blood flow is closely matched to myocardial oxygen demand (3), which is determined primarily by heart rate, wall tension, and contractility. Myocardial oxygen supply depends on coronary perfusion pressure (aortic diastolic pressure minus left ventricular end-diastolic pressure) and coronary blood oxygen content. Increases in heart rate and preload adversely affect both sides of the supply-demand relationship (Fig. 19-2) (4). In the awake resting man, blood flow to the left ventricle is approximately 70 mL·100 g^{-1}·min^{-1}, most of which occurs during diastole. This results in a basal myocardial oxygen consumption of 8 to 10·100 g^{-1}·min^{-1}. The endocardial region of the heart faces higher wall stresses and consumes approximately 20% more oxygen per unit mass than the epicardium (5). Myocardial flow and metabolism are coupled over a wide range of coronary perfusion pressures, resulting in relatively constant values of 70% and 30% for oxygen extraction ratio and coronary sinus oxygen saturation, respectively. The difference between basal coronary blood flow and maximal attainable blood flow, for any given level of myocardial metabolism, is termed the "coronary vascular reserve" (6). This reserve is accomplished by coronary dilation and is available to satisfy the increased myocardial oxygen demands of stress and exercise. In patients with a stenotic coronary artery, the coronary vasculature distal to the lesion may already be maximally dilated at rest. Coronary vascular reserve is therefore exhausted, and flow distal to the obstruction becomes pressure-dependent (7). In this situation, increasing myocardial oxygen demand precipitates ischemia, starting in the vulnerable subendocardium. On the other hand, a fall in myocardial metabolic requirements restores coronary vascular reserve, and flow once again becomes autoregulated (8).

Pharmacologic agents that dilate coronary resistance vessels uncouple the close relationship between flow and metabolism, leading to an inappropriately high global myocardial blood flow relative to myocardial oxygen needs (9). This indiscriminate coronary vasodilation can paradoxically

R. J. Bondy: Department of Anesthesia, McGill University Health Center and Royal Victoria Hospital, Montreal, Quebec H3A 1A1 Canada

J. E. Wynands: Division of Cardiac Anesthesiology, University of Ottawa Heart Institute, Ottawa, Ontario K1Y 4W7 Canada

B. H. Dorman: Department of Anesthesiology and Perioperative Medicine, Medical University of South Carolina, Charleston, South Carolina, 29425

J. G. Reves: Department of Anesthesiology, Duke University Medical Center, Durham, North Carolina 27710

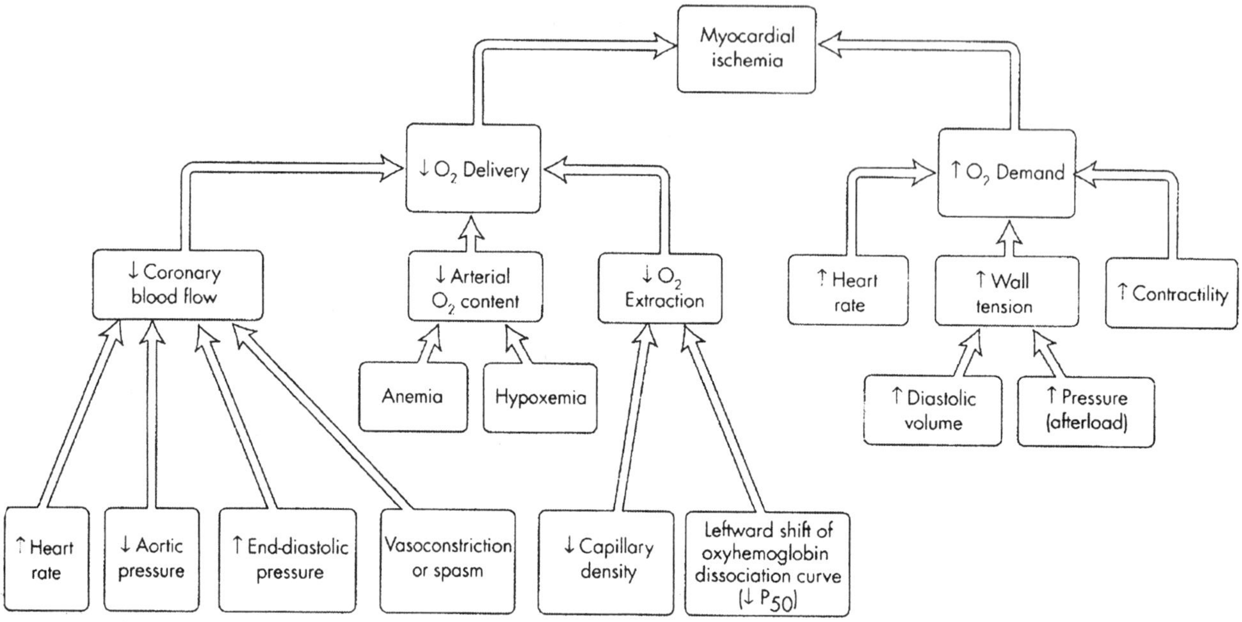

FIGURE 19-1. Conditions having detrimental influence on myocardial oxygen balance: mechanisms of myocardial ischemia. In normal hearts, myocardial oxygen supply (coronary blood flow) is matched to the prevailing myocardial oxygen demand via adjustments in vascular tone by local metabolic mechanisms. When the vasodilator reserve of the coronary bed is limited by a proximal stenosis, the myocardium becomes more vulnerable to ischemia (i.e., oxygen demand exceeds oxygen supply). The factors tending to promote this condition are presented in the figure. Several points to be made are as follows: (a) An increase in heart rate decreases myocardial oxygen delivery by decreasing coronary blood flow (via a shortening of the diastolic period), while it also increases myocardial oxygen demand. (b) An increase in preload reduces myocardial oxygen delivery (by reducing the pressure gradient for coronary blood flow), while it also increases myocardial oxygen demand (via an increase in wall tension). (c) A decrease in aortic pressure decreases myocardial oxygen delivery by decreasing coronary blood flow, but it decreases myocardial oxygen demand via a decrease in wall tension. Therefore, the net effect depends on the balance among these factors. Under conditions of restricted coronary vasodilator reserve, the most favorable hemodynamic situation is characterized by a low heart rate and preload, a normal aortic pressure, and a normal moderate inotropic state (97). P_{50}, Po_2 required for 50% saturation (42). (From Crystal GJ. Cardiovascular physiology. In: Miller RD, ed. *Atlas of anesthesia: vol VIII. Cardiothoracic anesthesia.* Philadelphia: Churchill Livingstone, 1999:1.1, with permission.)

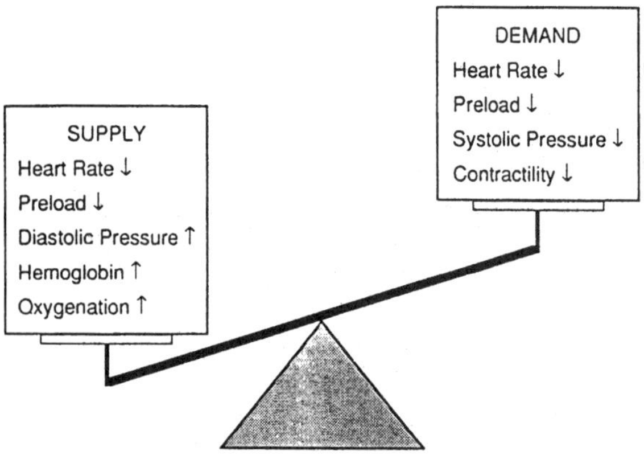

FIGURE 19-2. Myocardial oxygen balance: the determinants of myocardial oxygen supply and demand. (From Knopes KD, Leslie JB, London MJ. Pathophysiology and treatment of myocardial ischemia. *J Cardiothorac Anesth* 1990;4:51, with permission.)

lead to regional myocardial ischemia, referred to as "coronary steal," in patients with susceptible anatomy. Steal-prone anatomy is present when flow to an area of myocardium distal to a coronary obstruction is dependent on pressure in collateral vessels from an adjacent area of myocardium in which autoregulation is still intact. The presence of a hemodynamically significant stenosis in the artery proximal to where collateral flow originates minimizes the degree of coronary vasodilation required to induce steal.

The history of open heart surgery and myocardial revascularization has been extensively reviewed (1). Surgical treatment was frowned upon until well into the 1900s. Billroth claimed in 1883 that "A surgeon who would attempt such an operation [cardiac surgery] should lose the respect of his colleagues" (10). The prototype of the CABG operation was first described in 1910 by Carrel, who performed an aortocoronary artery graft on a dog, using a preserved length of carotid artery. In the 1930s and 1940s, Beck and others developed a multitude of surgical approaches to improve myocardial blood supply, including talcum powder poudrage, cardioomentopexy, coronary sinus ligation, and pericoronary neurectomy (11). In 1946 Vineberg described intracardiac implantation of the internal mammary artery (12). Seven years later, Gibbon reported the first successful use of a heart-lung machine for open heart surgery (13). This milestone, followed by the introduction of coronary angiography in 1958 by Sones, culminated in the development of aortocoronary bypass grafting by Favalaro in 1967 (14).

Advances in anesthesiology (15,16) have accompanied and contributed to the evolution of safe cardiopulmonary bypass and cardiac surgery. The first article concerning anesthesia for congenital heart palliative operations was published in 1946 by Harmel and Lamont (15), only 4 years after Griffith introduced curare into clinical practice. William McQuiston (16), an anesthetist working with the surgeon Potts, published important early observations on the use of hypothermia in 1950. The first monograph on cardiac anesthesia was published by Keown in 1956, the same year in which halothane was introduced. In 1967 the anesthetic experience with patients undergoing the Vineberg procedure was first reviewed (17). The "modern" era of cardiac anesthesia emerged in 1969 with Lowenstein's publication on high-dose morphine anesthesia for valve surgery (18). In the 1970s, Swan et al. (19) introduced the flow-directed pulmonary artery catheter, Lunn et al. (20) described high-dose fentanyl anesthesia for CABG surgery, and earlier (in 1977) the group in Alabama advocated a balanced anesthesia technique relying on diazepam, halothane, and fentanyl (21).

During the 1980s, three large randomized cooperative trials (22) were undertaken to compare surgical and medical treatments of CAD. Since then, percutaneous transluminal coronary angioplasty (PTCA) (23) evolved into a widespread alternative to conventional CABG surgery (24). More recently, a greater understanding of the natural history, biology, and progression of atherosclerosis (25) has developed, and a range of newer and less invasive therapeutic options has emerged, including beating-heart surgery, port-access bypass, therapeutic angiogenesis, and transmyocardial revascularization.

EPIDEMIOLOGY

Ischemic heart disease is the most prevalent form of cardiovascular disease in the United States. Among patients with CAD, 1.5 million per year will have an acute myocardial infarction, of whom approximately one third will die. Ischemic heart disease is responsible for 51% of deaths in men and 49% in women: It is the largest single cause of death in both genders. The morbidity, mortality, and health care costs related to cardiovascular disease are staggering; they have been reviewed by Mangano (27). Anesthesiologists should be aware of several significant epidemiologic and demographic trends in North America that will affect the surgical treatment of CAD and, more specifically, the profile of the typical cardiac surgery candidate in the future. The most significant pattern is the aging of the population, and the second is the growth of interventional cardiology (23). The persistence of CAD as a leading cause of morbidity and mortality (28) in North America, combined with the steady growth and rapid aging of the population and the relaxation of societal attitudes and restrictions toward treatment of the elderly, will have a major impact on the practice of cardiac anesthesia and surgery in the next decade. Demand for coronary revascularization procedures is increasing, and the profile of patients presenting for CABG surgery is constantly changing. The following data from a large tertiary-care institution illustrate this point. In a review of CABG surgery at the Cleveland Clinic, Lytle and Cosgrove (29) studied the characteristics of the first 1,000 patients undergoing primary elective CABG surgery during selected years from 1967 to 1990. The authors found that, "when compared to patients operated on in the early years of bypass surgery, patients today are older, less often men, and more likely to have triple-vessel disease, abnormal left ventricular function, severe angina, peripheral vascular disease, diabetes, and hypertension." The median age of surgical patients in their 1990 cohort was 65 years; 32% of these patients were older than 70 years of age. The same trends have continued during the 1990s. The importance of this demographic change is that older patients have a much higher rate of perioperative morbidity and mortality compared with younger patients, and noncardiac complications account for more than half of the deaths. This trend of older patients to experience poorer outcomes in general, and a much higher rate of debilitating noncardiac and neurologic complications in particular, poses a huge challenge to our specialty (30). Concerns over these perioperative outcomes and increased emphasis on quality assurance and cost containment have led to the publication of practice guidelines (31) and risk assessment programs (32) that are helpful in deciding who (24) should have surgery and what risk they represent.

Another major factor affecting the CABG population is PTCA and intracoronary stents; these are performed more often than bypass operations annually. Although the extraordinary growth in this area has not diminished the number of surgical revascularization procedures being performed, it has contributed in three ways to the rising proportion of high-risk patients undergoing bypass surgery. First, lower-risk patients undergoing PTCA are removed from the surgical pool. Second, up to 2% of PTCA procedures result in urgent or emergency operations, thus creating a new source of high-risk cases. Third, the ventricular function in patients who have undergone multiple catheter interventions is often reduced. The effect of all this on the changing profile and outcome of CABG surgery was clearly

TABLE 19-1. CORONARY ARTERY DISEASE (CAD)

Extent of CAD	Prognostic Weight (0–100)[a]
No CAD ≥50%	0
1 VD 50%–74%	19
>1 VD 50%–74%	23
1 VD (75%)	23
1 VD (≥95%)	32
2 VD	37
2 VD (both ≥95%)	42
1 VD, ≥95% proximal LAD	48
2 VD, ≥95% LAD	48
2 VD, ≥95% proximal LAD	56
3 VD	56
3 VD, ≥95% in at least one	63
3 VD, 75% proximal LAD	67
3 VD, ≥95% proximal LAD	74
Left main (75%)	82
Left main (≥95%)	100

Note: LAD, left anterior descending coronary artery; VD, vessel disease.
[a] The CAD index is hierarchical and that patients are assigned to the most severe category that applies. The higher the score, the higher the risk.
Source: Mark DB, Nelson CL, Califf RM, et al. Continuing evolution of therapy for coronary artery diseases: Initial results from the era of coronary angioplasty. *Circulation* 1994;89:2015, with permission.

demonstrated by Jones et al. (33). Hospital mortality more than doubled, from 1.2% to 3.1%, between 1981 and 1987. Another higher-risk group of patients that is expected to increase in the future is the patient with previous CABG surgery. The mortality rate in reoperated patients is significantly higher than in those undergoing primary operation, and this group of patients is expected to grow (34).

PREOPERATIVE EVALUATION

Preoperative evaluation of the cardiac surgery patient is the subject of Chapter 6 in this book. The following is a brief outline of our approach for patients with ischemic heart disease. In deciding whether a revascularization procedure is indicated, patients can be assigned a numeric prognostic score (35) (Table 19-1). This score is based on coronary anatomy and on ventricular function established with cardiac catheterization. Patients with the highest scores benefit the most from CABG surgery. In general, the more severe the atherosclerosis, the greater the benefit from surgery (24).

There have been a great number of methods proposed to identify patients at risk for death and complications after cardiac surgery (24,36–41). The overall risk of CABG surgery can be summarized in tabular form (Table 19-2) (42). One particularly popular method of forecasting the preoperative risk of CABG surgery was proposed by Parsonnet and coworkers in Table 19-3 (36). This risk scoring method assigns a numeric weight to various preoperative characteristics and is a way to compare the results of individual surgeons or institutions regarding operative mortality. One use of "risk adjustment" of a population permits better interpretation of mortality data. For example, cases with high Parsonnet scores would be expected to have higher mortality rate than those with a lower one.

The Veterans Administration Cardiac Surgery Risk Assessment Program (37), published in 1990, described the frequency and predictors of major complications after cardiac surgery in more than 10,000 patients. The authors reported that complications occurred in 15% of patients undergoing CABG surgery. Important predictors for the development of complications were previous heart surgery, surgical priority, old age, peripheral vascular disease, and elevated serum creatinine concentration. Patients experiencing one or more complications had an eight- to ten-fold increase in perioperative mortality. In another study from the Cleveland Clinic Foundation (38), a "clinical severity score" based on "easily retrievable clinical information" was developed. The authors identified 13 preoperative characteristics and assigned a total score to each patient by allocating values of 1 to 6 points for each of these risk factors. Higher scores correlated well with poor outcomes. A simpler

TABLE 19-2. PREOPERATIVE ASSESSMENT OF PATIENTS UNDERGOING CORONARY ARTERY BYPASS GRAFTING (CABG)

Determination	Outcome Predictor	Specific Physical Examination or Diagnostic Test
Coronary anatomy	Extent of disease and overall long-term survival	Coronary angiography
Cardiac function	Best predictor of outcome (EF >50%, good risk)	Ventricular angiogram
Renal function	If impaired, increases risk	Creatinine ≥2.0, increased risk
Emergency	Increases risk	History of failed PTCA or unstable angina
Reoperation	Increases risk	History of previous CABG
Central nervous system	Increases risk of stroke	History of TIA, symptomatic bruits, carotid Doppler study
Age and gender	Older and female, increased risk	History

Note: EF, ejection fraction; PTCA, percutaneous transluminal coronary angioplasty; TIA, transient ischemic attack.
Source: Clements F, de Bruijn N, Bennett-Guerrero E, et al: Anesthesia for cardiac surgery. In: Miller RD, ed. Anesthesia: subspecialty care, vol 5. Philadelphia: Churchill Livingstone, 1988:1.1, with permission.

TABLE 19-3. PARSONNET INDEX OF RISK FACTORS FOR PATIENTS UNDERGOING CORONARY ARTERY BYPASS GRAFTING (CABG)

Risk Factor	Assigned Weight
Female gender	1
Morbid obesity (≥1.5 × ideal weight)	3
Diabetes (unspecified type)	3
Hypertension (systolic BP >140 mm Hg)	3
Ejection fraction, % (actual value when available)	
Good (≥50)	0
Fair (30–49)	2
Poor (<30)	4
Age, yr	
70–74	7
75–79	12
≥80	20
Reoperation	
First	5
Second	10
Preoperative IABP	2
Left ventricular aneurysm	5
Emergency surgery after PTCA or catheterization complications	10
Dialysis dependency (PD or hemodialysis)	10
Catastrophic states (e.g., acute structural defect, cardiogenic shock, acute renal failure)[a]	10–50[b]
Other rare circumstances (e.g., paraplegia, pacemaker dependency, congenital HD in adult, severe asthma)[a]	2–10[b]
Valve surgery	
Mitral	5
PA pressure ≥60 mm Hg	8
Aortic	5
Pressure gradient >120 mm Hg	7
CABG at the time of valve surgery	2

Note: BP, blood pressure; HD, heart disease; IABP, intraaortic balloon pump; PA, pulmonary artery; PD, peritoneal dialysis.
[a] On the actual worksheet, these risk factors require justification.
[b] Values were predictive of increased risk of operative mortality in univariate analysis.
Source: From Parsonnet V, Dean D, Bernstein AD: A method of uniform stratification of risk for evaluating the results of surgery in acquired adult heart disease. *Circulation* 1989;79:3, with permission.

risk classification was described at the Montreal Heart Institute in Canada in 1993 (39).

In assessing the risk of complications in CABG surgery patients, three organ systems in addition to the heart are important. The most devastating noncardiac complication is neurologic (30). The incidence of perioperative stroke is generally about 2% to 3%, and the incidence for individual patients can be predicted using the nomogram in Fig. 19-3 (40). A neurologic risk minimization strategy is presented in algorithm form (42) in Fig. 19-4. Pulmonary complications are a second noncardiac concern after CABG surgery. Risk factors for the development of respiratory complications are presented in Table 19-4 (41). The third major organ system at risk involves the kidneys. The relation between postoperative mortality and rising creatinine concentration after surgery is presented in Fig. 19-5 (41). Methods to protect the kidney during CABG surgery have remained elusive. Recommendations regarding the use of diuretics, steroids, and dopamine remain controversial, although all have been proposed as renal-protective.

ANESTHETIC MANAGEMENT

The first step in anesthetic management involves a preoperative visit performed with three goals in mind. First, the anesthesiologist's usual thorough preoperative assessment must be performed with emphasis, as always, on coexisting medical disease and evaluation of the airway. Second, pertinent information obtained from the history, physical examination, and review of the chart and laboratory data must be analyzed to identify the patient with poor ventricular function and limited myocardial reserve (43) (Table 19-5), because this alters perioperative management and prognosis. Third, the preoperative visit is an opportunity to reduce the patient's understandable fear and anxiety by means of a reassuring and honest discussion of the next day's events. Questions concerning perioperative risk can be addressed using the information presented earlier in this chapter.

Noncardiac Premedication

Patients scheduled for CABG surgery can often benefit from pharmacologic anxiolysis in addition to the calming effect of the preoperative visit. The treatment must be individualized, taking into account age, body size, medical condition, ventricular function, concomitant medication, and level of preoperative anxiety. For most patients, the combination of oral diazepam (5 to 15 mg) and oral methadone (5 to 15 mg) provides effective sedation and analgesia. Patients should be given their usual cardiac medications also. All patients, regardless of ventricular function, normally are administered oxygen by mask with their premedication, to prevent hypoxia related to hypoventilation (44).

Once the sedative-hypnotic premedication is chosen, attention should be turned to other premedication that may optimize patient comfort and safety. For example, if an awake intubation is being contemplated, a drying agent will be most useful. For the patient who is at risk of regurgitation and aspiration, histamine-receptor antagonists are recommended. Antihistamines and steroids are indicated in a susceptible patient as prophylaxis against allergic reactions. Particular attention must be paid to insulin therapy for diabetic patients and to bronchodilator therapy for patients with obstructive lung disease.

Cardiac Premedication

Preoperative cardiac medication can influence perioperative hemodynamic stability and the incidence of ischemia. Slo-

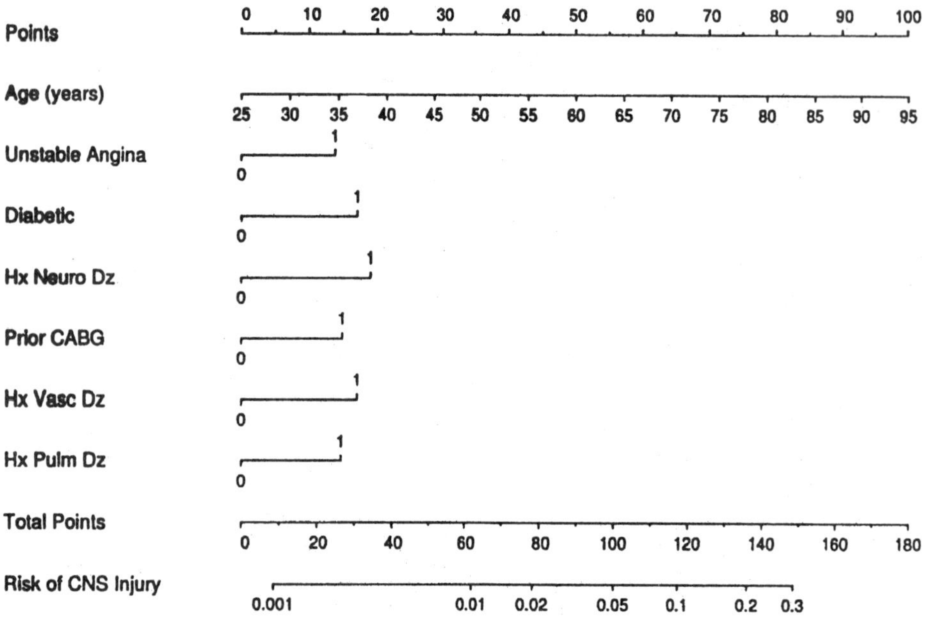

FIGURE 19-3. Nomogram using seven perioperative predictor variables to determine the risk of perioperative stroke. Strategies for brain protection begin with stratification or identification of patients at significant risk for central nervous system (CNS) injury. The nomogram is from the Multicenter Study of Perioperative Ischemia Research Group and is used to assess preoperative predictors of perioperative stroke in patients undergoing coronary artery bypass surgery. For each risk factor an individual risk score is determined on the point scale, and then the total number of points from the addition of all risk factors is used to predict CNS injury rate. The clinician is then able to assess the predicted risk of CNS injury for an individual patient. (From Newman MF, Wolman R, Kanchuger M, et al. Multicenter preoperative stroke risk index for patients undergoing coronary artery bypass graft surgery. *Circulation* 1996;94:II-74, with permission.)

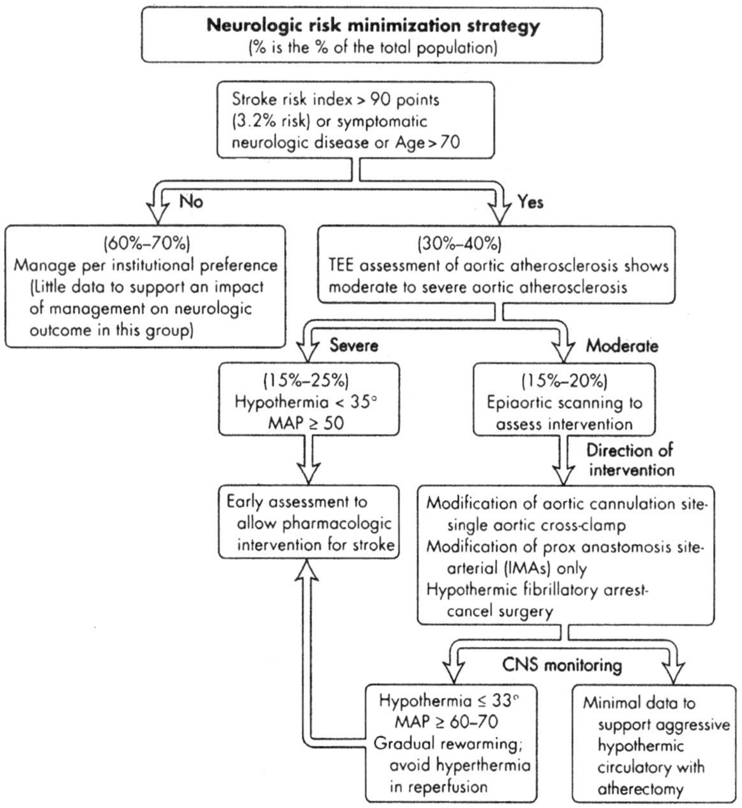

FIGURE 19-4. Neurologic risk minimization strategy. The neurologic outcome risk minimization strategy utilizing the Multicenter Study of Perioperative Ischemia stroke risk index as well as age and previous history of symptomatic neurologic disease stratifies patients into high- and low-risk groups and then, based on their transesophageal echocardiographic (TEE) and epiaortic echocardiographic assessment, determines their overall risk and potential management to reduce these risks. CNS monitoring is of greatest value in high-risk patients. CNS, central nervous system; IMA, internal mammary artery; MAP, mean arterial pressure. (From Clements F, de Bruijn N, Bennett-Guerrero E, et al. Anesthesia for cardiac surgery. In: Miller RD, ed. *Atlas of anesthesia: vol V. Subspecialty care.* Philadelphia: Churchill Livingstone, 1998:1.1, with permission.)

TABLE 19-4. SOME RISK FACTORS FOR RESPIRATORY COMPLICATIONS AFTER CARDIAC SURGERY[a]

Factor	Odds Ratio	95% CI
Current CHF	2.20	1.60–3.01
Emergency case	1.90	1.33–2.72
Reoperation	1.59	1.34–1.89
Preoperative serum Cr ≥1.9	1.56	1.11–2.20
COPD on medication	1.52	1.23–1.87
Aortic stenosis ≥2+	1.44	1.06–1.95
Prior vascular surgery	1.34	1.08–1.67
Mitral insufficiency ≥2+	1.32	1.03–1.70
Age/decade over 60	1.17	1.07–1.27

Note: CHF, congestive heart failure; CI, confidence interval; COPD, chronic obstructive pulmonary disease; CR, creatinine.
[a] All values significant to $p < .01$, except mitral insufficiency, $p = .027$; n = 4,170.
Source: From Higgins TL. Postoperative complications and ICU. In: Estafanous F, Barash P, Reves J, eds. *Cardiac anesthesia: principles and practice.* Philadelphia: Lippincott, 1994:373, with permission.

goff and Keats (45) and Chung et al. (46) studied the effects of preoperative β-blockade and calcium channel blockade. In Slogoff's study, only 3.4% of β-blocked patients had ischemia on arrival at the operating room, and only 1% of β-blocked patients had a peak heart rate greater than 109 beats/minute after induction. In contrast, the figures for patients not taking β-blockers were 15.4% and 10%, respectively. Consequently the incidence of prebypass ischemia in the β-blocked group was 34%, compared with 53% for the other patients. Many other studies have demonstrated the value of chronic or acute β-blockade in CABG patients. Interestingly, preoperative calcium channel blockade did not exhibit any similar protective effect. Chung's data corroborate these findings (46).

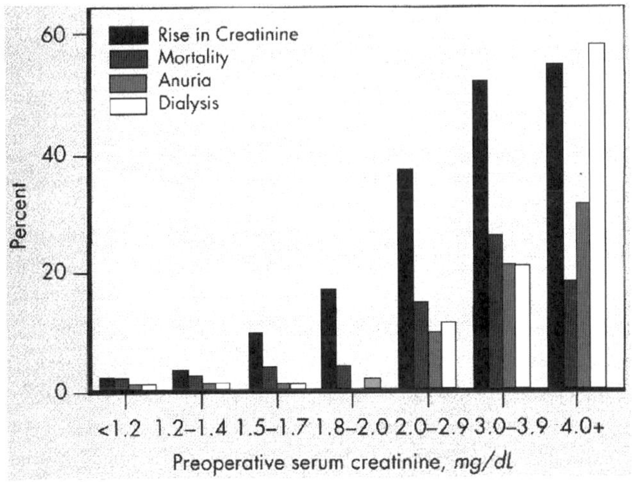

FIGURE 19-5. Relation between postoperative mortality and rising creatinine concentration after surgery. Marked increase is shown in all complications at increasing levels of preoperative serum creatinine. (From Higgins TL. Postoperative complications and ICU. In: Estafanous F, Barash P, Reves J, eds. *Cardiac anesthesia: principles and practice.* Philadelphia: JB Lippincott, 1994:373, with permission.)

TABLE 19-5. EVIDENCE OF IMPAIRED VENTRICULAR FUNCTION

Dyspnea
- At rest, with exertion, nocturnal, with angina, orthopnea

Edema
- Peripheral swelling, recurrent bronchitis or pneumonia, rales, hepatomegaly

Veins
- Distention and engorgement, hepatojugular reflux

Hypoperfusion
- Confusion (CNS), oliguria and increased serum creatinine and blood urea nitrogen (kidney), fatigue (muscle), angina (heart), anorexia (gut, CNS), cyanosis and poor capillary refilling (skin, mucous membranes)

Hypotension
- Especially with exertion (indicates ischemic dysfunction)
- With signs of sympathetic autonomic activity (tachycardia, diaphoresis)

Enlarged heart

Gallop rhythm
- S_3 indicates cardiac decompensation

Electrocardiogram
- Evidence of ischemia or infarction
- Hemodynamics during dysrhythmias

Data from laboratory examination of cardiac function
- Areas of hypokinesis, akinesis, dyskinesia, aneurysm of the ventricle
- Left ventricle end-diastolic pressures >15 mm Hg
- Ejection fraction <0.5
- Cardiac index <2.5 L/min/m^2

Source: From Shanewise JS, Hug CC Jr. Anesthesia for adult cardiac surgery. In: Miller R, ed. *Anesthesia,* 5th ed, vol 2. New York: Churchill Livingstone, 2000:1753, with permission.

Attempts have been made to extend the beneficial effects of these preoperative cardiac medications into the intraoperative period by means of prophylactic intravenous infusions. Thompson et al. (47) and Gallagher et al. (48) both attempted and failed to show a decrease in prebypass ischemia rates with prophylactic nitroglycerin infusions. In both studies, the patients given placebo had virtually the same ischemia rate as the treatment group. Controlling heart rate with esmolol or other longer-acting β-blockers may protect patients from ischemia. Newman et al., using bolus administration rather than continuous infusion, found that 1.0 and 1.5 mg/kg of esmolol given 1 minute before laryngoscopy significantly reduced peak heart rate and systolic blood pressure response to intubation (49), and heart rate is the single greatest predictor of development of ischemia.

The antihypertensive agent clonidine is another preoperative cardiac medication that has been used to attenuate undesirable intraoperative hemodynamic responses (50). Clonidine is a centrally acting α-adrenergic agonist that reduces sympathetic outflow from the central nervous system. Ghignone et al. (51) found that CABG patients given 5 μg/kg of oral clonidine 90 minutes before induction required 45% less fentanyl than the control group to achieve the same level of anesthetic depth and hemodynamic stability. Flacke et al. administered 200 to 300 mg of oral clonidine to patients 90 minutes before CABG surgery and repeated the dose intraoperatively by nasogastric tube. Perioperative treatment with clonidine reduced sufentanil requirements by 40% while improving hemodynamic control and reducing circulating catecholamine levels (52). The use of dexmedetomidine, a newer and more potent α-against, should have similar effects.

Monitoring

Monitoring for CABG surgery should begin on arrival in the operating room, once the patient is positioned comfortably and administered oxygen. Initial monitoring is established before vascular access is achieved and consists of automated noninvasive blood pressure measurement, pulse oximetry, and multiple-lead electrocardiography. Appropriate electrocardiographic lead selection and recording of baseline ST-segment morphology enhance detection of myocardial ischemia. In the study of London et al. (53), sensitivity for ischemia using a single lead was greatest with V_5 (75%) and V_4 (61%). Pairing of leads V_4 and V_5 increased the sensitivity to 90%, in contrast to the traditional combination of leads II and V_5, which yielded a sensitivity of 80%. Although few debate the importance of monitoring temperature, urine output, and beat-to-beat blood pressure for patients undergoing CABG surgery, considerable controversy still surrounds the use of the pulmonary artery catheter (54,55). Although it may be an acceptable practice to monitor only the central venous pressure in patients with normal ventricular function undergoing routine elective CABG surgery (56), there is no doubt that the pulmonary artery catheter can provide necessary information for evaluation of pulmonary artery pressure, right and left heart function, oxygen delivery and utilization, and myocardial ischemia. That the pulmonary artery catheter has never been shown to improve perioperative outcome may be related to incomplete use of the obtainable measured and derived data (57).

When faced with complicated cases in which circulatory instability is present or anticipated, insertion of the pulmonary artery catheter before, rather than after, induction of anesthesia should be considered. In these cases, significant hemodynamic deficits that are partially reversible with either volume loading or pharmacologic intervention may be found. Examples include inappropriately low filling pressures, abnormally elevated vascular resistances, and marked reductions in cardiac output and venous oxygen reserves. Pulmonary artery catheters that continuously measure and display mixed venous oxygen saturation may be particularly useful in the perioperative care of these high-risk patients (58). Intraoperative transesophageal echocardiography (TEE) for monitoring of patients during CABG surgery is useful. Valuable data concerning regional wall motion, intracardiac volume, and valve function can be obtained (59,60). TEE is also used to assist surgeons in evaluating the amount of atherosclerosis in the aorta, where to place clamps, and the aortic site of perfusion cannulation.

Principles of Anesthetic Management

The anesthesiologist's traditional approach to anesthesia for CABG in myocardial protection has emphasized the maintenance of hemodynamic stability (avoiding hypotension, hypertension, and tachycardia) and the optimization of oxygen-carrying capacity (avoiding hypoxia and anemia), thus preserving the delicate balance between myocardial oxygen supply and demand (Fig. 19-2). The problem of myocardial ischemia is much more complex than had been originally thought. It is now known that many patients with CAD experience frequent periods of electrocardiographic changes and myocardial hypoperfusion in the absence of an imbalance in correlates of oxygen supply and demand (61). Most of these ischemic episodes are not associated with hemodynamic instability. This phenomenon in awake patients is referred to as "silent ischemia" and has been extensively reviewed (62). Presumably it results from a primary reduction in myocardial blood flow. Persistent ischemia can ultimately precipitate life-threatening electrical or mechanical cardiac dysfunction and possibly perioperative myocardial infarction. Even if cell death is avoided, postischemic "stunning" (63) can lead to prolonged depression of contractile function. The three cornerstones of anesthetic management for patients undergoing CABG surgery remain prevention, detection, and treatment of perioperative myocardial ischemia, regardless of the cause.

Numerous studies have examined the incidence of intraoperative prebypass ischemia (defined as ischemia occurring between induction of anesthesia and onset of cardiopulmonary bypass) in patients undergoing CABG surgery. Some of the earliest studies are listed in Table 19-6. Depending on the means used to detect ischemia, the incidence range is 8% to 78%, with a mean in the 20% to 30% range. The association between prebypass ischemia and postoperative infarction has also been studied. Slogoff and Keats found that prebypass ischemia was one of three independent predictors of postoperative infarction (45,64–67). The incidence of postoperative infarction was almost three times higher in patients with prebypass ischemia (6.9%) than in those without prebypass ischemia (2.5%). Knight approached the problem by studying a group of CABG patients for 48 hours preoperatively with ambulatory electrocardiographic monitoring. Preoperative ischemic episodes occurred in 42% of the patients (68). Only 13% of these episodes were accompanied by angina, and only 25% were

TABLE 19-6. STUDIES OF PERIOPERATIVE MYOCARDIAL ISCHEMIA IN PATIENTS UNDERGOING CORONARY ARTERY BYPASS GRAFTING

Reference	No. of Patients	Monitor	Ischemia (%)
Slogoff et al., 1985–1990 (45, 64–67)	3,083	Electrocardiography (II, V_5)	32
Chung et al., 1988 (46)	92	Electrocardiography (II, V_5)	17
Thompson et al., 1988 (46)	20	Holter (II, CS_5)	50
Knight et al., 1988 (68)	50	Holter (CC_5, CM_5)	18
O'Connor et al., 1988 (98)	100	Holter (V_6 V_9)	8
Harrison et al., 1987 (99)	30	Holter (V_6 V_9)	13
Litak et al., 1987 (100)	27	Holter (V_6 V_9)	26
Kotter et al., 1987 (101)	312	ST trend analysis	12
Leung et al., 1989 (60)	50	Transesophageal echocardiography	20
Sonntag et al., 1982 (102)	9	Coronary lactate	78
Kleinman et al., 1986 (103)	22	Thallium scan	45
Bellows et al., 1984 (104)	24	Cardiokymography	33

Source: From Bondy RJ, Wynands JE. Anesthesia induction and maintenance strategies. In: Estafanous F, Barash PG, Reves JG, eds. *Cardiac anesthesia: principles and clinical practice.* Philadelphia: Lippincott, 1994:221, with permission.

associated with hemodynamic changes. Furthermore, only 18% of the patients subsequently developed intraoperative prebypass ischemia, but this incidence increased to 40% postoperatively. The majority of perioperative ischemic episodes were unrelated to hemodynamic aberrations, suggesting that more than maintenance of a stable hemodynamic profile is required. Although in Knight's study preoperative ischemia predicted intraoperative ischemia, neither preoperative nor intraoperative ischemia predicted the development of postoperative ischemia or infarction. The data suggest that intraoperative prebypass ischemia (most of which is nonhemodynamic) may simply recapitulate the preoperative pattern of ischemia, most of which is silent.

Leung et al. (60) examined the relation between TEE segmental wall motion abnormalities and outcome in 50 patients undergoing elective CABG surgery. Only postbypass abnormalities were significant predictors of adverse outcome. In fact, patients without a new segmental wall motion abnormality occurring after cardiopulmonary bypass had no major adverse outcome. In contrast, neither prebypass TEE ischemia, which occurred in 20% of the patients, nor prebypass electrocardiographic ischemia, which occurred in 7% of the patients, correlated with poor outcome. Furthermore, 73% of the echocardiographic ischemic episodes occurred without acute changes in heart rate, systemic blood pressure, or pulmonary artery pressure.

The studies by Knight (68) and Leung (60) and their colleagues have shown that prebypass ischemia is often unrelated to hemodynamic changes and may not be as strongly predictive of adverse outcome as was once thought. However, Buffington (69) suggested that it is dangerous to interpret this information as evidence that tight hemodynamic control in the prebypass period is totally unnecessary. On the contrary, safe passage of the patient through the peaks and valleys of induction, intubation, incision, sternotomy, dissection, and aortic cannulation requires attention to and attenuation of hemodynamic responses with special emphasis on prevention of tachycardia. In the original study of Slogoff and Keats, ischemia was significantly more frequent in patients who developed tachycardia, occurring in 40% of patients whose heart rate rose above 99 beats/minute (64). In a subsequent study, 63% of patients whose peak heart rate exceeded 109 beats/minute experienced ischemic episodes, compared with only 34% of the control group (45). Buffington observed that both heart rate and its relation to blood pressure are important (69,70). In a canine model of coronary stenosis, ischemia was absent if mean aortic blood pressure exceeded heart rate, that is, if the pressure-to-rate ratio exceeded unity. This concept is illustrated in Fig. 19-6. The blood pressure–heart rate quotient may be a more relevant hemodynamic correlate in anesthetized patients than the traditional heart rate–blood pressure product, which only estimates oxygen consumption.

Anesthetic Drug Selection

No single drug is suitable as the sole anesthetic agent for all patients undergoing CABG surgery (21,71–75). Numerous drug combinations can be used with equal efficacy to achieve hemodynamic stability and a low incidence of perioperative myocardial ischemia. The choice of anesthetic drugs is primarily determined by the patient's preoperative ventricular function, the desirability of early extubation, and the experience of the anesthesiologist with the anesthetic drugs.

Patients with good ventricular function can effectively be managed with a combination of hypnotics, opioids, and inhalational drugs. Appropriate doses for induction and maintenance are available in standard anesthesiology textbooks. If these drugs are administered rapidly or in large amounts, hypotension may occur. The importance of hemodynamic control in patients undergoing CABG surgery

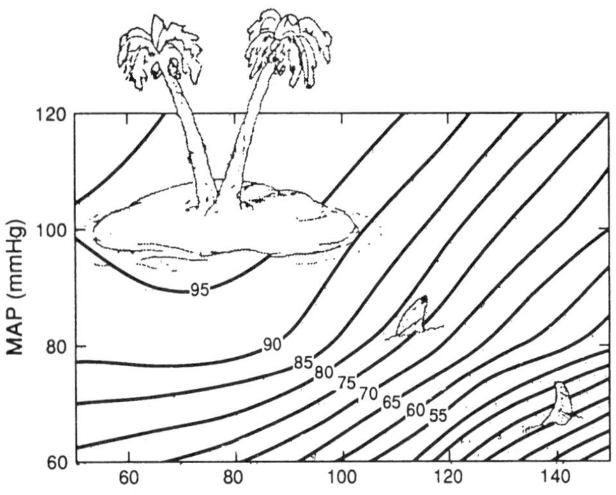

FIGURE 19-6. Relation between mean arterial pressure (MAP), heart rate, and normalized systolic contraction in an area of the heart supplied by a severely stenosed coronary artery. Each number is an isopleth of regional myocardial thickening during systole normalized as a percentage of the values obtained in the absence of stenosis. An "island of safety" is shown in the zone where ischemia is absent. (From Buffington CW. Hemodynamics and myocardial ischemia. *Anesthesiol Rev* 1990;17:11, with permission.)

has already been mentioned. Elevated myocardial oxygen demand, such as tachycardia caused by surgical stimulation in lightly anesthetized patients, can induce ischemia and is amenable to treatment with isoflurane and/or β-blockade. On the other hand, decreased myocardial oxygen supply, such as that caused by vasodilation from anesthesia in unstimulated patients, can also lead to ischemia and should be avoided. The effect of isoflurane on the hemodynamic determinants of myocardial oxygen balance appears to be more important in most patients than its direct effect on coronary tone. This conclusion was supported by Slogoff and Keats, who found that myocardial ischemia in CABG patients was no more frequent with isoflurane (66), even in patients with steal-prone anatomy (76), than with halothane, enflurane, or sufentanil regimens.

Patients with poor ventricular function present a more difficult anesthetic management problem. Reduced circulatory reserve may limit their ability to compensate for anesthetic-induced myocardial depression. Doses that are well tolerated by patients with good ventricular function may lead to diminished cardiac output, increased cardiac filling pressures, decreased systemic blood pressure, and a fall in coronary perfusion pressure in patients with poor ventricular function. This hemodynamic profile can initiate or aggravate myocardial ischemia.

Because the opioids do not cause direct myocardial depression in clinically relevant concentrations, they were historically used as the primary "anesthetic" drug in patients with severely impaired ventricular function. However, because opioids are incomplete anesthetics (77,78), patients managed with a pure opioid technique are at risk for awareness and recall of surgery. Modern anesthesia, even in patients with impaired ventricular performance, relies on hypnotics combined with opioids. Use of the bispectral (BIS) monitor to assess levels of consciousness is a useful adjunct (79). It is believed that most cardiac surgical cases can be kept at a BIS level of 60 or less without recall. The hypnotic drugs titrated to effect (e.g., midazolam, propofol) and/or inhalation anesthetics are useful to accomplish this goal.

Anesthetic Infusions and Drug Selections

The most rationale approach to the intravenous drug delivery for CABG surgery is to infuse the intravenous anesthetic drugs continuously (95). Repetitive bolus administration produces peaks and valleys in drug plasma and brain concentrations. To help decide which intravenous anesthetic drug is most appropriate to select, Hughes et al. performed computer simulations to study the time period required for central compartment drug concentrations to decline by 50% after termination of a continuous infusion (80). They labeled this new entity the "context-sensitive half-time" and found that it appears to differ markedly from the elimination half-life. In Fig. 19-7, the context-sensitive half-times predicted after termination of 1-minute, 1-hour, 3-hour, and 8-hour infusions are shown for each of the six drugs modeled. Because these predictions are based on pharmacokinetic determinations from bolus studies, they may misrepresent the actual case, but they do show the differences between elimination half-lives and drug clearances within the context of anesthetic practice.

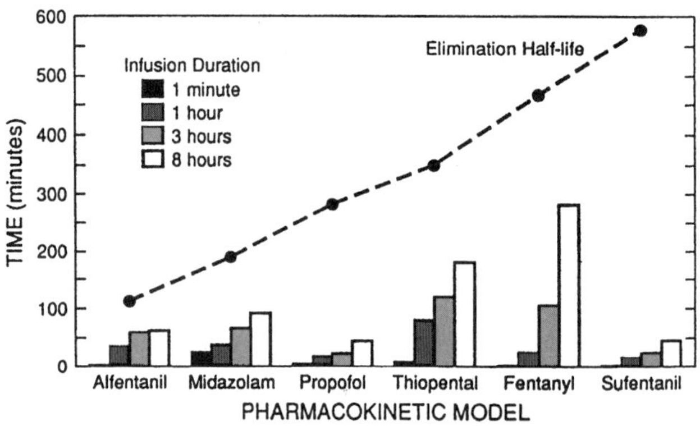

FIGURE 19-7. The context-sensitive half-times for six anesthetic drugs and four different intravenous infusion durations. The half-time is the time required for half of the drug concentration to disappear from the plasma after cessation of infusion. Note that the half-times are considerably shorter than the elimination half-lives. (From Hughes MA, Glass PS, Jacobs JR: Context-sensitive half-time in multicompartment pharmacokinetic models for intravenous anesthetic drugs. *Anesthesiology* 1992;76:334, with permission.)

The pharmacokinetics and pharmacodynamics of drug infusions are becoming better understood. This knowledge is being applied to computer-assisted continuous infusions of hypnotics and opioids for cardiac anesthesia (73,81). Computer-assisted continuous infusion (CACI) is a pharmacokinetic model–driven infusion device that uses pharmacokinetic parameters to deliver intravenous drugs according to concentration rather than dose, which is analogous to the way in which calibrated vaporizers are used to administer volatile anesthetics (73,82). These infusion devices may play a significant role in future anesthetic practice. Also, using previously published pharmacokinetic data for fentanyl, sufentanil, and alfentanil, Schafer and Varvel performed computer simulations to quantify the relation between narcotic infusion duration and the time required for recovery after termination of the infusion (83). As expected, the time required for narcotic concentration to decrease by a given percentage was found to increase with longer infusion duration. However, this effect peaked at 4 hours for alfentanil. Somewhat surprisingly, although sufentanil has longer distribution and elimination half-lives than alfentanil (Fig. 19-7), recovery from sufentanil infusions may be more rapid than recovery from alfentanil, and certainly from fentanyl infusions.

Intrathecal and Epidural Opiates

Intrathecal morphine used for postoperative analgesia in cardiac surgery was first described in 1980 by Mathews and Abrams, who reported prolonged pain relief with doses of 2 mg (84). Fitzpatrick and Moriarty investigated the analgesic and respiratory effects of intrathecal morphine in doses of 1 mg and 2 mg and compared this technique with a more traditional intravenous narcotic regimen (85). They found that the patients receiving intrathecal morphine had significantly lower pain scores, diminished requirements for supplemental analgesia, and higher postoperative peak expiratory flow rates. These findings conflicted with the results of Casey et al. (86), who administered intrathecal morphine in doses of 20 μg/kg in a double-blind and randomized fashion to 40 patients undergoing CABG surgery and found no clear benefit in postoperative analgesia and pulmonary function. This discrepancy can be explained by the fact that Casey had used a high-dose fentanyl technique (40 μg/kg), which may have saturated spinal opiate receptors, whereas the other studies relied primarily on inhalational anesthesia.

Experience with epidural opioids in cardiac anesthesia is limited. El-Baz and Goldin (87) described the effects of epidural morphine infusions in 60 patients anesthetized with a nonnarcotic technique for CABG. The epidural catheter was inserted between the third and fourth thoracic vertebrae before induction of anesthesia. The placement of epidural catheters before the administration of heparin was not associated with any neurologic complications. Epidural morphine was administered by infusion at a rate of 100 μg/hour, starting immediately on arrival to the intensive care unit. Effective analgesia was achieved in 80% of the epidural patients and was associated with a mean serum morphine level of only 2.5 ng/mL. Among patients receiving conventional intravenous opioids for postoperative pain, only 50% reported effective analgesia. This was achieved at the expense of a higher mean serum morphine level (17 ng/mL). Robinson et al. (88) administered lumbar epidural meperidine (Demerol) (1 mg/kg) to 10 patients after extubation on the morning after CABG surgery. Pain scores were significantly reduced for 6 hours. However, three patients exhibited somnolence, and two developed marked hypotension within minutes after the epidural injection. The hypotension may have been a result of partial sympathetic blockade caused by the local anesthetic properties of Demerol. The use of epidural local anesthetics is intriguing in view of findings that patients with CAD injected with thoracic epidural bupivacaine experienced angiographically proven coronary artery dilatation (89) and relief of angina (90). The use of epidural and intrathecal analgesia after CABG is still variable and being explored, as is the use of paravertebral analgesia, which has less chance of precipitating neurologic complications.

Supportive Intraoperative Care

The anesthesiologist not only safely provides adequate anesthesia during CABG surgery but is expected to support the cardiovascular and other organ systems. Most supportive therapy is designed to prevent or treat myocardial ischemia (Table 19-7), and when manipulation of the anesthesia (described earlier) is not successful, then the use of various pharmacologic drugs are indicated. Note that the table is designed to treat the determinants of myocardial oxygen supply and demand: A physiologic approach is used even though pharmacology is the means to that end. Hypotension usually responds to small intravenous boluses (25 to 100 μg) of phenylephrine. Sometimes norepinephrine infusions or bolus administrations of ephedrine are required to increase systemic vascular resistance. In cases of refractory hypotension in patients unresponsive to α-agonist therapy, arginine vasopressin (4 to 15 units/hour) can be used (91). Prompt treatment of hypotension is critical in patients with significant left main coronary disease and/or aortic stenosis. Despite careful drug titration, some patients may develop hypertension in response to laryngoscopy and intubation, which can be treated by increasing the depth of anesthesia with additional intravenous or inhalational anesthetics, by administering a β-adrenergic antagonist, or by giving nitroglycerin or sodium nitroprusside. If tachycardia occurs in response to noxious stimuli, it must be aggressively treated. For comparable increases in myocardial oxygen demand caused by either tachycardia or hypertension, tachycardia has been associated with a significantly higher incidence of myocardial ischemia (45,64,92). When tachycardia and

TABLE 19-7. INTRAOPERATIVE HEMODYNAMIC ABNORMALITIES AND MYOCARDIAL ISCHEMIA[a]

Abnormal Hemodynamic Profile	Treatment
Hypertension, tachycardia	IV nitroglycerin IV β-blockade Increased anesthetic depth Labetalol
Hypertension, normal heart rate	IV nitroglycerin Increased anesthetic depth SL nifedipine IV nicardipine IV β-blockade for reflex tachycardia
Normotension, tachycardia	R/O arrhythmia Check volume status, hematocrit Check anesthetic depth (change technique?) IV β-blockade IV nitroglycerin
Hypotension, tachycardia	R/O arrhythmia Check volume status, hematocrit } Specific, directed treatment Check contractile function } Calculate SVR } Check anesthetic depth IVα-agonist to support coronary perfusion pressure IV β-blockade once normotensive (with adequate contractile function) IV nitroglycerin once normotensive
Hypotension, bradycardia	R/O arrhythmia (i.e., junctional rhythm) Check volume status } Specific, directed treatment Check contractile function } Calculate SVR } IV ephedrine IV atropine IV epinephrine (infusion vs low-dose bolus) IV nitroglycerin once normotensive
Hypotension, normal heart rate	Check volume status } Specific, directed treatment Check contractile function } Calculate SVR } IVα-agonist for reduced SVR Volume and/or inotrope to correct specific abnormality IV nitroglycerin once normotensive

Note: R/O, rule out; SVR, systemic vascular resistance.
[a]Although a majority of episodes of intraoperative myocardial ischemia are not directly associated with hemodynamic changes, there are a number of hemodynamic abnormalities that can compromise the myocardial oxygen supply-demand relationship and directly precipitate ischemia (45). Deleterious hemodynamic abnormalities that are temporally associated with ischemia should be promptly diagnosed and treated. In the setting of an acute change in hemodynamic profile intraoperatively, the adequacy of oxygenation, ventilation, and volume status must be quickly confirmed and an arrhythmia or surgical factor (acute blood loss, cardiac manipulation) must be considered. Ideally, invasive cardiac monitoring with a pulmonary artery catheter or transesophageal echocardiography allows for prompt investigation of the cause of any hemodynamic alteration and appropriate, directed therapy. For example, hypotension can compromise coronary profusion and can be secondary to a reduction in preload, after load, contractile function, or an arrhythmia; appropriate management of volume status, systemic vascular resistance, inotropy, anesthetic depth, and heart rate and rhythm is necessary for optimal treatment of deleterious hemodynamic changes and subsequent resolution of intraoperative myocardial ischemia. Although nitroglycerin is the mainstay of treatment for ischemic heart disease, coronary perfusion pressure must be maintained and heart rate needs to be strictly controlled, because tachycardia has been shown to be directly associated with the development of ischemia.
Source: Adapted from Slogoff S, Keats AS. Does chronic treatment with calcium entry blocking drugs reduce perioperative myocardial ischemia? *Anesthesiology* 1988;68:676 and Dorman BH. Ischemic heart disease. In: Miller RD, ed. *Atlas of anesthesia,* vol 8. Philadelphia: Churchill Livingstone, 1999:4.1, with permission.

hypertension occur simultaneously, administration of intravenous β-blockers in addition to supplemental anesthesia and/or vasodilators should be considered. Incremental doses of either metoprolol (0.5 to 2 mg), propranolol (0.5 to 1.0 mg), or boluses of esmolol (1.0 to 1.5 mg/kg) are recommended (93). When tachycardia is associated with hypotension, information derived from the pulmonary artery catheter will be helpful in determining therapy. Bradycardia that occurs on induction is usually transient but responds to incremental doses of atropine (0.4 to 0.6 mg). When bradycardia is associated with hypotension, ephedrine (5 to 10 mg) is appropriate therapy. If myocardial ischemia is diag-

TABLE 19-8. FACTORS THAT PREDICT THE USE OF INOTROPIC DRUG SUPPORT AFTER CARDIOPULMONARY BYPASS[a]

Variable	Probability Value
Low ejection fraction	.002
Long duration of bypass	.004
Older age	.005
Longer duration of aortic cross-clamping	.009
Cardiac enlargement	.021
Female sex	.027

[a] Various preoperative and intraoperative factors associated with the use of inotropes were analyzed by logistic regression. The overall incidence of inotropic support in patients with ejection fraction less than 0.55 was approximately 60% to 70%.
Source: From Royster RL, Butterworth JF IV, Prough DS, et al. Perioperative and intraoperative predictors of inotropic support and long-term outcome in patients having coronary artery bypass grafting. *Anesth Analg* 1991;72:729, with permission.

nosed and associated with normal or elevated blood pressure, an infusion of nitroglycerin should be instituted. These interventions are made always with reliance on monitors that indicate myocardial ischemia and function. Care must be exercised in the use of these drugs not to cause greater imbalances in oxygen supply and demand.

Supportive management of the failing heart and circulation is sometimes required. The pharmacologic and technologic (mechanical) methods to support the failing circulation are presented elsewhere in this book, but it is important to know who is most likely to require this type of management during CABG. Royster et al. identified those patients most likely to require inotropic support (94). Factors most likely to predict the use inotropic drugs are presented in Table 19-8. Some of these factors are preoperative, and others are operative variables. Of course, the decision to intervene to support the heart or circulation depends on the individual patient's need as determined by measurement of cardiac output and other monitors of adequate circulation. Sole reliance on pharmacologic methods should always be done keeping in mind that several mechanical methods to support the circulation can spare the energy cost of excessive inotropic support.

SUMMARY

Patients undergoing CABG are at risk for myocardial ischemia and infarction before, during, and after surgery. They also can have other organ damage, and the role of the anesthesiologist is to minimize the risk of organ damage in addition to providing the patient adequate anesthesia. The appropriate use of monitors and selection of drugs and methods of drug delivery are all crucial decisions the cardiac anesthesiologist must make with each individual patient. Rational drug administration and appropriate monitoring are more important in this regard than the choice of anesthetic agent.

REFERENCES

1. Brewer LA. Open heart surgery and myocardial revascularization: historical notes. *Am J Surg* 1981;141:618.
2. Crystal GJ. Cardiovascular physiology. In: Miller RD, ed. *Atlas of anesthesia: vol VIII. Cardiothoracic anesthesia.* Philadelphia: Churchill Livingstone, 1999:1.1.
3. Sethna DH, Moffitt EA. An appreciation of the coronary circulation. *Anesth Analg* 1986;65:294.
4. Knopes KD, Leslie JB, London MJ. Pathophysiology and treatment of myocardial ischemia. *J Cardiothorac Anesth* 1990;4:51.
5. Katz AM, Katz PB. Homogeneity out of heterogeneity. *Circulation* 1989;79:712.
6. Hoffman JE. Maximal coronary flow and the concept of coronary vascular reserve. *Circulation* 1984;70:153.
7. Epstein SE, Cannon RO, Talbot TL. Hemodynamic principles in the control of coronary blood flow. *Am J Cardiol* 1985;56:4E.
8. Nathan HJ. Mechanisms of acute myocardial ischemia: pathophysiology of myocardial blood flow. *Anesth Clin North Am* 1991;9:455.
9. Becker LC. Conditions for vasodilator-induced coronary steal in experimental ischemia. *Circulation* 1978;57:1103.
10. Keown KK. History. In: Adriani J, ed. *Anesthesia for surgery of the heart.* Springfield, IL: Charles C Thomas, 1963.
11. Beck CS. The development of a new blood supply to the heart by operation. *Ann Surg* 1935;102:801.
12. Vineberg A. Development of anastomosis between coronary vessels and transplanted internal mammary artery. *Can Med Assoc J* 1946;55:117.
13. Gibbon JG. Development of the artificial heart and lung extracorporeal blood circuit. *JAMA* 1968;206:1983.
14. Favalaro RG. The present era of myocardial revascularization. *Int J Cardiol* 1983;4:331.
15. Harmel MH, Lamont A. Anesthesia in the surgical treatment of congenital pulmonic stenosis. *Anesthesiology* 1946;7:477.
16. McQuiston WO. Anesthesia in cardiac surgery. *Arch Surg* 1950;61:892.
17. Wynands JE, Sheridan CA, Kelkar K. Coronary artery disease and anesthesia. *Can Anaesth Soc J* 1967;14:382.
18. Lowenstein E, Hallowell P, Levine F, et al. Cardiovascular responses to large doses of intravenous morphine in man. *N Engl J Med* 1969;281:1389.
19. Swan HJ, Ganz W, Forrester CJ, et al. Catheterization of the heart in man with use of a flow-directed balloon-tipped catheter. *N Engl J Med* 1970;283:447.
20. Lunn JK, Stanley TH, Eiscle J, et al. High dose fentanyl anesthesia for coronary artery surgery. *Anesth Analg* 1979;58:390.
21. Reves JG, Samuelson PN, Lell WA, et al. Anesthesia for coronary artery surgery: An evolution in anesthetic management. *Alabama J Med Sci* 1977;14:394.
22. Rahimtoola SH. A perspective of three large multicenter randomized clinical trials of coronary bypass surgery for chronic stable angina. *Circulation* 1985;72:123.
23. Bittl JA. Advances in coronary angioplasty. *N Engl J Med* 1996;335:1290.
24. Jones RH, Kesler K, Phillips HR, et al. Long-term survival benefits of coronary artery bypass grafting and percutaneous transluminal angioplasty in patients with coronary artery disease. *J Thorac Cardiovasc Surg* 1996;111:1013.
25. Ross R. Atherosclerosis: an inflammatory disease. *N Engl J Med* 1999;340:115.

26. Rosengart TK. New approaches to the surgical therapy of coronary artery disease. *Am J Cardiol* 1999;83:40B.
27. Mangano DT. Perioperative cardiac morbidity. *Anesthesiology* 1990;72:153.
28. Gillum RF. Trends in acute myocardial infarction and coronary heart disease death in the USA. *J Am Coll Cardiol* 1993;23:1273.
29. Lytle BW, Cosgrove DM. Coronary artery bypass surgery. *Curr Probl Surg* 1992;29:746.
30. Arrowsmith JE, Grocott HP, Reves JG, et al. Central nervous system complications of cardiac surgery. *Br J Anaesth* 2000;84:378.
31. Eagle KA, Guyton RA, Davidoff R, et al. ACC/AHA Guidelines for coronary artery bypass graft surgery. *J Am Coll Cardiol* 1999;34:1262.
32. Higgins TL. Quantifying risk and assessing outcome in cardiac surgery. *J Cardiothorac Vasc Anesth* 1998;12:330.
33. Jones EL, Weintraub WS, Craver JM, et al. Coronary bypass surgery: is the operation different today? *J Thorac Cardiovasc Surg* 1991;101:108.
34. Machiraju VR. *Redo cardiac surgery in adults.* New York: CME Network, 1997.
35. Mark DB, Nelson CL, Califf RM, et al. Continuing evolution of therapy for coronary artery disease: Initial results from the era of coronary angioplasty. *Circulation* 1994;89:2015.
36. Bernstein AD, Parsonnet V. Bedside estimation of risk as an aid for decision-making in cardiac surgery. *Ann Thorac Surg* 2000;69:823.
37. Grover FL, Hammerstein KE, Burchfiel C. Initial report of the Veterans Administration Preoperative Risk Assessment Study for Cardiac Surgery. *Ann Thorac Surg* 1990;50:12.
38. Higgins TL, Estafanous FG, Loop FD, et al. Stratification of morbidity and mortality by preoperative risk factors in coronary artery bypass patients. *JAMA* 1992;267:2344.
39. Tremblay NA, Hardy JF, Perrault J, et al. The simple classification of the risk in cardiac surgery: the first decade. *Can J Anaesth* 1993;40:103.
40. Newman MF, Wolman R, Kanchuger M, et al. Multicenter preoperative stroke risk index for patients undergoing coronary artery bypass graft surgery. *Circulation* 1996;94:II-74.
41. Higgins TL. Postoperative complications and ICU. In: Estafanous F, Barash P, Reves J, eds. *Cardiac anesthesia: principles and practice.* Philadelphia: JB Lippincott, 1994:373.
42. Clements F, de Bruijn N, Bennett-Guerrero E, et al. Anesthesia for cardiac surgery. In: Miller RD, ed. *Atlas of anesthesia: vol V. Subspecialty care.* Philadelphia: Churchill Livingstone, 1998:1.1.
43. Hug CC. Anesthesia for adult cardiac surgery. In: Miller R, ed. *Anesthesia,* 3rd ed. New York: Churchill Livingstone, 1990:1605.
44. Marjot R, Valentine SJ. Arterial oxygen saturation following premedication for cardiac surgery. *Br J Anaesth* 1990;64:737.
45. Slogoff S, Keats AS. Does chronic treatment with calcium entry blocking drugs reduce perioperative myocardial ischemia? *Anesthesiology* 1988;68:676.
46. Chung F, Houston PL, Cheng DC, et al. Calcium channel blockade does not offer adequate protection from perioperative myocardial ischemia. *Anesthesiology* 1988;69:343.
47. Thompson IR, Mutch WA, Culligan JD. Failure of intravenous nitroglycerin to prevent intraoperative myocardial ischemia during fentanyl-pancuronium anesthesia. *Anesthesiology* 1984;61:385.
48. Gallagher JD, Moore RA, Jose AB. Prophylactic nitroglycerin infusions during coronary artery bypass surgery. *Anesthesiology* 1986;64:785.
49. Newman MF, Leslie JB, Maccioli GA, et al. Determination of optimal bolus esmolol for prevention of intraoperative hypertension and tachycardia. *Anesthesiology* 1989;71:285.
50. Maze M, Tranquilli W. Alpha-2 adrenoceptor agonists: defining the role in clinical anesthesia. *Anesthesiology* 1991;74:581.
51. Ghignone M, Quintin L, Duke PC, et al. Effects of clonidine on narcotic requirements and hemodynamic response during induction of fentanyl anesthesia and endotracheal intubation. *Anesthesiology* 1986;64:36.
52. Flacke JW, Bloor BC, Flacke WE, et al. Reduced narcotic requirement by clonidine with improved hemodynamic and adrenergic stability in patients undergoing coronary artery bypass surgery. *Anesthesiology* 1987;67:11.
53. London MJ, Hollenberg M, Wong MG, et al. Intraoperative myocardial ischemia: localization by continuous 12-lead electrocardiography. *Anesthesiology* 1988;69:232.
54. Mangano DT. Monitoring pulmonary arterial pressure in coronary artery surgery. *Anesthesiology* 1980;53:364.
55. Roizen MF, Berger DL, Gabel RA, et al. Practice guidelines for pulmonary artery catheterization. *Anesthesiology* 1993;78:380.
56. Bashein G, Johnson PW, Davis KB, et al. Elective coronary bypass surgery without pulmonary artery catheter monitoring. *Anesthesiology* 1985;63:451.
57. Tuman KJ, McCarthy RJ, Spiess BD, et al. Effect of pulmonary artery catheterization on outcome in patients undergoing coronary artery surgery. *Anesthesiology* 1989;70:199.
58. O'Connor JP, Townsend GE. Pro: perioperative continuous monitoring of mixed venous oxygen saturation should be routine during high-risk cardiac surgery. *J Cardiothorac Anesth* 1990;4:647.
59. Clements FM, de Bruijn NP. Perioperative evaluation of regional wall motion by transesophageal two-dimensional echocardiography. *Anesth Analg* 1987;66:249.
60. Leung JM, O'Kelly B, Browner WS, et al. Prognostic importance of postbypass regional wall motion abnormalities in patients undergoing CABG surgery. *Anesthesiology* 1989;71:16.
61. Shea MJ, Deanfield JE, Wilson R, et al. Transient ischemia in angina pectoris: frequent silent events with everyday activities. *Am J Cardiol* 1985;156:34E.
62. Epstein SE, Quyyumi AA, Bonow RO. Myocardial ischemia: silent or symptomatic. *N Engl J Med* 1988;318:1038.
63. Kloner RA, Przyklenk K, Patel B. Altered myocardial states: the stunned and hibernating myocardium. *Am J Med* 1989;86:14.
64. Slogoff S, Keats AS. Does perioperative myocardial ischemia lead to postoperative myocardial infarction? *Anesthesiology* 1985;62:107.
65. Slogoff S, Keats AS. Further observations on perioperative myocardial ischemia. *Anesthesiology* 1986;65:539.
66. Slogoff S, Keats AS. Randomized trial of primary anesthetic agents on outcome of coronary artery bypass operations. *Anesthesiology* 1989;70:179.
67. Slogoff S, Keats AS, David Y, et al. Incidence of perioperative myocardial ischemia detected by different electrocardiographic systems. *Anesthesiology* 1990;73:1074.
68. Knight AA, Hollenberg M, London MJ, et al. Perioperative myocardial ischemia: importance of the preoperative ischemic pattern. *Anesthesiology* 1988;68:681.
69. Buffington CW. Hemodynamics and myocardial ischemia. *Anesthesiology* Review 1990;17:11.
70. Buffington CW. Hemodynamic determinants of ischemic myocardial dysfunction in the presence of coronary stenosis in dogs. *Anesthesiology* 1985;63:651.
71. Reves JG, Sladen RN, Newman MF. Cardiac anesthetic: is it unique? *Anesth Analg* 1995;81:895.
72. Reves JG. Toward the goal of optimal cardiac anesthesia. *J Cardiothorac Vasc Anesth* 1999;13:1.
73. Theil DR, Stanley TEI, White WD, et al.. Midazolam and

fentanyl continuous infusion anesthesia for cardiac surgery: a comparison of computer-assisted versus manual infusion systems. *J Cardiothorac Vasc Anesth* 1993;7:300.

74. Bondy RJ, Wynands JE. Anesthesia induction and maintenance strategies. In: Estafanous F, Barash PG, Reves JG, eds. *Cardiac anesthesia: principles and clinical practice.* Philadelphia: JB Lippincott, 1994:221.
75. Shanewise JS, Hug CC Jr. Anesthesia for adult cardiac surgery. In: Miller R, ed. *Anesthesia,* 5th ed, vol 2. New York: Churchill Livingstone, 2000:1753.
76. Slogoff S, Keats AS, Dear WE, et al. Steal-prone coronary anatomy and myocardial ischemia associated with four primary anesthetic agents in humans. *Anesth Analg* 1991;72:22.
77. Wong KC. Narcotics are not expected to produce unconsciousness and amnesia. *Anesth Analg* 1983;62:625.
78. Hug CC. Does opioid "anesthesia" exist? *Anesthesiology* 1990; 73:1.
79. Sebel PS, Lang E, Rampil I, et al. A multi-center study of bispectral EEG analysis for monitoring anesthetic effect. *Anesth Analg* 1997;84:891.
80. Hughes MA, Glass PS, Jacobs JR. Context-sensitive half-time in multicompartment pharmacokinetic models for intravenous anesthetic drugs. *Anesthesiology* 1992;76:334.
81. Alvis JM, Reves JG, Govier AV, et al. Computer-assisted continuous infusions of fentanyl during cardiac anesthesia: comparison with a manual method. *Anesthesiology* 1985;63:41.
82. Glass PS, Shafer SL, Reves JG. Intravenous drug delivery. In: Miller R, ed. *Anesthesia,* 5th ed. New York: Churchill Livingstone, 2000:377.
83. Shafer SL, Varvel JR. Pharmacokinetics, pharmacodynamics and rational opioid selection. *Anesthesiology* 1991;74:53.
84. Mathews ET, Abrams LD. Intrathecal morphine in open heart surgery. Lancet 1980;2:543.
85. Fitzpatrick GJ, Moriarty DC. Intrathecal morphine in the management of pain following cardiac surgery. *Br J Anaesth* 1988; 60:639.
86. Casey WF, Wynands JE, Ralley FE, et al. The role of intrathecal morphine in the anesthetic management of patients undergoing coronary artery bypass surgery. *J Cardiothorac Anesth* 1987;1: 510.
87. El-Baz N, Goldin M. Continuous epidural infusion of morphine for pain relief after cardiac operations. *J Thorac Cardiovasc Surg* 1987;93:878.
88. Robinson RJ, Brister S, Jones E, et al. Epidural meperidine analgesia after cardiac surgery. *Can Anaesth Soc J* 1986;33:550.
89. Blomberg S, Emanuelson H, Kvist H, et al. Effects of thoracic epidural anesthesia on coronary arteries and arterioles in patients with coronary artery disease. *Anesthesiology* 1990;73:840.
90. Blomberg S, Emanuelson H, Ricksten S. Thoracic epidural anesthesia and central hemodynamics in patients with unstable angina pectoris. *Anesth Analg* 1989;69:558.
91. Argenziano M, Chen JM, Choudhri AF, et al. Management of vasodilatory shock after cardiac surgery: identification of predisposing factors and use of a novel pressor agent. *J Thorac Cardiovasc Surg* 1998;116:973.
92. Loeb HS, Saudye A, Croke RP, et al. Effects of pharmacologically induced hypertension on myocardial ischemia and coronary hemodynamics in patients with fixed coronary obstruction. *Circulation* 1978;57:41.
93. Reves JG, Croughwell ND, Hawkins E, et al. Esmolol for treatment of intraoperative tachycardia and/or hypertension in patients having cardiac operations. *J Thorac Cardiovasc Surg* 1990; 100:21.
94. Royster RL, Butterworth JF IV, Prough DS, et al. Perioperative and intraoperative predictors of inotropic support and long-term outcome in patients having coronary artery bypass grafting. *Anesth Analg* 1991;72:729.
95. Reves JG, Glass PSA, Jacobs JR. Alfentanil and midazolam: new anesthetic drugs for continuous infusion and an automated method of administration. *Mt Sinai J Med* 1989;56:99.
96. O'Connor JP, Ramsey JG, Wynands JE, et al. Anesthesia for myocardial revascularization. In: Kaplan J, ed. *Cardiac anesthesia,* 3rd ed. Philadelphia: WB Saunders Co, 1993:587.
97. Hug CC Jr, Shanewise JS. Anesthesia for adult cardiac surgery. In: Miller R, ed. *Anesthesia,* 4th ed. New York: Churchill-Livingstone, 1994:1757.
98. O'Connor JP, Ramsay JG, Wynands JE, et al. The incidence of myocardial ischemia during anesthesia for coronary artery bypass surgery in patients receiving pancuronium or vecuronium. *Anesthesiology* 1989;70:230.
99. Harrison L, Ralley FE, Wynands JE, et al. The role of an ultra short-acting adrenergic blocker (esmolol) in patients undergoing coronary artery bypass surgery. *Anesthesiology* 1987;66:413.
100. Litak CW, Ralley FE, Wynands JE, et al. Hemodynamic variables and the incidence of prebypass ischemia during sufentanil/ O_2/pancuronium anesthesia is patients undergoing coronary artery surgery. *J Cardiothorac Anesth* 1987;1:10.
101. Kotter GS, Kotrly KJ, Kalbfleisch JH, et al. Myocardial ischemia during cardiovascular surgery as detected by an ST segment trend monitoring system. *J Cardiothorac Anesth* 1987;1:190.
102. Sonntag H, Larsen R, Hilfiker O, et al. Myocardial blood flow and oxygen consumption during high-dose fentanyl anesthesia in patients with coronary artery disease. *Anesthesiology* 1982;56: 417.
103. Kleinman B, Henkin RE, Glisson SN, et al. Qualitative evaluation of coronary flow during anesthetic induction using thallium-201 perfusion scans. *Anesthesiology* 1986;64:157.
104. Bellows WH, Bode RH, Levy JH, et al. Noninvasive detection of peri-induction ischemic ventricular dysfunction by cardiokymography in humans: preliminary experience. *Anesthesiology* 1984;60:155.
105. Dorman BH. Ischemic heart disease. In: Miller RD, ed. *Atlas of Anesthesia,* vol VIII. Philadelphia: Churchill Livingstone, 1999: 4.1.

20

VALVULAR HEART DISEASE

PETER E. FRASCO
NORBERT P. DE BRUIJN

The perioperative management of patients with valvular heart disease is one of the more challenging tasks for anesthesiologists. Appropriate care begins with a thorough understanding of the etiology, clinical features, natural history, and pathophysiology of the specific valvular lesions. In an effort to approach the subject in a more useful fashion, we limit the discussion of the pathophysiology to "clinically important" information. In doing so, we present the reader with a baseline before presenting the anesthetic implications of the specific valvular lesions. We do not present a "recipe" approach to the anesthetic management of these disease processes. There are, unfortunately, few definitive studies that demonstrate the "best" anesthetic technique for patients with a specific valvular heart disease. Therefore, we highlight some of the aspects of anesthetic care as practiced by our group with the caveat that the choice of a particular agent is largely based on experience with that agent and that the important aspect of choosing anesthesia is not so much what the provider uses but how well he or she uses it. In addition, because we contend that the anesthesiologist must have a working knowledge of the surgical approach and technique in valve replacement or repair procedures, we highlight these aspects of operative care. Finally, because transesophageal echocardiography (TEE) is becoming more prevalent in the operating room, we present representative images depicting the various valvular lesions and appropriate adjuvant images.

DETERMINANTS OF MYOCARDIAL PERFORMANCE

Although anatomically the heart is a unit, the left and the right side of the heart function differently. The reduction of the right ventricular volume by a bellows action is obviously ideally suited to the ejection of large volumes against a low resistance, as is present in the pulmonary vasculature under normal conditions. The left ventricle, however, constricts primarily by contraction of the chamber with concentric inward motion of the ventricular walls and with very little shortening of the long axis (approximately 20%) (1). This chamber, by virtue of its thick wall and geometry, is therefore ideally suited to act as a pressure pump to eject blood against the relatively high resistance of the systemic circulation.

There are a number of terms and concepts that describe cardiac pump function and need further definition before specific valvular lesions are discussed. The determinants of cardiac output are (a) preload, (b) afterload, (c) contractility, and (d) heart rate. With the exception of heart rate, there has been much investigation and debate about the definitions of these variables. We limit the discussion to the most recent and "most acceptable" definitions.

Perhaps the most intuitively obvious, but least-understood, concept is contractility. If one reviews the literature, it rapidly becomes clear that there are as many definitions of contractility as there are authors (1–4). The concepts of dP/dt (the change in intraventricular pressure over time), E_{max} (5), and V_{max} (1,4) (the velocity contraction at zero force) have been used to measure and define the contractile state of the heart. To us, the following appears to be a reasonable working definition: Contractility is force developed during active myocardial contraction, independent of such extrinsic factors as preload or afterload. The problem has been to find a measurable parameter that is truly independent of the loading conditions of the ventricle (see later discussion). Contractility should not be confused with pump function, which describes the interaction of contractility, preload, and afterload.

Afterload is the load against which the ventricle must eject blood during systole and is best described as the force (or stress) per cross-sectional area in the ventricular wall during systole (6). This relationship, as it pertains to the sphere, is described by the law of Laplace:

$$\text{stress } (\Sigma) = P \times r/2h \qquad [20\text{-}1]$$

where P is ventricular transmural pressure, r is the ventricular radius (it is assumed in this model that the ventricle is

P. E. Frasco: Department of Anesthesiology, Mayo Clinic Scottsdale, Scottsdale, Arizona 85259
N. P. de Bruijn: Department of Anesthesiology, Duke University Medical Center, Durham, North Carolina 27710

a sphere, which is a modest oversimplification), and h is ventricular wall thickness. Obviously, the parameters that determine ventricular wall stress vary during the cardiac cycle; thus, afterload is not a static phenomenon, as suggested by the use of systemic (or pulmonary) vascular resistance.

Although there is much misunderstanding of the concept of preload, it is a simpler concept than afterload, and the misperceptions are mainly due to our inability to measure it accurately in the clinical setting.

The Frank-Starling relationship (i.e., within physiologic limits, stroke work is directly proportional to end-diastolic volume) defines preload as the initial myocardial fiber length. Clinically, end-diastolic pressure or pulmonary capillary wedge pressure (CPWP) is often used to approximate initial fiber length. These measurements, although related to initial myocardial fiber length, are dependent on the compliance of the ventricle. Disease processes such as hypertension, aortic stenosis, and hypertrophic cardiomyopathy decrease ventricular compliance, whereas aortic regurgitation may result in an increase in chamber compliance. End-diastolic volume represents a more accurate estimate of initial fiber length, but even this concept is based on many simplifications, including the conceptualization of the chamber as a sphere. If we examine the relationship between left ventricular end-diastolic pressure (LVEDP) and left ventricular end-diastolic volume (LVEDV), which is not linear, it is understandable that using pressures as a representation of initial fiber length is often invalid. However, in the absence of alternatives (see later discussion), measurement of filling pressures may be the only estimate of preload in certain clinical circumstances.

The introduction of echocardiography into the operating room represents a step forward in the monitoring of ventricular volume by allowing us to observe ventricular area changes.

The changing relationship between filling pressures and volume can frequently be observed in the operating room after discontinuation of cardiopulmonary bypass. In that procedure, large increases in pulmonary artery pressure may be accompanied by very small changes in left ventricular area because of the decreased compliance of the ventricle secondary to hypothermic cardiopulmonary bypass.

Myocardial ischemia and left ventricular hypertrophy are examples of commonly encountered states that may cause dysfunction of active relaxation and passive relaxation, respectively. Left ventricular diastolic function, partly an energy-dependent process and partly a passive function of the physical properties of the ventricular wall, is frequently affected by cardiac disease. The slope of the diastolic pressure-volume relationship, the change in ventricular volume per unit pressure change, represents ventricular compliance (Fig. 20-1).

Intraoperative echocardiography has brought a rough assessment of ventricular compliance to the clinical arena.

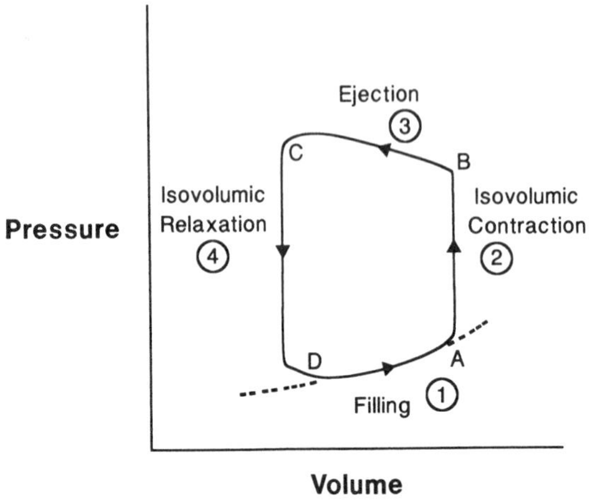

FIGURE 20-1. Pressure-volume relationship of a left ventricular contraction.

For the purpose of orientation to the function of the healthy heart, a description of the pressure-volume relationship in the left ventricle during each contraction cycle is useful (7,8). We limit ourselves to discussion of the left ventricular pressure-volume relationship, because it is better described than the right ventricular relation, mainly because the right ventricular geometry is complex and difficult to study.

Figure 20-1 shows a diagrammatic representation of the instantaneous left ventricular pressure-volume loop. Phase 1 represents diastolic filling of the left ventricle, which in itself consists of multiple phases. There is an initial passive rapid inflow of blood in early diastole as the mitral valve opens, which is followed by a phase of diminished filling (diastasis) and finally the contribution from active left atrial contraction, to reach point A (LVEDP and LVEDV). From this point, phase 2 (isovolemic contraction) begins, in which a steep rise in pressure is accompanied by only a minimal decrease in volume until the aortic valve opens at point B. At point B, left ventricular and aortic pressures are equal and blood enters the aorta, initiating phase 3 (the ejection phase). At point C, the end-systolic pressure-volume point, the aortic valve closes, ejection ceases, and phase 4 (isovolemic relaxation) begins. During this phase, there is little change in ventricular volume until the pressure falls below the left atrial pressure, point D, and the mitral valve opens again to start the next cycle. The area described by this loop represents left ventricular stroke work.

Many authors have examined the pressure-volume relationship both in animal models and in humans (9–11). One can examine the ventricle at various end-diastolic volumes (altering preload) while occluding the aorta (acute increase in afterload) so the ventricle can develop pressure but not eject blood (isovolemic pressure). The isovolemic pressures developed at each end-diastolic volume tend to form a straight line, the isovolemic pressure line (12).

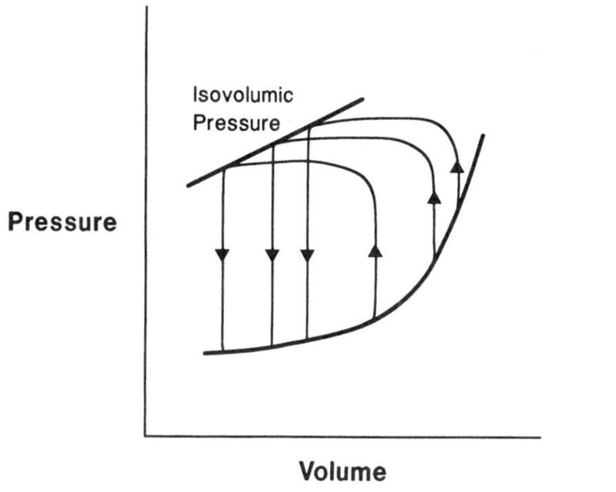

FIGURE 20-2. A series of pressure-volume loops illustrating the isovolumic pressure line.

In Fig. 20-2, the relationship between the isovolemic pressure line and the ejecting heart is shown: A series of contractions are shown at different end-diastolic volumes and arterial pressures (8). They illustrate that the end point of systolic contraction tends to approximate closely the isovolemic pressure line, independent of the initial end-diastolic volume (preload) and the aortic pressure, against which the heart is working (afterload), hence its description as a "load-independent" measure of contractility.

An increase in myocardial contractility, for example, by administration of a positive inotropic agent, shifts the isovolemic pressure line upward and to the left while the intercept of the line with the volume axis remains almost the same (Fig. 20-3) (9). Examination of Fig. 20-3 demonstrates that an increase in stroke volume can be produced at the same initial end-diastolic pressure (preload) and arterial pressure (afterload) (9). This end-systolic pressure-volume relationship has been postulated as a "pure" representation of the ventricular contractile state, because it is thought to be largely independent of the loading conditions of the ventricle. Recent investigations have demonstrated that the end-systolic pressure-volume relationship may not be as independent of preload and afterload as was initially thought (8,13).

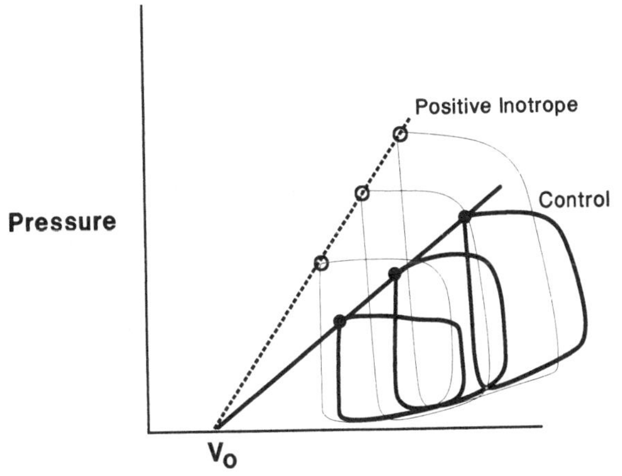

FIGURE 20-3. The effect of a positive inotropic intervention on the pressure-volume relationship.

Thinking about pressure-volume loops is useful in developing an understanding of the mechanical factors that determine ventricular performance and the interactions with pharmacologic agents in the perioperative care of patients with valvular heart disease.

DISEASES OF THE AORTIC VALVE

Aortic Valve

The aortic valve is situated between the left ventricle and the aorta and lies superior and anterior to the mitral valve. It consists of three fibrous semilunar leaflets that arise from the sinuses of Valsalva: the posterior or left coronary cusp (beneath the ostium of the left main coronary ostium), the anterior or the right coronary cusp (beneath the ostium of the right coronary artery), and the noncoronary leaflet.

Unlike the mitral and tricuspid valves, the aortic valve does not have a fibrous ring surrounding the valve leaflets and is thus supported by the base of the left ventricle and the aorta. The normal valve functions to prevent regurgitation from the aorta to the left ventricle by coaptation at the leaflet commissure during diastole.

The normal valve orifice area during systole is 2.1 to 3.6 cm^2 (14). In the absence of aortic stenosis or other obstruction to ejection, there is no measurable gradient between the left ventricle and the aorta.

Aortic Stenosis

Etiology

The most common causes of isolated aortic stenosis are calcification of congenital valve abnormalities (bicuspid and unicuspid valves), degenerative calcification of "normal" tricuspid valves, and isolated rheumatic disease of the valve (14–17). However, isolated aortic valve stenosis secondary to rheumatic disease is responsible for no more than 6% of all cases (15,16). There is a direct relationship between the number of cusps and the onset of significant stenosis: Patients with unicuspid valves develop stenosis sooner than patients with bicuspid valves (14,16). In addition, there may be a difference in the natural history of adults with the principal types of aortic stenosis, more rapid progression of obstruction being found in the degenerative calcific type than in the rheumatic or congenital types (14,16).

Clinical Features

Like many other valvular lesions, aortic stenosis is characterized by a relatively long asymptomatic period with a mean age of presentation of 63 years (18). The onset of any of the classic symptoms of angina, syncope, and congestive heart failure is associated with reduced survival rates (16, 19–21). The average duration of life after the onset of angina or syncope is approximately 3 years and of congestive heart failure, 1 to 2 years (14,19). The most common cause of mortality is sudden death; the next most common causes are congestive heart failure and bacterial endocarditis (14). It is rare for symptoms to develop before the valve area is reduced to 1 cm^2; however, some patients may tolerate an orifice area of 0.5 cm^2 without symptoms (14,16). Controversy surrounds the issue of whether patients with hemodynamically significant but asymptomatic aortic stenosis are best managed by surgical intervention (20,21). Specific criteria vary, but commonly referenced parameters cited as indications for operation are a valve area of less than 0.7 cm^2 and a peak systolic gradient of more than 50 mm Hg (14,16,19,22–26). It is apparent that the risk of sudden death is much greater in symptomatic patients, compared with those without symptoms (20,21,25). A recent study has demonstrated no difference in survival rates between asymptomatic patients with hemodynamically significant aortic stenosis undergoing aortic valve replacement or valvuloplasty and those patients with statistically similar degrees of aortic stenosis managed medically (20).

The physical examination for patients with aortic stenosis is notable for delayed upstroke of the carotid pulses and narrowed pulse pressure. Often, a prominent presystolic impulse at the apex is palpable. On auscultation, there is usually a normal S_1 followed by a systolic ejection click. The mid-systolic murmur of aortic stenosis is harsh and low pitched, and it is often described as "crescendo-decrescendo" or diamond shaped (27). The murmur is best heard at the right second intercostal space and along the left sternal border and may radiate to the carotids, but not to the axilla (14). The aortic component of the second heart sound may be delayed and diminished or absent in severe aortic stenosis (16,27).

Electrocardiographic (ECG) atrioventricular signs common in patients with aortic stenosis include left ventricular hypertrophy and atrioventricular and intraventricular conduction delays (14,16,19,27,28). ECG signs of left atrial enlargement and atrial fibrillation may suggest associated mitral valve disease.

Accurate assessment of patients with aortic stenosis has become possible with the advent of Doppler and two-dimensional (2D) echocardiography (29,30). These noninvasive techniques have assumed a major role in the timing of surgical treatment of aortic stenosis. 2D long-axis and short-axis views can provide clear definition of aortic valve structure and function. Differentiation among unicuspid, bicuspid, and tricuspid valves is possible. In addition, characterization of cusp mobility is possible. Doppler echocardiography and color flow mapping studies allow characterization of the hemodynamic abnormalities associated with aortic stenosis. Catheterization of patients with aortic stenosis is now performed in those patients with "echo-proven" aortic stenosis to determine whether the degree of stenosis is sufficient to produce the symptoms of angina, syncope, or congestive heart failure (23,30). In addition, because angina may occur in patients with aortic stenosis in the absence of coronary artery disease, catheterization is necessary to assess the contribution of coronary artery disease to the symptoms (23,31). The valve area can be calculated by the Gorlin formula (25,32).

$$\text{valve area} = \frac{\text{aortic valve flow (cm}^3\text{)/min)}}{44.5 \times (\text{mean pressure gradient [cm/sec]})^{-2}} \quad [20\text{-}2]$$

In the presence of low aortic flow (low cardiac output), valve area may be critically low despite a small pressure gradient. If the valve area decreases by a factor of two, then in the absence of a change in aortic flow, the transvalvular gradient must increase by a factor of four (32).

Pathophysiology

The dominant feature in the pathophysiology of aortic stenosis is obstruction to left ventricular ejection, which causes both a pressure overload on the left ventricle and a pressure gradient between the ventricle and the aorta. As the obstruction becomes more severe, the pressure gradient between the aorta and the left ventricle must increase to maintain forward flow. In addition, the systolic ejection interval increases, which helps to maintain flow across the stenosis. Wall stress (force per unit area), proportional to the radius of the chamber and the intraventricular pressure, but inversely proportional to the wall thickness, increases with outflow obstruction because of the dramatic increase in pressure. Systolic shortening decreases, end-systolic volume increases, and stroke volume must fall unless end-diastolic volume increases. Because it can take many years for the obstruction to become severe, the left ventricle can hypertrophy to compensate for the pressure overload. Concentric ventricular hypertrophy functions to maintain systolic wall stress at normal levels (wall thickness increases and chamber radius decreases or does not change). Thus, even in the presence of increased intraventricular pressure, stroke volume can be maintained as long as preload is adequate (16,33,34). However, this hypertrophy also causes decreased diastolic compliance (secondary to an increase in muscle mass and possibly an increase in muscle stiffness due to interstitial fibrosis), impaired myocardial oxygen balance, and eventually myocardial failure (25,35–37). It is this hypertrophy in response to the outflow obstruction, rather than the obstruction it-

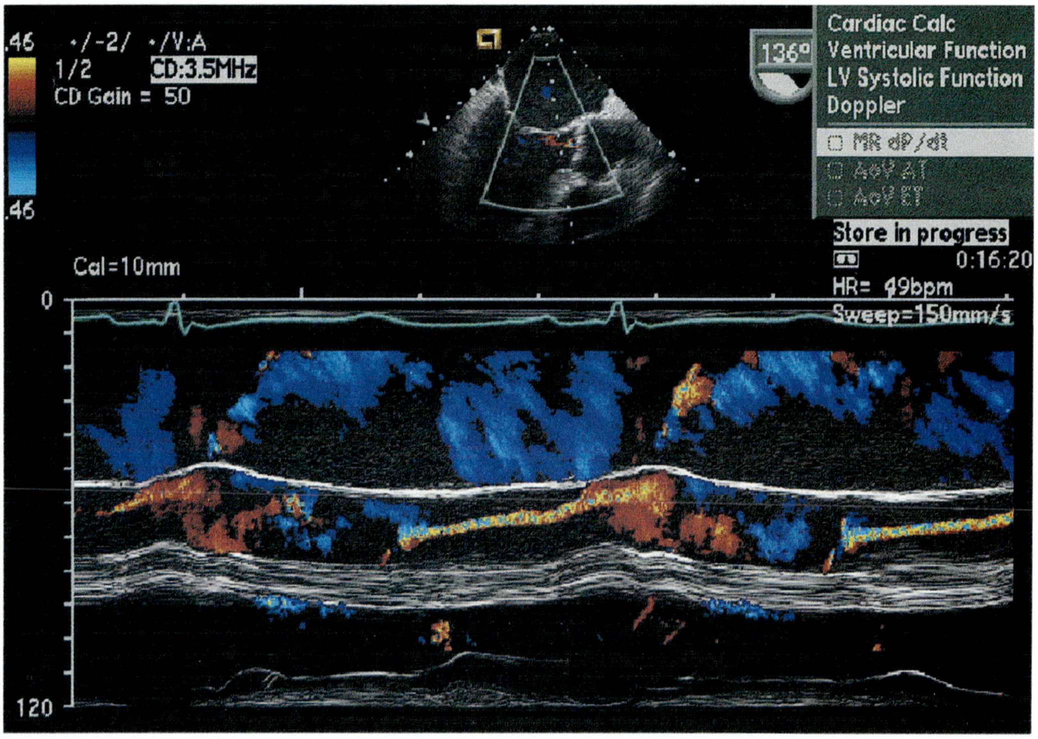

COLOR FIGURE 9-18. Color-M mode is extremely useful for timing of flow in the left ventricle outflow tract.

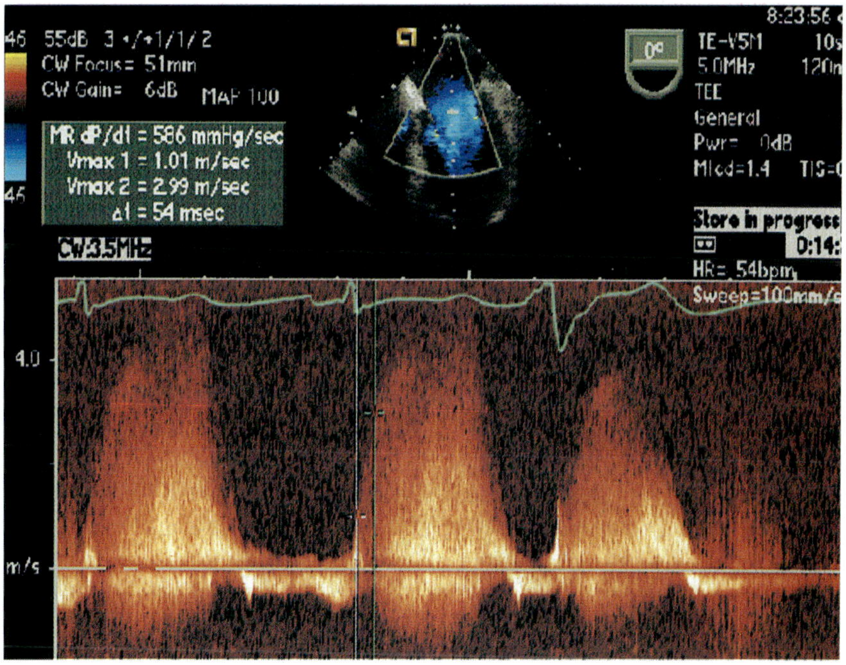

COLOR FIGURE 9-23. Dp/dt (change in pressure per change of time) is a load dependent index of contractility which may be calculated utilizing continuous wave Doppler interrogation of the mitral regurgitant jet.

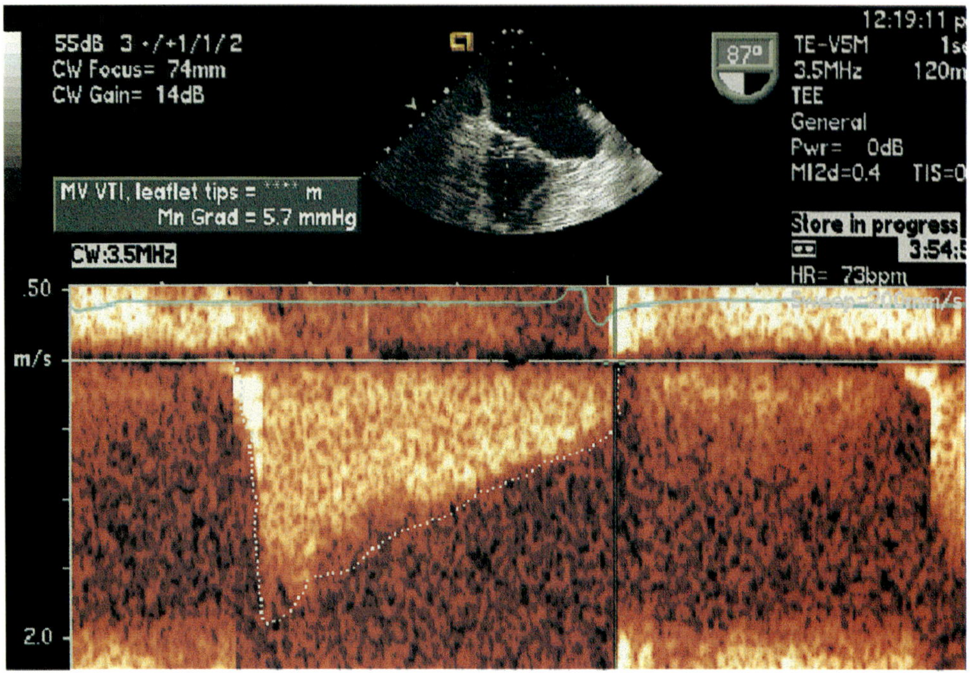

COLOR FIGURE 9-25. Continuous wave Doppler interrogation of the mitral inflow provides the mean gradient between the left atrium and ventricle.

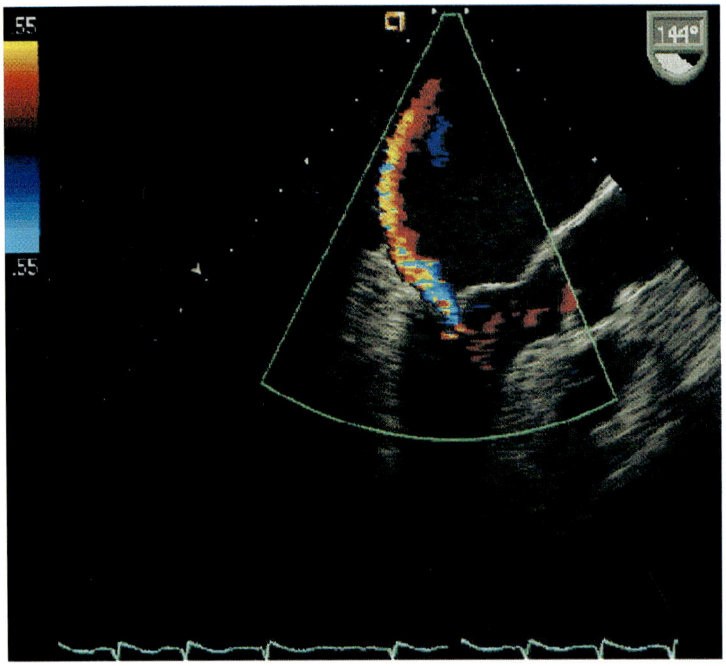

COLOR FIGURE 9-28. An eccentric mitral regurgitant jet hugs the left atrial wall (Coanda effect) leading to an underestimation of the severity of mitral regurgitation.

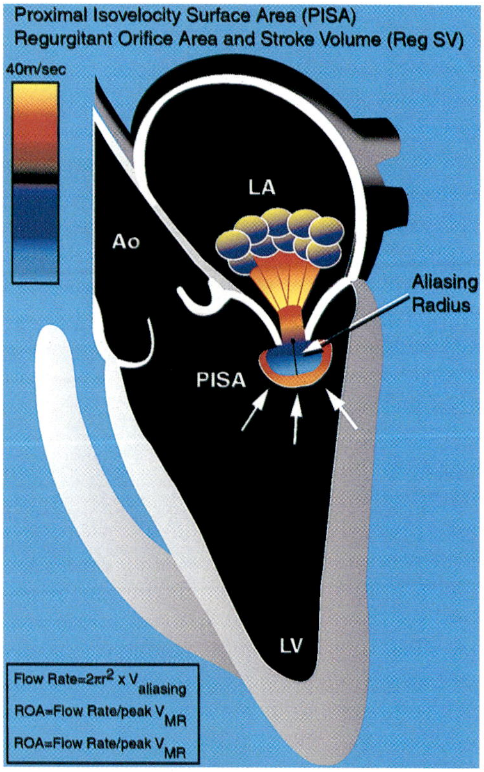

COLOR FIGURE 9-29. Proximal isovelocity surface area calculation of mitral regurgitation severity.

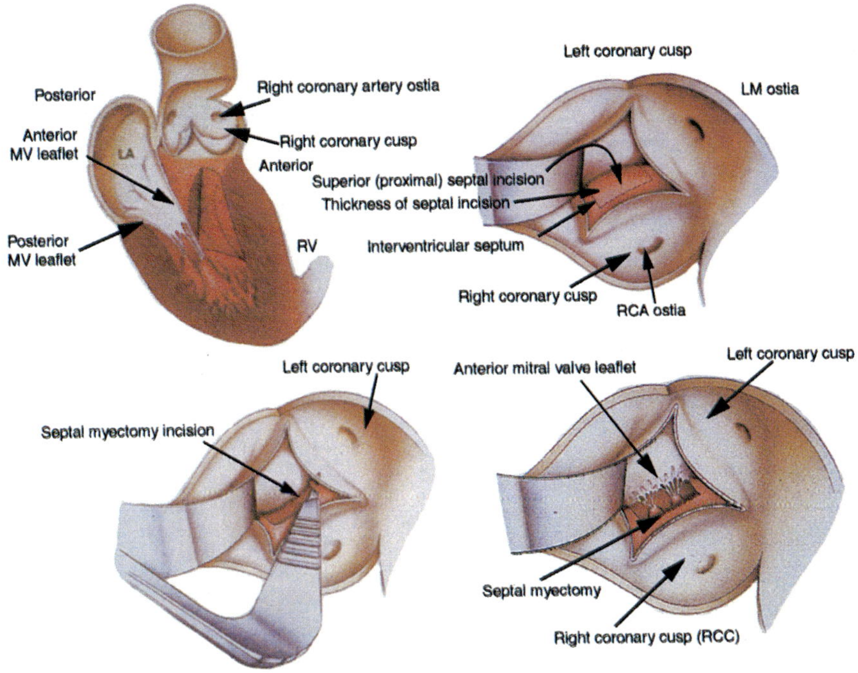

COLOR FIGURE 9-33. Surgical incisions involved in myectomy for hypertrophic obstructive cardiomyopathy (HOCM).

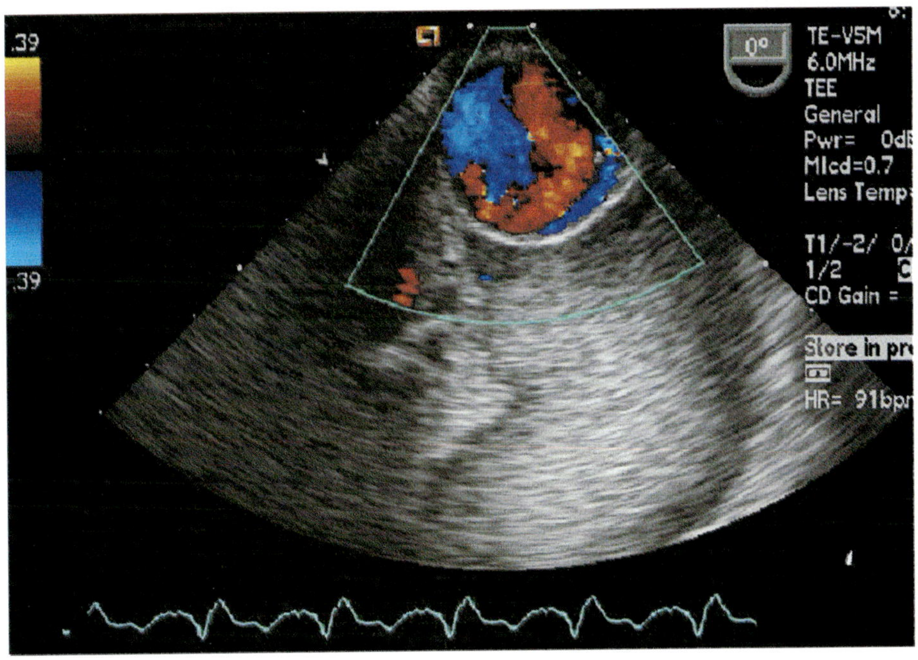

COLOR FIGURE 9-36. Color flow Doppler of the descending aorta.

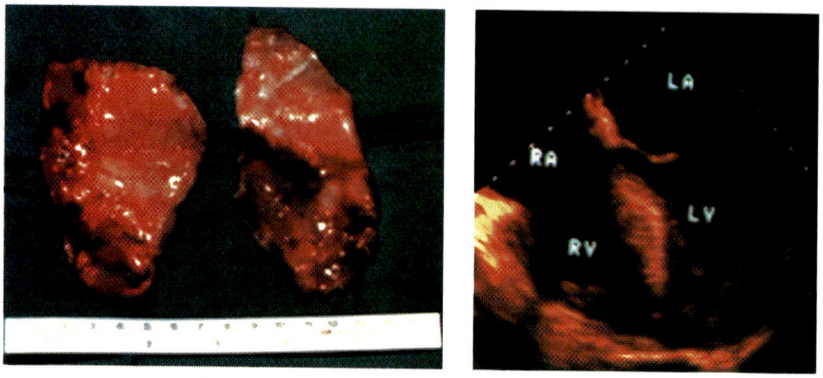

COLOR FIGURE 9-37. Heart is encased in a fibrotic and often calcified peal in patients with constrictive pericarditis.

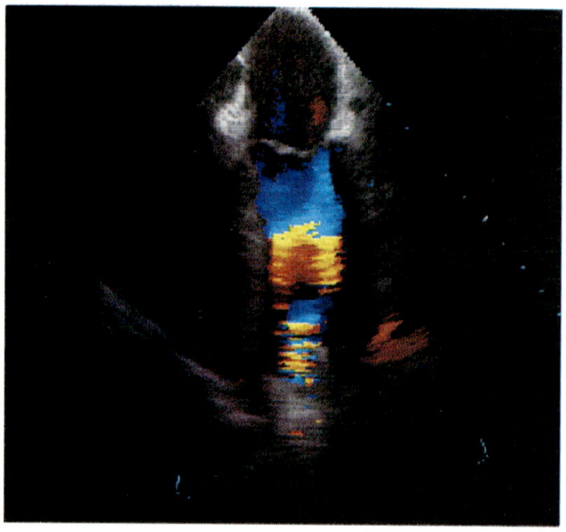

COLOR FIGURE 9-38 (right panel). Left ventricular assist device inflow cannula. (See left and right panels of Fig. 9.38 in black and white.)

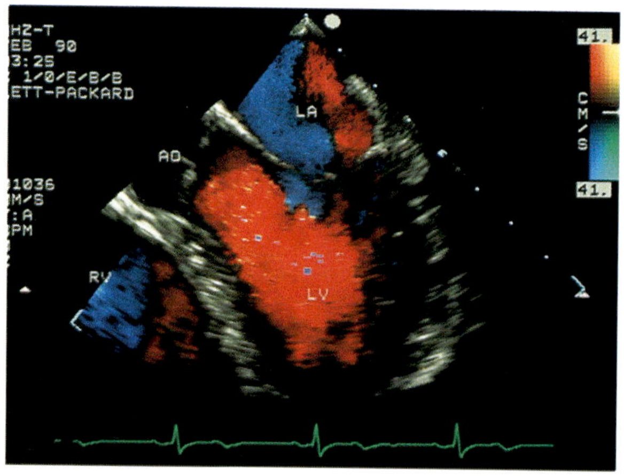

COLOR FIGURE 20-6. Two-dimensional transesophageal echocardiogram. The mitral valve is closed. Blood flow out of the left ventricle outflow tract can be observed. (LA, left atrium; LV, left ventricle; AO, aorta; RV, right ventricle.)

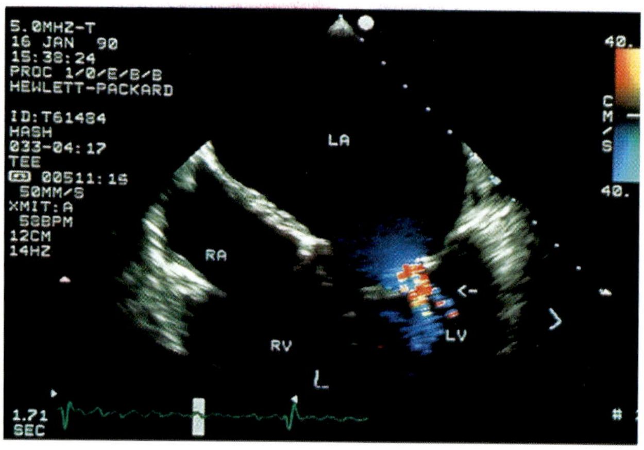

COLOR FIGURE 20-7B. With Doppler color flow mapping in the same patient as in A, a stenotic jet can be appreciated as a mosaic pattern distal to the mitral orifice during diastole.

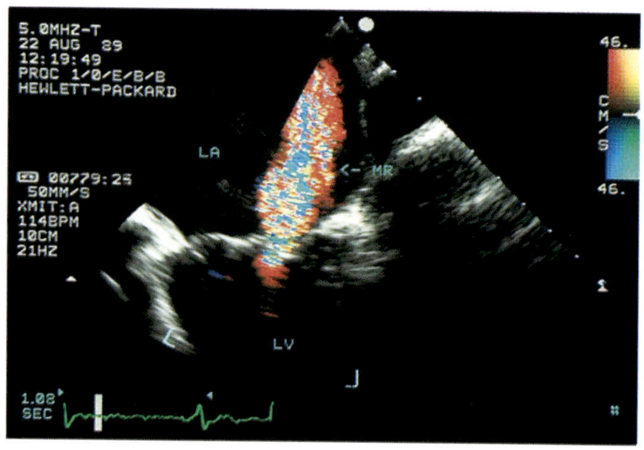

COLOR FIGURE 20-8. A close-up view of the mitral valve with a large systolic jet back into the left atrium, representing severe mitral regurgitation (*MR*). (LA, left atrium; LV, left ventricle.)

self, that is responsible for most of the symptoms seen in aortic stenosis.

Angina in patients with aortic stenosis frequently occurs in the absence of coronary artery disease. In the past, aortic stenosis was thought to be protective in the development of coronary artery disease (17). In fact, the prevalence of coronary artery disease in patients with aortic stenosis is no different from that in the general population (13). It is well known that angina, a symptomatic expression of myocardial ischemia, is reflective of inadequate myocardial oxygen supply relative to demand. In patients with aortic stenosis, myocardial ischemia may occur because of both inadequate supply and increased demand.

The hypertrophy that occurs in response to aortic outflow obstruction normalizes wall stress, which tends to preserve myocardial performance but may also cause a relative imbalance of myocardial oxygen supply and demand. The resting blood flow and myocardial oxygen consumption of the hypertrophic heart are proportionally normal for unit mass of heart muscle, but because myocardial mass is increased, global consumption is increased (37–39). In addition, the energy consumption for pressure work (isovolemic contraction) is proportionally greater than that needed for volume work (ejection) (40). The hypertrophic heart in aortic stenosis expends an increased fraction of energy in the development of the "additional" intraventricular pressure necessary to overcome the obstruction at the valvular level.

The left ventricular hypertrophy may also impair the myocardial blood supply. In response to hypertrophy, the epicardial vessels increase in cross-sectional area, but this increase is less than what is expected in proportion to the increase in myocardial mass (14,37,41). The myocyte-to-capillary ratio and intramyocyte distance increase in response to hypertrophy, which may result in increased susceptibility to ischemia (42). The hypertrophy may also cause a decrease in the coronary flow reserve (37,43). It has been shown that the resting myocardial blood flow in hypertrophic hearts secondary to outflow obstruction is near maximal. The absolute maximum level of coronary blood flow and coronary vascular resistance in patients with aortic stenosis in response to exertion is not statistically different from that in normal controls (39,43). Thus, a large fraction of coronary flow reserve is necessary to meet the demands of the hypertrophic heart, and during periods of increased demand, the normal response of increased flow does not occur (37,43). The combination of elevated LVEDP secondary to the hypertrophy-induced decrease in compliance and the lower diastolic aortic pressures results in a relative lowering of the diastolic coronary perfusion pressure (39, 43). In addition, because the systolic intraventricular pressure exceeds the aortic systolic pressure, any systolic coronary perfusion is greatly impaired. There is an abnormal flow pattern in the hypertrophic heart (38). The subendocardial-to-subepicardial flow ratio at rest favors subendocardial flow and normally increases during stress. In animal models of ventricular hypertrophy caused by aortic banding, this ratio actually decreases, thus making the subendocardium prone to ischemia (44).

The syncopal episodes that may accompany aortic stenosis generally occur while ventricular function is "normal," i.e., in the absence of frank ventricular failure. Symptoms occur during exertion or immediately after exertion. This syncope is probably not due to a low-output state, because it would be expected that during periods of low output, flow to the vital organs would be maintained. In fact, many patients with aortic stenosis have normal increases in cardiac output during exercise (33). It is also unlikely that dysrhythmias are the etiology of syncope. It is more likely that syncope in patients with aortic stenosis is the result of acute vascular dilation secondary to abrupt changes in the left ventricular systolic pressure. This baroreceptor response causes a decrease (instead of the normal increase) in the systemic vascular resistance in the nonexercising vascular beds, which when coupled to the normal decrease in systemic vascular resistance in the exercising muscle beds, leads to a profound level of vasodilation (16,33).

The myocardial hypertrophy affects both systolic (ejection) and diastolic (filling) functions. The importance of diastolic function lies in the development of adequate ventricular filling pressure and volume to sustain normal stroke volume. Therefore, diastolic dysfunction can be viewed as the inability to fill the ventricle without an increase in left atrial pressure. Ventricular diastole is composed of the rapid early filling phase (75%) and the late atrial contraction (25%). With hypertrophy, the ventricle stiffens and diastolic compliance decreases, leading to delayed ventricular relaxation (35) and delayed left ventricular filling (45,47) without an increase in left atrial pressure. As the hypertrophy becomes more severe, enhanced atrial contraction is necessary to compensate for the decreased compliance of the ventricle. In the later stages of the disease, the enhanced atrial contraction fails and cardiac output falls, unless left atrial pressure increases. Thus, unlike syncope and angina, the development of dyspnea may herald the onset of impaired contractility (14,33). However, in many cases, the signs and symptoms of heart failure represent what physiologists have termed "afterload mismatch," or hypertrophic response inadequate to generate adequate force to compensate for the increased left ventricular systolic pressure created by the stenosis (33,47). In this situation, the increased systolic pressure exceeds the decrease in the chamber radius-to-thickness ratio (*r:h*) that occurs in hypertrophy—wall stress increases and shortening decreases (48,49). Increased filling pressures are required to sustain cardiac output. The ventricle expands and the chamber dilates. Wall stress increases further, causing additional decreases in fiber shortening that ultimately lead to decreased cardiac output. In the later stages of the disease process, ventricular failure occurs because of frank myocardial damage and decreases in contractility. It is unclear whether these changes in ventricular performance regress after valve replacement surgery (34, 50–52). However, in patients with heart failure due to afterload mismatch, the hypertrophy may regress to within 20% of normal after successful valve replacement surgery (34,52).

Anesthetic Implications

It is clear that maintenance of cardiac output, avoidance of hypotension, prevention of ischemia, and control of autonomic responses to surgical stimulation are anesthetic goals for all patients undergoing surgery. In patients with valvular heart disease, these goals are both vitally important and at times difficult to achieve.

In general, patients with preserved left ventricular function will tolerate a heavy premedication before valve replacement surgery. Methadone with lorazepam is an effective oral combination. Large-bore intravenous access and arterial cannulation are requirements before surgery. Placement of a central venous introducer via the jugular vein is recommended in all patients. The necessity of pulmonary artery catheterization is debatable and depends on ventricular function, institutional bias, surgical preference, and nursing care in the postoperative care unit. The central venous (right atrial) pressure often underestimates the LVEDP because of the change in contractility that is associated with left ventricular hypertrophy. In addition, the PCWP may underestimate the LVEDP. Induction and maintenance of anesthesia can be achieved with continuous infusion of the lipophilic narcotics (fentanyl and sufentanil) with or without continuous infusion of midazolam, with the caveat that this combination may cause a decrease in systemic vascular resistance and subsequent hypotension (53). High-dose fentanyl techniques (50 to 75 mg/kg) may circumvent this problem but may require vasodilator therapy or supplemental anesthesia for breakthrough hypertension during sternotomy, sternal retraction, and aortic manipulation (54). Sufentanil in doses of 10 to 15 mg/kg may be a more complete anesthetic than fentanyl (55) and has been shown to decrease the requirement for the supplemental measures during the periods of peak stimulation listed previously. Choice of neuromuscular blocking agent largely depends on the resting heart rate and the expected change with induction of anesthesia (56). In the presence of β-blockade, the combination of vecuronium and fentanyl or sufentanil may lead to bradycardia. Pancuronium may be a better choice in these situations.

In patients with aortic stenosis, maintenance of sinus rhythm is particularly important. Because of the decreased compliance and increased chamber stiffness caused by the concentric hypertrophy, these patients are often dependent on the left atrial contribution to ventricular filling. The normal contribution of this atrial "kick" is approximately 20% of the diastolic filling. In patients with advanced cases of aortic stenosis, this may increase to 40% (33,36). Thus, supraventricular dysrhythmias, particularly atrial fibrillation and flutter, can cause dramatic reductions in cardiac output. These supraventricular dysrhythmias should be treated aggressively with synchronized DC cardioversion.

Patients with aortic stenosis are generally intolerant to extremes of heart rate. Tachycardia is potentially disastrous, because it may precipitate myocardial ischemia. Detection of ischemia may be difficult in these patients because of the ventricular hypertrophy and strain pattern often encountered with aortic stenosis. In addition, the hypertrophy can cause electrical instability, which may predispose the patient to ventricular ectopy. Low heart rates may not be tolerated well in patients with aortic stenosis, because stroke volume may be limited due to the fixed obstruction; thus, cardiac output may be "rate dependent." Therefore, it is preferable to maintain sinus rhythm at a ventricular rate of 60 to 80 beats/minute.

The concentric hypertrophy secondary to aortic stenosis induces a decrease in the compliance of the left ventricle. In addition, LVEDP and LVEDV are often increased (33, 36). The combination of these factors makes adequate preload essential to maintain output. The optimal level of preload may be difficult to predict in patients with a failing ventricle, because the ventricular function curve in these cases may be relatively flat. The central venous pressure is not an accurate measure of left ventricular filling, and therefore even with the risk of catheter-induced dysrhythmias, the pulmonary artery catheter may be an essential monitor of ventricular filling in patients with moderate to severe aortic stenosis who are undergoing surgical procedures associated with large intravascular volume shifts. However, the PCWP may underestimate the LVEDP, particularly in the poorly compliant ventricle.

Contractility is often maintained in the normal to supranormal range, except in advanced cases of aortic stenosis. In general, patients with advanced aortic stenosis may be intolerant to reductions in contractility as caused by β-adrenergic blockade. However, in the case of tachycardia, ischemia, and congenital heart failure in patients with aortic stenosis, β-blockade may improve ischemia, improve diastolic relaxation, and decrease filling pressures.

As previously noted, the hypertrophy that occurs in association with aortic stenosis may lead to a decrease in myocardial capillary reserve and to impaired subendocardial blood flow (17,37–39). The hypertrophy may also mask the ECG signs of myocardial ischemia. These factors, in combination with increased wall tension in the subendocardium compared with other regions, makes the subendocardium particularly prone to ischemia during hypotension. Any treatment of hypotension or tachycardia in patients with valvular heart disease, including aortic stenosis, must strike a balance between the hemodynamic consequences of the disease process and the need for coronary blood flow. Appropriate measures for the treatment of hypotension include volume, use of the Trendelenburg position, and small doses of α-adrenergic agonists such as phenylephrine (50 to 100 mg). Agents such as ephedrine may cause undue tachycardia, which as described, can be particularly dangerous in patients with aortic stenosis.

Afterload in patients with moderate to severe aortic stenosis is "fixed," caused by the obstruction at the valve itself. Further reductions in afterload, as caused by arterial vasodilators distal to the stenosis, do not improve cardiac output (35). This fact has led to the avoidance of major conduction anesthesia for noncardiac surgery in patients with aortic stenosis. In addition, the venodilation caused by spinal and epidural anesthesia reduces effective preload with a resultant reduction in cardiac output and hypotension. However, spinal and epidural anesthesia may be used in these patients in the appropriate surgical setting, provided that preload is effectively monitored and maintained. Epidural techniques may be preferable to spinal techniques because of the slower onset of sympathetic blockade in the former. In addition, any hypotension that occurs must be aggressively treated to prevent ischemia and/or failure.

Surgical Technique and Perioperative Problems

The aortic valve is approached via a median sternotomy. Aortic cannulation is followed by venous cannulation using either a single dual-stage or two single-stage cannulas (14). Cardiopulmonary bypass is instituted with an initial inflow temperature of 32°C to 34°C. Because cardioplegia can be difficult in these patients as a result of the concentric hypertrophy and the concomitant aortic insufficiency that often accompany the stenotic lesion, preparation is often made to deliver cardioplegic solution either directly into the coronary ostia or retrograde via the coronary sinus, in case antegrade aortic root needle delivery is inadequate (16). In general, the surgery is performed without a vent, but in cases in which the aortic valve is insufficient as well as stenotic, a vent may be placed from the left atrium through the mitral valve into the left ventricle (14). Inflow temperature is decreased to 25°C to 28°C after aortic cross-clamping and cardioplegic arrest. Protection of the myocardium in the severely hypertrophic ventricle can be difficult to accomplish. A transverse aortotomy is performed, avoiding the origin of the right coronary artery.

The diseased valve is resected by incising each leaflet away and parallel to its origin at the annulus; calcific matter in the annulus is excised. The presence of this calcium can make this part of the procedure very demanding. The prosthetic valve is then implanted by means of subanular or supraanular pledgeted sutures. The important issues in the choice of the prosthetic valve are discussed in Appendix 20-1.

After valve replacement and hypothermic cardiopulmonary bypass, the reduction in the transvalvular gradient, in general, will lead to reduction of end-systolic volume and therefore increased ejection fraction and cardiac output (16, 50). Vasodilator therapy can improve cardiac output in patients with increased afterload after cardiopulmonary bypass. Systolic dysfunction may exist before cardiopulmonary bypass or may be induced because of inadequate myocardial protection during cardiopulmonary bypass (16). In either case, inotropic drugs such as epinephrine, dobutamine, and dopamine may be used after cardiopulmonary bypass to augment stroke volume and cardiac output.

There is regression of the concentric hypertrophy in the first year after aortic valve replacement (34,36,52). However, in the immediate postoperative period, the ventricular compliance characteristics are essentially unchanged from those in the preoperative state. Therefore, the hemodynamic principles discussed previously (maintenance of adequate preload, sinus rhythm, and heart rate in the range of 60 to 90 beats/minute) apply in the immediate convalescent period.

In patients with preserved preoperative left ventricular function, hypertension after valve replacement is common because of the removal of the fixed obstruction. Vasodilators such as sodium nitroprusside and β-adrenergic blocking agents such as labetalol can be effective in treating this increase in blood pressure.

Early mortality rates, typically subsequent to arrhythmias secondary to left ventricular hypertrophy or congestive heart failure, vary from 3% to 6% (16,32,34,57,58). Mortality rate is increased with advanced age, in patients with New York Heart Association (NYHA) class IV symptoms, and in patients undergoing simultaneous mitral valve replacement and/or coronary artery bypass grafting (32,34). Regression of hypertrophy occurs in nearly all patients with normal preoperative left ventricular function (16,37–39). Reduction in left ventricular mass also occurs in many patients with left ventricular dysfunction secondary to afterload mismatch (14). However, in patients with reduced contractile function, hypertrophy rarely regresses and global ventricular function may worsen with time (14,16).

Transesophageal Echocardiographic Images

The aortic valve can be well visualized in the cross-sectional (short-axis) view using 2D echocardiography. The 2D image should be examined to view the three valve cusps that form the familiar Mercedes-Benz sign (Fig. 20-4). The cusps should be thin and should coapt during diastole. During systole, these cusps should open to the periphery of the aortic opening. Occasionally, the right or left coronary cusp can be seen to prolapse into the left ventricular outflow tract. Calcium deposits of the valve appear as bright echoes and are usually associated with valve thickening and poor motion. These deposits may cause a significant degree of masking, because the ultrasound does not penetrate calcium. Vegetations are irregular, and at times large growths are attached to the valve leaflets. They are not as bright, do

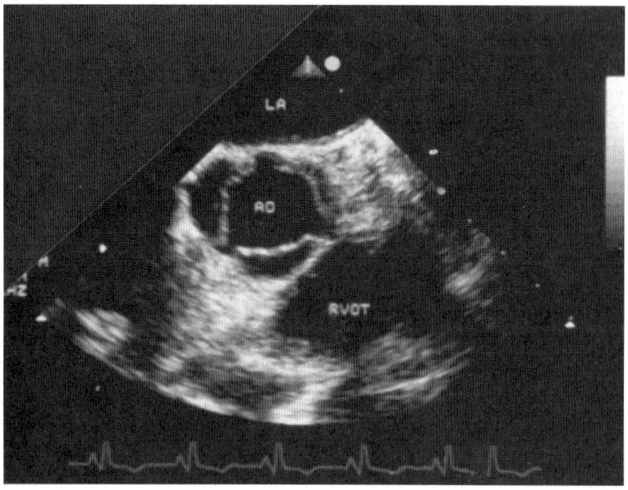

FIGURE 20-4. Two-dimensional transesophageal echocardiogram in the short-axis plane of the aortic valve. The cusp closest to the right ventricular outflow tract is the right coronary cusp; the most rightward cusp is the noncoronary cusp. (LA, left atrium; RVOT, right ventricular outflow tract; AO, aorta.)

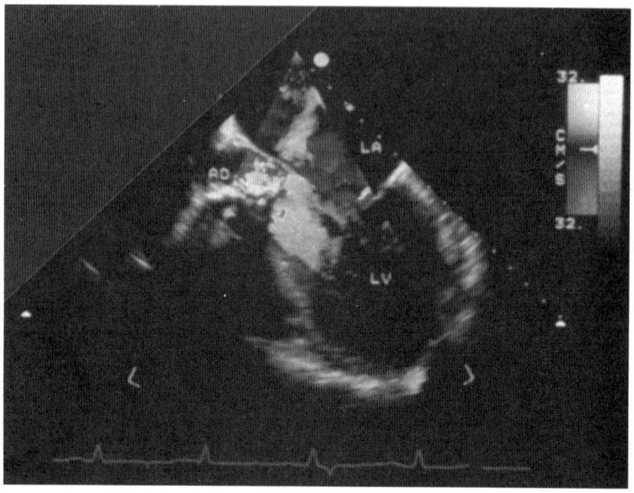

FIGURE 20-5. Long-axis view of the left ventricular outflow tract and the aortic valve, showing the blood flow in systole (red represents flow toward the transducer at the apex of the image). The mosaic in the aortic plane indicates turbulent flow. (AO, aorta; LA, left atrium; LV, left ventricle.)

not cause "shadowing" of posterior structures, and are as mobile as the calcium deposits.

Long-axis visualization of the valve can be difficult because of the anterior location of the aortic valve relative to the mitral valve, but Doppler color flow mapping in this plane is useful in examination of the function of the valve apparatus. The transducer is placed just behind the left atrium and angled anteriorly to bring the left ventricular outflow tract into view. In a functionally normal valve, the color flow image in the long-axis view is notable for deep hues (indicating laminar flow) of red (demonstrating flow toward the esophageal probe), originating in the left ventricular outflow tract (Fig. 20-5). In this view, the aortic and mitral valve can be displayed next to each other. Systole and diastole are indicated by the alternate opening and closing of the two valves.

Identification of aortic stenosis using TEE can be difficult, because it is virtually impossible to obtain a long-axis view of the aortic valve and aortic root to image the forward jet of turbulent flow. Chest wall echocardiography is superior in this regard. The best indication that stenosis is present is the observation of a large amount of turbulence (indicated by mosaically colored signal) just above the valve, as viewed in the short axis. In addition, a frequent finding is the appearance of a narrow jet of systolic flow in the left ventricular outflow tract, as if the red blood cells were "lining up" to pass through the stenotic valve.

Aortic Regurgitation

Etiology

The etiologies of aortic insufficiency can be classified as disease processes that cause (a) aortic root dilation, (b) damage to the leaflets, or (c) loss of commissural support, alone or in any combination (14,16). In addition, consideration must be given to whether the disease process causes chronic or acute aortic insufficiency. Aortic root dilation may cause valvular insufficiency by widening the commissures or stretching or bowing the leaflets. Idiopathic aortic root dilation occurs with some frequency (59). Approximately 80% of patients with Marfan syndrome develop aortic root dilation due to cystic medial necrosis (14). Root dilation may also occur in annuloaortic ectasis, syphilitic aortitis, ankylosing spondylitis, rheumatic arthritis, and osteogenesis imperfecta (60,61). In the recent past, rheumatic valvular disease causing leaflet damage was a common cause of aortic insufficiency. However, it is now an uncommon etiology of aortic insufficiency, except in the elderly population and in patients from countries in which rheumatic heart disease is still prevalent, often accompanied by mitral valve disease (60,61). Currently, congenital abnormalities (bicuspid aortic valve) and infective endocarditis are common etiologies of aortic insufficiency due to leaflet damage. Aortic dissection and blunt and penetrating chest trauma are the most common causes of acute aortic insufficiency. Aortic root dissection causes insufficiency in 30% of patients as a result of loss of commissural support and root dilation (59).

Clinical Features

In patients with chronic aortic insufficiency, there is a latent period of as long as 30 years between onset of "hemodynamic significance" and symptoms (62,63). The duration of the period of compensation to volume overload depends on the severity of the volume overload, coexisting valvular heart disease, and occurrence of additional damage to the valve (64). Patients may live without symptoms in the presence of significant regurgitation and ventricular dysfunction. For example, 81% of asymptomatic patients with normal left ventricular function were alive and without need for aortic valve replacement at 5 years (65). The 20-year survival rate of asymptomatic patients with "open" aortic insufficiency is 50% (19,63). The onset of symptoms heralds a rapid increase in mortality rates (64).

The most common presentation in chronic aortic regurgitation is dyspnea on exertion. In addition, patients often complain of episodic nocturnal dyspnea. Despite the presence of significant left ventricular hypertrophy, the occurrence of angina is not as common as in aortic stenosis (66). Myocardial ischemia may be more uncommon in patients with significant hypertrophy due to aortic regurgitation, because "volume work" is less expensive in terms of myocardial oxygen demand than the "pressure work" secondary to aortic stenosis (40). However, as with aortic stenosis, the subendocardial regions are the most susceptible to ischemia (14,16,64). Subendocardial ischemia may occur because of the decreased systemic diastolic pressure and increased LVEDP that accompany aortic regurgitation. The onset of right-sided heart failure and angina are poor prognostic indicators (16,62,64,67).

The physical examination in patients with chronic aortic regurgitation is notable for widened pulse pressure, which may be 100 mm Hg or more in hemodynamically severe cases. The diastolic pressure is usually less than 60 mm Hg. Auscultation is characterized by a normal or slightly diminished first heart sound. The second heart sound is usually normal; however, the A_2 component may be delayed or absent because the aortic valve does not close properly. The murmur of aortic regurgitation is best described as a high-pitched, decrescendo, "blowing" murmur peaking early in diastole and heard best at the left sternal border (64). In many cases, an additional mid-diastolic low-pitched murmur may be heard at the apex. This is known as the Austin Flint murmur (63).

The ECG findings are usually normal in patients with aortic regurgitation; however, in advanced cases, the signs of ventricular hypertrophy may be detected (68). Left bundle-branch block, first-degree atrioventricular block, and atrial fibrillation may be seen as well (64,68). The chest x-ray film demonstrates cardiomegaly (increased cardiothoracic ratio) due to the hypertrophy and dilation. Other findings include aortic root dilation and left atrial enlargement in the presence of associated mitral valve disease. In cases of acute aortic regurgitation, the chest x-ray finding is often normal; however, common findings include widening of the mediastinum and loss of the normal aortic contour.

Echocardiography has proven to be an invaluable tool in the diagnosis and assessment of aortic regurgitation. Both 2D and Doppler forms of echocardiography are useful.

Pathophysiology

As chronic aortic insufficiency progresses, the left ventricle is gradually exposed to increasing end-diastolic volume from regurgitation of blood from the incompetent valve. This "volume overloading" of the left ventricle induces hypertrophy of the wall of the ventricle such that the sarcomeres both elongate and replicate in series (69). This situation stands in contrast to the hypertrophy in aortic stenosis in which the sarcomeres thicken and replicate in parallel. As the left ventricular chamber dilates to accommodate the increased volume, wall stress as defined by the Laplace law would have to increase if intraventricular pressure remained the same (49,69). However, unlike the compensatory response in the presence of aortic stenosis, the increase in chamber diameter parallels the hypertrophy of the chamber wall, i.e., wall thickness is normal or increased in proportion to chamber radius (16,64,69,70). Therefore, the radius-to-wall-thickness ratio of radius to wall thickness (or volume to mass) tends to remain normal in the early stages of aortic insufficiency, and wall stress tends toward normal. The maintenance of a normal radius-to-thickness ratio defines the eccentric hypertrophy common in aortic insufficiency. In contrast, the concentric hypertrophy of aortic stenosis is marked by a decreased radius-to-thickness ratio because of the relative increase in wall thickness (16,64,70,71). This eccentric hypertrophy in volume-overload states counteracts the adverse effect of dilation on pressure work as long as a normal relationship of radius to wall thickness can be maintained. With progression of the disease, this ratio figures prominently in the development of ventricular dysfunction.

In the later stages of the disease, before any changes occur in the contractility of the ventricle, left ventricular dysfunction may occur secondary to inadequate hypertrophy to overcome the increased wall stress caused by progressive volume overload and chamber dilation (71). The radius-to-thickness ratio (see previous discussion) rises, which increases systolic wall stress (afterload). This phenomenon, in which the left ventricle is unable to maintain normal stroke volume against the systolic stress, represents "afterload mismatch," similar to what has been described in aortic stenosis (72). The normal compensatory response to progressive increases in afterload is for stroke volume to increase by an increase in end-diastolic volume (preload reserve) (72,73). In aortic regurgitation, preload reserve functions to maintain cardiac output. However, in the later stages of the disease process, this reserve is exhausted, and any changes in afterload may lead to impairment of ventricular performance in the absence of changes in contractility (16,64,72, 73).

The effect of chronic volume overloading of the left ventricle on intrinsic ventricular contractility has recently been elucidated (71,73,74). Many of the ejection-phase indexes of contractility (dP/dt, V_{max}) are dependent on the level of preload and afterload and thus are inadequate definitions of contractility. The end-systolic pressure-volume relationship is independent of the effects of preload and afterload (7–10). The relationship is nearly linear under varying conditions of load and can be described by its slope (E_{max}) and the intercept at the volume ordinate at a pressure of zero (V_0) (7–10). As volume overloading progresses, the intrinsic contractility eventually worsens, signified by a rightward shift of the end-systolic pressure-volume relationship and a decrease in the E_{max} (73). One should suspect a decrease in contractility in patients with aortic insufficiency in the presence of a decreased ejection fraction or a decrease in the mean velocity of fiber shortening (73,75,76).

In the presence of normal systolic function, the compliance (diastolic volume/diastolic pressure) of the left ventricular chamber increases so the end-diastolic volume can increase significantly with little or no change in the end-diastolic pressure. The increase in end-diastolic volume is determined by the regurgitant volume, which in turn is determined by (a) the area of the orifice, (b) the diastolic pressure gradient between the aorta and left ventricle, and (c) the length of diastole, which is inversely related to heart rate (63,64).

Patients often remain asymptomatic during exercise, even in the presence of decreased cardiac output, because the catecholamine-induced increase in heart rate shortens the diastolic interval, which decreases the regurgitant stroke volume and favors forward output (76–78). Venous return increases, which increases stroke volume by the Starling mechanism. However, if ventricular contractility is impaired, as in the later stages of the disease process, the increased venous return may increase the volume load on the heart with subsequent transmission of volume to the pulmonary vasculature. In addition, the increase in contractility and decrease in systemic vascular resistance lead to a net increase in forward flow. Thus, the physiologic effects of exercise are mostly beneficial to patients with aortic insufficiency (76–78).

The pathophysiologic response to acute aortic regurgitation is dramatically different (79). The presentation of severe diastolic volume overload to the left ventricle results in an abrupt increase in LVEDP with little or no change in the end-diastolic volume and fiber length (79). Because of the lack of compensatory hypertrophy, wall stress rises rapidly, total stroke volume does not increase, and forward stroke volume falls. The decrease in cardiac output causes a reflex activation of the sympathetic nervous system that leads to an increase in heart rate and systemic vascular resistance (79,80). These events may further decrease cardiac output, because the increase in heart rate generally fails to compensate for the increased systemic vascular resistance. The LVEDP rises rapidly and early, often exceeding the left atrial pressure early in diastole (79,80). This event leads to premature closure of the mitral valve, which may protect the pulmonary vasculature in the stages of acute aortic regurgitation (79,80). However, with time, even this protective mechanism fails, and pulmonary edema eventually develops.

Anesthetic Implications

The hemodynamic goals in the care of the patient with aortic regurgitation are based on the fact that in addition to the diameter of the aortic valve orifice, the mean diastolic aortic to left ventricular pressure gradient and the diastolic time determine the magnitude of regurgitant flow (64). Patients with aortic regurgitation often respond favorably to modest reductions in afterload, which reduce the diastolic pressure gradient and increase forward cardiac output. In general, patients with chronic aortic regurgitation and low cardiac output associated with normal to high arterial blood pressure and elevated LVEDP and patients with acute aortic regurgitation respond most favorably to afterload reduction. One must avoid significant reductions in the diastolic pressure (the driving pressure for coronary perfusion) to prevent a decrease in coronary perfusion pressure. Increases in afterload increase the diastolic pressure gradient and therefore increase regurgitant flow. In addition, it is necessary to avoid significant reductions in preload that may be caused by venodilators. Therefore, "pure" arteriolar vasodilators such as sodium nitroprusside may be preferred over those drugs that also cause venodilation.

Partial compensation for the regurgitation can be achieved by maintaining preload at an adequate level ("preload reserve") (72). The eccentric hypertrophy and chamber dilation render the left ventricular chamber more compliant than normal; therefore, large changes in left ventricular volume may result in only small changes in left atrial or PCWPs (72).

Theoretically, increases in heart rate should increase forward flow by decreasing the diastolic time. However, it is unclear whether increases in heart rate in the absence of increased contractility actually increase effective cardiac output (81,82). Brawley et al. (82) demonstrated that an increase in heart rate achieved by atrial pacing, in the absence of changes in contractility, had little effect on cardiac output. When heart rate was increased by isoproterenol infusion or exercise (both of which increased contractility), forward flow increased (82). It must be noted that a slow heart rate tends to increase the regurgitant fraction, causing left ventricular distention and increased wall tension.

Patients presenting for aortic valve replacement for chronic regurgitation are premedicated, monitored, induced, and maintained in much the same way as those presenting with stenotic lesions. The pulmonary artery catheter can help guide volume therapy; however, because of the chamber dilation, small changes in the PCWP may be associated with very large increases in LVEDV. Care must be taken during cardiopulmonary bypass to avoid left ventricular distention from retrograde pump flow through the incompetent valve. Venting of the left ventricle through the pulmonary vein may be used to decrease this distention. Also, because of the chronic decrease in systemic vascular resistance, mean arterial blood pressure may be low, despite normal pump flow. Use of inotropic agents should be considered in patients with preoperative left ventricular dysfunction and in situations in which myocardial protection during cardiopulmonary bypass is poor.

Patients with acute aortic regurgitation are often emergency cases and therefore may be at risk of aspiration of gastric contents during induction of anesthesia. Rapid-sequence induction with etomidate or ketamine and succinylcholine with supplemental boluses of narcotic may be appropriate in many cases, particularly in unstable patients. Alternatively, in patients who are hemodynamically stable, narcotic induction with a priming dose of nondepolarizing muscle relaxants followed by the intubating dose of the relaxant with application of cricoid pressure will often ensure adequate anesthesia and intubating conditions within 60 to 90 seconds. The PCWP will most often underestimate the LVEDP because of premature closure of the mitral valve (80). However, when acute aortic regurgitation is associated with pronounced aortic and ventricular dilation, mitral regurgitation may result (64,79,80). In these situations, the PCWP will overestimate the LVEDV. The hemodynamic concerns and management of bypass are similar to those for chronic aortic regurgitation.

Surgical Technique and Postoperative Problems

As in patients with aortic stenosis, patients with moderate to severe symptoms (NYHA class III or IV) secondary to aortic regurgitation merit aortic valve replacement (16,64, 68,83). Patients with acute aortic regurgitation also require surgery (16,64,68,83). However, left ventricular dysfunction may be quite extensive before the onset of symptoms (76). Therefore, attempts have been made to define criteria and indicators for surgery in the absence of symptoms (62, 67,68,83–85). These criteria have been defined through studies that have examined mortality and morbidity rates after aortic valve replacement. Factors that have been associated with increased postoperative morbidity and mortality rates include the following objective measures of left ventricular dysfunction: ejection fraction of less than 0.45, cardiac index of less than 2.2 L/minute, end-systolic diameter of more than 55 mm, fractional shortening of less than 25%, and end-diastolic radius-to-wall-thickness ratio of more than 4.0 (62,67,83–85). Therefore, surgery is probably indicated in patients with mild symptoms (NYHA class II) and an ejection fraction of less than 0.50 and in patients with decreasing ejection fraction as followed by echocardiography (16,64). Intervention with reasonable results is possible in these patients; however, successful outcome is more likely in the absence of these characteristics (86). It remains unclear what degree of left ventricular dysfunction places a patient in a higher risk group.

The surgical technique for replacement of the aortic valve replacement in patients with aortic regurgitation is similar to that for aortic stenosis, except for cases in which the disease process involves the ascending aorta. In these cases, most of which are secondary to aneurysmal disease, the surgical procedure generally involves primary repair of the aneurysm or resection of the aneurysmal segment with insertion of a synthetic graft. Under these circumstances, anastomoses to the coronary arteries must be performed by using either an additional synthetic graft from aorta to coronary ostia or direct anastomosis of aorta to coronary ostia (16,64).

Cardioplegia may be difficult in the presence of aortic regurgitation, because of leakage of the cardioplegic solution through the incompetent valve. In many cases, delivery through the coronary ostia may be necessary. An additional option is retrograde delivery of cardioplegic solution via the coronary sinus.

The immediate postoperative period after aortic valve replacement for aortic regurgitation is marked by a decrease in the LVEDP and LVEDV due to reduction or obliteration of the regurgitant contribution to preload (16,64). The ventricle must now accommodate an increase in afterload. Intraventricular pressure increases, but wall stress may not change because of the decrease in the chamber dilation (16, 64). Thus, it is particularly important to carefully monitor and maintain preload. TEE is particularly useful in this regard. It should be noted that the ventricle is now dependent on the normal filling sequence from the mitral valve; thus, atrial contribution to ventricular filling is important. Atrial fibrillation and other supraventricular arrhythmias should be aggressively treated. Modest reductions in heart rate may be better tolerated during the postoperative period. In patients with moderate to severe preexisting left ventricular dysfunction or in patients requiring prolonged cardiopulmonary bypass or those in whom myocardial protection is poor, inotropic support may be required, in the form of pharmacologic agents or an intraaortic balloon pump.

The perioperative mortality rate after aortic valve replacement in patients with symptomatic aortic regurgitation is between 2% and 15%, with an average of 6% (65,68,86). The long-term survival rate in patients undergoing aortic valve replacement for aortic regurgitation appears to be less than that in patients with aortic stenosis (16). For functional status after aortic valve replacement, preoperative contractile state and the radius-to-wall-thickness ratio appear to predict postoperative left ventricular performance, improvement in symptomatology, and survival (57,58,64,86). Prognosis is poor if surgery is delayed after the development of moderate to severe ventricular dysfunction (57,58,64,86). Patients who have normal left ventricular diastolic diameter after aortic valve replacement, in general, have preserved left ventricular function and a favorable radius-to-wall-thickness ratio before surgery (34,52).

Transesophageal Echocardiographic Images

The characteristics of the normal aortic valve during TEE are described under Aortic Stenosis. In patients with aortic regurgitation, there are a few characteristic findings. In the 2D long-axis view, regurgitant flow through the aortic valve appears to strike the anterior leaflet of the mitral valve, causing a characteristic flutter (87). The Doppler color flow images in patients with aortic regurgitation are distinguished by a high-velocity, often turbulent blue "jet," indicating flow away from the transducer probe (88). The jet of regurgitant flow often originates from the central portion of the valve where the leaflets are to coapt (87,88). However, when there is discrete damage or prolapse of a leaflet, an eccentric origin may be seen.

Attempts have been made to quantitate the degree of regurgitation by using Doppler color flow imaging (59, 87–90). Indexes that have been described include the width of the jet, the length of the jet extending into the left ventricle, and the area of the jet turbulence (59,88–91). These characteristics of the jet are subject to the imaging plane, loading conditions of the ventricle, and mitral inflow.

In general, the base or origin of the jet is fairly well defined, and its size at this point probably correlates most closely with the size of the valvular defect. In severe aortic regurgitation, the base of the jet is wider and more of the left ventricle fills in diastole than in mild regurgitation (91). The characteristic jet of the aortic regurgitation may have a velocity in excess of 3 m/second, which may cause frequency aliasing (91). Aliasing occurs when the flow velocity exceeds the rate at which the pulsed wave Doppler system can record it properly. It is depicted during color flow imaging as an apparent reversal of flow and, hence, color. Thus, flow toward the transducer appears blue and flow away from the transducer appears red. The color reversal may be the dominant feature of the examination and may actually help in the identification of abnormally high flow velocities.

DISEASES OF THE MITRAL VALVE

The mitral valve lies between the left atrium and the left ventricle. In the open position, there is a wide orifice, which allows unobstructed flow of the atrial blood volume into the ventricle. It is a bicuspid valve composed of two slender leaflets: a short but wide posterior leaflet and a long and narrow anterior leaflet. The leaflets insert into a fibrous annulus (92). The geometry of the annulus changes during ventricular systole to help maintain valve closure (93). The leaflets are attached via the chordae tendineae to the papillary muscles: a large anterior papillary muscle and a smaller posterior papillary muscle (93). Although the papillary muscles contract during systole, their function is not to facilitate valve closure but to prevent the leaflets from bulging into the left atrium. The normal mitral valve area is 4 to 6 cm^2 (92).

Mitral Stenosis

Etiology

Unlike the other valvular heart lesions, mitral stenosis is almost always caused by rheumatic fever, except for the rare cases of congenital mitral stenosis (94,95). Morphologically, the predominant feature is at least some degree of mitral commissural fusion and thickening of the leaflets (96). In older patients, frequently there is calcification of the leaflets and/or the mitral annulus (95).

Clinical Features

After the occurrence of the rheumatic fever (40% of patients are not aware that they have had rheumatic fever), there is generally a long latency period before any signs and symptoms appear (19,97–100). The literature quotes a range of 4 to 25 years, with the vast majority of patients being in the upper end of the range (19,101). After the onset of initial symptoms, it may take another 7 to 10 years for the patients to deteriorate to a state of cardiac disability (NYHA class IV) (98,101).

In most cases, the presenting symptom of mitral stenosis is the gradual onset of dyspnea (99). In other cases, atrial fibrillation or hemoptysis may precede any symptoms of shortness of breath (98,99).

Typically, the symptoms of dyspnea occur with exertion as the valve area decreases to less than 2 cm^2 (94,99). The exercise-induced increase in heart rate causes a decrease in the diastolic time for ventricular filling (99). Left atrial pressure increases during this interval. This increase in pressure is subsequently transmitted to the pulmonary vasculature and right side of the heart, generally leading to increased work of breathing and shortness of breath (102).

Patients with similar degrees of mitral stenosis may have very different symptoms and signs, depending on the particular hemodynamic pattern (100,101). In general, a reliable history of crescendo orthopnea, dyspnea, and nocturnal dyspnea, together with auscultatory findings of a loud first sound, opening snap, and a diastolic rumble with presystolic crescendo (if sinus rhythm is present), provide fairly secure evidence of some degree of mitral stenosis. Some patients present with hemoptysis, which varies from the typical pink frothy sputum of pulmonary edema to the frank red blood of pulmonary embolism and pulmonary infarction (101).

The natural history of mitral stenosis can be significantly modified by complications. The most frequent complication is atrial fibrillation (103). The loss of the atrial contribution to ventricular filling caused by atrial fibrillation is often the cause of initial symptoms of dyspnea.

The survival rate of patients with mitral stenosis is significantly affected by the presence of atrial fibrillation (97–99). Whereas the 10- and 20-year survival rates of patients with mitral stenosis in sinus rhythm are 46% and 29%, respectively, the rates for patients with mitral stenosis and atrial fibrillation are 20% and 10%, respectively (97). In general, the onset of atrial fibrillation signifies tight mitral stenosis (97).

Another frequent complication in patients with mitral stenosis is systemic arterial embolization, most commonly embolization to the brain. The rate for surgically untreated patients is about 10% to 15%, nearly 80% of whom have atrial fibrillation (104). Unfortunately, most of these embolic events (75%) involve the cerebral vasculature (99).

The ECG is often notable for P mitrale, which is indicative of left atrial enlargement (94,105). Atrial fibrillation may also be a prominent feature.

Chest radiographs may show left atrial enlargement, and pulmonary arterial and right ventricular enlargement may be present. There may be signs of pulmonary venous hypertension with frank alveolar pulmonary edema or more subtle Kerley B lines, interstitial pulmonary edema, and enlarged pulmonary veins (94,105). A calcified mitral valve may be visible on the chest radiograph, but there appears to be no good correlation between the intensity of the calcification and the severity of stenosis.

In patients less than 40 years of age in whom the incidence of coronary artery disease is low, use of 2D echocardiography with Doppler color flow mapping and spectral Doppler imaging to calculate the mitral valve pressure gradient and mitral valve area should be sufficient to decide whether surgical intervention or balloon valvuloplasty is indicated (94,106). In patients with atrial fibrillation, the echocardiogram should be scanned for evidence of left atrial thrombus, particularly in patients who are to undergo mitral balloon valvuloplasty. In practice, most patients also undergo cardiac catheterization.

Mitral stenosis is a surgically treated disease. The medical treatment has not significantly changed in decades, and the survival rate among patients who are medically treated is very poor: The 10-year survival rate is 44%, and the 20-year survival rate is 8% (8,98,100,107).

Pathophysiology

When the mitral valve area is reduced to less than 2 cm^2 by stenosis, a pressure gradient develops across the valve. It is generally believed that if the area is reduced to this degree, the left atrial pressure must be increased to maintain cardiac output (100,104,110). With progression of stenosis, increases in left atrial pressure are transmitted to the pulmonary vasculature with a resultant reduction in pulmonary compliance, increase in lung stiffness, and increased work of breathing (101). Symptoms at this level of stenosis are usually induced by exercise, and patients are often asymptomatic at rest (101).

With progression of stenosis to a valve area of 1.2 cm^2 or less, patients begin to experience progressive worsening of dyspnea on exertion, orthopnea, and/or paroxysmal nocturnal dyspnea (27,108). Left atrial pressure increases further to maintain ventricular filling and cardiac output. Eventually, this increase in left atrial pressure leads to left atrial enlargement. In most cases of pure mitral stenosis, this atrial enlargement is moderate (103). Left atrial dilation in time often leads to atrial dysrhythmias, most commonly atrial fibrillation (103). In this group of patients, in whom left ventricular filling is compromised already, rapid atrial fibrillation with the concomitant loss of the atrial kick is another insult that decreases the preload reserve and potentially decreases cardiac output (109). As valve area decreases to less than 1.0 cm^2, left atrial pressure and PCWP rise significantly such that capillary hydrostatic pressure is greater than the plasma oncotic pressure (94). Under these conditions, pulmonary edema is likely to occur, unless diastolic flow across the valve is decreased (101,102).

In patients with severe mitral stenosis, the pulmonary vascular resistance may be increased because of spasm of the pulmonary arterioles (102). This rise in pulmonary vascular resistance causes an increase in pulmonary arterial pressure and a subsequent reduction in cardiac output. This may help reduce the left atrial pressure below the pulmonary edema threshold (102). However, increased pulmonary artery pressure affects right ventricular pressure and function, subsequently leading to right ventricular hypertrophy and dilation and finally to tricuspid regurgitation. However, in the vast majority of patients with mitral stenosis, right ventricular function remains within normal limits (94,99,102). Elevated pulmonary artery pressures in the presence of mitral stenosis are a strong indication for surgery (110). There is often a dramatic reduction in the pulmonary artery pressures after successful mitral valve replacement (111,112).

Abnormalities in left ventricular function are frequently encountered in patients with mitral stenosis (113). LVEDP is normal or low in these patients; however, in most patients, it may be elevated (113,114). Left ventricular pump function, expressed by ejection fraction, is frequently decreased. In almost half of these patients, the ejection fraction is mildly decreased, but in 15% of patients, it is moderately depressed (less than 0.4) (114). The etiology of this ventricular dysfunction is not well understood. Posterobasal hypokinesia is often encountered in patients with annular calcification, which may account, in part, for the ventricular dysfunction and may explain the tethering often seen by echocardiography after insertion of a prosthetic valve or a rigid ring in the mitral orifice. Left ventricular geometry is also distorted by fusion and shortening of the chordae tendineae of the heart and by retraction of the mitral valve apparatus. Other suggested etiologies include the abnormal pattern of diastolic filling as well as a decreased preload reserve due to the stenotic valve (115,116). Patients with some additional mild degree of aortic insufficiency may have preserved ventricular function, possibly because left ventricular geometry is maintained and because the reduction in left ventricular wall thickness is prevented in this subgroup of patients, thus keeping wall stress within normal limits (94). Ventricular function remains depressed in a number of patients, even after successful mitral valve surgery or balloon valvuloplasty.

Anesthetic Implications

The main problem in patients with mitral stenosis is the inability to adequately provide the left ventricle with adequate preload. Filling of the left ventricle through a restricted orifice requires not only an increased driving pressure but also increased time (109). Thus, rapid ventricular rates are poorly tolerated in mitral stenosis as diastolic time is shortened, leading to decreased time intervals for ventricular filling (108,109). Therefore, to provide the left atrium with enough time to fill the ventricle, it is important to maintain strict control of the heart rate. This may be a challenge because so many of these patients develop atrial fibrillation. It is not our practice to continue administration of digitalis on the morning of surgery because of our fear of digitalis toxicity in the face of the large and sometimes unpredictable changes in potassium levels during the course of the surgery. Some authors do advocate the continued use of digitalis during the immediate perioperative period. Procainamide can safely be given on the morning of surgery. In the event of acute onset of atrial fibrillation with a rapid ventricular response, appropriate therapy includes low doses of β-adrenergic blocking drugs such as propranolol and esmolol, verapamil, and DC cardioversion (94,102). It should be noted that in patients with longstanding atrial fibrillation, DC cardioversion may dislodge atrial thrombi and predispose the patient to systemic embolic events (94,104).

Preload is especially important in patients with mitral stenosis. Ventricular filling across the stenotic mitral valve is dependent on maintaining an adequate volume gradient across the valve. However, these patients have elevated left atrial pressure as well, and marked increases in central blood volume can exacerbate or precipitate right ventricular failure. If available, a pulmonary artery catheter with continuous mixed venous oximetry provides optimal monitoring both in the operating room and in the immediate postoperative period. Because of the pressure gradient across the mitral valve, the PCWP overestimates LVEDP, but PCWP may be useful as a trend monitor as long as heart rate is controlled. With increased heart rates, the PCWP may increase because of a reduction of diastolic filling while the LVEDP may remain unchanged or may decrease, resulting in an increase in the discrepancy between the PCWP and LVEDP. The central venous pressure may also be useful in assessing the right ventricular function.

The right side of the heart functions as a low-pressure, volume-displacement pump that functions to fill the left ventricle and maintain low systemic venous pressures. Mitral stenosis impairs ventricular filling, thereby impeding right-sided heart function. A consequence of the obstruction to ventricular filling is transmission of the left atrial pressure to the pulmonary vasculature. A cornerstone in the management of patients with mitral stenosis is prevention of conditions that will exacerbate pulmonary hypertension and possibly precipitate right ventricular dysfunction. Thus, avoidance of hypoxia, hypercarbia, hypothermia, acidosis, catecholamine release, and possibly nitrous oxide is particularly important. Therapy with both pulmonary-specific and/or systemic vasodilators in the absence of concurrent mitral regurgitation or severe pulmonary hypertension may be particularly difficult in these patients, because reduction of pulmonary artery pressures may lead to further underloading of the left ventricle with a resultant reduction in cardiac output.

Premedication is important in all patients, but particularly in those in whom control of anxiety is necessary to control heart rate. However, in patients with advanced mitral valve disease, conservative dosing is indicated, because these patients tend to be intolerant of narcotics and hypnotics. All patients should be on supplemental oxygen from the time of their premedication.

Although there are many methods to induce and maintain anesthesia in these patients, it is generally advisable to stay away from agents that decrease ventricular contractility or that increase heart rate. These patients often have very low cardiac outputs at rest and may be exquisitely sensitive to anesthetic agents. Our practice is to use a narcotic-based technique for induction and maintenance of anesthesia for mitral valve replacement procedures. This technique can also be useful in noncardiac surgery, although the doses of narcotic chosen should be reduced appropriately. In patients premedicated with lorazepam, it is seldom necessary to give more than minimal doses of sedative-hypnotics. The use of nitrous oxide has been associated with elevation of pulmonary artery pressures via increases in pulmonary vascular resistance. It is not clear whether nitrous oxide acts via a direct vasoconstrictive effect or via a sympathomimetic effect (117–119). A relatively recent study has implicated a reduction of pulmonary blood flow as the cause of the increase in pulmonary vascular resistance (118).

Because of the tenuous nature of the response to loading conditions and heart rate, treatment of hypotension in the patient with moderate to severe mitral stenosis can be a difficult problem. Decreases in systemic vascular resistance are poorly tolerated because of (a) the fixed resistance to output at the level of mitral valve and (b) the reflex tachycardia. Excessive volume administration and the Trendelenburg position may worsen congestive failure. Agents such as ephedrine may increase heart rate and worsen ventricular function. Treatment with α-adrenergic agonists, such as phenylephrine, may cause pulmonary vasoconstriction, which may precipitate right ventricular dysfunction. If pharmacologic therapy is indicated, a decision must be made about whether the tachycardia often associated with ephedrine and epinephrine is potentially more dangerous than the pulmonary vasoconstriction seen with the α-agonists.

There are a few concerns in the patient presenting for mitral valve surgery. After mitral valve replacement, pulmonary artery pressures and pulmonary vascular resistance should decrease, whereas cardiac output should increase. In patients with persistent elevation of right-sided pressures, irreversible changes in the pulmonary vasculature may have occurred. These patients often fail to improve symptomatically after mitral valve replacement. However, immediately after mitral valve replacement and cardiopulmonary bypass, both left and right ventricular dysfunctions are common. Certainly, avoidance of those conditions that exacerbate pulmonary hypertension is especially important in the immediate postbypass period. In addition, treatment with inotropes, preload augmentation, afterload reduction, vasodilators, and mechanical assist devices may be necessary. In patients with severe pulmonary hypertension, the pulmonary artery catheter is particularly useful in the management of post–cardiopulmonary bypass right ventricular dysfunction (which may be more common than left-sided failure in these patients). Amrinone may be useful after mitral valve replacement because of its combined vasodilator and inotropic effects. In addition, the heart rate changes associated with catecholamines in combination with vasodilators are less likely to occur with amrinone. In a small study of 12 patients undergoing mitral valve replacement, the use of amrinone was associated with an increase in cardiac output, a decrease in pulmonary artery pressures, and no increase in heart rate (120). An alternate therapeutic plan for the management of post–mitral valve replacement right-sided heart failure has been described in which prostaglandin E_1 (30 to 150 ng/kg/minute) is infused via a right-side central line and high-dose norepinephrine (up to 1 mg/kg/minute) is infused via a left atrial line (121). The prostaglandin E_1 acts to dilate the pulmonary vasculature, causing a reduction in the pulmonary artery pressures while the norepinephrine counteracts any peripheral arterial effects of the prostaglandin.

In a few patients in whom there is a large discrepancy between the pulmonary artery catheter reading and the actual left atrial pressure, insertion of a left atrial catheter by the surgeon may be helpful in providing direct pressure measurements. The most serious complication of direct left atrial pressure monitoring is, of course, the potential for the introduction of air into the left side of the heart. The potential for bleeding at removal of the catheter is another possible complication.

Many patients with chronic atrial fibrillation spontaneously convert to sinus rhythm after valve replacement, even though the conversion is often short-lived. Intraoperative and postoperative care of these patients is much easier if sinus rhythm can be maintained for some time after surgery. A continuous infusion of procainamide may help stabilize sinus rhythm for a few hours after surgery.

Surgical Technique and Postoperative Problems

Indications for surgery include NYHA class III or IV symptoms, valve areas of less than 1.0 cm^2, and/or occurrence of embolic events (94,102).

There are three surgical options in patients with mitral stenosis: percutaneous balloon valvotomy (122), open commissurotomy (123), and mitral valve replacement (94,102). Open commissurotomy is performed via a median sternotomy or a lateral thoracotomy (123). Cardiopulmonary bypass is instituted and the aorta is cross-clamped, as in replacement surgery. After the left atrium is opened, typically from the interatrial septum, the pliability of the valve leaflets is assessed to judge whether it is suitable for commissurotomy. A stab wound is made in the commissure right at the mitral annulus and followed by extension of the incision toward the valve orifice. If chordae are fused, they may be separated (94,123).

It is thought that the long-term results of open mitral commissurotomy are poor and that most patients will eventually require mitral valve replacement, although the lag time between commissurotomy and valve replacement may be substantial (94).

The conduct of surgery for mitral valve replacement is typical of cardiac surgical procedures requiring median sternotomy, bicaval and aortic cannulation, and hypothermic (24°C to 28°C) cardiopulmonary bypass (94,124). The technique of mitral valve replacement begins with left atriotomy from behind the intraatrial sulcus, followed by resection of the mitral valve apparatus either completely or in part. The chordae are typically excised, but the papillary muscles are left in place. The new valve may be sewn into place by using either a continuous suture or interrupted simple or mattress sutures. Generally, all the sutures are first placed in or above the mitral annulus and then passed through the sewing ring of the valve (124). The valve is then lowered into position and tied in place. During closure of the left atrium, the valve is made incompetent by placing a Foley catheter through it to prevent left ventricular dilation. The heart must be de-aired before the atrium is finally closed completely, to minimize air emboli to the coronary and cerebral circulation.

The most frequently seen problem in the immediate postoperative period in patients with mitral stenosis after mitral valve repair or replacement is the management of supraventricular arrhythmias, notably atrial fibrillation (see previous discussion).

One of the more severe complications in patients who have undergone mitral valve replacement is atrioventricular rupture near the posterior wall of the left ventricle

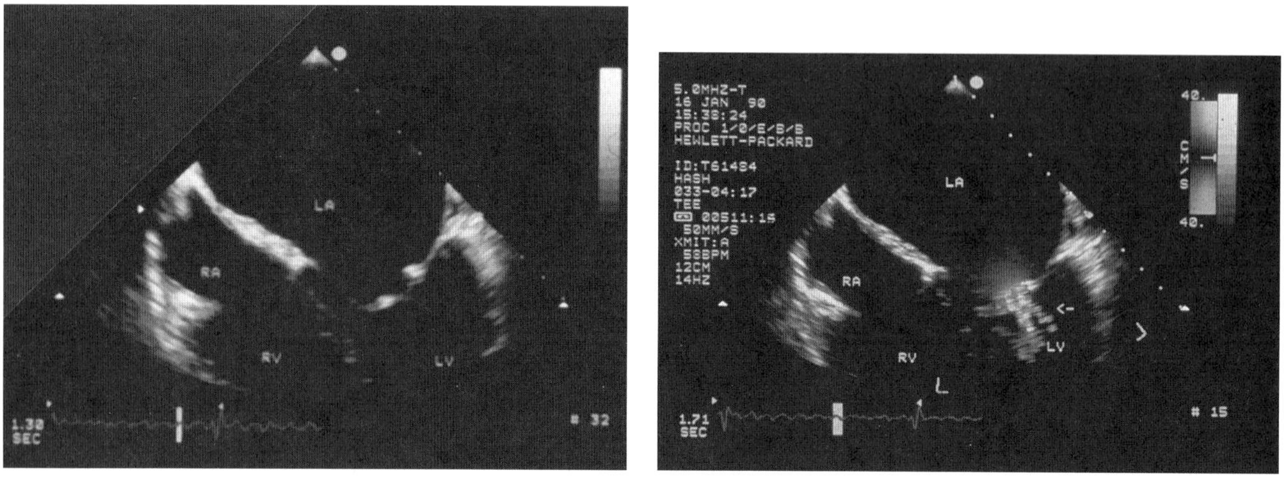

A B

FIGURE 20-7. **A:** Long-axis view of a stenotic mitral valve during diastole; the obstructed flow pushes the valve toward the left ventricle, a phenomenon known as "doming." The tips of the mitral leaflets show enhanced echodensity, probably due to fibrosis or calcification. (LA, left atrium; LV, left ventricle; RA, right atrium; RV, right ventricle.) **B:** With Doppler color flow mapping in the same patient as in **A**, a stenotic jet can be appreciated as a mosaic pattern distal to the mitral orifice during diastole.

(124–126). The cause of this complication, which carries a very high mortality rate, may be undue strain placed on the annulus during excision of the native valve or strain on the atrioventricular region if the heart is luxated out of the pericardial cradle after the prosthetic device is in place (124–126). Avoidance of elevated LVEDP during replacement surgery may reduce the likelihood of this event, which may be more common in patients with particularly poor ventricular compliance (124).

In addition, parts of the native mitral apparatus not excised may cause interference with the functioning of a mechanical prosthetic device. In the era of intraoperative echocardiography, this complication should be diagnosed in the operating room in almost all cases. The same is true of periprosthetic leaks of significant size. These should be diagnosed in the operating room and immediately repaired (see later discussion).

Postoperative bleeding and cardiac tamponade are risks in all patients who have undergone cardiac surgery. After mitral valve surgery, the atriotomy is a frequent site of postoperative bleeding.

Intraoperative Echocardiography

The main uses of intraoperative echocardiography in the patient with mitral stenosis are detection of thrombus in the left atrium and left atrial appendage, evaluation of the valve with regard to the suitability for repair, and evaluation of the operative result, either repair or replacement (Fig. 20-7; See Color Figs. 20-6 and 20-7B between pages 560 and 561).

The mitral valve is probably the valve most suitable for evaluation by TEE, because it is situated close to the esophageal transducer, directly in the line of the ultrasound beam, and can be evaluated from above, as if viewed from the left atrium. Evaluation of prosthetic mitral valves is generally difficult to accomplish by means of transthoracic ultrasound techniques, because the ultrasound is unable to penetrate the metal and plastic of which these valves are made. Looking at the valve through a "window" in the left atrium makes it possible to diagnose perivalvular leaks or inappropriate flow patterns through the valve with great sensitivity and accuracy.

In systole, the valve leaflets can be seen to have their closure point well into the left ventricle, below the level of the mitral annulus. The point of apposition is not the margin of the two leaflets, but a line about 1 mm inside the margin.

Doppler color flow mapping of the normal mitral valve demonstrates an acceleration of flow as blood enters the funnel-like structure of the valve. Otherwise, there is no evidence of turbulence in any phase of the cardiac cycle (91).

Enhanced echodensity in one or both mitral leaflets and in the mitral annulus is frequently seen in mitral stenosis, indicating fibrosis or calcification. The mitral valve orifice may appear small during diastole. Frequently, there may be decreased mobility of one or both leaflets (94). Doppler color flow mapping may be difficult to perform in the presence of calcification of the mitral valve, which often masks the stenotic jet (91). Also, because of the large size of the left atrium, the jet is almost always in the far field, which leads to degradation of the image quality. A phenomenon known as "doming" may occur during diastole, in which the blood appears to "line up" in front of the small orifice, pushing the leaflets down into the ventricle and giving them a conical, or dome, shape (94).

The left atrium is almost always enlarged, and there may be evidence of thrombus in the left atrial cavity itself or in the left atrial appendage. The slow blood flow in the atrium creates a foglike pattern on 2D echocardiography, known as "swirling" or "clouding." The left ventricle often appears underfilled.

After mitral valve commissurotomy and after cardiopulmonary bypass has been discontinued, the mitral valve should be checked critically for regurgitation or residual stenosis. If a prosthetic valve has been inserted, motion of the ball or leaflets should be unimpeded and the valve should close completely. Doppler color flow mapping should be used to detect any perivalvular leaks or abnormal transprosthetic flow patterns (91).

Mitral Insufficiency

Etiology

In contrast to mitral stenosis, mitral regurgitation has a complex pathogenesis and may be caused by a number of disease processes affecting the different components of the valve apparatus (95). These disease processes result in defects in the annulus, leaflets, or commissures; defects in the chordae or papillary muscles; or defects in left atrial or ventricular function (95). The most common cause of mitral regurgitation is rheumatic heart disease, but it may also be caused by mitral valve prolapse, myocardial ischemia, or infective endocarditis.

In the case of rheumatic mitral regurgitation there is progressive thickening of the leaflets, which retract and appear to fold back onto themselves (96). In addition, there may be elongation of the chordae, which may result in prolapse (96). Eventually, these elongated chordae may rupture. In almost all cases, there is dilation of the annulus with distortion of annular geometry (96,127).

Myxomatous degeneration of the valve leaflets is generally the cause of mitral valve prolapse. The collagen in the leaflets is replaced by mucopolysaccharides, leading to loss of fibrous support and causing one or both of the leaflets to "balloon" above the mitral annulus during systole (128, 129). This causes further strain on the chordae and progressive mitral insufficiency (96,130–132).

Not only do the components of the mitral valve need to function properly, but appropriate function of the ventricular wall is also necessary to ensure competence. Myocardial ischemia leading to papillary muscle or ventricular wall dysfunction may thus be responsible for mitral regurgitation in about 10% of patients who undergo coronary artery surgery (133). The posterior papillary muscle is more commonly affected in ischemia-related or infarction-related mitral regurgitation (95).

Acute mitral regurgitation is generally caused by one or more of three conditions: (a) rupture of a chorda tendinea, (b) rupture of a papillary muscle, or (c) myocardial ischemia or infarction leading to papillary muscle dysfunction (102, 110).

Clinical Features

In most patients, mitral insufficiency develops slowly, often over many years (45,110,128,134). As with mitral stenosis, the diagnosis of mitral insufficiency can often be made on the basis of the history and physical examination findings.

The natural history of mitral regurgitation is variable, due to the wide range of etiologies (128). However, as in mitral stenosis, patients with mild to moderate mitral regurgitation may function for many years without evidence of symptoms or progressive disease. Often an intercurrent event, such as the onset of atrial fibrillation, is necessary to initiate cardiac decompensation, even in patients with severe mitral regurgitation (128). Mitral valve prolapse frequently leads to elongation and eventually rupture of chordae tendineae, probably because of the abnormal strain on these structures (95,130). Rupture or elongation of the chordae will, of course, worsen the amount of mitral regurgitation and probably accelerate clinical deterioration (132,135). In patients with ischemic mitral regurgitation, the presence of symptoms is sometimes episodic and may occur only in the presence of myocardial ischemia (136). It may also appear at the time of cardiac catheterization but disappear hours or days later, for example, under anesthesia in the operating room. Unlike mitral stenosis, in which progressive pulmonary vascular hypertension and right-sided heart dysfunction are the main causes of morbidity and disability, left ventricular dysfunction is the major hemodynamic consequence of long-standing, chronic mitral regurgitation (110, 128).

As the mitral regurgitation becomes moderate to severe, the natural history progresses, as it does in patients with other forms of rheumatic heart disease; this is related in part to the degree of regurgitation, rapidity of onset, and status of left atrial and ventricular function (134). Early symptoms reflect low cardiac output and include malaise and easy fatigability. Symptoms of pulmonary congestion or dyspnea are rare, because the left atrium dilates and protects the pulmonary circulation from the regurgitant blood flow (128,134).

The characteristic finding on auscultation is a holosystolic murmur, loudest at the apex and radiating to the left axilla and the base of the left lung.

The ECG findings are normal in most patients with mitral regurgitation, although there may be evidence of left atrial enlargement or atrial fibrillation (105).

In severe mitral incompetence, the chest radiograph findings are notable for left atrial enlargement. Left atrial enlargement is a more frequent finding in mitral regurgitation than in mitral stenosis (105). The left ventricle can usually be seen to be enlarged as well. Pulmonary vascular redistribution may not be evident, even in patients with severe, chronic mitral regurgitation. On the other hand, in patients with acute mitral insufficiency, pulmonary vascular redistribution is almost always present and frank pulmonary edema is often present (105).

Combined 2D and Doppler echocardiography is most useful to document the presence, morphology, and severity of mitral regurgitation. Unless risk factors are present for coronary heart disease, the echocardiogram should provide sufficient information to warrant a decision about surgical intervention; however, most patients undergo left-sided and right-sided heart catheterization to further describe the hemodynamic qualities of mitral regurgitation (105,134). 2D echocardiography allows visualization of the valve leaflets, chordae, and papillary muscles. A frequent finding is incomplete closure of the mitral valve leaflets (105,134). In addition, the status of the left atrium (e.g., enlargement, presence of thrombi) and the left ventricle (e.g., dilation, eccentric hypertrophy) may be assessed (105,134). Doppler echocardiography is used in the assessment of mitral regurgitation to measure abnormal blood flow. Both color and pulsed wave Doppler techniques may be used. Both modalities allow spatial estimation and grading of the severity of the regurgitation. TEE results in images of exceptional quality in patients with mitral valve pathology. A number of factors influence the size and configuration of the regurgitant jet, including the volume of the jet, the pressure gradient between the ventricle and atrium, the size of the orifice, the size of the left atrium, the loading conditions of the ventricle, and the heart rate and rhythm.

Left ventriculography can verify the presence and amount of mitral regurgitation and often provides some information about the morphology of the mitral valve. As with Doppler color flow techniques, the estimate of the amount of regurgitation by observing contrast regurgitation is semiquantitative at best. More quantitative information about the regurgitant fraction can be obtained by calculation of forward output and stroke volume.

Contrast ventriculography and Doppler color flow echocardiography use a similar grading scale of 1+ to 4+ for quantification of the amount of regurgitation (105,134). In 1+, or mild regurgitation, either the Doppler jet or a small amount of contrast material enters the atrium from the ventricle and is cleared by the subsequent cardiac cycle. With increasing regurgitation, more contrast material or Doppler flow enters the atrium and less is cleared until in 4+, or severe regurgitation, the entire atrium is filled with contrast medium, and clearance of the medium is significantly reduced (88,134).

Pathophysiology

In mitral insufficiency, a fraction of the LVEDV is ejected backward into the low-pressure left atrium, instead of into the higher resistance aorta. This results in left ventricular and left atrial volume overload, which eventually leads to left ventricular and left atrial dilation. This chronic regurgitation occurs in both the ejection phase and the isovolemic contraction phase of ventricular systole. Similar to aortic regurgitation, the magnitude of the regurgitant fraction is determined by the size of the orifice, the pressure gradient between the left atrium and ventricle, and the relative compliance of these chambers.

In long-standing mitral regurgitation, there may be an increase in left ventricular compliance, so LVEDV may be increased without a significant rise in end-diastolic pressure. However, in the early stages of the disorder, hemodynamic compensation occurs through more complete emptying of the left atrium and then in the later stages, through left ventricular dilation (71). In addition, because afterload (systolic wall tension) is reduced by means of ejection into the left atrium by reduction of systolic ventricular pressure and radius (102), less energy is expended for development of tension during contraction, and cardiac output can be maintained. The volume overload also results in only small increases in myocardial oxygen consumption (40), which may be important in preservation of ventricular function, as measured by elevated ejection phase indexes, such as ejection fraction and mean velocity of fiber shortening (71). With progression of the disease and subsequent development of symptoms, these compensatory mechanisms are overcome, and those indexes of contractility and function begin to decline to normal levels. Therefore, normal values for these indexes may actually indicate impaired myocardial function (102,110).

The left atrium in patients with chronic mitral regurgitation is typically large and compliant. This dilation and the resultant increase in compliance account for the variability in the presence of *v* waves in the PCWP trace and may obscure the diagnosis of mitral regurgitation. The large compliant atrium can accommodate large regurgitant volumes without significant increases in pressure. The large *v* waves classically described for mitral regurgitation are, therefore, more common in acute mitral regurgitation. The compliant left atrium is also the reason that severe pulmonary hypertension is seen less frequently in these patients than in patients with mitral stenosis or acute mitral regurgitation.

Total cardiac output may be within the normal reference range to elevated; however, forward cardiac output is usually decreased in patients with moderately severe to severe mitral regurgitation. The amount of regurgitation, or the regurgitant fraction, is dependent on (a) the pressure gradient between the left ventricle and atrium, (b) the duration of ventricular ejection, and (c) the size of the mitral orifice, which is dependent on the status of the left ventricle. In the presence of a dilated left ventricle or impaired contractile function, the mitral valve orifice is increased in size, and as a consequence, regurgitation is worsened, which leads to a cycle of further damage to the left ventricle and increased regurgitation (102).

If acute mitral regurgitation is present, the compensatory changes in the compliance of the left ventricle and left atrium do not occur, and the sudden increase in left atrial pressure is transmitted to the pulmonary circulation. Subsequently, the LVEDP and pulmonary pressures are significantly elevated, and the acute symptoms of biventricular failure dominate the clinical presentation.

Anesthetic Implications

The eccentric hypertrophy, left ventricular chamber dilation, left atrial enlargement, and rarely, pulmonary hypertension associated with chronic mitral regurgitation determine the hemodynamic responses to anesthetic management in patients undergoing surgery. The guiding principle in the management of patients with regurgitant lesions is based on findings in studies of mitral regurgitation in animal models and patients, in which manipulation of preload, afterload, and contractility causing a decrease in LVEDV result in a decrease in regurgitant volume (137).

In patients with moderate to severe mitral regurgitation who are undergoing surgical procedures that may be associated with modest to large volume shifts, preload should be carefully monitored and optimized by using a pulmonary artery catheter or TEE. It may be difficult, at times, to balance the need for adequate preload against the risk of overdistension of the ventricle, which actually may cause further stretching of the annulus and increased regurgitation. In general, the size of the *v* wave of the PCWP (if present) waveform correlates with the regurgitant fraction, and this may help guide therapy.

As in aortic regurgitation, the fraction of stroke volume that is "regurgitated" is dependent on the size of the valve orifice, the duration of ventricular ejection (determined by the heart rate), and the pressure gradient across the valve. Afterload can be manipulated to reduce the pressure gradient to obtain the best possible forward flow. Optimally, afterload, as expressed by systemic vascular resistance and wall tension, should be kept low to decrease the regurgitant fraction. As forward flow increases due to the reduction of impedance to ventricular ejection, the diastolic volume and heart size decrease as well. These events contribute to the reduction of the orifice size, which is a major factor in decreasing the regurgitant flow (137). However, dramatic reduction of afterload with the use of vasodilators may cause a profound decrease in the diastolic blood pressure, which may impair coronary perfusion.

The duration of diastole is inversely related to the heart rate. Thus, bradycardia causes a relative increase in diastolic time and favors an increase in the regurgitant fraction. A faster heart rate, by increasing the duration of ventricular ejection, may augment forward flow and decrease the regurgitant volume. However, some doubt has recently been expressed about this concept (137). Generally, it is a good practice to maintain the heart rate at the preoperative level, provided the patient functions well at this rate.

Many patients with long-standing mitral regurgitation develop atrial fibrillation. A substantial number of these patients convert to normal sinus rhythm after mitral valve repair or replacement, although the vast majority revert to atrial fibrillation within a matter of hours. In our experience, a continuous infusion of procainamide may help preserve sinus rhythm for a longer time, thus optimizing the hemodynamic conditions after discontinuation of cardiopulmonary bypass into the immediate postoperative period.

More than in any other valvular heart procedure, maintenance of optimal myocardial performance is crucial, because mitral valve replacement with excision of the subvalvular apparatus (chordae) has the highest operative mortality rate and the poorest postoperative outcome of all left-sided valvular lesions. The anesthesiologist's task is preservation of myocardial contractility and optimization of loading conditions. After undergoing valve replacement, the patient with mitral regurgitation is at risk of perioperative pump failure, because the low-impedance pathway for left ventricular ejection is now closed. Therefore, afterload is increased while preload may be decreased. Many of these patients need some inotropic support in the form of dopamine or epinephrine. In patients with pulmonary hypertension, amrinone is our drug of choice for treatment of right-sided heart failure because of its potent pulmonary (and systemic) arterial vasodilatory effects, combined with inotropic actions. There are indications that preservation of the mitral apparatus, either by repairing the mitral valve or by sparing part of the mitral valve apparatus during mitral valve replacement, enhances myocardial performance (134).

Surgical Technique and Postoperative Problems

The approach to the mitral valve in mitral insufficiency is generally the same as in mitral stenosis, with the exception of cases of ischemic mitral regurgitation in the presence of a left ventricular aneurysm, in which the mitral valve may be approached through the aneurysm. Mitral valve replacement is technically the same as in mitral stenosis procedures, but mitral valve repair has gained popularity in the last decade. Frequently, mitral regurgitation is caused by a combination of dilation of the posterior aspect of the mitral annulus and elongation of chordae to one or both leaflets. This allows the leaflets to prolapse above the annular plane and into the left atrium.

Carpentier described a surgical technique to repair this mitral valve, consisting of resection of the redundant part of the posterior mitral valve leaflet, shortening of one or more sets of chordae tendineae, and insertion of a semirigid ring, which restores the geometry of the mitral annulus. Intraoperative 2D echocardiography and Doppler color flow mapping have been instrumental before repair in making an appropriate assessment of the valve to identify likely candidates, and after repair to immediately evaluate the hemodynamic result of the surgical intervention (91,138).

The hospital mortality rate after mitral valve replacement is probably higher than the mortality rate after mitral valve repair procedures (134) (the mortality rate for repairs approaches 0%, whereas the mortality rate for replacement appears to be between 2.7% and 6.9%) (139,140). The usual cause of postoperative death is associated with acute or subacute congestive heart failure (134,139,140). Two recent studies identified residual mitral regurgitation after mitral valve procedures as a major factor determining the incidence of congestive heart failure, death, and reoperation (91,138). Postoperative problems are essentially the same as in patients with mitral stenosis: atrial fibrillation, bleeding, and tamponade.

Long-term survival rates in patients leaving the hospital alive are from 70% to 75% after mitral valve replacement (139–141). The cumulative incidence of event-free long-term survival (free of thromboembolism, reoperation, endocarditis, and major hemorrhage) is 56% (141).

Intraoperative Echocardiography

In this area of increased interest in mitral valve repair, intraoperative echocardiography is a timely development. 2D TEE can provide the surgeon with a dynamic image of the (pathologic) anatomy of the mitral valve, including the subvalvular apparatus in a working heart under varied loading conditions. Doppler color flow imaging allows direct visualization of the pathophysiology of the valve about to be replaced or repaired, but it is particularly useful in the immediate evaluation of the surgical result after repair (See Color Fig. 20-8 between pages 560 and 561). Recent work has shown that acceptance of more than mild residual mitral regurgitation after mitral valve repair is related to a significant increase in the incidence of death, congestive heart failure, and the need for reoperation (138). Evaluation of the repaired valve immediately after discontinuation of cardiopulmonary bypass may lead to a decision to reinstitute bypass and revise the repair or replace the valve.

Evaluation of a replaced mitral valve for the presence of perivalvular leaks and function of the prosthesis is a particularly important use for TEE. Indeed, in approximately 11% of cases in our series, the findings of intraoperative echocardiography resulted in a major change in the operative plan (e.g., a procedure different from the one planned, reinstitution of bypass for re-repair or replacement of the valve) (138).

DISEASES OF THE TRICUSPID VALVE

Tricuspid Valve Anatomy

The tricuspid valve separates the right ventricle from the right atrium. The valve apparatus consists of the three leaflets (anterior, posterior, and septal), the annulus, two papillary muscles, and the chordae tendineae (which connect the papillary muscles to the free edges of the leaflets). The normal tricuspid valve area is approximately 7 to 9 cm^2 (142).

The tricuspid annulus is particularly important in the normal function of the valve. Tsakiris et al. have demonstrated that the tricuspid annulus shortens (i.e., the circumference decreases) by 25% during normal atrial systole, thereby contributing to normal valve closure (143). The annulus may dilate when right ventricular dilation secondary to pulmonary hypertension of right ventricular failure occur, preventing normal valve closure (144).

Tricuspid Stenosis

Etiology

The most common cause of tricuspid stenosis is rheumatic heart disease (143,145). Therefore, tricuspid stenosis is a rare disorder in developed countries. In addition, isolated stenosis of the tricuspid valve is extremely rare. Tricuspid stenosis is generally associated with concurrent disease of the mitral and aortic valves (143–147). However, the incidence of tricuspid stenosis in patients with left-sided rheumatic heart disease is variable (147).

Nonrheumatic causes of tricuspid stenosis include tumors that involve the right side of the heart (including right atrial myxomas), Löffler endocarditis, carcinoid syndrome, constrictive pericarditis, congenital disease of the tricuspid valve, and iatrogenic events (e.g., catheter entanglement, surgical annuloplasty for tricuspid regurgitation) (148).

Clinical Features

In general, the clinical history of tricuspid stenosis is largely dictated by the presence of the associated mitral and aortic disease (146). Nearly two thirds of patients with tricuspid valve disease are middle-aged women (146). Presenting symptoms include dyspnea, fatigue secondary to right ventricular failure, and systemic venous hypertension (144). The signs and symptoms of venous hypertension are often out of proportion to the symptoms of dyspnea.

Noninvasive assessment of hemodynamic events is possible, because jugular venous contours reflect right atrial pressure events. Examination of the jugular venous pulse is notable for dominant *a* waves in patients in sinus rhythm and slow *y* descent (shallow slope of the downward limb of the *v* wave) (149). Auscultation reveals a high-pitched, mid-diastolic murmur that increases with inspiration and is maximal at the lower left sternal edge. ECG signs of right atrial enlargement (large P waves in leads II, III, and aVF) may aid in the diagnosis of tricuspid stenosis.

Pathophysiology

Significant tricuspid stenosis probably occurs when the valve orifice decreases to less than 2 cm^2 and the transtricuspid pressure gradient is more than 2 mm Hg (144,150).

Right atrial pressure increases because of the obstruction. Subsequently, right ventricular filling pressure and right ventricular stroke volume decrease. Because tricuspid regurgitation often coexists with stenosis, right ventricular volumes may be low, normal (if the dominant lesion is stenosis), or increased (when significant regurgitation occurs).

The obstruction of the level of the tricuspid valve produces the two dominant hemodynamic abnormalities: (a) restriction of the heart's ability to increase cardiac output in response to increases in demand and (b) systemic venous hypertension.

Anesthetic Implications

There is little written about the appropriate management of tricuspid stenosis during anesthesia. General medical management of this disease is directed toward reduction of systemic venous hypertension and amelioration of congestive heart failure by the use of inotropic agents, diuretics, and vasodilator therapy. However, right-sided heart output depends on normal preload; therefore, care must also be taken to maintain adequate preload while avoiding volume overload in the perioperative fluid management of these patients. In general, patients with tricuspid stenosis respond favorably to increases in contractile state. These patients are similar to patients with aortic stenosis in that maintenance of sinus rhythm is particularly important. Atrial fibrillation and other supraventricular dysrhythmias can lead to a dramatic reduction in cardiac output due to elimination in effective right atrial contraction and subsequent reduction of right ventricular end-diastolic volume. Reduction of pulmonary artery pressure has little impact on the degree of forward flow in tricuspid stenosis.

There are no specific, absolute contraindications to the use of major conduction anesthesia in patients with tricuspid stenosis. However, because these patients frequently have abnormal aortic and mitral valves, caution is advised before spinal or epidural anesthesia is instituted, because systemic vasodilation may lead to dramatic hypotension in the presence of mitral and/or aortic stenosis.

Surgical Technique

In lieu of operative procedures to correct tricuspid stenosis, closed tricuspid valve balloon commissurotomy may be performed (151). Surgical correction of tricuspid stenosis necessitates bicaval cannulation, regardless of the type of procedure (147,148). The technique for open commissurotomy involves separation of the fused anterior and septal leaflets and the fused posterior and septal leaflets (147,148). The anterior-posterior leaflet apposition is left undisturbed, because separation of these leaflets may lead to an excessive amount of tricuspid regurgitation.

In the presence of extensive valvular and annular calcification, replacement of the valve may be necessary. In general, tissue valves are preferred in patients older than 50 years (147,148). In younger patients, low-profile, mechanical prosthetics are preferred for reasons of durability. The Björk-Shiley (tilting disk) valve has been used sparingly after reports of sudden thrombosis and strut fracture. According to Kirklin et al. (147), the ideal replacement prosthesis is a stent-mounted semilunar homograft. A large heterograft (porcine) device may be used in lieu of the human homograft (147).

Tricuspid Regurgitation

Etiology

As with tricuspid stenosis, the most common etiology worldwide for tricuspid regurgitation is rheumatic heart disease (152). Again, isolated involvement of the tricuspid valve is extremely rare. Tricuspid regurgitation may be seen as an additional, primary lesion in rheumatic heart disease, but it is most commonly a functional lesion, that is, the result of annular dilation due to pulmonary hypertension secondary to end-stage left-sided rheumatic valve disease (usually mitral stenosis), chronic congestive heart failure, or chronic cor pulmonale (144,153).

Acute infective endocarditis involving the tricuspid valve is extremely rare, except in intravenous drug abusers (153, 154). Tricuspid valve function rapidly declines secondary to destruction of the leaflet tissue or chordae. Vegetations may often embolize to the pulmonary vasculature, leading to pulmonary hypertension that often raises the mortality and morbidity rates for tricuspid regurgitation (154). Other less common causes of tricuspid regurgitation include tricuspid valve prolapse, Ebstein anomaly, severe chest trauma, carcinoid syndrome, thyrotoxicosis, Marfan syndrome, and right ventricular infarction leading to papillary muscle dysfunction (143,153).

Clinical Features

The clinical history of tricuspid regurgitation is most often dictated by the accompanying left-sided rheumatic valve lesions. Isolated tricuspid regurgitation leading to volume overload of the right ventricle is often well tolerated for long periods (154). However, when tricuspid regurgitation is the result of left-sided valvular disease and pulmonary hypertension, symptoms of biventricular failure may develop quickly (148). Hepatic congestion, ascites, and edema may dominate the clinical picture.

Examination of the jugular venous contour reveals a large *v* wave with a rapid *y* descent. The *v* wave may be so prominent as to be confused with the carotid pulse (155). Cardiac examination findings are notable for a right ventricular lift suggestive of right ventricular hypertrophy. A holosystolic murmur that often increases with inspiration is best heard over the lower sternum and xiphoid. The ECG signs of right atrial and ventricular enlargement often accompany the physical signs, although atrial fibrillation is commonly associated with tricuspid regurgitation. Echocardiography demonstrates enlargement of the right atrium and ventricle (148,156,157). In many cases, dilation of the inferior vena cava, hepatic veins, and coronary sinus may be seen. Doppler examination of the tricuspid apparatus demonstrating a systolic jet in the right atrium is considered diagnostic for tricuspid regurgitation (157).

Pathophysiology

Tricuspid regurgitation causes a reversal of the normal flow pattern on the right side of the heart. During ventricular systole, decreased flow into the right atrium and reversal of flow from the atrium into the ventricle occur. When pulmonary artery pressure is normal, this volume overload of the right ventricle caused by primary tricuspid regurgitation can be tolerated for long periods before symptoms intervene. In addition, right atrial pressure increases minimally because of the compliance of the atrium and venae cavae. However, when pulmonary hypertension and/or left ventricular failure is the cause of functional tricuspid regurgitation, the afterload stress on the right ventricle, coupled with annular dilation and regurgitation, leads to reduced ejection performance on the right ventricle (148,152). The reduced right-sided heart output and pulmonary blood flow eventually lead to further left-sided failure due to underloading of the left ventricle. In addition, in the presence of right ventricular failure and chamber enlargement, the shift of the intraventricular septum toward the left ventricular chamber may impair left ventricular filling and ejection.

In general terms, there is a direct relationship between the level of right ventricular pressure (and subsequently pulmonary artery pressure) and the regurgitant fraction. Thus, medical management of patients with tricuspid regurgitation is aimed at reduction of pulmonary hypertension.

Anesthetic Implications

Certain principles for the safe anesthetic management of tricuspid regurgitation apply, regardless of the presence or absence of pulmonary hypertension. However, when pulmonary hypertension is part of the clinical picture, it tends to be the more dominant consideration. Additionally, because tricuspid regurgitation is most commonly a functional lesion secondary to aortic or mitral valve disease, considerations for these left-sided processes may be more important.

In some respects, the management of tricuspid regurgitation is similar to that for other regurgitant lesions. In general, it is prudent to maintain normovolemia or mild hypervolemia to preserve right ventricular stroke volume and left-sided filling pressure. Because of high compliance of the right atrium, the central venous pressure is a poor indicator of the intravascular volume status.

In the presence of pulmonary hypertension, it is necessary to avoid increases in pulmonary vascular resistance. Hypercarbia and hypoxia are particularly deleterious. In addition, overinflation of the lungs or high ventilatory pressures may increase pulmonary vascular resistance and reduce right-sided filling pressures. Halothane and ketamine may be good choices. Ultimately, left and right ventricular function determines the choice of a particular agent. It should be noted that the central venous pressure may not be a reliable index of regurgitation or of intravascular volume. In addition, the accuracy of thermodilution cardiac output measurements in the presence of tricuspid regurgitation has been questioned because of the possibility of recirculation of the cold indicator (158). However, in a recent study, tricuspid regurgitation did not limit the utility of thermodilution cardiac output determinations (159).

Surgical Technique and Postoperative Problems

Similar to operations to correct tricuspid stenosis, procedures for the excision, repair, or replacement of an incompetent tricuspid valve require bicaval cannulation and usually are approached via median sternotomy (142,147,160).

In cases of isolated tricuspid regurgitation due to endocarditis, the tricuspid valve may be excised to control the infection without replacement (161). Because tricuspid valve excision has a hospital mortality rate of nearly 10%, this procedure is reserved for habitual intravenous drug abusers and for those in whom reinfection is likely (154, 162).

Under certain conditions, including ruptured chordae tendineae and functional tricuspid regurgitation, the regurgitant valve may be repaired with annuloplasty (148). The DeVega annuloplasty essentially involves placement of two encircling purse-string sutures to narrow the annulus (163). The Carpentier technique uses excision of any flail portion of the valve and a prosthetic rigid, cloth-covered ring to reduce the valve orifice (164). With either technique, it is important to avoid manipulation of the area near the ventricular septum, which contains the conduction tissue.

Considerations for the type of prosthetic device for tricuspid valve replacement are similar to those for tricuspid stenosis (see previous discussion).

Because of the proximity of the atrioventricular node and bundle to the tricuspid annulus, complete heart block or slow ventricular response to atrial fibrillation may develop early in the postoperative period in 5% to 9% of patients and is much more likely to occur after combined mitral and tricuspid procedures (160).

Anticoagulation with warfarin is continued for the first 3 months postoperatively in patients who receive tissue valves, because of the risk of thromboembolism (147). The risk of thromboembolic events is greater for prosthetic devices in the tricuspid position because of the low pressure and low flow velocity on the right side of the heart (147). In addition, because of the bellows-shaped configuration of the right ventricle, the tricuspid prosthesis can often become compressed between the intraventricular septum and the right ventricular free wall, resulting in valve obstruction.

Transesophageal Echocardiographic Images

TEE with combined 2D and Doppler color flow imaging has proved useful in the intraoperative management of functional tricuspid regurgitation (156). However, because the right ventricle and therefore the tricuspid valve are in an anterior location, transthoracic imaging is superior to the transesophageal approach (165). Tricuspid regurgitation is characterized by a systolic, mosaically colored jet originating in the right ventricle and directed toward and into the right atrium.

Preoperative grading of tricuspid regurgitation in the presence of mitral valve disease has been shown to be important in determining whether to replace or repair the tricuspid valve after the mitral valve procedure (87,156). Patients with moderate to severe functional tricuspid regurgitation may be best managed by operative correction, whereas patients with mild functional tricuspid regurgitation may be better served with nonsurgical management after mitral valve procedures (148,156).

Infective Endocarditis

Infective endocarditis is an infection of the endocardium or of a cardiac valve, distal structures such as atrioventricular fistulas or vascular prostheses may be involved as well.

In approximately three quarters of patients, the lesion is localized on an acquired valvular anomaly or on a congenital defect.

In adult cardiac surgical patients, to whom we will limit this discussion, we most often encounter lesions on bicuspid aortic valves, prolapsing or floppy mitral valves, and calcific aortic stenosis or calcified mitral annulus.

It is thought that the increased blood flow velocity across the above-mentioned lesions causes the infective agents to settle just beyond the orifice. Adherence of platelets and fibrin in the same area facilitates the implantation of the bacteria. Thus, in subacute bacterial endocarditis, the vegetations will be found downstream from the lesion, for example, on the atrial surface of the mitral valve in patients with mitral regurgitation.

Bacteremia is thought to be a necessary condition for the development of infective endocarditis, although opinions are changing with regard to what procedures might cause significant bacteremia. Dental procedures, for instance, are no longer regarded by some to constitute a significant risk.

In our practice, most surgical patients with bacterial endocarditis appear to have a history of either intravenous narcotic abuse or cardiac prosthetic valves.

The most prevalent organisms causing bacterial endocarditis are streptococcus, enterococcus, and *Staphylococcus aureus*, but almost any species of microorganism can cause infective endocarditis.

The manifestations of infective endocarditis are, to some extent, dependent on the causing organism. The more virulent the organism, the more prominent the systemic toxicity, valve damage, and metastatic symptoms; less virulent organisms may cause a more benign, subacute, clinical picture.

Most patients with subacute bacterial endocarditis present with fever, often with afternoon and evening peaks, as well as with a heart murmur. Other, not uncommon, symptoms are low back pain, myalgia, and arthralgia.

Signs include proximal subungual hemorrhages, Osler nodes, and petechiae, particularly on the anterior upper trunk. A substantial percentage of patients have splenomegaly. Embolic phenomena, such as hemiplegia (30% to 50% of patients have some neurologic complication), pleuritic pain, flank pain with hematuria, blindness, and others, may precipitate awareness of the diagnosis.

Acute bacterial endocarditis has similar signs and symptoms, which are however much more fulminant.

Almost all patients with bacterial endocarditis have normocytic, normochromic anemia, most show leukocytosis and histiocytes may be found. Proteinuria is common. Most patients have positive blood cultures, although positive cultures may be late in developing if the patient is being treated with antibiotics.

As far as prosthetic valve endocarditis is concerned, mechanical prostheses have relatively high early risk—as high as 3% in the first year—of endocarditis. Interestingly, aortic (freehand) homografts have no risk of early infection. The long-term risk of prosthetic valve endocarditis remains significantly higher for mechanical valves than for bioprostheses and homografts. Prosthetic endocarditis occurs most often at the interface between the annulus and the sewing ring. Frequently, an annular abscess exists. The abscess often destroys some of the sutures, causing partial dehiscence of the valve with a subsequent perivalvular leak. Most abscesses are seen in the aortic annulus. Aortic valve endocarditis occasionally results in the formation of an aneurysm of the sinus of Valsalva, which may rupture into a cardiac chamber, most frequently a right-sided chamber.

Mitral valve endocarditis may be as restricted as a small vegetation on a leaflet without hemodynamic consequence or as serious as rupture of the chordae tendineae and perforation of one or both leaflets with severe mitral regurgitation. Because of the often short duration of the mitral regurgitation, these patients very often remain in normal sinus rhythm, greatly simplifying the intraoperative and postoperative management. The location of annular abscesses may cause electrophysiologic complications, however, in the form of right or left bundle-branch block or significant prolongation of the PR interval.

The surgical treatment of the cardiac complications of

bacterial endocarditis has greatly improved the outcome. Even though the operative mortality rate may be in the order of 15% to 20%, the mortality rate of patients treated medically is 75% to 80%.

Surgical treatment of prosthetic valve endocarditis has a relatively high risk of recurrence, in contrast to surgery for native valvular endocarditis. Prosthetic device endocarditis carries a 6-month mortality rate of up to 50%. The insertion of freehand aortic homografts, even in operations on already infected valves, has a 6-month mortality rate of approximately 20%.

APPENDIX 20-1

Issues in Selection of Prosthetic Valves

The type of prosthetic valve chosen depends mostly on the age of the patient, the size of the valve (particularly the sewing ring) in relation to the size of the orifice, and surgical preference. Tissue valves such as the Carpentier-Edwards porcine heterograft require no long-term anticoagulation but have a life span shorter than that of the mechanical valves. Mechanical prosthetic valves in use today include the St. Jude rotating disk, the Starr-Edwards ball valve, and the Hall-Kaster, Medtronic, and Björk-Shiley tilting disk valve. The mechanical valves have a longer life span and the reoperation interval is longer, compared with the tissue valves. However, these devices require long-term anticoagulation with warfarin.

Need of long-term anticoagulation is perhaps the single most important consideration in choosing between a mechanical prosthesis and a biologic device. The lack of need for long-term anticoagulation of the bioprosthesis has great advantages over the lifelong anticoagulation necessary in patients with mechanical devices (27,111,163–168). The actual incidence of thromboembolic events may be similar for patients with mechanical devices, compared with patients who have biologic valves (169). However, most of the patients who receive biologic devices are not on anticoagulation therapy. Anticoagulation with warfarin is started in all patients immediately after surgery, regardless of the type of prosthetic valve. Therapy is usually discontinued in the second postoperative month in patients receiving tissue valves. However, in patients with significant left atrial enlargement, the risk of thromboembolic events is high enough, after insertion of bioprosthesis in the mitral position, to warrant continued anticoagulation.

The other issue is the durability of the mechanical, compared with the biologic, prostheses. Long-term durability of the bioprostheses has been particularly disappointing in younger individuals when they are used in the mitral position (27,111,166–168). The mechanical valves have greater durability, excellent flow characteristics, and a low incidence of mechanical valve failure. However, one such type of failure deserves mention. The Björk-Shiley tilting disk valve is no longer sold in the United States because of the occurrence of outlet strut fracture (213 reports in 83,000 prostheses) in one particular model (the 60° convexoconcave valve).

REFERENCES

1. Burns J, Covell J, Ross JJ. Mechanics of isotonic left ventricular contraction. *Am J Physiol* 1973;224:725.
2. Braunwald E, Sarnoff S, Stainsby W. Determinants of duration and mean rate of ventricular ejection. *Circ Res* 1958;6:319.
3. Grossman W, Braunwald E, Mann T, et al. Contractile state of the left ventricle in man as evaluated from end-systolic pressure-volume relations. *Circulation* 1977;56:845.
4. Mason D, Braunwald E, Covell J, et al. Assessment of cardiac contractility. *Circulation* 1971;44:47.
5. Alpert B, Benson L, Olley P. E_{max} during exercise in children with left-sided cardiac disease. *Am J Cardiol* 1980;45:467.
6. Noble N. Left ventricle load, arterial impedance and their interrelationship. *Cardiovasc Res* 1979;13:183.
7. Rankin J, McHale P, Arentzen C, et al. Three dimensional dynamic geometry of the left ventricle in the conscious dog. *Circ Res* 1976;39:304.
8. Foex P, Francis C, Cutfield G, et al. The pressure-length loop. *Br J Anaesth* 1988;60:65S.
9. Suga H, Sagawa K, Shoukas A. Load independence of the instantaneous pressure-volume relation of the canine left ventricle and effects of epinephrine and heart rate on the ratio. *Circ Res* 1973;32:314.
10. Taylor R, Covell J, Ross JJ. Volume-tension diagrams of ejecting and isovolumic contractions in the left ventricle. *Am J Physiol* 1966;211:674.
11. Weber K, Janicki J, Hefner L. Left ventricular force-length relations of isovolumic and ejecting contraction. *Am J Physiol* 1976; 231:337.
12. Mehmed H, Stockins B, Ruffman K, et al. The linearity of the end-systolic pressure-volume relationship and its sensitivity for assessment of left ventricular function. *Circulation* 1981;63: 1216.
13. Way B, Victory J, LeWinter M, et al. Hysteresis of left ventricular end-diastolic pressure dimensions relationships after acute pressure-loading in the dog. *Cardiovasc Res* 1986;20:490.
14. Giuliani E, Fuster V, Shub C, et al. Acquired valvular heart disease: aortic valvular stenosis. In: Giuliani E, Fuster V, Gersh B, et al., eds. *Cardiology: fundamentals and practice.* St. Louis, MO: Mosby–Year Book, 1991:1505.
15. Normand J, Loire R, Zambartas C. The anatomical aspects of adult aortic stenosis. *Eur Heart J* 1988;9[Suppl E]:31.
16. Kirklin J, Barratt-Boyes B. Aortic valve disease. In: Kirklin J, Barratt-Boyes B, eds. *Cardiac surgery. Morphology, diagnostic criteria, natural history, techniques, results and indications.* New York: John Wiley and Sons, 1986.
17. Anderson M, Kelsy JJ, Edwards J. Clinical and pathological considerations in cases of calcific aortic stenosis. *JAMA* 1952; 149:9.
18. Frank S, Johnson A, Ross JJ. Natural history of valvular aortic stenosis. *Br Heart J* 1973;35:41.
19. Rappaport E. Natural history of aortic and mitral valve disease. *Am J Cardiol* 1975;35:221.
20. Pellikka P, Nishimura R, Bailey K, et al. The natural history of adults with asymptomatic, hemodynamically significant aortic stenosis. *J Am Coll Cardiol* 1990;15:1012.
21. Braunwald E. On the natural history of severe aortic stenosis. *J Am Coll Cardiol* 1990;15:1018.

22. Craver J, Goldstein J, Jones E, et al. Clinical, hemodynamic, and operative descriptors affecting outcome of aortic valve replacement in elderly versus young patients. *Ann Surg* 1984;199:733.
23. Craver J, Weintraub W, Jones E, et al. Predictors of mortality, complications, and length of stay in aortic valve replacement for aortic stenosis. *Circulation* 1988;78[Suppl 3, Pt 2]:I85.
24. Tamari I, Borer J, Goldberg H, et al. Hemodynamic changes during retrograde left-heart catheterization in patients with aortic stenosis. *Cardiology* 1991;78:171.
25. Danielsen R, Nordrehaug J, Vik-Mo H. Clinical and haemodynamic features in relation to severity of aortic stenosis in adults. *Eur Heart J* 1991;12:791.
26. Kern M, Deligonul U. Interpretation of cardiac pathophysiology from pressure waveform analysis: I. The stenotic aortic valve. *Cathet Cardiovasc Dis* 1990;21:112.
27. Barlow J, Pocock W, Marchand P, et al. The significance of late systolic murmurs. *Am Heart J* 1963;66:443.
28. Thompson R, Mitchell A, Ahmed M, et al. Conduction defects in aortic valve disease. *Am Heart J* 1979;98:3.
29. Marx G. Noninvasive assessment of aortic valve disease. In: Emery R, Arom K, eds. *The aortic valve.* Philadelphia: Hanley & Belfus, 1989:39.
30. Currie P, Seward J, Reeder G, et al. Continuous-wave Doppler echocardiographic assessment of severity of calcific aortic stenosis: a simultaneous Doppler-catheterization correlation in 100 patients. *Circulation* 1985;71:1162.
31. Miller FJ. Aortic stenosis: most cases no longer require invasive hemodynamic study. *J Am Coll Cardiol* 1989;13:551.
32. Reynolds T. The determination of aortic valve area by the Gorlin formula: what the cardiac sonographer should know. *J Am Soc Echocardiogr* 1990;3:331.
33. Jorgensen C. The pathophysiology of aortic stenosis. In: Emery R, Arom K, eds. *The aortic valve.* Philadelphia: Hanley & Belfus, 1989:9.
34. Pantley G, Rahimtoda S. Effects of successful, uncomplicated valve replacement on ventricular hypertrophy, volume and performance in aortic stenosis and in aortic incompetence. *J Thorac Cardiovasc Surg* 1978;75:383.
35. Diver D, Royal H, Aroesty J, et al. Diastolic function in patients with aortic stenosis: influence of left ventricular load reduction. *J Am Coll Cardiol* 1988;12:642.
36. Ritter M, Hess O, Murakami T, et al. Left ventricular systolic series elastic properties in aortic stenosis before and after valve replacement. *Cardiovasc Res* 1988;22:759.
37. Smucker M, Tedesco C, Manning S, et al. Demonstration of an imbalance between coronary perfusion and excessive load as a mechanism of ischemia during stress in patients with aortic stenosis. *Circulation* 1988;78:573.
38. Neill W, Fluri-Lundeen J. Myocardial oxygen supply in left ventricular hypertrophy and coronary artery disease. *Am J Cardiol* 1979;44:747.
39. Bertrand M, Lablanche J, Tilmant P, et al. Coronary sinus blood flow at rest and during isometric exercise in patients with aortic valve disease: mechanism of angina pectoris in presence of normal coronary arteries. *Am J Cardiol* 1981;47:199.
40. Sarnoff S, Braunwald E, Welch GJ, et al. Hemodynamic determinants of oxygen consumption of the heart with special reference to the tension-time index. *Am J Physiol* 1958;192:148.
41. Alyono D, Anderson R, Parrish D, et al. Alterations of myocardial blood flow associated with experimental canine left ventricular hypertrophy secondary to valvular aortic stenosis. *Circ Res* 1986;58:47.
42. Naeye R, Liedtke A. Consequences of intramyocardial arterial lesions in aortic valvular stenosis. *Am J Pathol* 1976;85:569.
43. Hoffman J. Maximal coronary flow and the concept of coronary reserve. *Circulation* 1984;70:199.
44. O'Keefe JJ, Shub C, Rettje S. Risk of noncardiac surgical procedures in patients with aortic stenosis. *Mayo Clin Proc* 1989;64:400.
45. Smith V, Schulman P, Karimeddini M, et al. Rapid ventricular filling in left ventricular hypertrophy: II. Pathologic hypertrophy. *J Am Coll Cardiol* 1985;5:869.
46. Fifer M, Borow K, Colan S, et al. Early diastolic left ventricular function in children and adults with aortic stenosis. *J Am Coll Cardiol* 1985;5:1147.
47. Ross JJ. Afterload mismatch and preload reserve—a conceptual framework for the analysis of ventricular failure. *Prog Cardiovasc Dis* 1976;18:255.
48. DePace N, Ren J, Iskandrian A, et al. Correlation of echocardiographic wall stress and left ventricular pressure and function in aortic stenosis. *Circulation* 1983;67:854.
49. Douglas P, Reichek N, Hacnkey K, et al. Contribution of afterload, hypertrophy, and geometry to left ventricular ejection fraction in aortic stenosis, pure aortic regurgitation and idiopathic dilated cardiomyopathy. *Am J Cardiol* 1987;59:1398.
50. Cody RJ, Stephens D, Walker H, et al. Early post-operative changes in left ventricular dimensions and mass following valve replacement in adults with aortic stenosis. *J Cardiovasc Surg* 1981;22:19.
51. Cutilletta A. Regression of myocardial hypertrophy: III. Alterations in left ventricular performance. *J Mol Cell Cardiol* 1982;14:695.
52. Monrad E, Hess O, Murakami T, et al. Time course of regression of left ventricular hypertrophy after aortic valve replacement. *Circulation* 1988;77:1345.
53. West J, Estrada S, Heerdt M. Sudden hypotension associated with midazolam and sufentanil [Letter]. *Anesth Analg* 1987;66:693.
54. Waller J, Hug C, Nagle D, et al. Hemodynamic changes during fentanyl-oxygen anesthesia for aortocoronary bypass operation. *Anesthesiology* 1981;55:212.
55. Bovill J, Sebel P, Fiolet J, et al. The influence of sufentanil on endocrine and metabolic responses to cardiac surgery. *Anesth Analg* 1983;62:391.
56. Larach D, Hensley FJ, Martin D, et al. Hemodynamic effects of muscle relaxant drugs during anesthetic induction in patients with mitral or aortic valvular heart disease. *J Cardiothorac Vasc Anesth* 1991;5:126.
57. Scott W, Miller D, Haverich A, et al. Determinants of operative mortality for patients undergoing aortic valve replacement. Discriminant analysis of 1479 operations. *J Thorac Cardiovasc Surg* 1985;89:400.
58. McGoon D. Valve replacement: a comparative analysis of long-term results. In: Vogel J, ed. *Cardiovascular medicine.* New York: Raven Press, 1982:277.
59. Roman M, Devereux R, Niles N, et al. Aortic root dilatation as a cause of isolated, severe aortic regurgitation: prevalence, clinical and echocardiographic patterns, and relation to left ventricular hypertrophy and function. *Ann Intern Med* 1987;106:800.
60. Waller B. Rheumatic and nonrheumatic conditions producing valvular heart disease. *Cardiovasc Clin* 1986;16:3.
61. Edwards J. Manifestations of acquired and congenital diseases of the aorta. *Curr Probl Cardiol* 1979;3:1.
62. Yousof A, Mohammed M, Shuhaiber H, et al. Chronic severe aortic regurgitation: a prospective follow-up of 60 asymptomatic patients. *Am Heart J* 1988;116:1262.
63. Hegglin R, Scheu H, Rothlin M. Aortic insufficiency. *Circulation* 1968;38[Suppl 5]:77.
64. McGoon M, Fuster V, Shub C, et al. Acquired valvular heart

disease. Aortic regurgitation. In: Giuliani E, Fuster V, Gersh B, et al., eds. *Cardiology: fundamentals and practice.* St. Louis, MO: Mosby–Year Book, 1991:1524.
65. Bonow R, Rosing D, Kent K. Timing of operation for chronic aortic regurgitation. *Am J Cardiol* 1982;50:325.
66. Timmerman P, Willems J, Piessens J, et al. Angina pectoris and coronary artery disease in severe aortic regurgitation. *Am J Cardiol* 1988;61:826.
67. Louagie Y, Brohet C, Robert A, et al. Factors influencing postoperative survival in aortic regurgitation: analysis by Cox regression model. *J Thorac Cardiovasc Surg* 1984;88:225.
68. Samuels D, Curfman G, Friedlich A, et al. Valve replacement for aortic regurgitation: long term follow-up with factors influencing the results. *Circulation* 1979;60:647.
69. Grossman W, Jones D, McLaurin L. Patterns of hypertrophy in the human left ventricle. *J Clin Invest* 1975;56:56.
70. Grant C, Greene D, Bunnell I. Left ventricular enlargement and hypertrophy: a clinical and angiocardiographic study. *Am J Med* 1965;39:895.
71. Spotnitz H, Antunes M. Effect of aortic and mitral regurgitation of left ventricular structure and function. In: Karp R, ed. *Advances in cardiac surgery.* St. Louis, MO: Mosby–Year Book, 1990:85.
72. Ricci D. Afterload mismatch and preload reserve in chronic aortic regurgitation. *Circulation* 1982;66:826.
73. Osbakken M, Bove A, Spann J. Left ventricular function in chronic aortic regurgitation with reference to end-systolic pressure, volume and stress relations. *Am J Cardiol* 1981;47:193.
74. Niles N, Borer J, Kamen M, et al. Preoperative left and right ventricular performance in combined aortic and mitral regurgitation and comparison with isolated aortic or mitral regurgitation. *Am J Cardiol* 1990;65:1372.
75. Mehmel H, Olshausen KV, Schuler G, et al. Estimation of left ventricular myocardial function by the ejection fraction in isolated, chronic, pure aortic regurgitation. *Am J Cardiol* 1984;54:610.
76. Huxley R, Gafney F, Corbett J, et al. Early detection of left ventricular dysfunction in chronic aortic regurgitation as assessed by contrast angiography, echocardiography, and rest and exercise scintigraphy. *Am J Cardiol* 1983;51:1542.
77. Kawanishi D, McKay C, Chandraratna P, et al. Cardiovascular response to dynamic exercise in patients with chronic symptomatic mild-to-moderate and severe aortic regurgitation. *Circulation* 1986;73:62.
78. Dehmer G, Firth B, Hillis L, et al. Alterations in left ventricular volumes and ejection fraction at rest and during exercise in patients with aortic regurgitation. *Am J Cardiol* 1981;47:17.
79. Morganroth J, Perloff J, Zeldis S, et al. Acute severe aortic regurgitation: pathophysiology, clinical recognition, and management. *Ann Intern Med* 1977;87:223.
80. Perloff J. Acute severe aortic regurgitation: recognition and management. *J Cardiovasc Med* 1983;2:209.
81. Firth B, Dehmer G, Nicod P, et al. Effect of increasing heart rate in patients with aortic regurgitation. Effect of incremental atrial pacing on scintigraphic, hemodynamic and thermodilution measurements. *Am J Cardiol* 1982;49:1860.
82. Brawley R, Morrow A. Direct determinants of aortic blood flow in patients with aortic regurgitation: effects of alterations of heart rate, increased ventricular preload or afterload, and isoproterenol. *Circulation* 1967;35:32.
83. O'Rourke R, Crawford M. Timing of valve replacement in patients with chronic aortic regurgitation [Editorial]. *Circulation* 1980;61:493.
84. Gaasch W, Carroll J, Levine H, et al. Chronic aortic regurgitation: prognostic value of left ventricular end-systolic dimension and end-diastolic radius/thickness ratio. *J Am Coll Cardiol* 1983;1:775.
85. Forman R, Firth B, Barnard M. Prognostic significance of preoperative left ventricular ejection fraction and valve lesion in patients with aortic valve replacement. *Am J Cardiol* 1980;45:1120.
86. Clark D, McAnulty J, Rahimtoola S. Valve replacement in aortic insufficiency with left ventricular dysfunction. *Circulation* 1980;61:411.
87. Goldman M, Fuster V, Guarino T, et al. Intraoperative echocardiography for the evaluation of valvular regurgitation: experience in 263 patients. *Circulation* 1986;74[Suppl 1]:143.
88. Cujec B, David T, Wilansky S, et al. Colour flow imaging in severe mitral and aortic regurgitation. *Can J Cardiol* 1988;4:341.
89. Grayburn P, Handshoe R, Smith M, et al. Quantitative assessment of the hemodynamic consequences of aortic regurgitation by means of continuous wave Doppler recordings. *J Am Coll Cardiol* 1987;10:135.
90. Goldman M, Packer M, Horowitz S, et al. Relation between exercise-induced changes in ejection fraction and systolic loading conditions at rest in aortic regurgitation. *J Am Coll Cardiol* 1984;3:924.
91. deBruijn N, Clements F, Kisslo J. Transesophageal applications of color flow imaging. *Echocardiography* 1987;4:557.
92. DuPlessis L, Marchand P. The anatomy of the mitral valve and its associated structures. *Thorax* 1964;19:221.
93. Frater R. Functional anatomy of the mitral valve. In: Ionescu M, Cohn L, eds. *Mitral valve disease: diagnosis and treatment.* London: Butterworth-Heineman, 1985:127.
94. Brandenburg R, Giuliani E, Nishimura R, et al. Acquired valvular heart disease: mitral stenosis. In: Giuliani E, Fuster V, Gersh B, et al., eds. *Cardiology: fundamentals and practice.* St. Louis, MO: Mosby–Year Book, 1991:1543.
95. Davies M. The pathology of the mitral valve. In: Ionescu M, Cohn L, eds. *Mitral valve disease: diagnosis and treatment.* London: Butterworth-Heineman, 1985:27.
96. Roberts W. Morphologic features of the normal and abnormal mitral valve. *Am J Cardiol* 1983;51:1005.
97. Olesen K. The natural history of 271 patients with mitral stenosis under medical treatment. *Br Heart J* 1962;24:349.
98. Rowe J, Bland E, Sprague H, et al. The course of mitral stenosis without surgery: ten- and twenty-year perspectives. *Ann Intern Med* 1960;52:741.
99. Selzer A, Cohn K. Natural history of mitral stenosis: a review. *Circulation* 1972;45:878.
100. Wilson J, Greenwood W. The natural history of mitral stenosis. *Can Med Assoc J* 1954;71:3223.
101. Wood P. An appreciation of mitral stenosis. *Br Med J* 1954;1:1051.
102. Braunwald E, Turi Z. Pathophysiology of mitral valve disease. In: Ionescu M, Cohn L, eds. *Mitral valve disease: diagnosis and treatment.* London: Butterworth-Heineman, 1985:3.
103. Bailey G, Braniff B, Hancock E, et al. Relation of left atrial pathology to atrial fibrillation in mitral valvular disease. *Ann Intern Med* 1968;69:13.
104. Coulshed N, Epstein E, McKendrick C, et al. Systemic embolism in mitral valve disease. *Br Heart J* 1974;32:26.
105. Bloomfield P, Boyle J, Parisi A. Non-invasive investigations for the diagnosis of mitral valve disease. In: Ionescu M, Cohn L, eds. *Mitral valve disease: diagnosis and treatment.* London: Butterworth-Heineman, 1985;53.
106. Effron M, Alderman E, Popp R. Preoperative invasive testing in mitral stenosis: indications based on assessment of diagnostic yield. *Am J Cardiol* 1983;51:1116.

107. Grant R. After-histories for ten years of a thousand men suffering from heart disease. *Heart* 1933;6:275.
108. Reichek N, Shelburne J, Perloff J. Clinical aspects of rheumatic valvular disease. *Prog Cardiovasc Dis* 1973;15:491.
109. Thompson M, Shaver J, Leon D. Effect of tachycardia on atrial transport in mitral stenosis. *Am Heart J* 1977;94:297.
110. Gorlin R. Natural history, medical therapy and indications for surgery in mitral valve disease. In: Ionescu M, Cohn L, eds. *Mitral valve disease: diagnosis and treatment.* London: Butterworth-Heineman, 1985;105.
111. Starr A, Grunkemeier G, Lambert L, et al. Mitral valve replacement. *Circulation* 1976;54[Suppl III]:111.
112. Teoh K, Ivanov J, Weisel R. Determinants of survival and valve failure after mitral valve replacement. *Ann Thorac Surg* 1990; 49:643.
113. Heller S, Carlton R. Abnormal left ventricular contraction in patients with mitral stenosis. *Circulation* 1970;42:1099.
114. Kennedy J, Yarnell S, Murray J, et al. Quantitative angiocardiography: IV. Relationships of left atrial and ventricular pressure and volume in mitral valve disease. *Circulation* 1970;41:817.
115. Braunwald E, Ross JJ. Applicability of Starling's law of the heart to man. *Circ Res* 1964;14-15:II169.
116. Silverstein D, Hansen D, Ojiambo H, et al. Left ventricular function in severe pure mitral stenosis as seen at the Kenyatta National Hospital. *Am Heart J* 1980;99:727.
117. Schulte-Sasse U, Hess W, Tarnow J. Pulmonary vascular responses in patients with normal and high pulmonary vascular resistance. *Anesthesiology* 1982;57:9.
118. Heerdt P, Caldwell R. The mechanism of nitrous oxide-induced changes in pulmonary vascular resistance in a dog model of left atrial outflow obstruction. *J Cardiothorac Anesth* 1989;3:568.
119. Rorie D, Tyce G, Sill J. Increased norepinephrine release from dog pulmonary artery caused by nitrous oxide. *Anesth Analg* 1986;65:560.
120. Hess W. Effects of amrinone on the right side of the heart. *J Cardiothorac Anesth* 1989;3[Suppl 2]:38.
121. D'Ambra M, LaRaia P, Philbin D, et al. Prostaglandin E_1. A new therapy for refractory right heart failure and pulmonary hypertension after mitral valve replacement. *J Thorac Cardiovasc Surg* 1985;89:567.
122. Lock J, Khalilullah M, Shrivastava S, et al. Percutaneous catheter commissurotomy in rheumatic mitral stenosis. *N Engl J Med* 1985;313:1515.
123. Lower R, Ducey K. Open mitral valvotomy. In: Ionescu M, Cohn L, eds. *Mitral valve disease: diagnosis and treatment.* London: Butterworth-Heineman, 1985:153.
124. Ionescu M, Chidambaram, M. Operative techniques for mitral valve replacement. In: Ionescu M, Cohn L, eds. *Mitral valve disease: diagnosis and treatment.* London: Butterworth-Heineman, 1985:191.
125. Katske G, Golding L, Tubbs R, et al. Posterior midventricular rupture after mitral valve replacement. *Ann Thorac Surg* 1980; 27:130.
126. Bjjrk V, Henze A, Rodriguez L. Left ventricular rupture as a complication of mitral valve replacement. Surgical experience with eight cases and a review of the literature. *J Thorac Cardiovasc Surg* 1977;73:13.
127. Roberts W, Eways E. Clinical and anatomic observations in patients having mitral valve replacement for pure mitral regurgitation and simultaneous tricuspid valve replacement. *Am J Cardiol* 1991;68:1107.
128. Selzer A, Katayama F. Mitral regurgitation: clinical patterns, pathophysiology and natural history. *Medicine* 1972;51:337.
129. Edwards J. Pathology of mitral incompetence. In: Silver M, ed. *Cardiovascular pathology.* New York: Churchill Livingstone, 1983:575.
130. Devereux R, Perloff J, Reichek N, et al. Mitral valve prolapse. *Circulation* 1976;54:3.
131. Johnson A, Daily P, Peterson K, et al. Functional evaluation of the porcine heterograft in the mitral position. *Circulation* 1975; 50,51[Suppl 1]:1.
132. Mills P, Rose J, Hollingsworth J, et al. Long-term prognosis of mitral-valve prolapse. *N Engl J Med* 1977;297:13.
133. Hickey M, Smith L, Muhlbaier L, et al. Current prognosis of ischemic mitral regurgitation. Implications for future management. *Circulation* 1988;78[Suppl 3, Pt 2]:I51.
134. Fuster V, McGoon M, Callahan M, et al. Acquired valvular heart disease: D. Mitral regurgitation. In: Giuliani E, Fuster V, Gersch B, et al., eds. *Cardiology: fundamentals and practice.* St. Louis, MO: Mosby–Year Book, 1991:1556.
135. Wilcken D, Hickey A. Lifetime risk for patients with mitral valve prolapse of developing severe valve regurgitation requiring surgery. *Circulation* 1988;78:10.
136. Rankin J, Hickey M, Smith L, et al. Ischemic mitral regurgitation. *Circulation* 1989;79[Suppl 6, Pt 2]:I116.
137. Yellin E, Yoran C, Frater R, et al. Dynamics of acute experimental mitral regurgitation. In: Ionescu M, Cohn L, eds. *Mitral valve disease: diagnosis and treatment.* London: Butterworth-Heineman, 1985:11.
138. Sheikh K, deBruijn N, Rankin J. The utility of transesophageal echocardiography and Doppler color flow imaging in patients undergoing cardiac valve operations. *J Am Coll Cardiol* 1990; 15:363.
139. Cohn L, Allred E, Cohn L, et al. Early and late risk of mitral valve replacement: a 12 year concomitant comparison of the porcine bioprosthetic and prosthetic disc mitral valves. *J Thorac Cardiovasc Surg* 1985;90:872.
140. Dalby A, Firth B, Forman R. Preoperative factors affecting the outcome of isolated mitral valve replacement: a 10 year review. *Am J Cardiol* 1981;47:826.
141. McGoon M, Fuster V, McGoon D, et al. Aortic and mitral valve incompetence: long-term follow-up (10 to 19 years) of patients treated with the Starr-Edwards prosthesis. *J Am Coll Cardiol* 1984;3:930.
142. Hauck A, Freeman D, Ackerman D, et al. Surgical pathology of the tricuspid valve: a study of 363 cases spanning 25 years. *Mayo Clin Proc* 1988;63:851.
143. Tsakiris A, Mair D, Seki S, et al. Motion of the tricuspid valve annulus in anesthetized intact dogs. *Circ Res* 1975;36:43.
144. Wooley C. Rediscovery of the tricuspid valve. *Curr Probl Cardiol* 1981;6:1.
145. Finnegan P, Abrams L. Isolated tricuspid stenosis. *Br Heart J* 1973;35:1207.
146. Gutner R. Trivalvular rheumatic stenosis: documentation of disease progression by serial cardiac catheterization. *Am J Med Sci* 1980;280:185.
147. Kirklin J, Barratt-Boyes B. Tricuspid valve disease. In: Kirklin J, Barratt-Boyes B, eds. *Cardiac surgery. Morphology, diagnostic criteria, natural history, techniques, results and indications.* New York: John Wiley and Sons, 1986:447.
148. Giuliani E, McGoon D, Callahan M, et al. Acquired valvular heart disease: tricuspid valve disease. In: Giuliani E, Fuster V, Gersh B, et al., eds. *Cardiology: fundamentals and practice.* St. Louis, MO: Mosby–Year Book, 1991:1580.
149. Kern M, Deligonul U. Interpretation of cardiac pathophysiology from pressure waveform analysis. II. The tricuspid valve. *Cathet Cardiovasc Diagn* 1990;21:278.
150. Killip TI, Lucas D. Tricuspid stenosis: physiologic criteria for diagnosis and hemodynamic abnormalities. *Circulation* 1957; 16:3.
151. Bethencourt A, Median A, Hernandez E, et al. Combined percutaneous balloon valvuloplasty of mitral and tricuspid valves. *Am Heart J* 1990;119:416.

152. Sbar S, Daicoff G, Nightingale D, et al. Chronic tricuspid insufficiency. *South Med J* 1973;66:917.
153. Waller B. Etiology of pure tricuspid regurgitation. *Cardiovasc Clin* 1987;17:53.
154. Cannon N, Cabbs C. Infective endocarditis in drug addicts. In: *Infective endocarditis.* Baltimore: University Park Press, 1976: 111.
155. Pepine C, Nichols W, Selby J. Diagnostic tests for tricuspid insufficiency: how good? *Cathet Cardiovasc Diagn* 1979;5:1.
156. Chopra H, Nanda N, Fan P, et al. Can two-dimensional echocardiography and Doppler color-flow mapping identify the need for tricuspid valve repair? *J Am Coll Cardiol* 1989;14:1266.
157. Wong M, Matsumura M, Katsuzama S, et al. The value of echocardiography in the treatment of tricuspid regurgitation in patients with mitral valve replacement. *J Thorac Cardiovasc Surg* 1990;99:1003.
158. Lipkin D, Poole-Wilson P. Measurement of cardiac output during exercise by the thermodilution and direct Fick techniques in patients with chronic congestive heart failure. *Am J Cardiol* 1985;56:321.
159. Hamilton M, Stevenson L, Woo M, et al. Effect of tricuspid regurgitation on the reliability of the thermodilution cardiac output technique in congestive heart failure. *Am J Cardiol* 1989; 64:945.
160. McGrath L, Gonzalez-Lavin L, Bailey B, et al. Tricuspid valve operations in 530 patients. Twenty-five-year assessment of early and late phase events. *J Thorac Cardiovasc Surg* 1990;99:124.
161. Arbulu A, Thomas N, Wilson R. Valvulectomy without prosthetic replacement: a lifesaving operation for tricuspid Pseudomonas endocarditis. *J Thorac Cardiovasc Surg* 1972;64:103.
162. Stern H, Sisto D, Strom J, et al. Immediate tricuspid valve replacement for endocarditis: indications and results. *J Thorac Cardiovasc Surg* 1986;91:163.
163. Vega ND. La annulaplastia selectiva, regulable y permanente. Una tecnica orginal para el tratamiento de la insuficiencia tricuspide. *Rev Esp Cardiol* 1972;25:555.
164. Carpentier A, Deloche A, Hanania G, et al. Surgical management of acquired tricuspid valve disease. *J Thorac Cardiovasc Surg* 1976;67:53.
165. Pye M, Pringle S, Cobbe S. Reference values and reproducibility of Doppler echocardiography in the assessment of the tricuspid valve and right ventricular diastolic function in normal subjects. *Am J Cardiol* 1991;67:269.
166. Arom K, Nicoloff D, Kersten T. St. Jude Medical prosthesis: valve related deaths and complications. *Ann Thorac Surg* 1987; 43:591.
167. Beaudet R, Poirier N, Doyle D, et al. The Medtronic-Hall cardiac valve: 7 1/2 years' clinical experience. *Ann Thorac Surg* 1986;42:644–652.
168. Duncan J, Cooley D, Reul G, et al. Durability and low thrombogenicity of the St. Jude Medical valve at 5-year follow-up. *Ann Thorac Surg* 1986;42:500.
169. Rahimtoola S. Valvular heart disease: a perspective. *J Am Coll Cardiol* 1983;1:199.

Cardiac Anesthesia: Principles and Clinical Practice, Second Edition, edited by Fawzy G. Estafanous, Paul G. Barash, and J.G. Reves. Lippincott Williams & Wilkins, Philadelphia

21

CONGENITAL HEART DISEASE

WILLIAM J. GREELEY
FRANK H. KERN
SCOTT R. SCHULMAN

The extremes of physiologic and biologic trespass of patients are never greater in clinical medicine than during surgery for congenital heart disease in neonates, infants, and children. Providing safe and effective anesthetic management requires the proper application of the knowledge concerning the young patient and congenital heart disease. Proper application also requires an understanding of the complex surgical operations and cardiopulmonary bypass (CPB) technology, and their effects on the patient. These factors, which are the substance of pediatric cardiovascular anesthesia, are indispensable to optimal anesthetic management. What was once viewed primarily as a technical challenge has evolved into an exciting and demanding area in anesthesiology, in which patient care is based on sound physiologic principles. The challenge is to understand these principles and to apply them to the anesthetic management of patients with congenital heart disease.

A thorough understanding of pediatric cardiovascular anesthesia requires much time, experience, and attention. However, many of the requisite principles and skills are learned by providing anesthetic care for adult patients undergoing cardiac surgery. Although the disease states and surgical operations are vastly different for children and adults, the principles involved are more similar than different.

The practice of pediatric cardiovascular anesthesia changed throughout the 1980s. The movement in pediatric cardiovascular surgery away from palliation and toward early infant repair is a direct attempt to limit the increased morbidity and mortality rates associated with long-term medical management and the sequelae of multiple palliative operations (1,2). Young age is no longer considered a risk factor at some institutions. Early corrective surgery is expected to decrease the incidence of the chronic complications of congenital heart disease, such as the problems associated with ventricular overload, cyanosis, and pulmonary vascular obstructive disease (2). With the continued improvement in surgical techniques and the early treatment of congenital heart disease, specific organ systems such as the brain, heart, and lungs will be spared the detrimental effects of chronic cyanosis and ventricular dysfunction. Thus, we are entering an era in which elective surgical repair of the neonate will become commonplace. Excellence in anesthetic care is expected. Ideally, despite the complexity of the patients and the physiologic trespasses of the surgical procedures and CPB, anesthetic care should be consistently safe and should never contribute substantially to morbidity or mortality rates (3).

Because this clinical area has grown more complex and sophisticated, we must be able to understand, interpret, and apply our new concepts and skills in the care of patients. This cannot be accomplished without a sound working knowledge of all the multidisciplinary principles involved in pediatric cardiovascular anesthesia. To this end, this chapter introduces the reader to the principles governing pediatric cardiovascular anesthesia. The first discussion provides an overview of the unique features of the pediatric patient, congenital heart disease, and the surgical procedures, which are essential to understanding the anesthetic management of children undergoing cardiac surgery. The second discussion addresses the perioperative anesthetic management of open heart procedures, and the last discussion covers closed heart procedures, anesthesia for noncardiac surgery in the patient with congenital heart disease, and finally surgical outcome.

UNIQUE FEATURES OF PEDIATRIC CARDIAC ANESTHESIA

Although many of the anesthetic management principles that govern modern pediatric cardiovascular anesthesia are based on those of the adult cardiac patient, several differ-

W. J. Greeley: Department of Anesthesiology and Pediatrics, University of Pennsylvania and Department of Anesthesiology and Critical Care Medicine, Children's Hospital of Philadelphia, Philadelphia, Pennsylvania 19104

F. H. Kern and S. R. Schulman: Department of Anesthesiology and Pediatrics, Duke University School of Medicine and Pediatric Intensive Care Unit, Duke University Medical Center, Durham, North Carolina 27710

TABLE 21-1. UNIQUE CHARACTERISTICS OF PEDIATRIC CARDIAC ANESTHESIA

- Patient
  - Normal organ system development and maturational changes of infancy
    - Cardiovascular: blood flow patterns of circulation at birth, myocardial compliance, systemic and pulmonary vasculature
    - Pulmonary: respiratory quotient, closing capacity, chest compliance
    - Central nervous system: brain growth, cerebral blood flow, autonomic regulation
    - Renal: glomerular filtration rate, creatinine clearance
    - Hepatic: liver blood flow, microsomal enzyme activity
  - Disease-growth interrelationship
    - Effects of systemic disease alter somatic and organ growth
    - Compensatory ability of developing organs and organ recovery
  - Immunologic immaturity of the infant
  - Obligatory miniaturization i.e., small patient size and body surface area
- Congenital heart disease
  - Diverse anatomic defects and physiologic changes
  - Altered ventricular modeling due to myocardial hypertrophy and ischemia
  - Chronic sequelae of congenital cardiac disease
- Surgical procedures
  - Diversity of operation
  - Frequent intracardiac and right ventricular procedures
  - Use of deep hypothermia and circulatory arrest during repair
  - Trend toward repair in early infancy
  - Evolution of surgical techniques to avoid residua and sequelae
  - Trend toward wider application of certain operations

ences make pediatric cardiovascular management unique (Table 21-1). Broadly speaking, certain characteristics of the patient, congenital heart disease, and surgery account for these unique features, some of which are reviewed later. These differences are due to healthy organ system maturation in the developing neonate and infant, the pathophysiologic processes in congenital heart disease, the diversity of surgical repairs, and the use of specialized bypass techniques such as deep hypothermia and total circulatory arrest.

The Pediatric Patient

Recognition of the changes associated with growth and development is fundamental to understanding the pediatric patient. The cardiovascular system changes markedly at birth because of dramatic alteration in blood flow patterns (4). During fetal life, blood flow returning to the heart bypasses the unventilated, fluid-filled lungs. Blood is then preferentially shunted across the patent foramen ovale into the left atrium, or it passes from the right ventricle across the patent ductus arteriosus to the systemic circulation. At the time of birth, physiologic closure of the patent ductus arteriosus and the foramen ovale initiates normal adult circulatory patterns. All blood returning to the right atrium is diverted to the lung, and all pulmonary venous blood returns to the left atrium and is pumped via the left ventricle to the body. Certain congenital heart defects or pulmonary disease can disrupt this normal adaptation process, creating a transitional circulation in which right-to-left shunting across the foramen ovale or the patent ductus arteriosus persists. Under such circumstances, continued transitional circulation leads to severe hypoxemia, acidosis, and hemodynamic instability, which are poorly tolerated in the neonate. Nevertheless, in the initial treatment of some forms of cyanotic congenital heart disease, prolongation of this transitional circulation is actually beneficial, permitting pulmonary blood flow and postnatal viability. An example of the latter is pulmonary atresia, in which pulmonary blood flow is temporarily supplied by the patent ductus arteriosus. Closure of the patent ductus arteriosus results in absent pulmonary blood flow, hypoxemia, and death. Patency can be maintained with the administration of prostaglandin E_1.

Another difference in the cardiovascular system of infants is the decreased compliance of the neonatal myocardium, compared with the mature myocardium. Various cellular synthetic functions are occurring in immature myofiber. Large nuclei, mitochondria, and surface membranes dominate the ultrastructure of the newborn myofibers (5). This effectively reduces the functional contractile mass of the heart, resulting in a ventricle with low compliance. The transverse tubular system necessary for calcium uptake and release is also poorly formed, thereby decreasing myocardial contractile function. This limits augmentation of stroke volume; consequently, these patients are highly dependent on heart rate and adequate circulating blood volume to maintain cardiac output. Furthermore, the response to inotropic drugs is limited and sensitivity to β-adrenergic blockade is heightened (Fig. 21-1) (6). Obviously, these changes in the cardiovascular system of the young patient affect anesthetic management.

The pulmonary vasculature undergoes significant change during the first year of life. These changes are largely characterized by regression of the hypertrophic, medial smooth-muscle layer in the pulmonary arteries, which exists *in utero,* resulting in a concomitant drop in pulmonary vascular resistance. In the immediate newborn period, the large decrease in pulmonary vascular resistance is the result of lung expansion and the vasodilatory effects of a higher partial arterial oxygen pressure (Pao_2) than *in utero.* Further decline in pulmonary vascular resistance throughout the first month of life is attributable to regression of the smooth-muscle layer in the pulmonary arterioles. A corresponding fall in pulmonary artery pressure occurs as pulmonary vascular resistance declines. Acute physiologic stress in the newborn period, such as hypoxemia or acidosis, can increase both pulmonary artery pressure and pulmonary vascular resistance. Under these conditions, right-sided heart pressures become greater than left-sided heart pressures, producing

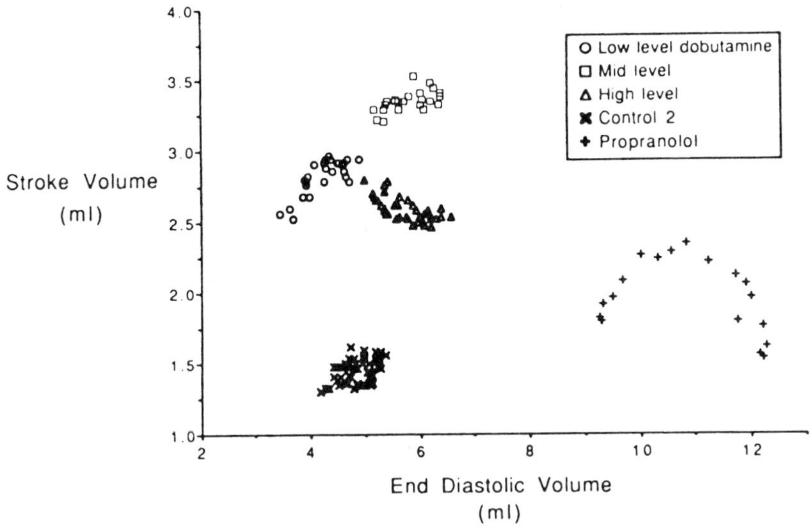

FIGURE 21-1. Cardiac function curves in the newborn lamb during dobutamine and propranolol infusions. Note that the propranolol curve is shifted downward and to the right, consistent with decreased contractility. Note that contractility (end-systolic pressure-volume ratio) changes very little in response to varying levels of β-adrenergic stimulation. (From Teitel DF, Klautz R, Steendijk P, et al. The end-systolic pressure-volume relationship in the newborn lamb: effects of loading and inotropic interventions. *Pediatr Res* 1991;29:473, with permission.)

right-to-left shunting across the patent ductus arteriosus and foramen ovale, exacerbating hypoxemia and acidosis. In contrast, left-to-right shunts, such as used with a ventricular septal defect, produce intimal changes in the pulmonary vasculature and delay regression of medial muscle hypertrophy. This results in persistent elevation of pulmonary artery pressure and pulmonary vascular resistance. It can be seen that control of pulmonary vascular resistance, pulmonary artery pressure, and pulmonary blood flow within the neonatal period becomes essential. The presence of elevated pulmonary artery pressure in the neonate and infant adds complexity to the perioperative anesthetic management and significantly increases the risk of mortality.

The developmental and maturational changes in the liver and kidneys of the young infant have particular effects on the pharmacology of intravenous anesthetic agents. During the first month of life, glomerular filtration rate and creatinine clearances are reduced. Therefore, renal elimination of ionized drugs, such as the nondepolarizing neuromuscular blockers, is reduced. There is also a decreased ability to excrete sodium and water. The neonatal liver has immature microsomal enzyme systems, which demonstrate delayed drug clearance of certain opioid and sedative drugs in pediatric cardiovascular patients (7,8). With maturation of hepatic enzyme systems and closure of the ductus venosus, which increases hepatic blood flow, drug clearance significantly improves during the first month of life (8). Thereafter, patients with cardiovascular disease demonstrate the usual age-related changes in drug clearance, namely increased clearance of narcotics and sedatives throughout childhood and decreasing clearance toward normal adult levels during adolescence. As a result, dosing of intravenous anesthetic agents in the patient younger than 1 month is complex and unpredictable. After 1 month of age, the pharmacokinetic processes of infants become mature, and drug clearance and elimination become more predictable, rendering anesthetic drug dosing easier.

Another obvious and practical difference between adult and pediatric cardiac surgery patients is the obligatory miniaturization: Infants and children are small. Anatomically, these patients have small upper and lower airways, small veins and arteries, and a decreased body surface area, compared with those of adult patients. The anesthetic implications of this miniaturization are several. First, invasive monitoring is often technically difficult. These children cannot be monitored by conventional invasive monitoring, as can the adult patient; for example, the pulmonary artery catheter and 64-element transesophageal probe cannot be used. In children, clinical observation, noninvasive and minimally invasive methodologies, and clinical experience are substituted. Intracardiac catheters are used for pressure measurements and epicardial echocardiography may be substituted for less sophisticated transesophageal probes in smaller infants. CPB is yet another example. Several studies have demonstrated a heightened inflammatory response to CPB in young patients, compared with adults (9,10). This effect is related to the disproportionate exposure to the nonendothelialized surfaces of the CPB circuit per body surface area in neonates and infants, compared with adults (Table 21-2). Greater damage to formed blood elements and plasma proteins occurs in children, resulting in the activation of the mediators of inflammation.

Congenital Heart Disease

The marked anatomic and physiologic differences between congenital heart disease and acquired adult cardiac disease also account for differences in anesthetic management between these two patient groups. The spectrum of intracardiac shunts, valve stenoses, disrupted great artery connec-

TABLE 21-2. MAJOR PHYSIOLOGIC DIFFERENCES OF CARDIOPULMONARY BYPASS IN CHILDREN VERSUS ADULTS

	Adults	Children
Hemodilute ECF by:	13%	60%
Temperature (°C)	28–32	15–20
Pump flow (ml · kg^{-1} · min^{-1})	50	0–200
Mean arterial pressure (mm Hg)	≥30	20 ?
$Paco_2$ (mm Hg)	30–45	20–80

Note: ECF, extracellular fluid; $Paco_2$, partial pressure of arterial oxygen.

TABLE 21-3. CLASSIFICATION OF CONGENITAL HEART DEFECTS

Physiologic Classification	Comments
Shunts	
Left to right	Volume-overloaded ventricle
Ventricular septal defect	Develop congestive heart failure
Atrial septal defect	
Patent ductus arteriosus	
Arteriovenous canal	
Right to left	
Tetralogy of Fallot	Pressure-overloaded ventricle
Pulmonary atresia	Cyanotic
Eisenmenger complex	Hypoxemic
Mixing lesions	Variable pressure and volume-loaded
Transposition of the heart arteries	Usually cyanotic
Tricuspid atresia	
Anomalous venous return	
Univentricular heart	
Obstructive lesions	Ventricular dysfunction
Interrupted aortic arch	Pressure-overloaded ventricle
Aortic stenosis	Ductal dependence
Pulmonic stenosis	
Hypoplastic left heart	
Coarctation	
Mitral stenosis	
Regurgitant lesions	Volume-overloaded ventricle
Ebstein anomaly	Develop congestive heart failure
Other secondary causes	

tions, and the absence of one or more chambers of the heart complicate a uniform anesthetic approach to patients with congenital heart disease. Moreover, some myocardial changes result from ventricular remodeling and increased cardiac work, which are chronically incurred by these defects. Functionally, these myocardial changes place the ventricles at great risk of intraoperative ischemia and failure. Therefore, an understanding of the isolated defect, associated myocardial changes, and hemodynamic consequences is fundamental to planning an appropriate anesthetic. Too often, because of the complexity and diversity of the defects, the attention of the anesthesiologist, cardiologist, and surgeon is focused on the specific anatomic defect while the physiologic changes are ignored. It is imperative that the anesthesiologist not only understand the anatomy but also comprehend its hemodynamic and functional consequence on both the heart and other organ systems. Although an isolated heart defect may be identified, the entire cardiopulmonary system is usually affected. One is managing a disease process, not an isolated defect. These cardiovascular effects are briefly reviewed here.

Compared with the adult who has acquired cardiac disease, the newborn with congenital heart disease has an array of marked structural and physiologic alterations. The structural alterations comprise a long list of malformations that can be grouped by defining the physiologic derangements. Identification and classification on the basis of physiology provide an organized framework for the intraoperative and postoperative management of children with complex congenital cardiac defects. In general, congenital heart lesions fit into one of four categories: shunts, mixing lesions, outflow obstruction, or regurgitant lesions (Table 21-3). Each lesion has a specific effect on pulmonary blood flow and ventricular function, which is manifest as cyanosis, congestive heart failure, or problems with pulmonary artery hypertension.

Shunt Lesions

Shunts are intracardiac connections between chambers or extracardiac connections between the aorta and pulmonary artery, such as a patent ductus arteriosus. The direction of blood flow through the shunt depends on the relative resistances on either side of the shunt. The resistance to flow depends on the pulmonary and systemic vascular beds and on the shunt orifice (11). Blood flows via the shunt in the direction of least resistance. Therefore, vascular resistance is a major determinant of shunt flow. The effect of a shunt lesion on the cardiovascular system depends on its size and its direction, either right to left or left to right. Left-to-right shunts occur when the pulmonary vascular resistance is less than the systemic vascular resistance and blood flow is preferentially directed toward the lungs, resulting in increased pulmonary blood flow. In patients with large left-to-right shunts and low pulmonary vascular resistance, pulmonary blood flow can be enormous. This results in three pathophysiologic problems: (a) volume overload of the pulmonary circulation, (b) increased cardiac work for the left ventricle, which is required to increase stroke volume and heart rate to ensure adequate systemic perfusion, and (c) excessive pulmonary blood flow leading to progressive elevation in pulmonary vascular resistance. The ability of the left ventricle to increase cardiac output is limited in infancy by virtue of its immature structure, so large left-to-right shunts may outstrip the capacity of the left heart to maintain adequate systemic perfusion, and congestive heart failure results. Prolonged exposure to increased pulmonary blood flow results in progressive elevations in pulmonary vascular resistance. Over time, fixed changes in pulmonary arterioles may occur, leading to pulmonary vascular obstructive disease. Table 21-3 lists the common left-to-right shunt lesions.

Right-to-left shunts occur when pulmonary vascular or right ventricular outflow tract resistance exceeds systemic vascular resistance, thereby reducing pulmonary blood flow. The systemic circulation receives an admixture of deoxygenated blood via the shunt and manifests clinically as cyanosis and hypoxemia. Pure right-to-left shunting due to raised pulmonary vascular resistance is seen both in Eisenmenger complex and in persistent pulmonary hypertension of the newborn with atrial and ductal-level shunting. More commonly, pulmonary vascular resistance is low and a more complex lesion with obstruction to pulmonary outflow exists, producing right-to-left shunting. Defects such as tetralogy of Fallot or pulmonary atresia with a ventricular septal defect are classic right-to-left shunts. The shunting occurs through the ventricular septal defect because of pulmonary outflow obstruction. Cardiac output is generally normal with right-to-left shunting lesions, unless hypoxemia is severe and oxygen delivery to tissue is inadequate. Thus, there are two pathophysiologic problems: (a) reduced pulmonary blood flow, resulting in systemic hypoxemia and cyanosis, and (b) an increased impedance to right ventricular ejection, resulting in pressure overload, ventricular dysfunction, and failure of the right ventricle.

Mixing Lesions

Mixing lesions constitute the largest group of cyanotic congenital heart defects (see Table 21-3). In these defects, the connections between the pulmonary and systemic circulations are so large that they are essentially a common chamber. The pulmonary-to-systemic flow ratio (Qp : Qs) is independent of shunt size and totally dependent on vascular resistance or outflow obstruction. In patients with no outflow obstruction, flow to the systemic or pulmonary circulation is dependent on vascular resistance alone, such as in univentricular hearts or a double-outlet right ventricle. Because systemic vascular resistance exceeds pulmonary vascular resistance, the tendency is toward excessive pulmonary blood flow and the predominant pathophysiologic process is left-to-right shunting. These patients have increased pulmonary blood flow, increased cardiac output, and a gradual elevation of pulmonary vascular resistance. In patients with a mixing lesion and left ventricular outflow obstruction, pulmonary blood flow is so excessive that systemic perfusion may be impaired. In patients with mixing lesions and right ventricular outflow obstruction such as a single ventricle with subpulmonic stenosis, the systemic-to-pulmonary blood flow can vary from balanced to significantly decreased pulmonary blood flow and hypoxemia, depending on the degree of obstruction. Typical mixing lesions include truncus arteriosus, univentricular heart, total anomalous pulmonary venous return, pulmonary atresia with large ventricular septal defect, and single atrium.

Obstructive Lesions

Obstructive lesions may be severe or mild. Severe lesions will present in the newborn period with a pressure-overloaded, diminutive, or dilated and profoundly dysfunctional ventricle retrograde to the obstruction. These lesions include critical aortic stenosis, critical pulmonic stenosis, coarctation of the aorta, interrupted aortic arch, or hypoplastic left-sided heart syndrome. In left-sided obstructive defects, systemic perfusion depends on patent ductus arteriosus flow, and coronary perfusion is supplied by retrograde flow from the descending aorta. In right-sided lesions, pulmonary blood flow is ductal dependent, and right ventricular function is impaired. Pathophysiologic problems in left-sided heart obstructive lesions include (a) profound left ventricular failure, (b) impaired coronary perfusion with an increased incidence of ventricular ectopy, (c) systemic hypotension, and (d) patent ductus arteriosus–dependent systemic circulation. The pathophysiologic problems of right-sided heart obstructive lesions include (a) right ventricular dysfunction, (b) decreased pulmonary blood flow, (c) systemic hypoxemia, and (d) patent ductus arteriosus–dependent pulmonary blood flow. Milder forms of outflow obstruction remain clinically asymptomatic for many years, for example, in mild to moderate aortic stenosis or asymptomatic coarctation of the aorta.

Regurgitant Lesions

Regurgitant lesions are uncommon as primary congenital defects. Ebstein malformation of the tricuspid valve is the only purely regurgitant defect. However, regurgitant lesions are frequently associated with an abnormality of valve structure, such as a complete or partial atrioventricular canal defect, truncus arteriosus, or tetralogy of Fallot with an absent pulmonary valve. The pathophysiologies of regurgitant lesions are (a) volume-overloaded circulation and (b) progression toward ventricular dilation and failure.

When one considers the incidence of the various heart defects, another perspective is gained. Three uncomplicated left-to-right shunts (ventricular septal defect, atrial septal defect, patent ductus arteriosus) and two obstructive lesions (pulmonary stenosis and coarctation) constitute 60% of all the congenital heart defects. Mixing lesions, complicated obstructive defects, and right-to-left shunting lesions account for the vast majority of the remaining 40%. Interestingly, the latter group of defects are more difficult to manage, are more labor intensive, and have a significantly higher morbidity and mortality. This is because of the complexity of the cardiovascular abnormalities in patients with these defects.

The chronic effects of congenital heart disease are a consequence of the imposed hemodynamic stress of the defect or the residua and sequelae that follow cardiac surgery. These effects continue to alter normal growth and development of the cardiovascular system and other organ systems throughout life. Because complete surgical cures are rarely achieved, abnormalities before and after repair produce long-term effects on the cardiac function of patients with congenital heart disease. Although the overall outlook for these patients is good, every defect has associated myocardial changes and every repair leaves certain obligatory abnormalities (12). Many of the abnormalities are trivial. Others affect ventricular function, central nervous system growth, the conduction system of the heart, or pulmonary blood flow. Under these circumstances, the long-term quality of life is affected. Abnormalities of ventricular performance at rest and with exercise can be detected in patients with chronic volume-overloaded or pressure-overloaded circulation and complex cyanotic lesions (13). These abnormalities in ventricular function are the consequences of altered ventricular loading conditions, repeated episodes of myocardial ischemia, and residua or sequelae of surgical treatment (e.g., ventriculotomy, altered coronary artery supply, and inadequate myocardial protection).

Chronic effects on the pulmonary circulation are associated with certain forms of congenital heart disease and lead to important pathologic sequelae. In the setting of a large left-to-right shunt such as a ventricular septal defect, increased pulmonary blood flow causes shear stress and an increase in pulmonary artery luminal pressure. The normally aligned pulmonary artery endothelial cells that control vascular tone and metabolic activity become fragmented, swollen, and malaligned because of elevated pressure and shear forces. Damaged endothelial cells release proteases and stimulate local release of vasoactive substances. The released metabolites break down and invade the smooth-muscle layer of the pulmonary arteries, stimulating smooth-muscle development and an elastin breakdown. This process is implicated as a major cause of changes in compliance of the pulmonary vascular bed (14). Clinically, this is manifest by pulmonary artery hypertension and the Eisenmenger physiology of fixed elevations in pulmonary vascular resistance. Before irreversible pulmonary vascular obstructive disease develops, the pulmonary artery circulation remains reactive and prone to hypertensive crisis and acute right ventricular failure. With the recent surgical trend toward early repair, the occurrence of Eisenmenger syndrome has been greatly reduced.

Patients with chronic cyanotic conditions redistribute organ perfusion to the heart, brain, and kidney by decreasing flow to the splanchnic circulation, skin, muscle, and bone. Chronic cyanosis is associated with increased work of breathing in an attempt to increase oxygen uptake and delivery and with the formation of arteriovenous collaterals in an attempt to improve pulmonary blood flow. The most dramatic long-term complications are the decreased rate of somatic growth, increased metabolic rate, and increased hemoglobin concentration seen in children with unrepaired defects.

In summary, congenital heart defects are diverse in nature and arise early in embryogenesis. The resultant hemodynamic forces have both direct and indirect developmental consequences, which in turn influence function. The disturbances can primarily be considered in terms of their effects on pulmonary blood flow, ventricular function, and pulmonary artery pressure and can be functionally classified into shunting, mixing, obstructive, and regurgitant lesions. Consequently, patient assessment should take into account the net effect of shunting, the presence or absence of obstruction, the functional status of the ventricles, and the state of the pulmonary vasculature. These factors predominantly influence anesthetic and surgical management and should be assessed when one evaluates the patient with congenital heart disease. The status of the pulmonary circulation and the right ventricle is prominently affected by congenital heart disease and strongly influences survival.

Surgical Procedures and Special Techniques

The broad objectives for congenital heart surgery are (a) physiologic separation of the circulation, (b) relief of outflow obstruction, (c) preservation or restoration of ventricular mass and function, and (d) normalization of life expectancy. The surgical procedures available to accomplish these objectives are complex and diverse. Compared with adult cardiac operations, these repairs involve more intracardiac surgery. In general, operations performed for congenital heart defects can be divided into palliative and complete repairs (15). The type and timing of repair depend on the age of the patient, the specific anatomic defect, and the experience of the surgeon (Table 21-4). Palliation in infancy is usually performed in individuals who are missing anatomic parts, such as in pulmonary atresia (absent right ventricle and pulmonary artery), tricuspid atresia (absent right ventricle and tricuspid valve), hypoplastic left-sided heart syndrome (absent mitral valve and small left ventricle), univentricular heart (absent right ventricle or left ventricle), or mitral atresia (absent left ventricle). These palliative procedures can be further subdivided into those that will increase pulmonary blood flow, those that decrease pulmonary blood flow, and those that increase mixing. Palliations that increase pulmonary blood flow include shunts (central or Blalock-Taussig), outflow patch, or enlargement of the ventricular septal defect. Those that decrease pulmonary blood flow include pulmonary artery banding, ligation of a patent ductus arteriosus, or closure of atrial septal defects or ventricular septal defects. Those that improve intracardiac mixing include atrial septostomy (e.g., balloon, blade, or Blalock-Hanlon). With the improvements in surgical technique coupled with the advancements in anesthetic and

TABLE 21-4. SURGICAL REPAIR OPTIONS IN INFANCY

Palliation
- Pulmonary atresia
- Tricuspid atresia
- Ebstein malformation
- Hypoplastic left heart syndrome
- Univentricular heart
- Mitral atresia

Corrective repair
- Aortic stenosis
- Total anomalous pulmonary venous return
- Cor triatriatum
- Patent ductus arteriosus
- Pulmonary stenosis
- Mitral stenosis
- Aortopulmonary window
- Coarctation
- Interrupted aortic arch
- Atrial septal defect

Palliation or corrective repair
- Atrioventricular canal defect
- Double-inlet right ventricle
- Double-outlet right ventricle
- Tetralogy of Fallot
- Truncus arteriosus
- Transposition of the great vessels
- Ventricular septal defects

technologic support, repair in early infancy is the preferred approach.

Critical congenital heart disease is associated with early death, abnormal coronary artery angiogenesis, myocardial hypertrophy, pulmonary vascular changes, and secondary changes in the brain and kidney (2,16,17). The movement in pediatric cardiovascular surgery away from palliation and toward early infant repair is a direct attempt to limit the increased morbidity and mortality rates associated with long-term medical management and the sequelae of multiple palliative operations (1). No longer is young age considered a risk factor at some institutions. Early corrective surgery is expected to decrease the incidence of the chronic complications of congenital heart disease, such as the problems associated with ventricular overload, cyanosis, and pulmonary vascular obstructive disease (2). With the continued improvement in surgical techniques and the early treatment of congenital heart disease, specific organ systems, such as the brain, heart, and lungs, will be spared the detrimental effects of chronic cyanosis and ventricular dysfunction. We are entering an era in which elective surgical repair of the neonate will become commonplace.

Currently, repair in infancy can be offered for a number of congenital heart defects, as shown in Table 21-4. These defects include total anomalous pulmonary venous return, interrupted aortic arch, coarctation of the aorta, aortic stenosis, and pulmonary stenosis. Ventricular septal defects, atrioventricular septal defects, tetralogy of Fallot, truncus arteriosus, and transposition of the great vessels can be repaired in early infancy or palliated early, with total correction later in life. However, infant repair remains the treatment of choice in some centers.

Another trend seen in pediatric cardiovascular surgery is the continued evolution of standard techniques to decrease long-term morbidity and enhance survival rates. For example, the long-term problems of right ventricular dysfunction and failure associated with the Mustard or Senning procedure for repair of transposition of the great arteries has encouraged many surgical groups to perform the arterial switch procedure in the neonatal period (18). With the arterial switch procedure, it is believed that a normal anatomic correction will have more favorable long-term results. A second example of the continuing evolution of technique is surgery for tetralogy of Fallot. Long-standing pulmonary insufficiency after right ventricular outflow repair for tetralogy of Fallot is associated with right ventricular dysfunction and failure. Preservation of the pulmonary valve at initial repair by means of a combined transatrial and transpulmonary approach during correction or the early insertion of a pulmonary homograft in the setting of pulmonary insufficiency are techniques being used to avoid the long-term problems of right ventricular dysfunction and failure (19).

The broader application of certain surgical procedures initially designed for a specific defect is another example of the evolution of congenital heart surgery. For example, the Fontan operation, which was originally devised for tricuspid atresia, is now being extended to such complex lesions as univentricular hearts and hypoplastic left-sided heart syndrome. However, with this wider application for complex defects that were once considered inoperable, the morbidity and mortality rates have increased for the Fontan procedure. The bidirectional Glenn operation and the fenestrated Fontan procedure are newer surgical approaches evolving to improve survival among patients with these more complex lesions. As the incisions in the myocardium become smaller and sutures more precisely placed, and as the great artery surgical techniques are improved, the complications of ventricular dysfunction, arrhythmias, and residual obstruction should decline.

One final difference unique to congenital heart surgery is related to CPB support. Because of the complexity of repair in small patients, surgery often requires significant alterations in the bypass techniques, such as deep hypothermic CPB and total circulatory arrest (20). Many operations are undertaken in this setting of extreme biologic conditions of temperature and perfusion. These specialized techniques are discussed later. Current methods of CPB management in neonates and infants involve extensive alterations in temperature, hemodilution, systemic perfusion pressure, and flow (see Table 21-2). Despite widespread use of these techniques during bypass, their physiologic effects on major organ system function are only now being investigated.

In summary, some unique features must be considered when one cares for children with congenital heart disease. These features include the patient's growth and development, the pathophysiology of congenital heart disease, the surgical procedures, and the CPB techniques. These differences between children and adults, coupled with the fundamental knowledge of adult cardiac and pediatric anesthetic principles, underlie the approach to the operative management of these patients.

PERIOPERATIVE ANESTHETIC MANAGEMENT

Preoperative Period

Preoperative Evaluation

Caring for children with congenital heart disease presents the anesthesiologist with a wide spectrum of anatomic and physiologic abnormalities. Patients range from the young, healthy, asymptomatic child with a small atrial septal defect to the newborn with hypoplastic left-sided heart syndrome that requires aggressive preoperative hemodynamic and ventilatory support. Intertwined with the medical diversity of these patients is the psychological aspect, in both the patient and the parents. Preparation of the patient and the family is time consuming, but omitting or compromising this aspect of patient care is a major deterrent to a successful outcome. Cardiac surgeons, cardiologists, anesthesiologists, intensivists, and nurses must work as a team in preparing the patient and the family for surgery and postoperative recovery. This team-oriented approach not only prepares the patient and family but also prevents errors and omissions in preoperative, intraoperative, and postoperative care. The preoperative visit offers the family the opportunity to meet the surgeon and anesthesiologist and begin preparing the patient and family for surgery.

The preoperative evaluation should always start with a careful history and physical examination. Although the history should concentrate on the cardiopulmonary system, 25% of patients with congenital heart disease have associated noncardiac congenital anomalies (21). The most common are genitourinary and musculoskeletal defects, but airway and pulmonary anomalies are frequent. Certain syndromes, such as Charge syndrome, are associated with choanal atresia. Tracheomalacia and thymic hypoplasia are associated with aberrant right subclavian arteries and aortic arch anomalies. Tetralogy of Fallot with absent pulmonary valve is associated with compression of the main bronchus and abnormal distal pulmonary vessels that form tufts that intertwine with and compress distal pulmonary bronchi, resulting in respiratory distress and wheezing due to extrinsic airway obstruction. Trisomy 21 is associated with upper and lower airway abnormalities, as well as cervical neck instability. Delineating these problems in the preoperative period allows for a carefully prepared anesthetic plan.

Parents should be questioned about the general health and activity of their child. Fundamentally, a child's general health and activity reflect the child's cardiorespiratory reserve. One must determine whether the child has normal or impaired exercise tolerance. Is the child gaining weight appropriately or exhibiting signs of failure to thrive on the basis of cardiac failure? Does the child exhibit signs of congestive heart failure (e.g., diaphoresis, poor feeding, and recurrent respiratory infections)? Is there progressive cyanosis or a new onset of cyanotic spells? Any intercurrent illness, such as a recent upper respiratory tract infection or pneumonia, must be ascertained. This may require delaying surgery because of the negative impact that airway reactivity and elevations in pulmonary artery pressure have on surgical outcome. Recurrent pneumonia is frequently associated with pulmonary overcirculation.

A thorough history must delineate previous surgical interventions. Shunts, patches, and conduits all affect the selected surgical and anesthetic approaches. For example, the presence or surgical creation of a left Blalock-Taussig shunt negates the use of the left radial artery for continuous monitoring of arterial pressure in that extremity. One should obtain a list of current medications, previous anesthetic problems, or family history of anesthetic difficulties.

In the modern era of echocardiography and cardiac catheterization, physical examination rarely contributes additional information about the underlying cardiac lesion. However, it is extremely useful in assessing the overall clinical condition of the child. An ill-appearing, cachectic child in respiratory distress has a limited cardiorespiratory reserve, and excessive premedication or a prolonged inhalational induction could result in significant hemodynamic instability. Physical examination should include palpation of the liver and fontanelle. This is a good means of assessing intravascular volume. A large, congested liver is frequently found in children with right-sided heart failure. A nonpalpable liver edge and sunken fontanelle are signs of intravascular volume depletion. Auscultation of the lungs is valuable as a baseline examination for comparison with intraoperative changes. An examination of the distal extremities and pulses provides an assessment of potential sites for indwelling venous and arterial catheters, and it limits the time spent searching in the operating room.

Laboratory evaluation should particularly focus on hematocrit, arterial blood gas analysis, and electrolytes. An elevated hematocrit indicates the chronicity of relative hypoxemia. Elevations of more than 60% may predispose to capillary sludging and secondary end-organ damage, including stroke (22). For this reason, children with hematocrit levels of more than 55% should have intravenous fluids initiated the night before surgery to maintain adequate hydration. If the hematocrit level is more than 65% in older children, plans for taking a unit of blood should be considered before CPB is initiated.

Echocardiography with Doppler color flow imaging is

an invaluable tool that provides a noninvasive means of assessing intracardiac anatomy, blood flow patterns, and estimates of physiologic data. For uncomplicated heart defects such as an atrial septal defect, patent ductus arteriosus, and coarctation of the aorta, echocardiography obviates the need for an invasive cardiac catheterization. Accurate interpretation of anatomic and physiologic changes requires a skilled echocardiographer as well as a well-integrated and interactive team.

Cardiac catheterization still remains the "gold standard" for assessing anatomy and physiologic function in patients with congenital heart disease. Important catheterization data for the anesthesiologist include the following:

1. Location, size (restrictive versus nonrestrictive), and direction (Qp:Qs) of intracardiac shunting.
2. Pulmonary and systemic arterial pressures.
3. Ventricular and atrial pressures with specific attention to left and right ventricular end-diastolic pressure.
4. Oxygen saturation data.
5. Intracardiac chamber size.
6. Pulmonary vascular resistance.
7. Valvular anatomy and function.
8. Anatomy and function of previously created shunts.
9. Anatomic distortion of systemic or pulmonary arterial vessels, particularly as it relates to previously placed shunts.
10. Coronary artery anatomy.
11. Obstructive gradients at valves or previously created baffles or conduits.

A careful review of the cardiac catheterization data and understanding its effects on the operative and anesthetic plan are essential. Because not all the medical problems can be evaluated and corrected preoperatively, the surgeon, cardiologist, and anesthesiologist must discuss potential management problems. Any needs for further evaluation or intervention should be addressed before entering the operating room. Appropriate communication and cooperation will maximize patient care and facilitate perioperative clinical management.

Premedication

The optimal premedication achieves adequate sedation, has a minimal effect on respiratory and hemodynamic function, and can be administered in a nontraumatic fashion. In children with complex congenital heart disease, a heavy premedication is advocated. It improves oxygen saturation, diminishes myocardial oxygen consumption, and promotes a more satisfactory induction. Many premedication combinations have been used, including rectal barbiturates; the combination of a rectal barbiturate and an intramuscular opioid; and a combination of oral medications including an opioid, a barbiturate, and/or a benzodiazepine. Rectal barbiturates are effective; however, reports of apnea, bradycardia, and a respiratory depression in 1% to 2% of patients mandate close observation by skilled personnel (23). Apnea and bradycardia are poorly tolerated in the child with congenital heart disease and may result in significant morbidity and mortality. Unless personnel with airway expertise can provide continuous human surveillance, this technique should not be used in patients with congenital heart disease. Intramuscular medications cause pain and agitation, which generally result in increased myocardial oxygen consumption and arterial desaturation at the time of injection. Because this usually occurs before arrival into the operating room and skilled observation is not readily available, a better method of administration may be necessary. Oral administration of a combined sedative, opioid, and amnestic agent is an effective premedication for children with heart disease. Generally, children younger than 6 months of age do not require a premedication. In children between the ages of 6 months and 9 months, pentobarbital (2 to 4 mg/kg), diazepam (0.1 to 0.2 mg/kg), or midazolam (0.3 to 0.5 mg/kg) may be administered orally. A calm, cooperative, sedated child is the usual result. Children older than 9 months of age receive a more potent oral premedication. In our institution, several oral regimens are popular and effective: (a) diazepam 0.1 mg/kg, pentobarbital 2 to 4 mg/kg, and meperidine 2 to 3 mg/kg; (b) pentobarbital 2 to 4 mg/kg and meperidine 2 to 3 mg/kg, or (c) midazolam 0.2 mg/kg and meperidine 2 to 3 mg/kg. If extubation is planned at the end of the operation, premedication is generally withheld in children younger than 9 months of age; children older than 9 months of age receive oral midazolam (0.3 to 0.5 mg/kg) 1 hour before arrival in the operating room.

Another approach is to allow a parent to accompany the patient to the operating room and remain during the induction of anesthesia until the patient loses consciousness. In our practice, premedication can be reduced or eliminated when a parent accompanies the child into the operating room. In our experience with this protocol, we have never had an untoward event involving the patient or parent.

Intraoperative Period

Operating Room Preparation

Advanced, careful preparation of the operating room is essential. The anesthesia machine must have the capacity to provide air as well as oxygen and nitrous oxide, to help balance pulmonary and systemic blood flows. Intravenous tubing must be free of air bubbles to prevent paradoxical air embolism. Resuscitative drugs labeled and ready for administration should include calcium gluconate or calcium chloride, sodium bicarbonate, atropine, phenylephrine, lidocaine, and epinephrine. An inotropic infusion, usually of dopamine, should be premixed and ready for administration in high-risk patients, but additional infusions are made available if there is a strong suspicion for their need. For all pediatric patients, certain anesthetic drugs are made available for emergencies (thiopental, ketamine, succinylcholine, and atropine). These drugs are selected because of the potential for airway reactivity, hypotension, or bradycardia during anesthetic induction. In pediatric cardiac anesthesia, many of the patients have high endogenous catecholamines as an adaptive response to their underlying cardiac disease and have limited reserves. Therefore, the need for predrawn syringes of these drugs is critical. A well-premedicated patient can minimize these untoward events.

In congenital heart surgery, one must be able to rapidly alter body temperature for cooling and rewarming. A heating-cooling water mattress and an efficient room cooling-heating system are important in the operative management of infants and small children.

Physiologic Monitoring

The monitoring used for any particular patient depends on the condition of the patient and on the type and extent of the surgical procedure. The perioperative monitoring techniques available are listed by the specific organ system monitored in Table 21-5. Noninvasive monitoring is usually placed before induction of anesthesia. This includes a seven-lead electrocardiography (ECG) system, pulse oximeter, precordial stethoscope, and appropriately sized noninvasive blood pressure cuff (either oscillometric or Doppler). As in adult patients, myocardial ischemia is monitored by the appropriate evaluation of ST-segment T waves from the surface ECG. Additional monitoring includes an indwelling arterial catheter, a central venous catheter, temperature monitors, and esophageal stethoscope. All are standard items for CPB surgery. Foley catheters are used in neonates and infants undergoing hypothermic circulatory arrest and reoperative procedures. They can be electively withheld in older children or less complex procedures, unless the patient has renal insufficiency.

TABLE 21-5. MONITORING OF ORGAN SYSTEMS

- Cardiopulmonary system
  - Esophageal stethoscope
  - Electrocardiogram
    - Standard seven-lead system, ST-segment T-wave analysis, esophageal electrocardiographic lead
  - Pulse oximeter
  - Automated oscillatory or Doppler blood pressure
  - Capnograph
  - Ventilator parameters
  - Indwelling arterial catheter
  - Central venous pressure catheter
  - Pulmonary artery catheter
  - Transthoracic pressure catheter
    - Left or right atrium, pulmonary artery
  - Echocardiography with Doppler colorflow imaging
    - Epicardial: any complex defect; weight <30 kg
    - Transesophageal: weight >30 kg, assessment of aortic or mitral valve and left ventricular function only
- Central nervous system
  - Peripheral nerve stimulator
  - Processed electroencephalogram
  - Specialized
    - Cerebral blood flow: xenon clearance methodology
    - Cerebral blood flow velocity: transcranial Doppler
    - Cerebral metabolism: near-infrared spectroscopy, oxygen consumption measurements
- Temperature
  - Nasopharyngeal, recta, esophageal, tympanic
- Coagulation
  - Activated clotting time
  - Clot formation rate and strength
    - Thromboelastogram
- Renal function
  - Foley catheter

Continuous monitoring of arterial pressure is performed through an indwelling intraarterial catheter. In young children, cannulation of the radial artery with a 22-gauge catheter is preferred. In older children and adolescents, a 20-gauge catheter may be substituted. Care must be taken to ensure that previous or currently planned operative procedures, such as a previous radial artery cutdown, subclavian flap of the aorta for coarctation repair, or a classic Blalock-Taussig shunt, do not interfere with the selected site of arterial pressure monitoring. Other sites available for cannulation include the ulnar, femoral, and axillary arteries. Cannulation of the posterior tibial and dorsalis pedis arteries is not usually performed for complex operative procedures. Peripheral arterial catheters, principally of the lower extremities, function poorly after CPB and do not reflect central aortic pressure when distal extremity temperature remains low (24).

Myocardial and cerebral preservation are principally maintained through hypothermia; therefore, the accurate and continuous monitoring of body temperature is crucial. Rectal and nasopharyngeal (or tympanic) temperatures are monitored, as they accurately reflect core and cerebral temperatures, respectively. Monitoring of esophageal temperature is a good reflection of cardiac and thoracic temperatures.

Pulse oximetry and capnography provide instantaneous feedback concerning adequacy of ventilation and oxygenation. They are useful in balancing shunt flow and providing feedback about surgically created shunts and pulmonary arterial bands. Peripheral vasoconstriction in patients undergoing deep hypothermia and circulatory arrest renders digital oxygen-saturation probes less reliable. A tongue sensor has been advocated for the newborn to provide a more central measure of oxygen saturation with less temperature-related variability (25). A second pulse oximeter probe may be placed as a backup before surgery begins in patients undergoing deep hypothermia, as probe dysfunction is not uncommon during weaning from CPB.

Percutaneous central venous access for pressure monitoring and drug infusion is usually a standard procedure for effective intraoperative management, even in the smallest infants. Placement and complications of central venous catheterization have recently been reviewed. Potential sites, in order of usefulness and success rate, are right internal jugular vein, left internal jugular vein, right external jugular vein, left external jugular vein, left subclavian vein, and right or left femoral vein. The potential complications, in order of occurrence, are arterial puncture, hematoma at the puncture site, bleeding, and catheter malposition. Because these catheters may be used for an extended time in the postoperative period for inotropic infusions and nutritional support, a sterile technique should be assiduously applied. Intracardiac lines (right atrial, left atrial, or pulmonary arterial) or transvenous pulmonary artery catheters should be used on an individual basis. Since the introduction of intraoperative Doppler echocardiography, intraoperative monitoring lines can be selectively placed on the basis of right ventricular or left ventricular function or the concomitant elevations in pulmonary artery pressure. As a general guideline, transvenous pulmonary artery catheters may be placed using the internal jugular approach in children weighing more than 7 kg. A 5F catheter is used in patients weighing 7 to 25 kg, and a 7F catheter for children heavier than 25 kg. For infants weighing less than 7.0 kg, percutaneous placement of a pulmonary artery catheter can be difficult and intracardiac lines placed surgically are preferred.

In neonates and small infants, certain circumstances dictate the need for continuous information regarding left and right atrial and/or pulmonary artery pressure monitoring. For example, in neonates with pulmonary artery hypertension or in children undergoing a Fontan operation, these measurements are particularly useful. With the Fontan procedure, there is no right ventricle pumping blood to the lungs. Adequacy of flow through the pulmonary bed depends on maintaining a pressure gradient from the right atrium to the left atrium. Intracardiac right atrial and left atrial pressure monitoring is valuable in intraoperative and postoperative management of patients.

Specialized Monitoring

Intraoperative Echocardiography

Recently, newer techniques for monitoring patients during pediatric cardiovascular surgery have been introduced. The most promising of these techniques is echocardiography with Doppler color flow imaging. Several reports have described intraoperative Doppler echocardiography during congenital heart surgery (26–30). Transesophageal echocardiography (TEE) is the preferred approach in adults, but probe size and restricted views may limit its use in infants and small children. TEE has been successfully employed in infants in whom a smaller probe was used. By means of TEE, the significant morphologic, color, and pulsed wave Doppler features of congenital heart defects can be consistently defined. Compared with the epicardial approach, this method allows the continuous monitoring of the heart without disruption of surgery. Early limitation in views have been virtually eliminated with clinical experience and improved biplane images. Pediatric biplane TEE probes have extended the patient-size limits to neonates between 2.5 and 3.0 kg (31). Potential hazards of TEE that merit particular vigilance include descending aorta and airway compression due to probe size or during probe flexion in small neonates and infants.

The second technique for intraoperative echocardiographic analysis in children is the epicardial approach (16, 31,32). This approach requires that a clean, short-focused 5.0- or 7.0-MHz transducer be passed over the anesthesia screen, into a sterile sheath, where it then can be placed on the epicardial surface of the heart. This technique best facilitates the probe manipulations necessary for thorough interrogation of the major structures and dynamic function of the heart. The advantage of this approach is that all views can be obtained in any size patient. Among the disadvantages are the need for sufficient operator skill and experience for manipulations (33), the need to interrupt surgery to manipulate the probe, and any deleterious impact of direct myocardial mechanical manipulation. With the current TEE capabilities, epicardial imaging is rarely employed.

Prebypass Doppler echocardiography precisely defines anesthetic and surgical management plans. Because of the unrestricted epicardial approach in anesthetized patients, new findings are frequently discovered and management plans changed accordingly. Postbypass Doppler echocardiography evaluation enables immediate assessment of the quality of the surgical repair as well as assessment of cardiac function by examining ventricular wall motion and systolic thickening (34). Residual structural defects after CPB can be immediately diagnosed and repaired in the same operative setting, to avoid the patient's leaving the operating room with significant residual structural defects that will require reoperation at a later time (Fig. 21-2). The identification of patients with new right and left ventricular dysfunction after CPB, as determined by a change in wall motion or systolic thickening, allows for immediate and more thoughtful pharmacologic interventions when guided by Doppler echocardiography. Postbypass ventricular dysfunction and residual structural defects identified by Doppler echocardiography are associated with an increased incidence of reoperation and higher morbidity and mortality rates. Thus, this monitoring tool is helpful in assessing surgical outcome and in identifying operative risk factors. Whether early identification of these abnormalities, which directs specific early intraoperative medical and surgical interventions, will improve outcome remains to be determined.

Specialized Central Nervous System Monitoring

Processed electroencephalography (EEG), transcranial Doppler echocardiography, cerebral blood flow, and jugular venous saturation measurements have provided important information during pediatric cardiovascular surgery. These

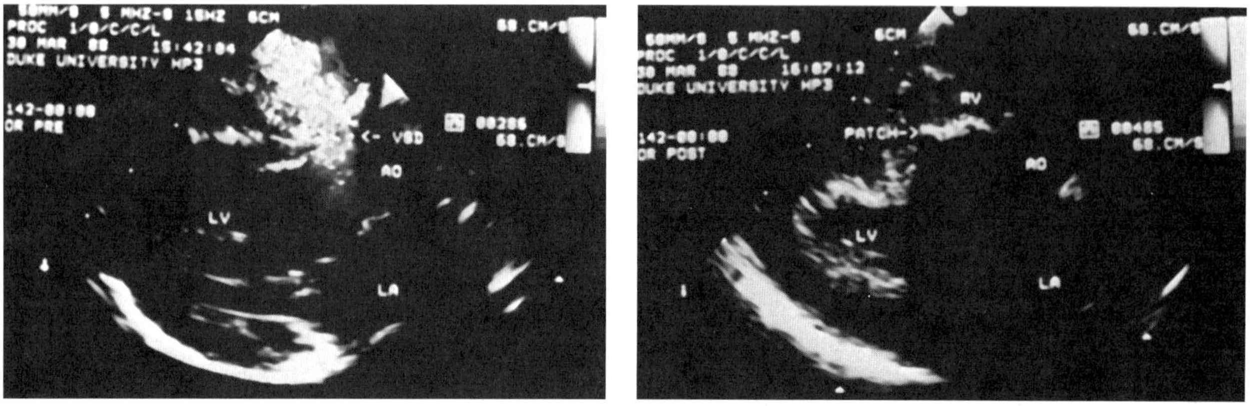

A B

FIGURE 21-2. Echocardiogram with a Doppler flow map in the long-axis view, **(A)** illustrating a residual ventricular septal defect (*VSD*) due to patch dehiscence after initial repair. Turbulent flow through the VSD (*arrow*) appears as a mosaic of white particles. This finding necessitated immediate reinstitution of CPB and re-repair. A second Doppler flow map in the long-axis view **(B)** illustrates patch closure (*arrow*) of the VSD after re-repair. Note the absence of turbulent flow with the loss of the mosaic of white. (LV, left ventricle; LA, left atrium; Ao, aorta.)

new techniques are particularly helpful in monitoring physiologic function of the central nervous system during deep hypothermic bypass and total circulatory arrest. For example, during deep hypothermia and before total circulatory arrest, the processed EEG can identify residual cerebral electrical activity (35). Because residual electrical activity during arrest is associated with ongoing cerebral metabolism, producing an isoelectric state may prevent ischemic injury to the brain during the period of deep hypothermic circulatory arrest (DHCA). Isoelectric silence can then be induced by barbiturate therapy. The EEG may also be useful in detecting the level and depth of anesthesia.

Transcranial Doppler imaging for measuring blood flow velocity in the middle cerebral artery during cardiac surgery is a new technique that has a number of potential useful applications. Although the absolute measurement of blood flow velocity and cerebral blood flow using transcranial Doppler imaging is poor, trend analysis and correlative changes of measured velocity with cerebral blood flow changes are good (36,37). Blood flow velocity trends during deep hypothermic CPB and $PaCO_2$ changes parallel the observations of direct cerebral blood flow measurements reported by others (38). Indeed, the trends of cerebral blood flow velocity during deep hypothermia and after total circulatory arrest are remarkably similar to actual cerebral blood flow measurements under similar conditions (39). Despite the potential lack of accuracy of transcranial Doppler imaging for absolute measurements, it appears to have value for trend analysis of cerebral hemodynamics.

Perhaps the greatest value of transcranial Doppler imaging is in the detection of emboli, both air and particulate, during cardiac surgery (Fig. 21-3) (32). This monitor can detect and semiquantitate air emboli. Awareness of risk periods for air emboli during cardiac surgery may influence practice patterns and thereby reduce the number and amount of these events. Whether transcranial Doppler imaging can reduce the neuropsychological sequelae associated with CPB remains to be determined. However, for children in whom the preponderance of surgical procedures either are on an open ventricle or are to repair an aorta or septal defect, the potential value is great for the transcranial Doppler imaging to detect and then reduce air emboli. At present, transcranial Doppler imaging is limited to selected research institutions. As reports of its value and utility increase, more widespread use is anticipated.

Cerebral blood flow studies using xenon clearance technology have improved the understanding of cerebrovascular

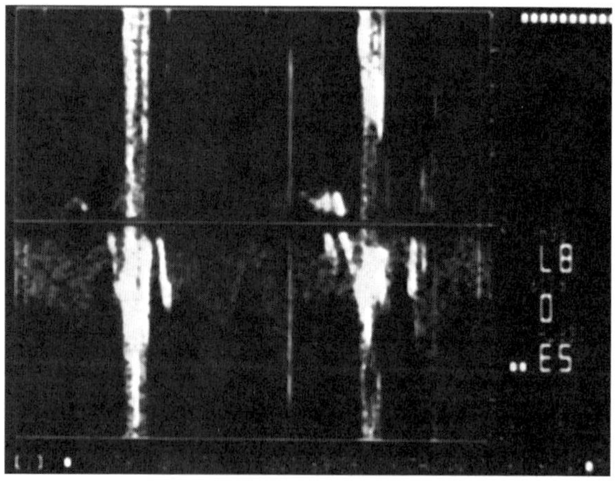

FIGURE 21-3. Transcranial Doppler of the middle cerebral artery during cardiopulmonary bypass in an infant. Note the opaque echogenic densities, which represent the detection of air emboli immediately after release of the aortic cross-clamp and initiation of left ventricular ejection.

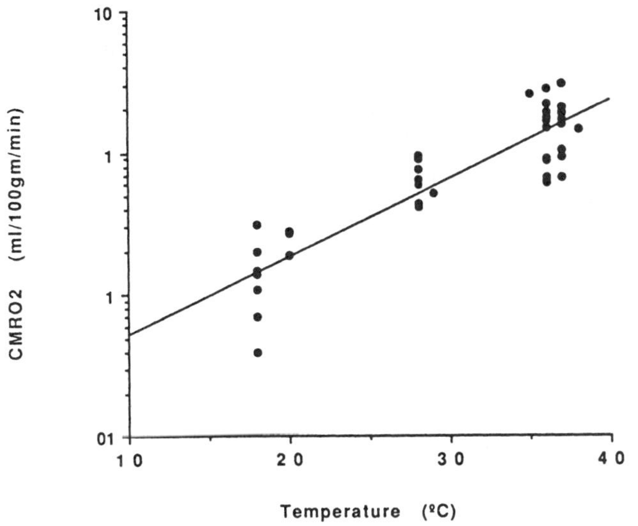

FIGURE 21-4. The logarithmic relationship of cerebral metabolism (CMRO2) and temperature in infants over the temperature range of 18°C to 37°C. The average exponential equation is CMRO2 = 0.0100e·1314·T; (r^2 = 0.76, r = 0.87, p = .001). (From Greeley WJ, Kern FH, Ungerleider RM, et al. The effect of hypothermic cardiopulmonary bypass and total circulatory arrest on cerebral metabolism in neonates, infants, and children. *J Thorac Cardiovasc Surg* 1991;101:783, with permission.)

dynamics during CPB in young children, particularly during deep hypothermia and after periods of circulatory arrest (10). Recent xenon-133 cerebral blood flow studies have enabled several investigative groups to provide new information on these questions regarding cerebral blood flow and CPB. During CPB, temperature, anesthetic depth, cerebral oxygen consumption ($CMRo_2$), and $Paco_2$ are the major factors that regulate cerebral blood flow (Fig. 21-4). Factors that do not influence cerebral blood flow (within the usual bounds of common practice) are blood pressure, pump flow, and age. Blood pressure (20 mm Hg) and pump flow (1.61 minute/m^2) do not affect cerebral blood flow because the brain is able to autoregulate; that is, changes in cerebral vascular resistance increase or decrease to change cerebral blood flow in response to the metabolic needs of the brain. Decreased cerebral blood flow occurs with increased anesthetic depth and lowered temperature because the $CMRo_2$ is reduced and the brain requires less oxygen delivery (cerebral blood flow). Cerebral blood flow varies directly with $Paco_2$ during CPB. Although autoregulation is preserved under most circumstances of CPB, under some conditions and in some patients, it is not. Autoregulation during CPB is lost with profound hypothermia (22°C)(40) and when pH-stat blood gas management is used (33), meaning that cerebral blood flow is pump flow–dependent and perfusion pressure–dependent. Autoregulation also appears to be impaired with total circulatory arrest. Loss of autoregulation requires changes in customary CPB management; for example, perfusion should be at higher flows, perfusion pressure should be maintained at higher levels, and possibly alpha-stat blood gas management should be used. More experience with these specialized central nervous system monitoring techniques, currently confined to some research programs, is expected to improve anesthetic and surgical management. This is important, because the last major area of morbidity associated with cardiac surgery is neurologic in origin.

Induction and Maintenance of Anesthesia

The principles of intraoperative management of cardiothoracic surgical procedures are based on the pathophysiology of the disease process and the effects of the various anesthetic and other pharmacologic interventions on a particular patient's condition. Selecting an induction technique depends on the degree of cardiac dysfunction, the cardiac defect, and the degree of sedation provided by the premedication. In children with a good cardiac reserve, induction techniques can vary, as long as induction is careful and well monitored. The execution of anesthetic induction is more important than the anesthetic technique in patients who have reasonable cardiac reserves. A wide spectrum of anesthetic induction techniques with a variety of agents has been used safely and successfully; these include halothane, halothane–nitrous oxide, and intravenous or intramuscular ketamine, fentanyl, or thiopental (41). Ketamine has been the most popular anesthetic induction agent in patients with cyanotic conditions, because it increases systemic vascular resistance and cardiac output and does not exacerbate right-to-left shunting. Ketamine can be given intravenously or intramuscularly. An intramuscular injection may result in pain, agitation, and subsequent arterial desaturation. Inhalational inductions are generally well received and well tolerated by most children, and it is the preferred approach. An inhalational induction with halothane can easily and safely be performed, even in cyanotic patients such as those with tetralogy of Fallot. In these patients, who are at risk of right-to-left shunting and systemic desaturation, oxygenation is well maintained with a good airway and adequate ventilation, despite halothane-induced hypotension (42). Skilled airway management and efficiency of ventilation are essential, and they take precedence over drug selection during anesthetic induction. Although it is essential to understand the complexities of shunts and vascular resistance changes, airway and ventilation effects on the cardiovascular system are of primary importance during the induction of anesthesia. Although the choice of an induction agent in patients with complex congenital heart disease can be chosen on the basis of sound pharmacologic and physiologic principles, skilled airway management and effective ventilation usually dictate success.

After anesthetic induction, intravenous access is established. A nondepolarizing muscle relaxant is usually administered, and an intravenous opioid and/or inhalational agent is chosen for maintenance anesthesia. Nasotracheal intubation is usually selected because most patients require a period of postoperative mechanical ventilation, and the nasal route provides greater stability and patient comfort compared with an oral endotracheal tube. An FiO_2 of 1.0 is administered, and anesthetic depth is increased just before intubation to avoid desaturation during intubation. If the child arrives in the operating room with an endotracheal tube in place, it is our practice to change it. Inspissated secretions in a tube with a small internal diameter can cause significant obstruction to gas flow. During periods of bypass in which humidified ventilation is discontinued, significant endotracheal tube obstruction can occur. This can be minimized by starting with a new endotracheal tube.

Because of the diverse array of congenital heart defects and surgical procedures, an individualized anesthetic management plan is essential. The maintenance of anesthesia in these patients depends on the age and condition of each patient, the nature of the surgical procedure, the duration of CPB, and the need for postoperative ventilation. The choice of a particular anesthetic agent is less important when the appropriate monitoring and observance of the physiologic guidelines, already mentioned, are used. In patients with complex defects requiring preoperative inotropic and mechanical ventilatory support, a carefully controlled hemodynamic induction and maintenance anesthetic with a potent opioid is generally chosen. In patients with an isolated atrial septal defect or ventricular septal defect, a potent inhalational agent is preferred as the principal anesthetic agent. This allows for early postoperative extubation and a less prolonged period of intensive care monitoring. More important than the specific anesthetic techniques and drugs is the skilled execution of the anesthetic plan, which accommodates the patient's response to drugs, the changes associated with surgical manipulation, and the early recognition of intraoperative complications.

The reported changes in blood pressure and heart rate for the inhalational agents in healthy children are observed in pediatric cardiac surgical patients as well. Although both halothane and isoflurane decrease blood pressure and heart rate in neonates, infants, and children, the vasodilatory properties of isoflurane may improve overall systemic perfusion, compared with halothane (31). Despite improved cardiac reserve with isoflurane, the incidence of laryngospasm, coughing, and desaturation during induction of anesthesia limits its use in children with congenital heart defects (43). Potent inhalational agents as primary anesthetics should be reserved for the child with adequate cardiovascular reserve who is a candidate for early postoperative extubation. In these patients, the myocardial depression and hypotension associated with inhalational agents are well tolerated. Examples include the closure of an atrial septal defect or ventricular septal defect, excision of a discrete subaortic membrane, simple pulmonic or aortic stenosis with good ventricular function, ligation of a patent ductus arteriosus, and repair of coarctation of the aorta.

Children with complex congenital heart disease and limited cardiac reserve demand an anesthetic technique that provides hemodynamic stability. Inhalational agents are less well tolerated as a primary anesthetic in patients who have limited cardiac reserve, particularly after CPB. Fentanyl and sufentanil are excellent induction and maintenance anesthetics for this group of patients. Low to moderate doses of these opioids can be supplemented with incremental doses of inhalational anesthetics or benzodiazepines. The advantage to adding a second drug to a primary opioid anesthetic is a shortened time of postoperative mechanical ventilation and preservation of intraoperative hemodynamic stability. Clearly, postoperative mechanical ventilation is required when a high-dose opioid technique is used. The hemodynamic effect of fentanyl at a dose of 25 mg/kg with pancuronium, given to infants in the postoperative period after operative repair of a congenital heart defect, shows no change in left atrial pressure, pulmonary artery pressure, pulmonary vascular resistance, and cardiac index; however, it shows a small decrease in systemic vascular resistance and mean arterial pressure (44). Higher doses of fentanyl at 50 to 75 mg/kg with pancuronium result in a slightly greater fall in arterial pressure and heart rate in infants undergoing repair for complex congenital heart defects (45). Fentanyl has also been shown to block stimulus-induced pulmonary vasoconstriction and to contribute to the stability of the pulmonary circulation in neonates after congenital diaphragmatic hernia repair (46). Thus, the experience with fentanyl may be extrapolated to the operating room, where stabilizing pulmonary vascular responsiveness in newborns and young infants with reactive pulmonary vascular beds is crucial to weaning from CPB and to stabilizing shunt flow. The superiority of an opioid technique, compared with halothane, in critically ill neonates has recently been demonstrated.

Sufentanil and pancuronium provide the same cardiovascular stability as fentanyl and pancuronium in pediatric cardiovascular patients. Children receiving a sufentanil induction as a single dose of 5 to 20 mg/kg have a stable preintubation period (47). Intubation and other stimuli such as sternotomy do not produce clinically significant alterations in hemodynamics, although the changes are greater than with equipotent doses of fentanyl. Sufentanil as an infusion along with a benzodiazepine produces fewer alterations in heart rate and blood pressure. This has particular significance in infants in whom significant hemodynamic changes are poorly tolerated (48).

Acceptable anesthesia during CPB may be best accomplished by the continuous administration of an inhalational anesthetic via the vaporizer or the pump-oxygenator, by careful titration of small doses of opioids, or by the exact administration of an opioid and/or benzodiazepine by a continuous-infusion technique. If depth of anesthesia is accomplished by the administration of excessively large doses of opioids (e.g., fentanyl or sufentanil), postoperative mechanical ventilation will be necessary. However, residual levels of inhalational anesthetic drugs (e.g., enflurane or isoflurane) can produce transient myocardial depression at the termination of CPB.

Because of the widespread use of opioids for pediatric cardiac surgery and the availability of invasive monitoring, the pharmacokinetics and pharmacodynamics of these drugs have been well studied compared with other groups of pediatric surgical patients (49). In general, the clinical pharmacologies of fentanyl and sufentanil share the same age-related pharmacokinetic and pharmacodynamic features as those that have been demonstrated for other drugs in the pediatric population. For example, sufentanil has increased clearance in patients 1 month to 12 years of age, comparable adult clearance in adolescents (12 to 16 years of age), and decreased clearance in the neonatal period (newborn to 1 month) (50,51). Furthermore, sequential sufentanil anesthetics in neonates with congenital heart disease show marked increases in clearance and elimination between the first week and the third or fourth week of life. This is most likely a result of maturational changes in hepatic microsomal activity and improved hepatic blood flow from closure of the ductus venosus. The variability in clearance and elimination, coupled with limited cardiovascular reserve in the neonate during the first month of life, makes opioid dosing difficult in this age-group. Careful titration of 5 to 10 mg/kg fentanyl, titration of 1 to 2 mg/kg of sufentanil, or a continuous-infusion technique are the most reliable methods of achieving hemodynamic stability and an accurate dose response.

The benzodiazepines are important in the premedication of children undergoing cardiac surgery, and they are used intraoperatively as well. However, little is known about their pharmacokinetic and pharmacodynamic effects on the pediatric patient during cardiac surgery. Alfentanil, a new short-acting potent narcotic, has also been used for cardiac surgery in children. It shows great promise in selective pediatric cardiac anesthesia cases because of its rapid onset, short elimination half-life, and hemodynamic stability. Its hemodynamic profile shows no superiority to the other synthetic opioids, fentanyl and sufentanil.

Anticoagulation and Reversal

The contact of blood with the nonendothelialized surfaces of the CPB circuit initiates clot formation. To prevent coagulation during CPB, the patient must be adequately anticoagulated with heparin. In 1975, Bull devised a quantitative method for heparin administration using the activated clotting time as an end point (52). By maintaining activated clotting times of between 300 and 600 seconds, visible clot formation in the operative field and the pump-oxygenator was prevented. A more fastidious evaluation by means of a radioimmunoassay for fibrin monomers demonstrated the presence of fibrin monomer when activated clotting times were maintained between 300 and 400 seconds (53). Therefore, it may be preferable to keep activated clotting times at 400 seconds or more for prolonged periods of CPB in both the adult and the pediatric populations.

Although it is now feasible to measure plasma heparin levels, generally there is a poor correlation between heparin levels and activated clotting time (54). Because the effect of heparin on coagulation is important, rather than the plasma heparin level, the activated clotting time remains the preferred monitor of effective coagulation during CPB. However, heparin levels may be helpful, after heparin reversal with protamine, to assess residual heparin activity or the presence of heparin rebound.

For initiating bypass, heparin is generally administered in an initial bolus dose of 300 to 400 U/kg (3 to 4 mg/kg), which will maintain an activated clotting time level of 400 seconds or longer. Heparin is administered before cannulation of the great vessels, either by direct injection into the right atrium or through a functioning central line. In either case, care must be taken to ensure that heparin enters the central circulation. Blood should be aspirated before injection, and an activated clotting time of longer than 400 seconds should be documented before initiating CPB. Periodic measurement of the activated clotting time is performed throughout CPB to ensure an adequate degree of anticoagulation.

Cardiopulmonary Bypass Management

Management of CPB for congenital heart surgery differs from adults in (a) the use of more extreme perfusion techniques and (b) the extent of the inflammatory reaction to extracorporeal circulation. Heretofore, a major cause of morbidity and mortality in the young patient has been attributed to the effects of CPB. Recent refinements in the technology of CPB and safer application of perfusion techniques have reduced these risks to an acceptable level.

Pediatric patients are exposed to biologic extremes, including deep hypothermia (15°C to 20°C), hemodilution (three-fold to four-fold dilution of circulating blood volume), low perfusion pressures (20 to 30 mm Hg), wide variation in pump flow rates (ranging from highs of 200 $mL \cdot kg^{-1} \cdot minute^{-1}$ to total circulatory arrest and wide-ranging blood pH management, e.g., controlled (alpha-stat, pH-stat) and uncontrolled (post–total circulatory arrest or post–low-flow CPB, when pH can be extremely and unpredictably low) (see Table 21-2). These unphysiologic parameters significantly alter cerebral regulatory function and probably affect neurologic outcome. In addition to these prominent changes, subtle variations in glucose supplementation, cannula placement, presence of aortopulmonary collaterals, patient age, and brain mass may also affect cerebral preservation during CPB.

Adult patients are rarely, if ever, exposed to these biologic extremes. Temperature is rarely lowered below 25°C, hemodilution is more moderate, perfusion pressure is generally maintained at 30 to 80 mm Hg, flow rates are maintained at 50 to 65 $mL{\cdot}kg^{-1}{\cdot}minute^{-1}$, and pH management strategy is less influential because of moderate hypothermic temperatures and rare use of circulatory arrest. Variables such as glucose requirements and brain mass are more consistent in adults. Venous and arterial cannulas are larger and less deforming of the atria and aorta, and their placement is more predictable. Although superficially similar, the conduct of CPB in children is considerably different from that in adults. Therefore, one would expect marked physiologic differences in cerebral response to CPB in the child.

In any patient, three externally controlled factors are managed during CPB: perfusion rate, temperature, and hemodilution. During pediatric CPB, the alteration of these factors is significantly greater than in adults. Perfusion is regulated by adjusting the pump flow rate of the CPB circuit. Recommendations for optimal pump flow rates for children have historically been based on the patient's body mass and on maintaining efficient organ perfusion as determined by arterial blood gases, acid-base balance, and whole-body oxygen consumption during CPB (38,69). This rate is maintained at a higher level in infants and children because of their higher metabolic rate and the need for increased oxygen delivery. Usually, pump flow rate is adjusted to 2.4 to 2.6 $L{\cdot}minute^{-1}{\cdot}m^{-2}$ in neonates and small infants, and to 2.2 to 2.4 $L{\cdot}minute^{-1}{\cdot}m^{-2}$ in older children at moderate hypothermic temperatures (28°C to 30°C) (70). With deep hypothermia (18°C to 20°C) further reductions in flow rate are tolerated, allowing some flexibility and variation in CPB management. Because of the noncompliant cardiovascular system in children, perfusion can be accomplished at low mean arterial perfusion pressures (20 to 30 mm Hg).

The second factor that is externally controlled during CPB is hemodilution. Hemodilution effects are great in neonates and infants because of the large priming volume of the CPB circuit. In neonates, the dilutional effect from the CPB circuit is 20-fold to 40-fold greater compared with that of adults. As a consequence, blood levels of plasma proteins, formed blood elements, and drugs are significantly lowered. These dilutional changes affect oncotic pressure, tissue water, and physiologic processes such as coagulation, and they alter anesthetic drug biodisposition. In children with polycythemia and in whom repair is to take place at cold temperatures, the hemodilution effects of the priming solution can be used advantageously to decrease blood viscosity. The priming solutions used in pediatric CPB assumes greater importance than in adults because of the large prime volume-to-blood-volume ratio. In adults the priming volume is equivalent to 25% to 33% of the patient's blood volume, whereas in neonates and infants the priming volume exceeds the patient's blood volume by 200% to 300%. Therefore, care must be taken to achieve a physiologically balanced prime. For neonates and infants, blood must be added to the priming solution. Most institutions use packed red blood cells in their prime solution, although some institutions use whole blood. The main disadvantage of whole blood, over packed red blood cells, is its much higher glucose load in the prime. Hyperglycemia may increase the risk of neurologic injury if brain ischemia occurs. The advantage of adding whole blood to the priming solution is maintaining a higher level of blood plasma products (e.g., fibrinogen, albumin). The appropriate level of hemodilution for a given hypothermic temperature, however, is not well defined. Ideally, during CPB the hematocrit level is maintained between 18% and 22%. Most centers maintain hematocrit levels at 20 5 2% during deep hypothermia (15°C to 20°C) and allow the hematocrit level to drift as low as 15% before transfusing additional red blood cells. This range of hematocrit levels allows an adequate supply of oxygen to reach the body tissues and at the same time provides optimal blood viscosity for the cold perfusion temperatures. To achieve this low hematocrit level in neonates and young children, one should add packed red blood cells to the priming solution to avoid excessive hemodilution. To achieve a hematocrit level of 20 5 2% in neonates and infants, one should add banked blood to the priming solution. A calculation of the mixed hematocrit on CPB (the hematocrit of the total priming volume plus the patient's blood volume) can be calculated using the following formula:

$$\text{HCTCPB} = \text{f[(BVpt)(HCTpt)|BVpt} + \text{TPV] a [1|2]}$$

where HCTCPB is the mixed HCT (TPV + BVpt), BVpt equals patient's blood volume (weight in kilograms × estimated blood volume in cubic centimeters per kilogram), TPV equals total priming volume, and HCTpt equals starting hematocrit level of the patient (54).

This calculation allows an estimate of the hematocrit of the patient using an asanguineous prime and is therefore useful for older children and adolescents. In neonates and infants, the perfusionist must add blood to the pump prime to achieve a desired hematocrit level during hypothermic CPB. The following formula estimates the amount of red blood cells that must be added to achieve this hematocrit.

$$\text{Added RBCs(cc)} = (\text{BVpt} + \text{TPV})(\text{HCTdesired}) - (\text{BVpt})(\text{HCTpt})$$

where Added RBCs equal cubic centimeters of packed red blood cells added to the prime volume, BVpt equals patient's blood volume, TPV equals total priming volume, HCTdesired equals the desired hematocrit on CPB, and HCTpt equals starting hematocrit level of the patient.

The third factor externally controlled during CPB is temperature of the perfusate. The goal of temperature reduction during CPB management is to reduce the metabolic rate of the body so that flow can be reduced to execute an optimal repair. Reducing the demand for oxygen reduces the need for its supply and minimizes tissue ischemia. Surgical repair of congenital heart defects takes place over a wide range of temperatures, varying from 15°C to 20°C for repair of a ventricular septal defect in infancy to normothermia for the repair of an atrial septal defect. During the periods of cooling and rewarming, organs are at high risk of developing ischemia because the flow may be inadequate for the changing metabolic demands of the tissues being perfused. Accelerated rates of cooling (1°C/minute) have been associated with a lower developmental quotient (55). Therefore, extraordinary vigilance is required during these phases of cooling and rewarming. Uneven cooling and rewarming of core and body surface temperatures suggest inadequate perfusion, the cause of which must readily be identified and corrected. Preliminary studies suggest that during the usual conditions of moderate hypothermic bypass (25°C to 32°C) in children, organ perfusion—particularly cerebral blood flow—appears to be maintained despite the lower perfusion pressures (37). Maintenance of pressure-flow autoregulation and $Pa{CO_2}$ responsivity is achieved (56). During deep hypothermia and after a period of total circulatory arrest, regulation of organ perfusion may change. Neonates and small infants who weigh less than 8 to 10 kg and require extensive repair of complex congenital heart defects may be optimally repaired by using deep hypothermic CPB at 15°C to 20°C with DHCA. Surgical repair is more exacting with this technique because of the bloodless, cannula-free operative field, in which CPB time is shortened and organ protection is maximized. DHCA depends on the reduction of organ metabolism by temperature reduction, which confers enhanced organ protection (57,58). Biochemical reactions are temperature dependent; hypothermia reduces oxygen consumption, thereby prolonging the "safe period" of circulatory arrest.

Because the brain is the organ system most vulnerable to ischemia, there has been concern about the safety of DHCA, specifically about the effect of DHCA on brain structure and function (59). Despite the routine clinical application of DHCA, now into its third decade, the technique is largely empirical and mechanisms of cellular integrity and protection are poorly understood (35). Both the duration of the arrest period and the quality of perfusion techniques appear to influence cerebral metabolism (Figs. 21-5 and 21-6) (60).

Several recent studies address the importance of thorough brain cooling. Bellinger and associates demonstrated that accelerated rates of cooling (1°C/minute) during CPB with alpha-stat regulation is associated with a lower developmental quotient in neonates undergoing DHCA (55). A recent study describes four patients who, despite having achieved nasopharyngeal and rectal temperatures at 18°C, had significantly higher cerebral oxygen extraction and cerebral metabolic rates than their cohorts. Three of these patients developed significant neurologic dysfunction, despite a relatively short period of circulatory arrest. Unexpectedly high jugular O_2 extraction and brain metabolism, despite hypothermic temperatures, were noted. It is most likely that inadequate cerebral perfusion resulted in inefficient brain cooling that maintained temperature gradients throughout the brain (61).

Evidence for temperature gradients between superficial temperature measurements and deep brain structures can be found in the literature on animals. Studies in the rat demonstrate temperature gradients of 2°C to 6°C between deep brain structures and the temporalis muscle in a study using a four-vessel occlusion model of cerebral ischemia (62). Significant differences in neuronal function, histopathology, free fatty acid, and excitatory neurotransmitter release were demonstrated on the basis of regional differences in brain temperature (62,63). Animal studies also suggest regional differences in the distribution of brain blood flow

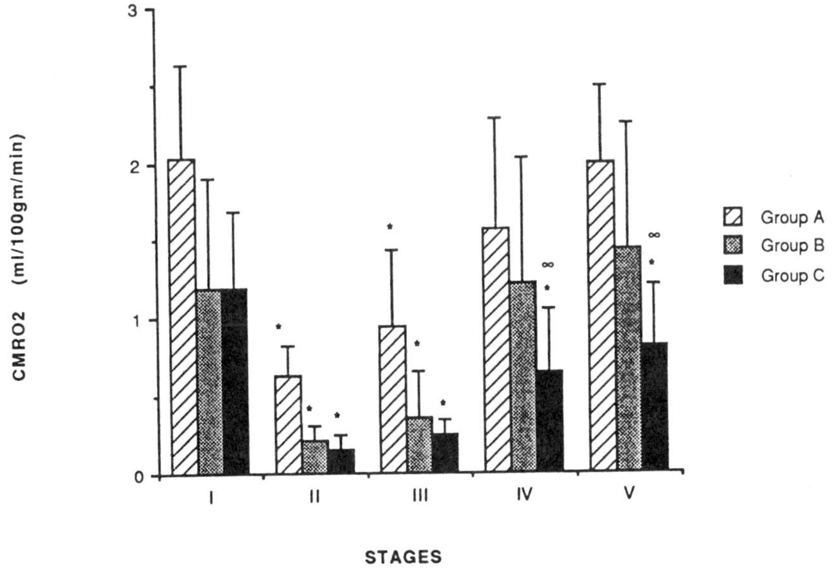

FIGURE 21-5. Bar chart of the changes in cerebral metabolic rate for oxygen ($CMRo_2$) before, during, and after cardiopulmonary bypass in neonates and infants. Group A underwent repair using moderate hypothermic bypass at 28°C to 32°C; group B, using deep hypothermic bypass with continuous flow at 18°C to 22°C; and group C, using deep hypothermic circulatory arrest at 18°C. Stage I, prebypass; stages II and III, during hypothermic bypass; stage IV, rewarmed on bypass; and stage V, after bypass. Note the reduction in cerebral metabolism in all groups during hypothermic CPB and the impaired cerebral metabolism after deep hypothermic circulatory arrest (group C). (Mean data 5 standard deviation; *, p = .001, stages II, III, IV, and V versus I; 1, p = .01; group C versus A and B.) (From Greeley WJ, Kern FH, Ungerleider RM, et al. The effect of hypothermic cardiopulmonary bypass and total circulatory arrest on cerebral metabolism in neonates, infants, and children. *J Thorac Cardiovasc Surg* 1991;101:783, with permission.)

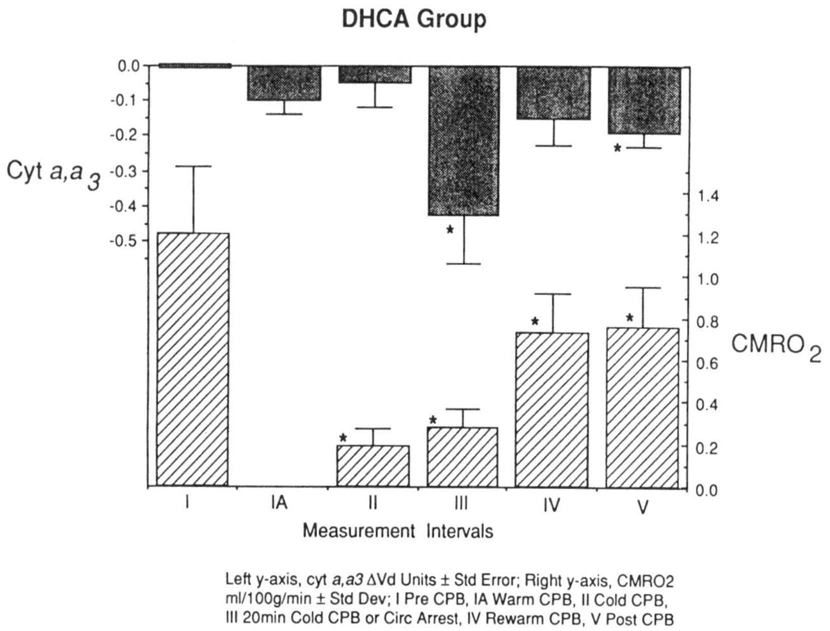

FIGURE 21-6. Bar graph of variations in cytochrome oxidase (cytochrome aa_3) near-infrared (NIR) signals and cerebral metabolic rate for oxygen ($CMRo_2$) in hypothermic bypass with patients undergoing deep hypothermic circulatory arrest (DHCA). Each point of cyt a,a3 represents mean 5 standard error in six patients; $CMRo_2$ values are mean 5 standard deviation. Negative values in cyt, a,a3 represent relative decreases in quantity of oxidized enzyme. (*, $CMRo_2$ and cyt a,a3 significantly different from control; p = .05.) (From Greeley W, Bracey V, Ungerleider R, et al. Recovery of cerebral metabolism and mitochondrial oxidation state are delayed after hypothermic circulatory arrest. *Circulation* 1991; 82:412, with permission.)

during hypercarbia. Deep brain structures (thalamus, brainstem, and cerebellum) receive a significantly greater percentage of cerebral blood flow than do cortical structures (64).

The earliest clinical investigations examining the effect of DHCA on the brain are controversial, and the results conflicting (65–70). This is largely because of methodological difficulties in evaluating neuropsychological outcome. In general, previously reported neuropsychological examinations in this age-group have been cursory and short term; evaluation of intraoperative cerebral pathophysiologic responses was lacking; survival was taken as the sole objective end point; and the quality of life was not examined (87). The earliest laboratory studies investigating DHCA consistently demonstrated two findings: (a) the reduction of oxygen and ATP requirements during deep hypothermia and the prompt recovery of ATP stores after DHCA and (b) the cerebral damaging effect of DHCA as a function of time of the arrest period (71–74).

More recently, a number of more sophisticated studies examining the outcome after DHCA had been performed. In a recent randomized clinical trial comparing the incidence of brain injury after DHCA or low-flow CPB, DHCA was demonstrated to have longer EEG recovery times and a higher incidence of clinical seizures in the early postoperative period (75). The DHCA group also had a higher incidence of neurologic abnormalities and poor motor function at 1 year of age, and poor expressive language and motor development at 2½ years, particularly in those who exhibited early postoperative seizures. Recent reports from the same clinical trial have shown that the DHCA cohort has continued to have worse motor coordination and planning and speech abnormalities at 4 years of age (76–78). Of interest, both the DHCA and the low CPB groups have lower cognitive and motor performance compared to that of a general population. This latter finding suggests factors outside DHCA and low-flow bypass, but within the perioperative period, are associated with poor neuropsychological development.

A recent clinical study has suggested pH-stat blood gas management strategy during CPB to be associated with an improved neuropsychological outcome in children (77). This study was a retrospective developmental study with a core of patients who have undergone surgery for transposition of the great artery. The authors found a strong positive correlation between arterial Pco_2 during cooling before circulatory rest and developmental score. This suggested that children undergoing an alpha-stat blood gas management strategy had a worse developmental outcome than those in which a pH-stat strategy was employed. In a recent randomized clinical trial of neonates undergoing cardiac surgery using DHCA, pH-stat management was noted to have faster EEG recovery times and fewer postoperative seizures compared to an alpha-stat bypass group (79,80). Therefore, the beneficial effect of pH-stat management clinically remains preliminary.

Certain experimental studies have also suggested the superiority of pH-stat strategy. In one recent study, pH-stat animals had greater cerebral blood flow during cooling and better recovery of cerebral ATP and intracellular pH after arrest and reperfusion (81). Brain water content was also less in the pH-stat group. These studies suggested that pH-stat CPB may have protective mechanisms due to an increased rate of brain cooling. In a more recent experimental study comparing pH-stat and alpha-stat CPB on cerebral oxygenation blood flow, cerebral protective effect of pH-stat management was demonstrated and indicated that the kinetics of cerebral deoxygenation might contribute to the mechanism of protection (82–84). Clearly more work needs to be done in this area before pH-stat is definitively recommended (85). However, preliminary experimental and clinical studies suggest a superiority of this technique in certain patient groups, particularly those with aortopulmonary collateral circulation.

Because of the potential for neurologic dysfunction after DHCA, some institutions use low-flow deep hypothermic CPB as an alternative technique. Because low-flow bypass can produce ischemia if flow is too low and because it lengthens the CPB time, compared to DHCA, serious concerns over this technique have also arisen.

Other factors such as surface cooling, anesthetic agents, and cerebral protective agents may influence and modify the effects of deep hypothermic CPB and DHCA. The potential use of certain pharmacologic agents such as anesthetic drugs, barbiturates, lidocaine, or calcium channel blockers is unknown. There are no clinical studies in children systematically examining the influence of these pharmacologic agents on cerebrovascular physiology or neurologic outcome. Therefore, the use of these agents remains entirely speculative and unfounded. Clearly, further study of the long-term effects of DHCA on neuropsychological outcome in children is necessary. Fundamental questions regarding deep hypothermic CPB with low-flow versus DHCA also need to be further addressed. Equally important, the manner in which the patient is cooled and rewarmed may affect outcome and merits further investigation, even before the testing of pharmacologic drugs.

Discontinuation of Cardiopulmonary Bypass

During weaning from CPB, an assessment of the requisite filling pressures can be made by temporarily increasing preload before terminating CPB. Myocardial contractility is assessed by direct visualization and, more quantitatively, by intraoperative echocardiography, either transesophageal or epicardial. If specific concerns of left-sided heart function are raised, monitoring the pulmonary artery wedge pressure or placing an intracardiac catheter in the left atrium can be performed by the surgeon. After adequate heart rate (by epicardial pacing if required), rhythm, preload, contractility, warming, and acid-base status have been achieved, the patient can be weaned from bypass. This is best accomplished by slowly filling the heart by clamping the venous return line and reducing the arterial inflow until adequate blood volume is achieved. Blood volume is assessed by directly visualizing the heart and measuring right atrial or left atrial filling pressures. When filling pressures are adequate, the arterial inflow is stopped. In small patients, the inflow is stopped by clamping the venous return cannula and turning off the arterial inflow immediately after adequate blood volume is achieved, thus abruptly terminating CPB. The arterial cannula is left in place so a slow infusion of residual pump blood can be used to optimize filling pressures and perfusion. Myocardial function is assessed by direct cardiac visualization and by placement of a transthoracic left atrial catheter, a percutaneous internal jugular catheter, or a transthoracic right atrial catheter, or by intraoperative epicardial echocardiography.

During the repair of complex congenital heart defects, the anesthesiologist and surgeon may be confronted with a patient who is difficult to wean from CPB. Under these circumstances, the problem, for example, a residual defect requiring repair or a functional abnormality requiring pharmacologic support, is often difficult to assess. In patients who are difficult to wean from CPB, an etiology must be determined immediately. Interventions must be made quickly and rationally based on available clinical information. The diverse causes of an inability to wean from CPB in children include (a) poor surgical result with a residual defect requiring re-repair, (b) pulmonary artery hypertension, and (c) right or left ventricular dysfunction. An intraoperative "cardiac catheterization" is done to assess isolated pressure measurements from the various chambers of the heart; catheter pullback measurements are taken to evaluate residual pressure gradients across valves, repaired sites of stenosis, and conduits; and oxygen saturation data are obtained in a search for residual shunts (86). Alternatively, epicardial echocardiography with Doppler color flow or TEE has been used to provide an intraoperative "picture" of structural or functional abnormalities, for evaluation of the postoperative cardiac repair (87). Doppler echocardiography is helpful in this circumstance, providing an additional method of rapidly diagnosing functional and structural abnormalities and assisting the anesthesiologist and surgeon in selecting the appropriate medical or surgical therapy. If structural abnormalities are found, the patient can be placed back on CPB, and residual defects can be repaired before the patient leaves the operating room (see Fig. 21-2). Leaving the operating room with a significant residual structural defect adversely affects survival and increases patient morbidity (87,88). For the anesthesiologist, Doppler echocardiography can rapidly identify specific wall motion or systolic thickening abnormalities due to ischemia or intramyocardial air. The technique directs specific pharmacologic interventions and provides a means of assessing their results (Fig. 21-7).

Left ventricular dysfunction can be treated by optimizing preload and heart rate, increasing coronary perfusion pressure, correcting ionized calcium levels, and adding inotropic support. Inotropic support is usually begun with calcium supplementation (10 to 30 mg/kg) and dopamine (5 to 15 $mg{\cdot}kg^{-1}{\cdot}minute^{-1}$). If function remains poor, a second drug is usually added. For left ventricular dysfunction, a more potent inotrope is administered, such as epinephrine at a dose of 0.03 to 0.05 $mg{\cdot}kg^{-1}{\cdot}minute^{-1}$ and titrated

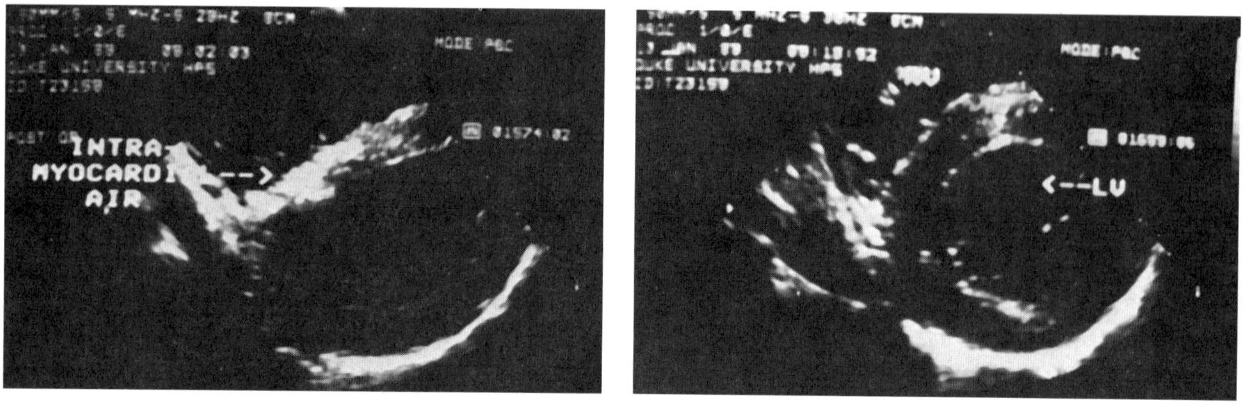

A B

FIGURE 21-7. **A:** A two-dimensional echocardiogram in the short-axis view across the ventricles demonstrating the presence of intramyocardial air (*arrow*) in the ventricular septum and right ventricular wall. The intramyocardial air appears as a dense "snowy" echogenic area. Note the associated wall motion abnormality appearing as flattening of the ventricular septum. **B:** The patient was treated with phenylephrine, which increased systemic and coronary perfusion pressure, resulting in clearance of the air and the echogenic density and the restoration of normal left ventricular wall motion and configuration. (From Greeley WJ, Kern FH, Ungerleider RM, et al. Intramyocardial air causes right ventricular dysfunction after repair of a congenital heart defect. *Anesthesiology* 1990;73:1042, with permission.)

to effect. Dobutamine may be used as an alternative second-line drug; however, dobutamine in conjunction with dopamine may produce significant sinus tachycardia in neonates and infants. This effect may be related to structural similarities between dobutamine and isoproterenol (89). Amrinone in conjunction with epinephrine may improve left ventricular contractility and reduce systemic afterload (90,91). This combination is highly effective for left ventricular dysfunction. If very high doses of inotrope are required, consideration for mechanical circulatory support with extracorporeal membrane oxygenation (ECMO) or a left ventricular assist device should be strongly considered.

Pulmonary artery hypertension is most effectively treated with ventilatory manipulations. The goal is to reduce pulmonary vascular resistance by regulating Pa_{CO_2}, pH, Pa_{O_2} (alveolar), Pa_{O_2} (arterial), and lung volumes. Arterial carbon dioxide tension is a potent mediator of pulmonary vascular resistance (this is especially true in the newborn). Reducing Pa_{CO_2} to 20 mm Hg and increasing pH to 7.60 produces a consistent and reproducible reaction in pulmonary vascular resistance in infants with pulmonary artery hypertension (25). Similarly, manipulation of serum bicarbonate to achieve a pH of 7.50 to 7.60 while maintaining a Pa_{CO_2} of 40 mm Hg has equal salutary effects on pulmonary vascular resistance (112,113). Because increasing Fi_{O_2} reduces pulmonary vascular resistance in patients with intracardiac shunts, by inference, this is probably a direct pulmonary vasodilatory effect of the alveolar, rather than arterial, P_{O_2} (26).

Adjusting lung volumes through ventilatory mechanics also plays a major role in controlling pulmonary artery hypertension. After CPB, lung compliance is reduced and closing capacity exceeds functional residual capacity. Airway closure occurs before end-exhalation, resulting in areas of lung that are perfused yet underventilated (92,93). These segments of lung become increasingly hypoxemic, and secondary vasoconstriction occurs. The result is elevated pulmonary vascular resistance and reduced pulmonary blood flow. Maintaining lung volumes with large tidal volume ventilation will restore functional residual capacity and decrease pulmonary vascular resistance (94). Therefore, not only are hyperventilation and alkalosis important, but achieving and maintaining lung volumes are crucial. Care must be taken to avoid excessive positive end-expiratory pressure or high mean airway pressure, as either may result in alveolar overdistension, compression of capillaries in the alveolar wall and interstitium, and elevated pulmonary vascular resistance, or reduced pulmonary blood flow (95). Therefore, high tidal volume ventilation with inspiratory-to-expiratory (I:E) ratios of 1:3 or longer may be necessary to optimize lung volumes and reduce pulmonary vascular resistance during weaning from CPB.

Drug therapy for pulmonary artery hypertension is of limited benefit. Amrinone, isoproterenol, prostaglandin E_1, and tolazoline have some effect on pulmonary vascular resistance. Amrinone reduces pulmonary vascular resistance and may increase right ventricular contractility. Myocardial oxygen consumption is not significantly increased, and heart rate is not elevated (96–101). Isoproterenol increases myocardial oxygen consumption, increases heart rate, and reduces systemic arterial pressure, all of which may reduce coronary perfusion and contribute to right ventricular ischemia (102,103). This is especially true if pulmonary pressures remain high and right ventricular subendocardial perfusion is impaired. Prostaglandin E_1 has been used to treat pulmonary hypertensive crisis with varying degrees of success (104,105). Severe systemic vasodilation with tolazoline (an α-blocker) has limited the use of this drug for post-CPB therapy (106). In our neonatal cardiac experience, we have had greater success with ventilatory manipulations and amrinone in conjunction with a catecholamine to improve right ventricular coronary perfusion pressure than with other therapeutic modalities. A hemofiltering system used after CPB has dramatically reduced the incidence of pulmonary hypertensive crises in some centers (107).

Right ventricular dysfunction can be treated by reducing pulmonary vascular resistance with ventilatory manipulations, increasing coronary perfusion pressure with phenylephrine or epinephrine and reducing pulmonary artery pressure with amrinone or isoproterenol (32,90,91). The right ventricle is most dependent on systolic pressure for coronary perfusion. Therefore, drug therapy must maintain systemic perfusion pressure. prostaglandin E_1 or tolazoline may result in substantial systemic hypotension and be counterproductive (105).

Use of Modified Ultrafiltration

One important factor effecting the morbidity and motility rates after cardiac surgery in children is effects of CPB. During the initiation of CPB, considerable hemodilution occurs. This hemodilution is the result of the priming volume required for the CBP circuit. Under many circumstances, this hemodilutional effect is intentional, decreasing blood viscosity and thereby preventing sludging when the patient is cooled to temperatures below 20°C. After CPB, hemodilution is associated with tissue edema and organ dysfunction. Because blood elements are exposed to the nonendothelialized circuitry of CPB, there is also a significant inflammatory response as result of CPB. Both these effects of hemodilution and inflammation are exaggerated in neonates, infants and young children due to their disproportionate exposure to the circuit relative to their body size. This inflammatory response leads to an increase in capillary permeability, leading to an overall increase in total body edema postoperatively.

Efforts to reduce the hemodilution and inflammatory effects CPB included reducing priming volume, perioperative antiinflammatory and diuretic therapies, and the use of postoperative peritoneal dialysis. The technique of modified ultrafiltration (MUF) was first used clinically as an alternative method to reduce the adverse effects of CPB in children (108).

The technique of MUF is performed after CPB is complete and allows filtration of both the patient and remaining contents of the CPB circuit including the venous reservoir (109–111). Using the MUF technique, an ultrafilter is interposed in the CPB circuit between the aortic arterial line and the venous cannula, which is located in the right atrium. After weaning from CPB, the blood is removed from the patient via the aortic cannula and fed through the ultrafilter along with blood from the venous reservoir and oxygen. The outlet of the ultrafilter is fed to the right atrium of the patient. Blood flow through the ultrafilter approximates 200 mL/minute, which is maintained by a roller pump. Suction is applied to the filter port of the ultrafilter, resulting in an ultrafiltration rate of 100 to 150 mL/minute. A constant left atrial or right atrial pressure is maintained, achieving continued hemodynamic stability in the patient. Ultrafiltration is carried out with end points either being time (15 to 20 minutes) or achieving a hematocrit value of approximately 40% (110).

Ultrafiltration appears to offer two major advantages. First, total body water is reduced as a direct result of removing the ultrafiltrate (108). This effect counteracts the hemodilution effects associated with the institution of CPB. In addition, the hematocrit is raised after CPB enhancing oxygen delivery to the tissues. Secondly, MUF has been shown to remove some of the deleterious vasoactive substances associated with inflammatory response to CPB (112,113). This effect is mediated by reducing circulating cytokines, which are associated with capillary leak syndrome. Examination of the ultrafiltrate shows that it contains low-molecular-weight, inflammatory mediators including C3a, C5a, interleukin-6A, interleukin-8A, tumor necrosis factor, myocardial depressant factor, and various other cytokines. Several studies have shown that compared to control patients, patients that have MUF after CPB have substantially less increase in total body water, less compliment and interleukin release, require less blood transfusions, and show a faster recovery of systolic blood pressure (108,110,114).

In a clinical study examining the effect of MUF on left ventricular systolic function in children, MUF was associated with an increase in intrinsic left ventricular systolic function and a decrease in end-diastolic pressure, thereby improving left ventricular compliance (115). In an experimental study, MUF has also been demonstrated to improve cerebral blood flow, cerebral metabolic activity, and cerebral oxygen delivery after DHCA (116). This latter effect acutely improves cerebral metabolism after DHCA and may reduce and reverse the known deleterious effects of DHCA on brain function after CPB. In another clinical study further defining the benefits of MUF, MUF was demonstrated to reduce postoperative blood use, chest tube drainage, plural effusions, and hospital stay in patients after cavopulmonary operations (117).

An alternative to MUF is conventional filtration during rewarming period of CPB. In an experimental model examining MUF versus conventional ultrafiltration, modified ultrafiltration was alone effective in reducing weight gain and myocardial edema and was associated with improving left ventricular function (118). Possible complications of modified ultrafiltration include air embolus, patient cooling during ultrafiltration, and bleeding (110). These theoretical and technical potential complications appear not to be of substantial concern. It is the view of most groups that the benefits of MUF far exceed the risk (111).

In summary, MUF is a safe adjunct reversing the deleterious effects of hemodilution and the inflammatory response associated with CPB in children. Perioperative blood loss and blood use is significantly reduced when MUF is used. MUF also improves left ventricular function and systolic blood pressure and increases oxygen delivery. Pulmonary compliance and brain function after CPB are also improved. Therefore, the use of MUF is becoming more routine in pediatric patients after CPB.

Mechanical Circulatory Assistance in Pediatric Patients

Mechanical circulatory assistance for the failing heart is achieving wide application in adult cardiac patients. Three modalities are currently available for circulatory support in children. These include the intraaortic balloon pump, ECMO, and ventricular assist devices. Indications of the need for mechanical circulatory support in the congenital heart patient include (a) inability to wean from CPB due to primary ventricular dysfunction (i.e., correctable residual anatomic defects have been eliminated), (b) failure of selective surgical interventions used to reduce volume or pressure load on an unaccepting ventricle (e.g., placing a small hole in an atrial septal defect patch to allow a dysfunctional right ventricle to shunt blood right to left at the atrial level and reduce its volume load), (c) successful weaning from bypass but escalating inotropic support because of an evolving picture of ventricular dysfunction, and (d) severe pulmonary artery hypertension despite maximal ventilatory support, systemic alkalinization, and inotropy. Care must be taken to ensure that the problem is functional and not anatomic. Inotropic and ventricular assistance cannot overcome a poor operative result. Intraoperative echocardiographic studies have shown an enhanced mortality rate if the patient leaves the operating room with a residual anatomic defect. Echocardiography and/or pressure monitoring may be used to localize the ventricular dysfunction to a right, left, or biventricular problem. Saturation monitoring or intraoperative echocardiography may be used to confirm that residual ventricular septal defects or atrial septal defects are eliminated. Once anatomic defects are eliminated and functional problems identified, mechanical circulatory assistance can be considered.

Mechanical circulatory assistance includes the intraaortic balloon pump, ECMO, and ventricular assist devices in children. Selecting the appropriate technology is based on the patient's underlying disease, size, heart rate, and degree of hypoxemia (Fig. 21-8).

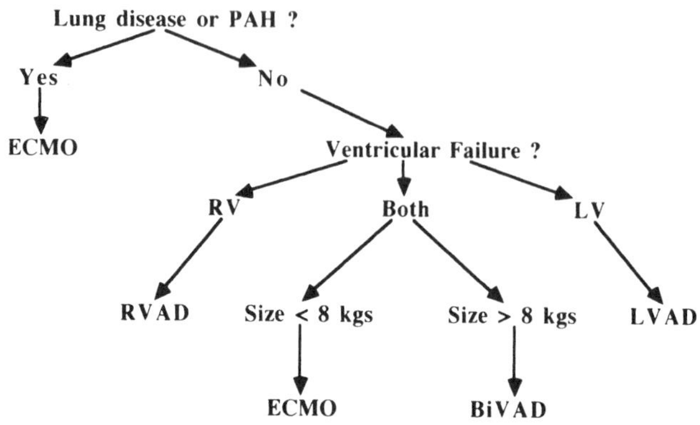

FIGURE 21-8. Decision algorithm for the selection of the appropriate circulatory assist device in infants and children. (PAH, pulmonary artery hypertension.)

Intraaortic Balloon Pump

The intraaortic balloon pump is an important adjunct in the management of adult patients with moderate to severe left ventricular dysfunction. The device consists of a long narrow balloon, which is positioned in the descending aorta just distal to the left subclavian artery. The balloon inflates during diastole and displaces blood from the thoracic aorta. Proximal aortic blood displacement results in increased aortic root pressure and augmented coronary blood flow. Blood that is displaced distally improves systemic perfusion by augmenting mean arterial pressure. During systole, the balloon is deflated, allowing the left ventricle to eject blood into a relatively empty, low-resistance descending aorta, and systemic afterload is reduced. The net result is a decrease in myocardial wall tension, reduced myocardial oxygen consumption, and augmented coronary perfusion.

Precise function of the intraaortic balloon pump depends on synchronizing inflation and deflation with the cardiac cycle. Either the arterial waveform or the ECG can be used. When it is timed to the arterial waveform, balloon inflation is set to begin at the dicrotic notch. If inflation begins earlier, left ventricular ejection will be compromised by balloon inflation. Deflation begins when the arterial trace reaches its nadir. If deflation begins too soon, the descending aorta may not fully evacuate its blood volume, resulting in reduction in mean arterial pressure and reduced coronary augmentation. If deflation is delayed, the left ventricle must pump against an increased resistance.

Despite the overwhelming success of balloon counterpulsation in adults, pediatric use of the balloon pump has been disappointing. The intraaortic balloon pump has not improved outcome in children younger than 5 years of age when used for postoperative myocardial dysfunction, or in older patients after Fontan procedures (119). In children more than 5 years of age undergoing a nonpalliative procedure (e.g., corrective repair), some success has been reported with intraaortic balloon pump assistance for postoperative left ventricular dysfunction. Several factors contributed to the unfavorable results of intraaortic balloon pumps in children. These include (a) higher heart rates in children, (b) increased aortic elasticity, (c) presence of aortopulmonary collaterals in cyanotic patients, (d) palliative rather than complete repairs, and (e) a higher incidence of right ventricular and biventricular dysfunction.

A miniature intraaortic balloon pump has been developed by the group at the University of Utah (120). It has been used successfully in small animals. Although the device has been in development for some time, no devices are commercially available; therefore, its clinical efficacy in comparison with ECMO and ventricular assist devices remains unknown.

Extracorporeal Membrane Oxygenation

In the early 1970s, case reports of the successful application of prolonged CPB in adults with trauma or combined cardiac and respiratory failure began to appear in the literature (121–123). These early reports led to a trial, sponsored by the National Institutes of Health, of ECMO for acute respiratory failure in the adult patient (124). The overall survival rate for both groups was less than 10%, and the ECMO trial was considered a failure. This early experience diminished the enthusiasm for this technology, and its application became limited to neonates with acute respiratory failure, in whom a clear improvement in survival was easily demonstrated (125–127).

ECMO was a profound failure in the adult population because of the strict criteria used for entry into the study. The average ECMO patient spent more than 9 days on maximal ventilatory support before randomization (124). Pathologic evaluation demonstrated a high incidence of pulmonary fibrosis and hyaline membrane formation (128).

These findings are crucial and extremely relevant to congenital heart patients. Mechanical circulatory assistance is used to rest a "stunned" myocardium that is capable of recovery. Therefore, mechanical circulatory assistance should be considered early, before irreversible damage occurs. Mechanical circulatory support is not salvage therapy; rather, it is a next level of support, just as a more potent inotrope (such as epinephrine) would be if dopamine were insufficient. Complications from prolonged cardiogenic shock in patients unresponsive to extended periods of maximal medical management may not be reversible and may increase the likelihood of ECMO-related complication and failure.

Before ECMO is initiated, the patients must be heparinized. Generally 100 to 150 U/kg of heparin is given and the activated clotting time is maintained between 180 and 220 seconds via a continuous heparin infusion. Once the patient is on ECMO, blood products are transfused to maintain a hematocrit of 40% to 45% and a minimum platelet count of 50,000 to 70,000, and fibrinogen levels of 150 to 200 mg/dL are maintained with cryoprecipitate. After ECMO has begun, hemodynamics stabilize and inotropic support can be reduced.

Published reports of congenital heart patients requiring ECMO for postoperative circulatory support due to intractable cardiac failure or severe pulmonary vasoactive crisis demonstrate an overall survival rate of 59% (129,130). When patients were successfully weaned from CPB and ECMO was begun in the postoperative period, 42 of 57 (74%) of children survived. Mortality rate was significantly greater for patients who could not wean from CPB and for whom ECMO support was instituted in the operating room. In this group, only 2 of 14 patients survived (14%). Complications from ECMO therapy were considerable and included hemorrhage (48%), renal insufficiency (29%), neurologic injury (17%), arrhythmias (17%), infectious complications (10%), and ECMO circuit problems (10%).

Although ECMO is an extremely effective means of support, the high mortality rate associated with weaning directly from CPB to ECMO is disturbing. Reasons include severe ventricular dysfunction and recalcitrant hemorrhage. Recovery from severe ventricular dysfunction is predicated on the concept that the myocardium sustained a transient injury and is capable of recovery with time (i.e., stunned myocardium). ECMO is used to decrease ventricular wall tension, increase coronary perfusion pressure, and maintain systemic perfusion with oxygenated blood. If left ventricular function is severely impaired, left ventricular end-diastolic pressure may remain high and endocardial perfusion may be impaired. Left atrial venting may reduce left ventricular end-diastolic pressure and improve myocardial recovery. Hemorrhage, however, remains a troublesome problem, due to the need for heparin on ECMO.

Ventricular Assist Devices

An alternative approach is to use a ventricular assist device. This device supports only the circulation. It does not include oxygenators and therefore requires significantly less anticoagulation (131), which minimizes hemorrhagic complications. Compared with ECMO, ventricular assist devices may be a preferred means of circulatory support for children unable to wean from CPB because of primary left ventricular dysfunction. Ventricular assist devices allow direct control of left atrial filling pressure; therefore, left ventricular end-diastolic pressure can be minimized, allowing for a greater likelihood of left ventricular recovery.

There are two types of ventricular assist devices: pulsatile and nonpulsatile. Pulsatile devices are sophisticated pumps, initially designed as permanent artificial implantable hearts. These pumps are durable, cause minimal blood trauma, and can be used for prolonged periods. Their most common function today is as a bridge to cardiac transplantation. Because of the lack of availability, high cost, and sophistication, these devices are not commonly used for postbypass ventricular support of the stunned myocardium. Typical devices include the Jarvik-7, and the Donachy/Thoratec pump.

Nonpulsatile continuous-flow pumps are less expensive and are commercially available. The most widely used device is the centrifugal pump, in which blood is moved by its entrainment against spinning blades or cones. An example is the Bio-Medicus pump. Centrifugal pumps require direct heart cannulation. A left ventricular assist device requires a left atrial venous cannula and an aortic cannula. Wire-reinforced cannulas are preferred, because kinking can result in marked reduction in cardiac output and/or ventricular distention. The cannulas are secured in place and connected via polyvinyl chloride tubing to the ports on the pump head.

The left ventricular assist device is activated and flow rates increased, until the patient is completely weaned from CPB and the left ventricular assist device is providing full circulatory support. A left and right atrial line is strongly recommended for monitoring during left ventricular assist. Maintaining low left atrial pressures reduces left ventricular end-diastolic pressure and may improve left ventricular recovery. In addition, there is no venous reservoir in the centrifugal pump system; therefore, pressure monitoring is essential to ensuring adequate intravascular volume to sustain pump flow rates and prevent pumping air. Low left atrial pressures may result from hypovolemia or right ventricular failure. A right atrial pressure monitor helps differentiate volume problems from right ventricular dysfunction. If right atrial pressures are high and left ventricular filling pressures are low, significant right ventricular failure is present. Supporting the right ventricle with inotropes such as dopamine, amrinone, isoproterenol, or prostaglandin E_1 may be helpful. However, if right ventricular dysfunction is prominent, biventricular support is considered. Right ventricular support is instituted with a right ventricular assist device. A wire-reinforced right atrial cannula and main pulmonary artery cannula are placed. These cannulas are connected to a second centrifugal pump. Management of a biventricular system is more complicated. Flows need to be adjusted independently to unload the right ventricle, maintain adequate blood return to the left atrium, and ensure effective systemic flows and perfusion pressure. Generally, left atrial pressures are maintained at 5 to 10 mm Hg, and right atrial pressures at 5 to 12 mm Hg. Pressures of less than 5 mm Hg in the left atrium are treated by increasing the patient's intravascular volume. Left atrial pressure monitoring is even more critical in neonates and infants because flow through the ventricular assist device is measured by an inline electromagnetic flow probe, which is inaccurate at flow rates below 500 mL/m^2.

Once the patient is stabilized on the ventricular assist device, heparin is reversed and any residual coagulopathy treated with fresh whole blood and component therapy. Due to prolonged multiple bypass runs, a severe coagulopathy is usually present. Treatment with platelets, fresh-frozen plasma, and cryoprecipitate is commonly required. Once bleeding is controlled, low-dose heparin is administered to maintain an activated clotting time of 120 to 180 seconds.

Published experience with ventricular assist devices is limited to adults. The overall survival rate from the Combined Registry of the International Society for Heart Transplantation and the American Society for Artificial Internal Organs reports a 24% survival rate in 451 patients receiving a ventricular assist device for postcardiotomy cardiogenic shock (132). This is consistent with the experience at the Cleveland Clinic, which reported an overall 23% survival rate. Survival rates for right ventricular assist devices, left ventricular assist devices, and biventricular assist devices were 22%, 23%, and 25%, respectively, in the Cleveland Clinic series (133).

At Boston Children's Hospital, a Bio-Medicus centrifugal pump has been used in six patients. In two patients, ventricular assist devices were used preoperatively for stabilization of cardiomyopathy myocarditis. One patient improved and was successfully weaned from a left ventricular assist device, and the other went on to transplant. In children with postcardiotomy cardiogenic shock, four patients received ventricular assist devices (two left ventricular assist devices and two right ventricular assist devices). All four recovered myocardial function and were weaned from ventricular assistance. Three of the four patients survived. In contrast, ECMO was used in eight patients with postcardiotomy cardiogenic shock, and only two patients (25%) survived for longer than 30 days. Although this is a small number of patients, it does raise the concern that ECMO may be less effective than a ventricular assist device for a stunned myocardium. Bleeding and absence of left-sided venting are the most likely causes. By reducing left ventricular end-diastolic pressure, ventricular assist devices may be more effective in maximizing myocardial recovery.

Blood Conservation During Cardiac Surgery

Modern pediatric cardiac anesthesia should include the principles and practice of blood conservation. An awareness of the need for blood conservation and the application of autotransfusion techniques makes it possible to perform open heart surgery without blood components, even in small children. Because the transfusion of blood products is associated with numerous complications (hemolytic and febrile reactions, bacterial infection, and disease transmission, e.g., viral hepatitis, cytomegalovirus, human immunodeficiency virus, and other viruses), transfusion is to be assiduously avoided unless specifically indicated by an impairment in tissue oxygenation or by documented coagulopathies with clinically significant bleeding. The decline in the quantity and quality of donor blood products has created tremendous supply difficulties for blood banks. Therefore, all efforts of blood conservation during cardiac surgery should be routinely employed by all members of the operative team, intraoperatively as well as postoperatively.

Techniques of blood conservation begin in the preoperative period. This can be accomplished in two ways: (a) maximizing preoperative hemoglobin and hematocrit levels by nutritional support of patients and (b) preoperatively storing the patient's own blood, to be used for later transfusion. The latter technique requires the collection of autologous blood 7 to 28 days before cardiac surgery and is usually limited to older children and adolescents. The most crucial measures of conserving blood occur intraoperatively. First, removal of autologous blood before CPB and reinfusion after bypass can reduce the requirements for blood in some older children. Another technique is the practice of controlled hemodilution during CPB, which not only enhances blood flow during hypothermic conditions but more importantly decreases the number of red cells lost during surgery. Next, a surgical technique that pays meticulous attention to hemostasis during surgery will result in decreased blood loss. Another important intraoperative blood conservation technique is the use of autologous autotransfusion devices during cardiac surgery. "Cell Savers" (Cell Saver-Haemonetics, Braintree, MA; BRAT-Kardiothor, Arvada, CO) for collecting, centrifuging, washing, and returning red blood cells to the patient are very effective. These blood-scavenging devices help to process mediastinal bloodshed in selective redo operations or to process red blood cells that remain in the oxygenator at the conclusion of bypass. These cell-saving techniques can yield 0.5 to 2.0 units of packed red blood cells per patient. Another blood-conserving technique is hemofiltration, which is included in the bypass circuitry and has the ability to remove excess fluid from the circulation near the termination of CPB. Finally, intraoperative blood conservation techniques include the careful monitoring of heparinization and its reversal with protamine. Inadequate reversal of heparin effect will prolong clotting time and unnecessarily increase the rate of bleeding in children. In general, other standard coagulation tests usually show a prolonged partial thromboplastin time and prothrombin time, hypofibrinogenemia, and dilution of other procoagulants as well as a prolonged bleeding time in many pediatric patients with and without significant bleeding (Table 21-6). The platelet count is reduced to a greater extent than can be accounted for by hemodilution alone, and this probably reflects platelet activation by the nonendothelialized surfaces of the CPB circuit and pump-oxygenator.

The most common reason for persistent bleeding is platelet dysfunction and reduced platelet number. Under these circumstances, administration of platelets is warranted. After platelets have been given and if bleeding is still present, reassessment and a second platelet infusion or the administration of cryoprecipitate is considered. In some neonates and infants, a diffuse coagulopathy with relatively severe reductions in factor activity (including fibrinogen) and platelet number is present after CPB. Moreover, prebypass fibrinogen less than 100 mg/dL has been noted in some neonates, which signifies a marked fibrinogen deficiency and may be an important contributing factor to post-CPB hemorrhage (see Table 21-6). The reduced prebypass fibrinogen level most likely reflects reduced fibrinogen synthesis by the liver due to hepatic immaturity and/or reduced function because of poor systemic perfusion.

TABLE 21-6. SURGICAL OUTCOME AND CONGENITAL HEART DEFECTS

Correction	Correction ?	Palliation
Patent ductus arteriosus	Ventricular septal defect	Conduits
Atrial septal defect	Coarctation	Transplantation
	Transposition of the great arteries	Definitive shunts
	Tetralogy of Fallot	Pulmonary atresia + ventricular septal defect
	Pulmonary stenosis	
	Aortic stenosis	
	Tricuspid atresia	
	Truncus arteriosus	

Source: From Stark J. Do we really correct congenital heart defects? *J Thorac Cardiovasc Surg* 1989;97:1, with permission.

In neonates, the increased incidence of bleeding and the escalating dilutional effects of selective component therapy on the remaining procoagulants in small patients have made bleeding a difficult problem. In a preliminary study, fresh whole blood (24 hours old) has been shown to be effective in establishing hemostasis after CPB in neonates (134). Fresh whole blood may be used under these circumstances in neonates. Recently, the beneficial effect of high-dose aprotinin therapy on blood loss and coagulation patterns during cardiac surgery in adult patients has been shown (135). This same group has also shown the effectiveness of aprotinin in infants and children for congenital heart surgery in very preliminary work. Although the drug is promising, controlled trials of aprotinin have not yet begun in children.

The techniques of blood conservation must be continued in the immediate postoperative period. Isolated coagulation abnormalities are often present in the uncomplicated postoperative cardiac patient (Table 21-7). Usually, these coagulation abnormalities self-correct during the first postoperative day and are not associated with excessive bleeding. Therefore, the routine administration of blood products to correct laboratory coagulation abnormalities in the absence of bleeding is never clinically indicated. Administration of blood products should not be made unless there is clinical evidence of bleeding or unless a specific defect has been identified and a specific component therapy employed. The routine use of blood products for volume replacement is to be avoided; lactated Ringer's or saline solution can be satisfactorily administered at a reduced cost without the hazards associated with transfusion.

TABLE 21-7. COAGULATION PROFILE IN NEONATES DURING CARDIOPULMONARY BYPASS (CPB)

Assay	Pre-CPB	1 min on CPB	Cold CPB	Warm CPB	Post-Protamine	ICU
Fibrinogen	200 ± 59[a]	92 ± 18	94 ± 21	107 ± 24	142 ± 28[a]	183 ± 33
Factor II	56 ± 13	30 ± 7	32 ± 8	33 ± 7	48 ± 10	60 ± 33
Factor V	68 ± 20[a]	15 ± 4	17 ± 5	22 ± 7	39 ± 11[a]	46 ± 10
Factor VII	54 ± 11[b]	26 ± 5	27 ± 6	28 ± 5	41 ± 8[b]	53 ± 16
Factor VIII	48 ± 20[c]	0	0	0	32 ± 15[c]	72 ± 45
Factor IX	31 ± 13	20 ± 8	23 ± 5	31 ± 4	31 ± 9	40 ± 12
Factor X	52 ± 10[a]	31 ± 7	31 ± 7	34 ± 8	46 ± 10	47 ± 16
Platelets (k/mm^3)	225 ± 54[a]	65 ± 17	45 ± 8	93 ± 28[a]	120 ± 29	
Antithrombin 3	49 ± 22	30 ± 12	29 ± 15	32 ± 13	57 ± 28	68 ± 23
Heparin (units)	0.02 ± 0.03	0.41 ± 0.08	0.42 ± 0.08	0.42 ± 0.08	0.04 ± 0.04	0.07 ± 0.06
Activated clotting time (seconds)	168 ± 20	>700	>700	>700	151 ± 31	

Note: Fibrinogen, factors II, V, VII, VIII, IX, and X, and antithrombin 3 are shown in percentage activity.
[a] $p < .0001$.
[b] $p < .002$.
[c] $p < .005$.

ANESTHESIA FOR CLOSED HEART OPERATIONS

Early corrective repair in infancy and less palliation have significantly reduced the number of noncorrective closed heart operations. Corrective closed heart procedures include patent ductus arteriosus ligation and repair of coarctation of the aorta. Noncorrective closed heart operations include pulmonary artery banding, extracardiac shunts such as the Blalock-Taussig shunt, and atrial septectomy. All of these procedures are performed without CPB. Venous access, intraarterial monitoring, and pulse oximetry are invaluable tools in the intraoperative management.

Patent ductus arteriosus ligation is performed through a left thoracotomy. The physiologic management is that of a simple shunt. Patients with a large patent ductus arteriosus and low pulmonary vascular resistance generally present with excessive pulmonary blood flow and congestive heart failure. Neonates and premature infants also run the risk of having a large diastolic pulmonary artery runoff. Their diastolic pressures can be so low that coronary and cerebral perfusion are impaired. Thus, patients range from the asymptomatic healthy young child to the sick ventilator-dependent premature infant on inotropic support. The former patient allows for a wide variety of anesthetic techniques and planned extubation in the operating room. The latter patient requires a carefully controlled anesthetic and fluid management plan. Generally, a trial of medical management with indomethacin and fluid restriction is attempted in the premature infant before surgical correction is performed. In the premature infant, transport to the operating room can be particularly difficult and tedious, requiring great vigilance to avoid extubation, excessive patient cooling, or venous access disruption. These factors can be minimized by performing ductal ligation in the neonatal intensive care unit. Intraoperatively, retractors may interfere with cardiac filling and ventilatory management, so hypotension, hypoxemia, and hypercarbia may occur. Complications include inadvertent ligation of the left pulmonary artery or descending aorta, recurrent laryngeal nerve damage, and excessive bleeding due to inadvertent patent ductus arteriosus disruption. After ductal ligation, worsening pulmonary compliance and increased ventilatory support are common, and an increase in left ventricular afterload should be anticipated, particularly if left ventricular dysfunction exists preoperatively.

Coarctation of the aorta is a narrowing of the descending aorta near the insertion of the ductus arteriosus. Obstruction to left ventricular outflow is the result, and this may range from severe obstruction with compromised systemic perfusion to mild upper extremity hypertension as the only manifestations. Associated anomalies of both the mitral and the aortic valves can occur. In the young infant with severe coarctation, systemic perfusion depends on right-to-left shunting across the patent ductus arteriosus. In these circumstances, left ventricular dysfunction is highly common, and prostaglandin E_1 is often necessary to provide systemic perfusion from the patent ductus arteriosus to the pulmonary artery. Generally, a peripheral intravenous tube and an indwelling arterial catheter (left upper extremity) are recommended for intraoperative and postoperative management. In patients with left ventricular dysfunction, a central venous catheter may be placed intraoperatively for pressure monitoring and inotropic support. The surgical approach is through a left thoracotomy, in which the aorta is cross-clamped and the coarctation repaired with an onlay prosthetic patch or a subclavian artery flap. Occasionally in older children, resection of the coarctation with an end-to-end anastomosis is performed. Once the aorta is cross-clamped, vasodilation with potent inhalational anesthesia is achieved to control the increased afterload. Intravascular volume loading with 20 mL/kg crystalloid is given just before removal of the clamp. The anesthetic concentration is then decreased, and the blood pressure is allowed to rise. Postrepair rebound hypertension is common because of heightened baroreceptor activity and often requires medical therapy. Intraoperatively, hypertension is best treated with β-blockade with esmolol or α-blockade or β-blockade with labetalol. Propranolol is useful in older patients, but it can cause severe bradycardia in infants and young children. Sodium nitroprusside does not appear to be useful, except in very high doses. Captopril or a combination of a β-blocker and hydralazine is begun in the convalescent stage of recovery in patients with persistent hypertension.

The placement of extracardiac shunts without CPB is managed like other shunt lesions, by balancing pulmonary and systemic blood flows by altering Pa_{CO_2}, Pa_{O_2}, and ventilatory dynamics, as discussed previously. Central shunts are usually performed through a median sternotomy, and Blalock-Taussig shunts may be performed through a left or right thoracotomy. For patients in whom pulmonary blood flow is critically low, partial cross-clamping of the pulmonary artery required for the distal anastomosis causes further reduction of pulmonary blood flow and desaturation. Pulse oximetry is helpful in monitoring the adequacy of pulmonary blood flow. Under rare circumstances, in which severe desaturation and bradycardia occur with cross-clamping, CPB is required for repair. Intraoperative complications include bleeding and severe systemic oxygen desaturation during chest closure, signifying shunt kicking. Pulmonary edema may result in the early postoperative period as a result of the creation of a large surgical shunt. Placing the patient on room air, increasing the Pa_{CO_2}, and adding positive end-expiratory pressure help to decrease pulmonary blood flow. Under such circumstances, early extubation is inadvisable.

Pulmonary artery banding is used to restrict pulmonary blood flow in infants who are deemed uncorrectable for either anatomic or physiologic reasons. These patients are generally in failure with reduced systemic perfusion and excessive pulmonary blood flow. The surgeon places a restrictive band across the main pulmonary artery to reduce flow. Band placement is very imprecise and requires careful assistance from the anesthesia team to accomplish successfully. Many approaches have been suggested. One approach is to place the patient on a 21% inspired oxygen concentration and to maintain the Pa_{CO_2} at 40 mm Hg to simulate the postoperative state. Observation of an elevation of systemic blood pressure by 10 mm Hg is suggestive of an appropriate band size. Pulmonary artery banding is also used for the management of transposition, in which the pulmonary artery is banded to increase left ventricle pressure in anticipation of an arterial switch procedure.

Blalock-Hanlon atrial septectomy is now an uncommon procedure for enlarging an intraatrial connection. This procedure is done by occluding caval flow and creating an intraatrial communication through the atrial septum. Balloon atrial septostomies (Rashkind procedure) and blade septectomies performed in the cardiac catheterization laboratory have almost replaced surgical intervention.

Procedures in the cardiac catheterization suite increasingly require general anesthesia. Commonly, cardiac catheterizations in uncooperative or mentally retarded children, prolonged electrophysiologic studies or pathway ablation procedures, interventional procedures for aortic or pulmonary stenosis, and coarctation or umbrella closures of an atrial septal defect or patent ductus arteriosus require anesthetic support. Problems in anesthetizing children in the cardiac catheterization laboratory include reduced access to the patient, a dark room necessitated by the need for fluoroscopy, and positioning that requires the patient's arms to be above the head for lateral fluoroscopy. Complications encountered in the cardiac laboratory include arrhythmias and heart block, hypercyanotic spells in patients at risk of right-to-left shunting, catheter-induced changes in blood flow patterns (e.g., aortic insufficiency, aortic stenosis, mitral regurgitation, and mitral stenosis), catheter-related accidents such as ventricular or atrial puncture, and dye-related myocardial depression in the patient with poor myocardial reserve. Resuscitative drugs and inotropic support must be available to aggressively treat these problems. The extent of monitoring should be chosen on the basis of the procedure and the child's cardiovascular status. Arterial line monitoring is indicated in patients with decreased myocardial reserve or with hemodynamically significant arrhythmias. Hemodynamic cardiac catheterizations require keeping the patient on room air and normocarbic to accurately measure intracardiac shunts and pulmonary artery pressures. Avoiding agents such as nitrous oxide when measuring pulmonary artery pressures is helpful, as it may increase pulmonary artery pressures.

ANESTHESIA FOR NONCARDIAC SURGERY

Improved survival and the ability to correct or palliate all forms of congenital heart defects have resulted in an ever-expanding population of adults and children with congenital heart lesions requiring anesthesia for noncardiac surgery. The greater anesthetic risks in these patients have recently been shown (136). The guiding principle is that true correction is rarely achieved. Except for atrial septal defect or patent ductus arteriosus closure, some residual abnormalities exist in almost all patients with congenital heart disease, no matter how early or how skillfully the initial repair is performed. These abnormalities may be a residual anatomic defect (abnormal valve, residual shunt), a residual physiologic problem (hypertension after coarctation repair, persistent ventricular dysfunction), or a complication of the surgical repair itself (heart block, ventricular dysfunction after mngfftriculotomy). Clearly, these problems need to be elucidated and anticipated before the child is taken to the operating room. A consultation with the pediatric cardiologist caring for the patient is the best source of this information. The anesthesiologist must be familiar with the anatomic defect, the anatomic repair or palliation, residual defects, and the anticipated physiologic response to anesthesia before considering anesthesia for these children. A careful and thoughtful perioperative approach based on the principles outlined previously is necessary. The type of monitoring depends on the severity of the child's illness and the hemodynamic derangements anticipated by the surgical procedure. In most cases, routine monitoring (e.g., ECG, noninvasive blood pressure cuff, precordial stethoscope, temperature, and pulse oximetry) is sufficient. In patients with residual defects, care must be taken to remove air bubbles from intravenous tubing to prevent paradoxical air emboli. Most patients will require subacute bacterial endocarditis prophylaxis.

In summary, the anesthetic management of children undergoing cardiac surgery requires a sound understanding of the basic principles of cardiovascular anesthesia. Knowledge of the pediatric patient, the variable pathophysiology of congenital heart disease, the surgical procedures, and special techniques such as DHCA are also essential for safe and effective anesthetic practice. Perioperative anesthetic care is necessary for the successful management of these patients. With the improvement in anesthetic drugs, the modes of delivering drugs, advanced monitoring techniques, and innovative surgical approaches, the quality of life and overall survival rates for patients with congenital heart disease should continue to improve.

REFERENCES

1. Turley K, Tucker WY, Ebert PA. The changing role of palliative procedures in the treatment of congenital heart disease. *J Thorac Cardiovasc Surg* 1980;79:194.
2. Castaneda AR, Mayer JEJ, Jonas RA, et al. The neonate with critical congenital heart disease: repair—a surgical challenge. *J Thorac Cardiovasc Surg* 1989;39.
3. Hickey PR, Hansen DD, Norwood WI. Anesthetic complications in surgery for congenital heart disease. *Anesth Analg* 1984; 63:657.
4. Rudolph AM. *Congenital diseases of the heart.* Chicago: Mosby–Year Book, 1974.
5. Legato MJ. Ultrastructural changes during normal growth in the dog and rat ventricular myofiber. In: Lieberman M, Sano T, eds. *Developmental and physiological correlates of cardiac muscle.* New York: Raven Press, 1975.
6. Teitel DF, Klautz R, Steendijk P, et al. The end-systolic pressure-volume relationship in the newborn lamb: effects of loading and inotropic interventions. *Pediatr Res* 1991;29:473.
7. Morselli PL, Franco-Morselli R, Bossi L. Clinical pharmacokinetics in newborns and infants. Age-related differences and therapeutic implications. *Clin Pharmacokinet* 1980;5:485.
8. Greeley WJ, de Bruijn NP. Changes in sufentanil pharmacokinetics within the neonatal period. *Anesth Analg* 1988;67:86.
9. Kirklin JK, Westaby S, Blackstone EH, et al. Complement and the damaging effects of cardiopulmonary bypass. *J Thorac Cardiovasc Surg* 1983;86:845.
10. Greeley W, Bushman G, Kong D, et al. Effects of cardiopulmonary bypass on eicosanoid metabolism during pediatric cardiovascular surgery. *J Thorac Cardiovasc Surg* 1988;95:842.
11. Berman W. The hemodynamics of shunts in congenital heart disease. In: Johansen KM, Burggren WW, eds. *Cardiovascular shunts: phylogenetic ontogenetic, and clinical aspects.* New York: Raven Press, 1985.
12. Engle MA, Perloff JK. *Congenital heart disease after surgery: benefits, residua, and sequelae.* New York: Yorke Medical Books, 1983.
13. Graham T. Ventricular performance in adults after operation for congenital heart disease. *Am J Cardiol* 1982;50:612.
14. Haworth SG. Normal pulmonary vascular development and its disturbance in congenital heart disease. In: Godman MJ, ed. *Paediatric cardiology,* vol 4. New York: Churchill Livingstone, 1981.
15. Arciniegas E. *Pediatric cardiac surgery.* Chicago: Mosby–Year Book, 1985.
16. Becu L, Somerville J, Gallo A. "Isolated" pulmonary valve stenosis as part of more widespread cardiovascular disease. *Br Heart J* 1976;38:472.
17. Newburger J, Silbert A, Buckley L, et al. Cognitive function and age at repair of transposition of the great arteries in children. *N Engl J Med* 1984;310:1495.
18. Castaneda AR, Trusler GA, Paul MA, et al. The early results of treatment of simple transposition in the current era. *J Thorac Cardiovasc Surg* 1988;95:14.
19. Pacifico AD, Sand ME, Bargeron LM, et al. Transatrialtranspulmonary repair of tetralogy of Fallot. *J Thorac Cardiovasc Surg* 1987;93:919.
20. Barratt-Boyes BG, Simpson MM, Neutze JM. Intracardiac surgery in neonates and infants using deep hypothermia. *Circulation* 1980;62:73.
21. Rashkind WJ. Historical aspects of surgery for congenital heart disease. *J Thorac Cardiovasc Surg* 1982;84:619.
22. Richardson JP, Clark CP. Tetralogy of Fallot. Risk factors associated with complete repair. *Br Heart J* 1976;38:926.
23. Laishley KS, O'Callaghan AS, Lerman J. Effects of dose and concentration of rectal methohexitone for induction of anaesthesia in children. *Can Anaesth Soc J* 1986;33:427.
24. Stern DH, Gerson J, Allen FB. Can we trust the direct radial artery pressure immediately following cardiopulmonary bypass? *Anesthesiology* 1985;62:557.
25. Jobes JR, Nicolson SC. Monitoring of arterial hemoglobin oxygen saturation using a tongue sensor. *Anesth Analg* 1988;67: 186.
26. Gussenhoven EJ, van Herwerden LA, Roelandt J, et al. Intraoperative two-dimensional echocardiography in congenital heart disease. *J Am Coll Cardiol* 1987;9:565.
27. Hagler DJ, Tajik AJ, Seward JB, et al. Intraoperative two-dimensional Doppler echocardiography. A preliminary study for congenital heart disease. *J Thorac Cardiovasc Surg* 1988;95:516.
28. Ungerleider RM, Kisslo JA, Greeley WJ, et al. Intraoperative prebypass and postbypass epicardial color flow imaging in the repair of atrioventricular septal defects. *J Thorac Cardiovasc Surg* 1989;98:90.
29. Ritter SB, Thys DM. Pediatric transesophageal color flow imaging: smaller probes for smaller hearts. *Echocardiography* 1989; 6:431.
30. Muhiudeen IA, Roberson DA, Silverman NH, et al. Intraoperative echocardiography in infants and children with congenital cardiac shunt lesions: transesophageal versus epicardial echocardiography. *J Am Coll Cardiol* 1990;16:1687.
31. Murray D, Vandewalker G, Matherne P, et al. Pulsed Doppler and two-dimensional echocardiography: comparison of halothane and isoflurane on cardiac function in infants and small children. *Anesthesiology* 1987;67:211.

32. Greeley WJ, Kern FH, Ungerleider RM, et al. Intramyocardial air causes right ventricular dysfunction after repair of a congenital heart defect. *Anesthesiology* 1990;73:1042.
33. Murkin JM, Farrar JK, Tweed WA, et al. Cerebral autoregulation and flow/metabolism coupling during cardiopulmonary bypass: the influence of $Paco_2$. *Anesth Analg* 1987;66:825.
34. Greeley W, Stanley T, Ungerleider R, et al. Intraoperative hypoxemic spells in tetralogy of Fallot: an echocardiographic analysis of diagnosis and treatment. *Anesth Analg* 1989;68:815.
35. Hickey PR, Wessel DL. Anesthesia for treatment of congenital heart disease. In: Kaplan JA, eds. *Cardiac anesthesia.* Miami, FL: Grune & Stratton, 1987.
36. Lindegaard KF, Lundar T, Wiberg J, et al. Variations in middle cerebral artery blood flow investigated with noninvasive transcranial blood velocity measurements. *Stroke* 1987;18:1025.
37. van der Linden J, Wesslén O, Ekroth R, et al. Transcranial Doppler-estimated versus thermodilution-estimated cerebral blood flow during cardiac operations. *J Thorac Cardiovasc Surg* 1991;102:95.
38. Lundar T, Lindberg H, Lindegaard KF, et al. Cerebral perfusion during major cardiac surgery in children. *Pediatr Cardiol* 1987; 8:161.
39. Hillier S, Burrows F, Bissonnette B, et al. Cerebral hemodynamics in neonates and infants undergoing cardiopulmonary bypass and profound hypothermic circulatory arrest: assessment by transcranial Doppler sonography. *Anesth Analg* 1991;72:723.
40. Greeley WJ, Ungerleider RM, Smith LR, et al. The effects of deep hypothermic cardiopulmonary bypass and total circulatory arrest on cerebral blood flow in infants and children. *J Thorac Cardiovasc Surg* 1989;97:737.
41. Laishley RS, Burrows FA, Lerman J, et al. Effects of anesthetic induction on oxygen saturation in cyanotic congenital heart disease. *Anesthesiology* 1986;65:673.
42. Greeley WJ, Bushman G, Davis DP, et al. Comparative effects of halothane and ketamine on systemic arterial oxygen saturation in children with cyanotic heart disease. *Anesthesiology* 1986; 65:666.
43. Friesen RH, Lichtor JL. Cardiovascular effects of inhalational induction with isoflurane in infants. *Anesth Analg* 1983;62:411.
44. Hickey PR, Hansen DD, Wessel DL, et al. Pulmonary and systemic hemodynamic responses to fentanyl in infants. *Anesth Analg* 1985;64:483.
45. Hickey PR, Hansen DD. Fentanyl- and sufentanil-oxygenpancuronium anesthesia for cardiac surgery in infants. *Anesth Analg* 1984;63:117.
46. Hickey PR, Hansen DD, Wessel DL, et al. Blunting of stress responses in the pulmonary circulation of infants by fentanyl. *Anesth Analg* 1985;64:1137.
47. Moore RA, Yang SS, McNicholas KW, et al. Hemodynamic and anesthetic effects of sufentanil as the sole anesthetic for pediatric cardiovascular surgery. *Anesthesiology* 1985;63:725.
48. Kern FH, Ungerleider RM, Jacobs JR, et al. Computerized continuous infusion of intravenous anesthetic drugs during pediatric cardiac surgery. *Anesth Analg* 1991;72:487.
49. Besunder JB, Reed MD, Blumer JL. Principles of drug biodisposition in the neonate. A critical evaluation of the pharmacokinetic-pharmacodynamic interface (part I). *Clin Pharmacokinet* 1988;14:189.
50. Greeley W, de Bruijn N, Davis D. Sufentanil pharmacokinetics in pediatric cardiovascular patients. *Anesth Analg* 1987;66:1067.
51. Davis PJ, Cook DR, Stiller RL, et al. Pharmacodynamics and pharmacokinetics of high-dose sufentanil in infants and children undergoing cardiac surgery. *Anesth Analg* 1987;66:203.
52. Bull BSJ, Korpman RA, Huse M, et al. Heparin therapy during extracorporeal circulation. I. Problems inherent in existing heparin protocols. II. The use of a dose response curve to individualize heparin and protamine dosage. *J Thorac Cardiovasc Surg* 1975;69:674.
53. Young JA, Kisker CT, Doty DB. Adequate anticoagulation during cardiopulmonary bypass determined by activated clotting time and the appearance of fibrin monomer. *Ann Thorac Surg* 1978;26:321.
54. Greeley WJ, Kern FH. Anesthesia for pediatric cardiac surgery. In: Miller RD, ed. *Anesthesia.* New York: Churchill Livingstone, 1990.
55. Bellinger D, Wernovsky G, Rappaport L, et al. Rapid cooling of infants on cardiopulmonary bypass adversely affects later cognitive function. *Circulation* 1988;78:A358.
56. Kern FH, Ungerleider RM, Quill TJ, et al. Cerebral blood flow response to changes in arterial carbon dioxide tension during hypothermic cardiopulmonary bypass in children. *J Thorac Cardiovasc Surg* 1991;101:618.
57. Field J, Fuhrman F, Martin A. Effect of temperature on the oxygen consumption of brain tissue. *J Neurophysiol* 1944;7:117.
58. Bigelow W, Callaghan J, Hopps J. General hypothermia for experimental intracardiac surgery. *Ann Surg* 1950;132:531.
59. Greeley WJ. Con: deep hypothermic circulatory arrest must be used selectively and discretely. *J Cardiothorac Vasc Surg* 1991; 5:638.
60. Kirklin JW, Barratt-Boyes BG, eds. *Cardiac surgery.* New York: John Wiley and Sons, 1986.
61. Greeley WJ, Kern FH, Ungerleider RM, et al. The effect of hypothermic cardiopulmonary bypass and total circulatory arrest on cerebral metabolism in neonates, infants, and children. *J Thorac Cardiovasc Surg* 1991;101:783.
62. Busto R, Dietrich WD, Globus MY, et al. Small differences in the intra-ischemic brain temperature critically determine the extent of ischemic neuronal injury. *J Cereb Blood Flow Metab* 1987;7:729.
63. Okada Y, Tanimoto M, Yoneda K. The protective effect of hypothermia on reversibility in the neuronal function of the hippocampal slice during long-lasting anoxia. *Neurosci Lett* 1988;84:277.
64. Hansen N, Brubakk A, Bratlid D, et al. The effects of variations in $Paco_2$ on brain blood flow and cardiac output in the newborn piglet. *Pediatr Res* 1984;18:1132.
65. Dickinson D, Sambrooks J. Intellectual performance in children after circulatory arrest with profound hypothermia in infancy. *Arch Dis Child* 1979;54:1.
66. Clarkson P, Barton M, MacArthur A, et al. Developmental progress after cardiac surgery in infancy using hypothermia and circulatory arrest. *Circulation* 1980;62:855.
67. Wells F, Coghill S, Caplan H, et al. Duration of circulatory arrest does influence the psychological development of children after cardiac operation in early life. *J Thorac Cardiovasc Surg* 1983;86:823.
68. Wright J, Hicks R, Newman DC. Deep hypothermic arrest: observation on later development in children. *J Thorac Cardiovasc Surg* 1979;86:466.
69. Blackwood M, Hakalkse K, Steward D. Developmental outcome in children undergoing surgery with profound hypothermia. *Anesthesiology* 1986;65:437.
70. Ferry PC. Impairment of cerebral function following cardiac and other major surgery. *Eur J Cardiothorac Surg* 1989;3:216.
71. Ferry PC. Neurologic sequelae of open-heart surgery in children. An "irritating question." *Am J Dis Child* 1990;144:369.
72. Norwood WI, Norwood CR, Castaneda AR. Factors influencing survival and successful weaning from clinical ventricular bypass with local heparinization and blood filtration: an analysis in 21 consecutive patients. *Trans Am Soc Artif Intern Organs* 1979;25:176.

73. Norwood W, Norwood C, Castaneda AR. Cerebral anoxia: effect of deep hypothermia and pH. *Surgery* 1979;86:203.
74. Treasure T, Naftel D, Conger K, et al. The effect of hypothermic circulatory arrest time on cerebral function, morphology, and chemistry: an experimental study. *J Thorac Cardiovasc Surg* 1983;86:761.
75. Newburger JW, Jonas RA, Wernovsky G, et al. A comparison of the perioperative neurologic effects of hypothermic circulatory arrest versus low-flow cardiopulmonary bypass in infant heart surgery. *N Engl J Med* 1993;329:1057.
76. Bellinger DC, Jonas RA, Rappaport LA, et al. Developmental and neurologic status of children after heart surgery with hypothermic circulatory arrest or low-flow cardiopulmonary bypass. *N Engl J Med* 1995;332:549.
77. Bellinger DC, Rappaport LA, Wypij D, et al. Patterns of developmental dysfunction after surgery in infancy to correct transposition of the great arteries. *J Dev Behav Pediatr* 1997;18:75.
78. Wernovsky G, Wypij D, Jonas RA, et al. Postoperative course and hemodynamic profile after the arterial switch operation in neonates and infants: a comparison of low-flow cardiopulmonary bypass versus circulatory arrest. *Circulation* 2995;92:2226.
79. Jonas RA, Bellinger DC, Rappaport LA, et al. Relation of pH strategy and developmental outcome after hypothermic circulatory arrest. *J Thorac Cardiovasc Surg* 1993;106:362.
80. du Plessis AJ. Neurologic complications of cardiac disease in the newborn. *Clin Perinatol* 1997;24(4):807.
81. Kawata H, Flackler JK, Aoki M, et al. Recovery of cerebral blood flow and energy state after hypothermic circulatory arrest versus low flow bypass in piglets. *J Thorac Cardiovasc Surg* 1993; 102:671.
82. Kurth CD, O'Rourke MM, O'Hara IB, et al. Brain cooling efficiency with pH-stat and alpha-stat cardiopulmonary bypass in newborn pigs. *Circulation* 1997;96[Suppl 9]:II358.
83. O'Rourke MM, Nork KM, Kurth CD. Altered brain oxygen extraction with hypoxia and hypotension following deep hypothermic circulatory arrest. *Acta Neurochirurg* 1997;70:78.
84. Kurth CD, O'Rourke MM, O'Hara IB. Comparison of pH-stat and alpha-stat cardiopulmonary bypass on cerebral oxygenation and blood flow in relation to hypothermic circulatory arrest in piglets. *Anesthesiology* 1998;89(1):110.
85. Greeley WJ, Ungerleider RM. Assessing the effect of cardiopulmonary bypass on the brain. *Ann Thorac Surg* 1991;52:417.
86. Gold JP, Jonas RA, Lang P, et al. Transthoracic intracardiac monitoring lines in pediatric surgical patients: a ten year experience. *Ann Thorac Surg* 1986;42:185.
87. Ungerleider RM, Greeley WJ, Kisslo J. Intraoperative echocardiography in congenital heart disease surgery: preliminary report on a current study. *Am J Cardiol* 1989;63:3F.
88. Ungerleider RM, Greeley WJ, Sheikh KH, et al. Routine use of intraoperative epicardial echocardiography and Doppler color flow imaging to guide and evaluate repair of congenital heart lesions. A prospective study. *J Thorac Cardiovasc Surg* 1990; 100:297.
89. Bohn DJ, Poirer CS, Edmonds JF. Efficacy of dopamine, dobutamine, and epinephrine during emergence from cardiopulmonary bypass in children. *Crit Care Med* 1980;8:367.
90. Hines R, Barash PG. Right ventricular failure. In: Kaplan JA, ed. *Cardiac anesthesia,* vol 2. New York: Grune & Stratton, 1987.
91. Lawless S, Burckart G, Diven W. Amrinone pharmacokinetics in neonates and infants. *J Clin Pharmacol* 1988;28:283.
92. Mansell A, Bryan C, Levinson H. Airway closure in children. *J Appl Physiol* 1972;33:711.
93. Zapletal A, Paul T, Samenek M. Pulmonary elasticity in children and adolescents. *J Appl Physiol* 1976;40:953.
94. Hammond JW, Wolfe WG, Moran JF, et al. The effect of positive end expiratory pressure on regional ventilation and perfusion in the normal and injured primate lung. *J Thorac Cardiovasc Surg* 1976;72:680.
95. Jenkins J, Lynn A, Edmonds J, et al. Effects of mechanical ventilation on cardiopulmonary function in children after open-heart surgery. *Crit Care Med* 1985;13:77.
96. Benotti JR, Grossman W, Braunwald E. Effects of amrinone on myocardial energy metabolism and hemodynamics in patients with severe congestive heart failure due to coronary disease. *Circulation* 1980;62:28.
97. Rich R, Ganz R, Levy P. Hemodynamic effects of hydralazine, nifedipine and amrinone in primary pulmonary hypertension. *Am J Cardiol* 1983;52:1104.
98. Konstam MA, Cohen SR, Salem DN. Effect of amrinone on right ventricular function: predominance of afterload reduction. *Circulation* 1986;74:359.
99. Konstam MA, Cohen SR, Weiland D. Relative contribution of inotropic and vasodilator effects of amrinone-induced hemodynamic improvement in congestive heart failure. *Am J Cardiol* 1986;57:242.
100. Hess W, Arnold B, Veit S. The hemodynamic effects of amrinone in patients with mitral stenosis and pulmonary hypertension. *Eur Heart J* 1986;7:800.
101. Wessel DL, Triedman JK, Wernovsky G. Pulmonary and systemic hemodynamics of amrinone in neonates following cardiopulmonary bypass. *Circulation* 1989;[Suppl 2]:II488.
102. Schwartz RL, Garrett JR, Karp RB, et al. Experience with profound hypothermia and circulatory arrest in the treatment of aneurysms of the aortic arch. Aortic arch replacement for acute arch dissections. *J Thorac Cardiovasc Surg* 1982;84:649.
103. Molloy DW. Effects of noradrenaline and isoproterenol on cardiopulmonary function in a canine model of acute pulmonary hypertension. *Chest* 1985;88:432.
104. Heymann MA, Hoffman JIE. In: Weir EK, Reeves JT, eds. *Pulmonary hypertension.* 1984.
105. D'Ambra M, LaRaia P, Phellan D. A new therapy for refractory right heart failure and pulmonary hypertension after mitral valve replacement. *J Thorac Cardiovasc Surg* 1985;89:567.
106. Drummond WH, Gregory GA, Heymann MA, et al. The independent effects of hyperventilation, tolazoline and dopamine on infants with persistent pulmonary hypertension. *J Pediatr* 1981;98:603.
107. Nakik SK, Knight A, Elliott MA. A successful modification of ultrafiltration for cardiopulmonary bypass in children. *Perfusion* 1991;6:41.
108. Naik SK, Knight A, Elliott MJ. A prospective randomized study of a modified technique of ultrafiltration during pediatric open-heart surgery. *Circulation* 1991;84[Suppl III]:422.
109. Elliott JJ. Ultrafiltration and modified ultrafiltration in pediatric open-heart operations. *Ann Thorac Surg* 1993;56(6):1518.
110. Ungerleider RM. Effects of cardiopulmonary bypass and use of modified ultrafiltration. *Ann Thorac Surg* 1998;65:S35.
111. Darling E, Nanry K, Shearer I, et al. Techniques of paediatric modified ultrafiltration: 1996 survey results. *Perfusion* 1998; 13(2):93.
112. Journois D, Pouard P, Greeley WJ, et al. Hemofiltration during cardiopulmonary bypass in pediatric cardiac surgery. *Anesthesiology* 1994;81:1181.
113. Wang MJ, Chiu IS, Hsu CM, et al. Efficacy of ultrafiltration in removing inflammatory mediators during pediatric cardiac operations. *Ann Thorac Surg* 1996;61(2):651.
114. Friesen RH, Campbell DN, Clarke DR, et al. Modified ultrafiltration attenuates dilutional coagulopathy in pediatric open-heart operation. *Ann Thorac Surg* 1997;65(6):1787.
115. Davies MJ, Nguyen K, Gaynor JW, et al. Modified ultrafiltra-

tion improves left ventricular systolic function in infants after cardiopulmonary bypass. *J Thorac Cardiovasc Surg* 1998;115(2):361.

116. Skaryak LA, Kirshbom PM, DiBernardo LR, et al. Modified ultrafiltration improves cerebral metabolic recovery after circulatory arrest. *J Thorac Cardiovasc Surg* 1995;109(4):744.
117. Koutlas TC, Gaynor JW, Nicolson SC, et al. Modified ultrafiltration reduces postoperative morbidity after cavopulmonary connection. *Ann Thorac Surg* 1997;64:37.
118. Daggett CW, Lodge AJ, Scarborough JE, et al. Modified ultrafiltration versus conventional ultrafiltration: a randomized prospective study in neonatal piglets. *J Thorac Cardiovasc Surg* 1998;115(2):336.
119. Pollock JC, Charlton MD, Williams WG, et al. Intraaortic balloon pumping in children. *Ann Thorac Surg* 1980;29:522.
120. Fukumasu F, Blaylock R, Veasy LG. Intra-aortic balloon pumping device for infants. *Clin Cardiol* 1979;2:348.
121. Hill JD, O'Brien TG, Murray JJ. Extracorporeal oxygenation for acute post-traumatic respiratory failure (shock-lung syndrome): use of the Bramson membrane lung. *N Engl J Med* 1972;286:629.
122. Bartlett RH, Gazzaniga AB, Fong SW, et al. Prolonged extracorporeal support in man. *J Thorac Cardiovasc Surg* 1974;68:918.
123. Pyle RB, Helton WC, Johnson FW. Clinical use of the membrane oxygenator. *Arch Surg* 1975;110:966.
124. Zapol WM, Snider MT, Hill JD. Extracorporeal membrane oxygenation in severe respiratory failure: a randomized prospective study. *JAMA* 1979;242:2193.
125. Bartlett RH, Andrews AF, Toomasian JM. Extracorporeal membrane oxygenation for newborn respiratory failure: 45 cases. *Surgery* 1982;92:425.
126. Bartlett RH, Roloff DW, Cornell RG. Extracorporeal circulation in neonatal respiratory failure: a prospective randomized study. *Pediatrics* 1985;76:479.
127. Toomasian JM, Snedecor SM, Cornell RG, et al. National experience with extracorporeal membrane oxygenation for newborn respiratory failure: data from 715 cases. *ASAIO Trans* 1988;34:140.
128. Gille JP, Bagniewski AM. Ten years of use of extracorporeal membrane oxygenation (ECMO) in the treatment of acute respiratory insufficiency. *ASAIO Trans* 1976;22:102.
129. Kanter KR, Pennington G, Weber TR, et al. Extracorporeal membrane oxygenation for postoperative cardiac support in children. *J Thorac Cardiovasc Surg* 1987;93:27.
130. Weinhaus L, Canter C, Noetzel M, et al. Extracorporeal membrane oxygenation for circulatory support after repair of congenital heart defects. *Ann Thorac Surg* 1989;48:206.
131. Magovern GJ, Park SB, Maher TD. Use of the centrifugal pump without anticoagulants for postoperative left ventricular assist. *World J Surg* 1985;9:25.
132. Miller CA, Pae WE, Pierce WS. Combined registry for the clinical use of mechanical ventricular assist devices, postcardiotomy cardiogenic shock. *ASAIO Trans* 1990;36:43.
133. Golding LAR. Postcardiotomy mechanical support. *Semin Thorac Cardiovasc Surg* 1991;3:29.
134. Manno CS, Hedberg KW, Kim HC, et al. Comparison of the hemostatic effects of fresh whole blood, stored whole blood, and components after open heart surgery in children. *Blood* 1991;77:930.
135. Strafford MA, Henderson KH. Anesthetic morbidity in congenital heart disease patients undergoing noncardiac surgery. *Anesthesiology* 1991;75:A1056.

Cardiac Anesthesia: Principles and Clinical Practice, Second Edition, edited by Fawzy G. Estafanous, Paul G. Barash, and J.G. Reves. Lippincott Williams & Wilkins, Philadelphia © 2001.

22

SURGICAL AND DEVICE THERAPY FOR CARDIAC ARRHYTHMIAS

LYNDA E. ROSENFELD
JOHN A. ELEFTERIADES

The inadequacy of pharmacologic therapy for the treatment of arrhythmias and the development of surgical procedures and devices to manage both bradyarrhythmias and tachyarrhythmias made the operating room a common venue for the treatment or cure of electrophysiologic problems during the 1980s and early 1990s. Since that time, the advent of catheter-based radiofrequency techniques and the simplification of device implantation has moved many of these procedures to the electrophysiology laboratory. However, anesthesia involvement continues to be important, not only in these procedures but also in newer operative techniques to treat arrhythmias and when these often complex patients undergo other, nonelectrical surgery. This chapter reviews the various operations and devices used to treat bradyarrhythmias and tachyarrhythmias and provides some perspective of their history.

PACEMAKER THERAPY

The initial use of an electrical pacemaker to stimulate a nonbeating human heart has been attributed to an Australian anesthesiologist, Mark C. Lidwill, who used a plunge electrode in the ventricle and an external electrical power source to resuscitate a stillborn infant sometime before 1929 (1). It was not until more than 20 years later that Zoll developed the concept of transcutaneously pacing the heart using a totally external system (2). Although initially abandoned as too painful for chronic use, such systems have recently had a resurgence, being used in emergency situations and in the operating room for backup support during permanent pacemaker implantation or generator changes in patients who are pacemaker dependent or patients with left bundle-branch block who require placement of a pulmonary artery catheter (3).

A totally indwelling system, consisting of an epicardial lead and an implanted generator, was first used by Senning in 1958 (4). By 1961, Furman et al. (5) had reported the use of a transvenous endocardial lead system, and the modern age of pacemaker therapy began.

Today, pacemaker systems are of six types: four temporary and two permanent; they are as follows:

1. Temporary transvenous pacing. A transvenous pacing wire is inserted percutaneously, usually via the internal jugular or the subclavian veins but also via the femoral or brachial veins, and is connected to an external pacing device. Ventricular pacing, accomplished by seating the pacing wire in the trabeculae at the right ventricular apex, is usually quite reliable. Atrial or dual-chamber pacing can be achieved using specially designed atrial pacing wires or by placing a catheter in the coronary sinus, but these configurations have generally been less reliable. Recently, active fixation temporary pacing leads have become available and may make atrioventricular (AV) synchrony more achievable on an emergency basis. Temporary transvenous pacing wires can be inserted under electrocardiographic (ECG) or fluoroscopic guidance.
2. Temporary epicardial pacing. Epicardial pacing wires may be sutured to the surface of the heart during cardiac surgery. These wires, which are externalized, are designed to be detached with traction and are removed before hospital discharge. Temporary atrial and ventricular epicardial wires are very useful in the early postoperative period, facilitating rhythm diagnosis and atrial, ventricular, or dual-chamber pacing as needed. Overdrive atrial pacing using temporary epicardial wires has proven to be an excellent treatment for postoperative atrial flutter (6).
3. Temporary transcutaneous pacing. Such pacing has proven to be life-sustaining when used as a bridge to

L. E. Rosenfeld: Department of Internal Medicine and Pediatrics, Yale University School of Medicine; and Cardiac Electrophysiology Laboratory, Yale-New Haven Hospital, New Haven, Connecticut 06510

J. A. Elefteriades: Department of Cardiovascular Surgery, Yale University School of Medicine; and Department of Cardiothoracic Surgery, Yale-New Haven Hospital, New Haven, Connecticut 06510 more reliable and less painful forms of temporary pacing during emergency situations. It has also served as a backup system for patients felt to be at high risk for symptomatic bradyarrhythmias. Large adhesive electrodes are applied to the chest and back and are connected to a generator that can provide high-output impulses, often more than 100 mA. Discomfort is related to the cutaneous application of current and the associated stimulation of muscle contraction.

4. Temporary transesophageal pacing. The esophagus lies just behind the left atrium, so placing a flexible electrode in the esophagus can facilitate the diagnosis of arrhythmias and permit atrial pacing (7). It is usually not feasible to pace the ventricle from this location. This technique has found particular application in the pediatric population, in which atrial arrhythmias predominate and transvenous catheter placement may be problematic.
5. Permanent epicardial pacing. Although the initial permanent pacing systems used epicardial leads, pacing thresholds are generally higher and lead longevity and reliability are less than with transvenous systems. Therefore, today such systems are usually used primarily in very small infants (8), in situations such as tricuspid atresia where transvenous access to the right ventricle is not possible or desirable (9), when pacing systems are implanted at the time of other cardiac surgery, or in the setting of recurrent infection when an extravascular pacing system is desirable.
6. Permanent transvenous pacing. Because of the excellent pacing thresholds obtained with transvenous leads and their long-term reliability, this is the preferred method of permanent pacemaker implantation today. Generally, the subclavian or cephalic veins are used for access, but the internal jugular, axillary, and rarely the femoral veins have been used.

Although ventricular pacing, which is insensitive to native beats, is all that is necessary to maintain life, improved lead technology, which has made stable atrial and nonapical ventricular leads a reality, as well as the development of sophisticated generators have made possible a wide selection of pacing system options. Pacemakers have also been used to recognize and terminate tachyarrhythmias (10–13). More recently, antitachycardia pacing has been an important component of complex devices that also provide bradycardia pacing, cardioversion, and defibrillation (14,15). The ability to program implanted pacemakers transcutaneously using an external device has greatly reduced the need for surgical revision of pacing systems and has permitted the modification of pacing characteristics to meet changing needs of patients (16). Although the increasing complexity and flexibility of pacemakers has been a great boon to patients, it has led to confusion. In an attempt to improve communication and understanding, the Intersociety Commission of Heart Disease (ICHD) Resources published a code for pacemaker identification in 1974, which was revised in 1981 (17).

The ICHD code uses five letters to describe pacemaker capabilities (Table 22-1), which are usually shortened to a three-letter code, and if indicated, the letter R is added to denote responsiveness to a sensor, most commonly a piezoelectric ceramic crystal sensitive to motion. The first letter in the code denotes the chamber paced: A, atrium; V, ventricle; or D, dual, or both atrium and ventricle. Next is the chamber sensed: A, V, D, or O (neither chamber). The third letter indicates the mode of pacemaker response: I, or inhibited by intrinsic output from the sensed chamber(s); T, triggered to fire by output from the sensed chamber(s); D, triggered to fire from the ventricle by atrial output but inhibited by ventricular output; O, "blind" to intrinsic output from the sensed chamber. R, which indicates "reverse" functions, is applicable to antitachycardia pacemakers and indicates that the pacemaker is silent at slow intrinsic heart rates but fires for fast rates. The fourth code letter indicates whether the pacemaker is not programmable (O); program-

TABLE 22-1. FIVE POSITION PACEMAKER CODE (ICHD)

Position	I	II	III	IV	V
Category	Chamber(s) paced	Chamber(s) sensed	Mode of response(s)	Programmable functions	Special tachyarrhythmia functions
Letters used	V- Ventricle	V- Ventricle	T- Triggered	P- Programmable (rate and/or output)	B- Bursts
	A- Atrium	A- Atrium	I- Inhibited	M- Multiprogrammable	N- Normal rate competition
	D- Double	D- Double	D- Double[a]		S- Scanning
			O- None		
		O- None	R- Reverse	O- None	E- External
Manufacturer's designation only	S- Single chamber	S- Single chamber			

[a] Atrial triggered and ventricular inhibited.
Source: From Parsonnet V, Furman S, Smyth NPD. A revised code for pacemaker identification. *PACE* 1981;4:400, with permission.

mable only for rate and/or output (P); or multiprogrammable (M) for a variety of parameters. The last letter in the code applies to antitachycardia functions: O, no antitachycardia features; B, able to deliver bursts of impulses; N, normal rate competition seen in "dual-demand" pacemakers; S, able to deliver timed extrasystoles; and E, the antitachycardia functions are externally controlled by application of a magnet or a radiofrequency signal.

Using the ICHD code, a variety of pacing modalities can be described. These include the following:

AOO or VOO. The first implanted pacemakers took this form. These single-chamber devices continuously pace at their programmed rate, regardless of any intrinsic rhythm. Thus, pacemaker output can fall within the vulnerable period of the atrium or ventricle, theoretically placing the patient at risk for atrial or ventricular tachycardia or fibrillation, depending on the chamber paced. For this reason, although these modes, as well as DOO pacing, are used on a temporary basis and may be useful in the operating room when cautery is in use, they are usually not employed chronically at this time.

AAT or VVT. These single-chamber devices were developed in an attempt to deal with the risks of asynchronous (AOO or VOO) pacing. They sense intrinsic activity and are triggered to fire by native output—during the P wave or QRS complex—at a time when the atrium/ventricle will be refractory and unresponsive, eliminating the risk of firing during the vulnerable period. They will also fire if no intrinsic output occurs from the sensed chamber during a preset period, preventing bradycardia.

AAI or VVI. These single-chamber devices are inhibited by output from their sensed chamber and fire if no intrinsic output occurs during a preset interval. AAI pacemakers can be used in patients with sinus node dysfunction and intact AV conduction, but they are not commonly implanted in the United States because of concern that concomitant AV block may develop. VVI pacing requires the placement of only one lead, and it is useful when only rare backup pacing is required or when the patient is in atrial fibrillation. AAI or VVI pacemakers that incorporate a sensor permit heart rate responsiveness to either activity or a change in a measured physiologic parameter.

Patients who are in sinus rhythm and have intact ventriculoatrial conduction can "entrain" their atria during ventricular pacing. This results in the perpetuation of pacing and the continued loss of AV synchrony. Adverse hemodynamic effects can result not only from the loss of the atrial contribution to ventricular systole but also from baroreceptor-mediated reflex peripheral vasodilation (18,19), producing "pacemaker syndrome." In some patients, units with programmable hysteresis, requiring a longer time to elapse before the first paced beat but then pacing at a faster rate, have reduced the amount of pacing and have ameliorated this problem. In other patients, dual-chamber pacing to maintain AV synchrony has been necessary.

Although VVI pacing may be adequate to prevent life-threatening bradycardia, there is increasing evidence that atrial (in patients with only sinus node dysfunction) or DDD pacing is associated with a better overall prognosis and a reduced incidence of atrial fibrillation (20–23).

VDD. These devices incorporate an atrial sensing electrode in the proximal portion of a ventricular lead. Thus, they provide rate responsiveness and maintain AV synchrony over a wide range of heart rates. Although they preserve the simplicity of a single-lead system, they cannot pace the atrium, and at lower rates, they revert to VVI pacing. VDD pacemakers are optimally employed in patients with intact sinus node function and AV block.

DVI. These pacemakers preceded DDD pacemakers. They pace both chambers, but because they pace the atrium asynchronously, they may produce atrial fibrillation. They do prevent pacemaker-mediated tachycardia however (24,25). DVI and more commonly DDI (which senses but does not track the atrium) pacing has been used by the newest DDD pacemakers at the time of "mode switching" when an atrial tachyarrhythmia is recognized. This prevents high ventricular rates due to tracking of the atrial tachycardia or fibrillation by the pacemaker and permits greater flexibility in programming.

DDD. In the 1993 Survey of Pacing in the United States, the most commonly used pacing modes were DDD and DDDR, representing more than 63% of implants and replacing VVI pacing, which was the most commonly used mode in a similar 1989 survey (26). Initial experience with these devices, which pace and sense both the atrium and the ventricle, was complicated by instability of the atrial lead and the development of pacemaker-mediated or endless loop tachycardias (24,25,27–30). New, steroid-eluting active fixation atrial leads and programming modifications have obviated these problems in most patients. DDDR programming has restored chronotropic responsiveness to patients with sinus node dysfunction and has been particularly useful in active children and young adults.

Beginning in 1984, and most recently in 1998 (31), guidelines for permanent cardiac pacemaker implantation were issued by the Joint Task Force on Practice Guidelines (Committee on Pacemaker Implantation) of the American College of Cardiology and the American Heart Association. Indications for pacemaker implantation have been classified as class I, indicating general agreement that a permanent pacemaker should be implanted; class II, situations in which such devices are frequently implanted but opinions diverge; and class III, situations in which there is general agreement that pacemakers are not indicated. A number of situations for bradycardia pacing were examined, and it is useful to view them in the context of the 1993 Survey of Pacing in the United States (26), which found that more than 52% of primary pacemaker implants were for sinus node dysfunction, 33% for abnormalities of AV conduction, 5% for drug-induced bradycardia, and 3% for tachyarrhythmias. A brief review of the Task Force's class I and II guidelines follows.

1. AV block associated with myocardial infarction. In this situation, indications for permanent pacing may be based on prognosis, rather than specific symptoms. The need for temporary pacing during an acute myocardial infarction does not always mandate permanent pacing. Definite indications for pacing include persistent symptomatic advanced second-degree heart block or complete heart block, with block in the distal conduction system; and transient advanced infranodal block associated with bundle-branch block. Although the presence of persistent symptomatic advanced block at the level of the AV node, seen most often in patients with inferior myocardial infarctions, is a class I indication, asymptomatic persistent advanced AV block is a less clear-cut (class II) indication.
2. Acquired AV block in adults. Absolute indications for pacing include complete heart block at the level of either the AV node or the distal conduction system, whether it is chronic or intermittent, if associated with symptoms due to bradycardia; arrhythmias or other conditions that require treatment with drugs that produce symptomatic bradycardia; documented asystole lasting at least 3 seconds or escape rates of less than 40 beats/minute in awake asymptomatic patients; AV nodal ablation; postoperative AV block not expected to recover; and muscular diseases such as myotonic muscular dystrophy, Kearns-Sayre syndrome, Erb's limb-girdle dystrophy, and peroneal muscular atrophy. The presence of second-degree AV block at any level, either chronic or intermittent, if associated with symptoms is also considered a class I indication for placement of a permanent pacemaker. Acceptable but not universally agreed-upon indications include asymptomatic permanent or intermittent complete heart block at any level with a ventricular response of 40 beats/minute or more; asymptomatic type 2 second-degree AV block identified incidentally at an electrophysiology study done for other reasons; first-degree AV block with symptoms of pacemaker syndrome, alleviated by temporary pacing; and marked first-degree AV block (more than 300 milliseconds) in the setting of left ventricular dysfunction and symptoms of congestive heart failure.
3. Chronic bifascicular and trifascicular block. Class I indications include bifascicular block associated with intermittent complete heart block or type II second-degree AV block. Syncope without other causes occurring in the presence of bifascicular or trifascicular block without documented complete heart block is a class II indication, as is an HV interval measured to be 100 milliseconds or longer, and nonphysiologic pacing-induced infra-His block.
4. Sinus node dysfunction. There is general agreement that if associated with symptomatic bradycardia, even in the presence of necessary drugs, documented sinus node dysfunction is an indication for permanent pacemaker placement. Similarly, evidence of chronotropic incompetence is a class I indication for pacing. Sinus node dysfunction with heart rates of less than 40 beats/minute in situations in which an association between bradycardia and symptoms has not been documented is considered a class II indication, as are mild symptoms in the presence of heart rates of less than 30 beats/minute while awake.
5. Carotid sinus hypersensitivity and neurovascular syncope. The presence of recurrent syncope associated with spontaneous episodes of carotid sinus stimulation or the production of more than 3 seconds of asystole with light carotid sinus pressure in the absence of drugs affecting AV conduction are class I indications for permanent pacing. Recurrent syncope without clear provocation but documentation of a hypersensitive cardioinhibitory response—reproduced by a tilt-table test—was felt by some on the panel to merit permanent pacing. Pacing may also be appropriate in patients with unexplained syncope if significant abnormalities of sinus or AV node function are documented at the time of electrophysiologic testing.
6. The indications for pacing in children are complex and take into consideration associated structural heart disease and previous cardiac surgery. Generally, agreed-on indications include sinus node dysfunction with symptoms corresponding to "age-inappropriate" bradycardia; advanced second- or third-degree AV block with symptomatic bradycardia, congestive heart failure, or a low-output state; congenital heart block with a wide complex escape rhythm, with ventricular dysfunction, or in infants with ventricular rates of less than 50 to 55 beats/minute (less than 70 beats/minute if congenital heart disease is present); advanced second- or third-degree AV block that persists 7 days after cardiac surgery or is not expected to recover; and sustained pause-dependent ventricular tachycardia that is demonstrated to be responsive to pacing. Pacing is commonly used but not universally agreed upon in the following circumstances: bradytachycardia syndrome requiring treatment with drugs other than digitalis; congenital heart block with an average rate of less than 50 beats/minute or evidence of exit block of the escape rhythm in children more than 1 year of age; long-QT syndrome with 2:1 or third-degree AV block; and asymptomatic bradycardia in patients with congenital heart disease. Also, transient postoperative complete

heart block that reverts to normal sinus rhythm with residual bifascicular block; and congenital heart block in an asymptomatic child with an acceptable escape rhythm and normal ventricular function.

There are also a number of newer indications for pacing, which include the following:

Atrial Fibrillation. There is increasing evidence that dual-chamber pacing may be helpful in preventing the recurrence of atrial fibrillation, particularly in patients with relative bradycardia or sinus node dysfunction (31,32). In patients with intraatrial conduction delay, multisite or biatrial pacing has also been advocated, both to prevent atrial fibrillation and to provide hemodynamic benefit (33,34).

Hypertrophic Cardiomyopathy with Obstructive Symptoms. Preexcitation of the right ventricle, accomplished by pacing at the right ventricular apex with a short PR interval, may reduce symptoms of obstruction by pulling the septum away from the free wall of the left ventricle at the time of ventricular contraction (31,32,35). Because these patients have an increased risk of sudden death, protection from ventricular arrhythmias has been combined with right ventricular preexcitation in the form of a dual-chamber implantable defibrillator.

Congestive Heart Failure. More normal ventricular activation and improved ventricular function have been demonstrated with high septal pacing in some patients (32). Dual-chamber pacing has been used to optimize the PR interval and enhance AV synchrony in others with marked PR prolongation and congestive heart failure (31,32). Recently, hemodynamic benefit has been demonstrated with biventricular pacing, particularly in patients with a pronounced left bundle-branch block (34). This has been accomplished either with epicardial systems or with leads introduced transvenously and advanced into the branches of the coronary sinus to pace the left ventricle.

Many pacemaker complications, most notably infection, lead malfunction, venous thrombosis, pocket erosion, and pulmonary embolism (36), occur late after implantation and may necessitate revision or removal of the pacemaker system. Complications seen at the time of implantation include air embolism and pneumothorax associated with subclavian puncture, as well as profound or symptomatic bradyarrhythmias. Bradycardia may be exacerbated by the use of local lidocaine anesthesia, which may suppress subsidiary pacemakers in patients with heart block (37). The availability of a transcutaneous pacemaker may be crucial in patients without an indwelling temporary pacing lead. One may also see tachyarrhythmias (atrial fibrillation or flutter; ventricular tachycardia) related to lead manipulation. Less common emergencies include vascular damage and cardiac perforation with tamponade.

Although uninfected but malfunctioning leads can usually be left in place, if sutured securely, the retention of infected leads or fragments is associated with a mortality rate of about 25% (38). Further, as pacing indications have broadened and the systems have become more complex, the need to remove leads has increased. Although active fixation leads, especially if they are infected, can often be removed by unscrewing them, scar tissue—most notably in the area of the clavicle/first rib—and neoendothelialization of tined leads may make their removal difficult after 6 to 8 weeks (39). A number of systems including chronic traction, snares, and telescoping sheaths have been used to extract such leads (39,40). The recent addition of laser technology has improved the efficacy and safety of percutaneous lead extraction (41). However, such procedures can be associated with arrhythmias, cavity invagination, perforation, vascular injury, or embolization of incompletely removed lead fragments, and cardiopulmonary bypass may be required (42).

Lastly, patients with pacemakers frequently require other operations or procedures, and the presence of a functioning pacemaker merits special consideration. The use of electrocautery can cause temporary or permanent pacemaker malfunction. Sensed as high-frequency electrical activity, cautery can inhibit or trigger pacemaker output, reprogram or permanently damage the generator, and cause reversion to the "fallback mode," which if not recognized can be misinterpreted as pacemaker malfunction (43,44). Such problems can be minimized by using a handheld cautery device for only brief periods, placing the dispersive (return) plate for the electrocautery so that it is close to the active tip but oriented perpendicular to the axis of the generator and pacemaker lead, and avoiding electrocautery near the pacemaker generator (44). Alternatively, a doughnut magnet may be placed over the generator or a programmer may be used to temporarily place the pacemaker in the AOO, VOO, or DOO mode to "blind" it to the cautery.

Interference with pacemaker function can be produced by magnetic resonance imaging (45–47), lithotripsy, cardioversion, defibrillation, electroconvulsive therapy, transcutaneous nerve stimulation, and diathermy (44). Appropriate programmers should be available in the operating room to allow correction of any induced abnormalities, and pacemakers should be interrogated after such procedures, even if they appear to be functioning correctly.

ANTITACHYCARDIA DEVICE THERAPY

Most antitachycardia devices are used to treat ventricular arrhythmias, although a small number of experimental antitachycardia pacemakers and devices have been used to treat supraventricular tachycardias as well as atrial fibrillation and flutter. In the United States, approximately 500,000 people are victims of sudden cardiac, mainly arrhythmic, death annually. These patients, if they can be identified before their event, as well as a much larger group of patients potentially at risk for such events (48,49), are candidates for implantable antitachycardia devices. These devices, known as implantable cardioverter defibrillators (ICDs), although originally designed to give only a defibrillating shock, can now provide tiered therapy, including defibrillating shocks, lower energy cardioverting shocks, antitachycardia pacing, and rate-responsive single- or dual-chamber bradycardia pacing (14,15).

Programmed electrical stimulation of the heart and pacing techniques have been used to study and treat ventricular tachycardia since the 1970s (50,51). Although antiarrhythmic drug therapy has played a central role in the treatment of both ventricular tachycardia and ventricular fibrillation (51), it has been recognized that drug intolerance and ineffectiveness will leave a large group of patients inadequately protected and that drugs may exacerbate arrhythmia risk. This has led to the development of surgical and device therapy for these arrhythmias. Michel Mirowski must be credited with the vision and perseverance to develop a totally implantable system (the ICD) that recognizes ventricular tachycardia and fibrillation and treats these rhythms automatically with shocks delivered to the heart (52–55).

Antitachycardia pacemakers, initially developed as "freestanding" devices are small implantable units that have been used to identify a tachyarrhythmia (supraventricular or ventricular), usually by rate criteria, and deliver burst pacing or programmed stimulation in an attempt to terminate the arrhythmia (10–12). Their use has been limited, however, by their efficacy in only a select group of patients with hemodynamically stable arrhythmias that are reliably terminated by these techniques, as well as by the concern that they could accelerate a stable rhythm into an unstable very rapid tachycardia, or in the ventricle, ventricular fibrillation (56). These concerns have resulted in incorporation of antitachycardia pacing techniques into the newer ICDs that provide tiered therapy (Fig. 22-1) (14,15). When compared with either empirical treatment of sustained ventricular arrhythmias, which carries up to a 40% 1-year recurrence rate, and drug therapy guided by electrophysiologic testing,

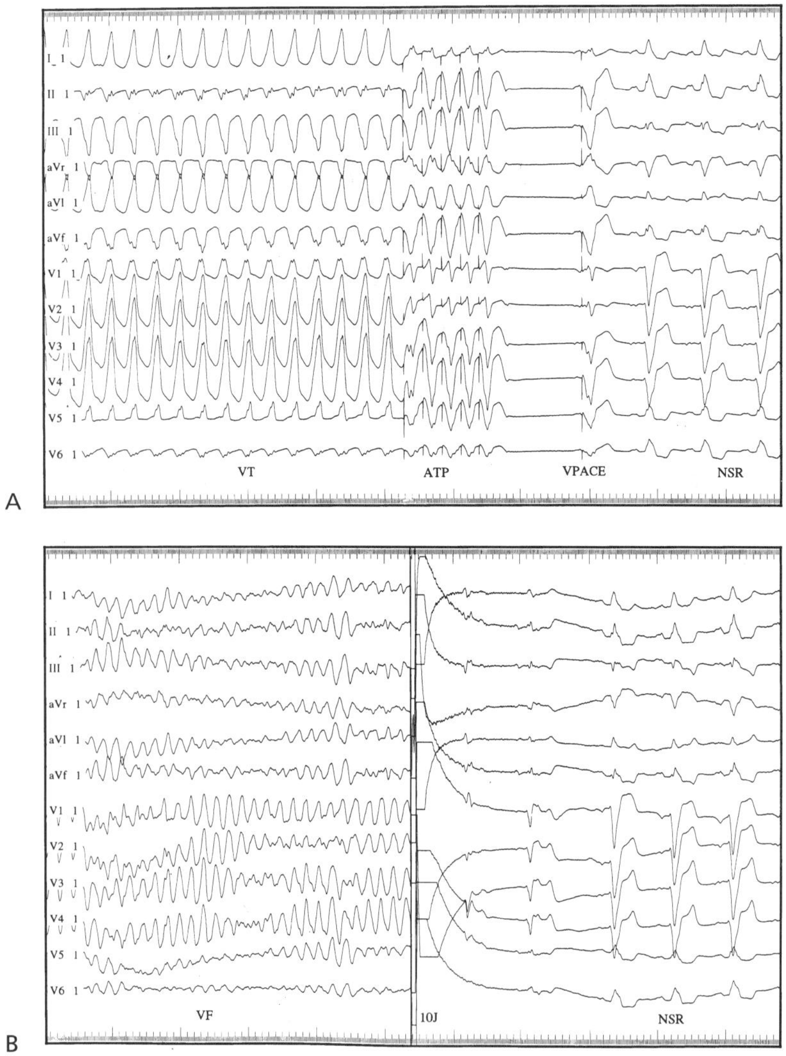

FIGURE 22-1. A: Antitachycardia pacing and **(B)** defibrillation by an implantable cardioverter defibrillator. **A:** Ventricular tachycardia (*VT*) is terminated by five beats of antitachycardia pacing (*ATP*), producing sinus rhythm (*NSR*) following a single beat of bradycardia pacing (*VPACE*). **B:** Induced ventricular fibrillation (*VF*) is terminated by a 10-J shock and sinus rhythm (*NSR*) results.

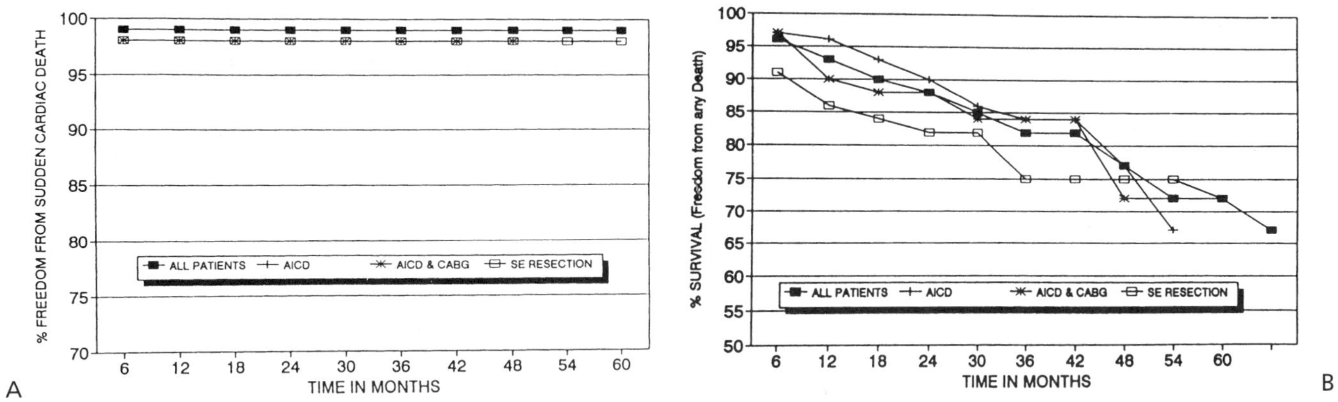

FIGURE 22-2. **A:** Excellent and comparable freedom from sudden cardiac death in a group of patients with life-threatening ventricular arrhythmias treated with a defibrillator, a defibrillator and coronary artery revascularization, or map-guided subendocardial resection. **B:** Overall survival rates for these groups do not differ significantly and are quite good when compared to survival rates in comparable patients with reduced left ventricular function, although there is a continuing attrition due primarily to nonsudden cardiac death. (From Geha AS, Elefteriades JA, Hsu J, et al. Strategies in the surgical treatment of malignant ventricular arrhythmias. *Ann Surg* 1992;216:309, with permission.)

which is associated with a 10% to 20% annual incidence of symptomatic arrhythmia recurrence, the ICD, with only a 1% to 2% annual sudden death rate (57,58), provides dramatically effective therapy. ICDs do not, however, prevent arrhythmia recurrences; rather, they treat them very effectively. This is the reason—that is, to minimize frequent device discharges—almost 50% of patients with ICDs require concomitant antiarrhythmic drug therapy (59).

There has been some concern that reporting only sudden cardiac death rates overestimates the benefit of ICD therapy. Although the small percentage of patients suffering severe adverse events at the time of device implantation has been virtually eliminated with the development of transvenous ICD systems (60), late nonsudden cardiac deaths do occur and overall survival rates may be considerably less than sudden death survival rates (Fig 22-2). Such deaths may be related to the frequent or incessant occurrence of even appropriately treated arrhythmias or to intractable heart failure (61,62). Nonetheless, a survival advantage may still accrue, even in those with poor ventricular function (62,63), and the ICD has been advocated as a bridge to cardiac transplant. The Multicenter Automatic Defibrillator Implantation Trial study has led to the prophylactic use of ICDs in patients with coronary artery disease, a reduced ejection fraction (less than 35%), and asymptomatic nonsustained ventricular tachycardia, who are found to be at high risk for sustained symptomatic ventricular arrhythmias (by virtue of the results of an electrophysiologic study) (48). This study demonstrated a clear survival advantage for devices as compared to conventional medical therapy in this patient group (Fig. 22-3).

The component parts of the original ICD systems included the following (64):

1. The ICD itself, which was rather large (220 g) and necessitated implantation in the abdomen. Newer devices have been significantly miniaturized (70 g) and are usually placed in the left pectoral region. The ICD contains the energy source and the circuitry that serves as the "brains" of the system.
2. A bipolar electrode system, either endocardial or epicardial, that monitors heart rate.
3. A separate electrode system used for shock delivery. This

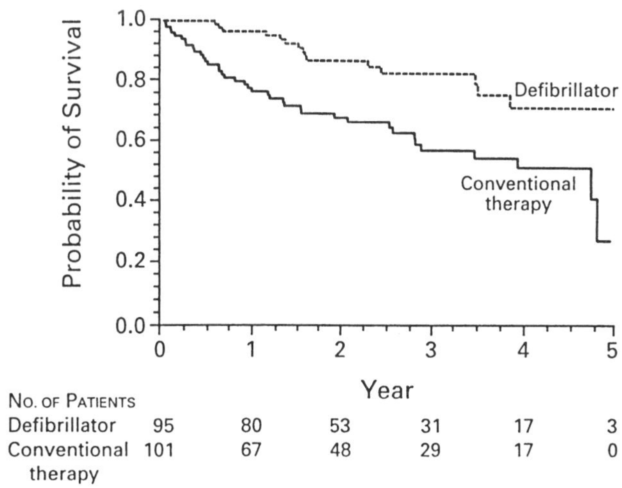

FIGURE 22-3. The Multicenter Automatic Defibrillator Implantation Trial Study demonstrated improved survival rates in the group receiving prophylactic defibrillators, as compared to those treated conventionally ($P = .009$). (From Moss AJ, Hall WJ, Cannom DS, et al. Improved survival with an implanted defibrillator in patients with coronary disease at high risk for ventricular arrhythmia. *N Engl J Med* 1996;335:1933, with permission.)

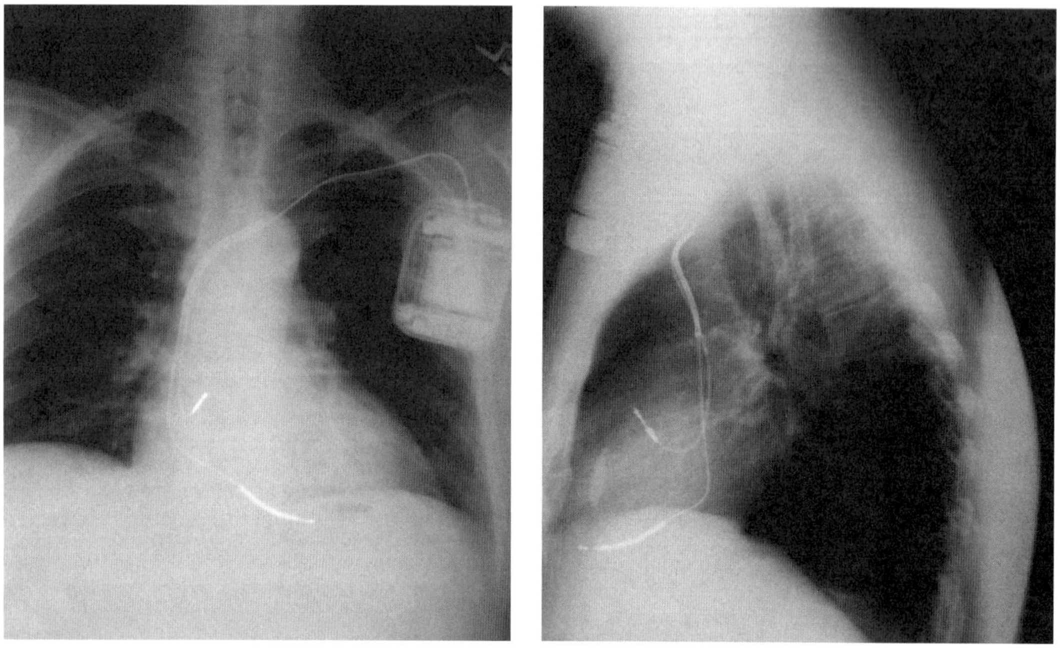

A B

FIGURE 22-4. **A:** Posteroanterior and **(B)** lateral chest radiographs of a patient with an endovascular atrioventricular (dual-chamber) implantable cardioverter defibrillator (ICD) lead system. The ICD generator is seen in the left infraclavicular area.

system initially consisted of either an endovascular spring electrode that terminated freely in the right atrium and a titanium mesh patch electrode positioned over the left ventricular apex or two patch electrodes straddling the mass of ventricular muscle.

Although the components of these earlier systems continue to function well in many patients in conjunction with newer ICD generators, they required extensive surgery (a thoracotomy or sternotomy) for implantation. Today, ICDs are almost always implanted prepectorally using a transvenous approach by electrophysiologists rather than surgeons. The sensing and shocking systems are usually combined in a single endocardial lead, and an additional atrial pacing/sensing lead is added if indicated. A left subclavian or cephalic vein approach is used most commonly (Fig. 22-4). ICD implantations are typically done with local anesthesia and conscious sedation in the operating room or electrophysiology laboratory (60,65).

The achievement of an adequate defibrillation threshold (the amount of energy required to convert an episode of induced ventricular fibrillation) with a miniaturized transvenous ICD system has become a reality primarily because of two developments. The characteristics of the defibrillating waveform are critical in determining how effective it is in converting ventricular fibrillation, and biphasic waveforms are considerably more effective than the monophasic waveforms delivered by the original ICDs (66–68). In addition, the can of the ICD has been made active or "hot" and has been incorporated into the defibrillating circuit. This has reduced the impedance of the circuit and increased the efficacy of the defibrillating shock (69), lowering achievable defibrillation thresholds even further.

In the operating room or electrophysiology laboratory, the surgeon and/or the electrophysiologist and the anesthesiologist must cooperate closely to implant an ICD system that will function appropriately and reliably. Once the lead or leads have been positioned, pacing thresholds must be determined and defibrillation thresholds measured. After adequate sedation is obtained, the device itself is used to induce ventricular fibrillation. Appropriate recognition and conversion of ventricular fibrillation with less energy than can be maximally delivered by the ICD must be documented. Although the determination of adequate defibrillation thresholds is essential, other intraoperative testing may include, when appropriate, measurement of low-energy cardioversion thresholds and documentation of the efficacy of antitachycardia pacing modalities. The presence of a standard external backup defibrillator with sterile external paddles or adhesive pads and the personnel to operate such a device are essential to the safe performance of these tests. Although there initially was some concern that defibrillating the patient several times during ICD implantation might produce myocardial damage, this has generally not been the case (70–72).

When high defibrillation thresholds or defibrillation thresholds within 10 J of the maximum output (usually 29 to 34 J) of the implanted ICD are accepted, there is an increased incidence of clinical device failure and arrhythmic death (73,74). If inadequate defibrillation thresholds are obtained, reversal of the defibrillating lead polarity, repositioning of the lead, placement of a subcutaneous patch or array, or very rarely use of an epicardial system may be necessary. High or inadequate defibrillation thresholds may be associated not only with the particular lead system, but also with body habitus, underlying cardiac diagnosis, myocardial mass, and the use of antiarrhythmic drugs such as amiodarone or class IC drugs such as flecainide (73,75,76).

When ICD implantation is performed at the time of other cardiac surgery, testing is done after rewarming, the termination of CBP, decannulation, and documentation of adequate hemostasis. More commonly, placement of the ICD may be deferred and is performed as a separate procedure while the patient is recovering from the initial cardiac surgery.

Because most ICDs still recognize ventricular tachycardia and fibrillation primarily by rate criteria, information with regard to ventricular tachycardia cycle length, the potential for significant sinus tachycardia and rapid supraventricular arrhythmias, and antiarrhythmic drug effects on tachycardia cycle length is critical for appropriate device programming. Equally important is knowledge about the need for dual-chamber or ventricular bradycardia pacing and the responsiveness of the arrhythmia to antitachycardia pacing, both in the baseline state and in the presence of antiarrhythmic drugs. Attention must also be given to the patient's hemodynamic valvular and vascular status to determine whether other therapy such as surgical or interventional revascularization, in addition to antiarrhythmic therapy, is indicated to optimize quality of life and survival (77).

Complications associated with ICD implantation have generally been limited, particularly with the newer nonthoracotomy devices. Frequent device discharges, most commonly for rhythms other than sustained ventricular tachycardia or fibrillation, remain a problem and may occur in up to 20% of patients (78). Such discharges may be "device appropriate but patient inappropriate" for rhythms such as atrial fibrillation with a rapid ventricular response or sinus tachycardia, or they may be due to system malfunctions such as lead fractures (79–81). Infection is a serious complication of ICD implantation, which occurs in 2% to 6% of cases (59,82) and usually requires explantation of the entire system. Other less common complications include coronary artery or graft erosion or the development of constrictive physiology related to epicardial defibrillating patches and the development of venous thrombosis or skin erosion at the generator site (83,84). In addition, a percentage of devices have reached "end of life" prematurely and have required early replacement.

Currently available ICD generators have a life expectancy of about 5 to 7 years. Generator replacement requires a small incision to open the device pocket, explant the device, and implant the new one. Adequacy of sensed electrograms, defibrillation thresholds, and pacing thresholds, as well as the integrity of the system, must again be tested. This is also routinely done with local anesthesia and intravenous sedation.

As with patients with pacemakers, those with ICDs often undergo surgery for other reasons. Electrocautery is sensed by these devices as a very rapid rhythm and may cause cessation of bradycardia pacing, spurious device discharges, and device reprogramming. This is the reason we routinely inactivate antitachycardia (but not necessarily bradycardia pacing) functions of ICDs in the operating room or at the time of procedures such as endoscopy, interrogating and reactivating them when the procedure is completed. This approach requires the availability of equipment and personnel for external cardioversion or defibrillation or urgent reactivation of the device. Certain devices, in addition, do permit temporary inactivation of their antitachycardia functions with a doughnut magnet. When abdominal or thoracic surgery is performed, attention must also be given to maintaining the integrity of the ICD leads and pocket.

An internal automatic atrial defibrillator (atrioverter) is currently under development (85,86). The evolution of this device has benefited from the technological gains and clinical experience achieved with the ICD, but it presents a number of unique challenges.

The practicality of internal electrical conversion of atrial fibrillation gained prominence in the early 1990s with the work of Levy et al. (87). These authors used high-energy (200 to 300 J) shocks delivered through a standard electrode catheter positioned at the tricuspid anulus (cathode) and a back-plate (anode) to convert 91% of their patients to sinus rhythm. This system also required a ventricular electrode to permit synchronization of the shock to the R wave and thus prevent inadvertent ventricular fibrillation.

Subsequently, a number of authors (88–90) have demonstrated that a totally internal defibrillating system can convert atrial fibrillation with relatively low-energy shocks of 5 J or less. This is particularly important because atrial fibrillation is not a life-threatening arrhythmia and usually does not produce syncope. Thus, the discomfort associated with such shocks must be tolerable to the awake patient. Utilization of biphasic shocks and an electrode system that spans the greatest mass of the atria with one lead in the right atrium and another in the coronary sinus has helped to reduce the energy requirements for internal atrial defibrillation (85,86,88).

Early recurrence of atrial fibrillation after effective conversion and subsequent delivery of multiple shocks has also been a problem with these devices and thus concomitant antiarrhythmic therapy is often required with the atrioverter (86).

The possibility that the atrioverter could inadvertently deliver a shock during the ventricular vulnerable period and produce ventricular fibrillation while the patient is in an unmonitored setting remains a concern (86). A separate ventricular pacing and sensing lead that permits R-wave synchronization of the shock and backup bradycardia pacing, if necessary, has reduced this risk. In an effort to reduce this risk further, the present systems are also designed to prevent delivery of shocks after very short RR intervals (86) and have sometimes been programmed to require external activation in a monitored setting before therapy is delivered. This concern would be ameliorated if there were a single device that could combine atrial and ventricular cardioversion, defibrillation, antitachycardia pacing, and complex bradycardia pacing. Such a device would be extremely complex and would have to take into consideration the differing optimal vectors for defibrillation of the atria and ventricles but increasingly would appear to be an achievable goal.

ARRHYTHMIA SURGERY

The concepts that surgical techniques can be used to interrupt, isolate, or extirpate reentrant arrhythmia circuits or to isolate, destroy, or remove foci of abnormal automatic rhythms come directly from basic animal laboratory work (91–96). Translation of this information to the operating room has further enhanced our understanding of arrhythmia mechanisms and has saved patients' lives. However, the development of radiofrequency ablation techniques and the flexibility of the newer defibrillators have moved the venue of definitive arrhythmia therapy to the electrophysiology laboratory and in recent years, heve dramatically reduced the need for and frequency of arrhythmia surgery. Thus, several of the procedures described in this section are presented to provide a historical perspective and to highlight the knowledge gained from them.

Surgery for Ventricular Tachycardia

Most surgery to treat ventricular tachycardia has been performed on patients with coronary artery disease, before myocardial infarction, and myocardial scar, usually associated with aneurysm formation.

Animal models have demonstrated that in this situation, monomorphic ventricular tachycardia originates in areas at the border of the scar in which damaged but viable cells produce an electrically inhomogeneous milieu suitable for the initiation of reentry (91–96). Both in animals (97) and in humans (98–100), mapping studies have associated the areas of earliest electrical activation during ventricular tachycardia with the site of tachycardia origin. Specific electrogram characteristics such as fractionation and the presence of continuous electrical activity have also been used to localize the reentrant circuit. Pathological studies have identified a "peel," or area of thickened white scar, on the endocardial surface of hearts of patients with prior infarction and clinical ventricular tachycardia (101). Removal of this tissue is associated with cure of the tachycardia.

Although Couch reported a case of ventricular aneurysm, associated ventricular tachycardia, and subsequent aneurysm excision in 1959 (102), surgical therapy of ventricular tachycardia did not become a reality until the late 1970s, when Guiraudon et al. described the encircling ventriculotomy (103), and Harken, Josephson, and colleagues reported the efficacy of map-guided endocardial resection (98, 104,105).

As described by Guiraudon et al. (103), the encircling endocardial ventriculotomy was achieved by opening the ventricle through the thinned area of a myocardial scar and making a full-thickness endocardial incision outlining the observed area of scarring, sparing the epicardium and superficial coronary vessels. The incision was repaired with a running suture, and the area of scarring was thus electrically isolated from the remainder of the ventricle by a barrier of fibrous scar.

Although electrical isolation of the reentrant circuit was thought to be important to the success of this procedure (106), subsequent studies demonstrated a significant decrease in blood flow to the encircled region, which suggested that ischemic damage also played a role (107). When it was recognized that this effect could contribute to clinically important myocardial dysfunction, and when the papillary muscles were involved, mitral regurgitation (108,109), the encircling ventriculotomy was abandoned in favor of a more limited map-guided procedure.

The procedure of map-guided endocardial resection actually began in the electrophysiology laboratory, where whenever possible preoperative transvenous endocardial catheter mapping of ventricular tachycardia was performed (110). This was done to define whether one or more tachycardias were inducible and to localize their sites of origin. This procedure was necessary because some patients were not inducible in the operating room, perhaps because of anesthetic effects (111) or the mechanical effects of surgically opening the area of ventricular scarring (110). For preoperative mapping to be performed, the patient had to have one or more hemodynamically stable monomorphic tachycardias that could be initiated and preferably terminated with pacing techniques.

Patients undergoing operative endocardial resection also underwent cardiac catheterization to identify any need for associated coronary artery revascularization and to demonstrate the dimensions of the aneurysm as well as the presence of adequate residual contractile myocardium. We have prophylactically inserted an intraaortic balloon pump to optimize hemodynamics and stabilize patients during the immediate postoperative period (77).

As with ICD implantation, intraoperative map-guided endocardial resection requires the understanding and cooperation of the operative team: the surgeon, electrophysiologist, and anesthesiologist. The chest is opened, the heart is exposed, and the patient is placed on normothermic bypass. The electrophysiologist then uses programmed stimulation to induce ventricular tachycardia. Epicardial mapping, looking for the earliest tachycardia exit site from the endocardium, is then performed. Although epicardial and endocardial mapping were initially executed using a handheld probe (59,112), they have since been facilitated by sophisticated computers that use an array of electrodes that may be configured as a "sock" to fit over the ventricle or a "balloon" that is inserted through the mitral valve into the left ventricular cavity, permitting simultaneous mapping of many points during a single beat of ventricular tachycardia (113). Epicardial mapping may localize the site of tachycardia origin, or the epicardial exit site of the tachycardia may in fact be some distance from its true endocardial origin (114). This procedure is done, however, because if the ventricle is opened, it may not be possible to reinduce ventricular tachycardia and perform endocardial mapping. The endocardial electrode balloon attempts to avoid this problem by permitting endocardial mapping before the ventricle is opened. When the ventricle is opened, this is done through the area of scar, and using the map developed, an area of interest is identified and removed. Actual endocardial peel may extend beyond this area and the purpose of endocardial mapping is to limit myocardial resection, preserving ventricular function and integrity. Reinduction of ventricular tachycardia is then attempted to assess the adequacy of the resection. If tachycardia remains inducible, further mapping and resection are performed. Cryoablation has been used as an adjunct to endocardial resection in an attempt to preserve structures such as the papillary muscles and mitral valve (Fig. 22-5) (77). It has also been used to encircle and isolate tachycardia foci (115). Laser photocoagulation (116) and direct application of radiofrequency energy have been used in conjunction with catheter mapping as well. Postoperative electrophysiologic studies are performed in these patients to assess whether the tachycardia remains inducible and requires additional treatment, such as an ICD (117).

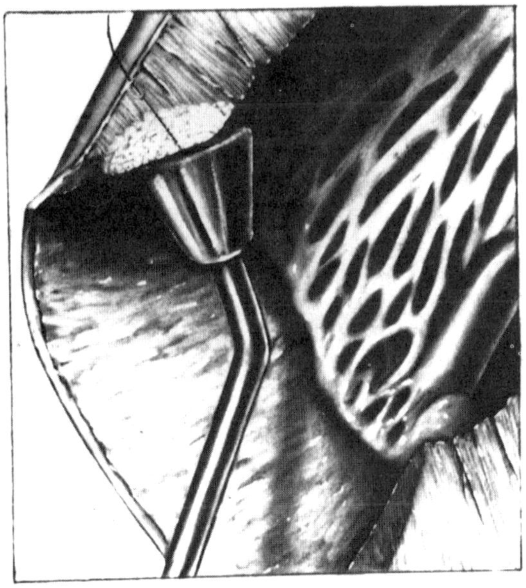

FIGURE 22-5. The use of cryoablation as an adjunct to map-guided subendocardial resection for the treatment of refractory ischemic ventricular tachycardia. Note the white cryoablation lesion at the end of the cryoprobe. (From Cox JL. Anatomic-electrophysiologic basis for the surgical treatment of refractory ischemic ventricular tachycardia. *Ann Surg* 1983;198:119, with permission.)

Map-guided subendocardial resection has a cure rate of 80% or more (59,105,112,118) and an operative mortality rate of about 10% (59,112,118). Failure of this technique to cure ventricular tachycardia has been associated with the presence of multiple morphologically distinct spontaneous tachycardias with disparate sites of origin, the absence of a discrete aneurysm, an inferior site of origin, and a right bundle-branch morphology (118). Nevertheless, the success of map-guided endocardial resection has been considerably better than that of blind aneurysmectomy (50%) (119–122), which would be expected to leave behind the arrhythmogenic focus in the border zone adjacent to the aneurysm. Similarly, coronary artery revascularization alone does not reliably prevent the recurrence of ventricular tachycardia (123), although it may be curative in patients without previous myocardial infarction or scar and normal ventricular function who experience ventricular fibrillation on the basis of severe ischemia.

Although the availability of ICDs and the developing experience with catheter-based radiofrequency ablation of ischemic ventricular tachycardia have significantly reduced the attractiveness of map-guided subendocardial resection, it must be remembered that subendocardial resection, like catheter ablation, is a potentially curative procedure while an ICD is palliative. Patients with incessant ventricular tachycardia or other indications for aneurysmectomy, such as congestive heart failure, emboli originating from the aneurysm, or angina thought to be due to the aneurysm, may be candidates for this procedure.

Although most patients undergoing surgery for ventricular tachycardia have had atherosclerotic coronary artery disease, these techniques have been applied to other disease states as well (124). Right ventricular dysplasia is a condition that affects primarily the right ventricular musculature and results in loss of muscle and its replacement with fatty and fibrous tissue (125). It is associated with sudden death and recurrent sustained ventricular tachycardia. Mapping studies can localize the site of tachycardia origin to these abnormal areas of muscle; however, this is a progressive disease, and map-guided resection of existing sites of tachycardia is unlikely to be curative in the long term. This led to a procedure in which the entire right ventricle was disarticulated from the heart (126), isolating it and preventing the spread of ventricular tachycardia to the left ventricle. Although this procedure has been curative, it has also been associated with a high incidence of right-sided heart failure. It has largely been supplanted by the use of ICDs.

Ventricular tachycardia developing after repair of tetralogy of Fallot is another model of a reentrant rhythm due to scar. The tachycardia usually maps to the subendocardium of the right ventricular outflow tract to the site of the previous ventriculotomy. Catheter-based radiofrequency techniques have been used to treat postoperative ventricular tachycardia in patients not requiring surgery for other reasons. However, map-guided resection or cryoablation of areas of early electrical activation in this region may be curative and may be incorporated into reoperations performed for hemodynamic reasons (127). More recently, in an effort to minimize the risk of such late postoperative ventricular arrhythmias, a transatrial approach has been used for the primary repair of tetralogy of Fallot (128).

It has been recognized that a syndrome of incessant ventricular tachycardia in infants less than 1 year old may be due to the presence of small myocardial tumors, most often hamartomas and rhabdomyomas (129–133). These tumors, which may be too small to be identified on contrast studies or by echocardiographic techniques, can be localized by mapping studies and identified visually at the time of operation. Excision or cryoablation terminates the ventricular tachycardia. Congenital nonischemic aneurysms of the left ventricle can also be the source of recurrent ventricular tachycardia in children and young adults (134) and map-guided surgery has also been used in their treatment.

Surgery for Arrhythmias due to Accessory Connections

The development of a surgical approach to treat arrhythmias associated with accessory connections represented an elegant step from the laboratory to the bedside, confirming the anatomic substrate for the macro-reentrant arrhythmias related to the Wolff-Parkinson-White and related syndromes. Catheter-based radiofrequency techniques have further amplified our understanding of these pathways and have virtually eliminated the need for a surgical approach to accessory connections (135,136). Today, such surgery is rarely performed except in refractory cases or those in which concomitant cardiac surgical procedures are required. Thus, the following description is provided largely to give a historical perspective.

The Wolff-Parkinson-White syndrome refers specifically to AV (Kent) fibers with manifest anterograde conduction that produces overt preexcitation on the surface ECG (a short PR interval and a delta wave). The most common arrhythmia associated with such connections is orthodromic supraventricular tachycardia, which utilizes the normal AV node in the anterograde direction and the accessory pathway in the retrograde direction. The QRS complex during orthodromic tachycardia is narrow unless rate-related aberration develops. Less commonly, antidromic tachycardia may be seen, which uses the accessory pathway in the anterograde direction and the AV node for its retrograde limb. Such tachycardias appear totally preexcited with a very bizarre QRS complex. Anterogradely conducting AV connections can also serve as "innocent" bystanders during atrial fibrillation or flutter and produce very rapid, potentially life-threatening, preexcited rhythms.

Concealed accessory connections conduct only in the retrograde direction and thus are not seen on the surface ECG. Although they cannot result in antidromic supraventricular tachycardia or rapid preexcited atrial fibrillation or flutter, they can participate in orthodromic supraventricular tachycardia, which may be quite frequent and symptomatic.

Although most accessory connections are now treated using radiofrequency techniques, the surgical interruption of an AV connection (bundle of Kent), described by Cobb et al. (137) in the late 1960s, represented a major advance in our understanding of this condition and provided a cure for a previously incurable disorder. Their patient underwent preoperative electrophysiologic evaluation and localization of the accessory connection. Epicardial mapping to further localize the accessory pathway was then performed in the operating room. This was routinely done before the institution of cardiopulmonary bypass unless the induced arrhythmias produced unacceptable hemodynamic instability. In a patient with anterograde conduction over the accessory connection, mapping at multiple sites along the ventricular aspect of the AV groove identified the site of earliest ventricular activation, representing the ventricular insertion of the pathway. Retrograde mapping of the atrial aspect of the pathway was then performed during ventricular pacing or optimally during orthodromic supraventricular tachycardia. The patient described by Cobb et al. had a right-sided accessory pathway, and although the patient was on cardiopulmonary bypass but in sinus rhythm, an incision was made transecting the communication between the atrium and the ventricle on the ventricular side of the right AV groove. As this incision was made, preexcitation was lost. After the incision was closed, mapping was repeated to eliminate the possibility of residual accessory pathway conduction or the presence of a second previously obscured accessory connection.

Although Sealy et al. (138) modified this technique to use a supravalvular, or atrial, approach to the pathway, the incision itself was quite localized and initial complete success rates were only in the range of 60%. Cox et al. (139) made several important advances in this operation. In 1983, they developed a computerized mapping system that used a belt of electrodes placed on either the atrial or the ventricular side of the AV groove. This greatly facilitated the mapping process, virtually eliminating the need for cardiopulmonary bypass during mapping and making it possible to map brief episodes of tachycardia if it proved difficult to induce the arrhythmia in the operating room. These authors also pioneered the concept that accessory connections may be formed by bands of tissue or that several discrete connections may be present. To deal with this, they identified four anatomic regions (Fig. 22-6), and if a pathway was localized to one of these regions, they extended their dissection to

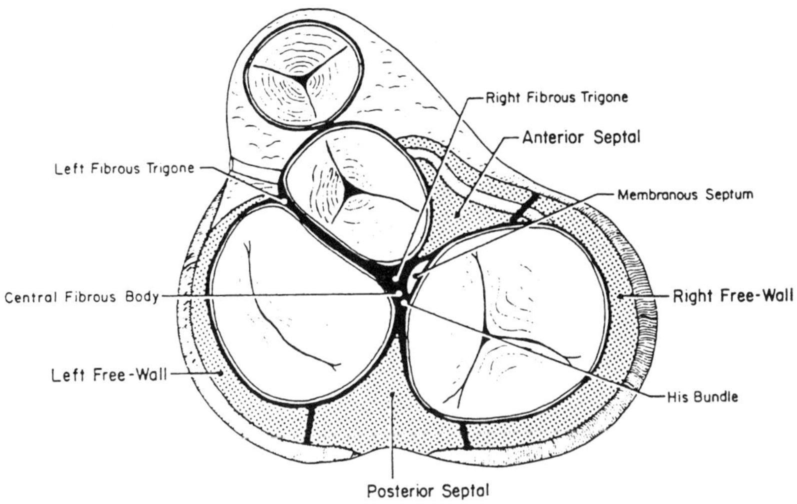

FIGURE 22-6. The heart as viewed from above with the atria removed. The anatomic boundaries of the four quadrants of dissection (anterior septal, right free wall, posterior septal, and left free wall) used to surgically ablate accessory connections are identified. (From Cox JL, Gallagher JJ, Cain ME. Experience with 118 consecutive patients undergoing operation for the Wolff-Parkinson-White syndrome. *J Thorac Cardiovasc Surg* 1985;90:490, with permission.)

include the entire area. Further, they squared off the edges of the incisions to disrupt any residual fibers of the connection that might persist after the initial dissection. Subsequently, cryoablation has been used to aid in this process. With these modifications, a success rate of virtually 100% was achieved with an operative mortality rate of less than 1% in the absence of other cardiac abnormalities.

With this technique, all dissections were performed under cardioplegic arrest and the AV groove was approached using an endocardial supraanular incision (139). Care was taken to preserve structures located in the AV fat pads, including the coronary arteries and the coronary sinus, and especially with posteroseptal pathways to avoid the normal conduction system (140). Inadvertent permanent complete heart block occurred in less than 1% in the series by Cox et al (139). After repairing the dissection and rewarming the heart, they repeated mapping studies to confirm the complete extirpation of the accessory connection and the absence of other anomalous pathways.

In an effort to eliminate the need for cardiopulmonary bypass, Guiraudon and colleagues developed an epicardial procedure for the transection of accessory connections (141–144). When initially reported, this procedure had no associated mortality rate and a success rate comparable to that of the endocardial approach (142). These authors have also made an association between the identification of posterior accessory connections and the presence of a coronary sinus diverticulum (145). Resection of such a diverticulum, or more commonly today, radiofrequency ablation in the diverticulum, is associated with the loss of accessory pathway conduction.

The Ebstein anomaly of the tricuspid valve is the congenital heart defect most commonly associated with accessory AV connections. Pressley et al. (146) have documented the feasibility of performing ablative surgery with or without associated tricuspid valve replacement or repair in these patients. To prevent emboli, repair of associated atrial septal defects or patent foramina is done during a brief period of ventricular fibrillation. Sinus rhythm is then restored and the ablative procedure is performed using an endocardial approach during normothermic cardiopulmonary bypass. This, in turn, is followed by tricuspid valve surgery. Eighty-two percent of the patients in the Pressley et al. study had no arrhthmias or clinically insignificant arrhythmias postoperatively; 5% had persistent AV connections.

Surgery for AV Nodal Reentrant Arrhythmias

The surgical approach to arrhythmias due to AV nodal reentry has been almost completely replaced by catheter-based radiofrequency ablation techniques (147). However, important information about the mechanisms of these arrhythmias, their anatomic substrate, and the feasibility of ablative procedures, whether surgical or catheter based, was gained in the operating room.

The most common form of regular macro-reentrant supraventricular tachycardia in adults is AV nodal reentrant tachycardia (148). Such tachycardia depends on the functional dissociation of two or more pathways located in or around the AV node and exhibiting AV nodal or decremental conduction characteristics. In the typical form of AV nodal reentrant tachycardia, conduction in the anterograde direction occurs over a slow AV nodal pathway while the retrograde limb of the circuit is completed using a fast AV nodal pathway; the reverse is true in the atypical form of AV nodal reentrant tachycardia.

In the past, total destruction of the AV node had been used to treat intractable forms of this tachycardia, but this had the disadvantage of leaving the patient pacemaker dependent (149). However, while doing such a surgical procedure, Pritchett et al. (149) fortuitously observed that they

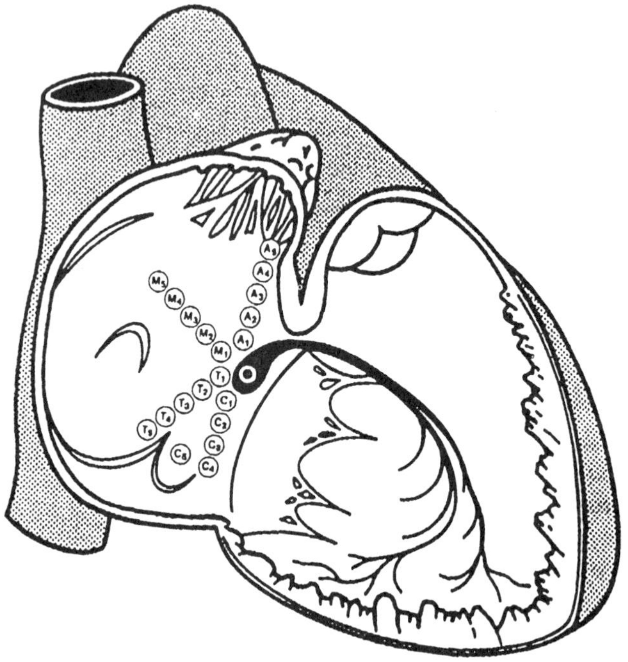

FIGURE 22-7. A template of the right atrial septum used during ice mapping performed in preparation for surgical modification of the atrioventricular (AV) node in patients with AV nodal reentrant tachycardia. *A, M, T,* and *C* denote mapping arrays. In most patients, the anterograde slow pathway was localized posterior and inferior to the compact AV node (*array C*) while the retrograde fast pathway was anterior or superior to the compact AV node (*A1* and *T*). (From Keim S, Werner P, Jazayeri M, et al. Localization of the fast and slow pathways in atrioventricular nodal reentrant tachycardia by intraoperative ice mapping. *Circulation* 1992;86:919, with permission.)

were able to abolish AV nodal tachycardia in a patient while preserving AV nodal conduction. This observation led to the concept of modifying the AV node by injuring one or the other of the pathways, most commonly the slow pathway, or the approaches to this structure, preventing the reentrant tachycardia but preserving normal AV conduction.

Intraoperative mapping of the atrial septum and surrounding areas has revealed the AV nodal region to be complex and somewhat variable but has added considerably to our knowledge of its structure. Intraoperative ice-mapping studies (Fig. 22-7) (150), as well as previous electrical mapping studies (151), have localized slow pathway tissues to an area posterior and inferior to the compact AV node along the tricuspid valve anulus while tissue with fast pathway characteristics has been found anterior or superior to the compact AV node. The anatomic distinction of these pathways and an intervening area of tissue with intermediate electrical characteristics makes possible the preservation of normal AV nodal conduction after surgery or catheter-based radiofrequency ablation of one pathway.

Although unusual today, surgical modification of the AV node is sometimes used in combination with other necessary surgical procedures. Cox et al. (152) and others (153) have advocated cryoablation rather than surgical dissection to modify the AV node. Sinus rhythm is monitored during the delivery of cryolesions, and if marked PR prolongation or heart block occurs, the ablation is terminated at that location and the area irrigated with warm saline, generally with reversal of the conduction defect. Reversal is obviously not possible once a surgical lesion has been made.

Surgery for Atrial Fibrillation

Atrial fibrillation is the most common sustained arrhythmia seen in clinical practice; it is estimated to be present in about 10% of the population more than 60 years of age (154). Although many patients are maintained in atrial fibrillation for long periods with acceptable clinical results, this approach has the disadvantages of increasing the risk of thromboemboli and potentially worsening hemodynamics as a result of the loss of organized atrial contraction. Some patients have unacceptable symptoms related to atrial fibrillation, and others such as those with hypertrophic cardiomyopathy or severe congestive heart failure may be incapacitated by this rhythm. Pharmacologic therapy aimed primarily at maintaining sinus rhythm and if that fails at controlling the ventricular response to the atrial fibrillation has frequently been unrewarding. AV nodal ablation, or less reliably modification, has provided a nonpharmacologic means of rate control but does not eliminate the hemodynamic or embolic complications of atrial fibrillation, and AV node ablation renders the patient pacemaker dependent. These problems have led to a surgical approach to this arrhythmia, and although catheter-based radiofrequency ablation techniques to deal with atrial fibrillation are being aggressively pursued, they remain investigational at this time.

Guiraudon pioneered the surgical treatment of atrial fibrillation with the "corridor operation"(155). This operation was based on the perhaps incorrect concept that the site of origin of atrial fibrillation could not be identified and therefore could not be ablated, removed, or excluded, and that a critical mass of tissue is required to maintain atrial fibrillation (155,156). In this procedure, most of the atria were surgically excluded and a corridor of tissue, one believed to be too small to maintain atrial fibrillation, was left connecting the sinus and AV nodes. The corridor procedure was initiated by establishing cardiopulmonary bypass, cross-clamping the aorta, and infusing cardioplegia solution. A horseshoe incision was next used to disconnect the left atrium along its attachment to the atrial septum, and a second horseshoe incision was extended from the tricuspid anulus anteroseptally and posteroseptally to the tricuspid anulus anterior to the coronary sinus. Seven of nine patients remained in sinus rhythm after this procedure, but four required pacemakers because of sinus node dysfunction, and in seven, the excluded atria were either in atrial fibrillation

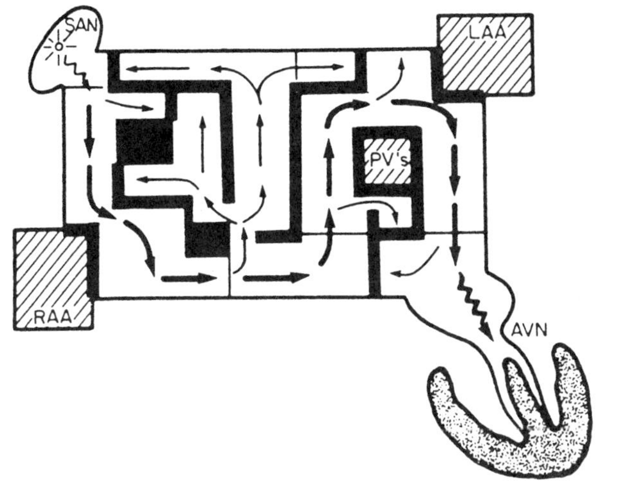

FIGURE 22-8. The maze procedure. The atria are divided into small areas of tissue, too small to support the macro-reentrant circuits needed to sustain atrial fibrillation but oriented to direct electrical impulses from the sinus node (*SAN*) to the atrioventricular node (*AVN*). The left (*LAA*) and right (*RAA*) atrial appendages are excised and the pulmonary veins (*PVs*) are isolated. (From Cox JL, Schuessler RB, D'Agostino HJ Jr, et al. The surgical treatment of atrial fibrillation. III. Development of a definitive surgical procedure. *J Thorac Cardiovasc Surg* 1991;101:569, with permission.)

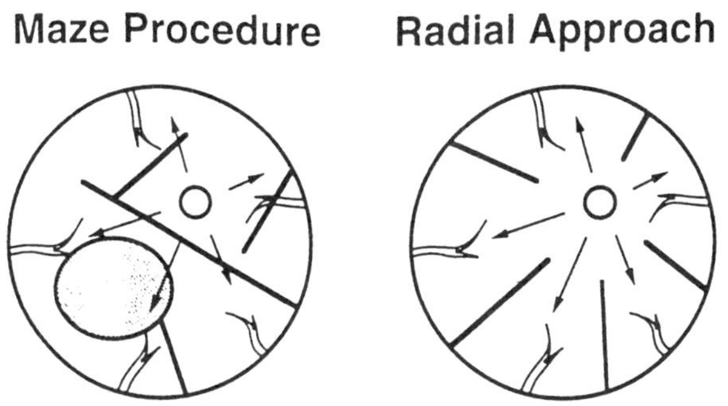

FIGURE 22-9. A schematic demonstrating the difference between the maze procedure and the radial approach. The large circle denotes the atria, bounded by the atrioventricular anular margins. The small circle represents the sinus node. The larger inner circle represents excluded areas of the atria in the maze procedure. Arrows indicate the activation wave front from the sinuatrial node to the anular margins. (From Nitta T, Lee R, Schuessler RB, et al. Radial approach: a new concept in surgical treatment for atrial fibrillation. I. Concept, anatomic and physiologic bases and development of a procedure. *Ann Thorac Surg* 1999;67:27, with permission.)

or flutter or were quiescent. Thus, this operation probably did not reduce the risk of thromboemboli substantially and did not restore atrial contractile function (155).

In an attempt to improve these limitations, Cox et al. (157,158) developed the maze procedure. It is based on the additional hypothesis that to prevent atrial fibrillation, all potential pathways for atrial macro-reentry must be interrupted (Fig. 22-8). Thus, multiple surgical incisions would be made in such a way that an impulse originating in the sinus node would be directed toward the AV node, but the entire atrium would be activated by impulses traveling along confined pathways throughout the atria, with no pathway large enough to sustain the reentrant circuits necessary for atrial fibrillation. To accomplish this as an open procedure, aortic, superior, and inferior vena caval cannulations are achieved. Although the initial dissection of the cavae is performed with the heart beating, the complex "maze" of atrial incisions is made while the patient is on cardiopulmonary bypass and the heart is arrested with cardioplegia. Both atrial appendages are excised. The final incisions are made after rewarming. In theory, after this operation, atrial fibrillation cannot be maintained unless the refractory period of the atrial myocardium is so short that macro-reentrant circuits can be supported in the small areas of tissue between the incisions. All seven patients initially described remained in a sinus or paced rhythm postoperatively, and there were no intraoperative deaths. Most interestingly, initially it was felt that atrial contractility, as measured by Doppler studies and magnetic resonance imaging, appeared to be preserved, effectively resolving the limitations of the corridor procedure. Further experience has confirmed the safety and electrical efficacy of this procedure, but there has been some concern about the efficiency of left atrial mechanical function after this operation. Recently this procedure has been further modified by Cox et al (159,160). It can be performed as a "minimally invasive" procedure, reducing the surgical risk further and a radial pattern rather than a maze of atrial incisions is made. In the "radial" procedure (Fig 22-9), all incisions radiate from the sinus node to the AV anular margins to permit a more physiologic atrial activation sequence and to minimize damage to the atrial blood supply (159, 160), hopefully more effectively preserving atrial contractile function.

SUMMARY

Surgical and device therapy of bradyarrhythmias and tachyarrhythmias has evolved substantially during the past 30 years. Although many procedures, such as the ablation of accessory connections, have moved from the operating room to the electrophysiology laboratory, other challenges will take their place. Newer, nonoperative techniques have all used concepts that originated in the laboratory, but developed in the operating room, to deliver better patient care and have provided the surgeon, electrophysiologist, and anesthesiologist with an exciting environment in which to work together.

REFERENCES

1. Mond HG, Sloman JG, Edwards RH. The first pacemaker. *PACE* 1982;5:278.

2. Zoll PM. Resuscitation of the heart in ventricular standstill by external electric stimulation. *N Engl J Med* 1952;247:768.
3. Madsen JK, Meibom J, Videbak R, et al. Transcutaneous pacing: experience with the Zoll noninvasive pacemaker. *Am Heart J* 1988;116:7.
4. Lagergren H. How it happened: my recollection of early pacing. *PACE* 1978;1:140.
5. Furman S, Schwedel JB, Robinson G, et al. Use of an intracardiac pacemaker in the control of heart block. *Surgery* 1961;49: 98.
6. Waldo AL, MacLean WAH, Karp RB, et al. Continuous rapid atrial pacing to control recurrent or sustained supraventricular tachycardias following open heart surgery. *Circulation* 1976;54: 245.
7. Gallagher JJ, Smith WM, Kerr CR, et al. Esophageal pacing: a diagnostic and therapeutic tool. *Circulation* 1982;65:336.
8. Kugler JD, Danford DA. Pacemakers in children: an update. *Am Heart J* 1989;117:665.
9. Taliercio CP, Vlietstra RE, McGoon MD, et al. Permanent cardiac pacing after the Fontan procedure. *J Thorac Cardiovasc Surg* 1985;90:414.
10. Griffin JC, Mason JW, Ross DL, et al. The treatment of ventricular tachycardia using an automatic tachycardia terminating pacemaker. *PACE* 1981;4:582.
11. Saksena S, Pantopoulos D, Parsonnet V, et al. Usefulness of an implantable antitachycardia pacemaker system for supraventricular or ventricular tachycardia. *Am J Cardiol* 1986;58:70.
12. Fisher JD, Johnston DR, Furman S, et al. Long-term efficacy of antitachycardia pacing for supraventricular and ventricular tachycardias. *Am J Cardiol* 1987;60:1311.
13. Barold SS, Wyndham CRC, Kappenberger LL, et al. Implanted atrial pacemakers for paroxysmal atrial flutter. *Ann Intern Med* 1987;107:144.
14. Leitch JW, Gillis AM, Wyse DG, et al. Reduction in defibrillator shocks with an implantable device combining antitachycardia pacing and shock therapy. *J Am Coll Cardiol* 1991;18:145.
15. Bardy GH, Troutman C, Poole JE, et al. Clinical experience with a tiered-therapy, multiprogrammable antiarrhythmia device. *Circulation* 1992;85:1689.
16. Billhardt RA, Rosenbush SW, Hauser RG. Successful management of pacing system malfunctions without surgery: the role of programmable pulse generators. *PACE* 1982;5:675.
17. Parsonnet V, Furman S, Smyth NPD. A revised code for pacemaker identification. *PACE* 1981;4:400.
18. Johnson AD, Laiken SL, Engler RL. Hemodynamic compromise associated with ventriculoatrial conduction following transvenous pacemaker placement. *Am J Med* 1978;65:75.
19. Alicandri C, Fouad FM, Tarazi RC, et al. Three cases of hypotension and syncope with ventricular pacing: possible role of atrial reflexes. *Am J Cardiol* 1978;42:137.
20. Rosenqvist M, Brandt J, Schuller H. Long-term pacing in sinus node disease: effects of stimulation mode on cardiovascular morbidity and mortality. *Am Heart J* 1988;116:16.
21. Sasaki Y, Furihata A, Suyama K, et al. Comparison between ventricular inhibited pacing and physiologic pacing in sick sinus syndrome. *Am J Cardiol* 1991;67:771.
22. Hesselson AB, Parsonnet V, Bernstein AD, et al. Deleterious effects of long-term single-chamber ventricular pacing in patients with sick sinus syndrome: the hidden benefits of dual-chamber pacing. *J Am Coll Cardiol* 1992;19:1542.
23. Lamas GA, Orav EJ, Stambler BS, et al. Quality of life and clinical outcomes in elderly patients treated with ventricular pacing as compared with dual-chamber pacing. *N Engl J Med* 1998;338:1097.
24. Hayes DL, Holmes DR Jr, Vlietstra RE. Early experience with a universal (DDD) pacing device. *Mayo Clin Proc* 1983;58:301.
25. Rubin JW, Frank MJ, Boineau JP, et al. Current physiologic pacemakers: a serious problem with a new device. *Am J Cardiol* 1983;52:88.
26. Bernstein AD, Parsonnet V. Survey of cardiac pacing and defibrillation in the United States in 1993. *Am J Cardiol* 1996;78: 187.
27. Den Dulk K, Lindemans FW, Bar FW, et al. Pacemaker related tachycardias. *PACE* 1982;5:476.
28. Littleford PO, Curry RC Jr, Schwartz KM, et al. Pacemaker-mediated tachycardias: a rapid bedside technique for induction and observation. *Am J Cardiol* 1983;52:287.
29. Elmqvist H. Prevention of pacemaker mediated arrhythmias. *PACE* 1983;6:382.
30. Amikam S, Andrews C, Furman S. "Pseudo-endless loop" tachycardia in an AV universal (DDD) pacemaker. *PACE* 1984; 7:129.
31. Gregoratos G, Cheitlin MD, Conill A, et al. ACC/AHA guidelines for implantation of cardiac pacemakers and antiarrhythmia devices. *J Am Coll Cardiol* 1998;31:1175.
32. Glikson M, Espinosa RE, Hayes DL. Expanding indications for permanent pacemakers. *Ann Intern Med* 1995;123:443.
33. Saksena S, Prakash A, Hill M, et al. Prevention of recurrent atrial fibrillation with chronic dual-site right atrial pacing. *J Am Coll Cardiol* 1996;28:687.
34. Barold SS, Cazeau S, Mugica J, et al. Permanent multisite cardiac pacing. *PACE* 1997;20:2725.
35. Fananapazir L, Epstein ND, Curiel RV, et al. Long-term results of dual-chamber (DDD) pacing in obstructive cardiomyopathy. *Circulation* 1994;90:2731.
36. Phibbs B, Marriott HJL. Complications of permanent transvenous pacing. *N Engl J Med* 1985;312:1428.
37. Kosowsky BD, Mufti SI, Grewal GS, et al. Effect of local lidocaine anesthesia on ventricular escape intervals during permanent pacemaker implantation in patients with complete heart block. *Am J Cardiol* 1983;51:101.
38. Rettig G, Doenecke P, Sen S, et al. Complications with retained transvenous pacemaker electrodes. *Am Heart J* 1979;98:587.
39. Myers MR, Parsonnet V, Bernstein AD. Extraction of implanted transvenous pacing leads: a review of a persistent clinical problem. *Am Heart J* 1991;121:881.
40. Byrd CL, Schwartz SJ, Hedin N. Intravascular techniques for extraction of permanent pacemaker leads. *J Thorac Cardiovasc Surg* 1991;101:989.
41. Wilkoff BL, Byrd CL, Love CJ, et al. Pacemaker lead extraction with the laser sheath: Results of the pacing lead extraction with the excimer sheath (PLEXES) trial. *J Am Coll Cardiol* 1999;33: 1671.
42. Brodman R, Frame R, Andrews C, et al. Removal of infected transvenous leads requiring cardiopulmonary bypass or inflow occlusion. *J Thorac Cardiovasc Surg* 1992;103:649.
43. Furman S, Hayes DL, Holmes DR Jr. *A practice of cardiac pacing.* Mount Kisco, NY: Futura Publishing, 1986:457.
44. Sager DP. Current facts on pacemaker electromagnetic interference and their application to clinical care. *Heart Lung* 1987; 16:211.
45. Achenbach S, Moshage W, Diem B, et al. Effects of magnetic resonance imaging on cardiac pacemakers and electrodes. *Am Heart J* 1997;134:467.
46. Lauck G, Von Smekal A, Wolke S, et al. Effects of nuclear magnetic resonance imaging on cardiac pacemakers. *PACE* 1995;18:1549.
47. Gimbel JR, Johnson D, Levine PA, et al. Safe performance of magnetic resonance imaging on five patients with permanent cardiac pacemakers. *PACE* 1996;19:913.
48. Moss AJ, Hall WJ, Cannom DS, et al. Improved survival with an implanted defibrillator in patients with coronary disease at

high risk for ventricular arrhythmia. *N Engl J Med* 1996;335:1933.
49. Anderson JL, Hallstrom AP, Epstein AE, et al. Design and results of the antiarrhythmics vs implantable defibrillators (AVID) registry. *Circulation* 1999;99:1692.
50. Josephson ME, Horowitz LN, Farshidi A, et al. Recurrent sustained ventricular tachycardia. 1. Mechanisms. *Circulation* 1978;57:431.
51. Mason JW, Winkle RA. Electrode-catheter arrhythmia induction in the selection and assessment of antiarrhythmic drug therapy for recurrent ventricular tachycardia. *Circulation* 1978;58:971.
52. Mirowski M, Mower MM, Staewen WS, et al. Standby automatic defibrillator. *Arch Intern Med* 1970;126:158.
53. Mirowski M, Mower MM, Reid PR. The automatic implantable defibrillator. *Am Heart J* 1980;100:1089.
54. Mirowski M, Reid PR, Mower MM, et al. Successful conversion of out-of-hospital life-threatening arrhythmias with the implanted automatic defibrillator. *Am Heart J* 1982;103:147.
55. Mirowski M. The automatic implantable cardioverter-defibrillator: an overview. *J Am Coll Cardiol* 1985;6:461.
56. Rosenfeld LE. Device therapy of ventricular tachyarrhythmias. In: Cleman MW, Cabin HS, eds. *Cardiology clinics.* Philadelphia, PA: WB Saunders, 1988:437.
57. Kelly PA, Cannom DS, Garan H, et al. The automatic implantable cardioverter-defibrillator: efficacy, complications and survival in patients with malignant ventricular arrhythmias. *J Am Coll Cardiol* 1988;11:1278.
58. Lehmann MH, Steinman RT, Schuger CK, et al. The automatic implantable cardioverter defibrillator as antiarrhythmic treatment modality of choice for survivors of cardiac arrest unrelated to myocardial infarction. *Am J Cardiol* 1988;62:803.
59. Geha AS, Elefteriades JA, Hsu J, et al. Strategies in the surgical treatment of malignant ventricular arrhythmias. *Ann Surg* 1992;216:309.
60. Fitzpatrick AP, Lesh MD, Epstein LM, et al. Electrophysiological laboratory, electrophysiologist-implanted nonthoracotomy-implantable cardioverter/defibrillators. *Circulation* 1994;89:2503.
61. Kim SG, Fisher JD, Furman S, et al. Benefits of implantable defibrillators are overestimated by sudden death rates and better represented by the total arrhythmic death rate. *J Am Coll Cardiol* 1991;17:1587.
62. Tchou PJ, Kadri N, Anderson J, et al. Automatic implantable cardioverter defibrillators and survival of patients with left ventricular dysfunction and malignant ventricular arrhythmias. *Ann Intern Med* 1988;109:529.
63. Newman D, Sauve MJ, Herre J, et al. Survival after implantation of the cardioverter defibrillator. *Am J Cardiol* 1992;69:899.
64. Mower MM, Reid PR, Watkins L Jr, et al. Automatic implantable cardioverter-defibrillator structural characteristics. *PACE* 1984;7:1331.
65. Kleman JM, Castle LW, Kidwell GA, et al. Nonthoracotomy-versus thoracotomy-implantable defibrillators. Intention-to-treat comparison of clinical outcomes. *Circulation* 1994;90:2833.
66. Fain ES, Sweeney MB, Franz MR. Improved internal defibrillation efficacy with a biphasic waveform. *Am Heart J* 1989;117:358.
67. Bardy GH, Ivey TD, Allen MD, et al. A prospective randomized evaluation of biphasic versus monophasic waveform pulses on defibrillation efficacy in humans. *J Am Coll Cardiol* 1989;14:7288.
68. Winkle RA, Mead RH, Ruder MA, et al. Improved low energy defibrillation efficacy in man with the use of a biphasic truncated exponential waveform. *Am Heart J* 1989;117:122.
69. Haffajee C, Martin D, Bhandari A, et al. A multicenter, randomized trial comparing an active can implantable defibrillator with a passive can system. *PACE* 1997;20:215.
70. Ehsani A, Ewy GA, Sober BE. Effects of electrical countershock on serum creatine phosphokinase (CPK) isoenzyme activity. *Am J Cardiol* 1976;37:12.
71. DiCola VC, Freedman GS, Downing SE, et al. Myocardial uptake of technetium-99m stannous pyrophosphate following direct current transthoracic countershock. *Circulation* 1976;54:980.
72. Frame R, Brodman R, Furman S, et al. Clinical evaluation of the safety of repetitive intraoperative defibrillation threshold testing. *PACE* 1992;15:870.
73. Epstein AE, Ellenbogen KA, Kirk KA, et al. Clinical characteristics and outcome of patients with high defibrillation thresholds. *Circulation* 1992;86:1206.
74. Marchlinski FE, Flores B, Miller JM, et al. Relation of the intraoperative defibrillation threshold to successful postoperative defibrillation with an automatic implantable cardioverter defibrillator. *Am J Cardiol* 1988;62:393.
75. Troup PJ, Chapman PD, Olinger GN, et al. The implanted defibrillator: relation of defibrillating lead configuration and clinical variables to defibrillation threshold. *J Am Coll Cardiol* 1985;6:1315.
76. Guarnieri T, Levine JH, Veltri EP, et al. Success of chronic defibrillation and the role of antiarrhythmic drugs with the automatic implantable cardioverter/defibrillator. *Am J Cardiol* 1987;60:1061.
77. Elefteriades JA, Biblo LA, Batsford WP, et al. Evolving patterns in the surgical treatment of malignant ventricular tachyarrhythmias. *Ann Thorac Surg* 1990;49:94.
78. Winkle RA, Mead RH, Ruder MA, et al. Long-term outcome with the automatic implantable cardioverter-defibrillator. *J Am Coll Cardiol* 1989;13:1353.
79. Chapman PD, Troup P. The automatic implantable cardioverter-defibrillator: evaluating suspected inappropriate shocks. *J Am Coll Cardiol* 1986;7:1075.
80. Mittleman RS, Mack K, Rastegar H, et al. Inappropriate shocks and elevation of defibrillation thresholds in a patient with automatic defibrillator patch Silastic erosion and titanium mesh fraying. *PACE* 1991;14:1452.
81. Nunain SO, Roelke M, Trouton T, et al. Limitations and late complications of third-generation automatic cardioverter-defibrillators. *Circulation* 1995;91:2204.
82. Kelly PA, Wallace S, Tucker B, et al. Postoperative infection with the automatic implantable cardioverter defibrillator: clinical presentation and use of the gallium scan in diagnosis. *PACE* 1988;11:1220.
83. Marchlinski FE, Flores BT, Buxton AE, et al. The automatic implantable cardioverter-defibrillator: efficacy, complications, and device failures. *Ann Intern Med* 1986;104:481.
84. Almassi GH, Chapman PD, Troup PJ, et al. Constrictive pericarditis associated with patch electrodes of the automatic implantable cardioverter-defibrillator. *Chest* 1987;92:369.
85. Lau C-P, Tse H-F, Lok N-S, et al. Initial clinical experience with an implantable human atrial defibrillator. *PACE* 1997;20:220.
86. Wellens HJJ, Lau C-P, Luderitz B, et al. Atrioverter: An implantable device for the treatment of atrial fibrillation. *Circulation* 1998;98:1651.
87. Levy S, Lauribe P, Dolla E, et al. A randomized comparison of external and internal cardioversion of chronic atrial fibrillation. *Circulation* 1992;86:1415.
88. Murgatroyd FD, Slade AKB, Sopher SM, et al. Efficacy and tolerability of transvenous low energy cardioversion of paroxys-

mal atrial fibrillation in humans. *J Am Coll Cardiol* 1995;25:1347.
89. Schmitt C, Alt E, Plewan A, et al. Low energy intracardiac cardioversion after failed conventional external cardioversion of atrial fibrillation. *J Am Coll Cardiol* 1996;28:994.
90. Cooper RAS, Johnson EE, Kanter RJ, et al. Internal cardioversion in two patients with atrial fibrillation refractory to external cardioversion. *PACE* 1996;19:872.
91. Boineau JP, Cox JL. Slow ventricular activation in acute myocardial infarction: a source of re-entrant premature ventricular contractions. *Circulation* 1973;48:702.
92. Waldo AL, Kaiser GA. A study of ventricular arrhythmias associated with acute myocardial infarction in the canine heart. *Circulation* 1973;47:1222.
93. Sherlag BJ, El-Sherif N, Hope R, et al. Characterization and localization of ventricular arrhythmias resulting from myocardial ischemia and infarction. *Circ Res* 1974;35:372.
94. El-Sherif N, Sherlag BJ, Lazzara R, et al. Re-entrant ventricular arrhythmias in the late myocardial infarction period. 1. Conduction characteristics in the infarction zone. *Circulation* 1977;55:686.
95. Boineau JP, Cox JL. Rationale for a direct surgical approach to control ventricular arrhythmias. *Am J Cardiol* 1982;49:381.
96. Cox JL. Anatomic-electrophysiologic basis for the surgical treatment of refractory ischemic ventricular tachycardia. *Ann Surg* 1983;198:119.
97. Wit AL, Allessie MA, Bonke FIM, et al. Electrophysiologic mapping to determine the mechanism of experimental ventricular tachycardia initiated by premature impulses. *Am J Cardiol* 1982;49:166.
98. Horowitz LN, Harken AH, Kastor JA, et al. Ventricular resection guided by epicardial and endocardial mapping for treatment of recurrent ventricular tachycardia. *N Engl J Med* 1980;302:589.
99. Horowitz LN, Josephson ME, Harken AH. Epicardial and endocardial activation during sustained ventricular tachycardia in man. *Circulation* 1980;61:1227.
100. Josephson ME, Horowitz LN, Farshidi A. Continuous focal electrical activity. *Circulation* 1978;57:659.
101. Hochman JS, Platia EB, Bulkley BH. Endocardial abnormalities in left ventricular aneurysms. *Ann Intern Med* 1984;100:29.
102. Couch OA Jr. Cardiac aneurysm with ventricular tachycardia and subsequent excision of aneurysm. *Circulation* 1959;20:251.
103. Guiraudon G, Fontaine G, Frank R, et al. Encircling endocardial ventriculotomy: a new surgical treatment for life-threatening ventricular tachycardias resistant to medical treatment following myocardial infarction. *Ann Thorac Surg* 1978;26:438.
104. Harken AH, Josephson ME, Horowitz LN. Surgical endocardial resection for the treatment of malignant ventricular tachycardia. *Ann Surg* 1979;190:456.
105. Josephson ME, Harken AH, Horowitz LN. Endocardial resection: a new surgical technique for the treatment of recurrent ventricular tachycardia. *Circulation* 1979;60:1430.
106. Ungerleider RM, Holman WL, Stanley TE III, et al. Encircling endocardial ventriculotomy for refractory ischemic ventricular tachycardia. I. Electrophysiological effects. *J Thorac Cardiovasc Surg* 1982;83:840.
107. Ungerleider RM, Holman WL, Stanley TE III, et al. Encircling endocardial ventriculotomy for refractory ischemic ventricular tachycardia. II. Effects on regional myocardial blood flow. *J Thorac Cardiovasc Surg* 1982;83:850.
108. Ungerleider RM, Holman WL, Calcagno D, et al. Encircling endocardial ventriculotomy for refractory ischemic ventricular tachycardia. III. Effects on regional left ventricular function. *J Thorac Cardiovasc Surg* 1982;83:857.
109. Ostermeyer J, Breithardt G, Borggrefe M, et al. Surgical treatment of ventricular tachycardias. *J Thorac Cardiovasc Surg* 1984;87:517.
110. Josephson ME, Horowitz LN, Spielman SR, et al. Role of catheter mapping in the preoperative evaluation of ventricular tachycardia. *Am J Cardiol* 1982;49:207.
111. Hunt GB, Ross DL. Comparison of effects of three anesthetic agents on induction of ventricular tachycardia in a canine model of myocardial infarction. *Circulation* 1988;78:221.
112. Haines DE, Lerman BB, Kron IL, et al. Surgical ablation of ventricular tachycardia with sequential map-guided subendocardial resection: electrophysiologic assessment and long-term follow-up. *Circulation* 1988;77:131.
113. Ideker RE, Smith WM, Wallace AG, et al. A computerized method for the rapid display of ventricular activation during the intraoperative study of arrhythmias. *Circulation* 1979;59:449.
114. Spielman SR, Michelson EL, Horowitz LN, et al. The limitations of epicardial mapping as a guide to the surgical therapy of ventricular tachycardia. *Circulation* 1978;57:666.
115. Caceres J, Akhtar M, Werner P, et al. Cryoablation of refractory sustained ventricular tachycardia due to coronary artery disease. *Am J Cardiol* 1989;63:296.
116. Selle JG, Svenson RH, Sealy WC, et al. Successful clinical laser ablation of ventricular tachycardia: a promising new therapeutic method. *Ann Thorac Surg* 1986;42:380.
117. Platia EV, Griffith LSC, Watkins L Jr, et al. Treatment of malignant ventricular arrhythmias with endocardial resection and implantation of the automatic cardioverter-defibrillator. *N Engl J Med* 1986;314:213.
118. Miller JM, Kienzle MG, Harken AH, et al. Subendocardial resection for ventricular tachycrdia: predictors of surgical success. *Circulation* 1984;70:624.
119. Harken AH, Horowitz LN, Josephson ME. Comparison of standard aneurysmectomy and aneurysmectomy with directed endocardial resection for the treatment of recurrent sustained ventricular tachycardia. *J Thorac Cardiovasc Surg* 1980;80:527.
120. Sami M, Chaitman BR, Bourassa MG, et al. Long term follow-up of aneurysmectomy for recurrent ventricular tachycardia or fibrillation. *Am Heart J* 1978;96:303.
121. Mason JW, Stinson EB, Winkle RA, et al. Surgery for ventricular tachycardia: efficacy of left ventricular aneurysm resection compared with operation guided by electrical activation mapping. *Circulation* 1982;65:1148.
122. Mason JW, Stinson EB, Winkle RA, et al. Relative efficacy of blind left ventricular aneurysm resection for the treatment of recurrent ventricular tachycardia. *Am J Cardiol* 1982;49:241.
123. Garan H, Ruskin JN, DiMarco JP, et al. Electrophysiologic studies before and after myocardial revascularization in patients with life-threatening ventricular arrhythmias. *Am J Cardiol* 1983;51:519.
124. Fontaine G, Guiraudon G, Frank R, et al. Surgical management of ventricular tachycardia unrelated to myocardial ischemia or infarction. *Am J Cardiol* 1982;49:397.
125. Marcus FI, Fontaine GH, Guiraudon G, et al. Right ventricular dysplasia: a report of 24 adult cases. *Circulation* 1982;65:384.
126. Nimkhedkar K, Hilton CJ, Furniss SS, et al. Surgery for ventricular tachycardia associated with right ventricular dysplasia: disarticulation of right ventricle in 9 of 10 cases. *J Am Coll Cardiol* 1992;19:1079.
127. Downar E, Harris L, Kimber S, et al. Ventricular tachycardia after surgical repair of tetralogy of Fallot: results of intraoperative mapping studies. *J Am Coll Cardiol* 1992;20:648.
128. Dietl CA, Cazzaniga ME, Dubner SJ, et al. Life-threatening arrhythmias and RV dysfunction after surgical repair of tetralogy of Fallot. *Circulation* 1994;90[Pt 2]:II7.

129. Garson A Jr, Gillette PC, Titus JL, et al. Surgical treatment of ventricular tachycardia in infants. *N Engl J Med* 1984;310:1443.
130. Garson A Jr, Smith RT Jr, Moak JP, et al. Incessant ventricular tachycardia in infants: myocardial hamartomas and surgical cure. *J Am Coll Cardiol* 1987;10:619.
131. Zeigler VL, Gillette PC, Crawford FA Jr, et al. New approaches to treatment of incessant ventricular tachycardia in the very young. *J Am Coll Cardiol* 1990;16:681.
132. Case CL, Gillette PC, Crawford FA. Cardiac rhabdomyomas causing supraventricular and lethal ventricular arrhythmias in an infant. *Am Heart J* 1991;122:1484.
133. Filiatrault M, Beland MJ, Neilson KA, et al. Cardiac fibroma presenting with clinically significant arrhythmias in infancy. *Pediatr Cardiol* 1991;12:118.
134. Fellows CL, Bardy GH, Ivey TD, et al. Ventricular dysrhythmias associated with congenital left ventricular aneurysms. *Am J Cardiol* 1986;57:997.
135. Jackman WM, Wang X, Friday KJ, et al. Catheter ablation of accessory atrioventricular pathways (Wolff-Parkinson-White syndrome) by radiofrequency current. *N Engl J Med* 1991;324:1605.
136. Calkins H, Sousa J, El-Atassi R, et al. Diagnosis and cure of the Wolff-Parkinson-White syndrome or paroxysmal supraventricular tachycardias during a single electrophysiologic test. *N Engl J Med* 1991;324:1612.
137. Cobb FR, Blumenschein SD, Sealy WC, et al. Successful surgical interruption of the bundle of Kent in a patient with Wolff-Parkinson-White syndrome. *Circulation* 1968;38:1018.
138. Sealy WC, Wallace AG. Surgical treatment of Wolff-Parkinson-White syndrome. *J Thorac Cardiovasc Surg* 1974;68:757.
139. Cox JL, Gallagher JJ, Cain ME. Experience with 118 consecutive patients undergoing operation for the Wolff-Parkinson-White syndrome. *J Thorac Cardiovasc Surg* 1985;90:490.
140. Sealy WC, Mikat EM. Anatomical problems with identification and interruption of posterior septal Kent bundles. *Ann Thorac Surg* 1983;36:584.
141. Guiraudon GM, Klein GJ, Gulamhusein S, et al. Surgical repair of Wolff-Parkinson-White syndrome: a new closed-heart technique. *Ann Thorac Surg* 1984;37:67.
142. Guiraudon GM, Klein GJ, Sharma AD, et al. Surgery for Wolff-Parkinson-White syndrome: further experience with an epicardial approach. *Circulation* 1986;74:525.
143. Guiraudon GM, Klein GJ, Sharma AD, et al. Closed-heart technique for Wolff-Parkinson-White syndrome: further evidence and potential limitations. *Ann Thorac Surg* 1986;42:651.
144. Guiraudon GM, Klein GJ, Sharma AD, et al. Surgical ablation of posterior septal accessory pathways in the Wolff-Parkinson-White syndrome by a closed heart technique. *J Thorac Cardiovasc Surg* 1986;92:406.
145. Guiraudon GM, Guiraudon CM, Klein GJ, et al. The coronary sinus diverticulum: a pathologic entity associated with the Wolff-Parkinson-White syndrome. *Am J Cardiol* 1988;62:733.
146. Pressley JC, Wharton JM, Tang ASL, et al. Effect of Ebstein's anomaly on short- and long-term outcome of surgically treated patients with Wolff-Parkinson-White syndrome. *Circulation* 1992;86:1147.
147. Jackman WM, Beckman KJ, McClelland JH, et al. Treatment of supraventricular tachycardia due to atrioventricular nodal reentry by radiofrequency catheter ablation of slow-pathway conduction. *N Engl J Med* 1992;327:313.
148. Akhtar M. Supraventricular tachycardias. In: Josephson ME, Wellens HJJ, eds. *Tachycardias: mechanisms, diagnosis, treatment.* Philadelphia, PA: Lea & Febiger, 1984:137.
149. Pritchett ELC, Anderson RW, Benditt DG, et al. Reentry within the atrioventricular node: surgical cure with preservation of atrioventricular conduction. *Circulation* 1979;60:440.
150. Keim S, Werner P, Jazayeri M, et al. Localization of the fast and slow pathways in atrioventricular nodal reentrant tachycardia by intraoperative ice mapping. *Circulation* 1992;86:919.
151. Ross DL, Johnson DC, Denniss AR, et al. Curative surgery for atrioventricular junctional ("AV nodal") reentrant tachycardia. *J Am Coll Cardiol* 1985;6:1383.
152. Cox JL, Holman WL, Cain ME. Cryosurgical treatment of atrioventricular node reentrant tachycardia. *Circulation* 1987;76:1329.
153. Wood DL, Hammill SC, Porter C-BJ, et al. Cryosurgical modification of atrioventricular conduction for treatment of atrioventricular node reentrant tachycardia. *Mayo Clin Proc* 1988;63:988.
154. Cox JL, Boineau JP, Schuessler RB, et al. Successful surgical treatment of atrial fibrillation. *JAMA* 1991;266:1976.
155. Leitch JW, Klein G, Yee R, et al. Sinus node-atrioventricular node isolation: long-term results with the "corridor" operation for atrial fibrillation. *J Am Coll Cardiol* 1991;17:970.
156. Cox JL, Schuessler RB, Boineau JP. The surgical treatment of atrial fibrillation. I. Summary of the current concepts of the mechanisms of atrial flutter and atrial fibrillation. *J Thorac Cardiovasc Surg* 1991;101:402.
157. Cox JL, Schuessler RB, D'Agostino HJ Jr, et al. The surgical treatment of atrial fibrillation. III. Development of a definitive surgical procedure. *J Thorac Cardiovasc Surg* 1991;101:569.
158. Cox JL. The surgical treatment of atrial fibrillation. IV. Surgical technique. *J Thorac Cardiovasc Surg* 1991;101:584.
159. Nitta T, Lee R, Schuessler RB, et al. Radial approach: A new concept in surgical treatment for atrial fibrillation I. Concept, anatomic and physiologic bases and development of a procedure. *Ann Thorac Surg* 1999;67:27.
160. Nitta T, Lee R, Watanabe H, et al. Radial approach: A new concept in surgical treatment for atrial fibrillation. II. Electrophysiologic effects and atrial contribution to ventricular filling. *Ann Thorac Surg* 1999;67:36.

Cardiac Anesthesia: Principles and Clinical Practice, Second Edition, edited by Fawzy G. Estafanous, Paul G. Barash, and J.G. Reves. Lippincott Williams & Wilkins, Philadelphia © 2001.

23

CARDIAC AND LUNG TRANSPLANTATION

MATTHEW BIGHAM
MARC L. DICKSTEIN
CHARLES W. HOGUE, JR.

CARDIAC TRANSPLANTATION

The technical feasibility of heart transplantation was demonstrated in 1905 and later with the pioneering work by Demikhov in the 1940s and Lower and Shumway in the early 1960s (1–3). In 1964 Hardy et al. reported the first attempt at human cardiac transplantation using a chimpanzee xenograft (4). This was followed in 1967 by the first report of human-to-human cardiac transplantation by Christiaan Barnard (5). Widespread use of this procedure, however, was thwarted by poor clinical results that led to a moratorium on clinical transplantation in the 1970s. Enhanced knowledge of the immunologic basis of rejection, introduction of transvenous endomyocardial biopsy, and the clinical availability of cyclosporine have all contributed to increasing numbers of cardiac transplantation operations (Fig. 23-1) (6–8). Cardiac transplantation is now an accepted treatment for a variety of end-stage cardiac diseases.

Patient Management before Cardiac Transplantation

An improved understanding of the pathophysiology of heart failure has led to a paradigm shift in the pharmacologic approach to chronic heart failure. This shift was born out of the appreciation that the compensatory responses to reduced cardiac output are inherently damaging over time. Initially, compensatory responses are beneficial because they mainly serve to increase ventricular preload and hence maintain stroke volume. However, with prolonged activation, these same compensatory mechanisms cause deleterious ventricular remodeling, exacerbate ventricular dysfunction, increase symptoms of heart failure, and increase the risk of sudden death (9,10). Therefore, rather than focusing on the pharmacologic restoration of systolic function (e.g., positive inotropes), therapy is now targeted at the interruption of the neurohumeral and immunologic pathways that are activated in response to heart failure (11,12).

Several neurohumeral pathways are activated as a homeostatic response to reduced cardiac output. The predominant effect is the increase in plasma concentrations of ligands that cause vasoconstriction (9,10). Epinephrine, norepinephrine, renin, angiotensin, and vasopressin all cause systemic vascular resistance (SVR) to increase in an attempt to restore blood pressure to its normal range. In addition, constriction of capacitance vessels and intravascular volume expansion by the kidneys serve to increase venous return and hence ventricular preload. Although these pathways are of obvious benefit during acute decreases in cardiac output, chronic activation leads to deleterious effects over time. Chronic elevations of circulating catecholamines lead to down-regulation of expression and function of β-adrenoceptor and α_2-adrenergic receptors (12). As a result, the responsiveness to β-adrenergic receptor agonists is reduced and myocardial catecholamines are depleted (13,14). In fact, the degree to which circulating catecholamines are elevated has been shown to be an independent prognostic indicator for mortality (15). Further, elevations in left ventricular afterload pose a continued stress for ventricular remodeling and thereby contribute to the vicious cycle of depressed systolic function, ventricular dilatation, and increased wall stress. Moreover, chronic elevations in left atrial pressure along with the resultant pulmonary hypertension pose a considerable afterload stress to the right ventricle, leading to right-sided heart failure (16).

There is mounting evidence that the immune system plays a role in the progression of heart failure. Several cytokines, namely plasma tumor necrosis factor-α, soluble tumor necrosis factor-receptor II, and interleukins-1, -2 and -6, are elevated in patients with heart failure (9,17). A recently proposed mechanism by which activation of the immune system occurs in heart failure involves endotoxin

M. Bigham and C. W. Hogue, Jr: Department of Anesthesiology, Washington University School of Medicine, St. Louis and Division of Cardiothoracic Anesthesia, Barnes-Jewish Hospital, St. Louis, Missouri 63110

M. L. Dickstein: Department of Anesthesiology, Columbia University College of Physicians and Surgeons and Division of Cardiothoracic Anesthesia, Columbia-Presbyterian Hospital, New York, New York 10032

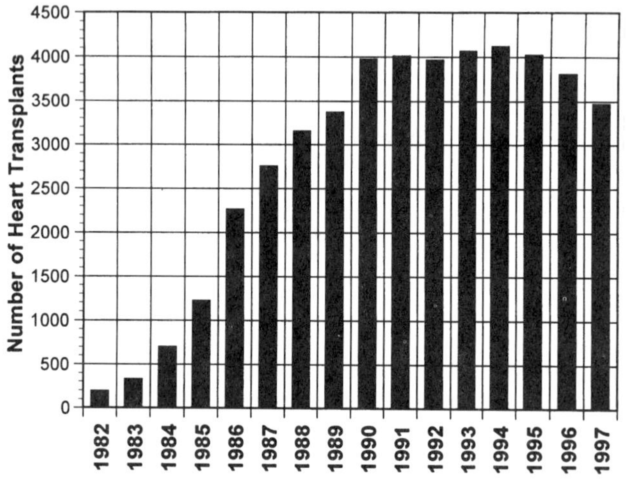

FIGURE 23-1. Number of cardiac transplantation operations performed worldwide. The number reached a plateau in the early 1990s and peaked in 1994 at 4,117 procedures per year. (From Hosenpud JD, Bennett LE, Keck BM, et al. The registry of the international society of heart and lung transplantation: fifteenth official report—1998. *J Heart Lung Transplant* 1998;17:656, with permission.)

that is released as a result of intestinal edema (18). Cytokines have been shown to depress myocyte function by altering excitation-contraction coupling via a nitric oxide synthase pathway, and they have also been associated with myocardial apoptosis (19–21). It has been speculated that therapies targeted at modulating the immunologic response to heart failure represent an important frontier that is just starting to be explored (22).

Current recommendations for the medical treatment of mild to moderate heart failure include the use of β-adrenergic receptor blockers, angiotensin-converting enzyme (ACE) inhibitors, and diuretics. The goals of treatment are to reduce circulating catecholamines, reduce ventricular afterload, and relieve pulmonary venous congestion. Acute administration of β-blockers is surprisingly well tolerated, and chronic use has been associated with improved ejection fraction, decreased left ventricular mass, decreased hospitalizations and mortality, and improved quality of life (23–26). In addition to the effects of β-blocker therapy on the cardiovascular system, there is additional evidence that its benefits may result in part from enhancement of immune system function (27). ACE inhibitors are well-established first-line agents in the treatment of heart failure, with impressive reductions in both symptoms and mortality (28). Although loop diuretics are typically the first choice for patients with mild to moderate heart failure, the addition of spironolactone has the added benefit of more complete suppression of the renin-angiotensin-aldosterone system (29). The roles of other pharmacologic therapies, such as digoxin, calcium channel blockers, and anticoagulants, remain controversial (30–34). Vasodilators such as isosorbide dinitrate and hydralazine are typically reserved for patients who are either intolerant of ACE inhibitors or have refractory symptoms (35).

Patients with congestive heart failure have a high incidence of sudden death; hence, considerable attention has been focused on the reduction of fatal arrhythmias (36). An important risk factor for sudden death is the presence of nonsustained ventricular tachyarrhythmias on Holter examination (37). Prophylactic treatment with amiodarone has been shown to be efficacious in this population, although the mechanisms by which benefit is conferred remain unclear (38,39). For example, in patients with ischemic cardiomyopathy, the increased survival seen with amiodarone is thought to result from its lowering of resting heart rate rather than suppression of ventricular arrhythmias *per se* (40). Implantable cardiac defibrillators reduce the incidence of sudden death in patients with impaired ventricular function and inducible sustained ventricular tachyarrhythmias, but they are of limited benefit to patients without inducible tachyarrhythmias (41,42). Surgical ablation of aberrant conduction pathways is recommended for patients with bundle branch reentry ventricular tachycardia that is refractory to medical therapy (36).

At the point at which patients are being considered for heart transplantation therapy, the therapeutic focus is on restoration of hemodynamic stability, end-organ perfusion, and symptomatic relief as a bridge to transplantation. Typically, symptoms tend to wax and wane but are present despite aggressive medical therapy. Often, patients exhibit signs of renal, hepatic, and respiratory insufficiency and require periodic hospitalization and positive inotropic support. Continuous home infusions of dobutamine or milrinone are becoming more popular because they allow for restoration of end-organ perfusion and symptomatic relief in an outpatient setting, but their use may be associated with risk for mortality (43,44). Exercise training has also been shown to be an important component in the armamentarium against heart failure with notable improvements in quality of life scores (45). Patients with end-stage heart disease have a high incidence of clinical depression, and therapy directed at improvement in quality of life takes on paramount concern (46,47).

Surgical Approaches to Heart Failure

Although heart transplantation is considered the definitive surgical treatment of impaired heart function, the severe shortage of donor hearts has led to considerable exploration of alternative surgical strategies. One such strategy is aimed at improving blood flow to regions of hibernating myocardium with the expectation of recruitment of dormant myocytes and hence improved ventricular function (48). Several studies have confirmed the benefits of coronary revascularization for patients in whom there is evidence of reversible chronic left ventricular dysfunction on positron emission tomography, or dobutamine echocardiography (49–52). However, even the majority of patients with ischemic cardiomyopathy are not candidates for revascularization because of extensive scarring or inoperable coronary vascular disease. Another strategy is aimed at improving the pumping efficiency of the impaired ventricle through repair of the regurgitant mitral valve (53). Even if mitral regurgitation is not causative, its correction retards further ventricular dilatation and also confers significant symptomatic relief through reduction in pulmonary venous congestion.

Other strategies involve more radical and currently unproven surgical approaches to alter myocardial mechanics (54). Dynamic cardiomyoplasty wraps the heart with a latissimus dorsi muscle flap that is stimulated to contract coincidentally with ventricular systole. Although it was hoped that this would reduce transmyocardial pressure and hence afterload, studies have shown that systolic augmentation is minimal and benefit is likely conferred through the restriction of further chamber dilatation (55,56). Because of mixed results, interest in this procedure is quickly waning (57). Another radical approach to the dilated ventricle, the partial left ventriculectomy, involves resection of a portion of the anterior wall of the left ventricle. The rationale for this procedure is that it reduces ventricular dimensions, and hence wall stress (58). Although early reports were encouraging, more recent data show a high failure rate and significant improvement in only a minority of patients (59,60). A related procedure (Dor procedure) involves resection of a nonfunctional akinetic anterior wall in the hope of affecting the progression of cardiac dilatation that follows anterior myocardial infarction (61).

Mechanical assist devices have become established surgical therapy for the heart transplantation candidate who is deemed unlikely to survive until a donor heart becomes available. Typically, the device is implanted in the setting of hemodynamic instability, deterioration in renal function, or respiratory failure that is refractory to medical therapy. Intraaortic balloon counterpulsation devices have been shown to be beneficial in both ischemic and nonischemic cardiomyopathies, but they are associated with high rates of infectious, bleeding, and thrombotic complications (62, 63). Left ventricular assist devices (LVAD) provide either pulsatile or steady flow and can be external or implantable. External devices are limited to several days' use and therefore are reserved for situations in which ventricular function is expected to rapidly return (i.e. myocardial stunning) or to temporize until the patient can be transferred to a center that is capable of placing an implantable device. Implantable LVADs are used to support the circulation for weeks to months. Although they were first intended as a bridge to transplantation, it is likely that future implantable devices will eventually take on the role of definitive therapy for end-stage heart failure (64).

Several devices are undergoing clinical trials, and two implantable LVADs have been approved by the U.S. Food and Drug Administration (FDA) for clinical use: Novacor (Baxter Healthcare Corporation, Oakland, CA) and Heartmate (ThermoCardiosystems, Woburn, MA). Both have a pumping chamber situated in the abdominal wall, with an inflow cannula attached to the left ventricular apex and an outflow cannula passed through the diaphragm to the ascending aorta. Both serve to decompress the left ventricle and, as a result, have favorable effects on ventricular remodeling; in fact, there have been several reports of successful explantation of the LVAD with restoration of adequate ventricular function (65,66). As a bridge to transplantation, ventricular assist has the advantage of improving end-organ perfusion, decreasing systemic catecholamines, improving exercise tolerance, and decreasing symptoms of heart failure (67). Further, the new generation of electrical LVADs allow for patients to be discharged from the hospital and managed on an outpatient basis. However, patients are at higher risk for elevated pretransplantation panel reactive antibody titers, which connotes greater difficulty in successful cross-matching with a donor heart (68). The success of the LVAD means that more and more recipients will require concomitant LVAD explantation at the time of heart transplantation.

Selection of the Heart Transplant Recipient

To ensure fair allocation of the limited number of available donor hearts, the selection of patients for cardiac transplantation is made by a multidisciplinary transplantation committee composed of physician, nursing, and nonmedical representatives. Patient eligibility varies among institutions but generally follows the guidelines listed in Table 23-1. The major indications for transplantation are end-stage heart disease due to idiopathic and ischemic dilated cardiomyopathy although the other myocardial diseases such as viral myocarditis, metabolic and toxic cardiomyopathies, and metabolic disorders are observed (Fig. 23-2).

Patients considered for transplantation undergo an extensive assessment that includes cardiac catheterization to evaluate for pulmonary hypertension and coronary angiography to determine the inoperable nature of coronary artery disease. Endomyocardial biopsy is recommended for patients with cardiomyopathy not related to coronary artery disease that is of less than 6 months' duration (2). The transplantation evaluation also includes extensive laboratory testing of thyroid function, fasting glucose determination, assessments for renal and hepatic disease, blood typing and antibody screen, human leukocyte antigen (HLA) typing, viral titers, fungal serology, pulmonary function testing, echocardiography, and a 12-lead electrocardiogram. Other laboratory testing is based on individual indications. Determination that the chance of survival in 1 year is 75% or less requires clinical judgment. Reduced serum sodium concentration, pulmonary capillary wedge pressure greater than 25 mm Hg, and plasma norepinephrine concentration

TABLE 23-1. PATIENT SELECTION CRITERIA AND CONTRAINDICATIONS FOR CARDIAC TRANSPLANTATION

Selection criteria
End-stage cardiac disease refractory to medical or surgical treatment
Prognosis for 1-yr survival ≤75%
Age <55 to 65 yr
Limited systemic disease
Compliant with existing treatments
Psychosocial stability
Absolute contraindications
Irreversible pulmonary hypertension (>6 Wood units)
Systemic infection
Irreversible renal and/or hepatic dysfunction
Relative contraindications
Severe chronic obstructive pulmonary disease
Severe peripheral or cerebral vascular disease
Peptic ulcer disease
Insulin-dependent diabetes with end-organ dysfunction
Untreated malignancy
Recent pulmonary infarction
Active diverticulitis
Any systemic illness with limited survival
Cardiac cachexia
Current substance abuse
Psychiatric disorder that could limit compliance
Absence of psychosocial support

greater than 600 pg/mL are associated with poor survival, but left ventricular ejection fraction less than 20% and/or maximal oxygen consumption of 10 mL/kg/minute or less have been suggested to be the strongest predictors of poor prognosis (2,69–74).

The age limits for cardiac transplantation have gradually increased, with greater emphasis placed on physiologic rather than chronologic age (75). Surgical outcomes are comparable between younger and carefully selected older patients and, in fact, the latter group may experience fewer episodes of rejection (75,76). A fixed pulmonary vascular resistance (PVR) of greater than 6 Woods units or a transpulmonary gradient (mean pulmonary artery pressure − pulmonary capillary wedge pressure) of more than 15 mm Hg is considered an absolute contraindication to transplantation (2,77–79). The basis for this restriction is the limited ability of the right ventricle of the transplanted heart to acutely adapt to an elevated afterload. During the preoperative evaluations, attempts are made to demonstrate the reversibility of elevated PVR by administering pulmonary vasodilators such as oxygen, nitric oxide (NO), calcium channel blockers, prostaglandin E_1, or sodium nitroprusside, often with inotropic drugs (2,79). Cardiac transplantation of larger donor hearts has been recommended for patients with mild increases in PVR (3 to 6 Woods units) (2). Recent pulmonary infarction (less than 6 weeks) is considered a contraindication for transplantation due to the increased risk of cavitation and abscess formation (80). Diseases likely to be exacerbated by immunosuppression, such as active infections or diabetes mellitus, are reasons to exclude potential transplantation patients, although the use of cyclosporine has reduced steroid requirements after transplantation, allowing liberalization of these criteria. Patients who are medically noncompliant, have continued substance abuse, have severe psychiatric disturbances, or lack a psychosocial support network are not considered for transplantation (81–84).

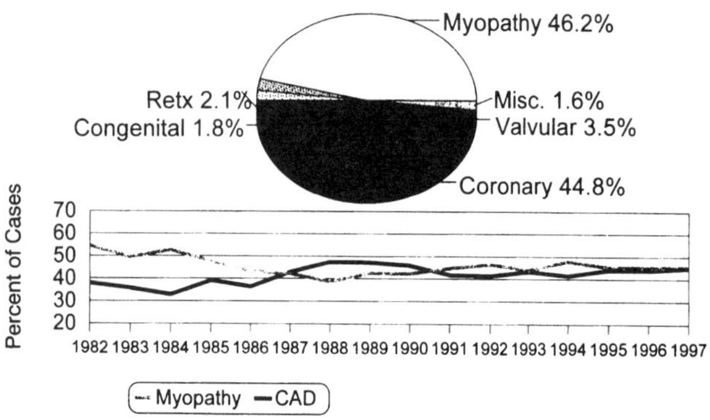

FIGURE 23-2. Indications for cardiac transplantation. The frequency of ischemic cardiomyopathy as an indication for transplantation increased in the late 1980s due to a general liberalization of selection criteria. (From Hosenpud JD, Bennett LE, Keck BM, et al. The registry of the international society of heart and lung transplantation: fifteenth official report—1998. *J Heart Lung Transplant* 1998;17:656, with permission.)

Available organs for cardiac transplantation are distributed based on recipient status criteria established by the United Network for Organ Sharing (UNOS), length of time on the transplantation waiting list, and distance between the donor and the recipient. According to the UNOS criteria, a status I recipient is one who requires support with any of the following: total artificial heart, LVAD, right ventricular assist device, intraaortic balloon pump, or ventilator. Status I is also granted for prospective recipients who require intensive care unit admission and inotropic drugs. Patients not meeting status I criteria are classified as status II. The number of patients with dilated cardiomyopathy continues to rise owing to the general aging of the population and, possibly, more effective therapies that extend life (85). At the same time, the number of available donors has reached a plateau (8). These trends have led to an increase in the waiting time for transplantation and an increase in the number of status I patients who cannot be weaned from inotropic support or mechanical assist devices (86–89). In 1988, 12.5% of patients waited longer than 1 year for cardiac transplantation; by 1994, this figure had increased to 45.4% (89).

Brain Death

The National Organ Transplantation Act provided the impetus in the 1980s for the establishment of Required Request Laws, whereby hospitals are required to request organ donation from families of potential donors (2,90,91). However, enhanced awareness of organ donation has not resulted in complete capture of all potential donors, in part because of psychological barriers related to defining brain death in patients whose life is maintained solely by advanced medical technology (92). In 1981 the President's Commission for the Study of Ethical Problems in Medicine and Biomedical Research provided national guidelines for defining brain death (2,92–94). These guidelines are largely based on earlier recommendations from the Harvard Committee, and later from the National Institutes of Health, the Model Brain Act, and the Uniform Brain Death Act (2,92,95–98). In the United States, brain death is defined as irreversible loss of cortical and brainstem function. The determination is made by physical examination, including apnea testing, once metabolic and pharmacologic causes, hypothermia, and other potentially reversible causes of coma are excluded (99). Confirmatory diagnostic testing is not required except when deemed necessary by examining physicians (99). The diagnosis of brain death requires that the criteria be fulfilled on two separate examinations at least 6 hours apart in adults (2,92,94).

Donor Selection and Management

Once brain death has been established, and after consent from the family has been obtained, the suitability of the organs for transplantation is determined. Because of the shortage of organs for heart transplantation, donor selection criteria have gradually become more lenient, especially with respect to age. Generally, patients 55 years of age or younger are considered as potential donors. The past history for potential donors must exclude prior cardiac arrest, hemodynamic instability requiring large doses of vasoactive drugs, preexisting cardiac disease, cardiac trauma, septicemia, noncerebral malignancy, and positive testing for hepatitis B and C or human immunodeficiency virus (HIV). The patient's height, weight, ABO blood group, and cause of death are collected by the local organ procurement agency for matching of potential recipients. Secondary evaluation is performed to exclude contraindications for heart donation, especially cardiac disease. Echocardiography and occasionally coronary angiography are more often considered for male donors older than 45 years of age and women older than 50 years or when the potential donor has risk factors for coronary artery disease. The final decision for suitability for heart donation occurs at the time of organ explantation, when the heart is inspected for evidence of prior myocardial infarction, trauma, coronary artery calcifications, or other abnormalities.

General care of the organ donor is supportive, including the correction of electrolyte abnormalities, maintenance of oxygenation and ventilation, and correction of anemia. Broad-spectrum antibiotics are given after the donor has had urine, blood, and pulmonary cultures. Hemodynamic instability is common in brain-dead patients, necessitating close monitoring of arterial pressures and often cardiac filling pressures before and during organ harvesting. Increased sympathetic outflow resulting from intracranial hypertension requires aggressive treatment with sodium nitroprusside or other vasodilators to avoid myocardial ischemic injury (2,100). More often, the management of increased intracranial pressures with diuretics results in hypovolemia, whereas brainstem injury may lead to vasomotor dysfunction. Hypotension is initially treated with the administration of crystalloids, but, when there is no response, phenylephrine or other vasoconstrictors are considered. Caution is taken, however, because high catecholamine requirements in the heart transplant donor have been associated with graft dysfunction after transplantation (101). The presence of persistent hemodynamic instability warrants further assessment of cardiac preload and function with a pulmonary artery catheter or even transesophageal echocardiography (TEE). Hypothalamic-pituitary dysfunction may accompany brain death resulting in low levels of circulating thyroid hormones. The administration of triiodothyronine (T_3) in some situations may allow for a decrease in vasoactive drug dosages, but this treatment remains controversial (102–104). Centrally mediated hypothermia may also be present in the brain-dead patient and should be aggressively treated with forced-air warming devices to avoid cardiac arrhythmias. Diabetes insipidus may require administration of vasopressin at 0.8 to 1.0 U/hour to maintain urine output less than 100 mL/hour (105).

Induction and Maintenance of Anesthesia for Heart Transplantation

On the day of surgery, the preoperative evaluation of patients undergoing heart transplantation is similar to the evaluation performed for any patient with heart failure. Special attention is required to the airway, vascular access, the potential for ischemia on induction, and end-organ impairment secondary to chronic hypoperfusion. Important points in the clinical history include cause of heart failure, previous anesthetic experiences, previous cardiac surgery (and previous exposure to aprotinin), presence of angina, the ability to lie flat, current medications, and allergies. Physical examination may reveal jugular venous distention, hepatojugular reflex (reflecting degree of right-sided heart failure), an S_3 gallop, laterally displaced point of maximal impulse (reflecting left ventricular failure and cardiomegaly), and pulmonary rales (106). Serum creatinine and liver function tests, including coagulation profiles, are important to identify patients with impaired renal and liver function. Serum electrolytes, specifically sodium, potassium, and magnesium, are often low as a consequence of either alterations in the renin-angiotensin system or aggressive diuretic therapy (107). Results from the most recent heart catheterization study should be available to document the transpulmonary gradient, PVR, the pulmonary vascular response to vasodilators (in patients with pulmonary hypertension), cardiac output, valvular function, and left ventricular filling pressure.

In order to minimize ischemic time of the donor heart, coordination of the timing of the harvest and implant procedures is essential. Hence, close communication with the donor team is required to ascertain the time of visualization (i.e., final determination of the acceptability of that heart for transplantation), the cross-clamp time (which marks the start of graft ischemia), and the estimated travel time back to the transplantation site. Patients who have had previous cardiac surgery, and especially those with ventricular assist devices in place, require more time for native heart explantation. Typically, intravenous and radial artery catheters are placed in prospective recipients in advance of visualization of the donor heart; on final acceptance of the donor heart, anesthesia is induced and surgery commences. Most centers place pulmonary artery catheters in heart transplant recipients. The decision to place the catheter before or after induction of anesthesia is based on the clinical status of the patient as well as the above-described timing issues (108). Pulmonary artery pressure, transpulmonary gradient, and PVR all convey information about right ventricular afterload and therefore are important parameters to monitor. In addition, TEE is extremely useful for assessment of graft function (especially right ventricular function), volume status, the presence of intracardiac air, and the presence of a patent foramen ovale in the transplanted heart (109).

The induction and maintenance of anesthesia may be associated with hemodynamic instability as a result of negative inotropic actions, negative chronotropic actions, and vasodilatory effects of induction agents; a reduction in the resting sympathetic tone; and the reduction in venous return that accompanies the transition from spontaneous to positive pressure ventilation. In general, induction agents are selected that are relatively devoid of negative inotropic or chronotropic effects. Although many successful induction regimens have been reported, narcotic-based inductions with a hypnotic tend to be favored (108,110,111). Patients treated with ACE inhibitors may have a higher risk of hypotension on induction (112). Moreover, bolus administration of vasoactive agents used to counteract changes in vascular resistance take considerably longer to have their desired effects, because circulation time is more than doubled in patients with congestive heart failure (113). Maintenance with small expired concentrations of potent volatile anesthetic agents is desirable to decrease the incidence of intraoperative awareness and hasten the time to extubation, although one retrospective review found no difference in outcome when comparing narcotic versus inhalational agents for maintenance of anesthesia (114). It is likely that the choice of anesthetic agent is less important than the management of the hemodynamic perturbations that follow.

Surgical Procedures

Orthotopic cardiac transplantation involves replacement of the diseased recipient's heart; with heterotopic transplantation, the donor heart is "piggy-backed" to the recipient's (Fig. 23-3). The latter procedure is reserved for a small subset of patients with increased pulmonary artery pressure and/or a small donor heart that precludes orthotopic transplantation (2,115). The traditional method of orthotopic cardiac transplantation is performed by excising the aorta and pulmonary artery above their respective valves and then excising the atria at the atrioventricular groove (Fig. 23-3A). This procedure leaves a cuff of the recipient's atrium to anastomose to the donor's heart. The bicaval technique is an alternative surgical method that leaves a small recipient left atrial cuff and involves direct anastomosis of the vena cava to the donor atrium (Fig. 23-3B). The latter technique is thought to better preserve atrial contractility, sinus node function, and atrioventricular valve function. Compared with the standard procedure, preliminary experience with the bicaval technique has shown that this method results in a lower incidence of atrial arrhythmias and conduction abnormalities, improved right ventricular performance, a lower frequency of atrioventricular valve dysfunction (especially tricuspid regurgitation), improved left ventricular ejection fraction, and better long-term survival (116–120).

Separation from Cardiopulmonary Bypass

Standard principles govern preparation for separation from cardiopulmonary bypass (CPB), such as normothermia, adequate depth of anesthesia, adequate muscle relaxation, resumption of ventilation, assessment of cardiac function and rhythm, and optimization of SVR. As in all open chamber procedures, attempts are made to evacuate all intracardiac air in order to avoid systemic air embolism. Typically, air bubbles migrate into the pulmonary veins and are expelled during resumption of ventilation. Efforts to de-air the cardiac chambers are evaluated by TEE; air in the ventricular chamber usually rests in the apex and layers out along the intraventricular septum and is seen as densely echogenic foci in these locations (121). An 18-gauge needle may be inserted into the LV apex to facilitate expulsion of air, and an aortic vent may be used during reestablishment of pulmonary circulation (122). Because air preferentially enters the right coronary artery due to its nondependent position, a sudden change in heart rhythm or right heart function may be the first sign of air emboli.

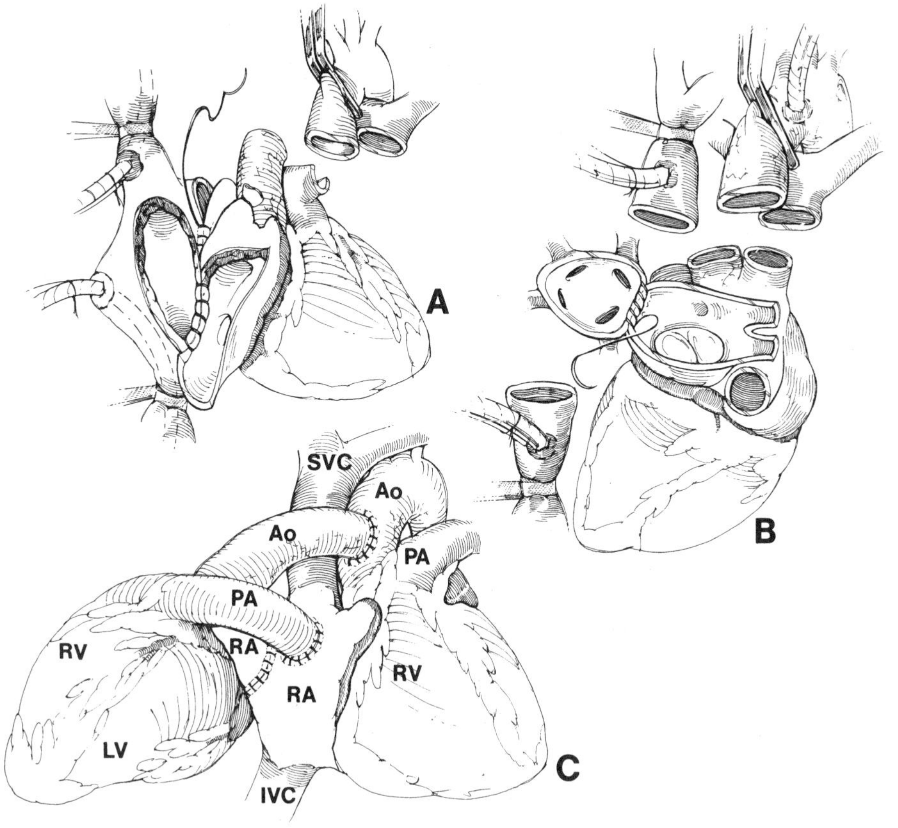

FIGURE 23-3. Surgical methods for cardiac transplantation. The traditional approach **(A)** involves anastomosis of the donor atrium to remnant atrial cuffs of the recipient as well as anastomoses of the great vessels. The bicaval technique **(B)** involves complete excision of the recipient's heart with end-to-end vena caval anastomoses along with the anastomoses of the aorta and pulmonary artery. Heterotopic cardiac transplantation **(C)** is performed by anastomosis of the donor and recipient atria and end-to-side anastomosis of the donor and recipient aortas. The donor's pulmonary artery is connected to either the recipient's right atrium or the recipient's pulmonary artery, depending on the adequacy of the donor's right ventricular function.

Usually the transplanted heart requires only moderate amounts of isoproterenol for chronotropic support, but not infrequently graft failure or profound systemic vasodilation complicates separation from CPB. The most common cause of inability to separate from CPB during heart transplantation is right-sided heart failure. The cause of right-sided heart failure after heart transplantation is thought to be sudden exposure of the unconditioned donor right ventricle to excessive afterload stress imposed by high PVR preexistent in the recipient. Refractory vasodilation may require norepinephrine, epinephrine, or vasopressin infusions to restore adequate vascular tone and optimize right ventricular myocardial perfusion (123). Occasionally, biventricular failure may result from damage to the heart before its harvest or from inadequate graft preservation during the harvest procedure (124).

Treatment of right-sided heart failure in this setting includes pulmonary vasodilation, augmentation of contractile strength, maintenance of adequate perfusion pressure, and optimization of preload. Pulmonary vasodilators such as nitroglycerin, sodium nitroprusside, prostacyclin, and prostaglandin E_1 reduce right ventricular afterload but also cause systemic hypotension (125,126). Inhaled NO has the advantage that its vasodilatory effects are confined to the pulmonary vasculature, owing to rapid binding and inactivation by hemoglobin (127). Positive inotropic drugs, such as dobutamine and milrinone, are especially effective when used together to augment right ventricular contractility while also reducing PVR (128,129). However, it is important that reductions in SVR caused by these "inodilators" be counteracted so as to maintain adequate perfusion pressure, because right ventricular ischemia has been shown to be a consequence of acute pulmonary hypertension (130). In addition to increasing perfusion pressure, raising systemic blood pressure serves to augment right ventricular systolic function via direct ventricular interactions; in other words, as left ventricular systolic pressure increases, there is greater transmission of forces across the septum to raise the right ventricular systolic pressure (131). However, the use of adrenergic agonists to raise perfusion pressure may also worsen pulmonary hypertension (132). Administration of norepinephrine directly into the left atrium to minimize delivery to the pulmonary vasculature is not effective in attenuating the pulmonary vascular response (126,133). Lastly, the central venous pressure should be high enough to maximize right ventricular Starling forces but not so high that intraventricular septal bowing encroaches on left ventricular filling (134). Acute right ventricular chamber dilation may also exacerbate tricuspid insufficiency and thereby decrease the efficiency of forward flow. In cases of refractory right-sided heart failure, right ventricular assist may be necessary to unload the ventricle and deliver adequate blood volume across the pulmonary bed (135,136).

Postoperative Management

With the exception of a few special considerations, the postoperative care of the cardiac transplantation patient is similar to that of other cardiac surgical patients. The lungs are mechanically ventilated until the patient is hemodynamically stable and normothermic and there is no evidence of other complications including excessive mediastinal bleeding. Reduced systolic and diastolic performance is often present after transplantation (137). As mentioned, right ventricular dysfunction is especially prevalent and this condition is an important cause of poor outcome. Because of the lack of autonomic nervous system innervation, the transplanted heart beats at the intrinsic rate of the donor's sinus node, usually 90 to 110 beats/minute (138). Reflex tachycardia caused by hypotension or stress responses is also necessarily delayed in the transplanted heart, and chronotropic responses are dependent on circulating catecholamine levels (139). Further, only drugs with direct sympathetic or parasympathetic agonist effects are effective. Perioperatively, bradycardia is reported to occur in more than 50% of transplantation patients in some series, necessitating continued chronotropic support after surgery with catecholamines (e.g., isoproterenol, dobutamine) or cardiac pacing (117). Permanent pacemaker insertion may be required in as many as 25% of patients (140). Cardiac arrhythmias are common, and their presence may be an indicator of acute rejection. The management of ventricular and atrial arrhythmias is similar to that in other cardiac surgical patients, including electrical cardioversion when the arrhythmia is associated with hemodynamic instability.

Infection is an important source of morbidity for the immunocompromised transplant recipient (2,8). Bacterial infections are the most likely cause of infections perioperatively, with opportunistic organisms becoming a dominant source of morbidity after 1 month (141–143). Prophylactic antibiotic regimens vary among institutions. The cause of any temperature greater than 38°C is aggressively sought by culturing of blood, sputum, and urine. To reduce the incidence of catheter-related sepsis, indwelling vascular catheters should be discontinued as early as possible or replaced with new catheters when they are still necessary. The lungs are the most common source of infection, and lung infections may be identified by chest radiography (2,142, 143). Empiric antibiotics may be indicated until culture results are available to guide therapy. Further diagnostic testing depends on the patient's clinical presentation.

Protocols for immunosuppression also vary among institutions. Induction of immunosuppression is started before the start of surgery with high doses of corticosteroids, cyclosporine, and azathioprine. Cytolytic therapy with OKT3 or antilymphocyte antibodies may also be used. Maintenance immunosuppression therapy often includes tapered doses of prednisone, azathioprine, and cyclosporine. The use of such three-drug regimens minimizes toxicity of individual drugs, especially nephrotoxicity, and hypertension associated with cyclosporine (144). Chronic immunosuppressive therapy with only cyclosporine and azathioprine allows for eventual discontinuance of prednisone (145). Immunosuppressive drugs and their toxicities are listed in Table 23-2.

Cardiac allograft rejection is categorized as hyperacute, acute, or chronic. Hyperacute rejection is a rare event that is caused by preformed antibodies from the recipient against donor antigens, often antibodies formed by prior exposure from blood transfusion or pregnancy (146). On reperfusion, the allograft immediately becomes cyanotic and nonfunctional. The prognosis for hyperacute rejection is poor despite intensive treatment with steroids, plasmapheresis, anticoagulation, and often insertion of a ventricular assist device (147). Acute rejection results from T lymphocytes directed at donor HLA antigens. Acute rejection occurs within the first 3 months after transplantation, often in the postoperative period (148). It is manifested as fever, arrhythmias, reduced ventricular performance, and pulmonary congestion. Endomyocardial biopsies are used for the diagnosis of and surveillance for acute rejection (149). Right ventricular biopsies are typically performed every 7 to 10 days after transplantation; the frequency is eventually reduced to every 3 to 6 months during the first year, after which they are performed only when there is suspicion of rejection (2). Rejection episodes are treated with an increased dose of methylprednisolone for several days (150). In cases of refractory rejection, high-dose steroids and additional therapy with OKT3 or antilymphocyte globulin and possibly tacrolimus, mycophenolate mofetil, or methotrexate are given (2, 151–153).

Chronic rejection is usually manifested as diffuse, concentric stenosis of the graft's coronary arteries (154). This process, termed allograft arteriopathy or vasculopathy, can be demonstrated in 42% of transplant recipients by angiography and in 75% of recipients by intracoronary artery ultrasound (IVUS) (155,156). Early diagnosis of the condition may allow for more effective treatment. The most sensitive method for diagnosis is IVUS, but improved results with noninvasive methods are encouraging, especially with dobutamine stress echocardiography (157,158). The latter techniques have low sensitivity but high specificity compared with IVUS (157,158). Allograft vasculopathy is believed to be secondary to immunologically mediated endothelial injury, but other recipient factors (e.g., dyslipidemia, diabetes, hypertension) and donor factors (e.g., older donor age, donor hypertension) may also play a role (154,159). The optimal treatment strategy for this condition is not clear. The introduction of cyclosporine has not changed the frequency of the condition, but preliminary data with newer second-generation immunosuppressants (e.g., rapamycin) suggest that these drugs may have a beneficial effect on

TABLE 23-2. IMMUNOSUPPRESSANT DRUGS, SIDE EFFECTS, AND PERIOPERATIVE IMPLICATIONS

Drug	Common Doses	Mechanism	Side Effects
Corticosteroids	*Cardiac treatment:* Methylprednisolone, 125 mg/kg × 3 doses; prednisone, 1 mg/kg/day tapered to 0.4 mg/kg then 0.2 mg/kg/day *Lung treatment:* Methylprednisolone, 500 mg before reperfusion; prednisone, 0.5 mg/kg/day × 3 mo then taper to 0.15 mg/kg/day (or equivalent)	Inhibit cytokine gene transcription and secretion from monocytes; ?lysis of lymphocytes	Hyperglycemia, hyperlipidemia, hypertension, myopathy, osteoporosis, avascular necrosis of the hip, cataracts, CNS effects (e.g., excitement, euphoria)
Azathioprine	*Preoperatively:* 4 mg/kg PO; 2 mg/kg IV *Postoperatively:* 1–3 mg/kg/day PO (adjusted to keep white blood count >4,000 cells/mm^3)	Intereferes with purine metabolism; blocks lymphocyte proliferation.	Leukopenia, thrombocytopenia, macrocytic anemia, hepatotoxicity, pancreatitis, nausea, acute increased nondepolarizing muscle relaxant requirements
Cyclosporine	*Preoperatively:* 4–10 mg/kg PO *Postoperatively:* 1–2 mg/kg/day IV (adjust for PO) then 5 mg/kg/day PO adjusted to trough level of 250–350 ng/mL	Inhibits lymphocyte IL-2 gene transcription; blunts lymphocyte proliferation	Nephrotoxicity, hypertension, neurotoxicity (tremor, headache, seizures), gingival hyperplasia, hirsutism, potentiation of nondepolarizing muscle relaxants
Tacrolimus	Adjusted to trough level of 10–20 g/mL	Inhibits lymphocyte IL-2 gene transcription; blunts lymphocyte proliferation	Nephrotoxicity, hypertension, hyperglycemia, neurotoxicity
Mycophenolate mofetil	1.0–1.5 g b.i.d.	Interferes with purine metabolism; blocks lymphocyte proliferation	Leukopenia, anemia, diarrhea, dyspepsia, emesis
Monoclonal antilymphocyte antibodies (OKT3)	5 mg/day *Pretreatment:* 8 mg/kg methylprednisolone, acetaminophen, antihistamines (1–4 hr before first few doses)	Depletes CD3 lymphocytes by phagocytosis; modulates T-lymphocyte interactions with antigen-presenting cells	Cytokine release syndrome with first dose—hypotension, pulmonary edema; azotemia, leukopenia, aseptic meningitis
Antilymphocyte globuin (ALG) or antithymocyte globulin (ATG)	10–30 mg/kg/day	Depletes lymphocytes by lysis or opsonization and phagocytosis	Leukopenia, thrombocytopenia, fever, allergic response to horse serum, serum sickness

Note: CNS, central nervous system; IL-2, interleukin 2.

neointimal hyperplasia and smooth muscle cell growth and could thereby be beneficial in reducing vascular responses to injury (160). Nonimmunologic therapies that have been suggested for allograft vasculopathy include diltiazem and pravastatin (161,162).

Outcomes

Perioperative mortality after cardiac transplantation is reported to be between 5% and 13% (163). The 1-year survival rate after cardiac transplantation is 79%, and the time to 50% survival (survival half-time) is 8.7 years (8). After the first year, survival declines linearly at 4% per year, with a survival half-time of 11.4 years (8). Risk factors for mortality after heart transplantation include prior transplantation, age, need for ventricular assist devices, mechanical ventilation of the lungs, recipient and donor age, donor ischemic time, and performance of transplantation at a center performing fewer than nine transplantations per year (8). Primary allograft failure and infection account for most early deaths after transplantation, but allograft coronary arteriopathy becomes the major cause of death 1 year after transplantation (2,154,163).

Anesthesia for the Patient with Prior Cardiac Transplantation

Patients who have previously undergone cardiac transplantation may require surgery for a variety of illnesses related and unrelated to transplantation (164). Both regional and general anesthesia can be used, depending on usual considerations of the procedure and the patient's condition. Decisions regarding the need for invasive patient monitoring and the choice of anesthetic drugs are based on similar considerations as for other patients. However, the perioperative care of the transplantation patient must take into account the unique physiology of the transplanted heart and the condition of the cardiac allograft. Patients with prior transplantation also require evaluation for several conditions that are common after transplantation and for adverse effects of immunosuppressive therapy (see Table 23-2).

Denervation of the transplanted heart results in impairment of autonomic reflex responses to stress and exercise. Normally, the onset of exercise is accompanied by synchronous increases in heart rate and stroke volume that combine to increase cardiac output in accordance with metabolic demands. In the transplanted heart, chronotropic responses to exercise and stress are delayed and the peak rate is attenuated (165,166). In addition to denervation, sinus nodal dysfunction may contribute to blunted chronotropic responses in the early posttransplantation period (167,168). The chronotropic responses to exercise do, however, improve by 6 months after transplantation (Fig. 23-4) (169). The latter finding might be explained by the β-adrenergic supersensitivity that occurs after transplantation is presynaptic in origin (170).

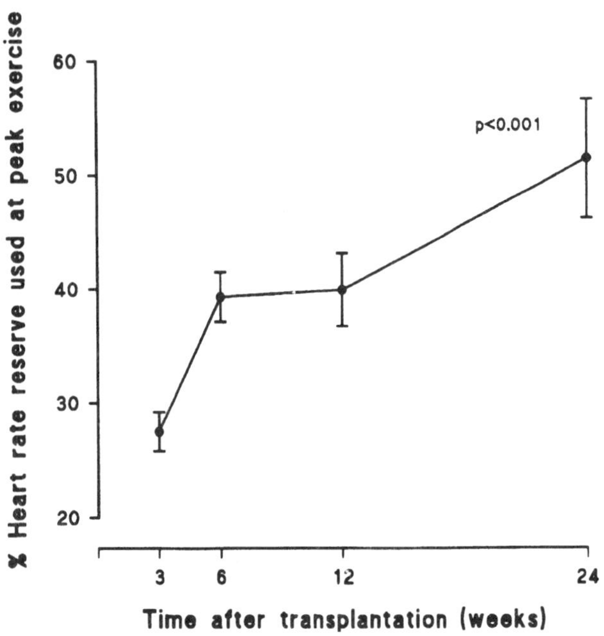

FIGURE 23-4. Peak heart rate during exercise at different time points after cardiac transplantation. There is a significant increase in chronotropic response to exercise 24 months after transplantation. (From Scott CD, Dark JH, McComb JM. Evolution of the chronotropic response to exercise after cardiac transplantation. *Am J Cardiol* 1995;76:1292, with permission.)

Although evidence of reinnervation has been demonstrated several years after transplantation, the clinical importance of these findings is not clear (171–173). The absence of meaningful cardiac autonomic input to the heart has important implications for pharmacologic responses perioperatively. Drugs with cardiac actions that depend on autonomic reflexes (e.g., atropine, digoxin, pancuronium) are ineffective in altering heart rate. For the same reason, opioid-induced bradycardia is absent. Drugs that are direct agonists to β-adrenergic receptors (e.g., epinephrine, isoproterenol) are chosen when treating bradycardia. Heart rate responses to vasodilation and vasoconstriction are also absent. Therefore, the normal increases and decreases in heart rate caused respectively by afterload reduction (e.g., with sodium nitroprusside, nicardipine) or increased blood pressure (e.g., with phenylephrine) do not occur. Similarly, cardiac output may be reduced more than usual when isoflurane is administered because the negative inotropic effects of this drug are not offset by reflex tachycardia. The β-adrenergic agonist effects of norepinephrine are also more apparent in the absence of reflex slowing of the heart rate when blood pressure is raised (174). β-Adrenergic supersensitivity enhances the response of the transplanted heart to epinephrine, norepinephrine, isoproterenol, and dobutamine, whereas drugs whose effects rely on the release of catecholamines from adrenergic nerves (indirectly acting drugs such as ephedrine and dopamine) may have reduced efficacy (170,174–176).

Patients with prior cardiac transplantation who are undergoing subsequent surgery require a careful evaluation of right and left ventricular function. Allograft rejection is manifested as reduced ventricular systolic function (148). Clinical evidence of congestive heart failure should be sought during the preoperative assessment. Elevations of cardiac filling pressures and PVR that are present before cardiac transplantation decline to the upper-normal range over the first 2 weeks after surgery, and the continued presence of elevations of these pressures requires investigation. Diastolic dysfunction with preserved systolic function, however, is common in the transplanted heart, and this condition may also manifest with signs of heart failure and elevated left ventricular end-diastolic pressure (177,178). Allograft coronary artery vasculopathy can also contribute to ventricular dysfunction (154,163). Diagnosis of the latter is problematic: typical angina may be absent due to denervation, noninvasive cardiac testing is insensitive for diagnosis, and coronary angiography may underestimate the extent of the condition (157,158,179–181).

Cardiac transplant recipients are susceptible to a variety of other illnesses, including cyclosporine-related renal dysfunction. The nephrotoxic effects of cyclosporine appear to be greatest during the first 6 months after transplantation, when dosage is the highest (181,182). Systemic hypertension is also common after transplantation because of increased SVR that results from cyclosporine and, to a lesser extent, fluid retention from treatment with steroids (183). Other conditions common in patients receiving long-term immunosuppressant drugs include an increased incidence of lymphoproliferative malignancies, bone marrow suppression, and complications from steroid therapy such as diabetes mellitus, avascular necrosis of the hip, and osteoporosis (2).

LUNG AND HEART-LUNG TRANSPLANTATION

The first successful heart-lung transplantation was reported by Reitz et al. in 1982 (184). Successful single-lung transplantation was reported in 1983, followed by reports of successful *en bloc* double-lung transplantation in 1988 and bilateral, sequential single-lung transplantation in 1989 (185–187). These landmarks were the culmination of more than 30 years of experimental and preliminary clinical investigations that had previously resulted in survival until hospital discharge of only a single patient (188–192). Eventual successes are attributed to improvements in the methods of preventing and treating three major complications of transplantation: infection, airway complications, and rejection. Today, lung transplantation is no longer considered experimental; rather, it is a therapeutic option for a variety of end-stage pulmonary illnesses. The number of lung transplantation operations has grown considerably over the last 10 years (a cumulative total of 4,777 single- and 3,278 double-lung transplantations were reported as of March 1998), but the indications are relatively unchanged (Fig. 23-5) (8). In contrast to lung transplantation, heart-lung transplantation is less frequently performed (151 procedures in 1997, compared with 241 in 1989) (8). Congenital heart disease complicated by Eisenmenger's syndrome and primary pulmonary hypertension (PPH) are the most common indications for heart-lung transplantation (8).

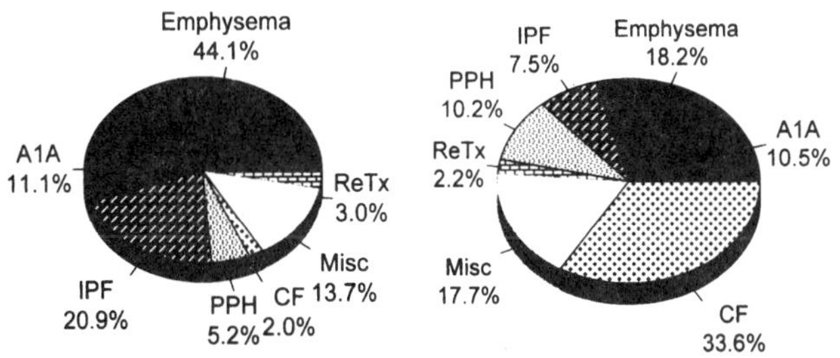

FIGURE 23-5. Indications for **(A)** single- and **(B)** bilateral lung transplantation for adults. A1A, α_1-antitrypsin; ReTx, retransplantation; CF, cystic fibrosis; PPH, primary pulmonary hypertension; IPF, idiopathic pulmonary fibrosis. (From Hosenpud JD, Bennett LE, Keck BM, et al. The registry of the international society of heart and lung transplantation: fifteenth official report—1998. *J Heart Lung Transplant* 1998;17:656, with permission.)

Selection of Recipients for Lung Transplantation

Candidates for lung transplantation are those with advanced lung disease who have failed alternative medical treatments and who have a high risk of death within 2 to 3 years (193, 194). General guidelines for recipient selection are listed in Table 23-3, although the ultimate selection criteria vary among institutions. Age guidelines usually require the patient to be younger than 50 to 55 years for bilateral lung transplantation, 60 to 65 years for single-lung transplantation, or 45 to 50 years for heart-lung transplantation (193,

TABLE 23-3. GUIDELINES FOR RECIPIENT SELECTION FOR LUNG TRANSPLANTATION

General indications	
End-stage lung disease	
Failure of medical treatment or no alternative available	
Life expectancy less than 2–3 yr	
Ability to walk and undergo rehabilitation	
Sound nutritional status (~80% to 120% of ideal body weight)	
Stable psychosocial profile and likely adherence to postoperative care	
Disease-specific indications	
COPD	FEV_1 <25% of predicted value after bronchodilators
	Clinically significant hypoxemia, hypercapnia, Pulmonary hypertension
	Frequent exacerbations or declining lung function
Cystic fibrosis	FEV_1 <30% of predicted value
	Hypoxemia, hypercapnia or rapidly declining lung function
	Weight loss
	Frequent exacerbations
Idiopathic pulmonary fibrosis	Vital capacity <60%–65% of predicted
	Resting hypoxemia
	Progression of disease
	Pulmonary hypertension
Pulmonary hypertension	NYHA functional status class III or IV
	Mean right atrial pressure >10 mm Hg
	Mean pulmonary artery pressure >50 mm Hg
	Cardiac index is <2.5 L/min/m^2
Contraindications	
Unstable clinical status	
Untreatable or poorly controlled infection (lung or extrapulmonary)	
Active cancer	
Vital organ dysfunction, including significant coronary artery disease, renal insufficiency (creatinine clearance <50 mL/min), hepatic dysfunction (portal hypertension, coagulopathy)	
Continued tobacco abuse	
Continued substance abuse	
Poorly controlled psychiatric illness likely to lead to noncompliance with medical therapy	

Note: COPD, chronic obstructive pulmonary disease; FEV_1, forced expiratory volume in 1 second; NYHA, New York Health Association

194). Decisions regarding lung transplantation are individualized for patients who are ventilator dependent, have had prior chest surgery or prior pleurodesis, have other poorly controlled medical conditions, are colonized with highly antibiotic-resistant bacteria, or have a high level of allosensitization (8,195,196). Severe coronary artery disease with impaired left ventricular function is considered a contraindication to lung transplantation, but such patients may be considered for heart-lung transplantation. Timing of candidacy for lung or heart-lung transplantation is critical, because the median waiting time for organs is typically 18 months (193). Disease-specific indications for lung transplantation are based on general physiologic parameters associated with poor prognosis (Table 23-3) (193,194, 197–200). For example, for patients with emphysema, the 3-year survival rate declines to 60% to 70% when the 1-second forced expiratory volume (FEV_1) is less than 30% of the predicted value (193,197,198). Because the death rate while waiting for lung transplantation is highest for patients with idiopathic pulmonary fibrosis (IPF), a 90-day credit is given for this diagnosis on listing for transplantation (193,194,201,202).

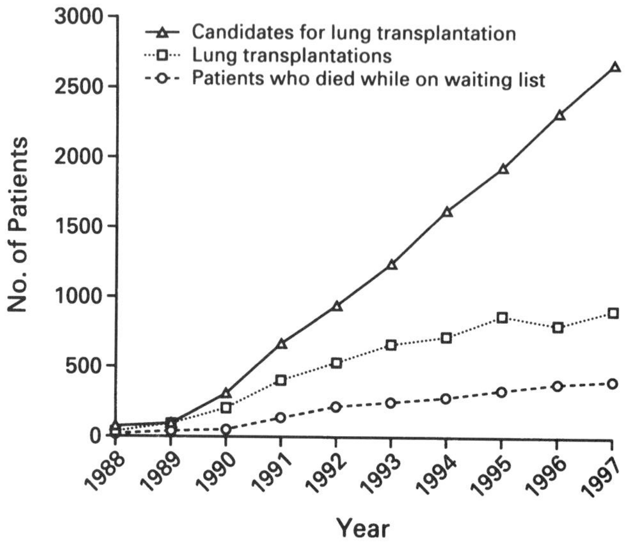

FIGURE 23-6. Number of patients undergoing lung transplantation in the United States. The number of procedures has reached a plateau owing to the limited availability of donor lungs, despite a growing number of candidates for the procedure. (Reproduced with permission.)

Donor Selection

Patients meeting criteria for brain death (see earlier discussion) are considered as donors for lung transplantation when they meet the general guidelines summarized in Table 23-4. Patients are excluded from organ donation when there is septicemia, HIV infection, tuberculosis, viral hepatitis, substance abuse, malignancy, or other severe medical conditions. Thoracic dimensions between donor and recipient are approximated based on the chest radiograph or predicted lung volumes (193). The discrepancy between the number of donor lungs and the number of candidates awaiting transplantation continues to grow (Fig. 23-6). The use of marginal donors (e.g., donors with localized opacity on chest radiography, those with an arterial oxygen tension of less than 300 mm Hg on 100% oxygen) is increasingly employed without compromising the results (203). Donor selection for heart-lung transplantation must meet both these criteria and those previously outlined for cardiac transplantation.

TABLE 23-4. GENERAL GUIDELINES FOR SELECTING SUITABLE DONORS FOR LUNG TRANSPLANTATION

Age ≤65 y
Absence of significant lung disease with <30 pack-years of tobacco use
Clear chest radiograph
Peak airway pressures <30 cm H_2O
Pao_2 >300 mm Hg with Fio_2 of 100%
Satisfactory bronchoscopic examination

Note: Fio_2, fraction of inspired oxygen; Pao_2, arterial partial pressure of oxygen.

Preoperative Evaluation

Preparation of the patient immediately before transplantation includes a focused history and physical examination. The patient's airway is carefully inspected for ease of placement of a double-lumen endobronchial tube, and the patient is evaluated for evidence of bronchospasm or right ventricular dysfunction. Previously completed diagnostic test results should also be reviewed, although varying intervals of time will have elapsed between the preliminary testing and transplantation. Particular attention is given to pulmonary function test results, ventilation-perfusion scan findings, assessments of right and left ventricular function, and cardiac catheterization data including intracardiac pressures and pulmonary artery pressures. Patients awaiting transplantation are enrolled in intensive pulmonary rehabilitation programs, and the patient's tolerance of physical activity provides an index of any deterioration in physical status since preoperative diagnostic testing. Comprehensive medical records are kept for each transplantation candidate, and review of these records can provide valuable information regarding the patient's current overall condition.

Despite the intensive preparation before transplantation, notification of donor lung availability invariably evokes a great deal of anxiety in the patient. The use of premedication is individualized but is tempered by concerns of respiratory depression in a patient with end-stage lung disease and by the fact that the procedure may always be canceled until the point of donor organ visualization. In the latter case, the patient is discharged from the hospital. Small doses of short-acting benzodiazepines (e.g., 0.5 to 1 mg midazolam) can be used judiciously. Patients typically have recently ingested food or liquids, necessitating premedication with metoclopramide, a histamine$_2$-antagonist, and/or a nonparticulate antacid. In preparing the patient, a large-bore intravenous catheter and an intraarterial catheter are placed. Epidural catheters are usually inserted before surgery unless contraindicated. Controversy persists regarding the use of an epidural catheter in a patient who may potentially require anticoagulation for CPB. Arguments in favor of preoperative epidural catheter placement include the fact that CPB usually is not necessary for patients with obstructive lung disease or for older cystic fibrosis patients. Further, the time interval between catheter placement and heparinization is long enough to allow adequate clot formation should bleeding occur during epidural placement.

Surgical Procedure

Single-lung transplantation offers technical advantages and maximizes the use of organs for multiple recipients. This procedure is performed via a posterolateral thoracotomy with the patient in the lateral decubitus position. Choosing the side for transplantation depends on ventilation-perfusion distribution (the lung with worse function is preferred for transplantation), whether there was prior surgery, and donor factors. End-to-end bronchial anastomosis using a tissue wrap of omentum was an initial approach to improve collateral blood flow to the bronchus, but this method has been supplanted by the telescoping anastomosis, wherein cartilaginous areas of the donor and recipient are intussuscepted (204–206). Direct bronchial artery revascularization is technically possible but is not routinely used because of the added complexity of the procedure and because its benefits have not been clearly defined (207,208).

Single-lung transplantation has been used for IPF, PPH, and chronic obstructive pulmonary disease (COPD) (8,193, 194,209–213). Normalization of pulmonary artery pressure and resolution of right ventricular hypertrophy and dysfunction are observed early after transplantation for patients with pulmonary hypertension (212–215). Nonetheless, this surgical approach has limitations. PVR is high in the remaining diseased lung of patients with PPH; as a result, the newly transplanted lung receives most of the pulmonary perfusion while ventilation is evenly distributed. Pulmonary artery pressures and oxygenation can be labile perioperatively, but others have reported no difference in early oxygenation and weaning from mechanical ventilation between patients receiving single- versus double-lung transplantation for PPH (216,217). Less functional recovery and a higher 15-month mortality rate were reported for patients with PPH who received single-lung transplantation, but more recent data suggest that actuarial survival is no different between single- versus double-lung transplantation for this disease (217,218). For patients with COPD, single-lung transplantation is associated with a lower rate of early complications compared with double-lung transplantation (209). Overdistention of the native, compliant, emphysematous lung, compromising ventilation of the new lung, was an initial concern with single-lung transplantation for COPD, but this phenomenon is infrequently observed (209,219).

Bilateral lung transplantation was initially performed via a median sternotomy using CPB for the *en bloc* implantation of both lungs and the trachea (220). Bilateral sequential lung transplantation, in which the right and left lungs are separately implanted using methods similar to those of single-lung transplantation, is now the preferred technique (221,222). Surgical access is via bilateral anterior thoracotomy with or without lower transverse sternotomy ("clamshell" incision). Bilateral sequential lung transplantation offers several advantages, including avoidance of CPB (one-lung ventilation performed to contralateral lung during implantation of each single lung) and improved healing of the bronchial compared with a tracheal anastomosis.

Bilateral sequential lung transplantation is the preferred technique for patients with cystic fibrosis or bronchiectasis, in whom removal of both lungs is needed to avoid bacterial contamination of the newly transplanted lung. Bilateral sequential lung transplantation using lobes from two living compatible adult donors is a newer option for extremely ill patients with cystic fibrosis who are unlikely to survive the wait for a cadaver donor (223). As discussed previously, there is uncertainty regarding the most appropriate method of transplantation for patients with PPH or IPF, with some centers now favoring bilateral sequential lung transplantation for these conditions (217–219). Bilateral lung transplantation for patients with COPD is associated with improved lung function and slightly improved 1- to 4-year survival, compared with single-lung transplantation (224–226). Since single-lung transplantation is a simpler operation, the decision to perform single versus bilateral lung transplantation is individualized based on donor and recipient factors but the former procedure may be advantageous for more complicated patients.

Heart-lung transplantation in the past was used for patients with PPH or Eisenmenger's syndrome, but single- or bilateral sequential lung transplantation is now used for both conditions (227,228). Combined heart-lung transplantation is indicated for patients who need lung transplantation and have uncorrectable congenital heart anomalies, impaired left ventricular function, and/or coronary disease. Heart-lung transplantation is usually performed through a median sternotomy, but the clamshell incision is a suitable alternative.

Intraoperative Management

The monitoring of patients undergoing lung transplantation is similar to that used for patients undergoing cardiac surgery. A pulmonary artery catheter with continuous mixed venous oximetry can facilitate rapid interpretation of intraoperative and postoperative changes in cardiac output, arterial oxygenation, oxygen consumption, and hemoglobin concentration when used in conjunction with other monitors and laboratory data. TEE is routinely used in lung transplantation for assessment of left and right ventricular function and evaluation of vascular anastomoses.

Pulmonary hypertension and/or hypoxemia during transplantation may warrant the use of NO, although this drug has not yet received FDA approval. Methods used to deliver NO (by physicians sanctioned by the FDA) include a simple delivery system using an H-size NO cylinder (2, 200 ppm at 2,000 psi) attached via a two-stage pressure regulator to deliver flows of 1/16 to 1 L/minute. Chemiluminescence methods are used to measure NO and nitrogen dioxide concentrations. Administration of NO via an H-size cylinder attached to the breathing circuit has the potential to deliver an hypoxic gas mixture. Care must be taken to measure inspired oxygen concentrations distal to the site where NO is delivered. A commercially available system (INOvent, Datex-Ohmeda, Madison, WI) has two NO cylinders (1,963 L per cylinder, 800 ppm at 2,000 psi) and a system to deliver and measure set concentrations (0.1 to 100 ppm) of NO. The delivery is flow independent, unlike the previous simple cylinder–pressure regulator setup. Furthermore, the INOvent measures oxygen and nitrogen dioxide concentrations. The setup of the INOvent requires calibration of a low and a high concentration before use (requiring 5 minutes or longer), and the device and circuit adapters are much more complicated than those of the the simple NO cylinder–pressure regulator setup.

The timing of patient preparation and anesthesia induction depends on the progress of donor lung procurement. Frequent communication with the transplantation coordinator who is tracking donor harvest progress is essential. Most often, the patient is prepared and anesthesia induced only after organ visualization. Lung transplantation is an emergency procedure necessitating consideration of a rapid-sequence induction or awake intubation for patients in whom difficulty in securing the airway may be anticipated. The goals of the anesthetic induction, therefore, are to minimize hemodynamic and respiratory compromise and prevent aspiration. Typically, while the patient is breathing 100% oxygen, 2 to 4 μg/kg fentanyl is given and anesthesia is induced with either etomidate and thiopental supplemented with a skeletal muscle relaxant and volatile anesthetics. When the patient is adequately anesthetized, a left-sided double-lumen tube is placed and its position is confirmed by fiberoptic bronchoscopy. Maintenance of anesthesia is with a combination of opioids, benzodiazepines, nondepolarizing muscle relaxants, and volatile anesthetics. Nitrous oxide is not used during lung transplantation because of the frequent requirement of high inspired oxygen concentrations, concerns for expansion of pneumothorax or intracardiac air introduced during pulmonary venous anastomosis, and the need to avoid potential increases in PVR.

Induction of anesthesia in patients with COPD is often complicated by sudden hypotension. Although the usual causes of hemodynamic instability must be excluded, hypotension in this group of patients is commonly caused by dynamic airway collapse leading to increased intrathoracic pressures or self-controlled end-expiratory pressure ("auto-PEEP") (Fig. 23-7). The higher intrathoracic pressure reduces venous return and may also compress vascular structures and the heart to reduce stroke volume. This condition should always be anticipated. Its treatment consists in opening the breathing circuit to the atmosphere to allow for more complete exhalation. If blood pressure does not promptly increase after this maneuver, other causes of hypotension should be considered. Intermittent ventilation of the patient

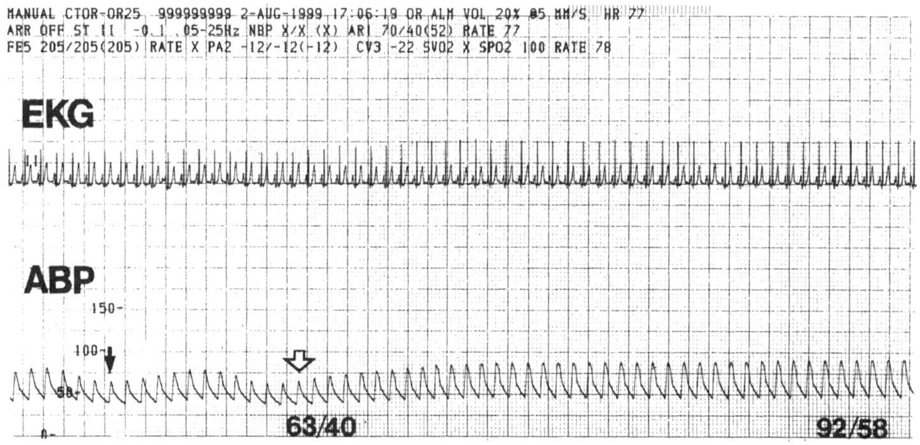

FIGURE 23-7. A representative hemodynamic tracing demonstrating hypotension from self-controlled end-expiratory pressure ("auto-PEEP") that developed with positive-pressure ventilation during induction of anesthesia in a patient with severe emphysema. The tracing (running at 5 mm/sec) demonstrates profound variation in arterial blood pressure (ABP) during inspiration *(small black arrow)*, which improves on disconnection of the patient from the ventilator circuit and opening of the airway to the atmosphere. The following maneuver resulted in an increase in blood pressure from 63/40 to 92/58 mm Hg.

may be required until the pleurae are opened. Tension pneumothorax is a rarer cause of hemodynamic instability during anesthesia induction, but it can occur in any patient with end-stage lung disease receiving positive-pressure ventilation or as a result of central venous cannulation. Falling oxygen saturation, increasing peak airway pressures, and hypotension not responsive to the usual treatments should prompt aggressive exclusion or treatment of tension pneumothorax. Negative inotropic effects of anesthetics, hypoxemia, hypercarbia, and increased sympathetic responses to stimulation can all contribute to increased PVR and right ventricular dysfunction during anesthesia induction, particularly for patients with pulmonary hypertension. After ensuring the adequacy of oxygenation and ventilation, further treatment is aimed at reducing right ventricular afterload with pulmonary vasodilators, increasing myocardial contractility, and ensuring adequate perfusion to the right ventricle. Patients with preexisting pulmonary hypertension are especially prone to right ventricular dysfunction. Anesthesia induction and maintenance in such patients should be slow, and histamine-releasing drugs should be avoided. The patient should not be stimulated until anesthesia is adequate and hypotension is avoided. Consideration of a narcotic-based induction should be given for this group of patients. In the lung transplant recipient who presents *in extremis*, it may even be necessary to consider CPB before or during the induction of anesthesia.

Anesthesia for patients with cystic fibrosis or bronchiectasis requires several special considerations. Because of the presence of thick, copious secretions, these patients benefit from the initial placement of a single-lumen endotracheal tube and bronchoscopy for systematic suctioning of pulmonary segments. Next, a left-sided double-lumen endobronchial tube is placed. During surgery in patients with cystic fibrosis, the dissection for explantation of the native lungs is often difficult. The result is a large surface area of abraded pleura that can lead to excessive bleeding, especially if CPB is needed. Patients with cystic fibrosis are also prone to reduced SVR leading to hypotension. The cause of the latter has not been proven, but it is suspected that dissection and compression of the septic lung results in the release of bacteria and other pyrogens, leading to a systemic inflammatory state.

CPB is used electively for patients with preexisting pulmonary hypertension and for those undergoing heart-lung transplantation. In addition to increasing the complexity of surgery, the use of CPB during lung transplantation may exacerbate lung graft dysfunction, resulting in a longer period of mechanical ventilation and increased duration of hospitalization (229–231). Insofar as patients having hemodynamic and oxygenation difficulties are more likely to require urgent CPB than others, it is difficult to separate the effects of CPB on patient outcomes from those of the lung allograft condition that necessitated bypass. Clinically, before proceeding with lung explantation, a trial of pulmonary artery cross-clamping is performed, especially for patients with limited right ventricular function or elevated pulmonary arterial pressures or both. First, the surgeon ensures that the pulmonary artery catheter is not in the operative lung. During clamping of the pulmonary artery, right ventricular function is evaluated with TEE and by observation of the hemodynamic response. Clinical judgment dictates whether CPB should be instituted, but this support is more likely for patients developing mixed venous oxygen desaturation and reduced cardiac output (229,232). Reduction in PVR with the use of NO has been reported to help avoid unplanned CPB in these situations (233). Despite these measures, unplanned CPB is necessary in 17% to 41% of patients—mostly for patients with restrictive lung disease and less often for those with COPD, although predicting which patients will require CPB unexpectedly is difficult (229,232,234). Early graft dysfunction during bilateral sequential lung transplantation is a challenging development. Increased capillary permeability and pulmonary hypertension associated with graft dysfunction result in pulmonary edema when the entire cardiac output perfuses the first-transplanted lung while the contralateral pulmonary artery is clamped. In some instances, the timely use of CPB is a more prudent approach than attempting to avoid CPB "at all costs."

Use of CPB during cardiac operations is known to activate the coagulation and fibrinolytic systems, leading to excessive nonsurgical bleeding after longer procedures (235, 236). These perturbations lead to consumption of coagulation factors and platelets as well as the breakdown of fibrin clot. Not surprisingly, blood transfusion requirements are higher for patients undergoing lung transplantation when CPB is used (231). The extent of blood loss is affected by the difficulty of dissection, the presence of extensive scarring, and collateral blood flow. Patients with cystic fibrosis or bronchiectasis are particularly prone to higher blood loss during lung transplantation. Aprotinin may be useful in reducing blood loss in these circumstances (237,238). Otherwise, treatment is with transfusion of platelets and/or fresh-frozen plasma as needed to correct specific deficiencies of coagulation factors.

The implantation of the donor lung proceeds in a posterior to anterior fashion, usually from the bronchial to the pulmonary artery, and then the pulmonary vein-atrial anastomosis. Near the time of completion of the latter, the lung is reexpanded by hand ventilation and the pulmonary artery clamp is opened slightly to flush out air from the vascular tree of the donor lung. Attention should be focused on the TEE to ensure adequate de-airing. On completion of the pulmonary vein-atrial anastomosis and de-airing of the pulmonary vascular tree, ventilation to the donor lung is reestablished and the pulmonary artery and left atrial clamps are removed. Severe hypotension is commonly seen at this point; it is probably caused by the presence of vasodilators (e.g., PGE_1, nitroprusside) in the preservative solution and loss of blood volume in the allograft vascular bed. To minimize postperfusion hypotension, a rapid infusion of crystalloid (5–10 mL/kg) along with a potent vasoconstrictor (e.g., phenylephrine) should precede removal of the vascular clamps. Generally, on ventilation and reperfusion of the donor lung, an immediate improvement in pulmonary airway compliance is noted concurrent with a reduction of pulmonary artery pressures. Positive end-expiration pressure (5 cm H_2O) is added to the circuit to enhance reexpansion and to possibly limit alveolar edema. After a short interval (e.g., 5 minutes) of ventilation to both lungs, an arterial blood gas determination is obtained to ensure adequate oxygenation and ventilation. For bilateral sequential lung transplantation, once the patient is stabilized, one-lung ventilation is instituted to the newly transplanted lung and the remaining lung is dissected and removed.

Careful surveillance is required during transplantation of the second lung for adequacy of oxygenation and for the development of signs of pulmonary edema or evidence of early graft dysfunction. Early graft dysfunction is a complication of lung transplantation that occurs in 15% to 35% of recipients and varies in magnitude from mild pulmonary infiltrates to florid adult respiratory distress syndrome (193). The mortality rate has been reported to be 16%, making this condition the most common cause of early mortality (239,240). The cause of early graft dysfunction is thought to be ischemia-reperfusion injury resulting from oxygen-derived free radicals and inflammatory cytokines leading to increased capillary permeability and alveolar edema (241,242). Graft dysfunction usually becomes apparent in the operating room, and hypoxemia, pulmonary hypertension, worsened pulmonary compliance, and production of copious amounts of pink-brown secretions in the endobronchial tube characterize it. Treatment is aimed at optimizing oxygenation. In the past, severe forms of transplanted lung dysfunction have required extracorporeal membrane oxygenation (ECMO), but the use of NO has reduced the frequency of need for extracorporeal oxygenation for this condition (240,243,244). Laboratory investigations have shown that capillary permeability after transplantation is directly related to donor lung inflation volume at the time of harvest (245). Use of low lung inflation volumes before donor lung explantation (i.e., donor trachea clamped at functional residual capacity) has contributed to a lower frequency of graft dysfunction. Experimentally, inhalation of NO reduces allograft dysfunction, possibly because of its effects of reducing neutrophil aggregation, adhesion, and resultant oxygen-derived free radical production (246–248). Novel methods of donor lung preservation and gene therapy show promise as potential strategies for attenuating reperfusion injury (248–253).

Technical difficulties with the vascular anastomosis are unusual but should, nonetheless, be excluded when the pulmonary arterial pressures are elevated or early graft dysfunction is suspected. A pressure gradient can be measured across the anastomosis with the use of a pulmonary artery catheter by palpating the location of the catheter tip and advancing the catheter across the anastamosis (254). However, when the arterial anastomosis is in question, direct pressure measurements should be obtained proximal and distal to the anastomosis, through the use of a small-bore needle attached to a pressure tubing passed off the sterile field. Pulmonary arterial and venous anastomosis can also be evaluated with TEE (255–257). Narrowed pulmonary veins along with turbulent flow on color Doppler flow examination and loss of normal phasic flow patterns are TEE manifestations of venous obstruction (257).

Incomplete de-airing before completion of the venous-atrial anastomosis can lead to coronary air embolism and myocardial ischemia. Varying degrees of "microbubbles" can be seen in most patients with TEE after release of the pulmonary venous cross-clamp. Regional and global myocardial dysfunction detected with the TEE, along with ST segment elevation/depression, are observed in severe cases. These changes are usually transient and typically respond to intravenous nitroglycerin and vasopressors. The acute reduction in pulmonary pressures after lung transplantation may lead to a sudden decrease in cavity size of the hypertrophied right ventricle, resulting in right ventricular outflow tract obstruction (258). This rare complication can be detected with TEE and is treated by increasing the ventricular preload.

At the completion of surgery, a single-lumen endotracheal tube is placed. Careful inspection of the upper airway with a laryngoscope is required before removal of the double-lumen endobronchial tube. Upper airway edema, common due to large crystalloid infusion and extended operative times, may complicate placement of the new endotracheal tube. In this situation, consideration is given to either using an endobronchial tube exchanger or, rarely, leaving the double-lumen endobronchial tube in place.

Postoperative Management

Patient management issues after lung transplantation include ventilatory support, optimization of hemodynamics, immunosuppression, and the management of complications including early graft dysfunction, rejection, infections, and airway complications. The care after surgery of the heart-lung transplant recipient combines these aims with the previously outlined management after heart transplantation. Full ventilatory support with the lowest fraction of inspired oxygen that is compatible with adequate oxygenation is employed until the patient meets standard criteria for weaning. Rarely, patients with COPD who have undergone single-lung transplantation require independent lung ventilation using a double-lumen endobronchial tube because overdistention of the native lung compromises oxygenation/ventilation (259). Independent lung ventilation may need to be started in the operating room using a intensive care unit–type ventilator. The transplanted lung is ventilated with tidal volumes of 8 to 10 mL/kg and low levels of PEEP, and the rate is adjusted to maintain normocapnia and pH. The native lung is ventilated with tidal volumes of 2 to 3 mL/kg and a lower rate. This condition typically improves with restoration of spontaneous ventilation. Patients with PPH often have episodes of pulmonary hypertension and oxygen desaturation after surgery with minimal stimulation (especially after single-lung transplantation). Heavy sedation with an opioid and a benzodiazepine and full ventilatory support may need to be maintained for 24 to 48 hours after surgery. Because of the interruption of lymphatic drainage and the increased capillary permeability, alveolar edema in the newly transplanted lung is a persistent threat. Generally, fluids are minimized to the lowest level of ventricular filling pressure needed to maintain hemodynamics and urine output. Postoperative analgesia facilitates deep breathing and early ambulation. Epidural narcotics given via an indwelling catheter are used in the early postoperative period for these purposes. Consideration should be given to placing an epidural catheter after surgery for patients who did not have one inserted before the procedure, although any persistent coagulopathy must first be corrected.

Immunosuppressant drugs are started before lung transplantation, and this regimen is continued for 5 to 10 days. Drugs chosen for this induction phase of immunosuppression usually consist of a corticosteroid, cyclosporine, and azathioprine with or without lymphocyte depletion therapy (e.g., OKT3, antithymocyte globulin), but there is little evidence regarding superiority of any particular protocol (193,260,261). Maintenance therapy is with two or three drugs. Steroids are tapered or even discontinued in some protocols. Tacrolimus and mycophenolate mofetil offer new options, and preliminary data comparing these newer drugs with traditional immunosuppressants are encouraging (11, 262,263). Drugs employed for immunosuppression and their toxicities are listed in Table 23-2. Specific anesthetic interactions include a modest increase in the dose of nondepolarizing muscle relaxants after acute azathioprine administration and a potentiation of neuromuscular blockade by cyclosporine (264,265).

Despite current immunosuppression regimens, at least one episode of acute rejection occurs in most recipients (193,194), typically during the first 100 days after lung transplantation, after which the risk persists at a lower rate (239). Mild forms of acute rejection may be subclinical in some patients, but it is usually manifested by nonspecific symptoms such as fever, malaise, cough, dyspnea, leukocytosis, and declining oxygenation (266,267). Interstitial changes, alveolar densities, and pleural effusions are common, but chest radiologic findings are insensitive for its detection (268). Acute rejection episodes are associated with a reduction of 10% or more in forced vital capacity and FEV_1 (269,270). Differentiating acute rejection from infection based on clinical diagnosis, radiologic findings, or spirometry is difficult, and misdiagnosis can lead to incorrect treatment or unnecessary subjection of patients to augmented immunosuppression. Histologic analysis of transbronchial biopsy specimens is the preferred method for diagnosis of rejection (193,194,266,267). Acute rejection is treated with methylprednisolone (15 mg/kg/day intravenously for 3 days) and by optimization of other immunosuppressant drugs. Repeat transbronchial biopsy is recommended after episodes of acute rejection to confirm the efficacy of treatment (193,266,267). Persistent or recurrent rejection is treated aggressively, because its occurrence is an important risk factor for bronchiolitis obliterans syndrome (BOS) (271).

For a variety of reasons, including constant allograft exposure to the external environment and prior colonization of the upper respiratory tract or sinuses, heart-lung and lung transplantation patients are more susceptible to infections than are recipients of other transplanted organs (193). The most common infection is bacterial pneumonia, which is reported to occur in 10% of lung allograft recipients, most often during the first 2 weeks after transplantation (272, 273). Infection caused by cytomegalovirus (CMV) is the second most common infection after lung transplantation (271,274). This virus can be acquired via reactivation of latent infection, transmission from the donor lung, or blood transfusion (193). Infection from CMV is unusual the first 2 weeks after transplantation. It is most often manifested as pneumonitis, and its presentation can be confused with acute rejection (193,275).

All patients receive broad-spectrum prophylactic antibiotics for several days; this therapy is adjusted based on the results of donor and recipient bronchial cultures. For patients with cystic fibrosis, prophylactic antibiotics are chosen based on preoperative culture and sensitivity results, and aerosolized colistin or tobramycin is also given. The routine use of prophylactic acyclovir has reduced the frequency of herpes simplex infections (193). Trimethoprim-sulfamethoxazole is given for prevention of *Pneumocystis carinii* infection (inhaled pentamidine is an alternative for patients with sulfa allergies). Treatment of bacterial infection is guided by culture and sensitivity findings. Empiric therapy should include antibiotics active against gram-negative bacteria, especially *Pseudomonas* species. Ganciclovir is used to treat CMV infections. Other less common infections in heart-lung and lung transplant recipients include other viruses (e.g., herpes simplex, adenovirus, influenza, parainfluenza) and fungi (e.g., *Candida, Aspergillus*) (193,194).

Airway complications are less common with modern surgical techniques compared with early experiences with lung transplantation. These complications include airway dehiscence, stenosis, and bronchomalacia, and their presence is associated with significant morbidity. These conditions are manifested as cough, wheezing, dyspnea, pulmonary infiltrates on radiologic examination, and airflow obstruction with spirometric testing (193). Diagnosis of airway complications is by bronchoscopic examination, although computer tomographic scan results can be complementary (276). The management is individualized from a variety of methods, including bronchial dilation, stenting, and laser removal of granulation tissue (277,278).

Outcomes

Actuarial survival is not different after single versus bilateral lung transplantation (time to 50% survival, 3.6 and 4.5 years, respectively) (8). Overall, the 1-, 2-, and 3-year survival rates for patients undergoing lung transplantation are 72%, 63%, and 56%, respectively, with survival highest for patients with COPD and lowest for patients with IPF, PPH, or retransplantation (8,193,194). Survival after heart-lung transplantation is lower, with the time to 50% survival being 2.6 years (8). The most common causes of early death are infection and graft dysfunction, whereas infection and rejection are the main causes of late mortality. Mortality after lung transplantation is lower in the period since 1994 than it was during the period 1988–1990 (8). There are limited data regarding whether lung transplantation improves survival compared with the natural history of the diseases, but this appears to be the case for patients with cystic fibrosis or IPF (279). BOS is the main obstacle to long-term survival (193,194).

In addition to survival, lung transplantation leads to improvements in lung function, exercise capacity, and quality of life (193,194). Oxygenation improves early after lung transplantation, but peak improvements in lung function are delayed for at least 3 months after surgery. Pulmonary function increases after both single and bilateral lung transplantation to near-normal values, but the improvements depend on the underlying diagnosis and the procedure. After single-lung transplantation for COPD, FEV_1 reaches 45% to 60% of predicted, with the donor lung accounting for 60% to 80% of ventilation (193). Lung function after bilateral transplantation for COPD recovers to near-normal values. Pulmonary hemodynamics improve early after transplantation for PPH, and there is a sustained improvement in right ventricular function detectable by 3 months after surgery (212–215).

Surgery in the Patient with Prior Lung Transplantation

Several special considerations exist for the perioperative care of patients with a prior lung transplantation who require surgery for other conditions. Lung transplantation results in complete lung denervation, and there is no evidence that reinnervation occurs even after long-term follow-up (280). Therefore, the cough reflex is intact proximal to the airway anastomosis (usually bronchial) but absent in the transplanted lung. Mucociliary function is also impaired, further contributing to reduced clearance of secretions (281). Airway hyperreactivity in the transplanted lung has not been a clinical problem, but there is a concern for denervation hypersensitivity of muscarinic receptors after lung transplantation (193,282–285). Exercise and isocapnic hyperventilation do not appear to appreciably increase airway reactivity in the transplanted lung, but increased airway resistance after methacholine challenge has been demonstrated, although the data are inconsistent (11,282–285). Hypoxic pulmonary vasoconstriction remains intact after lung transplantation, and denervation does not effect central respiratory control (286). Hypercapnia and a blunted response to carbon dioxide persists for up to 1 week after transplantation for patients with preoperative carbon dioxide retention, but these abnormalities normalize by 1 week postoperatively (287). Transplantation does not affect the ventilatory response to isocapnic hypoxia (288).

The preoperative evaluation of the lung transplantation patient includes review of recent pulmonary function studies, assessing for a history of past or ongoing rejection episodes, as well as airway complications or infections. The presence or absence of bronchiolitis obliterans should be especially noted. BOS is a manifestation of chronic allograft rejection that is the major cause of late mortality (8,289, 290). The diagnosis of BOS is based on spirometric evidence of airflow limitations after exclusion of other causes such as airway complications or infection (193,194). The time-course of BOS is variable, with some patients demonstrating periods of stability interspersed with the overall progressive decline (291). Once detected, BOS is treated by augmentation of immunosuppressive therapy and with measures aimed at improving airflow obstruction (193, 194). Other aspects of perioperative management are individualized based on the presence of these complications. Current medication use is also evaluated, and consideration is given to providing supplemental steroid doses to prevent perioperative addisonian crisis, depending on the operative procedure. Toxicity of immunosuppressant drugs must be sought (e.g., cyclosporine-associated renal dysfunction, neurotoxicity, hypertension). In light of the interruption of lymph flow of the transplanted lung, administration of fluids should be carefully regulated to the minimum volume needed to maintain stable hemodynamics, oxygen delivery, and urine output. Special precautions to avoid iatrogenic infections are warranted in these immunocompromised patients. Other perioperative considerations depend on the status of the transplanted lung and whether the patient has undergone single- or double-lung transplantation. Patients with single-lung transplantation have persistent disease in the native lung. Ventilation and perfusion to the transplanted lung depend on the preexisting disease and whether there is rejection. For patients with COPD who have undergone single-lung transplantation, overdistention of the compliant, native lung leading to ventilation-perfusion mismatch deserves consideration; if severe, this condition can ameliorated with independent lung ventilation. The possibility of pulmonary vascular hyperreactivity in the patient with PPH who has received a single lung transplant should be considered. In these situations, drugs and physiologic factors that can provoke pulmonary vasoconstriction (e.g., hypercapnia, ketamine, nitrous oxide) should be avoided.

REFERENCES

1. Carrel A, Guthrie CC. The transplantation of veins and organs. *Am Med* 1905;10:1101.
2. Fleischer KJ, Baumgartner WA. Heart Transplantation. In: Edmunds LH Jr, ed. *Cardiac surgery in the adult.* St. Louis: McGraw-Hill, 1997:1410.
3. Lower RR, Shumway NE. Studies on the orthotopic homotransplantation of the canine heart. *Surg Forum* 1960;11:18.
4. Hardy JD, Chavez CM, Kurrrus FD, et al. Heart transplantation in man. *JAMA* 1964;188:114.
5. Barnard CN. A human cardiac transplant: an interim report of a successful operation performed at Groote Schuur Hospital, Capetown. *S Afr Med J* 1967;41:1271.
6. Caves PK, Stinson EB, Billingham ME, et al. Percutaneous endomyocardial biopsy in human heart recipients. *Ann Thorac Surg* 1973;16:325.
7. Oyer PE, Stinson EB, Jamieson SA, et al. Cycolsporin A in cardiac allografting: a preliminary experience. *Transplant Proc* 1983;15:1247.
8. Hosenpud JD, Bennett LE, Keck BM, et al. The registry of the international society of heart and lung transplantation: fifteenth official report—1998. *J Heart Lung Transplant* 1998;17:656.
9. Ferrari R, Ceconi C, Curello S, et al. The neuroendocrine and sympathetic nervous system in congestive heart failure. *Eur Heart J* 1998;19:F45.
10. Mann DL. Basic mechanisms of disease progression in the failing heart: the role of excessive adrenergic drive. *Prog Cardiovasc Dis* 1998;48:1.
11. Middlekauff HR, Mark AL. The treatment of heart failure: the role of neurohumoral activation. *Intern Med* 1998;37:12.
12. Bristow M, Kantrowitz N, Ginsburg R, et al. Beta-adrenergic function in heart muscle disease and heart failure. *J Mol Cell Cardiol* 1985;17:41.
13. Chidsey CA, Braunwald E, Morrow AG. Catecholamine excretion and cardiac stores of norepinephrine in congestive heart failure. *Am J Med* 1965;39:442.
14. Anker SD. Catecholamine levels and treatment in chronic heart failure. *Eur Heart J* 1998;19:F56.
15. Valdemarsson S, Bergdahl A, Edvinsson L. Relationships between plasma levels of catecholamines and neuropeptides and the survival time in patients with congestive heart failure. *J Intern Med* 1994;235:595.
16. Kawaguchi A, Gandjbakhch I, Pavie A, et al. Cardiac transplant recipients with preoperative pulmonary hypertension: evolution of pulmonary hemodynamics and surgical options. *Circulation* 1989;80:III-90.
17. Lommi J, Pulkki K, Koskinen P, et al. Haemodynamic, neuroendocrine and metabolic correlates of circulating cytokine concentrations in congestive heart failure *Eur Heart J* 1997;18:1620.
18. Niebauer J, Volk HD, Kemp M, et al. Endotoxin and immune activation in chronic heart failure: a prospective cohort study [see comments]. *Lancet* 1999;353:1838.
19. Haque R, Kan H, Finkel MS. Effects of cytokines and nitric oxide on myocardial E-C coupling. *Basic Res Cardiol* 1998;93:86.
20. Finkel MS, Oddis CV, Jacob TD, et al. Negative inotropic effects of cytokines on the heart mediated by nitric oxide. *Science* 1992;257:387.
21. Pulkki KJ. Cytokines and cardiomyocyte death. *Ann Med* 1997;29:339.
22. Sasayama S, Matsumori A, Matoba Y, et al. Immunomodulation: a new horizon for medical treatment of heart failure. *J Card Fail* 1996;2:S287.
23. Andersson B, Lomsky M, Waagstein F. The link between acute haemodynamic adrenergic beta-blockade and long-term effects in patients with heart failure: a study on diastolic function, heart rate and myocardial metabolism following intravenous metoprolol. *Eur Heart J* 1993;14:1375.
24. Constant J. A review of why and how we may use beta-blockers in congestive heart failure. *Chest* 1998;113:800.
25. Goldstein S. Clinical studies on beta blockers and heart failure preceding the MERIT-HF Trial. Metoprolol CR/XL Randomized Intervention Trial in Heart Failure. *Am J Cardiol* 1997;80:50J.
26. Heidenreich PA, Lee TT, Massie BM. Effect of beta-blockade on mortality in patients with heart failure: a meta-analysis of randomized clinical trials. *J Am Coll Cardiol* 1997;30:27.
27. Maisel AS. Beneficial effects of metoprolol treatment in congestive heart failure: reversal of sympathetic-induced alterations of immunologic function. *Circulation* 1994;90:774.
28. Garg R, Yusuf S. Overview of randomized trials of angiotensin-converting enzyme inhibitors on mortality and morbidity in patients with heart failure. Collaborative Group on ACE Inhibitor Trials [published erratum appears in *JAMA* 1995 Aug 9; 274(6):462] [see comments]. *JAMA* 1995;273:1450.
29. Anonymous. Effectiveness of spironolactone added to an angiotensin-converting enzyme inhibitor and a loop diuretic for severe chronic congestive heart failure (the Randomized Aldactone Evaluation Study [RALES]). *Am J Cardiol* 1996;78:902.
30. Riaz K, Forker AD. Digoxin use in congestive heart failure: current status. *Drugs* 1998;55:747.
31. Young JB, Gheorghiade M, Uretsky BF, et al. Superiority of "triple" drug therapy in heart failure: insights from the PROVED and RADIANCE trials. Prospective Randomized Study of Ventricular Function and Efficacy of Digoxin. Randomized Assessment of Digoxin and Inhibitors of Angiotensin-Converting Enzyme [see comments]. *J Am Coll Cardiol* 1998;32:686.
32. Moser M. Angiotensin-converting enzyme inhibitors, angiotensin II receptor antagonists and calcium channel blocking agents: a review of potential benefits and possible adverse reactions. *J Am Coll Cardiol* 1997;29:1414.
33. Cohn JN, Ziesche S, Smith R, et al. Effect of the calcium antagonist felodipine as supplementary vasodilator therapy in patients with chronic heart failure treated with enalapril: V-HeFT III. Vasodilator-Heart Failure Trial (V-HeFT) Study Group. *Circulation* 1997;96:856.
34. Koniaris LS, Goldhaber SZ. Anticoagulation in dilated cardiomyopathy [see comments]. *J Am Coll Cardiol* 1998;31:745.
35. Baker DW, Konstam MA, Bottorff M, et al. Management of heart failure: I. Pharmacologic treatment [see comments]. *JAMA* 1994;272:1361.
36. Stevenson WG, Sweeney MO. Pharmacologic and nonpharmacologic treatment of ventricular arrhythmias in heart failure. *Curr Opin Cardiol* 1997;12:242.
37. Doval HC, Nul DR, Grancelli HO, et al. Nonsustained ventricular tachycardia in severe heart failure: independent marker of increased mortality due to sudden death. GESICA-GEMA Investigators [see comments]. *Circulation* 1996;94:3198.
38. Hammill SC, Packer DL. Amiodarone in congestive heart failure: unraveling the GESICA and CHF-STAT differences [Editorial]. *Heart* 1996;75:6.

39. Pinto JV Jr, Ramani K, Neelagaru S, et al. Amiodarone therapy in chronic heart failure and myocardial infarction: a review of the mortality trials with special attention to STAT-CHF and the GESICA trials. Grupo de Estudio de la Sobrevida en la Insuficiencia Cardiaca en Argentina. *Prog Cardiovasc Dis* 1997; 40:85.
40. Nul DR, Doval HC, Grancelli HO, et al. Heart rate is a marker of amiodarone mortality reduction in severe heart failure. The GESICA-GEMA Investigators. Grupo de Estudio de la Sobrevida en la Insuficiencia Cardiaca en Argentina—Grupo de Estudios Multicentricos en Argentina. *J Am Coll Cardiol* 1997;29: 1199.
41. Moss AJ, Hall WJ, Cannom DS. Improved survival with an implanted defibrillator in patients with coronary disease at high risk for ventricular arrhythmia. Multicenter Automatic Defibrillator Implantation Trial Investigators [see comments]. *N Engl J Med* 1996;335:1933.
42. Bigger JT Jr, Whang W, Rottman JN, et al. Mechanisms of death in the CABG Patch trial: a randomized trial of implantable cardiac defibrillator prophylaxis in patients at high risk of death after coronary artery bypass graft surgery. *Circulation* 1999;99:1416.
43. Miller LW, Merkle EJ, Jennison SH. Outpatient use of dobutamine to support patients awaiting heart transplantation. *J Heart Lung Transplant* 1994;13:S126.
44. Cesario D, Clark J, Maisel A. Beneficial effects of intermittent home administration of the inotrope/vasodilator milrinone in patients with end-stage congestive heart failure: a preliminary study. *Am Heart J* 1998;135:121.
45. Belardinelli R, Georgiou D, Cianci G, et al. Randomized, controlled trial of long-term moderate exercise training in chronic heart failure: effects on functional capacity, quality of life, and clinical outcome. *Circulation* 1999;99:1173.
46. Dracup K, Walden JA, Stevenson LW, et al. Quality of life in patients with advanced heart failure. *J Heart Lung Transplant* 1992;11:273.
47. Stevenson LW. Inotropic therapy for heart failure [Editorial; comment]. *N Engl J Med* 1998;339:1848.
48. Baker DW, Jones R, Hodges J, et al. Management of heart failure: III. The role of revascularization in the treatment of patients with moderate or severe left ventricular systolic dysfunction. *JAMA* 1994;272:1528.
49. Pagano D, Townend JN, Littler WA, et al. Coronary artery bypass surgery as treatment for ischemic heart failure: the predictive value of viability assessment with quantitative positron emission tomography for symptomatic and functional outcome. *J Thorac Cardiovasc Surg* 1998;115:791.
50. Hausmann H, Topp H, Siniawski H, et al. Decision-making in end-stage coronary artery disease: revascularization or heart transplantation? *Ann Thorac Surg* 1997;64:1296.
51. Trachiotis GD, Weintraub WS, Johnston TS, et al. Coronary artery bypass grafting in patients with advanced left ventricular dysfunction. *Ann Thorac Surg* 1998;66:1632.
52. Marwick TH, Zuchowski C, Lauer MS, et al. Functional status and quality of life in patients with heart failure undergoing coronary bypass surgery after assessment of myocardial viability. *J Am Coll Cardiol* 1999;33:750.
53. Bolling SF, Pagani FD, Deeb GM, et al. Intermediate-term outcome of mitral reconstruction in cardiomyopathy. *J Thorac Cardiovasc Surg* 1998;115:381.
54. Kass DA. Surgical approaches to arresting or reversing chronic remodeling of the failing heart. *J Card Fail* 1998;4:57.
55. Lehmann A, Faust K, Boldt J, et al. Dynamic cardiomyoplasty in patients with end-stage heart failure: anaesthetic considerations. *Br J Anaesth* 1999;82:140.
56. Schreuder JJ, van der Veen FH, van der Velde ET. Left ventricular pressure-volume relationships before and after cardiomyoplasty in patients with heart failure. *Circulation* 1997;96:2978.
57. Delahaye F, Jegaden O. Cardiomyoplasty in severe heart failure: where do we stand? [Editorial; comment]. *Eur Heart J* 1998; 19:202.
58. Dickstein ML, Spotnitz HM, Rose EA, et al. Heart reduction surgery: an analysis of the impact on cardiac function [see comments]. *J Thorac Cardiovasc Surg* 1997;113:1032.
59. Batista RJ, Verde J, Nery P. Partial left ventriculectomy to treat end-stage heart disease. *Ann Thorac Surg* 1997;64:634.
60. McCarthy JF, McCarthy PM, Starling RC, et al. Partial left ventriculectomy and mitral valve repair for end-stage congestive heart failure. *Eur J Cardiothorac Surg* 1998;13:337.
61. Robicsek F. Surgical repair of extensive myocardial infarction: ventricular aneurysmectomy according to Dor with exclusion-closure of ventricular septal perforation and mitral replacement: a case report. *J Heart Valve Dis* 1996;5:561.
62. Rosenbaum AM, Murali S, Uretsky BF. Intra-aortic balloon counterpulsation as a "bridge" to cardiac transplantation: effects in nonischemic and ischemic cardiomyopathy. *Chest* 1994;106: 1683.
63. Lazar JM, Ziady GM, Dummer SJ, et al. Outcome and complications of prolonged intraaortic balloon counterpulsation in cardiac patients. *Am J Cardiol* 1992;69:955.
64. Oz MC, Argenziano M, Catanese KA, et al. Bridge experience with long-term implantable left ventricular assist devices: are they an alternative to transplantation? *Circulation* 1997;95: 1844.
65. Dipla K, Mattiello JA, Jeevanandam V, et al. Myocyte recovery after mechanical circulatory support in humans with end-stage heart failure [see comments]. *Circulation* 1998;97:2316.
66. Mancini DM, Beniaminovitz A, Levin H, et al. Low incidence of myocardial recovery after left ventricular assist device implantation in patients with chronic heart failure [see comments]. *Circulation* 1998;98:2383.
67. Levin HR, Oz MC, Chen JM, et al. Reversal of chronic ventricular dilation in patients with end-stage cardiomyopathy by prolonged mechanical unloading. *Circulation* 1995;91:2717.
68. Tsau PH, Arabia FA, Toporoff B, et al. Positive panel reactive antibody titers in patients bridged to transplantation with a mechanical assist device: risk factors and treatment. *ASAIO J* 1998;44:M634.
69. Stevenson LW, Tillisch JH, Hamilton M, et al. Importance of hemodynamic response to therapy in predicting survival with ejection fraction $<$ 20 percent secondary to ischemic or nonischemic dilated cardiomyopathy. *Am J Cardiol* 1990;66:1348.
70. Lee WH, Packer M. Prognostic importance of serum sodium concentration and its modification by converting enzyme inhibition in patient with severe heart failure. *Circulation* 1986;73: 257.
71. Mancini DM, Eisen H, Kussmaul W, et al. Value of peak exercise oxygen consumption of opitmal timing of cardiac transplantation in ambulatory patients with heart failure. *Circulation* 1991;3:778.
72. Unverferth DV, Magorien RD, Moeschberger ML, et al. Factors influencing the one-year mortality of dilated cardiomyopathy. *Am J Cardiol* 1984;54:147.
73. Keogh AM, Barone DW, Hickie JB. Prognostic guides in patients with idiopathic or ischemia dilated cardiomyopathy assessed for cardiac transplantation. *Am J Cardiol* 1990;65:903.
74. Cohn JN, Johnson GR, Sabetai R, et al. Ejection fraction, peak exercise oxygen consumption, cardiothoracic ratio, ventricular arrhythmias, and plasma norepinephrine as determinants of prognosis in heart failure. *Circulation* 1993;87[Suppl VI]:VI-5.

75. Carrier M, Emergy RW, Riley JE, et al. Cardiac transplantation in patients over 50 years of age. *J Am Coll Cardiol* 1986;8:285.
76. Renlung DG, Gilbert EM, O'Connell JB, et al. Age-associated decline in cardiac allograft rejection. *Am J Med* 1987;83:391.
77. Erickson KW, Costanzo-Nordin MR, O'Sullivan EJ, et al. Influence of preoperative transpulmonary gradient on late mortality after orthotopic heart transplantation. *J Heart Transplant* 1990;9:526.
78. Kormos RL, Thompson M, Hardesty RL, et al. Utility of preoperative right heart catheterization data as a predictor of survival after heart transplantation. *J Heart Transplant* 1990;9:391.
79. Addonizio LJ, Gersony WM, Robbins RC, et al. Elevated pulmonary vascular resistance and cardiac transplantation. *Circulation* 1987;76[Suppl V]:52.
80. Young JN, Yazbeck J, Esposito G, et al. The influence of acute preoperative pulmonary infarction on the results of heart transplantation. *J Heart Transplant* 1986;5:20.
81. Caplan AL. Equity in the selection of recipients for cardiac transplants. *Circulation* 1987;75:10.
82. Herrick CM, Mealey PC, Tischner LL, et al. Combined heart failure transplant program: advantages in assessing medical compliance. *J Heart Transplant* 1987;6:141.
83. Freeman AM, Folks DG, Sokol RS, et al. Cardiac transplantation clinical correlates of psychiatric outcome. *Psychosomatics* 1988;2:47.
84. Olbrisch ME, Levenson JL. Psychological evaluation of heart transplantation candidates: an international survey of process, criteria, and outcomes. *J Heart Lung Transplant* 1991;10:948.
85. American Heart Association. *Heart and stroke facts: statistical supplement.* Dallas, Texas: American Heart Association, 1998.
86. Stevenson LW, Warner SL, Steimle AE, et al. The impending crisis awaiting cardiac transplantation: modeling a solution based on selection. *Circulation* 1994;89:450.
87. Stevenson LW, Hamilton MA, Tillisch JH. Decreasing survival benefit from cardiac transplantation for outpatients as the waiting list lengthens. *J Am Coll Cardiol* 1991;18:919.
88. Mudge GH, Goldstein S, Addonizio LJ, et al. Task Force 3: recipient guidelines/prioritization. *J Am Coll Cardiol* 1993;22: 21.
89. *1995 Annual report of the US Scientific Registry of Transplant Recipients and the Organ Procurement and Transplant Network: transplant data, 1988–1994.* Richmond, VA: United Network for Organ Sharing; and Rockville, MD: Division of Organ Transplantation, Bureau of Health Resources Development, Health Resources and Services Administration, US Department of Health and Human Services, 1995.
90. National Task Force on Organ Transplantation: *Final report.* Rockville, MD: Office of Organ Transplantation, Health Resources and Services Administration, US Department of Health and Human Services, 1986.
91. *Omnibus Budget Reconciliation Act of 1986,* Public Law 99-509.
92. Van Norman GA. A matter of life and death: what every anesthesiologist should know about the medical, legal, and ethical aspects of declaring brain death. *Anesthesiology* 1999;91:275.
93. President's Commission for the Study of Ethical Problems in Medicine and Biomedical and Behavioral Research. *Defining death.* Washington, DC, US Government Printing Office, 1981.
94. Guidelines for the determination of death: report of the medical consultants on the diagnosis of death to the President's Commission for the Study of Ethical Problems in Medicine and Biomedical Research and Behavioral Research. *JAMA* 1981;246: 2184.
95. Report of Ad Hoc Committee of the Harvard Medical School to Examine the Definition of Brain Death: a definition of irreversible coma. *JAMA* 1968;205:337.
96. Mohandas A, Chou SN. Brain death: a clinical and pathological study. *J Neurosurg* 1971;44:1.
97. *Uniform Brain Death Act.* Approved at Annual Conference of National Conference of Commissioners of Uniform State Laws, Washington, DC, July 28–August 4, 1978.
98. McGaman B, Hirsh HL: Brain death: legal issues. *Heart Lung* 1979;8:1098.
99. Norton DJ. Clinical application of brain death protocols. *J Neurosci Nurs* 1992;24:354.
100. Frilman NF, Jeffers WA. Effect of progressive sympathectomy on hypertension produced by increased intracranial pressure. *Am J Physiol* 1940;128:662.
101. Rose AG, Novitzky D, Cooper DK. Myocardial and pulmonary histopathologic changes. *Transplant Proc* 1988;20:29.
102. Novitzky D. Heart transplantation, euthyroid sick syndrome, and triiodothyronine replacement. *J Heart Lung Transplant* 1992;11:S196.
103. Novitzky D, Cooper DKC, Reichart B. Hemodynamic and metabolic responses to hormonal therapy in brain-dead potential organ donors. *Transplantation* 1987;43:852.
104. Randell TT, Hockerstedt KA. Triiodothyronine treatment in brain-dead multiorgan donors: a controlled study. *Transplantation* 1992;54:736.
105. Davis FD. Coordination of cardiac transplantation: patient processing and donor organ procurement. *Circulation* 1987;75:29.
106. Butman SM, Ewy GA, Standen JR, et al. Bedside cardiovascular examination in patients with severe chronic heart failure: importance of rest or inducible jugular venous distension. *J Am Coll Cardiol* 1993;22:968.
107. Dei Cas L, Metra M, Leier CV. Electrolyte disturbances in chronic heart failure: metabolic and clinical aspects. *Clin Cardiol* 1995;18:370.
108. Berberich JJ, Fabian JA. A retrospective analysis of fentanyl and sufentanil for cardiac transplantation. *J Cardiothorac Anesth* 1987;1:200.
109. Suriani RJ: Transesophageal echocardiography during organ transplantation. *J Cardiothorac Vasc Anesth* 1998;12:686.
110. MacGillivray RG, Rocke DA, Mahomedy AE. Midazolam for induction of anaesthesia in patients with limited cardiac reserves: a comparison with etomidate. *S Afr Med J* 1988;73:101.
111. Hensley FA Jr, Martin DE, Larach DR, et al. Anesthetic management for cardiac transplantation in North America—1986 survey. *J Cardiothorac Anesth* 1987;1:429.
112. Coriat P, Richer C, Douraki T, et al. Influence of chronic angiotensin-converting enzyme inhibition on anesthetic induction. *Anesthesiology* 1994;81:299.
113. Campione KM. Heart to head circulation time. *Illinois Medical Journal* 1972;141:75.
114. Demas K, Wyner J, Mihm FG, et al. Anaesthesia for heart transplantation: a retrospective study and review. *Br J Anaesth* 1986;58:1357.
115. Nakatani T, Frazier OH, Lammermeier DE, et al. Heterotopic heart transplantation: a reliable option for a select group of high-risk patients. *J Heart Transplant* 1989;8:40.
116. Angerman CE, Spes CH, Tammen A, et al. Anatomic characteristics and valvular function of the transplanted heart: transthoracic versus transesophageal echocardiographic findings. *J Heart Transplant* 1990;9:331.
117. Jacquet L, Ziady G, Stein K, et al. Cardiac rhythm disturbance early after orthotopic heart transplantation: prevalence and clinical importance of observed abnormality. *J Am Coll Cardiol* 1990;16:832.
118. El-Gamel A, Yonan NA, Grant S, et al. Orthotopic heart transplantation: a comparison between the standard and the bicaval Wythenshawe technique. *J Thorac Cardiovasc Surg* 1995;109: 721.

119. Deleuze PH, Benvenuti C, Mazzuotelli JP, et al. Orthotopic cardiac transplantation with direct caval anastomosis: is it the optimal procedure? *J Thorac Cardiovasc Surg* 1995;109:731.
120. Aziz T, Burgess M, Khafagy R, et al. Bicaval and standard techniques in orthotopic heart transplantation: medium-term experience in cardiac performance and survival. *J Thorac Cardiovasc Surg* 1999;118:115.
121. Orihashi K, Matsuura Y, Sueda T, et al. Pooled air in open heart operations examined by transesophageal echocardiography. *Ann Thorac Surg* 1996;61:1377.
122. Bugge M, Lepore V, Dahlin A. The de-airing clamp in cardiac surgery. *Eur J Cardiothorac Surg* 1997;11:189.
123. Mets B, Michler RE, Delphin ED, et al. Refractory vasodilation after cardiopulmonary bypass for heart transplantation in recipients on combined amiodarone and angiotensin-converting enzyme inhibitor therapy: a role for vasopressin administration. *J Cardiothorac Vasc Anesth* 1998;12:326.
124. Bittner HB, Kendall SW, Chen EP, et al. The combined effects of brain death and cardiac graft preservation on cardiopulmonary hemodynamics and function before and after subsequent heart transplantation. *J Heart Lung Transplant* 1996;15:764.
125. Armitage JM, Hardy RL, Griffith BP. Prostaglandin E_1: an effective treatment of right heart failure after orthotopic heart transplantation. *J Heart Transplant* 1987;6:348.
126. D'Ambra MN, LaRaia PJ, Philbin DM, et al. Prostaglandin E_1: a new therapy for refractory right heart failure and pulmonary hypertension after mitral valve replacement. *J Thorac Cardiovasc Surg* 1985;89:567.
127. Rich GF, Murphy GD Jr, Roos CM, et al. Inhaled nitric oxide: selective pulmonary vasodilation in cardiac surgical patients. *Anesthesiology* 1993;78:1028.
128. Orime Y, Shiono M, Hata H, et al. Effects of concomitant usage of milrinone and catecholamine for weaning from cardiopulmonary bypass. *Jpn J Thorac Cardiovasc Surg* 1998;46:803.
129. Pamboukian SV, Carere RG, Webb JG, et al. The use of milrinone in pre-transplant assessment of patients with congestive heart failure and pulmonary hypertension. *J Heart Lung Transplant* 1999;18:367.
130. Vlahakes GJ, Turley K, Hoffman JI. The pathophysiology of failure in acute right ventricular hypertension: hemodynamic and biochemical correlations. *Circulation* 1981;63:87.
131. Chow E, Farrar DJ. Effects of left ventricular pressure reductions on right ventricular systolic performance. *Am J Physiol* 1989;257:H1878.
132. Barman SA. Effect of catecholamines on pulmonary circulation at elevated vascular tone. *J Appl Physiol* 1995;78:1452.
133. Lee R, Neya K, Svizzero TA, et al. Norepinephrine infusion following cardiopulmonary bypass: effect of infusion site. *J Surg Res* 1995;58:143.
134. Bemis CE, Serur JR, Borkenhagen D, et al. Influence of right ventricular filling pressure on left ventricular pressure and dimensions. *Circ Res* 1974;34:498.
135. Fonger JD, Borkon AM, Baumgartner WA, et al. Acute right ventricular failure following heart transplantation: improvement with prostaglandin E1 and right ventricular assist. *J Heart Transplant* 1986;4:317.
136. Esmore DS, Spratt PM, Branch JM, et al. Right ventricular assist and prostacyclin infusion for allograft failure in the presence of high pulmonary vascular resistance. *J Heart Transplant* 1990; 9:136.
137. Stinson EB, Caves PK, Griepp RB, et al. The transplanted heart in the postoperative period. *Surg Forum* 1983;24:189.
138. Urelsky BF. Physiology of the transplanted heart. *Cardiovascular Clin* 1990;20:23.
139. Griepp RB, et al. Hemodynamic performance of the transplanted human heart. *Surgery* 1971;70:88.
140. Montero JA, Anguita M, Concha M, et al. Pacing requirements after orthotopic heart transplantation: incidence and related factors. *J Heart Lung Transplant* 1992;11:799.
141. Hosenpud JD, Herschberger RE, Pantely GA, et al. Late infection in cardiac allograft recipient: profiles, incidence and outcome. *J Heart Transplant* 1987;10:80.
142. Gentry LO, Zeluff BJ. Diagnosis and treatment of infection in cardiac transplant patients. *Surg Clin North Am* 1986;66:459.
143. Mammana RB, Petersen EA, Fuller JK, et al. Pulmonary infections in cardiac transplant patients: modes of diagnosis, complications, and effectiveness of therapy. *Ann Thorac Surg* 1983;36: 700.
144. Olivari MT, Kubo SH, Braunlin EA, et al. Five-year experience with triple-drug immunosuppressive therapy in cardiac transplantation. *Circulation* 1990;82:IV-276.
145. Price GD, Olsen SL, Taylor DO, et al. Corticosteroid-free maintenance immunosuppression after heart transplantation: feasibility and beneficial effects. *J Heart Lung Transplant* 1992; 11:403.
146. Weil R, Clarke DR, Iwaki Y, et al. Hyperacute rejection of a transplanted human heart. *Transplantation* 1981;32:71.
147. Olsen SL, Wagoner LE, Taylor DO, et al. Treatment of vascular rejection in the 1990's: The Utah experience. *Circulation* 1992; 86:2500.
148. Baumgartner WA, Reitz BA, Oyer PE, et al. Cardiac homotransplantation. *Curr Probl Surg* 1979;16:1.
149. Billingham ME. Endomyocardial biopsy detection of acute rejection in cardiac allograft recipients. *Heart Vessels* 1985;1:86.
150. Miller LW. Treatment of cardiac allograft rejection with intravenous corticosteroids. *J Heart Transplant* 1990;9:283.
151. Griepp RB, Stinson EB, Dong EJ, et al. The use of antithymocyte globulin in human heart transplantation. *Circulation* 1972; 45:147.
152. Haverty TP, Sanders M, Sheahan M. OKT3 treatment of cardiac allograft rejection. *J Heart Lung Transplant* 1993;12:591.
153. Olsen SL, O'Connell JB, Bristow MR. Methotrexate as an adjunct in the treatment of persistent mild cardiac allograft rejection. *Transplantation* 1990;50:773.
154. Hosenpud J, Morris TE, Shipley GD, et al. Cardiac allograft vasculopathy. *Transplantation* 1996;61:939.
155. Yeung AC, Davis SF, Hauptmann PJ. Incidence and progression of transplant coronary artery disease over 1 year: results of a multicenter trial with us of intravascular ultrasound. *J Heart Lung Transplant* 195;14:5215.
156. Costanzo MR, Naftel DC, Pritzker MR, et al. Heart transplant coronary artery disease detected by coronary angiography: a multi-institutional study of preoperative donor and recipient risk factors. *J Heart Lung Transplant* 1998;17:744.
157. Fang JC, Rocco T, Jarcho J, et al. Noninvasive assessment of transplant associated arterial sclerosis. *Am Heart J* 1998;135: 980.
158. Spes CH, Klauss V, Mudra H, et al. Diagnostic and prognostic value of serial dobutamine stress echocardiography for noninvasive assessment of cardiac graft vasculopathy: a comparison with coronary angiography and intravascular ultrasound. *Circulation* 1999;100:509.
159. Libby P, Salomon RN, Payne DD, et al. Functions of vascular wall cells related to development of transplantation: associated with coronary arteriosclerosis. *Transplant Proc* 1989;21:3677.
160. Gregory CR, Huang X, Pratt RE, et al. Treatment with rapamycin and mycophenolic acid reduces arterial intimal thickening produced by mechanical injury and allow endothelial replacement. *Transplantation* 1995;59:655.
161. Schroeder JS, Gao SZ, Alderman EL, et al. A plenary study of

diltiazem in the prevention of coronary disease in heart transplant recipients. *N Engl J Med* 1993;328:164.
162. Kobashigawa JA, Katznelson S, Laks H, et al. Effect of pravastatin on outcomes after cardiac transplantation. *N Engl J Med* 1995;333:621.
163. Robbins RC, Barlow CW, Oyer PE, et al. Thirty years of cardiac transplantation at Stanford University. *J Thorac Cardiovasc Surg* 1999;117:939.
164. Bailey PL, Stanley TH. Anesthesia for patients with a prior cardiac transplantation. *J Cardiothorac Anesth* 1990;4:38.
165. Pope SE, Stinson EB, Daughters GT, et al. Exercise response of the denervated heart in long term cardiac transplant recipients. *Am J Cardiol* 1980;46:213.
166. Quigg RJ, Rocco MB, Gauthier DF, et al. Mechanism of attenuated peak heart rate response to exercise after orthotopic heart transplantation. *J Am Coll Cardiol* 1989;14:338.
167. Mackintosh AF, Carmichael DJ, Wren C, et al. Sinus node function in the first three weeks after cardiac transplantation. *Br Heart J* 1982;48:584.
168. Heinz G, Hirschl M, Buxbaum P, et al. Sinus node dysfunction after orthotopic cardiac transplantation: postoperative incidence and long term implications. *Pacing Clin Electrophysiol* 1992;15:731.
169. Scott CD, Dark JH, McComb JM. Evolution of the chronotropic response to exercise after cardiac transplantation. *Am J Cardiol* 1995;76:1292.
170. Gilbert EM, Eiswerth CC, Mealey PC, et al. Beta adrenergic supersensitivity of the transplanted human heart is pre-synaptic in origin. *Circulation* 1989;79:344.
171. Kontos HA, Thames MD, Lower RR. Responses to electrical and reflex autonomic stimulation in dogs with cardiac transplantation before and after reinnervation. *J Thorac Cardiovasc Surg* 1970;59:382.
172. Fallen EL, Kamath MV, Ghista DN, et al. Spectral analysis of heart rate variability following human heart transplantation: evidence for functional reinnervation. *J Auton Nerv System* 1988;23:199.
173. Bernardi L, Valle F, Leuzzi S, et al. Non-respiratory components of heart rate variability in heart transplant recipients: evidence of autonomic reinnervation? *Clin Sci* 1994;86:537.
174. Cannom DS, Rider AK, Stinson EB, et al. Electrophysiologic studies in the denervated transplanted human heart: II. Response to norepinephrine, isoproterenol and propranolol. *Am J Cardiol* 1975;36:859.
175. Borow KM, Neuman A, Arensman FW, et al. Left ventricular contractility and contractile reserve in humans after cardiac transplantation. *Circulation* 1985;71:866.
176. Donald DE, Shepherd JT. Supersensitivity to L-norepinephrine of the denervated sinoatrial node. *Am J Physiol* 1965;208:255.
177. Paulus WJ, Bronzwaer JF, Felice H, et al. Deficient acceleration of left ventricular relaxation during exercise after heart transplantation. *Circulation* 192;86:1175.
178. Hullin R, Asmus F, Ludwig A, et al. Subunit expression of the cardiac L-type calcium channel is differently regulated in diastolic heart failure of the cardiac allograft. *Circulation* 1999;100:155.
179. Stark RP, McGinn AL, Wilson RF. Chest pain in cardiac-transplant recipients. *N Engl J Med* 1991;324:1791.
180. Smart FW, Ballantyne CM, Cocanougher B, et al. Insensitivity of noninvasive test to detect coronary artery vasculopathy after heart transplant. *Am J Cardiol* 1991;67:243.
181. Myers BD, Sibley R, Newton L, et al. The long-term course of cyclosporine-associated chronic nephropathy. *Kidney Int* 1988;33:590.
182. Miller LW, Pennington DG, McBride LR. Long-term effects of cyclosporine in cardiac transplantation. *Transplant Proc* 1990;22:15.
183. Frist WH, Stinson EB, Oyer PE, et al. Long-term hemodynamic results after cardiac transplantation. *J Thorac Cardiovasc Surg* 1987;94:685.
184. Reitz BA, Wallwork JL, Hunt SA, et al. Heart-lung transplantation: successful therapy for patients with pulmonary vascular disease. *N Engl J Med* 1982;306:557.
185. Toronto Lung Transplantation Group. Unilateral lung transplantation for pulmonary fibrosis. *N Engl J Med* 1986;314:1140.
186. Patterson GA, Cooper JD, Goldman B, et al. Technique of successful clinical double-lung transplantation. *Ann Thorac Surg* 1988;45:626.
187. Pasque MK, Cooper JD, Kaiser LR, et al. Improved technique for bilateral lung transplantation: rationale and initial clinical experience. *Ann Thorac Surg* 1990;49:785.
188. Metras D. Henri Metras: a pioneer in lung transplantation. *J Heart Lung Transplant* 1992;11:1213.
189. Hardin CA, Kittle CF. Experiences with transplantation of the lung. *Science* 1954;119:97.
190. Hardy JD, Webb WR, Dalton ML Jr, et al. Lung homotransplantation in man: report of the initial case. *JAMA* 1963;186:1065.
191. Veith FJ, Kamholz SL, Mollenkoff FP, et al. Lung transplantation 1983. *Transplant* 1983;35:271.
192. Derom F, Barbier F, Ringoir S, et al. Ten-month survival after lung homotransplantation in man. *J Thorac Cardiovasc Surg* 1971;61:835.
193. Trulock EP. Lung transplantation. *Am J Respir Crit Care Med* 1997;155:789.
194. Arcasoy SM, Kotloff RM. Lung transplantation. *N Engl J Med* 1999;340:1081.
195. Low DE, Trulock EP, Kaiser LR, et al. Lung transplantation of ventilator-dependent patients. *Chest* 1992;101:8.
196. Flume PA, Egan TM, Westerman JH, et al. Lung transplantation for mechanically ventilated patients. *J Heart Lung Transplant* 1994;13:15.
197. Anthonisen NR. Prognosis in chronic obstructive pulmonary disease: results from multicenter trials. *Am Rev Respir Dis* 1989;140:S95.
198. Seersholm N, Kok-Jensen A. Survival in relation to lung function and smoking cessation in patients with severe hereditary alpha1-antitrypsin deficiency. *Am J Respir Crit Care Med* 1995;151:369.
199. Kerem E, Reisman J, Corey M, et al. Prediction of mortality in patients with cystic fibrosis. *N Engl J Med* 1992;326:1187.
200. Cooper JD. Current status of lung transplantation. *Transplant Proc* 1991;23:2107.
201. Hayden AM, Robert RC, Kriett JM, et al. Primary diagnosis predicts prognosis of lung transplant candidates. *Transplantation* 1993;55:1048.
202. D'Alonzo GE, Barst RJ, Ayres SM, et al. Survival in patients with primary pulmonary hypertension: results from a national prospective registry. *Ann Intern Med* 1991;115:343.
203. Sundaresan S, Semenkovich J, Ochoa L, et al. Successful outcome of lung transplantation is not compromised by the use of marginal donor lungs. *J Thorac Cardiovasc Surg* 1995;109:1075.
204. Cooper JD, Pearson FG, Patterson GA, et al. Technique of successful lung transplantation in humans. *J Thorac Cardiovasc Surg* 1987;93:173.
205. Calhoon JH, Grover FL, Gibbons WJ, et al. Single lung transplantation: alternative indications and technique. *J Thorac Cardiovasc Surg* 1991;101:816.
206. Miller JD, DeHoyos A, and The University of Toronto and Washington University Lung Transplant Programs. An evalua-

tion of the role of omentopexy and of early perioperative corticosteroids administration in clinical lung transplantation. *J Thorac Cardiovasc Surg* 1993;105:247.

207. Daly RC, Tadjkarimi S, Khaghani A, et al. Successful double-lung transplantation with direct bronchial artery revascularization. *Ann Thorac Surg* 1993;56:885.
208. Patterson GA. Airway revascularization: is it necessary? *Ann Thorac Surg* 1993;56:807.
209. Low DE, Trulock EP, Kaiser LR, et al. Morbidity, mortality, and early results of single versus bilateral lung transplantation for emphysema. *J Thorac Cardiovasc Surg* 1992;103:1119.
210. Trulock EP, Cooper JD, Kaiser LR, et al. The Washington University–Barnes Hospital experience with lung transplantation. *JAMA* 1991;266:1943.
211. Levine SM, Gibbons WJ, Bryan CL, et al. Single lung transplantation for primary pulmonary hypertension. *Chest* 1990;98:1107.
212. Pasque MK, Trulock EP, Kaiser LR, et al. Single-lung transplantation for pulmonary hypertension: three-month hemodynamic follow-up. *Circulation* 1991;84:2275.
213. Pasque MK, Trulock EP, Cooper JD, et al. Single lung transplantation for pulmonary hypertension: single institution experience in 34 patients. *Circulation* 1995;92:2252.
214. Kramer MR, Valantine HA, Marshall SE, et al. Recovery of the right ventricle after single-lung transplantation in pulmonary hypertension. *Am J Cardiol* 1994;73:494.
215. Ritchie M, Waggoner AD, Dávila-Román VG, et al. Echocardiographic characterization of the improvement in right ventricular function inpatients with severe pulmonary hypertension after single-lung transplantation. *J Am Coll Cardiol* 1993;22:1170.
216. Levine SM, Jenkinson SG, Bryan CL, et al. Ventilation-perfusion inequalities during graft rejection in patients undergoing single lung transplantation for primary pulmonary hypertension. *Chest* 1992;101:401.
217. Gammie JS, Keenan RJ, Pham SM, et al. Single- versus double-lung transplantation for pulmonary hypertension. *J Thorac Cardiovasc Surg* 1998;115:397.
218. Bando K, Armitage JM, Paradis IL, et al. Indications for and results of single, bilateral, and heart-lung transplantation for pulmonary hypertension. *J Thorac Cardiovasc Surg* 1994;108:1056.
219. Levine SM, Anzueto AR, Gibbons WJ, et al. Graft position and pulmonary function after single lung transplantation for obstructive lung disease. *Chest* 1993;103:444.
220. Patterson GA, Cooper JD, Goldman B, et al. Technique of successful clinical double-lung transplantation. *Ann Thorac Surg* 1988;45:626.
221. Pasque MK, Cooper JD, Kaiser LR, et al. Improved technique for bilateral lung transplantation: rationale and initial clinical experience. *Ann Thorac Surg* 1990;49:785.
222. Egan TM, Detterbeck FC. Technique and results of double lung transplantation. *Chest Surg Clin North Am* 1993;3:89.
223. Starnes VA, Barr ML, Schenkel FA, et al. Experience with living-donor lobar transplantation for indications other than cystic fibrosis. *J Thorac Cardiovasc Surg* 1997;114:917.
224. Patterson GA, Maurer JR, Williams TJ, et al. Comparison of outcomes of double and single lung transplantation for obstructive lung disease. *J Thorac Cardiovasc Surg* 1991;101:623.
225. Levy RD, Ernst P, Levine SM, et al. Exercise performance after lung transplantation. *J Heart Lung Transplant* 1993;12:27.
226. Sundaresan RS, Shiraishi Y, Trulock EP, et al. Single or bilateral lung transplantation for emphysema? *J Thorac Cardiovasc Surg* 1996;112:1485.
227. Aeba R, Griffith BP, Hardesty RL, et al. Isolated lung transplantation for patients with Eisengmenger's syndrome. *Circulation* 1993;88:452.
228. Lupinetti FM, Bolling SF, Bove EL, et al. Selective lung or heart-lung transplantation for pulmonary hypertension associated with congenital cardiac anomalies. *Ann Thorac Surg* 1994;57:1545.
229. DeHoyos A, Demajo W, Snell G, et al. Preoperative prediction for the use of cardiopulmonary bypass in lung transplantation. *J Thorac Cardiovasc Surg* 1993;106:787.
230. Aeba R, Griffith BP, Kormos RL, et al. Effect of cardiopulmonary bypass on early graft dysfunction in clinical lung transplantation. *Ann Thorac Surg* 1994;57:715.
231. Egan TM, Detterbeck FC, Mill MR, et al. Improved results of lung transplantation for patients with cystic fibrosis. *J Thorac Cardiovasc Surg* 1995;109:224.
232. Triantafillou AN, Pasque MK, Huddleston CB, et al. Predictors, frequency and indications for cardiopulmonary bypass during lung transplantation in adults. *Ann Thorac Surg* 1994;57:1248.
233. Myles PS, Venema H. Avoidance of cardiopulmonary bypass during bilateral sequential lung transplantation using inhaled nitric oxide. *J Cardiothorac Vasc Anesth* 1995;9:571.
234. Hirt SW, Haverich A, Wahler T, et al. Predictive criteria for the need of extracorporeal circulation in single-lung transplantation. *Ann Thorac Surg* 1992;54:676.
235. Despotis GJ, Joist JH, Hogue CW Jr, et al. More effective suppression of hemostatic system activation in patients undergoing cardiac surgery by heparin dosing based on heparin blood concentration rather than ACT. *Thromb Haemostat* 1996;76:902.
236. Stibbe J, Kluft C, Brommer EJP, et al. Enhanced fibrinolytic activity during cardiopulmonary bypass in open-heart surgery in man is caused by extrinsic (tissue-type) plasminogen activator. *Eur J Clin Invest* 1984;14:375.
237. Gu YJ, de Haan J, Brenken UP, et al. Clotting and fibrinolytic disturbance during lung transplantation: effect of low-dose aprotinin. *J Thorac Cardiovasc Surg* 1996;112:599.
238. Jaquiss RD, Huddleston CB, Spray TL. Use of aprotinin in pediatric lung transplantation. *J Heart Lung Transplant* 1995;14:302.
239. Bando K, Paradis IL, Komatsu K, et al. Analysis of time-dependent risks for infection, rejection, and death after pulmonary transplantation. *J Thorac Cardiovasc Surg* 1995;109:49.
240. Date H, Triantafillou AN, Trulock EP, et al. Inhaled nitric oxide reduces human allograft dysfunction. *J Thorac Cardiovasc Surg* 1996;111:913.
241. Kaplan JD, Trulock EP, Cooper JD, et al. Pulmonary permeability after lung transplantation: a positron emission tomographic study. *Am Rev Respir Dis* 1992;145:954.
242. Qayumi AK, Jamieson WRE. Pathophysiology of reperfusion injury in organ transplantation. In: Dad DK, ed. *Pathophysiology of reperfusion injury.* Boca Raton, FL: CRC Press, 1993:325.
243. Whyte RI, Deeb GM, McCurry KR, et al. Extracorporeal life support after heart or lung transplantation. *Ann Thorac Surg* 1994;58:754.
244. Adatia I, Lillehei C, Arnold JH, et al. Inhaled nitric oxide in the treatment of postoperative graft dysfunction after lung transplantation. *Ann Thorac Surg* 1994;57:131.
245. Haniuda M, Hasegawa S, Shiraishi T, et al. Effects of inflation volume during lung preservation on pulmonary capillary permeability. *J Thorac Cadiovasc Surg* 1996;112:85.
246. Okabayashi K, Triantafillou AN, Yamashita M, et al. Inhaled nitric oxide improves lung allograft function after prolonged storage. *J Thorac Cardiovasc Surg* 1996;112:293.

247. Bacha EA, Hervé P, Murakami S, et al. Lasting beneficial effect of short-term inhaled nitric oxide on graft function after lung transplantation. *J Thorac Cardiovasc Surg* 1996;112:590.
248. Murakami S, Bacha EA, Hervé P, et al. Inhaled nitric oxide and pentoxifylline in rat lung transplantation from non-heart beating-donors. *J Thorac Cardiovasc Surg* 1997;113:821.
249. Clark SC, Sudarshan C, Khanna R, et al. Controlled reperfusion and pentoxifylline modulate reperfusion injury after single lung transplantation. *J Thorac Cardiovasc Surg* 1998;115:1335.
250. Yamashita M, Schmid RA, Fujino S, et al. Nicorandil, a potent adenosine triphosphate-sensitive potassium-channel opener, ameliorates lung allograft reperfusion injury. *J Thorac Cardiovasc Surg* 1996;112:1307.
251. Okubo K, Kosaka S, Isowa N, et al. Amelioration of ischemia-reperfusion injury by human thioredoxin in rabbit lung. *J Thorac Cardiovasc Surg* 1997;113:1.
252. Eppinger MJ, Ward PA, Bolling SF, et al. Regulatory effects of interleukin-10 on lung ischemia-reperfusion injury. *J Thorac Cardiovasc Surg* 1996;112:1301.
253. Boasquevisque CHR, Mora BN, Bernstein M, et al. Ex vivo liposome-mediated gene transfer to lung isografts. *J Thorac Cardiovasc Surg* 1998;115:38.
254. Despotis GJ, Karanikolas M, Triantafillou AN, et al. Pressure gradient across the pulmonary artery anastomosis during lung transplantation. *Ann Thorac Surg* 1995;60:630.
255. Haydock DA, Trulock EP, Kaiser LR, et al. Management of dysfunction in the transplanted lung: experience with 7 clinical cases. *Ann Thorac Surg* 1992;53:635.
256. Leibowitz DW, Smith CR, Michler RE, et al. Incidence of pulmonary vein complications after lung transplantation: a prospective transesophageal echocardiographic study. *J Am Coll Cardiol* 1994;24:671.
257. Hausmann D, Daniel WG, Mügge A, et al. Imaging of pulmonary artery and vein anastomoses by transesophageal echocardiography after lung transplantation. *Circulation* 1992;86:II-251.
258. Gorscan J III, Reddy SCB, Armitage JM, et al. Acquired right ventricular outflow tract obstruction after lung transplantation: diagnosis by transesophageal echocardiography. *J Am Soc Echocardiogr* 1993;6:324.
259. Smiley RM, Navedo AT, Kirby T, et al. Postoperative independent lung ventilation in a single-lung transplant recipient. *Anesthesiology* 1991;74:1144.
260. Griffith BP, Hardesty RL, Armitage JM, et al. Acute rejection of lung allografts with various immunosuppressive protocols. *Ann Thorac Surg* 1992;54:846.
261. Kriett JM, Smith CM, Hayden AM, et al. Lung transplantation without the use of antilymphocyte antibody preparation. *J Heart Lung Transplant* 1994;13:915.
262. Griffith BP, Bando K, Hardesty RL, et al. A prospective randomized trial of FK506 versus cyclosporine after human pulmonary transplantation. *Transplantation* 1994;57:848.
263. Keenan RJ, Konishi H, Kawai A, et al. Clinical trial of tacrolimus versus cyclosporine in lung transplantation. *Ann Thorac Surg* 1995;60:580.
264. Dretchen KL, Morgenroth VH, Standaert FG, et al. Azathioprine: effects on neuromuscular transmission. *Anesthesiology* 1986;45:604.
265. Crosby E, Robblee JA. Cyclosporine-pancuronium interaction in a patient with a renal allograft. *Can J Anesth* 1988;35:300.
266. Trulock EP, Ettinger NA, Brunt EM, et al. The role of transbronchial lung biopsy in the treatment of lung transplant recipients: an analysis of 200 consecutive procedures. *Chest* 1992; 102:1049.
267. Guilinger RA, Paradis IL, Dauber JH, et al. The importance of bronchoscopy with transbronchial biopsy and bronchoalveolar lavage in the management of lung transplant recipients. *Am J Respir Crit Care Med* 1995;152:2037.
268. Millet B, Higenbottam TW, Flower CDR, et al. The radiographic appearances of infection and acute rejection of the lung after heart-lung transplantation. *Am Rev Respir Dis* 1989;140: 62.
269. Otulana BA, Higenbottam T, Ferrari L, et al. The use of home spirometry in detecting acute lung rejection and infection following heart-lung transplantation. *Chest* 1990;97:353.
270. Becker FS, Martinez FJ, Brunsting LA, et al. Limitations of spirometry in detecting rejection after single-lung transplantation. *Am J Respir Crit Care Med* 1994;150:159.
271. Bando K, Paradis IL, Similo S, et al. Obliterative bronchiolitis after lung and heart-lung transplantation: an analysis of risk factor and management. *J Thorac Cardiovasc Surg* 1995; 110:4.
272. Paradis IL, Williams P. Infection after lung transplantation. *Semin Respir Infect* 1993;8:207.
273. Deusch E, End A, Grimm M, et al. Early bacterial infections in lung transplant recipients. *Chest* 1993;104:1412.
274. Keenan RJ, Lega ME, Dummer JS, et al. Cytomegalovirus serologic status and postoperative infection correlated with risk of developing chronic rejection after pulmonary transplantation. *Transplantation* 1991;51:433.
275. Ettinger NA, Bailey TC, Trulock EP, et al. Cytomegalovirus infection and pneumonitis: impact after isolated lung transplantation. *Am Rev Respir Dis* 1993;147:1017.
276. Semenkovich JW, Glazer HS, Anderson DC, et al. Bronchial dehiscence in lung transplantation: CT evaluation. *Radiology* 1995;194:205.
277. Higgins R, McNeil K, Dennis C, et al. Airway stenoses after lung transplantation: management with expanding stents. *J Heart Lung Transplant* 1994;13:774.
278. Colt H, Janssen JP, Dumon JF, et al. Endoscopic management of bronchial stenosis after double lung transplantation. *Chest* 1992;102:10.
279. Hosenpud JD, Bennett LE, Keck BM, et al. Effect of diagnosis on survival benefit of lung transplantation for end-stage lung disease. *Lancet* 1998;351:24.
280. Higenbottam TM, Jackson M, Woolman P, et al. The cough response to ultrasonically nebulized distilled water in heart-lung transplantation patients. *Am Rev Respir Dis* 1989;140:58.
281. Herve P, Silbert D, Cerrina J, et al., and the Paris-Sud Transplant Group. Impairment of bronchial mucociliary clearance in long-term survivors of heart/lung and double-lung transplantation. *Chest* 1993;103:59.
282. Herve P, Picard N, Ladurie MLR, et al. Lack of bronchial hyperresponsiveness to methacholine and to isocapnic dry air hyperventilation in heart/lung and double-lung transplant recipients with normal lung histology. *Am Rev Respir Dis* 1992;145:1503.
283. Higenbottam T, Jackson M, Rashdi T, et al. Lung rejection and bronchial hyperresponsiveness to methacholine and ultrasonically nebulized distilled water in heart-lung transplantation patients. *Am Rev Respir Dis* 1989;140:52.
284. Glanville AR, Burke CM, Theodore J, et al. Bronchial hyperresponsiveness after human cardiopulmonary transplantation. *Clin Sci* 1987;73:299.
285. Maurer JR, McLean PA, Cooper JD, et al. Airway hyperreactivity in patients undergoing lung and heart/lung transplantation. *Am Rev Respir Dis* 1989;139:1038.
286. Robin ED, Theodore J, Burke CM, et al. Hypoxic pulmonary vasoconstriction persists in the human transplanted lung. *Clin Sci* 1987;72:283.

287. Trachiotis GD, Knight SR, Hann M, et al. Respiratory responses to CO_2 rebreathing in lung transplant recipients. *Ann Thorac Surg* 1994;58:1709.
288. Sanders MH, Owens GR, Sciurba FC, et al. Ventilation and breathing pattern during progressive hypercapnia and hypoxia after human heart-lung transplantation. *Am Rev Respir Dis* 1989;140:38.
289. Sundaresan RS, Trulock EP, Mohanakumar T, et al., and the Washington University Lung Transplant Group. Prevalence and outcome of bronchiolitis obliterans syndrome after lung transplantation. *Ann Thorac Surg* 1995;60:1341.
290. Bando K, Paradis IL, Komatsu K, et al. Analysis of time-dependent risks for infection, rejection and death after pulmonary transplantation. *J Thorac Cardiovasc Surg* 1995;109:49.
291. Nathan SD, Ross DJ, Belman MJ, et al. Bronchiolitis obliterans in single-lung transplant recipients. *Chest* 1995;107:967.

24

CARDIAC REOPERATIONS

MICHAEL G. LICINA
JEAN-PIERRE YARED
FAWZY G. ESTAFANOUS

Cardiac reoperations have evolved from an anesthetic and surgical challenge to routine patient management (1). This is the result of increased experience and new methods of anesthetic, surgical, and postoperative management, which have led to better outcomes despite the higher risk factors associated with reoperations. In general, patients presenting for reoperations are older and have progression of their initial disease process such as cardiac, pulmonary, and renal dysfunction, atherosclerosis, and diabetes mellitus. The surgeries are usually more complex and time-consuming. Such complexity includes releasing adhesions during dissection of the heart and major vascular structures and finding suitable conduits and graft material for patients who have already had saphenous vein or thoracic artery harvesting. It is therefore not surprising to find that reoperations are associated with increased mortality and morbidity. This chapter reviews the evolution of cardiac reoperations such as coronary artery bypass grafting (CABG), valve repair/replacement, aortic surgery, placement of a ventricular assist device, and transplantation. Overall, the incidence of reoperations at the Cleveland Clinic (CCF) has remained relatively constant at about 25%, although the absolute number of cases has increased (Fig. 24-1). Interestingly, the mortality rates for both primary operations and reoperations decreased from 1993 to 1999 (Fig. 24-2).

CORONARY ARTERY BYPASS GRAFTING REOPERATIONS

Since the late 1950s, surgeons have used various techniques to improve blood supply to the myocardium. These techniques include the Beck's procedure (creation of adhesions between the pericardium and the heart), the Vinberg procedure (internal thoracic artery implanted into the myocardium), and aortocoronary bypass grafts using venous segments (saphenous vein) or arterial segments (internal thoracic, radial, or epigastric artery). Newer, experimental techniques include the use of epicardial lasers to enhance myocardial blood supply. These procedures have been accomplished with and without the use of cardiopulmonary bypass (CPB). Roughly every fifth patient undergoing CABG will eventually need a reoperation because of recurrent angina and deteriorating myocardial function (2). The reasons include poor technical results, early graft thrombosis, and progressive atherosclerosis of either the grafts or native vessels (3–9). In that regard, arterial grafts often are patent at the time of reoperation because they have better long-term patency rates than vein grafts (4,9). Recent developments in noninvasive and invasive cardiology have modified the indications and selection of patients for reoperation. Now one expects the patients presenting for CABG reoperation to be older and to have progression of associated diseases such as diabetes mellitus, renal dysfunction, and cerebrovascular disease, as well as more advanced cardiac disease. Moreover, patients presenting for both primary and reoperation surgery are frequently undergoing more complex procedures, as shown by the increased frequency of "extended CABG" surgery (i.e., CABG combined with valve, vascular, or ventricular outflow tract or aneurysm surgery). At CCF, extended CABG procedures are increasing in frequency, from 13.8% in 1993 to 21.8% in 1999. CABG reoperations increased from 2.7% in the late 1970s to 26% in 1993; since then, the frequency has remained stable (Fig. 24-3).

Risk Factors

At CCF, a severity scoring system was developed to measure the risk of CABG operations (10). A score was assigned for each significant preoperative risk factor for morbidity or mortality, as determined by logistic regression analysis. Risk factors have weights from 1 to 6 assigned to them, based

M. G. Licina: Department of Anesthesiology, Health Science Center of the Ohio State University and Department of Cardiac Anesthesia, The Cleveland Clinic Foundation, Cleveland, Ohio 44195

J. P. Yared: Department of Cardiac Anesthesia, The Cleveland Clinic Foundation, Cleveland, Ohio 44124

F. G. Estafanous: Division of Anesthesiology and Critical Care Medicine, The Cleveland Clinic Foundation, Cleveland, Ohio 44195

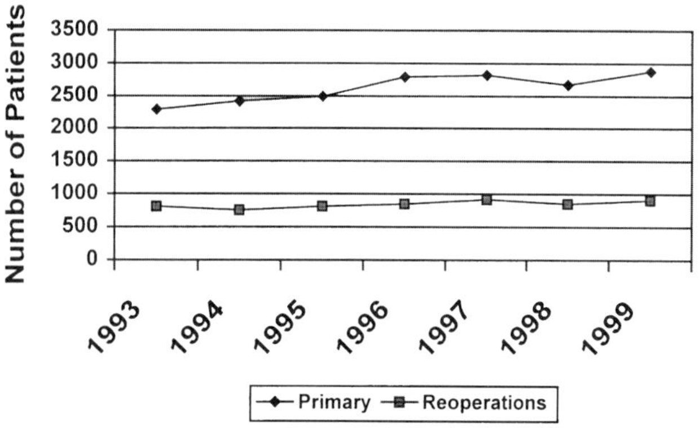

FIGURE 24-1. Number of primary cardiac operations versus cardiac reoperations.

TABLE 24-1. CLEVELAND CLINIC SEVERITY SCORING SYSTEM

Preoperative Factors	Score
Emergency case	6
Serum creatinine	
≥141 and ≤167 μmol/l (≥1.6 and ≤1.8 mg/dL)	1
≥168 μmol/l (≥1.9 mg/dL)	4
Severe left ventricular dysfunction	3
Reoperation	3
Operative mitral valve insufficiency	3
Age >65 and <74 yr	1
Age >75 yr	2
Prior vascular surgery	2
Chronic obstructive pulmonary disease	2
Anemic (hematocrit >0.34)	2
Operative aortic valve stenosis	1
Weight <65 kg	1
Diabetes: oral or insulin therapy	1
Cerebrovascular disease	1

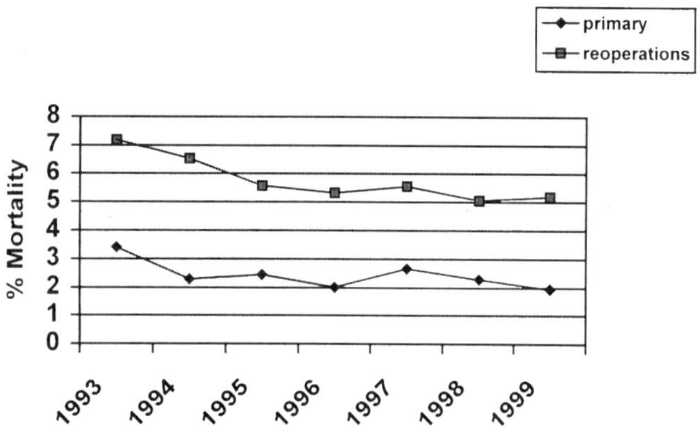

FIGURE 24-2. Comparison of mortality rates: cardiac primary operation versus cardiac reoperation.

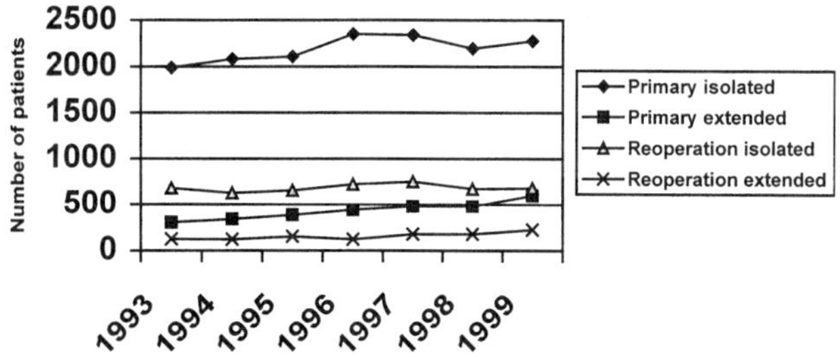

FIGURE 24-3. Number of coronary artery bypass grafting (CABG) cases: isolated CABG versus extended CABG (i.e., CABG plus another cardiac procedure).

on both odds ratio and clinical importance. The total risk score for the patient is the sum of all preoperative risk factors. Reoperation *per se* carries a risk score of 3, accounting for the increased surgical risk associated with reoperations (Table 24-1).

Figure 24-4 lists the severity scores for four groups of patients: primary isolated CABG (first-time CABG only), primary extended CABG (first-time extended CABG), redo isolated (reoperation for grafts only), and redo extended (reoperation for extended CABG). The severity scores for all groups increased from 1993 to 1999, and there is some indication that the severity scores of the redo groups are increasing at a greater rate than those of the primary groups. Higher scores reflect the higher risk of the reoperative procedure itself and the progression of organ dysfunction, particularly left ventricular dysfunction.

Evaluation of specific preoperative risk factors from 1993 to 1999 showed an increasing incidence of the following parameters in each of the four subgroups: advanced age, preoperative left ventricular dysfunction (ejection fraction less than 35%), and cerebrovascular disease (history of cerebrovascular accidents or previous vascular surgery) (Figs. 24-5 and 24-6). Of note, the prevalence of octogenarians doubled in all four groups from 1993 to 1999. Despite the higher risk in patients with advanced age, the long-term results in these patients are good and age should not be a contraindication to reoperative CABG surgery (11). In contrast, factors such as female gender, low body weight (less than 65 kg), pharmacologically treated diabetes mellitus, and preoperative renal insufficiency showed minimal change. Emergency CABG reoperations had a high operative mortality rate (17%) and poor postoperative functional results (12). Urgent operations saw a four-fold decline in

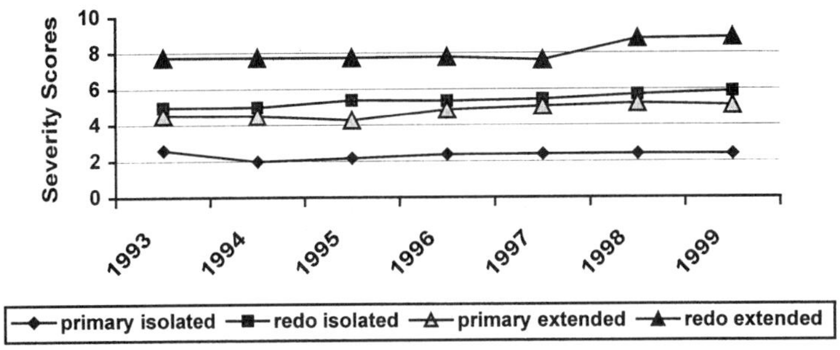

FIGURE 24-4. Severity scores according to type of coronary artery bypass grafting (CABG) surgery each year.

incidence from 1993 to 1999 in all four groups, and fewer patients had preoperative insertion of intraaortic balloon pumps. This decline is probably the result of better catheterization laboratory rescue techniques, such as thrombolysis, balloon angioplasty, coronary artery stenting, atherectomy, and valvuloplasty.

Other studies support the predictive value of the scoring system in use at CCF but, additionally, stress the importance of left main coronary artery stenosis, unstable angina (New York Health Association class III or IV), and an interval shorter than 1 year since the initial revascularization procedure as independent risk factors for mortality (2, 13–18).

Morbidity and Mortality

Overall, the morbidity and mortality rate of CABG reoperations is higher than that of the comparable primary operations, but the incidence is decreasing in both groups: the rate for isolated reoperation in 1999 was approaching that of the 1993 primary operation (Fig. 24-7). In Fig. 24-7, national mortality data for primary isolated CABG published by the Society of Thoracic Surgeons is plotted and follows the same decline as for the CCF groups.

The changing trends in morbidity affect isolated and extended surgery similarly. The definition of morbidity is listed in Table 24-2. For the sake of simplicity, only data comparing primary isolated versus isolated reoperations are presented. The morbidity rates for the extended groups fol-

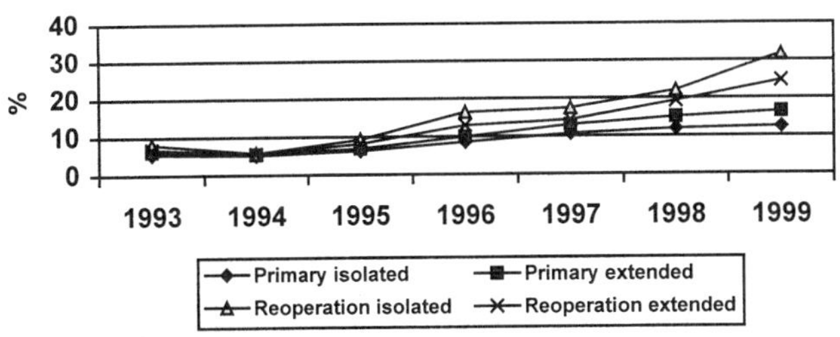

FIGURE 24-5. Incidence of severe left ventricular dysfunction in the coronary artery bypass grafting (CABG) groups.

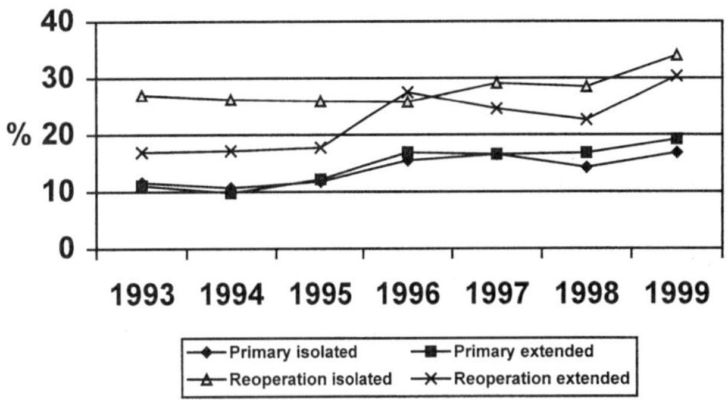

FIGURE 24-6. Coronary artery bypass grafting (CABG) with age greater than 75 years.

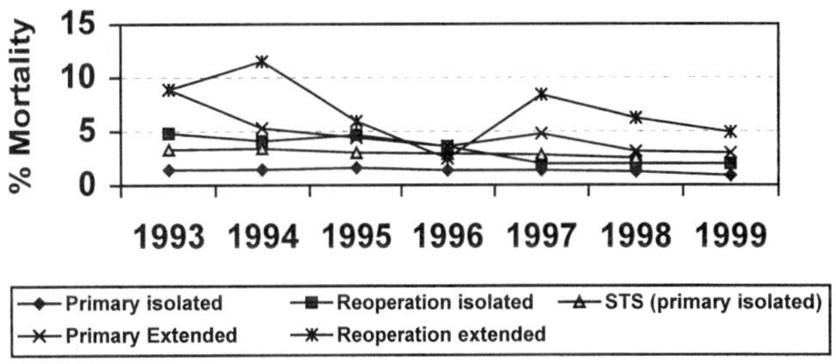

FIGURE 24-7. Mortality rate for patients undergoing coronary artery bypass grafting (CABG).

TABLE 24-2. CLEVELAND CLINIC DATABASE DEFINITIONS OF MORBIDITIES

System	Definition of Morbidity
Pulmonary	Total intubation time >72 hr
Renal	Anuria or dialysis started in ICU
Cardiac	Low cardiac output despite inotropic drugs, or postoperative MI requiring mechanical assistance
Infection	Sepsis, mediastinitis, pneumonia in ICU
Neurologic	Focal or global deficit
Death	Death in hospital
Overall morbidity	One or more of the above six morbidities

Note: ICU, intensive care unit; MI, myocardial infarction.

lowed a similar pattern. The incidence of respiratory failure decreased by about 40% for primary isolated CABG and 38% for isolated reoperations. The isolated reoperation group had a decrease in the incidence of postoperative renal failure and cardiac morbidity of 40% and 14%, respectively; whereas there was no change in the primary group. The incidence of intraaortic balloon pump insertion in the operating room declined in both groups, but more so in the reoperation group. The use of inotropes in all groups remained the same (39% primary, 59% reoperation) despite the increasing severity scores of the patients. This could be a result of better anesthetic and surgical techniques or better myocardial preservation. The surgical techniques used include minimally invasive surgery, surgery without CPB, and the use of arterial conduits (19,20). The use of retrograde cardioplegia has improved myocardial preservation (21). The type of inotropes used is changing over time. Epinephrine is still the primary agent used. The use of milrinone and norepinephrine has increased, with a concomitant decrease in the usage of dopamine and dobutamine. Perhaps this represents increased use of a pharmacologic balloon pump to avoid the insertion of an intraaortic balloon pump with its associated vascular complications in a high-risk vascular disease population. The recognition of this vascular disease is a result of the increased use of transesophageal echocardiography (TEE) and epiaortic echocardiography to reveal ascending aortic atheroma. No notable change was observed in the incidence of neurologic morbidity or serious wound infection. The absence of increase in the incidence of such complications in itself reflects improved outcome, because it occurred concomitantly with an increase in severity score of the patient.

Intraoperative Course

Analysis of intraoperative data reveals several interesting points that may have been instrumental in improving the outcomes reported here. The incidence of multiple CPB pump runs decreased by 20% in all groups. The duration of CPB and aortic cross-clamping remained about the same,

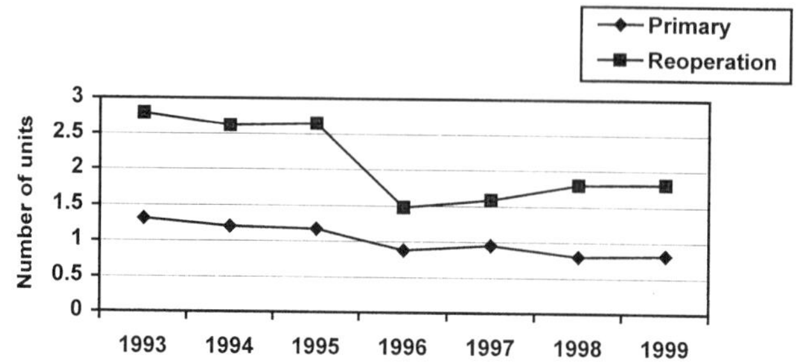

FIGURE 24-9. Number of transfusions per coronary artery bypass grafting (CABG) patient.

with the reoperations requiring about 10% more time than primary operations. Interestingly, the use of circulatory arrest increased by 30% in the reoperation groups, reflecting the inability to dissect out the aorta and the increased recognition of atheroma in the ascending aorta by means of TEE and epiaortic echocardiography.

The incidence of return to the operating room for bleeding/tamponade decreased in all groups by 40%. Intraoperative use of packed red blood cells declined despite a lower preoperative hematocrit in patients undergoing reoperation (41.1% in 1993 versus 38.4% in 1999). The number of blood transfusions per patient and the percentage of patients transfused decreased by 35%. This was not due to acceptance of a lower hematocrit, because the average hematocrit on admission to the intensive care unit (ICU) increased from 29% in 1993 to 31% in 1999. These observations suggest that the incidence of surgical bleeding decreased or that blood conservation techniques improved, or both (Figs. 24-8 and 24-9).

The usage of ϵ-aminocaproic acid (EACA) increased dramatically in both primary and redo CABG operations, whereas the use of aprotinin remained low: 0.31% in the primary operation group and 1.29% in the reoperation group (Fig. 24-10).

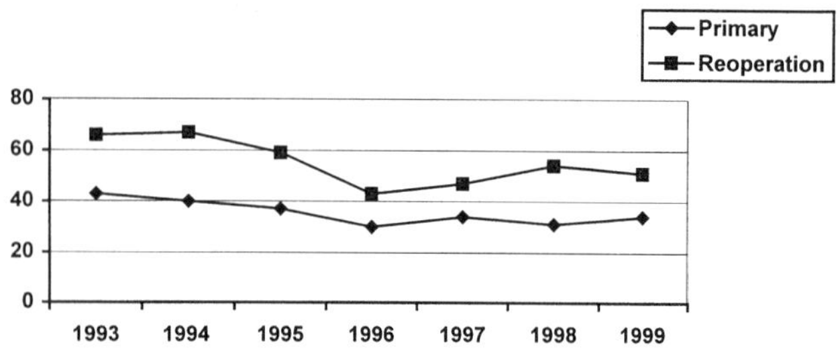

FIGURE 24-8. Percentage of coronary artery bypass grafting (CABG) patients receiving red blood cell transfusions.

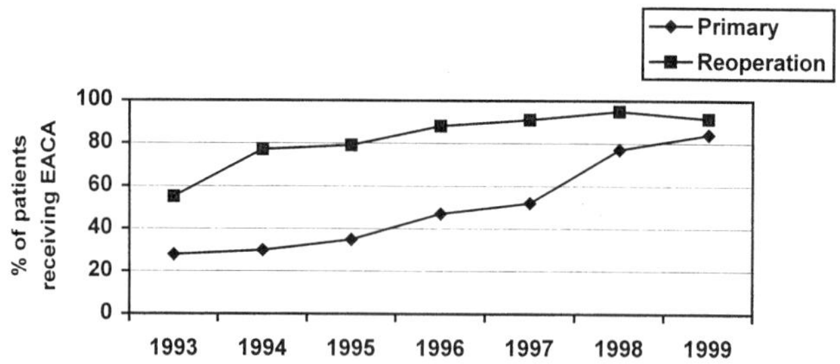

FIGURE 24-10. ϵ-Amino caproic acid (EACA) use in coronary artery bypass grafting (CABG) patients.

TABLE 24-3. AORTIC VALVE REOPERATION RISK FACTORS

Older age
Female sex
Coronary artery disease
Endocarditis
Severe left ventricular dysfunction

CARDIAC VALVE REOPERATIONS

Lytle reviewed the first 1,000 valve reoperations performed at the CCF from 1958 to 1984 (22). Risk factors included age, number of reoperations, type and number of valves being replaced, and left ventricular dysfunction. Patients undergoing first single-valve reoperation had a mortality rate of 32% if they were 70 years of age or older. The mortality was 17% if the patients were between the ages of 60 to 70 years, and 4% if they were younger than 60 years.

Additional risk factors for aortic valve reoperation included endocarditis, female gender, and number of coronary vessels with 70% or greater stenosis (Table 24-3). The mortality rate for first aortic valve reoperations was 11%, with 69% of these deaths related to myocardial dysfunction.

Additional risk factors for mitral valve reoperations included old age, severe left ventricular dysfunction, preoperative shock or cardiac arrest, previous aortic or tricuspid valve surgery, and type of mitral valve procedure. For example, risk for repair of a periprosthetic leak was greater than that for mitral valve replacement, which in turn was greater than the risk for a mitral valve–conserving procedure (Table 24-4). There was a 10% in-hospital mortality rate among first mitral valve reoperation patients, mainly due to myocardial dysfunction (36%). In general, mitral valve reoperation was associated with a higher risk than aortic valve surgery.

Risk factors for first multiple-valve reoperations were ascites and diabetes. One exception was that patients undergoing mitral valve replacement and a tricuspid valve operation were at decreased risk. The mortality rate in that group was 14% (60% due to myocardial causes).

TABLE 24-4. MITRAL VALVE REOPERATION RISK FACTORS

Older age
Severe left ventricular dysfunction
Previous aortic or tricuspid valve operations
Type of procedure
Periprosthetic leak repair
Valve replacement
Mitral valve-conserving procedure
Coronary artery bypass grafting

TABLE 24-5. REPEAT REOPERATION RISK FACTORS

Older age
Coronary artery bypass grafting

Mortality increased with each additional procedure and with each additional risk factor. Risk factors for this group included rereplacement of prosthesis, concomitant CABG operation, and increased age (Table 24-5). The mortality rate for second reoperations was 15%; for third reoperations, it was 44%.

One of the major risks of reoperation was catastrophic hemorrhage associated with sternal reentry. This complication occurred in 36 of 1,000 valve reoperations and was associated with a 33% mortality rate.

A multicenter study looked at 2,246 valve reoperations performed from 1963 to 1992 at three institutions (23). The patients included in the study ranged from high-risk moribund patients to elective well patients. The risk-unadjusted mortality rate was 10.8%, neurologic deficit at discharge was 1.1%, and length of stay was 10 days. Risk factors included advanced age, severity and acuity of cardiac function impairment, extent of valvular disease, coexisting morbid conditions, number of previous heart operations, and concomitant procedures. The mortality rate for elective, low-risk patients undergoing their first reoperation was 1.3%, with a rate of neurologic deficit of 0.3% and a postoperative length of stay of 7 days. The authors found that mitral valve reoperations had a higher mortality rate than aortic valve reoperations, similar to Lytle's findings. Again, age and preoperative left ventricular function were important risk factors.

Data from 1993 to 1999 for 3,695 primary isolated valve operations and 1,320 isolated valve reoperations done at CCF reveal overall mortality rates of 1.38% and 5.76%, respectively. The mortality rate after isolated aortic valve reoperations was 3.1% for patients younger than 70 years of age and 6.72% for older patients. In contrast, Lytle's earlier paper (22) at the same institution showed that aortic valve reoperation was associated with mortality rates of 8.25% and 44% for patients younger and older than 70 years of age, respectively. Thus there has been marked improvement in mortality, especially among older patients. Patients undergoing mitral valve reoperation had an overall mortality rate of 3.54%. The rate was 2.43% for those younger than 70 years of age, and 6.54% for those older than 70. Again, patient outcomes have improved, compared with Lytle's earlier data, in which there was an overall 10% mortality rate.

Assessment of preoperative risk factors shows that, compared with patients undergoing primary valvular surgery, the reoperation group had a higher prevalence of risk factors: patients in this group were older and had a higher incidence of vascular disease (13% versus 3.7%), severe left ventricular dysfunction (7.8% versus 4.8%), and history of preoperative congestive heart failure (57% versus 31%). Between 1993 and 1999, the incidence of severe left ventricular dysfunction in the reoperation group increased from 3.37% to 12.62%. The incidence of emergency operation decreased by 50% in both groups.

Evaluation of data at CCF between 1993 and 1999 shows a clear trend toward reduced need for intraoperative blood transfusions in both groups, lower incidence of returns to the operating room for bleeding, and decreased requirement for circulatory arrest. In more than 90% of both primary and valvular reoperations ϵ-aminocaproic acid (EACA) was used. Aprotinin was administered in 3.7% of the reoperations and in 0.4% of the primary valve operations. The incidence of morbidity remained constant during the 1993–1999 period. In particular, cardiac morbidity stayed low (2.58%) despite an increasing incidence of preoperative severe left ventricular dysfunction, one of the risk factors for mortality previously described. The risk-unadjusted postoperative length of stay in the reoperation group decreased from 15 to 10.86 days, whereas in the primary group it remained constant at 7.8 days. Therefore, over time, the operative results improved despite the fact that patients presented with more risk factors.

Figure 24-11 shows the decreased mortality rates for isolated aortic and mitral valve reoperations done at CCF over time.

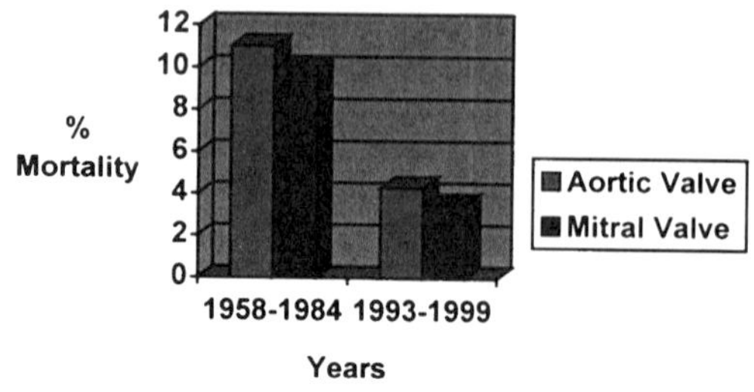

FIGURE 24-11. Mortality rates for aortic and mitral valve reoperations.

HEART TRANSPLANTATION

From 1993 to 1999, 507 heart transplantation operations were performed at CCF, of which 56% were reoperations. In the reoperation heart transplantation group of 286 patients, 190 patients (66%) had implanted ventricular assist devices. Mechanical assistance was provided by preoperative extracorporeal membrane oxygenation (ECMO) in 9 reoperation patients. Evaluation of preoperative risk factors showed that patients undergoing reoperation were older (55.6 versus 52.83 years of age) and had a higher incidence of stroke (11% versus 5%). As expected, almost all transplantation patients had severe left ventricular dysfunction. Intraoperative data showed that the reoperation group had more prolonged durations of CPB (131 versus 119 minutes) and aortic cross-clamping (119 versus 72 minutes). Almost all patients required pharmacologic hemodynamic support. Intraoperative blood transfusions were twice as frequent in the reoperation group. The postoperative morbidity rate was also twice as high in the reoperation group (27% versus 14%). This was the consequence of a two-fold higher incidence of respiratory failure, renal failure, neurologic morbidity, major transfusions, and return to the operating room for bleeding. There was a four-fold increase in serious wound infections and a slight increase in cardiac morbidity. The overall mortality rate was 4% for the primary group versus 5.9% for the reoperation heart transplantation group. Postoperative length of stay was slightly longer for the reoperative group: 17.7 versus 16.2 days.

VENTRICULAR ASSIST DEVICES

From 1993 to 1999 there were three main types of left ventricular assist devices inserted at the CCF: the pneumatic

TABLE 24-6. INCIDENCE OF MORBIDITIES ASSOCIATED WITH A VENTRICULAR ASSIST DEVICE (%)

Event	Primary Heartmate	Reoperation Heartmate	Primary Novacor	Reoperation Novacor
Preoperative CVA	3	7	3	4
Overall morbidity	83	95	97	96
Cardiac	83	95	97	96
Respiratory	48	67	63	60
Renal	17	27	20	20
Neurological	8	12	30	16
Infection	23	45	47	48
Return to OR for bleeding	27	23	23	16
Major transfusions	27	46	23	24
Mortality	16	35	23	24

Note: CVA, cerebrovascular accident; OR, operating room.

and electric Heartmate (Thermo Cardiosystems, Woburn, MA) and the Novacor (Baxter Healthcare Corporation, Oakland, CA) devices. A total of 202 devices were implanted, 72% of which were Heartmate (56% for patients with prior cardiac surgery) and 38% of which were Novacor devices (45% for patients with prior cardiac surgery). As would be expected for both devices, the reoperation groups had markedly higher rates of mortality, morbidity, and transfusion (Table 24-6). Differences in the incidence of mortality and morbidity were observed among devices, especially in neurologic outcome. The Novocor group had a higher incidence of cerebrovascular accidents that prompted a change in the design of the inflow cannula.

AORTIC SURGERY

A total of 665 aortic surgeries without associated cardiac operation were done from 1993 to 1999 at CCF. Of these, 189 were reoperations (28%). Preoperative history of congestive heart failure was twice as frequent in the reoperation group compared with the primary group. The primary group had a higher incidence of emergency surgery (27% versus 12%). Intraoperatively, the reoperation group required more transfusions (81% versus 67%) and more inotropic support (64% versus 50%) than the primary group. Postoperatively, the reoperation group had higher incidences of perioperative myocardial infarction (3.7% versus 1.05%) and overall cardiac morbidity (6.35% versus 2.94%). Other morbidity rates stayed unchanged, but mortality in the reoperation group was higher (12.17% versus 8.82%).

SURGICAL MANAGEMENT

Surgical experience with the large number of reoperations done at CCF has led to changes in surgical practice that may explain the improved outcomes observed. For instance, in order to permit rapid establishment of CPB in case of prebypass catastrophic events, the surgeons frequently expose or cannulate either the femoral or subclavian vessel before sternal opening. When sternotomy or surgical dissection results in uncontrollable hemorrhage, or when myocardial ischemia occurs secondary to interruption of flow or embolization from a diseased but patent aortocoronary graft, this approach allows rapid reestablishment of hemodynamic stability and preservation of end-organ function. Ligation of these old diseased grafts is frequently done to prevent this type of myocardial injury (24,25). The use of the oscillating saw and blunt dissection under the sternum have decreased the risk of hemorrhage. Moreover, alternative surgical approaches, such as a thoracotomy rather than a median sternotomy, allow the surgeon to avoid injuries potentially associated with the midsternal approach. This is beneficial in mitral valve procedures and certain CABG operations.

The decrease in cardiac morbidity along with a decrease in use of the intraaortic balloon pump can be attributed to better surgical technique, including better myocardial preservation and the use of TEE (26). Myocardial preservation is accomplished via both antegrade and retrograde blood cardioplegia and administration of cardioplegia through the proximal end of coronary grafts after the distal anastomosis is completed. The use of internal thoracic arteries, radial arteries, and inferior epigastric arteries has led not only to better long-time patency but to improved intraoperative patency in CABG reoperations where no veins may be available for grafting (27–30). However, shortage of conduits and more advanced coronary artery disease increase the risks for incomplete revascularization in this group of patients. The use of TEE and epicardial echocardiography to identify ascending aortic atheromas allows the surgeon to select alternative cannulation sites when appropriate, thereby decreasing the potential for atherosclerotic embolization. Furthermore, increased ability to detect such atheromas has led to an increase in the instances in which it is preferable to avoid aortic cross-clamping. This explains why the incidence of circulatory arrest has increased over the past 6 years. TEE is also used to ascertain adequate evacuation of air from the heart before separation from CPB, thereby decreasing the potential for air embolism. TEE also confirms the adequacy of the surgical procedure and helps detect potential surgical problems (26).

Performing cardiac surgery without CPB is very useful in certain CABG reoperations because it allows avoidance of full anticoagulation and may decrease risks of postoperative bleeding. Non-CPB technology may have additional benefits since it avoids the excessive inflammatory response and potential embolic complications associated with extracorporeal circulation. To date, however, there are no published studies on this matter.

CPB equipment has improved, perhaps leading to a decrease in blood product administration. Heparin-coated cannulas (Carmeda Duraflo: Bacter Healthcare Corp., Irvine, CA) are associated with reduced activation of the complement system (31,32). Newer CPB circuits require smaller priming volumes, resulting in less hemodilution. In addition, the use of hemoconcentrators to remove excess fluids has decreased blood utilization. Ultrafiltration has been advocated for infants and children undergoing repair of congenital heart disease. It may result in improved left ventricular function (33). However, at the present time, there is no evidence of improved outcome in adults (34). The technology is expensive and is not currently used in adult cardiac surgery at CCF. Moreover, although hypothermic CPB was routinely used in 1993, especially for reoperations, the tendency has shifted toward normothermia or mild to moderate hypothermia for all cases except those involving circulatory arrest The change in temperature management may have improved hemostatic function and could explain in part the reduction in the use of blood transfusions (see Chapter 14).

Surgical experience in preventing hemorrhage and controlling post-CPB bleeding, along with the use of EACA, has decreased the amount of blood transfusions and the incidence of return to the operating room for hemostasis. Aprotinin has been advocated in this role, but its usage at CCF is minimal (35–38). Nevertheless, the rates of transfusion and of return to the operating room for bleeding decreased dramatically, perhaps in part because of the increasing use of EACA. In a recent review of 72 trials (39), aprotinin and other lysine analogs (EACA) decreased the frequency of surgical reexploration and allogeneic blood transfusion but did not increase the risk of myocardial infarction. Desmopressin use was found to reduce perioperative blood loss slightly but was associated with a 2.4-fold increase in myocardial infarction.

ANESTHETIC MANAGEMENT

In addition to the standard requirement for adequate analgesia, amnesia, and immobility, anesthetic success depends on adequate intravenous access, adequate monitoring with a pulmonary artery catheter and/or TEE, and prompt identification and treatment of problems such hemorrhage, low cardiac output, myocardial ischemia, and arrhythmias. Such problems may not be amenable to medical treatment, and the surgeon should be promptly informed about persistent hypotension, ischemia, and arrhythmias so that the proper surgical intervention (e.g., establishment of CPB) can be implemented promptly. When ventricular or paroxysmal atrial tachycardia or fibrillation occurs during dissection of the heart during reoperation, it is often impossible to adequately apply internal defibrillation paddles, and it is necessary in these situations to use external pads or paddles. Reoperations for which a thoracotomy approach is selected to avoid the risks associated with median sternotomy require the use of single-lung ventilation to facilitate surgical exposure. Any anesthetic technique can be used without influencing patient outcome as long as the anesthesiologist is aware of the potential side effects of the agents used, particularly in view of the higher incidence of impaired left ventricular dysfunction in the reoperation group of patients. There is a trend toward "fast-tracking" of patients to allow for earlier extubation, and these techniques can be used in the reoperation population equally. Postinduction corticosteroids are administered to cardiac surgical patients by many anesthesiologists. Steroids modulate the inflammatory response to CPB and facilitate fast-track recovery (40,41). Dexamethasone decreases the incidence of postoperative shivering, fever, and atrial fibrillation and facilitates early endotracheal extubation (42,43). The use of the pulmonary artery catheter with the TEE is controversial and currently under scrutiny, but it is important to note that the TEE is

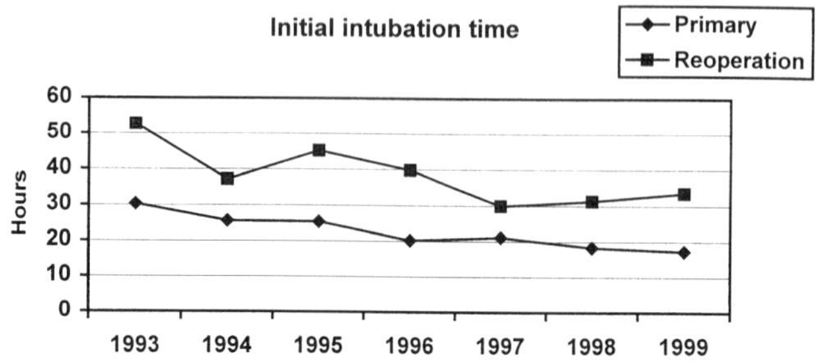

FIGURE 24-12. Initial intubation times.

an intraoperative monitor, whereas the pulmonary artery catheter is a perioperative monitor, which is useful in the ICU. Adequate intravenous access is vital in these operations, because there is high risk of catastrophic hemorrhage. It is not uncommon for hemorrhage to result from laceration of the brachiocephalic vein or, less commonly, the superior vena cava. Control of hemorrhage and repair of the laceration usually require ligation or clamping of the brachiocephalic vein or super vena cava. This results in a temporary or permanent inability to deliver fluids and drugs via upper extremity venous access.

POSTOPERATIVE MANAGEMENT

The literature as well as the data presented in this chapter associate reoperations with increased mortality and morbidity. It is therefore not surprising to find that reoperations are associated with increased intubation time and longer durations of ICU and hospital length of stay. However, the decreasing trends observed for mortality and morbidity are paralleled by a trend toward earlier extubation and shorter ICU and hospital length of stay. The figures show data for all CABG and valve patients (Figs. 24-12 through 24-14). The shorter ICU length of stay occurred while the rate of readmission to the ICU remained stable, at an average of 6.83% for primary operations and 9.4% for reoperations.

It is apparent from these data that fast-track recovery is

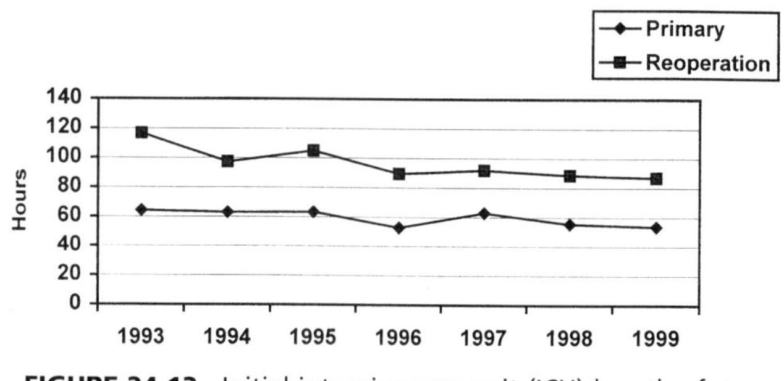

FIGURE 24-13. Initial intensive care unit (ICU) length of stay.

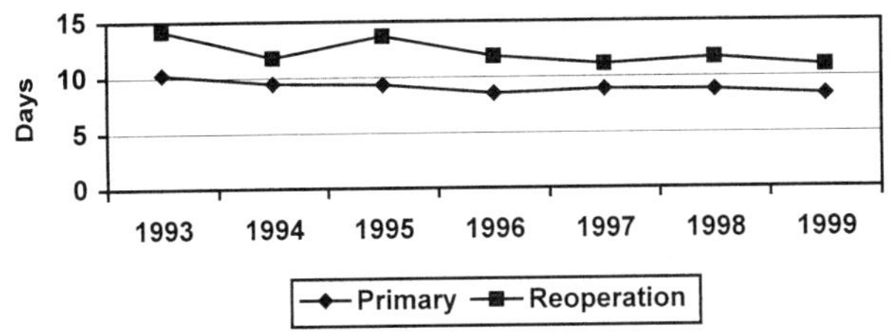

FIGURE 24-14. Postoperative hospital length of stay.

applicable to reoperations provided that patients are selected appropriately. Postoperative management is discussed in greater detail in Chapter 17.

CONCLUSIONS

Improvement in the management of reoperations is continuing. The results presented in this chapter indicate a marked improvement in morbidity and mortality of reoperation patients over the last 30 years. These improvements are occurring regardless of the type of reoperation. Reoperations are becoming very common to the practicing cardiac anesthesiologist. The management of these patients has become routine. Keys to the successful management of these patients include communication with the surgeon about the surgical plan, adequate venous access, intraoperative use of lysine analogs, and the use of TEE.

REFERENCES

1. Camann WR, Wojtowicz SR, Mark JB. Reoperation for coronary artery bypass grafting: anesthetic challenge. *J Cardiothorac Anesth* 1987;1:458.
2. Christensen JT, Schmuziger M, Simonet F. Reoperative coronary artery bypass procedures: risk factors for early mortality and late survival. *Eur J Cardiothorac Surg* 1997;11:129.
3. Schaff HV, Orszulak TA, Gersh BJ, et al. The morbidity and mortality of reoperation for coronary artery disease and analysis of late results with use of actuarial estimate of event-free interval. *J Thorac Cardiovasc Surg* 1983;85:508.
4. Loop FD, Lytle BW, Gill CC, et al. Trends in selection and results of coronary artery reoperations. *Ann Thorac Surg* 1983; 36:380.
5. Reardon MJ, Conklin LD, Reardon PR, et al. Coronary artery bypass conduits: a review of current status. *J Cardiovasc Surg* 1997;38:201.
6. Buche M, Dion R. Current status of the inferior epigastric artery [Review]. *Semin Thorac Cardiovasc Surg* 1996;8:10.
7. Shapira OM, Alkon JD, Aldea GS, et al. Clinical outcomes in patients undergoing coronary artery bypass grafting with preferred use of the radial artery. *J Card Surg* 1997;12:381.
8. Del Rizzo DF, Fremes SE, Christakis GT, et al. Coronary bypass with arterial conduits. *Cardiovasc Surg* 1998;6:81.
9. Buxton BF, Komeda M, Fuller JA, et al. Bilateral internal thoracic artery grafting may improve outcome of coronary artery surgery: risk-adjusted survival. *Circulation* 1998;98[Suppl 19]:II-1.
10. Higgins TL, Estafanous FG, Loop FD, et al. Stratification of morbidity and mortality outcome by preoperative risk factors in coronary artery bypass patients. *JAMA* 1992;267:2344.
11. Christenson JT, Simonet F, Schmuziger M. The influence of age on the results of reoperative coronary artery bypass grafting. *Coron Artery Dis* 1997;8:91.
12. Lemmer JH Jr, Ferguson DW, Rakel BA, et al. Clinical outcome of emergency repeat coronary artery bypass surgery. *J Cardiovasc Surg (Torino)* 1990;31:492.
13. Lytle BW, Loop FD, Cosgrove DM, et al. Fifteen hundred coronary reoperations: results and determinants of early and late survival. *J Thorac Cardiovasc Surg* 1987;93:847.
14. Loop FD, Stewart RL, Lytle BW, et al. Reoperation for myocardial revascularization. *World J Surg* 1978;2:719.
15. Lytle BW, Loop FD. Coronary reoperations. *Surg Clin North Am* 1988;68:559.
16. Loop FD. A 20-year experience in coronary artery reoperation. *Eur Heart J* 1989;10:78.
17. Loop FD, Lytle BW, Cosgrove DM, et al. Reoperation for coronary atherosclerosis. *Ann Surg* 1990;212:378.
18. Salomon NW, Bigelow JC, Metzdorff MT. Reoperative coronary surgery. *J Thorac Cardiovasc Surg* 1990;100:250.
19. Doty JR, Salazar JD, Fonger JD, et al. Reoperative MIDCAB grafting: 3-year clinical experience. *Eur J Cardiothorac Surg* 1998; 13:641.
20. Allen KB, Matheny RG, Robison RJ, et al. Minimally invasive versus conventional reoperative coronary artery bypass. *Ann Thorac Surg* 1997;64:616.
21. Goldman SM, Sutter FP, Priest BP, et al. Continuous retrograde cardiac perfusion decreases risk of reoperative coronary artery bypass grafting. *Angiology* 1997;48:433.
22. Lytle BW, Cosgrove DM, Taylor PC, et al. Reoperations for valve surgery: perioperative mortality and determinants of risk for 1,000 patients, 1958–1984. *Ann Thorac Surg* 1986;42:632.
23. Piehler JM, Blackstone EH, Bailey KR, et al. Reoperation on prosthetic heart valves: patient-specific estimates of in-hospital events. *J Thorac Cardiovasc Surg* 1995;109:30.
24. Keon WJ, Heggtveit HA, Leduc J. Perioperative myocardial infarction caused by atheroembolism. *J Thorac Cardiovasc Surg* 1982;84:849.
25. Walts AE, Fishbein MC, Sustaita H, et al. Ruptured atheromatous plaques in saphenous vein coronary artery bypass grafts: a mechanism of acute, thrombotic, late graft occlusion. *Circulation* 1982;65:197.
26. Savage RM, Lytle BW, Aronson S, et al. Intraoperative echo is indicated in high risk coronary artery bypass surgery. *Ann Thorac Surg* 1997;64:368.
27. Akhter M, Lajos TZ, Grosner G, et al. Reoperations with the right gastroepiploic artery without cardiopulmonary bypass. *J Card Surg* 1997;12:210.
28. Taggart DP. Arterial or venous conduits for redo coronary artery bypass grafting? *Heart* 1998;80:1.
29. Jones JW, Schmidt SE, Miller R, et al. Suitability and durability of multiple internal thoracic artery coronary artery bypasses. *Ann Surg* 1997;225:785; discussion 1997;225:791.
30. Dougenis D, Brown AH. Long term results of reoperations for recurrent angina with internal mammary artery versus saphenous vein grafts. *Heart* 1998;80:9.
31. Muehrcke DD, McCarthy PM, Kottke-Marchant K, et al. Biocompatibility of heparin-coated extracorporeal bypass circuits: a randomized, masked clinical trial. *J Thorac Cardiovasc Surg* 1996; 112:472.
32. McCarthy PM, Yared JP, Foster RC, et al. A prospective randomized trial of Duraflo II heparin-coated circuits in cardiac reoperations. *Ann Thorac Surg* 1999;67:1268.
33. Chaturvedi RR, Shore DF, White PA, et al. Modified ultrafiltra-

tion improves global left ventricular systolic function after open-heart surgery in infants and children. *Eur J Cardiothorac Surg* 1999;15:742.
34. Tassani P, Richter JA, Eising GP, et al. Influence of combined zero-balanced and modified ultrafiltration on the systemic inflammatory response during coronary artery bypass grafting. *J Cardiothorac Vasc Anesth* 1999;13:285.
35. Smith CR. Management of bleeding complications in redo cardiac operations. *Ann Thorac Surg* 1998;65[Suppl 4]:S2; discussion 1998;65[Suppl 4]:S27.
36. Goldstein DJ, DeRosa CM, Seldomridge JA, et al. Is aprotinin indicated for reoperative valvular surgery? *J Heart Valve Dis* 1997; 6:888.
37. Belisle S, Hardy JF. Hemorrhage and the use of blood products after adult cardiac operations: myths and realities. *Ann Thorac Surg* 1996;62:1908.
38. Hardy JF, Belisle S, Couturier A, et al. Randomized, placebo-controlled, double-blind study of an ultra-low dose aprotinin regimen in reoperative and/or complex cardiac operations. *J Card Surg* 1997;12:15.
39. Levi M, Cromheecke ME, de Jonge E, et al. Pharmacological strategies to decrease excessive blood loss in cardiac surgery: a meta-analysis of clinically relevant endpoints. *Lancet* 1999;354: 1940.
40. Engelman RM, Rousou JA, Flack JE. Fast-track recovery of the coronary bypass patient. *Ann Thorac Surg* 1994;58:1742.
41. Jansen NJG, van Oeveren W, Broek L. Inhibition by dexamethasone of the reperfusion phenomena in cardiopulmonary bypass. *J Thorac Cardiovasc Surg* 1991;102:515.
42. Yared JP, Starr NJ, Hoffman-Hogg L, et al. Dexamethasone decreases the incidence of shivering following cardiac surgery: a randomized, double-blind, placebo controlled study. *Anesth Analg* 1998;87:795.
43. Yared JP, Starr NJ, Torres FK, et al. Effects of single dose, post-induction dexamethasone on recovery after cardiac surgery. *Ann Thorac Surg* 2000;69:1420.

Cardiac Anesthesia: Principles and Clinical Practice, Second Edition, edited by Fawzy G. Estafanous, Paul G. Barash, and J.G. Reves. Lippincott Williams & Wilkins, Philadelphia © 2001.

25

ANESTHESIA FOR MINIMALLY INVASIVE CARDIAC SURGERY

RANDALL M. SCHELL
STEVEN R. GUNDRY
KATHERINE P. GRICHNIK

"Cardiac surgery will never again be accused of being the boring 'routine sternotomy, pump and sew' . . . . "

Hani Shennib, M.D. (1)

"We have successfully made cardiac surgery more painful for the surgeon than the patient."

Denton Cooley, M.D. (2)

OVERVIEW

Definition of Minimally Invasive Cardiac Surgery

The traditional surgical model for cardiac surgery has relied on cardiopulmonary bypass (CPB), myocardial protection with an arrested heart, and the median sternotomy incision. Recently, cardiac surgery has enjoyed an explosion of innovative techniques and technology that allow many cardiac procedures to be performed through small incisions with or without CPB (2–4). These "new" ways to perform coronary artery bypass graft (CABG) surgery, valvular heart surgery, and congenital heart surgery—termed "minimally invasive cardiac surgery" (MICS)—have been developed in an attempt to decrease trauma to patients, improve postoperative recovery, and decrease costs. It has been estimated that approximately 25% of cardiac surgery will be performed through minimal access by the year 2000, with other estimates as high as 50% (5,6).

Despite the great interest in these procedures by cardiac surgeons, media, and patients alike, a consensus definition of MICS is still not available. Is "minimally invasive" defined, as many cardiac surgeons believe, by the avoidance of CPB, or does it simply refer to the size or location of the incision (i.e., smaller incision, avoidance of median sternotomy)? (6) Simplistically, MICS techniques can be divided into two groups: (a) beating heart cardiac surgery without CPB and (b) Port-Access cardiac surgery requiring video assistance and closed-chest CPB (7). Vanermen (3) defined four categories of less invasive cardiac surgery: (a) direct coronary artery surgery via sternotomy on the beating heart (no CPB); (b) limited or modified approaches using conventional techniques and instruments with either conventional CPB or the EndoCPB endovascular CPB system; (c) minimally invasive direct coronary artery bypass on the beating heart via a parasternal or left anterior small thoracotomy; and (d) true Port-Access surgery, in which all surgical acts are performed through ports and the heart is arrested with the Endoaortic Clamp catheter (see later discussion). Common abbreviations used to describe MICS are listed in Table 25-1.

Although reducing incision size and avoiding median sternotomy may be important, most cardiac surgeons believe that mitigation of CPB is the most important factor to reduce morbidity in MICS (6), and that the avoidance of CPB appears to have the greatest potential to minimize procedural costs.

Minimally Invasive Coronary Artery Bypass Graft Surgery

There are multiple variations in the way CABG surgery and valvular heart surgery are performed in a minimally invasive manner (Fig. 25-1). Minimally invasive coronary artery bypass (MICAB) grafting has been defined as a grafting operation performed through smaller and less painful incisions with or without use of CPB. However, MICAB may utilize CPB; may be performed through a median sternotomy (8, 9), partial sternotomy, or thoracotomy (10) (or abdominal

R. M. Schell: Department of Anesthesiology, Loma Linda University and Loma Linda University Medical Center, Loma Linda, California 92354

S. R. Gundry: Department of Surgery, Loma Linda University and Department of Cardiothoracic Surgery, Loma Linda University Medical Center, Loma Linda, California 92354

K. P. Grichnik: Department of Anesthesiology, Duke University Medical Center, Durham, North Carolina 27710

TABLE 25-1. COMMON ABBREVIATIONS USED IN MINIMALLY INVASIVE CARDIAC SURGERY

Abbreviation	Definition
MICS	Minimally invasive cardiac surgery
MICAB	Minimally invasive coronary artery bypass
OPCAB	Off-pump coronary artery bypass
MIDCAB	Minimally invasive direct coronary artery bypass
MIDCABG	Minimally invasive direct coronary artery bypass graft
MITACAB	Minimally invasive thoracoscopically assisted coronary artery bypass
VADCAB	Video-assisted direct coronary artery bypass
LAST	Left anterior small thoracotomy
PACAB	Port-Access coronary artery bypass (also called Port-CAB, Port-CABG)

TABLE 25-2. COMPARISON OF BEATING AND ARRESTED HEART TECHNIQUES

Technique	Advantages	Disadvantages
Beating heart surgery	Avoids CPB Small incisions	Field movement Target limitation No intracardiac procedures
Arrested heart (e.g., Port-Access)	Small incisions Security of CPB Motionless field Intracardiac procedures possible	Requires CPB

Note: CPB, cardiopulmonary bypass.
Source: From Fontana GP. Minimally invasive cardiac surgery. *Chest Surg Clin North Am* 1998;66:875, with permission.

incision [11]); may utilize thoracoscopic assistance (12); or may be performed totally thoracoscopically with special instruments using endovascular equipment on the beating or the arrested heart (Port-Access) (13), among other possibilities. Nevertheless, some generalizations of the most common MICAB procedures can be made. When CPB is not used and coronary artery anastomoses are performed on the nonarrested heart, this procedure is often referred to under the broad heading "beating heart surgery" or "off-pump" coronary artery bypass (OPCAB). Beating heart surgery performed via median sternotomy is frequently referred to as OPCAB.

MIDCAB is an acronym for "minimally invasive direct coronary artery bypass" and is strictly defined as CABG surgery where the anastomosis is performed under "direct" vision without sternotomy, CPB, or cardioplegia (14). In practice, this usually refers to harvesting of the left internal mammary artery (LIMA) and performance of a single-vessel anastomosis with the left anterior descending (LAD) coronary artery through a small anterior left thoracotomy at the fourth intercostal space on the beating heart. "Hybrid" refers to procedures in which minimally invasive coronary bypass is combined with transcatheter procedures (stents, angioplasty) for the treatment of multivessel disease (15). Transmyocardial laser revascularization, in which transmural cardiac channels are created in an attempt to establish blood flow from the ventricular cavity to the myocardial vascular network (16), may also immediately follow MIDCAB or OPCAB (17). Less-invasive techniques that use CPB have emerged as an extension of videoscopic and endovascular surgery. Port-Access surgery uses specialized equipment (Heartport Inc., Redwood City, CA), borrowing techniques from laparoscopy, thoracoscopy, and microsurgery to provide a still heart and bloodless field in which to perform coronary anastomoses through small thoracotomy (18). Beating and arrested heart techniques are compared in Table 25-2. In summary, MICAB encompasses OPCAB, MIDCAB, Port-Access, and ministernotomy techniques of coronary revascularization.

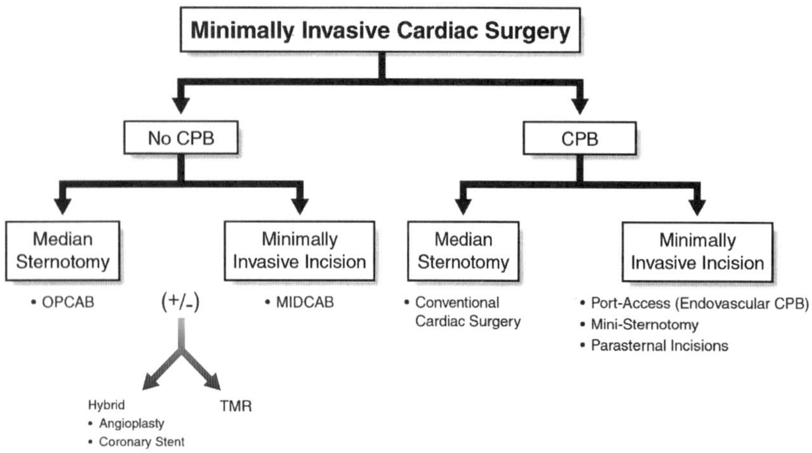

FIGURE 25-1. Variations in the way in which coronary artery bypass surgery and valvular heart surgery are performed. Minimally invasive surgery may avoid the median sternotomy incision or cardiopulmonary bypass (CPB). OPCAB, off-pump coronary artery bypass; MIDCAB, minimally invasive direct coronary artery bypass; TMR, transmyocardial revascularization (laser).

Minimally Invasive Intracardiac/Valvular Heart Surgery

CPB is a requisite for open heart surgery. Therefore, efforts to decrease the invasiveness of valvular heart surgery have focused primarily on reducing the size of the incision or avoiding median sternotomy (2,19). In 1996, Carpentier et al. (20) successfully performed the first video-assisted mitral valve repair through a minithoracotomy incision. Several months later, Chitwood et al. (21) performed a direct-vision micromitral repair, also through a minithoracotomy. Others soon followed with additional mitral valve repairs and aortic valve procedures through a right-sided parasternal incision and through modified median sternotomy (ministernotomy) (22–25). The Port-Access technology has also been used to provide endovascular aortic occlusion, cardioplegia delivery, left ventricular decompression, and femoral bypass for mitral valve operations while avoiding sternotomy (13).

The new millennium will undoubtedly bring new advances to supplant current management techniques in this rapidly changing and advancing frontier of MICS. Today, surgical and anesthetic management for these "new" procedures vary widely between institutions. Technologic advances that occur on an almost daily basis may make older management strategies obsolete. An example is the use of mechanical devices that allow stabilization of the epicardial surface of the heart in "beating heart" procedures, thereby reducing myocardial movement at the operative site and negating the need for pharmacologic induced bradycardia or decreased inotropy. The newest advances in industry or surgical techniques may be advertised or published on the World Wide Web in advance of standard textbooks or journals. Therefore, abstracts published on the Web and commercial websites of interest are listed in the references and at the end of this chapter.

History of Development

The first efforts to perform coronary artery bypass on the beating heart were in the 1960s (Fig. 25-2) (26). The first LIMA to LAD coronary artery anastomosis was effected through a left anterior thoracotomy on a beating heart without CPB support. CPB was in its infancy and was associated with well-recognized morbidity. However, the 1970s and 1980s saw major improvements in perfusion techniques and methods of myocardial protection that resulted in the abandonment of "off-pump" techniques by most cardiac surgeons. The morbidity of CPB was accepted in order to provide a still, bloodless anastomotic site for revascularization. In developing countries where resources were scarce, CABG surgery without CPB continued. Benetti in Argentina, Buffolo in Brazil, and others (27,28) performed CABG surgery in selected patients via a median sternotomy but without CPB. As a result of pharmacologic advances, new technology, and concern about the detrimental effects of CPB, coronary revascularization without CPB was reintroduced in the 1990s as an alternative to the conventional approach. Less invasive techniques of cardiac surgery have emerged as an extension of videoscopic and endovascular surgery.

Benetti and colleagues (29) were the first to describe thoracoscopic harvesting of the LIMA and anastomosis with the LAD through a small anterior left thoracotomy. Subramanian and Stelzer (30) used the same surgical approach but harvested the LIMA under direct observation (MIDCAB). Since then, many centers have reported increasing experience with minimally invasive coronary revascularization on a beating heart through a limited thoracotomy incision (10) and via median sternotomy. Industry responded to interest in beating heart surgery with specialized instrumentation to assist in retraction (LIMA Lift; CardioThoracic Systems, Cupertino, CA) and epicardial stabilization (Octopus 2, Medtronic, Minneapolis, MN). These technologic advances made beating heart surgery technically easier, resulting in rapid and wide acceptance of OPCAB. In 1996 the Heartport Port-Access system received approval by the U.S. Food and Drug Administration. This system was developed in response to the concept that successful coronary revascularization and intracardiac procedures rely on the use of CPB with cardioplegic arrest but could be performed

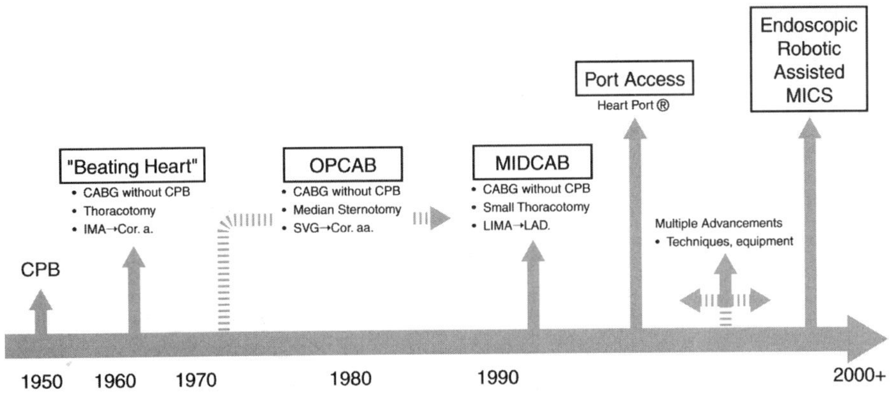

FIGURE 25-2. Abbreviated history of minimally invasive cardiac surgery. CABG, coronary artery bypass graft; Cor.A., coronary artery; CPB, cardiopulmonary bypass; LIMA, left internal mammary artery; MIDCAB, minimally invasive direct coronary artery bypass; IMA, internal mammary artery; MICS, minimally invasive cardiac surgery; OPCAB, off pump coronary artery bypass; SVG, saphenous vein graft.

through smaller incisions. The Port-Access system has been successfully employed clinically in single-vessel and multivessel coronary revascularization and in valve surgery (13). Endoscopic, robotic-assisted MICS may sound futuristic, but it has been successfully performed (31).

Reason for Interest in Minimally Invasive Cardiac Surgery

There has been tremendous enthusiasm on the part of patients, industry, and the press for CABG surgery that is "less traumatic," avoids CPB with its potential pathology, and may reduce cost and length of hospital stay. Economic demands followed by patient demands appear to be the most important driving force for the expansion of MICAB (6), rather than improvement in long-term outcome. Myocardial revascularization is the most common major surgery performed in the United States, and techniques have been "perfected" that result in low perioperative mortality with excellent long-term results (e.g., graft patency). It is unlikely, therefore, that any current developments in minimally invasive myocardial revascularization will lead to an improvement in the long-term results as compared with current conventional techniques. Ideally, the minimally invasive approach must, therefore, not only reproduce the current results associated with conventional surgery but also reduce the morbidity associated with those conventional procedures (32). What is the problem with "standard" techniques of cardiac surgery? Is it the pump or the incision (Table 25-3)? The potential deleterious effects of CPB, such as neurologic injury, coagulopathy, and systemic inflammatory response, are well known (Fig. 25-3). Off-pump MICS (OPCAB, MIDCAB) should avoid many of these complications. Does a smaller incision warrant increased technical difficulty of coronary anastomosis or valvular heart surgery? Although some call MICS a "triumph of technique over reason," the demand for MICS, whether spurred on by avoidance of CPB, economic issues, competition with cardiologists, media, industry, or patients, is likely to increase.

TABLE 25-3. POTENTIAL DELETERIOUS EFFECTS OF CARDIOPULMONARY BYPASS (CPB) AND THE MEDIAN STERNOTOMY INCISION

Complications of CPB	Complications of Median Sternotomy
Stroke	Mediastinitis
Neuropsychologic dysfunction	Sternal dehiscence
Systemic inflammatory response	Chest wall instability
Coagulopathy	Wound pain
Acute renal failure	
"Pump lung"	
Aortic dissection	
Systemic embolization	

The cardiac anesthesiologist, therefore, must be familiar with required alterations in surgical and anesthetic management.

MYOCARDIAL REVASCULARIZATION WITHOUT CPB: PERIOPERATIVE CONSIDERATIONS

Overview of Anesthetic Management for Beating Heart Surgery

The range of minimal-access cardiac surgery approaches has many implications in intraoperative management for the anesthesiologist (7,33–40). Management of the patient undergoing beating heart surgery is arguably more complex not only for the surgeon but also for the cardiac anesthesiologist. However, like surgical techniques, management strategies vary among institutions and evolve as more experience is gained. An overview of major differences between beating heart surgery and "standard" CABG via median sternotomy with CPB and their implications are summarized in Table 25-4. Systemic perfusion and ventricular function must be maintained while the surgeon manipulates and operates on the beating heart, with periods of complete target coronary artery occlusion of approximately 8 to 28 minutes for each vessel (41,42). Mechanical manipulation of the heart and myocardial ischemia may result in extreme hemodynamic instability and dysrhythmias. Detection of myocardial ischemia is complicated by the positioning of the heart within the chest that is required for coronary anastomosis, which may alter electrocardiographic (ECG) vectors and move the heart away from the esophagus and the transesophageal echocardiography (TEE) probe. Although mechanical stabilizers have decreased the need for pharmacologic methods of reducing cardiac motion, the anesthesiologist may occasionally be requested to slow the heart rate or to provide short periods of pharmacologically induced cardiac standstill with intravenous adenosine. Single-lung ventilation techniques are occasionally requested for MICS procedures that use thoracotomy incisions or thoracoscopy. If defibrillation and pacing capabilities are desired for MICS performed via thoracotomy, it must be provided by means that do not require direct epicardial contact. Because CPB with a pump oxygenator is not used, reduced doses of heparin are usually administered. Exposure of the entire body of the patient, including the groin for possible CPB access and legs for saphenous vein graft, may result in hypothermia and often necessitates active warming measures. Lastly, if MICS procedures are to compete with catheter-based techniques and conventional methods of coronary revascularization, cost containment issues—including an anesthetic technique that allows rapid emergence with a minimum of postoperative mechanical ventilation—must be considered. There are limited data to indicate the "best" monitors and anesthetic management techniques for each type of mini-

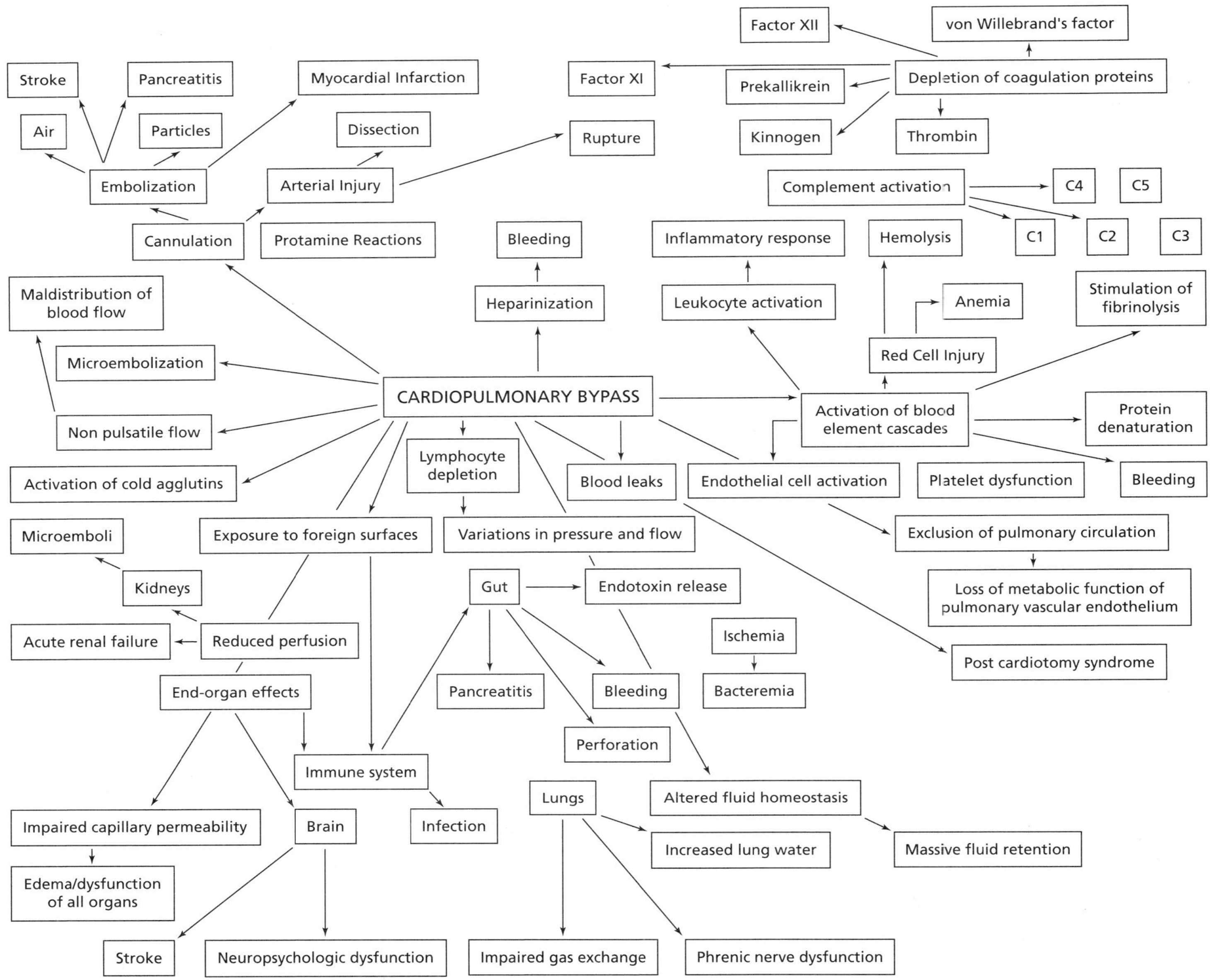

FIGURE 25-3. The "explosion" of adverse events triggered by cardiopulmonary bypass. (From Elefteriades JA. Mini-CABG: a step forward or backward? *J Cardiothorac Vasc Anesth* 1997;11:661, with permission.)

TABLE 25-4. DISTINCTIVE ASPECTS OF BEATING HEART SURGERY[a]

Factor	Implications
Potential for extreme hemodynamic instability and dysrythmias	*Monitoring choices:* TEE, PA catheter, CVP, ECG, continuous CO *Understand management options:* ischemic preconditioning, coronary shunt, conversion to CPB, circulatory support systems (right heart, left heart), inotropes Should standby CPB be required?
Requirement for "quiet" surgical field	Mechanical stabilizers used Pharmacologically induced bradycardia; avoid vagolytic anesthetic choices One-lung ventilation occasionally required/requested
Poor access to epicardium (MIDCAB)	Defibrillation and pacing capabilities, if desired, must be provided by means that do not require direct epicardial contact if surgery is performed via thoracotomy
CPB not used	Reduced doses of heparin; reversal with protamine optional Hypothermia possible; active warming measures encouraged
Variation in incision site/postoperative pain	Postoperative pain management; varies based on incision site (thoracotomy, median sternotomy)
Cost-containment issues	"Fast-track" or "appropriately timed extubation" especially important Anesthetic choices and postoperative pain management should meet the "fast-track" goals Is standby CPB (primed or nonprimed) required?

Note: CO, cardiac output; CPB, cardiopulmonary bypass; CVP, central venous pressure; ECG, electrocardiogram; MIDCAB, minimally invasive direct coronary artery bypass; PA, pulmonary artery; TEE, transesophageal echocardiography.
[a] Compared with "standard" coronary artery bypass graft surgery via median sternotomy with CPB.

mally invasive procedure. Therefore, recommendations are based on current research and the institutional and personal experience of those involved in the care of these patients.

OPCAB: Median Sternotomy

Overview of Surgical Strategy

With the growing experience in MICS surgery, three groups of potential candidates for beating heart surgery are emerging: (a) patients who require one or two grafts and who have failed or are not candidates for angioplasty; (b) those patients requiring coronary revascularization not amenable to angioplasty, who might be at high risk with CPB (e.g., previous cerebrovascular accident, renal insufficiency); and (c) candidates for conventional bypass surgery who can

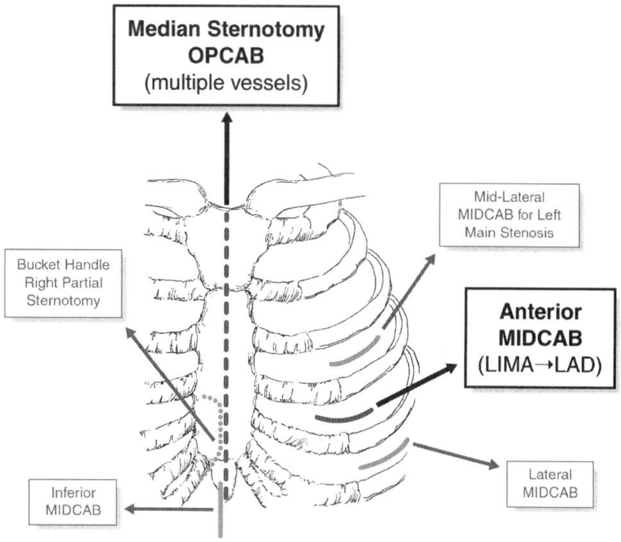

FIGURE 25-4. Incision sites for access to various target coronary arteries in minimally invasive coronary artery bypass graft surgery.

safely undergo multivessel OPCAB. Although CABG on the beating heart can be performed through several different incisions (median sternotomy, partial sternotomy, anterior thoracotomy, posterior thoracotomy, or subxiphoid incision) (Fig. 25-4), this latter group of patients with multivessel coronary artery disease who are also candidates for conventional CABG appears to be growing most quickly, with median sternotomy the incision of choice (OPCAB) (2). The advantages and disadvantages of OPCAB are listed in Table 25-5. Shennib et al. (6) reported in 1997 that 81% of cardiac surgeons surveyed would rather eliminate CPB

TABLE 25-5. ADVANTAGES AND DISADVANTAGES OF OFF-PUMP STERNOTOMY CORONARY ARTERY BYPASS GRAFT SURGERY (OPCAB)

Advantages	Disadvantages
Obviates morbidity of cardiopulmonary bypass	Complete sternotomy necessary
Cost-effective	Surgery technically more difficult
Extends indications for surgery to patients who are not candidates for routine approaches	Approach to the posterior ventricular wall difficult
Capability of multivessel, multiconduit bypass	
Use of standard operative techniques	
No aortic manipulation	
Familiar exposure	

Source: From Gayes JM. The minimally invasive cardiac surgery voyage. *J Cardiothorac Vasc Anesth* 1999;13:119, with permission.

from the conduct of cardiac surgery than eliminate a median sternotomy. The median sternotomy approach allows the cardiac surgeon to offer the benefits of avoiding CPB to a much larger group of patients than does MIDCAB through a minithoracotomy. With currently available instrumentation and mechanical stabilization, OPCAB via median sternotomy allows access to all coronary vessels. It is relatively easy to bypass the more accessible coronary arteries such as the LAD, diagonal, right coronary artery (RCA), or posterior descending coronary artery. The greater dilemma is how to revascularize the lateral surface of the heart (marginal arteries) without CPB. More than 75% of cardiac surgeons (6) report that anastomosis to the marginal arteries is the most challenging anastomosis through a sternotomy incision without the use of CPB. The cardiac manipulations necessary to adequately expose these vessels behind the heart may result in extreme hemodynamic compromise, and CPB may be required at some institutions.

After median sternotomy (or partial sternotomy), the IMA and saphenous vein are prepared for grafting. Minimally invasive video-assisted removal of the saphenous vein using an endoscopic vein harvesting system (Ceres SV System, CardioThoracic Systems, Cupertino, CA; and Guidant Corporation, Menlo Park, CA) is performed at some centers (7,43). CPB is usually available, but the aortic and venous cannulas are not placed. Although OPCAB can be performed without any new equipment, it is made easier by technology that physically immobilizes the target coronary artery (OP-CAB, CardioThoracic Systems; Octopus Stabilizer, Medtronic) (Fig. 25-5). According to Benetti, the territory of the LAD should be revascularized first; this is different from what normally happens during conventional coronary surgery and ensures the best function of the anterior and septal myocardial walls. The RCA should be revascularized after the LAD territory, leaving the marginal branches for last. The revascularized heart can better tolerate the manipulation required to reach the marginal branches. When saphenous vein grafts are used, the proximal anastomosis should be performed first, so as to provide adequate

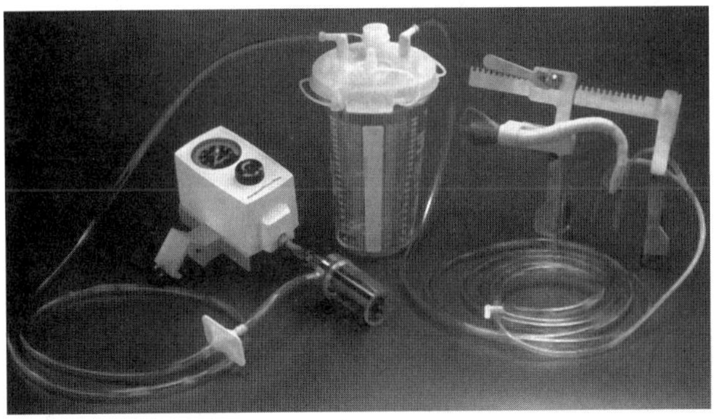

FIGURE 25-5. The Octopus (Medtronic Corporation) mechanical stabilization system.

TABLE 25-6. INDICATIONS AND CONTRAINDICATIONS FOR OFF-PUMP CORONARY ARTERY BYPASS GRAFT SURGERY (OPCAB)

Indications	Contraindications
Presence of ischemic heart disease	Intracardiac surgery (i.e., valve surgery) also required
Contraindication to cardiopulmonary bypass	Severely calcified coronary arteries
"Graftable" coronary artery (adequate size)	Intramyocardial course of coronary arteries
Significant stenosis in lumen diameter (>50%)	Physiologic intolerance to cardiac manipulation

blood flow to the revascularized vessel immediately after completion of the anastomosis and to allow adequate debubbling and washout of debris or particles from the venous graft. Anastomosis of the arterial or venous conduit to the target site is performed on the beating heart during a period of target coronary artery occlusion. This may result in hemodynamic instability and dysrhythmias. Reperfusion is accomplished and graft flow ensured by one of several methods.

Preoperative Assessment

In general, patients with multivessel coronary artery disease who are candidates for conventional coronary surgery with CPB via midline sternotomy may benefit from OPCAB. Indications and contraindications for OPCAB are listed in Table 25-6. Coronary arteries that are severely calcified, are small, or take an intramyocardial course may make OPCAB untenable. The proximal circumflex and marginal branches are difficult to reach and expose and require repositioning of the heart. Physiologic tolerance of the heart to manipulation is unpredictable.

Preoperative assessment is initially the same as for patients undergoing any type of myocardial revascularization. The anesthesiologist should review indices of left ventricular function, the patient's exercise tolerance, and the presence or absence of comorbid conditions. Patient selection criteria are continually being reevaluated. Obesity, chronic obstructive pulmonary disease (COPD), and dysrhythmias can increase the difficulty of OPCAB. Obesity and COPD with associated large lung volumes may make surgical exposure difficult. Atrial fibrillation and dysrhythmias with associated irregular or fast heart rate can make sewing on the beating heart more difficult, although mechanical stabilization has obviated much of this problem. Previous CABG surgery (reoperation [44]), recent myocardial infarction (45), and depressed myocardial function (46) are not absolute exclusion criteria. Myocardial function may be better preserved by performing CABG without CPB (47). Patients with associated renal or hepatic insufficiency, previous cerebrovascular accidents, hematologic/coagulation disorders, or Jehovah's Witness faith (for whom blood transfusion is not an option) are ideal candidates for OPCAB. Also, patients with aortic calcification and severe peripheral vascular disease are ideal candidates because of the associated risks of either aortic or femoral cannulation.

Importance of Catheterization Data

The catheterization data and the order of revascularization should be reviewed with the surgeon preoperatively. The anesthesiologist can then anticipate and plan for likely difficulties. The degree of stenosis, presence or absence of collateral vessels, and vessels involved (e.g., marginal, RCA) are especially important to the anesthesiologist. If the degree of stenosis is greater than 95%, then target vessel occlusion is usually well tolerated. If the level of stenosis is less than 95%, then vessel occlusion may more frequently cause hemodynamic decompensation and dysrhythmias (48). The assumption is that the myocardial territory subtended by a coronary vessel with a high degree of stenosis may have developed collateral vessels, so that interruption of coronary flow during off-pump anastomosis would be well tolerated (49). A vessel with lesser degrees of stenosis (e.g., <75%) (50) may be supplying more critical amounts of oxygenated blood, so that occlusion during coronary anastomosis may result in myocardial ischemia in the at risk-territory, hemodynamic compromise, and dysrhythmias. Evidence from MICAB surgery and angioplasty support this concept. During percutaneous transluminal coronary angioplasty, patients with coronary lesions less than 80% occluded had an increased incidence of arrhythmia during coronary artery balloon occlusion (51). During MIDCAB procedures, areas of regional myocardial ischemia, as evidenced by regional wall motion abnormalities on TEE, typically occurred only with lesions of less than 75% (50).

Premedication

Laboratory evaluation is similar to that for conventional CABG surgery. However, hematology workup is often limited to a type and screen to limit costs, and patients are usually admitted on the same day of surgery. β-Blockers such as atenolol may be administered for 1 or 2 days before surgery to aid in the control of perioperative tachycardia. The preoperative use of clonidine (0.3 mg PO) (52) and aggressive sedation may decrease the amount of endogenous catecholamine release, potentially decreasing the amount of β-blockade required intraoperatively. However, the use of large doses of long-acting benzodiazepines (e.g., diazepam [Valium]) and scopolamine that might preclude "fast-track" goals should probably be avoided.

Intraoperative Management for OPCAB

The operating room is configured as for standard CABG surgery (Fig. 25-6). The CPB pump is often set up but not

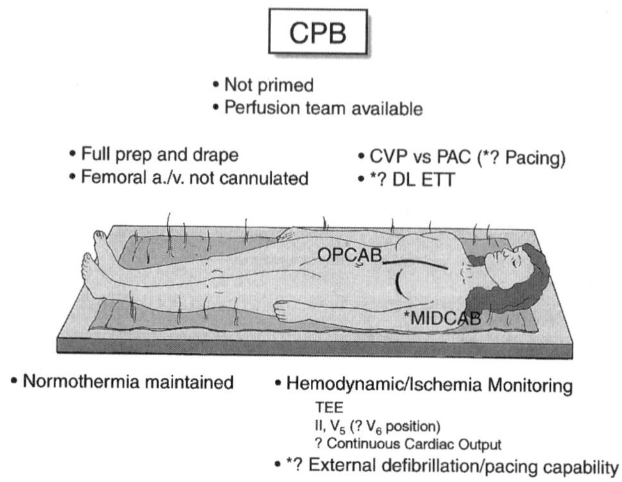

FIGURE 25-6. Operating room configuration for minimally invasive coronary artery bypass graft surgery.

primed, and the perfusion team is immediately available. Most programs performing OPCAB (more than 90% [6]) have the perfusionist on standby and always available; a small number have the perfusionist on standby only during high-risk cases. The patient is positioned supine and prepared and draped for conventional CABG to facilitate sternotomy, vein harvest, and access to the groin vessels for either cannulation or intraaortic balloon pump (IABP) implantation should it becomes necessary. The femoral artery and vein are not usually cannulated prophylactically. The temperature in the operating room should be warm, and normothermia should be maintained. It may not be possible to use a warm-air blanket because the patient's entire body is exposed, including the legs, for possible femoral cannulation and vein harvesting. A new warm-air blanket (Sterile Cardiac Access Blanket, Augustine Medical Inc., Eden Prairie, MN) is available that lies around rather than over the patient. Because CPB is not used, prophylactic antiinflammatory (solumedrol) and antifibrinolytic (ϵ-aminocaproic acid [Amicar]) agents may not be administered.

Selection of Monitors

There are several opinions regarding the necessary invasiveness of monitoring appropriate for MICS (33). The first view is that "minimally invasive monitoring" should accompany MICS unless there is a specific indication for more intensive monitoring (53). Standard monitors might then include an arterial catheter, central venous pressure catheter, and possibly TEE to help detect myocardial ischemia and guide the administration of myocardial depressant drugs. The use of a pulmonary artery (PA) catheter in addition to the other monitors is often based on institutional preference or an unacceptable level of left ventricular dysfunction. The opposing view is that more intensive monitoring is required for one or more of the following reasons: the heart cannot be directly visualized (MIDCAB, not OPCAB); frequent and multiple manipulations of the heart with likely accompanying hemodynamic instability are required to obtain optimal exposure of targeted vessels; and multiple episodes of induced myocardial ischemia are possible and can be detected and therefore treated earlier during target coronary artery occlusion. Standard monitors might then include those previously mentioned plus automated multilead continuous ST-segment analysis monitoring, TEE, and a PA catheter (with or without mixed venous oxygen saturation or continuous cardiac output capability). One author with considerable experience in anesthetic management for MICS suggested that the most reliable measurement of myocardial function during the 7- to 10-minute distal coronary artery anastomosis is continuous cardiac output (7). Pulse-contour analysis and continuous thermodilution cardiac output measurements are two options (54–56).

Anesthetic Choice

The anesthetic management goals of hemodynamic stability, provision of a relatively quiet operative field (e.g., slow heart rate), and early emergence and extubation can be achieved by a wide variety of anesthetic techniques for which there is considerable institutional variation. Any balanced anesthetic technique that provides smooth induction and timely conditions for extubation can be used. A "high-dose" regimen of fentanyl or sufentanyl that does not allow early emergence and extubation is not well suited for shorter-duration MICAB procedures. Propofol has been shown to be safe and effective for cardiac and thoracic surgical procedures (57–59). The opioid remifentanil provides at least as good attenuation of the stress response in CABG patients as does fentanyl (60), has little effect on myocardial contractility (61,62), and can be used safely in patients with decreased left ventricular function (62). It allows early tracheal extubation and may have a lower incidence of postoperative confusion when compared with fentanyl (63). Total intravenous anesthesia (propofol/remifenantil) and inhalational anesthesia with supplemental intravenous opioids are anesthetic options. Because CPB is sometimes required, the use of nitrous oxide is omitted to avoid possible air embolism (39). The vagolytic properties of pancuronium and its long duration of action make it less desirable, although not contraindicated (35), as the choice for neuromuscular blockade. A propofol infusion may be used to maintain anesthesia if the patient is transported to the angiography suite immediately after surgical revascularization for evaluation of graft patency or for planned coronary angioplasty or coronary stent placement of other target coronary arteries (hybrid procedure).

Management During Coronary Artery Anastomosis and Vessel Occlusion

After median sternotomy, the mammary artery and saphenous vein are prepared for grafting. Ventilation with decreased tidal volumes can provide better conditions for LIMA harvest. Some institutions use a double-lumen tube and single-lung ventilation to facilitate surgical exposure both for takedown of the mammary artery and for positioning of the heart. A nitroglycerin infusion (approximately 0.2 to 2.0 μg/kg/minute) is often used throughout the procedure, providing it does not negatively affect hemodynamic stability. A reduced dose of heparin is used, compared with conventional CABG with CPB; it is administered before distal transection of the IMA and occlusion of the target coronary artery. Heparin must be administered before snaring of the target coronary artery to prevent clot formation in the vessel. Heparin doses are usually 100 to 200 U/kg intravenously, with the end point for heparin monitoring being an activated clotting time (ACT) of at least 200 (41) or 250 (64) seconds. Two situations are necessary for performing a coronary anastomosis on the beating heart: a stable and still site of the anastomosis and a bloodless field.

Stabilization Techniques

Pharmacologic Stabilization. There are pharmacologic, mechanical/physical, and "physiologic" methods of reducing myocardial movement during coronary anastomosis (Table 25-7). Early attempts to provide a relatively stable and still site of coronary anastomosis relied on pharmacologic agents (Table 25-8) to reduce contractility and induce bradycardia. If pharmacologically induced bradycardia is desirable, the β-blocker esmolol, which decreases myocardial oxygen requirements, decreases heart rate, and may attenuate regional ischemia during vessel occlusion (65), is frequently used (38,66–68). Metoprolol, 0.5 to 1.0 mg intravenously every 5 minutes titrated to a heart rate of 60 beats/minute, is an economical alternative to esmolol. However, its long half-life does not allow discontinuation of β-blockade if extreme hemodynamic instability is encountered. Esmolol has a serum half-life of only about 9 minutes and provides rapidly titratable β-blockade. It is typically administered to a heart rate of 50 to 60 beats/minute, start-

TABLE 25-7. METHODS OF REDUCING MYOCARDIAL MOVEMENT DURING CORONARY ANASTOMOSIS IN MINIMALLY INVASIVE CORONARY ARTERY BYPASS GRAFT SURGERY

Category	Method
Mechanical	Suction type (Octopus Stabilizer, Medtronic Corp., Minneapolis, MN)
	Pressure plate type (Access Ultima System, Cardiothoracic Systems, Cupertino, CA)
Pharmacologic	Esmolol, metoprolol
	Diltiazem, verapamil
	Adenosine
	Neostigmine, edrophonium
"Physiologic"	Vagal nerve stimulation

TABLE 25-8. PHARMACOLOGIC THERAPIES TO REDUCE MOVEMENT AT THE ANASTOMOTIC SITE DURING MINIMALLY INVASIVE CORONARY ARTERY BYPASS GRAFT SURGERY

Drug	Dose	Comment
Esmolol	50–150 μg/kg/min	Serum half-life, 9 min
Adenosine	0.2–0.3 mg/kg	Causes 15–30 sec of asystole
Verapamil	5-mg doses titrated to desired heart rate	May cause unacceptable hypotension
Diltiazem	0.1 mg/kg/hr	May cause unacceptable hypotension
Neostigmine	1–3 mg bolus	Will reverse muscle paralysis; muscarinic side effects (i.e., salivation, bronchospasm)

Source: Adapted from Krucylak PE. Intraoperative considerations during minimal-access cardiac surgery. *Semin Thorac Cardiovasc Surg* 1999;11:116, with permission.

ing with 10- to 30-mg intravenous boluses followed by an intravenous infusion (2.5 g per 250 mL of 5% dextrose in water [D5W]) at approximately 50 to 150 μg/kg/minute (69). The use of esmolol alone may not provide a sufficient reduction in heart rate and optimization of surgical conditions in approximately 40% of the patients (70). Diltiazem (71), verapamil (9), adenosine (72), and neostigmine (71) have also been used, alone or in combination with esmolol, to induce bradycardia. The calcium channel blockers diltiazem and verapamil can cause vasodilation and hypotension. Esmolol has been shown to be similar to verapamil with regard to hemodynamic effects during myocardial revascularization without CPB in pigs, but esmolol demonstrated superior antiarryhthmic effects (73).

The induction of transient ventricular asystole with the endogenous nucleotide adenosine has proved quite useful when the surgeon has difficulty controlling bleeding at the operative site secondary to cardiac motion or desires brief asystole to place partial aortic clamps. Periods of cardiac standstill lasting 5 to 12 seconds may be accomplished by administration of a rapid intravenous bolus of adenosine (0.2 to 0.3 mg/kg). Once asytole occurs, a suture (or aortic clamp) is placed and sinus rhythm resumes spontaneously or, if necessary, temporary epicardial pacing may be initiated (Fig. 25-7). Persantine (5 mg) has been administered before occlusion of the target vessel to potentiate the effects of adenosine (53). However, the high cost of adenosine still limits its usefulness. Vagal nerve stimulation has also been used to produce ventricular pauses (74). Anticholinesterases such as neostigmine (0.5 mg IV boluses) (71) or edrophonium (5 mg IV boluses) can induce bradycardia without

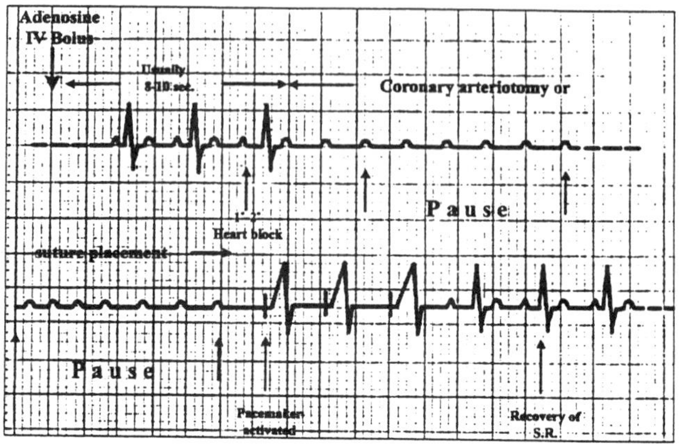

FIGURE 25-7. Effects of adenosine. (From Robinson MC, Gross DR, Zeman W, et al. Minimally-invasive coronary artery bypass grafting: a new method using an anterior mediastinotomy. *J Card Surg* 1995:529, with permission.)

decreasing cardiac contractility. The accumulation of acetylcholine at muscarinic and nicotinic receptors results in decreased heart rate, the potential side effect of bronchospasm in patients with reactive airways, and reversal of muscle paralysis if neuromuscular blockade is used. A small dose of a short-acting opioid (remifentanil, sufentanil, fentanyl) can also be effective in producing moderate slowing of the heart rate. The use of pharmacologic stabilization combined with physical manipulation of the heart often results in a reduced cardiac index and systemic hypotension. A phenylephrine or norepinephrine infusion is occasionally necessary to maintain systemic blood pressure and augment coronary perfusion pressure during the coronary anastomosis (34,38).

Mechanical Stabilization. Occluding sutures were used as the first method of mechanical target coronary artery stabilization. Anastomotic site movement was reduced by pulling up the occluding sutures in opposite directions along the course of the artery. Good stabilization of the segment of coronary artery including the arteriotomy can be achieved by this method without apparent injury to the target coronary artery or coronary endothelium (75). However, use of occluding sutures as a stabilizing device can only partially reduce the movements of the epicardial surface. The more recent development of mechanical devices that reduce myocardial movement (Octopus 2, Medtronic; OPCAB Access Ultima System, CardioThoracic Systems) has greatly decreased the requirement for pharmacologic modes of myocardial stabilization. The Octopus stabilizer uses a series of suction cups on two fixed arms that allow adherence to the epicardium on either side of the target vessel (Fig. 25-8). It provides excellent immobilization, limiting motion in an area of about 1 × 1 mm without compressing the heart, and allows mechanical traction for centering the site of anastomosis within the operative field (2,

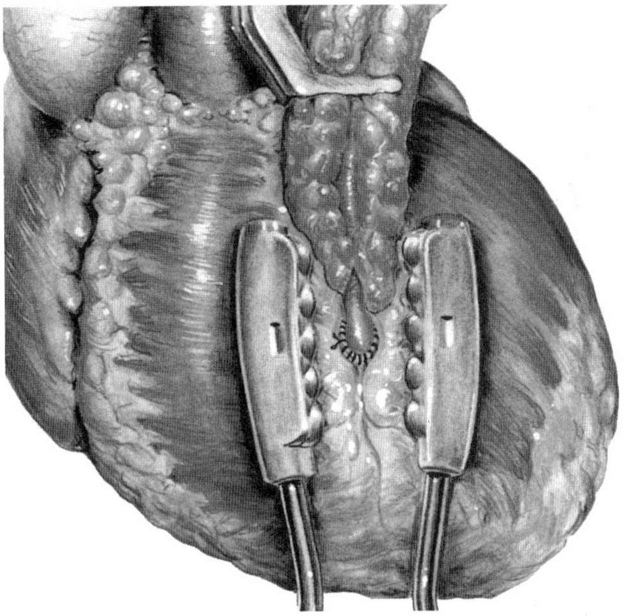

FIGURE 25-8. The Octopus (Octopus 2, Medtronic Inc, Minneapolis, MN) uses a series of suction cups on two fixed arms that adhere to the epicardial surface and reduce myocardial motion at the anastomotic site during off-pump coronary artery bypass graft surgery.

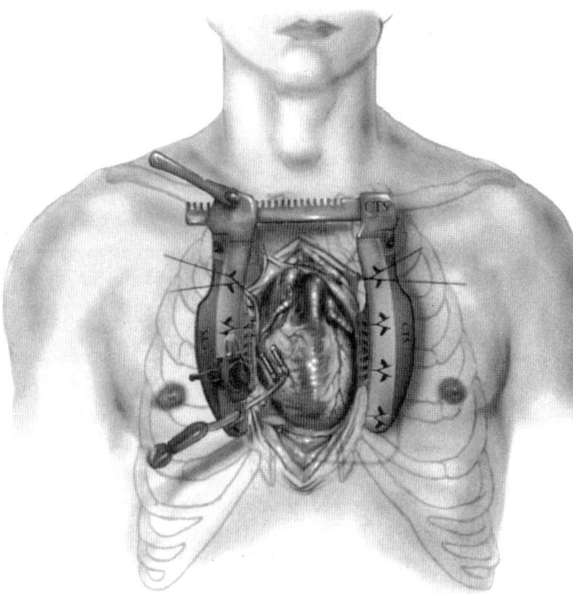

FIGURE 25-9. Pressure-plate stabilizing devices such as the CTSR Access Ultima System (CardioThoracic Systems, Cupertino, CA) reduce epicardial motion at the site of coronary anastomosis during off-pump coronary artery bypass graft surgery.

76,77). Other pressure-plate-type stabilizing devices (Fig. 25-9), such as the OPCAB Access Ultima System, do not adhere to the epicardium but are low-profile devices that do not interfere with the use of surgical instruments and provide excellent visualization of the targeted coronary artery. In one study (78), the pressure-plate-type device resulted in a small decrease in left ventricular end-systolic and end-diastolic dimensions, but cardiac function remained unchanged until occlusion of the target coronary artery (LAD).

A comparison of pharmacologic versus mechanical stabilization of the heart demonstrates clear advantages for the use of mechanical devices (7). These advantages include superior limitation in cardiac motion, better preservation of hemodynamic parameters (79), better access to the RCA and marginal branches (2,80), and improved anastomotic patency rates (81–84). Occasionally, a combination of mechanical stabilization and pharmacologic intervention may be necessary to produce optimal immobilization of the surgical site (2).

Bloodless Field Techniques

A bloodless field is needed for optimal view and access to the arteriotomy edges. This can be accomplished by means of external occluding sutures, blowing devices, intravascular occluders, deep-bite pledgeted snares, or a combination of these techniques. The majority of cases are performed with encircling sutures or retractotapes, with or without Teflon or rubber bolsters, to interrupt blood flow (2). However, this may cause hematomas, plaque disruption, and distal ischemia. The introduction of atraumatic coronary shunts (Fig. 25-10) (FloCoil Shunt, CardioThoracic Systems) may be of value not only in maintaining a near-bloodless field but also in providing blood flow to the myocardium fed by the coronary vessel during the anastomosis, relieving distal ischemia (85–87). Air or mist blowers (Aries CO_2 Blower/Mister, CardioThoracic Systems) facilitate dispersion and soft-tipped fine suction collection of residual blood in the field. Blowing devices can provide a localized wash-out of the remaining blood in the anastomotic site by using either filtered gas (O_2, CO_2, air) or a mixture of gas and sterile saline solution. These devices may be handheld or attached to a variety of retractor systems.

Hemodynamic Alterations with Cardiac Manipulation

Episodes of hypotension and decreased cardiac output are not infrequent during MICAB. Most hemodynamic problems occur because of surgical manipulation of the heart, myocardial ischemia, or decreased preload. The hemodynamic alterations in the mechanically displaced diseased human heart have not been completely elucidated. Right heart dysfunction appears to be the cause of hemodynamic instability in displaced normal animal hearts (88), whereas right as well as left ventricular dysfunction appears to be the cause of hemodynamic instability in diseased human hearts (89). After identification of the target coronary artery, the heart and mechanical stabilization device are manipu-

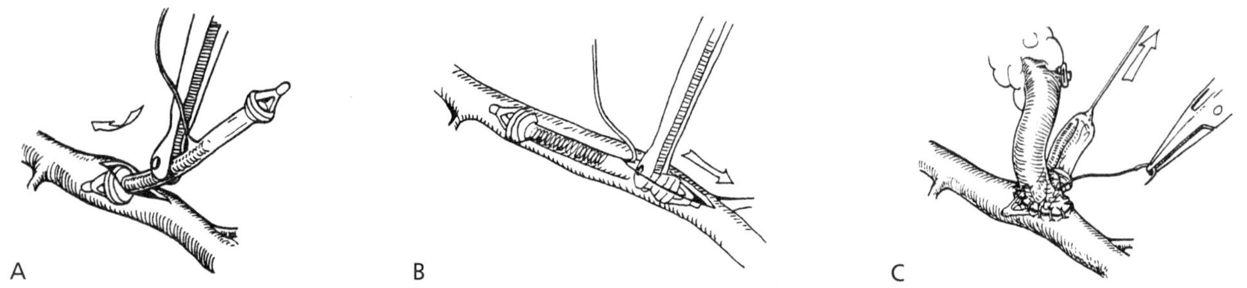

FIGURE 25-10. Coronary shunts (FloCoil Shunt, CardioThoracic Systems, Inc, Cupertino, CA) can provide distal blood flow during the period of coronary occlusion necessary for off-pump coronary artery bypass graft surgery. **A:** Insertion of coil end tip of shunt. **B:** Insertion of non-coil tip of shunt. **C:** Shunt removal.

lated into optimal position (Fig. 25-11). Adequate exposure of the target vessels without hemodynamic compromise remains the most important element in OPCAB. These manipulations may result in hemodynamic compromise requiring inotropic/chronotropic therapy or maneuvers to increase preload (e.g., Trendelenburg position).

The exposure of the LAD, in general, requires little or no rotation of the heart and is often performed first. Revascularization of the posterior and lateral surfaces is more difficult (88–91). The RCA and marginal arteries are often left to revascularize last because of increased potential for hemodynamic compromise. The heart may be positioned almost vertically in the chest to expose posterior cardiac vessels. Occlusion of the proximal RCA is not always well tolerated,

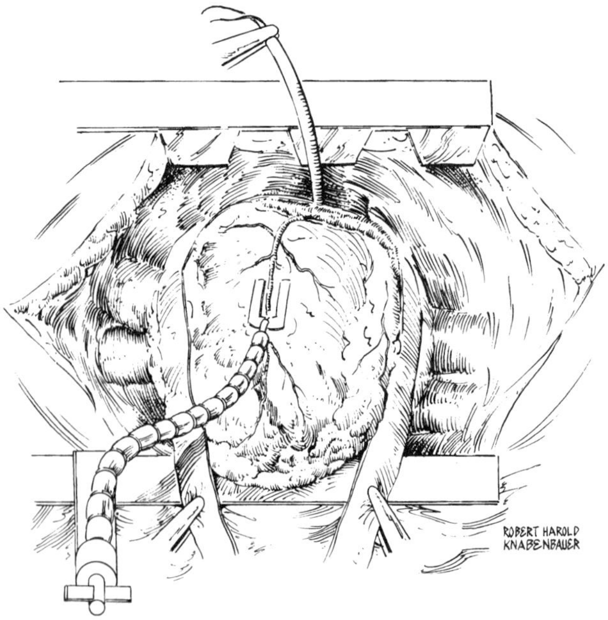

FIGURE 25-11. Manipulation of the heart and placement of a pressure-plate-type mechanical stabilizer is performed in preparation for off-pump coronary artery bypass graft surgery.

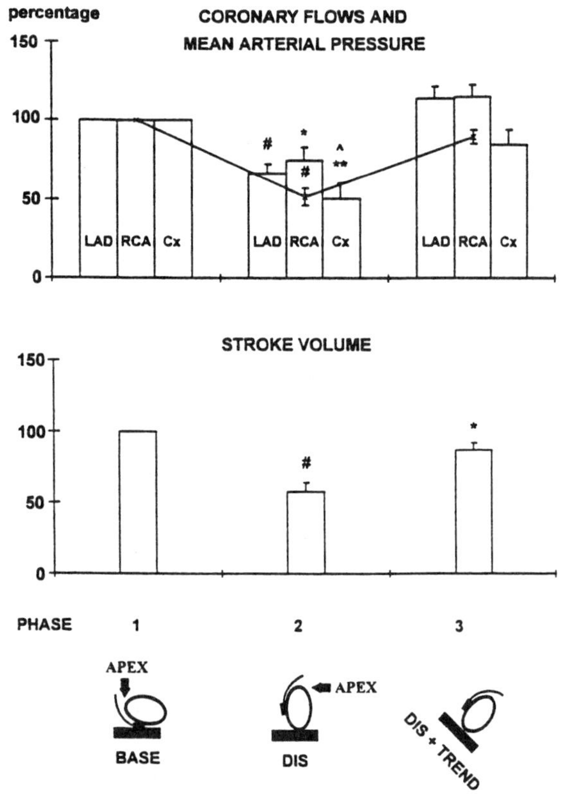

FIGURE 25-12. Relative changes in hemodynamic parameters during verical displacement of the beating porcine heart by the Medtronic Octopus Tissue Stabilizer and the effect of head-down tilt. BASE, pericardial control position; Cx, circumflex cornary artery; DIS, displacement of the heart by the Octopus; DIS + TREND, Trendelenburg maneuver (20° head-down tilt) while the heart remains 90° retracted; LAD, left anterior descending cornary artery; RCA, right coronary artery; X, mean arterial pressure. Statistical comparison with control values: *, $p < .05$; **, $p < .01$; #, $p < .001$; , $p = .046$ versus combined relative value of LAD and RCA flows. (From Grundeman PF, Borst C, van Herwaarden JA, et al. Vertical displacement of the beating heart by the Octopus tissue stabilizer: Influence on coronary flow. *Ann Thorac Surg* 1998;65:1348, with permission.)

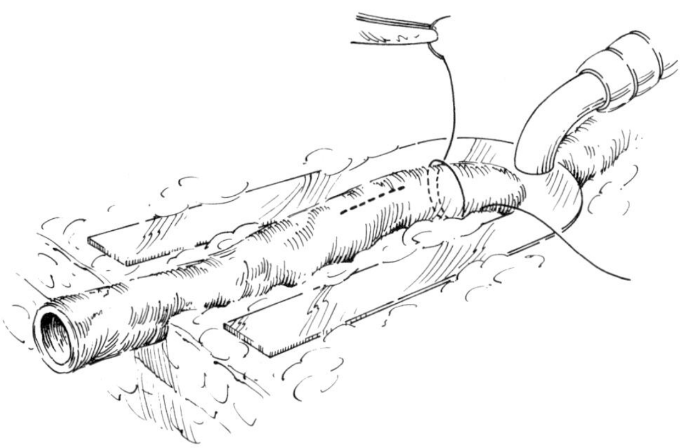

FIGURE 25-13. With the mechanical stabilizer in place, a test occlusion of the target coronary artery is performed by upward traction of the proximal occluding suture before arteriotomy *(dotted line)* and anastomosis.

and rhythm disturbances may result. For surgical access to circumflex branches (marginal arteries) through sternotomy, the beating heart needs to be displaced anteriorly (92,93). This displacement results in hemodynamic changes, including decreased mean arterial pressure, cardiac index, stroke volume, mixed venous oxygen saturation, and coronary flow and increased superior vena cava and PA occlusion pressures (89,92). Right as well as left ventricular dysfunction appears to be of concern. However, Grundeman et al. (92) demonstrated that the borderline circulatory status during displacement was markedly improved to almost baseline status by blood volume redistribution using the Trendelenburg maneuver. At the same time, coronary blood flow returned to baseline values (Fig. 25-12).

Management of Myocardial Ischemia and Hemodynamic Complications

Management of Ischemia. With the mechanical stabilization device in place and pharmacologic therapy optimized, a test occlusion (approximately 3 to 5 minutes) of the target coronary artery is usually performed before coronary arteriotomy and anastomosis to see whether the patient can tolerate OPCAB (Fig. 25-13). Coronary revascularization without CPB requires local occlusion of the target vessel for approximately 10 minutes during anastomosis (approximately 8 to 20 minutes), which may induce variable periods of regional myocardial ischemia, dysrhythmias, and hemodynamic instability (Fig. 25-14). It has been estimated that one-third of the patients will show signs of ischemia during the period of vessel occlusion (32,94). However, many years of coronary angioplasty have demonstrated that occlusion of a coronary artery for a short period is generally well tolerated. Prophylactic antiischemic therapies including calcium channel blockers (diltiazem, 2 to 5 mg IV loading dose over 10 to 15 minutes and infusion of 50 mg per 250 mL saline

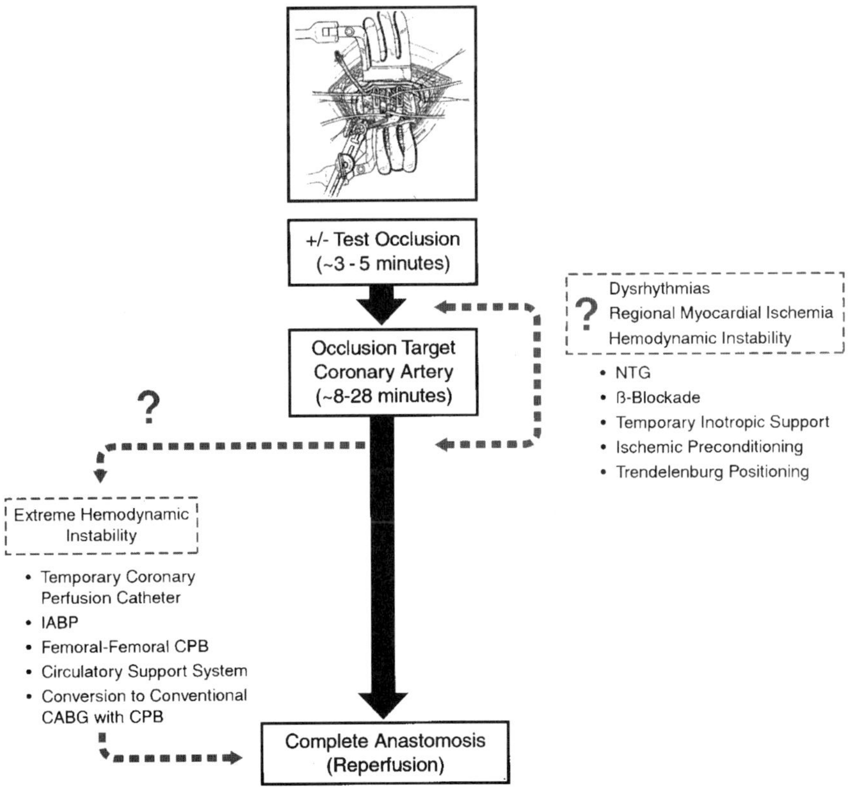

FIGURE 25-14. Management of possible hemodynamic and ischemic complications encountered during coronary occlusion for minimally invasive coronary artery bypass graft surgery.

or D5W at 2.0 to 4.0 mg/hour), β-blockers, and nitrates are used by some institutions performing MICAB.

Detection of myocardial ischemia is complicated by the frequent and multiple cardiac manipulations required to obtain optimal exposure of targeted vessels. As a result, conventional methods for monitoring intraoperative ischemia become less useful. Accurate TEE interpretation of new regional wall motion abnormalities is difficult if not impossible with the apex of the heart elevated perpendicular to the thoracic cavity and away from the esophagus and the TEE transducer. The use of mechanical stabilizers on the surface of the heart may appear as areas of hypokinesis or akinesis on TEE. Inspection of the anterior surface of the heart via a gastric short-axis view by TEE before stabilizer application is necessary to give a true picture of anterior wall function (33). Although multilead continuous ST-segment trend analysis is a good monitor of ischemia, ECG vector direction and amplitude may be altered by cardiac manipulation (7). In one study, ECG changes associated with temporary occlusion of the LAD during anastomosis were not a reliable predictor for perioperative myocardial infarction (95). Continuous cardiac output may be a useful monitor of myocardial function during distal coronary artery anastomosis (7, 54,56).

If ischemia is detected by either ST-segment changes, increase in pulmonary capillary occlusion pressure, development of significant "V" waves, regional wall motion abnormalities on TEE, or hemodynamic instability, steps are taken to ameliorate ischemia with nitroglycerin, β-blockade, or ischemic preconditioning. Ischemic preconditioning refers to the capacity of the myocardium to develop resistance to myocardial infarction caused by repeated episodes of ischemia (96–100). Ischemic preconditioning during beating heart surgery may be accomplished by occluding the target coronary by upward traction on the proximal and distal stay-sutures for approximately 3 to 5 minutes, followed by reperfusion for 3 to 5 minutes, and repeated several times (96). Once ischemic preconditioning has been performed, the myocardial protection that it confers lasts for at least 1 hour but dissipates by 2 hours (97). Adenosine has been proposed as a mediator of the ischemic preconditioning phenomenon (Fig. 25-15).

The use of ischemic preconditioning has declined or been completely abandoned (35) as the time necessary to create the coronary anastomosis has decreased with experience and with the use of mechanical stabilizers. Potential benefits of this maneuver may be reduced by the presence of chronic coronary artery narrowing, collateral vessels, and the confounding influences of anesthesia (101). Buffolo et al. (9) and Tasdemir et al. (102) described more than 3,000 cases of CABG without CPB; neither reported the use of ischemic preconditioning. The perioperative myocardial infarction rate was comparable to that in patients for whom CPB and cardioplegia were used (9). However, there remain some patients who poorly tolerate even a short period of regional ischemia, in whom ischemic preconditioning may have some usefulness (2).

Management of Hemodynamic Complications. Dilemmas regarding not only the appropriate degree of hemodynamic monitoring but also the intraoperative management of hypotension continue. Prophylactic doses of nitroglycerin can enhance hypotension and therefore may need to be discontinued. In contrast to the pharmacologically induced bradycardia and decreased inotropy often used in the past, the new mechanical stabilizers may instead require chronotropic and inotropic support (e.g., dobutamine, dopamine) to help maintain cardiac output. Blood volume redistribution, accomplished by simply placing the patient in Trendelenburg position, can markedly improve hemodynamic status (92).

If extreme hemodynamic instability is encountered (Fig. 25-14), placement of an IABP, institution of femoral-femoral bypass, use of a temporary coronary artery perfusion catheter (87,103), or conversion to traditional CABG with CPB may be required.

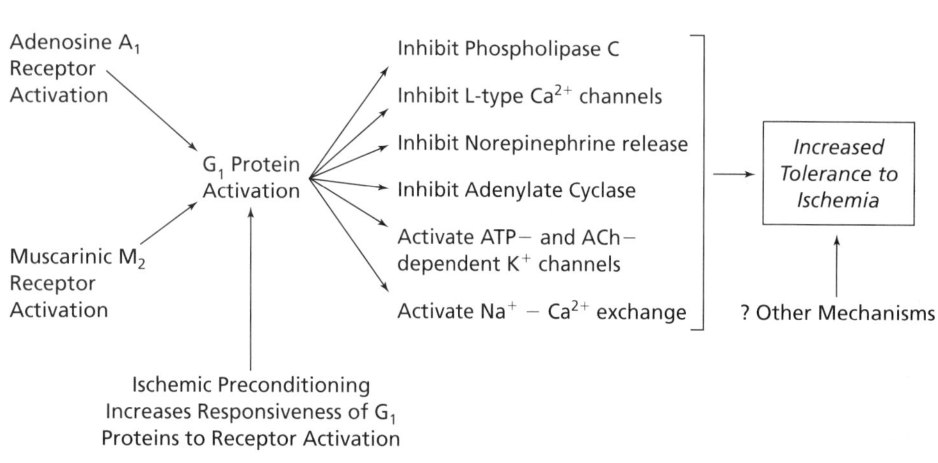

FIGURE 25-15. Proposed receptor and molecular mechanisms of ischemic preconditioning. ATP, adenosine triphosphate; Ach, acetylcholine. (From Jacobsohn E, Young CJ, Aronson S, et al. The role of ischemic preconditioning during minimally invasive coronary artery bypass surgery. *J Cardiothorac Vasc Anesth* 1997;11:790, with permission.)

Temporary coronary perfusion may be accomplished via either an intracoronary cannula with oxygenated blood supplied from the femoral artery (87,103) or an intraluminal coronary shunt (CTS FloCoil, CardioThoracic Systems; Intravascular Arteriotomy Cannulae, Medtronic DLP, Grand Rapids, MI) (Fig. 25-10). The intraluminal coronary shunts are designed to permit coronary artery blood flow and help prevent backflow of blood at the anastomotic site. By means of temporary intraluminal shunts, both functional alterations and rhythm disturbances can be decreased (85) during completion of the coronary anastomosis. Placement of shunts may be particularly useful in patients with a low degree of stenosis of the RCA when there is little likelihood of collateral circulation (104). However, the potential for endothelial damage with intracoronary shunts exists (105).

Right ventricular dysfunction is responsible for many of the hemodynamic changes induced by mechanical tilting of the heart. A right heart circulatory support system with a pulsatile pump and a catheter draining blood from the right atrium and returning it to the PA has been used experimentally during revascularization of the coronary arteries of the inferior and posterior wall (88,90,91). Left ventricular assist devices have also been used to maintain acceptable hemodynamic conditions (106,107).

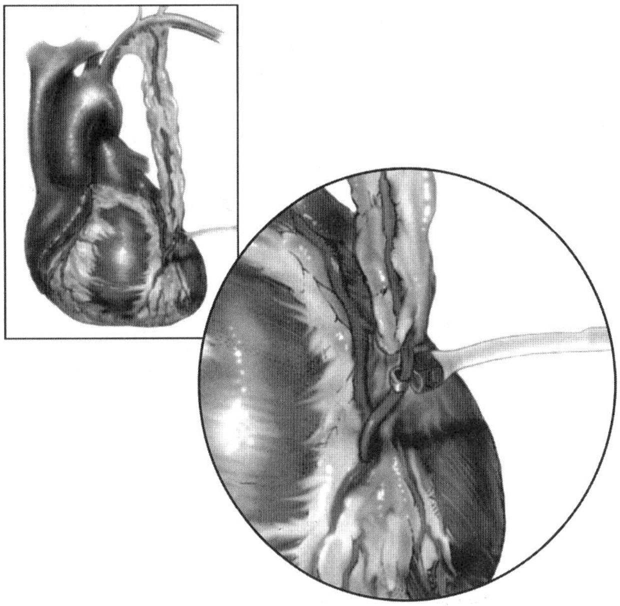

FIGURE 25-16. A coronary flow probe can be used to assess graft patency (CTS Coronary FloMeter System, CardioThoracic Systems, Inc., Cupertino, CA).

Reperfusion and Evaluation of Graft Patency

With completion of the coronary anastomosis, reperfusion is allowed. Reperfusion arrythmias may occur, especially if the native vessel was not severely occluded (33). Lidocaine (1 mg/kg) is administered at some institutions just before reperfusion in an attempt to reduce reperfusion dysrhythmias. Heparin is usually reversed with protamine. However, some choose to avoid protamine because of its potential associated side effects and allow the residual heparin to be metabolized and its effect terminated over time.

Anastomotic quality is a critical issue in minimally invasive coronary surgery. Surgeons traditionally have relied on crude and unreliable techniques, such as probing the anastomosis, absence of hemodynamic compromise, or absence of ECG abnormalities, as methods of determining the quality of the grafts. Graft patency may be assessed in the operating room by multiple techniques, including Doppler flow ultrasound (108,109), contrast echocardiography (110), or thermal imaging (111). Flow-measuring devices (CTS Coronary FloMeter System, Cardiothoracic Systems) (Fig. 25-16) can be used to detect technical failure at the anastomotic site early and to identify low-flow situations resulting from poor runoff or vasospasm. Flow probes provide a continuous flow tracing and measurements of mean flow through the coronary graft. Flow through the coronary graft occurs during diastole, with a short systolic peak. Absence of diastolic flow in a graft is indicative of an occluded graft. In a graft that has some degree of stenosis, the flow is predominantly diastolic but with taller systolic peaks. Although flow parameters and flow tracing morphology can be used to detect a severely stenosed anastomosis (more than 75%), lesser degrees of stenosis may go undetected with this technique (108). The increase of the diastolic component of the flow velocity pattern is considered a demonstration of patency of the anastomosis, even if little can be said about its quality.

Contrast echocardiography with an albumin-based ultrasound agent and TEE has been used intraoperatively to assess myocardial perfusion after MICS. Delivery of the ultrasound contrast material can be seen in the area supplied by the graft (110). Angiography is universally considered the "gold standard" technique. However, it is costly, time-consuming, and invasive. Angiography can be performed in the operating room (112) or after transport to the cardiac catheterization suite. A propofol infusion can provide maintenance of anesthesia if transport to the catheterization laboratory is necessary (34). Immediate postprocedure coronary angiography enables angioplasty, coronary stent, or reoperation if the graft is occluded.

Postoperative Management

Postoperative management issues for the anesthesiologist include the decision for early extubation and the treatment of postoperative pain. The avoidance of CPB alleviates the problems of hypothermia, electrolyte abnormalities, coagulation disturbances, interstitial edema, and anemia that might preclude early extubation. Moreover, cost savings and improved patient satisfaction promote fast-track early extubation in most patients undergoing MICS, including those with decreased left ventricular function. A goal of

"90/90"—or 90% of the patients extubated either in the operating room or within the first 90 minutes postoperatively—is attainable (7). Early extubation should be avoided in the setting of persistent myocardial ischemia, hypothermia, severe global myocardial dysfunction, or coexisting pulmonary disease (53). The use of active warming devices intraoperatively helps prevent hypothermia and facilitates emergence and extubation.

Leg pain from saphenous vein dissection during CABG is stated by many patients to be more painful than the median sternotomy incision. Although epidural or intrathecal opioid techniques have been used for pain management for cardiac surgery (113–116), many avoid neuraxial pain management techniques because of the potential risk of epidural/spinal hematoma formation in anticoagulated patients (117). Although MICS techniques use reduced doses of heparin, successful completion of the coronary grafts may not be attainable without CPB, and therefore full systemic anticoagulation is required.

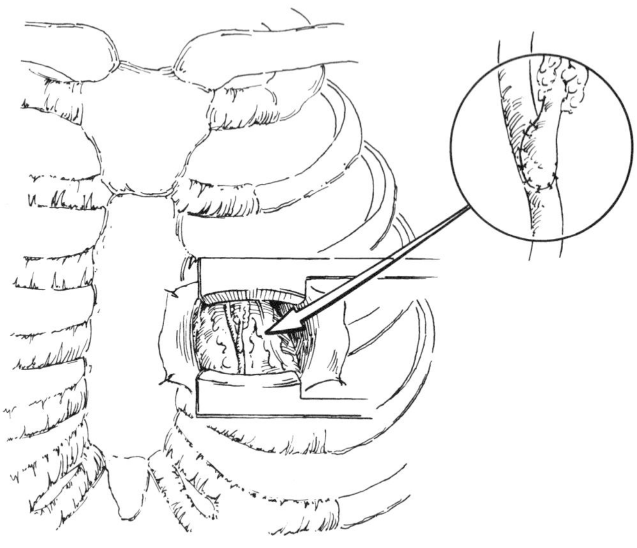

FIGURE 25-17. Minimally invasive direct coronary artery bypass (MIDCAB) usually refers to a single-vessel anastomosis performed between the left internal mammary artery and the left anterior descending coronary artery on the beating heart through a small anterior left thoracotomy under direct vision.

MIDCAB: Minithoracotomy

Overview of Surgical Strategy

MIDCAB is strictly defined as CABG surgery on the beating heart where the anastomosis is performed under "direct" vision without sternotomy, CPB, or cardioplegia (10,14). Keyhole and left anterior small thoracotomy (LAST) surgery are also terms used to describe this surgical procedure. The proposed benefits of anterior thoracotomy over median sternotomy include a reduction in sternal infection, reduced musculoskeletal injury, and possibly decreased pain in the postoperative period (118,119). However, the minithoracotomy approach does not allow access to multiple target vessels as OPCAB does. In practice, MIDCAB usually refers to coronary revascularization on the beating heart in a patient with one- or two-vessel coronary artery disease. Most commonly, the LIMA is harvested with or without thoracoscopic assistance (12,120,121), and a single vessel anastomosis is performed with the LAD on the beating heart through a small anterior left thoracotomy at the fourth intercostal space with or without removal or dislocation of the third and fourth costal cartilages (Fig. 25-17).

The right IMA may occasionally be used to bypass the RCA through a small right anterior thoracotomy. Coronary bypass performed with a small lateral thoracotomy to graft the obtuse marginal to the descending thoracic aorta with a vein or arterial conduit and grafting of the gastroepiploic artery to the inferior surface of the heart would also be considered MIDCAB procedures. The H-graft technique, which consists of anastomosing a vascular conduit from the intact IMA to the native coronary artery, has been proposed to minimize the dissection of the IMA and allow for future use if a more distal anastomosis is necessary (35,122). MIDCAB retains the benefits of IMA grafting and may avoid the potential problems of median sternotomy, aortic cross-clamping (no proximal graft anastomosis), and CPB. Occasionally, femoral-femoral CPB is used.

Simplistically, an 8- to 12-cm incision is made in the fourth intercostal space and a retraction device (LIMA Lift) is installed to spread the fourth and fifth ribs, creating a window that exposes the entire length of the LIMA. Dissection of the LIMA is then performed either directly or with thoracoscopic assistance with or without one-lung ventilation. The LAD is identified after opening of the pericardium, the mechanical coronary stabilization device is placed, and a brief test occlusion of the LAD is performed after heparinization (100 to 200 U/kg). The hemodynamic consequences of test occlusion of the LAD help determine whether ischemic preconditioning, femoral-femoral bypass, or conversion to median sternotomy with or without CPB is necessary. With the mechanical stabilizer in place and a tourniquet or snare around the proximal vessel or an intraluminal occluding device, a still and bloodless field is obtained. The IMA is anastomosed to the LAD, the stabilizer and occluding sutures are removed, the thoracotomy is closed, and a chest drain placed. An immediate postprocedure angiogram is frequently performed (38), or patency and flow are assessed intraoperatively by some other method (Doppler flow).

A MIDCAB procedure with a single-vessel bypass immediately followed in the cardiac catheterization suite by an angioplasty or stent procedure of other target vessels (hybrid operation [6,15,111,123]), or MIDCAB with the addition of transmyocardial revascularization by laser (124), is occasionally performed. Although MIDCAB continues to be performed, there has been a transition from MIDCAB to OPCAB. OPCAB allows improved anastomotic conditions and access to multiple vessels for grafting and eliminates the need for both one-lung ventilation and induced bradycardia (7).

Indications for MIDCAB

In the current era, few patients with single-vessel coronary artery disease are referred for operation regardless of the surgical approach taken. Natural history studies of medically treated patients with single-vessel coronary artery disease demonstrate good long-term prognosis. The exception is the subgroup with severe proximal LAD stenosis. Observational studies suggest that angioplasty may provide a slightly better long-term survival benefit than bypass surgery in patients with single-vessel coronary artery disease (125). Indications for MIDCAB may then be limited to the few patients who need interventional therapy but are not suitable candidates for coronary angioplasty due to their anatomy, such as those who have undergone one or more failed angioplasties and those who elect surgical revascularization (126). In 1998, Riess et al. (15) described three groups of patients who are candidates for MIDCAB: (a) patients with a significant proximal LAD stenosis not suitable for coronary balloon angioplasty, (b) patients with one- to three-vessel coronary disease and severe concomitant diseases, and (c) patients with coronary multivessel disease including significant stenoses in the circumflex artery and the RCA or the left main stem treatable by balloon angioplasty but a significant proximal LAD lesion not suitable for percutaneous transluminal coronary angioplasty.

Selection criteria for MIDCAB are continually being reevaluated (34). Some institutions are performing MIDCAB for patients with impaired left ventricular function, recent myocardial infarction (45), or reoperation and for those deemed "too sick" for CPB, for whom, should complications arise, CPB would not be used (H. Greenspun, M.D., *personal communication*). However, MIDCAB is typically performed on patients who have discreet single-vessel disease and require LIMA-to-LAD grafting. Morbid obesity, severe COPD, and atrial fibrillation (difficulty controlling heart rate and an irregular heart rhythm) make the surgical and anesthetic care of these patients more difficult. In patients in whom the coronary arteries are running under subepicardial tissue or even intramyocardially, it can be impossible to locate them and perform an anastomosis of good quality. It may become necessary to convert to a median sternotomy, which gives a better view and easier access to CPB if needed. Moreover, if the degree of stenosis is less than 95%, vessel occlusion during anastomosis can cause increased incidence of hemodynamic decompensation and arrythmias (48). Some surgeons (50) believe MIDCAB should be performed only for coronary stenosis greater than 75% or if collateral vessels are present to the area of myocardium at risk from vessel occlusion. The myocardium may not be well adapted to ischemia with lesser degrees of coronary stenosis and with poor collateralization. Sudden interruption of the remaining coronary blood flow may not be well tolerated. Conditions for MIDCAB are optimal if there is a good-caliber LAD target artery, free of disease at the middle level, with high-grade proximal lesions. Intraoperatively, the vessel must be on the surface of the heart and be free of calcification or atheroma at the proposed level of anastomosis (32). With MIDCAB, the long-term advantages of IMA grafting can be achieved with minimal surgical access trauma in selected patients.

Intraoperative Management

Differences from OPCAB: Median Sternotomy

Many of the management issues for MIDCAB are similar to those for OPCAB (median sternotomy). However, MIDCAB blends aspects of both thoracic and cardiac anesthesia practice. The surgical incision is a minithoracotomy rather than a median sternotomy. This minithoracotomy incision does not allow good direct visualization of the heart surface to assess myocardial function. Moreover, access to the epicardial surface of the heart is limited if pacing, defibrillation, or conventional CPB becomes necessary. Postoperative pain management must focus on techniques to relieve pain from the thoracotomy incision rather than median sternotomy and pain from saphenous vein dissection. Lastly, it becomes even more important to ensure patency of the single-vessel anastomosis immediately after the procedure.

Anesthetic Management

Anesthetic as well as surgical approaches to MIDCAB evolve with experience. Initially, anesthetic management often included PA catheters with pacing capability, double-lumen endotracheal tubes for one-lung ventilation, and the use of pharmacologically induced bradycardia/asystole to provide a "still" heart during coronary anastomosis (39,67,127). Surgical experience and industry development of specialized surgical equipment for MIDCAB, including coronary stabilizers and retraction devices, have decreased the complexity of anesthetic technique for MIDCAB. The use of a PA catheter, need for pharmacologically induced bradycardia/asystole, and requirements for single-lung ventilation have decreased dramatically (7,35). The need for temporary pacing techniques also appears to be reduced (35).

As with OPCAB, the operating room is configured as for a conventional CABG surgery, although the CPB pump is often set up but not primed and the perfusion team is immediately available (Fig. 25-6). The patient is positioned supine with or without elevation of either side of the chest. The patient is typically placed in a right lateral decubitus position (30° from the horizontal plane) with the arm secured above the head (29). This position allows good access to the left hemithorax and also to the groin if femoral vessel cannulation for CPB becomes necessary. The presence of an intramyocardial LAD or other anatomic considerations may preclude MIDCAB and necessitate full sternotomy with CPB. Therefore, the chest, femoral area, and legs are prepared and draped. Keeping the MIDCAB patient warm is frequently a challenge. Techniques to achieve temperature homeostasis such as a forced-air warming blank, warm circulating water mattress, airway warming or heat/moisture exchanger, and a warm operating room should be considered. The V_5 lead of the ECG is usually placed somewhat closer to a V_6 position to avoid interfering with the surgical incision, and external defibrillation pads are placed on the patient.

In the early experience, as many as 35% of patients required transvenous pacing during MIDCAB (66). Therefore, a pacing PA catheter with atrioventricular pacing was considered necessary. Mechanical stabilizing devices have dramatically reduced the need for pharmacologically induced bradycardia/asystole (35,36). With less use of negatively inotropic and negatively chronotropic medications, the need for pacing should also be decreased. In one series, only 1 of 60 patients required pacing (35). Percutaneous defibrillator/pacing pads (Zoll Pacing Pads, Zoll Medical Corp, Burlington, MA) are mainly for defibrillation or cardioversion, because it is difficult to place internal paddles through the small thoracotomy incision. They can also be used for external pacing of the heart if necessary. If a PA catheter is placed to monitor filling pressures, cardiac output (e.g., continuous cardiac output), or mixed venous oxygen saturation or to provide pacing capability, it is important that it be flow-directed into the right PA if the left lung is to be collapsed.

One-lung ventilation during the minithoracotomy approach can improve visualization of the anastomotic site and may be especially useful early in a surgeon's experience or during the video-assisted approach to MIDCAB surgery (128). However, reducing the tidal volume, increasing the respiratory rate, and retracting the ipsilateral lung usually allow adequate visualization of the anastomotic site and negate the need for one-lung ventilation (OLV). One-lung ventilation may be more helpful for procedures on the RCA, for bilateral MIDCABs, and when there is hyperinflation of the lungs (COPD) or scarring of the left lung (53). A Univent endobronchial blocker (Fuji Systems Corporation, Tokyo, Japan) may offer some advantages over a standard double-lumen endotracheal tube. The Univent can be inserted on a prophylactic basis and used only if one-lung ventilation is required; it eliminates the need for endotracheal tube exchange to a single-lumen tube at the end of the surgery if postoperative ventilation is necessary (129). If OLV is used, the left lung should be reinflated before closure to ensure that the IMA graft is not kinked (130).

Clearly, the most critical aspect of the anesthesia is management of LAD ischemia without the support of CPB. Monitoring techniques and the management of hemodynamic and ischemic complications related to mechanical stabilization and temporary coronary occlusion are similar to those discussed for OPCAB. Although patients with a totally occluded LAD usually tolerate temporary coronary occlusion during the LIMA-to-LAD anastomosis, many patients develop worsening of their baseline anterior wall dysfunction as diagnosed by TEE (36). In others, TEE findings do not change from baseline; the assumption is that such patients have adequate collateral blood flow. Pharmacologic therapy with esmolol or phenylephrine may not be necessary in more than 75% of patients (36), especially if a mechanical stabilizer is used. The regular use of ischemic preconditioning has been abandoned by many (35). The groin vessels may be accessed if CPB is required.

LIMA patency is by far the most important determinant of survival and event-free survival after coronary revascularization (131). Because it is so extremely important that the single graft in the case of MIDCAB remain patent, patients often undergo angiography in the operating room (132) or are transported to the angiography suite for immediate coronary angiography enabling angioplasty/stent or reoperation if the graft is occluded. Angioplasty or stenting of other coronary vessels (hybrid procedure) can also be performed at that time (15,133,134). A propofol infusion may be used to maintain anesthesia for transport and during the interventional procedure. Graft patency can also be assessed in the operating room by thermal imaging, Doppler flow, or contrast echocardiography.

Pain management after minithoracotomy for MIDCAB is controversial. The immediate postoperative thoracotomy pain after MIDCAB may be higher than the pain after conventional CABG with sternotomy. Although overall pain levels after cardiac operations by either conventional or minimally invasive techniques are relatively low, in one study patients having a lateral minithoracotomy experienced more pain during the first 2 postoperative days, after which pain levels were lower (135). The same concerns for neuraxial pain management techniques in patients who are partially anticoagulated or may require full anticoagulation if CPB is required apply for MIDCAB. Intravenous opioids, ketoralac, epidural analgesia, and intrathecal opioids have all been used with some success (36). Pain management techniques often used with thoracotomy for lung surgery, intrapleural analgesia (136), intercostal nerve blocks, and thoracic epidural analgesia (137) have also been used for minithoracotomy for MIDCAB. Intercostal nerve blocks are uniquely well suited to providing 6 hours of analgesia (138). Thoracic epidural blocks may be placed before or after the procedure (35). Although there are reports showing the safety of epidurals with regard to risk of epidural hematoma for conventional CABG procedures, they are often placed hours or days before systemic anticoagulation (117). Potential benefits that have been attributed to thoracic epidural analgesia include improved graft flow and decreased stress response after MIDCAB (137,139) and better pain control than with continuous intercostal nerve block (140). A more novel approach to pain management for MIDCAB is the use of paravertebral blocks or paravertebral catheters on the side of the minithoracotomy (Roy Greengrass M.D., *personal communication, 1999*). This would avoid many of the potential problems of thoracic epidural analgesia, including the risk of epidural hematoma and sympathetic blockade.

Outcome Measures: MIDCAB and OPCAB

Are we reproducing the results of conventional CABG surgery? Are we significantly reducing the morbidity of the procedure? These are two important questions that must be asked when evaluating outcome after MIDCAB or OPCAB. The largest series with the longest follow-up times are from South America and represent primarily procedures performed through a median sternotomy (8,9). Moreover, much of the material is observational data only, and from relatively small series of patients. Mortality, graft patency, perioperative comorbidity (e.g., central nervous system), and economic issues are of importance.

Mortality

Two of the largest series of OPCAB are from South America. Benetti performed 1,420 OPCAB procedures via median sternotomy with no reported in-hospital deaths and a 97% survival rate at 5 years (45). Buffolo performed 1,274 OPCAB procedures with a reported 2.5% mortality rate (9). Moshkovitz, in Israel, reported on 220 OPCAB patients. The operative mortality rate was 3.2% with 93% actuarial survival at 1 year. A calcified aorta, nonuse of the IMA, reoperation, and diabetes mellitus were independent predictors of unfavorable events (141). Tasdemir, in Turkey, reported on a very large OPCAB study group of 2,052 patients. The operative mortality rate was 1.9%. Associated hypertension, poor quality of the LAD graft, and ungrafted circumflex coronary artery were predictors of early mortality (102). Pfister performed 220 OPCAB procedures and compared them with 220 on-pump control operations. There was no statistical difference between groups in mortality (1.4% and 2.4%, respectively) (142).

Fewer patients have undergone MIDCAB. Subramanian et al. reported on 199 MIDCAB procedures with an operative mortality rate of 3.8% (14). Calafiore et al. reported on 434 patient who underwent the LAST procedure (MIDCAB). The operative mortality rate was 1.1% (81). Although studies of OPCAB/MIDCAB with large series of patients including patient control groups with long-term follow-up are not presently available, observational data suggests that MIDCAB and OPCAB can be performed safely with regard to early mortality.

Graft Patency

In 1996, approximately two-thirds of cardiac surgeons did not believe one could achieve the same quality of anastomosis on the beating heart as with CPB. Moreover, 75% of the surgeons polled were either slightly or very uncomfortable with performing MICAB. Not only did most surgeons believe the quality of the anastomosis was inferior when performed on the beating heart, the majority (64%) did not routinely evaluate the anastomosis to prove anastomotic patency (6). It must be remembered that there are three components that account for patency of the coronary artery anastomoses: the technical skill of the surgeon, the quality of the artery being grafted, and the quality of the conduit used. The introduction of mechanical stabilizers has greatly reduced epicardial surface motion, thereby improving anastomotic conditions and decreasing the technical difficulties associated with OPCAB/MIDCAB. These devices were not available when many of the earlier studies were reported. Gundry et al. (143) reported on 107 OPCAB procedures performed between 1989 to 1990 and compared them with 112 conventional CABG operations. Although survival and cardiac death rates were similar between the two groups groups at 7-year follow-up, reintervention (coronary catheterization, angioplasty, second coronary bypass) was greatly increased among the OPCAB patients (143). Subramanian et al. reported an increase in the LIMA-to-LAD (MIDCAB) anastomosis patency rate from 89% to 97% with the routine use of mechanical stabilization (14). Calafiore et al. noted an increase in early anastomotic patency rates from 92.5% to 98.9% after mechanical stabilization was introduced in 1996 (81). The fact that the minimal-access operation is technically feasible is not enough to justify widespread use if the quality of the anastomosis is compromised. Prospective and controlled studies that use immediate postprocedure angiography will help answer this question. Early graft patency by either conventional procedures or MICS is usually 90% or greater. Late graft patency of the LIMA graft performed by conventional technique is 80% or greater in most series and greater than 90% in some. The late patency of the grafts performed by MIDCAB is unknown (144). However, early observational studies suggest that acceptable graft patency can be obtained in experienced hands and with the use of mechanical stabilization techniques.

Comorbidity

Avoiding CPB has the potential for decreasing perioperative central nervous system injury, the systemic inflammatory response, transfusion requirements, and renal injury.

The risk of stroke and neuropsychologic injury after CPB is well known (145). CPB with its attendant alterations in cerebral perfusion (146) and systemic embolization have been blamed for these complications. OPCAB avoids CPB and MIDCAB (LIMA-to-LAD anastomosis) avoids CPB as well as manipulation of the ascending aorta for placement of proximal grafts. Studies have documented a reduced number of cerebral microemboli (147,148) and decreased release of S100 (149,150), an astroglial-specific protein released into blood after brain injury, in off-pump versus on-pump cases. Cerebral function measured by cognitive tests and auditory evoked potentials (151,152) demonstrated an advantage for off-pump surgery. In one large study, Buffolo et al. reported a 3.8% stroke rate among patients undergoing conventional operations (689 patients) compared with 1.1% among patients (378 patients) operated on via median sternotomy without CPB (9). Another small study found no difference in early neurologic outcome assessed by neurologic examination and neuropsychologic testing in patients subjected to CABG with or without CPB (153).

The exposure of the patient's blood to the foreign surfaces of the CPB apparatus results in a systemic inflammatory response and alterations in coagulation. The release of inflammatory mediators appears to be less with OPCAB (154–160). Reported rates of requirement for blood transfusion for conventional cardiac surgery and MICS vary widely. Reported transfusion rates for MIDCAB/OPBCAB range from approximately 2% to approximately 25% (8, 10,102,142,161). One study comparing OPCAB with conventional CABG demonstrated a 27.3% rate of transfusion in the former group, versus 45.4% in the latter (142).

CPB is a nonphysiologic mode of perfusion that may contribute to renal damage after cardiac surgery. Loef et al. (et al.) studied parameters of glomerular function (microalbuminuria), tubular function (fractional excretion of sodium), and renal damage (*N*-acetyl D-glucosaminidase [NAG]) in patients undergoing conventional CABG with CPB and CABG without CPB. They demonstrated that CPB induces renal damage at both the glomerular and the tubular level, and the avoidance of CPB was associated with improved indices of renal function (162).

Economics

Economics is the major driving force in changing the management of conventional cardiac surgery (163) and for the interest in MICS (6). The potential economic advantages of MICS include less patient trauma with reduced need for extended intensive care unit stay, reduced lengths of stay, and avoidance of the costs of extracorporeal circulation equipment. The MIDCAB procedure is associated with reduced hospital stay (approximately 2 days versus approximately 5 days) may offer a cost advantage of $5,000 to $10,000 (164–168).

The effects of beating heart surgery performed via median sternotomy and minithoracotomy on outcomes such as mortality, comorbidity, time needed to resume normal activities, postprocedure pain, and cost of medical care will remain uncertain until more patients undergo this procedure and long-term follow-up results have been reported. A registry for patients undergoing MIDCAB and its variations has been established (http://www.heartnet.org) and will be helpful in determining the safety and efficacy of this technique.

CARDIAC SURGERY USING CPB BUT WITH MINIMALLY INVASIVE ACCESS OR INCISION

Port-Access Cardiac Surgery

Overview of Surgical Strategy

The Port-Access system provides the convenience of CPB and hypothermic cardiac arrest without requiring sternotomy. The Port-Access model borrows techniques from laparoscopy, thoracoscopy, and microsurgery to make it possible to operate in a quiet and bloodless field. It uses an endovascular CPB system of catheters and cannulas (Fig. 25-18), many placed percutaneously, and instruments that are task-specific to graft coronary vessels or perform mitral valve surgery. Equipment used in Port-Access surgery can be viewed on the World Wide Web at www.heartport.com/surgprod/stop.php3. This Port-Access approach to cardiac surgery is currently used at more than 100 centers throughout the world, but it requires specialized equipment as well as training of the surgeon, anesthesiologist, and perfusionist. The theory behind the system is the avoidance of sternotomy with its associated risk of mediastinal wound infection and thorax instability and the ability to perform true

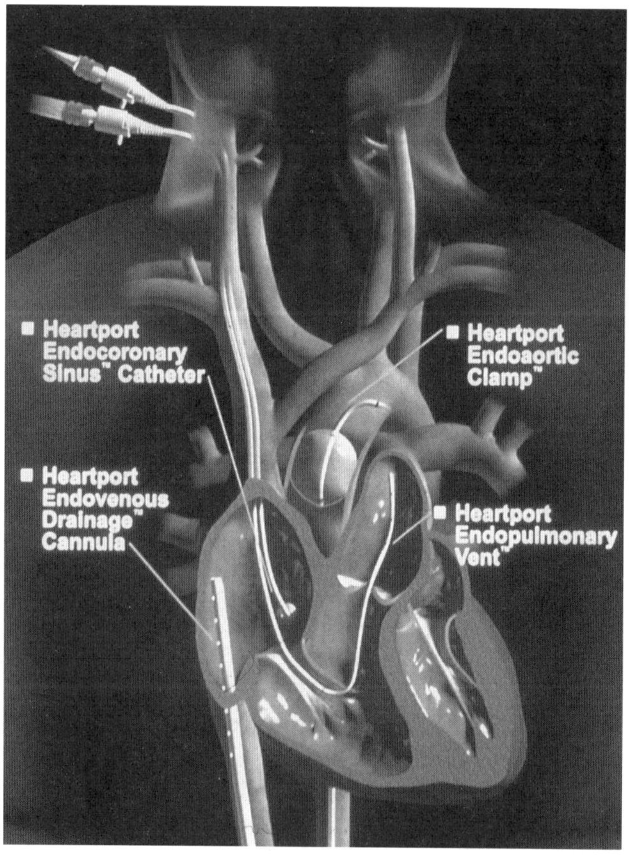

FIGURE 25-18. The Heartport Port-Access (Heartport Inc., Redwood City, CA) endovascular cardiopulmonary bypass system of catheters and cannulas.

Port-Access cardiac surgery through very small ports without a major thoracotomy. The consequences of this kind of surgery are less atrial manipulation, which may reduce the incidence of postoperative atrial fibrillation; less aortic manipulation; avoidance of the need to clamp the aorta externally; the ability to perform PA venting as in conventional CPB procedures; and the ability to work on the arrested heart using antegrade or retrograde application of cardioplegia, allowing precise anastomosis for MICAB. The underlying premise is that a smaller incision causes less postoperative pain, resulting in a quicker overall recovery.

After percutaneous placement of a catheter in the coronary sinus to provide retrograde cardioplegia, and often in the PA to provide venting capability, a minithoracotomy on the left for CABG or on the right for mitral valve surgery is performed. After the surgeon obtains adequate exposure, the venous drainage cannula for CPB is inserted through the femoral vein, and then the arterial inflow cannula is inserted through a femoral artery. An inflatable balloon on the end of the Endoaortic Clamp (Heartport) catheter is advanced through the arterial inflow catheter. This will be used to provide intravascular occlusion of the aorta ("soft clamp"), antegrade cardioplegia, and aortic venting capability. The venous drainage cannula is positioned in the right atrium and the balloon-tipped catheter in the ascending aorta with the assistance of TEE and fluoroscopy. CPB and hypothermia can then be initiated. To arrest the heart, the balloon-tipped catheter in the ascending aorta is inflated and antegrade or retrograde cardioplegia is administered. The coronary anastomosis or valve surgery is performed using instruments passed through ports in the chest, with or without a small additional chest incision. After completion of surgery, the Endoaortic Clamp is deflated and the patient is weaned from CPB.

This Port-Access system has been successfully employed clinically in single and multivessel coronary revascularization, in valvular repair or replacement, and for repair of atrial septal defect (169–173). A multicenter international registry designed to collect, analyze, and report relevant clinical data and track clinical outcomes of patients undergoing Port-Access procedures was launched in 1997 and is accessible on the World Wide Web (www.heartport.com, PAIR, Port Access International Registry, PAIR Data Update).

Indications for Port-Access MICS

The Port-Access technology allows access to all epicardial surfaces of the heart and intracardiac structures through a minimal incision. Applications of the Port-Access technology include CABG (single and multivessel), valves (repair or replacement), atrial septal defect repair, combined procedures, and redo procedures.

If the iliac or femoral arteries manifest atherosclerotic change, the procedure, which requires femoral cannulation, may be contraindicated because of potential retrograde aortic dissection (172,173). An aorta with mural thrombi or atheromatous plaque is not suitable for the procedure because the technique requires retrograde perfusion. However, a new aortic cannula that allows antegrade CPB is available (EndoDirect System, Heartport); it is placed percutaneously into the ascending aorta under vision. Preoperative screening for peripheral vascular disease has been recommended (13).

Intraoperative Management

Port-Access surgery demands an expanded role for the anesthesiologist before, during, and after CPB. Bilateral radial arterial catheters are usually placed to monitor for possible dislocation of the balloon of the Endoaortic Clamp, which may then occlude the right brachiocephalic artery, and a left-sided double-lumen endotracheal tube is positioned to provide single-lung ventilation during surgical exposure. TEE has an important role during Port-Access procedures (Table 25-9) (174). The aorta should be interrogated for evidence of plaque, dissection, or hematoma which might exclude the use of retrograde perfusion and an IABP if required. The presence of aortic valve insufficiency excludes the use of antegrade cardioplegia.

The anesthesiologist is responsible for inserting both the endopulmonary vent and the endocoronary sinus catheters through introducer sheaths placed in the internal jugular vein (175). The Endocoronary Sinus catheter, if required (176), is usually placed first with the aid of TEE and fluoroscopy (40,175,177), In experienced hands, only TEE may be required. The zero-degree, four-chamber orientation and especially the modified bicaval view allow visualization of the coronary sinus to help engage the coronary sinus catheter into the coronary sinus (178). Monitoring of the distal tip pressure of the coronary sinus catheter also allows one

TABLE 25-9. ROLE OF TRANSESOPHAGEAL ECHOCARDIOGRAPHY (TEE) DURING PORT-ACCESS PROCEDURES

Goals of TEE Examination	Comments
Evaluate aortic plaque	Exclude use of IABP
Evaluate aortic dissection and hematoma	Exclude use of retrograde perfusion
Rule out aortic valve insufficiency	Exclude use of antegrade cardioplegia
Role out ASD or patent foramen ovale	Change approach during mitral valve surgery
Check positions of cannulas	Confirm position
Evaluate valvular and myocardial function	Aid in terminating CPB

Note: ASD, atrioseptal defect; CPB, cardiopulmonary bypass; IABP, intra-aortic balloon pump.
Source: From Krucylak PE. Intraoperative considerations during minimal-access cardiac surgery. *Semin Thorac Cardiovasc Surg* 1999; 11:116, with permission.

to confirm proper position of the coronary sinus catheter in the coronary sinus. With inflation of the balloon within the coronary sinus, the pressure tracing becomes ventricularized, an easy trace to differentiate from the central venous pressure trace and one that occurs only after balloon inflation. The coronary sinus catheter is routinely used during mitral valve repair or replacement and in patients with aortic insufficiency and optionally during other procedures. To prevent clot formation on or in the catheter, a single dose of heparin (approximately 5,000 U) is administered intravenously. The catheter should be seen in the right atrium by 30 cm and sometimes less in smaller patients. Monitoring of distal tip pressure provides a direct indication should the tip be advanced from the right atrium across the tricuspid valve (179).

The Endopulmonary Vent (Heartport) may be used to return blood to the CPB machine that is not drained by the femoral venous catheter and to decompress the left ventricle. Fluoroscopy, TEE, and monitoring of the pressure waveform as it is flow-directed into the PA may help ensure proper positioning. With adequate venous drainage, the Endopulmonary Vent catheter may not be necessary (176). Moreover, it precludes the use of a thermodilution PA catheter, which can be valuable in the management of these cases.

After systemic heparinization, an Endovenous Drainage cannula is placed into the femoral vein, and the arterial inflow cannula is placed in the femoral artery. A guidewire is advanced from the femoral vein to the right atrium, visualized by TEE, and the Heartport Endovenous Drainage cannula advanced into the right atrium with the tip at the superior caval atrial junction. The Endoaortic Clamp is advanced over a guidewire and positioned in the ascending aorta with the tip slightly above the sinotubular ridge, as seen by TEE. Simultaneous measurements of the aortic root pressure and radial arterial pressure should be equal. Extracorporeal circulation can then be initiated. The Endo-CPB system (180,181) is graphically demonstrated in Fig. 25-19. Venous return is

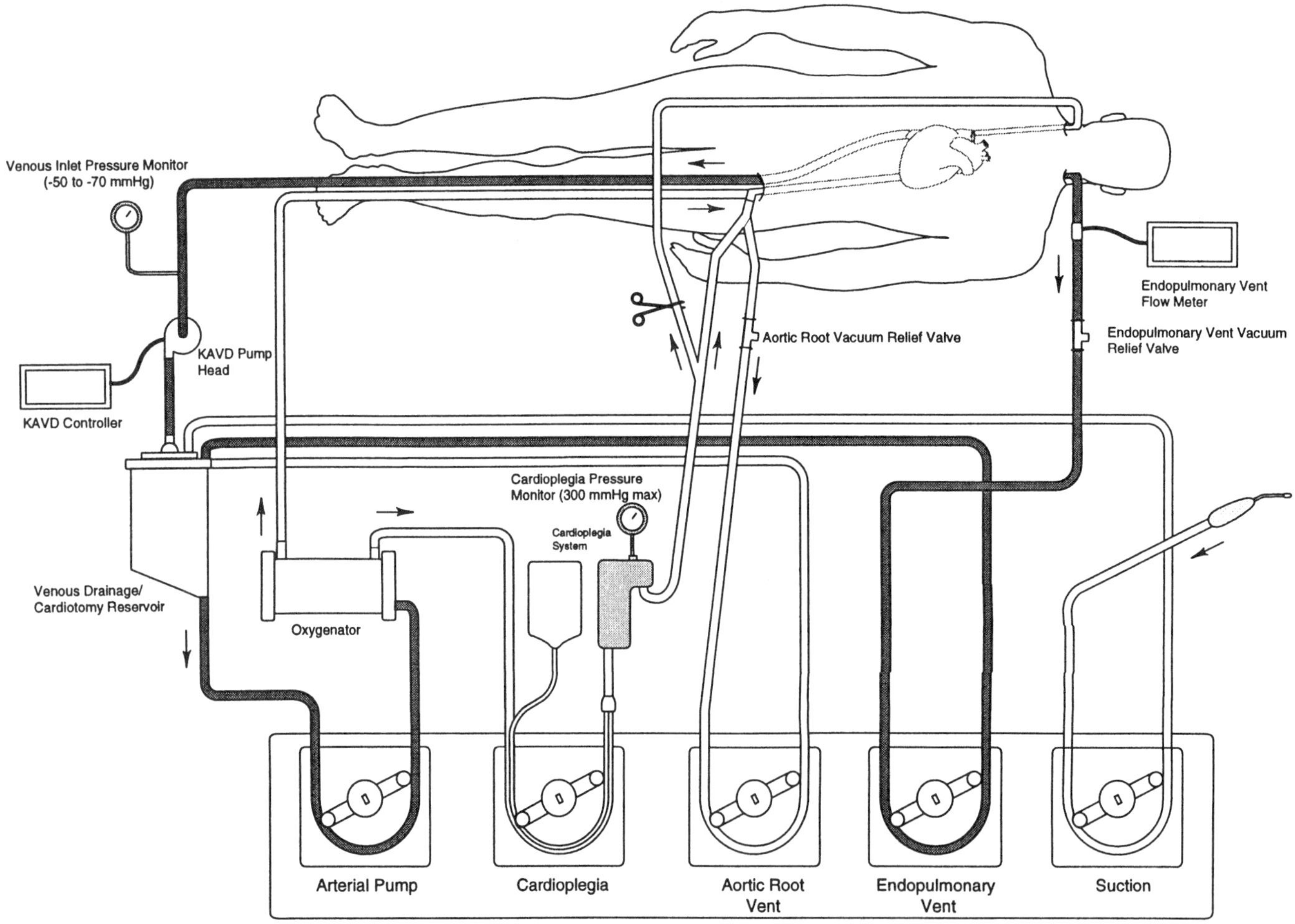

FIGURE 25-19. Extracorporeal circulation for Port-Access cardiac surgery. (From Toomasian JM, Peters WS, Siegel LC. Extracorporeal circulation for port-access cardiac surgery. *Perfusion* 1997; 12:83, with permission.)

augmented by a centrifugal pump rather than relying solely on gravity drainage. Conventional femoral venous cannulation without augmentation can support only 75% to 80% of the normal cardiac output (180). Therefore, a centrifugal kinetic-assisted venous drainage (KAVD) pump is placed between the venous cannula and the venous reservoir to completely decompress the heart for total cardiopulmonary support. With the Endoaortic Clamp balloon inflated, cardioplegia may be administered antegrade through the Endoaortic Clamp catheter or retrograde into the coronary sinus via the Endocoronary Sinus catheter.

During CPB, the anesthesiologist must monitor adequacy of venous return and position of the Endoaortic Clamp balloon. Inadequate venous return is indicated by the following: venous pump flow remaining low despite adequate negative inlet pressure on the centrifugal pump, inadequate decrease of central venous pressure, excessive pulmonary vent catheter flow (more than 5% of total bypass flow [180]) and not decreasing, radial artery pressure remaining pulsatile, TEE showing a nonempty right ventricle, and lack of right atrial and ventricular decompression as demonstrated by video-assisted thoracoscopy. The Endovenous Drainage catheter may need to be repositioned. Because cephalad migration of the Endoaortic Catheter balloon can occlude the right brachiocephalic artery or other arch vessels and compromise cerebral blood flow, it is imperative to continuously monitor its position. There are several proposed methods to achieve this goal. Potential migration of the Endoaortic Clamp may be detected by abnormal position on visualization with TEE or fluoroscopy, altered flow in the carotid artery by carotid ultrasound or in intracranial arteries by transcranial Doppler ultrasound, comparison of the aortic root pressure with the systemic arterial pressure, and comparison of right and left radial arterial pressures. After completion of surgery, the endoaortic balloon is deflated and the patient is separated from CPB.

Results of Port-Access Surgery

The proposed advantages of Port-Access surgery include less postoperative pain, decreased hospitalization and rehabilitation periods, and reduced health care costs. Port-Access surgery is still in its early stages of development, and these potential advantages remain unsubstantiated by well-controlled prospective investigations. Moreover, Port-Access cardiac surgery does not avoid the known problems associated with conventional hypothermic CPB, is technically challenging, requires specialized expertise from surgeons and anesthesiologists, and increases operating room use.

Hypotheses that need to be tested include the following: (a) Can femoral bypass and port-facilitated surgery be performed with equal risk of morbidity and mortality and short- and long-term graft patency (CABG) as conventional cardiac surgery with median sternotomy? and (b) Does this approach result in less pain, shorter length of stay, and decreased costs?

Early clinical results from an international registry (Port-Access International Registry, PAIR), individual centers, and multiinstitutional studies are encouraging (13,169,172, 182–184). The PAIR data on more than 1,000 patients from 121 centers (182,183) demonstrate that Port-Access CABG and mitral valve operations can be performed safely, with morbidity and mortality rates equal or to better than those associated with open-chest operations (Society of Thoracic Surgeons database). Although some have criticized the method of data collection (volunteer entrance of patients from multiple institutions), the operative mortality rate for Port-Access CABG and valve replacement/repair compared favorably with that for conventional cardiac surgery via sternotomy (183). The incidence of postoperative atrial fibrillation was decreased. Successful completion of the surgery without conversion to sternotomy occurred in approximately 95% of the cases. Some concerns have been expressed regarding a risk of aortic dissection from femoral arterial cannulation and retrograde perfusion and neurologic complications. Early in the experience, several cases of aortic dissection were reported. With proper patient screening (exclusion of patients with significant aortoiliac occlusive disease) and improved placement techniques and equipment, the incidence has been significantly reduced. The stroke rate was 2.2% in the largest Port-Access subgroup (CABG), which is comparable to the rate for patients in the STS registry. Long-term graft patency rates for the Port-Access group have yet to be reported (169).

Several studies comparing incision pain after Port-Access versus conventional cardiac surgery with median sternotomy demonstrated an advantage for the port-facilitated technique (185,186). However, this technique may increase operating room time, increase perfusion expenses, and increase overall cost despite facilitating early postoperative hospital discharge (171,186–188).

The Port-Access approach is slowly gaining acceptance for a variety of indications, including multivessel revascularization and valve operations. However, the equipment cost is high and hinders its wide acceptance (1).

Conventional Surgery via Limited Incisions

The most uncomplicated approach to MICS is to use smaller incisions, avoid full sternotomy, and use conventional instruments and cannulas. These surgical approaches have included partial upper, middle, and lower sternotomy; parasternal incisions; and a variety of thoracotomies. Essentially all major adult cardiac procedures, including CABG, aortic valve replacement, mitral valve repair or replacement, multivalve procedures, and septal myectomy, have been performed through these approaches (2,21–23,25,189,190). Cannulation for CPB may be performed through the primary incision or via the femoral artery and vein.

From the anesthesiologist's viewpoint, this type of MICS often requires little deviation from conventional anesthetic management. The limited incision decreases the ability to access the epicardium if pacing or defibrillation/cardioversion becomes necessary. Defibrillator-pacemaker pads allow for defibrillation, cardioversion, and external pacing if the surgeon cannot introduce the defibrillation paddles or pacemaker wires through the limited access. Only rarely is one-lung ventilation necessary (191). The anesthesiologist may not be able to directly observe myocardial contractility and ventricular filling, as is possible with median sternotomy cases, and therefore must rely on hemodynamic monitoring and TEE to guide separation from CPB. The anesthetic goals should be similar to the surgical goals; early tracheal extubation, ambulation, and hospital discharge.

According to its proponents, this minimally invasive approach results in less pain, faster recovery, and better cosmetic result. However, operative times may be longer, morbidity and mortality rates do not appear to be decreased, the length of hospital stay varies by only 1 or 2 days, and patients do not necessarily report less postoperative pain (192).

OTHER MINIMALLY INVASIVE PROCEDURES IN CARDIAC SURGERY

Minimally Invasive Congenital Heart Surgery

The impetus for minimally invasive congenital cardiac surgery is similar to that for adult surgery: to avoid the known long-term morbidity of sternotomy and thoracotomy and to reduce postoperative pain, respiratory dysfunction, and length of hospital stay (Fontana, 1998). Burke (193) and Fontana (2) have recently reviewed this topic.

To reduce the trauma of pediatric surgery, initial efforts were devoted to video-assisted endoscopic instrumentation and technique development. Applications were then developed for simple extracardiac lesions (e.g., ligation of patent ductus arteriosus [PDA], ligation of systemic-to-PA collaterals, division of complete vascular ring), intraoperative endoscopy, surgery through small incisions, and, ultimately, potentially endoscopic open heart surgery. Repair of atrial septal defects, ventricular septal defects, and tetralogy of Fallot have all been reported using a variety of minimally invasive approaches (193–195).

Anesthetic management should limit the need for prolonged unplanned postoperative mechanical ventilation. Limited incisions provide limited access to the epicardial surface if pacing or defibrillation is required. Femoral bypass may be used.

Minimally Invasive Saphenous Vein Dissection

Standard open-incision saphenous vein harvesting may be the major source of postoperative pain for many patients undergoing routine CABG. With minimally invasive vein harvesting, subcutaneous tissue is tunneled under photo-optical view using specially designed instruments (Guidant Corporation, Menlo Park, CA). Carbon dioxide is insufflated along the course of the vein to aid in its visualization and dissection. Up to 10 to 20 L of carbon dioxide may be insufflated during this 20- to 60-minute procedure (7,196). Increases in end-tidal carbon dioxide concentration may be noted, especially if the ventilatory tidal volume is reduced to assist IMA dissection, which often occurs concurrently with saphenous vein harvest. Carbon dioxide embolization has occurred during carbon dioxide insufflation (K. Grichnik, M.D., *personal communication, 1999*). Minimally invasive techniques may decrease postoperative leg edema and requirement for wound care, decrease postoperative pain, and result in increased mobility compared with traditional open methods (196–198).

INTERNET SITES OF INFORMATION ON MICS

Technologic advances in MICS are occurring on an almost daily basis. In some cases, distribution of information on the World Wide Web (Internet) may provide a more "up-to-date" information source. Information about and pictures of commercial equipment used to perform beating heart surgery can be found at www.medtronic.com (In-Cardia systems for MICS) and www.cardioth.com (CTS, Cardiothoracic Systems). Information about and pictures of equipment to perform Port-Access surgery as well as data from the Port-Access international registry can be found at www.heartport.com. A MIDCAB registry where data about MIDCAB can be collected and reviewed in real time is at www.heartnet.org. The web site for the new International Society for Minimally Invasive Cardiac Surgery (ISMICS) is www.ismics.org. This site includes abstracts from recent meetings. The official peer review journal of the ISMICS is *The Heart Surgery Forum.*

ETHICAL QUESTIONS AND FUTURE

More than 20 years ago, before MICS, Eugene Braunwald warned that "an industry is being built around" bypass surgery. In 1996, the most common response by cardiac surgeons, when asked what they thought would be the most important driving force for the expansion of MICAB, was economic demands. Widespread media coverage is already spurring patient demand for MICS procedures. Patients, surgeons, cardiologists, industry, investors, and third-party payers all have an interest in MICS. Some surgeons who do these procedures may have financial interests in the companies promoting them or other incentives for wanting to influence the treatment choice patients make in consultation with their cardiologists (199).

> "Under any circumstances, surgeons should refuse to compromise the clinical outcome of an operation just to satisfy a desire to be innovative or to improve their image among their peers or the public. The choice of operative technique must fit the patient. Whenever possible, surgeons should choose the simple approach and avoid unproven innovations."
>
> Denton A. Cooley, M.D. (192)

There are many possible options for coronary artery revascularization—catheter-based therapies, conventional CABG, MIDCAB, hybrid procedure, OPCAB, and Port-Access CABG surgery—with little definitive data to support one option over another. How can a patient provide a truly informed consent under these circumstances? A study that assessed patient preferences for consequences of three coronary revascularization procedures (angioplasty, conventional CABG, and MICAB surgery) identified the risk of repeat revascularization as the most important concern (62%), followed by postprocedure pain (22%), time to recovery of physical functioning (8%), time in hospital (4%), and body appearance (4%). Respondents preferred angioplasty to conventional CABG and MICS if the 3-year risk of repeat revascularization with angioplasty were to decline to less than 28% and 21%, respectively (200). Long-term outcome data for the various methods of MICS will help resolve this issue in the future.

Endoscopic robotic-assisted CABG with computer elimination of tremor and motion scaling (201), laser albumin welding of vessels (202), and one-shot coronary anastomosis devices (203,204) all seem futuristic but are currently being investigated.

REFERENCES

1. Shennib H. Facts and myths of minimally invasive cardiac surgery: current trends in thoracic surgery IV. Introduction. *Ann Thorac Surg* 1998;66:997.
2. Fontana GP. Minimally invasive cardiac surgery. *Chest Surg Clin North Am* 1998;8:871.
3. Vanermen H. What is minimally invasive cardiac surgery? *J Card Surg* 1998;13:268.
4. Shennib H. Evolving strategies in minimally invasive coronary artery surgery. *Int J Cardiol* 1997;62[Suppl 1]:S81.
5. Glenville B. Minimally invasive cardiac surgery. *BMJ* 1999;319:135.
6. Shennib H, Mack MJ, Lee AGL. A survey on minimally invasive coronary artery bypass grafting. *Ann Thorac Surg* 1997;64:110.
7. Gayes JM. The minimally invasive cardiac surgery voyage. *J Cardiothorac Vasc Anesth* 1999;13:119.
8. Benetti FJ, Naselli G, Wood M, et al. Direct myocardial revascularization without extracorporeal circulation: experience in 700 patients. *Chest* 1991;100:312.
9. Buffolo E, de Andrade JCS, Branco JNR, et al. Coronary artery bypass grafting without cardiopulmonary bypass. *Ann Thorac Surg* 1996;61:63.
10. Calafiore AM, Giammarco GD, Teodori G, et al. Midterm results after minimally invasive coronary surgery (LAST operation). *J Thorac Cardiovasc Surg* 1998;115:763.
11. Lajos TZ, Akhter M. Combined minimally invasive approach with right gastroepiploic artery, offpump. *Heart Surgery Forum* 1999. Available at: http://www.hsforum.com/abstracts/C14.asp.
12. Duhaylongsod FG, Mayfield WR, Wolf RK. Thoracoscopic harvest of the internal thoracic artery: a multicenter experience in 218 cases. *Ann Thorac Surg* 1998;66:1012.
13. Reichenspurner H, Welz A, Gulielmos V, et al. Port-Access cardiac surgery using endovascular cardiopulmonary bypass. *J Card Surg* 1998;13:275.
14. Subramanian VA, McCabe, Geller CM. Minimally invasive coronary artery bypass grafting: two-year clinical experience. *Ann Thorac Surg* 1997;64:1648.
15. Riess F-C, Schofer J, Kremer P, et al. Beating heart operations including hybrid revascularization: initial experiences. *Ann Thorac Surg* 1998;66:1076.
16. Grocott HP, Newman MF, Lowe JE, et al. Transmyocardial laser revascularization: an anesthetic perspective. *J Cardiothorac Vasc Anesth* 1997;11:206.
17. Trehan N, Mishra Y, Mehta Y, et al. Transmyocardial laser as an adjunct to minimally invasive CABG for complete myocardial revascularization. *Ann Thorac Surg* 1998;66:1113.
18. Stevens JH, Burdon TA, Peters WS. Port-Access coronary artery bypass grafting: a proposed surgical method. *J Thorac Cardiovasc Surg* 1996;111:567.
19. Cohn LH, Adams DH, Couper GS, et al. Minimally invasive cardiac valve surgery improves patient satisfaction while reducing costs of cardiac valve replacement and repair. *Ann Surg* 1997;226:421.
20. Carpentier A, Loulmte D, Carpentier A. First open heart operation (mitral valvuloplasty) under videosurgery through a minithoracotomy. *C R Acad Sci Ser III Sci Vie* 1996;319:219.
21. Chitwood WR, Elbeery JR, Chapman WHH, et al. Video-assisted minimally invasive mitral valve surgery: the "micromitral" operation. *J Thorac Cardiovasc Surg* 1997;113:413.
22. Cosgrove DM III, Sabik JF. Minimally invasive approach for aortic valve operations. *Ann Thorac Surg* 1996;62:596.
23. Massetti M, Babatasi G, Lotti A, et al. Less invasive cardiac operations through a median sternotomy: 100 consecutive cases. *Ann Thorac Surg* 1998;66:1050.
24. Weinschelbaum E, Stutzbach P, Machain A, et al. Valve operations through a minimally invasive approach. *Ann Thorac Surg* 1998;66:1106.
25. Gundry SR, Shattuck OH, Razzouk AJ, et al. Facile minimally invasive cardiac surgery via ministernotomy. *Ann Thorac Surg* 1998;65:1100.
26. Kolessov VL. Mammary artery-coronary anastomosis as a method of treatment for angina pectoris. *J Thorac Cardiovasc Surg* 1967;54:535.
27. Ankeney JL. To use or not to use the pump oxygenator in coronary bypass operations. *Ann Thorac Surg* 1975;19:108.
28. Trapp WG, Bisarya R. Placement of coronary artery bypass graft without pump oxygenator. *Ann Thorac Surg* 1975;19:1.
29. Benetti FJ, Ballester C, Sani G, et al. Video-assisted coronary bypass surgery. *J Card Surg* 1995;10:620.
30. Subramanian V, Stelzer P. Clinical experience with minimally invasive coronary artery bypass grafting (CABG). *Eur J Thorac Cardiovasc Surg* 1996;10:1058.
31. Stephenson ER, Sankholkar S, Ducko CT, et al. Robotically assisted microsurgery for endoscopic coronary artery bypass grafting. *Ann Thorac Surg* 1998;66:1064.
32. Elefteriades JA. Mini-CABG: a step forward or backward? *J Cardiothorac Vasc Anesth* 1997;11:661.
33. Krucylak PE. Intraoperative considerations during minimal-access cardiac surgery. *Semin Thorac Cardiovasc Surg* 1999;11:116.
34. Gayes JM, Emery RW. The MIDCAB experience: a current

look at evolving surgical and anesthetic approaches. *J Cardiothorac Vasc Anesth* 1997;11:625.
35. Maslow AD, Park KW, Pawlowski J, et al. Minimally invasive direct coronary bypass grafting: changes in anesthetic management and surgical procedure. *J Cardiothorac Vasc Anesth* 1999; 13:417.
36. Heres EK, Marquez J, Malkowski MJ, et al. Minimally invasive direct coronary artery bypass: anesthetic, monitoring, and pain control considerations. *J Cardiothorac Vasc Anesth* 1998;12:385.
37. Hultman J. Anaesthesia and monitoring for minimally invasive cardiac surgery with special reference to minimally invasive direct coronary artery bypass surgery. *Perfusion* 1998;13:259.
38. Schaff HV. New surgical techniques: implications for the cardiac anesthesiologist. Mini-thoracotomy for coronary revascularization without cardiopulmonary bypass. *J Cardiothorac Vasc Anesth* 1997;11:6.
39. Gayes JM, Emery RW, Nissen MD. Anesthetic considerations for patients undergoing minimally invasive coronary artery bypass surgery: mini-sternotomy and mini-thoracotomy approaches. *J Cardiothorac Vasc Anesth* 1996;10:531.
40. Chaney MA, Nikolov MP, Tuchek M, et al. An institution's initial experience with Port-Access minimally invasive cardiac surgery. *J Cardiothorac Vasc Anesth* 1998;12:617.
41. Boonstra PW, Grandjean JG, Mariani MA. Improved method for direct coronary grafting without CPB via anterolateral small thoracotomy. *Ann Thorac Surg* 1997;63:567.
42. Stanridge RL, Hadjinikolaou LK, Cohen AS, et al. Minimally invasive coronary revascularization through parasternal incisions without cardiopulmonary bypass. *Ann Thorac Surg* 1997;63: S53.
43. Allen KB, Shaar CJ. Endoscopic saphenous vein harvesting. *Ann Thorac Surg* 1997;64:265.
44. Fanning WJ, Kakos GS, Williams TE Jr. Reoperative coronary artery bypass grafting without cardiopulmonary bypass. *Ann Thorac Surg* 1993;55:486.
45. Benetti JF, Mariani MA, Ballester C. Direct coronary surgery without cardiopulmonary bypass in acute myocardial infarction. *J Cardiovasc Surg* 1996;37:391.
46. Moshkovitz Y, Sternik L, Paz Y, et al. Primary coronary artery bypass grafting without cardiopulmonary bypass in impaired left ventricular function. *Ann Thorac Surg* 1997;63:S44.
47. Akins CW, Boucher CA, Pohost GM. Preservation of interventricular septal function in patients having coronary artery bypass grafts without cardiopulmonary bypass. *Am Heart J* 1984;107: 304.
48. Westaby S. Coronary surgery without cardiopulmonary bypass. *Br Heart J* 1995;73:203.
49. Borst C, Jansen EWL, Grundeman PF. Less invasive coronary artery bypass grafting: without cardiopulmonary bypass and via reduced surgical access. *Heart* 1997;77:302.
50. Westaby S, Benetti FJ. Less invasive coronary surgery: consensus from the Oxford meeting. *Ann Thorac Surg* 1996;62:924.
51. Airaksinen KEJ, Ikaheimo MJ, Huikuri HV. Stenosis severity and the occurrence of ventricular ectopic activity during acute coronary occlusion during balloon angioplasty. *Am J Cardiol* 1995;76:346.
52. Subramanian VA. MIDCAB Approach for single vessel coronary artery bypass graft. In: Cox JL, Sundt TM III, eds. Operative techniques in cardiac and thoracic surgery. A comparative atlas. Vol 3, Number 1 February 1998. Philadelphia: WB Saunders, 1998; Vol. 3.
53. Pawlowski J, Haering JM, Communale ME, et al. Minimally invasive anesthesia should accompany minimally invasive surgery. *J Cardiothorac Vasc Anesth* 1997;11:536.
54. Buhre W, Weyland A, Kazmaier S, et al. Comparison of cardiac output assessed by pulse-contour analysis and thermodilution in patients undergoing minimally invasive direct coronary artery bypass grafting. *J Cardiothorac Vasc Anesth* 1999;13:437.
55. Godie O, Thiel C, Reichenspurner P, et al. Less invasive continuous beat-to-beat hemodynamic monitoring during minimally invasive coronary surgery. *Heart Surgery Forum* 1999. Available at: http://www.hsforum.com/abstracts/O20.asp.
56. Zollner C, Polasek J, Kilger E, et al. Evaluation of a new continuous thermodilution cardiac output monitor in cardiac surgical patients: a prospective criterion standard study. *Crit Care Med* 1999;27:293.
57. Mulligan KR, Coppel DG, Johnston JR, et al. Propofol anesthesia for major thoracic surgery. *J Cardiothorac Vasc Anesth* 1990; 4:323.
58. Myles PS, Buckland MR, Weeks AM, et al. Hemodynamic effects, myocardial ischemia, and timing of tracheal extubation with propofol-based anesthesia for cardiac surgery. *Anesth Analg* 1997;84:12.
59. Sherry KM, Sartain J, Bell JH, et al. Comparison of the use of a propofol infusion in cardiac surgical patients with normal and low cardiac output states. *J Cardiothorac Vasc Anesth* 1995;9: 368.
60. Mollhoff T, Herregods L, Blake D, et al. Remifentanil versus fentanyl in patients undergoing CABG surgery. *Anesthesiology* 1999;91:A144.
61. Sprung J, Ogletree-Hughes M, Moravec C. Effects of remifentanil on contractility of failing human ventricular muscle. *Anesthesiology* 1999;91:A416.
62. Larbuisson R, Van Dyck M, Herregods L, et al. Remifentanil is as well tolerated as fentanyl in patients with poor LV function during CABG surgery. *Anesthesiology* 1999;91:A417.
63. Cheng DC, Newman MF, Duke P, et al. A prospective randomized, double-blind controlled trial of remifentanil and fentanyl in fast tract CABG surgery: efficacy and resource utilization. *Anesthesiology* 1999;91:A142.
64. Grandjean JG, Mariani MA, Ebels T. Coronary reoperation via small laparotomy using right gastroepiploic artery without CPB. *Ann Thorac Surg* 1996;61:1853.
65. Labovitz AJ, Barth C, Castello R, et al. Attenuation of myocardial ischemia during coronary occlusion by ultrashort-acting beta adrenergic blockade. *Am Heart J* 1991;121:1347.
66. Wasnick JD, Acuff T. Anesthesia and minimally invasive thoracoscopically assisted coronary artery bypass: a brief clinical report. *J Cardiothorac Vasc Anesth* 1997;11:552.
67. Greenspun HG, Adourian UA, Fonger JD, et al. Minimally invasive direct coronary artery bypass (MIDCAB): surgical techniques and anesthetic considerations. *J Cardiothorac Vasc Anesth* 1996;10:507.
68. Abramson DC, Pivalizza EG, Gottschalk LI. Drug management for coronary revascularization without cardiac standstill: the use of high-dose esmolol. *J Cardiothorac Vasc Anesth* 1995;9:184.
69. Jacobsohn E, Ferdinand F, Albertucci M, et al. Minimally invasive CABG: anesthetic technique and outcome. *Anesth Analg* 1997;84:S91.
70. Robinson MC. Identification and management of coronary arteries: immobilization and control. In: Emery RW, Arom KV, Fonger JD, et al., eds. *Techniques for minimally invasive direct coronary artery bypass (MIDCAB) surgery.* Philadelphia: Hanley & Belfus, 1997:79.
71. Hesselvik JF, Ortega RA, Shemin RJ. The use of neostigmine to decrease the heart rate in a patient undergoing minimally invasive coronary artery bypass surgery. *J Cardiothorac Vasc Anesth* 1997;11:883.
72. Robinson MC, Thielmeier KA, Hill BB. Transient ventricular asystole using adenosine during minimally invasive and open sternotomy coronary artery bypass grafting. *Ann Thorac Surg* 1997;63:S30.

73. Rajeck A, Podesser A, Kupilik N, et al. Effect of β-blockers versus calcium channel blockers in myocardial revascularization without cardiopulmonary bypass in pigs. *Br J Anaesth* 1996;76: A39.
74. Ronson RS, Puskas JD, Velez DA, et al. Controlled intermittent asystole for off-pump coronary surgery does not cause myocardial or neural injury. *Heart Surgery Forum* 1999. Available at http://www.hsforum.com/abstracts/C37.asp.
75. Perrault LP, Menasche P, Bidouard J-P, et al. Snaring of the target vessel in less invasive operations does not cause endothelial dysfunction. *Ann Thorac Surg* 1997;63:751.
76. Borst C, Jansen EWL, Tulleken CAF, et al. Coronary artery bypass grafting without cardiopulmonary bypass and without interruption of native coronary flow using a novel anastomosis site restraining device ("Octopus"). *J Am Coll Cardiol* 1996; 27:1356.
77. Spooner TH, Dyrud PE, Monson BK, et al. Coronary artery bypass on the beating heart with the Octopus: a North American experience. *Ann Thorac Surg* 1998;66:1032.
78. Jurmann MJ, Menon AK, Haeberle L, et al. Left ventricular geometry and cardiac function during minimally invasive coronary artery bypass grafting. *Ann Thorac Surg* 1998;66:1082.
79. Jurmann MJ, Menon A, Guggenberger H, et al. Pharmacologic versus mechanical stabilization of the heart during minimally invasive coronary artery bypass: effects on left ventricular geometry and hemodynamics. *Circulation* 1997;96:I680.
80. Diegeler A. Coronary bypass surgery without cardiopulmonary bypass using the Medtronic Octopus II Device. *Heart Surgery Forum* 1999. Available at: http://www.hsforum.com/abstracts/C101.asp.
81. Calafiore AM, Vitolla G, Mazzei V, et al. The LAST operation: techniques and results before and after the stabilization era. *Ann Thorac Surg* 1998;66:998.
82. Carrier M, Poirier NC, Lesperance J, et al. Quantitative angiographic assessment of coronary anastomoses performed without cardiopulmonary bypass. *Heart Surgery Forum* 1999. Available at: http://www.hsforum.com/abstracts/C89.asp.
83. Boonstra PW, Grandjean JG, Mariani MA. Local immobilization of the left anterior descending coronary artery for minimally invasive coronary bypass grafting. *Ann Thorac Surg* 1997;63: 576.
84. Pagni S, Paquish NK, Senior DG, et al. Anastomotic complications in minimally invasive coronary bypass surgery. *Ann Thorac Surg* 1997;63:564.
85. Alhes JM, Menon AK, Ziemer G. Myocardial function during MIDCAB revascularization: early clinical experience with temporary intraluminal shunts. *Heart Surgery Forum* 1999. Available at: http://www.hsforum.com/abstracts/C151.asp.
86. Spiliopoulos S, Mehlhorn U, Raji R, et al. Epicardial coronary flow measurements during intraluminal shunting in a simulated porcine MIDCAB model. *Heart Surgery Forum* 1999. Available at: http://www.hsforum.com/abstracts/C83.asp.
87. Coulson A, Bakhsahp S, Quarnstrom J, et al. Temporary coronary artery perfusion catheter during minimally invasive coronary surgery. *Chest* 1998;113:514.
88. Autschbach R, Sharonil R, Krakor R, et al. Right ventricular support during beating heart surgery. *Heart Surgery Forum* 1999. Available at: http://www.hsforum.com/abstracts/C109.asp.
89. Edgerton JR, Mathison M, Akin JJ, et al. Hemodynamic changes in the displaced human heart during beating heart surgery. *Heart Surgery Forum* 1999. Available at: http://www.hsforum.com/abstracts/C118.asp.
90. Mack M, Akin J, Mullangi C, et al. Effect of mini-pump flow rate during right heart support for off-pump bypass. *Heart Surgery Forum* 1999. Available at: http://www.hsforum.com/abstracts/C93.asp.
91. Dekker AL, Geskes GG, Cramers AA, et al. The Enabler right heart support system for posterior and inferior wall access during beating heart surgery in sheep. *Heart Surgery Forum* 1999. Available at: http://www.hsforum.com/abstracts/O26.asp.
92. Grundeman PF, Borst C, van Herwaarden JA, et al. Vertical displacement of the beating heart by the octopus tissue stabilizer: influence on coronary flow. *Ann Thorac Surg* 1998;65:1348.
93. Soltoski P, D'Ancona G, Salerno TA, et al. Improving the exposure of the posterior coronary arteries during off-pump coronary artery bypass. *Heart Surgery Forum* 1999. Available at: http://www.hsforum.com/abstracts/C22.asp.
94. Rivetti LA, Gandria SMA. Initial experience using an intraluminal shunt during revascularization of the beating heart. *Ann Thorac Surg* 1997;63:1742.
95. Matin M. Do intraoperative ECG abnormalities correlate with perioperative infarction in MIDCAB surgery? *Heart Surgery Forum* 1999. Available at: http://www.hsforum.com/abstracts/C110.asp.
96. Jacobsohn E, Young CJ, Aronson S, et al. The role of ischemic preconditioning during minimally invasive coronary artery bypass surgery. *J Cardiothorac Vasc Anesth* 1997;11:787.
97. Lawson CS, Downey JM. Preconditioning: state of the art myocardial protection. *Cardiovasc Res* 1993;27:542.
98. Hawaleshka A, Jacobsohn E. Ischaemic preconditioning: mechanisms and potential clinical applications. *Can J Anaesth* 1998; 45:670.
99. Zarro DL, Palanzo DA, Sadr FS. Myocardial preconditioning using adenosine: review and clinical experience. *Perfusion* 1998; 13:145.
100. Niroomand F, Kubler W. Hibernating, stunning, and ischemic preconditioning of the myocardium: therapeutic implications. *Clin Invest* 1994;72:731.
101. Cope DK, Impastat WK, Cohen MV, et al. Volatile anesthetic protection of the ischemic rabbit myocardium from infarction. *Anesthesiology* 1997;86:699.
102. Tasdemir O, Vural KM, Karagoz H, et al. Coronary artery bypass grafting on the beating heart without the use of extracorporeal circulation: review of 2052 cases. *J Thorac Cardiovasc Surg* 1998;116:68.
103. Borges MF, Spohn PK, Coulson AS. Arrhythmia/ischemia management during minimally invasive cardiac operation. *Ann Thorac Surg* 1997;64:843.
104. Lima LE, Nataf P, Gandjbakhch I, et al. Thoracoscopic IMA dissection and direct suture (La Pitie technique). In: Emery RW, Arom KV, Fonger JD, et al., eds. *Techniques for minimally invasive direct coronary artery bypass (MIDCAB) surgery.* Philadelphia: Hanley & Belfus, 1997:55.
105. Perrault LP, Carrier M, Cartier R, et al. Endovascular versus extravascular devices for control of the target vessel in beating heart CABG: what's best for the endothelium? *Heart Surgery Forum* 1999. Available at: http://www.hsforum.com/abstracts/C88.asp.
106. Peterzen B, Lonn U, Babi'c A, et al. Anesthetic management of patients undergoing coronary artery bypass grafting with the use of an axial flow pump and a short-acting β-blocker. *J Cardiothorac Vasc Anesth* 1999;13:431.
107. Waldenberger FR, Haisjackl M, Holinski S, et al. Centrifugal pumps as left ventricular assist for coronary revascularization on a beating heart. *Artif Organs* 1998;22:698.
108. Jaber SF, Koenig SC, BhaskerRao B, et al. Role of graft flow measurement technique in anastomotic quality assessment in minimally invasive CABG. *Ann Thorac Surg* 1998;66:1087.
109. Walpoth BH, Bosshard A, Genyk I, et al. Transit-time flow

measurement for detection of early graft failure during myocardial revascularization. *Ann Thorac Surg* 1998;66:1097.

110. Jacobsohn E, Aronson S, Young CJ, et al. On-line contrast echocardiographic assessment of myocardial perfusion: its role in minimally invasive coronary artery bypass procedures. *J Cardiothorac Vasc Anesth* 1997;11:517.
111. Emery RW, Emery AM, Flavin TF, et al. Revascularization using angioplasty and minimally invasive techniques documented by thermal imaging. *Ann Thorac Surg* 1996;62:591.
112. Lazzara RR, McLellan BA, Kidwell FE, et al. Intraoperative angiography during minimally invasive direct coronary artery bypass operations. *Ann Thorac Surg* 1997;64:1725.
113. Cheney MA. Intrathecal and epidural anesthesia and analgesia for cardiac surgery. *Anesth Analg* 1997;84:1211.
114. Swanton BJ, Moriarty DC. Anticoagulation and intrathecal opioids in cardiac surgery: a large case series without resultant neurological complication. *Anesth Analg* 1997;84:SCA44.
115. Kirno K, Friberg P, Grzegorczyk A, et al. Thoracic epidural anesthesia during coronary artery bypass surgery: effects on cardiac sympathetic activity, myocardial blood flow and metabolism, and central hemodynamics. *Anesth Analg* 1994;79:1075.
116. Sanchez R, Nygard E. Epidural anesthesia in cardiac surgery: is there an increased risk? *J Cardiothorac Vasc Anesth* 1998;12:170.
117. Vandermeulen EP, Van Aken H, Vermylen J. Anticoagulants and spinal-epidural anesthesia. *Anesth Analg* 1994;79:1165.
118. Calafiore AM, Angellini GD, Bergsland J, et al. Minimally invasive coronary artery bypass grafting. *Ann Thorac Surg* 1996;62:1545.
119. Hensley FA. Minimally invasive revascularization surgery: here to stay? *J Cardiothorac Vasc Anesth* 1996;10:445.
120. Acuff TE, Landreneau RJ, Griffith BP, et al. Minimally invasive coronary artery bypass grafting. *Ann Thorac Surg* 1996;61:135.
121. Benetti FJ, Ballester CB. Use of thoracoscopy and a minimal thoracotomy, in mammary–coronary artery bypass to left anterior descending artery, without extracorporeal circulation. *J Cardiovasc Surg* 1995;36:159.
122. Cohn WE, Suen HC, Weintraub RM, et al. The "H" graft: an alternative approach for performing minimally invasive direct coronary artery bypass. *J Thorac Cardiovasc Surg* 1998;115:148.
123. Angellini GD, Wilde P, Salerno TA, et al. Integrated left small thoracotomy and angioplasty for multivessel coronary artery revascularization. *Lancet* 1996;347:757.
124. Saatvedt K, Dragsund M, Nordstrand K. Transmyocardial laser revascularization and coronary artery bypass grafting without cardiopulmonary bypass. *Ann Thorac Surg* 1996;62:323.
125. Jones RH, Kesler K, Phillips HR III, et al. Long-term survival benefits of coronary artery bypass grafting and percutaneous transluminal angioplasty in patients with coronary artery disease. *J Thorac Cardiovasc Surg* 1996;111:1013.
126. Hartz RS. Minimally invasive heart surgery. *Circulation* 1996;94:2669.
127. Wasnick JD, Hoffman WJ, Acuff T, et al. Anesthetic management of coronary bypass via minithoracotomy with video assistance. *J Cardiothorac Vasc Anesth* 1995;9:731.
128. Landreneau RJ, Mack MJ, Acuff TA, et al. "Keyhole" coronary artery bypass surgery. *Ann Surg* 1996;224:459.
129. Gayes JM. Pro: one-lung ventilation is best accomplished with the Univent endobronchial blocker. *J Cardiothorac Vasc Anesth* 1993;7:103.
130. Duncan S, Fonger JD. Operative MIDCAB nursing. In: Emery RW, Arom KV, Fonger JD, et al., eds. *Techniques for minimally invasive direct coronary artery bypass (MIDCAB) surgery.* Philadelphia: Hanley & Belfus, 1997:119.
131. Loop FD. Internal thoracic artery grafts-biologically better coronary arteries. *N Engl J Med* 1996;334:263.
132. Elbeery JR, Brown PM, Chitwood WR Jr. Intraoperative MIDCABG arteriography via the left radial artery: a comparison with Doppler ultrasound for assessment of graft patency. *Ann Thorac Surg* 1998;66:51.
133. Wittmer T, Cremer I, Boonstar P, et al. Myocardial hybrid revascularization with minimally invasive direct coronary artery bypass grafting and staged coronary angioplasty. *Heart Surgery Forum* 1999. Available at: http://www.hsforum.com/abstracts/C9.asp.
134. Izzat MB, Yim AP, Mehta D, et al. Staged minimally invasive direct coronary artery bypass and percutaneous angioplasty for multivessel coronary artery disease. *Int J Cardiol* 1997;62[Suppl 1]:S105.
135. Walther T, Falk V, Metz S, et al. Pain and quality of life after minimally invasive versus conventional cardiac surgery. *Ann Thorac Surg* 1999;67:1643.
136. Mehta Y, Swaminathan M, Mishra Y, et al. A comparative evaluation of intrapleural and thoracic epidural analgesia for postoperative pain relief after minimally invasive direct coronary artery bypass surgery. *J Cardiothorac Vasc Anesth* 1998;12:162.
137. Ganapathy S, Dobkowski WB, Murkin JM, et al. Thoracic epidural analgesia (TEA) increases graft flow and reduces cortisol release in minimally invasive coronary bypass surgery (MIDCABG). *Anesthesiology* 1999;91:A130.
138. Westaby S. Coronary surgery without cardiopulmonary bypass: rationale and evolution of technique. In: Emery RW, Arom KV, Fonger JD, et al., eds. *Techniques for minimally invasive direct coronary artery bypass (MIDCAB) surgery.* Philadelphia: Hanley & Belfus, 1997:3.
139. Ganapathy S, Boyd WD, Dobkowski W, et al. Thoracic epidural analgesia improves post-anastomotic graft flow in MIDCAB. *Heart Surgery Forum* 1999. Available at: http://www.hsforum.com/abstracts/C123.asp.
140. Ganapathy S, Boyd WD, Morgan J, et al. Thoracic epidural analgesia offers improved postoperative analgesia following MIDCAB. *Heart Surgery Forum* 1999. Available at: http://www.hsforum.com/abstracts/C124.asp.
141. Moshkovitz Y, Lusky A, Mohr R. Coronary artery bypass without cardiopulmonary bypass: analysis of short-term and mid-term outcome in 220 patients. *J Thorac Cardiovasc Surg* 1995;110:979.
142. Pfister AJ, Zaki MS, Garcia JM, et al. Coronary artery bypass without cardiopulmonary bypass. *Ann Thorac Surg* 1992;54:1085.
143. Gundry SR, Romano MA, Shattuck OH, et al. Seven-year follow-up of coronary artery bypasses performed with and without cardiopulmonary bypass. *J Thorac Cardiovasc Surg* 1998;115:1273.
144. Mack MJ, Osborne JA, Shennib H. Arterial graft patency in coronary artery bypass grafting: what do we really know? *Ann Thorac Surg* 1998;66:1055.
145. Roach GW, Kanchuger M, Mora Mangano C, et al. Adverse cerebral outcomes after coronary bypass surgery. *N Engl J Med* 1996;335:1857.
146. Schell RM, Kern F, Greeley W, et al. Cerebral blood flow and metabolism during cardiopulmonary bypass. *Anesth Analg* 1993;76:849.
147. Bhasker-Rao B, VanHimbergen D, Edmonds HL Jr, et al. Evidence for improved cerebral function after minimally invasive bypass surgery. *J Card Surg* 1998;13:27.
148. Schneider F, Falk V, Diegeler A, et al. Significant reduction of cerebral microembolism during off-pump CABG operations. *Heart Surgery Forum* 1999. Available at: http://www.hsforum.com/abstracts/C102.asp.
149. Anderson RE, Hiansson L-O, Vaage J, et al. Release of S100 during coronary bypass grafting is reduced by off-pump surgery.

Heart Surgery Forum 1999. Available at: http://www.hsforum.-com/abstracts/C143.asp.

150. Leger Ph, Dequen L, Fellahi JL, et al. Release of S100 protein after coronary artery bypass grafting with and without cardiopulmonary bypass. *Heart Surgery Forum* 1999. Available at: http://www.hsforum.com/abstracts/C41.asp.
151. Murkin JM, Boyd WD, Ganapathy S, et al. Postoperative cognitive dysfunction is significantly less after coronary artery revascularization without cardiopulmonary bypass. *Heart Surgery Forum* 1999. Available at: http://www.hsforum.com/abstracts/C77.asp.
152. Grimm M, Czerny M, Wolner E. Coronary artery bypass grafting without cardiopulmonary bypass is beneficial for cognitive brain function: a prospective randomized study. *Heart Surgery Forum* 1999. Available at: http://www.hsforum/abstracts/C74.asp.
153. Malheiros SMF, Brucki SMD, Babbai AA, et al. Neurological outcome in coronary artery surgery with and without cardiopulmonary bypass. *Acta Neurol Scand* 1995;92:256.
154. Gu YJ, Mariani MA, van Oeveren W, et al. Reduction of the inflammatory response in patients undergoing minimally invasive coronary artery bypass grafting. *Ann Thorac Surg* 1998;65:420.
155. Fransen E, Maessen J, Dentener M, et al. Systemic inflammation present in patients undergoing CABG without extracorporeal circulation. *Chest* 1998;113:1290.
156. Kilger E, Pichler B, Goetz AE, et al. Procalcitonin as a marker of systemic inflammation after conventional or minimally invasive coronary artery bypass grafting. *Thorac Cardiovasc Surg* 1998;46:130.
157. Ganapathy S, Murkin JM, Boyd W, et al. MIDCAB reduces release of proinflammatory cytokines compared to conventional bypass surgery. *Heart Surgery Forum* 1999. Available at: http://www.hsforum.com/abstracts/C126.asp.
158. Diegeler A. The humoral immune response in coronary artery bypass grafting: conventional versus "off-pump" surgery. *Heart Surgery Forum* 1999. Available at: http://www.hsforum.com/abstracts/C100.asp.
159. Wildhirt SM, Schulze C, Conrad N, et al. Reduction of cytokine induced expression of cell adhesion molecules after off-pump coronary artery bypass grafting. *Heart Surgery Forum* 1999. Available at: http://www.hsforum.com/abstracts/C113.asp.
160. Gulielmos V, Dill HM, Eller M, et al. A prospective randomized clinical trial comparing inflammatory response parameters in patients undergoing minimally invasive and conventional coronary artery bypass surgery. *Heart Surgery Forum* 1999. Available at: http://www.hsforum.com/abstracts/C52.asp.
161. Puskas JD, Wright CE, Ronson RS, et al. Clinical outcomes and angiographic patency in 100 consecutive off-pump coronary bypass patients. *Heart Surgery Forum* 1999. Available at: http://www.hsforum.com/abstracts/C36.asp.
162. Loef BG, Henning RH, Navis G, et al. Beating heart coronary artery surgery avoids renal damage as compared to surgery with cardiopulmonary bypass. *Anesthesiology* 1998;89:A297.
163. Cheng DCH. Fast-track cardiac surgery: economic implications in postoperative care. *J Cardiothorac Vasc Anesth* 1998;12:72.
164. Doty JR, Fonger JD, Nicholson CF, et al. Cost analysis of current therapies for limited coronary artery revascularization. *Circulation* 1997;96[Suppl II]:II-16.
165. Zenati M, Domit TM, Saul M, et al. Resource utilization for minimally invasive direct and standard coronary artery bypass grafting. *Ann Thorac Surg* 1997;63:S84.
166. King RC, Reece TB, Hurst JL, et al. Minimally invasive coronary artery bypass grafting decreases hospital stay and cost. *Ann Surg* 1997;225:805.
167. Del Rizzo DF, Boyd WD, Novick RJ, et al. Safety and cost-effectiveness of MIDCABG in high-risk CABG patients. *Ann Thorac Surg* 1998;66:1002.
168. Novitzky D. The cost benefit of myocardial revascularization without cardiopulmonary bypass. *Heart Surgery Forum* 1999. Available at: http://hsforum.com/abstracts/C127.asp.
169. Ribakove GH, Miller JS, Anderson RV, et al. Minimally invasive port-access coronary artery bypass grafting with early angiographic follow-up: initial experience. *J Thorac Cardiovasc Surg* 1998;115:1101.
170. Fann JI, Pompili MF, Stevens JH, et al. Port-Access cardiac operations with cardioplegic arrest. *Ann Thorac Surg* 1997;63:S35.
171. Gulielmos V, Wagner FM, Waetzig B, et al. Clinical experience with minimally invasive coronary artery and mitral valve surgery with the advantage of cardiopulmonary bypass and cardioplegic arrest using the port access techniquc. *World J Surg* 1999;23:480.
172. Reichenspurner H, Gulielmos V, Wunderlich J, et al. Port-access coronary artery bypass grafting with the use of cardiopulmonary bypass and cardioplegia arrest. *Ann Thorac Surg* 1998;65:413.
173. Mohr FW, Falk V, Diegeler A, et al. Minimally invasive Port-Access mitral surgery. *J Thorac Cardiovasc Surg* 1998;115:567.
174. Applebaum RM, Cutler WM, Bhardwaj N, et al. Utility of transesophageal echocardiography during port-access minimally invasive cardiac surgery. *Am J Cardiol* 1998;82:183.
175. Siegel LC, St. Goar FG, Stevens JH, et al. Monitoring considerations for port-access cardiac surgery. *Circulation* 1997;96:562.
176. Ortega RA, Hesselvik JF. Reducing the risk of perforation of the right ventricle during port-access minimally invasive cardiac procedures. *Anesthesiology* 1999;90:1233.
177. Clements F, Wright SJ, deBruijn N. Coronary sinus catheterization made easy for Port-Access minimally invasive cardiac surgery. *J Cardiothorac Vasc Anesth* 1998;12:96.
178. Clements F, deBruijn NP. Coronary sinus catheterization for port-access minimally invasive cardiac surgery. *J Thorac Cardiovasc Anesth* 1999;13:377.
179. Siegel LC. Coronary sinus catheterization for minimally invasive cardiac surgery. *Anesthesiology* 1999;90:1232.
180. Toomasian JM, Peters WS, Siegel LC. Extracorporeal circulation for port-access cardiac surgery. *Perfusion* 1997;12:83.
181. Groh MA, Fallen DM. Alteration of the traditional extracorporeal bypass circuit to accommodate Port-Access minimally invasive cardiac procedures using endovascular based cardiopulmonary bypass. *Artif Organs* 1998;22:775.
182. Port-Access International Registry. Available at: http://www.heartport.com or http://www.ctsnet.org/journal/ats/67/51/.
183. Galloway A, Shemin R, Glower D, et al. First report of the port access international registry. *Ann Thorac Surg* 1999;67:51.
184. Siegel LC, Glower DD, Galloway AC, et al. Multi-variable modeling of duration of ICU stay in port-access minimally invasive cardiac surgery. *Anesthesiology* 1999;91:A129.
185. Stafford Smith M, Gerstle LJ, Funk BL, et al. Heart-Port versus median sternotomy: postoperative visual analogue pain scores. *Heart Surgery Forum* 1999. Available at: http://www.hsforum.-com/abstracts/V6.asp.
186. Watson DR. The clinical and financial impact of port-access mitral valve surgery. *Heart Surgery Forum* 1999. Available at: http://www.hsforum.com/abstracts/V13.asp.
187. Chaney MA, Fluder EM, Tuchek JM, et al. Port-access coronary artery bypass grafting facilitates early postoperative hospital discharge yet increases cost. *Heart Surgery Forum* 1999. Available at: http://www.hsforum.com/abstracts/C64.asp.
188. Glower DD, Davis RD, Landolfo KP, et al. Comparison of

minimally invasive port-access to sternotomy or thoracotomy for redo-mitral operation. *Heart Surgery Forum* 1999. Available at: http://www.hsforum.com/abstracts/V5.asp.

189. Doty DB, DiRusso GB, Doty JR. Full-spectrum cardiac surgery through a minimal incision: mini-sternotomy (lower half) technique. *Ann Thorac Surg* 1998;65:573.
190. Letsou GV, Reardon MJ. Minimally invasive valve surgery. *Curr Opin Cardiol* 1998;13:105.
191. Hearn CJ, Kraenzler EJ, Wallace LK, et al. Minimally invasive aortic valve surgery: anesthetic considerations. *Anesth Analg* 1996;83:1342.
192. Cooley DA. Minimally invasive valve surgery versus the conventional approach. *Ann Thorac Surg* 1998;66:1101.
193. Burke RP. Minimally invasive pediatric cardiac surgery. *Curr Opin Cardiol* 1999;14:67.
194. Bauer M, Redcepagic S, Alexi-Meskishvilli V, et al. Minimally invasive approaches for correction of congenital heart defects. *Heart Surgery Forum* 1999. Available at: http://www.hsforum.-com/abstracts/P4.asp.
195. del Nido PJ, Nicholson I. Minimal sternotomy for complex congenital heart surgery. *Heart Surgery Forum* 1999. Available at: http://hsforum.com/abstracts/P2.asp.
196. Morris RJ, Butler MT, Samuels LE. Minimally invasive saphenous vein harvesting. *Ann Thorac Surg* 1998;66:1026.
197. Nahata SK, Genovesi MH, Torrillo L, et al. Endoscopic saphenous vein harvesting decreases leg wound infections in CABG patients. *Heart Surgery Forum* 1999. Available at: http://www.hsforum.com/abstracts/C2.asp.
198. Copoolse R, Rees W, Warni KH. Minimally invasive vein harvesting (MIVH) in a series of 1400 cardiac bypass patients. *Heart Surgery Forum* 1999. Available at: http://www.hsforum.-com/abstracts/C98.asp.
199. Klaidman S. Should smart operators mix business and surgery. *Ann Thorac Surg* 1998;66:1119.
200. Hornberger J, Bloch DA, Hlatky MA, et al. Patient preferences in coronary revascularization. *Am Heart J* 1999;137:1153.
201. Shennib H, Bastawisy A, Mack MJ, et al. Computer-assisted telemanipulation: an enabling technology for endoscopic coronary artery bypass. *Ann Thorac Surg* 1998;66:1060.
202. Hamawy AH, Phillips AB, Lauto A, et al. Laser welding with albumin solder for vascular anastomosis: ideal conditions for minimally invasive coronary bypass. *Heart Surgery Forum* 1999. Available at: http://www.hsforum.com/abstracts/I7.asp.
203. Nataf P, Hinchliffe P, Manzo S, et al. Facilitated vascular anastomoses: the one-shot device. *Ann Thorac Surg* 1998;66: 1041.
204. Morota T, Burfeind WR, Huang CT. The proximal one-shot anastomotic device: short term results. *Heart Surgery Forum* 1999. Available at: http://www.hsforum.com/abstracts/O14.asp.

Cardiac Anesthesia: Principles and Clinical Practice, Second Edition, edited by Fawzy G. Estafanous, Paul G. Barash, and J.G. Reves. Lippincott Williams & Wilkins, Philadelphia © 2001.

26

ANESTHESIA FOR PULMONARY AND MEDIASTINAL SURGERY

MARK BANOUB
ERIK J. KRAENZLER

DIAGNOSIS AND STAGING OF LUNG CANCER

Clinical Manifestations

Most patients who develop lung cancer have a previous history of smoking and therefore often have chronic bronchitis and cough. Retention of secretions distal to a tumor predisposes the patient to infection. In patients with chronic obstructive pulmonary disease (COPD), an acute exacerbation of chronic bronchitis can cause a change in the quality and quantity of sputum. Failure to clear the sputum within 2 weeks of antibiotic therapy should lead one to suspect a neoplasm. Hemoptysis may affect up to 50% of patients. Dyspnea develops early in up to 60% of patients and is usually associated with increased cough, sputum, atelectasis, and pneumonia distal to the tumor. Chest pain, if present, is usually mild, nonspecific, dull, and intermittent, occurring on the side of the tumor. Shoulder pain may result from a tumor at the apex of the lung invading the brachial plexus such as Pancoast tumor. This pain is frequently mistaken for osteoarthritis or cervical spondylitis. A unilateral localized wheeze that does not clear with bronchodilation and coughing is highly suggestive of a tumor. If a large tumor is occluding the carina or the trachea, severe dyspnea and stridor may also develop.

Pleural effusion may result from lymphatic obstruction by neoplasm or from malignant extension of the tumor to the surface of the lung. Previous pleuritic chest pain may disappear with the accumulation of pleural effusion. Hoarseness of voice may occur secondary to recurrent laryngeal nerve paralysis. Phrenic nerve involvement by the tumor leads to paralysis of the corresponding hemidiaphragm, which can be seen as an elevated diaphragm on radiographs or fluoroscopy. Obstruction of the superior vena cava by a tumor or lymph nodes results in dyspnea, dysphagia, stridor, redness and edema of the face, dilated veins across the upper chest and neck, and periorbital edema. The occurrence of superior vena cava obstruction is a serious complication and can be life-threatening due to the potential for airway obstruction.

Chest wall metastasis to the ribs and vertebrae can result in local tenderness and pleuritic chest pain. Horner syndrome may occur from involvement of the cervical sympathetic and first thoracic sympathetic ganglia. Pericarditis, pericardial effusion, cardiac dysrhythmias, and even tamponade may occur as a result of tumor extension to the pericardium.

Common extrathoracic sites of metastases are lymph nodes, brain, bone, liver skin, and suprarenal glands. Bone metastases are usually osteolytic and occur primarily in the ribs, vertebrae, humerus, and femur. Hepatic metastases presenting as asymptomatic enlargement of the liver are usually a late sign. Jaundice occurs infrequently and is also a late feature. The kidneys and renal system can be involved with bronchogenic carcinoma, particularly that of the small cell type.

Approximately 2% of patients with bronchial carcinoma seek medical advice because of paraneoplastic syndromes not caused by tumor spread. Metabolic manifestations usually result from the secretions of endocrine-like substances by the tumor. Cushing syndrome occurs most often in patients with small cell carcinoma of the lungs. Significant amounts of adrenocorticotropic hormone have been found in tumor tissue and in these patients' blood. Excessive antidiuretic hormone production is most often seen in patients with small cell carcinoma of the lung. The patient may have anorexia, nausea, vomiting, hyponatremia, neurologic disturbances, seizures, and relative hypertonicity of the urine. Carcinoid syndrome may result from production of serotonin by the tumor. Patients have elevated urinary levels of 5-hydroxyindoleacetic acid. Hypercalcemia, not associated with bone metastasis, may occur from secretion of a

M. Banoub: Division of Anesthesia and Critical Care Medicine, The Cleveland Clinic Foundation, Cleveland, Ohio 44195; and Department of Anesthesia, St. Vincent Mercy Medical Center, Toledo, Ohio 43608

E. J. Kraenzler: Department of Cardiothoracic Anesthesiology, Ohio State University; and Department of Cardiothoracic Anesthesiology, The Cleveland Clinic Foundation, Cleveland, Ohio 44195

parathyroid hormone–like polypeptide by the tumor. Hypercalcemia is usually accompanied by hypophosphatemia and most often occurs with squamous cell carcinoma of the bronchus. Calcium levels return to the normal range after successful tumor resection. Paraneoplastic myopathy may appear as a myasthenia-like syndrome. Polymyositis is another manifestation and results from primary degeneration of the muscle fibers and more prominent muscle wasting. Paraneoplastic neuropathy may be sensory, motor, or a combination of both. Patients may have pain and paresthesias, then complete sensory loss of extremities, weakness, and muscle wasting. Histologically, loss of neurons occurs in the dorsal root ganglia, along with selective degeneration of nerve roots and spinal cord. Subacute cerebellar degeneration results in a rapidly progressing degeneration of cerebellar function, ataxia, and lack of coordination, as well as vertigo, nystagmus, or dysarthria. The cause and pathogenesis of these neuropathies are unclear. However, the current hypothesis is that they are caused by immune responses to substances produced by the tumor cells. Patients with paraneoplastic neurologic syndromes have circulating antineuronal antibodies in their blood and cerebrospinal fluid. Symptoms may improve with tumor resection, chemotherapy, radiotherapy, and plasma exchange (1).

The most frequent skeletal manifestation is clubbing of the fingers. This is sometimes associated with generalized hypertrophic pulmonary osteoarthropathy, characterized by periosteal proliferation and new bone formation at the ends of long bones. Dermatologic manifestations include acanthosis nigricans, scleroderma, and other dermatoses. Vascular manifestations such as thrombophlebitis may be the first indication of a bronchial tumor. Normocytic and normochromic anemia, porphyria, erythrocytosis, and leukocytosis have been reported. Other nonspecific symptoms, such as weight loss, weakness, anorexia, lethargy, malaise, and fever, may also occur.

Physical Examination

The examiner should focus on the chest, looking for signs of congestion, atelectasis, pleural effusion, and cervical lymphadenopathy. Patients who cannot tolerate lying supine because of a choking sensation may have significant airway obstruction from a mediastinal mass. One should look for clinical signs of brain metastasis, Horner syndrome, evidence of vocal cord paralysis, clubbing of the fingers, cyanosis, and pulmonary osteoarthropathy. The patient's respiratory patterns and respiratory rate should be observed. If the patient has central cyanosis, usually the arterial saturation is 80% or less, with an arterial tension ($Pa{O_2}$) of about 50 mm Hg, indicating severely limited respiratory reserve. Careful auscultation of breath sounds may reveal crackles, rales, wheezing, and rhonchi. Deviation of the trachea may indicate a mediastinal mass, hemothorax, pneumothorax, or fibrothorax.

Laboratory Tests

The blood count may reveal polycythemia, reflecting prolonged smoking and hypoxemia. Leukocytosis may indicate active infection. Liver enzymes may be elevated, indicating possible hepatic metastasis. If the patient has elevated alkaline phosphatase levels, the source of that enzyme may be the liver, bone, or both. If other hepatic enzymes, particularly the γ-glutamyltransferase or 5′-aminopeptidase, are elevated, the elevated alkaline phosphatase level is probably of hepatic origin.

Most patients who are symptomatic from bronchogenic carcinoma have abnormal chest radiograph results, which frequently antedate the first sign or symptom of lung cancer by 7 months or more (2). The radiograph may reveal the tumor, secondary changes in lung parenchyma distal to an obstructed airway, or other abnormalities caused by intrathoracic and extrapulmonary tumor spread, which may influence anesthetic management. Tracheal deviation may lead to difficult intubation. Mediastinal masses indicate the potential for airway obstruction during induction and controlled ventilation. Bullae may rupture at any time during the procedure and can cause tension pneumothorax and/or ineffective ventilation. Consolidation and atelectasis can cause rapid desaturation and difficult ventilation. Pleural effusion increases $\dot{V}/\dot{Q}$ mismatch and decreases lung compliance. A computed tomography (CT) scan of the chest is helpful in delineating the presence or absence of a hilar lymph node and extrapulmonary spread of the disease. Based on the CT scan, if mediastinal nodes are suspected, cervical mediastinoscopy or parasternal mediastinotomy may be performed to determine the extent of tumor spread. To rule out distant metastasis, one should perform investigations such as bone scans and CT scans of the brain, liver, and upper abdomen.

Physiologic Assessment of Respiratory and Cardiac Function

Patients undergoing thoracotomy for lung resection usually have a long-standing history of smoking and varying degrees of underlying lung disease. Therefore, they have decreased pulmonary reserve and are at an increased risk of operative and postoperative morbidity and mortality. The aim of the preoperative evaluation of pulmonary functional reserve is to determine the patient's ability to tolerate thoracotomy and lung resection. One must realize that carcinoma of the lung has a 100% mortality rate within 5 years if not surgically treated, with an average survival length of 18 months. Therefore, every effort should be made to give the patient the benefit of surgical resection while undertaking an acceptable operative risk.

Arterial Blood Gas Analysis

Arterial carbon dioxide tension ($Pa{O_2}$) of more than 45 mm Hg is considered by many to represent patients who are at a higher risk for operative complications (3). Attempts should be made to correct all potentially reversible conditions. Persistent hypercarbia indicates high risk for lung resection and is an indication to perform further testing such as split-lung function tests. Hypoxemia, on the other hand, is not a consistent criterion for increased risk. The change in PaO_2 after thoracotomy and lung resection varies. Some tumors may have already completely occluded a bronchus and the blood supply to the corresponding lung segments. In effect, these patients have already had a functional resection, and removal of that part of the lung is followed by no further change in PaO_2 concentration. Other patients may show an actual improvement in PaO_2 concentration after thoracotomy and lung resection if the tumor was obstructing a bronchus resulting in atelectasis and infection. Removal of that lung segment, with the concomitant ligation of its pulmonary artery, will eliminate the physiologic shunt, resulting in an increased PaO_2 level.

Spirometry

Spirometry is performed on all patients having lung resection. The most important measurements to observe on a spirometry report are the forced vital capacity (FVC), FEV_1, and $FEV_{1\%}$. Normally, an individual can exhale 80% of the vital capacity in 1 second. Measurements of peak expiratory flow rates are usually effort dependent and therefore highly variable depending on patient cooperation. Maximum mid-expiratory flow rate, also known as forced expiratory flow (FEF), is a good indicator of small airway disease and is largely independent of patient effort. Abnormal results indicating higher operative risk include an FVC of less than 50%, a predicted FEV_1 of less than 2 L, and an FEV_1/FVC ratio of less than 50%.

Maximum Breathing Capacity

Several studies have found that the maximum breathing capacity, frequently known as the maximum voluntary ventilation, is a good predictor of the risk in pulmonary resection (4). This test is effort dependent and requires the patient to breathe as fast and as deeply as possible for 6 to 12 seconds. The maximum volume that can be breathed in 1 minute is then calculated. Besides being effort dependent, this test also has the unique value of assessing the entire cardiorespiratory system as well as the patient's cooperation and motivation. Thus, the predictive value of the maximum breathing capacity is somewhat similar to an exercise test.

Lung Volume Determination

The functional residual capacity (FRC) is the volume of gas that remains in the lung at the end of normal expiration when no airflow exists and when alveolar pressure equals airway pressure. The FRC can be measured using the nitrogen washout method, the helium dilution method, or body plethysmography. After measuring the FRC by one of these methods, one can calculate the residual volume by using the following formula: Residual volume = FRC − expiratory reserve volume. A ratio of residual volume to total lung capacity of more than 50% is recognized as a factor of increased risk. Also, the relationship of the FRC to the closing capacity is important in the pathogenesis of airway closure (Fig. 26-1). Pulmonary function criteria suggesting higher risk in pulmonary resective surgery includes an FVC value of less than 50% of predicted value, an FEV_1 of less than 2 L, FEV_1/FVC ratio of less than 50%, a maximum ventilatory ventilation value of less than 50% of predicted value, residual volume/total lung capacity of more than 50%, diffusing capacity of less than 50% of predicted value, and an arterial carbon dioxide tension ($PaCO_2$) of more than 45 mm Hg (5). Several studies have shown the diffusing lung capacity for carbon monoxide and the predicted postoperative diffusing lung capacity were good predictors of postoperative complications, including death and respiratory failure. No specific level of diffusing lung capacity for carbon monoxide has been established that constitutes a prohibitive surgical risk. However, many believe that a diffusing lung capacity for carbon monoxide of less than 50% to 60% of the predicted value is an indication for further testing with split-lung function tests before undertaking major pulmonary resection.

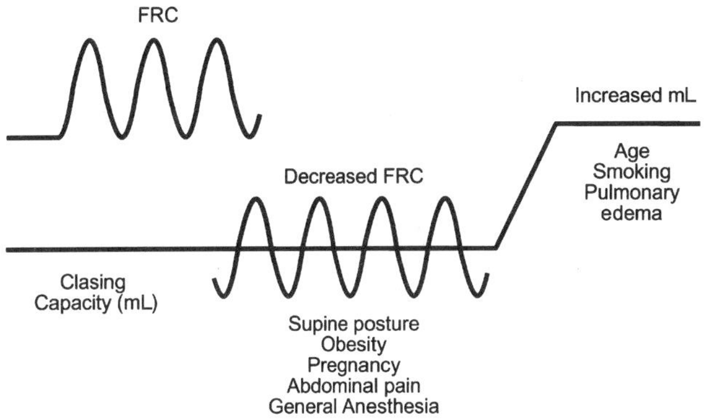

FIGURE 26-1. Relationship between closing volume and functional residual capacity.

Flow-Volume Loops

The flow-volume loop is a forced expiratory maneuver that displays the same information as a spirometer in graphic form, with flow rates expressed in liters per second on the vertical axis and lung volume in liters on the horizontal axis (Fig. 26-2). The shape of the flow-volume loop and its position on the x-axis and y-axis differentiate obstructive lung disease from restrictive lung disease from normal lung function. Flow-volume loops are useful to differentiate in-

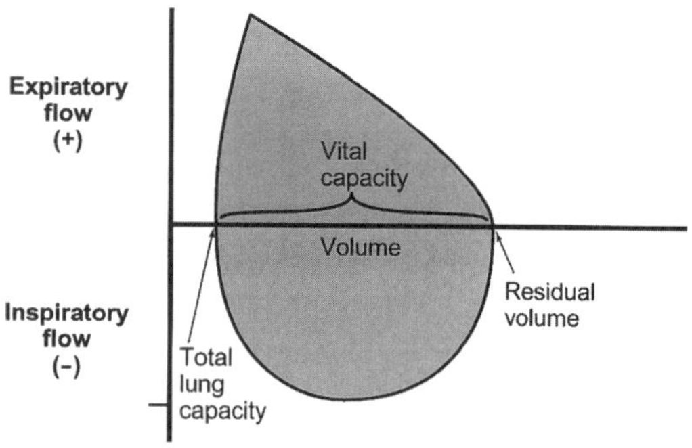

FIGURE 26-2. Flow-volume loop showing normal pulmonary function.

trathoracic from extrathoracic airway obstruction (Fig. 26-3). The shape and peak air flow rates during expiration at high lung volumes near the total lung capacity are effort dependent and indicate the patency of large airways. Effort-independent expiration occurs at the lower lung volumes and is best measured by the maximum mid-expiratory flow rate between 25% and 75% of the vital capacity, which is referred to as FEF 25% to 75% ($FEF_{25\%-75\%}$). Patients with obstructive airway disease such as asthma, bronchitis, and emphysema usually have a reduction in FEV_1/FVC ratio and $FEF_{25\%-75\%}$. Patients with restrictive lung diseases are characterized by a reduction in both FVC and FEV_1 with a normal FEV_1/FVC ratio.

Split-Lung Function Studies

Patients whose test results put them at high risk for lung resection should proceed to the split-lung function studies. In this phase, one attempts to predict the postoperative lung function remaining after pulmonary resection. The involved lung tissue may not be contributing much to the existing lung function, and removal of that part of the lung may not cause further deterioration in pulmonary function tests. The goal of these tests is to estimate postoperative lung function. The contribution of the lung that is to be removed

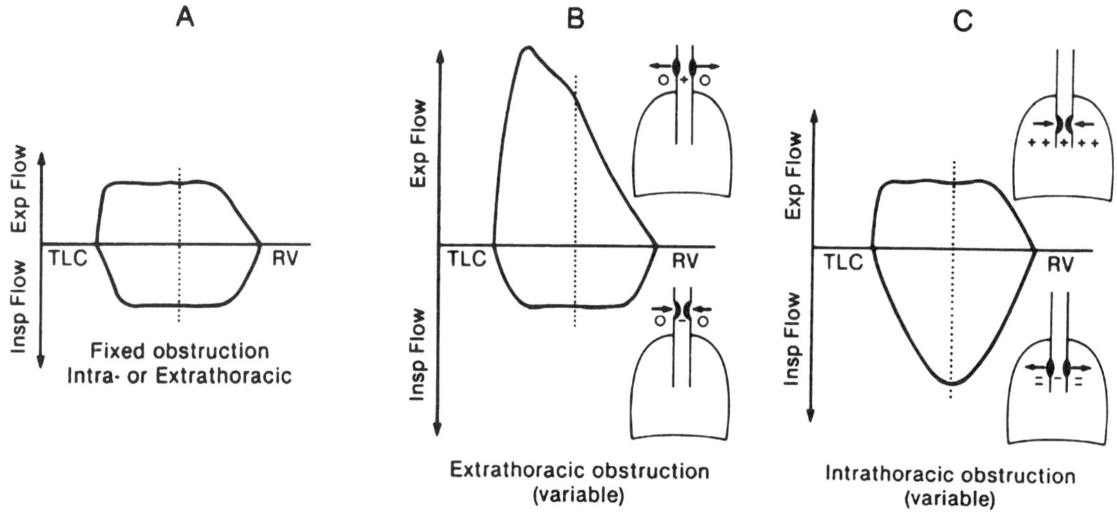

FIGURE 26-3. Maximal inspiratory and expiratory flow-volume curves in **(A)** fixed obstruction (intrathoracic or extrathoracic), in which airway diameter does not change with either inspiration or expiration, **(B)** extrathoracic variable obstruction, and **(C)** intrathoracic variable obstruction. The dotted line indicates 50% of the vital capacity (VC): The ratio of expired to inspired flow at this point is the mid-VC ratio and is normally 0.0 to 1.0. **A:** With a fixed obstruction, both expiratory (*exp*) and inspiratory (*insp*) flows are equally altered and the mid-VC ratio remains normal. **B:** With a variable extrathoracic obstruction, forced expiration results in a slightly positive (+) intratracheal pressure that is more than the pressure around the airway (atmospheric or 0), resulting in a decrease of the obstruction (airway dilates). During forced inspiration when pressure around the airway (0) exceeds the intratracheal pressure (−), the obstruction is increased (airway narrows). Because the expiratory curve is normal and the inspiratory curve is altered, the mid-VC ratio is much greater than normal. **C:** With a variable intrathoracic obstruction, forced expiration results in a very positive (+ +) pleural pressure that is greater than the slightly positive (+) intratracheal pressure, resulting in an increase of the obstruction (airway narrows). During forced inspiration, the intratracheal pressure (−) is greater than the pleural pressure (− −), thus decreasing the obstruction (airway dilates). Because the inspiratory curve is normal and the expiratory curve is attenuated, the mid-VC ratio is much less than normal. A normal flow-volume curve is a composite of the expiratory curve in Fig. 26-3B and the inspiratory curve in Fig. 26-3C. (TLC, total lung capacity; RV, residual volume.) (From Benumof JL, ed. *Anesthesia for thoracic surgery,* 2nd ed. Philadelphia: WB Saunders, 1995, with permission.)

to total lung function can be predicted using radioisotope ventilation scans, perfusion scans, or a combination of both. Using a xenon-133 (^{133}Xe) ventilation scan and technetium-99 (^{99}Tc) macroaggregate perfusion scan, split pulmonary functions can be estimated. Radioactive scanning yields data on regional perfusion, regional ventilation, and regional lung volumes, from which one can estimate the percentage of lung function contributed by the lung segment to be removed. One is then able to calculate the predicted pulmonary function after pneumonectomy as follows: Predicted postoperative FEV_1 = (preoperative FEV_1) × (perfusion [%] to remaining lung). For example, if the preoperative FEV_1 were 1.5 L and the perfusion to the lung that is to remain after resection is 60%, the predicted postoperative FEV_1 would be 900 mL. To calculate the predicted pulmonary function after lobectomy, the loss of function equals (preoperative FEV_1) (number of functional segments in lobe to be resected/total number of segments in both lungs). A lower limit of 800 mL has been suggested as the minimal predicted postoperative FEV_1 that will be tolerated. This is based on the observation that patients with COPD and an FEV_1 value less than 800 mL have significant reduction in their level of daily function and that patients with COPD start retaining CO_2 and develop hypercapnia when their FEV_1 value is less than 800 mL (6). The question has arisen as to whether the predicted FEV_1 as a percentage of the normal FEV_1 expected for that patient should be used rather than an absolute value of 800 mL. Those in favor argue that a short, elderly woman may not need as large a post-pneumonectomy FEV_1 value as a tall, young man. A proposed cutoff value is a predicted FEV_1 of at least 30% of that predicted for a particular patient based on age, sex, weight, and height (7).

Kearney et al. prospectively reported on 331 patients who underwent thoracic surgery in an attempt to further clarify the value of preoperative testing and how it relates to postoperative complications. They reported that preoperative hypercarbia ($Pa{CO_2} \geq 45$ mm Hg), desaturation on exercise oximetry to less than 90%, and a preoperative FEV_1 value of less than 1 L were not predictive of complications.

Univariate predictors of complications included an age of 60 years or more, male sex, history of smoking, a pneumonectomy procedure, and a low predicted postoperative FEV_1 value of less than 1 L. For each 0.2-L decrease in predicted FEV_1, the odds ratio for complications was 1.46 (8). Patients at low risk for complications have been suggested as having an FEV_1 value of more than 60% the predicted value, diffusing lung capacity for carbon monoxide of more than 60% of predicted value, a postoperative FEV_1 value of more than 40% the predicted value, a postoperative FEV_1 value of more than 800 mL, a postoperative diffusing lung capacity for carbon monoxide or more than 40%, and a $V{O_2}max$ during exercise of more than 15 mL/kg/minute (9).

Dales et al. (10) reported that patients 75 years old or older had twice as many complications as those younger than 50 years. Current cigarette smoking and the presence of lung cancer doubled the complication rate. The incidence of respiratory complications was 21% in patients with a normal FEV_1 compared to a 50% incidence of patients with an FEV_1 of less than 60% of predicted value. A doubling of the complications was noted in patients with an FVC of less than 60% when compared to patients with an FVC of more than 80%. The absolute value of predicted FEV_1 was not significantly associated with pulmonary complications (10).

Assessment of Cardiovascular Function in Patients Having Thoracic Surgery

Patients who are to undergo thoracotomy and lung resection frequently have a long-standing history of smoking and underlying COPDs, which can lead to pulmonary arterial hypertension and its sequelae. Pulmonary arterial hypertension results from an increase in pulmonary vascular resistance (PVR) caused by a reduction of cross-sectional area of pulmonary vasculature. This reduction results from the destruction of the alveolar septa and from hypoxemia-induced pulmonary vasoconstriction. Over time, pulmonary hypertension can lead to right ventricular hypertrophy, cor pulmonale, and eventually right ventricular failure. The normal pulmonary vascular bed can tolerate an increase in cardiac output of 250% without an increase in pulmonary artery pressure. In contrast, even a small augmentation of cardiac output causes a large increase in pulmonary artery pressure in patients with a restricted pulmonary vascular bed. Therefore, during the preoperative assessment of these patients, one must look for signs and symptoms of pulmonary hypertension, right ventricular and right atrial hypertrophy, cor pulmonale, and congestive heart failure. These patients will have prominent neck veins, a right-sided S_4 gallop, and dependent edema. The chest radiograph results may reveal dilation of the main pulmonary vessels, attenuation of peripheral pulmonary vasculature, hyperinflated lungs, flattened diaphragms, and loss of the airspace behind the sternum indicating right ventricular hypertrophy.

Preoperative Preparation of the Patient for Thoracic Surgery

The preoperative preparation should focus on the treatment of reversible conditions so the patient is in optimal condition for surgery. Prophylactic measures, such as optimization of bronchodilator therapy, hydration, and chest physical therapy, should be started preoperatively and continued intraoperatively and postoperatively in an effort to help optimize outcome and reduce morbidity. Patient education will help ensure optimal postoperative compliance and performance and includes cessation of smoking and training in incentive spirometry. Bronchodilation and control of infection and secretions when indicated and weight reduction when appropriate should also be considered.

Cessation of smoking for at least 4 to 8 weeks before surgery is associated with decreased incidence of postoperative respiratory complications. Cessation of smoking for 12 to 48 hours preoperatively does not decrease the incidence of postoperative respiratory complications but may still have a salutary effect by decreasing the concentration of carboxyhemoglobin, increasing the blood's O_2-carrying capacity, and shifting the oxyhemoglobin curve to the right. Other beneficial effects of smoking cessation several weeks before surgery are terminating the stimulus for bronchoconstriction, decreasing sputum production, and improving ciliary activity.

Chronic wheezing is often seen in patients with COPD because of airflow obstruction from bronchial smooth-muscle contraction, accumulation of secretions, and mucosal edema. Severe acute wheezing represents a medical emergency, and elective surgery should be postponed until proper treatment has been instituted and the condition resolved. Bronchodilators should be administered to patients who have airflow obstruction, and the response to such therapeutic intervention should be quantified by repeated pulmonary function tests. Most patients are treated with inhaled β_2-adrenergic agonists and/or parasympatholytic agents. Ipratropium bromide (Atrovent) is a synthetic analog of atropine that shares its bronchodilator properties but is poorly absorbed from the tracheobronchial tree. The drug is most effective in COPD patients in whom it is at least as potent a bronchodilator as the adrenergic agents. Administration of inhibitors of phosphodiesterase such as aminophylline leads to the accumulation of intracellular cyclic adenosine monophosphate by inhibition of its enzymatic breakdown. In addition, aminophylline improves diaphragmatic contractility and the patient's resistance to fatigue (11). Aminophylline has a relatively low toxic-therapeutic ratio, and therapeutic blood levels are 5 to 20 μg/mL. The combination of aminophylline and β_2-adrenergic agonists can lead to tachycardia, ventricular dysrhythmias, and myocardial ischemia and should therefore be used with caution. Steroids can be used to decrease mucosal edema and to suppress inflammation in the tracheobronchial tree. They are slow to act and are of questionable benefit in patients with acute bronchospasm. Beclomethasone can be used in an aerosolized form. Cromolyn sodium stabilizes mast cell membranes, preventing their degranulation and release of chemical mediators responsible for bronchospasm, edema, and inflammation. This drug is most useful in the prevention of bronchospastic attacks but has no role in the treatment of an acute episode of asthma. Montelukast sodium (Singulair) is a selective and orally active leukotriene receptor antagonist that inhibits the cysteinyl-leukotriene receptor. The cysteinyl leukotrienes are products of arachidonic acid metabolism and are released from mast cells found in the human airway. Occupation of cysteinyl-leukotriene receptors has been correlated with the pathophysiology of asthma including airway edema and smooth-muscle contraction. Montelukast sodium is indicated for the prophylaxis and chronic treatment of asthma.

Acute and chronic infections should be vigorously treated before surgery. A change in the color and quantity of sputum produced by a patient with COPD may indicate infection. Humidification of bronchial secretions can also be accomplished by the use of an ultrasonic nebulizer or a respiratory humidifier. In addition, mucolytic agents such as acetylcysteine or an oral expectorant such as potassium iodide can be of benefit to patients with viscous secretions. Mobilization of secretions is achieved by a combination of deep breathing, vigorous coughing, postural drainage, and optimal hydration and chest percussion.

Monitoring During Thoracic Anesthesia

The degree of invasiveness in monitoring should be individualized according to the extent of surgery and the patient's underlying cardiovascular and respiratory condition. Standard monitors are applied and include blood pressure cuff, electrocardiogram (ECG), pulse oximetry, and end-tidal CO_2, temperature, and listening to breath sounds. Airway pressures should be monitored to reflect alterations in the airway resistance, lung compliance, and position of double-lumen tubes. The end-tidal CO_2 usually correlates well with Pa_{CO_2}, with end-tidal CO_2 about 4 to 6 mm Hg less than the Pa_{CO_2}. Both usually follow the same trend. Widening of the gap between the end-tidal CO_2 value and the Pa_{CO_2}, as determined by arterial blood gases, indicates an increase in dead space ventilation ($\dot{V}/\dot{Q}$ less than 1.0). An increase in shunt leads to only a small increase in the gap between end-tidal CO_2 and Pa_{CO_2}, as determined by arterial blood gases. Valuable information can be obtained by continuous observation of the shape of the capnograph. An increasing slope of the curve and failure to reach a plateau indicate increased airway resistance and a prolonged expiratory phase. Any significant change in the value of end-tidal CO_2 that cannot be explained by changes in the minute ventilation should be confirmed by measuring arterial blood gases.

Radial arterial catheters are indicated in most patients undergoing thoracotomy. Blood gas analysis can then be facilitated in patients who undergo one-lung ventilation. It is important to determine baseline arterial blood gases and to obtain intermittent samples during surgery, particularly when pulse oximetry and end-tidal CO_2 start showing unfavorable changes. Central venous pressure (CVP) monitoring may also be indicated depending on the magnitude of the intended resection and the physiologic status of the patient. The CVP reflects the relationship among the patient's blood volume, venous tone, and right ventricular performance. Requirements for CVP to reflect left ventricular preload accurately include (a) normal left ventricular compliance, (b) normal mitral valve, (c) normal PVR, and (d) normal right ventricular compliance and normal tricuspid valve. Therefore, a CVP catheter is frequently sufficient in patients without significant cardiac disease or pulmonary hypertension for monitoring intravascular volume and for the infusion of fluids and blood. The CVP can be monitored through an external or internal jugular catheter. The disadvantage of using the external jugular vein during thoracotomy is that the catheter often becomes obstructed when the patient is turned to the lateral decubitus position. If a subclavian technique is chosen, one may consider placement on the same side of surgery to avoid the potential development of a pneumothorax on the dependent side. The subclavian vein is also at risk for technical problems such as occlusion when the patient is placed in the lateral decubitus position.

A pulmonary artery catheter can be considered to monitor left-sided filling pressures, to estimate the coronary perfusion pressure, and to measure cardiac output. This is indicated in patients with severe cardiovascular disease, coronary artery disease, valvular heart disease, significant pulmonary hypertension, and congestive heart failure. The information obtained from the pulmonary artery catheter can also be of great assistance in the postoperative management. More than 90% of pulmonary artery catheters float to and locate in the right lung (12). During a right thoracotomy with the patient in the left lateral decubitus position, the pulmonary artery catheter is then in the nondependent or operative lung. This lung is either collapsed if one-lung ventilation is employed or is in zone 1 or 2 if the up lung is ventilated. When the pulmonary artery catheter is in zone 1 and/or 2 of the lung, the pressure recorded during the wedging of the catheter is more reflective of airway pressure than of left atrial pressure, particularly if a large tidal volume, positive end-expiratory pressure (PEEP), or constant positive airway pressure (CPAP) is applied to the up lung. Also, if hypotension and decreased cardiac output occur occur, perfusion to the nondependent lung will decrease, which may lead to total or near-total collapse of the pulmonary veins. Airway pressure will be higher than pulmonary venous pressure, and the pressure that is recorded by the pulmonary artery catheter will be airway pressure, not left atrial pressure. Conversely, when left thoracotomy is performed and the pulmonary artery catheter is in the right dependent lung, which is well perfused and functioning in zone 3, the pressures obtained when the pulmonary artery catheter is wedged will truly reflect left atrial pressure.

When measuring the cardiac output with the patient in the lateral decubitus position, one should again consider the position of the pulmonary artery catheter. When the catheter is in the upside lung and the lung is collapsed, and when the pulmonary blood flow is distorted from surgical manipulations and hypoxic pulmonary vasoconstriction (HPV), measurements of cardiac output and $S\text{v}O_2$ will be inaccurate because of stagnated blood flow. In summary, when the pulmonary artery catheter is in the nondependent lung, which is either collapsed or ventilated with large tidal volume, PEEP, or CPAP, the pulmonary artery wedge pressure (PAWP) may not reflect left atrial pressure. When the pulmonary artery catheter is in the dependent lung and presumably in the zone 3 region, PAWP should accurately reflect left atrial pressure, even when PEEP is applied to the dependent lung.

The Lateral Decubitus Position

The lateral decubitus position is commonly employed during thoracic surgery. The advantages of using the lateral decubitus position are (a) it permits the most complete access to the hemithorax, (b) the length of the intercostal incision can be easily extended anteriorly and posterior as needed, (c) the patient can be tilted forward or backward, providing optimal access to the ipsilateral mediastinum, pericardium, hilum of the lung, and descending thoracic aorta, and (d) it permits intraoperative pericardial control of the hilar vessels when needed. The disadvantages of the lateral decubitus position are (a) the opposite hemithorax is relatively inaccessible, (b) alterations in ventilation distribution and $\dot{V}/\dot{Q}$ mismatches due to gravity are more likely to occur, (c) the dependent lung is exposed to the risk of contamination through the tracheobronchial tree with blood and/or purulent material, (d) the dependent lung has a decreased FRC, which promotes airway closure, and atelectasis, and (e) positioning injuries caused by abnormal pressure to muscles, eyes, ears, and stretching of nerves are more likely than if the patient were supine.

An additional complication while utilizing the lateral decubitus position includes unwanted movement of the double-lumen tube. Flexion of the neck moves the endotracheal tube distally, whereas extension of the neck leads to movement of the endotracheal tube proximally and risks extubation. Proper location of endotracheal and double-lumen tubes must be determined after anesthesia induction and again immediately after the lateral decubitus position has been established. We routinely use fiberoptic endoscopy to reconfirm the position of these tubes.

The lateral decubitus position is inherently unstable and places the relaxed, anesthetized patient at considerable risk for pressure and stretch damage. Complications of surgical positioning are usually attributed to abnormal pressure, stretch, or both. In the lateral decubitus position, compression is the leading cause of brachial plexus injury. Ischemia of the intraneural vasonervosum is the principal cause of positional nerve injuries. Compression of the brachial plexus may occur when the lower shoulder and arm are allowed to remain directly under the rib cage after turning the patient into the lateral position. A properly placed axillary roll reduces the risk of compression injury to the brachial plexus. An entrapment neuropathy of the suprascapular nerve is an infrequent, easily overlooked source of pain after a surgical

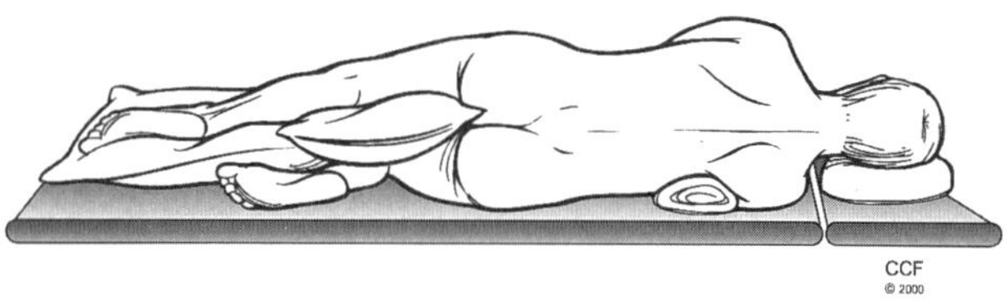

FIGURE 26-4. Patient properly positioned for a lateral thoracotomy.

procedure in the lateral decubitus position. Stretch of the nerve apparently occurs by circumduction of the upper extremity across the chest or by lateralization of the neck toward the opposite shoulder. The median and ulnar nerves can also be damaged if allowed to hang over the edge of the operating table. The radial nerve is susceptible to damage in the lateral position if the extended dependent arm is pushed cephalad against the vertical bar of the anesthesia screen, thereby compressing the nerve between the humerus and the bar. The common peroneal nerve (lateral popliteal nerve) is the most frequently injured nerve in the lower extremity. Damage occurs if the patient is placed in the lateral position on a poorly padded operating table and the nerve is compressed as it courses around the lateral aspect of the proximal fibula. The sciatic nerve may be injured in an emaciated patient if compressed between the operating table and the ischiopubic ramus or if tight hip straps or strap buckles are used. Properly positioned patients have their head supported, an axillary role in place, and pillows between their legs with the bottom leg slightly flexed at the hip and knee (Fig. 26-4).

Vascular complications such as venous thrombosis can occur in the lateral decubitus position, but no more often than in any other surgical position, provided venous occlusion or stasis is avoided. Hyperabduction of the arm that is up, as might occur when it is suspended from the anesthesia screen, has resulted in peripheral gangrene. Periodic palpation of the pulse in the abducted arm, particularly in an elderly or diabetic patient, is suggested to prevent this complication. The upper arm can also be monitored by a pulse oximeter placed on a finger.

Rotation of the head in an elderly arthritic patient has been suggested as a cause of central nervous system damage caused by occlusion of the vertebral artery. A history of vascular disease, including coronary artery disease or transient ischemic attacks, should alert the anesthesiologist to this possibility.

The lateral decubitus position places the dependent eye at risk of damage and permanent blindness from retinal artery thrombosis. Controlled or prolonged hypotension may reduce retinal perfusion and accentuate the possibility of thrombosis. This complication is preventable by proper padding and support around the lower eye with foam and sponge headrests to protect the eye from being compressed against the hard surface of the operating table.

Physiology of Lateral Decubitus Position

The distribution of perfusion is altered in the lateral decubitus position. The contraction of the right ventricle imparts kinetic energy to the blood in the main pulmonary artery. Some of the kinetic energy is dissipated in climbing a vertical hydrostatic gradient toward the portions of the lung higher than the heart level. The absolute pressure in the pulmonary arteries decreases by 1 cm H_2O per centimeter of vertical distance up to the lung (Fig. 26-5). Moving from the cephalad to the more caudad portions of the lung, the vessel diameters progressively increase. The distending transmural pressure is equal to the pressure inside the vessel minus the intrapleural pressure. The pleural pressure increases by 0.25 cm of H_2O per centimeter of lung dependency. Therefore, the pressure outside the vessel—that is,

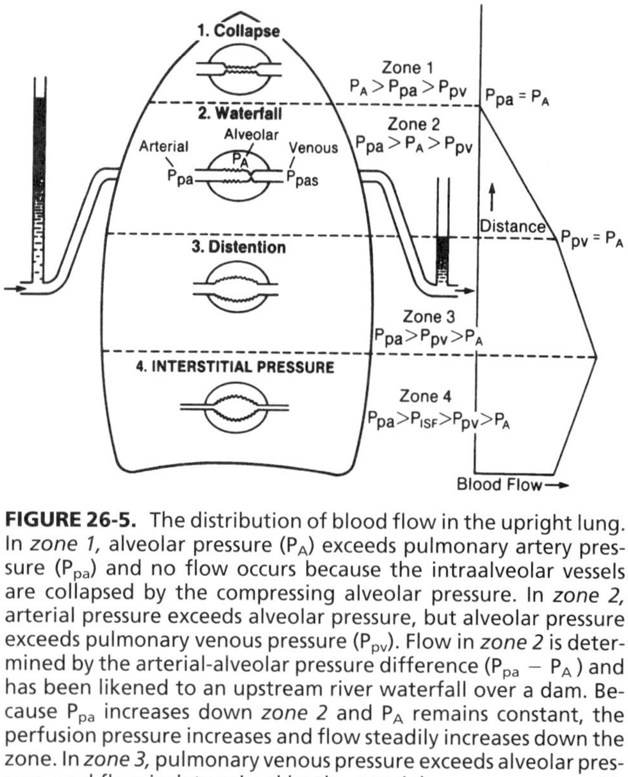

FIGURE 26-5. The distribution of blood flow in the upright lung. In *zone 1,* alveolar pressure (P_A) exceeds pulmonary artery pressure (P_{pa}) and no flow occurs because the intraalveolar vessels are collapsed by the compressing alveolar pressure. In *zone 2,* arterial pressure exceeds alveolar pressure, but alveolar pressure exceeds pulmonary venous pressure (P_{pv}). Flow in *zone 2* is determined by the arterial-alveolar pressure difference ($P_{pa} - P_A$) and has been likened to an upstream river waterfall over a dam. Because P_{pa} increases down *zone 2* and P_A remains constant, the perfusion pressure increases and flow steadily increases down the zone. In *zone 3,* pulmonary venous pressure exceeds alveolar pressure, and flow is determined by the arterial-venous pressure difference ($P_{pa} - P_{pv}$), which is constant down this portion of the lung. However, the transmural pressure across the wall of the vessel increases down this zone as the caliber of the vessels increases (resistance decreases), and therefore flow increases. Finally, in *zone 4,* pulmonary interstitial pressure becomes positive and exceeds both pulmonary venous pressure and alveolar pressure. Consequently, flow in *zone 4* is determined by the arterial-interstitial pressure difference ($P_{pa} - P_{15f}$). (From Benumof JL, ed. *Anesthesia for thoracic surgery,* 2nd ed. Philadelphia: WB Saunders, 1995, with permission.)

the pleural pressure (P_{pl})—increases at a slower rate than the pulmonary artery pressure (P_{pa}) the and pulmonary venous pressure (P_{pv}). Therefore, the transmural distending pressure, which is P_{pa} minus P_{pl} and P_{pv} minus P_{pl}, increases going down the lungs from zone 1 to zone 2 and then zone 3. Vessel radii increase, vascular resistance decreases, and blood flow increases moving down the lung. Therefore, lung perfusion depends on gravity, with the dependent lung regions receiving more perfusion than the nondependent regions. The apicis of the lung may have no perfusion at all. A decrease in the cardiac output and pulmonary arterial pressure results in an increase in the extent of zone 1, whereas an increase in cardiac output and pulmonary arterial pressure leads to a decrease in the extent of zone 1.

The distribution of ventilation is also altered when the patient goes from the supine to the lateral decubitus position. The lung is a physical elastic structure resembling a plastic bag filled with semifluid contents. It is enclosed within a chest cavity. Because of the effect of gravity, the top of the lung tends to collapse inward, and the lower dependent part tends to push outward toward the chest wall. The tendency of the top of the lung to collapse inward creates a negative intrapleural pressure as the lung tries to pull away from the chest wall and relatively more positive pressure at the dependent part, where the lung is trying to bulge outward against the chest wall. The magnitude of this pressure gradient depends on the lung's density, which is one quarter that of water. The intrapleural pressure gradient in centimeters of water is about one quarter the height of the upright lung, which is 30 cm. Therefore, the difference between the intrapleural pressure at the bottom of the lung and that at the top is equal to 30/4, or 7.5 cm H_2O. The intrapleural pressure therefore increases by 0.25 cm H_2O per 1 cm of lung dependency. If the intraalveolar pressure is the same throughout the lung, the transpulmonary distending pressure, which is equal to the alveolar pressure minus intrapleural pressure, decreases from the top of the lung toward the bottom. That is, more distending force is pulling the alveoli open at the top of the lung than at its base. The intrapleural pressure is at least negative at the dependent basilar lung regions, so the alveoli in these regions are more compressed and are considerably smaller than the alveoli at the apex of the lung. Approximately a four-fold alveolar volume difference exists between the lung's most dependent part and the lung's most apical part (Fig. 26-6). The dependent small alveoli are on the steep portion of their compliance curve, whereas the nondependent alveoli are on the relatively flat, noncompliant portion of the curve. Therefore, in the upright position, most of the tidal volume is preferentially distributed to the dependent alveoli, because they expand more per unit pressure change than the nondependent alveoli.

Both blood flow and ventilation increase linearly moving down the normal upright lung. Because blood flow increases from a very low value and increases more rapidly than the

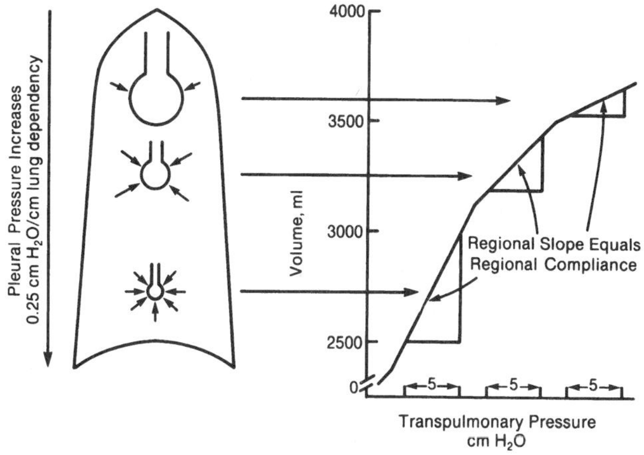

FIGURE 26-6. Pleural pressure increases 0.25 cm H_2O every centimeter down the lung. The increase in pleural pressure causes a four-fold decrease in alveolar volume. The caliber of the air passages also decreases as lung volume decreases. When regional alveolar volume is translated over to a regional transpulmonary pressure–alveolar volume curve, small alveoli are on a steep (*large slope*) portion of the curve, and large alveoli are on a flat (*small slope*) portion of the curve. Because the regional slope equals regional compliance, the dependent small alveoli normally receive the largest share of the tidal volume. Over the normal tidal volume range (lung volume increases by 500 mL from 2,500 [normal functional residual capacity] to 3,000 mL), the pressure-volume relationship is linear. Lung volume values in this diagram relate to the upright position. (From Benumof JL, ed. *Anesthesia for thoracic surgery,* 2nd ed. Philadelphia: WB Saunders, 1995, with permission.)

increase in ventilation moving down the lung, the ventilation/perfusion ($\dot{V}/\dot{Q}$) ratio decreases rapidly at first, then more slowly. Figure 26-7 shows the calculated ventilation, blood flow, $\dot{V}/\dot{Q}$ ratio, and alveolar O_2 tension (Pao_2) and alveolar CO_2 tension ($Paco_2$) and for horizontal slices of the lung. One can see that Pao_2 is highest at the apex of the lung, 132 mm Hg, and lowest at the base of the lung, 89 mm Hg. The $\dot{V}/\dot{Q}$ ratio is equal to 1 in the region of zone 2 in the area between the third and fourth ribs. The $\dot{V}/\dot{Q}$ ratio is 0.63 at the base of the lung and 3.3 at the apex of the lung. In keeping with the regional $\dot{V}/\dot{Q}$ ratio, the bottom of the lung is relatively hypoxic and hypercarbic compared with the top of the lung. Other nongravitational important determinants of PVR and blood flow distribution include cardiac output, alveolar hypoxia, lung volume flow, and alternative nonalveolar pathways of blood flow through the lung. These relationships change depending on whether the patient is awake, anesthetized, spontaneously breathing or having his or her ventilation monitored, and having his or her chest open or closed.

Patient Awake, Spontaneously Breathing

In the lateral decubitus position, while the patient is still awake and spontaneously breathing, the distributions of ventilation and perfusion are as follows: Gravity causes a

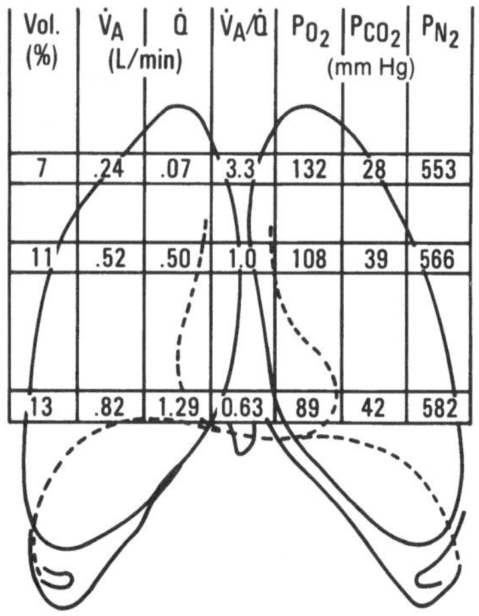

FIGURE 26-7. Ventilation/perfusion ($\dot{V}/\dot{Q}$) ratio and the regional composition of alveolar gas. PN_2 has been obtained by what remains from the total gas pressure (which, including water vapor, equals 760 mm Hg). The volumes (*vol* [%]) of the three lung slices are also shown. Compared with the top of the lung, the bottom of the lung has a low $\dot{V}/\dot{Q}$ ratio and is relatively hypoxic and hypercarbic. (From Benumof JL, ed. *Anesthesia for thoracic surgery,* 2nd ed. Philadelphia: WB Saunders, 1995, with permission.)

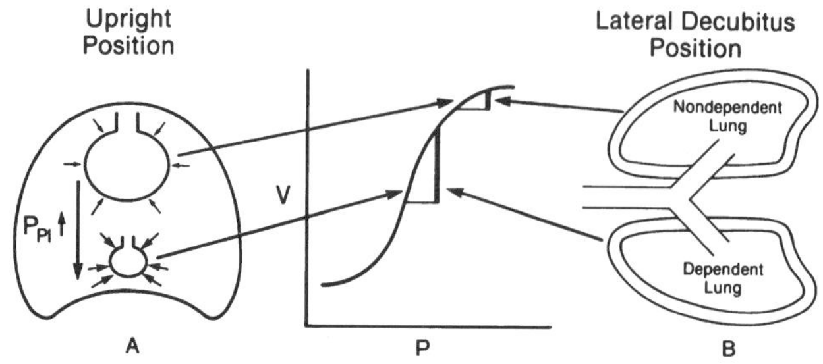

FIGURE 26-9. Pleural pressure in the awake patient (closed chest) is most positive in the dependent portion of the lung, and alveoli in this region are therefore most compressed and have the least volume. Pleural pressure is least positive (most negative) at the apex of the lung, and alveoli in this region are therefore least compressed and have the largest volume. When these regional differences in alveolar volume are translated over to a regional transpulmonary pressure–alveolar volume curve, the small dependent alveoli are on a steep (*large slope*) portion of the curve and the large nondependent alveoli are on a flat (*small slope*) portion of the curve. In this diagram, regional slope equals regional compliance. Thus, for a given and equal change in transpulmonary pressure, the dependent part of the lung receives a much larger share of the tidal volume than the nondependent part of the lung. In the lateral decubitus position **(right)**, gravity also causes pleural pressure gradients and therefore similarly affects the distribution of ventilation. The dependent lung lies on a relatively steep portion and the upper lung lies on a relatively flat portion of the pressure-volume curve. Thus, in the lateral decubitus position, the dependent lung receives most of the tidal ventilation. (From Benumof JL, ed. *Anesthesia for thoracic surgery,* 2nd ed. Philadelphia: WB Saunders, 1995, with permission.)

vertical gradient in distribution of pulmonary blood flow in the lateral decubitus position for the same reason it does in the upright position (Fig. 26-8). The vertical hydrostatic gradient is less than it is in the upright position because the distance from the most dependent to the most nondependent part of the lung is less. Consequently, there is less zone 1 and more zone 2 and 3 blood flow in the lateral decubitus position compared with that in the upright position. Nevertheless, blood flow to the dependent lung is still significantly greater than blood flow to the nondependent lung. When the right lung is up, it receives approximately 45% of total blood flow, whereas the left dependent lung receives 55% of the total blood flow. Normally in the upright position, the right lung receives 55% of the total blood flow because of its larger size, whereas the left lung receives 45% of total blood flow. When the left lung is up, it receives approximately 35% of the total blood flow, whereas 65% goes to the right dependent lung. As in the upright position, ventilation is also relatively increased in the dependent lung zones (Fig. 26-9). In addition, in the lateral decubitus position, the dome of the lower diaphragm is pushed higher into the chest than the dome of the upper diaphragm and is therefore more stretched and sharply curved than the upper diaphragm. This gives the lower diaphragm more efficiency during spontaneous ventilation. Thus, in the lateral decubitus position with an awake, spontaneously breathing patient, the lower lung is better ventilated than the upper lung, regardless of the side on which the patient is lying, and $\dot{V}/\dot{Q}$ is still a good match.

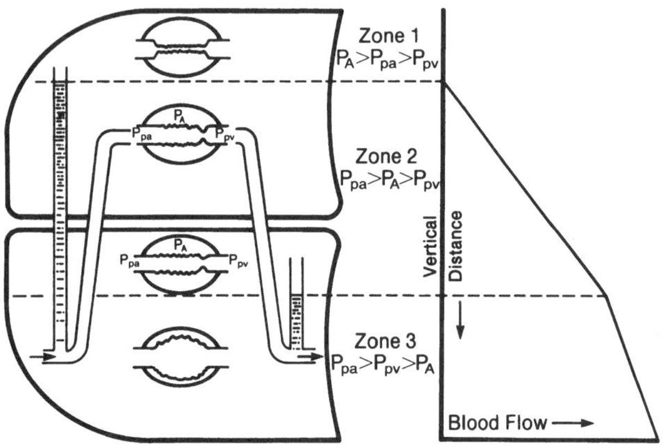

FIGURE 26-8. The effects of gravity on the distribution of pulmonary blood flow in the lateral decubitus position. Vertical gradients in the lateral decubitus position are similar to those in the upright position and cause the creation of zones 1, 2, and 3. Consequently, pulmonary blood flow increases with lung dependency and is largest in the dependent lung and least in the nondependent lung. (From Benumof JL, ed. *Anesthesia for thoracic surgery,* 2nd ed. Philadelphia: WB Saunders, 1995, with permission.)

Patient Anesthetized, Chest Closed

In the anesthetized, spontaneously breathing patient in the lateral decubitus position, the dependent lung continues to receive relatively more perfusion than the nondependent

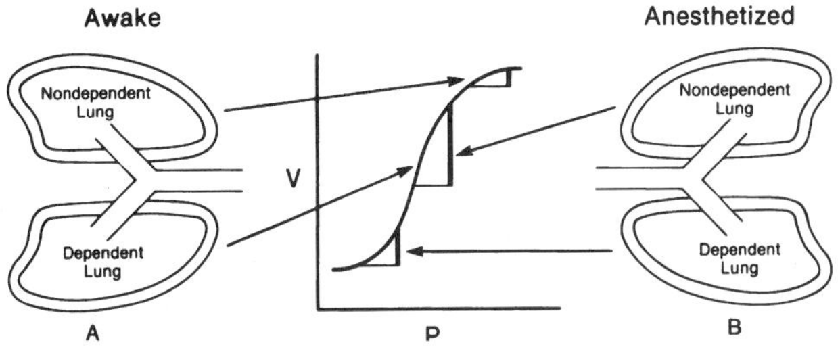

FIGURE 26-10. The **(left)** distribution of ventilation in the awake patient (closed chest) in the lateral decubitus position and the **(right)** distribution of ventilation in the anesthetized patient (closed chest) in the lateral decubitus position. The induction of anesthesia has caused a loss in lung volume in both lungs, with the nondependent (up) lung moving from a flat noncompliant portion to a steep compliant portion of the pressure-volume curve and the dependent (down) lung moving from a steep compliant part to a flat, noncompliant part of the pressure-volume curve. Thus, the anesthetized patient in a lateral decubitus position has the majority of the tidal ventilation in the nondependent lung (where there is the least perfusion) and the minority of the tidal ventilation in the dependent lung (where there is the most perfusion). (From Benumof JL, ed. *Anesthesia for thoracic surgery,* 2nd ed. Philadelphia: WB Saunders, 1995, with permission.)

lung. The distribution of ventilation, however, does change after the induction of anesthesia (Fig. 26-10). With the induction of general anesthesia, FRC decreases. Both lungs share in the loss of lung volume and move to a lower location on the pressure-volume curve. The dependent lung now occupies the low flat portion of the curve and is therefore less compliant. The nondependent lung, initially in the noncompliant part, now moves to the steep, compliant, part of the curve. Other factors that contribute to the decrease in FRC of the dependent lung include its compression by the weight of the mediastinum and the abdominal contents. Therefore, with the induction of anesthesia, little change occurs in perfusion distribution, whereas significant change occurs in ventilation distribution. Now the nondependent lung receives most of the ventilation but is still less perfused, whereas the dependent lung receives less ventilation but continues to be more perfused. This leads to an increase in both the amount of shunt (dependent lung has a low $\dot{V}/\dot{Q}$ ratio) and the amount of dead space ventilation (nondependent lung has a $\dot{V}/\dot{Q}$ ratio of more than 1).

Patient Anesthetized, Paralyzed, Mechanically Ventilated

This causes further deterioration in the $\dot{V}/\dot{Q}$ relationship. Perfusion continues to be more to the dependent lung because of gravitational effects. There is even more distribution of ventilation to the nondependent lung compared with the previous stage. In addition to the decrease in the FRC of both lungs, with the lower dependent lung compromised more than the nondependent lung, another factor appears with the institution of mechanical ventilation. The highly curved, actively contracting diaphragm in the lower hemithorax no longer confers any advantage in ventilation, as it does in the awake, spontaneously breathing patient, because it is no longer actively contracting (13). In addition, the weight of the abdominal viscera physically restricts expansion of the lower lung. This leads to further preferential distribution of ventilation to the nondependent, less perfused lung. In summary, the anesthetized patient in the lateral decubitus position has an unfavorable $\dot{V}/\dot{Q}$ ratio that is more severe with muscle relaxation and controlled ventilation than with spontaneous breathing. The application of PEEP to both lungs restores their FRC. The lower lung returns to a steeper, more favorable part on the pressure-volume curve, and the upper lung resumes its original position on the flat, unfavorable portion of the curve. This restores most ventilation to the lower lung. This is important when trying to optimize oxygenation during one-lung ventilation, as discussed in the following sections.

Patient Anesthetized, Chest Open

Two phenomena occur in a spontaneously ventilating patient with an open chest that can lead to significant impairment in ventilation: mediastinal shift and paradoxical respiration (Fig. 26-11). Mediastinal shift is the up-and-down

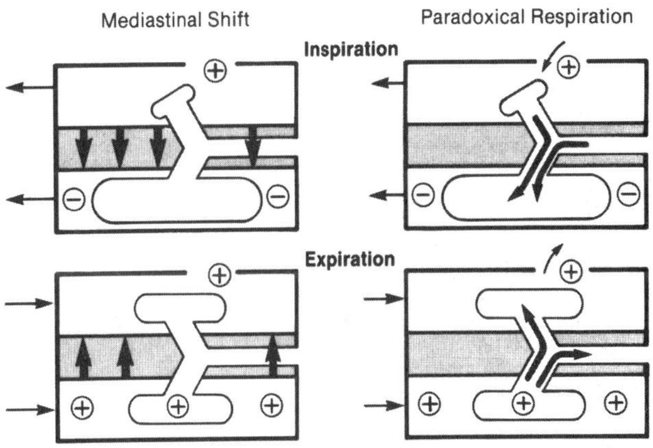

FIGURE 26-11. Mediastinal shift and paradoxical respiration in the spontaneously ventilating patient with an open chest and placed in the lateral decubitus position. The open chest is always exposed to atmospheric pressure (+). During inspiration, negative pressure (−) in the intact hemithorax causes the mediastinum to move vertically downward (mediastinal shift). In addition, during inspiration, movement of gas from the nondependent lung in the open hemithorax into the dependent lung in the closed hemithorax and movement of air from the environment into the open hemithorax cause the lung in the open hemithorax to collapse (paradoxical respiration). During expiration, relative positive pressure (+) in the closed hemithorax causes the mediastinum to move vertically upward (mediastinal shift). In addition, during expiration, the gas moves from the dependent lung to the nondependent lung and from the open hemithorax to the environment; consequently, the nondependent lung expands during expiration (paradoxical respiration). (From Benumof JL, ed. *Anesthesia for thoracic surgery,* 2nd ed. Philadelphia: WB Saunders, 1995, with permission.)

movement of the mediastinum with respiratory movements caused by changes in the intrapleural pressure in the dependent hemithorax. An amount equal to the downward inspiratory displacement of the mediastinum decreases the tidal volume in the dependent lung during inspiration. This leads to significant impairment in ventilation to the lower lung. Mediastinal shift can also cause circulatory changes such as decreased venous return and reflexes because of sympathetic activation, resulting in a clinical picture similar to shock. The patient is hypotensive, pale, cold, and clammy, with dilated pupils. Local anesthetic infiltration of the pulmonary plexus at the hilum and of the vagus nerve can diminish these reflexes. However, more practically, controlled positive-pressure ventilation abolishes the ventilatory and circulatory changes associated with mediastinal shift.

Paradoxical respiration refers to the movement of air between the dependent lung and the nondependent lung during respiration, along with movement of air from the ambient atmosphere in and out of the open chest cavity. In combination with mediastinal shift, it leads to further impairment in ventilation. Paradoxical respiration may be prevented either by manual collapse of the upper lung or more often by controlled positive-pressure ventilation. Because of mediastinal shift and paradoxical respiration, controlled positive-pressure ventilation is the best way to provide adequate gas exchange during thoracotomy.

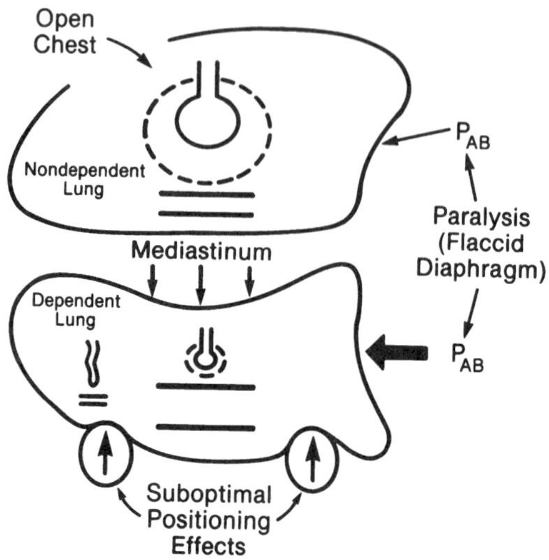

FIGURE 26-12. Summary of ventilation/perfusion relationships in the anesthetized patient in the lateral decubitus position, with an open chest, paralyzed, and suboptimally positioned. Nondependent lung is well ventilated (*large dashed lines*) but poorly perfused (*small perfusion vessel*), and the dependent lung is poorly ventilated (*small dashed lines*) but well perfused (*large perfusion vessel*). In addition, the dependent lung may also develop an atelectatic shunt compartment (*left side of the lower lung*) because of the circumferential compression of this lung. (From Benumof JL, ed. *Anesthesia for thoracic surgery,* 2nd ed. Philadelphia: WB Saunders, 1995, with permission.)

Effects of Surgical Manipulation

With the onset of surgical manipulations, compliance and distribution of ventilation to the upper lung significantly decreases. End-tidal CO_2 and CO_2 elimination from the upper lung decrease greatly. Changes in $Paco_2$ are minimal. Surgical manipulations mechanically restrict the expansion of the upper lung and counteract its tendency to be over ventilated. The anesthetized, paralyzed patient in the lateral decubitus position with an open chest may have a considerable $\dot{V}/\dot{Q}$ mismatch (Fig. 26-12). The nondependent lung receives greater ventilation and less perfusion and has a $\dot{V}/\dot{Q}$ ratio of more than 1. The dependent lung has more perfusion and less ventilation and a low $\dot{V}/\dot{Q}$ ratio and therefore acts as a physiologic shunt. Effects of gravity mainly determine the blood flow distribution. Causes of poor ventilation of the dependent lung are (a) loss of FRC because of induction of general anesthesia, (b) compression of the dependent lung by the mediastinum, (c) upward shift of the abdominal contents facilitated by paralysis of the diaphragm, (d) suboptimal positioning effects, (e) impaired ciliary clearance of mucus, and (f) absorption atelectasis from the use of high Fio_2. Consequently, two-lung ventilation under these circumstances may result in an increased alveolar-to-arterial Po_2 difference and less than optimal oxygenation. A group of patients receiving differential lung ventilation using 10 cm H_2O PEEP to the dependent lung while the nondependent lung was ventilated with zero end-expiratory pressure (ZEEP) was compared to another group intubated with a single-lumen tube and mechanically ventilated with ZEEP to both lungs. Selective PEEP applications to the dependent lung resulted in an adequate Pao_2 at a lower inspired O_2 concentration and a smaller degree of shunt at the end of surgery than when both lungs were ventilated with ZEEP. The explanation is that PEEP to the lower lung increases the FRC of that lung, moving it to a steeper, more favorable portion on its pressure-volume curve and leading to improved distribution of ventilation to the dependent lung. Even if the increase in PVR caused by the application of PEEP results in shifting blood flow from the dependent to the nondependent lung, that portion of cardiac output diverted to the nondependent lung still participates in gas exchange as long as the upper lung is being ventilated or exposed to CPAP.

Indications and Techniques for One-Lung Ventilation

The absolute indications for one-lung ventilation include situations in which it is necessary to prevent the spillage and consequent spread of blood or pus from one lung to the other or to allow for control of the airway in patients with bronchial pleural fistula, giant unilateral lung cysts, or major tracheobronchial disruptions. In rare situations, it is also necessary to provide one-lung ventilation in patients having unilateral pulmonary lavage. With the introduction of video-assisted thoracic surgery, another absolute indication for one-lung ventilation has evolved. Some have performed video-assisted thoracic surgery with unilateral insufflation of the thorax and others with high-frequency jet ventilation; however, the surgical field is far from optimal. Both of these techniques do not provide a collapsed, quiet, lung that facilitates video-assisted thoracic surgery. In our institution, video-assisted thoracic surgery is an absolute indication for one-lung ventilation, which provides optimal lung collapse, allowing for efficient surgery with a low conversion rate to an open thoracotomy.

The remaining indications for one-lung ventilation are relative with high-priority surgical procedures being thoracic aortic aneurysm repair and major pulmonary resections. Most operations that are performed in the thoracic cavity can be facilitated by one-lung ventilation. In such instances, the lung can be collapsed to allow for better access to organs such as the esophagus, pericardium, mediastinum, and pleural. The surgeons then have no need to compress and retract the lung that inherently would lead to less trauma to the lung. An additional benefit of one-lung ventilation for relative indications is that in most instances, the surgeons are able to operate more efficiently if they are not otherwise exerting their time and efforts by trying to keep the lung out of their surgical field.

Several techniques are available to provide one-lung ventilation, with the most common being double-lumen endotracheal tube. Double-lumen tubes are available with either left- or right-directed bronchial lumina and come in sizes 28F, 32F, 35F, 37F, 39F, and 41F. Tube-size recommendations can be based on gender and height. A 39F is recommended for men 165 cm or less in height, and a 41F is recommended for men taller than 165 cm. A 35F is recommended for women 160 cm or less in height, with a 37F being used for women who are taller than 160 cm (14). Another way to estimate double-lumen–tube size is to review the chest radiograph for physical anatomy of the airways. Brodsky et al. (15) reported measuring the width of the trachea at the level of the clavicles and correlated this width to choose an appropriately sized left-directed double-lumen tube. If the trachea measured more than or equal to 18 mm, a 41F tube was placed; for more than or equal to 16 mm, a 39F; for more than or equal to 15 mm, a 37F; and for a tracheal diameter of less than 15 mm, a 35F double-lumen tube was used. The average tracheal width for men was 21 mm, and for women, it was 17 mm. All double-lumen tubes selected using this measurement technique were successfully placed (15). In the past, physicians have also estimated the diameter of the main bronchi by considering the diameter of the small finger. The largest size double-lumen tube that can comfortably pass through the glottis should be used, because this leads to more accurate positioning, less chance of dislodgment, and less chance of too distal advancement of the tube. In addition, using the larger size tube minimizes airflow resistance and allows for easy passage of suction catheters and fiberoptic bronchoscopes. Also, the smaller the tube, the greater is the volume of air needed to inflate the bronchial cuff. This may result in higher lateral pressures against the bronchial wall, which may increase the risk of airway trauma, ischemia of the bronchial wall, and cuff herniation proximally into the carina, leading to obstruction of the opposing lung's ventilation.

The preferred bronchial direction of the double-lumen tube, either right or left, varies. Many anesthesiologists prefer to use left-sided double-lumen tubes whenever possible because of their ease of placement and a larger "margin of safety" for their proper placement. The length of the left main bronchus in men is approximately 49 mm, and in women, 44 mm, whereas the length of the right main bronchus is only 19 mm in men and 15 mm in women. Benumof et al. (16) describe the "margin of safety" as the length of the tracheal bronchial tree over which a double-lumen tube may be moved or positioned without obstructing a conducting airway. The average margin of safety for positioning a left-sided double-lumen tube was 16 to 19 mm and for right-sided tubes was only 1 to 9 mm (16). This margin of safety also improves as the tube size becomes larger, such that the margin of safety for a 41F double-lumen tube is better than that for a 35F double-lumen tube. Because of the potential for easier placement and better margin of safety, Benumof and colleagues recommend using a left-sided double-lumen tube whenever possible. Our preference is to direct the double-lumen tube away from the site of surgery whenever possible. When the double-lumen tube is directed to the opposite side of surgery, the need for possible repositioning of the tube during surgery, such as for pneumonectomy, is eliminated and the potential for the tube to be dislodged by surgical manipulation of the airway is also greatly reduced. By using right-sided double-lumen tubes more frequently, one can diminish the degree of difficulty due to unfamiliarity with the device. Campos et al. recently described 40 patients undergoing left thoracotomy (17). Twenty patients were managed with left-sided double-lumen tubes and 20 with right-sided double-lumen tubes. The tube size was determined by measuring the width of the trachea from the preoperative chest radiograph, as described by Brodsky et al. (15). Time to properly position the left-sided double-lumen tubes was 2 minutes, compared to 3½ minutes for the right-sided double-lumen tubes. Five malpositions occurred with right-sided double-lumen tubes, compared to two for the left-sided double-lumen tubes, which was not statistically significant. They reported equally good surgical exposure with both right- and left-sided double-lumen tubes and there were no upper-lobe obstructions in either group. The authors concluded that right-sided double-lumen tubes presented no increased risk of complications for left-sided surgery and should not be abandoned. The anatomy of the airway should be known before placement of any device into the airway, including double-lumen tubes. Before using a right-sided double-lumen tube, the operator should confirm adequate length of the right main bronchus, because a short right main or anomalous right upper-lobe bronchus make the use of a right-sided double-lumen tube extremely difficult or impossible. Tumors in the airway as well as external compression by tumors or the aorta will also influence the bronchial direction of the double-lumen tube.

Proper positioning of the double-lumen tube is essential for successful and efficient one-lung ventilation. Proper double-lumen tube placement should be confirmed by auscultation followed by fiberoptic bronchoscopy to ensure proper positioning. The left and right lung fields are initially auscultated to confirm that the double-lumen tube is indeed in the trachea and end-tidal CO_2 is observed. To confirm the proper position of a left-sided double-lumen tube, one performs systematic auscultation of the lungs along with double-lumen tube lumen clamping. In a systematic fashion, the left lung is auscultated, followed by clamping of the left bronchial lumen. Lung sounds should now be decreased or absent on the left. The clamp remains in place and breath sounds should now be heard on the right. The clamp is next moved to occlude the right lumen and eliminate breath sounds on the right. Breath sounds should now be heard on the left, confirming, in this example, a properly positioned left-sided double-lumen tube. We prefer to have left-sided double-lumen tubes positioned in the bronchus such that the inflated cuff of the bronchial lumen is in the middle of the left main bronchus. This position is then confirmed and optimized with a fiberoptic bronchoscopy passed through the tracheal lumen of the left-sided double-lumen tube (Fig. 26-13). In placing a right-sided double-lumen tube, one follows the same initial sequence of auscultation as that for a left-sided double-lumen tube except for fiberoptic confirmation of placement. After confirmation by auscultation that the right-sided double-lumen tube is in the right main bronchus, the fiberoptic bronchoscope is passed into the bronchial lumen and is positioned to view through the ventilation slot. The right upper-lobe bronchus should be in view. In many cases, this indeed is not in view initially and the double-lumen tube should be gradually withdrawn until the right upper-lobe bronchus comes into view (Fig. 26-14). Both the tracheal and the bronchial cuffs should be deflated before movement of the double-lumen tube. Proper positioning of the ventilation slot for the right upper lobe is of paramount importance when using right-sided double-lumen tubes to avoid obstruction of the right upper bronchus. Although use of fiberoptic bronchoscopy is key to this effort, the patient must have the proper airway anatomy for right-sided double-lumen tube use. If the patient has an anatomic variance in which there is a high takeoff of the bronchus to the right upper lobe, use of a right-sided tube would be contraindicated. This anomaly occurs in approximately 1 out of every 250 patients (18).

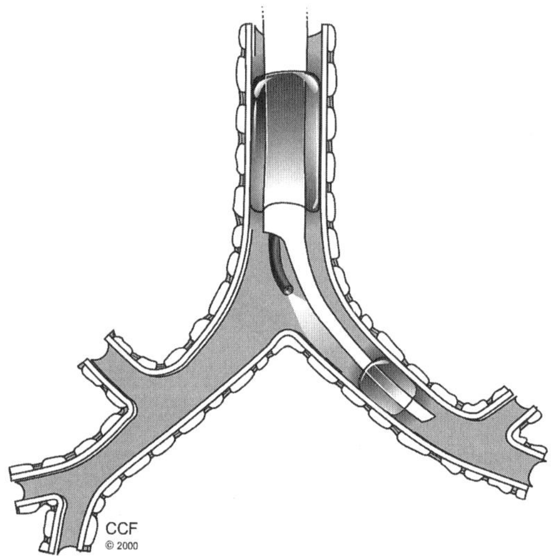

FIGURE 26-13. Recommended positioning for left-sided double-lumen endotracheal tubes.

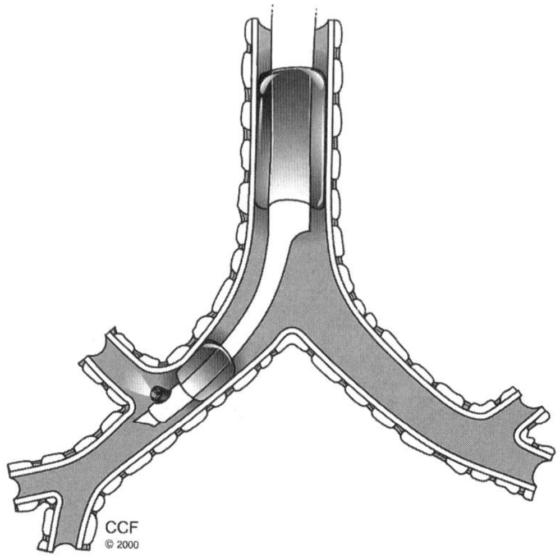

FIGURE 26-14. Recommended positioning for right-sided double-lumen endotracheal tubes.

Auscultation followed by fiberoptic bronchoscopy offers great confidence that a double-lumen tube is properly positioned. In situations in which the leak of fluid from one lung to the other would be catastrophic, confirmation that the bronchial cuff has achieved a watertight seal should be considered. During unilateral bronchopulmonary lavage and when there is a risk of contamination of one lung by spillage of blood or purulent material, an adequate cuff seal and complete functional separation of two lungs must be confirmed with absolute certainty. This can be done using the air bubble method. The tracheal lumen is clamped and its suction port opened. An intravenous extension tube is connected to the suction port of the tracheal lumen, and

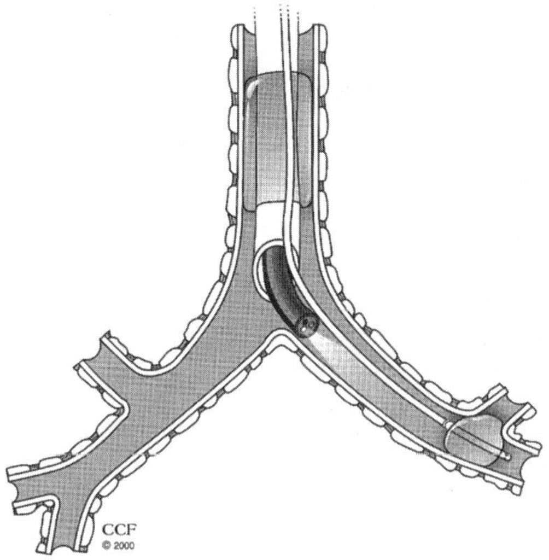

FIGURE 26-15. Recommended positioning of a left-sided bronchial blocker.

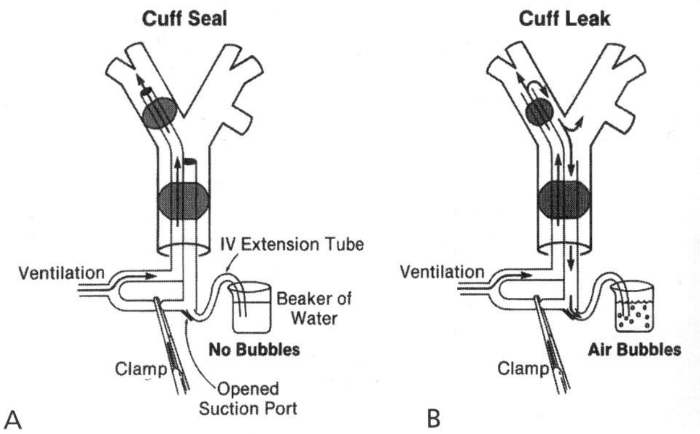

FIGURE 26-16. The air bubble detection method for checking adequacy of the seal of the left endobronchial cuff of a left-sided double-lumen tube. **A:** When the left lung is selectively ventilated or exposed to any desired distending pressure, and the left cuff is adequately sealed, no air will escape around the left cuff and out the open right suction port, and thus, no bubbles will be observed passing through the beaker of water. **B:** When the left lung is ventilated or exposed to any desired distending pressure and the left endobronchial cuff is not adequately sealed, air will escape around the left cuff and out the open right suction port, and thus, air bubbles will be observed passing through the beaker of water. (From Benumof JL, ed. *Anesthesia for thoracic surgery,* 2nd ed. Philadelphia: WB Saunders, 1995, with permission.)

its other end is submerged in a beaker of water. Both cuffs are inflated to achieve an adequate seal. Positive-pressure ventilation is then applied to the bronchial lumen. No bubbles should appear in the beaker, as this would indicate air leaking around the bronchial cuff entering the trachea (Fig. 26-15).

Bronchial blockers may also be used to provide one-lung ventilation. For this purpose, we commonly use a Baxter Fogarty (Fogarty-Baxter Healthcare Corporation, McGraw Park, IL) cava occlusion catheter with a 10-mL balloon (model CV 1012). Bronchial blockers are always directed toward the side of surgery and are most commonly positioned outside of a single-lumen endotracheal tube. Laryngoscopy is performed; the bronchial blocker is placed into the trachea followed by the single-lumen tube. To facilitate passage of the bronchial blocker into the desired main-stem bronchus, the tip of the bronchial blocker is bent into the shape of a hockey stick. The angle of the bend should be about 45° and start 3 cm from the tip of the bronchial blocker. This angle in the bronchial blocker will then be used to deflect off of the carina as the bronchial blocker is rotated to direct it into the desired main stem bronchus with the guidance provided by fiberoptic bronchoscopy. We recommend positioning the left-sided bronchial blocker so the inflated balloon expands into the upper-lobe bronchus. This positioning will help to decrease the incidence of the bronchial blocker becoming malpositioned (Fig. 26-16). A right-sided bronchial blocker is similarly positioned such that the balloon inflates up into the upper-lobe bronchus. Our preference is to avoid using right-directed bronchial blockers, because the short length of the right main bronchus, when compared to that of the left, allows for it to become easily dislodged.

Bronchial blockers may also be placed directly through a single-lumen tube in situations such as a difficult airway or if the need for one-lung ventilation occurs unexpectedly during surgery. In this situation, the cap to a Portex (Concord/Portex, Keene, NH) fiberoptic bronchoscopy swivel adapter is modified by cutting off the tip, thereby leaving a hole through which a lubricated bronchial blocker can be inserted (Fig. 26-17). The bronchial blocker can then be positioned into the appropriate bronchus with the guidance of fiberoptic bronchoscopy. A newer device, the Arndt bronchial blocker (Cook Critical Care, Bloomington, IN), provides a bronchial blocker with a small port along its center, which contains a monofilament guide loop. This device is used through the lumen of a single-lumen tube. The guide loop is passed over a pediatric fiberoptic bronchoscope, the fiberoptic bronchoscope is directed into the desired main bronchus and the bronchial blocker is then advanced into position (Fig. 26-18).

Another technique for achieving one-lung ventilation is an endotracheal tube with a movable endobronchial blocker, the Univent tube (Univent, Fuji Systems Corporation, Tokyo, Japan). This tube consists of an endotracheal tube with a small channel bored throughout the anterior wall that transmits an endobronchial blocker having a low-pressure, high-volume cuff. The Univent tube is inserted into the trachea then turned 90° toward the side in which the thoracotomy is to be carried out. The blocker is pushed downward, into the targeted main bronchus (Fig. 26-19). Fine adjustments of the blocker's position are carried out using fiberoptic bronchoscopy. The bronchial blocker has

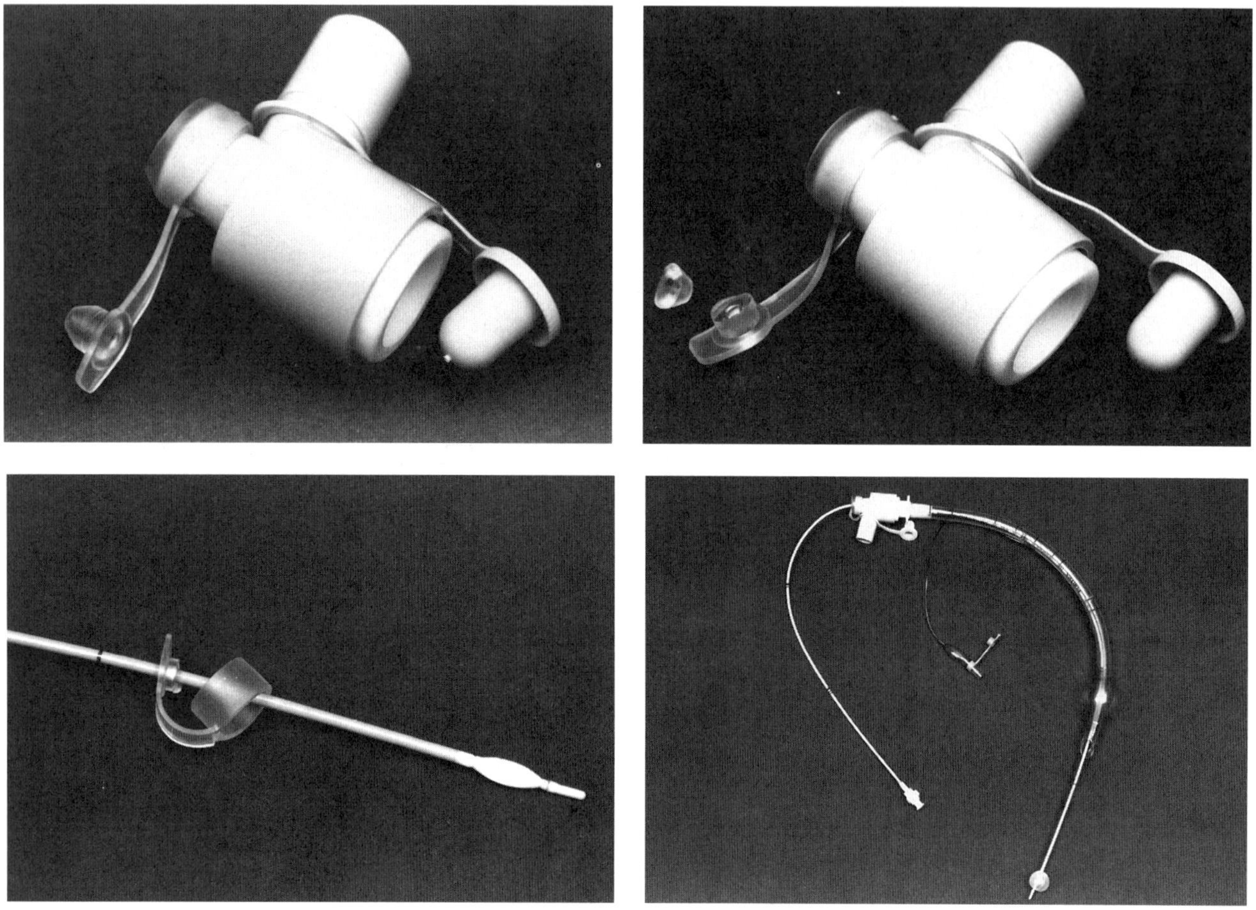

FIGURE 26-17. Top left: Portex swivel adapter. **Top right:** Portex swivel adapter with tip of plunger cut off. **Bottom left:** Bronchial blocker passed through plunger and cap of swivel adapter. **Bottom right:** Bronchial blocker passed through Portex swivel adapter and endotracheal tube.

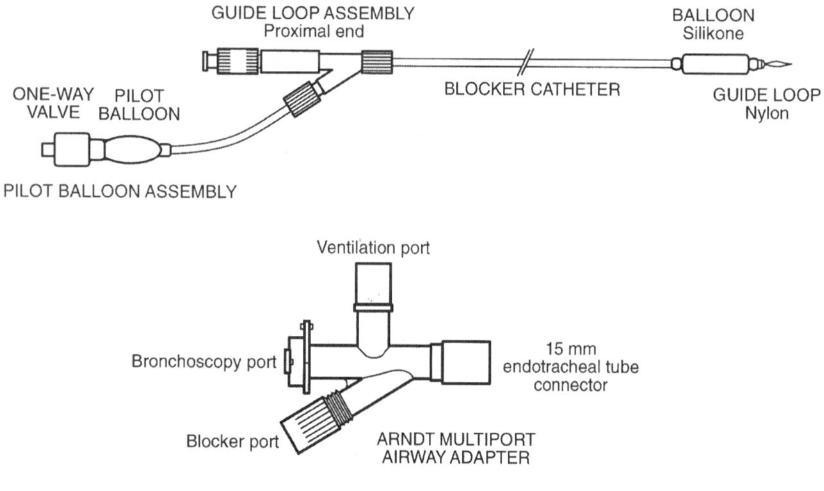

FIGURE 26-18. Arndt endobronchial blocker with multiport airway adapter.

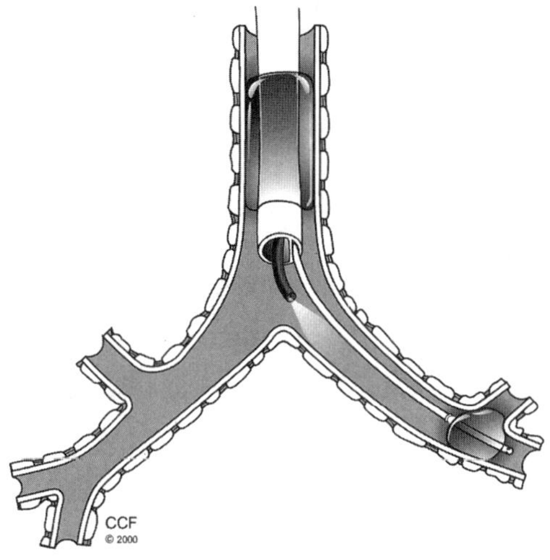

FIGURE 26-19. Recommended positioning for the Univent tube.

a small lumen, which allows the escape of air and potentially the administration of oxygen. One should exercise caution when administering oxygen through this port because of the potential for development of high airway pressures distal to the port of the Univent's bronchial blocker.

Diligent management of the various bronchial blocker devices and the use of fiberoptic bronchoscopy are essential to help ensure their success. We recommend placing the bronchial blocker deep into the main bronchus such that when the balloon is inflated, under direct vision, it slightly protrudes into either the left or the right upper bronchus. This positioning will give some stabilization to the bronchial blocker and decrease its potential to become malpositioned. Bronchial blockers should be inflated when the patient is supine or immediately after the patient has been positioned to allow for optimal lung collapse. One may also choose to deflate both lungs, inflate the bronchial blocker, and then resume ventilation in an effort to optimize lung collapse. The administration of 100% oxygen is commonly required and in addition to preventing hypoxemia also aids to collapse of the operative lung by absorption atelectasis. During surgery, hypoxemia can be initially addressed by the judicious application of PEEP to the dependent lung, followed by brief deflations of the bronchial blocker to allow for one or two small tidal volumes to the operative lung. The clinician must be aware that manipulation of the bronchial blocker increases the risk for malposition.

Most simplistically, one-lung ventilation can be obtained by main stem intubation with a single-lumen tube. This technique has been the mainstay in pediatric thoracic surgery on small infants for whom other devices are much too large. In adults, this simple technique can also be used for situations when one-lung ventilation is required on short notice or when the airway has been difficult to secure. Rapid surgery is important because even with positive-pressure ventilation, blood flow through the collapsed lung often leads to hypoxemia. Disadvantages of single-lumen endobronchial intubation include inability to suction the manipulated lung or to reexpand it if hypoxemia develops intraoperatively, unless the tube is pulled back into the trachea. Instantaneous unilateral endobronchial intubation using a single-lumen endotracheal tube can be a lifesaving measure in patients with massive pulmonary hemorrhage. In these patients, because of the anatomic structure of the tracheobronchial tree, left-sided endobronchial intubation is not easily accomplished blindly. Turning the head to the right after the tube has passed through the vocal cords, then rotating the tube 180°, and then advancing it results in a 92% success rate in "blind" intubation of the left main bronchus (19).

High-frequency ventilation is an alternative mode of ventilation that has been used to provide a quiet operative field during thoracic surgery. This type of ventilation has the advantage of not requiring one-lung ventilation; however, it does require modified endotracheal tubes, special equipment, and a totally intravenous anesthetic technique. Although high-frequency ventilation is able to provide a quiet nonmoving field, the lungs are nearly fully inflated and occasionally can become overdistended due to airtrapping—all of which can make surgical conditions less than optimal.

The success and efficient establishment of one-lung ventilation by any device or technique is facilitated by the frequent use of fiberoptic bronchoscopy. Although auscultation can roughly confirm the proper position of these devices, a fiberoptic examination allows for fine-tuning. In a study by Smith and coworkers (20), bronchoscopy findings after confirmation of double-lumen tube placement by auscultation revealed less than satisfactory positioning in 48% of patients. In 17% of patients, herniation of the bronchial cuff over the carina was noted, requiring repositioning of the double-lumen tube (20). Regardless of which technique is used to achieve one-lung ventilation, patient repositioning and neck extension and flexion can cause the device employed to become malpositioned. Flexion of the neck leads to distal migration of the tip of the endotracheal and endobronchial lumina up to 3.5 cm. This can lead to difficulty in ventilating the lung and to obstruction of an upper-lobe bronchus. Extension of the neck can lead to proximal migration of the tube and possibly to extubation of the bronchus. Fiberoptic bronchoscopy should therefore be performed while the patient is supine and again after repositioning. Failure of one-lung ventilation intraoperatively is also frequently remedied by the use of fiberoptic bronchoscopy and should remain available during surgery.

Complications of one-lung ventilation include faulty device placement, hypoxia, hypercarbia, trauma, and difficulty clearing secretions. As addressed previously, the key to proper placement of the device to provide one-lung ventilation is confirmation by auscultation followed by fiberoptic bronchoscopy. Hypoxemia is addressed by the use of 100% oxygen during the period of one-lung ventilation and the judicious use of PEEP and CPAP, which will be detailed later in this chapter. Choosing smaller size tubes and only repositioning double-lumen tubes with both the bronchial and tracheal cuffs deflated can decrease trauma to the vocal cords, trachea, and bronchi. Although clinically unproven, it also seems reasonable that vocal cord trauma could potentially be decreased by earlier removal of double-lumen tubes. If a patient is unable to be extubated before leaving the operating room, our preference is to change the double-lumen tube to a single-lumen tube under direct vision, thereby allowing for easier ventilation, better patient comfort, and more efficient secretion control. Changing the double-lumen tube to a single-lumen tube may also be accomplished over a longer tube exchanger that has been developed specifically for this purpose. In patients with extreme tongue and upper-airway edema, the double-lumen tube should remain in place. Usually overnight ventilation with the patient's head elevated to 45° allows the edema to subside, and then the tube can be exchanged or the patient can be safely extubated.

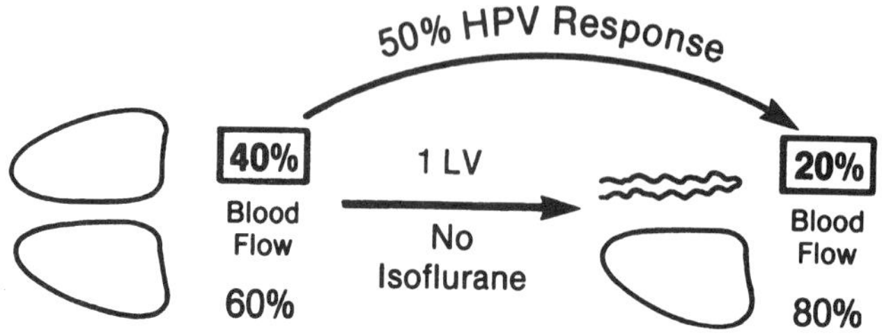

FIGURE 26-20. **A:** With two-lung ventilation, the nondependent lung–to–dependent lung blood flow ratio is 40%:60%. **B:** When two-lung ventilation is converted to one-lung ventilation (as indicated by atelectasis of the nondependent lung), the hypoxic pulmonary vasoconstriction response decreases the blood flow to the nondependent lung by 50%, so the nondependent lung–to–dependent lung blood flow ratio is now 20%:80%. (From Benumof JL, ed. *Anesthesia for thoracic surgery,* 2nd ed. Philadelphia: WB Saunders, 1995, with permission.)

Oxygenation During One-Lung Ventilation

Hypoxic Pulmonary Vasoconstriction

If one lung or part of a lung is made hypoxic by either atelectasis or ventilation with a hypoxic gas mixture, active vasoconstriction of the pulmonary artery supplying that hypoxic segment occurs, leading to the diversion of blood to the better ventilated, nonhypoxic lung segments. This is a protective mechanism that decreases the amount of shunt and improves the arterial oxygenation in the presence of regional lung hypoxia. The phenomenon is known as HPV. When fully operational and in the absence of inhibiting factors, a single-lung HPV response can decrease blood flow to that lung by 50%. When a patient is in the lateral decubitus position, the dependent lung receives 60% of the cardiac output, whereas the nondependent lung receives about 40% of the cardiac output. If the nondependent lung is not ventilated and made atelectatic, a maximal HPV response can decrease its blood supply by 50%. As a result, the dependent lung receives 80% of the cardiac output, and the upside atelectatic lung receives only 20% of the cardiac output (Fig. 26-20). Therefore, the arterial oxygen tension ($Pa{O_2}$) observed during regional lung hypoxia is much higher than would be expected if no HPV response were present. The main stimulus for development of HPV is a decrease in alveolar oxygen tension ($PA{O_2}$). Mixed venous oxygen tension ($P\bar{v}{O_2}$), indirectly influences the HPV response. The hypoxia-sensitive site in the lung is thought to be an extravascular receptor on the arterial side of the pulmonary vasculature, functionally closer to the alveoli than to the responding vessel (21).

Hemodynamic variables can influence the magnitude of HPV. Increases in pulmonary vascular pressures can mechanically open and recruit closed vessels in hypoxic lung regions, overcoming part of the active pulmonary vasoconstriction (22). HPV is optimal when the pulmonary vascular pressure is within the normal range and is decreased with either high or low pressures. An increase in cardiac output can also mask the HPV response by recruiting pulmonary vessels or by increasing $P\bar{v}{O_2}$. HPV is decreased by hypocapnia but is not increased by hypercapnia (23). HPV is maximal at normal pH levels. It is decreased by acidosis or alkalosis, whether induced by metabolic or respiratory means. The chemical mediators of HPV have also been the subjects of considerable research. Calcium channel blockers were found to attenuate HPV. In addition, potentiators of calcium channels have been found to augment HPV. Some evidence indicates that calcium agonists also act on mast cells or basophils to inhibit the release of vasoactive substances, which have been proposed as mediators of pulmonary vasoconstriction (24). Most systemic vasodilator drugs inhibit HPV including nitroglycerin, sodium nitroprusside, and dobutamine. These agents preferentially vasodilate the hypoxic lung and therefore inhibit HPV. Calcium channel blockers including nifedipine, minoxidil, and verapamil have been shown to inhibit HPV. β-Agonists such as isoproterenol, ritodrine, salbutamol, and glucagon inhibit HPV. Aminophylline and hydralazine did not inhibit HPV in canines. Vasoconstrictors such as dopamine, epinephrine, and phenylephrine inhibit HPV by causing preferential vasoconstriction in the normoxic lung, thereby increasing flow to the hypoxic lung (25).

Extensive studies have been performed to examine the effect of inhalation and intravenous anesthetics on HPV.

Findings on the effect of anesthetics on HPV differ according to the type of experimental preparation used. In the *in vitro* and *in vivo* nonintact preparations, the inhalation agents are found to have a significant inhibitory effect on HPV. However, in the more physiologic *in vivo* intact and human studies, inhalation agents only cause a slight decrease in HPV. Nitrous oxide (N_2O) seems to cause a small but somewhat consistent inhibition of HPV. All intravenous anesthetics studied to date have no effect on HPV. The potent, volatile anesthetics inhibit HPV to various degrees. When compared to intravenous anesthesia, 1-MAC halothane inhibited HPV, causing a small increase in shunt of 7% to the nondependent lung, and 1-MAC isoflurane produced an insignificant 2% increase in shunt. This study concluded that the use of halogenated agents was not a clinically significant issue (26). Isoflurane is known to allow for better oxygenation than halothane and has also been shown to be superior to enflurane (27). Another study showed that oxygenation during one-lung ventilation with propofol anesthesia was greater than with either isoflurane or sevoflurane. This same study showed that the effects on oxygenation with isoflurane were similar to those with sevoflurane (28). Desflurane has also been shown to have the similar effects as isoflurane on arterial oxygenation during one-lung ventilation (29). Although the volatile anesthetics produce a small decrease in oxygenation during one-lung ventilation, they have several desirable properties during thoracic surgery. They decrease airway irritability and obtund airway reflexes in patients who usually have reactive airway disease. Using volatile agents allows for the elimination of N_2O and the administration of high inspired O_2 concentration. And finally, volatile agents are rapidly eliminated and produce less postoperative respiratory depression than opioids.

Blood Flow Distribution in the Lateral Decubitus Position

Blood flow to the nondependent, nonventilated lung is decreased in patients in the lateral decubitus position because of passive mechanical mechanisms such as gravity and surgical interference with blood flow and with the institution of one-lung ventilation, the nondependent lung becomes atelectatic and HPV ensues, diverting the blood to the dependent lung. HPV starts shortly after pulmonary hypoxia occurs and usually takes 20 to 30 minutes to reach maximal intensity. In the lateral decubitus position, 60% of the blood flow goes to the dependent lung and 40% to the nondependent lung. With the institution of one-lung ventilation, a total uninhibited HPV response is capable of diverting half the blood flow from the nondependent lung to the dependent lung. This results in 20% of the cardiac output flowing through the atelectatic nondependent lung and 80% through the dependent lung. The shunt fraction would therefore be 20% of cardiac output. However, these shunt fractions are influenced and altered by the amount of disease in the nondependent lung. If the nondependent lung is severely diseased, a fixed reduction in the blood flow to this lung may already exist preoperatively and the collapse of such a diseased lung may not cause further significant increase in the shunt fractions. Not surprisingly patients who have the greatest decrease in PaO_2 with the institution of one-lung ventilation are those who have healthy lungs and are undergoing thoracotomy for nonpulmonary disease. The HPV response is maximal when PVR is normal and is decreased by either high or low pulmonary vascular pressure. The HPV response is also maximal when the $P\bar{v}O_2$ level is normal and is decreased by either a high or a low $P\bar{v}O_2$ level. The intraoperative use of vasoactive drugs can interfere with or modify the HPV response. Agents such as sodium nitroprusside and nitroglycerin inhibit HPV by causing more vasodilation in the nondependent lung, thereby increasing the shunt. Vasopressors such as phenylephrine also decrease shunt because of preferential vasoconstriction in the dependent lung, which acts to increase blood flow to the nondependent lung and thereby increases the shunt flow. Hypocapnia and respiratory alkalosis directly inhibit HPV response in the atelectatic lung. On the other hand, hypercapnia and respiratory acidosis do not enhance HPV. Hypercapnia can actually interfere with the efficiency of the HPV response by inducing vasoconstriction and increasing PVR in the dependent lung, thereby decreasing its ability to receive the blood diverted to it from the nondependent lung.

Blood flow to the dependent lung is increased when the patient is in the lateral decubitus position because of the passive effect of gravity and surgical manipulation of the upside lung and the development of HPV in the upside lung. However, the development of atelectasis and areas with a low $\dot{V}/\dot{Q}$ ratio in the dependent lung can interfere with arterial oxygenation during one-lung ventilation. During two-lung ventilation in the anesthetized paralyzed patient in the lateral decubitus position, the fraction of tidal volume delivered to the dependent lung is about 35% to 40% less than that delivered to the nondependent lung. The FRC of the dependent lung is also decreased to about one half the FRC of the nondependent lung (30). An additional 10% decrease in the FRC of the dependent lung occurs consistently when the nondependent pleura is opened (31). The dependent lung is compressed by the weight of the mediastinum, by chest rolls on the operating table below, and cephalad displacement of the diaphragm by the intraabdominal viscera. In addition, varying degrees of interstitial edema from the gravity-induced elevation of pulmonary capillary hydrostatic pressure can result in further decreases in the dependent lung's FRC and compliance. The decrease in the dependent lung's FRC is actually improved when one-lung ventilation is instituted, leading to the diversion of the entire tidal volume to the dependent lung. Areas of absorption atelectasis can occur in regions of low $\dot{V}/\dot{Q}$ ratios when they are exposed to a high inspired oxygen concentration. Areas of atelectasis and low $\dot{V}/\dot{Q}$ ratio can therefore develop intraoperatively in the dependent lung (32).

Maximizing Oxygenation in the Lateral Decubitus Position

The basic principles for the initial management of the patient on one-lung ventilation include (a) initially administering 100% oxygen, (b) starting one-lung ventilation with a relatively large tidal volume of 8 to 12 mL/kg, (c) adjusting respiratory rate to keep Pa_{CO_2} about 40 mm Hg, (d) continuously monitoring oxygenation and ventilation with pulse oximetry and end-tidal CO_2 concentrations, and (e) facilitating pulmonary vasodilation in the dependent lung to promote the diversion of blood from the nondependent lung. With the institution of one-lung ventilation, the initial tidal volume should be about 10 mL/kg, which can be adjusted upward or downward by monitoring airway pressure, end-tidal CO_2, and arterial blood gases. Using an excessively high tidal volume to the dependent lung can lead to increases in airway pressure and PVR and diversion of blood back to the nondependent lung (33). An excessively small tidal volume to the dependent lung can lead to a further decrease in FRC, airway closure, and development of atelectasis. Atelectasis in the dependent lung impairs the effectiveness of HPV in the nondependent lung and the ability to maintain adequate arterial oxygenation. The respiratory rate should be adjusted to maintain near baseline CO_2 tension. The change from two-lung ventilation to one-lung ventilation usually causes no problem with CO_2 elimination because of the very high diffuseness of CO_2 across the alveolar membrane. Hypocapnia should be avoided because it can directly dilate the pulmonary vessels in the nondependent lung, thus interfering with its HPV. In patients with elevated baseline Pa_{CO_2}, mild to moderate hypercapnia may be well tolerated. Arterial pH monitoring may serve as a useful guide.

Because the dependent lung often has a decreased volume during one-lung ventilation, an attempt can be made to improve oxygenation by applying PEEP to the ventilated lung. The application of PEEP to the dependent lung results in recruitment of closed alveoli and airways, increased FRC, and finally compliance, but it has the potential disadvantage of increasing PVR in that lung, leading to the diversion of some blood back toward the nondependent lung. The application of PEEP may have a variable effect on Pa_{O_2} if the nondependent lung is totally collapsed and hypoxic. The net result would be the balance between the beneficial effects of increasing dependent lung compliance and the deleterious effects of the redistribution of blood to the dependent lung. Some patients have an improved Pa_{O_2}, some have no change, and some have decreased oxygenation. Patients who have a relatively normal dependent lung may have decreased oxygenation if PEEP is applied to the dependent lung without CPAP to the nondependent lung (Fig. 26-21). A level of PEEP of more than 5 cm H_2O is seldom needed and may be harmful if the level of PEEP compresses the pulmonary artery in the dependent lung, thereby diverting blood flow to the nondependent lung and increasing shunt. The application of CPAP to the nonventilated, nondependent lung is the single most important measure to improve oxygenation during one-lung ventilation (Fig. 26-22). CPAP should be applied during the deflation phase of a larger tidal volume. In human (34) and dog (35) studies, O_2 insufflation below zero airway pressure did not significantly improve Pa_{O_2} because of the inability to overcome critical opening pressures of collapsed alveoli. The three essential features of a CPAP system are an oxygen source, a pressure monitor, and a variable pop-off valve (Fig. 26-23). An anesthesia reservoir bag may be part of the CPAP system, which allows delivery of independent tidal breaths or sighs to the nondependent lung. In most CPAP systems, an O_2 flow rate of 5 to 10 L/minute creates a CPAP of 5 to 20 cm H_2O.

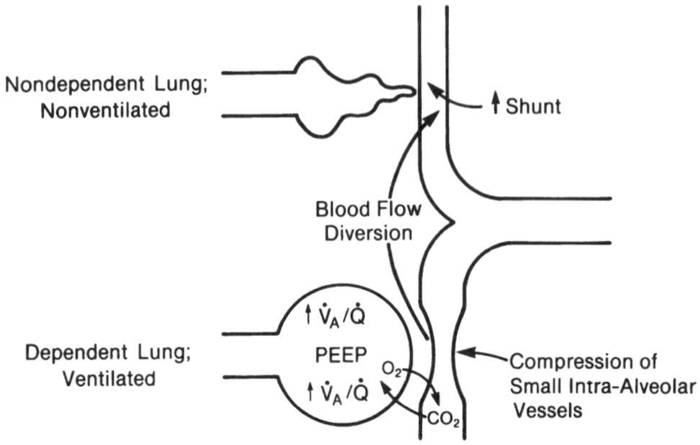

FIGURE 26-21. Selective positive end-expiratory pressure (PEEP) to the ventilation-dependent lung can increase dependent lung ventilation-perfusion ration (↑V_A/Q). However, dependent lung PEEP can also cause compression of the small intraalveolar vessels in the dependent lung, causing blood flow diversion to the nonventilated nondependent lung, thereby increasing the shunt through the nonventilated nondependent lung. Therefore, the overall arterial oxygenation effect of dependent lung PEEP will be a trade-off between the good effect of an increase in dependent lung V_A/Q and the bad effect of increased nonventilated lung blood flow. (From Benumof JL, ed. *Anesthesia for thoracic surgery,* 2nd ed. Philadelphia: WB Saunders, 1995, with permission.)

In summary, the most effective initial step to improve arterial oxygenation would be to apply 5 to 10 cm of CPAP to the nondependent lung. If not sufficient, the next step would be to apply 5 cm H_2O of PEEP to the dependent lung (Fig. 26-24). If arterial oxygenation remains subopti-

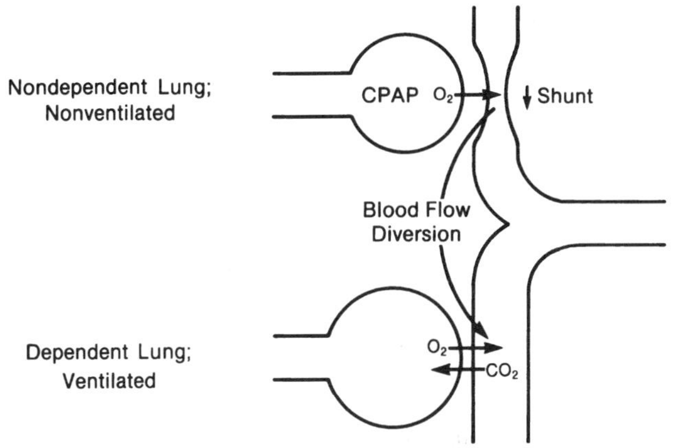

FIGURE 26-22. Selective continuous positive airway pressure (CPAP) to the nonventilated nondependent lung (static distention without tidal movement) allows this lung to participate in oxygen uptake and markedly decreases the shunt through the nonventilated nondependent lung. Even if the nonventilated nondependent lung CPAP causes blood flow diversion to the ventilated dependent lung, the diverted flow still can participate in oxygen uptake and CO_2 elimination in the ventilated dependent lung. Usually 5 to 10 cm H_2O of nondependent lung CPAP is all that is clinically needed, and this amount of CPAP does not cause any significant surgical interference. (From Benumof JL, ed. *Anesthesia for thoracic surgery,* 2nd ed. Philadelphia: WB Saunders, 1995, with permission.)

mal, which would be extremely unusual, one should reassess and optimize the position of the double-lumen tube with fiberoptic bronchoscopy. The patient's hemodynamic status should also be evaluated and optimized. A decrease in mixed venous oxygen saturation ($S\bar{v}O_2$) can magnify the effect of any shunt on arterial oxygenation. If hypoxemia is still present, nondependent lung CPAP should then be increased to

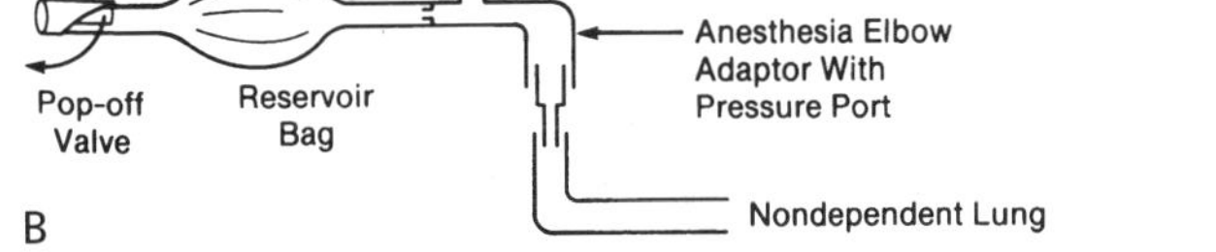

FIGURE 26-23. Two **(A and B)** nondependent lung continuous positive airway pressure (CPAP) systems with reservoir bags. Both of these systems contain an oxygen source, some type of pressure relief valve, and a pressure manometer to measure the CPAP. The presence of a reservoir bag allows for intermittent positive-pressure breathing and sighing, if desired. (From Benumof JL, ed. *Anesthesia for thoracic surgery,* 2nd ed. Philadelphia: WB Saunders, 1995, with permission.)

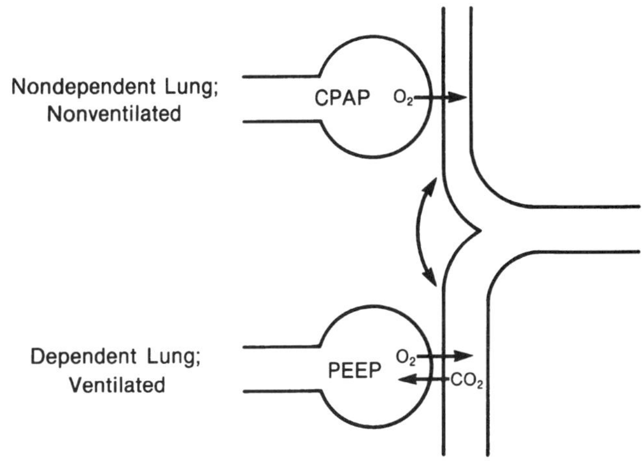

FIGURE 26-24. Differential lung continuous positive airway pressure (CPAP)/positive end-expiratory pressure (PEEP) during one-lung ventilation allows for the entire lung to participate in oxygen uptake and markedly reduces the shunt during one-lung ventilation. With differential lung CPAP/PEEP, the distribution of blood flow is not critically important because all of the lung can participate in oxygen uptake. (From Benumof JL, ed. *Anesthesia for thoracic surgery,* 2nd ed. Philadelphia: WB Saunders, 1995, with permission.)

10 cm H_2O (Fig. 26-25). If hypoxemia still persists after differential CPAP/PEEP, which would be extremely rare, the nondependent lung may be intermittently ventilated with positive pressure and 100% O_2. Finally, clamping or ligation of the pulmonary artery of the nonventilated lung will eliminate most of the $\dot{V}/\dot{Q}$ mismatch (Fig. 26-26).

Anesthetic Techniques

Thoracic surgery can be performed with a patient under general or regional anesthesia or a combination of both. Most thoracotomies are performed under general anesthesia with controlled ventilation. General anesthesia can be induced with thiopental (3 to 5 mg/kg), etomidate (0.3 mg/kg), or propofol (2 to 3 mg/kg). In most patients in whom extubation is planned at the end of the procedure or shortly thereafter, we usually use opioids to supplement the inhala-

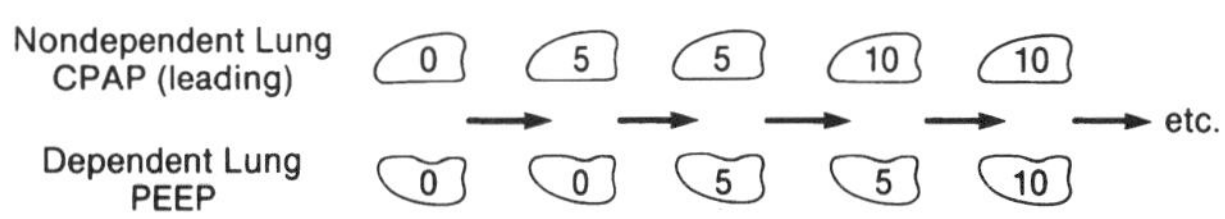

FIGURE 26-25. A search for optimal nondependent lung continuous positive airway pressure (CPAP) and dependent lung positive end-expiratory pressure (PEEP) is performed by leading with nondependent lung CPAP and following with dependent lung PEEP. Leading with nondependent lung CPAP removes the deleterious arterial oxygenation blood flow diversion effects of dependent lung PEEP. (From Benumof JL, ed. *Anesthesia for thoracic surgery,* 2nd ed. Philadelphia: WB Saunders, 1995, with permission.)

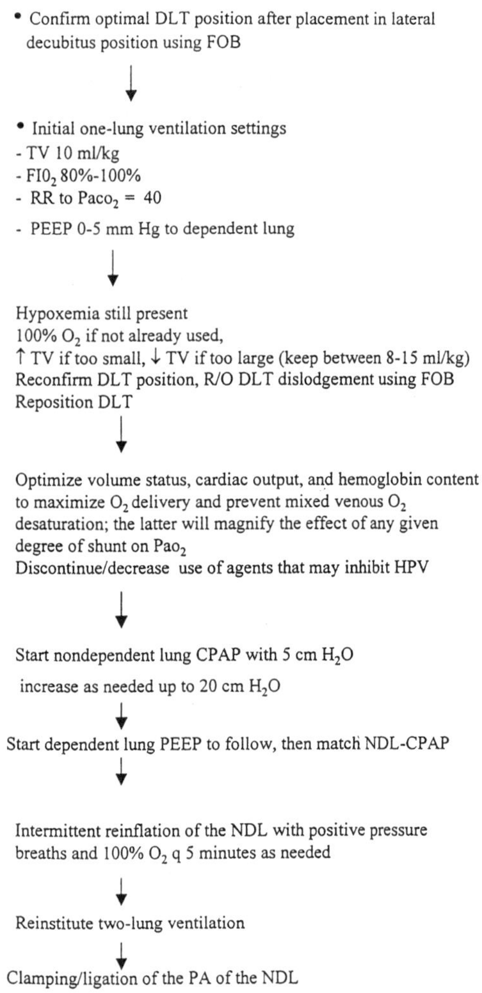

FIGURE 26-26. Algorithm for managing one-lung ventilation.

tion anesthetic. After the induction of general anesthesia, controlled manual ventilation by mask is started using an oxygen/inhalation anesthetic mixture. N_2O can be used during the induction phase and during preparation, draping, and positioning of the patient but is eliminated once one-lung ventilation is instituted to allow the use of 100% O_2. N_2O should not be used in patients who have marginal preoperative oxygenation or in those with large bullae or very emphysematous lungs. A muscle relaxant is then administered, followed by fentanyl (3 to 5 μg/kg) or sufentanil (1 μg/kg) to help attenuate the hemodynamic response to laryngoscopy and intubation. Intravenous lidocaine (1.5 mg/kg) may also be used before intubation. The trachea is then intubated with a single-lumen or double-lumen tube, as indicated by the surgical procedure. Position of the endotracheal tube is confirmed by auscultation, observing the CO_2 capnograph waveform and, if indicated, by fiberoptic bronchoscopy. During the maintenance phase, we routinely use inhalation anesthetic agents, usually isoflurane or sevoflurane in 100% O_2, supplemented with intermittent dosing of opioids prior to emergence. Any residual neuromuscular blockade is reversed using a combination of anticholinergic and anticholinesterase agents. The presence of adequate muscle strength is confirmed with the use of a nerve stimulator.

Epidural anesthesia, paravertebral block, intercostal nerve blocks, and field blocks have been used for various procedures on the thorax, including thoracotomy. Field block consists of local infiltration of the skin and muscles surrounding the area of resection. Intercostal nerve blocks anesthetize the intercostal nerve in the intercostal groove on the lower margin of the ribs. Paravertebral blocks consist of blocking the intercostal nerves as they emerge from the intervertebral foramen. A separate injection is made for each spinal nerve. A paravertebral block anesthetizes the intercostal nerve posteriorly so that all its distribution is effectively anesthetized. Resection of a portion of the rib, resection of adjacent ribs, resection of costal cartilages, and surgery on the sternum can be performed with the use of field blocks, intercostal nerve blocks, and paravertebral blocks.

General anesthesia combined with an epidural catheter is our most common anesthetic management plan for patients having thoracic surgery. Potential advantages of epidural anesthesia include a reduction in cardiac preload and afterload, higher postoperative pulmonary flow rates and improved oxygenation, optimal postoperative pain control, decreased incidence of venous thromboembolism, better suppression of the stress response, and a positive effect on postoperative nitrogen balance. Potential disadvantages include the time required to establish the block, increased fluid requirements needed to avoid a decrease in arterial blood pressure, and the potential for technical complications such as epidural hematoma. Advantages of general anesthesia are ease of administration, satisfactory relaxation, ability to control the depth of anesthesia, and usually good hemodynamic stability. Disadvantages of general anesthesia include the central depression of respiration that can extend into the postoperative period and lack of postoperative pain control. A combination of epidural anesthesia with light general anesthesia seems to offer a method of anesthesia that maximizes the benefits of each.

The advantages of combined epidural and general technique for thoracic anesthesia include control of the airway, light anesthesia, prompt awakening, adequate control of respiration with quickly reversible apnea, and efficient postoperative analgesia. Airway control is the customary and safest method of anesthesia for thoracic surgery. The application of topical analgesia to the larynx and the trachea during a combined technique helps provide a tranquil airway with the patient under light general anesthesia. This can be accomplished by laryngeal spray under direct vision, superior laryngeal nerve blocks, or transtracheal injection of 2 to 4 mL of 4% lidocaine. Gradual establishment of the epidural block with small incremental doses of local anesthetic appears to minimize sympathectomy-related hypotension. After the institution of a successful epidural block, anesthesia is induced with a small amount of thiopental, such as 2 mg/kg. The trachea may be intubated with the patient under deep inhalation anesthesia, succinylcholine, or a short-acting, nondepolarizing muscle relaxant. Anesthesia is maintained with O_2/N_2O inhalation anesthetic mixture and if necessary small intermittent doses or a continuous infusion of opioids. During one-lung ventilation, 100% O_2 is most commonly used. The epidural catheter can be used for the maintenance and/or postoperative analgesia with the use of either intermittent doses of local anesthetic, morphine, or a continuous infusion of epidural fentanyl, sufentanil, or a mixture of dilute local anesthetic solution and an opioid.

Pain Management for Thoracic Surgery

Pain after thoracotomy is one of the most severe and complex types of pain to manage. Pain after thoracotomy is generated by injury and inflammation of the skin, muscle, ribs, vertebrae, chest wall, pulmonary parenchyma, pleura, pericardium, and diaphragm. One or more chest tubes also cause pain at their entry sites, as well as within the thorax and shoulder region that is often overlooked. The pain impulses are sent to the brain by three pathways. Impulses from the chest wall and pleura travel along the intercostal nerves, the phrenic nerve conducts impulses from the diaphragm, and the vagus nerve routes impulses from the lung, mediastinum, and mediastinal pleura to the central nervous system. Pain impulses from six to seven dermatomes are commonly involved in a lateral thoracotomy. On a microscopic level, pain impulses are carried by slow-conducting A-delta, unmyelinated C fibers and thinly myelinated, faster conducting A-delta fibers.

Patients with inadequate pain relief are unable to cough effectively, breath deeply, and ambulate and are at increased risk for retaining secretions that will eventually lead to airway closure, atelectasis, and possibly pneumonia. To adequately control postoperative pain, one must consider the multiple sites from which the pain is generated, as well as the multiple techniques available.

Many techniques and agents are available to provide postoperative analgesia. Opioids are effective and can be given intramuscularly, intravenously as a bolus or by patient-controlled delivery, intrathecally, or in the epidural space. Local anesthetics can be administered directly into the wound as a peripheral nerve block, intercostal block, epidural block, or intrapleurally. Other means of pain relief include cryoanalgesia and transcutaneous nerve stimulation. Other agents that have been used successfully to improve pain relief include systemic nonsteroidal antiinflammatory drugs (NSAIDs), ketamine, and clonidine.

Having an analgesic technique in place and functioning before the surgical stimulus may also be beneficial and is referred to as preemptive analgesia. The basis for this concept is that in response to noxious stimuli, changes may be induced in central neural function, which contribute to pain long after the offending stimuli have been removed or the peripheral injury has heeled. The administration of opioids or local anesthetics before noxious stimulation may prevent or decrease the development of such injury-induced spinal hyperexcitability, potentially leading to less postoperative pain (36).

Advantages of Epidural Analgesia

Although there is much controversy regarding the level at which epidural catheters are placed and which agents should be used, there is little controversy regarding their overall effectiveness. Advantages of the epidural technique are multiple and include (a) no surgical intervention is required, (b) the same technique can be used for multiple procedures, (c) opioids can be used in combination or alone, (d) local anesthetics can be used in varied concentrations depending on the desired effect or site of insertion, (e) lipophilic or hydrophilic options can be used, (f) multiple sties of insertion are useful, (g) effects are reversible, (h) patient-controlled delivery can be used, (i) continuous as well as dynamic pain relief can be provided to respond to patient activity, (j) placement can be done preoperatively, intraoperatively, or postoperatively, and (k) the catheter can be maintained in place for several days.

Improving outcome is another potential advantage of epidural anesthesia and analgesia. In patients with refractory myocardial ischemia, initiation of thoracic epidural blockade of the cardiac sympathetic innervation (T1-5) resulted in rapid relief of chest pain and reduced ST-segment changes. These benefits were probably due to increased myocardial oxygen delivery and decreased myocardial oxygen demand (37). Postoperative morbidity including congestive heart failure and myocardial infarction has been shown to be lower in high-risk patients receiving general anesthesia in combination with an epidural local anesthetic than in those receiving general anesthesia alone. Epidural anesthesia with local anesthetics improves blood flow to the lower extremities, which may improve graft patency in patients having vascular surgery. Coagulation is also influenced, as epidural anesthesia has been shown to increase fibrinolytic activity and lessen the postoperative aggregation of platelets. Systemically absorbed local anesthetics can also directly inhibit platelet aggregation. Patients undergoing hip replacements with a lumbar epidural dosed with local anesthetic have a lower incidence of deep venous thrombosis and pulmonary embolism when compared to patients receiving general anesthesia alone (38).

Postoperative pulmonary function can be improved by

the epidural administration of local anesthetics in patients with underlying pulmonary disease, upper-abdominal and thoracic incisions, and in the elderly and obese. The diaphragmatic dysfunction after thoracic or upper-abdominal surgery results from reflex inhibition of the phrenic nerve and is not significantly altered by relief of pain. This improvement in pulmonary function most likely results from the neural blockade of this inhibitory reflex. Bowel function returns more rapidly when postoperative analgesia is provided with epidural local anesthetics rather than systemic opioids. Experimental evidence suggests that this is multifactorial and occurs because of pain relief, the systemic absorption of local anesthetic, blockade of sympathetic innervation of the bowel, and a reduction in the requirement for postoperative systemic opioids. Epidural anesthesia and analgesia also effectively blunts the surgical stress response including the systemic release of neuroendocrine hormones and the local release of cytokines (38). A large metaanalysis of 65 randomized, controlled trials reviewed the effectiveness of various modalities for postoperative pain management. They reported that when compared to systemic opioids, epidural opioids decreased the incidence of atelectasis and had a weak tendency to reduce the incidence of pulmonary infections and overall pulmonary complications. When compared to systemic opioids, epidural local anesthetics increased PaO_2 level and decreased the incidence of pulmonary infections and overall pulmonary complication rate (39).

Disadvantages of Epidural Anesthesia and Analgesia

To provide epidural anesthesia and analgesia, one must have a patient who is willing to undergo the procedure, have the appropriate equipment, be skilled in the technique, have the time to perform the technique, be able to manage the catheter intraoperatively as well as postoperatively, and be prepared to deal with potential complications and side effects. The most common complication encountered during placement of the catheters is accidental dural puncture, which has an incidence of 0.16% to 1.3%. Postdural puncture headache after dural puncture ranges in incidence from 16% to 86%. Paresthesias and neurologic injury are much less frequent, with a reported incidence rate of 0.01% to 0.001%. Most are self-limited and do not require treatment. Puncture of epidural vessels occurs in 3% to 12% of cases, although the formation of a symptomatic epidural hematoma occurs in less than 1 in 100,000 patients. Patients at increased risk for an epidural hematoma are those on anticoagulants or with coagulation disorders. An extremely rare but devastating complication is paraplegia, which can potentially occur after the formation of an epidural hematoma. Infection, subarachnoid cannulation, subdural cannulation, and backache are also potential complications. The risk of complications secondary to catheter placement appears equal in thoracic and lumbar locations. Complications from the accidental intrathecally or intravascular injection of a local anesthetic include dysrhythmias, cardiovascular collapse, or a high spinal blockade. Using a test dose of local anesthetic with epinephrine before use of the catheter may reduce these specific complications. When concentrations of bupivacaine of more than 0.15% are used postoperatively, 37% to 80% of patients will experience some degree of motor and/or autonomic blockade. Complications from such blockade include hypotension, urinary retention, impaired ambulation, and pressure necrosis. Preliminary evidence suggests that complications resulting from postoperative analgesia with local anesthetics can be reduced if the catheter is placed in the thoracic versus the lumbar region. This would seem logical for thoracic surgery, as less anesthetic agents would be needed to obtain the desired effect.

Complications from the epidural administration of opioids include pruritus (14% to 100%), nausea (11% to 100%), urinary retention (15% to 90%), sedation (3.3%), and respiratory depression (less than 1%). The incidence of complications varies with morphine having the highest incidence of side effects and fentanyl having the lowest. The incidence of these side effects is also dose dependent. Other risk factors for respiratory depression include concomitant use of parenteral opioids, age of more than 70 years, debilitated patients, and patients with poor pulmonary function. By adding a local anesthetic to an opioid infusion, the amount of opioid used can be decreased by up to 33% (40).

Contraindications

Patient refusal is the most common contraindication to epidural anesthesia and analgesia. Explanation of the risks and benefits of epidural analgesia at the time of informed consent can minimize this contraindication. We obtain consent for epidural placement before all thoracic procedures. This can be particularly useful for the "brief" thoracoscopy that turns into a thoracotomy, for which we are then able to place a lumbar epidural catheter and dose it before emergence. Patients with ongoing sepsis or infection at the proposed insertion site are generally not candidates for epidural catheter placement. Coagulation status is important in the decision to use an epidural catheter. In general, patients who have received thrombolytic therapy within the past 24 hours, have known coagulopathies, have a platelet count of less than 50,000, or are anticoagulated with heparin or Coumadin are not candidates for epidural analgesia. Patients who are fully anticoagulated on heparin should have the infusion discontinued 6 hours before the planned procedure. A partial thromboplastin time in the reference range is desirable. Patients who have been on Coumadin should have a prothrombin time within the reference range before needle insertion. Patients treated with low-dose subcutaneous unfractionated heparin can have an epidural catheter placed 6 hours after the last dose, without measuring a partial thromboplastin time and sooner if the partial thromboplastin time is within the reference range. Patients treated with low-molecular-weight heparin warrant additional caution, as these agents have higher bioavailability and longer durations of action compared to unfractionated heparin. The American Society of Regional Anesthesia (ASRA) states that the monitoring of the inhibitory activity to activated factor X (factor Xa inhibition) is not recommended, because it is not predictive of the risk of bleeding. For patients receiving 1 mg/kg of enoxaparin twice daily, the ASRA recommends a delay of 24 hours before needle placement. Review of the literature and case reports regarding the use of low-molecular-weight heparin suggests that further study is indicated (41). For patients who will be anticoagulated after placement of the epidural catheter, normalization of the coagulation status should be verified before catheter removal and should not be restarted for at least 1 hour after removal. For postoperative pain relief, opioid without local anesthetic may be preferred to allow for continuous neurologic monitoring. Short-acting local anesthetics may be preferred if their use is deemed necessary. The use of aspirin or NSAIDs by themselves is not necessarily a contraindication to epidural techniques and would seem low risk. Theoretically, a midline approach has a lower risk of epidural venous plexus injury than a paramedian approach and therefore may be preferable. Avoidance of threading the catheter in more than 5 cm into the epidural space may also decrease the risk of bleeding secondary to venous injury.

Site of Insertion and Technique

Optimally, the insertion site for the epidural catheter is in the middle of the dermatomal field of the surgical incision. Easily recognized landmarks include the prominence of C-7 and the angle of the scapula, which corresponds to the level of the spine of T-7. The advantages of thoracic insertion site versus lumbar include (a) a 30% lower dose requirement of local anesthetic for selective thoracic blockade, (b) sparing of lower lumber and sacral segments with earlier ambulation, (c) potentially lower incidence of urinary retention and need for bladder catheterization, (d) a more intense block of upper-thoracic segments, (e) less hypotension due to less sympathetic blockade, and (f) the ability to obtain segmental thoracic anesthesia (42). The disadvantages of thoracic placement include potential difficulty with catheter placement, along with a more developed venous plexus, which can cause additional technical difficulties. The sitting position is preferred, with the patient's feet supported by a stool, the neck flexed, and the arms crossed in front of his or her body or resting on a pillow. An attendant should be observing and stabilizing the patient on the opposite side of the bed from the anesthesiologist. A simple and effective way to decide in which inner space to place your needle is to identify the space that coincides with the superior aspect of the incision. We prefer the median approach for T3-4 and T4-5 catheter placement. The steep angles of the thoracic spines from T-5 to T-9 are best navigated by the paramedian approach. The epidural space can then again be entered by the median approach below T-9. Loss of resistance with air or saline is used by many to access the epidural space. We find the hanging drop method particularly effective for thoracic epidural catheter placement. This technique takes advantage of the transmission of negative intrathoracic pressure to the thoracic epidural space. Seeing the fluid disappear into the hub of the needle is a dramatic sign that you have entered the epidural space. Easy threading of the catheter is also consistent with being in the epidural space. The catheter should be threaded into the epidural space 3 to 5 cm. To secure the catheter, we use four ¼-inch sterile strips, each of which are applied first to the catheter and then rolled onto the skin. The entry site is covered with a sterile transparent dressing and 2-inch plastic tape is used to secure the catheter on its entire way up the back onto the shoulder. In an effort to decrease disconnects, a loop is made with the catheter before reaching the shoulder and the hub is also taped to the catheter.

Delivery

Agents can be given either as a bolus or by continuous infusion. We use a bolus technique followed by an infusion. The advantages of continuous infusions are (qqa) less rostral spread when compared to bolus dosing thereby minimizing side effects, (b) providing continuous analgesia without peaks and troughs as seen with bolus dosing, (c) allowing the use of shorter acting opioids and dilute local anesthetics to minimize side effects, (d) lower risk of infection with less manipulation of the system, (e) less attendants required versus repeatedly injecting the catheter and monitoring the patient after each injection, and (f) allows for patient-controlled analgesia. Disadvantages of the continuous infusion technique include (a) the need for a sophisticated pump and (b) early recognition of catheter migration may be more difficult to diagnose compared to a bolus technique in which the catheter is aspirated before each medication delivery.

Agents

Opioids and local anesthetics can be used alone or in combination in the epidural space. Combining fentanyl with bupivacaine has been shown to have a significant opioid sparing effect. It appears that a combination of a lower dose of opioid and a lower concentration of local anesthetic may minimize overall side effects while providing effective analgesia. The basis for this combination effect is that opioids are able to produce analgesia by binding to opiate receptors in the substantia gelatinosa (Rexed laminae I and III) while local anesthetics are able to provide analgesia by blocking impulse transmission at the nerve roots and dorsal root ganglia. Fentanyl has been used extensively to provide analgesia after thoracic surgery. It takes effect 10 minutes after dosing and has a duration of 2 to 3 hours. It is very lipid soluble with an octanol-to-water coefficient of 813. In the thoracic region, a bolus dose of 50 to 100 μg is given, followed by an infusion of 0.5 to 1.5 μg/kg/hour. Fentanyl is effective when given intravenously, by a lumbar epidural catheter or by a thoracic epidural catheter. When the lumbar route is used, larger doses are required to produce similar analgesia, which also leads to more side effects. There seems to be little justification to use fentanyl in the lumbar epidural space for thoracic procedures. Epinephrine (3.33 μg/mL) added to fentanyl for thoracic epidural administration was shown to decrease fentanyl requirements and lower serum levels of fentanyl. There were no differences in side effects; however, only 34 patients were in the study (43).

Sufentanil is a highly lipid soluble opioid with an octanol-to-water coefficient of 1,778. It starts to take effect 5 minutes after administration and has a duration of 1 to 5 hours. In the thoracic region, a bolus dose of 20 to 40 μg is followed by an infusion of 5 μg/hour. The high lipid solubility of sufentanil requires that it be administered in the dermatomal region of the surgical incision.

Morphine is the most widely used analgesic agent. It is not lipid soluble and has an octanol-to-water coefficient of 1.4. After thoracic dosing of 2 to 4 mg, it starts to take effect in 40 to 60 minutes and has a duration of 12 to 24 hours. Up to 5 mg can be administered into the lumbar region, followed by an infusion of 0.5 to 1.5 mg/hour depending on the patient's age. The onset of action in the thoracic region is faster than with lumber administration, although the duration of action is similar. Disadvantages of using morphine include its slower onset and a higher incidence of delayed respiratory depression as compared to either fentanyl or sufentanil. Major advantages are that it can be given in the lumbar region and its low lipid solubility allows it to spread rostrally, which provides effective pain relief for thoracotomy incisions.

Inadequate Analgesia and Management

When a patient reports inadequate analgesia, the catheter is initially checked to be intact and in place. The catheter is then dosed with 3 mL of 1.5% lidocaine with epinephrine 1:200,000. If no sensory block is obtained, the catheter can be replaced or the patient is started on an alternative mode of pain management such as intravenous patient-controlled anesthesia. If a unilateral block is obtained, the catheter should be withdrawn 1 to 2 cm and bolused with 3 to 5 mL of 1.5% lidocaine without epinephrine. One may also consider the addition of fentanyl at 25 to 50 μg, which can be repeated in 30 minutes. If you obtain a bilateral sensory block, the catheter is in proper position. Several options exist and include a bolus of 25 to 50 μg of fentanyl and/or a bolus of 3 to 6 mL of 0.25% bupivacaine. You may also increase the rate of infusion by 2 mL/hour and consider other agents such as ketorolac, 15 to 30 mg intravenously every 6 to 8 hours, with a maximum duration of 5 days due to its potential for renal dysfunction. Chest tubes that extend into the apex of the thorax can cause extreme pain, which is difficult to control with an epidural catheter. Withdrawal of the chest tube so that it no longer puts pressure on the apex remedies this problem.

Patients with epidural catheters should be on a nursing floor that is familiar with the technique and able to monitor patients for side effects such as respiratory depression. Daily examination of the catheter insertion site is essential. Optimally, a pain management service should coordinate the delivery of postoperative epidural analgesia.

What We Do at the Cleveland Clinic Foundation

Upon the patient entering the operating room or induction room, monitors are applied and an intravenous line is started. An arterial line may be started or a blood pressure cuff is used. Small amounts of intravenous midazolam are used for light sedation (0.5 to 2.0 mg intravenously). The patient is then placed in the sitting position for epidural placement. Thoracic placement is preferred. Patients who have thoracic epidurals are awake during placement. The sites chosen are generally from T-4 to T-6. Although some clinicians promote the hanging drop technique, others prefer loss of resistance with either air or saline. Success rates have been similar for both techniques. Catheters are threaded into the epidural space 3 to 5 cm. A 3-mL test dose of 1.5% lidocaine with epinephrine, 1:200,000 is administered. If we are unable to access the thoracic epidural space, we place a lumbar epidural catheter at that same sitting. For patients who refuse catheters while awake, we offer a lumbar catheter after induction, but before incision. For the unexpected thoracotomy, we place a lumbar catheter after completion of surgery before emergence from anesthesia.

For an unexpected wet tap, one may convert to an intrathecal technique and simply inject an agent such as morphine (0.4 to 0.8 mg) or fentanyl (10 to 25 μg). These patients will then require monitoring of their respiratory rate and level of sedation for the next 24 hours. Our preference is to withdraw the needle and move to another site that is at least two inner spaces away and then reattempt catheter placement. If technical difficulty persists, the patient is managed with intravenous patient-controlled anesthesia. Catheters are dosed with opioid after placement and then started on an infusion. For thoracic catheters, we use bupivacaine or ropivacaine with fentanyl, morphine or hydromorphone. The dosing scheme is based on age as follows:

First choice: bupivacaine 0.1% + fentanyl 5 μg/mL infusion

Patient Age (yr)	Bupivacaine Load 0.25%–0.5% (mL)	Fentanyl Load After 15 min (μg)	Infusion Rate (mL/hr)	PCA Dose (mL) 15-min delay
15–44	5–8	100	6	4
45–65	4–6	100	5	3
66–75	4–5	75	3	2
76+	3–4	50	2	2

Second choice: bupivacaine 0.1% + morphine 0.05 mg/mL infusion

Patient Age (yr)	Bupivacaine Load 0.25%–0.5% (mL)	Morphine Load After 15 min (μg)	Infusion Rate (mL/hr)	PCA Dose (mL) 20-min delay
15–44	5–8	4	6	2.5
45–65	4–6	3	5	2
66–75	4–5	2	3	1.5
76+	3–5	1	2	1

For lumbar catheters, we utilize morphine (0.05 mg/mL). The dosing scheme is as follows:

Patient Age (yr)	Morphine Load (mg)	Infusion Rate (mL/hr)	PCA Dose (mL) 15-min delay
15–44	5	8	3
45–65	4	6	2.5
66–75	3	5	2
76+	2	3	1.5

For thoracic surgery, we frequently combine several techniques to provide the best possible analgesia. Each of these techniques individually provides some degree of pain relief; however, when combined, the result is more than the sum of its parts. The epidural catheter placed preoperatively is the main focus of our pain relief strategy. Fentanyl is given intravenously during induction up to 3 μg/kg. After induction, the epidural catheter is bolused, after which the infusion is started. Before chest closure, the surgeons or anesthesiologists administer an intercostal nerve block. The incision, including two inner spaces above, two inner spaces below the incision, as well as the chest tube insertion sites, are blocked using 0.5% bupivacaine.

Treatment of Side Effects

Stopping the present epidural infusion for 2 hours and then resuming the infusion at 1/2 to 1/3 of the initial rate initially addresses postoperative sedation. If using a fentanyl and bupivacaine combination, one may consider decreasing the concentration of fentanyl. For patients at high risk for respiratory depression such as those who are more than 75 years old, have severe COPD, or have CO_2 retention, we frequently decrease the initial fentanyl concentration to 2 μg/mL. Respiratory depression is treated by administering naloxone. For severe or life-threatening respiratory depression, up to 1 mg of naloxone may be given, and intubation followed by controlled ventilation may be required. For milder forms of respiratory depression, naloxone should be administered in divided doses of 20 to 40 μg. Infusions of naloxone are also effective and can be started at 1 μg/kg/hour. Consideration should also be given to residual benzodiazepines for which the administration of flumazenil, 0.2 to 1.0 mg intravenously, would be appropriate. If the patient cannot be closely monitored on the regular nursing floor, he/she should be transferred to an intensive care unit.

Nausea and vomiting are initially treated with prochlorperazine, 5 to 10 mg intravenously or orally every 6 hours as needed. Severe nausea is effectively treated by the administration of ondansetron, 4 mg intravenously. Pruritus can initially be treated with nalbuphine, 5 mg intravenously. Other agents to consider include diphenhydramine, 25 to 50 mg intravenously every 8 hours as needed, and/or a naloxone drip, which can be started at 20 μg/hour. For continued pruritus despite these interventions, the opioid, if morphine, can be switched to fentanyl. If the opioid is fentanyl, removing the fentanyl and treating the patient with bupivacaine alone can address continued pruritus. Urinary retention is generally not a problem, as our patients have thoracic catheters in place. Lumbar catheters with morphine have a low incidence of urinary retention, which can be treated by a naloxone infusion of 1 μg/kg/hour. The rate of urinary retention is most likely underestimated, as our patients frequently have urinary catheters in place for a day or two postoperatively.

Epidural catheters may easily remain in place for up to 5 days postoperatively. In general, they are discontinued several hours after chest tube removal, after which time the patient is managed with oral analgesics. Adequate pain relief after thoracic surgery is essential for an optimal postoperative course. Epidural techniques form the cornerstone of our pain management strategy for thoracic surgery. Thoracic catheters are preferred, through which fentanyl and bupivacaine are given in combination. Lumbar catheters are also effective and can be used with morphine. The overall scheme also includes small amounts of intravenous opioid at induction, as well as intercostal nerve blocks with bupivacaine before chest closure. Any remaining deficiencies in pain relief can be addressed with the judicious use of ketorolac.

ANESTHESIA FOR PATIENTS WITH MEDIASTINAL MASSES

Anesthesia for patients with mediastinal masses may be associated with significant respiratory and cardiovascular complications. Several reports of death or severe life-threatening complications have been reported during anesthesia for patients with mediastinal masses (44–48). The mediastinum can be divided into superior, anterior, middle, and posterior mediastinal regions. Anatomic structures of major importance are at the junction of superior, middle, anterior, and posterior mediastinal regions. These structures include the superior vena cava, tracheal bifurcation, main pulmonary artery, aortic arch, and part of the heart's superior surface.

Pathology

Many types of tumors have been reported in the various mediastinal regions (Fig. 27-27). In adults, 97% of mediastinal tumors are malignant, and 3% are benign. About 80% of the malignant tumors are metastatic bronchogenic carcinomas, and 17% are lymphomas. In children, 87% of mediastinal masses are malignant, and of these, 40% are lymphomas. Different types of tumors in children and in adults, according to their location in the mediastinum, are shown in Table 26-1.

Signs and Symptoms

Patients with mediastinal masses may have the signs or symptoms listed in Table 26-2. Symptoms arise from the encroachment by the mediastinal tumor on important mediastinal structures. These include (a) progressive airway obstruction caused by compression of the distal trachea and the bronchi, (b) loss of lung volume, (c) compression of the pulmonary artery or the heart, (d) superior vena cava obstruction, (e) involvement of the recurrent laryngeal nerves or sympathetic chain, and (f) spinal cord compression from intraspinal extension of neurogenic tumors of the posterior mediastinum.

Preoperative examination and evaluation of patients should focus on signs and symptoms of compression or involvement of the vital structures in the mediastinum. In one large series, clinical manifestations observed, in descending order of frequency, included (a) cough and pain, 40% each; (b) weight loss and fever, 24% each; (c) dyspnea and dysphagia, 20% each; (d) superior vena cava obstructions, 16%; (e) tracheal deviations, 12%; (f) Horner syndrome, 7%; (g) spinal cord compression, 5%; and (h) cyanosis, mediastinal widening, and hoarseness, 3% each. In 20% of patients, no signs were found (49).

The incidence of complications is related to the size of

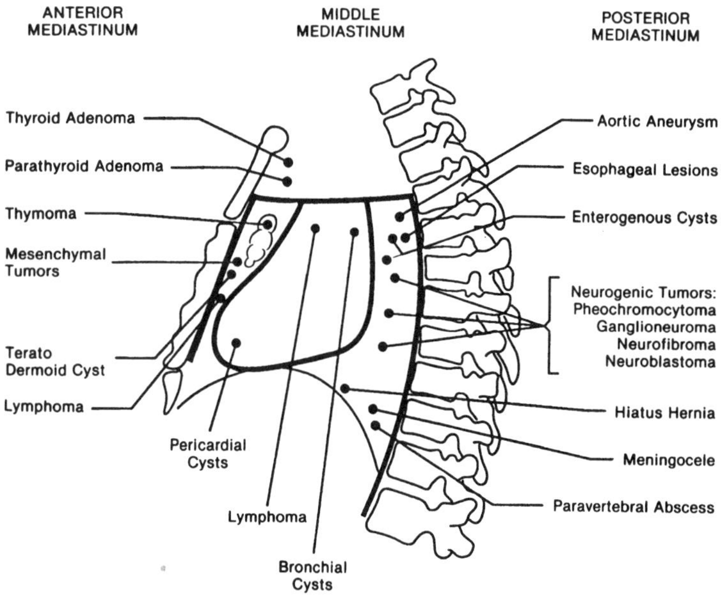

FIGURE 26-27. The location of commonly occurring mediastinal tumors.

TABLE 26-1. MEDIASTINAL MASS LOCATION

Superior	Anterior	Middle	Posterior
Children			
Lymphoma	Lymphoma	Lymphoma	Neurogenic tumors
Thymoma	Teratoma	Tuberculous nodes	Esophageal duplication cysts
Retrosternal thyroid	Cystic hygroma		
Parathyroid tumor	Thymoma		Diaphragmatic hernia (Bochdalek)
	Pericardial cysts		
	Diaphragmatic hernia (Morgagni)		
Adults			
Lymphoma	Lymphoma	Lymphoma	Neurogenic tumors
Thymoma	Metastatic carcinoma	Metastatic carcinoma	Lymphoma
Retrosternal thyroid	Teratoma	Teratoma	Hernia (Bochdalek)
Metastatic carcinoma	Bronchogenic cyst	Bronchogenic cyst	Aortic aneurysm
Parathyroid tumors	Aortic aneurysm	Aortic aneurysm	
Zenker's diverticulum	Pericardial cyst	Pericardial cyst	
Aortic aneurysm			

Source: From Pullerits, Holzman R. Anaesthesia for patients with mediastinal masses. *Can J Anaesth* 1989;36:681, with permission.

the mediastinal mass and extent of disease within the thoracic cavity. Of a large group of patients with mediastinal Hodgkin disease, 10% had acute life-threatening airway complications during staging laparotomy. Some of these patients were asymptomatic and showed no airway compression on chest radiographs (50). The severity of the patient's preoperative respiratory symptoms therefore may be unrelated to the degree of respiratory or cardiovascular compromise that may be encountered during anesthesia. This is true even in the asymptomatic patient. Patients who show mediastinal masses on chest radiographs should have a CT scan to delineate the tumor's exact location and extent. The anesthesiologist should examine the CT scan and evaluate the extent of compression of the airway, heart, and vascular structures.

In the asymptomatic patient who has a mediastinal mass on chest radiograph and CT scan, a series of noninvasive studies should be performed to detect or rule out occult airway or cardiac involvement. Upright and supine flow-volume loops are simple, noninvasive, and sensitive studies for the diagnosis of occult airway obstruction. The dynamic nature of this study makes it an extremely sensitive tool for evaluating obstructive lesions of major airways. The inspiratory limb of the flow-volume loop is useful in diagnosing extrathoracic airway obstruction, whereas the expiratory limb is sensitive to intrathoracic airway obstruction (Fig. 26-3). Maximal inspiratory and expiratory flow-volume loops obtained with the patient in upright and supine positions enable the functional degree of impairment to be quantitated and help distinguish fixed from variable intrathoracic airway obstruction. Echocardiography in the upright and supine position can also reveal encroachment of tumor on

TABLE 26-2. CLINICAL FINDINGS IN PATIENTS WITH MEDIASTINAL MASSES

History	Physical Examination	Laboratory
Airway		
Cough	Decreased breath sounds	Chest radiograph (posteroanterior and lateral to look for tracheal deviation or compression)
Cyanosis	Wheezing	
Dyspnea	Stridor	
Orthopnea	Cyanosis	Flow-volume loops, supine and sitting
Cardiovascular		
Fatigue	Neck or facial edema	Chest radiographic changes in cardiac silhouette
Faintness	Jugular distention	
Headache	Papilledema	Echocardiogram, supine and sitting
Shortness of breath and orthopnea	Blood pressure changes or changes in pallor with postural changes	
Cough	Pulsus paradoxus	

Source: From Pullerits J, Holzman R. Anaesthesia for patients with mediastinal masses. *Can J Anaesth* 1989;36:681, with permission.

the heart and intrathoracic vessels. Venography may be used to evaluate the patency of the superior or inferior vena cava. The degree of tracheal compression found on CT scan is a general predictor of whether anesthetic difficulty with the airway may be expected. In one series, all five patients who developed total or near-total airway obstruction during induction or emergence from anesthesia had greater than a 50% decrease in tracheal cross-sectional area, as measured by CT scan (44). A disproportionate reduction in maximal expiratory flow should alert the physician to the presence of tracheomalacia and its inherent risk of precipitating dynamic airway collapse after extubation of the trachea.

Flexible fiberoptic bronchoscopy with topical anesthesia performed preoperatively is another method of evaluating dynamic airway obstruction. It allows assessment of the functional anatomy of the entire airway and the response of the airway to variations in intrathoracic pressure. During the procedure, the patient should be changed from the supine to the sitting to the semiprone and prone positions, because airway obstruction may change with the patient's position. This is important to know preoperatively; if airway obstruction occurs intraoperatively, one will know the best position in which to maintain a patent airway.

In 1976, Piro et al. (50) recommended emergency prebiopsy radiation therapy to prevent development of life-threatening complications in patients with mediastinal masses. In a subsequent study from the same institution, a tissue diagnosis could not be obtained in 8 of 19 irradiated patients. However, the lack of histologic diagnosis before treatment did not change the treatment course; seven patients received empiric therapy based on their presumed diagnosis, resulting in absence of relapse in four. In the remaining 11 patients, a histologic diagnosis was possible even after radiotherapy and was found to confirm the presumed prebiopsy diagnosis. If the tumor does respond to therapy or chemotherapy, it is usually radiosensitive and is most likely to be lymphatic in origin. Some of the patients who were empirically treated subsequently developed relapses, and a tissue biopsy was obtained at the time of the relapse. The initial presumed diagnosis was confirmed. The authors at this institution therefore concluded that the lack of histologic diagnosis before therapy did not compromise or alter patient outcomes (51). Currently, the intense investigation of these tumors before treatment would be hampered or eliminated by preoperative radiation.

Transcarinal aspiration of a large cystic subcarinal mass can be performed via fiberoptic bronchoscopy. It should be possible to use this technique preoperatively in patients who have cystic subcarinal masses to decrease the size of the mass before induction of anesthesia. Other tissue diagnostic techniques that can be employed successfully while avoiding the administration of general anesthesia include percutaneous needle aspiration of the hilum and mediastinum and thoracoscopy.

Pathophysiology of Mediastinal Masses with Important Anesthetic Implications

Both symptomatic and asymptomatic patients have developed severe, life-threatening airway obstruction after induction of general anesthesia. The presence or absence of symptoms or the severity of the patient's preoperative respiratory symptoms do not reliably predict the degree of respiratory compromise that could be encountered during anesthesia (52). However, most patients who have severe respiratory symptoms do have significant decreases in the tracheal cross-sectional area (44). Difficulties have occurred during induction of anesthesia, after intubation, after the administration of muscle relaxants, during emergence from anesthesia, and after extubation. Anesthesia in the supine patient leads to several factors that can contribute to airway obstruction. This obstruction can occur distal to a properly placed endotracheal tube and therefore can lead to difficulty with ventilation, even after easy intubation. Several factors that lead to airway compromise include the following:

- In the supine position, anesthesia and muscle paralysis lead to decreased dimensions of the rib cage, cephalad displacement of the diaphragm's dome, and a reduction in the thoracic volume, which limits the space available of the trachea (53).
- At low lung volumes, the decreased tracheal distending pressure can lead to its collapse, particularly in the presence of tracheomalacia.
- It is well known that spontaneous ventilation is preferred over positive-pressure ventilation in patients with mediastinal masses. Airway obstruction has occurred after the administration of muscle relaxants in patients who were doing well during spontaneous ventilation. With spontaneous ventilation, the negative intrapleural pressure exerts a distending force on the airway, thus offsetting their tendency to collapse. This factor is immediately abolished with the administration of muscle relaxants. A decrease in tracheal distending pressure is also caused by the action of inhalation agents, which reduces intercostal muscle tone and promotes mechanical instability of the rib cage (54). The supine position also causes an increase in central blood volume, which can further increase tumor blood volume and tumor skin. Edema, bleeding, and hematoma formation in the tumor as a result of surgical biopsy can also further contribute to airway compromise.
- Physiologic PEEP is normally created by the glottic mechanism, which increases the tracheal distending pressure and reduces the possibility of dynamic collapse. This protective mechanism is abolished with the insertion of an endotracheal tube.
- Rapid respirations and cough during awakening from anesthesia may promote dynamic collapse of a tracheal segment.
- Infants and small children may have obstructive symptoms earlier than adults because of their smaller airway

size, leading to great increases in airway resistance with relatively small decreases in airway dimensions.

Compression of the main pulmonary artery is relatively rare, partly because of the protective effect of the aorta. Compression of the pulmonary trunk or one of the main pulmonary arteries can result in sudden hypoxemia, hypotension, and cardiac arrest. This was reported to result in the death of a 6-year-old child undergoing a cervical lymph biopsy (55). Another report describes a 14-year-old girl with a large dermoid cyst in the anterior mediastinum that required cardiopulmonary bypass to maintain arterial oxygenation and to counteract severe compression of the pulmonary artery by tumor during anesthesia (56). Syncope during forced Valsalva maneuvers, such as occurs with a bowel movement, should alert the physician to the possibility of cardiovascular compression. Autopsy reports describe involvement of the pericardium, myocardium, and pulmonary arteries by lymphomatous tumors in patients who died on the induction of anesthesia. The patient assuming the supine position, the induction of anesthesia, the decrease in the chest cavity's size, and the tumor's gravitational effects on the heart and pulmonary artery are important factors contributing to the severe reduction in right ventricular output, hypotension, and severe hypoxemia observed in these patients before cardiac arrest.

Superior vena cava syndrome results from extrinsic compression or thrombosis of the superior vena cava. Of patients with superior vena cava syndrome, 87% have associated bronchial carcinoma, 10% have malignant lymphoma, and 3% have benign causes such as central venous hyperalimentation, mediastinal fibrosis, and multinodular goiter. The clinical features of superior vena cava syndrome and its anesthetic implications are discussed in detail later in this chapter.

Anesthetic Management

All patients, including the pediatric group, should have an intravenous line in place before the induction of anesthesia. Patients with masses compressing the pulmonary artery may be relatively asymptomatic while awake but may develop severe life-threatening hypoxemia requiring emergency extracorporeal bypass after anesthetic induction or even mild sedation. If preoperative echocardiography or cardiac catheterization reveals compression of the heart and pulmonary artery or pericardial involvement with tumor, standby cardiopulmonary bypass should be available. The pump team should be in the operating room, the pump should be primed and ready to run, the patient's groin should be prepared and draped, and the cannulation sites should be in the sterile field. If a disaster occurs, cardiopulmonary bypass can then be immediately initiated. In patients with significant cardiovascular or airway compression, cardiopulmonary bypass can be instituted by cannulating the femoral artery and vein using local anesthesia before the induction of general anesthesia.

If at all possible, local anesthesia is the method of choice for patients with anterior mediastinal masses. This is usually feasible in patients having cervical lymph node biopsies. Mediastinoscopy has also been successfully performed using local anesthesia. Premedication should be light or omitted because of concerns about potential airway obstruction. Anticholinergic agents should be administered to help reduce secretions, because difficulties with intubation and the need for fiberoptic bronchoscopy are likely. The patient is transported to the operating room with the head up to minimize airway edema. This is particularly useful if there is associated superior vena cava syndrome. Adequate intravenous access should be secured in the lower extremities if concurrent superior vena cava obstruction exists. Intraarterial catheters, central venous lines, or pulmonary artery catheters may be indicated in selected patients based on the findings on preoperative evaluation, severity of the symptoms, and degree of cardiovascular and respiratory compromise. If superior vena cava syndrome is present, central venous access and pulmonary artery catheters should be inserted via the femoral vein.

Patients who are symptomatic in the supine position are best maintained in the sitting or semisitting position during induction of anesthesia. The most important aspect in the anesthetic management of these patients is the maintenance of spontaneous ventilation throughout the procedure. One should decide whether to perform fiberoptic bronchoscopy and intubation with the patient awake based on the patient's preoperative evaluation and the degree of symptoms. If the patient is asymptomatic in the supine position and the chest radiograph and CT scan do not reveal airway obstruction or compression, awake fiberoptic bronchoscopy probably is not necessary. The equipment, however, should be immediately available and ready to use if difficulties arise. If the patient is symptomatic in the supine position, or if airway compression is seen on chest radiograph, or preoperative CT scan or the flow-volume loop is abnormal, awake fiberoptic bronchoscopy before induction of anesthesia should be considered. Fiberoptic bronchoscopy with the patient awake can then be performed to evaluate the patency of the entire airway down to the level of the bronchi. If no significant compression is seen, intubation can be done after induction of anesthesia. If any airway compression is seen on fiberoptic bronchoscopy, one should decide on the technique of intubation considering several options. If the compression is confined to the thoracic trachea and ends high above the carina, an armored single-lumen tube can be placed so its tip is past the level of obstruction. If obstruction and compression are present at the level of the carina down to one or the other main bronchi, endobronchial intubation is recommended. One can accomplish this using a single-lumen tube guided by the fiberoptic bronchoscopy toward the side not significantly compressed. Alternatively, one can use a double-lumen tube. For example, if total or near-total compression and occlusion of the right main bronchus are present, a left-sided endobronchial intubation using a double-lumen tube can be guided by the fiberoptic bronchoscopy into the left main bronchus. Both these methods adequately ventilate the left lung. One may decide to perform the intubation after inhalation induction of anesthesia. In that case, after the patient is anesthetized while maintaining spontaneous ventilation, the fiberoptic bronchoscopy, jacketed with an armored endotracheal tube, can be used to visualize the patient's airway down to the main bronchi. This might reveal previously unsuspected airway obstruction and/or compression that have developed after induction. The fiberoptic bronchoscope should be used to place the tip of the armored endotracheal tube distal to the most distal site of airway compression.

Fiberoptic bronchoscopy is extremely valuable in the management of patients with anterior mediastinal masses. Older children and young adults with the use of adequate local anesthesia and judicious sedation can tolerate awake fiberoptic bronchoscopy. When dealing with younger children, however, awake fiberoptic bronchoscopy is difficult and heavy sedation or general anesthesia are usually required before securing the airway, even if the patient is symptomatic. Inhalation induction followed by maintenance with spontaneous ventilation is required for optimal safety and the avoidance of airway obstruction. A mixture of 80% helium and 20% O_2 is useful in patients with significant airway compromise. This gas mixture has a low density and therefore provides less resistance and less turbulence when flowing through areas of airway narrowing and compression. Although increasing the concentration of inspired O_2 in the mixture increases the density of inspired gas and may offset some of its advantages, clinical improvement has been reported with a mixture containing up to 50% O_2.

Equipment that must be available in the operating room while caring for a patient with mediastinal mass includes the following:

- Different-size armored single-lumen tubes and different sizes of double-lumen tubes.
- Different-size fiberoptic bronchoscopes, including pediatric sizes.
- Local anesthetics to topicalize the airway.
- Standby rigid bronchoscopy setup with a surgeon or endoscopist experienced in performing this technique.
- Sanders jet ventilator with attachment to fit onto rigid bronchoscope.
- Standby cardiopulmonary bypass, as well as the necessary personnel for selected patients.
- Sternal saw to open the chest immediately if airway obstruction occurs and cannot be quickly overcome.

Standby rigid bronchoscopy should always be available when caring for patients with mediastinal masses. A surgeon or endoscopist experienced in using a rigid bronchoscope must be available in the room at the time of induction. If airway obstruction occurs during induction or surgery, several measures can be taken. The FiO_2 should be increased to 1.0. The patient's position should be quickly altered in an effort to relieve airway obstruction. The endotracheal tube should then be advanced more distally into the airway in an effort to bypass the obstruction. The fiberoptic bronchoscope should then be introduced into the airway to help diagnose the problem and potentially act as a stylet to pass the endotracheal tube past the level of the obstruction. At this time, the surgical team should make final preparations to initiate cardiopulmonary bypass. If airway obstruction and ventilation remain impossible, the rigid bronchoscope should be inserted into the airway past the level of the obstruction or into the opposite lung to allow for jet ventilation with the Sanders injector. If the chest is open, the surgical team should attempt to lift the mass off of the airway in an effort to relieve obstruction. When all of these measures fail to relieve airway obstruction, cardiopulmonary bypass must be initiated to save the patient. In one instance when all of the above measures failed to relieve the obstruction, the main bronchus was surgically opened and intubated with a standard single-lumen tube. A sterile anesthesia circuit was then connected to the endotracheal tube directly through the surgical incision and ventilation was reestablished.

Difficulties can occur during emergence from anesthesia as frequently as they can occur with induction. Coughing, straining, and bucking on an endotracheal tube with an increase in intrathoracic pressure can precipitate airway obstruction in these patients. Deep extubation while breathing spontaneously has been recommended unless contraindicated. Alternative measures include administering lidocaine or small doses of opioids titrated to the respiratory rate to allow the patient to awaken smoothly with the endotracheal tube in place. My personal preference is to extubate patients very fully awake. Fiberoptic bronchoscopy can be performed after surgery to determine airway patency. With the patient spontaneously ventilating, tracheomalacia involving the trachea's intrathoracic portion can result in dynamic airway collapse during expiration, whereas tracheomalacia of the trachea's extrathoracic part results in dynamic collapse of the trachea during inspiration. Therefore, the recommended technique is to introduce the fiberoptic bronchoscope into the airway at the end of surgery. The endotracheal tube, whether a single- or double-lumen tube, should then be slowly and gradually withdrawn, with the fiberoptic bronchoscope inside serving as a stylet. Careful evaluation of dynamic airway collapse can then be done under direct vision. If the trachea collapses with respiration, the patient should remain intubated.

After diagnostic procedures such as mediastinoscopy, bronchoscopy, and thoracoscopy, in which the mediastinal mass has not been resected, or even after removal of the mass, severe respiratory failure requiring intubation and ventilation may occur. This may result from (a) tumor swelling caused by edema or hemorrhage as a result of partial resection or biopsy, (b) tracheomalacia, causing dynamic airway collapse, (c) laryngospasm, bronchospasm, and airway edema, particularly in patients with superior vena cava syndrome, (d) abnormal response to muscle relaxants in patients with malignancies, and (e) postoperative pulmonary edema after airway obstruction (57). All patients must therefore be closely monitored in the first few postoperative hours and in most cases overnight admission to the ICU is warranted.

SUPERIOR VENA CAVA SYNDROME

Superior vena cava obstruction occurs in approximately 6% to 7% of patients with lung carcinoma (58). Its causes include bronchial carcinoma (87% of patients), malignant lymphoma (10%), and benign conditions (32%). Benign causes include central venous hyperalimentation, pacemaker catheter-induced thrombosis of the superior vena cava, idiopathic mediastinal fibrosis, mediastinal granulomas, or multimodular goiter. Venous distention is most prominent in the recumbent position, but the veins usually do not collapse in the normal manner with the patient upright. The severity of symptoms depends on the rapidity with which the vena cava becomes occluded. If the occlusion develops rapidly, all clinical manifestations are more prominent. With slower occlusion, signs and symptoms may be insidious in onset. With complete obstruction, the venous distention is more than it would be if there were partial occlusion. If the azygous vein is occluded or if the superior vena cava is occluded caudal to the point of entry of the azygous vein, the signs and symptoms of superior vena cava syndrome are more severe. Survival correlates with the development of cerebral or airway compromise (59).

Superior vena cavography proved to be an excellent guide for the design of patient management programs. Radiography of the superior vena cava appears useful in defining those types of obstruction in which an increased likelihood exists for the development of cerebral or airway symptoms, which strongly correlate with survival. Radiography also appears useful in defining the location of obstruction and in planning the surgical management. The risks of surgery are increased in patients with superior vena cava obstruction. Venous pressure is high, and patients are at increased risk of bleeding. Treatment consists of irradiation and chemotherapy for those with incomplete obstruction and a patent azygous system. Thrombectomy is effective only in those with acute intraluminal thrombosis. Once the thrombotic material has organized, little can be done surgically to open the superior vena cava. Patients who have near-total or total obstructions of the superior vena cava with obstruction or reversal of azygous vein blood flow are at a high risk of developing cerebral and airway compromise.

Anesthetic Management

Preoperative evaluation of the patient with superior vena cava syndrome should include a careful assessment of the airway. Edema of the mouth, oropharynx, hypopharynx, larynx, and trachea should be expected and can be as severe or more severe than the degree of external edema and swelling of the face and neck. Recurrent laryngeal nerve involvement, fibrosis, and external compression of the airway can cause further airway compromise. The patient should be transported in the semisitting position with the head up to minimize airway edema and to facilitate venous drainage from the head and neck. Venous access should be inserted in the lower extremities. An arterial line should be inserted in all patients. A central venous line or a pulmonary artery catheter should be inserted via the femoral vein. Premedication should be limited to an anticholinergic agent. The method chosen for induction of anesthesia and intubation depends on the preoperative airway evaluation, as with patients who have mediastinal masses. Anesthesia may need to be induced with the patient in the sitting position and breathing spontaneously. If significant airway edema is present, awake fiberoptic bronchoscopy and intubation with an armored endotracheal tube should be performed (Fig. 26-28).

ANESTHESIA FOR PATIENTS WITH MYASTHENIA GRAVIS

Myasthenia gravis is a disorder of the muscular system caused by destruction of the nicotinic acetylcholine receptors at the neuromuscular junction by immunoglobulin G (IgG) antibodies. Myasthenia gravis is frequently associated with other autoimmune disorders, such as Graves disease. Histologic studies of the endplate area show loss of synaptic folds and widening of the synaptic clefts (60). The number of acetylcholine receptors is decreased, and therefore, the endplates have reduced sensitivity to acetylcholine. The prevalence of myasthenia gravis is 1 out of 20,000 to 30,000 in the population worldwide. Female-to-male ratio is 6:4. Onset is usually slow and insidious, and any group of skeletal muscles can be initially affected. However, most patients initially have ocular manifestations. If the disease remains localized to the eyes for 2 years, the likelihood of progression to generalized myasthenia gravis is low. Of the patients with myasthenia gravis, 33% have bulbar symptoms such as difficulty swallowing and clearing secretions, which predisposes them to the risk of aspiration during anesthesia. Skeletal muscle involvement is characterized by weakness and easy fatigability that improves with rest. The disease is characterized by remissions and relapses. The Osserman classification characterizes patients based on their symptoms. Type 1 patients have involvement of extra ocular muscles only. Type 2a patients have mild skeletal muscle weakness with sparing

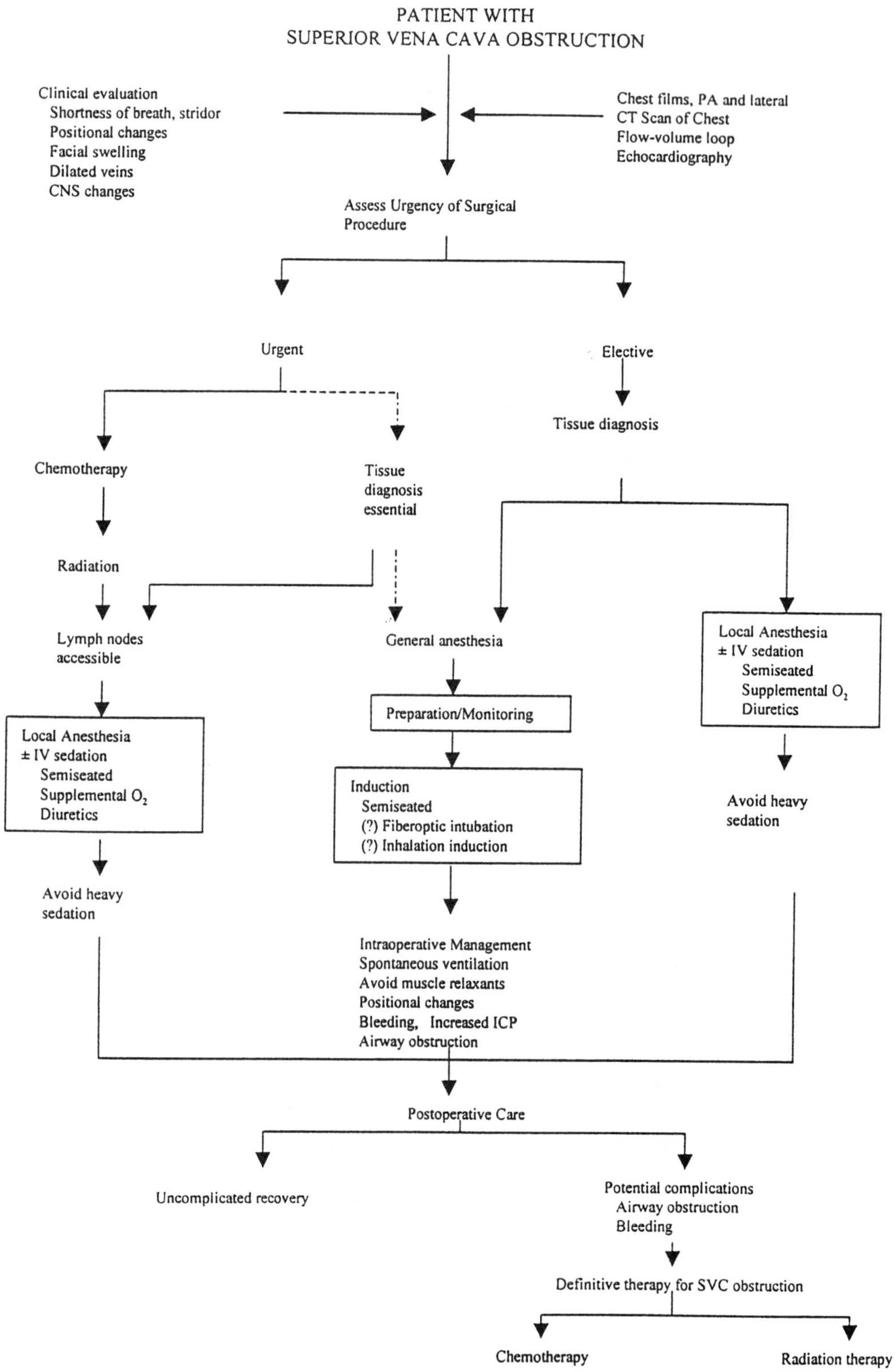

FIGURE 26-28. Flow chart for management of patients with superior vena cava obstruction.

of the muscles of respiration. Type 2b patients have more severe skeletal muscle weakness with bulbar involvement. Type 3 patients have an acute onset of symptoms with rapid deterioration of bulbar and skeletal muscles. Type 4 myasthenia is late, severe involvement of bulbar and skeletal muscles.

Treatment

The pharmacologic treatment of myasthenia gravis includes anticholinesterases to increase the amount of acetylcholine at the neuromuscular junction. The accurate titration of the correct dose of anticholinesterases is necessary in these patients. Undertreatment can lead to muscle weakness or a myasthenic crisis. Overtreatment can cause excessive muscarinic side effects from anticholinesterase and may cause a cholinergic crisis because of excessive accumulation of acetylcholine at the motor endplate, leading to a depolarizing type of muscle weakness. Because the autoimmune mechanism is implicated in the pathogenesis of myasthenia gravis, therapy with corticosteroids and immunosuppressants have been used. With corticosteroids, the usual dose is prednisone, 1 mg/kg every other day. Immunosuppressant drugs that have been used include azathioprine, cyclophosphamide, and cyclosporine. Plasmapheresis has also been used in the treatment of severe myasthenia gravis and myasthenic crisis, as well as in the preparation of patients for surgery. It is followed by a dramatic decrease in the titer of acetylcholine-receptor antibodies.

The surgical treatment for myasthenia gravis is thymectomy by a transcervical or transsternal approach. Of the patients who have myasthenia gravis, 75% have abnormalities of the thymus glands (85% of the glands show hyperplasia; 15% show thymomas). The response to surgery is usually encouraging (61). Approximately 20% of patients demonstrate complete remission; 40% show marked clinical improvement and decreased requirements for anticholinesterase drugs; 20% demonstrate clinical improvement with no change of medication dosage; and 6% show no improvement clinically and continue to require the same preoperative doses of anticholinesterases.

In the past, most patients underwent a transsternal thymectomy. This was followed by an incidence of postoperative mechanical ventilation ranging from 10% to 50%. Transcervical thymectomy is now increasing in popularity and has a postoperative mechanical ventilation rate of 0% to 9% (62). Although the transsternal route can perform a more complete removal of thymus tissue, the morbidity rate appears to be greater than by the transcervical route. Results in terms of clinical improvement and remission rate after transcervical thymectomy are reported to be equally as good as those after transsternal thymectomy.

Anesthetic Management

Preoperative vital capacity, peak inspiratory force, and maximum breathing capacity should be measured in every patient. Those with abnormal test results indicating impaired respiratory function should have complete pulmonary function tests performed, including blood gas analysis. Chest radiographs and CT scans of the chest should be reviewed to assess the presence and size of the thymic tumor and its possible interference with airway management. A preoperative ECG should be performed, because myasthenia gravis may be associated with myocardial degenerative changes. Fluid and electrolyte imbalances may be present if the patient has been receiving steroid preparations and should be corrected before surgery.

The patient's usual medications should be reviewed for drugs that can interfere with neuromuscular function and may therefore potentiate the response to muscle relaxants. Drugs that potentially can cause muscle weakness in myasthenia gravis patients include (a) calcium channel blockers, (b) aminoglycoside antibiotics, (c) triethylenethiophosphoramide (thiotepa), and (d) antidysrhythmic drugs such as quinidine and procainamide. Preoperatively, we continue all medications and the patient's usual dose of Mestinon is given with a sip of water. Patients receiving systemic steroids should have steroid supplementation administered on the day of surgery, followed by a gradual steroid tapering. Our preference is to avoid premedication with opioids; however, a small dose of oral or intramuscular benzodiazepine can be considered.

Standard monitors are applied in addition to radial arterial and internal jugular central venous lines. The arterial lines will allow for beat-to-beat blood pressure monitoring and for blood gas analysis intraoperatively as well as postoperatively. The central line aids in fluid status evaluation and is particularly helpful for administering vasoactive agents intraoperatively. The nerve stimulator is used to record single-twitch, train-of-four tetanic stimulation and posttetanic facilitation.

The response of patients with myasthenia gravis to succinylcholine can be unpredictable. Most authors report an increased resistance of myasthenic patients to succinylcholine. The phase II block also tends to appear early. A dose of 1 to 1.5 mg/kg has been reported to result in phase II block, with a recovery time ranging from 4 to 87 minutes (63). Therefore, we prefer to avoid the use of succinylcholine in these patients. If the patient has an anatomically difficult airway or a full stomach, we recommend an awake fiberoptic intubation. Patients with myasthenia gravis are extremely sensitive to nondepolarizing muscle relaxants, and they act as if they are already partially curarized. Atracurium or rocuronium are our preferred agents because of their short elimination half-life. After induction, the twitch monitor is turned on at 1 twitch/second and the chosen muscle relaxant is given in increments of 20% of the usual intubating dose. Halogenated agents have some muscle-relaxing properties as well and must be taken into consideration when managing myasthenia gravis patients.

Leventhal et al. (64) described the predictors of the need

for postoperative mechanical ventilation in patents with myasthenia gravis undergoing transsternal thymectomy with halogenated anesthesia without use of muscle relaxants. The predictive accuracy under these conditions was found to be 80%. Although their scoring system was not intended to be an absolute rule, it can help the clinician focus on important patient characteristics. The decision to extubate the trachea early should be individualized. When the Leventhal et al. criteria were tested in patients undergoing transcervical thymectomy with the same anesthetic technique, the predictive accuracy of the scoring system was found to be only 13% (65).

Anesthesia may be induced with thiopental, etomidate, or propofol, followed by the administration of a halogenated drug, preferably sevoflurane or desflurane. An O_2/N_2O mixture of 30%/70% can be used. Anesthesia is allowed to deepen using an inhalation agent. We usually avoid the use of muscle relaxants whenever possible. If a muscle relaxant is used, our first choice is atracurium or rocumonium. The initial dose being 20% of the usual intubating dose. We then administer fentanyl (1 to 2 μg/kg) and lidocaine (1.5 mg/kg) to blunt the hemodynamic response to laryngoscopy and intubation. Airway management can be done with a single-lumen tube; however, this is dependent on the practice of the surgical team, as some surgeons request a double-lumen tube and one-lung ventilation.

After the procedure, the patient is allowed to awaken, and we usually plan an immediate extubation in the operating room. Patients more commonly requiring postoperative extubation include those who have had myasthenia gravis for more than 6 years, those who have COPD in addition to myasthenia gravis, those who take more than 750 mg/day of pyridostigmine, and those who have a preoperative FEV_1 value of less than 2.9 L. Before extubation, adequate suctioning from the tracheobronchial tree is important in these patients. Neuromuscular transmission is monitored using train-of-four tetanic stimulation and posttetanic facilitation. If a nondepolarizing muscle relaxant has been used, it should be reversed using neostigmine and atropine. Criteria for extubation include a tidal volume of 6 to 7 mL/kg, the ability to generate a negative inspiratory force of at least -20 cm H_2O, a vital capacity of 15 mL/kg, and the ability to sustain a head lift for 5 seconds. Postoperative pain management is with intravenous patient-controlled anesthesia and NSAIDs.

The improvement after thymectomy may take weeks, months, or years. Therefore, these patients may continue to need their anticholinesterase for a varying period after thymectomy. Dose requirements may change unpredictably in the early postoperative period. If residual muscle weakness is present and the patient is not yet able to take oral medications postoperatively, an equivalent parenteral intravenous or intramuscular dose of the patient's usual daily maintenance dose is given. The ratio of oral-to-intravenous pyridostigmine is 30:1. Therefore, a 60-mg oral dose of pyridostigmine would be equivalent to 2 mg of intravenous pyridostigmine.

MYASTHENIC SYNDROME (LAMBERT-EATON SYNDROME)

Lambert-Eaton syndrome is a condition that results from an association between carcinomatous conditions and most commonly small cell carcinoma of the lungs, as well as motor neuropathy. Clinically, it resembles myasthenia gravis. Patients complain of weakness of the proximal muscles, which unlike in patients with myasthenia gravis, improves with exercise. The syndrome is caused by the decreased release of acetylcholine at the neuromuscular junction. The serum of these patients contains IgG antibodies that are directed against voltage-dependent calcium channels (66). The cells of small cell carcinoma of the lung and other malignancies possess calcium channels that may serve as the antigenic stimulus for the production of these antibodies. The destruction of the presynaptic calcium channels at the nerve terminal by immune-mediated complement activation results in decreased release of acetylcholine. Patients with Lambert-Eaton syndrome have developed respiratory failure while being treated with verapamil. Lambert-Eaton syndrome has also been reported to occur in conjunction with subacute cerebellar degeneration in a patient with small cell carcinoma of the lung. Antibodies directed against cerebellar Purkinje cell proteins were detected in the serum (67). Lambert-Eaton syndrome may also be associated with other autoantibodies, such as antithyroid, antigastric, or antiskeletal muscle antibodies. Electromyogram shows a significant reduction in the amplitude of the compound muscle action potential, which improves greatly after exercise.

Patients with Lambert-Eaton syndrome symptoms do not respond well to anticholinesterases. However, 4-aminopyridine, guanidine, and germine increase repetitive nerve firing, and the synaptic release of acetylcholine improves the symptoms. Patients with Lambert-Eaton syndrome are extremely sensitive to the effects of all muscle relaxants, both depolarizers and nondepolarizers. The possibility of Lambert-Eaton syndrome should be considered in all patients with known malignant disease and those undergoing diagnostic procedures for suspected lung carcinoma. Clinical improvement after plasma exchange suggests that a humoral factor may be the cause but additional mechanisms have also been proposed. A patient with chronic muscle weakness undergoing lobectomy for adenocarcinoma of the lung showed an immediate improvement of the initially reduced neuromuscular twitch response on the ligation of the pulmonary vein. Because the half-life of IgG is about 21 days, a factor—or factors other than IgG—must have been involved, at least partially, in the myasthenic syndrome observed in that patient. The authors therefore suggested that a humoral factor with an ultrashort half-life that affects neuromuscular function may be produced by the tumor (68).

Patients with Lambert-Eaton syndrome also manifest prominent symptoms of autonomic dysfunction involving the mucous membranes (dry mouth and dry eyes), skin (decreased sweating), peripheral blood vessels (orthostatic hypotension and lightheadedness), bladder and bowel (constipation and difficulty with micturition), and sexual organs (impotence). Autonomic dysfunction may also be subclinical, demonstrable only with formal autonomic testing. Autonomic abnormalities affect both cholinergic (nicotinic as well as muscarinic) and adrenergic functions. Suggested mechanisms include a defect in the release of acetylcholine and noradrenaline neurotransmitters (perhaps by the same autoimmune mechanism responsible for muscle weakness) and a lack of functional antagonism between the cholinergic and adrenergic systems. The autonomic dysfunction and muscle weakness usually improve after surgery or chemotherapy, but regression may be incomplete. Immunosuppressive therapy with corticosteroids, azathioprine, and plasmapheresis seems to provide the most satisfactory long-term improvement when tumor therapy alone is not successful.

TRACHEAL RESECTION AND TRACHEOBRONCHIAL RECONSTRUCTION

Patients with tracheal tumors, carinal tumors, or traumatic tracheobronchial disruptions require resection of the trachea or main bronchi and tracheobronchial reconstruction. The surgical management of these patients poses major challenges for the anesthesiologist. The most challenging aspects of this procedure are (a) to manage the induction of anesthesia without precipitating airway obstruction and (b) to design an effective plan for ventilating the lungs during the resection and reconstruction that does not interfere with surgical exposure and allows adequate ventilation and oxygenation. After the procedure, the patient ideally should be breathing spontaneously and be extubated in the operating room or shortly thereafter. An inflated cuff and positive-pressure ventilation adjacent to the suture line may interfere with its healing and cause its disruption. Patients with large intratracheal or carinal masses are at an extremely high risk for developing total airway obstruction at the induction of anesthesia. These patients may undergo laser-debulking procedures before surgical resection.

Surgical techniques may include resection and primary anastomosis, the insertion of a T-tube stent, or resection and reconstruction with prosthetic material. Therapeutic adjuncts may include radiotherapy (preoperatively or postoperatively), radioactive seed implantation, and preoperative laser debulking. Surgery on the trachea and right main bronchus is usually done through a right thoracotomy to avoid the interference posed by the aortic arch. However, if the left main bronchus is involved or left pulmonary resection may be done, a left thoracotomy would be performed. The surgical procedure requires extensive hilar dissection, mobilization of the lungs, and possibly opening of the pericardium. The omentum may be mobilized through an abdominal incision to wrap the anastomosis or to cover defects in the tracheobronchial tree. The large thoracoabdominal exposure substantially increases heat loss and fluid requirements. To decrease tension on the anastomosis at the conclusion of surgery, one may have to maintain the patient's neck in a flexed position by suturing the skin and soft tissues of the chin to the anterior chest wall.

Preoperatively, patients are carefully evaluated for airway patency and cardiopulmonary reserve. Unless airway obstruction is imminent, requiring emergency surgery, pulmonary function studies should also be obtained. Flow-volume loops are very helpful in detecting and determining the presence of fixed or variable intrathoracic or extrathoracic obstruction. Preoperative optimization of pulmonary function as needed with antibiotics and bronchodilators should be achieved. All considerations that apply to patients with airway obstruction resulting from extrinsic compression by mediastinal masses also apply to patients with intrinsic obstruction of the airways. Preoperative arterial blood gas values should be obtained. Because a significant degree of mucosal edema frequently contributes to airway obstruction in these patients, preoperative steroids and diuretics may be beneficial.

In addition to standard monitoring, radial artery and central venous lines are utilized. The arterial line allows for beat-to-beat blood pressure monitoring along with blood gas analysis. The central line allows for central pressure measurement and the administration of vasoactive agents.

Some patients have such severe airway obstruction that induction of anesthesia would precipitate total airway obstruction. Cardiopulmonary bypass may be initiated through the femorofemoral approach with these patients under local anesthesia before anesthetic induction. The routine use of cardiopulmonary bypass during carinal resection has been advocated but caries a high risk of intrapulmonary hemorrhage due to heparinization as well as cardiopulmonary bypass–related pulmonary dysfunction. Intrapulmonary hemorrhage is a serious risk however, because of excessive lung manipulations in the presence of total heparinization. Therefore, cardiopulmonary bypass should be used only in selected patients when absolutely necessary.

Induction of anesthesia follows the same guidelines as discussed in the section on anesthesia for patient with mediastinal masses. The anesthesiologist must know precisely the site and the size of the lesion, as well as the degree of airway lumen compromise before induction of anesthesia. The anesthesiologist should carefully review the chest radiographs, tomograms, CT scans, flow-volume loops, and results of bronchoscopy or bronchography done preoperatively. The major challenge during surgery for tracheobronchial resections and reconstruction is the method used for ventilation. The options include (a) high-frequency ventilation to one or both lungs, (b) a single-lumen tube above or below the site of the lesion, (c) a single endobronchial tube or two endobronchial tubes: one into each main-stem bronchus distal to the area of resection, (d) high-frequency or low-frequency jet ventilation, and (e) cardiopulmonary bypass.

High-frequency positive-pressure ventilation usually employs a respiratory rate of 60 to 100 breaths/minute administered with a volume-cycled ventilator. It does not depend on gas entrainment. Inspiration is active, and expiration is passive. High-frequency jet ventilation uses jet pulsations at a rate of 100 to 400 breaths/minute. It depends on gas entrainment. Again, inspiration is active, and expiration is passive. High-frequency jet ventilation has the disadvantage of depending on gas entrainment for ventilation. It tends to result in distal aspiration of blood and tumor debris. With high-frequency positive-pressure ventilation however, a continuous flow of gas occurs to the outside, which protects against distal aspiration of blood and debris. High-frequency positive-pressure ventilation provides adequate oxygenation and ventilation by the generation of eddy flows in the airway. It may lead to better distribution of gas flow compared with conventional mechanical ventilation. Airway pressure during high-frequency positive-pressure ventilation is continuously positive, with low, mean, and peak pressures. Intrapleural pressure is continuously subatmospheric, with minimal effect on pulmonary and systemic hemodynamics. The principle advantage of high-frequency positive-pressure ventilation in tracheobronchial resection is the ability to deliver ventilation through small catheters located either in the airway or even passing through standard endotracheal tubes. These catheters provide less interference with the surgical technique than standard-size single-lumen or double-lumen tubes. After the trachea has been incised, the jet ventilation catheters can be passed into one or both bronchi, providing independent ventilation to both lungs.

High-frequency positive-pressure ventilation is likely to be beneficial in patients undergoing (a) carinal resections, (b) sleeve pneumonectomies or sleeve upper-lobe resections, (c) tracheal reconstruction supported by Montgomery T tubes, and (d) tracheal resections (Fig. 26-29). For left-sided sleeve pneumonectomy, endobronchial intubation with a small catheter passing through the endotracheal tube provides the surgeon with an unobstructed field of vision. The catheter is passed through the operative field and guided by the surgeon into the left main bronchus. The continuous outflow of gas through the open bronchus during high-frequency positive-pressure ventilation minimizes the distal aspiration of blood and debris. Ventilation of the right lung with high-frequency positive-pressure ventilation via a thin catheter inside the right main bronchus eliminates the problem of right upper-lobe collapse associated with the use of right-sided endobronchial tubes (Fig. 26-30). Independent high-frequency jet ventilation to each lung can be delivered as depicted in Fig. 26-31. This is particularly advantageous when a large carinal tumor significantly obstructs one or both bronchi, preventing delivery of adequate tidal volume to either lung. In this situation, a catheter could be passed into one or both bronchi under fiberoptic bronchoscopic guidance. Another useful application of this technique is if the two lungs are asymmetrically diseased. In this situation, a high-frequency jet ventilation catheter is introduced into each main-stem bronchus. Each is connected to a high-

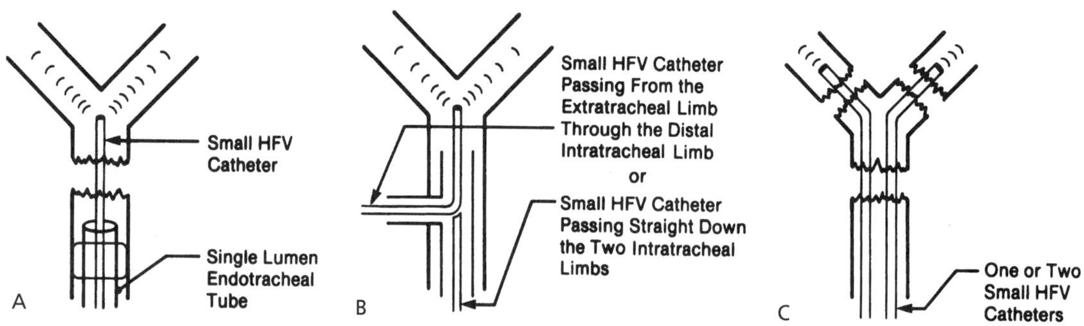

FIGURE 26-29. The three types of airway surgery aided by small high-frequency ventilation (HFV) catheters are tracheal resections, tracheal reconstructions that require support by a Montgomery T tube and carinal procedures (e.g., sleeve pneumonectomy, carinal resections). With tracheal resection **(A)**, a simple HFV catheter can be passed beyond the point of airway interruption, but above the tracheal carina, and used to ventilate both lungs with HFV. With tracheal reconstructions supported by a Montgomery T tube **(B)**, the small HFV catheter can be passed from either the extraluminal limb or the proximal intraluminal trachea limb to the distal intraluminal tracheal limb and can be used to ventilate both lungs with HFV. With carinal procedures **(C)**, one or two HFV catheters can be passed into one of the main bronchi, or both, and can be used to ventilate one or both of the lungs with HFV. (From Benumof JL, ed. *Anesthesia for thoracic surgery,* 2nd ed. Philadelphia: WB Saunders, 1995, with permission.)

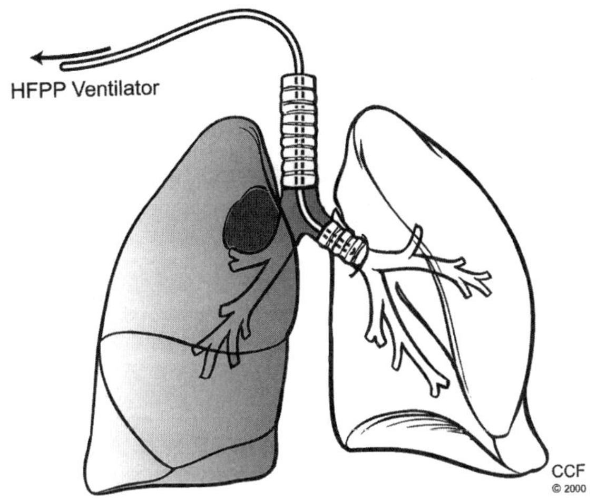

FIGURE 26-30. High-frequency ventilation through a catheter positioned in the left main bronchus to allow for right sleeve pneumonectomy.

frequency ventilator, and the ventilators are adjusted separately according to the compliance of each lung. The presence of even two high-frequency jet ventilation catheters through the surgical field does not significantly interfere with surgical exposure. Patients who have a significant degree of tracheal stenosis may not accommodate a large enough endotracheal tube to permit adequate ventilation. Several solutions exist for this problem. First, one can use a specially made, long endotracheal tube that has a small internal diameter—for example, a long size-5 oral endotracheal tube that would pass through the tracheal lesion. Ventilation of an adult through this size endotracheal tube obviously requires very high airway pressures and is not particularly effective. Second, one can use high-frequency positive-pressure ventilation through a small catheter passing through the stenotic area. One must ensure, however, that enough space exists between the stenotic lesion and the catheter to allow for the adequate outflow of gas; otherwise, barotrauma will occur. Third, the surgeon first can perform laser resection of the stenotic lesion to increase airway diameter. The choice of endotracheal tube after laser debulking no longer depends on the tracheal diameter, but on the method of ventilation chosen.

High-frequency positive-pressure ventilation is also useful during tracheobronchial reconstructive surgery in patients undergoing sleeve pneumonectomy, sleeve lobectomies, and tracheal reconstruction. For example, a patient undergoing a right upper-sleeve lobectomy is ventilated through a regular single-lumen tube until the right main bronchus and the right upper lobe are resected. The single-lumen tube is then advanced into the left main bronchus, and unilateral intermittent positive-pressure ventilation is continued to the left lung. At the same time, high-frequency jet ventilation is delivered to the right intermediate bronchus to ventilate the residual right, middle, and lower lobes and thereby maintain better oxygenation.

When planning to use conventional ventilation and conventional endotracheal tubes during tracheobronchial reconstructive surgery, one must have several different sizes of armored endotracheal tubes available, some of them still sterile. The management technique depends on the lesion's location and its distance from the carina. For resection of high tracheal lesions, an armored single-lumen tube is placed above the lesion after induction of general anesthesia. Spontaneous ventilation is maintained and 100% O_2 used. If the stenosis is mild, the single-lumen tube can be passed through the narrow segment into the distal trachea. If the area of obstruction is bypassed, mechanical positive-pressure ventilation can be safely used. The surgeon may help by guiding the single-lumen tube past the area of stenosis when the trachea is open. Another method involves passing a second tube through the field into the distal trachea after the trachea has been transected below the lesion. That tube is then connected via a second set of sterile anesthesia hoses and Y piece to the anesthesia machine. The single-lumen tube's tip distal to the cuff can be cut to allow the tube to remain above the carina if the distal segment of the trachea is short. A repair of a high tracheal lesion is usually done through a cervical incision, possibly combined with a median sternotomy. After excision of the tracheal lesion and placement of the posterior tracheal suture line, the second distal endotracheal tube or endobrachial tube is removed from the trachea. The first endotracheal tube is advanced past the anastomotic line and reconnected to the anesthesia circuit, and the anastomosis is completed.

The resection of a more distal lesion can be performed through a right thoracotomy incision. A single-lumen tube is placed with its tip above the lesion. If sufficient length of trachea distal to the area of resection is available, a Foley catheter with its tip cut off just distal to the balloon may be used as a single-lumen endotracheal tube. It is inserted by the surgeon and maintained in place above the carina, thereby avoiding endobronchial intubation and the need for one-lung ventilation. If the distal tracheal stump is very short, a single-lumen endotracheal tube must be advanced into an endobronchial location. The bronchus of the dependent lung must be intubated. Because the procedure is usually done through a right thoracotomy, left endobronchial and left lung ventilation are usually used. If oxygenation is inadequate, the degree of shunt can be decreased by temporarily clamping the pulmonary artery of the atelectatic side (Fig. 26-32). When the posterior suture line has been completed, the distal endobronchial tube or Foley catheter is removed, and the original orotracheal tube is advanced across the suture line into the bronchus of the dependent lung. The anterior suture line is then completed. The endotracheal tube is then pulled proximally so its tip lies above the suture line.

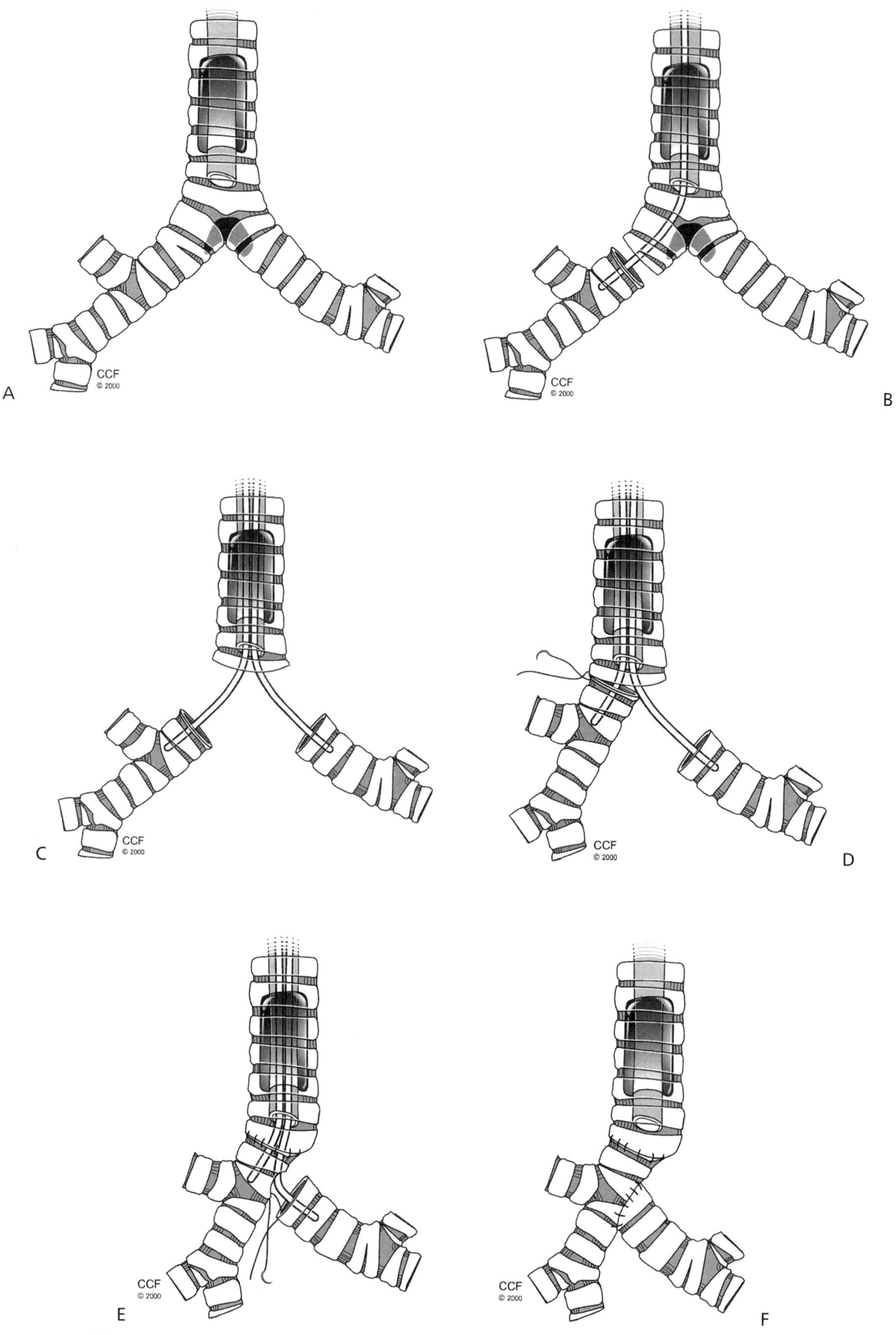

FIGURE 26-31. The use of high-frequency jet ventilation catheters for the management of carinal resection.

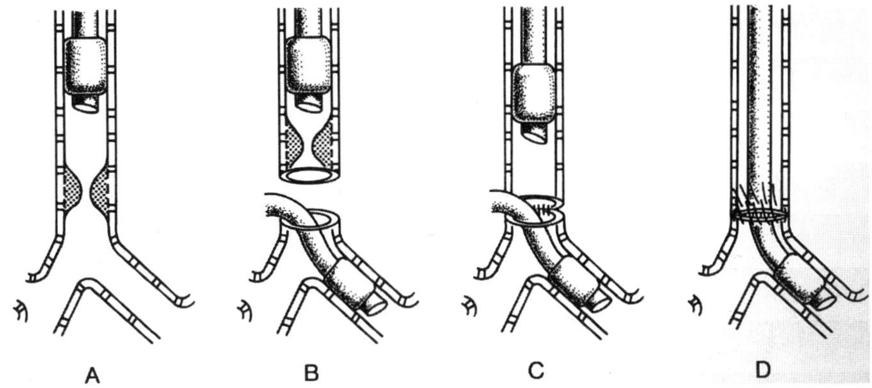

FIGURE 26-32. Airway management and surgical procedure for resection of a low tracheal lesion. **A:** Initial intubation above the lesion. **B:** Left endobronchial intubation distal to the lesion after the trachea has been opened. **C:** Placement of sutures for the posterior anastomosis. **D:** The endobronchial tube has been removed, and the original endotracheal tube has been advanced distal to the anterior anastomosis into an endobronchial position. (From Benumof JL, ed. *Anesthesia for thoracic surgery,* 2nd ed. Philadelphia: WB Saunders, 1995, with permission.)

For carinal resections (Fig. 26-33), a single-lumen tube is inserted through the larynx. After the carina is resected, the surgeon places a second single-lumen tube into the bronchus of the dependent lung, usually the left. Again, this is connected by a set of sterile anesthesia hoses and a Y piece to the anesthesia machine. The left lung is now ventilated through the endobronchial tube, whereas the right lung is temporarily collapsed while the right main bronchus is attached to the trachea. After the right main bronchus and the trachea have been reattached, the original translaryngeal endotracheal tube is advanced past the suture line into the right main bronchus. The left endobronchial tube is then removed, and the left main bronchus is attached to the trachea by an end-to-side anastomosis. The endotracheal tube is then pulled proximally so its tip is above both anastomotic lines. Alternatively, once the carina is resected, one can independently ventilate each lung through the distal bronchial stumps. The surgeon places a single-lumen tube into each bronchial stump. A plastic Y connector is used to divide the tidal volume from the anesthesia machine between the two endotracheal tubes. A good air seal can be achieved by using stay sutures to pull the bronchial stump up against the distal end of the inflated cuff. As the posterior layer of the anastomosis is being done, ventilation is maintained through the accessible distal bronchi. When is it time to anastomose the lateral wall of one bronchus to the trachea, the corresponding endobronchial tube is then removed and one-lung ventilation is used for a limited period. As the anastomosis of the anterior wall nears completion, ventilation from above is restored. When the anastomosis of one side is complete, that side is then ventilated and the other endobronchial tube is removed; then the other anastomosis is started. Once the anastomosis is complete, ventilation through the trachea is reestablished.

Low-frequency jet ventilation has been used successfully for maintaining normal ventilation during tracheal resection. Intermittent O_2 jets at pressures of 40 to 60 psi can be delivered with a Saunders injector into the lungs via a small-bore catheter, which can be passed through a single-lumen tube past the site of surgical resection. After resection of the stenotic area, the endotracheal tube is advanced into the distal trachea or into a bronchus until the anastomosis is complete. After this, the tube is pulled proximally above the suture line (Fig. 26-34).

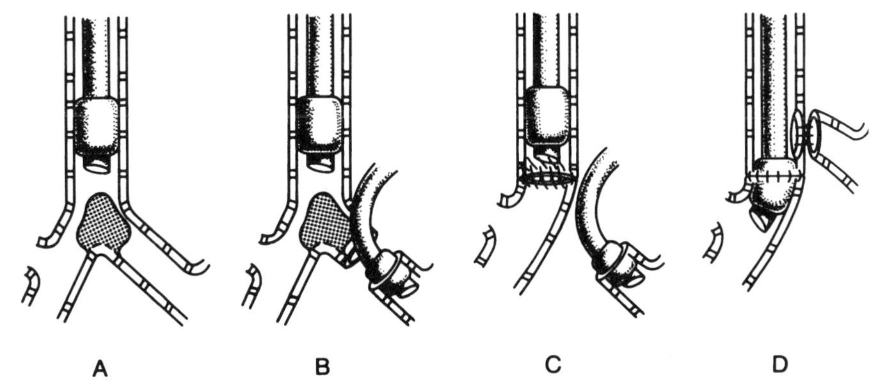

FIGURE 26-33. Airway management and surgical procedure for resection of a carinal lesion. **A:** Initial intubation above the lesion. **B:** Left endobronchial intubation distal to the lesion after the left main bronchus has been severed. **C:** The trachea is anastomosed to the right main bronchus. **D:** The left endobronchial tube has been removed to allow for anastomosis between the trachea and the left main bronchus, during which ventilation is accomplished via the original endotracheal tube. (From Benumof JL, ed. *Anesthesia for thoracic surgery,* 2nd ed. Philadelphia: WB Saunders, 1995, with permission.)

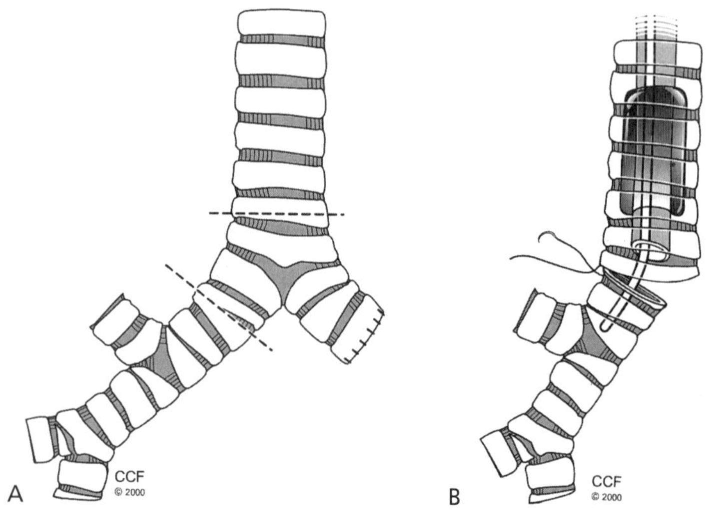

FIGURE 26-34. The use of a single-lumen tube and high-frequency jet ventilation catheter for left pneumonectomy and carinal resection.

ANESTHESIA FOR PATIENTS WITH BRONCHOPLEURAL FISTULA

Various surgical and pathologic conditions can cause bronchopleural fistula. Bronchopleural fistula can result from pneumonectomies or lobectomies because of a breakdown in the bronchial suture line. This can be caused by faulty surgical technique, excessive dissection and devascularization of the bronchial stump, excessively long bronchial stumps or infection. Certain patients are more predisposed to develop air leaks after lung resection, including those with cancer, those who are malnourished and debilitated and in poor general condition, immunosuppressed patients, those receiving steroid therapy, diabetic patients, those receiving preoperative or postoperative radiation and/or chemotherapy, and those undergoing pulmonary resection for tuberculosis. Failure of the remaining lung to expand after lung resection to fill the postoperative space also predisposes the patient to the development of bronchopleural fistula. A continued air leak can lead to infection in the pleural space and dehiscence of the bronchial stump (69). Traumatic bronchopleural fistulas may result from disruption of the airway followed by communication with the pleural cavity. A bronchopleural fistula may be caused by rupture of a lung abscess into the pleura or rupture of an empyema into the bronchus and by barotrauma in patients on mechanical ventilation.

Management

A bronchopleural fistula occurring early after resection is usually the result of a technical error. Early resuturing of the bronchial stump can be successful. If the fistula develops later after surgery, establishment of adequate dependent drainage and the reduction of the pleural space constitute the first step in therapy. Many small fistulas will close spontaneously. If the lung expands to fill the thoracic cavity, the leak can usually be controlled with chest tube drainage alone. A persistent airspace indicates a leak from a larger bronchus, usually requiring surgical treatment. Sepsis should be controlled with antibiotics and adequate chest drainage. Surgical options include (a) decortication if the lung is trapped by a thick purulent layer, (b) shortening of an excessively long bronchial stump, with or without resection of additional lung tissue, (c) closure of the bronchopleural fistula with a pedicled muscle flap, usually in the form of an intercostal flap, (d) thoracoplasty to obliterate the pleural space, usually combined with a pedicled muscle flap to cover the bronchial stump, and (e) performing flexible fiberoptic bronchoscopy and using fibrin glue to seal the communication between the bronchus and the pleural space.

Patients with a bronchopleural fistula may come under the anesthesiologist's care either in the intensive care unit when they have respiratory failure and sepsis requiring difficult ventilator management or in the operating room when they are undergoing various surgical procedures related or unrelated to the bronchopleural fistula. The most difficult aspects of caring for these patients are maintenance of adequate ventilation and oxygenation and protection of the contralateral lung from spillage of purulent material. Several methods have been developed to improve the ventilation of patients with a bronchopleural fistula using conventional intermittent positive-pressure ventilation. Chest tubes with unidirectional valves have been used to prevent air leakage to the outside during inspiration. This is hampered by the frequent malfunction of the valve because of interference by blood and pus inside the chest tube. One-lung ventilation to the healthy lung with collapse of the diseased lung with the aid of a double-lumen tube is a good method for intraoperative management of these patients. However, for prolonged periods in the intensive care unit, this usually predisposes the collapsed lung to infection. The use of high-frequency ventilation to treat patients with a bronchopleural fistula has therefore been attempted, with several conflicting reports regarding its efficacy (70,71) high-frequency jet ventilation may be of benefit only in some patients with a bronchopleural fistula. It appears to be less effective when patients have bilaterally diseased noncompliant lungs. Because the air leak improves with the decrease in peak and mean airway pressures, it is recommended that when high-frequency jet ventilation is used in patients with a bronchopleural fistula, both tracheal pressures and air flow through the leak should be measured and compared with values obtained during conventional mechanical ventilation. The lowest airway pressures that will allow adequate oxygenation and CO_2 elimination will be most advantageous in ventilating these patients. A disadvantage of high-frequency jet ventilation, however, is that it does not isolate the two lungs, allowing for possible contamination of the contralateral lung by spillage of purulent material from the affected side, particularly if an empyema or lung abscess is present.

Intraoperative management of patients with a bronchopleural fistula therefore requires different management of ventilation than in the intensive care unit setting. If an empyema is present, it should be drained first under local anesthesia and a chest tube should be placed before induction of anesthesia. This decreases the amount of pus in the pleural cavity, decreases the chance of flooding the contralateral lung, and provides a protective measure against the development of a tension pneumothorax. The period of induction is difficult and challenging. Application of positive pressure by a mask or a mechanical ventilator can lead to loss of most of the tidal volume through the fistula and to inadequate ventilation. Also, if no chest tube is placed or it is malfunctioning, or if a predisposing valvular mechanism exists, a tension pneumothorax may result. The ideal but often difficult approach is an awake intubation using a double-lumen tube with the patient breathing spontaneously. The bronchial lumen should be on the side opposite to the bronchopleural fistula. Once the tube has been positioned, the healthy lung should be isolated immediately by inflating the bronchial cuff and testing the adequacy of the cuff's seal by using the water bubble test described previously. Placing the head slightly up and the affected side in a 30° dependent position helps decrease the likelihood of contamination of the healthy lung. In patients with a normal airway, we prefer a rapid-sequence induction without ventilation, placement of a double-lumen tube through the glottis with immediate introduction of the fiberoptic bronchoscopy, and passage of the bronchial lumen of the double-lumen tube into the uneffected lung. Both cuffs are then inflated and ventilation is resumed to only the uneffected lung. When a double-lumen tube cannot be used, as in pediatric patients or those with difficult airway anatomy, lung separation can be achieved by endobronchial placement of a single-lumen tube or by an endotracheal single-lumen tube used in combination with a bronchial blocker.

ANESTHETIC IMPLICATIONS OF SPONTANEOUS PNEUMOTHORAX

Patients who develop spontaneous pneumothorax are usually young, healthy, and sometimes athletic with no preexisting lung disease and no prior lung resections. Surgical treatment for spontaneous pneumothorax includes pleurectomy, chemical pleurodesis, or apical resection of a bleb. Surgical treatment is indicated in patients with spontaneous pneumothorax in the following situations: (a) failure of the pneumothorax to resolve with chest tube drainage and suction, which indicates that a bronchopleural fistula has formed; (b) if a second ipsilateral or a first contralateral spontaneous pneumothorax occurs; and (c) if the patient's lifestyle is such that a recurrence might be life-threatening or highly inconvenient. The recurrence rate for spontaneous pneumothorax is 10% to 25%.

These patients are managed in a similar fashion as patients with a bronchopleural fistula. When patients with pneumothorax come to the operating room, they typically have a chest tube in place, and tension pneumothorax is not a major concern. Most patients can be managed with a single-lumen endotracheal tube. If the air leak is large, difficulty in ventilation may require measures to control the distribution of the tidal volume to the unaffected side. This can be achieved either with a double-lumen tube or a with a single-lumen tube advanced with the guidance of a fiberoptic bronchoscopy into the bronchus of the unaffected side. An arterial line would be useful for monitoring arterial blood gases if one-lung ventilation is employed.

ANESTHESIA FOR PATIENTS WITH SUPPURATIVE LUNG DISEASE

Single-lung abscess usually arises from suppurative inflammation distal to obstruction of a bronchus. Aspiration secondary to alcoholic stupor is probably the most common factor that precipitates lung abscess. Aspiration of teeth, foreign bodies, or blood produced by upper-airway procedures may be followed by collapse, infection, and then cavitation in the involved lung segment. Obstruction may also result from benign or malignant tumors or inspissated bronchial mucus. Infection and cavitation with abscess formation can also occur within a malignant tumor. Empyema results if a lung abscess located peripherally ruptures into the pleural cavity. Empyema may also follow pneumonia or result from infection of an undrained hemothorax or from residual clotted blood after drainage of a hemothorax by chest tube. Empyema has been described after diagnostic thoracentesis in patients with concurrent intraabdominal infections. Both lung abscesses and empyema can erode into a bronchus and cause a bronchopleural fistula or a bronchopleurocutaneous fistula.

Patients usually complain of fevers, chills, prostration, local pleuritic chest pain, cough, and leukocytosis. When the abscess or empyema ruptures into a bronchus, patients expectorate a large amount of foul-smelling, purulent sputum. Hemoptysis is a common feature, particularly when an abscess ruptures into the bronchus. Patients may be ill, debilitated, and have a toxic appearance. Physical examination reveals evidence of consolidation, fremitus, and rales, which frequently have a consonating or resonating quality. An empyema results in dullness to percussion over the lower chest. Chest radiographs in the presence of a lung abscess reveal the presence of an air-fluid level and perhaps an underlying tumor. If an empyema from a bronchopleural fistula is present, an air-fluid level should be detected in the pleural cavity on the upright chest radiograph. Bronchoscopy should be performed routinely in all patients with proven or suspected lung abscess. During bronchoscopy, a foreign body may be removed, a tumor may be detected, or a mucous plug may be removed.

Patients with simple empyema without abscess may be treated by repeated thoracentesis, chest tube drainage, or open drainage and rib resection. Early open drainage and rib resection is the treatment of choice for postoperative empyema and empyema that occurs in immunocompromised patients because it leads to a high success rate. Thoracoscopy and irrigation of the empyema cavity with antibiotic-containing solution has been used with good results. Intraoperatively, positive pressure applied to the affected lung can result in tearing of the fibrin deposits on the visceral pleura, thus enabling the maximal possible reexpansion of the lung.

Intraoperative isolation of the lungs is mandatory to prevent flooding and contamination of the healthy side by purulent material. In addition, one-lung ventilation greatly facilitates exposure when thoracoscopy is being performed for the treatment of empyema. If a bronchopleural fistula is present, management of ventilation should proceed according to the guidelines described in the previous section. At the end of the surgical procedure, the lung is reexamined and the surgeon carefully checks for air leaks.

ANESTHESIA FOR PATIENTS WITH BULLOUS LUNG DISEASE

Cysts of the lung can be classified as bronchogenic, postinfectious, infantile, or emphysematous. They may occur in association with COPD, may be diffuse and bilateral, or may be an isolated finding. Bullae are thin wall spaces filled with air that result from the destruction of the alveolar septa. The wall of the bulla is composed of visceral pleura, connective tissue septa, or compressed lung tissue. In general, bullae represent an area of end-stage emphysematous destruction of the lung. They result in a significant increase in the physiologic dead space and the amount of wasted ventilation; that is, they represent areas of high $\dot{V}/\dot{Q}$ ratio. Bullous lung disease may be seen in elderly patients with a long history of smoking and widespread COPD. Bullae may also be seen in relatively young patients with inborn defects in their connective tissue structure, such as α_1-antitrypsin deficiency. Some bullae have poor communication with the bronchial system, whereas others have wide communication with the tracheobronchial tree. Bullae cause compression of the adjacent healthy lung tissue and can lead to significant impairment of pulmonary function. Patients may require surgery for the removal of one or more unilateral or bilateral bullae, or they may require surgery for other unrelated conditions. In either case, bullae pose challenges for anesthetic management.

Preoperatively, one should assess the state of the nonbullous lung areas. Postoperative recovery rates and pulmonary function in patients with giant bullae and generalized emphysema are not as good as those in patients with well-demarcated bullae without underlying lung disease (72). Pulmonary function tests and ventilation and perfusion scans have been suggested to select patients who are likely to benefit from bullectomy. Surgical treatment of giant bullae is beneficial only to patients in whom the space occupied by the bullae inhibits ventilation of potentially functional and perfused lung. Suggestive evidence includes crowding of pulmonary vessels on radiographic studies and the presence of perfusion on a perfusion scan. If bullous emphysema is only the end-stage manifestation of generalized degenerative changes in the entire lung, excision of the bullae will have little beneficial effect. Patients who have an FEV_1 value of less than 35% of the normal value, and more importantly, those who show evidence of delay in ^{133}-Xe washout in all lung regions, generally have poor results after bullectomy. Patients with an FEV_1 value of more than 45% of normal value and relatively normal washout of ^{133}-Xe from the basal portions of the lungs generally experience good results after bullectomy (73).

The anesthetic management involves several specific ventilation hazards. These patients usually have severely diseased lungs and impaired respiratory reserve. Bullae not communicating with a major airway can grow and rupture if N_2O is used, leading to pneumothorax or tension pneumothorax. Communicating bullae can enlarge with positive-pressure ventilation and then rupture. Also, bullae are very compliant, and if the communication with the airway is large, most of the tidal volume can be wasted in the bulla, resulting in poor ventilation, hypoxemia, hypercarbia, and acidosis. The communication with the airway may act as a one-way valve, resulting in airtrapping, rapid enlargement in size, and compression of surrounding lung tissue, resulting in further impairment of pulmonary function and gas exchange, followed by development of a tension pneumothorax. Patients may require a variable period of postoperative mechanical ventilation, and the weaning process may be difficult.

Anesthetic Technique

A combined technique using a thoracic epidural catheter with general anesthesia and one-lung ventilation with 100% O_2 is commonly employed. Spontaneous ventilation should be maintained as long as possible, at least until the chest is open. A double-lumen tube is necessary to allow separation of both lungs, and in the event of unilateral disease, the tidal volume can be directed toward the unaffected side. One should remain constantly aware of the potential for pneumothorax. The development of a pneumothorax in the dependent, ventilated lung represents a life-threatening, catastrophic complication. A pneumothorax should be suspected if one detects decreasing breath sounds, appearance of wheezing, hypotension, desaturation, and deviation of the trachea to one side. The dependent hemithorax optimally should be accessible during the surgical procedure. It should be prepared and draped in such a way that if a pneumothorax developed, rapid placement of a chest tube would be possible. One should use positive-pressure ventilation with the lowest possible inspiratory pressure necessary to provide adequate ventilation. Pressure-regulated ventilation should also be considered as a technique to help keep the airway pressures as low as possible. If a pneumothorax develops, a chest tube inserted for its drainage, in effect, constitutes a bronchopleurocutaneous fistula that would produce severe problems in ventilation. Some advocate that general anesthesia be induced only after the surgeon has prepared the operative field and draped the patient. If the patient's condition suddenly deteriorates during induction, the surgeon can immediately open the chest. Sequential one-lung ventilation with a double-lumen tube may facilitate removal of bilateral bullae. The bullectomy should be performed on the more severely affected lung first while the better lung supports gas exchange. When the roles of the lungs are switched, the function and gas exchange capability of the postbullectomy lung should have improved. If hypoxemia develops during one-lung ventilation, application of CPAP to the nonventilated lung during the deflation phase of a large tidal breath usually improves arterial oxygenation.

VOLUME REDUCTION SURGERY FOR EMPHYSEMA

Dr. Otto Brantigan reported the concept of volume reduction surgery for the treatment of emphysema more than 40 years ago. He described volume reduction surgery as an operation directed at restoration of a physiologic principle, rather than the removal of pathologic tissue. Brantigan realized that the circumferential pull holding open the bronchioles was greatly impaired and lost on expiration, which resulted in airway obstruction. He noted that patients with emphysema had an overextended thorax due to voluminous lungs that occupied a space larger than normal, which interfered with the normal motion of the chest on inspiration and expiration. As a result, the diaphragm becomes flattened, the chest becomes barrel-shaped, and the intercostal muscles are in a state of overstretch, which causes them to become less effective. The method of operation was to remove the most useless and functionless areas of lung tissue to reduce the lung volume so that it would fill the pleural space on full expiration. One side of the chest was operated on at a time and at least 3 months was allowed before surgery was performed on the remaining hemithorax. This procedure was postulated to normalize the shape of the thorax, thereby allowing the diaphragm to dome and to decrease the stretch on the intercostal muscles, all to increase the circumferential, outward, elastic pull, on the small airways. The result is a decrease in airway obstruction and the subjective degree of dyspnea. In 1959, Brantigan presented 33 patients who had volume reduction surgery for emphysema (74). Patients were 16 to 69 years old. There were six postoperative deaths (18%), with two of these deaths being related to technical errors. No deaths were reported after the second operation on the contralateral side. All patients who survived the operation improved subjectively, although no objective data were presented. This procedure never gained widespread acceptance due to the relatively high mortality rates and few objective data available.

Cooper revisited volume reduction surgery in 1995 (75). Twenty patients with severe COPD were selected for surgery on the basis of having a distended thorax with significant functional limitation, despite maximum medical therapy. None of the patients had giant bullae or α_1-antitrypsin disease, and none of them were current smokers. There were 11 men and 9 women with a mean age of 56 years (range 37 to 76 years). Fourteen required oxygen with exertion and five also required oxygen at rest. Two patients were on the lung transplant waiting list and another four had been referred to their institution for transplantation. Patients were evaluated preoperatively, as well as 3 and 6 months after operation. The approach was through a median sternotomy and surgery was performed on the more severely affected lung first. Excision was directed to those portions of lung that remained distended despite one-lung ventilation indicating areas of airtrapping. The goal was to reduce overall lung volume by 20% to 30%. Excision was accomplished using surgical staplers lined with strips of bovine pericardium for buttressing in an effort to reduce air leaks. The lung volume was reduced to produce a shape that would fill the thorax and not leave a residual airspace. All attempts were made to stop remaining air leaks. No early or late deaths occurred in this series of patients. Hospital stay ranged from 6 to 49 days, with a mean of 15 days. Prolonged air leak (more than 7 days) was present in 11 patients. Four patients required reexploration: one for bleeding, one for a persistent apical airspace, and two for sudden massive bilateral air leak. Preoperatively, the mean FEV_1 value was 0.77 L (25% of predicted value), and the postoperative FEV_1 value was 1.4 (44% of predicted value) representing an 82% improvement. Significant improvements were also noted in FVC, total lung capacity, residual volume, and trapped gas. Oxygen was required on 14 of the 20 patients preoperatively, which decreased to 4 of the 20 patients postoperatively. The mean grade of dyspnea preoperatively was 2.9, indicating the need to stop for breath after walking 100 yards, and postoperatively was 0.8, indicating shortness of breath with hurried walking.

Volume reduction surgery remains a current treatment modality for patients with emphysema. Patients considered for surgery are those with dyspnea despite maximal medical therapy. Preoperative evaluation includes pulmonary function tests, arterial blood gas tests, 6-minute walk, chest x-ray, dynamic CT scan, ventilation-perfusion scans, lung volume by nitrogen washout, lung volume by body plethysmography (body box), echocardiography with pulmonary artery pressure estimation, and cardiac catheterization as clinically indicated. Good candidates for volume reduction surgery have the following characteristics: heterogeneous disease on CT scan (good targets for excision), flattened diaphragms and widened intercostal spaces on chest x-ray, evidence of trapped gas determined by the discrepancy between residual lung volumes obtained by nitrogen washout and body box, little or no movement of the diaphragm on dynamic CT scan, a $PaCO_2$ of less than 50 mm Hg, and a pulmonary artery mean pressure of less than 35 mm Hg. Patients are not considered for surgery if they are active smokers. Once accepted for lung reduction surgery, patients are enrolled into a preoperative 6-week course of pulmonary rehabilitation.

The surgical approach is by either median sternotomy or bilateral video-assisted thoracotomy. The thoracoscopic approach was associated with a lower mortality rate, particularly in those older than 65 years (76). Our surgical approach is bilateral video-assisted thoracoscopy. The patient is supine with rolls placed behind the shoulders, along the spine, and behind the pelvis. The arms are positioned on arm boards out to the side or above the surgical field secured to an ether screen. Targeted areas of diseased lung are identified as those that remain distended after the institution of one-lung ventilation. Surgical staplers are lined with bovine pericardium to decrease postoperative air leaks. The goal is to resect 20% to 30% of the preoperative total lung volume.

All current medications are continued until the morning of surgery. If the patient has been on steroids, a supplemental dose is given on the morning of surgery. All inhalers should be administered before induction of anesthesia. An antisialagogue, such as glycopyrrolate 0.2 mg, is the only premedication given routinely to help reduce secretions, which can interfere with one-lung ventilation. Preoperative administration of opioids and benzodiazepines is avoided.

Standard monitors are applied and a large-bore intravenous line is started. An arterial line is placed and a baseline arterial blood gas analysis is obtained. For anxiolysis, a small amount of midazolam may be given before placement of the epidural catheter. For placement of thoracic epidural catheters, patients are in the sitting position with their legs on a stool next to the operating room table. Catheters are placed at the T3-6 level. Hanging drop or loss of resistance techniques are used to access the epidural space. Catheters are tested using 3 mL of 1.5% lidocaine with epinephrine 1/200,000. After placement of the epidural catheter, the patient is returned to the supine position for central line placement via the right internal jugular vein. Pulmonary artery catheters may be considered for patients with ventricular dysfunction or pulmonary hypertension.

Before induction, any patient on bronchodilators self-administers a dose from his or her own inhaler. During induction, patients are at risk for severe hypotension and airtrapping. The hypotension can be due to several factors including hypovolemia and hyperinflation of the lungs, which can decrease venous return and directly compress the heart. After adequate preoxygenation, we proceed with a rapid induction and intubation, using such agents as sodium pentothal or amidate and succinylcholine. We commonly administer a fluid bolus before induction, which has helped decrease the incidence of hypotension. Before intubation, mask ventilation is avoided, which tends to be ineffective and may lead to airtrapping. Hypotension during induction is treated with volume administration and phenylephrine or ephedrine. Pneumothorax must also be quickly ruled out and treated when hypotension does not respond to aggressive treatment with volume and vasopressors. Immediately after intubation, the patient is placed on mechanical ventilation with an inspiration-to-expiration (I-to-E) ratio of 1 to 3 or 1 to 4 to allow for complete exhalation.

Lung separation is best achieved using double-lumen tubes. We strive to use the largest tube that the patient will safely accommodate, which is generally size 39F or 41F for men and 37F or 39F for women. Because of the faint and distant breath sounds, the early use of fiberoptic bronchoscopy is required to confirm and optimize placement of the double-lumen tube. The fiberoptic bronchoscopy should remain available throughout the case should the double-lumen tube need to be repositioned. Inspired FIO_2 is adjusted to maintain a PaO_2 of more than 60 mm Hg or at the preoperative value. Ventilation is adjusted to maintain a $PaCO_2$ at preoperative levels, most commonly between 45 and 60 mm Hg. To facilitate ventilation, I-to-E ratios are usually 1 to 3 to 1 to 4. The addition of small amounts of PEEP to the nonoperative lung may help to prevent airway collapse and facilitate ventilation. Patients are frequently managed with an FIO_2 value of 1.0 and small amounts of

CPAP can be applied to the operative lung to maintain oxygenation. It is not uncommon to have significant difficulty with ventilation intraoperatively with a resultant increase in $PaCO_2$. Permissive hypercapnea is generally tolerated provided that the pH remains ≥ 7.29. The utilization of intraoperative pressure-regulated ventilation has decreased our incidence of inadequate ventilation. Before anesthesia machines capable of pressure ventilation, we utilized intensive care unit ventilators when conventional ventilation became inadequate.

Anesthesia is maintained using inhalation agents such as sevoflurane or desflurane and muscle relaxants such as rocuronium or cisatracurium. Any benzodiazepines or opioids used to supplement the anesthetic should be limited and given at the beginning of the case. We commonly use a small amount of midazolam (less than 0.03 mg/kg) and fentanyl (less than 3 μg/kg) intravenously. After induction, the thoracic epidural is bolused with fentanyl followed by an infusion of fentanyl (5 μg/mL) and bupivacaine (0.1%). One may also consider dosing the epidural catheter with 0.25% bupivacaine, after which the patient will require less intravenous and inhalation agents. Warmed fluids, heating blankets, and heated circuits are all used to help maintain the patient's temperature during surgery.

Intraoperative hypotension is usually due to hypovolemia that can be exacerbated by airtrapping. Administering volume, vasopressors, and relaxation of any traction on the hilum or compression on the heart usually alleviates hypotension. When hypotension is not readily reversible despite intervention, we have used transesophageal echocardiography to assist in making the proper diagnosis (e.g., hypovolemia or cardiac dysfunction) and guiding our therapy. Intraoperative gas exchange impairments more frequently involve carbon dioxide elimination versus oxygenation. The administration of 100% oxygen and the proper balance of CPAP and PEEP usually adequately control oxygenation. Relative hypoventilation resulting in elevated $PaCO_2$ is initially treated by checking the double-lumen tube for proper placement and cuff inflation, adjusting the I-to-E ratio (1 to 3 to 1 to 5), administering bronchodilators, and accepting permissive hypercapnia. When this proves ineffective, alternative modes of ventilation such as pressure-regulated volume control and pressure-controlled ventilation are instituted. Pulmonary hypertension may be encountered and is most effectively treated by optimizing oxygenation and ventilation and ensuring adequate anesthesia. Agents such as nitroglycerin, sodium nitroprusside, prostaglandin, and/or milrinone are occasionally required for severe pulmonary hypertension.

After completion of the bilateral resection, the patient is returned to two-lung ventilation. A "trial of extubation" is attempted, provided that the patient did not require alternative modes of ventilation, excessive fluid administration, has adequate reversal of muscle relaxants, and has a temperature of more than 35°C. If a trial of extubation is unsuccessful, the double-lumen tube is changed to a single-lumen tube before transfer to the intensive care unit. In general, our preference is to spend no more than 30 minutes in the operating room deciding whether the patient can be extubated, can remain extubated, or requires reintubation before transfer to the intensive care unit. When postoperative ventilation is required, patients are sedated with agents such as propofol and/or fentanyl with the addition of a muscle relaxant as clinically indicated. The modes of ventilation used most commonly include pressure-regulated volume control or pressure-controlled ventilation when full support is required and pressure support is used for weaning. The goal is to extubate all patients as soon as possible and to avoid barotrauma and its potential consequences such as air leaks.

ANESTHESIA FOR MEDIASTINOSCOPY

Mediastinoscopy is performed most frequently to determine the resectability and the stage of lung cancer or the diagnosis of mediastinal and hilar masses. The goal is to detect the presence of lymph node metastasis that would make the disease incurable by surgery. Biopsies are usually obtained. In patients with carcinoma of the left lung, spread to the subaortic lymph nodes often occurs. In some instances, these are more easily accessible by performing anterior mediastinoscopy through a small incision at the third left intercostal space (Chamberlain operation).

The technique has also been modified for the examination of the anterior mediastinum and the thymus and to perform transcervical thymectomy. To reach the anterior mediastinum, the surgeon passes the instrument anterior to the innominate vessels, in contrast to classic mediastinoscopy, in which the mediastinoscope is passed posterior to the innominate vessels.

Preoperatively, these patients should be carefully assessed for the degree of airway obstruction and the severity of pulmonary dysfunction. Patients known to have mediastinal masses on chest radiograph or CT scan should be managed as previously discussed. In these patients, mediastinoscopy should be performed under local anesthesia if at all possible. The possibility of a thymoma should be considered in patients undergoing mediastinoscopy as part of a diagnostic workup for an anterior mediastinal mass. Even if symptoms of myasthenia are absent, the patient may be in a premyasthenic state (occult myasthenia gravis) and may respond dramatically to nondepolarizing muscle relaxants.

All patients receive the usual monitors of noninvasive blood pressure cuff, ECG, pulse oximetry, and temperature, as well as constant auscultation of heart sounds and breath sounds. The innominate artery can become pinched and occluded by the mediastinoscope, leading to total cessation of blood flow to the right upper extremity and right carotid circulation. Transient ischemic attacks after mediastinoscopy have been reported. Most patients are monitored with an arterial line. Major alterations in pressure lasting 15 to 360 seconds occur from compression of innominate artery or the aorta. It is therefore recommended that patients have a blood pressure cuff on the left arm and a right radial arterial line. If the right radial artery cannot be cannulated, a pulse oximeter should be placed on a finger of the patient's right hand.

The surgical technique involves a small suprasternal notch incision followed by passage of the mediastinoscope in the plane anterior to the trachea and behind the innominate vessels. To examine the anterior mediastinum, the surgeon passes the mediastinoscope anterior to the innominate vessels. The potential for injury to many vital structures therefore exists.

Most patients having mediastinoscopy are under general anesthesia. Induction is usually accomplished by intravenous agents, followed by introduction of an inhalation agent. If no real threat of airway compression by an extrinsic mass exists, a muscle relaxant can be administered. If a mediastinal mass is present, spontaneous ventilation should be maintained. Otherwise, mechanical ventilation is preferred during mediastinoscopy to decrease the risk of venous air embolism. If the patient is breathing spontaneously, the negative intrapleural pressure can lead to a greater risk of air embolism resulting from injury to the venous structures in the mediastinum. The tip of the mediastinoscope is exposed to negative intrapleural pressure, and therefore, air is sucked in from the atmosphere through the mediastinoscope into the mediastinum. Another advantage for administering muscle relaxants and controlling ventilation is to prevent the patient from sudden cough or movement during the procedure, which can significantly increase the risk of injury to intrathoracic structures by the rigid mediastinoscope. Anesthesia is usually maintained by a volatile agent $+/-N_2O$ supplemented with small doses of opioid as needed. Alternatively, total intravenous anesthesia can be achieved with infusions of propofol and short-acting opioids such as alfentanil or remifentanil. Most patients are extubated in the operating room after reversal of neuromuscular blockade. If the results of the mediastinoscopy are negative, some surgeons proceed directly with the planned lung resection, which requires changing the patient from the supine to the lateral decubitus position. The mortality rate from mediastinoscopy is less than 0.5% and the overall complication rate does not surpass 2.5% (78).

Complications include massive hemorrhage, so a large-bore intravenous line should always be placed for these cases. If superior vena cava obstruction is present, intravenous lines must be secured in the lower extremity. If the hemorrhage is caused by a tear in a vein and the intravenous lines are in the upper extremity, new lines must be placed in the lower extremity to resuscitate the patients effectively. Otherwise, all infused fluids and drugs can escape into the mediastinum through the torn vessel. Typed and cross-matched blood should be available for all patients and immediately accessible. Support of the circulation and infusion of blood, crystalloids, colloids, and pharmacologic agents are necessary. Hemorrhage can be temporarily controlled by packing the surgical wound using a sponge forceps or a small pack. Emergent median sternotomy may be required to control life-threatening hemorrhage.

Massive hemorrhage has resulted from laceration of the pulmonary artery when it was biopsied unintentionally during mediastinoscopy. Perforation of an unsuspected thoracic aortic aneurysm has also been reported. If the laceration is to a major vein in the mediastinum, air embolism is a serious threat, particularly if the patient is breathing spontaneously. Prompt recognition is important. The condition should be suspected by a change in the quality of the heart sounds heard through an esophageal stethoscope or by a precordial Doppler monitor, (b) hypotension and perhaps tachycardia, (c) cardiac dysrhythmias, or (d) a decrease in end-tidal CO_2 and an increase in end-tidal nitrogen concentrations. Immediate measures to treat air embolism include (a) stop administering N_2O; (b) immediately reposition the patient into the left lateral position to help trap intravascular air in the right atrium; bring the head down to the horizontal or head-down position to decrease further aspiration of air; (c) raise the intrathoracic venous pressure above atmospheric by inflating the patient's lungs using positive-pressure ventilation and PEEP; (d) if a central venous catheter is present, attempt to aspirate air; and (e) maintain pharmacologic support of the circulation and the right ventricle while all these measures are being instituted.

During surgery the mediastinoscope can impinge upon the innominate artery causing a decrease in cerebral perfusion. A right hemispheric stroke manifesting as left hemiparesis can result. If cessation or a decrease in flow is detected by a change in the right radial waveform, the surgeon should be immediately alerted to change the mediastinoscope's position. Compression of the aortic arch and the great vessels can also result in the initiation of autonomic reflexes such as bradycardia and hypotension. The loss of the right radial pulse during mediastinoscopy may be mistaken for cardiac arrest. Mediastinoscopy under local anesthesia might be advantageous for patients with obstructive disease of the carotid artery, so that the patient's level of consciousness can be continually evaluated.

Airway complications may also occur intraoperatively, the most common of which being direct compression. An abrupt increase in airway pressures should alert the clinician to check for external compression or bending of the single-lumen tube and to alert the surgeon for repositioning of the mediastinoscope. More distal advancement of the endotracheal tube should also be considered to relieve airway obstruction. Initial use of an armored endotracheal tube will greatly reduce intraoperative complications caused by compression of the airway.

Pneumothorax may also occur and can be unilateral or

bilateral. The use of positive-pressure ventilation can result in a rapid increase in the size of pneumothorax, leading to a tension pneumothorax. This complication should be suspected with increasing difficulty providing ventilation, an increase in peak airway pressure, deviation of the trachea, hypotension, and dysrhythmias. Injury to the recurrent laryngeal nerve may also occur during mediastinoscopy, which can be permanent. Upper-airway obstruction occurs if the nerve is damaged bilaterally. If injury to the recurrent laryngeal nerve is suspected, the vocal cords should be visualized while the patient is breathing spontaneously during extubation. Unilateral nerve injury without airway obstruction is treated conservatively. Laceration of the esophagus presents as postoperative chest pain, mediastinitis, and sepsis. Esophagoscopy should be performed, followed by surgical repair. Other complications of mediastinoscopy include chylothorax resulting from laceration of the thoracic duct and tumor seeding into the incision line.

ANESTHETIC CONSIDERATIONS FOR BRONCHOSCOPY

Bronchoscopy is frequently performed for the diagnosis and treatment of chest diseases. Diagnostic indications usually fall under three categories: (a) preoperative evaluation of patients for thoracic surgery; (b) determination of the etiology, site, and extent of acute changes such as hemoptysis, inhalation burn injuries, or abnormal chest radiograph results; and (c) diagnosis of chest-related signs and symptoms resistant to medical treatment, such as persistent cough, wheezing, atelectasis, or unresolved pneumonia. Therapeutic indications for bronchoscopy include the removal of foreign bodies, control of hemoptysis, laser airway surgery, placement of double-lumen endotracheal tubes, removal of secretions, and performance of bronchial toilet in patients with respiratory failure on mechanical ventilation in the intensive care unit. The choice between rigid bronchoscopy or flexible fiberoptic bronchoscopy generally depends on the indications. Some procedures and maneuvers are better performed via the rigid bronchoscope, whereas others are better suited to the flexible bronchoscope.

Rigid bronchoscopy is commonly employed for foreign body removal, airway dilation, placement of stents, and laser resection of masses within the airway. The carina and subcarinal area can also be palpated with the bronchoscope to assess the resectability of a bronchogenic carcinoma. The rigid bronchoscope has also been used to emergently overcome airway obstruction, which can occur in patients with mediastinal masses. Flexible fiberoptic bronchoscopy is used for visualization of the airway, removal of secretions, diagnostic bronchoalveolar lavage, biopsies, delivery of fibrin glue sealants for treatment of bronchopleural fistulas, and small foreign body removal with snares passed through the suction port. Flexible fiberoptic bronchoscopy also plays a key role in securing the difficult airway.

Flexible fiberoptic bronchoscopy can be easily performed under local anesthesia with sedation in spontaneously breathing patients, including children. It can also be performed under general anesthesia with or without an endotracheal tube in place. Rigid bronchoscopy, on the other hand, is very uncomfortable but can be performed with patients under local anesthesia and sedation. The technique for rigid bronchoscopy may cause excessive stress on the teeth and mouth, as well as excessive extension of the cervical spine. Therefore, it is almost always performed using general anesthesia.

Bronchoscopy can be performed with adequate topical anesthesia of the airway. Inadequate anesthesia will render bronchoscopy difficult and it can also lead to significant trauma resulting from unexpected patient movement. Topical local anesthetics should be applied to the nose, mouth, and oropharynx. Various nerve blocks to the superior laryngeal, glossopharyngeal, and recurrent laryngeal nerves may be achieved by transmucosal application or percutaneous injection of a local anesthetic. Inhalation of a nebulized local anesthetic could cover the entire mucous membrane of the mouth, pharynx, larynx, trachea, and proximal bronchi.

The nose can be anesthetized using 0.5% tetracaine with epinephrine, administering 4% lidocaine with epinephrine, or applying 10% cocaine pledgets containing 3 to 4 mL of cocaine. In addition, the nasal mucosa can be anesthetized by passing nasopharyngeal airways covered with a generous amount of lidocaine jelly. The mouth, pharynx, and oropharynx are anesthetized by spraying the mouth with tetracaine or lidocaine. In addition, the patient can gargle with 2% viscous lidocaine. The glossopharyngeal nerve can be blocked intraorally by injecting a local anesthetic into the midpoint of the posterior pillar of the fauces, which blocks the distribution of the glossopharyngeal nerve to the oropharynx.

The superior laryngeal branch of the vagus nerve is easily blocked as it traverses the thyrohyoid membrane. A small, 2.5-cm, 25-gauge needle is walked off the inferior border of the greater cornu of the hyoid bone near its tip, and 3 mL of local anesthetic is infiltrated both superficial and deep to the thyrohyoid membrane. Penetration of the membrane by the needle is felt as a slight loss of resistance. The process is then performed on the opposite side. This produces anesthesia of the inferior aspect of the epiglottis and laryngeal mucosa as far down as the vocal cords. To block the recurrent laryngeal nerve, a 20- or 22-gauge needle is introduced in the midline through the cricothyroid membrane. Entry of the needle into the trachea is identified by the aspiration of air, and most patients will cough slightly. Rapid injection of 3 to 5 mL of 4% lidocaine produced dramatic cough in most patients. This spreads the local anesthetic up and down the trachea and results in excellent topical anesthesia.

Another method of producing topical anesthesia of the

larynx and the trachea involves (a) spraying the mouth and oral cavity, (b) performing laryngoscopy, and (c) spraying the epiglottis, larynx, and the vocal cords with a local anesthetic. Bronchoscopy proceeds, during which the larynx and trachea are further sprayed as needed. A disadvantage of using the transtracheal route is that bleeding can occur into the trachea. This may be undesirable when performing diagnostic bronchial washing and lavage, because the presence of blood may confuse the diagnostic picture. The entire mucosa from the mouth to the bronchi can be anesthetized by a single technique using a nebulized local anesthetic solution. An O_2 tank is connected via O_2 tubing to an atomizer containing the local anesthetic solution, either 0.5% tetracaine with epinephrine or 4% lidocaine. Oxygen flowing through the atomizer creates a fine, dense mist that is inhaled by the patient continuously through a mouth piece or intermittently using 10 seconds of spraying alternating with 10- to 20-second pauses. Adequate anesthesia requires at least 15 minutes of topical administration of the mist.

Over 15 minutes in a 70-kg patient, the total dose of tetracaine should not exceed 100 mg (1 to 2 mg/kg), and of lidocaine 400 mg (5 to 6 mg/kg). Additional intravenous lidocaine may help suppress the cough reflex and decrease the incidence of cardiac dysrhythmias. However, one must be careful not to produce toxic serum levels. In the presence of significant liver disease, decreased hepatic lidocaine clearance can predispose patients to lidocaine toxicity, particularly in the elderly. Patients undergoing endoscopic manipulation of the airway should be pretreated with an anticholinergic agent. This prevents excessive salivation and allows for optimal effect of topical anesthesia. Glycopyrrolate is preferred because it lacks central nervous system side effects and has less potential for unwanted tachycardia. Sedation is essential for patients having bronchoscopy under local anesthesia. Supplemental oxygen should be given. Premedication with benzodiazepines is useful in producing anxiolysis and also in increasing the threshold for central nervous system toxicity from local anesthetics. Sedation should be titrated carefully to the desired effect, particularly in elderly debilitated patients and those with significant underlying respiratory compromise. Useful medications include diazepam, midazolam, morphine, fentanyl, alfentanil, and meperidine. After the procedure, the patient should not eat or drink for several hours until protective airway reflexes have returned.

In preparation for general anesthesia, the preoperative evaluation should focus on the patient's diagnosis and underlying pulmonary function. Pulmonary function tests should be evaluated and the degree of airway obstruction assessed. Respiratory infection and bronchospasm should be treated preoperatively. Premedication should to include an antisialagogue such as glycopyrrolate. Monitoring should include noninvasive blood pressure cuff, ECG, pulse oximetry, end-tidal CO_2 monitor, temperature, and precordial stethoscope. Additional monitoring is dictated by the patient's underlying medical condition. Induction technique depends on the patient's degree of airway obstruction, symptoms, and overall medical condition. Most frequently, intravenous induction is with barbiturates, etomidate, or propofol. Further management is dependent on whether a rigid or flexible bronchoscopy is to be performed. Flexible fiberoptic bronchoscopy is usually performed with the patient intubated and the bronchoscope passed through the inside of the endotracheal tube. This reduces the endotracheal tube's functional internal diameter, thereby greatly reducing the area available for ventilation. Therefore, ventilation should be preferentially controlled. The fiberoptic bronchoscope passes though a self-sealing diaphragm of an elbow connector attached to the single-lumen tube, and ventilation occurs between the bronchoscope and the wall of the endotracheal tube. Because of the increased resistance to exhalation caused by the bronchoscope, high distal PEEP and barotrauma may occur. One must therefore eliminate all PEEP from the anesthesia circuit and use longer periods of exhalation such as an I-to-E ratio of 1 to 3 to 1 to 4. In addition, one should use the largest possible endotracheal tube that can be passed atraumatically through the glottis (8.5 to 9.0 outside diameter for adult men and 7.5 to 8.0 outside diameter in adult women). Most commonly, 100% oxygen is delivered along with an inhalation agent. Unless contraindicated, the patient is paralyzed and ventilation controlled. In awake spontaneously breathing patients, the suction channel of the adult fiberoptic bronchoscope can be used as a conduit to help oxygenate patients. Oxygen flow through the suction channel also helps to keep the tip clear of secretions and improve visibility. During rigid bronchoscopy, intermittent positive-pressure ventilation (intermittent positive-pressure ventilation) can be delivered by connecting the standard anesthesia circuit to the ventilating side arm of the rigid bronchoscope. Positive pressure can be administered by squeezing the bag or using the anesthesia ventilator. Ventilation is possible only when the eyepiece of the rigid bronchoscope is in place and air still leaks because of the absence of a tight seal. To compensate for the leak, high gas flows should be used, or the pharynx and larynx could be packed with gauze. We have found this technique to be cumbersome and inefficient, as it impedes the surgeon's work. Our standard mode of ventilation is by low-frequency, manual jet ventilation with a Saunders injector that is connected to the side of the rigid bronchoscope (Fig. 26-35). This method involves the use of jet Venturi ventilation during rigid bronchoscopy. Oxygen from a high-pressure (50 psi) source is delivered to a port built into the rigid bronchoscope or to a steel needle that lies inside the lumen of the bronchoscope. The driving pressure is adjusted to the desired level using a pressure regulator. When the in-line on/off valve is manually activated, a jet of O_2 flows into the rigid bronchoscope at high velocity, creating a negative pressure and therefore entraining air developing a Venturi effect. The Venturi jet and the entrained

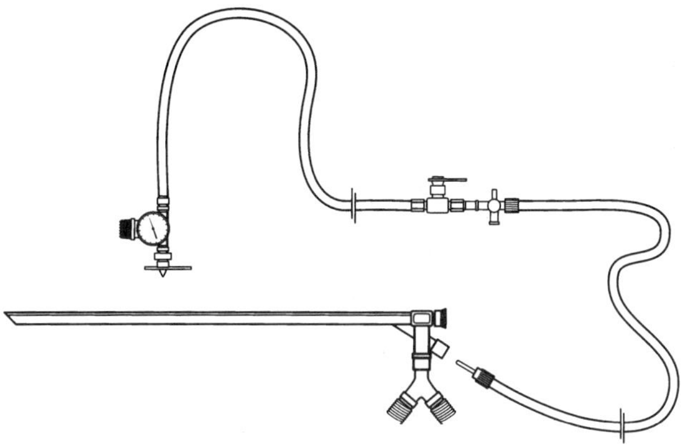

FIGURE 26-35. Components required for jet ventilation through a rigid bronchoscope with a Sanders injector.

gas produce a positive pressure at the bronchoscope's tip, resulting in expansion of the lungs subsequent to delivery of tidal volume. The amount of pressure generated into the trachea depends on (a) the driving force as determined at the level of the pressure-regulator valve, (b) the diameter of the jet port or needle, and (c) the diameter, length, and type of bronchoscope. Careful observation of the patient's chest movements are necessary to ensure adequate tidal volumes. A tracheal pressure of 30 cm H_2O usually results in normocarbia in patients with healthy lungs and chest wall compliance. The pressure generated at the tip of the bronchoscope is not influenced by the volume or compliance of the lungs. However, the effective tidal volume and alveolar ventilation depend on lung compliance. If the lungs are noncompliant, a large amount of tidal volume will escape between the bronchoscope and the tracheal wall, resulting in poor alveolar ventilation. During insertion of the suction catheter or biopsy forceps into the lumen of the bronchoscope, the generated inflation pressure increases. As long as no tight fit exists between the bronchoscope and the inside of the airway, barotrauma will be unlikely. If the fit is tight, the driving pressure should be reduced. In children and infants, the starting driving pressure should be approximately 0.5 psi/lb adjusted according to chest expansion.

High-frequency jet ventilation can be applied using a commercial high-frequency jet ventilator connected to a rigid bronchoscope. high-frequency jet ventilation rates of 150 to 300 breaths/minute have resulted in blood gases comparable to those of intermittent low-frequency manual jet ventilation (78). However, during bronchoscopy in patients with bronchial stenosis, high-frequency jet ventilation with rates higher than 300 breaths/minute resulted in a decrease in arterial oxygenation and an increase in Pa_{CO_2} in some patients. The intratracheal pressures generated during high-frequency jet ventilation are lower than those obtained with low-frequency mechanical jet ventilation. Therefore, in the presence of bronchial stenosis when the bronchoscope's tip in the main-stem bronchus above the area of stenosis, better blood gases are obtained with low-frequency manual jet ventilation than with high-frequency jet ventilation. This is probably because the higher pressures generated with low-frequency jet ventilation provide ventilation of the opposite lung through the side vents of the rigid bronchoscope, even when it is present in a main-stem bronchus. High-frequency jet ventilation, however, produces acceptable blood gases when the bronchoscope's tip is above the carina. Advantages of the high-frequency jet ventilation include less movement of the tracheobronchial tree and therefore better surgical conditions, particularly in procedures involving use of the laser. Because the tidal volumes generated with high-frequency jet ventilation are small, chest movements are not observed.

Complications during rigid bronchoscopy include trauma, which is much less likely during flexible fiberoptic bronchoscopy. Dental trauma or laceration of the mucosa of the larynx, trachea, or bronchi can occur with a rigid bronchoscope, which may result in pneumomediastinum or pneumothorax. Perforation of the esophagus has also occurred. The extreme hyperextension of the neck required for the passage of the rigid bronchoscope can lead to injury of the cervical spine or a vasovagal reaction. Patients with insufficient cerebral circulation may even have a cerebrovascular accident because of the occlusion of the vertebral arteries. One must ensure that the patient does not move or cough during rigid bronchoscopy, which can precipitate serious injury. The patient should be kept paralyzed and deeply anesthetized. Intravenous lidocaine can help suppress the cough reflex.

Intraoperative laryngospasm and bronchospasm can occur during bronchoscopy. Establishing deep levels of anesthesia and/or adequate topical anesthesia of the airway before starting any airway manipulations can help reduce their incidence. Even in patients who are under general anesthesia, topical application of lidocaine can help decrease the incidence of these complications. Remifentanil has a particular advantage in that it can provide a deep level of opioid effect while permitting rapid emergence without residual respiratory depression. Continuous infusions of propofol and remifentanil are also useful for procedures of short duration. β-Blockers such as esmolol are also beneficial in blunting the intense hemodynamic response that can occur during rigid bronchoscopy and mediastinoscopy. After bronchoscopy, airway obstruction can result from subglottic edema, mechanical activation of irritative cough, and mechanical trauma to the airway resulting in mucosal edema. Bleeding into the airway may be responsible for airway obstruction, particularly after tumor biopsy. Airway edema after bronchoscopy can be improved by administering humidified oxygen and racemic epinephrine.

Hypoxemia can occur during bronchoscopy from many sources, including inadequate oxygenation and ventilation, inadequate F_{IO_2} decreased FRC, atelectasis, and airway closure. During rigid bronchoscopy, inadequate ventilation may result from a large leak along the space between the bronchoscope and the tracheal wall or from an excessively prolonged period of apnea. Hypoxemia is prevented with supplemental O_2 administration to spontaneously breathing patients or use of a high FiO_2 in anesthetized patients. Monitoring of O_2 saturation by pulse oximetry is mandatory. Judicious use of suction during bronchoscopy should help decrease the loss of lung volume. At the end of rigid bronchoscopy, it is beneficial to intubate the patient with a single-lumen tube to provide larger tidal volumes and PEEP to reexpand the lungs. The single-lumen tube can then be gently suctioned before extubation.

ANESTHETIC CONSIDERATIONS FOR THORACOSCOPY

Thoracoscopy has been used successfully for both diagnostic and therapeutic purposes. Thoracoscopy is able to treat and diagnose recurrent or persistent pleural effusions, obtain fluid for cytology, drain persistent empyema not adequately drained by a chest tube, drain and evacuate multiloculated empyema, obtain pleural biopsy, and perform pleurodesis for recurrent spontaneous pneumothorax by instilling talc powder or tetracycline in the pleural space. One may also diagnose and stage intrathoracic tumors, biopsy mediastinal masses, or small peripheral lung lesions.

Thoracoscopy does not mandate general anesthesia, as several options exist depending on the proposed procedure. Thoracoscopy for the evaluation of pleural diseases has been successfully completed under local and/or regional anesthesia. Regional anesthesia is accomplished by performing intercostal nerve blocks two spaces above and two spaces below the intercostal space to be used, usually the sixth. The intercostal block should be performed as posteriorly as possible to provide adequate anesthesia to the parietal pleura. Traction on the lung and the hilum may precipitate coughing, which a stellate ganglion block can prevent. Local or regional anesthetic techniques are not suitable for more invasive procedures and perfect patient comfort is not guaranteed. In our institution, general anesthesia is most commonly employed. General anesthesia for thoracoscopy depends on the procedure's expected duration and the underlying patient condition. A one-lung ventilation technique greatly facilitates visualization of the operative field. If thoracoscopy is being performed for the drainage of an empyema, one-lung ventilation is absolutely indicated. Complete functional separation of the two lungs must be ensured to prevent spillage and contamination of the dependent ventilated lung by purulent material.

Thoracoscopy is usually performed with the patient in the lateral decubitus position. A small incision is made at the level of the sixth intercostal space. A mediastinoscope is inserted, which allows for visualization of the entire hemithorax. During thoracoscopy, a pneumothorax is created when the incision is made into the parietal pleura. The partial collapse of the lung allows for visualization of the hemithorax. The pneumothorax is usually limited and well tolerated because the intercostal muscles and the skin form a seal around the thoracoscope, thus limiting the amount of lung collapse.

Invasive monitoring is not routinely required during thoracoscopy but may be indicated based on the patient's cardiovascular condition. Pulse oximetry, however, and other routine monitors should be used. When local or regional anesthesia is used, O_2 supplementation should be provided. An arterial line should be considered if one-lung ventilation is utilized. Morbidity and mortality rates are minimal after thoracoscopy.

ANESTHETIC CONSIDERATIONS FOR MINIMALLY INVASIVE THORACIC SURGERY

Minimally invasive thoracic surgery is more commonly referred to as video-assisted thoracic surgery. With the introduction of high-quality imaging cameras and specialized endoscopic instruments and staplers, video-assisted thoracic surgery has become an accepted and popular modality to operate within the thoracic cavity. The advantages of video-assisted thoracic surgery over open thoracotomy include less morbidity, less pain, shorter hospital stay, and a more cosmetic incision. These advantages were reported by Landreneau et al. (79), who described 138 patients, 81 of which had video-assisted thoracic surgery and 57 patients who had limited lateral thoracotomy for resection of peripheral lung lesions. No video-assisted thoracic surgery patient had an epidural catheter or an intercostal nerve block. Patients who underwent video-assisted thoracic surgery had lower pain scores, less opioid use, better shoulder use at 3 weeks, and a hospital stay of 5 days compared to 7.5 days for the limited lateral thoracotomy patients (79). During video-assisted thoracic surgery, the surgeons are able to avoid rib spreading, which can lead to rib fractures and costochondral dislocation. They are also able to spare major muscles when compared to open thoracotomy. The disadvantages for video-assisted thoracic surgery are primarily surgical and include difficulty with target identification, loss of palpation, technical complexity, difficult hemorrhage control, potentially increased operating room time, and increased use of disposable items. Target identification has been enhanced with the use of percutaneous hook wires passed into the lesion, percutaneous staining of the lesion, and by the use of intraoperative intrathoracic ultrasound. The increased operating room time and increased use of disposable items can be justified if the use of video-assisted thoracic surgery is associated with a lower morbidity rate, a shorter hospital stay, and a reduction in total costs.

Indications for video-assisted thoracic surgery can be categorized as either diagnostic or therapeutic. The diagnostic indications include pleural effusions, solitary pulmonary nodules, lung biopsy, lung and esophageal cancer staging procedures, diagnosis of mediastinal tumors, and pericardial effusion. The therapeutic indications include pleurodesis, pulmonary resections, pericardial window, thymectomy, resection of mediastinal masses and cysts, sympathectomy, Heller myotomy, vagotomy, antireflux procedures, and repair of diaphragmatic hernias. Various pulmonary resections have been successfully performed using video-assisted thoracic surgery, including bleb and wedge resections, lobectomy, and even pneumonectomy. The absolute contraindications to video-assisted thoracic surgery are dense adhesions and inability to tolerate one-lung ventilation, both of which are necessary for adequate visualization. Previous thoracotomy or video-assisted thoracic surgery can cause adhesions that limit the surgeon's view of the operative field and are considered relative contraindications.

Both surgical and anesthesia teams should be fully prepared to perform an open thoracotomy because conversion may be required. The patient is positioned in the lateral decubitus position with an axillary roll. Preoperative evaluation should be as thorough as that for an open thoracotomy. The patient's pulmonary status should be optimized and may include cessation of smoking, chest physiotherapy, bronchodilators, and steroids as indicated. Cardiovascular and other coexisting diseases should also be investigated and optimized. Although the overall surgical goal is to remain minimally invasive, our preoperative evaluation and preparation have not been minimized or reduced.

On the day of surgery, all current medications are continued, and any utilized inhalers accompany the patient to the operating room. The preoperative medication includes a drying agent such as glycopyrrolate to help facilitate one-lung ventilation and a sedative such as midazolam. Standard monitors are applied with the ECG patches placed so that they will not need to be replaced after the patient is in the lateral thoracotomy position. Large-bore intravenous and radial arterial lines are placed, preferably in the dependent arm, which limits intraoperative technical problems. If planned, an epidural catheter is placed before induction usually with the patient sitting. Induction agents include thiopental, propofol, or etomidate. Muscle relaxation is accomplished with shorter acting agents such as succinylcholine followed by rocuronium or cisatracurium. Most commonly, maintenance is with sevoflurane, desflurane, or isoflurane. If an epidural catheter is present, the infusion is started immediately after the patient is positioned.

One-lung ventilation is essential for video-assisted thoracic surgery and is commonly provided by the use of double-lumen tubes. Because of the ease of positioning, left double-lumen tubes are most commonly used to provide one-lung ventilation. Immediately after placement, auscultation should be performed to determine the direction of the bronchial lumen. After auscultation, fiberoptic bronchoscopy should be used to confirm and optimize the position of the double-lumen tube. Fiberoptic bronchoscopy should also be performed after the patient is in his or her final lateral decubitus position. We use a Velcro strap device to secure double-lumen tubes that are easy to undo, should repositioning of the double-lumen tube be necessary intraoperatively. To provide ample time for lung deflation, one-lung ventilation is established immediately after the patient is in the lateral decubitus position. This will also allow the anesthesiologist to determine whether the patient will tolerate one-lung ventilation, to diagnose and correct any problems, to determine airway pressures, and to make any necessary ventilation adjustments.

Pain management depends on the expected extent of the surgery and the likelihood of conversion to open thoracotomy. The analgesic plan may include local infiltration, intercostal nerve blocks, NSAIDs, intravenous patient-controlled analgesia, and epidural analgesia. Our surgical team infiltrates port access sites and wounds with 0.25% bupivacaine before making an incision. For diagnostic and therapeutic video-assisted thoracic surgery, in which three to four surgical ports will be used, the patient will have wound infiltration and intercostal nerve blocks by the surgical team. Before emergence, ketorolac will be given intravenously and the patient will have a patient-controlled analgesia opioid until the chest tubes have been removed. For less extensive procedures with a low likelihood for conversion, an epidural catheter is usually not inserted. Instead, the pain management plan will include local anesthetic infiltration, intercostal nerve blocks, NSAIDs and intravenous patient-controlled analgesia, provided the lesion is peripheral and less than 3 cm in diameter. The likelihood for conversion to an open thoracotomy is greater with centrally located lesions and those that are larger than 3 cm. In these patients, an epidural is placed before induction. We usually start a local anesthetic/opioid infusion immediately after the patient has been positioned. Catheters are placed in the thoracic epidural space from T-4 to T-10. For a video-assisted thoracic surgery lobectomy, an epidural catheter is placed preoperatively due to its relatively high potential for conversion to open thoracotomy.

The overall conversion rate to thoracotomy has been reported to be 1.4% to 24% (80,81). Our conversion rate has decreased over time due to increasing surgical experience, refinement of endoscopic instruments, and better patient selection. The reasons for conversion include bleeding, dense adhesions, tumor adhesion to chest wall or hilum, stapler misfire, larger operation required for cure, technical failure of one-lung ventilation, or inability of the patient to tolerate one-lung ventilation.

ANESTHESIA FOR ESOPHAGEAL SURGERY

The most frequently encountered disorders of the esophagus are tumors, hiatal hernia, benign strictures, achalasia, diverticula, foreign bodies, perforations, and tracheoesophageal fistulas. Clinical suspicion of esophageal disease arises from the history and physical examination results. Patients are usually evaluated by barium swallow under cinefluoroscopy followed by esophagoscopy and tissue biopsy.

Esophagoscopy

Esophagoscopy may be performed for diagnostic and/or therapeutic indications. The diagnostic workup of an esophageal lesion will include tissue biopsy, cytology, and brushings obtained by flexible esophagoscopy. With esophagoscopy, foreign bodies can be removed, strictures can be dilated, stents can be placed, and esophageal varices can be sclerosed. Esophagoscopy can be performed using a flexible fiberoptic endoscope or an open-tube rigid esophagoscope. Rigid esophagoscopy is particularly valuable for removal of larger foreign bodies and examination and management of massive esophageal bleeding.

The anesthetic management for fiberoptic esophagoscopy most commonly includes topical anesthesia of the mouth and pharynx combined with light sedation. However, in pediatric patients, general anesthesia and endotracheal intubation are usually required. The patient should not be allowed to eat or drink for several hours until protective airway reflexes have returned. Rigid esophagoscopy is usually performed under general anesthesia with endotracheal intubation and muscle relaxation. An anticholinergic agent is useful as a premedication to minimize airway secretions and decrease the vagal response to gastric distention. All patients must be viewed as having a full stomach because of the risk of regurgitation of contents from the esophageal pouch proximal to the area of stenosis or obstruction. Either awake endotracheal intubation or rapid-sequence induction should be performed. To facilitate passage of the esophagoscope, it may be necessary to temporarily deflate the endotracheal tube cuff. A smaller than usual single-lumen tube should be used to prevent compression of the esophagus, which may also be caused by an overinflated endotracheal cuff. Total relaxation should be maintained to prevent patient movement and coughing during passage of the rigid esophagoscope, which can result in significant tissue trauma. The patient's esophagus should be thoroughly suctioned and emptied of all food particles and secretions. Patients should be extubated when fully awake with adequate protective airway reflexes. Potential complications of esophagoscopy include perforation of the esophagus, pneumothorax, pneumomediastinum, pneumoperitoneum, subcutaneous emphysema, hemorrhage, cardiac dysrhythmias, and aspiration pneumonia.

Esophagectomy and Esophagogastrectomy

Patients with esophageal lesions such as strictures or malignancy usually have a long history of dysphagia and poor feeding. They therefore have clinical manifestations of severe malnutrition, weight loss, cachexia, anemia, electrolyte imbalances, and hypoalbuminemia. Optimization of the nutritional status preoperatively has been shown to lower mortality and morbidity rates and decrease the incidence of wound sepsis (82). Organ toxicity and the anesthetic implications of cancer chemotherapy agents must be considered. Frequently used drugs include doxorubicin (Adriamycin), bleomycin, and mitomycin C. All antineoplastic agents can depress erythropoiesis, leukocyte, and platelet production, and the proliferation of gastrointestinal tract epithelium. Adriamycin can result in cardiac toxicity. Acute cardiac toxicity from Adriamycin consists of supraventricular and ventricular dysrhythmias, abnormal conduction patterns, and ST-segment T-wave changes. These acute changes usually resolve 1 to 2 months after cessation of therapy. Adriamycin may also result in a dose-dependent cardiomyopathy and congestive heart failure. The total cumulative dose of Adriamycin is usually limited to a maximum of 300 mg/m^2 to avoid this complication. Cardiomyopathy and congestive heart failure from Adriamycin are usually irreversible. Adriamycin-induced cardiomyopathy is monitored by obtaining an endomyocardial biopsy and by determining the ejection fraction using a multiple-gated acquisition nuclear scan. Echocardiography is helpful in determining overall cardiac function. Bleomycin is also used for esophageal cancer and can result in pulmonary toxicity. Clinical manifestations include cough, dyspnea, and rales, which may progress to severe hypoxemia at rest with a radiologic picture similar to that seen in adult respiratory distress syndrome, followed by pulmonary fibrosis. Predisposing factors include age of more than 20 years, dose greater than 400 U, underlying pulmonary disease, and prior or concomitant radiation therapy. A high concentration of oxygen can predispose the patient to pulmonary toxicity from bleomycin. Duration of the sensitivity of these patients to O_2 after the conclusion of bleomycin therapy is still unknown. The lowest FiO_2 necessary to maintain adequate arterial saturation should be used intraoperatively and postoperatively. Mitomycin C can also cause pulmonary toxicity and lung fibrosis (83).

Surgical Approach to Esophageal Surgery

The surgical approach depends on the location and size of the lesion. Patients with tumors of the lower third of the esophagus are treated by esophagogastrectomy through either a left-sided thoracotomy or a transhiatal esophagogastrectomy, along with a gastric pull-through technique. Patients with lesions of the middle third of the esophagus are treated by a combined laparotomy and right-sided thoracotomy. Those with lesions of the upper third of the esophagus may be treated in the supine position with a combined laparotomy and cervical incision. Esophagogastrectomy with colon interposition is used for lesions in the upper third of the esophagus when insufficient stomach length exists to perform an esophagogastrectomy. A midline laparotomy is performed to mobilize the colon. An esophagectomy is performed through a right thoracotomy. The colon is passed in the retrosternal space and anastomosed to the cervical esophagus.

Preoperative medication is given according to the patient's general condition to allay anxiety. These patients are frequently elderly and debilitated and have limited cardiorespiratory reserve. Preoperative sedatives and respiratory depressants should be used cautiously. An anticholinergic agent may be helpful, particularly if an awake intubation is to be performed. Monitoring should include a noninvasive blood pressure cuff, ECG, temperature, pulse oximetry, and CO_2 monitoring. Additional monitoring includes radial arterial and central venous lines. If there is a concern regarding cardiac function and/or congestive heart failure, a pulmonary artery catheter should be inserted. At least two large-bore 14- or 16-gauge peripheral intravenous lines should be started in anticipation of at least moderate blood loss and evaporative fluid loses from the abdominal and/or thoracic cavities being open to air. Fluid warmers should be used from the start of the operation. Knowledge of the surgical procedure is needed to guide line placement. For patients having an anastomosis performed in the left side of the neck, central access is limited to the right side of the neck and the right subclavian region. Some surgeons also like to free drape the left arm and have it in the surgical field. The left arm can then be positioned in front of the patient for the thoracotomy and then moved to the left side to facilitate the cervical anastomosis. In such instances, it is best to avoid the left arm for intravenous and arterial line placement due to the high probability of intraoperative technical problems. An epidural catheter is placed preoperatively and is located at the center of the proposed dermatomal field of surgery.

If a proximal esophageal pouch is present, it should be emptied before the induction of general anesthesia. All patients are managed as if they had a full stomach with awake intubation or rapid-sequence induction. Surgical exposure for esophageal surgery is greatly facilitated by one-lung ventilation. Significant hypoxemia frequently develops during one-lung ventilation and may persist as long as the lung is collapsed. The application of CPAP to the nondependent lung with or without the application of PEEP to the dependent lung and an FiO_2 of 1.0 is frequently required.

Anesthesia is maintained with volatile agents, intermittent boluses or a continuous infusion of opioids, and a nondepolarizing muscle relaxant. Bradycardia and hypotension may result from stimulation of the carotid sinus reflex during neck dissection and mobilization of the esophagus. This is easily reversed with atropine. Compression or occlusion of the inferior vena cava resulting in decreased venous return and hypotension may occur during surgical manipulation around the distal end of the esophagus. Significant intraoperative hemorrhage leading to severe hypotension may occur rapidly.

Transhiatal esophagectomy without thoracotomy is also performed by some surgeons in patients with benign or malignant disease. The esophagus is approached through both a left cervical and an abdominal incision. Blunt manual dissection of the esophagus through the diaphragmatic hiatus is done. Wide swings in hemodynamic responses are frequently observed during this procedure. Significant arterial hypotension is often seen during manual dissection of the esophagus and when the stomach is brought up through the posterior mediastinum. Most commonly, this hypotension is due to impaired venous return and manual compression of the heart. Diligent fluid management is required in these cases to minimize intraoperative hemodynamic instability. Because of the large magnitude of surgery, advanced age, and the usual concomitant debilitation and cardiorespiratory impairment, these patients are usually ventilated for several hours postoperatively.

Postoperative complications include pleural effusions, wound infection, pneumonia, and anastomotic leak resulting in mediastinitis, sepsis, hydrothorax, or pyrothorax. The decrease in FRC due to surgical manipulation and trauma, anesthesia, and postoperative incisional pain results in airway closure, atelectasis, and pulmonary impairment. An effective regimen for postoperative pain control is essential to facilitate deep breathing, coughing, and adequate participation in chest physiotherapy regimens, as well as to encourage early ambulation. Postoperative analgesia can be most effectively achieved by infusing local anesthetic and opioid mixture through a thoracic or lumbar epidural catheter.

ANESTHESIA FOR PATIENTS WITH A ZENKER DIVERTICULUM

A Zenker diverticulum is an outpouching of the pharyngeal mucosa that develops most commonly at the level of the cricoid cartilage. It is believed to result from weakness or neuromuscular dysfunction of the cricopharyngeus muscle. Patients complain of food sticking in the throat, difficulty with swallowing, noisy swallowing, regurgitation of food, and bouts of coughing when lying supine. A compressible swelling may develop as the sac enlarges. Recurrent pneumonia and lung abscess may result from aspiration. Diagnosis is confirmed with a barium swallow. Compromised cardiovascular pulmonary and nutritional states are frequently encountered in patients with a Zenker diverticulum (84). Malnutrition, hypoproteinemia, and muscle wasting may result from long-standing dysphagia.

Oral premedications are not suitable because the tablets may lodge in the pouch or be aspirated to the lungs. The risk of regurgitation of the contents of the diverticulum into the lungs during induction of anesthesia and intraoperatively is a major concern for the anesthesiologist. The contents of the pouch usually have an alkaline pH level, and therefore, chemical pneumonitis is unlikely. H_2-receptor antagonists, antacids, and metoclopramide will have no effect on the contents of the pouch. Regurgitation and aspiration may occur during the induction of anesthesia, during intubation, or even after successful intubation because of the seepage of fluid around the single-lumen tube cuff during surgical manipulation. Measures to minimize the risk of aspiration include overnight fasting and preoperative emptying of the pouch by manual external pressure. If there is any doubt as to the safety of rapid-sequence induction with the inherent risk of aspiration, the airway should be secured by awake fiberoptic bronchoscopy. Topical anesthesia of the airway for awake intubation should be limited to the supraglottic region of the airway, but not both. This leaves part of the airway responsive, and protected against aspiration. Transtracheal injection, which blocks the recurrent laryngeal nerve, is not advised.

Cricoid pressure may be helpful in some patients but may be deleterious and precipitate regurgitation and aspiration in others. This is based on the size of the pouch and the location of the opening of the pouch. Careful preoperative examination of the barium swallow and conferring with the surgeon are helpful in determining whether cricoid pressure will be effective or harmful. If the sac is large, extending down into the mediastinum with its orifice at the level of the cricoid cartilage, it is likely that cricoid pressure will obliterate the opening and protect against regurgitation. If the sac is small and the opening is higher than the level of cricoid cartilage, the application of cricoid pressure may actually squeeze the sac, resulting in regurgitation of its contents into the hypopharynx and increasing the likelihood of aspiration (Fig. 26-36). Some authors have suggested that the best protection during anesthetic induction in patients with a Zenker diverticulum is not by the use of awake intubation or cricoid pressure, but by conducting a smooth induction with a 30° upward head tilt. The avoidance of coughing and straining is critical. After adequate preoxygenation, an intravenous hypnotic supplemented with opioids and/or lidocaine with or without mask ventilation with O_2, N_2O, and inhalation anesthetic mixture usually result in a smooth induction. A nondepolarizing muscle relaxant is administered and endotracheal intubation performed after complete relaxation has been achieved. The cuff of the single-lumen tube must be promptly inflated to provide adequate sealing of the airway. Perforation of the diverticulum is a potential complication. Great care and gentleness should be exercised when inserting a nasogastic tube. Our preference is to place the nasogastric tube with surgical assistance after incision.

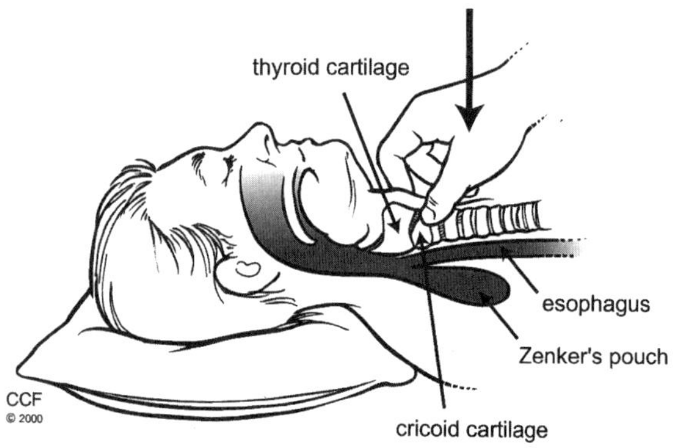

FIGURE 26-36. A Zenker diverticulum with the opening of the pouch at the level of the cricoid cartilage.

Alternatively, the procedure can be performed under regional anesthesia using deep and superficial cervical plexus blocks. Decreasing the risk of aspiration, by preserving protective airway reflexes, is one advantage of regional anesthesia. An awake, alert patient is able to cooperate with the surgeon and to swallow on command, allowing the surgeon to view the pathology in action. After repair of the diverticulum with the incision still open, the patient is fed small spoonfuls of gelatin so the surgeon can ensure the adequacy of correction under direct vision. No anesthetic complications were reported in one series of 58 cases performed under regional anesthesia (85).

ANESTHESIA FOR PATIENTS WITH MASSIVE HEMOPTYSIS

Massive hemoptysis, defined as coughing of more than 600 mL of blood in 24 hours, is associated with more than a 50% mortality rate. Patients who bleed at a rate of more than 150 mL/hour for 4 hours or more are considered as having exsanguinating hemoptysis. Life is threatened by exsanguination as well as asphyxiation (86). Etiology includes chronic infection, particularly tuberculosis, and bronchiectasis and iatrogenic pulmonary artery perforation. The likelihood of massive endobronchial hemorrhage after the insertion of a pulmonary artery catheter is increased by subsequent heparinization. Risk factors for pulmonary artery rupture from pulmonary artery catheter placement include female patients, preexisting pulmonary hypertension, hypothermia, coagulopathy, and anticoagulation.

Pulmonary resection has been shown to be the most effective way to stop bleeding in most patients. Those who can tolerate a resection benefit from removal of the bleeding lung parenchyma, because there is a high incidence of repeated bleeding. The bleeding site must be identified by bronchoscopy. Rigid bronchoscopy may be required because the lens of the fiberoptic bronchoscopy becomes easily obscured with blood. In addition, the suction channel of the flexible fiberoptic bronchoscopy is narrow and does not permit rigorous suctioning of blood and blood clots. However, flexible fiberoptic bronchoscopy is useful when bleeding is not excessive and when visualization of the upper-lobe bronchi is needed. Iced saline lavage of the bronchus is helpful in managing massive hemorrhage. The affected bronchus can also be packed with gauze or occluded using a bronchial blocker. If the bleeding site cannot be identified by bronchoscopy, bronchial angiography or pulmonary angiography may be needed. Embolization of the bronchial and intercostal arteries has also been used to stop hemoptysis.

The goals of anesthetic management are to prevent contamination of the nonbleeding lung, prevent asphyxiation, and correct hypovolemia. Large-bore intravenous lines and infusion of fluids and blood should proceed at the same time as other therapeutic measures. An intraarterial line should be placed for monitoring of blood pressure and frequent measurement of arterial blood gases. Supplemental O_2 should be given if the patient is not yet intubated. The bleeding lung should be placed in the dependent position to prevent drowning of the nonbleeding lung. Lung separation is to be achieved as soon as possible. Cough suppressants should not be used until the lungs are completely separated.

The best method to achieve lung separation is with the use of a double-lumen tube. However, placement and positioning of a double-lumen tube may be technically difficult in such an emergency situation in which large quantities of blood are in the airway. An alternative method is to use a single-lumen tube advanced into the bronchus of the nonbleeding lung. If bleeding is from the left side, intubation of the right main bronchus can be achieved by blindly advancing the single-lumen tube. If bleeding is from the right side, a fiberoptic bronchoscopy is used to advance the single-lumen tube tube into the left main bronchus. The third option is insertion of a bronchial blocker into the main-stem bronchus of the bleeding lung. The patient can be intubated awake or after rapid-sequence induction with cricoid pressure. Visualization of the larynx will be obscured by blood. Air bubbles exiting from the trachea may be the only guide to the glottic opening. Adequate suction must be available. Performing the intubation in the semiupright position may decrease the amount of blood pooling in the upper airway, minimize cough, and help improve the field of vision.

All patients with massive hemoptysis must be regarded as having a full stomach. If one elects to perform a rapid-sequence induction, rather than an awake intubation, cricoid pressure must be used. Because of the likely hypovolemia, ketamine or etomidate are the preferred induction agents. Because of the ability to suction and ventilate each lung individually, a double-lumen tube is the preferred method for lung separation. Once the airway has been established, the patient is placed in the lateral decubitus position in preparation for resection of the bleeding lung segment. Because the bleeding lung has to be placed in the nondependent position, it is mandatory to achieve complete separation of the lungs to protect the dependent, nonbleeding lung.

COMPLICATIONS UNIQUE TO THORACIC SURGERY AND THEIR MANAGEMENT

Herniation of the Heart

Herniation of the heart is the most dreaded complication after thoracotomy. It is rapidly and uniformly fatal if not immediately diagnosed and treated. Even with rapid intervention, the mortality rate is 50%. Herniation of the heart occurs more often after a right pneumonectomy in which the adjacent pericardium has been disrupted. It is particularly likely to occur after a radical intrapericardial pneumonectomy in which the pericardium has been opened to gain better access to the pulmonary vessels. Cardiovascular collapse occurs as a result of herniation of the heart and the great vessels into the pericardial defect, leading to acute angulation of the great vessels and decreased cardiac output. Rapid return of cardiac output and blood pressure follow the return of the heart to its normal position. The risk of cardiac herniation is decreased if the defect in the pericardium is closed with pleural tissue or prosthetic material. Cardiac herniation may also occur after the creation of a pericardial window for the relief of a pericardial tamponade.

Precipitating factors include repositioning the patient at the end of pneumonectomy from the lateral decubitus position to the supine position, application of suction to the chest tube on the side of the pneumonectomy, rigorous coughing, placing the patient with the resected hemithorax in the dependent position, and positive-pressure ventilation of the remaining lung. Cardiac herniation may also occur without any precipitating factors. The clinical features are sudden and severe cardiovascular collapse, evidence of superior vena cava obstruction, distended neck veins, facial flushing and edema, new axis change on the ECG, and unusual bulging contour of the heart on chest radiography (snow cone sign). Diagnosis must depend on a very high index of suspicion. It must be differentiated from other causes of sudden, severe cardiovascular collapse, such as tension pneumothorax, cardiac tamponade, dysrhythmias, pulmonary emboli, and massive intrathoracic hemorrhage. Immediate surgical exploration is mandatory. Temporary measures that can be undertaken while transporting the patient to the operating room include placing the patient with the side to be operated on up to allow the heart to fall back by the effect of gravity into the pericardial sac, decreasing airway pressure and PEEP to the remaining lung, and injecting air into the empty hemothorax. It must be emphasized that these are only temporary measures and should not delay definitive emergency surgical intervention. The surgical procedure consists of reexploring the thorax and repairing the pericardial defect by primary closure, an autograft, or prosthetic material. Anesthesia is induced with etomidate or ketamine, succinylcholine, and 100% oxygen.

Cardiac Dysrhythmias

Supraventricular dysrhythmias, particularly atrial fibrillation, atrial flutter, and atrial tachycardia, commonly occur after pneumonectomy. The incidence of atrial fibrillation ranges from 10% to 20% after lobectomy and up to 40% after pneumonectomy. The incidence of atrial fibrillation is higher when the surgical procedure includes lymph node resection. Atrial fibrillation develops within the first 3 postoperative days in 82% of patients (87). In a review of 236 consecutive patients undergoing pneumonectomy at the Mayo Clinic, supraventricular dysrhythmias occurred in 22% of the patients. Atrial fibrillation was the most common, accounted for 64% of dysrhythmias; supraventricular tachycardia accounted for 23%; and atrial flutter for 13%. Twenty-five percent of the patients with supraventricular tachydysrhythmias died within 30 days after their pneumonectomy, compared to a 7% mortality rate in patients without dysrhythmias (88). More encouraging results have recently been reported by Cardinale and colleagues, who prospectively evaluated 233 patients who underwent thoracotomy for lung cancer resection. They reported an incidence of atrial fibrillation of 12% with a peak occurrence on postoperative day two. Atrial fibrillation occurred more frequently in patients who were older (63 years versus 58 years) and in those who had systemic hypertension and/or lymph node dissection. Atrial fibrillation was successfully terminated by amiodarone treatment within 48 hours. The overall mortality rate for patients who developed atrial fibrillation was similar to that for those without atrial fibrillation (87).

Factors predisposing patients to supraventricular dysrhythmias after pulmonary resection include (a) cardiac contusion and edema caused by blunt trauma, dissection, and retraction around the heart; (b) increase in PVR due to the reduction in the pulmonary vascular bed, which increases PVR; (c) inadequate postoperative analgesia, leading to increased sympathetic tone; and (d) postoperative hypoxemia, hypercarbia, respiratory acidosis, and electrolyte imbalances.

Prophylactic digitalization has been recommended for some patients before pneumonectomy to decrease postoperative supraventricular dysrhythmias (89). We do not however routinely digitalize patients before pneumonectomy. We use prophylactic digitalization only in selected patients undergoing pneumonectomy or if multiple premature supraventricular beats start to occur during the course of pulmonary resection. Although there is no firm evidence to support this practice, anecdotal reports suggest that patients treated with digoxin who subsequently develop atrial fibrillation have better rate control and are more easily cardioverted. This is in agreement with other authors who have reported a decrease in postoperative cardiac complications, including dysrhythmias, congestive heart failure, and death with prophylactic digitalization (90). Amar et al. prospectively studied supraventricular dysrhythmias and the prophylactic use of diltiazem and digoxin in patients having pneumonectomy. Postoperatively, patients were given an appropriate intravenous loading dose of either diltiazem or digoxin and were orally maintained on this treatment for 30 days. Patients treated with digoxin had an incidence of supraventricular dysrhythmia similar to that in untreated controls. Patients who received diltiazem had a 14% incidence of supraventricular dysrhythmia compared to 31% for those patients treated with digoxin. The development of supraventricular dysrhythmia did not correlate with tumor stage, right-sided operation, or intrapericardial operations but was associated with a longer hospital stay (91).

Supraventricular dysrhythmias resulting in hemodynamic instability require emergent cardioversion. Atrial flutter is particularly sensitive to cardioversion and may respond to low energy levels, such as 25 joules. Patients with supraventricular tachycardia could be treated with carotid sinus massage, edrophonium (2 to 10 mg), phenylephrine (50 to 100 mg), verapamil (2.5 to 10 mg), or β-blockers (e.g., propranolol and esmolol). Adenosine has also been an effective drug for the rapid termination of supraventricular tachycardia. Patients with atrial fibrillation should be treated with verapamil, digitalis, or cardioversion. Those with atrial flutter are treated with verapamil, propranolol, or cardioversion. In addition, any underlying predisposing factor such as hypoxemia, hypercarbia, acidosis, and electrolyte imbalances should be promptly corrected.

Right-Sided Heart Failure

Acute cor pulmonale and right-sided heart failure can follow lung resection. Removal of lung parenchyma decreases the total pulmonary vascular cross-sectional area, resulting in an increase in PVR and right ventricular afterload. Preoperative cardiopulmonary assessment can be helpful in predicting postoperative right-sided heart failure. If temporary unilateral occlusion of the main pulmonary artery on the affected side results in an increase in mean pulmonary artery pressure to more than 30 to 40 mm Hg, the risk of acute cor pulmonale postoperatively is greatly increased. Patients who were originally assessed as having adequate right ventricular reserve may still develop postoperative right-sided heart failure because of transient postoperative conditions that lead to further increases in PVR. For example, the development of postoperative pneumonia leading to HPV in a portion of the lung will further increase PVR, leading to additional right ventricular strain. Hypercarbia, acidosis, increases in airway pressure during mechanical ventilation, and the application of high levels of PEEP can also be deleterious. Clinically, patients with right-sided heart failure have distended neck veins, hepatomegaly, peripheral edema, right-sided S_3 or S_4 gallops, and dysrhythmias. Large P waves (P pulmonale) are seen on the ECG. Chest radiography may reveal cardiomegaly and right ventricular enlargement. A pulmonary artery catheter would measure elevated right-sided pressures that may become equal to or greater than left-sided pressures. Echocardiography is helpful in differentiating right-sided heart failure from cardiac tamponade.

Whereas volume expansion is the basic treatment of right ventricular failure when PVR is normal, in patients with an elevated PVR volume, expansion could be deleterious due to excessive increase in right ventricular end-diastolic pressure, wall stress, and metabolic demands. Right ventricular ischemia may develop resulting in further deterioration of right ventricular function. The first line of treatment should be a reduction of pulmonary hypertension with a vasodilating agent. Nitroglycerin, calcium channel blockers, hydralazine, and sodium nitroprusside have all been used, but they are selective to the pulmonary circulation and will lower the systemic blood pressure. Infusion of prostaglandin E_1 is also effective in dilating the pulmonary vasculature and reducing PVR. Inotropic agents that cause an increase in cardiac function along with vasodilation such as milrinone or dobutamine should also be considered. Phosphodiesterase inhibitors such as milrinone and amrinone improve both systolic and diastolic myocardial function and are extremely beneficial in this clinical setting. Inhaled nitric oxide may also be useful, as it causes dose-dependent pulmonary arterial and venous vasodilation. The I-NOvent System (Ohmeda) is currently available and can deliver 0 to 80 parts per million of nitric oxide. Inhaled nitric oxide in the range of 5 to 40 parts per million can be given and its effects are proportionately greater with increasing degrees of pulmonary vasoconstriction (92). It produces selective pulmonary artery vasodilation, leading to a decrease in right ventricular afterload, which may improve right ventricular function. Significant hypotension generally does not occur, as nitric oxide is rapidly inactivated by rapidly binding to hemoglobin.

In patients with normal pulmonary artery pressure, right ventricular wall stress is low compared with that of the left ventricle. Pulmonary hypertension often leads to the dilation of the thin-walled right ventricle and an increase in right ventricular muscle mass. The increase in O_2 demand may not be met by a corresponding increase in coronary blood flow. Subendocardial ischemia may occur, resulting in decreased myocardial contractility. Maintenance of an adequate coronary perfusion pressure is extremely important. Therapy with inodilator agents such as milrinone or dobutamine may pose a risk if arterial hypotension results in a reduction in right ventricular O_2 supply that exceeds the concomitant decrease in right ventricular wall stress and O_2 demand. In such a situation, norepinephrine, dopamine, or phenylephrine should be added to maintain an adequate systemic arterial pressure.

Postpneumonectomy Pulmonary Edema

Pulmonary edema after lung resection occurs in approximately 3% to 5% of patients undergoing pneumonectomy and has a mortality rate of 30% to 100%. It appears 2 to 3 days after an otherwise uncomplicated postoperative period. There seems to be no correlation to age, gender, lung function, comorbid conditions, blood loss, or anesthetic technique. Within 12 hours of the onset of dyspnea and hypoxemia, virtually all patients require positive-pressure ventilation. To make the diagnosis, one should ensure that there is no clinical or radiological evidence of aspiration, bacterial pneumonia, heart failure, thromboembolism, bronchopleural fistula, or other causes of adult respiratory distress syndrome such as shock or overwhelming sepsis. Therefore, postpneumonectomy edema is primarily a diagnosis of exclusion. The radiological detection of interstitial pulmonary edema may precede the onset of symptoms by 12 to 24 hours (93).

Zeldin et al. reported 10 cases from different centers and identified right pneumonectomy, large perioperative fluid load, and high urine volumes as risk factors for the development of postpneumonectomy edema (94). They recommended the judicious use of intravenous fluids. Other factors such as endothelial damage, lymphatic interruption, ventilatory volotrauma, right ventricular dysfunction, and vasoactive mediators have also been implicated. Deslaurius et al. (93) reviewed the records of 291 consecutive patients who underwent pneumonectomy for lung cancer. Postpneumonectomy edema developed in 13 (4.5%) of the patients. Nine patients had a right pneumonectomy while four had a left pneumonectomy. Eventually, 85% of the patients died of respiratory or multiorgan failure. The extent and duration of surgery and lymph node dissection were significant risk factors for the development of postpneumonectomy edema. The duration of surgery was 184 minutes for patients with postpneumonectomy edema and 144 for patients without postpneumonectomy edema. Right- or left-sided operation did not have statistical significance. These authors reported probable factors contributing to postpneumonectomy edema as increased capillary pressure and filtration pressure, reduced lymphatic capacity for interstitial fluid resorption, and hyperinflation of the contralateral lung. Possible factors were reported as right ventricular dysfunction and excessive analgesia. For prophylaxis, they recommend (a) total positive fluid balance during the first 24 hours, including the intraoperative period, not to exceed 20 mL/kg of crystalloid solution; (b) for low blood pressure, consideration should be given to an inotrope, (c) to reduce catecholamine release, adequate pain control should be provided, and (d) the mediastinum should be kept in a relatively central position to prevent overexpansion of the residual lung. The treatment for established postpneumonectomy edema was supportive and included intubation, mechanical ventilation with the lowest possible airway pressures, PEEP, and nutrition through a feeding jejunostomy.

Mathisen et al. (95) reported more encouraging results in 10 consecutive patients who developed severe adult respiratory distress syndrome after pulmonary resection who were treated with inhaled nitric oxide. There were six men and four women with an average age of 58 years. Five of the 10 patients received preoperative radiation. Two patients had lobectomy and eight underwent pneumonectomy (five left sided and three right sided). The median number of days from operation to diagnosis of adult respiratory distress syndrome was 2.5. The median length of stay in the intensive care unit was 26 days, median intubation was 24 days, and the median hospital stay was 31 days. All patients with signs of adult respiratory distress syndrome were managed with diuresis, early intubation, mechanical ventilation, and aspiration bronchoscopy. Steroids were given to five patients at the initiation of nitric oxide therapy. Nitric oxide therapy was initiated immediately after the diagnosis of adult respiratory distress syndrome and the dose varied between 5 and 20 parts per million. The inhalation of nitric oxide produced an immediate increase in PaO_2 in all patients ranging from 9% to 85%. Seven of 10 patients survived, translating into a 30% mortality. The three deaths in this series were ultimately related to sepsis. Before the utilization of nitric oxide, this same institution reported a mortality rate of 86% in patients who developed adult respiratory distress syndrome after pneumonectomy.

Pneumothorax

Many factors cause and predispose the patient to the development of pneumothorax in relation to thoracic surgery. These include COPD, emphysema, asthma, barotrauma from mechanical ventilation with high airway pressures, high levels of PEEP, the use of jet ventilation, the occlusion of chest tubes with tissues or blood clots, and the unrecognized, unintentional entry to the pleural space. Pneumothorax may also occur as a complication from central line placement or from diagnostic procedures, such as thoracoscopy, bronchoscopy, and percutaneous needle lung biopsy. Difficult to treat causes of pneumothorax include rupture of a bronchial stump or tracheobronchial anastomosis and bronchopleural fistula resulting from infection or poor tissue healing. Tension pneumothorax develops when air continues to enter the hemithorax while not being effectively decompressed. It develops more rapidly if the patient is receiving positive-pressure ventilation and PEEP but may also occur in spontaneously breathing patients.

The diagnosis requires a high index of suspicion. Signs and symptoms include respiratory distress, increased work of breathing, decreased breath sounds, decreased chest movement on one or both sides, wheezing, increased airway pressure, decreased PaO_2 and arterial oxygen saturation (SaO_2), and increased $PaCO_2$. In addition, tension pneumothorax should be suspected if the trachea and mediastinum are deviated to the contralateral side. If not rapidly relieved, a tension pneumothorax will lead to hypotension and cardiovascular collapse. A chest radiograph reveals the diagnosis.

Treatment of a simple pneumothorax is by insertion of a chest tube. In a spontaneously breathing asymptomatic patient, a chest tube is inserted if the pneumothorax occupies 15% or more of the hemithorax. In spontaneously breathing patients who are symptomatic, a chest tube should be inserted regardless of the size of the pneumothorax. A pneumothorax of any size in patients who are mechanically ventilated requires the placement of a chest tube. Tension pneumothorax must be rapidly relieved by the emergency placement of a chest tube, usually in the fifth or sixth intercostal space. In dire situations, emergency decompression of the thorax with a 14-gauge intravenous catheter may be lifesaving until a chest tube can be inserted. A 14-gauge intravenous catheter is inserted on one or both sides in the second intercostal space at the anterior axillary line. An escaping hiss of decompressed air is easily heard when the chest cavity is entered.

Torsion of Residual Lobe

After pulmonary resection, the remaining lobes of the lungs are no longer tightly packed together in the thoracic cavity and they acquire increased mobility. This can lead to torsion of a lobe. The right middle lobe and the lingula are at greater risk of torsion after right upper or left upper lobectomy, respectively (96). Torsion of a lobe leading to occlusion of its bronchus produces a large intrapulmonary shunt, which can result in respiratory decompensation in patients with borderline reserve. If left uncorrected, the entire lobe may also infarct. Chest radiography reveals a density consistent with atelectasis that does not respond to the usual therapeutic measures of chest physiotherapy and deep breathing. If suspected, bronchoscopy should be performed followed by immediate surgical reexploration in an attempt to salvage the lobe. If a pulmonary infarction has developed and lung tissue is not viable, the lobe should be removed. This problem can be greatly reduced by surgical inspection of the operative hemithorax after a breath has been administered. Adjacent lobes may have their leading edges stapled together such that torsion will no longer be possible. A pleural tent in which the overall size of the thorax cavity is reduced can also address excessive space in the thorax.

Phrenic Nerve Injury

The phrenic nerve originates from C-3, C-4, and C-5 and passes into the chest anterior to the hilum of the lung to enter the diaphragm. It is at risk of damage during thoracotomy, particularly if mediastinal dissection is extensive or if the nerve is involved by tumor. Phrenic nerve paralysis may result in acute respiratory failure and the inability to wean the patient from mechanical ventilation. In patients who are breathing spontaneously, the chest radiograph reveals an elevated hemidiaphragm on the corresponding side. Patients with adequate pulmonary reserve who have had limited lung resection may tolerate unilateral diaphragmatic paralysis without difficulty. Patients who already have undergone extensive lung resection do not tolerate unilateral injury of the phrenic nerve on the side opposite to the resection. No patient tolerates a bilateral phrenic nerve injury.

Phrenic nerve injury should be suspected in patients who have relatively clear chest radiographs, have adequate gas exchange, but cannot be weaned from the ventilator. Paradoxical movements of the diaphragm on fluoroscopy confirm diagnosis. Atelectasis and pneumonia frequently ensue once the patient is allowed to breathe spontaneously, resulting in respiratory failure requiring prolonged mechanical ventilation. Return of function frequently occurs 2 to 9 months after injury. If paralysis persists, the diaphragm can be paced via an implantable phrenic nerve stimulator or diaphragmatic plication can be considered.

Recurrent Laryngeal Nerve Injury

The left recurrent laryngeal nerve is at more risk of injury during hilar lymph node dissection. Unilateral recurrent laryngeal nerve injury is either asymptomatic or results in hoarseness. The contralateral unaffected cord can usually cross the midline and compensates for the paralyzed cord. Bilateral partial injury of the recurrent laryngeal nerve causes spasm of the adductor muscles of the vocal cords, resulting in upper-airway obstruction after extubation. Immediate reintubation is necessary, followed by a tracheostomy until recovery occurs. Return of function usually requires 2 to 9 months. After unilateral injury, if return of function is incomplete, the affected vocal cord can be augmented with injectable gel foam or Teflon to improve its function. Bilateral complete recurrent laryngeal nerve injuries result in both vocal cords, assuming a cadaveric position and exposing the patient to the risk of aspiration. Again, a tracheostomy is required.

Spinal Cord Injury

Paraplegia may follow thoracotomy even if the thoracic aorta was not clamped during the procedure. Direct interruption of an intercostal artery supplying a major spinal cord radicular branch may cause spinal cord ischemia. An epidural hematoma causing spinal cord compression and paraplegia is a rare complication of pneumonectomy. Surgical dissection may create an opening between the epidural and pleural spaces. Blood can then enter the epidural space and compress the spinal cord, resulting in paraplegia.

Brachial Plexus Injury

The brachial plexus is vulnerable to injury during thoracic surgery. Suspension of the arm from an ether screen with the arm hyperextended can result in stretch and damage to the brachial plexus. Extreme abduction, external rotation, and extension of the arm on an arm board can also result in excessive stretch and injury to the brachial plexus. In the lateral decubitus position, the brachial plexus on the downside can be damaged from excessive pressure if an axillary roll is not properly placed.

Injuries Related to Lateral Decubitus Position

Careful positioning of the patient in the lateral decubitus position is mandatory to prevent injury. The brachial plexus is susceptible to damage by excessive stretch or compression during anesthesia, particularly in the lateral decubitus position. Hyperextension and external rotation of the arm results in excessive stretch of the nerve roots around the head of the humerus. Excessive rotation of the neck to the contralateral side worsens the situation. The brachial plexus may also be injured by compression on the dependent side from improper placement of the axillary roll. The radial nerve may be injured because of excessive pressure as it crosses the spiral groove behind the humerus, resulting in wrist drop. The ulnar nerve can be injured as it passes behind the elbow. The sciatic nerve can be compressed as it emerges from the pelvis. The common peroneal nerve is injured as it curves around the neck of the fibula, resulting in foot drop. Necrosis of the external ear may result if the ear is folded under the head. Excessive pressure on the downside eye is a catastrophic complication and can lead to blindness from impairment of retinal artery blood flow.

Hemorrhage

Major postoperative hemorrhage occurs in about 3% of patients with pulmonary resections. It is associated with a high mortality rate even with prompt surgical reexploration. The source of bleeding may be a bronchial or intercostal vessel, large raw exposed surface areas, or slipped ligatures around the pulmonary artery or pulmonary veins. Surgical dissection of adhesions between the visceral and parietal pleura results in large raw surface areas, increasing the potential for hemorrhage. Drainage of more than 200 mL/hour of blood with a hematocrit value of more than 20% from the chest tube blood despite correction of any coagulation deficiency is an indication for immediate surgical reexploration. The chest tubes must be kept patent, because obstruction by a clot may result in excessive amounts of blood accumulating in the chest unnoticed for a considerable time. Large-bore intravenous lines must be inserted if not already present. Aggressive resuscitation with crystalloids, colloids, and blood products should proceed while the patient is being transferred to the operating room. Coagulopathies are worked up with laboratory tests and perhaps thromboelastography and specific therapy is provided by the transfusion of platelets, fresh-frozen plasma, or cryoprecipitate, as indicated by the results of coagulation studies. Ketamine or etomidate are favorable induction agents. Positive-pressure ventilation may be poorly tolerated until hypovolemia has been corrected.

REFERENCES

1. Weissman DE, Gottschall JL. Complete remission of paraneoplastic sensory neuropathy: a case associated with small-cell lung cancer responsive to chemotherapy, plasma exchange, and radiotherapy. *J Clin Apheresis* 1989;5:3.
2. Rigler LG. The earliest roentgenographic signs of carcinoma of the lung. *JAMA* 1966;195:655.
3. Wait J. Preoperative pulmonary evaluation. *Am J Med Sci* 1995; 310:118.
4. Boysen PG, Block AJ, Moulder PV. Relationship between preoperative pulmonary function and complications after thoracotomy. *Surg Gynecol Obstet* 1981;152:813.
5. Mohr DN, Lavender RC. Preoperative pulmonary evaluation. Identifying patients at increased risk for complications. *Postgrad Med* 1996;100:241.
6. Olsen GN. Pulmonary function evaluation of the lung resection candidate: a prospective study. *Am Rev Respir Dis* 1975;111:379.
7. Gass GD, Olsen GN. Preoperative pulmonary function testing to predict postoperative morbidity and mortality. *Chest* 1986;89: 127.
8. Kearney DJ, Lee TH, Reilly JJ, et al. Assessment of operative risk in patients undergoing lung resection. Importance of predicted pulmonary function. *Chest* 1994;105:753.
9. Ferguson MK. Preoperative assessment of pulmonary risk. *Chest* 1999;115:59S.
10. Dales RE, Dionne G, Leech JA, et al. Preoperative prediction of pulmonary complications following thoracic surgery. *Chest* 1993; 104:155.
11. Aubier M. Aminophylline improves diaphragmatic contractility. *N Engl J Med* 1981;305:249.
12. Benumof JL. Where pulmonary arterial catheters go: intrathoracic distribution. *Anesthesiology* 1977;46:336.
13. Rehder K, Hatch DJ, Sessler AD, et al. The function of each lung of anesthetized and paralyzed man during mechanical ventilation. *Anesthesiology* 1972;37:16.
14. Slinger PD. Fiberoptic bronchoscopic positioning of double-lumen tubes. *J Cardiothorac Anesth* 1989;3:486.
15. Brodsky JB, Macario A, Mark JB. Tracheal diameter predicts double-lumen tube size: a method for selecting left double-lumen tubes. *Anesth Analg* 1996;82:861.
16. Benumof JL, Partridge BL, Salvatierra L, et al. Margin of safety in positioning modern double-lumen endotracheal tubes. *Anesthesiology* 1987;67:729.
17. Campos JH, Massa FC, Kernstine KH. The incidence of right upper-lobe collapse when comparing a right-sided double-lumen tube versus a modified left double-lumen tube for left-sided thoracic surgery. *Anesth Analg* 2000;90:535.
18. Stene R, Rose M, Weinger MB, et al. Bronchial trifurcation at the carina complicating use of a double-lumen tracheal tube. *Anesthesiology* 1994;80:1162.
19. Kubota H. Selective blind endobronchial intubation in children and adults. *Anesthesiology* 1987;67:587.
20. Smith GB, Hirsch NP, Ehrenwerth J. Placement of double-lumen endobronchial tubes. *Br J Anaesth* 1986;58:1317.
21. Bjertnaes LJ, Hauge A, Torgrimsen T. The pulmonary vasoconstrictor response to hypoxia: the hypoxia sensitive site studied with a volatile inhibitor. *Acta Physiol Scand* 1980;109:447.
22. Miller FL, Chen L, Malmkvist G, et al. Mechanical factors do not influence blood flow distribution in atelectasis. *Anesthesiology* 1989;70:481.
23. Benumof JL, Wahrenbrock EA. Blunted hypoxic pulmonary vasoconstriction by increased lung vascular pressures. *J Appl Physiol* 1975;38:846.
24. Ahmed T, Abraham WM. Role of calcium-channel blockers in obstructing airway disease. *Chest* 1985;88:142S.
25. Benumof JL. One-lung ventilation and hypoxic pulmonary vasoconstriction: implications for anesthetic management. *Anesth Analg* 1985;64:821.
26. Benumof JL, Augustine SD, Gibbons JA. Halothane and isoflurane only slightly impair arterial oxygenation during one-lung ventilation in patients undergoing thoracotomy. *Anesthesiology* 1987;67:910.
27. Slinger P, Scott WA. Arterial oxygenation during one-lung ventilation. A comparison of enflurane and isoflurane. *Anesthesiology* 1995;82:940.
28. Abe K, Shimizu T, Takashina M, et al. The effects of propofol, isoflurane, and sevoflurane on oxygenation and shunt fraction during one-lung ventilation. *Anesth Analg* 1998;87:1164.
29. Pagel SP, Fu JL, Damask MC, et al. Desflurane and isoflurane produce similar alterations in systemic pulmonary hemodynamics and arterial oxygenation in patients undergoing one-lung ventilation during thoracotomy. *Anesth Analg* 1998;87:800.
30. Hedenstierna G, Baehrendetz S, Klingstedt C, et al. Ventilation and perfusion of each lung during differential ventilation with selective PEEP. *Anesthesiology* 1984;61:369.
31. Larsson A, Malmkvist G, Werner O. Variations in lung volume and compliance during pulmonary surgery. *Br J Anaesth* 1987; 59:585.
32. Dantzker DR, Wagner PD, West JB. Instability of lung units with low V/Q ratios during O_2 breathing. *J Appl Physiol* 1975; 38:886.
33. Benumof JL, Rogers SN, Moyce PR, et al. Hypoxic pulmonary vasoconstriction and whole-lung PEEP in the dog. *Anesthesiology* 1979;51:503.
34. Capan LM, Turndorf H, Chandrakant P, et al. Optimization of arterial oxygenation during one-lung anesthesia. *Anesth Analg* 1980;59:847.
35. Alfery DD, Benumof JL, Trousdale FR. Improving oxygenation during one-lung ventilation: the effects of PEEP and blood flow restriction to the nonventilated lung. *Anesthesiology* 1981;55:381.
36. Katz J. Pre-emptive analgesia: evidence, current status and future directions. *Eur J Anaesthesiol* 1995;12:8.
37. Blomberg S, Emanuelsson H, Ricksten SE. Thoracic epidural anesthesia and central hemodynamics in patients with unstable angina pectoris. *Anesth Analg* 19898;69:558.
38. Liu S, Carpenter RL, Neal JM. Epidural anesthesia and analgesia. Their role in postoperative outcome. *Anesthesiology* 1995;82: 1474.
39. Ballantyne JC, Carr DB, deFerranti S, et al. The comparative effects of postoperative analgesic therapies on pulmonary outcome: cumulative meta-analyses of randomized, controlled trials. *Anesth Analg* 1998;86:598.
40. Burgess FW, Anderson M, Colonna D, et al. Thoracic epidural analgesia with bupivacaine and fentanyl for postoperative thoracotomy pain. *J Cardiothorac Vasc Anesth* 1994;8:420.
41. Sternlo JE, Hybbinette CH. Spinal subdural bleeding after attempted epidural and subsequent spinal anaesthesia in a patient

on thromboprophylaxis with low molecular weight heparin. *Acta Anaesthesiol Scand* 1995;39:557.

42. O'Connor CJ. Thoracic epidural analgesia: physiological effects and clinical applications. *J Cardiothorac Vasc Anesth* 1993;7:595.
43. Baron CM, Kowalski SE, Greengrass R, et al. Epinephrine decreases postoperative requirements for continuous thoracic epidural fentanyl infusions. *Anesth Analg* 1996;82:760.
44. Azizkhan RG, Dudgeon DL, Buck JR, et al. Life-threatening airway obstructions a complication to the management of mediastinal masses in children. *J Pediatr Surg* 1985;20:816.
45. Bray RJ, Fernandes FJ. Mediastinal tumor causing airway obstruction in anaesthetized children. *Anaesthesia* 1982;37:571.
46. DeSoto H. Direct laryngoscopy as an aid to relieve airway obstruction in a patient with a mediastinal mass. *Anesthesiology* 1987;67:116.
47. Ferrari LR, Bedford RF. General anesthesia prior to treatment of anterior mediastinal masses in pediatric cancer patients. *Anesthesiology* 1990;72:991.
48. John RE, Narang VS. A boy with an anterior mediastinal mass. *Anaesthesia* 1988;43:864.
49. Adkins RB, Maples MD, Hainsworth JD. Primary malignant mediastinal tumors. *Ann Thorac Surg* 1984;38:648.
50. Piro AJ, Weiss DR, Hellman S. Mediastinal Hodgkin's disease: a possible danger for intubation anaesthesia. *Int J Radiat Oncol Biol Phys* 1976;1:415.
51. Loeffler JS, Leoplod KA, Recht A, et al. Emergency prebiopsy radiation for mediastinal masses: impact on subsequent pathologic diagnosis and outcome. *J Clin Oncol* 1986;4:716.
52. Pullerits J, Holzman R. Anaesthesia for patients with mediastinal masses. *Can J Anaesth* 1989;36:681.
53. Bergmans NA. Reduction in resting and end-expiratory position of the respiratory system with induction of anesthesia and neuromuscular paralysis. *Anesthesiology* 1982;57:14.
54. Jones FG, Faithfull D, Jordan C, et al. Rib cage movement during halothane anaesthesia in man. *Br J Anaesth* 1979;51:399.
55. Levin H, Bursztein S, Heifetz M. Cardiac arrest in a child with an anterior mediastinal mass. *Anesth Analg* 1985;64:1129.
56. Hall KD, Friedman M. Extracorporeal oxygenation for induction of anesthesia in a patient with an intrathoracic tumor. *Anesthesiology* 1975;42:493.
57. Price SL, Hecker BR. Pulmonary oadema following airway obstruction in a patient with Hodgkin's disease. *Br J Anaesth* 1987;59:518.
58. Dyet JF, Naghissi K. Role of venography in assessing patients with superior caval obstruction caused by bronchial carcinoma for bypass operation. *Thorax* 1980;35:628.
59. Stanford W, Doty DB. The role of venography and surgery in the management of patients with superior vena cava obstruction. *Ann Thorac Surg* 1986;41:158.
60. Engel AG. Myasthenia gravis and myasthenic syndromes. *Ann Neurol* 1984;16:519.
61. Hankins JR, Mayer RF, Satterfield JR, et al. Thymectomy for myasthenia gravis: fourteen year experience. *Ann Surg* 1985;201:618.
62. Eisenkraft JB, Papatestas AE, Kahn CH, et al. Predicting the need for postoperative mechanical ventilation in myasthenia gravis. *Anesthesiology* 1986;65:79.
63. Wainwright AP, Brodrick PM. Suxamethonium in myasthenia gravis. *Anaesthesiology* 1987;42:950.
64. Leventhal SR, Orkin FK, Hirsch RA. Prediction of the need for postoperative mechanical ventilation in myasthenia gravis. *Anesthesiology* 1980;53:26.
65. Eisenkraft JB. Myasthenia gravis and thymic surgery—anesthetic considerations. In: Gothard JWW, ed. *Bailliere's clinical anaesthesiology.* London: Balliere Tindall, 1987.
66. Pancrazio JJ, Viglione MP, Tabbara IA, et al. Voltage-dependent ion channels in small cell lung cancer cells. *Cancer Res* 1989;49:5901.
67. Tanaka K, Tanaka M, Miyatake T, et al. Antibodies to brain proteins in a patient with subacute cerebellar degeneration and Lambert-Eaton myasthenic syndrome. *Tohoku J Exp Med* 1987;153:161.
68. Irita K, Satoh M, Akata T, et al. Lambert-Eaton myasthenic syndrome. *Can J Anaesth* 1990;37:944.
69. Steiger Z, Wilson RF. Management of bronchopleural fistulas. *Surg Gynecol Obstet* 1984;158:267.
70. Albelda SM, Hanson-Flaschen JH, Taylor E, et al. Evaluation of high-frequency jet ventilation in patients with bronchopleural fistulas by quantification of the airleak. *Anesthesiology* 1985;63:551.
71. Bishop MJ, Benson MS, Sato P, et al. Comparison of high-frequency jet ventilation with conventional mechanical ventilation For bronchopleural fistula. *Anesth Analg* 1987;66:833.
72. FitzGerald MX, Keelan PJ, Cugell DW, et al. Long term results of surgery for bullous emphysema. *J Thorac Cardiovasc Surg* 1974;68:566.
73. Nakahara K, Nakaoka K, Ohno K, et al. Functional indications for bullectomy of giant bulla. *Ann Thorac Surg* 1983;35:480.
74. Brantigan OC, Mueller E, Kress MB. A surgical approach to pulmonary emphysema. *Am Rev Respir Dis* 1959;80:194.
75. Cooper JD, Chardak WM, Andersen MN, et al. Bilateral pneumectomy (volume reduction) for chronic obstructive pulmonary disease. *J Cardiovasc Surg* 1995;109:106.
76. Kotloff RM, Tino G, Bavaria JE, et al. Bilateral lung volume reduction surgery for advanced emphysema. A comparison of median sternotomy and thoroscopic approaches. *Chest* 1996;110:1399.
77. Kirschner PA. Cervical mediastinoscopy. *Chest Surg Clin North Am* 1996;6:1.
78. Vourch G, Fischler M, Michon F, et al. Manual jet ventilation vs high frequency jet ventilation during laser resection of tracheobronchial stenosis. *Br J Anaesth* 1983;55:973.
79. Landreneau RJ, Hazelrigg SR, Mack MJ, et al. Postoperative pain-related morbidity: video assisted thoracic surgery versus thoracotomy. *Ann Thorac Surg* 1993;56:1285.
80. DeCamp MM, Jaklitsch MT, Mentzer SJ, et al. The safety and versatility of video-thoracoscopy: a prospective analysis of 895 consecutive cases. *J Am Coll Surg* 1995;181:113.
81. Hazelrigg SR, Nunchuck SK, LoCicero J. Video assisted thoracic surgery study group data. *Ann Thorac Surg* 1993;56:1039.
82. Heatley RV, Williams RP, Lewis MH. Preoperative intravenous feeding—a controlled trial. *Postgrad Med J* 1979;55:541.
83. Selvin BL. Cancer chemotherapy: implications for the anesthesiologist. *Anesth Analg* 1981;60:425.
84. Thiagarajah S, Lear E, Keh M. Anesthetic implications of Zenker's diverticulum. *Anesth Analg* 1990;70:109.
85. Adams CF. Regional anesthesia for repair of Zenker's diverticulum. *Anesth Analg* 1990;70:676.
86. Garzon AA, Cerruti MM, Golding ME. Exsanguinating hemoptysis. *J Thorac Cardiovasc Surg* 1982;84:829.
87. Cardinale D, Martinoni A, Cipolla CM, et al. Atrial fibrillation after operation for lung cancer: clinical and prognostic significance. *Ann Thorac Surg* 1999;68:1827.
88. Gallagher C, Sladen RB, Lubarsky D. Thoracotomy: postoperative complications. *Probl Anesth* 1990;4:393.
89. Shields TW, Ujiki GT. Digitalization for prevention of arrhythmias following pulmonary surgery. *Surg Gynecol Obstet* 1968;126:743.
90. Burman SO. The prophylactic use of digitalis before thoracotomy. *Ann Thorac Surg* 1972;14:359.

91. Amar D, Roistacher N, Burt ME, et al. Effects of diltiazem versus digoxin on dysrhythmias and cardiac function after pneumonectomy. *Ann Thorac Surg* 1997;63:1374.
92. Frostell C, Fratacci MD, Wqin JC, et al. Inhaled nitric oxide: a selective pulmonary vasodilator reversing hypoxic pulmonary vasoconstriction. *Circulation* 1991;83:2038.
93. Deslaurius J, Aucoin A, Gregoire J. Postpneumonectomy pulmonary edema. *Chest Surg Clin North Am* 1998;8:611.
94. Zeldin RA, Normandin D, Landtwing D, et al. Postpneumonectomy pulmonary edema. *J Thorac Cardiovasc Surg* 1984;87:359.
95. Mathisen DJ, Kuo EY, Hahn C, et al. Inhaled nitric oxide for adult respiratory distress syndrome after pulmonary resection. *Ann Thorac Surg* 1998;66:1894.
96. Patterson GA, Cooper JD. Complications of thoracotomy. In: Marshall BD, Longnecker DE, Fairley HD, eds *Anesthesia for thoracic procedures.* Boston, MA: Blackwell Science, 1988.

Cardiac Anesthesia: Principles and Clinical Practice, Second Edition, edited by Fawzy G. Estafanous, Paul G. Barash, and J.G. Reves. Lippincott Williams & Wilkins, Philadelphia © 2001.

27

ANESTHESIA FOR THORACIC AORTIC SURGERY

MARK BANOUB

Surgical diseases of the thoracic aorta can be divided into four main groups: (a) aortic dissection, (b) aortic aneurysms, (c) traumatic aortic rupture, and (d) developmental anomalies (coarctation and vascular rings).

AORTIC DISSECTION

Acute dissection of the thoracic aorta is the most common catastrophic aortic condition encountered in clinical practice. Aortic dissection is usually a event of sudden onset in which blood leaves the normal aortic channel through a discrete point of entry (the intimal tear) and rapidly dissects the inner from the outer layer of the media to produce a false channel. The dissection usually proceeds distally, but it may extend proximally as well. Patients are considered to have an acute dissection when the process is less than 14 days old; dissection of longer duration is considered chronic. The mortality rate in untreated cases is as high as 1% per hour during the first 48 hours.

Pathogenesis

Aortic dissection is believed to begin with the formation of a tear in aortic intima that directly exposes an underlying diseased medial layer to the driving force (pulse pressure) of intraluminal blood. The diseased media is cleaved in two layers, thus dissecting the aortic wall. Driven by persistent intraluminal pressure, the dissection process extends a variable length along the aortic wall. Extension typically occurs antegrade, but sometimes retrograde, from the site of the intimal tear. The blood-filled space between the dissected layers of the aortic wall becomes the false lumen. An alternative theory suggests that dissection begins with rupture of a vasa vasorum within the aortic media, resulting in the development of an intramural hematoma. The hematoma then secondarily ruptures through the intimal layer, creating an intimal tear and aortic dissection.

M. Banoub: Division of Anesthesia and Critical Care Medicine, The Cleveland Clinic Foundation, Cleveland, Ohio 44195; and Department of Anesthesia, St. Vincent Mercy Medical Center, Toledo, Ohio 43608

Classification

Most classification schemes for aortic dissection are based on the fact that the vast majority of aortic dissections originate in one of two locations: the ascending aorta within several centimeters of the aortic valve and the descending aorta just distal to the origin of the left subclavian artery (1). Sixty-five percent of intimal tears occur in the ascending aorta, 20% in the descending aorta, 10% in the aortic arch, and 5% in the abdominal aorta (2) (Fig. 27-1). There are three major classification systems to define the location and extent of aortic involvement (Table 27-1 and Fig. 27-2):

1. DeBakey: types I, II, and III (3)
2. Stanford: types A and B
3. Anatomic types: proximal and distal

Dissections involving the ascending aorta, regardless of the location of the intimal tear, are called type A or proximal dissections and comprise DeBakey types I and II. The involvement of the ascending aorta is the crucial determinant of prognostic and therapeutic implications. In general, surgery is always indicated for dissections involving the ascending aorta, whereas medical management may be the appropriate initial therapy for uncomplicated distal dissections that do not involve the ascending aorta. Accordingly, because DeBakey types I and II involve the ascending aorta, they are grouped together for simplicity into the Stanford (type A) and anatomic (proximal type) classification systems. Proximal or type A dissections account for about two-thirds of the cases, whereas distal dissections make up the remaining one-third. Aortic dissection is also classified according to its duration, which is defined as the length of time from onset of symptoms to medical evaluation. An acute dissection is one that has been present for less than 2 weeks; a chronic dissection has been present for 2 weeks or longer. At diagnosis, about two-thirds of aortic dissec-

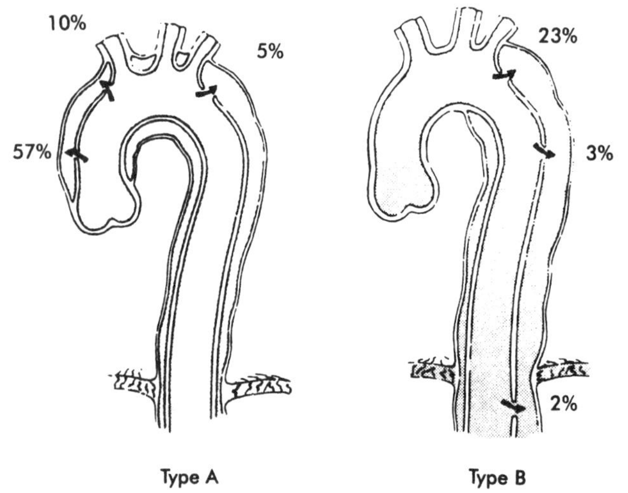

FIGURE 27-1. Classification of aortic dissections and distribution of the sites of the intimal tear. (From Ergin MA, Galla JD, Lansman S, et al. Acute dissections of the aorta. *Surg Clin North Am* 1985; 65:721, with permission.)

TABLE 27-1. COMMONLY USED CLASSIFICATION SYSTEMS TO DESCRIBE AORTIC DISSECTION

DeBakey system	
Type I	Originates in the ascending aorta, propagates at least to the aortic arch and often beyond it distally
Type II	Originates in and is confined to the ascending aorta
Type III	Originates in the descending thoracic aorta and extends distally down the aorta or, rarely, retrograde into the aortic arch and ascending aorta
Stanford system	
Type A	All dissections involving the ascending aorta, regardless of the site of origin
Type B	All dissections not involving the ascending aorta
Anatomic system	
Proximal	Includes DeBakey types I and II or Stanford type A
Distal	Includes DeBakey type III or Stanford type B

tions are acute and one-third are chronic. About 70% of patients with untreated aortic dissection die in the first 2 weeks after the onset of symptoms (2). Because mortality from dissection and the risk of progression decrease with time, therapeutic strategies for chronic dissections are quite different from those for acute dissections.

Etiology and Predisposing Factors

Multiple risk factors for aortic dissection have been identified, the most common being advanced age, systemic hypertension, congenital abnormalities of the aortic valve, and heredity disorders of connective tissue. Degeneration of collagen and elastin fibers in the aortic media is a chief predisposing factor in many cases.

Hereditary Connective Tissue Disorders and Marfan Syndrome

Cystic medial degeneration is an intrinsic feature of several hereditary defects of connective tissue, most notably the Marfan and Ehlers-Danlos syndromes. Patients with Mar-

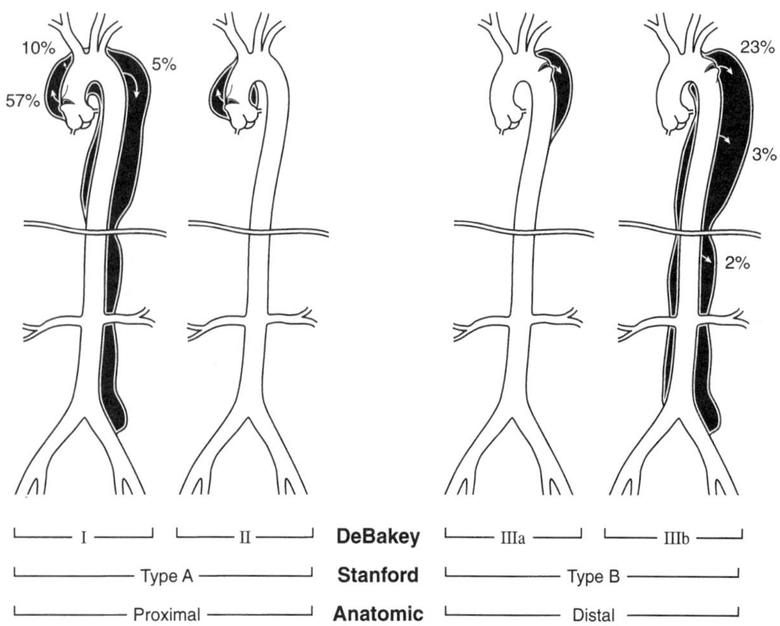

FIGURE 27-2. The three classification systems of aortic dissection and the frequency distribution of the different locations of the intimal tear. (Modified from Edmonds LH Jr, ed. *Cardiac surgery in the adult.* New York: McGraw-Hill, Health Professions Division, 1997:1129, with permission.)

fan syndrome are at risk for development of acute aortic dissections and aneurysms at a relatively young age. Marfan syndrome accounts for 6% to 9% of all aortic dissections (4).

Hypertension

Of the various factors implicated in the etiology of acute aortic dissections, arterial hypertension remains the most consistent. Hypertension is present in 75% of acute dissections and is more prevalent in patients with type B dissections (5). Hypertension accelerates the degenerative changes in the aging aorta, predisposes to the development of an intramural hematoma, and promotes progression of the dissection process (2).

Aortic Stenosis and Coarctation of the Aorta

Congenital aortic stenosis, bicuspid aortic valve, and coarctation of the aorta are well-established risk factors for proximal aortic dissection, especially in younger patients. Bicuspid aortic valve is found in 7% to 14% of proximal aortic dissections (5). The causative role of systemic hypertension is further supported by the finding that coarctation of the aorta predisposes to aortic dissection.

Pregnancy

About 50% of all aortic dissections in women younger than 40 years of age occur during pregnancy, typically in the third trimester, but occasionally in the early postpartum period (6). Increases in blood volume, cardiac output (CO), and blood pressure seen in late pregnancy may contribute to the risk. Women with Marfan syndrome and dilated aortic root are at very high risk for acute aortic dissection during pregnancy (7).

Iatrogenic Trauma

Iatrogenic aortic dissection is an uncommon but serious complication of invasive vascular procedures and cardiac surgery. Coronary angiography, percutaneous transluminal coronary angioplasty, intraaortic balloon insertion, and translumbar aortography have all been complicated by aortic dissections. The majority of catheter-induced dissections are retrograde and tend to decrease in size over time due to thrombosis of the false lumen; antegrade dissections, on the other hand, tend to persist on follow-up. Most iatrogenic catheter-induced aortic dissections can be treated medically with serial clinical examinations and noninvasive testing to identify progression and the need for surgical therapy (8). Aortic dissection may complicate cardiac surgical procedures that require cross-clamping or cannulation of the ascending aorta, such as valve replacement and/or coronary artery bypass grafting (CABG) (2). Dissection can arise at the site of ascending aortic cannulation, saphenous vein anastomosis, or aortic cross-clamping or as a result of direct arterial injury. Most of these dissections are discovered intraoperatively and repaired immediately, although 20% are not diagnosed until the postoperative period. Aortic valve replacement in patients with a bicuspid valve carries an increased risk of perioperative dissection. A distinct group of patients undergoing aortic valve replacement develop delayed aortic dissection several years after the procedure (9–11).

Other Rare Associations

Aortic dissection has been reported in association with Noonan syndrome, Turner syndrome, fibromuscular dysplasia, annuloaortic ectasia, cocaine use, polycystic kidney disease, giant cell aortitis, polyarteritis nodosa, systemic lupus erythematosus, trauma, syphilitic aortitis, cystinosis, Cushing syndrome, and pheochromocytoma.

Clinical Features

Aortic dissection most frequently affects patients in the fifth to the seventh decades of life and is more common in men. Because of the variable involvement of the aorta and its branches, aortic dissection may have diverse presentations resulting in difficulty with diagnosis. Despite major advances in diagnostic modalities, up to 50% of patients die without a correct premortem diagnosis. Therefore, a high index of clinical suspicion is imperative. Sudden or accelerated death may be the initial presentation, with the true diagnosis made only at autopsy. Severe pain is the most constant and dramatic symptom of aortic dissection; it is found in 74% to 90% of cases. The pain is typically of sudden onset and is maximum at its inception, in contrast to the pain of myocardial infarction, which usually has a crescendo-like onset. The pain is often described as tearing, ripping, or stabbing. An important characteristic is the tendency of the pain to migrate from its point of origin to other sites, generally following the path of dissection as it extends through the aorta. Such migratory pain is noted in 70% of cases (Fig. 27-3). The location of the initial pain can help predict the site of intimal tear. A pain in the anterior chest suggests ascending dissection, whereas interscapular pain is more frequently associated with descending dissection (Table 27-2). Acute dissection is painless in 15% to 20% of patients. Most of those presenting without pain are found to have chronic dissection. Differences in the characteristics of type A and type B aortic dissection are shown in Table 27-3. Manifestations of the intense neural and humoral responses to the severe pain include pallor, cold sweats, nausea, and vomiting. The patient may appear to be in shock despite an adequate and in many cases hypertensive arterial blood pressure.

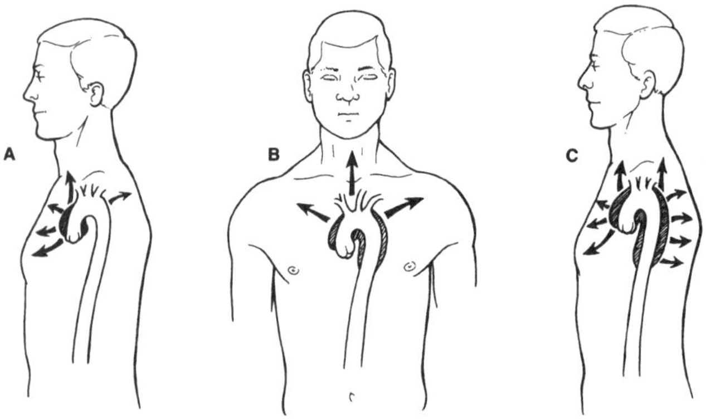

FIGURE 27-3. Migration of pain *(arrows)* from anterior chest **(A)** to the neck and shoulders **(B)** and to the back **(C)** as the false lumen extends from proximal to distal aorta.

Syncopy is the second most common presenting symptom of dissection. It usually results from rupture into the pericardial space that produces cardiac tamponade. Neurologic manifestations occur in 6% to 20% of all aortic dissections (12) and are more common with proximal dissections. Cerebral vascular accidents occur in 3% to 6% as a result of involvement of the innominate or left common carotid artery. A compromise of spinal cord perfusion may produce paraparesis or paraplegia.

Aortic regurgitation occurs in 50% to 66% of cases of proximal aortic dissection and may result from several mechanisms (Fig. 27-4). Severe aortic regurgitation is the most common cause of acute congestive heart failure (CHF) occurring in association with proximal aortic dissection. Rarely, CHF is caused by the large shunt resulting from rupture of the dissecting process into the right or left atrium or the right ventricle. Myocardial infarction occurs in 1% to 2% of patients as a result of compromise of the coronary ostia. The right coronary artery is more commonly affected, resulting in inferior myocardial infarction. Extension into the abdominal aorta may result in renal and mesenteric ischemia. Hematuria, oliguria, flank pain, and azotemia accompany significant renal involvement. Hematemesis and melena indicate intestinal ischemia and a very poor prognosis. Femoral pulse deficits and acute lower-extremity ischemia occur in 12% of cases (12). Differential or absent pulses accompanied by varying degrees of limb ischemia are among the best clinical signs of acute dissection and are present in about 40% of patients at the time of admission (12). Other clinical manifestations include pleural effusions, hemothorax, vocal cord paralysis, upper airway obstruction, dysphagia, rupture of the aneurysm into the tracheobronchial tree resulting in hemoptysis and asphyxia, superior vena cava (SVC) syndrome, Horner syndrome, and unexplained fever. Signs of pericardial involvement include jugular venous distention, paradoxic pulse, pericardial friction rub, and cardiac tamponade. Expansion of the false lumen and compression of adjacent structures may cause the SVC syndrome, vocal cord paralysis, tracheal or bronchial

TABLE 27-2. CLINICAL CLUES TO PROXIMAL VERSUS DISTAL AORTIC DISSECTION

Proximal	Distal
Initial pain in the anterior chest	Interscapular pain
Aortic diastolic murmur	Hypertension
Pericardial friction rub	Left pleural effusion
Decreased or absent blood pressure or pulses in the right arm	
Decreased right carotid artery pulsation	
Evidence of myocardial ischemia or infarction on electrocardiogram	
Marfan syndrome	
Congenital abnormality of the aortic valve	

Source: Topol EJ, ed. *Comprehensive cardiovascular medicine.* Philadelphia: Lippincott-Raven, 1998, with permission.

TABLE 27-3. CHARACTERISTICS OF TYPE A AND TYPE B AORTIC DISSECTION

Parameter	Type A	Type B
Frequency (%)	65–70	30–35
Average age (yr)	50–55	60–70
Associated hypertension (%)	50	80
Arterial pressure on admission	50% normal or elevated; 50% hypotensive	80% normal or elevated; 20% hypotensive
Pain	Anterior, substernal	Posterior, midscapular
Associated atherosclerosis	±	+
Aortic regurgitation (%)	50	10
Diastolic murmur (%)	50	10
Pericardial effusion	+ +	±
Pleural effusion	±	+ + (left pleura)
Syncope	+ +	Rare
Hemiparesis or hemiplegia	+	−
Paraparesis or paraplegia	±	+
Acute mortality (%)	90–95	40
Renal-intestinal infarction	+	+
Myocardial infarction	+	Rare

Note: +, frequency present; ±, sometimes present, sometimes absent; −, usually absent.
Source: Adapted from Ergin MA, Galla JD, Lansman S, et al. Acute dissections of the aorta: current surgical treatment. *Surg Clin North Am* 1985;65:721, with permission.

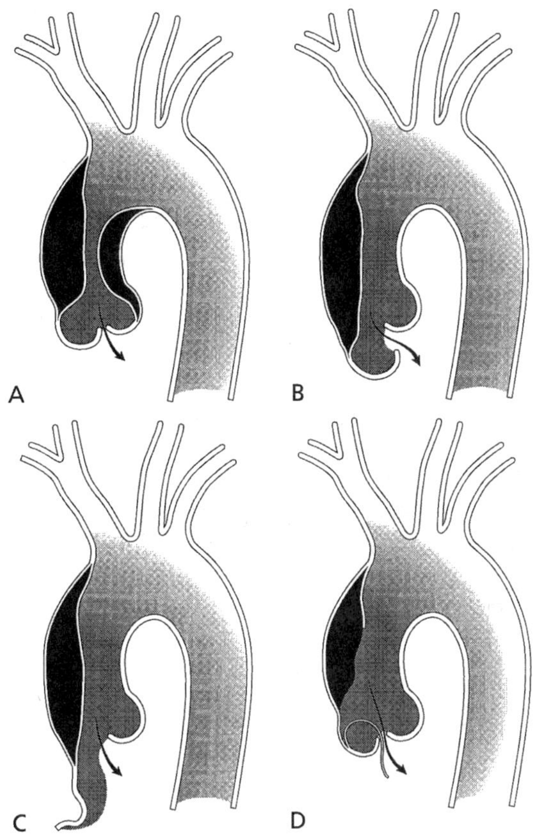

FIGURE 27-4. Mechanics of aortic regurgitation in proximal aortic dissection. **A:** An extensive or circumferential tear dilates the aortic root and annulus, causing failure of coaptation of aortic valve leaflets. **B:** With asymmetric dissection, pressure from the false lumen depresses one aortic leaflet below the coaptation line of the other leaflets. **C:** The annular support is disrupted, resulting in a flail aortic leaflet. **D:** Prolapse of a mobile intimal flap through the aortic valve during diastole, which prevents leaflet coaptation. (Redrawn from Braunwald E, ed. *Heart disease: a textbook of cardiovascular medicine,* 5th ed, vol 5. Philadelphia: WB Saunders Co, 1980:1557, with permission.)

compression, massive hemoptysis from erosion into the tracheobronchial tree, or hematemesis from erosion into the esophagus. Hypertension on admission is frequently present in patients with type B dissection and in some patients with type A dissection. Hypotension may be caused by cardiac tamponade, hypovolemia (due to loss of blood externally or into the false lumen), myocardial ischemia, or severe CHF. Disseminated intravascular coagulopathy occurs frequently owing to the activation and consumption of clotting factors and platelets in the false lumen.

Differential diagnosis includes myocardial infarction or ischemia, acute aortic regurgitation without dissection, nondissecting aortic aneurysm, pericarditis, musculoskeletal pain, and mediastinal tumors. Aortic dissection should always be considered in the differential diagnosis of a patient with unexplained syncopy, stroke, CHF, acute arterial occlusion, or an abnormal aortic contour on chest radiography, even in the absence of chest pain.

Cardiac tamponade (resulting from rupture of the aneurysm into the pericardial space) is responsible for 70% of the deaths occurring in the first 2 weeks.

Diagnosis

Because of its variable manifestations, the clinical diagnosis of aortic dissection must depend on a high index of suspicion. It is essential to confirm the diagnosis promptly and accurately (13). Sudden, severe migratory pain in a hypertensive patient, together with a pulse deficit and a new diastolic murmur, is highly suggestive of an acute dissection.

Laboratory Findings

Laboratory findings are nonspecific and may include leukocytosis, anemia, elevated serum lactate dehydrogenase, and elevated bilirubin due to blood sequestration in the false lumen. Serum creatine phosphokinase and aspartate transaminase are usually normal. Prolonged prothrombin time (PT) and partial thromboplastin time (PTT), thrombocytopenia, hypofibrinogenemia, and elevated fibrin split products indicate the presence of disseminated intravascular coagulopathy (14). Elevations of blood urea nitrogen and creatinine may be caused by renal malperfusion or preexisting renal impairment.

Electrocardiogram

The absence of acute ischemic electrocardiographic (ECG) changes in a patient with severe chest pain is highly suggestive of acute aortic dissection. Myocardial infarction is seen in 10% to 20% of patients with dissections due to obstruction of a coronary ostium. Underlying coronary artery disease (CAD) or hypertension may be manifested on the ECG by evidence of previous myocardial infarction, left ventricular hypertrophy, or strain (15). Heart block or pericarditic changes may be present.

Chest Radiograph

More than 80% of patients with aortic dissection have one or more of the following chest radiographic abnormalities: bulging of the descending thoracic aorta, deformity of the aortic knob, irregular aortic contour, loss of sharpness of the aortic shadow, enlargement of the cardiac shadow, displacement of the esophagus after passage of a nasogastric tube, widened mediastinum, tracheal or bronchial displacement, a pleural effusion, and aortic intimal calcifications separated by more than 6 mm from the edge of the aortic contour.

Diagnostic Imaging

The definitive diagnosis of aortic dissection requires the use of one or more diagnostic imaging techniques to delineate the following:

1. Presence of a dissection membrane separating the true and false lumens
2. Presence of ascending aortic involvement
3. Location of the intimal tear
4. Size of the aortic root and presence of aortic regurgitation
5. State of patency of the major aortic branches
6. Extent and patency of the false lumen
7. Presence of a reentry tear
8. Presence of pericardial effusion
9. State of the coronary circulation

Currently available and developing imaging techniques can answer most of these questions adequately. The extent of preoperative evaluation and the choice of diagnostic modality depend largely on the degree of surgical urgency and the hemodynamic stability of the patient. The most useful noninvasive and minimally invasive diagnostic tools are transthoracic echocardiography (TTE), transesophageal echocardiography (TEE), computed tomography (CT), and magnetic resonance imaging (MRI). Invasive imaging modalities include aortography and intravascular ultrasonography. The choice of a diagnostic test depends on institutional availability and experience and the hemodynamic stability of the patient.

Transthoracic Echocardiography

When a dilated aortic root, widened aortic wall, and linear undulating intimal flap are detected, the positive predictive value of TTE is 100%. Advantages of TTE are its portability, rapid on-line diagnosis, and the ability to evaluate aortic regurgitation and other valvular abnormalities, left ventricular function, regional wall motion abnormality (RWMA), pericardial effusion, and cardiac tamponade (16,17). TTE has a sensitivity of 60% to 85% and a specificity of 65% to 95% for diagnosis of aortic dissection. Its sensitivity is highest for dissections involving the ascending aorta but drops to only 30% to 50% for dissections of the descending aorta (18). Furthermore, image quality is often adversely affected by obesity, emphysema, mechanical ventilation, and small intercostal spaces.

Transesophageal Echocardiography

TEE has become an indispensable tool for the diagnosis, intraoperative management, and postoperative follow-up and is currently the preferred initial diagnostic method in patients with suspected acute aortic dissection (19). Two large, prospective studies demonstrated that the sensitivity of TEE for aortic dissection is 98% to 99% (19,20). Furthermore, TEE detected both aortic regurgitation and pericardial infusion in 100% of cases. The specificity of TEE is reported to be as high as 97% (19). Inclusion of biplane or multiplane transducers and confirmation of two lumens by the demonstration of differential color flow patterns have been suggested to reduce the possibility of false-positive TEE diagnosis. The echocardiographic finding considered diagnostic of an aortic dissection is the presence of an undulating intimal flap within the aortic lumen, separating the true and false channels. The sensitivity of TEE for 73% for detection of the site of intimal tear and 68% for the presence of thrombus in the false lumen (20). Color flow Doppler imaging significantly improves the sensitivity and specificity of TEE and TTE by localizing the entry site and delineating flow through the true and false lumens (21,22). In addition, TEE is extremely accurate in defining the presence and severity associated with aortic regurgitation, RWMAs that may be indicative of myocardial ischemia or infarction, and the presence of cardiac tamponade. Performing TEE in an awake, nonintubated patient with suspected acute aortic dissection could lead to dangerous increases in heart rate and blood pressure, which may lead to extension of the dissection or aortic rupture or both. Therefore, it is preferable to perform TEE after the induction of general anesthesia and intubation of the trachea, either in the intensive care unit or in the operating room. Vasodilators and β-blockers should be used to prevent and treat hypertension and tachycardia. If the TEE findings are considered definitive in a hemodynamically unstable patient, surgery could be performed without any further diagnostic studies.

Computed Tomography

CT with intravenous contrast enhancement is an accurate noninvasive screening test in patients with suspected aortic dissection (23). It reliably demonstrates the intimal flap, pericardial and pleural effusions, associated mediastinal hemorrhage, and involvement of the abdominal aorta. However, it often fails to demonstrate the site of entry or reentry, associated aortic regurgitation, or branch involvement. Because the CT equipment is not portable, its use in hemodynamically unstable patients is limited. Contrast-enhanced CT was found to have a sensitivity of 83% to 94% and a specificity of 87% to 100% in diagnosing acute aortic dissection (12,20). Ultrafast CT scanning with an electron beam, which provides superior image resolution (24), and spiral CT scanning, which permits three-dimensional display of the aorta and its branches (25), are both likely to improve the accuracy of CT in the diagnosis of aortic dissection (26) (Fig. 27-5). Using powerful computer image manipulation, spiral three-dimensional CT angiographic scanning can provide a clear definition of the aorta and its branches and may evolve to be the most accurate noninvasive diagnostic tool in the near future (27,28).

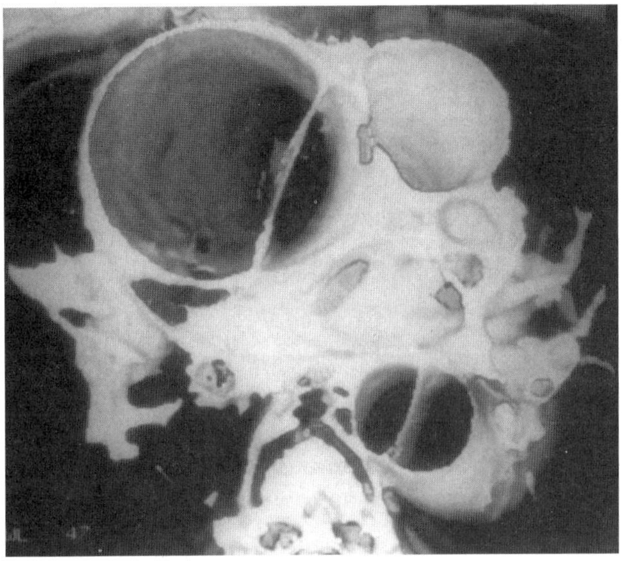

FIGURE 27-5. Three-dimensional spiral computed tomographic angiography in chronic type A dissection. An intimal flap is seen in both the ascending and descending aorta. (Courtesy of Dr. H. Adachi, Omiya Medical Center, Jicji Medical School, Omiya, Japan.)

Magnetic Resonance Imaging

The use of MRI has particular appeal in that it is entirely noninvasive and does not require the use of intravenous contrast material or ionizing radiation. MRI produces high-quality images in transverse, sagittal, and coronal planes. The left anterior oblique view displays the entire thoracic aorta in one plane (Fig. 27-6). It can determine the extent of dissection and the presence of branch vessel involvement. Both the sensitivity and specificity of MRI in diagnosis of aortic dissection were found to be 98%; the sensitivity was 88% for identifying the site of intimal tear, 98% for the presence of false-lumen thrombus, and 100% for the presence of pericardial effusion. Cine-MRI imaging has an 85% sensitivity for the detection of aortic regurgitation. Gated spin-echo MRI accurately demonstrates the site of the entry and the intimal flap and may become the optimal method for localizing the entry site location within all segments of the aorta (29,30). Major disadvantages include nonportability, the hostile MRI environment, and the presence of standard contraindications to MRI (e.g., pacemakers). MRI is not useful in hemodynamically unstable acute dissections; it is most valuable in stable patients, those with chronic dissections, and those who have been treated and are undergoing follow-up studies.

A

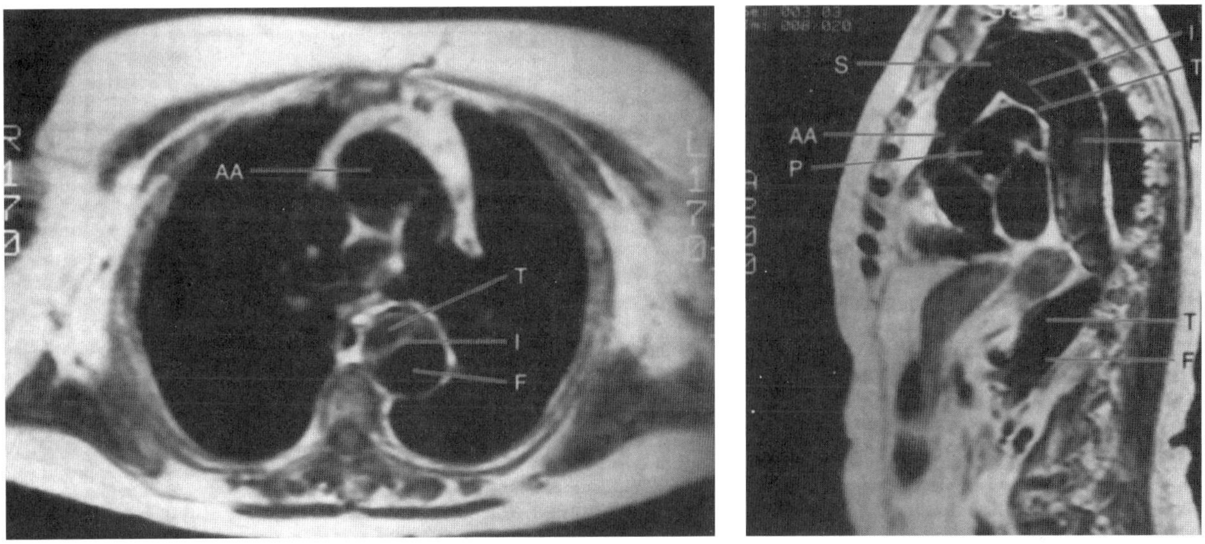

B

FIGURE 27-6. Magnetic resonance images in two planes in a patient with a distal aortic dissection. **A:** This image in the transverse plane through the upper thorax at the level of the pulmonary artery shows an intact ascending aorta (*AA*), but in the descending aorta it reveals an intimal flap (*I*) separating the true (*T*) and false (*F*) lumens. **B:** This image in the sagittal plane of the aorta shows the site of intimal tear (*S*) together with the intimal tear (*I*), which begins just distal to the takeoff of the left subclavian artery and spirals distally along the descending aorta. The true (*T*) and false (*F*) lumens are identified in both the descending thoracic aorta above and the abdominal aorta below. The ascending aorta (*AA*) is uninvolved by the dissection. Also seen here is the pulmonary artery (*P*) at its bifurcation. Notice that in both views the false lumen originates posteriorly and is wider than the true lumen. This pattern is typical in distal aortic dissections. (From Isselbacher EM, Cigarroa JE, Eagle KA. Aortic dissection. In: Creager M, ed. *Atlas of heart disease: vascular disease.* [Braunwald E, series ed.]. Philadelphia: Current Medicine, 1996, with permission.)

Aortography

Traditionally, aortography has been the definitive "gold standard" method of diagnosis in aortic dissection. Diagnosis is based on identification of the false and true lumens and the presence of an intimal flap. Other indirect signs considered suggestive of aortic dissection, especially if an intimal flap is visualized, include deformity of the true aortic lumen, thickening of aortic walls, branch vessel abnormalities, and aortic regurgitation. The false lumen is visualized in 87%, the intimal flap in 70%, and the site of intimal tear in 56% of cases. The sensitivity and specificity of aortography for the diagnosis of aortic dissection were reported to be 88% and 95%, respectively (19,31). Advantages include the ability to delineate the extent of dissection, including branch vessel involvement, the presence of aortic regurgitation, and patency of the coronary arteries. Disadvantages include limited sensitivity, inherent delay in diagnosis due to the time needed to complete the study, invasiveness, exposure to ionizing radiation, and the use of intravenous contrast agents. The development of catheter fenestration techniques has expanded the role of aortography from a diagnostic modality to one of therapeutic value in selected cases. Percutaneous fenestration of the dissecting intima has been used to relieve lower-extremity and acute mesenteric ischemia in patients with acute aortic dissection (32–34).

Intravascular Ultrasonography

Intravascular ultrasound is one of the most recent advances in the echocardiographic evaluation of aortic dissection. The catheter is inserted through the femoral artery and the aorta is imaged in a transverse plane through its short access, allowing the two lumens and the intimal flap to be detected. Intravascular ultrasonography, in combination with standard aortography, greatly improves the accuracy of diagnosis and could be useful in selected patients with suspected aortic dissection (35,36).

Coronary Angiography

The importance of assessing the status of coronary artery patency before the surgical repair of acute aortic dissection continues to be controversial. Two types of coronary artery involvement must be considered. The first is acute proximal coronary narrowing or occlusion as a result of the dissection process. The second is the possible presence of chronic atherosclerotic CAD, which, although generally independent of the dissection process, may complicate its surgical management. TEE can effectively define the patency of the proximal coronary artery in most cases (37). Aortography may also reveal such coronary artery involvement. However, a more comprehensive evaluation requires the performance of coronary angiography, which may be risky in patients with aortic dissection and often prolongs the time to operative repair by several hours. Proximal coronary obstruction resulting from dissection can usually be readily identified at the time of surgery. Chronic CAD is seen in about 25% of patients presenting with aortic dissection and is not well identified by any of the imaging modalities discussed previously. The impact of unrecognized CAD on outcome is not certain. Accordingly, some authors recommend avoiding preoperative coronary angiography unless a specific indication exists, such as a known history of CAD or the presence of ischemic ECG changes (38). Conversely, Creswell et al. reported good outcomes when performing combined aortic repair and CABG in patients with underlying CAD and recommended that all stable patients with acute proximal dissection undergo preoperative coronary angiography (39). While the debate continues, the current trend is to selectedly perform coronary angiography only in patients with acute aortic dissection (40).

Selecting an Imaging Modality

The diagnostic modalities differ in their ability to detect complications associated with dissection, and each has particular advantages and disadvantages (Table 27-4). Given the high early mortality rate of unoperated proximal aortic dissection, the selection of an imaging modality depends on accessibility and the time required to complete the study. MRI, although optimal in its accuracy, is usually unavailable on emergency basis and poses the risk of limited patient monitoring and accessibility during the lengthy procedure. TEE is readily available and can be completed quickly at the bedside or immediately preoperatively, making it ideal for evaluating unstable patients. In light of its accuracy, safety, speed, and convenience, TEE has become the procedure of choice in many institutions. Surgery could proceed based on echocardiographic findings alone (41). When TEE is not readily available, CT serves as an effective screening test. If dissection is detected, the patient may then be taken to the operating room, where TEE is performed. Although MRI is less practical than the other modalities in acute unstable dissections, it is well suited for stable or chronic dissections. MRI is also the test of choice for serial follow-up examinations of medically and surgically treated patients. Despite its relative disadvantages, aortography still plays an important role when clear definition of branch vessel anatomy is essential for management and when a definitive diagnosis is not made by one or more of the other, less invasive modalities. The presence or absence of a dissecting membrane in the ascending aorta must be ascertained with absolute certainty and should be differentiated from intramural hematoma. The demonstration of a dissection membrane is an absolute indication for operative replacement of the ascending aorta. In the absence of complicating factors, some authors recommend no further diagnostic evaluation, because the arch and coronary ostia can be examined during the operation. In patients with cardiovascular collapse and

TABLE 27-4. DIAGNOSTIC PERFORMANCE OF IMAGING MODALITIES IN THE EVALUATION OF SUSPECTED AORTIC DISSECTION

Diagnostic Performance	Angio	CT	MRI	TEE
Sensitivity	+ +	+ +	+ + +	+ + +
Specificity	+ + +	+ + +	+ + +	+ +/+ + +
Site of intimal tear	+ +	+	+ + +	+ +
Presence of thrombus	+ + +	+ +	+ + +	+
Presence of aortic insufficiency	+ + +	−	+	+ + +
Pericardial effusion	−	+ +	+ + +	+ + +
Branch vessel involvement	+ + +	+	+ +	+
Coronary artery involvement	+ +	−	−	+ +

Note: + + +, excellent; + +, good; +, fair; −, not detected; Angio, angiography; CT, computed tomography; MRI, magnetic resonance imaging; TEE, transesophageal echocardiography.
Source: Modified from Cigarro JE, Isselbacher EM, DeSanctis RW, et al. Diagnostic imaging in the evaluation of suspected aortic dissection: old standards and new directions. *N Engl J Med* 1993; 328:35, with permission. Copyright by the Massachusetts Medical Society.

a high likelihood of acute aortic dissection (i.e., severe chest pain without ECG changes and a new murmur of regurgitation or pulse deficit), immediate transfer to the operating room without confirmatory images is recommended (42). A TEE is performed immediately after induction of general anesthesia. If the diagnosis proves false or if the ascending aorta cannot be visualized, the patient may be transferred to the angiography facility for further evaluation (Fig. 27-7).

Initial Medical Management

At least 50% of untreated patients die within the first 48 hours, yielding a 1% per hour mortality risk for acute aortic dissection. All patients in whom there is a strong suspicion of acute aortic dissection should immediately be placed in an intensive care setting for hemodynamic monitoring and stabilization of blood pressure, cardiac rhythm, and urine output. The initial objectives are to control pain, reduce systemic blood pressure, and lower the rate of rise of aortic pressure (dP/dT) to the lowest level that is compatible with maintenance of adequate visceral, renal, and cerebral perfusion. In hypertensive patients, treatment consists of the use of an intravenous β-adrenergic blocking agent (most commonly propranolol) followed by the institution of an intravenous vasodilator (most commonly sodium nitroprusside) (Table 27-5). Alternatives to propranolol include intravenous esmolol, metoprolol, or atenolol. β-Blockade should

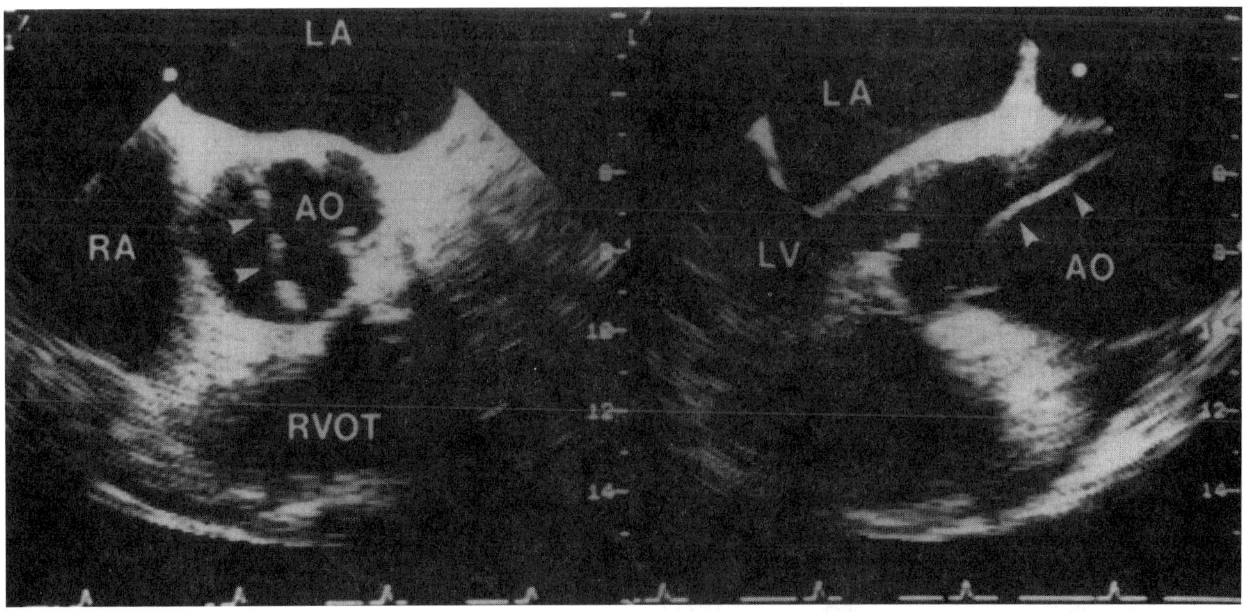

FIGURE 27-7. Transesophageal echocardiogram showing the dissection membrane *(arrows)* in the short **(left panel)** and long **(right panel)** view of a proximal dissection.

TABLE 27-5. PHARMACOLOGIC THERAPY FOR ACUTE AORTIC DISSECTION

Hypertensive patients
Sodium mitroprusside IV (2.5–5.0 μg/kg/min) with propranolol IV (1 mg every 4–6 hr)
Goal: systolic blood pressure in the range of 110 mm Hg (or the lowest level maintaining a urine output of 25–30 mL/hr) until oral medication is started.
Or IV esmilol, metoprolol, or atenolol (in place of propranolol)
Or IV labetolol (in place of sodium nitroprusside and a β-blocker)
Normotensive patients
Propranolol 1 mg IV every 4–6 hr or 20–40 mg orally every 6 hr (metoprolol, atenolol, or labetolol may be used in place of propranolol)

be instituted before afterload reduction, because the latter increases the velocity of left ventricular ejection and may propagate the dissection. Two large-bore intravenous catheters and an arterial line should be placed as early as possible in the intensive care unit. One suggested initial management algorithm for suspected acute aortic dissection is shown in Fig. 27-8.

Blood Pressure Reduction

The blood pressure should be reduced to the lowest level that is compatible with adequate vital organ perfusion. The target should be a systolic blood pressure of 100 to 120 mm Hg or a mean arterial pressure of 60 to 75 mm Hg if well

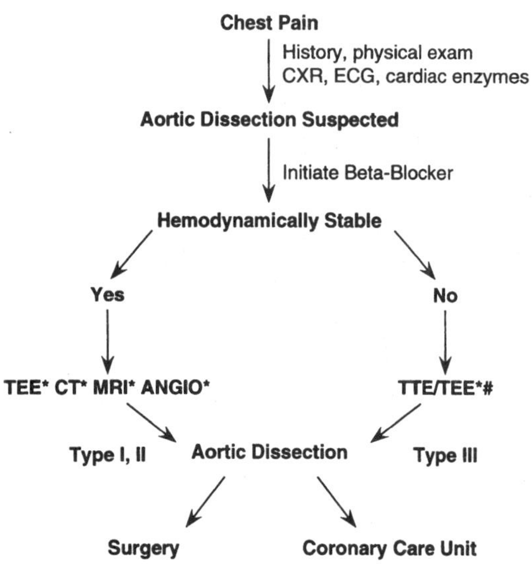

FIGURE 27-8. Initial management of suspected acute aortic dissection. *TEE, transesophageal echocardiography; CT, computed tomography; MRI, magnetic resonance and imaging; ANGIO, aortography; #, Aortogram or CT if TEE is not available, or rapid transfer to a tertiary facility.

as tolerated. To reduce dP/dT acutely, an intravenous β-blocker should be administered in incremental doses until there is a reduction of heart rate to 60 to 70 beats/minute. Propranolol 1 mg is given every 3 to 5 minutes until the desired effect is achieved (maximum dose, 0.15 mg/kg). Labetalol, which has both α- and β-adrenergic receptor blocking activity, may be especially useful because it effectively lowers both dP/dT and arterial pressure. The initial dose is 10 mg administered over 2 minutes, followed by 20 to 80 mg every 10 to 15 minutes (up to a maximum total dose of 300 mg) until heart rate and blood pressure are adequately controlled. Maintenance therapy may be achieved with a continuous intravenous infusion starting at 2 mg/minute and titrating up to 5 to 20 mg/minute (43). The ultrashort-acting β-blocker esmolol may be particularly useful in patients with labile blood pressure, especially if surgery is imminent, because it can be abruptly discontinued if necessary (44). When contraindications to the use of β-blockers (e.g., sinus bradycardia, second- or third-degree atrioventricular block, CHF, bronchospasm) exist, other agents to reduce arterial pressure and dP/dT should be considered. Calcium channel blockers have proved effective in managing hypertensive crises and are now used with increasing frequency in the treatment of aortic dissection. The combined vasodilator and negative inotropic effects of diltiazem and verapamil make these agents well suited for the treatment of aortic dissection. If the patient is still hypertensive after the institution of β-adrenergic or calcium channel blockade, vasodilator therapy is instituted, most commonly with sodium nitroprusside. Alternatively, the autonomic ganglion blocker trimethaphan or the vasodilating calcium channel antagonist nicardipine may be used. Refractory hypertension may result when the intimal flap compromises one or both renal arteries, thereby causing the release of large amounts of renin. In that situation, the most efficacious antihypertensive therapy may be the intravenous angiotensin-converting enzyme inhibitor enalapril.

Management of Cardiac Tamponade

Cardiac tamponade frequently complicates acute proximal aortic dissection and is one of the most common mechanisms of death in these patients. One retrospective series reported that pericardiocentesis in that setting may be followed by hemodynamic collapse and death (45). It may be that in such patients the rapid increase in CO and aortic pressure that follows pericardiocentesis may reopen the communication between the false lumen and the pericardial space, leading to recurrent hemorrhage and lethal cardiac tamponade. Therefore, when a patient with acute aortic dissection complicated by cardiac tamponade is relatively stable, the risk of pericardiocentesis probably outweighs the benefits, and every effort should be made to proceed as urgently as possible to the operating room for direct surgical repair of the aorta and intraoperative drainage of the hemopericardium. On the other hand, when the patient presents with electromechanical dissociation or cardiogenic shock, pericardiocentesis may be warranted. A prudent strategy in such a case may be to aspirate just enough pericardial fluid to raise the blood pressure to the lowest acceptable level (45). The presence of significant hypotension with suspected aortic dissection should also be treated by rapid volume expansion, given the possible presence of hypovolemia or cardiac tamponade. Before initiation of aggressive treatment for hypotension, pseudohypotension, which occurs when the arterial pressure is being measured in an extremity whose circulation is selectively compromised by the dissection, should be carefully excluded (40).

Definitive Therapy

The treatment of acute dissections of the aorta has evolved with the improvement in diagnostic tools, operative techniques, and pharmacologic means. It is now universally agreed that surgical therapy is superior to medical therapy for acute proximal dissection unless contraindicated by age or severe debilitating disease (46). Medical management of acute type A dissection still carries a very high mortality rate of 57% within the first 2 weeks of the event (46), whereas the rate after surgical treatment of acute type A dissection has decreased to less than 10% (47). Patients presenting with acute distal (type B) aortic dissection, on the other hand, are at lower risk of early death from complications of the dissection, compared with those patients with proximal dissection (48). The mortality rate for medically treated acute type B dissections has decreased to about 10% (49). Because studies indicate that the outcome is similar with medical surgical therapy in patients with uncomplicated distal dissection, most groups favor the medical management of such patients (50). Surgery is indicated for acute distal dissection in the presence of one or more of the following complications: progression with vital organ compromise, rupture or impending rupture, aneurysm formation, limb ischemia, continued pain, and poor response to medical therapy. Surgical therapy is recommended for all patients with Marfan syndrome with either proximal or distal dissection. Patients with chronic aortic dissection have, through self-selection, survived the early period of highest mortality and have a subsequent hospital survival rate of 90% whether treated medically or surgically. Accordingly, medical therapy is recommended for the management of all stable patients with chronic proximal dissection unless complicated by rupture, aneurysm formation, aortic regurgitation, arterial occlusion, extension, or recurrence of dissection (51) (Table 27-6).

TABLE 27-6. INDICATIONS FOR DEFINITIVE SURGICAL AND MEDICAL THERAPY IN AORTIC DISSECTION

Surgical
Treatment of choice for acute proximal dissection
Treatment for acute distal dissection complicated by the following:
Progression with vital organ compromise
Rupture or impending rupture (e.g., saccular aneurysm formation)
Aortic regurgitation (rare)
Retrograde extension into the ascending aorta
Dissection in the Marfan syndrome
Medical
Treatment of choice for uncomplicated distal dissection
Treatment for stable, isolated arch dissection
Treatment of choice for stable chronic dissection (uncomplicated dissection in patients presenting 2 weeks or longer after onset)

Anti-Impulse Therapy

The principles of medical therapy for acute aortic dissection are based on the observations linking progression of experimental dissections to mean arterial pressure and the rate of rise of the arterial pulse (dP/dT). Anti-impulse therapy aimed at reducing mean arterial pressure and myocardial contractility should be initiated immediately via a central venous line in patients with acute dissection. β-Adrenergic blockade is achieved with propranolol (2 to 10 mg IV) as tolerated. Labetalol combines selective α_1-adrenergic blockade with nonselective β-blockade and reduces the peripheral resistance without significantly changing the CO. It may be useful in patients who do not tolerate or respond to propranolol. Esmolol, a cardioselective β-blocking agent, is useful in the initial management of acute dissection. Its ultrashort half-life permits rapid achievement of stable blood levels, and its effects are easily titratable (25 to 300 μ/kg/minute). Further blood pressure reduction to a level compatible with adequate vital organ and peripheral perfusion is accomplished by the use of vasodilating agents, primarily sodium nitroprusside (0.5 to 5.0 μg/minute). Because nitroprusside increases the dP/dT if used alone, it should be started only after adequate β-blockade. Unlike sodium nitroprusside, the ganglion blocker trimethaphan decreases the dP/dT and can be used without prior β-blockade. Trimethaphan (0.2 to 6.0 mg/minute) may be the drug of choice for patients who cannot tolerate β-blockers.

Surgical Management

Surgical Treatment for the Repair of Acute Type A Aortic Dissections

Acute aortic dissection that originates in or extends to the ascending aorta is an absolute indication for emergency operation to prevent rupture into the pericardium. The presence of stroke or acute paraplegia does not contraindicate operation, because patients may experience significant recovery after the operative repair. The goals of surgical therapy are to prevent proximal and distal extension, excise the intimal tear, and replace the portion of the aorta that is most prone to rupture. Every attempt should be made to include the site of the intimal tear, because aortic dilatation and rupture occur most commonly at that site. Clinical evidence suggests that resection of the primary tear reduces the incidence of long-term complications (52). In most cases, graft replacement of the aortic segment containing the intimal tear achieves these goals. Ideally, resection of the intimal tear and repair of the involved aortic segment redirect flow back to the true lumen and convert the false lumen to a contained hematoma that, in the absence of additional distal tears, allows for complete healing. The operation does not remove the entire false channel in most patients; however, areas of actual or impending rupture of the false channel should be resected. In the presence of acute aortic incompetence resuspension of the detached commissures is frequently sufficient, but in some patients aortic valve replacement is necessary. The selection of the surgical procedure varies with the pathology.

Whenever possible the native aortic valve should be resuspended and valve replacement avoided. In the absence of phenotypic markers for connective tissue disorders, patients with involvement of ascending aorta and a normal aortic root may undergo simple tube graft replacement of the ascending aorta, resuspension of the aortic valve, and an open anastomosis with reconstitution of the downstream aorta. Patients with connective tissue disorders (especially Marfan syndrome) and those who have dilatation of the aortic annulus or the sinotubular junction require composite graft replacement of the aortic valve and ascending aorta reimplantation of the coronary arteries (Bentall procedure). An aortic valve–sparing operation has been described for patients with connective tissue disorders (e.g., Marfan syndrome) and a relatively normal aortic valve; the native aortic valve can be preserved while the ascending aorta, including the aortic sinuses, is replaced with a prosthetic graft (53,54). When the proximal dissection extends into the aortic arch, graft replacement of ascending aorta is extended into the lesser curvature of the aortic arch (55,56).

Less commonly, the dissection originates in the arch and propagates proximally as far as the aortic root. When the tear originates in the aortic arch, the site must be resected in conjunction with replacement of the ascending aorta. Most intimal tears in the aortic arch occur near the innominate artery, permitting aortic construction with a single suture line. In some cases it is necessary to replace the entire arch with reimplantation of the arch vessels (57).

Inadequate hemostasis has been the most significant technical difficulty in surgery for acute aortic dissection. The friable dissected aortic wall, together with the hemostatic derangements resulting from cardiopulmonary bypass (CPB) and disseminated intravascular coagulopathy, predisposes to excessive bleeding. Graft to aorta suture lines may be secured with Teflon felt, fibrin glue, or gelatin resorcinol fibrin biologic glue (56,58). In the United States, 25% glutaraldehyde has been used to toughen the dissected tissues with good preliminary results. The development of pliable double-velour prosthetic grafts that are presealed by collagen impregnation has eliminated the problem of bleeding from graft interstices (59).

Type A dissections are approached by a median sternotomy and are repaired using right artial-to-femoral arterial bypass, with selection of the strongest pulsating femoral artery for cannulation. Most commonly, deep hypothermic circulatory arrest (DHCA) is used to avoid cross-clamping of the friable aortic tissue and to permit an open distal anastomosis. In the presence of aortic incompetence, left ventricular distention must be prevented by placement of a vent, usually through the right superior pulmonary vein. Preservation of the native aortic valve is possible in 70% to 80% of patients with acute type A dissection (60,61). The competence of the aortic valve can be restored with either simple resuspension of the commissures and Teflon remodeling of the aortic root or with valve-preserving aortic root replacement (53). Preservation of the aortic valve in most series does not affect the immediate mortality or long-term survival rate. Postoperative freedom from valve replacement at 10 years varies between 80% and 90%. The presence of a dilated root frequently leads to failure and is one of the leading causes of reoperation (61). For patients with dilated aortic root, aortic annular ectasia, or Marfan syndrome, most authors recommend composite replacement of the aortic valve and ascending aorta with reimplantation of the coronary arteries to the graft (Bentall procedure) (61,62) (Fig. 27-9). In the presence of coronary ostial involvement, the repair of the ascending aorta represents a difficult technical challenge. Most authors recommend composite replacement of the aortic root and valve with the Cabrol modification of the Bentall procedure (63,64). The dissected coronary ostia are isolated on buttons of aortic tissue, which are reinforced with a collar of Teflon felt washer to buttress the dissection. Coronary perfusion is reconstituted with a separate tube graft, which is anastomosed end-to-end with the coronary orifices and side-to-side with the composite aortic root graft (Fig. 27-10). The alternative technique of oversewing the coronary ostia and performing saphenous vein aortocoronary bypass grafting produced poor long-term results (65).

In summary, the operation for the repair of acute type A aortic dissection is performed using CPB through a median sternotomy via right atrial-to-femoral arterial cannulation with or without DHCA. The aortic arch is included in the repair if it is the site of the intimal tear or aneurysm formation. The surgical procedure may consist of (a) isolated replacement of the ascending aorta with an interposition graft, (b) prosthetic graft replacement of the ascending aorta and

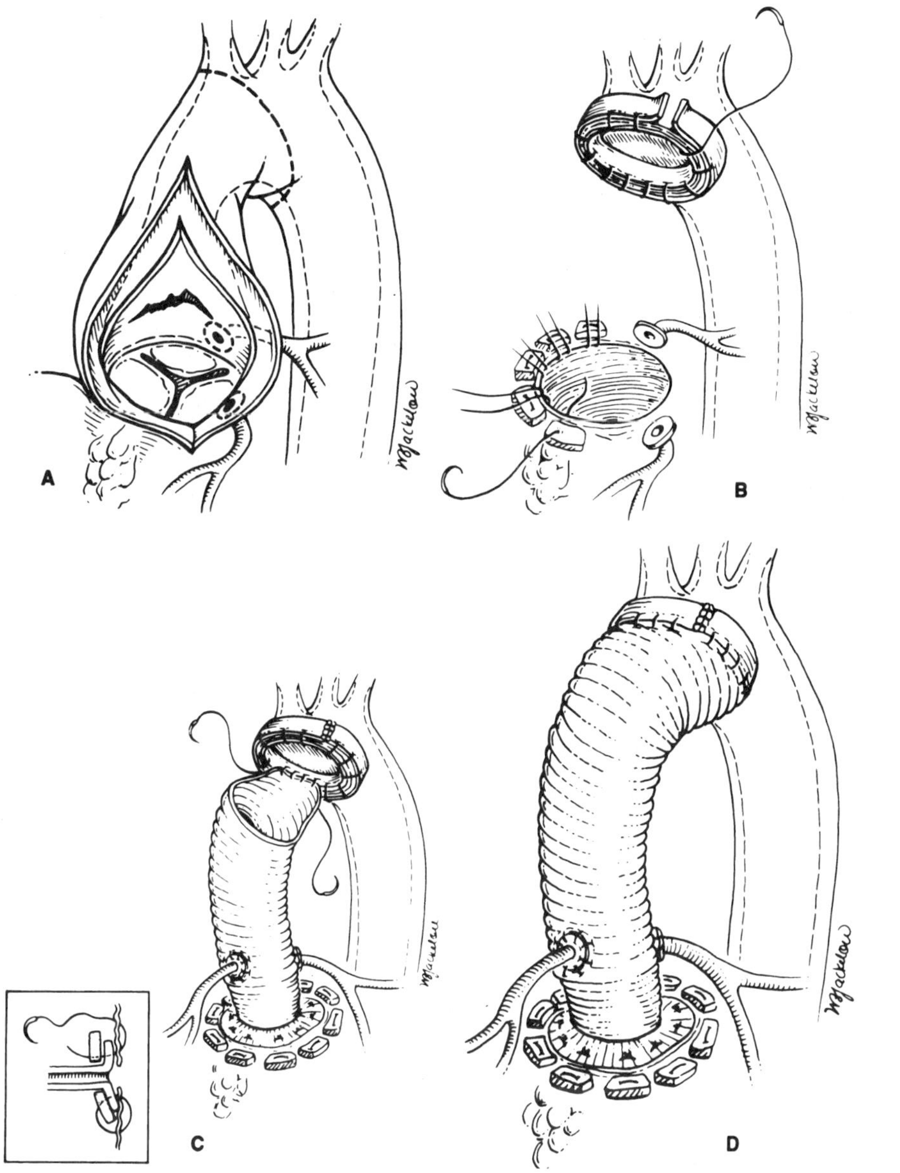

FIGURE 27-9. Modified Bentall procedure for composite replacement of the aortic valve and the ascending aorta and the proximal arch in type A dissection with a dilated root and aortic regurgitation or Marfan syndrome. The inset shows the details of the technique of coronary button anastomosis to the graft. A Teflon felt washer is incorporated into the anastomosis which yields a leakproof suture line at these critical anastomoses. Notice the reinforcing Teflon strip at the distal anastomosis, which has been tightened to further compress the false lumen and take the tension off the anastomosis.

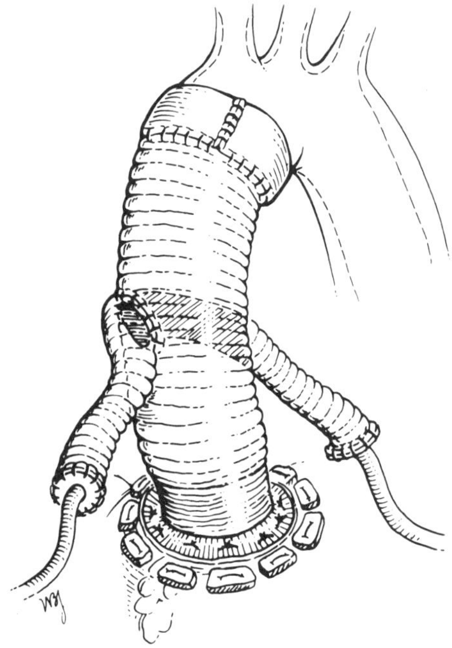

FIGURE 27-10. Cabrol modification of the Bentall procedure for composite replacement of the aortic root in acute type A dissection when the tear or dissection extends into the coronary orifices. Coronary buttons are dissected and reinforced with felt washers and anastomosed to a separate graft, which is connected to the composite graft. This technique allows tension-free anastomosis of the dissected coronary ostia and easy access for hemostasis.

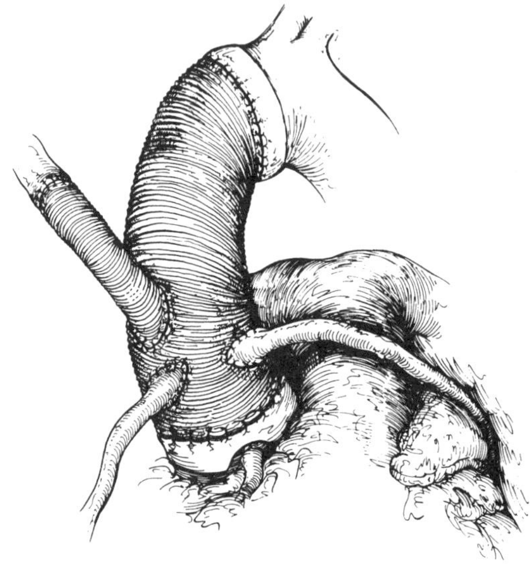

FIGURE 27-11. In certain circumstances ancillary concomitant procedures can be extensive, as illustrated here. This patient with a chronic type A dissection, severe coronary artery disease, and right cerebral hemispheric transient ischemic attacks required replacement of the entire ascending aorta as well as the proximal half of the transverse aortic arch. Aortic valve replacement was performed for irreparable valvular incompetence, and coronary artery bypass grafts were established to the left anterior descending and right coronary arteries. Occlusion of the innominate artery also required concomitant replacement of the proximal innominate artery with a separate Dacron tube graft. (From Miller DC. Surgical treatment of aortic dissections. In: Dudley H, Carter D, eds. *Rob and Smith's operative surgery.* St. Louis: CV Mosby, 1986:534, with permission.)

the aortic arch, (c) repair or replacement of the aortic valve and replacement of the ascending aorta with a tube interposition graft (although the long-term results of separate valve and graft replacement of the ascending aorta in patients with degenerative disease of the aortic wall are poor), or (d) replacement of the aortic valve and ascending aorta using a composite valve-graft conduit together with reanastomosis of the coronary ostia to the aortic graft (the Bentall or Cabrol procedure). In the presence of severe coexisting atherosclerotic CAD or unreconstructable coronary compromise resulting from the dissection process, concomitant CABG is performed with anastomosis of the vein graft to the ascending aortic Dacron graft (Fig. 27-11).

When the aortic arch is included in the procedure and when cross-clamping of the ascending aorta is not possible because of excessive friability of the aortic tissues, DHCA is required. In addition, many authors recommend performing the anastomosis between the distal end of the ascending aortic graft and the native aorta using an open anastomosis technique during a brief period of hypothermic circulatory arrest. Cardioplegia is achieved with the use of a cold hyperkalemic crystalloid or blood cardioplegic solution, which may be administered in one of several ways: (a) antegrade aortic root administration if the aorta can be cross-clamped and the aortic valve is competent, (b) direct coronary ostial administration after opening of the ascending aorta, or (c) retrograde administration through the coronary sinus.

Surgical Treatment of Chronic Type A Dissections

Indications for surgery in patients with chronic type A dissection include symptomatic or rapid expansion, dilatation of the distal false lumen, pain and compression symptoms, chronic aortic insufficiency, and dilatation of the aortic root beyond 5.5 cm. Chronic dissections usually require extensive aortic resection and reconstruction. Chronic type A dissection in most cases requires composite graft replacement of the aortic valve and root, but occasionally a valve-preserving replacement may be possible. Not infrequently the arch and part of the descending aorta must be replaced as well, because of significant aneurysmal dilatation. This is usually done in a staged fashion ("elephant trunk technique") (66) (Fig. 27-12).

Surgical Treatment for the Repair of Type B Dissections

Type B aortic dissection is approached by a left lateral thoracotomy with the hips swiveled to permit femoral cannula-

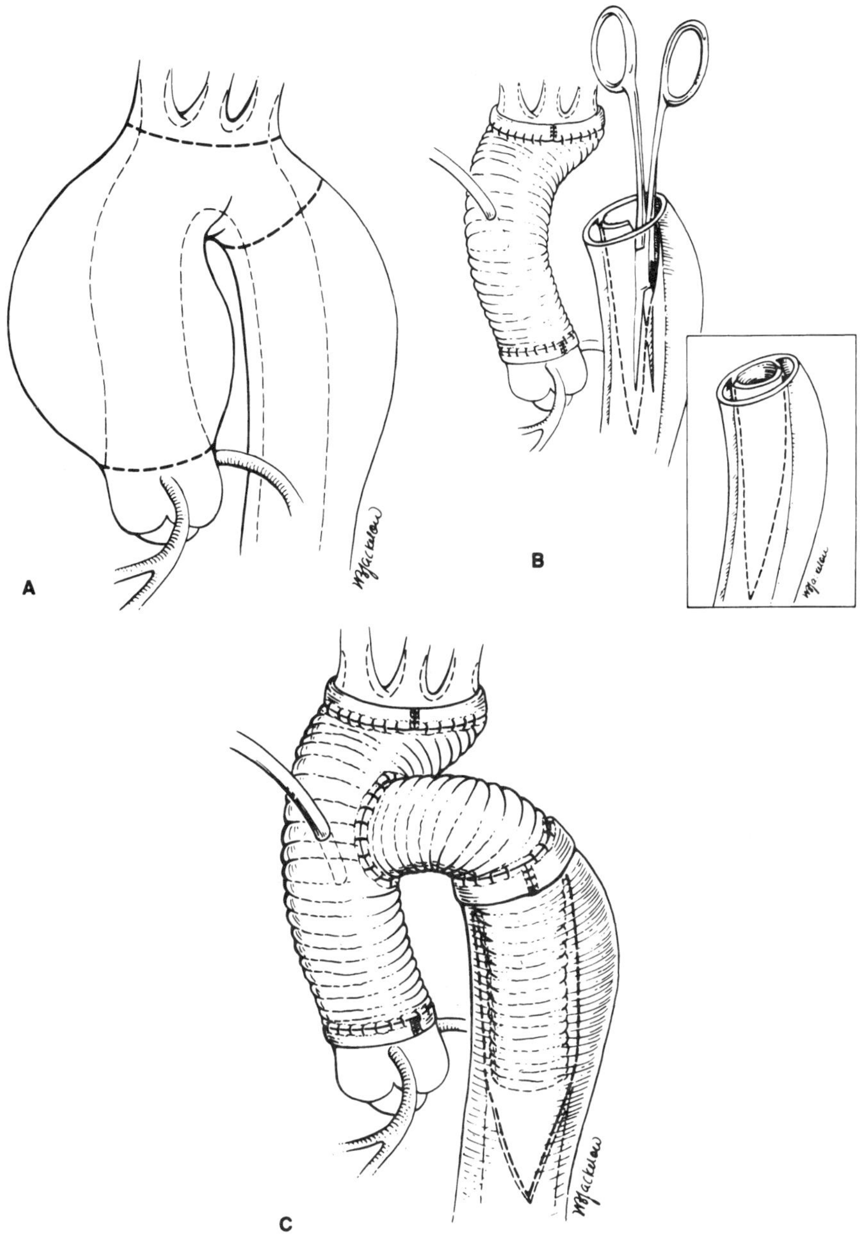

FIGURE 27-12. Chronic type A dissection with a competent aortic valve and dilatation of the ascending and descending aorta and the arch requiring replacement of these segments. Treatment with the modified "elephant trunk" method (66). **A:** Pathology showing the dilatation of the aorta; the dotted lines indicate the limits of the resection. **B:** Through median sternotomy, the ascending aorta and the arch are replaced, with preservation of the aortic valve. The arch anastomosis is made to the island of aortic tissue containing the origins of the brachiocephalic vessels during hypothermic circulatory arrest. At the completion of this anastomosis, an arterial cannula is inserted into the graft and hypothermic antegrade cerebral perfusion is started; the distal body is not perfused during the construction of the descending aortic anastomosis. This simple method of selective perfusion helps reduce the prolonged circulatory arrest time necessary for these complex repairs. In the descending aorta, the intimal flap is excised with long scissors, creating a generous communication between the false and true lumens. The inset shows the extent of the fenestration to ensure perfusion of both lumens. **C:** A separate graft is then anastomosed to the narrowest segment of the proximal descending aorta, allowing a length of the graft to hang down into the fenestrated area. The proximal end of this graft is connected to the ascending graft, and antegrade perfusion and warming of the entire body are carried out via the arterial cannula in the ascending aortic graft. In the second stage of the elephant trunk procedure, through a left thoracotomy the descending aorta is opened and the end of the graft in the descending aorta is controlled and sutured to normal-sized aorta distally.

tion. The segment containing the intimal tear and the dilated portion of the descending aorta is resected (Fig. 27-13). A graft is interposed, obliterating the proximal and distal false lumens and redirecting flow to the true lumen. As in type A dissection, suture lines are reinforced with Teflon strips (Fig. 27-14). Provision of distal body perfusion is advisable in most cases to reduce the risk of paraplegia, since repair of the dissected aorta may require prolonged periods of cross-clamping of the descending aorta (see Aneurysms of the Descending Thoracic and Thoracoabdominal Aorta). The length of the resected segment should be limited as much as possible to minimize the risk of paraplegia. The incidence of paraplegia is higher in patients with aortic dissection than in those with a nondissecting descending thoracic aortic aneurysms. DHCA may be required if the aortic arch must be replaced owing to retrograde extension of the dissection (67). In chronic type B dissection, it is necessary to replace the entire descending aorta in most patients and the thoracoabdominal aorta in some. Perfusion of vital organs may be dependent on the persistent false lumen, necessitating direction of flow into both true and false channels. Because of sufficient thickening and fibrosis of the aneurysmal aortic wall, tissue friability and suture line bleeding are less problematic than in chronic acute dissections. Anesthe-

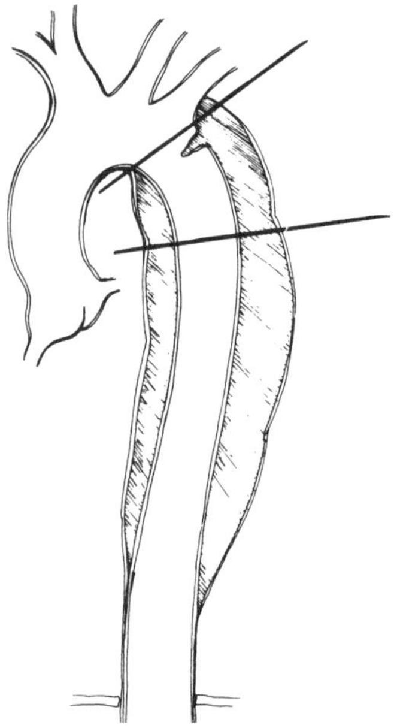

FIGURE 27-13. The surgical goal in a patient with an acute type B aortic dissection is to resect only a short segment of descending aorta containing the most severe degree of injury and replace it with a tubular Dacron graft. In the case of a patient with a chronic aortic dissection, the extent of graft replacement is tailored to the area of saccular aneurysm enlargement that has either produced symptoms or been documented to be expanding. Preservation of as many intercostal vessels as possible is advised, particularly in cases of acute type B dissection. (From Miller DC. Surgical treatment of aortic dissections. In: Dudley H, Carter D, eds. *Rob and Smith's operative surgery.* St. Louis: CV Mosby, 1986:535, with permission.)

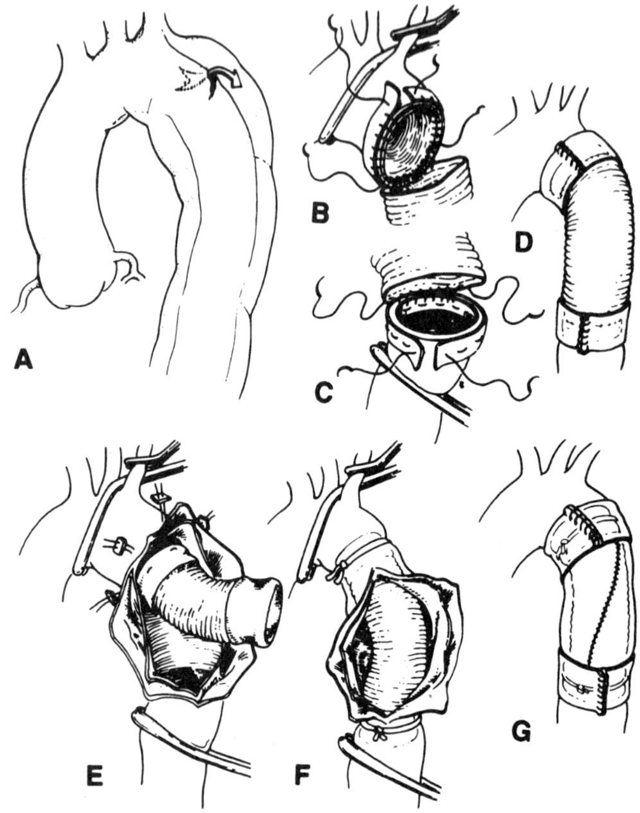

FIGURE 27-14. Surgical treatment of acute type B dissection. **A:** Pathology with the intimal tear in the initial segment of the descending aorta. **B** and **C:** Alternative techniques for preparing the proximal and distal cuffs, with single-strip felt reinforcement on the outside (shown for proximal anastomosis) or double-strip inside and outside felt reinforcement (shown for distal anastomosis) used as dictated by the local conditions. **D:** Both anastomoses are wrapped with wide strips of Teflon felt for further hemostasis with compression of the false lumen. **E** through **G:** Use of the intraluminal graft for both anastomoses is possible only if the intimal tear is located away from the left subclavian artery to allow room for safe fixation of the proximal ring. If the intraluminal graft is used, the aorta is closed around the graft and both ring ties are reinforced with a collar of Teflon felt.

sia management of descending thoracic aortic surgery is discussed in detail in the section entitled Aneurysms of the Descending Thoracic and Thoracoabdominal Aorta.

Management of Dissection-Related Acute Complications

Prevention and Treatment of Malperfusion Syndrome

Malperfusion syndrome is the second leading cause of death from acute dissection, after aortic rupture. Malperfusion may occur spontaneously (as in most patients presenting with cerebral symptoms and ischemic extremities), or it may develop during or after surgical treatment. Intraoperative malperfusion is detected in 13% of patients by TEE monitoring and can lead to catastrophic consequences (68). Monitoring of the right radial artery pressure during all phases of the operation ensures that there is adequate perfusion of the innominate artery (69). Monitoring of flow patterns in the true and false channels with TEE or epiaortic echo Doppler ultrasound may give the earliest warning of intraoperative malperfusion (68). At the completion of the surgical repair, perfusion is restarted antegrade through the true-lumen ascending aortic graft, and femoral retrograde perfusion is not used during the remainder of the surgical procedure (70). Detection of intraoperative malperfusion requires immediate action to correct the situation and prevent major neurologic injury. Treatment of persisting peripheral malperfusion is tailored to the particular patient. Lower-limb ischemia may be treated with a crossover graft. More serious instances of malperfusion (e.g., total occlusion of the aorta and visceral or renal ischemia) have been effectively treated with abdominal aortic fenestration (65). Surgical fenestration in the abdomen may be the procedure of choice in patients with type B dissection and malperfusion of the distal aortic branches who are otherwise not candidates for proximal repair of the dissection in the descending thoracic aorta (71). Radiologic transcatheter techniques that create controlled reentry tears in the abdominal aorta for reestablishment of flow to compromised branches provide alternatives to surgical fenestration (33,72).

Stroke and Paraplegia in Patients with Acute Dissection

About 5% to 6% of patients present with symptoms of stroke. The incidence of neurologic symptoms is as high as 42% when the tear is located in the aortic arch (73). Most strokes occur with type A dissection and are associated with carotid occlusion. With heparinization and CPB, an ischemic cerebral infarct could be converted to a hemorrhagic one, with catastrophic neurologic consequences (74). Nevertheless, the current consensus favors immediate repair of the ascending aorta, which results in total correction of cerebral malperfusion and improvement in neurologic outcome in many patients (65,74). Although stroke is a predictor of mortality and poor outcome, it is not a contraindication to surgery. Stroke-related mortality in one series of acute dissections was 14%, but neurologic recovery and satisfactory long-term outcomes were seen in 43% of cases (74). The incidence of paraplegia in acute dissection ranges from 2% to 6%, with most of the cases occurring in patients with acute type A dissection (12). In patients presenting with paraplegia, the possibility of neurologic recovery after surgery is slim. Nevertheless, urgent operation is still indicated to prevent other lethal complications.

Renal and Visceral Ischemia

The dissection involves the renal arteries in 60% of patients. Clinically important renal dysfunction occurs in only 5% to 8% of patients but carries a high risk of death (12). Prompt proximal repair of the dissection restores renal perfusion in most cases. Postoperative renal perfusion scans should be performed to determine the need for further treatment (e.g., aortic fenestration). In most patients renal function recovers, and the need for permanent dialysis is rare in survivors.

Evidence of compromised perfusion of other viscera is seen in 3% to 5% of patients and is associated with a high mortality rate. In the absence of frank intestinal necrosis, urgent treatment should be directed to the proximal aorta. A limited laparotomy may be indicated to determine the viability of the abdominal content in selected cases. Doppler examination of visceral and mesenteric blood flow can detect visceral malperfusion and determine the need for revascularization using catheter or surgical transcatheter fenestration or vascular bypass (32,75).

Marfan Syndrome

Aortic dissection occurs in 33% to 44% of patients with Marfan syndrome (76). Timely surgical treatment results in improved prognosis. The incidence of life-threatening events including acute dissections in Marfan patients rises with increasing diameter of the ascending aorta. Elective replacement of the ascending aorta before the occurrence of dissection results in less likelihood of aneurysmal dilatation of remaining aorta. Chronic β-blockade therapy for patients with Marfan syndrome may retard the dilatation of the aortic root (77). Close follow-up with aggressive surgical treatment of asymptomatic aortic dilatation is believed to reduce the incidence of acute dissection and late aortic complications (78). Surgery is indicated when the aortic root reaches 5 cm or twice the size of the normal aortic segment. The overwhelming majority of surgeons recommend that acute dissection in patients with Marfan syndrome is best treated with composite valve-graft replacement of the aortic root (Bentall procedure). The role of a valve-preserving aortic root replacement remains to be defined (63,79). The incidence of late reoperation was significantly higher (50%) in patients who did not receive a composite replacement at their initial operation (80). Bleeding and suture line complications are more common than in patients without an underlying connective tissue disorder. Meticulous attention to hemostasis and the strict control of blood pressure with vasodilators and anti-impulse therapy are extremely important in this patient population.

Aortic Dissection Complicating Cardiac Surgery

Ascending aortic dissection is a rare but catastrophic complication of cardiac surgery. It results from surgical injury to the aortic intima, usually in patients predisposed by cystic medial degeneration, long-standing hypertension, or advanced aortic atherosclerosis. The dissection frequently occurs at the site of the aortic cross-clamping or cannulation, at a proximal vein graft anastomosis, at an aortotomy suture line, or at the cardioplegia injection site. Intraoperative dissection is usually immediately recognized by the discoloration on the surface of the ascending aorta. In instances where compressed spectral array electroencephalographic (EEG) monitoring is used during CPB, flattening of the EEG waveforms of one or both cerebral hemispheres may be the first clue that acute aortic dissection involving the corresponding carotid artery has occurred. Sudden loss of the arterial line waveform is also highly suggestive. Murphy et al. stressed that the systolic blood pressure should be maintained at less than 110 mm Hg before cannulation and decannulation of the aorta. In addition, the aortic pressure should be lowered before the application and release of the aortic cross-clamp to decrease the possibility of intraoperative dissection (81). Acute intraoperative dissection results in a markedly increased operative mortality rate of up to 33%. The major causes of death are myocardial dysfunction due to ischemia or infarction and aortic rupture.

Acute dissection may also occur in the postoperative period and has a higher mortality rate (70% to 80%), which is attributed mostly to the delay in diagnosis and treatment (82). Postoperative dissection is frequently initiated during a period of hyperdynamic stress—for example, during emergence from anesthesia and extubation of the trachea. Manifestations include excessive mediastinal drainage, hemopericardium, hemothorax, severe chest pain, cardiac tamponade, and myocardial ischemia. Prompt diagnosis is the most important factor in successful management of both intraoperative and postoperative dissections. Echocardiography plays a major role in the diagnosis of intraoperative and postoperative aortic dissections.

In patients with persistent mediastinal hemorrhage, cardiac tamponade, new-onset aortic regurgitation, or loss of a carotid or upper-extremity pulse, prompt mediastinal exploration is the most expeditious way to establish the diagnosis and provide early definitive therapy. Aggressive therapy should be instituted to reduce the aortic blood pressure, heart rate, and dP/dT, followed by prompt surgical repair to prevent fatal propagation and aortic rupture. Surgical management techniques are similar to those for spontaneous ascending aortic dissection.

Anesthetic Management of Ascending Aortic Dissection

Preoperative Preparation and Monitoring

Anesthetic management of these patients usually starts in the intensive care unit during the diagnostic evaluation. Large-bore intravenous lines and an intraarterial line should be inserted as soon as the diagnosis of acute dissection is suspected. Monitoring of intraarterial pressure should be performed in the left upper extremity, because the innominate artery may be occluded by the aortic cross-clamp or included in the surgical repair, or both. However, some recommend also placing a right radial arterial catheter to detect the presence of a malperfusion state after the initiation of CPB. A femoral artery is acceptable for monitoring, however, one side is likely to be used for CPB arterial inflow. Central venous and pulmonary artery (PA) catheters are inserted to monitor filling pressures and CO and to administer vasoactive drugs. Diagnostic TEE is best performed after the induction of general anesthesia and intubation of the trachea. Sedatives and β-blockers can then be used more liberally to ablate the airway and hemodynamic responses associated with the TEE examination. Blood, fresh-frozen plasma, and platelets should be ordered for intraoperative use. The extent of preoperative preparation and the evaluation may be limited by the degree of hemodynamic instability. On arrival in the operating room, additional large-bore intravenous catheters are inserted. Rapid-infusion devices with efficient fluid warming capabilities are required. Intraoperative TEE should be used to monitor cardiac function and to evaluate aortic pathology and the success of surgical repair. Urine output is monitored with an indwelling catheter.

Intraoperative Anesthetic Management

The general principles of anesthetic management are similar to those for other cardiac procedures. Special emphasis is given to control of blood pressure and the rate of rise of aortic pressure (dP/dT), using β-blockers and vasodilators, which are maintained into the postoperative period. The anesthetic implications of the presence of aortic valve incompetence should be appreciated. Anesthesia concerns for patients with aortic insufficiency include the presence of impaired left ventricular function and the necessity for afterload reduction and avoidance of bradycardia. Inadequate myocardial protection may occur because of the presence of hypertrophied left ventricle and may contribute to the postbypass ventricular dysfunction. Intramyocardial catecholamines are depleted in patients with chronic aortic regurgitation (83). Inotropic support may be needed to successfully wean the patient from CPB. Because regurgitation occurs during diastole, a slower heart rate provides more opportunity for backward flow. Faster heart rates are therefore preferred to decrease the regurgitation time (84). Bradycardia and afterload increase the regurgitant fraction in the presence of significant aortic insufficiency. Intramyocardial catecholamines are also depleted in patients with chronic aortic incompetence, which may predispose to postbypass left ventricular dysfunction. Because of advances in surgical and anesthetic management, the operative mortality rate for ascending aortic surgery has decreased to 5% to 10% (85). Predictors of poor outcome include emergency surgery, advanced patient age, preoperative functional status, and cross-clamping time and duration of circulatory arrest.

Partial CPB under local anesthesia should be considered in hemodynamically unstable patients and in those who have had a previous sternotomy (86). Intraoperative TEE is routinely used to confirm the preoperative diagnosis of aortic dissection, locate the sites of intimal tears, identify the true and false lumens, and determine the extent of the dissection. In addition, TEE can assess the adequacy of retrograde CPB perfusion, detect the presence of malperfusion, and evaluate the presence and degree of aortic regurgitation. The detection of left ventricular distention by TEE is an indication for placement of a left ventricular vent. Also, TEE provides important information on the patency of the coronary ostia, the presence of RWMAs, global ventricular function, and the adequacy of aortic valve reconstruction. Comparison of right and left upper-extremity and femoral arterial pressures may allow early identification of a malperfusion syndrome. Monitoring of the cerebral circulation with transcranial Doppler ultrasound or a compressed spectral EEG may provide early detection of cerebral ischemia and malperfusion. During CPB, malperfusion may result from retrograde flow into the false lumen without a proximal entry site; this may cause the blind pocket phenomenon and occlude the true lumen. Anesthesia is often induced with etomidate, midazolam, fentanyl, and a nondepolarizing muscle relaxant and maintained with inhalation agents and intravenous narcotics.

Surgery for acute dissection is usually complicated by more blood loss than is seen in other cardiac surgical procedures. Difficulties with hemostasis result from friability of the aortic tissues, suture line bleeding, long CPB and DHCA durations, and activation of the coagulation antifibrinolytic cascades by the dissection process, resulting in disseminated intravascular coagulopathy. Intraoperative red blood cell (RBC) salvage techniques should be employed. Antifibrinolytic drugs (aprotinin, ϵ-aminocaproic acid [EACA], and tranexamic acid) were shown to significantly reduce bleeding. Because of concerns about thrombosis and renal dysfunction, aprotinin is better deferred until after circulatory arrest. Platelets, fresh-frozen plasma, and cryoprecipitate should be available. Advances in surgical technique, including the widespread use of Teflon felt and both fibrin and gelatin resorcinol fibrin biologic glue, collagen, or gelatin-impregnated graft have significantly decreased the incidence of excessive hemorrhage and operative mortality (87). Major causes of morbidity and mortality include hemorrhage, renal failure, myocardial infarction, left ventricular failure, and stroke. Ventricular dysrhythmias are reported to occur in 20% to 30% of patients. Excessive antihypertensive and anti-impulse therapy are continued after separation from CPB and in the intensive care unit.

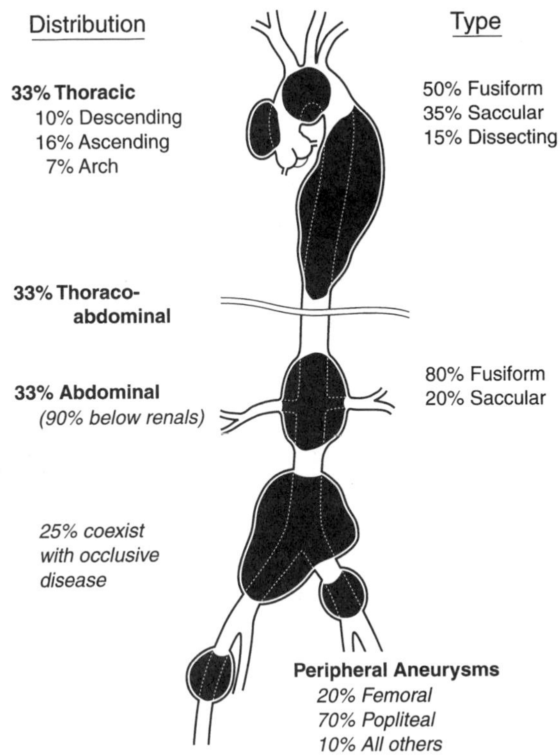

FIGURE 27-15. The distribution, frequency, and morphology of type A aortic aneurysms. Any aortic segment could be affected. (Modified from 1st edition.)

THORACIC AORTIC ANEURYSMS

Thoracic aortic aneurysms are less common than those of the abdominal aorta. They may involve the ascending aorta, the aortic arch, or the descending thoracic aorta. Descending thoracic aneurysms may extend distally to involve the abdominal aorta, creating what is known as a thoracoabdominal aneurysm. Sometimes the entire aorta is ectatic, with localized aneurysms seen at multiple sites in both the thoracic and abdominal regions. The cause, natural history, and treatment of thoracic aneurysms differ according to the segment involved.

Aneurysms of the Ascending Aorta

The ascending aorta includes the aortic annulus, aortic sinuses of Valsalva, ascending aorta, and ascending limb of the aortic arch; it terminates at the origin of the innominate artery.

Location and Distribution of Thoracic Aortic Aneurysms

Classification of aortic aneurysms is based on location, cause, and morphologic characteristics. Aneurysms of the ascending thoracic aorta occur between the annulus of the aortic valve and the origin of the innominate artery. Descending thoracic aneurysms begin distal to the origin of the left subclavian artery. Aneurysms of the aortic arch occur between the innominate artery and the left subclavian artery. Thoracoabdominal aortic aneurysms originate in the descending thoracic aorta but extend below the diaphragm to involve part or all of the abdominal aorta. Frequencies and distributions of aortic aneurysms are shown in Fig. 27-15. Morphologically, aneurysms are subdivided into (a) spindle-shaped fusiform aneurysms that circumstantially involve a segment of the aorta (typical of aneurysms resulting from aortic cystic medial degeneration and annuloaortic ectasia); (b) pouch-like saccular aneurysms that have localized involvement of part of the aortic circumference; and (c) dissecting aneurysms that have an intramural separation within the aortic medial layer. An autopsy study reported a prevalence of aortic aneurysms of more than 3.4%. Infrarenal abdominal aortic aneurysms are the most commonly encountered aneurysms. The thoracic aorta is involved in 30% to 40% of cases. Within the thoracic area, the anatomic distribution is as follows: 45% involve the ascending aorta, 35% involve the descending thoracic aorta, 10% involve the aortic arch, and 10% involve both the thoracic and abdominal aorta.

Etiology and Pathogenesis

Thoracic aortic aneurysms are estimated to develop at a rate of 6 new aneurysms per 1,000 person-years. The median age at presentation is 65 years for men and 77 years for women. The male-to-female ratio ranges from 1.1 : 1 to 1.7 : 1. Hypertension, congenitally bicuspid and unicuspid aortic valves, and the Marfan syndrome are important risk factors for the development of ascending aortic aneurysm. Generalized atherosclerosis and cigarette smoking also increase the risk of thoracic aortic aneurysms.

Cystic Medial Degeneration and Annuloaortic Ectasia

The most common cause of ascending aortic aneurysms is cystic degeneration in the medial layer of the aorta. These aneurysms are often associated with marked dilatation of the sinuses of Valsalva and the aortic annulus, a combination that has been termed annuloaortic ectasia. Aortic regurgitation develops because of loss of coaptation of the aortic valve leaflets, which are usually structurally normal. Annuloaortic ectasia is frequently present in patients who manifest the clinical stigmata of Marfan syndrome or other connective tissue disorders such as Ehlers-Danlos syndrome, but it may also be an idiopathic isolated condition. Intimal tears are frequently seen in the ascending aorta, and frank dissection may occur. Histologically, cystic medial degeneration is characterized by fragmentation and degeneration of the elastic fibers and smooth muscles in the medial layer of the aorta. The accumulation of basophilic amorphous material in the media imparts a cystic appearance; hence, the nomenclature. It results from abnormal synthesis of fibrillin, a glycoprotein that is a component of aortic elastic fibers (88).

Marfan Syndrome

Marfan syndrome is a common genetically determined disorder that results from a defect in chromosome 15, which affects fibrillin synthesis (89). Fibrillin and elastin represent the major components of the elastic fiber system. Histologically, the aorta demonstrates cystic medial degeneration, disruption of elastic fibers, and fibrosis of the media. Some 75% to 85% of patients with Marfan syndrome have aortic annular dilation that frequently results in aortic regurgitation, and one-third have significant mitral regurgitation (4). In addition to cardiovascular disease, Marfan syndrome is associated with ocular, pulmonary, musculoskeletal, and central nervous system (CNS) abnormalities.

Atherosclerosis

Atherosclerosis is the second most common cause of aneurysmal degeneration of the ascending aorta. These aneurysms are typically irregular, fusiform, or saccular, in contrast to the more uniformly fusiformed dilatation associated with cystic medial degeneration (90).

Chronic Dissecting Aneurysms

Patients who survive acute dissections usually develop chronic dilation of the ascending aorta. These aneurysms have a more rapid rate of expansion and a higher rate of rupture than other types of ascending aortic aneurysms (91).

Aneurysms Associated with Aortic Valve Disease

Aneurysms of the ascending aorta are commonly associated with the congenitally bicuspid aortic valve and may occur in the absence of significant valvular stenosis (92). The association of bicuspid valve with other congenital aortic abnormalities such as coarctation and acute dissection supports the presence of primary structural abnormality of the aortic wall (92,93).

Inflammatory and Infectious Aneurysms

The ascending aorta may be involved in systemic vasculitis such as giant cell or granulomatous arthritis, often in association with rheumatic diseases (94). Aneurysm formation is presumed to develop from medial destruction by the inflammatory process. Mycotic aneurysms, which are caused by primary bacterial infections of the ascending aorta, are rare. They are believed to develop most commonly after an episode of valvular endocarditis or from infection of an aortic jet lesion (95). An intraluminal clot in an atherosclerotic aneurysm may become infected after transient bacteremia. Before the advent of modern antibiotics, syphilis was the most common cause of aneurysms of the ascending aorta. Syphilitic infection produces aortitis and an obliterative endarteritis, resulting in the destruction of vasa vasorum and degeneration of the medial elastic fibers. Inflammatory changes surrounding the coronary ostium may lead to clinically significant coronary arterial obstruction.

Ehlers-Danlos Syndrome

One form of this uncommon inherited connective tissue disorder (type 4) is associated with life-threatening cardiovascular disease. Spontaneous arterial rupture is the most common cause of death. Aneurysms more commonly affect the abdominal than the thoracic aorta. As with Marfan syndrome, friable vascular tissue may complicate surgical treatment (96,97).

Chronic Traumatic Aneurysms

Although the ascending aorta is the site of rupture in approximately 20% of patients with blunt traumatic aortic injuries, only a few survive the initial insult because of acute cardiac tamponade and other associated injuries (98).

Pseudoaneurysms

The term pseudoaneurysm describes an aneurysmal dilatation that is not surrounded by all layers of the aortic wall. The wall usually consists of adventitia, portions of the media, and surrounding anatomic structures. Pseudoaneurysms may develop after trauma, infection, or surgical procedures. Postoperative pseudoaneurysms arise from sites of aortic cannulation or from aortic suture lines.

Natural History

Whatever the underlying cause, the development of an aneurysm is related to weakening of the wall of the artery. Once dilatation begins, enlargement tends to be progressive, because the lateral pressure increases with widening of the lumen (Bernoulli theorem). Furthermore, wall tension at constant arterial pressure increases with the increasing diameter (law of Laplace) (99). Systemic hypertension also enhances aneurysm formation. Subtle defects in collagen and elastin, combined with an accelerated breakdown of these molecules by an increase in proteolytic enzyme activity, play a significant role in the development of aortic aneurysms (100). Marfan syndrome patients with cystic medial degeneration have a 5-year survival rate of approximately 30%. The most common causes of death are complications of aortic root dilatation, aortic dissection, rupture, and CHF due to aortic regurgitation. Rupture is the most common cause of death in patients with atherosclerotic aneurysms.

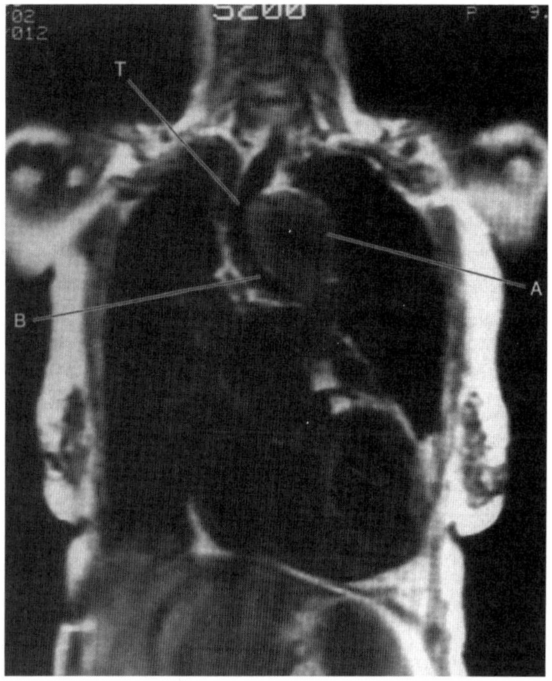

FIGURE 27-16. Magnetic resonance image in coronal projection of a large thoracic aortic aneurysm in an elderly woman who presented with a complaint of dyspnea and cough. In this view the markedly dilated aortic arch (*A*) compresses the trachea (*T*), causing rightward tracheal deviation. The aneurysm also compresses the left main stem bronchus (*B*). In addition, all four cardiac chambers are dilated, consistent with the patient's known idiopathic dilated cardiomyopathy.

Clinical Manifestations

At the time of presentation 40% of patients are asymptomatic, with the aneurysms typically discovered as incidental findings during routine physical examination or chest roentgenography (101). Symptoms arise from the cardiovascular consequences of the aneurysm or a local mass effect. CHF may develop as a result of aortic regurgitation. Myocardial ischemia or infarction may result from local compression of the coronary arteries by enlarged sinuses of Valsalva. A mural thrombus may develop in the aneurysm and produce embolic manifestations such as stroke, lower-extremity ischemia, renal infarction, or mesenteric ischemia (102). Occasionally patients present with disseminated intravascular clotting (103). SVC syndrome results from the obstruction of venous return caused by compression of SVC or innominate veins. Aneurysms of the arch or descending aorta may compress the trachea or left main stem bronchus, producing tracheal deviation, wheezing, cough, hemoptysis, recurrent pneumonia, and dyspnea. Symptoms may vary with patient position, usually being worse in the supine position (Fig. 27-16). Chest pain and back pain occur in 37% and 21% of nondissecting aneurysms, respectively, and result from the direct compression of other intrathoracic structures or from erosion into adjacent bone. Hoarseness of voice and dysphagia result from compression of the recurrent laryngeal nerve and esophagus, respectively. Stellate ganglion compression may result in Horner syndrome. Typically such pain is steady, deep, boring, and at times extremely severe. Pain from the ascending aortic aneurysm is usually precordial in location, whereas that from the aortic arch may radiate to the jaw or to the mandible. Aneurysms of the descending thoracic aorta commonly produce interscapular pain. The sudden onset of pain may reflect acute expansion and or impending rupture of the aneurysm. Other stigmata of atherosclerosis are frequently present in patients with thoracic aortic aneurysms. A significant percentage of patients (25% or more) have evidence of CAD, peripheral vascular disease, and cerebral vascular disease. About 10% have an associated abdominal aortic aneurysm.

As with abdominal aortic aneurysms, the most catastrophic consequence of thoracic aneurysms is leakage or rupture. Frank rupture is manifested by the sudden onset of severe pain associated with immediate death or severe hemodynamic collapse. Rupture occurs most commonly into the left intrapleural space or the intrapericardial space, manifesting as hypovolemia, hypotension, or cardiac tamponade. The distal arch and descending thoracic aorta may rupture into the adjacent esophagus, producing an aortoesophageal fistula that manifests as life-threatening hematemesis. Acute aneurysm expansion, which may herald rupture, usually produces similar pain. A contained rupture, resulting in a limited leak, manifests with pain and a variable degree of hemodynamic compromise.

Aneurysms of the Sinus of Valsalva

Although most aneurysms of the sinus of Valsalva are believed to be congenital, some occur secondary to medial degeneration, atherosclerosis, ankylosing spondylitis, Marfan syndrome, endocarditis, penetrating injury, or, rarely, syphilis (104). They are commonly associated with an intracardiac fistula and may rupture into an adjacent low-pressure cardiac chamber. Ventricular septal defects are present in 30% to 50% of patients with congenital sinus of Valsalva aneurysm (105). As many as 10% of patients have significant valvular or subvalvular pulmonary stenosis. Right coronary sinus aneurysms are the most common, accounting for 70% to 75% of cases. They frequently cause compression of the adjacent right ventricular outflow tract. The noncoronary sinus accounts for 20% to 25% of Valsalva sinus aneurysms. Those usually project into the right atrium, and rarely into the right ventricle. Conduction abnormalities, including complete heart block and right bundle branch block, may develop when the aneurysm ruptures into the right atrium adjacent to the tricuspid valve in close proximity to the atrioventricular node and conduction pathways. Aneurysms arising from the left coronary sinus are rare and can rupture into the left atrium or pericardium.

Presenting symptoms include sudden chest pain and CHF with tachycardia and dyspnea. Symptoms result from aortic regurgitation or rupture of the aneurysm into one of the cardiac chambers (Fig. 27-17). Physical examination reveals a hyperdynamic state accompanied by wide pulse pressure and a continuous murmur as a result of the intracardiac fistula and left-to-right shunt. Echocardiography can help determine the size and site of the aneurysm, and communication with a cardiac chamber can be identified by color flow Doppler ultrasonography. Cardiac catheterization, ventriculography, and aortography are useful in diagnosing this condition. Management is similar to that of other ascending aneurysms.

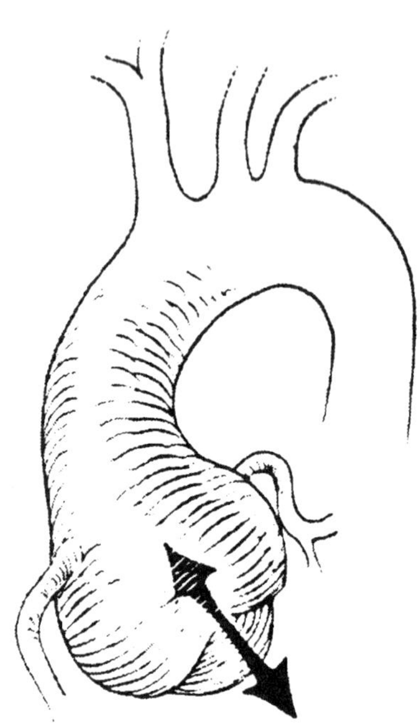

FIGURE 27-17. Drawing showing a sinus of Valsalva aneurysm producing aortic insufficiency in a 50-year-old man with Marfan syndrome. (From Crawford ES. Marfan's syndrome: broad spectral surgical treatment of cardiovascular manifestations. *Ann Surg* 1983;198:487, with permission.)

Annuloaortic Ectasia

The term annuloaortic ectasia was first used by Ellis et al. to describe a clinicopathologic condition seen in a subset of patients with thoracic aortic aneurysms in whom idiopathic dilatation of the proximal aorta and aortic annulus leads to pure aortic regurgitation (106). It typically manifests with the sudden onset of symptoms in the fourth decade, followed by progressively worsening aortic regurgitation. On physical examination, the diastolic murmur of aortic regurgitation is frequently detected to the right of the sternum. The acute or subacute development of symptoms and the presence of associated chest pain are more common in patients with annuloaortic ectasia than in those with primary aortic regurgitation.

Diagnostic Studies

Many asymptomatic aneurysms are discovered on routine chest radiography. Signs include a widened mediastinum, tracheal and esophageal displacement, and arterial wall calcifications. Ascending aneurysms may produce a convex contour of the right superior mediastinum, which may be difficult to distinguish from mediastinal tumor. Loss of retrosternal airspace is often present on lateral films (107). The ECG may be normal or may show evidence of left ventricular hypertrophy (increased QRS voltage) and strain (ST-segment depression and T-wave inversion). Evidence of coronary arterial disease or previous myocardial infarction may be present. Echocardiography is being used with increasing frequency in the diagnosis and management of ascending aortic aneurysms. A dilated aortic root or an ascending aneurysm may first be detected during echocardiographic evaluation of aortic regurgitation. TEE is a rapid and accurate imaging technique to differentiate ascending aortic aneurysms from aortic dissection and to detect the presence of intramural hematoma and intraluminal thrombus (108). However, up to 40% of the ascending aorta is not well visualized by TEE, and significant disease

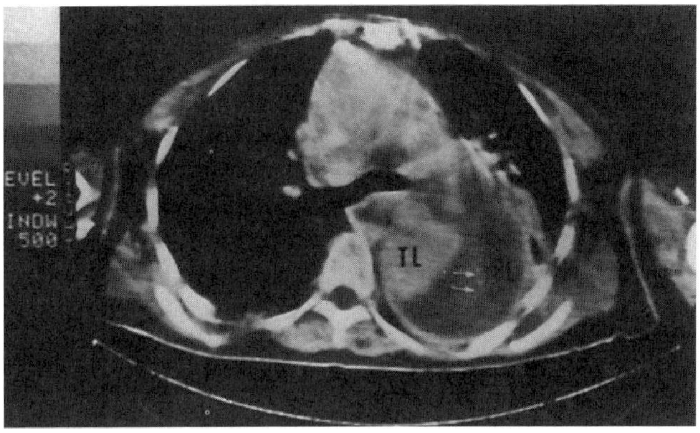

FIGURE 27-18. Computed tomogram with enhancement by intravenous injection of a water-soluble contrast medium in a patient with chronic aortic dissection. The true lumen at the midthoracic aorta level is deformed by the aneurysmally enlarged false lumen. The *arrows* indicate calcification within the aneurysm. (From Kirklin JW, Barratt-Boyes BG, eds. Acute aortic aneurysms. In: *Cardiac surgery,* 2nd ed. New York: Churchill Livingstone, 1993:1759, with permission.)

in the distal ascending aorta may not be accurately imaged (109). The combined use of TTE and TEE may overcome some of these limitations. CT scanning with intravenous contrast enhancement permits accurate evaluation of the extent and size of aortic aneurysms. CT scanning is complimentary to aortography, particularly when intraarterial thrombus or dissection is present (Fig. 27-18). Three-dimensional CT imaging may provide more information about the longitudinal extension and saccular outpouchings of the aneurysm. Magnetic resonance angiography may prove especially useful in defining the anatomy of aortic branch vessels and the direction and velocity of aortic flow, as well as limited imaging of coronary arteries. Functional nuclear magnetic imaging may also provide information about the coronary arteries and help in the evaluation of myocardial function (110).

Aortography is still the preferred modality for preoperative evaluation of thoracic aortic aneurysms. It provides precise definition of the anatomy of the aneurysm and the arch vessels. Aortography also documents the presence of aortic regurgitation, dilatation of the sinuses of Valsalva, and cephalad displacement of the coronary ostia. The characteristic angiographic pattern of annuloaortic ectasia is a dilated pear-shaped aorta; the aortogram reveals dilatation of the aortic sinus and ascending aorta that tapers to a more normal size at the level of the innominate artery. Pseudoaneurysms often appear as saccular expansions with an irregular contour (111). Coronary angiography is generally performed as part of the preoperative evaluation of patients with ascending aortic disease who are older 40 years of age or who have evidence of CAD. Ascending aortography and left ventriculography are usually performed in conjunction with coronary arteriography (112).

Preoperative Evaluation

Preoperative evaluation usually includes chest radiography, CT scanning or MRI, aortography, and coronary angiography. Echocardiography is useful to assess the presence and severity of aortic and other valvular disease and to evaluate left ventricular function. Mitral valve disease is frequently encountered in patients with aortic aneurysms and should be carefully evaluated preoperatively. Because of the high prevalence of carotid occlusive disease, carotid duplex imaging studies should be obtained in patients who are 65 years of age or older, those with an audible carotid bruit or history of stroke or transient ischemic events, and those with extensive peripheral vascular disease or CAD (113). Detection and treatment of significant carotid occlusive disease before ascending aortic surgery may reduce the incidence of perioperative stroke (114). Abdominal aortic aneurysms occur in 10% to 20% of patients with ascending aortic aneurysms. Therefore, the abdominal aorta is usually evaluated with ultrasonography, CT, or MRI (115). Severe chronic obstructive pulmonary disease is present is 20% to 30% of patients with thoracic aneurysms. Preoperative pulmonary function tests and arterial blood gas determinations should be obtained in patients with evidence of significant pulmonary disease. Cessation of smoking before surgery is desirable. Preoperative treatment with bronchodilators, chest physiotherapy, and corticosteroids may be indicated to treat bronchospasm and reversible airway obstruction. If infectious bronchitis is suspected, it should be treated preoperatively with antibiotics. Renal function should be evaluated preoperatively by appropriate testing (115).

Surgical Treatment of Ascending Aortic Aneurysms

Indications for Surgical Treatment

Symptomatic ascending aortic aneurysms require urgent operative intervention. Aortic leak, rupture, or dissection necessitates emergency surgical repair. Severe or symptomatic aortic regurgitation is often the primary indication for operation in patients with ascending aneurysms. Asymptomatic aneurysms greater than 6.0 cm in diameter and those that are expanding at a rate of more than 1 cm/year should be repaired electively, because the risk of rupture is higher for larger aneurysms (62,91,116). Patients with Marfan syndrome undergo aortic root replacement at an earlier stage, usually when the greatest diameter of the ascending aorta exceeds 5.0 to 5.5 cm (117,118) or when it has increased by more than 0.5 cm in the previous 6 months. An aorta that is twice the diameter of a normal segment is also an indication for surgery. Surgery should be considered even sooner in high-risk Marfan patients, such as those with a family history of aortic dissection and women planning pregnancy. In patients with symptomatic aortic stenosis or regurgitation, surgery may be required before the aorta dilates to 5 to 6 cm. Because the incidence of aortic dissection after aortic valve replacement is as high as 27% in patients with aortic diameters greater than 5 cm, those patients should have replacement of the ascending aorta at the time of valve replacement (119). Aneurysms of the sinus of Valsalva may develop or persist after replacement of the ascending aorta or aortic valve in patients with cystic medial degeneration and Marfan syndrome. Repair is indicated if intimal tears develop in the sinuses or if the diameter exceeds 6 cm (120). Pseudoaneurysms should be repaired as soon as they are discovered, because they have a tendency to progressively increase in size and may become adherent to the undersurface of the sternum and erode into adjacent cardiac chambers or the SVC. Emergency operations are frequently required and carry a high risk of operative mortality.

Choice of Operation

For patients with aneurysms confined to the ascending aorta who have a normal aortic annulus and sinuses with no evidence of Marfan syndrome, the ascending aorta is replaced with an interposition tube graft from the level of the supravalvular ridge to the origin of the innominate artery. Separate aortic valve replacement with a mechanical or biologic prosthesis can be performed when indicated. Patients with annuloaortic ectasia, including those with Marfan syndrome, most frequently undergo the Bentall operation, which consists of replacement of the ascending aorta and aortic valve with a composite graft containing a mechanical valve and a collagen- or gelatin-impregnated Dacron graft with reimplantation of the coronary arteries into the graft. Aortic root homographs can be used to replace the aortic valve, aortic sinuses, and ascending aorta. They are particularly valuable in the management of infective endocarditis and in patients for whom anticoagulation with warfarin derivatives is undesirable or contraindicated (121,122). Pulmonary root autografts are also used to replace the aortic valve and root (Ross operation). The more distal ascending aorta may be replaced with a Dacron graft if aneurysmal enlargement is present. Pulmonary autographs should not be used in patients with marked aortic root dilatation or in those with Marfan syndrome (123,124). In patients with aortic regurgitation and annuloaortic ectasia in whom the aortic leaflets are normal, annuloplasty is performed with resuspension of the aortic valve within the Dacron tube graft and reimplantation of the coronary arteries (125).

Management of Associated Conditions

Approximately 25% of patients undergoing ascending aortic aneurysm resection have significant CAD. Bypass grafting is performed at the time of aortic replacement, using the internal thoracic artery or saphenous vein grafts. Stenosis of major coronary arteries greater than 50% should be bypassed (115). Mitral valve disease is frequently encountered in patients with aortic aneurysms, particularly those with Marfan syndrome, in whom the incidence approaches 30%. Those with moderate to severe mitral regurgitation should undergo mitral valve repair or replacement at the time of aortic replacement (62,117). Gillinov et al. reported an 88% actuarial rate of freedom from significant mitral regurgitation at 5 years (126).

Surgical Technique

Most procedures are performed through a median sternotomy, which can be extended with a transverse T incision through the left third or fourth intercostal space to provide exposure of the distal aortic arch or the proximal descending aorta as required. Cannulation of the distal ascending aorta or the proximal arch for arterial inflow may be possible if these areas are disease free. Alternatively, the common femoral artery is exposed and cannulated. Venous drainage is achieved through right atrial or bicaval cannulation. A left ventricular venting catheter is inserted through the right superior pulmonary vein. A balloon-tipped coronary sinus catheter is placed for the administration of retrograde cardioplegia. Myocardial temperature is monitored by a thermistor probe placed in the anterior ventricular septum. CPB is established at an initial flow rate of 2.5 L/minute/m^2 with moderate systemic hypothermia (28°C) and hemodilution (hematocrit, 15% to 25%). If the aortic valve is competent, the initial dose of cardioplegia is given in an antegrade fashion through the aortic root and an additional dose is given retrograde into the coronary sinus (127). Additional retrograde cardioplegia is given every 20 to 30 minutes. When antegrade cardioplegia cannot be infused into the aortic root because of aortic valve incompetence, the arrest and cooling of the heart are achieved with retrograde cardioplegia alone. If adequate cooling of the myocardium to a temperature of 10° to 12°C cannot be achieved, the aorta is opened and additional cardioplegia solution is administered directly into the coronary ostia. After closure of the aortotomy but before removal of the cross-clamp, warm blood cardioplegia is infused through the coronary sinus while gentle suction is applied to a needle vent in the ascending aorta. In addition to myocardial protective effects, this maneuver facilitates removal of air from the aorta and coronary arteries (127).

The most commonly used prosthetic grafts are the woven, double-velour, collagen- or gelatin-impregnated Dacron grafts that are highly impervious to blood (59). The graft may be attached to a mechanical or a bioprosthetic valve.

Replacement of the Ascending Aorta

After establishing CPB, the aorta is clamped proximal to the origin of the innominate artery and the heart is vented and arrested by infusion of cardioplegia. An adequate cuff of nonaneurysmal aorta should be available proximal to the innominate artery and the aortic arch to facilitate a precise distal anastomosis with the aortic graft. If this is not possible, an open technique employing DHCA is used (see later discussion). Techniques for preserving the native aortic valve by its resuspension inside a Dacron tube graft or by aortic root remodeling using a scalloped Dacron tube graft have been described for patients with aortic regurgitation (125,129).

Composite Replacement of the Aortic Valve, Aortic Root, and Ascending Aorta

Bentall Operation. After establishing CPB, the aorta is clamped just proximal to the innominate artery, the heart is vented and arrested, the aorta is incised, and the aortic leaflets are removed. An appropriate-sized composite graft is sutured to the annulus. The coronary arteries are reimplanted into openings made in the Dacron graft. The distal anastomosis is then completed.

Cabrol Technique. Cabrol described the use of an 8- or 10-mm woven Dacron tube graft that is anastomosed end-to-end to buttons of aortic tissue surrounding the left and right coronary ostia. An opening is made in the midportion of this graft and is anastomosed side-to-side to a similar-sized opening in the aortic graft (128) (Fig. 27-19). Compression or kinking of this graft may result in myocardial ischemia or infarction.

Open Technique for Distal Anastomosis. If the clamp cannot be placed on the distal ascending aorta because of marked aneurysmal dilatation extending into the aortic arch or the presence of severe atherosclerosis or a thrombus, the distal anastomosis is performed by the open technique during a period of DHCA. CPB is established using bicaval and common femoral artery cannulation. The circulation is arrested when the nasopharyngeal temperature reaches 12° to 14°C, the esophageal temperature is 18° to 20°C, and, if monitored, an isoelectric EEG has been achieved for at least 5 minutes. The aorta is then opened. For aneurysms involving the proximal and inferior portions of the aortic arch, a single anastomosis is performed beneath the brachiocephalic vessels by beveling the graft and the aortic incision. If the disease involves the entire ascending aorta and arch, the aorta is transected beyond the origin of the left subclavian artery. The aortic graft is then anastomosed to the descending aorta. The brachiocephalic vessels are then reattached on an island of native aortic tissues to an opening in the Dacron graft. The use of special cerebral perfusion techniques during DHCA for operations on the aortic arch is discussed later. When the anastomosis is completed, slow antegrade perfusion of the body is begun through a cannula placed in the aortic graft. Reestablishing flow in the antegrade direction reduces the possibility of embolization into the brachiocephalic vessels of atherosclerotic debris or thrombus that may have fallen into the descending aorta. During the period of rewarming, other procedures such as coronary reimplantation, CABG, or mitral valve replacement or repair are performed (129).

The inclusion/wrap technique, in which the graft is sewn to the inside of the native aorta and aortic tissue is tightly wrapped around the graft, has been described to control bleeding. An open technique in which all aortic and coronary arterial anastomoses to prosthetic grafts are performed using full-thickness aortic tissue is preferred by many surgeons. The inclusion/wrap techniques have been associated with a substantial incidence of pseudoaneurysm formation at the coronary and aortic suture lines (80). Persistent communications between the aortic lumen and the perigraft space can produce large pseudoaneurysms with compression of the lumen of the aortic graft or the coronary ostia. The open technique is associated with a lower incidence of reoperation and of pseudoaneurysm formation (116). The availability of pliable aortic grafts that are impermeable to blood and the improvement in surgical and perfusion techniques

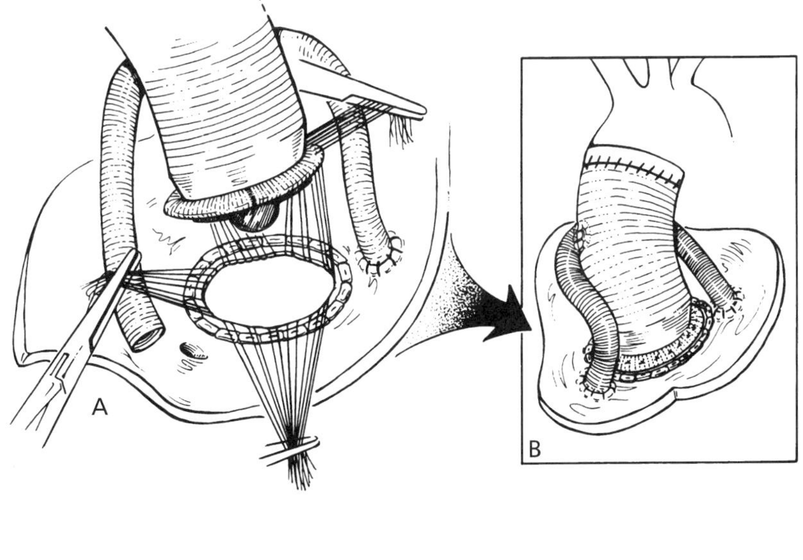

FIGURE 27-19. Cabrol technique of coronary reimplantation. **A:** An 8- or 10-mm woven Dacron tube graft is anastomosed end-to-end to the aortic tissue surrounding the left and right coronary ostia. **B:** An opening is made in the midportion of the graft, opposite a similar-sized opening in the aortic graft, and an anastomosis is performed.

have reduced the incidence of excessive hemorrhage and hence the need for the inclusion/wrap technique.

Anesthetic Management for Ascending Aortic Aneurysms

Preparation and Monitoring

Because the innominate artery is frequently obstructed by the aortic cross-clamp or may be involved in the surgical repair, arterial pressure is monitored by cannulation of the left radial, left brachial, left axillary, or left or right femoral artery. A central venous catheter and a PA catheter are inserted to measure cardiovascular hemodynamics and filling pressures and to administer drugs rapidly into the central circulation. The internal jugular vein is preferable, because the right subclavian vein can be distorted or compressed by an enlarging aneurysm and there is a possibility of accidentally puncturing the aneurysm when the subclavian approach is used. An oximetric PA catheter may be beneficial in patients with impaired ventricular function because it permits continuous measurement of mixed venous oxygen saturation. This provides an indication of the balance between oxygen delivery and oxygen consumption and may be particularly useful in the postoperative period, especially in patients with impaired myocardial function. In patients who are to undergo a Ross procedure, some anesthesiologists prefer not to place a PA catheter. Others place a pulmonary catheter initially and then withdraw it back into the SVC after the onset of CPB; the PA catheter is then readvanced distally after the repair has been completed. The usual noninvasive monitors should also be used along with the continuous monitoring of ECG leads II and V to detect dysrhythmias and myocardial ischemia. Continuous ST-segment analysis, if available, should be used. Core body temperature is monitored from the nasopharynx, esophagus, and urinary bladder. Intraoperative TEE is used to evaluate cardiac function and aortic valve pathology. The detection of extensive atherosclerotic changes or thrombus in the aneurysm by TEE may prevent the application of cross-clamping and dictate the use of DHCA. The presence of extensive atherosclerotic changes in the descending thoracic aorta (especially of mobile atheromas) may predispose to retrograde embolization into the cerebral circulation after the institution of CPB via femoral arterial inflow. In addition, TEE provides a wealth of information regarding the mechanism and severity of aortic regurgitation, and valvular function after replacement or repair. In patients with sinus of Valsalva aneurysm, TEE detects the presence of ventricular septal defect and aortocardiac fistula. In patients with a ruptured aneurysm, TEE provides information on the presence of cardiac tamponade and also detects the presence of myocardial ischemia resulting from embolization, kinking, or compression of the coronary arteries.

Because of the possibility of excessive blood loss, intraoperative cell salvage and rapid-transfusion devices with efficient fluid-warming capabilities should be available. Packed RBCs, fresh-frozen plasma, and platelets should be ordered; occasionally, cryoprecipitate is also required. As with all cardiac surgical procedures, the capabilities for rapid determination of arterial blood gases, electrolytes, hematocrit, and coagulation tests should be readily available. Point-of-care testing of PT and PTT is now readily available. The thromboelastogram and sonoclot may be helpful in evaluating whole-blood coagulation, platelet function, and fibrinolytic activity.

Anesthetic Management

In hemodynamically stable patients with nondissecting aneurysms, premedication with benzodiazepines provides amnesia and anxiolysis while opioids provide analgesia during placement of invasive monitors. The choice of anesthetic induction drugs depends on the degree of hemodynamic stability and myocardial function. Etomidate is frequently used because it maintains sympathetic tone and does not depress myocardial function. In patients who are hemodynamically unstable due to cardiac tamponade or aneurysm rupture, the careful titration of ketamine may be used. A rapid-sequence induction with succinylcholine and rapid intubation of the trachea should be used in patients presenting for emergency surgery; otherwise, muscle relaxation can be provided with a nondepolarizing neuromuscular blocker. Opioids are used to blunt the hemodynamic response to laryngoscopy and intubation, which is important to prevent expansion or rupture of the aneurysm. Esmolol, nitroglycerin, and lidocaine are used to blunt and modify the hemodynamic response to laryngoscopy and intubation. Anesthesia maintenance is usually with a combination of opioids, benzodiazepines, and volatile anesthetics. In good-risk patients who are candidates for early extubation, the total dose of narcotics should be limited, and propofol can be used in the postbypass and early postoperative periods. Many patients have acute or chronic left ventricular volume overload due to aortic regurgitation. Management goals include improvement of forward flow and CO, decrease in the regurgitant volume, and avoidance of excessive left ventricular distention and ischemia. Afterload reduction improves the forward flow and decreases the regurgitant fraction. However, the excessive reduction in the diastolic pressure may produce myocardial ischemia due to inadequate coronary blood flow. Bradycardia should be avoided because it prolongs the diastolic period and the time available for regurgitation. Myocardial catecholamines are depleted in patients with chronic aortic regurgitation, which may predispose them to post-CPB dysfunction.

Anesthetic Management of Special Problems with Ascending Aortic Surgery

Management of Ventilation and of the Airway

Ascending and transverse aortic arch lesions are repaired through a median sternotomy and do not require one-lung ventilation (OLV). Therefore, these patients are managed with a single-lumen endotracheal tube. A thoracic aortic lesion can compress and damage the trachea or major bronchi, leading to tracheomalacia, respiratory distress, and airway obstruction. Descending aortic aneurysms not infrequently produce compression of the left main stem bronchus (130,131). Less commonly, aneurysms of the ascending aorta and arch have been reported to cause compression of the trachea and right main stem bronchus (132,133). Symptoms of airway compression may be induced or exacerbated in the supine position. The presence of stridor, wheezing, cough, or tracheal deviation should raise suspicion of aortic impingement. Preoperative pulmonary function testing with flow-volume loops in the supine and erect position reveals an intrathoracic airway obstructive pattern. Radiographic studies, especially CT and MRI, are useful in delineating the location and degree of airway compromise. Rupture of an aneurysm by the forceful placement of an endotracheal tube has been reported (134). The use of fiberoptic bronchoscopy to detect the degree of airway compression and guide the placement of the endotracheal tube is recommended (132). In patients with severe airway compression, femorofemoral CPB is instituted with the use of local infiltrative anesthesia before the induction of general anesthesia. Anesthetic management of DHCA is discussed in the section entitled Aneurysms of the Aortic Arch.

Management of Excessive Bleeding

Several advances in surgical technique have substantially reduced the frequency and severity of perioperative bleeding. These include the use of collagen- or gelatin-impregnated Dacron grafts, incorporation of strips of Teflon felt into the suture lines, and the use of fibrin glue. Until recently, the average transfusion requirements were 4 to 6 units of packed RBCs, 10 to 14 units of fresh-frozen plasma, 20 units of platelets, and 10 units of cryoprecipitate (135). Blood conservation techniques include preoperative donation of autologous blood, intraoperative isovolumic hemodilution, the use of intraoperative cell salvage devices, the use of antifibrinolytic agents, and the collection and reinfusion of chest tube drainage postoperatively. With aggressive

thesiologists prefer to use other antifibrinolytic agents or to start aprotinin only after the period of circulatory arrest (see Deep Hypothermic Circulatory Arrest). In the presence of excessive bleeding, appropriate laboratory studies should be obtained to diagnose the cause of hemostatic dysfunction and to treat specific defects by the selective administration of fresh-frozen plasma, platelet concentrates, and cryoprecipitate as indicated.

Pulmonary Dysfunction

Noncardiogenic pulmonary edema and increased transpulmonary shunt may occur after replacement of the ascending aorta as a result of CPB-mediated lung injury (138). The alveolar-arterial oxygen gradient is increased, lung compliance is decreased, and an interstitial pattern is seen on chest radiography (139). A heparin-protamine reaction, low hematocrit, and the use of fresh-frozen plasma can exacerbate the injury. The administration of perioperative steroids has been advocated to reduce the inflammatory response, complement activation, and cytokine generation after CPB (140,141). Continuous ultrafiltration was shown to decrease pulmonary edema and to remove the vasoactive mediators from the circulation in pediatric cardiac patients (142,143). Treatment is primarily supportive, with close attention to fluid management, diuresis, and the appropriate use of ventilator settings to improve oxygenation and minimize barotrauma and volutrauma. Positive end-expiratory pressure (PEEP) and inverse-ratio ventilation are used to improve arterial oxygenation. In very severe cases, the use of extracorporeal membrane oxygenation may be required in the early postoperative period until lung function improves.

Postoperative Coronary Insufficiency

Myocardial ischemia may occur after aortic root replacement as a result of (a) technical problems with the coronary artery to aortic graft anastomosis (twisting, kinking, or stretching); (b) embolization of air and debris into the coronary circulation; or (c) compression of the coronary arteries

TABLE 27-7. CAUSES OF EARLY MORTALITY

Cause	Percentage of Cases
Cardiac failure	50–75
Multiple causes	15–31
Stroke	8–25
Pulmonary failure	8–25
Arrhythmia	8–35
Renal failure	10–18
Sepsis/multisystem organ failure	8–10
Bleeding	8–28

to 5%. Prolonged ventilation is required in 10% of patients, and 20% to 25% require inotropic support for longer than 6 hours postoperatively (62,144). Significant ventricular dysrhythmias occur in 25% to 33% of patients. In one series the incidences of heart block, new myocardial infarction, and renal failure were 7%, 3%, and 6%, respectively (146).

Perioperative Mortality

The hospital mortality rate ranged from 2% to 10% and averaged 3% to 5% in two reported series (144,145). The most frequent mode of early death is cardiac failure, followed by stroke and respiratory failure (Table 27-7). Aortic root replacement for endocarditis is associated with a significantly higher mortality rate (33% to 50%). Emergency operation is the strongest risk factor for early hospital mortality. After elective operations, the strongest predictors of early mortality are advanced age, prolonged duration of CPB, and impaired left ventricular function (144,145) (Table 27-8).

Aneurysms of the Aortic Arch

Etiology and Pathogenesis

Aneurysms of the aortic arch are often contiguous with aneurysms of the ascending or descending aorta. They may be caused by atherosclerotic disease, cystic medial degeneration, or acute or chronic dissection. The majority of arch aneurysms are extensions of ascending aortic atherosclerotic aneurysms into the proximal arch. Patients are frequently smokers with chronic obstructive pulmonary disease, chronic hypertension, and widespread arterial atherosclerotic disease. Aneurysms of the descending thoracic aorta may also extend to involve the distal aortic arch. Patients with Marfan syndrome and other congenital connective tissue abnormalities may also have aneurysms of the aortic arch. A small group of patients have mycotic, infectious, granulomatous, or inflammatory aneurysms (147).

TABLE 27-8. RISK FACTORS FOR EARLY MORTALITY

Factor	Probability
Emergency operation	.0000–<.0001
Duration of CPB	.002–.017
Age	.005–.034
Advanced NYHA class	.0001–.026
Previous aortic surgery	.001–.04
Arch involvement	.0026
Postoperative bleeding	.032
Previous or concurrent CABG	.001–.0014

Note: CABG, coronary artery bypass graft; CPB, cardiopulmonary bypass; NYHA, New York Health Association.

Clinical Manifestations

Many patients are asymptomatic, with the aneurysm discovered incidentally on chest radiography or CT scanning performed for unrelated problems. With progressive aneurysmal enlargement, there is compression or obstruction of adjacent mediastinal structures, including the SVC, innominate veins, PA, trachea, bronchi, lungs, and left recurrent laryngeal nerve. Symptoms may include dyspnea, stridor, hoarseness, hemoptysis, cough, and chest pain. Physical findings may include distended veins of the upper body, cardiovascular murmurs, hoarseness due to left vocal cord paralysis, abnormal pulsations of the anterior chest and suprasternal notch, pleural effusions, and CHF. Erosion and fistula formation may occur between the aneurysm and the great veins, PA, right atrium, or right ventricle, resulting in the typical hemodynamic changes of a large arteriovenous fistula including severe CHF. Rupture usually occurs into the pericardium, bronchial airway, or pleural cavity, resulting in death from cardiac tamponade, suffocation, or exsanguination.

Diagnosis

The aneurysm may first be discovered on routine chest radiography. An aortic arch aneurysm manifests as enlargement of the superior mediastinal silhouette or a left-sided shadow. Contrast-enhanced CT of the entire aorta and MRI are very useful methods for the evaluation and follow-up of aortic arch aneurysms (148). Newer technologies, such as ultrafast CT and three-dimensional CT scan reconstruction and contrast-enhanced MRI, are evolving methods for the preoperative evaluation and follow-up of thoracic aortic aneurysms (149,150). Echocardiography (TTE and TEE) is valuable in assessing the extent of transverse aortic arch aneurysms and provides additional valuable information regarding myocardial function and concomitant valvular abnormalities such as aortic insufficiency, the presence and extent of atheromatous changes, and mural thrombi in the aorta. Thoracic aortography allows visualization of the entire aorta and evaluation of the aortic valve and brachiocephalic vessels. Abnormalities of the branch vessels may be

arch and the proximal descending aorta are frequently approached through a left lateral thoracotomy and are facilitated by the use of OLV. Cannulation for CPB is through the femoral artery for arterial inflow. Venous drainage is achieved with the use of bicaval, right atrial, or femoral vein cannulation. When performed through the left lateral thoracotomy position, venous drainage could be obtained via cannulation of the PA. Hypothermia is induced by a combination of surface cooling (ice packs, cooling blankets) and core cooling through cold CPB perfusate at 10°C. Core temperature may be measured from the rectum, nasopharynx, esophagus, or tympanic membrane. Tympanic membrane measurements correlate best with actual brain temperature. Vasodilators (e.g., nitroprusside) are used to counteract cooling-induced vasoconstriction, which limits peripheral perfusion and further cooling and hence may result in the undesirable development of temperature gradients between different body regions. Rapid and incomplete cerebral cooling has been implicated in postoperative neurologic deficits after DHCA. Packing of the head in ice helps prevent brain rewarming during circulatory arrest.

The depth of cooling remains controversial, with most clinicians choosing to monitor EEG activity. Once the EEG is isoelectric (usually between 15° and 20°C nasopharyngeal temperature), the patient is cooled for another 10 minutes before DHCA is initiated to ensure adequate homogeneous cooling of the brain. Some surgeons advocate monitoring of jugular venous bulb oxygen saturation and termination of perfusion only after the saturation is greater than 95% (155). Surface cooling of the cranium is performed by packing the head with ice at the onset of cooling and throughout the DHCA period. Monitoring of brain stem activity with auditory evoked potentials has been suggested as a means for determining the optimal temperature for circulatory arrest (156). The period of safe arrest varies from patient to patient depending on multiple variables. It is generally accepted that 30 to 40 minutes of DHCA is well tolerated by most adult patients (155,157). Rewarming should not exceed 1°C core temperature rise per 3 minutes of bypass time. The temperature gradient between the circuit and the patient should not exceed 10°C. Vasodilators may be useful to improve peripheral perfusion. Termination of rewarming should occur when the nasopharyngeal temperature reaches 35°C. Myocardial protection is achieved with cold crystalloid or blood cardioplegia administered in an antegrade and/or retrograde manner.

Operative techniques have been modified to expedite arch repairs so that the period of circulatory arrest is kept to a minimum. The three great arch vessels can be anastomosed as a single unit to the prosthetic arch graft. This modification substantially decreases the number of anastomoses and the time required to complete the arch repair. Most surgeons favor the technique of open aortic repair, in which the distal anatamosis and arch vessel reimplantation are performed during circulatory arrest without aortic clamping (158). The aorta is then de-aired and CPB flow is gradually restarted. Great care must be taken to de-air the arch branches and to milk out all air, clot, and debris before the circulation to the brain is reestablished. The proximal end of the tube graft is then clamped, and the circulation is resumed to all parts of the body except the heart. Cannulation of the graft to provide antegrade flow may decrease the risk of embolization to the cerebral circulation. Systemic rewarming is started while the proximal arch anastomosis is being constructed. The heart is then restarted, myocardial function is assessed, and the patient is weaned from CPB in the usual manner.

Strategies for Cerebral Protection

Repair of aortic arch lesions requires interruption of the cerebral circulation. Hypothermia is the most essential ingredient of all cerebral protection strategies. Techniques used to preserve the integrity of the CNS include

1. Deep hypothermia and complete interruption of the cerebral circulation (DHCA)
2. DHCA along with retrograde cerebral perfusion (RCP)
3. Antegrade selective cerebral perfusion (SCP)

The use of pharmacologic adjuncts to protect the brain has been described, but their effectiveness remains controversial. Several of these techniques can be combined during the same procedure to allow for surgical repair of the aortic arch.

Hypothermia

Hypothermia exerts numerous effects on all body organs. Oxygen consumption decreases by approximately 7% for every 1°C decrease in temperature. Hypothermia decreases the energy needed to maintain cerebral cellular integrity (which amounts to 40% to 50% of the total cerebral metabolic rate for oxygen [$CMRO_2$]) as well as the energy needed to maintain electrical activity (50% to 60% of the total $CMRO_2$). The decrease in energy used is expressed as the Q10, which is the ratio of two $CMRO_2$ values measured at two temperatures that are 10°C apart. When electrical activity is present the Q10 between 28° and 18°C is about 1.5. But when cerebral electrical activity has been previously suppressed (e.g., by barbiturates) before induction of hypothermia, the Q10 is about 2.2 (159). Hypothermia reduces cerebral blood flow (CBF) and metabolism and offers protection in the face of ischemic and hypoxemic insults. The efficacy of hypothermia in protecting the brain during circulatory arrest cannot be entirely explained by metabolic suppression alone. In addition to metabolic suppression, hypothermia modifies the postischemic response to injury. Additional mechanisms of neuroprotection may include suppression of release of cytotoxic excitatory neurotransmitter and/or free oxygen radicals, reduction of postischemic edema, leukotriene production, and reduction of abnormal ion fluxes.

Brain regions appear to be affected differently by hypothermia, some (e.g., hippocampus) showing marked protection, whereas others (e.g., thalamic nuclei) are less protected (160). However, the use of DHCA may be associated with focal or global, transient or permanent CNS perturbations, raising concerns about its safety, especially when long durations of DHCA are required to treat complex lesions. In addition, there is evidence to suggest that deep hypothermia by itself can induce neuronal cell damage. Therefore there is renewed interest in the use of alternative techniques such as antegrade SCP, RCP, and low-flow hypothermic bypass (161). The use of DHCA results in metabolic deregulation and changes in membrane integrity and cellular function (162). In primates cooled to 20°C, CO and CBF are concomitantly reduced but the ratio of CBF/CO is increased (163). Furthermore, in contrast to other tissue beds, the oxygen extraction ratio in brain increases as CBF decreases under hypothermic conditions. It has been shown that even when nasopharyngeal temperatures are reduced to 15°C, severe cerebral hypoxia quickly develops once the circulation is arrested (164).

Deep hypothermia was shown to produce profound inhibition of cerebral metabolism in dogs. Michenfelder and Milde originally postulated that complete arrest of the cerebral circulation for as long as 30 minutes at 18°C would not result in permanent brain injury. However, careful studies using standardized tests of behavior and learning in young children revealed some loss of cognitive function after the use of DHCA in infancy, especially with prolonged intervals of circulatory arrest (165,166). Animal studies revealed that depression of $CMRO_2$ by hypothermia is less complete than initially predicted. In weaning puppies, the $CMRO_2$ was reduced only to 40% of control levels at 18°C. DHCA for 60 minutes at 18°C was followed by quantitative EEG changes and early behavioral dysfunction (167,168). Similarly, prolonged DHCA at 20°C in young piglets produced unequivocal behavioral sequelae, EEG changes, and histologic evidence of cerebral damage (169). Laboratory studies consistently showed a period of severe cerebral vasoconstriction and decreased CBF lasting for several hours after even short intervals of DHCA (no-reflow phenomenon). Whereas brain metabolism returns to normal after rewarming and termination of DHCA, the CBF remains significantly reduced, resulting in cerebral ischemia.

A large prospective study of infants undergoing repair of transposition of the great arteries using DHCA documented subclinical EEG evidence of seizures and subtle abnormalities in neurologic examination as late as 1 year after surgery, especially in those patients exposed to prolonged periods of DHCA (170,171). Brain imaging studies performed 1 to 4 years postoperatively revealed a disturbingly high incidence of focal injury (172). Long durations of DHCA during correction of congenital heart disease in infancy were shown to correlate with lower scores on intelligence tests later in childhood (165,173). A review of 200 adult patients who underwent DHCA during operations on the thoracic aorta revealed that 19% of survivors had diffuse temporary neurologic dysfunction manifesting as prolonged postoperative obtundation, confusion, agitation, or transient parkinsonism. These symptoms correlated with DHCA duration and advanced age. On the other hand, the duration of DHCA did not correlate with mortality or with permanent focal neurologic injury. Patients with advanced atheromatous aortic disease had a higher incidence of permanent focal neurologic injury, which is consistent with an embolic etiology.

It has been established unequivocally that colder temperatures at the time of DHCA confer a greater degree of protection. Too short a period of cooling may result in neurologic damage due to uneven and inadequate lowering of brain temperature (170). Packing the head in ice during prolonged intervals of circulatory arrest improves neurologic outcome. It is currently agreed that periods of arrest longer than 20 minutes require hypothermia to 12° to 15°C to ensure adequate cerebral protection. Durations of DHCA exceeding 40 to 50 minutes even at these lower temperatures raise concerns, and those exceeding 60 minutes are universally regarded as risky (155) (Fig. 27-20).

Infants who underwent DHCA had significantly lower CBF after reestablishment of perfusion than a similar group of infants cooled to equivalent temperatures without circulatory arrest (174). Moreover, CBF did not recover to prearrest values even after separation from CPB, in contrast to patients exposed to deep hypothermia without circulatory arrest, in whom CBF returned rapidly with rewarming to pre-CPB levels (174). Therefore, through mechanisms that are still unclear, DHCA appears to produce a persistent decrease in CBF. Burrows et al. (175) demonstrated a progressive rise in anterior fontanelle pressure during DHCA in infants. There was a direct correlation between the duration and lowest temperature of DHCA and the duration of increase in anterior fontanelle pressure. They also demonstrated a significant negative correlation between the return of cerebral function (as assessed using cortical evoked potentials) and anterior fontanelle pressure. Patients with the highest anterior fontanelle pressure had the greatest decrease in cortical evoked potential activity, indicating impairment of cerebral cortical function. Whether this corresponds to the same mechanism producing persistent decreases in CBF after DHCA is unclear (175). The inappropriate cerebral vascular occlusion that occurs after DHCA (no reflow) is now believed to be an important cause of neurologic injury. Because cerebral injury may occur during reperfusion or thereafter, an initial period of cold reperfusion after DHCA was suggested to decrease cerebral ischemic injury, which may result if rewarming is begun immediately after the resumption of perfusion (176). Current research is focusing on the role of the systemic inflammatory response, leukocyte aggregation, and cytokines in mediating neurologic injury.

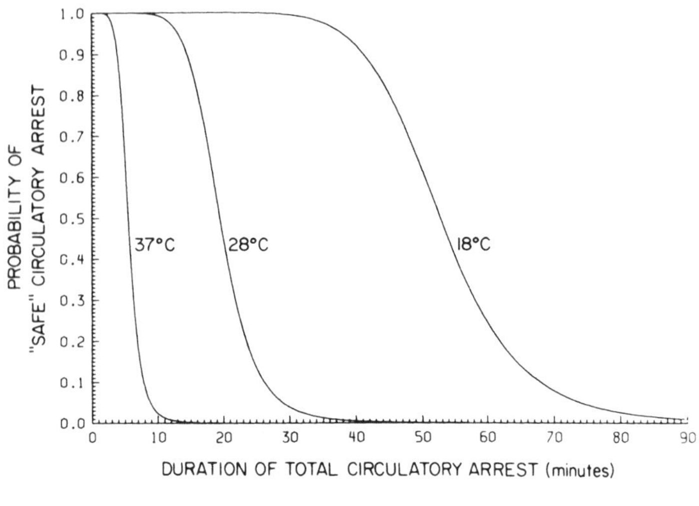

FIGURE 27-20. Informal estimate of the probability of "safe" total circulatory arrest (absence of structural or functional damage), according to the arrest time, at nasopharyngeal temperatures of 37°, 28°, and 18°C. (From Kirklin JW, Barratt-Boyes BG, eds. Hypothermia, circulatory arrest, and cardiopulmonary bypass. In: *Cardiac surgery,* 2nd ed, vol 1. New York: Churchill Livingstone, 1993:74, with permission.)

Monitoring the Brain during Deep Hypothermic Circulatory Arrest

Many centers monitor cerebral electrical activity by means of the EEG or of auditory evoked potentials (AEPs) and somatosensory evoked potentials (SSEPs) to assess the adequacy of cooling before DHCA. Cerebral electrical function may be assessed. Because the EEG represents cortical electrical activity, the presence of EEG silence does not ensure adequate cooling of deeper areas of the brain, such as the basal ganglia and the brain stem. Therefore, after EEG silence has been achieved cooling should be continued for additional 5 to 10 minutes to ensure adequate brain cooling. Cooling for a minimum duration of 20 to 30 minutes regardless of when EEG silence occurs has been suggested (152). It may be more prudent to rely on the disappearance of AEPs or SSEPs, which take somewhat longer to vanish with cooling, than on the EEG (152).

Monitoring of raw EEG data is usually impractical for routine intraoperative monitoring because it generates an enormous volume of data and requires continuous assessment by a highly skilled medical or paramedical specialist. Power spectral analysis converts EEG information from time domain to a frequency domain for a given segment of the EEG. The compressed spectral array displays serial power spectra plotted one above the other to give a mountain and valley presentation of the EEG pattern. Using computerized fast Fourier transformation, power spectra for several channels can be simultaneously recorded. It has been shown that the time needed for the return of EEG activity correlates with the duration of DHCA and with neurologic outcome.

Advanced applications of near-infrared technology can detect oxyhemoglobin, cytochrome aa_3 redox status, and cerebral blood volume, which allows the evaluation of brain oxygenation. A significant decrease in oxidative state of cytochrome aa_3 was noted in patients undergoing DHCA, compared with low-flow CPB (177). Transcranial Doppler ultrasonography has been used to assess the adequacy of cerebral perfusion during cooling and after rewarming and to detect the presence and quantity of cerebral emboli. Its routine use during DHCA is not yet established. Monitoring of jugular venous bulb saturation during DHCA has been described. Because oxygen extraction is an accurate reflection of total cerebral metabolic activity, cooling until the jugular venous oxygen saturation exceeds 95% has been suggested. Animal and human studies confirm the association between low cerebral venous saturation before circulatory arrest and poor neurologic outcome after DHCA (167, 178).

Surgical Technique for the Repair of Aneurysms of the Transverse Arch

Repair of the aortic arch under DHCA, first described by Griepp et al. (179), is usually performed through a median sternotomy. Less commonly, a left thoracotomy incision is used (180). Atrial or bicaval cannulation provides venous drainage, while arterial return is accomplished via the left femoral artery. In the presence of significant peripheral vascular or thoracoabdominal atheromatous disease precluding femoral arterial perfusion, an aortic antegrade cannula is used temporarily until a portion of the graft is anastomosed. Arterial flow is then established via the graft. Femoral vein-to-femoral artery bypass is used for left thoracotomy procedures. Patients are cooled to 15° to 20°C or until the EEG is isoelectric. Hemodilution is used to achieve a hematocrit of 20%. After completion of the arch segment, air is vented from the graft and the aorta with the patient in the head-down position. The graft is clamped, bypass flow is resumed, and rewarming is begun while the proximal aortic reconstruction is being completed. The period of circulatory arrest ideally should be less than 30 minutes. The brachiocephalic vessels are attached to the dome of the graft as a single patch. If disease extends distally to involve the descending aorta, the patient may be treated in a staged fashion using the elephant trunk procedure. Completion of the second stage of the elephant trunk operation by an endovascular technique has been described (181).

Results following DHCA

Despite the multitude of advances in surgical techniques and perioperative management, the surgical treatment of aortic arch disease is still associated with significant morbidity and mortality. Svensson et al. reported on 656 patients undergoing aneurysm repair with DHCA (254). He noted that arrest times longer than 40 minutes were associated with a higher incidence of stroke, and DHCA times longer 60 minutes were associated with increased mortality. Coselli et al. reported on 227 transverse arch aneurysms, half of which were treated with RCP. In-hospital and long-term mortality rates were 6% and 9%, respectively (182). Many reports have indicated that the safe arrest time can be extended by the use of cold RCP. Deeb et al. (183) reported an experience with 35 patients having a mean arrest time of 63 minutes. There was a single intraoperative death and two late deaths, and only one patient suffered a stroke (183).

Cerebroplegia

In an attempt to reduce neurologic injury associated with DHCA, the technique of selective cerebral asanguinous perfusion and regional cooling has been investigated. The antegrade infusion of cold oxygenated asanguinous cardioplegia solution into the cerebral circulation (cerebroplegia) was studied in animals during 2 hours of DHCA at 12° to 15°C (184). During rewarming after DHCA, EEG activity returned more rapidly in animals receiving cerebroplegia than in the control group (36 versus 117 minutes). Cerebral high-energy phosphate levels and intracellular pH also remained higher in the cerebroplegia-treated group. Animals subjected to antegrade cerebroplegia tended to have better preservation of neurologic function than those in the control group. External cranial cooling appeared to confer similar cerebral protective effects in that study (185). Wolfson et al. (186) reported better preservation of neurologic function in primates receiving cold saline cerebral perfusion compared with untreated controls. Independent of the substrate composition of such cerebroplegic solutions, the maintenance of lower brain temperatures and perhaps the washout of toxic metabolites are probably the more important mechanisms providing additional cerebral protection with this technique. Sanguinous cerebroplegia was also described in a series of 54 patients undergoing aortic arch surgery. The carotid arteries were continuously perfused with cold blood at 6° to 12°C during moderately hypothermic circulatory arrest of the rest of the body (187). The technique permitted more time to perform the aortic repair and was associated with a low incidence of neurologic complications (see Antegrade Selective Cerebral Perfusion). Prospective randomized trials are necessary to establish the role of various cerebroplegic solutions during cardiac and aortic surgical procedures requiring circulatory arrest.

Antegrade Selective Cerebral Perfusion

Initial efforts to protect the brain during circulatory arrest included the isolated cannulation of brachiocephalic vessels. Interest in antegrade SCP has been reawakened by the realization that the long periods of DHCA required for the repair of complex and extensive aneurysms are associated with a high incidence of neurologic injury. When combined with hypothermia, low-flow rates of antegrade SCP are sufficient to preserve cerebral integrity. Bachet et al. perfused the innominate and left carotid arteries with blood at 6° to 12°C (188). One technique of antegrade SCP involves the cannulation of one or more of the brachiocephalic or axillary arteries with small cannulas connected to a separate circuit with a dedicated heat exchanger. The systemic extracorporeal circulation continues to perfuse the patient via femoral cannulation with moderately cold (20° to 28°C) perfusate at a rate of 60 to 70 mL/kg/minute. Arterialized blood is drawn from the oxygenator through a separate pump and passed through the cardioplegia heat exchanger, which lowers the temperature further to approximately 15°C. The perfusate then passes through a 40-μm filter before perfusing the brachiocephalic arteries. Flow rates to the brain are controlled at 5 to 10 mL/kg/minute. Disadvantages of SCP include the need for a secondary bypass circuit and additional cannulation sites, cluttering of the surgical field by the additional cannulas, and embolization of atheromatous material. The simplified method of perfusing only the innominate artery relies on flow through an intact circle of Willis to protect the left side of the brain (189) (Fig. 27-21).

Because of the enhanced risk of embolization many surgeons are not enthusiastic about antegrade SCP, especially if it requires multiple cannulation sites. Another simplified technique for antegrade SCP has been described. An island of tissue on the superior wall of the aortic arch including the origins of the innominate artery, the left carotid artery, and, if possible, the left subclavian artery is isolated. A beveled graft of 18- to 20-mm Dacron is sewn into this island, and flow is established at a rate of 100 to 600 mL/minute with a perfusate temperature of 10°C. The flow rate is adjusted to achieve a radial artery pressure of 50 mm Hg. At the end of aortic reconstruction, the bevelled graft with its attached cerebral vessels is sewn to the rest of the aortic graft using a short interval of DHCA (152). When multiple cannulas are connected to a single roller pump head, the downstream flow cannot be independently determined without individual monitoring devices for each line. However, this is not of major concern because of the anatomic nature of the circle of Willis and distribution of CBF. The most recent reports using antegrade SCP recommend flow rates ranging from 500 to 1,000 mL/minute and perfusion

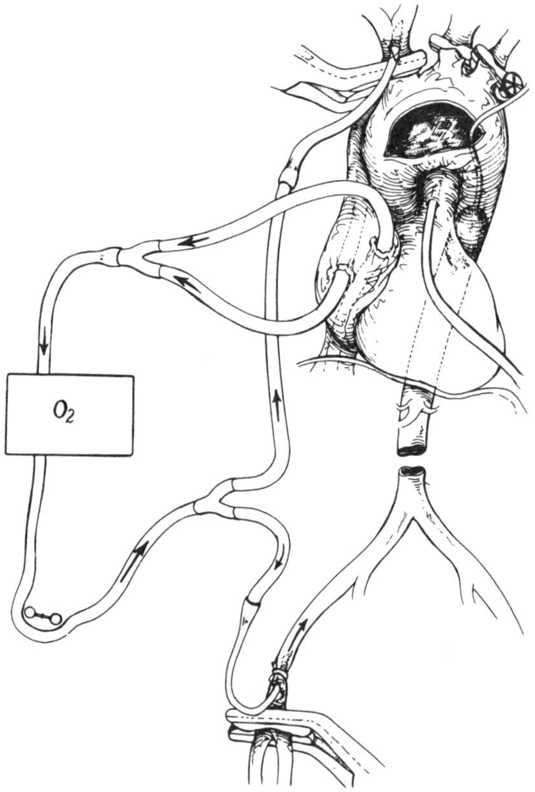

FIGURE 27-21. Transfemoral retrograde CPB with selective antegrade perfusion of the innominate artery. The patient is cooled by means of the heat exchanger in the oxygenator to the range of 24° to 28°C (nasopharyngeal). Cardiopulmonary bypass (CPB) flows are kept in the usual range, which varies between 30 and 50 mL/kg/minute. Subsequently, after clamping of the innominate artery and occlusion of the descending thoracic aorta, the flow rate can be reduced slightly. The absolute volume of flow delivered to the cerebral circulation is then dependent on the vascular resistance of the regional bed and is not controlled by the perfusionist using a separate pump head. The ascending aorta is clamped (temporarily), and the heart is arrested with crystalloid cardioplegia. An appropriately sized, low-porosity, very soft woven Dacron graft and a large aortic occlusion balloon catheter are then brought on to the field. The balloon catheter is placed through the graft. The innominate artery is occluded with a clamp; the left common carotid and left subclavian arteries are then also occluded. CPB flow is reduced to the range of 400 to 500 mL/minute, and the aneurysm is opened. Any laminated clot is quickly evacuated with gauze sponges, and the aortic occlusion balloon is threaded down into the proximal descending thoracic aorta and inflated. Pump flow is then increased back to baseline level. (From Miller DC. Surgical treatment of aneurysms and dissections involving the transverse aortic arch. In: Dudley H, Carter D, eds. *Rob and Smith's operative surgery.* St. Louis: CV Mosby, 1986:540, with permission.)

pressures of 40 to 70 mm Hg (190,194). Kazui recommended CBF rates of 10 mL/kg/minute to be delivered with the use of a dedicated roller pump separate from that perfusing the rest of the body (190). Monitoring of jugular bulb oxygen saturation or cerebral oxygenation by near-infrared spectroscopy could be used to provide feedback information that for adjustment of flow rates and perfusion pressures so that oxygen delivery is matched to cerebral oxygen extraction rates (155,191,192). Technologic advancements in the design of heart-lung machines, such as pressure-control modules and air detection systems, have increased the safety of extracorporeal circulation techniques and may decrease some of the risks associated with antegrade SCP.

It has been unequivocally demonstrated that low-flow hypothermic antegrade SCP provides better cerebral protection from global ischemia than either DHCA or RCP (168, 169,193). Good results have been reported with the use of antegrade SCP to permit open distal anastomosis during repair of acute aortic dissection (194–196). Several studies have demonstrated improved outcome of aortic arch surgery with the use of antegrade SCP (197). In one series of 100 patients, the incidence of stroke was 1% after aortic arch dissection repair using SCP (198). Matsuda et al. (191) operated on 34 patients with aortic arch aneurysms using SCP at 16° to 20°C with an average duration of 123 minutes. They reported a 9% mortality rate, a 3% incidence of stroke, and a 6% rate of transient neurologic symptoms. Kazui et al. had a 16% mortality rate in 80 patients with aortic arch aneurysms operated on with the use of SCP, with only one postoperative stroke (199). Another series reported a stroke rate of 5% in aortic arch aneurysms and dissections repaired with the use of SCP; mortality rates were 19% and 7%, respectively (200). Some of the cerebral complications encountered during the early experience with antegrade SCP were attributed in part to high cerebral perfusion pressures and cerebral edema (201). Kazui et al. recommended the use of cerebral perfusion pressures of 50 to 70 mm Hg (190). Antegrade SCP in conjunction with moderate systemic hypothermia (28°C) removes the time limits imposed by DHCA, thereby permitting the completion of complex repairs. It also avoids the excessively long extracorporeal perfusion times necessary to achieve profound cooling and rewarming, which reduces the hematologic and organ abnormalities that can occur with profound hypothermia and prolonged CPB.

Retrograde Cerebral Perfusion

Several investigators have suggested that RCP, which had previously been described as a treatment for catastrophic air embolism arising during CPB (202), may be useful in avoiding some of the disadvantages of DHCA (203–205). Ueda et al. described the technique of RCP by which arterialized blood is delivered to the cerebral vasculature during the period of systemic circulatory arrest (204). The CPB circuit is modified to allow the delivery of oxygenated blood in a retrograde direction into the cerebral venous system via the SVC (206,207) (Fig. 27-22). This can be accomplished with either bicaval cannulation or an isolated SVC cannula and a dual-stage right atrial cannula (208). Use of a retrograde cardioplegia cannula placed in the SVC permits monitoring of the infusion pressure through the end-lumen pres-

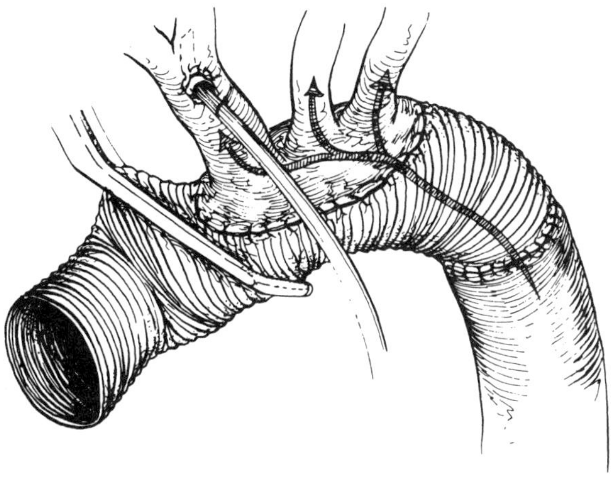

FIGURE 27-22. Once reperfusion of the cerebral vessels from both arterial cannulas has been accomplished, attention is directed at hemostasis of the end-to-end suture line containing the origins of the great vessels. Significant problems should be corrected at this time. The innominate arterial cannula can be removed either at this time or later, after completion of the proximal anastomosis. (From Miller DC. Surgical treatment of aneurysms and dissections involving the transverse aortic arch. In: Dudley H, Carter D, eds. *Rob and Smith's operative surgery.* St. Louis: CV Mosby, 1986:540, with permission.)

sure port. Flow rates for RCP ranging from 250 to 500 mL/minute are adjusted to achieve a perfusion pressure (measured in the SVC or internal jugular vein) of 15 to 30 mm Hg. The cerebral perfusate temperature is maintained at 15° to 18°C. Despite these cold temperatures, desaturated blood is seen returning from the arch vessels, indicating that the brain continues to consume oxygen. There is evidence to suggest that pulsatile flow provides more cerebral protective effects that nonpulsatile flow (209). An RCP pressure greater than 25 to 30 mm Hg results in cerebral edema, whereas pressures less than 20 mm Hg are ineffective (210). Potential problems with RCP include the presence of jugular venous valves, which may restrict rostral delivery of the perfusate to the brain (211). Because of increased cerebral venous pressure, cerebral edema and destruction of the blood-brain barrier may occur (212). Intracranial hemorrhage and focal cerebral infarcts are other potential complications (155,161,213). Surgical visibility may be impaired by blood spilling out of the aortic arch during RCP. This may necessitate intermittent rather than continuous RCP. Even at the minimum pressures required for effective retrograde flow, the development of cerebral edema limits the safe duration of RCP (213,214).

The actual mechanism by which RCP enhances cerebral protection in humans and the fraction of the retrograde perfusate that is actually delivered to the brain are uncertain. The possible mechanisms by which RCP may enhance cerebral protection during CA include (a) the maintenance of low cerebral temperatures via continuous delivery of a hypothermic perfusate (RCP does allow the brain to be better cooled and maintained at a lower temperature than the rest of the body, thus conferring better cerebral protection without the complications of profound total body cooling); (b) the continuous delivery of oxygen and substrate to the brain; and (c) decreased risk of embolization of air and atheromatous debris from open brachiocephalic vessels. RCP appears be effective in flushing air, blood, and particulate debris from the cerebral circulation, thereby mitigating the harmful effects of particulate emboli during aortic arch surgery. Some surgeons advocate the use of continuous or intermittent RCP in patients who are at high risk for embolization as a consequence of the presence of thrombi or debris in the aorta (155). Although the delivery of metabolic substrate during circulatory arrest has been one rationale for the use of RCP, existing experimental and clinical studies have not consistently demonstrated that RCP provides sufficient nutrient flow to support cerebral metabolism during DHCA. Animal and human studies have demonstrated significant gradients in oxygen saturation, partial pressure of oxygen (PO_2), partial pressure of carbon dioxide (PCO_2), and pH across the cerebral vascular bed, indicative of continued cerebral metabolic activity, during DHCA with RCP (215, 216). Clinical reports in small numbers of patients demonstrated that RCP used during circulatory arrest partially restored cerebral oxygenation and provided cerebral cortical blood flow that was 10% of baseline (217,218). The presence of CBF during DHCA and RCP in humans has also been verified with the use of radionuclide techniques and transcranial Doppler ultrasonography (211,219). Cheung et al. (216) demonstrated a progressive increase in oxygen extraction ratio across the brachiocephalic circulation during DHCA with RCP, suggestive of insufficient oxygen delivery and continued cerebral oxygen consumption. These observations are consistent with their earlier findings that RCP attenuated but did not prevent the decay in the amplitude of brain stem SSEPs during DHCA. The increase in oxygen extraction ratio paralleled the decrease in amplitude of brain stem SSEPs over time during DHCA and RCP (220). The depletion of high-energy phosphates and the decline of cerebral intracellular pH were shown to occur to a lesser degree with RCP than with DCHA alone (221). Although animal and human data suggest that the metabolic benefits of RCP are minimal, the technique still offers important beneficial effects such as the maintenance of brain cooling and the washout of particulate emboli, which are the major cause of permanent neurologic injury after aneurysm surgery (114).

Some animal studies indicate that RCP provides 10% to 50% of the CBF and 33% of the oxygen normally delivered during CPB while allowing 20% removal of CO_2 (222, 223). Some experimental models demonstrated cerebral tissue flow with RCP as high as 30% to 50% of that achieved with antegrade perfusion rates that were sufficient to support cerebral metabolic requirements. One study concluded that 60 minutes of RCP in dogs provided adequate cerebral metabolic support during DHCA (213). Intracellular pH mapping in dogs demonstrated that animals subjected to DHCA and RCP had a less profound decrease in cerebral intracellular pH than those subjected to DHCA without RCP (224). Other animal models failed to demonstrate a significant level of brain blood flow via RCP or the ability of RCP to sustain metabolic function during DHCA (214, 215,224–227). However, another dog study demonstrated that only 2% to 3% of the required capillary blood flow was provided with RCP (228). It was shown in a rabbit model (where the jugular venous system is valveless) that retrograde perfusion through the SVC reached the cerebral venous system but there was minimal flow through the capillaries; the authors speculated that venovenous and venoarterial shunting in the brain prevented adequate cerebral capillary flow during RCP (229).

Differences between animal and human venous anatomy must be taken into account when interpreting the results of these studies. It is unlikely that RCP rates that are sufficient to provide nutritive maintenance to the brain during antegrade CA can be clinically achieved. In humans, the majority of jugular venous valves are incompetent but in some cases they do interrupt RCP flow (222). With selective SVC perfusion in humans, less than 5% of the retrograde flow returns via the arch vessels, far too little to meet the ongoing metabolic demands of the brain even in the presence of hypothermia (169). Nevertheless, some uptake of oxygen and nutrients occurs during human RCP, since the blood returning to the arch is desaturated. A postmortem study in humans demonstrated that most of the retrograde flow is shunted away from the SVC to the inferior vena cava (IVC), mainly via the azygous system (230), but that some flow eventually reaches the brain via the vertebral veins. One human clinical study did show rapid cerebral uptake of a lipophilic tracer within several seconds after the initiation of RCP via the SVC. The technique of whole-body retrograde perfusion through the SVC and IVC increases the delivery of blood in a retrograde fashion to the brain. The increase in IVC pressure prevents diversion of SVC blood away from the cranium and increases collateral flow to the brain through the azygous and vertebral venous plexus. In addition it provides continuous retrograde perfusion to the abdominal visceral through the IVC and intermittent retrograde coronary perfusion through the coronary sinus. The initial flow rate of whole-body retrograde perfusion is usually 800 to 1,000 mL/minute. Once the venous capacitance vessels have been filled, a flow rate of 200 to 500 mL/minute is sufficient to maintain SVC pressure of 20 to 25 mm Hg (224,231).

Animal studies of the effect of RCP on neurologic outcome are inconclusive. One study in pigs showed RCP to reduce neurologic dysfunction and improve cerebral protection (232). Cerebral function was better preserved in pigs exposed to RCP at 20°C for 90 minutes than in those undergoing DHCA with ice packing of the head (169). Other pig studies showed RCP during profound hypothermia to be similar to DHCA alone and inferior to antegrade SCP (233,234).

The clinical efficacy of RCP in improving outcome during circulatory arrest in humans is also unclear. Some studies have demonstrated reduced rates of stroke and mortality in adults undergoing aortic operations using RCP (235–240); other clinical studies were inconclusive (232,241). The maximum safe duration that antegrade SCP can be interrupted when RCP is used and the mechanisms by which RCP prevents neuronal injury in this setting have not been established. A study of RCP in 228 patients showed poor results with 20% neurologic dysfunction and 50% mortality (223). The two factors that appeared to correlate with neurologic dysfunction were RCP duration greater than 60 minutes and cardiac ischemic time greater than 120 minutes. There was no neurologic dysfunction when the duration of RCP was less than 30 minutes, but significant neurologic damage occurred if RCP duration was greater than 100 minutes. An SVC pressure between 15 and 24 mm Hg was associated with the least risk for neurologic dysfunction (223). In a small series of 23 patients undergoing emergency and elective aortic operations using DHCA (15°C; mean arrest time, 21 minutes) and RCP, the mortality rate was 13% and the stroke rate was 4.3% (241). In a series of 103 patients undergoing repair of the ascending aorta and arch under moderately hypothermic systemic circulatory arrest (mean nasopharyngeal temperature, 23°C; mean arrest time, 27 minutes) and RCP at 10°C, the incidences of stroke (7.7%), seizures (3.8%), and death (7.7%) were similar to those reported in other series of DHCA with or without RCP. The authors suggested that it may not be necessary to cool the whole body to temperatures less than 20°C when continuous cold RCP is used (242).

At the present time it is difficult to conclusively recommend RCP or antegrade SCP routinely in all patients requiring aortic arch reconstruction. However, in complicated cases such as those requiring prolonged arrest time (more than 45 minutes), some adjunctive technique for cerebral perfusion is probably beneficial and warranted. Prospective randomized studies of DHCA with and without RCP and antegrade SCP are still needed to determine the role of these techniques in improving neurologic outcome (203).

Anesthetic Management of Aortic Arch Surgery

Anesthesia for the repair of aortic arch lesions requires understanding and application of the principles of CPB, myocardial and cerebral protection, hemodynamic monitoring and manipulation, and the prevention and treatment of hemorrhage and coagulopathy. The anesthesiologist should understand the physiology and the implications of deep hypothermia and circulatory arrest. In most cases the patient is supine and the surgery is performed through a median sternotomy. In some cases the procedure is done with the patient in the left lateral thoracotomy position. CPB is established via the femoral artery with venous drainage achieved through right atrial, bicaval, or femoral venous cannulation. Moderate or profound systemic hypothermia is used in association with variable periods of circulatory arrest. Surface cooling and rewarming via thermal blanket is used along with core cooling and rewarming through the CPB heat exchanger. The head should be packed in ice during core cooling and kept cold until the period of arrest is over. Core temperature is monitored from the esophagus, nasopharynx, or tympanic membrane. The nose, eyes, and earlobes should be covered and protected from frostbite. During cooling, hemodilution to a hematocrit of 20% partially counteracts the deleterious effects of hypothermia on blood viscosity, erythrocyte aggregation, and regional perfusion. The risk of hemorrhage is significant and may result from surgical bleeding, bleeding through graft porosity, and/or coagulopathy. Preparations for rapid volume resuscitation, massive blood transfusions, and RBC salvage should include placement of two or more large-bore intravenous catheters and automated rapid transfusion and cell saver systems in addition to the CPB pump. Six units of compatible blood should be present throughout the procedure. Platelets and fresh-frozen plasma should be immediately available (243). The blood pressure should be carefully monitored and controlled. In the presence of aortic dissection, the dP/dt_{max} must be minimized to that amount that is just sufficient to permit adequate tissue perfusion. β-Adrenergic receptor blocking agents, supplemented with vasodilators, are excellent for this purpose. The use of inotropic drugs in the presence of aortic dissection could be hazardous because of the increase in dP/dt_{max}. The anesthetic technique should allow for complete neurologic assessment within a few hours after surgery.

Monitoring

In addition to the standard routine monitors, invasive hemodynamic monitoring with an intraarterial line and Swan-Ganz catheter is required. The site of arterial line placement depends on the location and extent of the aortic pathology and the planned surgical procedure. In proximal aortic lesions, a left upper-extremity arterial line is used. Distal arch lesions necessitate placement of the arterial line in the right upper extremity. During antegrade SCP, the right radial or brachial arterial pressure reflects the cerebral perfusion pressure in the innominate and right common carotid arteries. A femoral arterial line monitors distal aortic pressure and the adequacy of the distal perfusion. Communication with the surgical team should be done before placement of the arterial line to determine which artery will be used for femoral cannulation. A Swan-Ganz catheter is placed to monitor CO and filling pressures and in some instances mixed venous oxygen saturation and right ventricular ejection fraction. TEE gives valuable information regarding ventricular function, preload, and the presence of aortic atherosclerotic disease. During RCP the venous pressure in the internal jugular vein is monitored through the site port of the Swan-Ganz introducer. Depending on local practice and the technique used for cerebral protection, some institutions insert a jugular venous bulb catheter to assess the degree of reduction in $CMRO_2$. Cerebral electrophysiologic monitoring using raw or processed EEG data, SSEPs, or AEPs is employed in some institutions. CBF velocity could be monitored by transcranial Doppler ultrasound. The EEG is useful to indirectly assess metabolic activity of the brain; temperature monitoring from clinically available sites is not a reliable indicator of brain temperature or the degree of metabolic suppression (244). Once the EEG becomes isoelectric, cooling should be continued for an additional 5 to 10 minutes to ensure homogenous cooling of deep portions of the brain, because it has been shown that the brain stem is very resistant to cooling (156). The subcortical wave of the SSEP may be a better indicator than the EEG of the temperature at which maximum $CMRO_2$ suppression and brain protection are achieved. Monitoring of the jugular venous oxygen saturation provides a measure of overall cerebral oxygen use during cooling and rewarming (245). Transcranial Doppler ultrasound may be useful to determine the adequacy of CBF during cooling and rewarming and to detect embolic events and cerebral malperfusion states (246, 247).

Premedication

For elective procedures, patients should receive their antihypertensive and antianginal agents before surgery, including β-blockers and calcium channel blockers. The use of angiotensin-converting enzyme inhibitors on the day of surgery has been associated with refractory hypotension after CPB. Sedative agents should be administered to prevent the increase in aortic wall stress that would result from anxiety-related hypertension and tachycardia. Commonly used sedatives include lorazepam 1 to 4 mg PO, midazolam 1 to 4 mg IV, and morphine 0.05 to 0.1 mg/kg IM. Patients who present for emergency repair of aortic aneurysm or dissection require meticulous hemodynamic management before and during anesthetic induction. β-Blocking agents and vasodilators are the main cornerstones of therapy.

Induction

Large-bore intravenous catheters and the arterial line should be placed before induction. All necessary hemodynamic, pressor, and vasodilatory drugs should be available in the operating room along with 6 units of blood before induction. The main goal during induction is to minimize the hypertensive response to laryngoscopy and intubation, which may result in rupture of an aneurysm or propagation of a dissection. In addition, myocardial ischemia should be prevented and treated. Patients presenting for emergency repair usually have a full stomach and require prophylaxis against aspiration and a rapid-sequence induction. Blunting of the hemodynamic response to laryngoscopy and intubation can be achieved with the use of moderate- to high-dose narcotics, lidocaine supplementation, short-acting β-blockers (e.g., esmolol), and boluses of nitroglycerin or nitroprusside. Providing small doses of muscle relaxants during narcotic infusion minimizes opioid-induced chest wall rigidity. Large doses of pancuronium are generally avoided during induction because of the drug's vagolytic and norepinephrine releasing effects, which produce hypertension and tachycardia. However, after intubation small doses of pancuronium for maintenance relaxation are usually well tolerated. In patients with poor myocardial function and those who are hemodynamically unstable, etomidate 0.2 to 0.3 mg/kg along with a small dose of narcotic preserves hemodynamic stability during induction. Anesthesia is maintained with inhalation agents, narcotics, and nondepolarizing muscle relaxants.

Airway Management

Lesions of the ascending and transverse aortic arch are managed with a single-lumen endotracheal tube. As discussed previously, aortic lesions may cause tracheal and bronchial deviation and compression. Repairs of lesions of the distal aortic arch and descending thoracic aorta require OLV. This is preferably provided through a left-sided double-lumen tube (DLT). However, caution must be exercised in recognizing the presence of left bronchial compression by the aneurysm. The tube should never be pushed blindly, and it should be placed under direct vision using fiberoptic bronchoscopy. In some instances a right-sided DLT may be required, but it is more difficult to position because of the easily obstructed orifice of the right upper lobe bronchus. Other options to provide OLV include the Univent tube (Fuji Systems Corp., Tokyo) or a bronchial blocker. The Univent tube consists of a single-lumen tube with a built-in bronchial blocker. The bronchial blocker can be directed to either main stem bronchus. It may be easier to insert and position properly in the trachea than a DLT, especially during a rapid-sequence induction. Fine adjustments of the blocker's position can be guided by the use of fiberoptic bronchoscopy. The bronchial blocker has a small lumen which allows the escape of gases and potentially the administration of oxygen and CPAP. Use of the Univent tube eliminates the need to exchange the DLT to a single-lumen endotracheal tube at the end of the surgical procedure, which may be extremely difficult and dangerous due to the development of airway edema in many patients. Disadvantages of the Univent tube include high bronchial cuff pressures and compromised ability to actively deflate, suction, or apply continuous positive airway pressure (CPAP) to the nondependent lung (248).

Physiologic Effects of Hypothermia

Hypothermia reduces oxygen consumption of tissues, thereby prolonging the period of anoxia that can be tolerated without permanent damage. Hypothermia causes a shift to the left of the oxygen dissociation curve, resulting in less oxygen availability to the tissues, an effect that is partially compensated by an increase in the amount of oxygen that is dissolved in plasma. Therefore, under hypothermic conditions a greater proportion of tissue oxygen requirements is supplied by the amount of oxygen that is dissolved in plasma, which is a function of the arterial oxygen tension (PaO_2). Glucose hemostasis is impaired. There is an increase in plasma insulin and catecholamine levels and decreased tissue responsiveness to insulin. Glucose use is decreased and glycogen stores are depleted. Hypothermia impairs hepatic and renal function. Drug metabolism and elimination are markedly slowed. Renal tubal function and urine output are diminished. In addition, hypothermia produces a slight degree of metabolic acidosis, which worsens during the period of circulatory arrest. Cerebral oxygen consumption is decreased as brain electrical activity decreases with hypothermia. EEG isoelectricity develops at 18° to 20°C (Fig. 27-23). Hypothermia produces a linear decrease in the minimal alveolar concentration of inhaled anesthetics. Deep hypothermia significantly increases blood viscosity. Hemodilution is beneficial for improving blood flow characteristics; during deep hypothermia, oxygen delivery is maximum at hematocrits between 18% to 22%. In addition, hypothermia produces a decrease in the number of platelets as well as impairment of platelet function. Thrombocytopenia persists even after rewarming. Coagulopathy and excessive bleeding are more commonly encountered after DHCA than after moderately hypothermic CPB. The transfusion of platelets and coagulation factors is frequently required. Cooling results in severe peripheral vasoconstriction, which may compromise the adequacy of further cooling of peripheral tissues and result in the development of internal temperature gradients. Vasodilators are commonly used during cooling to overcome the effects of hypothermia-induced vasoconstriction. In children undergoing repair of congenital heart disease, phentolamine 0.2 mg/kg (or phenoxybenzamine 0.5 mg/kg) is commonly used. In adults nitroprusside and nitroglycerin infusions are frequently used. Direct arterial vasodilators may result in a decrease in arterial oxygenation during OLV because of blunting of the hypoxic pulmonary vasoconstriction.

Glucose and Cerebral Ischemia

When cerebral oxygen delivery is inadequate, anaerobic glucose metabolism becomes the main source of adenosine triphosphate (ATP) production, resulting in intracellular lactic acidosis. Experimental studies have shown the deleterious effects of hyperglycemia in the presence of cerebral ischemic injury. Numerous animal studies have shown that hyperglycemia, at the time of an ischemic insult, increases the severity of neurologic injury. This is presumably caused by the lowering of intracellular pH that results from the continued anaerobic glycolysis and lactic acid production. Neurologic outcomes after cardiac arrest correlated negatively with elevated plasma glucose levels. Mild insulin-induced hypoglycemia has been shown to improve neurologic function in the

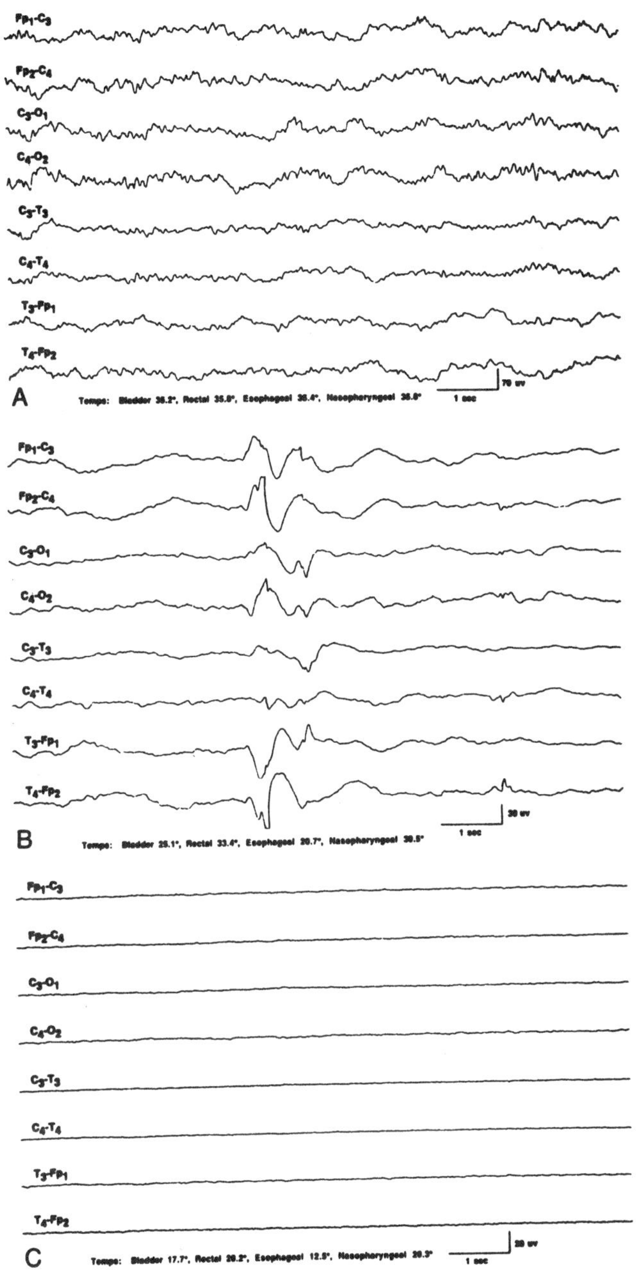

FIGURE 27-23. A: Electroencephalographic (EEG) activity at 35.8°C. Note depression of amplitude and slowing of background frequencies. **B:** EEG activity at 30.5°C. Note suppression burst pattern. **C:** EEG activity at 20.2°C. Note electrocerebral silence. (From Shenaq SA, Childres WF: Management of aortic aneurysms. *Semin Anesth* 1991;(2):108, with permission.)

setting of cerebral ischemia (249,250). Glucose-containing solutions should be avoided except to treat hypoglycemia. Whether mild to moderate hyperglycemia should be aggressively treated with insulin during CPB and DHCA is still controversial. Some human studies have challenged the recommendation that near-euglycemia be achieved during CPB (251). Metz and Keats reported no neurologic injury among 54 patients undergoing CABG managed with glucose-containing fluids (serum glucose, 700 mg/dL during bypass), compared with one stroke and one case of encephalopathy among 53 patients in whom glucose was avoided during CPB (glucose, 200 mg/dL) (252). A more detailed study of neuropsychologic performance found no correlation between serum glucose level during bypass (ranging from 103 to 380 mg/dL) and subsequent neuropsychologic deterioration (253). Nevertheless, the current consensus is to avoid hyperglycemia during periods of potential neurologic injury (e.g., CPB and DHCA).

Pharmacologic Cerebral Protection

Although profound hypothermia produces an isoelectric EEG and decreases cerebral oxygen requirements by up to 70%, it cannot provide total cerebral protection because of the potential for uneven brain cooling and the presence of residual electrical and metabolic activity. Further suppression of cerebral activity and metabolic rate can be accomplished with anesthetic agents such as sodium thiopental 5 to 40 mg/kg given during core cooling and before circulatory arrest. The efficacy of such intervention remains to be proven by well designed, prospective, randomized clinical trials. Calcium channel blockers and corticosteroids may modify postischemic cascades and have been used as adjuncts to achieve cerebral protection during DHCA, although their benefit has not been proven (254).

Barbiturates and Intravenous Anesthetics

The use of barbiturates to protect the brain during CPB and DHCA is controversial. Whereas barbiturates have been shown to protect the brain in cases of focal cerebral ischemia, they have not been shown to have an effect in cases of global ischemia or in the setting of DHCA. Barbiturates are most effective in ameliorating injury that results from temporary focal cerebral ischemia. During cardiac surgery barbiturates may be of benefit in ameliorating the sequelae of temporary focal lesions in situations where maximum metabolic suppression has not been achieved by hypothermia. Protection from permanent focal lesions has been demonstrated with prolonged (96 hours) therapy. In one study of 182 patients undergoing normothermic open cardiac chamber procedures, Nussmeier et al. reported that maintenance of EEG burst suppression with thiopental before and during CPB reduced the incidence of neurologic abnormalities, compared with untreated controls (255). In contrast, Zaidan et al. found no neurologic benefit to thiopental in patients undergoing CABG with moderate hypothermia using membrane oxygenators. The need for inotropes and the time to extubation were markedly prolonged in patients receiving thiopental (256). Short-term barbiturate therapy is probably of no benefit when modern CPB techniques including membrane oxygenators, arterial filters, and hypothermia are used (257). In experimental studies, normothermic deep pentobarbital anesthesia was associated with 30%

decrease in $CMRO_2$ and cerebral glucose use, compared with lightly anesthetized controls. However, similar values were achieved with hypothermia to 30°C. The addition of hypothermia to pentobarbital anesthesia decreases cerebral use of oxygen and glucose by 70%. Despite unproven benefits, some anesthesiologists still administer a moderate dose of thiopental (3 to 10 mg/kg) before circulatory arrest to provide an added degree of cerebral protection (258). In addition to the reduction in $CMRO_2$, barbiturates decrease the release of cytotoxic excitatory neurotransmitters and may influence transmembrane ionic fluxes in a favorable fashion. Etomidate has not been found to protect the brain in the setting of DHCA (259). Similarly, propofol and ketamine have not been shown to be useful for cerebral protection in the clinical setting (260).

Corticosteroids

A large dose of corticosteroids is often given before circulatory arrest, although experimental evidence for cerebral protection is equivocal. Their potentially useful properties include stabilization of the microcirculation during hypothermia, stabilization of cellular membranes, and prevention of lysosomal breakdown. The usual dose is 10 to 20 mg/kg of methyl prednisolone before circulatory arrest. An intense systemic inflammatory reaction—manifested by the release of chemical mediators such as cytokines, interleukins, and endothelin; the adhesion and aggregation of leukocytes; and widespread capillary leak—is known to occur with CPB and DHCA. There is increasing evidence to suggest that reperfusion injury is an important contributing mechanism to neurologic injury. Corticosteroids may have a salutary effect on these perturbations (261,262).

Diuretics

Mannitol (0.5 g/kg) is often given as an osmotic diuretic to protect renal function and to attenuate the cerebral edema and increased intracranial pressure that may follow DHCA. Mannitol may also function as a free radical scavenger. Furosemide also decreases brain edema, cerebrospinal fluid (CSF) production, and astroglial cellular fluid transport and results in relaxation of cerebral capacitance vessels.

Calcium Channel Blockers

The renewed interest in calcium channel blockers as cerebral protective agents is based on the knowledge that intracellular calcium increases after an ischemic insult owing to the breakdown of membrane ion pumps and hypoxia of the mitochondria and endoplasmic reticulum. The rapid increase in intracellular calcium paradoxically stimulates neuronal metabolism while further impeding substrate delivery by causing glial cell swelling and intracellular accumulation of sodium and water. The increase in intracellular calcium causes the uncoupling of oxidative phosphorylation at the mitochondrial level and initiates subsequent biochemical cascades, which lead to further cell injury. Calcium-induced direct vasoconstriction may also contribute to postischemic vasospasm and result in sludging of RBCs in the microvasculature. Verapamil and diltiazem are not useful because they have poor blood-brain barrier penetration. Nimodipine, which crosses the blood-brain barrier, was shown to be effective when given after an ischemic insult in the primate model, but has not been shown to improve neurologic outcome after cardiopulmonary arrest in humans (263,264).

Other Pharmacologic Agents

The prevention of reperfusion injury after DHCA has been suggested as a potentially effective approach to cerebral protection. Magnesium, oxygen free radical scavengers (mannitol and superoxide dismutase) catalase, and adenosine have been shown to ameliorate reperfusion injury, probably by antagonizing the effects of calcium. However, there is no evidence for a beneficial effect of these agents in DHCA. Lidocaine appears to have a beneficial effect on $CMRO_2$ even if the EEG is already flat. In very large doses, lidocaine and phenytoin slow the release of potassium from ischemic neurons; however, the clinical relevance of this effect is unknown (265,266).

Summary

In summary, pharmacologic brain protection using high doses of steroids and barbiturates is frequently used during DHCA despite the lack of studies supporting their protective effects against DHCA-related brain damage. The prevention of reperfusion injury and attenuation of the systemic inflammatory response have been suggested as potentially effective approaches to cerebral protection in the setting of DHCA. The current management of DHCA is based on the following principles:

1. Maintenance of adequate brain hypothermia using surface and core cooling
2. The use of appropriate hemodilution to a hematocrit of 20% at 20°C
3. The use of muscle relaxants to reduce whole-body oxygen consumption
4. Monitoring of EEG or evoked potentials and possibly jugular venous oxygen saturation to ensure adequate suppression of cerebral electrical and metabolic activity with hypothermia and perhaps anesthetic agents
5. Attenuation of the stress response, the systemic inflammatory response, and reperfusion injury
6. Avoidance of severe hyperglycemia before and after circulatory arrest
7. Limiting the duration of DHCA to 40 minutes or less. (If a longer period of arrest is required, a reperfusion period of 5 minutes every 20 to 30 minutes is recommended.)
8. Strong consideration of antegrade SCP or RCP for complex repairs and those that are likely to exceed 30 to 40 minutes

9. Consideration of the growing evidence suggesting that pH-stat may be preferable to alpha-stat blood gas management in cases of DHCA (see later discussion)
10. Prevention and treatment of coagulopathy with the use of antifibrinolytic agents, platelets, and coagulation factors. (The use of aprotinin during DHCA is controversial. See later discussion.)
11. Careful management of the reperfusion period, which is very important to prevent or minimize brain injury. (Because ultrafiltration removes the chemical mediators of the systemic inflammatory response, its use on resumption of CPB after circulatory arrest has been recommended [267–269].)

Bleeding and Hematologic Dysfunction

Thoracic aortic surgery represents a high risk of bleeding because of long bypass time and the effects of deep hypothermia on the clotting system. The risk of bleeding and coagulopathy is highest in patients with dissection or systemic infection (270). Because bleeding and coagulopathy are common causes of death during aortic arch repair, adequate preparations for massive transfusion and RBC salvage are required (243). A coagulation defect of multifactorial origin results from deep hypothermia and extracorporeal circulation. Platelet dysfunction and thrombocytopenia are the most common causes of hemostatic defects. *In vitro* platelet aggregation is abolished at temperatures lower than 33°C. Below 25°C, platelets are sequestered primarily in the liver and released back into the circulation during rewarming (271,272). Platelets are activated by and adhere to the foreign surfaces of the extracorporeal circuit. The platelet count usually decreases by 25% to 60% from baseline owing to dilution by the priming solution, fragmentation, aggregation, and blood loss. A platelet count lower than 40,000/mm^3 represents a risk factor for post-CPB hemorrhage. Protamine produces a transient decrease in platelet count by about 33% that starts minutes after injection and lasts for about 1 hour (273). The hypothermia causes a reversible change in platelet activity, with the platelets being less functional at low temperatures but returning to near-normal function when normothermia is restored (274).

With profound hypothermia there is also a reduction of coagulation factors, fibrinogen, and plasminogen of sufficient magnitude to result in bleeding diathesis. The transfusion of packed RBCs and cell-saver blood does not replenish the coagulation factors or platelets (275). Hypofibrinogenemia and elevated fibrin split products, seen after profound hypothermia and massive transfusion, further contribute to hemostatic dysfunction. Hypothermia increases fibrinolytic and antithrombin activities and decreases plasma concentrations of prothrombin and factor VII. The transfusion of large volumes of RBCs, fresh-frozen plasma, cryoprecipitate, and platelets is frequently required during procedures requiring DHCA. Use of a graft surrounding surgical technique (wrapping the remaining portions of the original aortic wall around the synthetic graft) helps to tamponade perigraft bleeding. The development of high-capacity automated transfusion devices such as the Level One and the Rapid Infusion System (Haemontics, Braintree, MA) has reduced the risk of intraoperative hemorrhagic death because they allow the rapid infusion of large volumes of warm fluids and blood products. Blood conservation strategies are beneficial and may reduce the quantity of allogenic transfusion requirements. An effective blood conservation strategy may include autologous preoperative donation, intraoperative acute isovolemic hemodilution, cell salvage, and use of antifibrinolytic agents as well as postoperative collection and retransfusion of chest tube drainage (276, 277).

Antifibrinolytics

Enhanced fibrinolytic activity occurs during CPB. The three antifibrinolytic agents that are currently in use have been shown to improve hemostasis after CPB to varying degrees. Ideally these agents should be administered before activation of the coagulation and fibrinolytic cascades by the bypass circuit. EACA is a synthetic analog of lysine that inhibits fibrinolysis by occupying the lysine binding sites and preventing the interaction of plasminogen with fibrin. Tranexamic acid is also a synthetic lysine analog with a similar mechanism of action, but is 6 to 10 times more potent than EACA. Aprotinin is a naturally occurring polypeptide that inhibits the actions of serine proteases (plasmin, kallikerin, and bradykinin) by reversibly binding to the active serine sites of these enzymes. In addition to inhibiting fibrinolysis, these agents preserve platelet function by inhibiting the deleterious effects of plasmin on platelet receptors (278). The inhibition of fibrinolysis reduces the production of fibrin degradation products, which have deleterious effects on hemostasis. The hemostatic effects of aprotinin are more complex than those of EACA and tranexamic acid. When administered during CPB, aprotinin inhibits the contact activation of the intrinsic coagulation pathway that results from exposure of blood to the bypass circuit. In addition, it decreases the release of tissue plasminogen activator and increases α_2-antiplasmin activity and the release of plasminogen activator inhibitor. Aprotinin blunts the CPB-induced inflammatory response and DHCA-related reperfusion injury by inhibiting the release of interleukins and tumor necrosis factor in a manner similar to methylprednisolone (279). In high doses, aprotinin also inhibits the effects of bradykinin and kallikerin. Platelet function is preserved through the prevention of plasmin-mediated platelet inhibition and the protection of platelet surface glycoprotein receptors (280). However, aprotinin may also predispose to thrombosis because of the inhibition of protein C and protein S, especially during low-flow states and DHCA (281).

When tranexamic acid was administered before CPB in a general population of cardiac surgery patients, chest tube drainage in the first 12 hours was reduced by 30% and the need for homologous blood transfusion within 5 days of surgery decreased from 41% to 22%. Royston et al. documented a greater than four-fold reduction in blood loss during repeat cardiac surgery with the use of aprotinin (282). Subsequent studies using high-dose aprotinin confirmed the conservation of blood products and a reduction in bleeding ranging from 30% to 50% (283,284). Concern has been raised regarding the safety of aprotinin use in association with DHCA because of reports of increased mortality, renal failure, myocardial infarction, and death (285–288). Surprisingly, animal and human studies suggest that aprotinin may improve neurologic outcome after DHCA through a yet unidentified mechanism. In an animal model, aprotinin was shown to preserve cerebral function after DCHA for 60 minutes at 15°C (289). A controlled study showed a significant reduction in the incidence of stroke among patients undergoing redo myocardial revascularization when aprotinin was added to the pump prime (290). However, the administration of aprotinin during DHCA has been associated with paradoxic bleeding (291), renal dysfunction, myocardial infarction, and death (285). Aprotinin is known to inhibit the protein C system and tissue plasminogen activator, both of which may be important in the prevention of intravascular coagulation during low-flow states or circulatory stasis (292). Postmortem findings suggest that the adverse effects of aprotinin result from widespread intravascular thrombosis (285). Aprotinin and heparin act synergistically to elevate the activated clotting time (ACT), so there is risk of underheparinization if ACT alone is used for anticoagulation monitoring. The ACT is less artificially elevated with the kaolin than the celite test (293). It has been anecdotally recommended to maintain a celite ACT of more than 750 seconds and a kaolin ACT of more than 500 seconds when aprotinin is being used (297). There are no studies to determine the safe ACT levels when aprotinin is used in the setting of DHCA.

Westaby et al. reported thrombosis-related death and paradoxically greater incidence of bleeding and coagulation defects in patients who underwent ascending aortic surgery with DHCA and high-dose aprotinin (291,294). Sundt et al. reported a 65% incidence of postoperative renal dysfunction, a 25% hemodialysis requirement rate, and a 20% perioperative myocardial infarction rate in a small group of patients receiving high-dose aprotinin during aortic surgery with DHCA. The mortality rate was 35% in aprotinin-treated patients, compared with 5% in matched controls (285). That series was done before the distorting effects of aprotinin on celite ACT were recognized, suggesting that insufficient heparinization may have resulted in the widespread platelet-fibrin thrombi noted on autopsy. When a celite ACT of more than 750 seconds was maintained, there was no adverse effect on early survival among patients receiving a high-dose aprotinin regimen during thoracic aortic surgery with DHCA. However, transient postoperative renal dysfunction was still commonly observed in aprotinin-treated patients (295). Rooney et al. (296) recommended withholding aprotinin until the recommencement of bypass flow after the period of circulatory arrest. Using a loading dose of 280 mg given into the bypass pump, followed by a 70 mg/hour infusion, they did not observe a high incidence of renal dysfunction. Goldstein et al. (297) demonstrated no significant difference in the incidence of neurologic complications, myocardial infarction, or death among 24 aprotinin-treated patients who underwent complex aortic procedures and DHCA, compared with the control group. However, they also confirmed a higher incidence of postoperative renal dysfunction in the aprotinin-treated group. They maintained an ACT of greater than 500 with kaolin or 750 seconds with celite activators. Okita et al. (298) demonstrated unacceptable clotting in patients undergoing arch repair using DHCA who had kaolin ACT values greater than 500 seconds. They suggested that a kaolin ACT of 500 seconds was still not enough to prevent intravascular coagulation in aprotinin-treated patients. Therefore, a reliable measure of adequate anticoagulation in aprotinin-treated patients undergoing DHCA is still unavailable. At present the use of antifibrinolytic agents during DHCA varies among institutions. Some avoid aprotinin altogether and use EACA or tranexamic acid instead; others administer aprotinin after the reinstitution of bypass flow after the arrest period.

Acid-Base Management During Aortic Arch Surgery

Profound hypothermia with or without circulatory arrest is routinely used during repair of congenital heart defects in children (299) and in aortic arch procedures in adults (300). Hypothermia is the major strategy used to reduce ischemic injury during cardiac operations. Within limits, as brain temperature decreases its tolerance to ischemia increases. By reducing the metabolic rate, hypothermia slows the rate of high-energy phosphate depletion and development of intracellular acidosis during cerebral ischemia. In this way hypothermia delays or prevents neuronal energy failure and terminal membrane depolarization during periods of greatly reduced or absent blood flow. Multiple additional mechanisms contribute to the protective effects of hypothermia. These include the reduction in endothelial and neutrophil activation, decreased excitatory neurotransmitter release, and a decrease in the severity of the no-reflow phenomenon. Furthermore, hypothermia has important effects on pH by altering the dissociation constant of water and various metabolic intermediates. The pH of neutrality of water at 37°C is approximately 6.8, whereas at 20°C it is 7.0. Because there is an inverse relationship between temperature and gas solubility, hypothermia produces an apparent metabolic alkalosis by rendering CO_2 more soluble. Two strategies have been proposed for acid-base management during hypothermic CPB. In pH-stat method, carbon dioxide is added to the pump oxygenator during the cooling phase to maintain an Pa_{CO_2} of 40 mm Hg and a pH of 7.4 corrected to the patient's hypothermic temperature. In the alpha-stat method, Pa_{CO_2} is maintained at 40 mm Hg when the sample is measured at 37°C and is not corrected for the patient's temperature. Both strategies have theoretic advantages and disadvantages.

The alpha-stat strategy is based on the premise that maintaining a neutral pH that is appropriate to the temperature of the cell best preserves cellular function. This is achieved by allowing the pH to rise naturally with cooling so that it is approximately 7.70 when measured at 20°C and 7.4 when measured at 37°C. Alpha-stat management results in a constant ratio (alpha) of dissociated to nondissociated imidazole group of histidine, which is an essential component of the protein buffer system. Whole-body oxygen consumption was shown in one study to be greater with the alpha-stat than the pH-stat strategy, which may reflect a higher enzymatic activity level (301). On the other hand, the leftward shift in the oxyhemoglobin dissociation curve caused by alkalosis and hypothermia restricts tissue oxygen extraction at a time when areas of the brain may still be quite warm and have a high metabolic rate. The lower CBF and the leftward shift of the oxyhemoglobin dissociation curve could lead to cerebral hypoxia and inadequate brain cooling. This is reflected by a decrease in the cytochrome aa_3 signal noted by infrared spectroscopy during alpha-stat cooling.

The goal of pH-stat management is to overcome hypothermia-induced alkalosis by adding CO_2 to the circuit to maintain a temperature-corrected pH of 7.4. This results in a pH and Pa_{CO_2} profile, when corrected to patient temperature, that is unchanged from that seen at 37°C. The more acidotic pH-stat strategy shifts the oxyhemoglobin dissociation curve to the right, increasing the availability of oxygen at the tissue level and balancing the shift to the left caused by hypothermia. The relative acidosis produced by pH-stat management also serves as a stimulus for cerebral vasodilation, resulting in a 1.5- to 2-fold increase in CBF at 26°C, compared with alpha-stat management (302). The pH-stat–induced cerebral vasodilatation results in loss of cerebral perfusion pressure/blood flow autoregulation and loss of the normal CBF/$CMRO_2$ coupling. Under pH-stat conditions, CBF exceeds metabolic requirements (luxury perfusion) and varies in a direct linear manner with changes in cerebral perfusion pressure (303). Whether the pH-stat–induced increase in CBF is beneficial or harmful depends on the clinical setting. Excessive CBF increases the delivery of microemboli and macroemboli to the cerebral circulation and may result in cerebral edema and intracranial hypertension. In patients with cerebral vascular atherosclerotic disease, there is the theoretic concern of diverting blood away from ischemic area (by intracerebral steal). On the other hand, the higher CBF promotes better brain cooling and may be useful under situations of decreased cerebral perfusion (e.g., after circulatory arrest).

It has been demonstrated that pH-stat management produces cerebral hyperemia, uncoupling of CBF and metabolism, and loss of cerebral pressure/flow autoregulation, resulting in a CBF that is dependent on the cerebral perfusion pressure. The potential dangers of excessive CBF include cerebral edema, increased intracranial pressure, and the increased delivery of emboli to the cerebral circulation.

It is currently accepted that alpha-stat is preferable to pH-stat management during routine moderately hypothermic CPB because it preserves electrochemical neutrality and cerebral autoregulation. Because CBF remains appropriately coupled to cerebral metabolic demands, the potential dangers of luxury perfusion are avoided (260). Studies of continuous moderately hypothermic CPB in adults either demonstrated no important differences between pH-stat and alpha-stat management (304,305) or favored the alpha-stat strategy or even more alkaline strategies (301,306). Murkin et al. randomly assigned 316 patients undergoing continuous CPB at 26° to 28°C to either alpha-stat or pH-stat management (307). Overall, there was no difference in neurologic or neuropsychologic outcomes between groups. However, in the subgroup of patients undergoing CPB for longer than 90 minutes, those managed with alpha-stat had a lower incidence of neuropsychologic abnormalities at 2 months postoperatively than did those managed with pH-stat (27% versus 44%). Presumably the slight advantage of alpha-stat management during continuous CPB at moderate hypothermia results from the lower CBF and consequently less cerebral embolization compared with the pH-stat technique.

Whereas several studies have shown no important difference in neurologic outcome between alpha-stat and pH-stat management of routine CPB with moderate hypothermia, blood gas management during DHCA is a more complicated and controversial issue. There is growing evidence that acid-base management during DHCA may have a significant impact on cerebral metabolic preservation and neurologic outcome and that pH-stat may be preferable to alpha-stat management, especially during the cooling phase of CPB before DHCA. Skaryak et al. studied 1-week-old piglets cooled to either 14° or 18°C during CPB and DHCA with pH or alpha-stat management (308). They measured CBF and $CMRO_2$ in conditions of normothermic bypass, before circulatory arrest, and after rewarming. $CMRO_2$ was lower at 14° than at 18°C, and the reduction in $CMRO_2$ was better sustained by pH-stat than by alpha-stat management to 14°C. Maintaining the pH-stat strategy throughout the bypass period caused profound acidosis with very low arterial and sagittal sinus pH and markedly increased Pa_{CO_2} values. They devised a switch strategy, using pH-stat during cooling and alpha-stat during maintenance of hypothermia and rewarming in an attempt to prevent excessive lowering of cerebral intracellular pH and impairment of intracellular enzyme function.

Watanabe et al. showed that recovery of brain pH and

PO_2 after DHCA was more complete in animals receiving alpha-stat compared with pH-stat management (309). In contrast, laboratory investigations in an immature piglet model demonstrated more rapid recovery of cerebral high-energy phosphate stores and intracellular pH with the pH-stat strategy after 1 hour of DHCA (310,311). Hiramatsu et al. demonstrated more rapid recovery of cerebral ATP levels when the pH-stat strategy was used both before and after DHCA (311). They compared cooling/rewarming strategies of pH/pH, alpha/alpha, pH/alpha, and alpha/pH for 1 hour of circulatory arrest. Cerebral high-energy phosphates and intracellular pH were measured by magnetic resonance spectroscopy, and CBF was measured with microspheres. CBF was greater and cytochrome aa_3 values were less reduced when pH-stat was used during cooling. Near-infrared spectroscopy demonstrated a greater reduction of cytochrome aa_3 values with alpha-stat cooling. During rewarming, cerebral intracellular pH recovered faster with the pH/pH strategy. Cerebral intracellular pH (pHi) continued to decrease during the first 40 minutes of warm reperfusion only when alpha-stat was applied during both the cooling and rewarming phases. Global and regional CBF values were greater when pH-stat was used for rewarming, regardless of the method used during cooling. Despite the marked difference in recovery rates of high-energy phosphates, no demonstrable differences in $CMRO_2$ or in the cerebral metabolic rate for glucose were apparent with the various cooling/rewarming strategies. It was shown in a piglet model that oxygen and glucose consumption are insensitive end points of recovery after DHCA (312,313).

Although Hiramatsu et al. did not correlate acute cerebral metabolic findings with neurologic outcome, others have reported a close relation between cerebral ATP stores and EEG recovery after circulatory arrest (314). Alkaline pH immediately before DHCA was shown to correlate with a delay in recovery of SSEPs (315). It has been shown that EEG activity and SSEPs in the period after CA are important indicators of cerebral function. Cortical evoked potentials may require several hours to return to normal, whereas the EEG and brain stem AEPs return to normal quickly on rewarming (315). Several investigators have reported a close correlation between EEG recovery and cerebral ATP stores. The reappearance latency of the EEG has been shown to correlate with the duration of arrest. The latency time for return of EEG activity was shown to correlate with histologic changes in piglets recovering from DHCA at 20°C. A prolonged recovery time for SSEPs was observed after DHCA in infants who had subsequently developed seizures (315). A more alkaline pH (alpha-stat) immediately before DHCA correlated with a delay in the recovery of SSEPs (315). A prospective clinical study of circulatory arrest in neonates revealed a correlation between longer EEG recovery time after DHCA and worse developmental outcome at 1 year of age (319).

Kirshbom et al. (316) observed no differences in recovery of CBF and $CMRO_2$ after DHCA between alpha-stat and pH-stat management in piglets. However, in animals with systemic-to-pulmonary collaterals, recovery was slightly better with pH-stat. Systemic-to-pulmonary collaterals (which are common in children with cyanotic heart disease) increase the risk of perioperative neurologic injuries by diverting blood away from the cerebral circulation, resulting in inadequate brain cooling (317). The hypercarbia of pH-stat management produces concurrent cerebral vasodilatation and pulmonary vasoconstriction, resulting in higher CBF and more effective brain cooling.

In a small retrospective study, cognitive developmental outcome in infants undergoing repair of transposition of the great arteries with DHCA was worse with alpha-stat than with pH-stat management (318). A shorter duration of cooling was also associated with worse neurologic and developmental outcome after DHCA (319). Jonas et al. proposed that the higher CBF associated with pH-stat management resulted in better cerebral cooling and hence better protection (318). An alternative explanation is that pH-stat management has some neuroprotective effect in itself. In animal studies, pH-stat management resulted in $CMRO_2$ levels that were 40% lower than those achieved with alpha-stat at equal degrees of hypothermia (308,320). The reduction in $CMRO_2$ may be caused by suppression of cerebral metabolism by the greater $PaCO_2$ of pH-stat management. As discussed earlier, most enzymatic reactions are pH dependent and many enzymes have pH optima that follow the predictions of the alpha-stat theory. The relatively acidic intracellular environment induced by the pH-stat strategy could decrease enzyme reaction rates, ATP consumption, and consequently $CMRO_2$. It is conceivable that the additional pH-stat–induced $CMRO_2$ reduction may further delay the onset of terminal membrane depolarization and thereby confer an extra measure of brain protection beyond that provided by hypothermia. Although membrane depolarization is the first step in the ischemic cascade, many subsequent events play critical roles in determining the final extent of neurologic injury. These include calcium influx, excitatory neurotransmitter release, and reperfusion injury. Whether hypothermic acid-base management alters any of these reactions (and consequently neurologic outcome) in the setting of complete global cerebral ischemia (e.g., DHCA) is not yet clear.

Several studies suggest that, independent of temperature and CBF changes, pH-stat management and hypercarbia decrease $CMRO_2$ and thereby increase the degree of metabolic suppression produced by profound hypothermia. Hindman et al. reported that pH-stat management reduced $CMRO_2$ by an additional 35% to 40% compared with alpha-stat during steady-state CPB at 17°C in rabbits (321). In their experiment, systemic arterial pressure, hemispheric CBF, and $CMRO_2$ were all greater with the alpha-stat than with the pH-stat strategy. The finding that alpha-stat management in animals resulted in greater CBF was not consistent with the known cerebral vasodilatory effect of hypercarbia and acidosis. It has been clearly demonstrated that pH-stat results in a higher CBF, compared with alpha-stat, at moderate hypothermia (25° to 27°C) in humans (322) and in animals (323). However, at profound hypothermia, cerebral pressure/flow autoregulation appears to be completely inhibited so that CBF varies directly with arterial blood pressure (324,325). Therefore, the higher CBF obtained with alpha-stat management in the Hindman study most likely resulted from the higher perfusion pressures achieved with that technique. When the arterial pressure and hence the CBF were equalized between the two groups with the use of vasoactive drugs, the $CMRO_2$ was lower in the animals treated with pH-stat than in those treated with alpha-stat. The researchers concluded that pH-stat–induced $CMRO_2$ reduction resulted from the additional suppression of cerebral metabolism by the greater $Pa{CO_2}$ of the pH-stat strategy. They postulated that pH-stat management creates a relatively acidic intracellular environment that decreases enzyme reaction rates, ATP consumption, and consequently $CMRO_2$. This process has been proposed as the mechanism by which hibernating species, which follow a pH-stat strategy, reduce oxygen consumption in nonessential organs to the lowest possible values.

Animal and human studies have demonstrated an alkaline shift in cerebral pHi with both alpha-stat and pH-stat cooling (312,326). Despite the extracellular acidosis associated with pH-stat and the high diffusability of CO_2 across cell membranes, pHi still showed an alkaline shift with pH-stat management, albeit to a lesser degree than with alpha-stat management (326,327). This is consistent with the important hypothesis proposed by Swain et al. that brain pHi is actively regulated to maintain an alpha-stat intracellular environment independent of blood pH (327). This effect decreases the rationale for the use of alpha-stat management: the cerebral intracellular enzyme system will be exposed to an alpha-stat environment anyway, regardless of the extracellular milieu during hypothermia. Therefore, it appears that preservation of intracellular enzyme function is not an important mechanism distinguishing the two pH management strategies in terms of subsequent recovery of cerebral function after circulatory arrest. After the onset of arrest, pHi decreases rapidly to less than 7.0. During pH-stat rewarming, the pHi recovers rapidly toward baseline, whereas alpha-stat reperfusion is associated with a further decrease in pHi followed by slow recovery to baseline. This observation suggests less reperfusion injury with pH-stat than with alpha-stat (328). The more acidic blood and extracellular fluid pH values associated with pH-stat may decrease reperfusion injury. Extracellular acidosis (pH 6.1 to 6.9) has been shown to improve cell survival in anoxic energy-depleted hepatocytes (329). Likewise, cell culture studies of neuronal hypoxia have shown reduced calcium influx and improved cell survival in the presence of a higher extracellular hydrogen ion concentration and a more acidic extracellular pH (330,331). Similar findings have been reported in studies of myocardial protection, where transient acidotic reperfusion (pH 6.4 to 6.8) was reported to attenuate reperfusion injury in the myocardium. The main mechanism seems to be inhibition of calcium influx through pH-dependent calcium channels during early reperfusion (332). Extracellular acidosis has also been shown to reduce excitatory neurotransmitter mediated neuronal toxicity by blocking *N*-methyl D-aspartate (NMDA) receptor–mediated calcium influx (333, 334).

In summary, the improved cerebral protection with pH-stat management results from several salutary effects, including (a) improved oxygen delivery due to an acidosis-related rightward shift of the oxyhemoglobin dissociation curve, (b) improved extent and homogeneity of brain cooling due to the higher CBF, (c) a decrease in reperfusion injury mediated by the more acidic blood and extracellular fluid pH, and (d) more rapid recovery of cerebral high-energy phosphate stores and pHi. *Therefore, contrary to earlier beliefs, the theoretic advantage of that alpha-stat strategy in providing a better milieu for cellular function may not hold true during DHCA arrest. The pH-stat strategy appears to provide better protection against cerebral ischemia during and immediately after DHCA* (311,327).

Aneurysms of the Descending Thoracic and Thoracoabdominal Aorta

Descending thoracic aneurysms start distal to the origin of the left subclavian artery. They can involve varying parts of the descending thoracic aorta and may extend to involve parts or all of the abdominal aorta. Crawford (335) proposed a classification for thoracoabdominal aortic aneurysms (TAAA), as shown in Fig. 27-24. Anesthetic management of these patients is extremely challenging because of the significant hemodynamic changes associated with the operation, patient positioning, OLV, and frequent coexisting cardiovascular disease, as well as the risk of spinal cord, renal, and amesenteric ischemic injuries. In addition, the anesthesiologist must be prepared for rapid and massive blood loss and coagulopathy.

Patient Positioning

The patient is positioned in the right lateral decubitus position. An axillary roll is placed under the patient's upper chest to prevent compression of the brachial neurovascular bundle. The left arm is placed in a splint to aid in brachial plexus protection (Fig. 27-25). Padding of the right knee helps to prevent compression of the peroneal nerve and subsequent foot drop. All bony prominences likewise should be padded to prevent neural compression.

Anesthetic Technique

Induction is usually performed by slow administration of a sleep dose of an intravenous anesthetic agent such as etomi-

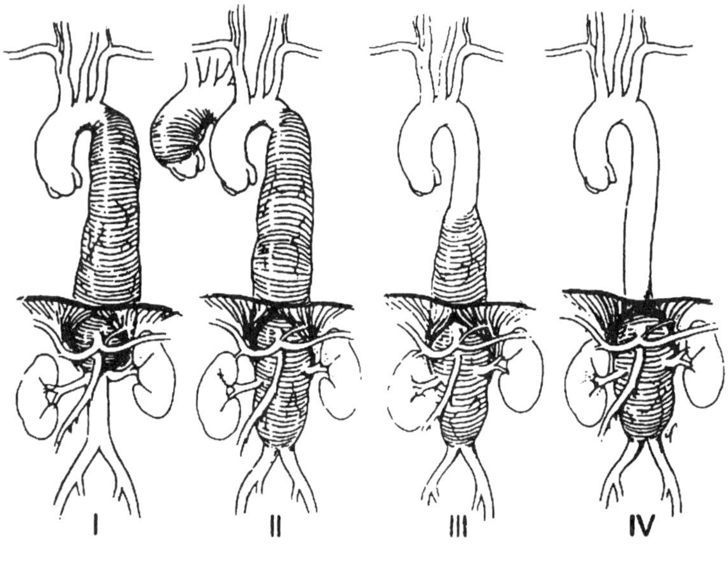

FIGURE 27-24. Drawing illustrating the Crawford classification of thoracoabdominal aortic aneurysms according to the extent of involvement of the thoracoabdominal aorta. Crawford type I, most or all of descending thoracic aorta, suprarenal abdominal aorta; type II, most or all of descending thoracic aorta, most or all of abdominal aorta; type III, distal descending thoracic aorta, varying segments of abdominal aorta including the renal and visceral arteries; type IV, most or all of abdominal aorta. (From Crawford ES, Coselli JS. Thoracoabdominal aneurysm surgery. *Semin Thorac Cardiovasc Surg* 1991;3:300, with permission; and Kuchoukos NT, Rokkas CK. Descending thoracic and thoracoabdominal aortic surgery for aneurysm or dissection: how do we minimize the risk of spinal cord injury? *Semin Thorac Cardiovasc Surg* 1993;5:47, with permission.)

date, midazolam, propofol, or thiopental followed by a neuromuscular blocking drug. Fentanyl or sufentanil is then added to blunt the hemodynamic response to laryngoscopy and intubation. This sequence avoids opioid-induced chest wall rigidity, which may cause hypercarbia and trigger sympathetically mediated hypertension and tachycardia (336). Maintenance of anesthesia is usually with inhalation agents and/or opioid infusions as determined by the cardiopulmonary and anesthetic/analgesic properties of these agents and the desired pharmacologic effect. Enflurane has been shown to increase CSF production and decrease CSF absorption and theoretically should be avoided to maximize spinal cord perfusion pressure (SCPP) (336).

Controversy exists regarding the use of epidural analgesia for surgery on the descending thoracic aorta. Combined general and epidural anesthesia has been described for abdominal aortic and thoracic surgery. The purported benefits of the combined technique include not only a decrease in postoperative pain but also reductions in adrenocortical stress response, protein catabolism, hypercoagulable state, immunosuppression, and pulmonary and myocardial morbidity. Epidural anesthesia/analgesia has also been shown to improve graft patency in peripheral vascular procedures (336). In a small, noncontrolled, nonrandomized study, epidural anesthesia blunted the increase in systemic vascular resistance and blood pressure associated with proximal aortic cross-clamping in patients undergoing descending thoracic and thoracoabdominal aneurysm repairs (337). One major concern about the use of epidural blockade relates to the potential risk of epidural hematoma in patients in whom anticoagulation is to be initiated. Several studies have indicated that the risk of epidural hematoma is minimal in patients receiving low doses of heparin during major vascular surgery. The American Society of Regional Anesthesia has published a consensus statement for the use of neuroaxial blockade in association with anticoagulation (*Regional Anes-*

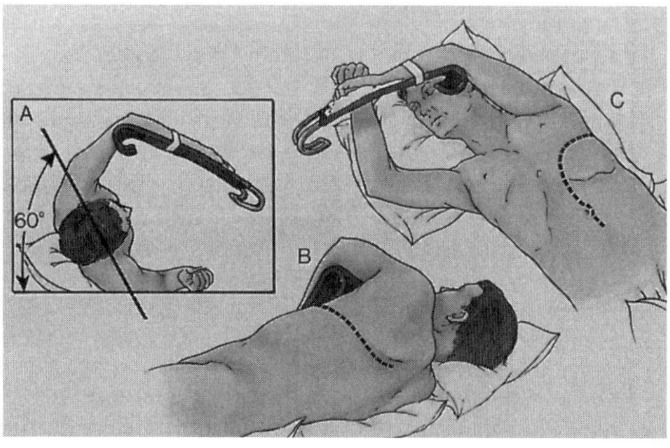

FIGURE 27-25. Positioning of the patient. **A:** The lateral position maintained at a 60° angle. **B:** A sixth intercostal incision. **C:** The incision extends across the costal arch as an upper abdominal incision. The left arm is supported on a plane. (From Crawford ES, Crawford J. *Disease of the aorta.* Baltimore: Williams & Wilkins, 1984:84, with permission.)

thesia and Pain Medicine 1998;23[Suppl], www.asra.com). Epidural anesthesia was associated with more pronounced intraoperative hypotension, especially after cross-clamp release in patients undergoing thoracic aortic repair. Well-controlled prospective, randomized trials are needed to substantiate the risks and benefits of combined epidural-general anesthesia compared with general anesthesia alone for thoracic aortic surgery. At our institution, we usually place a midthoracic epidural catheter before the induction of general anesthesia in patients undergoing elective thoracic aortic surgery. To avoid excessive sympathectomy-mediated intraoperative hypotension, we usually administer only the test dose of 3 to 5 mL of 1.5% lidocaine with 1:200,000 epinephrine together with an appropriate dose of a preservative-free morphine or fentanyl preparation before anesthesia induction. Before closure of the wound, after hemodynamic stability has been restored after aortic unclamping, we start an epidural infusion of a mixture of local anesthetic (bupivacaine or ropivacaine) plus an opioid (morphine, hydromorphine, or fentanyl). After the conclusion of surgery, the patient is transferred to the intensive care unit, intubated, and mechanically ventilated. Additional doses of intravenous sedative-hypnotics such as midazolam or diazepam and opioids are usually required after discontinuation of the volatile agents.

One-Lung Ventilation

During repair of the descending thoracic aorta a DLT is extremely helpful in providing OLV for several reasons: (a) it provides better visualization of the surgical field; (b) it reduces retraction and trauma to the left lung; (c) should intrapulmonary hemorrhage or rupture of the aneurysm into the left bronchus occur, the down (right) lung could be isolated and protected; and (d) it provides a quieter, more accessible surgical field, which helps speed the operation and decrease aortic cross-clamping time, thereby decreasing the likelihood of spinal cord and visceral ischemic injury.

Placement of a DLT in a patient with a descending thoracic aneurysm requires consideration of several clinical problems. Left endobronchial intubation using a left-sided DLT eliminates the concern about inadequate right upper lobe ventilation that is commonly seen if a right DLT tube is used. However, placement of a left-sided DLT can be difficult because of anatomic displacement of the left main bronchus by the aneurysm. In addition, there have been rare case reports of fatal hemorrhage occurring when a left-sided tube was forcefully placed into an aneurysm eroding into the left main stem bronchus. It is therefore preferable to place the left DLT under direct vision, using the fiberoptic bronchoscope as a stylet to ensure that the aneurysm has not narrowed or eroded the bronchus. After the DLT has been positioned, its proper location is confirmed by looking down the tracheal lumen and visualizing the upper edge of the endobronchial cuff at the carina.

When placement of a left DLT is not possible, other options include (a) the use of a single-lumen endotracheal tube and a left bronchial blocker or (b) the use of a right-sided endobronchial tube. Correct placement and maintenance of the right DLT is more difficult and requires the use of a fiberoptic bronchoscope to properly position the right upper lobe bronchus. After the initiation of OLV, PaO_2 may decrease rapidly and may require the application of CPAP to the upper lung. CPAP to the lung is the most effective means of maintaining arterial oxygenation. Careful observation of arterial oxygen saturation by pulse oximetry and frequent measurement of arterial blood gas levels are required during this phase of the operation (338). PEEP to the lower lung has variable results (339). PEEP to the dependent lung may improve PaO_2 if it increases the functional residual capacity of the down lung. On the other hand, if dependent-lung PEEP causes significant redistribution of blood flow to the upper lung, then PaO_2 will not improve and may actually decrease (338,340). Tidal volumes should be 8 to 12 mL/kg at the initiation of OLV, and the respiratory rate should be adjusted to maintain normocapnea. Inhalational anesthetic agents cause only slight inhibition of hypoxic pulmonary vasoconstriction (HPV) and usually do not result in clinically significant decreases in PaO_2 during OLV (340,341). Vasodilating agents that may be used to control hypertension, such as nitroglycerin and sodium nitroprusside, are potent inhibitors of HPV and can exacerbate hypoxemia during OLV (340). Whenever these agents are introduced or their infusion rates are changed during OLV, it is important to reassess the adequacy of arterial oxygenation. At the end of the procedure the DLT should be changed, if possible, to a single-lumen tube. However, marked facial and airway edema may be present after repair of a descending thoracic aneurysm, making this task very difficult or even impossible. If severe edema is present, the DLT should be left in place with the bronchial cuff deflated until the swelling resolves over the first or second postoperative day.

Pathophysiology of Aortic Cross-Clamping

Hemodynamic Effects

Clamping of the aorta causes hypertension in the proximal segment and hypotension in the distal segment. The degree of hypertension caused by the application of an aortic cross-clamp depends on the location of the clamp, the degree of collateralization, and the preocclusion aortic flow. Aortic clamping above a thoracic coarctation may result in no pressure changes proximal or distal to the clamp because of the presence of fully developed collateral flow. In the case of a thoracic aortic aneurysm of atherosclerotic origin where collateralization is minimal, a significant increase in blood pressure should be expected with application of the cross-clamp. Unlike clamping below the renal arteries, which usually produces only a small increase in blood pressure, supraceliac occlusion of the aorta can result in significant in-

TABLE 27-9. HEMODYNAMIC RESPONSE (MEAN ± STANDARD ERROR) TO AORTIC CLAMPING AND TO DECOMPRESSION WITH A TEMPORARY SHUNT IN EIGHT PATIENTS

Variable	Baseline (Period I)	Aorta Clamped (Period II)	Shunt Opened (Period III)
MAP (mm Hg)	90.3 ± 4.0	122.1 ± 4.1[a]	86.4 ± 4.4
MPAP (mm Hg)	21.3 ± 2.1	30.5 ± 3.1	19.9 ± 1.7
CVP (mm Hg)	7.0 ± 0.5	11.5 ± 2.2[a]	7.8 ± 1.5
PCWP (mm Hg)	9.6 ± 1.9	17.6 ± 2.4[a]	10.4 ± 1.9
CI (L/min/sq m)	2.66 ± 0.34	1.88 ± 0.25[a]	2.18 ± 0.24[a]
HR (beats/min)	85.2 ± 7.6	89.9 ± 11.8	86.6 ± 4.5
SVI (ml/beats/sq m)	34.0 ± 6.4	23.0 ± 3.8	26.0 ± 3.0
LVSWI (g. m/sq m)	35.6 ± 4.9	31.8 ± 4.6	25.8 ± 2.4[a]

Note: MAP, mean arterial pressure; MPAP, mean pulmonary arterial pressure; CVP, central venous pressure; PCWP, pulmonary capillary wedge pressure; HR, heart rate; SVI, stroke volume index; LVSWI, left ventricular stroke work index.
[a] Significant different from period I (baseline) value ($p < .05$).
Source: Nugent M, Oliver WC, Roseberg JN. Anesthesia for thoracic aortic surgery. In: Tarhan S, ed. *Cardiovascular anesthesia and prospective care.* Chicago: Year Book Medical Publishers, 1989, with permission.

creases in systemic vascular resistance, significant proximal hypertension, and increased myocardial systolic wall stress. Mean arterial pressure usually increases by approximately 40% after cross-clamping of the descending thoracic aorta. Arterial pressure below the cross-clamp decreases to approximately 15% of the values before cross-clamping, with distal aortic pressures ranging between 11 and 30 mm Hg. Further decreases of 30% to 60% in distal aortic pressures have been reported when nitroprusside is administered to return the proximal mean arterial pressure to the pre-cross-clamp levels (342,343). Central venous pressure usually increases slightly (by approximately 2 to 4 mm Hg), probably because of autotransfusion of blood from the lower extremities. Left atrial and pulmonary wedge pressures also have been reported to show a variable increase of 2 to 12 mm Hg with aortic cross-clamping (Table 27-9). These changes may be attenuated by the use of a temporary shunt or a left atrial-to-femoral bypass flow, as discussed later. TEE is helpful during thoracic surgery to monitor ventricular preload, contractile function, and valvular function and to detect RWMAs that may indicate myocardial ischemia.

In laboratory models, cross-clamping of the descending thoracic aorta was shown to increase coronary blood flow by approximately 40% (343,344). It was reported that cross-clamping of the descending thoracic aorta in dogs with normal coronary arteries did not alter the ratio of endocardial-to-epicardial blood flow and did not result in depletion of myocardial high-energy phosphates (343,344). This, however, may not be the case in patients with significant concomitant CAD.

The effect of cross-clamping of the descending thoracic aorta on venous return and CO has been reported to be variable. Normally, 22% of the CO goes to the renal circulation and 30% goes to the superior mesenteric and celiac trunks. With the application of a supraceliac or descending thoracic aortic vascular resistance, venous return and CO usually are not immediately affected, and blood pressure suddenly rises. Venous return is initially unimpeded and may actually initially increase with the application of the cross-clamp. Some animal studies and clinical reports have actually reported an increase in CO after cross-clamping of the thoracic aorta (345). This may be caused by the autotransfusion of volume from below the clamp into the active circulation. After arterial inflow suddenly stops at the time of aortic occlusion, the capacitance vessels below the clamp continue to discharge their contents into the right atrium until their pressure is equal to the right atrial pressure. Provided that the left ventricle is of good contractile function and capable of performing against the elevated afterload, CO may temporarily increase. Other mechanisms that have been suggested to explain the initial increase in CO include an aortic cardiac reflex causing an increase in contractility (346) and elimination of the slow-time-constant vascular beds (splanchnic circulation) from the circulation (345).

In order to maintain contractility and CO in the face of the increased afterload, the left ventricle dilates to increase its end-diastolic fiber length (i.e., the Starling mechanism and preload reserve are called upon). Therefore there is an increase in end-diastolic and end-systolic volumes and a decrease in ejection fraction (Table 27-10). If the left ventricle is of good compliance, a proportional increase in pulmonary capillary wedge pressure (PCWP) may not be seen. The increase in left ventricular end-diastolic dimensions can be seen more accurately with the use TEE. RWMAs are frequently seen on TEE after application of the aortic cross-clamp. These may reflect changes in myocardial function caused by increased afterload, or they may reflect myocardial ischemia caused by ventricular dilatation and decreased subendocardial blood flow. In patients with impaired left ven-

TABLE 27-10. EFFECT OF LEVEL OF AORTIC OCCLUSION ON CARDIOVASCULAR VARIABLES DURING VASCULAR SURGERY (% CHANGE)

	Level of Occlusion		
Variable	Supraceliac	Infraceliac-Suprarenal	Infrarenal
Mean arterial blood pressure	54	5[a]	2[a]
Pulmonary capillary wedge pressure	38	10[a]	0[a]
End-diastolic area	28	2[a]	9[a]
End-systolic area	69	10[a]	11[a]
Ejection area	−38	−10[a]	−3[a]
Abnormal wall motion (% of patients)	92	33	0
New myocardial infarction	8	0	0

[a] Significantly different ($p < .05$) from group undergoing aortic occlusion at the supraceliac level.
Source: Roizen MF. Anesthesia goals for surgery to relieve or prevent visceral ischemia. In: Roizen MF, ed. *Anesthesia for vascular surgery.* New York: Churchill Livingstone, 1990:177, with permission.

tricular function, hemodynamic decompensation may occur after occlusion of the thoracic aorta, resulting in severe left ventricular dilation and failure, significant increases in PCWP, and the appearance of V waves on the wedge tracing, indicative of acute functional mitral regurgitation. Acute episodes of ventricular failure can be treated with preload and afterload reduction. Shunt bypass flow can be instituted or increased. The increase in proximal aortic pressure stimulates the baroreceptors, resulting in reflex feedback slowing of the heart rate, decreased contractility, and peripheral vasodilatation in an attempt to limit the degree of rise in the blood pressure.

Although some reports describe an increase in CO in animals and humans with cross-clamping of the thoracic aorta, many previous studies have shown a decrease in CO with aortic occlusion (347). Likely explanations for the discrepancy in these results might be differences in intrinsic myocardial function, the efficacy of homeostatic reflex control mechanisms, the type of background anesthesia, and differences in the administration of vasodilators in these different reports. In clinical practice, the response of each patient is likely to depend on the interaction of these multiple factors.

Myocardial Effects

In the absence of impaired contractility or CAD, the heart can well tolerate the increased afterload. Left ventricular end-diastolic pressure and volume increase (preload reserve mechanism). Coronary perfusion pressure also increases. Myocardial ischemia or pump failure usually does not occur in isolated ventricle experiments in healthy hearts. However, serious deterioration of pump function could occur if the high afterload is superimposed on a diseased myocardium. In addition, myocardial ischemia could be precipitated during clamping if afterload elevation occurs in the presence of significant coronary artery stenosis (347). The high intracavitary pressures in conjunction with impaired coronary flow result in significantly decreased subendocardial blood flow. Roizen et al. found new and worsening RWMAs more frequently during supraceliac than during suprarenal or infrarenal aortic occlusion. These abnormalities did not resolve completely with moderation of the loading conditions of the ventricle (347).

Metabolic Changes

Cross-clamping of the descending thoracic aorta results in decreased total body oxidative metabolism and oxygen consumption as well as conversion to anaerobic metabolism by the ischemic body mass distal to the cross-clamp. Supraceliac cross-clamping of the aorta causes a 55% reduction in total-body oxygen consumption (348). Changes in mixed venous oxygen saturation depend on the therapeutic modality used to control the blood pressure. Arteriolar dilators tend to result in overperfused tissues proximal to the cross-clamp and increased mixed venous oxygen saturation. Nitroglycerin and preload reduction techniques, on the other hand, tend to maintain oxygen extraction ratio and mixed venous saturation at their levels before cross-clamping (349).

Cross-clamping of the descending thoracic aorta without the use of a shunt produces hypoperfusion and anaerobic metabolism in the splanchnic viscera and the lower extremity. In addition, the exclusion of the liver and kidneys from the circulation greatly attenuates the elimination of lactic acid. Lactate concentration rises promptly and progressively during high thoracic cross-clamping, presumably reaching the proximal circulation by way of collaterals (350). We recommend a continuous infusion of sodium bicarbonate at the rate of 0.2 to 0.3 mEq/kg/minute or 1.2 to 1.8 mEq/kg/hour throughout the period of aortic cross-clamping (351).

Unclamping of the Thoracic Aorta

The most consistent observation on release of the cross-clamp is an acute fall in systemic blood pressure. This is caused mostly by a decrease in SVR and a reactive hyperemia in the previously ischemic vascular beds. Whereas the release of an infrarenal aortic cross-clamp usually produces a modest decrease in blood pressure, the release of a supraceliac cross-clamp can result in profound hypotension. Before unclamping, vasodilators should be discontinued and intravascular volume should be increased. Transient vasopressor support is frequently required. Pulmonary capillary wedge pressure should be increased to about 2 to 4 mm Hg above the baseline value. Acidosis may contribute to hypotension by producing myocardial depression and systemic vasodilation. The level of vasoactive intestinal peptide measured in mixed venous blood doubles with reperfusion of the splanchnic organs after supraceliac cross-clamp release (349) and could contribute to hypotension by causing peripheral arterial vasodilation.

Total-body oxygen consumption increases with unclamping as tissues return to aerobic metabolism. Mixed venous oxygen saturation shows an abrupt decrease within minutes after unclamping but rapidly returns to control values (Fig. 27-26). Carbon dioxide is elevated in arterial and venous blood within moments of unclamping. This rapid increase is caused by the buffering of lactic acid and other organic acids that are washed out from the distal circulation after reperfusion. Ventilation should be increased before unclamping to eliminate the excess CO_2 load. Bolus administration of sodium bicarbonate at this stage can produce further increases in Pa_{CO_2} and worsening of intracellular acidosis. That is why it is preferable to administer bicarbonate gradually by an infusion during the entire period of cross-clamping rather than as a bolus injection after unclamping. Unclamping of the descending thoracic aorta after 45 minutes of occlusion results in a 4 mmol/L increase in serum lactate concentration that usually returns rapidly to normal after complete restoration of hepatic and renal blood flow (350). It is uncommon for significant lactate elevations to persist into the postoperative period unless hepatic and intestinal ischemic injury has occurred. Partial bypass and shunt techniques maintain near-adequate perfusion of most tissues below the cross-clamp and significantly reduce lactic acid production and accumulation.

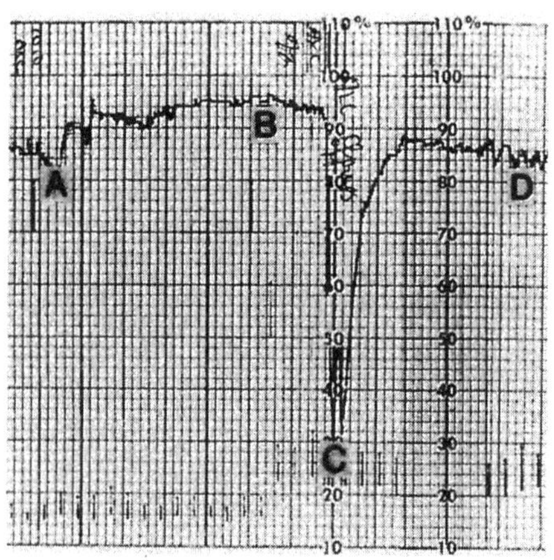

FIGURE 27-26. Continuous recording of mixed venous oxygen saturation from an oximetric pulmonary artery catheter during thoracoabdominal aortic aneurysm surgery. **A:** Aortic clamp applied. Oxygen saturation is 85% before clamping. **B:** Oxygen saturation increases to 96% in the patient during cross-clamping. **C:** Saturation falls to 30% transiently during unclamping. **D:** Return to preclamp values. (From Beattie C, Frank SM. Anesthesia for major vascular surgery. In: Rogers MC, Tinker JH, Covino BG, et al., eds. *Principles and practice of anesthesiology.* St. Louis: Mosby–Year Book, 1993:1939, with permission.)

Pharmacologic Management of the Period of Aortic Cross-Clamping

When the simple clamp-and-sew technique is employed without the use of temporary shunts or partial bypass techniques, significant pharmacologic interventions are necessary to treat proximal arterial hypertension and to protect the myocardium. Vasodilators, usually sodium nitroprusside, are routinely used to control proximal hypertension (352,353). Arterial vasodilators result in relative overperfusion of the proximal organs and exceedingly low pressures distal to the lowest clamp. This may contribute to the occurrence of spinal cord injury. Nitroprusside and other vasodilators should therefore be used with extreme caution. Because the distal half of the body is unavailable for oxidative metabolism, CO and oxygen delivery do not need to be maintained at the preclamp level. Interventions that would reduce CO therefore seem appropriate (354). Nitroglycerin is helpful in reducing preload and cardiac filling pressures. This limits ventricular dilatation and wall tension, which tend to increase in response to cross-clamping. Nitroglycerin alone is usually not sufficient to control proximal arterial hypertension during descending thoracic aortic cross-clamping; it is best used in combination with nitroprusside and deepening levels of anesthesia (355). Isoflurane, which mildly depresses contractility and causes vasodilatation of both resistance and capacitance vessels, has been safely used for anesthesia and blood pressure control in patients with good myocardial function undergoing thoracic aneurysm repair (356). Isoflurane-induced coronary steal is usually not of clinical concern. In the presence of a hyperdynamic state and good CO, an esmolol infusion can also be useful in reducing contractility, decreasing CO, and controlling proximal arterial pressure. It has the advantage of being short-acting, so that its effects do not persist after unclamping of the aorta. It should be carefully titrated to avoid inducing left ventricular decompensation and failure in the setting of a significantly increased afterload, especially in patients with impaired left ventricular function.

Before clamping of the aorta, it is helpful to keep the patient in a slightly hypovolemic state to help decrease the extent of arterial hypertension. Shortly before cross-clamp application, vasodilator therapy is started through a dedicated central line. During the period of cross-clamping, intravascular volume must be maintained and replenished with the use of crystalloids, colloids, and blood transfusions in order to raise the PCWP to above its baseline status by approximately 2 to 4 mm Hg. Because a large part of the vascular tree is excluded from the circulation, blood loss can be considerable during cross-clamping without the onset of hypotension and tachycardia. Observation of the surgical field is therefore of extreme importance. Aggressive fluid replacement should take into account the insensible surgical losses caused by exposure of the abdominal contents. Urine output ceases during supraceliac aortic cross-clamping and therefore is not a helpful guide in directing fluid therapy during that period.

Before unclamping, the infusions of vasodilator agents should be discontinued and the level of anesthesia slightly decreased. Ventilation should be increased in anticipation of an increased acid load from the distal circulation. Vasopressor substances, including phenylephrine hydrochloride (Neo-Synephrine) and dopamine, should be available to treat declamping hypotension. Even though each patient should be treated individually, the usual aim is to have a hematocrit of 28% to 32% at the end of surgery. Because of the frequently present concomitant CAD in these patients and the risk of spinal cord and splanchnic ischemia, lower hematocrit levels may cause inadequate oxygen delivery to vital organs. Persistent hypotension usually indicates hypovolemia. Blood volume replacement should be guided by monitoring of filling pressures and CO and by TEE. Other causes include myocardial dysfunction, hypocalcemia, acidosis, and persistent occult bleeding. If necessary, the surgeon can partially or totally reclamp the aorta until appropriate therapy is instituted.

Mechanical Methods to Protect the Myocardium

Five surgical techniques can be used to control upper- and lower-body blood flow during resection of a descending thoracic aneurysm: (a) simple aortic cross-clamping, (b) heparin-coated passive shunts, (c) centrifugal pump bypass flow, (d) partial CPB, and (e) DHCA. The goals for the use of distal aortic perfusion techniques include attenuation of proximal hypertension, reduction in myocardial wall stress, perfusion to the organs below the cross-clamp, prevention of metabolic acidosis, prevention of severe hypotension with aortic unclamping, and perhaps reduction of the incidence of paraplegia and renal insufficiency. There are no established criteria for the selection of one technique over another. Cross-clamping of the descending thoracic aorta produces substantial changes in ejection fraction, cardiac filling pressures, and volumes. Proximal mean arterial pressure and cardiac filling pressures increase while CO and ejection fraction decrease (357). Myocardial wall stress and oxygen consumption are substantially increased, which may be detrimental in patients with CAD. The use of distal perfusion stabilizes hemodynamics during and after cross-clamping, which may prevent myocardial ischemia and other cardiovascular complications, especially in patients with CAD or impaired ventricular function. Despite considerable research, controversy still exists about the value of distal perfusion adjuncts in reducing the incidence of renal failure, paraplegia, or cardiovascular complications (358, 359). Livesay et al. reported no reduction in the risks of TAAA repair with the use of distal perfusion (360). Similarly, in a large review of more than 1,500 patients, Svensson et al. failed to demonstrate improvement in outcome with the use of passive shunts or active bypass techniques (361). Cooley suggested that the risks of distal perfusion may be greater than simple aortic cross-clamping (362). Schepens et al. reported no improvement in 2- or 5-year survival after TAAA repair using left-sided heart bypass compared with simple cross-clamping (363). In their extensive experience, Crawford et al. reported a low incidence of paraplegia with a simple aortic cross-clamping of short duration (364). Svensson and Crawford recommended atriofemoral bypass for patients with fragile distal aortic arches and those with extensive aneurysms (365). There is evidence, mostly from unblinded, nonrandomized, and retrospective studies, to suggest satisfactory outcomes, low paraplegia rates, and minimal bleeding complications with distal perfusion techniques (366–369). In one study, the use of distal aortic perfusion to maintain a distal mean aortic pressure of 60 mm Hg or more was effective in preventing spinal cord ischemia unless the critical intercostal artery arose from the excluded aortic segment and was surgically ligated or destroyed (370). Najafi concluded that chronic localized aneurysms of the descending aorta that are amenable to expeditious reconstruction within 30 minutes can be managed with a simple clamp-and-sew technique. More extensive and complex repairs that are likely to require prolonged cross-clamping times should probably be managed with distal circulatory support (366). In some patients with certain anatomic relationships, left atrial-to-distal aorta or femoral artery bypass, in conjunction with staged replacement of an extensive TAAA, may be advantageous (371).

Simple Aortic Cross-Clamping

This technique consists of clamping the descending thoracic aorta proximal and distal to the aneurysm without the use of a shunt or pump. This is the simplest method for resection in the shortest period of time. Disadvantages of this technique are distal organ ischemia, proximal arterial hypertension, and metabolic acidosis. The longer the aortic cross-clamping time, the higher the incidence of ischemic complications. A cross-clamping time exceeding 30 minutes increases the risk of spinal cord injury (335,360,372). Several studies have shown that simple cross-clamping results in lower morbidity and mortality than shunt and bypass techniques, provided that surgery is expeditious (373).

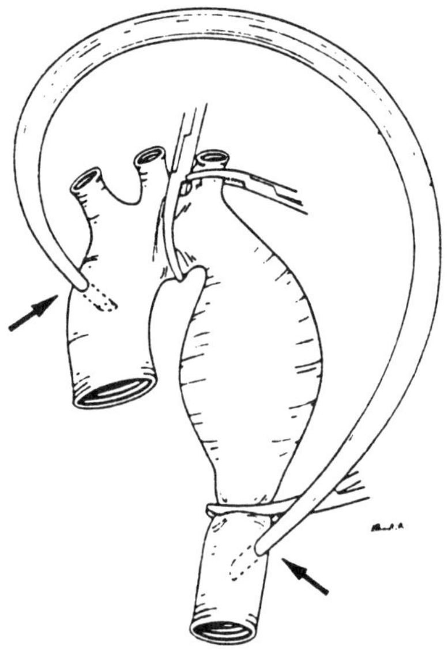

FIGURE 27-27. Figure showing the most common site of proximal aortic cross-clamping, between the left common carotid, the left carotid, and the left subclavian arteries. The arrows indicate the preferred sites for proximal and distal insertion for the Gott shunt. (From Verdant A, Page A, Cossette R. Surgery of the descending thoracic aorta: spinal cord protection with Gott shunt. *Ann Thorac Surg* 1988;46:147, with permission.)

Passive Shunts

Shunts are used to divert blood from proximal aortic sites to the distal aorta or femoral artery (Fig. 27-27). The shunts control proximal hypertension primarily by decreasing left ventricular afterload. They decrease the need for arterial vasodilators. Initial reports indicated that shunts did not decrease the incidence of paraplegia, which remained at approximately 7% to 16% (374). In addition, hemorrhage may occur at the site of shunt insertion (375). Some reports even suggested that the mortality rate was higher when the shunt was used, compared with simple aortic cross-clamping techniques (376). Passive shunts of small diameter provide inadequate proximal decompression and distal perfusion due to the lack of an interposed pump to enhance flow. Molina et al. (374) showed that paraplegia and renal damage can be avoided in dogs with the use of large shunts. For the shunt to be effective it has to carry 60% or more of the baseline descending aortic flow. The most commonly used shunt is the 9-mm heparin-coated conduit (Gott shunt), which does not require systemic anticoagulation. Placement of the proximal end of the shunt in the ascending aorta is associated with the highest flow rates and appears to be the preferred cannulation site (368). Use of the left subclavian artery for proximal cannulation should be avoided because it may cause flow reversal in the vertebral artery (from which the anterior spinal artery is derived) and in the internal mammary artery (which contributes to spinal cord blood supply through its anastomoses with the intercostal arteries) (377). A flow probe is useful to monitor proper shunt function and detect malposition, kinking, or dislodgement. Using a 9-mm shunt, Verdant reported a mean flow of 2.5 L/minute and a mean femoral artery pressure of 62 mm Hg (368). There was no paraplegia in a large, nonrandomized series of patients with TAAA managed with Gott shunts during short aortic-clamping (mean duration, 30 minutes) (378). Without precise knowledge of the spinal cord blood supply anatomy, shunting cannot consistently prevent paraplegia. The use of shunts has been associated with technical difficulties, bleeding, dislodgement, embolic stroke, and death (360).

Atriofemoral Centrifugal Bypass

The bypass is established from the left atrium to the left common femoral artery with an interposed Biomedicus (Minneapolis, MN) centrifugal pump (Fig. 27-28). The pump is nonocclusive and nontraumatic to blood cells and requires the use of minimal or no heparin provided that flow is greater than 800 mL/minute. Diversion of blood from the left atrium to the bypass on cross-clamping decreases left ventricular preload, CO, proximal aortic pressure, and left ventricular stroke work. The ACT is maintained between 150 to 200 seconds (379). With this technique, the need for vasodilators and sodium bicarbonate is almost eliminated, because proximal arterial hypertension, metabolic acidosis, and splanchnic organ ischemia do not occur. An intraarterial catheter is inserted into the other femoral artery to monitor blood pressure in the distal aortic segment. Bypass flow

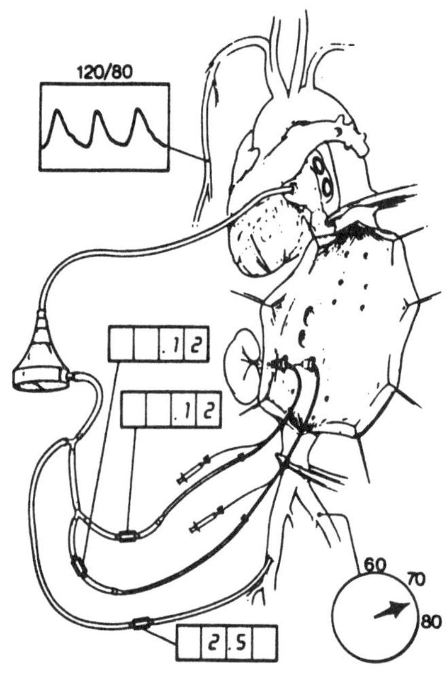

FIGURE 27-28. Left atrium-to-femoral artery bypass plus renal artery perfusion using the centrifugal pump. (From Shenaq SA, Childres WF. Management of aortic aneurysms. *Semin Anesth* 1991;(2):108, with permission.)

should be adjusted to maintain a distal mean aortic pressure of 60 to 70 mm Hg. Because about 50% of total CO goes to the organs below the diaphragm, pump flow is frequently set at 2 to 3 L/minute. Human and animal studies indicate that bypass flow rates of 25 to 40 mL/kg/minute are sufficient to normalize proximal aortic pressure, normalize left ventricular function, maintain distal aortic perfusion, and provide satisfactory renal and spinal cord blood flow (360). Adjustments in pump flow rates and circulating blood volume are guided by the careful interpretation of hemodynamic data, including ventricular filling pressures and end-diastolic area, measured with a PA catheter and TEE, respectively, along with proximal and distal aortic pressures.

Studies have shown an inconsistent reduction in perioperative complications with the use left atriofemoral centrifugal pump bypass during descending aortic clamping (363, 369). Importantly, spinal cord viability is not guaranteed with this technique, because the origin of the artery of Adamkowitz may be between the aortic clamps or the vessel may be surgically sacrificed. If the critical spinal cord blood flow has not been excluded by the surgical clamps and the anterior spinal artery is well developed, then distal aortic pressure will be very important in helping to prevent spinal cord ischemia during aortic cross-clamping. Laschinger et al. reported that a mean distal aortic pressure of at least 60 mm Hg was required to prevent or ameliorate spinal cord injury (380). Biglioli et al. found that left-sided heart bypass prevented the increase in CSF pressure associated with aortic cross-clamping but could not prove a reduction in the incidence of paraplegia comparison with the clamp-and-sew method (359). Katz et al. (381) reviewed a group of patients undergoing emergency repair of acute traumatic transection of thoracic aorta and reported a trend toward an increased rate of paraplegia in patients who were not shunted when the cross-clamping times exceeded 30 minutes. In another series, the risk of paraplegia was significantly lower (but not totally eliminated) in patients with dissections of the descending thoracic aorta when a shunt was used (8% versus 44%). This finding is in contrast to earlier reports suggesting that shunting procedures did not prevent paraplegia (see later discussions of spinal cord protection.) Cartier et al. suggested that left atriofemoral bypass was preferable to passive shunting and to the clamp-and-sew method in patients undergoing TAAA repair (382). Although earlier studies did not show a reduction in renal failure with the use of distal aortic perfusion, a more recent retrospective review of 832 patients undergoing TAAA repair suggested that left atriofemoral bypass may provide protection to the kidneys (383). Analysis of current evidence indicates that left atriofemoral centrifugal pump bypass may be useful in patients with poor left ventricular function, CAD, preexisting renal disease, or anticipated prolonged aortic cross-clamping time (359).

Partial Cardiopulmonary Bypass

Partial CPB has been used during thoracic aortic aneurysm repair with a femoral vein-to-femoral artery or right atrial-to-femoral artery bypass. The technique employs oxygenators and requires heparinization. On application of the cross-clamp, the institution of partial CPB results in reduction of venous return, preload, and CO, which helps control proximal hypertension. The arterial cannula in the femoral artery provides distal perfusion to the lower extremities, spinal cord, and splanchnic viscera. It is extremely helpful to have a second arterial cannula in the femoral artery to continuously monitor distal aortic arterial pressure. A flow rate of 25 to 40 mL/kg/minute is usually adequate to control proximal hypertension and maintain mean distal aortic pressure of 50 to 60 mm Hg. Ventilation of the lungs must be continued. With partial CPB, there is no correlation between complication rate and aortic cross-clamp duration. This technique has been proposed to lower the incidence of paraplegia, left ventricular failure, and renal failure. In one series of high-risk patients managed with partial CPB, the incidences of renal insufficiency and dialysis requirement were 7.8% and 2.2%, respectively (384). However, the mortality rate has been reported to be as high as 20%, leading to the recommendation that partial CPB be used only in patients who require a long duration of aortic cross-clamping (384). Several studies reported a substantial increase in blood loss and hemorrhagic complications with this technique (335,369). The increased bleeding is presumably caused by heparinization, CPB-related coagulopathy, and hemorrhage from surgical cannulation sites. The advent of heparin-bonded tubings and oxygenators decreases heparin requirements and may decrease bleeding complications.

Deep Hypothermic Circulatory Arrest

DHCA has been used to protect vital organs, especially the spinal cord, from ischemic injury during thoracic aortic clamping. The $CMRO_2$ at 37°C is 2.2 times that at 27°C. The decrease in spinal cord temperature by even a few degrees can significantly improve its tolerance to ischemia. In rabbits, a 3°C reduction in temperature doubled the duration of tolerable ischemia (385,386). Advantages of DHCA include minimal aortic dissection, avoidance of proximal aortic cross-clamping, and a bloodless surgical field. Deep hypothermia extends the tolerable ischemic time, thereby allowing the completion of complex repairs and the reimplantation of intercostal and lumbar arteries. The period of cerebral circulatory arrest should still be limited to 30 to 40 minutes to minimize the risk of cerebral injury. In a nonhomogeneous series of 51 patients with thoracic and thoracoabdominal aneurysms and dissections, the use of DHCA to 15°C resulted in a lower incidence of paraplegia (4.5%) and renal failure compared with simple cross-clamping, but pulmonary complications were similar. The incidence of stroke was 4.3%. A major disadvantage of DHCA is the substantial increase in blood loss and transfusion requirements (387).

Conclusions

Studies have not shown a consistent improvement in outcome with the use of distal aortic perfusion compared with the clamp-and-sew technique, provided that aortic occlusion time is less than 30 minutes (360,388). At present shunting and bypass procedures are employed selectively but not universally. Their use, however, makes the intraoperative anesthetic management of these patients easier by decreasing proximal arterial hypertension, providing renal perfusion, and minimizing metabolic acidosis as well as declamping hypotension. Advantages of distal perfusion techniques include (a) effective control of proximal hypertension while avoiding the deleterious effects of vasodilators; (b) provision of splanchnic and renal perfusion, which may reduce the incidence of renal insufficiency, gut ischemia and hepatic injury; (c) prevention of acidosis and declamping shock; (d) potential reduction in the incidence of disseminated intravascular coagulopathy; (e) ability to rapidly warm patients; (f) access for rapid volume infusion; (g) supplementary oxygenation with extracorporeal oxygenators; (h) maintenance of higher distal aortic pressures and SCPP; (i) potential reduction in the incidence of spinal cord ischemic injury; and (j) protection against myocardial ischemia by decreasing afterload and/or preload and left ventricular stroke work and systolic wall stress. The use of distal perfusion techniques is associated with some risks and disadvantages, which include (a) increased operative time, (b) interference and cluttering of the operative field, (c) shunt dislodgement, (d) technical difficulties with atrial or proximal aortic cannulation, (e) risk of air or particulate emboli including stroke, (f) risk of hemorrhage from cannulation sites, (g) the need for anticoagulation with some techniques, and (h) risk of atrial, ventricular, aortic, or femoral arterial injury (389).

Renal Ischemia and Protection During Thoracic and Thoracoabdominal Aortic Reconstructions

Acute renal failure after repair of thoracic aortic aneurysms results from multiple causes and has a serious negative effect on outcome. Whereas the incidence of renal insufficiency after infrarenal abdominal aortic reconstruction is approximately 2% to 5%, the incidence after thoracic or thoracoabdominal operations is 2.7% to 13.8% (389) but can be as high as 30% (390–393). Dialysis requiring renal failure occurs in approximately 6% of patients undergoing thoracoabdominal aortic reconstruction and is associated with a mortality rate of 30% to 60% (394,395). Ischemia-induced acute renal failure results from the 90% reduction in renal blood flow during thoracic aortic cross-clamping which is worsened by periods of intraoperative and postoperative hemodynamic instability. Proximal tubular cell damage may be mediated by the alteration in renal hemodynamics caused by activation of the renin-angiotensin and/or prostaglandin pathways and oxygen free radical release during reperfusion injury. The release of vasoactive compounds, bacterial translocation, and endotoxemia resulting from visceral hypoperfusion may add to organ dysfunction by initiating a systemic inflammatory response and having a deleterious effect on the vasculature and microcirculation. The use of distal perfusion techniques during thoracic aortic cross-clamping may theoretically ameliorate these reactions and reduce postoperative renal dysfunction (396). Risks factors for the development of acute renal failure (Table 27-11) include aortic cross-clamping time greater than 30 to 45 minutes, advanced age, preexisting renal impairment and renal artery occlusive disease, sustained perioperative hypotension and low CO, left ventricular dysfunction, and failure to use atriofemoral bypass intraoperatively (383,389). In addition, renal function may be impaired as a result of preoperative contrast angiography or perioperative medications (e.g., aminoglycoside antibiotics). So long as intravascular volume and hemodynamics are adequate, intraoperative urine output is not an reliable predictor of postoperative renal failure (397).

TABLE 27-11. RISK FACTORS FOR ACUTE RENAL FAILURE AFTER THORACIC AORTIC SURGERY

Aortic cross-clamping time >30–45 min
Sustained intraoperative and postoperative hypotension
Prolonged reduction in cardiac output
Left ventricular dysfunction
Preoperative renal dysfunction
Advanced age
Failure to use atriofemoral bypass intraoperatively

In view of the high mortality and morbidity rates associated with acute renal failure, every effort should be made to reduce its occurrence (Table 27-12). The most effective renal protective measures include minimization of the aortic cross-clamping time and maintenance of adequate intravascular blood volume, CO, and perfusion pressure (398,399). Elective surgery should be postponed for 24 hours after radiographic studies with nephrotoxic contrast media. Use of mannitol during and after arteriography was shown to reduce the risk of subsequent acute renal failure (397). Other potentially useful methods of renal protection are of uncertain benefit. All anesthetic agents decrease the glomerular flow rate by reducing renal blood flow and mean arterial pressure. Although there are no data to favor one anesthetic technique over another, it seems prudent to avoid agents that can potentially contribute to renal toxicity, such as enflurane and sevoflurane. The use of potent vasodilators (e.g., sodium nitroprusside) to manage proximal hypertension results in severe distal aortic hypotension and further reduction in renal perfusion pressure. Early studies of distal perfusion techniques such as passive shunts, femorofemoral and atriofemoral bypass did not yield conclusive evidence of renal protective benefit during prolonged aortic cross-clamping (394). A more recent retrospective review suggested that left atriofemoral bypass was protective to the kidneys (383).

TABLE 27-12. METHODS THAT MAY BE USEFUL FOR RENAL PROTECTION DURING THORACIC AORTIC SURGERY

Minimization of aortic cross-clamp time
Maintenance of adequate renal perfusion
Maintenance of intravascular volume
Maintenance of adequate ventricular function and cardiac output
Avoidance of prolonged intraoperative and postoperative hypotension
Maintenance of renal perfusion during clamping
Atriofemoral bypass
Selective renal artery perfusion
Minimization of distal hypotension during aortic cross-clamping
Decreasing renal metabolic rate
Cold perfusion of renal arteries
Furosemide
Systemic hypothermia
Decreasing reperfusion injury
Mannitol
Calcium channel blockers
Superoxide dismutase
Pharmacologic manipulation of renal blood flow
Low-dose dopamine
Mannitol
Furosemide
Fenoldepam
Prostaglandin E-1

Source: O'Connor CJ, Rothenberg DM. Anesthetic considerations for descending thoracic aortic surgery: part II. *J Cardiothorac Vasc Anesth* 1995;9:734, with permission.

Selective renal artery perfusion was described in patients undergoing TAAA repair with the use of left atrial-to-femoral artery bypass. The orifices of the exposed renal artery are cannulated with a 9F catheter and perfused with blood from the centrifugal pump using a Y-shaped connection (361,366,394). Cold renal perfusion and surface cooling may decrease the incidence of renal failure (400,401). The renal arteries are selectively perfused with cold blood or crystalloid solution, and the kidneys are covered with ice to achieve a local renal temperature of 15°C (402,403). Svensson et al. (404) used selective hypothermic perfusion to limit renal dysfunction in patients with renal artery occlusive disease. Systemic hypothermia during atriofemoral bypass is associated with improved renal outcome, compared with normothermia (361).

Despite the absence of strong scientific evidence indicating substantial clinical benefit, mannitol 0.25 to 0.5 g/kg is frequently administered before cross-clamping to protect the kidneys during aortic surgery (402). Mannitol induces an osmotic diuresis that helps maintain patency of the renal tubules. Additional renal protective effects include renal cortical vasodilation, decreased blood viscosity, decreased renin release, increased circulating blood volume, increased renal cortical blood flow and glomerular flow rate, scavenging of oxygen free radicals, and attenuation of endothelial cell swelling (405). Mannitol was ineffective in reversing the profound reduction in glomerular filtration rate and renal blood flow induced by 60 minutes of suprarenal aortic cross-clamping in dogs (406). In a randomized, controlled trial in patients undergoing aortic aneurysm surgery, mannitol 0.3 g/kg improved biochemical markers of renal dysfunction including serum creatinine and *N*-acetyl glucosaminidase (407). In general, loop diuretics are less effective than mannitol in experimental models of complete renal ischemia (408,409). Furosemide produces natriuresis, diuresis, and renal vasodilatation. By inhibiting tubular sodium reabsorption, loop diuretics eliminate a major component of tubular cell energy expenditure and thereby produce a substantial reduction in metabolic rate and oxygen requirement. This could theoretically improve renal tolerance to ischemia. However, available data do not support the presence of useful clinical renal protective benefits. The prophylactic use of loop diuretics was shown not to improve outcome or reduce the frequency of dialysis requirement in patients undergoing aortic surgery (410). Nevertheless, furosemide is commonly used in patients who remain oliguric despite a normal hemodynamic state. Its use may be helpful in converting established oliguric renal failure to nonoliguric renal failure.

Dopamine 1 to 3 μg/kg/min produces renal arteriolar dilatation, increases renal blood flow and glomerular flow rate, and inhibits sodium reabsorption, resulting in diuresis and natriuresis (411). The administration of dopamine after a period of renal ischemia in patients undergoing renal transplantation has been shown to increase renal blood flow, urine volume, and glomerular filtration rate (411). Although dopamine was shown to improve renal function in oliguric patients after CPB (412) and in patients undergoing orthotopic liver transplantation (413), so far it has not been shown to improve renal outcome during thoracic aortic surgery. Dopamine was found to be ineffective in reversing the renal injury produced by thoracic aortic cross-clamping (406). Despite the lack of conclusive evidence supporting its protective role, the prophylactic use of low-dose dopamine varies widely in clinical practice. Some use it routinely, whereas others limit its use to patients identified as being at high risk, such as those with preoperative renal dysfunction or prolonged cross-clamping time and those who remain oliguric after unclamping. Fenoldopam mesylate is a specific agonist of dopamine$_2$ (DA_2) receptors, increasing renal blood flow together with systemic arteriolar vasodilatation. It may prove to be more useful than dopamine as a renal protective agent during aortic cross-clamping (414).

Several other agents have been investigated for their renal protective effects. Pretreatment with calcium entry blockers was found to limit the degree of renal injury produced by experimental complete renal ischemia (415). Verapamil injected directly into the renal arteries may be protective after renal ischemia. Calcium entry blockers inhibit intracellular calcium influx during ischemia, thereby preventing mitochondrial calcium deposition and subsequent cellular destruction (416). Preoperative verapamil administration did not improve biochemical markers of renal outcome including serum creatinine and *N*-acetyl glucosaminidase (417). Additional clinical evidence is necessary before calcium entry blockers can be added to the routine management of patients undergoing aortic reconstruction.

Oxygen free radicals and neutrophils have been implicated in ischemic renal damage. Superoxide dismutase and allopurinol were found to reduce renal experimental ischemic injury when administered prophylactically (419). An imbalance between the vasodilator prostaglandin I_2 and the vasoconstrictor thromboxane A_2 appears to mediate changes in vascular tone in response to ischemic renal injury. Inhibition of thromboxane synthesis protects against tubular necrosis after experimental ischemia in animals (418). Oxygen free radical scavengers were also found to inhibit thromboxane synthesis, which may contribute to their renal protective effect observed in experimental models (419). Despite initial enthusiasm about the possible renal protective effects of angiotensin-converting enzyme inhibitors, human (394,420,421) and animal (422) studies found them not to be protective against renal ischemia. The phosphodiesterase inhibitor theophylline was found to improve renal inulin clearance after renal ischemia and nephrotoxic myoglobinuric injury in experimental animals. The mechanism of protection may be by antagonizing the effects of endogenous renal vasoconstrictors. Pentoxifylline has a phosphodiesterase inhibitory effect as well as a salutary effect on blood rheology. Other potentially protective agents include prostaglandin E_1, atrial natriuretic factor, and epidermal growth factor. The continuous infusion of prostaglandin E_1 was shown to improve renal blood flow, but, as with other experimental agents, its use remains speculative (361).

Mesenteric Ischemia and Protection

Cross-clamping of the descending thoracic aorta results in ischemia and reperfusion injury to the mesenteric circulation. Mucosal permeability was shown to increase during mesenteric ischemia and reperfusion (423). This results in increased fluid shifts, increase in intracellular volume, and depletion of intravascular fluid space (424). Bleeding abnormalities and depletion of coagulation factors were found to occur after supraceliac cross-clamping (425). Platelets and fibrinogen decreased while PT and PTT increased after aortic cross-clamping in dogs. This picture is consistent with diffuse intravascular coagulopathy. The severity of bleeding abnormalities correlates with increasing supraceliac cross-clamping time. These abnormalities persisted for 24 hours or longer after declamping. Cohen et al. (425) postulated that ischemia and reperfusion injury to the liver and mesenteric bed were responsible for the abnormal fibrinolysis and the decrease in concentrations of coagulation factors. Prolonged mesenteric ischemia results in marked metabolic acidosis requiring treatment with sodium bicarbonate. Irreversible ischemia and gangrene of the small or large bowel is rare. Upper gastrointestinal bleeding occurs in some patients as a result of mucosal damage caused by ischemia and reperfusion injury. To attenuate the effects of mesenteric hypoperfusion, rapid reimplantation of the celiac trunk and superior mesenteric artery is required. Short mesenteric ischemic time prevents excessive fluid shifts and decreases the likelihood of coagulopathy. Maintenance of perfusion of the gut, liver, and kidneys with the use of distal perfusion techniques lowers the severity of these complications. Transfusion of blood, fresh-frozen plasma, platelets, and cryoprecipitate is frequently needed to treat diffuse intravascular coagulopathy. Arterial blood gas levels should be monitored at regular intervals, and acidosis should be corrected with an intravenous continuous infusion of sodium bicarbonate, as described earlier. The use of distal aortic perfusion is helpful in decreasing metabolic acidosis and the need for sodium bicarbonate (382,426). Animal experiments demonstrated the beneficial effects of superoxide dismutase, allopurinol, glucagon, methylprednisolone, and prostacyclin in decreasing ischemic and reperfusion injury to the mesenteric circulation, but clinical information is still not available (427–429).

Spinal Cord Ischemia and Paraplegia After Thoracic and Thoracoabdominal Aortic Surgery

Paraplegia is the most devastating and, at present, not totally preventable complication after thoracoabdominal aortic operations. The cause of paraplegia is multifactorial. Several anatomic, physiologic, and technical factors have been implicated in contributing to ischemic and reperfusion injury to the spinal cord. Paraplegia is much more frequent after repair of extensive thoracoabdominal aneurysms that involve the entire descending thoracic aorta and most or all of the abdominal aorta. The most important factors contributing to the development of paraplegia include the presence of aortic rupture or dissection, long aortic cross-clamping time, the extent of the aneurysm, whether intercostal arteries were reimplanted, and the patient's age (360,390). In addition, perioperative hypotension has been implicated in the development of delayed-onset postoperative paraplegia. Increased CSF pressure after proximal aortic cross-clamping may decrease the effective perfusion pressure of the spinal cord and contribute to paraplegia (426).

Frequency of Spinal Cord Ischemic Injury

The incidence of this complication depends primarily on the type and extent of the aortic disease (3,372,392). Repair of coarctation of the aorta is followed by a low incidence of paraplegia (0.25% to 1.5%), presumably because of the presence of adequate collateral circulation to the spinal cord through well-developed radicular branches of the upper tho-

TABLE 27-13. INCIDENCE OF SPINAL CORD INJURY AFTER THORACOABDOMINAL AORTIC ANERUYSM SURGERY

Type and Extent of Aneurysm	Incidence of Paraplegia/ Paraparesis (%)	
	Without Dissection	With Dissection
Crawford type I: Most or all of the descending thoracic aorta and part of the abdominal aorta, but not below the renal arteries	6–10	21
Crawford type II: Most or all of the descending thoracic aorta and most or all of the abdominal aorta as far as the aortic bifurcation	17–21	40–60
Crawford type III: Distal descending thoracic aorta and varying segments of the abdominal aorta	2–9	14–22
Crawford type IV: abdominal aorta	0.5–2	—

Source: Compiled from Crawford ES, Crawford JL, Safi HJ, et al. Thoracoabdominal aortic aneurysms: preoperative and intraoperative factors determining immediate and long-term results of operations in 605 patients. *J Vasc Surg* 1986;3:389; and Gloviczki P, Bower TC. Visceral and spinal cord protection during thoracoabdominal aortic reconstructions. *Semin Vasc Surg* 1992;5: 163, with permission.

TABLE 27-14. IMPORTANT FACTORS AFFECTING THE INCIDENCE OF SPINAL CORD INJURY AFTER OPERATION ON THE DESCENDING THORACIC AND THORACOABDOMINAL AORTA

Duration of aortic cross-clamping
Extent of aortic disease
Extent of surgical resection
Presence of aortic dissection or rupture
Sacrifice of critical intercostal arteries
Method of managing proximal hypertension during aortic cross-clamping (vasodilators versus active or passive shunts)
Distal aortic pressure during cross-clamping
Cerebrospinal pressure and drainage
Patient's age
Degree and duration of intraoperative and postoperative hypotension
Perioperative hyperglycemia

racic intercostal arteries. Repair of acute traumatic aortic disruption is associated with a variable but substantially higher incidence of spinal cord injury, up to 24% (85,360, 381). Data by Crawford et al. clearly showed that there is a significant correlation between the extent of the aorta resected and the frequency of paraplegia (335). In one series the incidences were 60% and 17% for type II dissecting and nondissecting aneurysms, respectively, and 2% for type IV nondissecting aneurysms (Table 27-13).

Blood Supply of the Spinal Cord

The blood supply of the spinal cord consists of two posterior and one anterior spinal artery. All three arteries receive collateral supply from radicular branches of the intercostal and lumbar arteries (430). The upper portion of the spinal cord receives most of its blood supply via the vertebral arteries and a small portion via the descending deep cervical arteries. The lower half of the spinal cord is supplied entirely by branches of the intercostal, iliolumbar, and lateral sacral arteries. The anterior spinal artery has high resistance to blood flow and usually is not continuous but rather interrupted along its course. It receives multiple feeding branches from intercostal and lumbar arteries. One of these feeding branches is usually large and known as the artery of Adamkiewicz or the arteria radicularis magna (ARM). The ARM originates between T9 and T12 in 60% of patients (more commonly on the left side), between T5 and T8 in 12% to 15%, at L1 in 14%, at L2 in 10%, at L3 in 1.4%, and from L4–L5 in 0.2% of cases (431).

Etiology of Spinal Cord Ischemic Injury

Spinal cord injury after descending thoracic or thoracoabdominal aortic reconstruction correlates with the degree and duration of the ischemic state (Table 27-14). Perioperative hypotension is an important factor contributing to the development of paraplegia (432). Because of high arterial resistance, adequate flow through the spinal cord arterial bed requires a mean aortic pressure of 60 to 70 mm Hg (433). Prolonged intraoperative hypotension is associated with a substantial incidence of paraplegia (360). In addition, episodes of postoperative hypotension have been linked to the occurrence of paraplegia or paraparesis starting several days postoperatively in patients who have undergone successful and initially uncomplicated aortic reconstruction (360).

The duration of aortic cross-clamping is an important determinant of spinal cord ischemia. The duration of aortic occlusion has a significant direct correlation with the frequency of neurologic deficits of the lower extremities (360, 381). During the period of aortic clamping, the spinal cord cannot be perfused from the distal hypotensive aorta. Instead, its blood supply is provided through collateral circulation, which is better developed in the upper thoracic than in the lumbar segments (the watershed area of the spinal cord). Furthermore, it is postulated that retrograde bleeding from the intercostal arteries into the open aorta tends to drain blood away from the spinal cord, resulting in a steal phenomenon (434). This implies that large intercostal or lumbar arteries that are found to be patent and bleeding when the aorta is opened should probably be anastomosed to the graft. Simple aortic clamping for periods of less than 20 to 25 minutes appears to be safe for most patients.

CSF pressure increases after proximal aortic cross-clamping, presumably because of increases in central venous pressure and CSF production (431,435). The increase in CSF

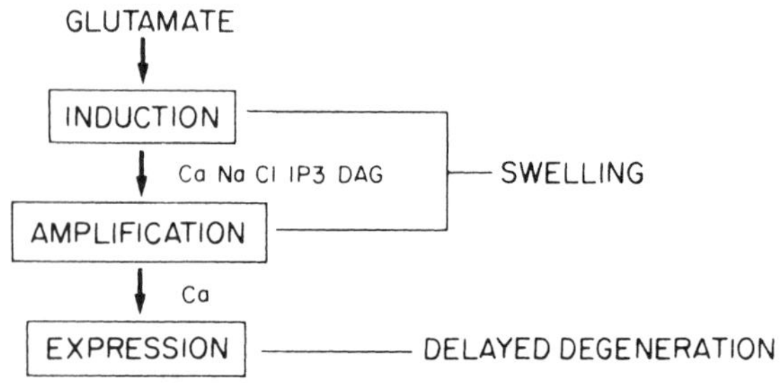

FIGURE 27-29. Three stages of glutamate toxicity. (From Kouchoukos NT, Rokkas CK. Descending thoracic and thoracoabdominal aortic surgery for aneurysm or dissection: how do we minimize the risk of spinal cord injury? *Semin Thorac Cardiovasc Surg* 1993; 5:47, with permission.)

TABLE 27-15. METHODS THAT ARE POTENTIALLY EFFECTIVE IN REDUCING THE FREQUENCY OF SPINAL CORD ISCHEMIC INJURY DURING THORACOABDOMINAL AORTIC SURGERY

Limited aortic cross-clamping time
Perfusion of the distal aorta using femorofemoral or atriofemoral bypass
Drainage of cerebrospinal fluid
Reimplantation of intercostal and lumbar arteries
Hypothermia (mild to profound, systemic or regional)
Pharmacologic protection

Source: Kouchoukos NT, Rokkas CK. Descending thoracic and thoracoabdominal aortic surgery for aneurysm or dissection: how do we minimize the risk of spinal cord injury? *Semin Thorac Cardiovasc Surg* 1993;5:47, with permission.

pressure decreases the effective SCPP, which is equal to the distal aortic arterial pressure minus the CSF pressure (436). Sacrifice of critical intercostal or lumbar arteries is probably an important determinant of paraplegia. However, Crawford et al. (388) were unable to show a beneficial effect of reimplantation of these vessels into the graft.

Evidence suggests that glutamate, an excitatory neurotransmitter and the major intracellular anion in the CNS, is an important mediator of neuronal death in conditions of hypoxia and ischemia (437). Glutamate appears to be a potent and rapidly acting neurotoxin. The transient release of only a small fraction of intracellular stores of glutamate into the extracellular space can initiate a lethal chain of events (438) (Fig. 27-29). Initially in the stage of induction, excessive buildup of extracellular glutamate causes intracellular derangements probably mediated by the toxic influx of extracellular calcium. Glutamate activates NMDA receptors, which results in the opening of membrane channels that are permeable to calcium ions (439). The buildup of intracellular calcium acts to amplify the intracellular derangements and promote the involvement of other neurons. As glutamate leaks from the injured cells, a positive feedback mechanism is created, leading to the continued stimulation of membrane receptors and further calcium influx. This process of amplification of the initial neurotoxic event is followed by excitotoxicity when a toxic level of intracellular calcium is reached. Destructive cascades are triggered and result in neuronal death as the final outcome.

Prevention of Spinal Cord Ischemic Injury

A number of adjunctive techniques and interventions have been used to reduce the frequency of paraplegia and are discussed in the following paragraphs (Table 27-15).

Aortic Cross-Clamping Time

The probability of ischemic spinal cord injury during occlusion of the thoracic aorta increases with the aortic cross-clamping time (Fig. 27-30). The maximum safe period that does not result in ischemic injury to patients is not known. Katz et al. (381) indicated a significant increase in neurologic deficits at approximately 20 to 25 minutes after descending thoracic aortic cross-clamping. Jex et al. (440) in another series found a sudden increase in paraplegia after 45 minutes of aortic cross-clamping in patients with descending thoracic aortic dissections who did not undergo shunting. Many surgeons prefer the rapid and simple technique of aortic clamping and rapid sewing of the graft to minimize cross-clamping time. The blind reimplantation of multiple intercostal arteries significantly prolongs total aortic cross-clamping time and may be one reason why it was found not to be protective in most cases (439).

Maintenance of Distal Aortic Perfusion

The maintenance of a distal aortic pressure of 60 to 70 mm Hg has been shown experimentally to have a protective effect on the spinal cord (370,433). Perfusion of the distal aorta via shunt or bypass techniques protects the spinal cord only if the ARM originates beyond the distal clamp. In addition to providing distal aortic perfusion, the use of a shunt or bypass reduces proximal aortic pressure and left ventricular afterload, thereby minimizing the need for vasodilator therapy. Experimental and clinical evidence indicates that the use of peripheral arterial vasodilators to treat proximal hypertension could be detrimental to spinal cord perfusion by shunting blood away from the high-resistance spinal cord collaterals. Sodium nitroprusside was found to have a deleterious effect on the incidence of paraplegia (425). In addition, sodium nitroprusside dilates the cerebral vessels and causes further increase in CSF pressure and decrease in SCPP. Bypass techniques employing a pump are superior to passive shunts because they permit more precise control of flow rate as well as proximal and distal aortic pressures (441,443). Left atrium-to-femoral artery bypass by means of a Biomedicus centrifugal pump has been used successfully for elective and emergency aortic reconstructions (441). These systems do not require an oxygenator and can be used with minimal or no heparinization (Fig. 27-31). Rapid

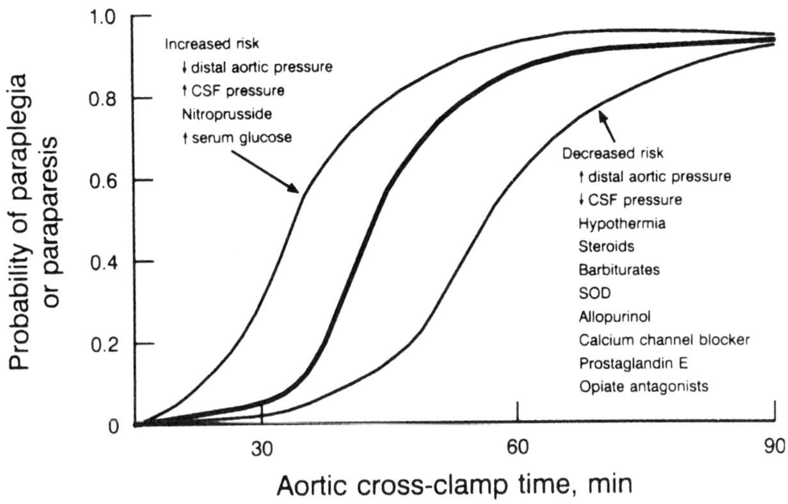

FIGURE 27-30. The probability of ischemic spinal cord injury during occlusion of the thoracic aorta. (From Gloviczki P, Bower TC. Visceral and spinal cord protection during thoracoabdominal aortic reconstructions. *Semin Vasc Surg* 1992;5:163, with permission.)

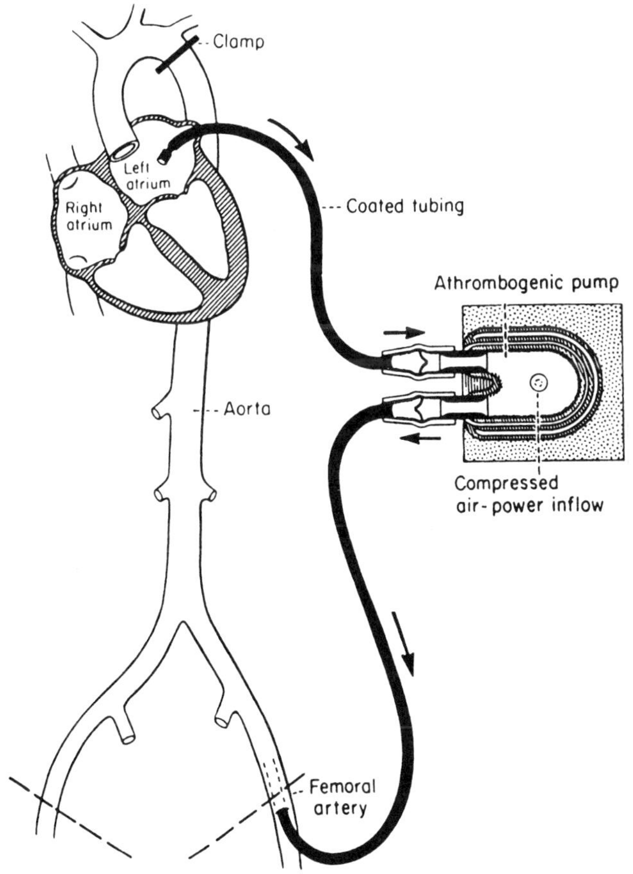

FIGURE 27-31. Diagram of nonthrombogenic left atrium-to-femoral artery bypass with pulsatile pump. (From Shenaq SA, Svensson LG. Paraplegia following aortic surgery. *J Cardiothorac Vasc Anesth* 1993;7:81, with permission.)

compensation for sudden volume changes is possible because all of the shed blood can be returned to the extracorporeal circuit. Reduction of cardiac preload and CO on application of the cross-clamp can be achieved by increasing venous drainage to the reservoir. In addition, this technique permits the induction and maintenance of mild hypothermia (33° to 35°C), which may have a protective effect on the spinal cord (389,442).

When intercostal artery reimplantation is performed in conjunction with a distal perfusion technique (shunt or bypass), the distal aortic clamp is repositioned proximally on completion of the distal aortic and intercostal artery anastomoses to reperfuse the spinal cord through the reimplanted intercostal arteries while the proximal anastomosis is being completed, thereby reducing spinal cord ischemic time.

The use of distal perfusion was shown to provide spinal cord protection in experimental animal models (434). In an experimental model of aortic cross-clamping, no significant changes were noted in spinal cord blood flow or SSEP in animals whose distal aortic pressures were maintained at 70 mm Hg or higher by the use of atriofemoral bypass (433, 443). However, results of the clinical studies in patients undergoing aortic reconstruction have been controversial. Katz et al. (381) were the first to report lowering of the rate of paraplegia in patients with acute upper traumatic transection of the descending thoracic aorta by the use of a shunting procedure to pressurize the distal aorta. The beneficial effect became apparent when the cross-clamping time exceeded 30 minutes. Several other studies also concluded that maintaining adequate distal aortic perfusion pressure directly influenced neurologic outcome (370,444). Using SSEP monitoring, Laschinger et al. (445) confirmed that a mean distal aortic pressure of at least 60 mm Hg was necessary to eliminate or reduce the risk of spinal cord injury during aortic occlusion. Other series of patients undergoing descending thoracic aortic surgery reported no decrease in paraplegia rate with the use of shunt or bypass techniques (382), except perhaps in patients with chronic dissection of the descending thoracic aorta (446). Some studies even suggest worsening of the neurologic outcome when distal perfusion techniques were employed (335). Crawford (447) recommended the selective use of atriofemoral bypass only in patients with limited cardiac reserve to decrease left ventricular afterload during cross-clamping. For extensive aneurysms, the use of bypass and segmental clamping would permit distal perfusion while the proximal anastomosis is being performed, thereby reducing spinal cord ischemic time. However, this gain in time is short, and the use of bypass also carries some risks. Bleeding from the aortic or left atrial cannulation site may occur. In one study, the use of distal perfusion techniques to maintain a distal aortic pressure of 60 mm Hg or higher was effective in preventing spinal cord ischemia unless the critical intercostal artery arose from the excluded aortic segment and was ligated or surgically destroyed (370). In contrast, several large clinical series showed no difference in the overall incidence of paraplegia with any of the surgical techniques used (simple clamp, shunt, and partial bypass) (360,448). In a prospective study, Crawford et al. (449) reported no difference in paraplegia rate between patients managed with SSEP monitoring plus temporary bypass to maintain a distal aortic pressure greater than 60 mm Hg and those in whom distal perfusion and SSEP monitoring were not used. Therefore, it appears that current clinical data do not support a consistent protective benefit of distal aortic perfusion techniques in reducing the rate of neurologic injury in the majority of cases.

Hypothermia

For every 1°C reduction in temperature from 37° to 22°C, oxygen consumption of neural tissues is decreased by about 5% to 7%. In a rabbit model, a reduction of 3°C doubled the duration of ischemia, which could be reversibly sustained (450). Various forms of hypothermia have been used to theoretically increase the tolerance of the spinal cord to ischemia. Mild to moderate hypothermia (28° to 34°C), DHCA, and local spinal cord cooling have been shown in experimental and human studies to be protective to the spinal cord (389,451–455). Animal studies demonstrate a reduction in clinical and histopathologic evidence of spinal cord injury with hypothermia. Hypothermic regional perfusion of the spinal cord is a technique in which the area of the aorta within the cross-clamps is perfused with iced solutions. The cold fluid is transported directly to the spinal cord by the intercostal and/or lumbar arteries. With an iced perfusate at 5°C, the spinal cord temperature can be reduced to 20°C with only a small (2°C) reduction in systemic temperature. The infusion of cold asanguinous Ringer's lactate solution at 5°C into an isolated aortic segment in dogs was shown to have a significant protective effect on the spinal cord (454). Likewise, in another animal experiment, hypothermic regional perfusion of the isolated aortic segment with cold blood was also found to decrease the incidence of spinal cord ischemic injury (422). Berguer et al. (456) showed that intrathecal perfusion of the spinal cord with cold saline completely prevented the development of paraplegia after aortic cross-clamping in the dog model. Davison et al. (457) described the infusion of iced saline at 4°C through an epidural catheter placed at the T11–T12 interspace. A subarachnoid thermistor catheter placed at L3–L4 was used to measure CSF temperature and pressure and to provide for CSF drainage. Of the 68 patients who underwent epidural cooling, 7 (10.3%) developed paraplegia or paresis, an incidence comparable to that previously reported from the same institution (458). The increase in intraspinal pressure resulting from fluid infusion decreases SCPP, which may counteract the potential benefit from hypothermia (459). Drainage of CSF through the subarachnoid catheter prevents the increase in CSF pressure and the consequent reduction in SCPP. Further studies are required to determine the best method of achieving regional spinal cord cooling and whether neurologic outcome during thoracic aortic surgery can be improved with that technique. In clinical practice it is beneficial to allow mild hypothermia (32° to 34°C) to occur before the application of the cross-clamp. This can easily be achieved if no attempt at warming of the patient is made and the ambient room temperature is kept cool (393). Rewarming of the room and of the patient should be started at the time of cross-clamp application to avoid excessive hypothermia, which increases the risk of dysrhythmias and coagulopathy. Ventricular fibrillation develops at about 28°C.

Kouchoukos et al. described the use of DHCA in conjunction with intercostal artery reimplantation to protect the spinal cord in patients with descending thoracic aortic aneurysms (455). Disadvantages include the need for full heparinization, which increases hemorrhagic complications; inherent CPB risks; and increased pulmonary complications (intrapulmonary hemorrhage and respiratory failure). Crawford et al. (460) reported significant mortality and morbidity (including paraplegia) with the use of DHCA in a large series of patients with complex and extensive descending thoracic aortic aneurysms. Nonetheless, the period of circulatory arrest did allow for technical accomplishments that could not have been completed within the time limits imposed by the other techniques.

Cerebrospinal Fluid Drainage

There is ample experimental evidence that CSF drainage improves effective SCPP, decreases reperfusion hyperemia, and improves neurologic outcome after thoracic aortic cross-clamping (426,461). However, the clinical role of CSF drainage alone in protecting the spinal cord during thoracoabdominal aortic reconstruction has been the subject of considerable debate (462). The SCPP is equal to the distal aortic pressure minus the CSF pressure. Although CSF drainage does lower intraspinal pressure and hence increases SCPP, the clinical reduction of the incidence of paraplegia has varied. One group of investigators evaluated the role of SCPP in producing spinal cord ischemia while monitoring SSEPs (463). Although SSEPs were absent for 40 minutes after aortic occlusion, normal physiologic function recovered when the SCPP was greater than 15 mm Hg. Conversely, permanent injury occurred after 20 minutes of ischemia when the SCPP was zero. They concluded that tolerable ischemic time depends on the SCPP and recommended that the SCPP be maintained at more than 15 mm Hg by either draining the CSF or using an adequate shunting procedure to pressure the distal aorta. Despite favorable results in a number of animal models (464–466), a prospective randomized study of 98 patients with high-risk thoracoabdominal aneurysms found no reduction in paraplegia with drainage of 50 mL of CSF (467). Similarly, another clinical study from the Mayo Clinic found no decrease in the incidence of paraplegia with the removal of a mean of 67 mL of CSF. Larger volumes of CSF may need to be removed to achieve a beneficial effect (468,469). Another study showed that CSF drainage was not effective in improving neurologic outcome when high doses of sodium nitroprusside were used to control proximal aortic hypertension (470).

Although CSF drainage alone does not appear to be effective in substantially reducing the incidence of paraplegia, it may prove to be useful in combination with other modalities. Svensson et al. (471,472) reported that the intrathecal administration of papaverine combined with CSF fluid drainage decreased the incidence of paraplegia. The beneficial effects of papaverine may be mediated by the vasodilatation of the spinal arteries, calcium channel blocking, and/or free radical scavenging properties. Spinal cord protection during aortic occlusion was also demonstrated with a combination of CSF fluid drainage and intrathecal tetracaine (473) and in conjunction with systemic methylprednisolone (474) and naloxone (475,476). The use of systemic steroids together with CSF drainage provided more protection against ischemic spinal cord injury than either steroids or CSF drainage alone (477). Hollier et al. (390,393,461) advocated the routine use of CSF pressure monitoring and drainage as part of a protocol that includes complete intercostal artery reimplantation, maintenance of proximal aortic hypertension, moderate hypothermia, high-dose barbiturates, mannitol, steroids, and calcium channel blocking agents. Using this technique, they reported no incidence of spinal cord dysfunction among 42 consecutive patients undergoing thoracoabdominal aortic reconstruction (393).

The intrathecal administration of Fluosol-DA (an oxygenated perfluorocarbon emulsion with the ability to enhance oxygen delivery to ischemic neuronal tissue) was shown to be associated with improved neurologic outcome in dogs undergoing cross-clamping of the descending thoracic aorta (478). This compound has the capacity to carry oxygen and carbon dioxide and to provide nutritional support to ischemic tissues (456,471,478–480).

Monitoring of Spinal Cord Function

SSEP monitoring has been used to detect spinal cord ischemia during aortic cross-clamping (433,481). Animal and small clinical studies showed good correlation between the duration of aortic clamping and the loss of SSEPs (482). Progressive prolongation of latency and a decrease in amplitude of the SSEPs is noticed within the first 10 minutes after the application of the proximal cross-clamp (482). Eventually the SSEPs are completely lost but, in the absence of permanent injury, the evoked response returns after unclamping (Fig. 27-32). Monitoring of SSEPs during aortic occlusion may show four patterns of response: (a) no change in SSEPs, (b) changes that return to normal within 30 minutes after unclamping, (c) changes with inconsistent return 30 minutes after unclamping, and (d) changes in latency and amplitude with no return to normality after unclamping. The incidence of paraplegia for each of these patterns of SSEP response was reported to be 13%, 27%, 20%, and 32%, respectively (449). In a study of 33 patients, Cunningham et al. showed that loss of the SSEP signal for longer than 30 minutes was associated with a 71% incidence of paraplegia, whereas aortic clamping with less than 30 minutes' loss of SSEP did not result in spinal cord injury (370). In children undergoing coarctation repair, the loss of SSEP signal for longer than 14 minutes was associated with postoperative neurologic deficit (444). Both of these studies also concluded that maintenance of adequate distal aortic perfusion pressure directly influenced neurologic outcome. Using SSEP monitoring, Laschinger et al. (445) suggested that a mean distal aortic pressure of at least 60 mm Hg was necessary to eliminate or reduce the risk of spinal cord injury during aortic occlusion.

Monitoring of SSEP has several limitations in the setting of aortic occlusion and reconstruction. These techniques monitor the posterior column (sensory function) of the spinal cord and not the anterior motor column, and therefore paraplegia may occur despite the presence of intact SSEPs (483). Factors other than spinal cord ischemia may influence their recording and sensitivity (e.g., general anesthesia, hypothermia, hypotension). Peripheral nerve ischemia resulting from aortic cross-clamping interferes with the interpretation of the SSEP recordings. Cunningham et al. (481) indicated that the loss of SSEPs due to ischemia of the spinal cord usually begins 3 to 4 minutes after aortic clamping and is maximum in 10 minutes, whereas the SSEP loss secondary to peripheral nerve ischemia usually occurs 20 minutes after the application of the cross-clamp. False-positive and false-negative results have been reported with the use of SSEP monitoring for detection of spinal cord ischemia. Paraplegia may still occur in the presence of normal SSEP tracings (484). Ischemic changes of the anterior motor portion of the spinal cord may be associated with

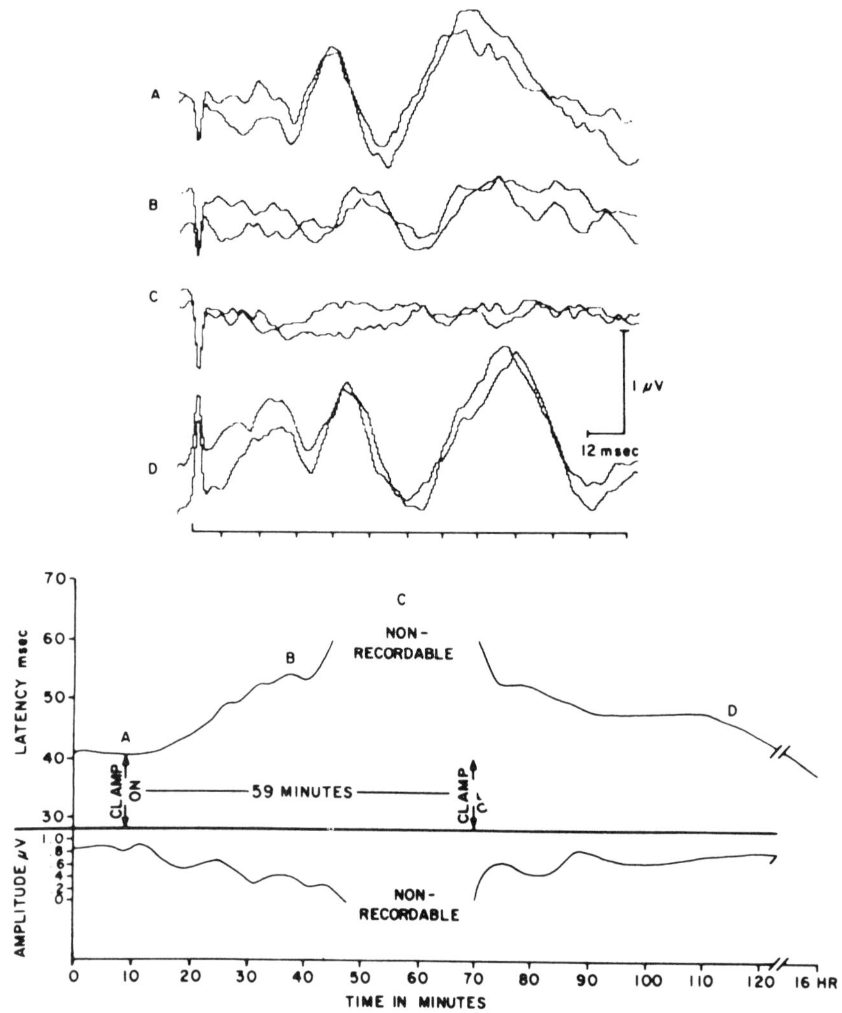

FIGURE 27-32. Bottom: Cross-clamping of the aorta produced a gradual prolongation of latency and diminution of amplitude of the sensory evoked potential. The response eventually was nonrecordable but rapidly returned and improved when the clamp was removed. **Top:** Superimposed consecutive trials of selected cephalic responses are shown at various times after clamping. The letters A and D of each response in the upper figure correspond to the letters in the graph below, indicating when each response was obtained. (From Shenaq SA, Svensson LG. Paraplegia following aortic surgery. *J Cardiothorac Vasc Anesth* 1993;7:81, with permission.)

complete motor loss (anterior spinal cord syndrome) despite the preservation of SSEPs and dorsal column functions (485). Paraplegia has been reported in patients in whom only transient episodes of reversible loss of SSEPs occurred (486). To overcome the problem of peripheral nerve ischemia associated with aortic clamping and the effect of peripheral neuropathy, the spinal cord can be stimulated by a flexible bipolar neural electrode inserted percutaneously into the epidural space. The use of a distal aortic perfusion technique prevents lower-limb and peripheral nerve ischemia, thereby facilitating SSEP recording. Monitoring of SSEPs has been used during exclusion and reperfusion of critical aortic segments for localization of the spinal cord blood supply and reimplantation of critical intercostal arteries to the aortic graft (370,487). In patients in whom distal aortic pressure was maintained at more than 60 mm Hg with a shunt or bypass and SSEPs were preserved, no intercostal artery reimplantation was performed and no paraplegia developed. In contrast, a prospective study by Crawford et al. (449) showed that the pattern of change in SSEPs and paraplegia rate were not influenced by the use of distal aortic perfusion.

The anesthetic technique must be modified to permit the satisfactory acquisition and interpretation of evoked potential waveforms. Isoflurane in concentrations of 0.5% to 1% permits the successful recording of SSEPs. Nitrous oxide was shown to decrease the amplitude of SSEPs, and its use together with a halogenated agent may cause significant depression of SSEPs (488). A predominantly intravenous anesthetic technique in conjunction with low to moderate doses of isoflurane is probably the best to use while monitoring SSEPs. The most important factor is the maintenance of a steady state of anesthesia to avoid rapid changes in anesthetic depth, especially during anticipated periods of greatest neurologic risk. Close communication with the technician performing the evoked potential monitoring is essential.

Motor Evoked Potentials

Because of the limitations of SSEPs, motor evoked potentials (MEPs) have been introduced to monitor the integrity of the anterior spinal cord. The motor cortex is stimulated transcranially with the use of electromagnetic or electrical energy, and the myogenic MEPs are recorded from the lower paravertebral muscles (426,489). Peripheral nerve ischemia does not appear to affect such measurement, as it does with SSEPs (489). Complete muscle relaxation cannot be used during MEP recording. However, MEPs can be monitored in the presence of a stable degree of partial neuromuscular blockade. MEP monitoring has been shown to be highly sensitive and specific for the detection of significant motor tract injury in numerous experimental studies (490, 491). Furthermore, changes in MEP have been shown to reliably predict neurologic outcome and paraplegia after ischemia or mechanical injury (492). Monitoring of spinal cord evoked potentials is another electrophysiologic modality that has been used for the early detection of spinal cord ischemia (493–495). The use of MEP monitoring alone or in conjunction with SSEP monitoring in patients undergoing aortic reconstruction awaits further clinical studies.

Localization of Spinal Cord Blood Supply and Reimplantation of Critical Intercostal Arteries

The most important artery supplying the distal thoracic and lumbar cord is the ARM or artery of Adamkiewicz, which originates from the T9 to T12 level in 60% to 70% of patients. However, clinical studies with preoperative spinal cord angiography have failed to identify this artery in a substantial number of patients, either because of technical problems or because the main intercostal artery was chronically occluded or stenosed (434,496). In one study, when the ARM was identified preoperatively and reimplanted into the aortic graft, the incidence of paraplegia was significantly lower than when revascularization of the spinal cord was incomplete (434). Williams et al. (496) were able to localize the origin of the ARM angiographically in 26 of 47 patients. They reported a lower incidence of paraplegia when the critical intercostal or lumbar artery was avoided altogether (i.e., was above or below the cross-clamped segment) than when the artery originated from the aneurysmal segment of the aorta and was reattached to the graft. Therefore it appears that, although preoperative identification of spinal cord arterial supply would be ideal, arteriography is frequently incomplete and time consuming. In addition, selective spinal cord angiography *per se* carries a small risk of paraplegia (434). In addition, clinical reports of paraplegia rates after the reimplantation of intercostal arteries are at present equivocal. The blind reimplantation of multiple intercostal arteries can significantly prolong aortic cross-clamping time and by this means may add to the risk of paraplegia and negate any beneficial effect of attaching the critical intercostal arteries to the graft. Hollier et al. (393) advocated the routine reimplantation of all patent intercostal arteries. In a prospective randomized study, Crawford et al. failed to confirm the benefit of intercostal artery reimplantation on postoperative paraplegia (467). However, an analysis of a subset of their patients showed that the paraplegia rate was significantly higher if patent intercostal arteries at T11, T12, or L1 were present and were not reimplanted. Further advancement in imaging techniques is required to provide precise anatomic details of the critical spinal cord blood supply.

Svensson et al. (480) described a method for intraoperative identification of the intercostal and lumbar arteries that contribute to the spinal cord blood supply (Fig. 27-25). They injected hydrogen-saturated saline into excluded segments of the aorta and into the ostia of the patent intercostal and lumbar arteries when the aortic aneurysm was opened. A platinum electrode was placed intrathecally to identify hydrogen-induced current impulses. When an artery supplying the spinal cord was injected with the hydrogen-saturated solution, the current elicited was recorded by the intrathecal platinum electrode. Important intercostal or lumbar arteries thus identified were reimplanted into the graft. Another means of preserving the intercostal arteries involves preservation of the posterior wall of the aorta from which the vessels arise. The graft is then cut obliquely and anastomosed to the posterior wall of the native aorta, thereby preserving the origin of the intercostal arteries. Svensson et al. (479) recommended the use of a multifaceted approach, including intrathecal papaverine, distal aortic perfusion, and preservation of the arteries localized by hydrogen-induced current impulse. When reliable localization of spinal cord blood supply is not available or not possible, some surgeons recommend the preservation and reimplantation of all large patent lower intercostal and lumbar arteries. In addition, retrograde bleeding into the open aorta should be minimized to prevent further compromise of spinal cord blood supply (steal phenomenon). Retrograde bleeding can be controlled by balloon occlusion catheters until these arteries are reimplanted into the graft and perfused.

Pharmacologic Spinal Cord Protection

A number of pharmacologic agents have been used both experimentally and in clinical studies in an attempt to reduce the incidence and severity of spinal cord ischemic injury (Table 27-16). Thiopental and hypothermia reduce tissue metabolism and spinal cord oxygen requirement, thereby increasing the tolerance of the spinal cord to ischemia. Studies have shown that hypothermia and thiopental produce similar spinal cord protection, increasing the tolerable ischemia time in animals (497). One human study reported that thiopental significantly decreased the incidence of paraplegia (498).

Corticosteroids have been used as protective agents against spinal cord ischemia. Suggestions for their mechanisms of protective action include stabilization of cell membranes, prevention of the release of chemical mediators, and scavenging of oxygen free radicals, which have been implicated in the development of ischemic injury (499,500). One canine study found that methylprednisolone enhanced the tolerance of the spinal cord to ischemia (499). This may be

TABLE 27-16. PHARMACOLOGIC AGENTS THAT MAY REDUCE THE FREQUENCY OR SEVERITY OF SPINAL CORD INJURY AFTER AN ISCHEMIC INSULT

Systemically administered agents
Steroids: methyl prednisolone
Barbiturates: thiopental
Opioid antagonists: naloxone
Oxygen free radical scavengers: superoxide dismutase, allopurinol
Calcium channel blockers: verapamil, flunarizine
N-Methyl D-aspartate (NMDA) receptor antagonists
Perfluorocarbon emulsions: Fluosol-DA
Magnesium
Gangliosides: GM-1
Poloxamer 188
Antiadhesion molecule monoclonal antibodies
Intrathecally administered agents
Papaverine
Magnesium
Tetracaine
Perflurocarbon emulsions: Fluosol DA

Source: Kouchouskos NT, Rokkas CK. Descending thorac and thoracoabdominal aortic surgery for aneurysm or dissection: how do we minimize the risk of spinal cord injury? *Semin Thorac Cardiovasc Surg* 1993;5:47, with permission.

related to the finding that neurologic outcome is improved in humans after spinal cord traumatic injury by high-dose corticosteroid therapy. However, a study by Woloszyn et al. (477) showed that steroids combined with CSF drainage provided spinal cord protection during aortic cross-clamping but steroids alone were ineffective. Therefore, at present the protective effect of steroids on spinal cord protection is at best equivocal. The use of steroids may result in significant hyperglycemia, which may in itself worsen neurologic outcome (see later discussion).

Calcium channel blockers reduce the cellular influx of calcium after ischemia and reperfusion. Calcium channel blockers were found in experimental studies to decrease the incidence of spinal cord ischemic injury (501–503). Naloxone in large doses has been found to be effective in the treatment of patients with traumatic spinal cord injury (504, 505). Robertson et al. (497) found that naloxone increased the duration of tolerable ischemia in the rabbit model. The mechanism of action of naloxone as a protective agent may include blocking of neuronal activities and reduction of tissue metabolism, either directly or indirectly. Because of these findings, some anesthesiologists are reluctant to use neuroaxial opioids to provide analgesia to these patients.

Oxygen free radical scavengers may exert a protective effect by counteracting the effects of oxygen free radicals produced during the ischemic interval. Some studies report success with the use of superoxide dismutase in reducing paraplegia associated with aortic cross-clamping (506–508). However, this result was not substantiated in a study by Svensson et al. (432), which failed to demonstrate a protective effect of allopurinol or superoxide dismutase in reducing the risk of paraplegia in baboons after aortic cross-clamping. Additional agents that may exert spinal cord protective effects include magnesium and prostaglandin E (507).

Intrathecal papaverine was used successfully in humans with encouraging initial results (471). It acts by dilating spinal cord blood vessels and improving the blood supply to the spinal cord. It is used in conjunction with CSF drainage. Intrathecal tetracaine also has been found to be effective, probably by reducing spinal cord metabolism or exerting membrane-stabilizing effects (473). An oxygenated perfluorocarbon (Fluosol-DA) administered intraarterially or intrathecally is associated with improved neurologic outcome in dogs after cross-clamping of the descending thoracic aorta (478). This compound has the capacity to carry oxygen and to provide nutritional support to ischemic areas.

Activation of NMDA receptors by glutamate released from nerve terminals in response to an ischemic insult is believed to be an important mechanism mediating neuronal cell death. Pharmacologic antagonism of NMDA receptor-mediated neurotoxicity may provide an effective approach for attenuation of the effects of spinal cord ischemia. The most extensively studied glutamate antagonist, MK-801, was shown to have protective effects after focal cerebral ischemia in cats (509). In a rabbit model of spinal cord ischemia, treatment with MK-801 increased the tolerable period of ischemia from 29 to 50 minutes (510). The clinical use of MK-801 is limited by its toxicity. Ketamine is an NMDA receptor antagonist, but its use for spinal cord protection during aortic surgery has not been studied. Magnesium administered systemically or intrathecally may improve neurologic outcome, possibly via antagonism of NMDA receptors (511,512).

Gangliosides are complex acidic glycolytics that are present in high concentrations in the CNS cells and are believed to block calcium activity and help stimulate growth of nerve cells and regeneration of damaged nervous tissues. One such ganglioside, GM-1, has been shown clinically to enhance the recovery of motor function after traumatic spinal cord injury (513). A copolymer (poloxamer 188) has been shown to improve CNS function after long periods of DHCA (514). Its role in the prevention of paraplegia remains to be examined. Research has also focused on monoclonal antibodies to prevent adhesions and transendothelial migration of activated leukocytes. Leukocytes potentiate neurologic injury by direct cytotoxic effect and by the mechanical occlusion of the microcirculation of the spinal cord (491). Monoclonal antibodies to an intracellular adhesion molecule on the endothelium (anti-CD-18) significantly reduced neurologic injury in a reversible spinal cord ischemic model in rabbits (394).

Hyperglycemia. Using a rabbit model, Drummond et al. (515) demonstrated that moderate elevation of the serum glucose concentration before and during a period of spinal cord ischemia is associated with markedly poor neurologic outcome. The adverse spinal cord effects appear to be similar to the findings in cerebral ischemia and may be the result of increased lactate production during or after the period of ischemia. Several studies have demonstrated that the provision of exogenous glucose exacerbates spinal cord ischemic damage in animal models (516,517). Therefore, it is best to avoid hyperglycemia in patients undergoing thoracoabdominal aortic reconstruction. Glucose should not be included in the intravenously administered fluids except when specifically indicated to treat hypoglycemia (517,518). Whereas some advocate the aggressive treatment of glucose concentrations higher than 150 mg/dL before aortic cross-clamping with intravenous insulin, such an approach has not been proven by prospective, randomized clinical studies to improve neurologic outcome.

Summary. Pharmacologic agents that have been experimentally shown to be effective in delaying the onset of paraplegia act primarily by one or more of five mechanisms: (a) stabilization of membrane damage that occurs as a result of ischemia (steroids and thiopental), (b) prevention of reperfusion injury secondary to calcium influxes (calcium channel blocking agents and magnesium), (c) counteraction of the effects of oxygen free radicals produced during the ischemic interval (oxygen free-radical scavengers, intrathecal papaverine), (d) optimization of the driving pressure or rheology in collateral arteries that supply the distal spinal cord (intrathecal papaverine, CSF drainage, oxygenated perfluorocarbon), and (e) provision of a direct source of supplemental oxygen delivery to the distal spinal cord (intravascular or intrathecal infusion of oxygenated perfluorocarbon).

Despite important advances in understanding of the etiology of the spinal cord ischemic injury and the development of methods to reduce its frequency, it seems unlikely that this complication can be totally eliminated or that any single intervention will substantially reduce its incidence after extensive resection of the thoracoabdominal aorta. Optimal protection of the spinal cord during aortic occlusion will require a multifaceted approach, combining pharmacologic agents with the rapid, precise identification and preservation or reimplantation of critical intercostal or lumbar arteries. In selected groups of patients, hypothermic protection with CPB or even DHCA may be a useful adjunct.

Endovascular Stent-Graft Repair of Aortic Aneurysms

The technique of endovascular aortic aneurysm repair has evolved from the minimally invasive method of transfemoral repair of infrarenal abdominal aortic aneurysms to more complex treatment of aortic disease including aneurysms of the descending thoracic aorta (519–521). The endovascular stent-graft is composed of a stainless steel endoskeleton of stent elements and a covering of woven Dacron. The diameter, length, taper, and curvature of the stent are based on measurements obtained from each patient's radiologic scanning results. The technique avoids or reduces the hemodynamic, hemorrhagic, and hemostatic derangements that may be associated with traditional open aneurysm surgery. Initially, endovascular repair was offered primarily to high-risk patients with significant coexisting cardiovascular and pulmonary impairments. Because of potentially lower morbidity and faster recovery, it is now being increasingly used in lower-risk patients as well. Endovascular repair may be performed in the operating room or, less preferably, at remote sites such as the radiology department or cardiac catheterization laboratory. Repair is usually done through the surgically exposed femoral or iliac artery or the lower abdominal aorta. The premeasured graft is inserted through an open arteriotomy under fluoroscopic control.

A variety of endovascular prostheses are undergoing various stages of trials in the United States. The two currently used grafts employ different methods to hold the graft in its proper position. The EVT graft (Endovascular Technologies Inc., Menlo Park, CA) uses hooks incorporated at the proximal and distal ends of the graft, which become embedded into the aortic wall when an intraluminal balloon is briefly inflated (522,523). The AneuRx graft (Medtronic AneuRx, Inc., Sunnyvale, CA) is composed of graft material covering a self-expanding metallic framework. It does not routinely require intraluminal balloon inflation during its deployment. The lateral pressure of the self-expanding graft on the aortic wall is sufficient to prevent any distal migration. During deployment of the AneuRx graft a balloon may or may not be transiently inflated. The inflation of the endovascular balloon is equivalent to a brief period of aortic cross-clamping. At present, aortic stent-grafts are most frequently used to repair infrarenal aortic aneurysms. The hemodynamic consequences of infrarenal endovascular balloon inflation are minimal compared with those of suprarenal, supraceliac, or thoracic aortic occlusion. More significant hemodynamic changes are likely to be encountered during stent-graft repair of the descending thoracic aorta.

Anesthetic Considerations for Endovascular Aortic Aneurysm Repair

Generally patients undergoing endovascular stent-graft aortic repair appear to have greater hemodynamic stability compared with those undergoing traditional open repair (524). Baxendale et al. demonstrated greater hemodynamic stability in patients undergoing endovascular infrarenal aortic repair under general anesthesia (525). However, marked changes in hemodynamic conditions, including sudden and severe hypotension and bradycardia, have been described, especially during balloon inflation for device deployment (526). Causes of hypotension include hemorrhage and loss of blood into the aneurysm sac after graft implantation, release of endothelial vasoactive substances, and/or an autonomic reflex in response to endovascular balloon inflation. In a series of 12 patients undergoing infrarenal aortic repair with an EVT endovascular graft under neuroaxial blockade (epidural or continuous spinal), 25% of patients had sudden severe bradycardia and hypotension necessitating immediate therapy (527). More recent experience suggests that deployment of the AneuRx self-expanding stent-graft usually is not associated with significant bradycardic events (528).

Other anesthetic considerations of endovascular aortic repair include the need for patient immobility and a quiescent surgical field, anticoagulation, invasive monitoring, the possible need for induced hypotension, the potential for sudden or insidious blood loss, impaired renal function, and unintentional hypothermia (529). Excessive blood loss may occur suddenly or insidiously, internally or externally, as a result of aneurysm leak or rupture or by continuous oozing at the endovascular access points. Accordingly, blood must be immediately available, and large-bore intravenous access must be obtained before the procedure. Because of the high incidence of CAD, careful monitoring and aggressive treatment of myocardial ischemia is essential. Conversion to open repair may be required in 2% to 20% of patients (average, 9%) due to technical difficulty with graft deployment or acute surgical complications such as aneurysm rupture or arterial injury (530,531). With increasing experience, the need for emergency conversion to open repair is decreasing to approximately 2% to 5% of cases but is still associated with increased morbidity and mortality in these high-risk surgical patients (528).

Hemodynamic Manipulations for Device Deployment

Some endovascular stents, especially the EVT graft, require alteration of blood pressure and flow through the aorta during graft deployment to avoid a windsock effect that may result in pushing the device distal to its intended placement site. Decreasing the mean arterial pressure to approximately 60 mm Hg and reducing the force of forward blood flow can minimize the windsock effect. The desired hypotension and decreased dP/dT can be achieved by the judicious use of β-blockers in combination with vasodilators or neuroaxial blockade-induced sympathectomy (528). In patients with significant coexisting atherosclerotic vascular disease of major organs (heart, brain, kidneys), induced hypertension should be avoided altogether or its duration minimized. A stent-graft that does not require hemodynamic manipulations for its deployment would be more desirable in such patients. Adenosine has been used to induce transient asystole for stent deployment during endovascular descending thoracic aortic repair. Transient asystole for 20 to 60 seconds can be induced with the use of 12 to 45 mg of adenosine (532,533). Thoracic aortic endovascular grafts have also been successfully deployed without the use of adenosine-induced asystole.

Preoperative Patient Evaluation and Preparation for Endovascular Aortic Repair

Vascular surgical patients frequently have associated comorbid conditions, including diabetes, pulmonary impairment (usually due to smoking), and atherosclerosis of the coronary, cerebral, renal, visceral, and peripheral vascular beds. Perioperative cardiac morbidity is a major risk in these patients. The severity and stability of cardiac disease and its treatment history must be clearly delineated. New guidelines for preoperative evaluation take into account the patient's functional capacity and coexisting diseases as well as surgery-specific cardiac risk classification. Traditional open aortic repair is considered to be a high-risk surgical procedure, whereas endovascular aortic repair appears to carry an intermediate surgical risk unless open conversion occurs (528). The framework and recommendations for preoperative evaluation should follow the guidelines proposed by the American College of Cardiology and the American Heart Association (534). Prophylactic coronary revascularization before noncardiac surgery is necessary only for a small subset of very high-risk patients. However, the perioperative use of β-blockers reduces the incidence of perioperative myocardial infarction, the frequency of postoperative ischemia, and the risk of death at 2 years postoperatively (535,536).

Intraoperative Anesthetic Management of Endovascular Aortic Repair

In addition to standard noninvasive monitoring, intraarterial pressure monitoring is required because of the potential for rapid and wide swings in blood pressure and also because of the frequent coexisting disease states. The radial artery is the most frequently used site, but other alternatives are acceptable depending on specific patient factors. In aneurysms involving the descending thoracic aorta that could encroach on the left subclavian artery, a right upper-extremity arterial line may be preferable. A central venous line is useful for hemodynamic monitoring and for the rapid administration of resuscitative drugs into the central circulation. A CVP that slowly drifts lower may be one of the earlier signs of occult bleeding. The placement of a PA catheter introducer sheath (8.5F or 9F) has the added advantage of providing large-bore intravenous access and would permit floating of a PA catheter if that becomes necessary. A PA catheter is useful in patients with severely impaired left ventricular function or significant renal impairment and in those who will be undergoing inflation of an intraluminal balloon in the descending thoracic aorta. Continuous computerized ST-segment monitoring improves the sensitivity for detection of intraoperative and postoperative myocardial ischemic events, which are strong predictors of myocardial infarction (537). Similarly, postoperative myocardial ischemia is a significant predictor of long-term myocardial infarction and cardiac death, suggesting that aggressive ST-segment monitoring should be continued into the postoperative period (538).

The anesthetic technique may consist of general anesthesia, regional anesthesia (epidural, spinal, or continuous spinal), or local anesthesia plus sedation (528). The choice of technique is influenced by multiple factors, including local customs and the experience of the surgical and anesthetic teams. Consideration should be given to the potential for intraoperative hemodynamic instability and the possible need to react rapidly to surgical complications. The anesthetic goals include analgesia, sedation, anxiolysis, patient immobility, and maintenance of hemodynamic stability.

General anesthesia was the most commonly used method during the initial experience with endovascular infrarenal aortic repairs because it provided the ability to rapidly convert to open surgical repair. With evolving experience, regional anesthesia (subarachnoid or epidural blockade) and even local anesthesia with sedation and monitoring are being increasingly used for endovascular aortic repairs. Central neuroaxial blockade was shown to improve short-term graft patency in peripheral vascular procedures, probably as a result of its favorable effects on the coagulation system (539,540). A variety of drugs have been used successfully for general anesthesia, including etomidate, thiopentone, propofol, potent synthetic opioids, nitrous oxide, volatile anesthetics, and muscle relaxants (525,529). In patients with severely impaired left ventricular function, etomidate together with a potent opioid such as fentanyl or sufentanil provides adequate hemodynamic stability. Advantages of regional anesthesia include minimization of systemic drug use, decreased afterload, continuation of pain relief into the postoperative period, and the improved ability to detect symptoms of myocardial ischemia in patients who can report the occurrence of chest pain. Central neuroaxial blockade was shown to reduce the postoperative hypercoagulable state, which may result in a decreased incidence of deep vein thrombosis and vascular graft occlusion (539,540).

Because of the variable and unpredictable duration of these procedures, epidural anesthesia is the most commonly used technique because it has the flexibility of providing anesthesia of indefinite duration. Careful titration of the dermatomal level helps minimize the sympathectomy-related hypotension. Continuation of epidural blockade beyond the operating room is an excellent method of providing postoperative analgesia. A normal coagulation profile must be assured before catheter placement and removal. Continuous spinal anesthesia using an intrathecally placed epidural catheter provides a more rapid onset of a more dense neuroaxial block than does epidural anesthesia. By the incremental titration of the dermatomal level, it can be associated with more hemodynamic stability than a single-dose spinal block. Its duration can be extended by repeat administration of small doses of local anesthetics. At our institution, we are reluctant to use a subarachnoid catheter to provide postoperative analgesia. Concern about postlumbar puncture headache is minimal in the geriatric population even after dural puncture with an 18-gauge Touhy needle.

Endovascular aortic stent repair, especially of the infrarenal segment, has also been performed under monitored anesthesia care. The surgical incision site in the groin is infiltrated with a local anesthetic together with the intravenous administration of a sedative-hypnotic agent (midazolam, propofol) and an opioid. Remifentanil is an ultrashort-acting opioid that is well suited for administration by a continuous infusion either alone or in combination with a sedative-hypnotic drug. The infusion of propofol in combination with fentanyl, alfentanil, or remifentanil is commonly used during monitored anesthesia care.

Drake et al. used general anesthesia in 103 patients undergoing endovascular repair of the descending thoracic aorta (541). The procedure was performed with the patient in the right lateral decubitus position, and TEE was used to guide proper stent placement. General anesthesia provides greater patient comfort when adenosine is used to induce sinus arrest and temporary interruption of CO during thoracic aortic stent deployment. The surgical team must be fully prepared to rapidly perform a left lateral thoracotomy in the event of a surgical emergency. OLV, achieved with the use of a DLT or a bronchial blocker, would help in surgical exposure and rapid proximal control of the aorta.

TRAUMATIC INJURY OF THE AORTA AND GREAT VESSELS

During blunt chest trauma, abrupt deceleration of the thorax applies a shearing force to the aortic wall that is greatest at the origin of the subclavian artery and, in the ascending aorta, at the level of the coronary ostia. Traumatic disruption of the aorta is immediately fatal in approximately 85% of cases. A minority of patients survive because of containment and tamponade of the hemorrhage by adjacent mediastinal structures. Often the adventitia remains intact and prevents immediate exsanguination, but sudden aortic rupture may develop later. Alternatively, an intimal tear may be produced, with subsequent formation of a dissecting aneurysm. Occasionally patients are asymptomatic and remain undiscovered after injury, only to present with chronic traumatic aneurysm formation several years later. Aortic rupture is encountered in one of every six patients dying from blunt chest trauma secondary to motor vehicle accidents. The most notorious cause and mechanism is steering wheel impact during a motor vehicle accident (542). Additional causes of aortic injury include penetrating trauma, crush injuries, large animal kicks, and falls from great heights. The most common sites of traumatic aortic rupture

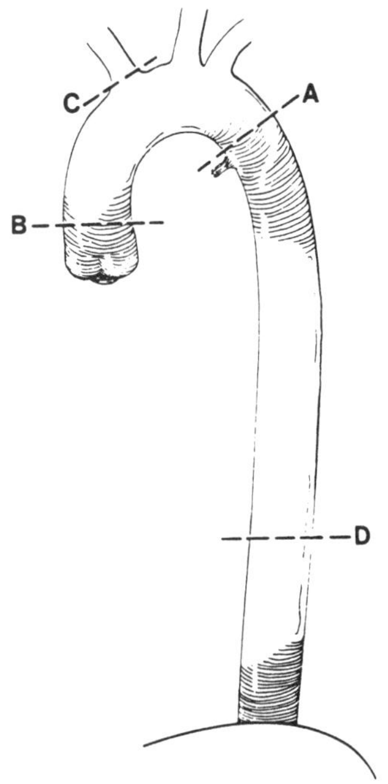

FIGURE 27-33. Sites of traumatic aortic disruption in descending order of frequency. **A:** Most common site adjacent to the ligamentum arteriosum. **B:** Ascending aorta. **C:** Avulson of the innominate artery from the aortic arch. **D:** Lower descending aorta. (From Stene JK, Grande CM, Bernhard WN, et al. Perioperative anesthetic management of the trauma patient: thoracoabdominal and orthopaedic injuries. In: Stene JK, Grande CM, eds. *Trauma anesthesia.* Baltimore: Williams & Wilkins, 1991:218, with permission.)

are (a) just distal to the origin of the left subclavian artery at the ligamentum arteriosum (80% to 90%), (b) at the root of the aorta (with possible dissection back to the coronary ostia, (c) at the innominate artery (avulsion from the aortic arch), and (d) at the aortic hiatus at the level of the diaphragm (Fig. 27-33).

Clinical findings of aortic rupture include the following diagnostic triad, which is seen in more than 50% of cases: (a) increased arterial blood pressure and pulse amplitude in the upper extremities, (b) decreased pressure and pulse amplitude in the lower extremities, and (c) a widened superior mediastinum on the chest radiograph (543) (Table 27-17). Additional symptoms in the conscious patient include retrosternal or interscapular pain, dysphagia due to esophageal compression, ischemic extremity pain, dyspnea, and hoarseness due to recurrent laryngeal nerve dysfunction. Associated injuries may include the steering wheel imprint on the chest wall, massive hemothorax, cardiac contusion, rib fractures, and tension pneumothorax (542). Diagnosis should be suspected in trauma victims when the chest radiograph shows a widened superior mediastinum (544). Aortography remains the definitive diagnostic procedure. The yield of positive aortography in acute trauma victims with widened mediastinum is approximately 17% (545). After

TABLE 27-17. COMMON CLINICAL AND RADIOGRAPHIC FEATURES OF AORTIC RUPTURE

Clinical Features	Radiographic Features
Increased arterial pressure and pulse amplitude of upper extremities	Widened mediastinum
Decreased arterial pressure and pulse amplitude of lower extremities	Unsharp aortic contours
Retrosternal or interscapular pain	Opacified pulmonary window
Hoarseness	Broadened paratracheal stripe
Systolic flow murmur over the precordium or medial to the left scapula	Displacement of the left main stem bronchus
Neurologic deficits in the lower extremities	Rightward deviation of the esophagus
	Sternal and/or upper rib fractures
	Left hemothorax

Source: Jackson J. Management of thoracoabdominal injuries. In: Capan LM, Miller SM, Turndorf H, eds. *Trauma: Anesthesia and intensive care.* Philadelphia: JB Lippincott, 1991:498, with permission.

confirming the diagnosis by angiography, surgical repair should be accomplished as soon as possible.

Surgical Management

The surgical approach is dictated by the location of the tear. Depending on the anatomy of the tear and the condition of the aorta, surgical repair may consist of excision and end-to-end anastomosis, patching, or replacement with a prosthetic vascular tube graft. The surgical repair may be performed with a simple clamp-and-sew technique, passive (Gott) shunt, partial CPB, or left-sided heart bypass. Although the simple clamp-and-sew technique is associated with many disadvantages, it offers some advantages, especially in fast and experienced hands. The use of partial CPB or atriofemoral bypass has been shown to reduce the incidence of paraplegia and neurologic complications, compared with passive shunts and simple clamp-and-sew technique (546–548). A left-sided heart bypass using the Biomedicus centrifugal pump allows the regulation of flow while requiring little or no systemic heparinization, which may lessen bleeding from associated injuries in the setting of traumatic aortic rupture (549). The use of partial CPB was shown to decrease mortality as well as the paraplegia rate in traumatic aortic rupture (546,550). Higher paraplegia rates ranging from 3% to 33% are observed after the repair of traumatic aortic rupture than after descending thoracic aneurysm repair. In addition to aortic cross-clamping time, other factors influence the incidence of paraplegia after traumatic aortic rupture. In patients treated without the use of distal aortic perfusion, the incidence of paraplegia has a strong positive correlation with aortic cross-clamping time longer than 30 minutes (551). Completion of the surgical repair within 30 minutes is frequently not feasible. Technical difficulties with complex tears and intraoperative cardiovascular instability frequently increase cross-clamping duration. Distal aortic perfusion attenuates hemodynamic and metabolic disturbances and confers spinal cord protection, especially during the longer cross-clamping times that are frequently required to repair traumatic aortic rupture (550).

Anesthetic Management

The usual anesthetic implications of patients with multiple trauma are applicable to those with acute traumatic aortic rupture. These include nothing-by-mouth (NPO) status; the need for full-stomach precautions; the presence of associated injuries, especially head and cervical spine injuries and pneumothorax; the need for large-bore intravenous access; the need for massive transfusions of blood and coagulation factors; and the susceptibility to intraoperative hypothermia. The possibility of acute alcohol intoxication should also be kept in mind. In addition to the usual routine monitors, intraoperative invasive hemodynamic monitoring should include a right radial arterial line in case of descending traumatic aortic rupture and a left radial arterial line in case of ascending traumatic aortic rupture. In all but the most emergent cases, PA catheterization is also desirable because proximal aortic occlusion imposes a severe afterload stress on the left ventricle and may precipitate left ventricular failure. In addition, monitoring of cardiac filling pressures guides intraoperative fluid management. Descending thoracic aortic tears are usually approached via a left thoracotomy. A DLT is highly desirable to facilitate surgical exposure and to isolate the dependent right lung from the parenchymal hemorrhage that frequently occurs in the left lung as a result of surgical retraction. This can be a particularly serious problem in patients who are heparinized for femorofemoral bypass.

Surgical technique may consist of a simple clamp-and-sew technique, the use of a Gott shunt, partial CPB, or the use of an atriofemoral left heart centrifugal pump bypass. When methods that provide distal perfusion are to be employed, an additional arterial line in the femoral artery is helpful to monitor distal aortic perfusion pressure. The prevention of renal, spinal cord, and mesenteric ischemia follows similar guidelines as discussed earlier. The use of full CPB and DHCA for spinal cord protection has been described (546). The induction of anesthesia depends on the patient's mental status and the degree of hemodynamic instability as well as other associated injuries. Useful induction agents include etomidate or ketamine together with succinylcholine and rapid intubation of the trachea. Hypertension should be prevented during induction and intubation in order to avoid the free rupture of a previously contained aortic tear. Maintenance of anesthesia is usually with a narcotic-oxygen-relaxant technique supplemented with low-dose volatile agents or benzodiazepines as tolerated by the patient's hemodynamic status. The patient remains intubated and ventilated postoperatively in the intensive care unit.

Injury is confined to the ascending aorta in fewer than 10% of patients with traumatic aortic rupture. These patients usually present with cardiac tamponade and may have concurrent involvement of the coronary arteries or the aortic valve. Repair of these lesions requires median sternotomy, CPB, and cardioplegia for myocardial preservation. Frequently, when aortic cross-clamping is not possible, DHCA is used.

Survival after traumatic avulsion of the arch vessels is extremely rare, but successful repairs have been reported. Total CPB is initiated using femoral artery cannulation. Profound hypothermia is achieved, and repair of the arch is completed during a period of DHCA (57). As discussed earlier, pharmacologic brain protection during DHCA is of unproven benefit. Although barbiturates do reduce cerebral metabolism, their cerebroprotective effect is not additive to that conferred by hypothermia alone (552). The risk of paraplegia in patients with acute traumatic aortic rupture ranges from 3% to 33% (381). In a retrospective clinical study of patients with traumatic aortic rupture, postoperative renal dysfunction was found to have occurred in 27% of the cases. Preservation of distal perfusion with the use of a shunt or partial bypass was associated with a lower incidence of postoperative renal dysfunction (553). The mortality rate may be as high as 30%, especially in patients with multiple associated injuries. Mortality is directly related to the injury severity score, the number of injured organ systems and the time from the accident to arrival at the emergency department, but it does not correlate directly with the time taken in the hospital to make a definitive diagnosis or to reach the operating room. Advanced age and preoperative hypotension are risk factors for intraoperative death (550,554).

DEVELOPMENTAL ANOMALIES

Coarctation of the Aorta

Coarctation of the aorta is a congenital narrowing of the aortic lumen near the attachment of the ductus arteriosus. It accounts for 6% to 8% of all congenital heart defects. Approximately 50% of coarctations are classified as simple. The remaining 50% are associated with other congenital defects, as follows: (a) bicuspid aortic valve, 15% to 85%; (b) mitral valve anomalies, 20% to 60%; (c) Turner syndrome, 50%; (d) patent ductus arteriosus (PDA), 20% to 100%; (e) ventricular septal defects, 40%; (f) cerebral aneurysms of the Circle of Willis, 10%. A PDA is present in almost 100% of neonates and in most infants with preductal coarctation.

Anatomy

Coarctation is produced by a ridge-like protrusion within the posterior and lateral aortic media. The lesion may be discrete near the ductus arteriosus, or it may be accompanied by extensive abnormalities of the aortic arch, aortic valve, and left ventricular outflow tract. The coarctation is described by its relationship to the ductus arteriosus as preductal, juxtaductal, or postductal. Lesions in patients who present in infancy are usually proximal to the ductus (preductal) and are characterized by poor collateral flow. Hypoplasia of the isthmus and transverse arch frequently accompanies preductal coarctation. The aortic wall is infiltrated with abnormal ductal tissue, which must be excised to avoid recoarctation (555,556). The introduction of prostaglandins to maintain ductal patency has significantly reduced mortality and morbidity in neonates with symptomatic coarctation (556). Juxtaductal and postductal coarctations are the most common forms; the patient usually present later in life. Clinical diagnosis is usually delayed because of the presence of abundant collateral blood flow that develops even prenatally. Collaterals develop between the subclavian artery and intercostal arteries later in childhood (Fig. 27-34).

Pathophysiology and Clinical Manifestations

Preductal coarctation is characterized by CHF manifesting in the neonatal period. Lower-body hypoperfusion develops as the ductus arteriosus starts to close. A large shunt from the PA into the descending aorta occurs in patients with preductal coarctation and a PDA, resulting in differential cyanosis of the lower extremities and sometimes of the left hand, while the right hand and lips remain pink. Poor distal body perfusion and systemic acidosis rapidly develop if the ductus arteriosus closes. The increased left atrial and left ventricular pressure may result in reopening of the foramen ovale and the development of a left-to-right interatrial shunt. Management in these infants must be aggressive, with diuresis, inotropic support, endotracheal intubation, and positive-pressure ventilation. The infusion of prostaglandin E_1 is essential to maintain ductal patency and restore the fetal blood flow pattern, thereby ameliorating left ventricular failure and improving distal body perfusion. Rapid surgical correction of the coarctation is necessary in these critically ill neonates. The spectrum of disease is differ-

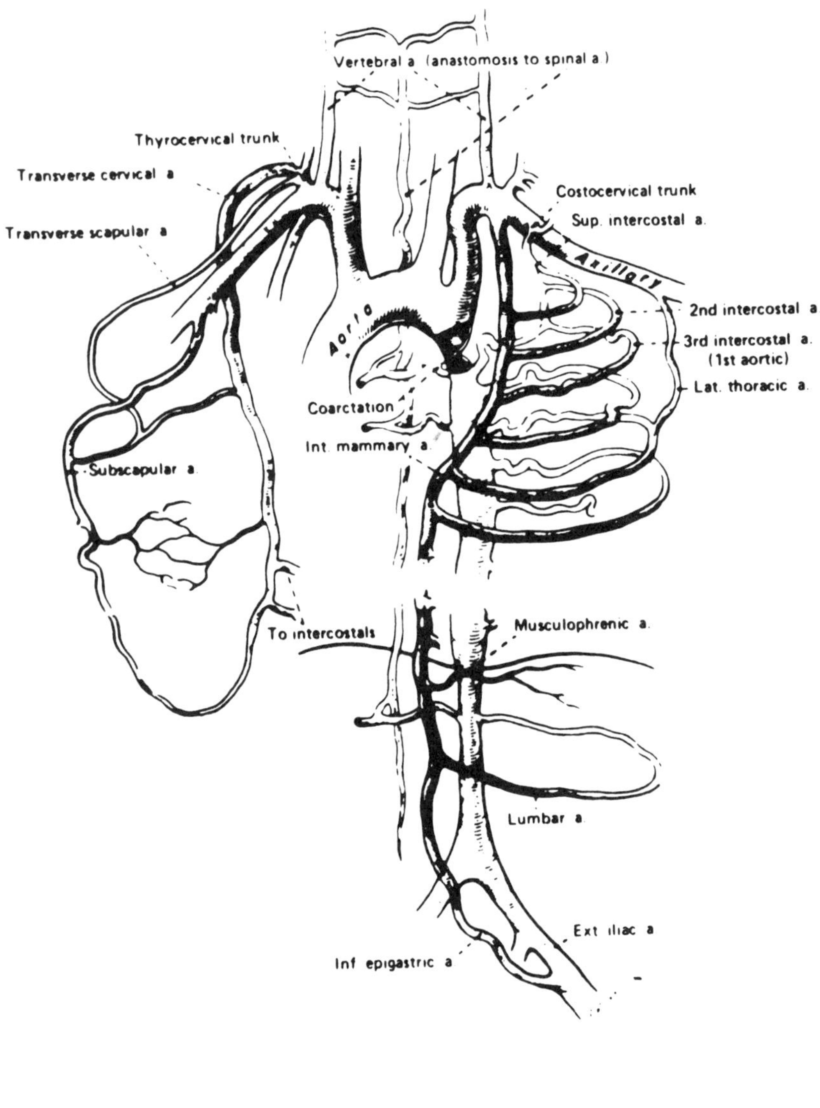

FIGURE 27-34. Collateral circulation in coarctation of the aorta. (From Davis PJ, Cook DR. Anesthesia for pediatric vascular lesions. In: Kaplan JA, ed. *Vascular anesthesia.* New York: Churchill Livingstone, 1991:494, with permission.)

ent in infants with isolated coarctation, compared with those with associated ventricular septal defect or other complex congenital cardiac lesions.

Postductal coarctation manifests later in childhood with less severe symptoms, such as headaches, epistaxis, or lower-extremity fatigue after exercise. A blood pressure gradient of 20 mm Hg or more between the upper and lower extremities is suggestive of coarctation. Diagnostic features include upper-extremity hypertension in conjunction with weak to absent lower-extremity pulses. Systolic hypertension above and hypotension below the coarctation are common in older infants and children. A systolic ejection murmur is commonly present along the left upper sternal border. A PDA is present in 20% of these patients. An extensive collateral circulation involving the periscapular, intercostal, transverse cervical, and internal mammary arteries develops with time. In patients with well-developed collaterals, the pressure difference between the upper and lower extremities may become apparent only with exercise. In addition to the afterload increase, an increase in plasma renin activity and an expanded extracellular fluid volume contribute to the hypertension (557).

Chest radiographic findings include left ventricular dilatation and cardiomegaly. Pulmonary edema and pleural effusions indicate the presence of CHF. Rib notching indicates the presence of tortuous collateral vessels along the inferior borders of the rib margins and is usually seen after the age of 5 years. *In utero* evidence of coarctation can be found as early as 18 weeks of gestation. The lesion is inferred from measurements of relative ventricular size, diminished aortic flow, and a greater than 2:1 flow ratio of tricuspid versus mitral valve (558).

Cardiovascular collapse was a frequent presentation in neonates before the introduction of prostaglandin therapy. More subtle neonatal presenting signs and symptoms include decreased femoral pulses (92%), proximal hypertension (44%), CHF (54%), tachypnea (50%), distal body cyanosis (32%), difficulty in feeding (23%), and listlessness (13%). Clinical recognition of coarctation beyond the neonatal period may be difficult. Femoral pulses may be present in patients with mild coarctation, PDA, or well-developed collaterals. A pressure gradient of more than 20 mm Hg between the upper and lower extremities is suggestive of coarctation (559). The presence of aortic regurgitation minimizes the pressure gradient. Continuous wave Doppler echocardiographic estimates of aortic gradients correlate well with angiographic findings (560). The ratio of blood flow velocity in the distal aortic arch to that in the proximal descending aorta is useful for the diagnosis of coarctation (561). Echocardiographic and Doppler criteria for the diagnosis of coarctation in the presence of PDA have also been established (562). Angiography is no longer required in most patients if echocardiographic and MRI findings are conclusive (562,563). Cardiac catheterization is performed to evaluate associated congenital heart defects and before balloon angioplasty (563). Experience with MRI as a diagnostic modality has increased. Advantages of MRI include definitive anatomic visualization, dynamic spatial-to-temporal flow assessment in all regions, the ability to analyze ductal and aortic flows independently, and good accuracy even in the presence of coexisting lung disease or chest wall deformities (564,565). Coarctation may be associated with several genetic syndromes. Frequently, coarctation and bicuspid aortic valve accompany Turner syndrome. The anomalous origin of one or both coronary arteries from the PA is seen very infrequently with coarctation and should be suspected if clinical deterioration occurs after uneventful repair (566).

Natural History

If left untreated, aortic coarctation has a very poor prognosis, with death occurring at the mean age of 34 years. Mortality results from CHF (25%), aortic rupture (21%), bacterial endocarditis (18%), and intracranial hemorrhage due to rupture of a cerebral aneurysm (12%). Other causes include hypertension and CAD.

Surgical Treatment

The optimal age to perform elective coarctation repair beyond the neonatal period is debated. Early repairs in patients younger than 1 year of age are associated with higher rates of early mortality and residual or recurrent coarctation. Correction later in childhood is associated with a higher incidence of residual hypertension and persistently increased risk of late cardiovascular mortality and morbidity. Evidence suggests that the best short and long-term results are achieved when repair is performed between the ages of 12 and 18 months (567). There are multiple therapeutic options for the correction of coarctation, each with its own advantages and disadvantages. The classic approach is resection of the stenosed area followed by an end-to-end anastomosis. This approach is associated with a high incidence of recurrent coarctation, especially if the repair is performed before the age of 1 year. Modifications of the classic end-to-end repair are gaining popularity, especially in neonates. Oblique anastomosis with anterior augmentation by subclavian flap angioplasty, left subclavian reimplantation, or subclavian end-to-side anastomosis allows for enlargement of the hypoplastic arch that is frequently seen in neonates. Old ductal tissue is excised, and left arm blood flow can be maintained.

Subclavian flap angioplasty was introduced as a technique for augmenting the aorta without a circumferential suture line, thereby preserving the natural ability of the aorta to grow. However, the incidence of restenosis was not entirely eliminated. Horner syndrome, subclavian steal, brachial plexus injury, and aneurysm formation are possible complication of subclavian flap angioplasty. Although it successfully decreases the incidence of recoarctation, subclavian flap angioplasty decreases blood flow velocity in the left brachial artery, potentially causing ischemia and claudication during exercise. Diminished growth and gangrene of the left arm have been described (568). Patch augmentation of the aorta with synthetic materials (Gore-Tex or Dacron) produces excellent early results but has largely been abandoned because of the high incidence of aneurysm formation at the site of repair, with the associated potential for acute rupture and sudden death (569). In some patients with severe, complex, or recurrent lesions, the insertion of a long segment tube graft maybe required to reconstruct the aorta.

Although initial reports of balloon angioplasty described good short-term results and reduced hospital costs, subsequent follow-up indicated a high incidence of recurrent or residual stenosis (570). Balloon dilatation relieves coarctation or recoarctation by circumferential tearing of the intimal and medial layers of the vessel wall. In 60% to 80% of interventions gradient reduction is satisfactory, there are no significant complications, and there is rapid healing of the vessel wall. The technique appears best suited to the child older than 1 year of age, although acute gradient reduction can also be achieved in neonates and infants. Long-term relief is obtained in 85% of those with initially successful procedures. In a patient who does not achieve a satisfactory hemodynamic or vascular outcome, open surgical repair can be employed with no increased risk and with good long-term outcome. Because of its relatively low morbidity and mortality, balloon angioplasty may become the first therapeutic modality for unoperated coarctation in children (with the exception of neonates and young infants) and in all patients with recoarctation after surgical repair (571). Risk factors for recurrence were young age (less than 1 year) at the time of angioplasty, tubular hypoplasia of the aortic arch, the presence of PDA, and a postangioplasty gradient more than 12 mm Hg (572). Compromise or total occlusion of the femoral artery through which the balloon was passed is common in patients younger than 1 year of age (573). This may be avoided by use of the transumbilical approach in neonates. Improvements in endovascular technique are being investigated and may improve the usefulness of balloon angioplasty for the repair of aortic coarctation. Intravascular ultrasound may be used to monitor the extent of vascular disruption and to assist in optimal positioning of the endovascular balloon (574). Experimental and clinical studies demonstrated the effectiveness of balloon-expandable stent placement in patients with coarctation or recoarctation. Stent placement may address some of the limitations of simple balloon angioplasty, including restenosis due to vessel recoil and aneurysm formation. The insertion of endovascular balloon-expandable stents has also been successful in patients with residual and recurrent stenosis and long tubular narrowing (575,576).

Perioperative and Anesthetic Management of Coarctation Repair

In addition to the routine noninvasive monitors, one or two intraarterial catheters are essential for continuous monitoring of the arterial blood pressure. The ideal sites of cannulation are the right radial artery and one of the femoral arteries. Alternatively, a single arterial catheter is used in the right radial or femoral artery and a blood pressure cuff placed on the alternate site. The left radial artery is avoided because of possible clamping of the left subclavian artery during the repair. Large-bore peripheral venous access is usually sufficient. In older and asymptomatic children with well-developed collaterals, the hemodynamic and metabolic changes associated with aortic cross-clamping are minimal. Indications for central venous access include (a) associated cardiovascular disease, (b) the anticipated use of CPB for the repair of associated congenital defects, (c) critically ill infant or neonate, and (d) patient requiring aggressive hemodynamic and inotropic therapy. Antihypertensive therapy with vasodilators and β-blockers could be safely administered through peripheral venous catheters.

Most procedures are performed via a left thoracotomy, but a midline approach may be required in neonates in the presence of significant arch hypoplasia or other cardiac defects requiring extensive intervention. General anesthesia with endotracheal intubation and controlled ventilation is required. Although OLV is beneficial in improving exposure, it is difficult to achieve in neonates and young children. If absolutely required, a single-lumen endotracheal tube is positioned above the carina and an endobronchial blocker is placed in the left main stem bronchus. Hyperventilation should be avoided because it decreases blood flow to the CNS, including the spinal cord. Although combined general and thoracic epidural anesthesia has been used with success (577), most clinicians are reluctant to place thoracic epidural catheters after the induction of general anesthesia in infants and young children, especially when paraplegia is a recognized risk of the surgical procedure. In neonates and young infants, analgesia could be provided from an epidural catheter placed via the caudal route and advanced toward the thoracic region. However, in skilled hands the use of thoracic epidural anesthesia and analgesia is still acceptable. Maintenance of anesthesia is usually by volatile anesthetics in conjunction with opioids. Nitrous oxide is usually avoided during the period of compression, retraction, and deflation of the left lung. In critically ill neonates and infants, the myocardial depressant effects of volatile anesthetics may not be well tolerated; this may necessitate their substitution with intravenous agents such as opioids and benzodiazepines. The use of ketamine is not advisable in the presence of severe proximal hypertension. In most cases early postoperative extubation is possible, except in critically ill neonates and infants.

The incidence of paraplegia after coarctation repair is relatively low, ranging from 0.4% to 1.0%. It is more common in patients with poorly developed collaterals. Maintenance of adequate lower body perfusion is important during the period of aortic clamping. Watterson et al. indicated that the mean arterial pressure in the descending aorta should be greater than the critical value of 45 mm Hg in children older than 1 year of age (578). Limiting the cross-clamping time, minimizing the number of intercostal arteries that are sacrificed, and avoiding hyperthermia reduce the risk of spinal cord ischemia. Spinal cord injury was reported in two infants and a 2-year-old child who had unintentional hyperthermia with temperatures of 39° to 40°C during or immediately after cross-clamping (579). Induction of mild hypothermia is an accepted method to reduce the risk of spinal cord ischemia in these patients. The temperature is allowed to drift to approximately 33° to 34°C by exposure to a cold operating room environment. Active rewarming with forced-warm-air blankets is commenced only after cross-clamp removal.

SSEPs and/or MEPs have been used to monitor spinal cord function during aortic cross-clamping in adults but are not commonly employed during aortic coarctation repair. Changes in SSEPs may reflect decreased blood flow to the spinal cord. Neuronal cell death may occur 15 to 45 minutes after loss of SSEPs (580). During cross-clamping, moderate hypertension in the proximal aorta should be accepted. The blood pressure should be allowed to rise to 20% to 30% above preoperative levels. An attempt to decrease proximal aortic pressure to near-normal levels will result in severe hypotension in the descending aorta and a marked decrease in spinal cord perfusion. Deepening the anesthetic level with volatile agents usually treats more severe proximal hypertension. If that is not sufficient, small doses of vasodilators and/or β-blockers are added. If a distal perfusion pressure of 45 mm Hg cannot be maintained, left-sided heart bypass or total CPB may be necessary to maintain adequate distal perfusion during the repair. Hypotension after the cross-clamp release is treated with fluid administration and small doses of vasoconstrictors. If necessary, blood is transfused to correct anemia and replace blood loss. Patients with well-developed collaterals experience mild hemodynamic changes and usually do not develop significant acidosis with clamping and unclamping. Most patients can be extubated at the end of the procedure, provided that they are hemodynamically stable, neuromuscular blockade is adequately reversed, and their temperature is greater than 35°C. However, because mild hypothermia is intentionally induced, the patient may still be hypothermic at the conclusion of surgery and may require active postoperative rewarming with forced-warm-air blankets before extubation. Multimodal postoperative pain management is achieved with the use of regional anesthetic techniques such as intercostal and paravertebral nerve blocks and intrathecal or epidural narcotics with or without local anesthetics together with intravenous opioids and nonsteroidal antiinflammatory drugs (NSAIDs).

Neonates and young infants presenting for coarctation repair are usually critically ill with CHF and respiratory insufficiency. Mechanical ventilation and infusions of prostaglandin E_1, inotropic agents, and sodium bicarbonate are typically started in the intensive care unit before arrival in the operating room. Pulmonary vascular congestion and interstitial edema decrease pulmonary compliance and interfere with gas exchange. The anesthetic technique usually involves the use of high-dose narcotics, oxygen, and muscle relaxants. In more hemodynamically stable infants, small doses of volatile anesthetics may be added as tolerated. Maintenance of adequate intravascular volume and oxygen carrying capacity by meticulous attention to blood and fluid replacement is essential. Mild hypothermia (34° to 35°C) is acceptable. Postoperative mechanical ventilation is continued until the CHF, acidosis, and pulmonary dysfunction have improved.

Postoperative Care

Postoperative hypertension is commonly seen after repair of aortic coarctation. Early hypertension (within the first 24 hours) results from catecholamine secretion, abnormal baroreceptor function, and the activity of the renin-angiotensin system (581). Control of blood pressure is achieved with β-blockers, angiotensin-converting enzyme inhibitors, and vasodilators such as sodium nitroprusside. If a thoracic epidural catheter has been placed, local anesthetic-induced sympathectomy is an effective persistent adjunct to lower the blood pressure. In 50% of patients, hypertension with a prominent diastolic component may be seen after the first postoperative day. It is associated with arteritis and increased levels of norepinephrine, angiotensin, and vasopressin together with a decreased concentration of atrial natriuretic factor (582). Pretreatment with β-blockers has been suggested to attenuate this hypertensive response.

A syndrome of mesenteric arteritis consisting of abdominal pain and distention, intestinal ileus, nausea, vomiting, and hypertension is reported to occur in 2% to 30% of patients 1 to 3 days after coarctation repair. The clinical picture is similar to that of patients with other sources of acute abdominal pain. Treatment consists of nasogastric decompression, intravenous fluids, and treatment of hypertension. Gastrointestinal bleeding is uncommon and can be minimized with a delay in feedings and administration of β-blockers. In addition to paraplegia, less severe, temporary or permanent neurologic complications may occur, including unilateral Horner syndrome, left recurrent laryngeal nerve injury (manifesting as stridor or hoarseness), and left phrenic nerve injury. Prolonged airway and ventilatory support may be required as a result of these nerve injuries. Recurrent laryngeal nerve complications are especially common in small premature infants.

Long-Term Results

Even after successful repair, long-term residual hypertension is reported in 17% to 50% of patients (583). A higher incidence of hypertension correlates with older age at the time of repair. Exercise-induced upper-body hypertension is associated with accelerated cardiovascular disease and premature mortality despite a good surgical repair (584). Abnormal baroreceptor function and stiffness of the proximal aorta are factors implicated in exercise-induced differential upper-body hypertension. Despite successful repair, intrinsic arterial pathophysiology contributes to long-term complications such as persistent hypertension, aneurysm formation (of the aorta, cerebral artery, and other arteries), and even aortic rupture. Decreased cardiac performance at peak exercise can be detected even after successful surgical repair. Residual left ventricular abnormalities include increased shortening fraction and left ventricular mass (585). Even in patients with residual gradients of less than 15 mm Hg and minimal or no systolic hypertension, persistent diastolic dysfunction with elevated left ventricular end-diastolic pressure has been reported (586). Decreased reactive hyperemia and a lower capacity for vascular relaxation were reported even after neonatal correction. The extent and severity of most residual cardiovascular abnormalities are directly proportional to the patient's age at the time of primary repair (586,587). Late cardiovascular complications include sudden death, premature cerebral vascular disease, and CAD. Treatment with cardioselective β-blockers may prevent accelerated cardiovascular disease. Restenosis occurs in almost 20% of the patients, especially those whose defect was repaired before 1 year of age. The surgical technique employed and the presence of residual ductal tissue at the site of resection affect the restenosis rate (588). Aneurysmal dilatation after repair may be related to cystic medial necrosis of the aorta. The incidence of aneurysm formation may be as high as 30% in patients who were treated with patch angioplasty. These patients are at risk of sudden death due to aortic rupture and must be monitored with repeat echocardiograms, chest radiographs, and CT scans (557).

Vascular Rings

Vascular rings are abnormalities of the great vessels and their branches that result in compression of the trachea and/or the esophagus, causing respiratory or feeding difficulties in infants. Congenital cardiac anomalies, including tetralogy of Fallot and transposition of the great vessels, are present in up to 20% of patients (589). The most common form of complete vascular ring is the double aortic arch with both arches remaining patent. Other variants include right aortic arch and retropharyngeal right subclavian artery with a left-sided ductus arteriosus. The common variants of complete vascular rings, in descending order of frequency, include a double aortic arch with both arches being patent, a right-sided aortic arch with a retropharyngeal right subclavian artery and a left-sided ductus arteriosus, right aortic arch with mirror-image branching and a left ligament arteriosum. The latter variant is almost always associated with cyanotic congenital heart disease. The most common variants of incomplete rings are the retropharyngeal right subclavian artery, anomalous innominate artery, and PA sling. Congenital cardiac anomalies are present in 50% to 80% of patients with PA sling.

Clinical Manifestations

Complete rings totally surround and compress the trachea and/or the esophagus, whereas incomplete rings produce only compressive manifestations. Symptoms include respiratory distress, dysphagia, wheezing, and cyanosis as early as the first day after birth. Infants are usually symptomatic by 3 months of age. Rarely, symptoms are first noted after 1 year of age. With tracheal obstruction, hyperinflation of the lungs progressively develops. Esophageal obstruction results in feeding difficulties and failure to thrive. Other respiratory symptoms include a harsh cry, inspiratory stridor, chronic cough, and recurrent bronchopneumonia (Table 27-18). The ECG and cardiac examination are usually normal unless there is associated congenital heart disease. The chest radiogram may show compression of the trachea, hyperinflation of the lungs, and/or the presence of atelectasis and pneumonia. The differential atelectasis of various lobes may indicate independent origin of the right upper bronchus from the trachea (bronchus suis). The esophagogram shows narrowing and compression in most malformations except the anomalous innominate artery. A pulsatile mass

TABLE 27-18. PRESENTATION OF COMPLETE AND INCOMPLETE VASCULAR RINGS

Finding	Symptoms	Postoperative Course
Left aortic arch with right descending aorta and right ductus	Dysphagia	Short
Double aortic arch	Severe symptoms: stridor, dyspnea, cough	Short-term postoperative tracheal obstruction
Right aortic arch with mirror-image branching	Congenitial heart disease (CHD) predominates	Depends on repair of CHD
Right aortic arch with anomalous left subclavian	Usually asymptomatic	Short
Left arch and right retroesophageal right subclavian	Usually asymptomatic	Short
Anomalous innominate	Tracheal compression	Patient may have tracheomalacia
Pulmonary artery sling	Obstructive emphysema or right lung atelectasis	May be prolonged

compressing the trachea is seen on bronchoscopy in the stridorous child with an anomalous innominate artery. Noninvasive methods have largely replaced angiography in the diagnosis of vascular rings. Echocardiography provides accurate diagnosis of the most common abnormalities. MRI is becoming the preferred technique for defining vascular anatomy. New technology permits three-dimensional modeling (590,591). A child with severe respiratory symptoms requires endotracheal intubation and mechanical ventilation until surgical repair is completed.

Surgical Repair

Surgical repair is required in the presence of significant symptoms or complications such as stridor, aspiration, atelectasis, or recurrent pneumonia. Complete vascular rings are surgically divided through a left posterolateral thoracotomy. A right thoracotomy is used when the patient has a left-sided aortic arch. Compression of the airway by an anomalous innominate artery is relieved by suspending the vessel from the underside of the sternum. Video-assisted thoracoscopic surgery has been most successful in situations where the ligamentum arteriosum completes the ring. The need to convert to open thoracotomy should always be anticipated (592). Repair of a PA sling is done through a median sternotomy. CPB may be required, especially when tracheal reconstruction is performed in an infant or young child. That procedure has a perioperative mortality rate of 40% to 50% (589).

Anesthetic Management

Vascular rings pose great challenges to anesthesia and airway management. In most cases, invasive measurement of arterial blood pressure is advisable. The site of cannulation depends on the anatomy of the vascular ring and the planned surgical procedure. Central venous catheters may be required if extensive surgical repair or CPB is required and for the infusion of inotropic drugs in critically ill patients. Large-bore intravenous access is important because of the potential for sudden and uncontrolled hemorrhage. The degree of tracheal compression should be known preoperatively by examination of the CT and MRI results. As with anterior mediastinal masses, severe airway compression and obstruction may occur with the administration of neuromuscular blocking agents. Therefore, an inhalation induction with preservation of spontaneous ventilation is recommended. The endotracheal tube should be advanced past the level of obstruction, and the ability to provide controlled positive-pressure ventilation should be confirmed before any neuromuscular blocking agents are administered. Satisfactory placement and positioning of an endotracheal tube may be particularly difficult in the presence of anomalous pulmonary arteries or bronchus suis. OLV, if essential, can be achieved by advancing the endotracheal tube into one main stem bronchus or by the use of a bronchial blocker. Ventilation with 100% oxygen may be required to maintain adequate arterial saturation in the presence of large areas of ventilation-perfusion mismatch. Maintenance of anesthesia is usually with volatile agents supplemented with opioids. In the presence of significant preoperative respiratory symptoms, tracheomalacia, or airway stenosis, postoperative intubation and mechanical ventilation are usually required. Postoperative analgesia can be provided by a thoracic epidural catheter placed directly or via the caudal canal. Epidural analgesia may improve postoperative respiratory function, especially in patients with preoperative pulmonary compromise.

Postoperative Management

Patients with minimal airway compromise and pulmonary dysfunction can usually be extubated immediately at the end of the procedure. Children with significant preoperative respiratory distress, airway stenosis, or tracheomalacia and those undergoing extensive surgical repairs usually require postoperative mechanical ventilation. Tracheostomy may be required to facilitate prolonged respiratory support. Surgical injury to the phrenic nerve, recurrent laryngeal nerve, or thoracic duct may complicate the postoperative course. Long-term results for most variants of vascular rings are excellent. Repair of a PA sling may be followed by postoperative vascular stenosis or airway obstruction or both. Follow-up care requires repeated ventilation-perfusion scans and/or bronchoscopy. Aortopexy may be required to relieve persistent airway obstruction. In a large series that included all types of vascular rings, an early mortality rate of 5% and an additional late mortality rate of 3.4% were reported (593).

ACKNOWLEDGMENTS

The author would like to express his profound gratitude to Dr. Fawzy G. Estafanous, Dr. Paul G. Barash, and Dr. J.G. Reves for the opportunity to contribute this chapter to their textbook. I also want to express my deep appreciation to my secretary, Tanya D. Callaway, and other office personnel who have helped in the preparation and publication of this chapter.

REFERENCES

1. Roberts WC. Aortic dissection: anatomy, consequences, and causes. *Am Heart J* 1981;101:195.
2. Spittell PC, Spittell JA Jr, Joyce JW, et al. Clinicave features and differential diagnosis of aortic dissection: Experience with 236 cases (1980 through 1990). *Mayo Clin Proc* 1993;68:642.
3. DeBakey ME, McCollum CH, Crawford ES, et al. Dissection and dissecting aneurysms of the aorta: twenty-year follow-up of five hundred twenty-seven patients-treated surgically. *Surgery* 1982;92:1118.
4. Marsalese DL, Moodie DS, Vacante M, et al. Marfan's syn-

drome: natural history and long-term follow-up of cardiovascular involvement. *J Am Coll Cardiol* 1989;14:422.
5. Larson EW, Edwards WD. Risk factors for aortic dissection: a necropsy study of 161 cases. *Am J Cardiol* 1984;53:849.
6. William GM, Gott VL, Brawley RK, et al. Aortic disease associated with pregnancy. *J Vasc Surg* 1988;8:470.
7. Elkayam U, Ostzaga E, Shotan A, et al. Cardiovascular problems in pregnant women with the Marfan syndrome. *Ann Intern Med* 1995;123:117.
8. Sakamoto I, Hyaashi K, Matsunaga N, et al. Aortic dissection caused by angiographic procedures. *Radiology* 1994;191:467.
9. Pieters FA, Widdershoven JW, Gerardy AC, et al. Risk of aortic dissection after aortic valve replacement. *Am J Cardiol* 1993;72:1043.
10. Albat B, Thevent A. Dissecting aneurysm of the ascending aorta occurring late after aortic valve replacement. *J Cardiovasc Surg (Torino)* 1992;33:272.
11. Still RJ, Hilgenbert AD, Akins CW, et al. Intraoperative aortic dissection. *Ann Thorac Surg* 1992;53:374.
12. Fann JI, Saris GE, Mitchell RS, et al. Treatment of patients with aortic dissection presenting with peripheral vascular complications. *Ann Surg* 1990;212:705.
13. O'Gara PT, DeSanctis RW. Acute aortic dissection and its variants: toward a common diagnostic and therapeutic approach. *Circulation* 1995;92:1376.
14. Scott J, Humphreys DR. Dissecting aortic aneurysm and disseminated intravascular coagulation. *BMJ* 1997;1:24.
15. Eagle KA, DeSanctis RW. Aortic dissection. *Curr Probl Cardiol* 1989;14:225.
16. Enia F, Ledda G, Lo Mauro R, et al. Utility of echocardiography in the diagnosis of aortic dissection involving the ascending aorta. *Chest* 1989;95:124.
17. Chia BL, Yan PC, Ee BK, et al. Two-dimensional echocardiography and Doppler color flow abnormalities in aortic root dissection. *Am Heart J* 1988;116:192.
18. Cigarroa JE, Isselbacher EM, DeSantis RW, et al. Diagnostic imaging in the evaluation of suspected aortic dissection: old standards and new directions. *N Engl J Med* 1993;328:35.
19. Erbel R, Engberding R, Daniel W, et al. Echocardiography in the diagnosis of aortic dissection. *Lancet* 1989;1:457.
20. Nienaber CA, von Kodolitsch Y, Nicolas V, et al. Definitive diagnosis of thoracic aortic dissection: the emerging role of noninvasive imaging modalities. *N Engl J Med* 1993;328:1.
21. Armstrong WF, Bach DS, Carey L, et al. Spectrum of acute dissection of the ascending aorta: a transesophageal echocardiographic study. *J Am Soc Echocardiogr* 1996;9:646.
22. Hashimoto S. Assessment of transesophageal Doppler echocardiography in dissecting aortic aneurysm. *J Am Coll Cardiol* 1989;14:1253.
23. Verdant A, Cossette R, Page A, et al. Aneurysms of the descending thoracic aorta: three hundred sixty-six consecutive cases resected without paraplegia. *J Vasc Surg* 1995;21:385.
24. Hamada S, Takamiya M, Kimura K, et al. Type A aortic dissection: evaluation with ultrafast CT. *Radiology* 1992;183:155.
25. Gomes MN, Davros WJ, Zemen RK. Preoperative assessment of abdominal aortic aneurysm: the value of helical and three-dimensional computed tomography. *J Vasc Surg* 1994;20:367.
26. Zemen RK, Berman PM, Silverman PM, et al. Diagnosis of aortic dissection: value of helical CT with multiplanar reformation and three-dimensional rendering. *AJR Am J Roentgenol* 1995;164:1357.
27. Hamada S, Takamiya M, Kimura K, et al. Type A aortic dissection: evaluation with ultrafast CT. *Radiology* 1992;183:155.
28. Rubin GD, Dake MD, Napel SA, et al. Three-dimensional spiral CT angiography of the abdomen: initial clinical experience. *Radiology* 1993;186:147.
29. Chung JW, Park JH, Kim HC, et al. Entry tears of thoracic aortic dissections: MR appearance on gated SE imaging. *J Comput Assist Tomogr* 1994;18:250.
30. Nienaber CA, von Kodolitsch Y, Brockhoff CJ, et al. Comparison of conventional and transesophageal echocardiography with magnetic resonance imaging for anatomical mapping of thoracic aortic dissection: a dual noninvasive imaging study with anatomical and/or angiographic validation. *Int J Imaging* 1994;10:1.
31. Mugge A, Daniel WG, Lass J, et al. False-negative diagnosis of proximal aortic dissection by computed tomography or angiography and possible explanations based on transesophageal echocardiographic findings. *Am J Cardiol* 1990;65:527.
32. Saito S, Arai H, Kim K, et al. Percutaneous fenestration of dissecting intima with a transseptal needle: a new therapeutic technique for visceral ischemia complicating acute aortic dissection. *Cathet Cardiovasc Diagn* 1992;26:130.
33. Faykus MH Jr, Hiette P, Koopot R. Percutaneous fenestration of a type I aortic dissection for relief of lower extremity ischemia. *Cardiovasc Intervent Radiol* 1992;15:183.
34. Williams DM, Brothers TE, Messina LM. Relief of mesenteric ischemia in type III aortic dissection with percutaneous fenestration of the aortic septum. *Radiology* 1990;174:450.
35. Weintraub AR, Erbel R, Gorge G, et al. Intravascular ultrasound imaging in acute aortic dissection. *J Am Coll Cardiol* 1994;24:495.
36. Yamada E, Matsumura M, Kyo S, et al. Usefulness of a prototype intravascular ultrasound imaging in evaluation of aortic dissection and comparison with angiographic study, transesophageal echocardiography, computed tomography, and magnetic resonance imaging. *Am J Cardiol* 1995;75:161.
37. Bellal RS, Nanda NC, Gatewood R, et al. Usefulness of transesophageal echocardiography in assessment of aortic dissection. *Circulation* 1991;84:1903.
38. Kern MJ, Serota AH, Callicoat P, et al. Use of coronary arteriography in the preoperative management of patients undergoing urgent repair of the thoracic aorta. *Am Heart J* 1990;119:143.
39. Creswell LL, Kouchoukos NT, Cox JL, et al. Coronary artery disease in patients with type A aortic dissection. *Ann Thorac Surg* 1995;59:585.
40. Braunwald E, ed. *Braunwald heart disease: a textbook of cardiovascular medicine,* 5th ed. Philadelphia: WB Saunders Co, Philadelphia, 1997.
41. Banning AP, Ruttley MST, Musumeci F, et al. Acute dissection of the thoracic aorta: transesophageal echocardiography is the investigation of choice. *BMJ* 1995;310:72.
42. Edmounds LH Jr, ed. *Cardiac surgery in the adult.* New York: McGraw-Hill, Health Professions Division, 1997.
43. Grubb BP, Sirio C, Zelis R. Intravenous labetalol in acute aortic dissection. *JAMA* 1987;258:78.
44. Fenner SG, Mahoney A, Cashman JN. Repair of traumatic transection of the thoracic aorta: esmolol for intraoperative control of arterial pressure. *Br J Anaesth* 1991;67:483.
45. Isselbacher EM, Cigarroa JE, Eagle KA. Cardiac tamponade complicating proximal aortic dissection: is pericardiocentesis harmful? *Circulation* 1994;90:2375.
46. Masuda Y, Yamada Z, Morooka N, et al. Prognosis of patients with medically treated aortic dissections. *Circulation* 1991;84[Suppl III]:III-7.
47. Miller DC. Surgical management of acute aortic dissection: new data. *Semin Thorac Cardiovasc Surg* 1991;3:225.
48. Doroghazi RM, Slater EE, DeSanctis RW, et al. Long-term survival of patients with treated aortic dissection. *J Am Coll Cardiol* 1984;3:1026.
49. Nienaber CA, von Kodolitsch Y. Metaanalyse zur Prognose der

thorakalen Aortendissektion: Letalitat im Wandel der letzten vier Jahrzehnte. *Herz* 1992;17:398.
50. Glower DD, Fann JI, Speier RH, et al. Comparison of medical and surgical therapy for uncomplicated descending aortic dissection. *Circulation* 1990;82[Suppl IV]:IV-39.
51. Haverich A, Miller DC, Scott WC, et al. Acute and chronic aortic dissections: determinants of long-term outcome for operative survivors. *Circulation* 1985;72[Suppl II]:II-22.
52. Bachet JE, Termignon JL, Dreyfus G, et al. Aortic dissection: prevalence, cause, and results of late reoperations. *J Thorac Cardiovasc Surg* 1994;108:199.
53. David TE, Feindel CM. An aortic valve-sparing operation for patients with aortic incompetence and aneurysm of the ascending aorta. *J Thorac Cardiovasc Surg* 1992;103:617.
54. David TE. When, why, and how should the native aortic valve be preserved in patients with annuloaortic ectasia or Marfan syndrome? *Semin Thorac Cardiovasc Surg* 1993;5:93.
55. Heinemann M, Laas J, Jurmann M, et al. Surgery extended into the aortic arch in acute type A dissection: indications, techniques, and results. *Circulation* 1991;84:III-25.
56. Laas J, Jurmann MJ, Heinemann M, et al. Advances in aortic arch surgery. *Ann Thorac Surg* 1992;53:227.
57. Ergin MA, O'Connor J, Guinto R, et al. Experience with profound hypothermia and circulatory arrest in the treatment of aneurysms of the aortic arch: aortic arch replacement for acute arch dissections. *J Thorac Cardiovasc Surg* 1982;84:649.
58. Seguin JR, Frapier JM, Colson P, et al. Fibrin sealant improves surgical results of type A acute aortic dissections. *Ann Thorac Surg* 1991;52:745.
59. Westaby S, Parry A, Giannopoulos N, et al. Replacement of the thoracic aorta with collagen-impregnated woven Dacron grafts: early results. *J Thorac Cardiovasc Surg* 1993;106:427.
60. Weinschelbaum EE, Schamun C, Caramutti V, et al. Surgical treatment of acute type A dissecting aneurysm, with preservation of the native aortic valve and use of biologic glue: follow-up to 6 years. *J Thorac Cardiovasc Surg* 1992;103:369.
61. Mazzucotelli JP, Deleuze PH, Baufreton C, et al. Preservation of the aortic valve in acute aortic dissection: long-term echocardiographic assessment and clinical outcome. *Ann Thorac Surg* 1993;55:1513.
62. Kouchoukos NT, Wareing TH, Murphy SF, et al. Sixteen-year experience with aortic root replacement: results of 172 operations. *Ann Surg* 1991;214:308.
63. Cabrol C, Pavie A, Mesnildrey P, et al. Long-term results with total replacement of the ascending aorta and reimplantation of the coronary arteries. *J Thorac Cardiovasc Surg* 1986;91:17.
64. Svensson LG, Crawford ES, Hess KR, et al. Composite valve graft replacement of the proximal aorta: comparison of techniques in 348 patients. *Ann Thorac Surg* 1992;54:427.
65. Borst HG, Laas J, Heinemann M. Type A aortic dissection: diagnosis and management of malperfusion phenomena. *Semin Thorac Cardiovasc Surg* 1991;3:238.
66. Borst GG, Frank G, Schaps D. Treatment of extensive aortic aneurysms by a new multiple-stage approach. *J Thorac Cardiovasc Surg* 1988;95:11.
67. Ergin MA, Galla JD, Lansman SL, et al. Hypothermic circulatory arrest in operations on the thoracic aorta: determinants of operative mortality and neurologic outcome. *J Thorac Cardiovasc Surg* 1994;107:788.
68. Kyo S, Takamoto S, Omoto R, et al. Intraoperative echocardiography for diagnosis and treatment of aortic dissection: utility of color flow mapping for surgical decision making in acute stage. *Herz* 1992;17:377.
69. Lass J, Heinemann M, Schaefers HJ, et al. Management of thoracoabdominal malperfusion in aortic dissection. *Circulation* 1991;84:11120.
70. Ergin MA, Phillips RA, Galla JD, et al. Significance of distal false lumen after Type A dissection repair. *Ann Thorac Surg* 1994;57:820.
71. Elefteriades JA, Hartleroad J, Gusberg RJ, et al. Long-term experience with descending aortic dissection: the complication-specific approach. *Ann Thorac Surg* 1992;53:11.
72. Williams DM, Andrews JC, Marx MV, et al. Creation of reentry tears in aortic dissection by means of percutaneous balloon fenestration: Gross anatomic and histologic considerations. *J Vasc Interv Radiol* 1993;4:75.
73. Carrel T, Pasic M, Vogt P, et al. Retrograde ascending aortic dissection: a diagnostic and therapeutic challenge. *Eur J Cardiothorac Surg* 1993;7:146.
74. Fann JI, Sarris GE, Miller DC, et al. Surgical management of acute aortic dissection complicated by stroke. *Circulation* 1989; 80:1257.
75. Elefteriades JA, Hammond GL, Gusberg RJ, et al. Fenestration revisited: a safe and effective procedure for descending aortic dissection. *Arch Surg* 1990;125:786.
76. Maddox BK, Sakai LY, Keene DR, et al. Connective tissue microfibrils: isolation and characterization of three large peps-resistant domains of fibrillin. *J Biol Chem* 1989;264:21381.
77. Shores J, Berger KR, Murphy EA, et al. Progression of aortic dilatation and the benefit of long-term β-adrenergic blockade in Marfan's syndrome. *N Engl J Med* 1994;330:1335.
78. Gott VL, Pyeritz RE, Cameron DE, et al. Composite graft repair of Marfan aneurysm of the ascending aorta: results in 100 patients. *Ann Thorac Surg* 1991;52:38.
79. Pasic M, von Segesser L, Carrel T, et al. Surgical treatment of cardiovascular complications in Marfan syndrome: a 27-year experience. *Eur J Cardiothorac Surg* 1992;6:149.
80. Carrel T, Pasic M, Jenni R, et al. Reoperations after operation on the thoracic aorta: etiology, surgical techniques, and prevention. *Ann Thorac Surg* 1993;56:259.
81. Murphy DA, Craver JM, Jones EL, et al. Recognition and management of ascending aortic dissection complicating cardiac surgical operations. *J Thorac Cardiovasc Surg* 1983;85:247.
82. Dagenais GR, Rouleau JR, Christen A, et al. Survival of patients with strongly positive exercise electrocardiogram. *Circulation* 1982;65:452.
83. Maurer W, Ablasser A, Tschada R, et al. Myocardial catecholamine metabolism in patients with chronic aortic regurgitation. *Circulation* 1982;66(2, Part 2):I139.
84. Laniado S, Yellin EL, Yoran C, et al. Physiologic mechanism in aortic insufficiency. *Circulation* 1982;66:226.
85. Svensson LG, Crawford ES, Hess KR, et al. Dissection of the aorta and dissecting aortic aneurysms: improving early and long-term surgical results. *Circulation* 1990;82:IV24.
86. Crawford ES, Kirklin JW, Naftel DC, et al. Surgery for acute dissection of ascending aorta: should the arch be included? *J Thorac Cardiovasc Surg* 1992;104:46.
87. Borst HG, Haverich A, Walterbusch G, et al. Fibrin adhesive: an important hemostatic adjunct in cardiovascular operations. *J Thorac Cardiovasc Surg* 1982;84:548.
88. Fuster V, Halperin JL. Aortic dissection: a medical perspective. *J Card Surg* 1994;9:713.
89. Dietz HC, Cutting GR, Pyeritz RE. Marfan syndrome caused by a recurrent de novo missense mutation in the fibrillin gene. *Nature* 1991;352:337.
90. Galloway AC, Covlin SB, LaMendola CL, et al. Ten year experience with 165 aneurysms of the ascending aorta and aortic arch. *Circulation* 1989;80:249.
91. Dapunt OE, Galla JD, Sadeghi AM, et al.The natural history of thoracic aortic aneurysms. *J Thorac Cardiovasc Surg* 1994; 107:1323.
92. Pachulski TR, Wienberg AL, Chan KL. Aortic aneurysm in

patients with functionally normal or minimally stenotic bicuspid aortic valve *Am J Cardiol* 1991;67:78.

93. Lindsay J Jr. Coarctation of the aorta, bicuspid aortic valve and abnormal ascending aortic wall. *Am J Cardiol* 1988;61:182.
94. Salisbury RS, Hazelman BC. Successful treatment of dissecting aortic aneurysm due to giant cell arteritis. *Ann Rheum Dis* 1989; 40:507.
95. Feigl D, Feigl A, Edwards JE. Mycotic aneurysms of the aortic root: a pathologic study of 20 cases. *Chest* 1986;90:553.
96. Pope FM, Narcisi P, Nicholls AC, et al. Clinical presentations of Ehlers Danlos syndrome type IV. *Arch Dis Child* 1988;63: 1016.
97. Raman J, Saldanha RF, Esmore DS, et al. The Bentall procedure: a surgical option in Ehlers-Danlos syndrome. *J Cardiovasc Surg* 1988;29:647.
98. Turney SZ. Blunt trauma of the thoracic aorta and its branches. *Semin Thorac Cardiovasc Surg* 1992;4:209.
99. Johansen K. Aneurysms. *Sci Am* 1982:247:110.
100. Greipp RB, Ergin MA, Lansmann SL, et al. The natural history of thoracic aortic aneurysms. *Semin Thorac Cardiovasc Surg* 1991:3:258.
101. Pressler V, McNamara JJ. Aneurysm of the thoracic aorta: review of 260 cases. *J Thorac Cardiovasc Surg* 1985;89:50.
102. Spittell JA Jr. Clinical aspects of aneurysmal disease. *Curr Probl Cardiol* 1980;5:1.
103. Fisher DF, Yawn DH, Crawford ES. Preoperative disseminated intravascular coagulation associated with aortic aneurysms. *Arch Surg* 1983;118:1252.
104. Amar D, Komer CA. Anesthetic implications of a ruptured aneurysm of the sinus of Valsalva. *J Cardiothorac Vasc Anesth* 1993;7:730.
105. Burakovsky VI, Podsolkov VP, Sabirow BOV, et al. Ruptured ocngenital aneurysm of the sinus of Valsalva: clinical manifestations, diagnosis and results of surgical corrections. *J Thorac Cardiovasc Surg* 1988;95:836.
106. Coselli JS, Crawford ES. Composite valve-graft replacement of aortic root using separate Dacron tube for coronary artery reattachment. *Ann Thorac Surg* 1989;47:558.
107. Guthaner DF. The plain chest film in assessing aneurysms and dissecting hematomas of the thoracic aorta. In: Taveras JN, Ferrucci JT, eds. *Radiology diagnosis-imaging-intervention.* Philadelphia: JB Lippincott, 1994:1.
108. Price WH, Wilson J. Dissection of the aorta in Turner's syndrome. *J Med Genet* 1983;20:61.
109. Konstadt SN, Reich DL, Quintana C, et al. The ascending aorta: how much does transesophageal echocardiography see? *Anesth Analg* 1994;78:240.
110. Mohiaddin RH, Longmore DB. Functional aspects of cardiovascular nuclear magnetic resonance imaging: techniques and application. *Circulation* 1993;88:264.
111. Guthaner DF. Angiography in assessing aneurysms and dissecting hematomas of the thoracic. In: Taveras JN, Ferrucci JT, eds. *Radiology diagnosis-imaging-intervention.* Philadelphia: JB Lippincott, 1994:1.
112. Israel DH, Sharma SK, Ambrose JA, et al. Cardiac catheterization and selective coronary angiography in ascending aortic aneurysm or dissection. *Cathet Cardiovasc Diagn* 1994;32:232.
113. Berens ES, Kouchoukos NT, Murphy S, et al. Preoperative carotid artery screening in elderly patients undergoing cardiac surgery. *J Vasc Surg* 1992;15:313.
114. Kouchoukos NT. Adjuncts to reduce the incidence of embolic brain injury during operations on the aortic arch. *Ann Thorac Surg* 1994;57:243.
115. Crawford ES, Svensson LG, Coselli JS, et al. Surgical treatment of aneurysm and/or dissection of the ascending aorta, transverse aortic arch, and ascending aorta and transverse aortic arch: factors influencing survival in 717 patients. *J Thorac Cardiovasc Surg* 1989;98:659.
116. Gott VL, Gillinov AM, Pyeritz RE, et al. Aortic root replacement: risk factor analysis of a seventeen-year experience with 270 patients. *J Thorac Cardiovasc Surg* 1995;109:536.
117. Gott VL, Cameron DE, Pyeritz RE, et al. Composite graft repair of Marfan aneurysm of the ascending aorta: results in 150 patients. *J Card Surg* 1994;9:482.
118. Gott VL, Caneron DE, Reitz BA, et al. Current diagnosis and prescription for the Marfan syndrome: aortic root and valve replacement. *J Card Surg* 1994;9[Suppl]:101.
119. Prenger K, Pieters F, Cheriex E, et al. Aortic dissection after aortic valve replacement: incidence and consequences for strategy. *J Card Surg* 1994;9:495.
120. Lawrie GM, Earle N, DeBakey ME. Long-term fate of the aortic root and aortic valve after ascending aneurysm surgery. *Ann Surg* 1993;217:711.
121. Albertucci M, Wong K, Petrou M, et al. The use of unstented homograft valves for aortic valve reoperations: review of a twenty-three-year experience. *J Thorac Cardiovasc Surg* 1994; 107:152.
122. Prager RL, Deschner W, Kong B, et al. Early experience with homograft aortic root replacement for complex aortic pathology. *Surgery* 1993;114:794.
123. Kouchoukos NT, Davila-Roman VG, Spray TL, et al. Replacement of the aortic root with a pulmonary autograft in children and young adults with aortic-valve disease. *N Engl J Med* 1994; 330:1.
124. Elkins RC. Pulmonary autograft: expanding indications and increasing utilizations. *J Heart Valve Dis* 1994;3:356.
125. David TE, Feindel CM, Bos J. Repair of the aortic valve in patients with aortic insufficiency and aortic root aneurysm. *J Thorac Cardiovasc Surg* 1995;109:345.
126. Gillinov AM, Hulyalkar A, Cameron DE, et al. Mitral valve operation in patients with the Marfan syndrome. *J Thorac Cardiovasc Surg* 1994;107:724.
127. Buckberg GD, Beyersdorf F, Allen BS, et al. Integrated myocardial management: background and initial application. *J Card Surg* 1995;10:68.
128. Cabrol C, Pavie A, Ganjbakch I, et al. Complete replacement of the ascending aorta with reimplantation of the coronary arteries. *J Thorac Cardiovasc Surg* 1981;81:309.
129. Downing SW, Kouchoukos NT. Ascending aortic aneurysm. In: Edmonds LH Jr, ed. *Cardiac surgery in the adult.* New York: McGraw-Hill, Health Professions Division, 1997:1165.
130. Mori M, Chuma R, Kiichi Y, et al. The anesthetic management of a patient with a thoracic aortic aneurysm that caused compression of the left mainstem bronchus and the right pulmonary artery. *J Cardiothorac Vasc Anesth* 1993;7:579.
131. Penner C, Myacher B, Light RB. Compression of the left main bronchus between a descending thoracic aortic aneurysm and an enlarged right pulmonary artery. *Chest* 1994;106:959.
132. Nishiwaki K, Komatsu T, Shimada Y, et al. Severe tracheal compression caused by false aneurysm arising from the ascending aorta: successful airway management using induced hypotension and bronchoscopy. *Anesthesiology* 1993;73:1047.
133. Gorman RB, Merritt WT, Greenspun H, et al. Aneurysmal compression of the trachea and right mainstem bronchus complicating thoracoabdominal aneurysm repair. *Anesthesiology* 1993;79:1424.
134. Cohen JA, Denisco RA, Richards TS, et al. Hazardous placement of a Robertshaw-type endobronchial tube. *Anesth Analg* 1986;65:10.
135. Svensson LG, Sun J, Nadolny E, et al. Prospective evaluation of minimal blood use for ascending aorta and aortic arch operations. *Ann Thorac Surg* 1995;59:1501.

136. Cohn LH, Rise RJ, Adams DH, et al. Reduced mortality and morbidity for ascending aortic aneurysm resection regardless of cause. *Ann Thorac Surg* 1996;62:463.
137. Sundt TM III, Kouchoukos NT, Saffitz JE, et al. Renal dysfunction and intravascular coagulation with aprotinin and hypothermic circulatory arrest. *Ann Thorac Surg* 1993;55:1418.
138. Edmonds LH Jr. Why cardiopulmonary bypass makes patients sick: strategies to control the blood-synthetic surface interface. *Adv Card Surg* 1995;6:131.
139. Marinelli WA, Ingbar DH. Diagnosis and management of acute lung injury. *Clin Chest Med* 1994;15:517.
140. Engelman RM, Rousou JA, Flack JE 3rd, et al. Influence of steroids on complement and cytokine generation after cardiopulmonary bypass. *Ann Thorac Surg* 1995;60:801.
141. Teoh KH, Bradley CA, Gualdie J, et al. Steroid inhibition of cytokine-mediated vasodilation after warm heart surgery. *Circulation* 1995;92(9 Suppl):II3.
142. Journois D, Pouard P, Greeley WJ, et al. Hemofiltration during cardiopulmonary bypass in pediatric cardiac surgery: effects on hemostasis, cytokines, and complement components. *Anesthesiology* 1994;81:1181.
143. Andreasson S, Gothberg S, Berggren AH, et al. Hemofiltration modifies complement activation after extracorporeal circulation in infants. *Ann Thorac Surg* 1993;56:1515.
144. Jault F, Nataf P, Rama A, et al. Chronic disease of the ascending aorta: surgical treatment and longterm results. *J Thorac Cardiovasc Surg* 1994;108:747.
145. Lewis CT, Cooley DA, Murphy MC, et al. Surgical repair of aortic root aneurysms in 280 patients. *Ann Thorac Surg* 1992; 53:38.
146. Moreno-Cabral CE, Miller DC, et al. Degenerative and atherosclerotic aneurysms of the thoracic aorta. *J Thorac Cardiovasc Surg* 1984;88:1020.
147. Crawford ES, Coselli JS. Replacement of the aortic arch. *Semin Thorac Cardiovasc Surg* 1991;3:194.
148. Bogaert J, Gewilling M, Rademakers F, et al. Transverse arch hypoplasia predisposes to aneurysm formation at the repair site after patch angioplasty for coarctation of the aorta. *J Am Coll Cardiol* 1995;26:521.
149. Graeter T, Schaefer C, Prokop M, et al. Three-dimensional vascular imaging: an additional diagnostic tool. *Thorac Cardiovasc Surg* 1993;41:183.
150. Thompson BH, Stanford W. Utility of ultrafast computed tomography in the detection of thoracic aortic aneurysms and dissections. *Semin Ultrasound CT MR* 1993;14:117.
151. Crawford ES, Coselli JS, Svensson LG, et al. Diffuse aneurysmal disease (chronic aortic dissection, Marfan, and mega aorta syndromes) and multiple aneurysm: treatment by subtotal and total aortic replacement emphasizing the elephant trunk operation. *Ann Surg* 1990;211:521.
152. Griepp RB, Ergin MA. Aneurysm of the aortic arch. In: Edmonds LH Jr, ed. *Cardiac surgery in the adult.* New York: McGraw-Hill, Health Professions Division, 1997:1197.
153. Dapunt OE, Galla JD, Sadeghi AM, et al. The natural history of thoracic aortic aneurysms. *J Thorac Cardiovasc Surg* 1994; 107:1323.
154. Shores J, Berger KR, Murphy EA, et al. Progression of aortic dilatation and the benefit of long-term beta-adrenergic blockade in Marfan's syndrome. *N Engl J Med* 1994;330:1335.
155. Ergin MA, Griepp EB, Lansman SL, et al. Hypothermic circulatory arrest and other methods of cerebral protection during operations on the thoracic aorta. *J Card Surg* 1994;9:525.
156. Guerit JM, Verhelst R, Rubay J, et al. The use of somatosensory evoked potentials to determine the optimal degree of hypothermia during circulatory arrest. *J Card Surg* 1994;9:596.
157. Raskin SA, Fuselier VW, Reeves-Viets JL, et al. Deep hypothermic circulatory arrest with and without retrograde cerebral perfusion. *Int Anesthesiol Clin* 1996;34:177.
158. Livesay JJ, Cooley DA, Duncan JM, et al. Open aortic anastomosis: improved results in the treatment of aneurysms of the aortic arch. *Circulation* 1982;66[Suppl I]:I-222.
159. Fox LS, Blackstone MD, Kirklin JW, et al. The relationship of whole body oxygen consumption to perfusion flow rate during hypothermic cardiopulmonary bypass. *J Thorac Cardiovasc Surg* 1982;83:239.
160. Onesti ST, Baker CJ, Sun PP, et al. Transient hypothermia reduces focal ischemia brain injury in the rat. *Neurosurgery* 1991; 29:369.
161. Swain JA, McDonald TJ, Griffith PK, et al. Low-flow hypothermic cardiopulmonary bypass protects the brain. *J Thorac Cardiovasc Surg* 1991;102:76.
162. Hochachka PW. Defense strategies against hypoxia and hypothermia. *Science* 1986;231:234.
163. Fox LS, Blackstone EH, Kirklin JW, et al. Relationship of brain blood flow and oxygen consumption to perfusion flow rate during profoundly hypothermic cardiopulmonary bypass. *J Thorac Cardiovasc Surg* 1984;87:658.
164. Hilberman M, Barlow CH, Haselgrove JC, et al. Cerebral mitochondrial oxygenation during CPB in dogs. *Anesthesiology* 1980; 53:693.
165. Bellinger DC, Jonas AR, Rapport LA, et al. Developmental and neurological status of children after heart surgery with hypothermic circulatory arrest or low-flow cardiopulmonary bypass. *N Engl J Med* 1995;332:549.
166. Wells FC, Coghill S, Caplan HL, et al. Duration of circulatory arrest does influence the psychological development of children after cardiac operation in early life. *J Thorac Cardiovasc Surg* 1983;86:823.
167. Mault JR, Ohtake S, Klingensmith MF, et al. Cerebral metabolism and circulatory arrest: effects of duration and strategies for protection. *Ann Thorac Surg* 1993;55:57.
168. Mezrow CK, Midulla PS, Sadeghi AM, et al. Quantitative electroencephalography: a method to assess cerebral injury after hypothermic circulatory arrest. *J Thorac Cardiovasc Surg* 1995; 109:925.
169. Midulla PS, Gandsas A, Sadeghi AM, et al. Comparison of retrograde cerebral perfusion to antegrade cerebral perfusion and hypothermic circulatory arrest in a chronic porcine model. *J Card Surg* 1994;9:560.
170. Bellinger DC, Wernovsky G, Rapaport LA, et al. Cognitive development following repair as neonates of transposition of the great arteries using deep hypothermic circulatory arrest. *Pediatrics* 1991;87:701.
171. Newburger JW, Jonas RA, Wernovsky G, et al. A comparison of the perioperative neurological effects of hypothermic circulatory arrest versus low flow cardiopulmonary bypass in infant heart surgery. *N Engl J Med* 1993;329:1057.
172. Jonas RA, Bellinger DC, Rappaport LA, et al. Relationship of pH strategy and developmental outcome after hypothermic circulatory arrest. *J Thorac Cardiovasc Surg* 1993;106:362
173. Oates RK, Simpson JM, Turnbull JAB, et al. The relationship between intelligence and duration of circulatory arrest with deep hypothermia. *J Thorac Cardiovasc Surg* 1995;110:786.
174. Greeley WJ, Ungerleider RM, Smith R, et al. The effects of deep hypothermic cardiopulmonary bypass and total circulatory arrest on cerebral blood flow in infants and children. *J Thorac Cardiovasc Surg* 1989;97:737.
175. Burrows FA, Hillier SC, McLeod ME, et al. Anterior fontanel pressure and visual evoked potentials in neonates and infants undergoing profound hypothermic circulatory arrest. *Anesthesiology* 1990;73:632.
176. Jonassen AE, Quaegebeur JM, Young WL, et al. Cerebral blood

flow velocity in pediatric patients is reduced after cardiopulmonary bypass with profound hypothermia. *J Thorac Cardiovasc Surg* 1995;110:934.
177. Greeley WJ, Bracey VA, Ungerleider RM, et al. Recovery of cerebral metabolism and mitochondrial oxidation state is delayed after hypothermic circulation arrest. *Circulation* 1991;84:400.
178. Hoka S, Tatebayashi E, Okamoto H, et al. Reduction of jugular venous oxygen saturation coincidental with electroencephalographic abnormality. *Anesth Analg* 1993;77:387.
179. Greipp R, Stinson E, Hollingsworth J, et al. Prosthetic replacement of the aortic arch. *J Thorac Cardiovasc Surg* 1975;70:1051.
180. Kieffer E, Koskas F, Walden R, et al. Hypothermic circulatory arrest for thoracic aneurysmectomy through left-sided thoracotomy. *J Vasc Surg* 1994;19:457.
181. Suto Y, Yasuda K, Shiiya N, et al. Stented elephant trunk procedure for an extensive aneurysm involving distal aortic arch and descending aorta. *J Thorac Cardiovasc Surg* 1996;112:1389.
182. Coselli J, Buket S, Djukanovic B. Aortic arch surgery: current treatment and results. *Ann Thorac Surg* 1995;59:19.
183. Deeb G, Jenkins E, Bolling S, et al. Retrograde cerebral perfusion during hypothermic circulatory arrest reduces neurologic morbidity. *J Thorac Cardiovasc Surg* 1995;109:259.
184. Robbins RC, Balaban RS, Swain JA. Intermittent hypothermic asanguinous cerebral perfusion (cerebroplegia) protects the brain during prolonged circulatory arrest. *J Thorac Cardiovasc Surg* 1990;99:878.
185. Crittenden MD, Roberts CS, Rosa L, et al. Brain protection during circulatory arrest. *Ann Thorac Surg* 1991;51:942.
186. Wolfson SK Jr, Icoz MV, Luber S. Preservation of conditioned responses in primates after total circulatory arrest with preferential cerebral hypothermia. *Surg Forum* 1965;16:409.
187. Bachet J, Guilmet D, Goudot B, et al. Cold cerebroplegia. *J Thorac Cardiovasc Surg* 1991;102:85.
188. Bachet J, Guilmet D, Goudot B, et al. Cold cerebroplegia: a new technique of cerebral protection during operations on the transverse aortic arch. *J Thorac Cardiovasc Surg* 1991;102:85.
189. Aoyagi S, Akashi H, Kubota Y, et al. Partial brachiocephalic perfusion in aortic arch replacement. *Jpn J Surg* 1993;23:331.
190. Kazui T, Inoue N, Yama O, et al. Selective cerebral perfusion during operation for aneurysms of the aortic arch: a reassessment. *Ann Thorac Surg* 1992;53:109.
191. Matsuda H, Nakano S, Shirakura R, et al. Surgery for aortic arch aneurysm with selective cerebral perfusion and hypothermic cardiopulmonary bypass. *Circulation* 1989;80[Suppl I]:I-243.
192. Katoh T, Esato K, Gohra H, et al. Evaluation of brain oxygenation during selective cerebral perfusion by near-infrared spectroscopy. *Ann Thorac Surg* 1997;64:432.
193. Mezrow CK, Gandsas A, Sadeghi AM, et al. Metabolic correlates of neurologic and behavioral injury after prolonged hypothermic circulatory arrest. *J Thorac Cardiovasc Surg* 1995;109:959.
194. Alamanni F, Agrifoglio M, Pompilio G, et al. Aortic arch surgery: pros and cons of selective cerebral perfusion. A multivariable analysis for cerebral injury during hypothermic circulatory arrest. *J Cardiovasc Surg* 1995;36:31.
195. Ando M, Nakajima N, Adachi S, et al. Simultaneous graft replacement of the ascending aorta and total arch for type A aortic dissection. *Ann Thorac Surg* 1994;57:699.
196. Kazui T, Yamada O, Komatzu S. Emergency graft replacement of the aortic arch for acute type A dissection. *J Cardiovasc Surg* 1992;33:211.
197. Alamanni F, Agrifoglio M, Pompilio G, et al. Aortic arch surgery: pros and cons of selective cerebral perfusion. A multivariable analysis for cerebral injury during hypothermic circulatory arrest. *J Cardiovasc Surg* 1995;36:31.
198. Kazui T, Kimura N, Komatsu S. Surgical treatment of aortic arch aneurysms using selective cerebral perfusion: experience with 100 patients. *Eur J Cardiothorac Surg* 1995;9:491.
199. Kazui T, Kimura N, Yamada O, et al. Surgical outcome of aortic arch aneurysms using selective cerebral perfusion. *Ann Thorac Surg* 1994;57:904.
200. Tabayashi K, Ohmi M, Togo T, et al. Aortic arch aneurysm repair using selective cerebral perfusion. *Ann Thorac Surg* 1994;57:1305.
201. First WH, Baldwin JC, Vaughn AS, et al. A reconsideration of cerebral perfusion in aortic arch replacement. *Ann Thorac Surg* 1986;42:273.
202. Mills NL, Ochsner JL. Massive air embolism during cardiopulmonary bypass: causes, prevention, and management. *J Thorac Cardiovasc Surg* 1980;102:85.
203. Safi HJ, Brien HW, Winter JN, et al. Brain protection via cerebral retrograde perfusion during aortic arch aneurysm repair. *Ann Thorac Surg* 1993;56:270.
204. Ueda U, Miki S, Kusuhara K, et al. Surgical treatment of the aneurysm or dissection involving ascending aorta and aortic arch utilizing circulatory arrest and retrograde perfusion. *J Jpn Assoc Thorac Surg* 1988;36:161.
205. Takamoto S, Matsuda T, Harada M, et al. Simple hypothermic retrograde cerebral perfusion during aortic arch surgery. *J Cardiovasc Surg* 1992;33:560.
206. Coselli JS. Retrograde cerebral perfusion via a superior vena caval cannula for aortic arch aneurysm operations. *Ann Thorac Surg* 1994;57:1668.
207. Bavaria JE, Woo YJ, Hall RA, et al. Retrograde cerebral and distal aortic perfusion during ascending and thoracoabdominal aortic operations. *Ann Thorac Surg* 1995;60:345.
208. Cope JT, Tribble RW, Komorowski B, et al. A simple technique for retrograde cerebral perfusion during circulatory arrest. *J Card Surg* 1996;11:65.
209. Mori A. Retrograde cerebral perfusion using pulsatile flow under conditions of profound hypothermia. *Ann Thorac Surg* 1993;56:1497.
210. Valk A, Kanten RA, Oosterheert M. Treating massive air embolism. *J Extracorp Technol* 1982;14:325.
211. Ganzel BL, Edmonds HL, Pank JR, et al. Neurophysiologic monitoring to assure delivery of retrograde cerebral perfusion. *J Thorac Cardiovasc Surg* 1997;113:748.
212. Yerlioghu ME, Wolfe D, Mezrow CK, et al. The effect of retrograde cerebral perfusion after particulate embolization to the brain. *J Thorac Cardiovasc Surg* 1995;110:1470.
213. Nojima T, Magara T, Nakjima Y, et al. Optimal perfusion pressure for experimental retrograde cerebral perfusion. *J Card Surg* 1994;9:548.
214. Yoshimura N, Okada M, Ota T, et al. Pharmacologic intervention for ischemic brain edema after retrograde cerebral perfusion. *J Thorac Cardiovasc Surg* 1995;109:1173.
215. Boeckxstaens CJ, Flameng WJ. Retrograde perfusion does not perfuse the brain in non-human primates. *Ann Thorac Surg* 1995;60:319.
216. Cheung AT, Bavaria JE, Pochettino A, et al. Oxygen delivery during retrograde cerebral perfusion in humans. *Anesth Analg* 1999;88:8.
217. Levy WJ, Levin SK, Bavaria JE. Cerebral oxygenation during retrograde perfusion. *Ann Thorac Surg* 1995;60:184.
218. Lin PJ, Chang CH, Tan PP, et al. Prolonged circulatory arrest in moderate hypothermia with retrograde cerebral perfusion: is the brain ischemic? *Circulation* 1996;94[Suppl II]:II-169.
219. Pagno D, Boivin CM, Faroqui MH, et al. Retrograde perfusion

through the superior vena perfuses the brain in human beings. *J Thorac Cardiovasc Surg* 1996;111:270.
220. Cheung AT, Bavaria JE, Weiss SJ, et al. Neurophysiologic effects of retrograde cerebral perfusion used for aortic reconstruction. *J Cardiothorac Vasc Anesth* 1998;12:252.
221. Winsborrow BG, Koslowski P, Figueiras CL, et al. ^{31}P spectroscopic imaging of pig brains during circulatory arrest. *Can J Appl Spect* 1994;39:135.
222. Usui A, Hotta T, Hiroura M, et al. Retrograde cerebral perfusion through a superior vena caval cannula protects the brain. *Ann Thorac Surg* 1992:53:47.
223. Usui A, Abe T, Murase M. Early clinical results of retrograde cerebral perfusion for aortic arch operations in Japan. *Ann Thorac Surg* 1996;62:94.
224. Watanabe T, Iijima Y, Abe K, et al. Retrograde brain perfusion beyond the venous valves: hemodynamics and intracellular pH mapping. *J Thorac Cardiovasc Surg* 1996;111:36.
225. Usui A, Oohara K, Liu T, et al. Determination of optimum retrograde cerebral perfusion conditions. *J Thorac Cardiovasc Surg* 1994;107:300.
226. Filgueiras CL, Ryner L, Ye J, et al. Cerebral protection during moderate hypothermic circulatory arrest: histopathology and magnetic resonance spectroscopy of brain energetics and intracellular pH in pigs. *J Thorac Cardiovasc Surg* 1996;112:1073.
227. Sakurada T, Kazui T, Tanaka H, et al. Comparative experimental study of cerebral protection during aortic arch reconstruction. *Ann Thorac Surg* 1996;61:1348.
228. Oohara K, Usui A, Murase M, et al. Regional cerebral tissue blood flow measured by the colored microsphere method during retrograde cerebral perfusion. *J Thorac Cardiovasc Surg* 1995; 109:772.
229. Katz MG, Khazin V, Steinmetz A, et al. Distribution of cerebral flow using retrograde versus antegrade cerebral perfusion. *Ann Thorac Surg* 1999;67:1065.
230. de Brux JL, Subayi JB, Pegis JD, et al. Retrograde cerebral perfusion: anatomic study of the distribution of blood to the brain. *Ann Thorac Surg* 1995;60:1294.
231. Yasuura K, Okamoto H, Ogawa Y, et al. Resection of aortic aneurysms without aortic clamp technique with the aid of hypothermic total body retrograde perfusion. *J Thorac Cardiovasc Surg* 1994;107:1237.
232. Safi HJ, Iliopoulos DC, Gopinath SP, et al. Retrograde cerebral perfusion during profound hypothermia and circulatory arrest in pigs. *Ann Thorac Surg* 1995;59:1107.
233. Filgueiras CL, Winsburrow B, Ye J, et al. A ^{31}P-magnetic resonance study of antegrade and retrograde cerebral perfusion during aortic arch surgery in pigs. *J Thorac Cardiovasc Surg* 1995; 110:55.
234. Ye J, Yang L, Del Bigio MR, et al. Neuronal damage after hypothermic circulatory arrest and retrograde perfusion in the pig. *Ann Thorac Surg* 1996;61:1316.
235. Lytle BW, McCarthy PM, Meaney KM, et al. Systemic hypothermia and circulatory arrest combined with arterial perfusion of the superior vena cava. *J Thorac Cardiovasc Surg* 1995;109: 738.
236. Bavaria JE, Woo YJ, Hall RA, et al. Retrograde cerebral and distal aortic perfusion during ascending and thoracoabdominal aortic operations. *Ann Thorac Surg* 1995;60:345.
237. Deeb GM, Jenkins E, Bolling SF, et al. Retrograde cerebral perfusion during hypothermic circulatory arrest reduces neurologic morbidity. *J Thorac Cardiovasc Surg* 1995;109:259.
238. Ueda Y, Miki S, Kusuhara K, et al. Surgical treatment of the aneurysm of dissection involving the ascending aorta and aortic arch utilizing circulatory arrest and retrograde cerebral perfusion. *J Jpn Assoc Thorac Surg* 1988;36:161.
239. Murase M, Maeda M, Koyama T, et al. Continuous retrograde cerebral perfusion for protection of the brain during aortic arch surgery. *Eur J Cardiothorac Surg* 1993;7:597.
240. Bavaria JE, Pochettino A. Retrograde cerebral perfusion (RCP) in aortic arch surgery: efficacy and possible mechanisms of brain protection. *Semin Thorac Cardiovasc Surg* 1997;9:222.
241. Pagano D, Carey JA, Patel RL, et al. Retrograde cerebral perfusion: clinical experience in emergency and elective aortic operations. *Ann Thorac Surg* 1995;59:393.
242. Moshkovitz Y, David TE, Caleb M, et al. Circulatory arrest under moderate systemic hypothermia and cold retrograde cerebral perfusion. *Ann Thorac Surg* 1998;66:1179.
243. Gilling-Smith GL, Worswick L, Knight PF, et al. Surgical repair of thoracoabdominal aortic aneurysm: 10 years' experience. *Br J Surg* 1995:82:624.
244. Livesay JJ, Cooley DA, Reul GJ, et al. Resection of aortic arch aneurysms: a comparison of hypothermic techniques in 60 patients. *Ann Thorac Surg* 1983;36:19.
245. Cook DJ, Oliver WC Jr, Orszulak TJ, et al. A prospective, randomized comparison of cerebral venous oxygen saturation during normothermic and hypothermic cardiopulmonary bypass. *J Thorac Cardiovasc Surg* 1994;107:1020.
246. Ergin MA, Griepp EB, Lansman SL. Hypothermic circulatory arrest and other methods of cerebral protection during opertions on the thoracic aorta. *J Card Surg* 1994;9:525.
247. Alamanni F, Agrifoglio M, Pompilio G, et al. Aortic arch surgery: pros and cons of selective cerebral perfusion. A multivariable analysis for cerebral injury during hypothermic circulatory arrest. *J Cardiovasc Surg* 1995;36:31.
248. Kelley JG, Gaba DM, Brodsky JB. Bronchial cuff pressures of two tubes used in thoracic surgery. *J Cardiothorac Vasc Anesth* 1992;6:190.
249. Lanier WL. Post-ischemic neurologic recovery and cerebral blood flow using a compression model of complete bloodless cerebral ischemia in dogs. *Resuscitation* 1988;16:271.
250. Lemay ER. Insulin administration protects neurologic function in cerebral ischemia in rats. *Stroke* 1988;19:411.
251. Lanier WL. Glucose management during cardiopulmonary bypass: cardiovascular and neurologic implications. *Anesth Analg* 1991;72:423.
252. Metz S, Keats AS. Benefits of a plasma containing solution for cardiopulmonary bypass. *Anesth Analg* 1991;72:428.
253. Frasco P, Croughwell N, Blumenthal J, et al. Association between blood glucose level during cardiopulmonary bypass and neuropsychiatric outcome. *Anesthesiology* 1991;75[Suppl]:55.
254. Svensson LG, Crawford ES, Hess KR, et al. Deep hypothermia with circulatory arrest: determinants of stroke and early mortality in 656 patients. *J Thorac Cardiovasc Surg* 1993;106:19.
255. Nussmeier NA, Arlung C, Slogoff S. Neuropsychological dysfunction after cardiopulmonary bypass: cerebral protection by a barbiturate. *J Cardiothorac Vasc Anesth* 1991;5:584.
256. Zaidan JR, Klochany A, Martin WA, et al. Effects of thiopental on neurological outcome following coronary artery bypass grafting. *Anesthesiology* 1991;74:406.
257. Topol EJ, Humphrey LS, Borkon AM, et al. Value of intraoperative left ventricular microbubbles detected by transesophageal two dimensional echocardiography in predicting outcome after cardiac operations. *Am J Cardiol* 1985;56:773.
258. Milewicz DM. Ultrasonic characterization of the aortic architecture in Marfan patients. *Circulation* 1995;91:1272.
259. Wauquier A. Brain protective properties of etomidate and flunarizine. *J Cereb Blood Flow Metab* 1982;2:53.
260. Murkin JM. Anesthesia, the brain and cardiopulmonary bypass. *Ann Thorac Surg* 1993;56:1461.
261. Altman DI, Young RSK, Yagel SK. Effects of dexamethasone in hypoxic ischemic brain injury in the neonatal rat. *Biol Neonate* 1984;46:149.

262. Bass E. Cardiopulmonary arrest: pathophysiology and neurologic complications. *Ann Intern Med* 1985;103:920.
263. Steen PA, Gisvold SE, Milde JH, et al. Nimodipine improves outcome when given after complete cerebral ischemia in primates. *Anesthesiology* 1985;62:406.
264. Wauquier A, Ashton D, Clincke G, et al. Calcium entry blockers as cerebral protecting agents comparative activity in tests of hypoxia and hyperexcitability. *Jpn J Pharmacol* 1985;38:1.
265. Cullen JP, Aldrete JA, Jankousky L. Protective action of phenytoin in cerebral ischemia. *Anesth Analg* 1979;58:165.
266. Astrup J, Moller-Sorensen P, Rahbek-Sorensen H. Inhibition of cerebral oxygen and glucose consumption in the dog by hypothermia, pentobarbital and lidocaine. *Anesthesiology* 1981;55:263.
267. Skaryak LA, Kirshbom PM, DiBernardo LR, et al. Modified ultrafiltration improves cerebral metabolic recovery asfter circulatory arrest. *J Thorac Cardiovasc Surg* 1995;109:744; discussion 751.
268. Ungerleider RM. Effects of cardiopulmonary bypass and use of modified ultrafiltration. *Ann Thorac Surg* 1998;65[Suppl 6]:S35; discussion S39,S74.
269. Elliot M. Modified ultrafiltration and open heart surgery in children. *Paediatr Anaesth* 1999;9:1.
270. Kurrek MM, Reed RL. Effect of hypothermia on enzymatic activity of thrombin and plasmin. *Surg Forum* 1987;38:221.
271. Holmson H, Karpatkin S. Metabolism of platelets. In: Williams WJ, Beutler E, Erslev AJ, et al., eds. *Hematology,* 3rd ed. New York: McGraw-Hill, 1983:1157.
272. Aster RH. Thrombocytopenia due to sequestration of platelets. In: Williams WJ, Beutler E, Erslev QJ, et al., eds. *Hematology,* 3rd ed. New York: McGraw-Hill, 1983:1338.
273. Heyns A. Kinetics and in vivo redistribution of 111 indium-labeled human platelets after intravenous protamine sulfate. *Thromb Heamost* 1980;44:605.
274. Valeri CR, Cassidy G, Khuri WS, et al. Hypothermia-induced reversible platelet dysfunction. *Ann Surg* 1987;205:175.
275. Thomas R, Hessel EA, Harker LA, et al. Platelet function during and after deep surface hypothermia. *J Surg Res* 1981;31:314.
276. Ereth MH, Oliver WC Jr, Sanatrach PJ. Perioperative interventions to decrease transfusion of allogeneic blood products. *Mayo Clin Proc* 1994;69:575.
277. Scott WJ, Kessler R, Wernly JA. Blood conservation in cardiac surgery. *Ann Thorac Surg* 1990;50:843.
278. Horrow JC, Van Riper DF, Strong MD, et al. The hemostatic effects of tranexamic acid and desmopressin during cardiac surgery. *Circulation* 1991;84:2063.
279. Hill GE, Alonso A, Stammers AH, et al. Aprotinin and methylprednisolone equally blunt cardiopulmonary bypass-induced inflammation in humans. *J Thorac Cardiovasc Surg* 1995;110:1658.
280. Taylor KM. Aprotinin therapy in cardiac surgery. *Ann Cardiac Surg* 1994:89.
281. Lu H, Soria C, Soria J, et al. Reversible translocation of glycoprotein Ib in plasmin-treated platelets: consequences for platelet function. *Eur J Clin Invest* 1993;23:785.
282. Royston D, Taylor KM, Bidstrup BP, et al. Effect of aprotinin on need for blood transfusion after repeat open heart surgery. *Lancet* 1987;2:1289.
283. Dietrich W, Barankay A, Dilthey G, et al. Reduction of homologous bolld requirements in cardiac surgery by intraoperative aprotinin application: clinical experience in 152 cardiac surgical patients. *Thorac Cardiovasc Surg* 1989;37:92.
284. Blauhut B, Gross C, Necek S, et al. Effects of high-dose aprotinin on blood loss, platelet function, fibrinolysis, complement, and renal function after cardiopulmonary bypass. *J Thorac Cardiovasc Surg* 1991;101:958.
285. Sundt TM, Kouchoukos NT, Saffitz JE, et al. Renal dysfunction and intravascular coagulation with aprotinin and hypothermic circulatory arrest. *Ann Thorac Surg* 1993;55:1418.
286. Westaby S, Forni A, Dunning J, et al. Aprotinin and bleeding in profoundly hypothermic perfusion. *Eur J Cardiothorac Surg* 1994;8:82.
287. Goldstein DJ, DeRosa CM, Mongero LB, et al. Safety and efficacy of aprotinin under conditions of deep hypothermia and circulatory arrest. *J Thorac Cardiovasc Surg* 1995;110:1615.
288. Regragui IA, Bryan AJ, Izzat MB, et al. Aprotinin use with hypothermic circulatory arrest for aortic valve and thoracic aortic surgery: renal function and early survival. *J Heart Valve Dis* 1995;4:674.
289. Aoki M, Jonas RA, Normura F, et al. Aprotinin enhances acute recovery of cerebral metabolism after circulatory arrest. *Proc Am Heart Assoc* 1992;117:324.
290. Levy JH, Pifarre R, Schaff HV, et al. A multicenter, double-blind, placebo-controlled trial of aprotinin for reducing blood loss and the requirement for donor-blood transfusion in patients undergoing repeat coronary artery bypass grafting. *Circulation* 1995;92:2236.
291. Westaby S, Forni A, Dunning J, et al. Aprotinin and bleeding in profoundly hypothermic perfusion. *Eur J Cardiothorac Surg* 1994;8:82.
292. Espana S, Estelles A, Griffin JH, et al. Aprotinin (Trasylol) is a competitive inhibitor of activated protein C. *Thromb Res* 1989;56:751.
293. Wendel HP, Heller W, Gallimore MJ, et al. The prolonged activated clotting time (ACT) with aprotinin depends on the type of activator used for measurement. *Blood Coagul Fibrinolysis* 1993;4:41.
294. Westaby S, Forni A, Dunning J, et al. Aprotinin and bleeding in profoundly hypothermic perfusion. *Eur J Cardiothorac Surg* 1994;8:82.
295. Regragui IA, Bryan AJ, Izzat B, et al. Aprotinin use with hypothermic circulatory arrest for aortic valve and thoracic aortic surgery: renal function and early survival. *J Heart Valve Dis* 1995;4:674.
296. Rooney SJ, Pagano D, Bognolo G, et al. Aprotinin in aortic surgery requiring profound hypothermia and circulatory arrest. *Eur J Cardiothorac Surg* 1997;11:373.
297. Goldstein DJ, DeRosa CM, Mongero LB, et al. Safety and efficacy of aprotinin under conditions of deep hypothermia and circulatory arrest. *J Thorac Cardiovasc Surg* 1995;110:1615.
298. Okita Y, Takamoto S, Ando M, et al. Coagulation and fibrinolysis system in aortic surgery under deep hypothermic circulatory arrest with aprotinin: the importance of adequate heparinization. *Circulation* 1997;96[Suppl 9]II-376.
299. Newberger JW, Jonas RA, Wernovsky G, et al. A comparison of the perioperative neurologic effects of hypothermic circulatory arrest versus low-flow cardiopulmonary bypass in infant heart surgery. *N Engl J Med* 1993;329:1057.
300. Ergin MA, Galla JD, Lansman SL, et al. Hypothermic circulatory arrest in operations on the thoracic aorta: determinants of operative mortality and neurologic outcome. *J Thorac Cardiovasc Surg* 1994;107:788.
301. Willford DC, Moores WY, Ji S, et al. Importance of acid-base strategy in reducing myocardial and whole body oxygen consumption during perfusion hypothermia. *J Thorac Cardiovasc Surg* 1990;100:699.
302. Murkin JM, Farrar JK, Tweed WA, et al. Cerebral autoregulation and flow/metabolism coupling during cardiopulmonary bypass: the influence of $PaCO_2$. *Anesth Analg* 1987;66:825.
303. Henriksen L. Brain luxury perfusion during cardiopulmonary bypass in human: a study of cerebral blood flow response to

changes in CO_2, O_2 and blood pressure. *J Cereb Blood Flow Metab* 1986;6:366.

304. Baraka AS, Baroody MA, Haroun ST, et al. Effect of alpha stat versus pH stat strategy on oxyhemoglobin dissociation and whole-body oxygen consumption during hypothermic cardiopulmoary bypass. *Anesth Analg* 1992;74:32.
305. Rogers AT, Prough DS, Roy RC, et al. Cerebrovascular and cerebral metabolic effects of alterations in perfusion flow rate during hypothermic cardiopulmonary bypass in man. *J Thorac Cardiovasc Surg* 1992;103:363.
306. Tuppurainen T, Settergren G, Stensved P. The effect of arterial pH on whole body oxygen uptake during hypothermic cardiopulmonary bypass in man. *J Thorac Cardiovasc Surg* 1989;98: 769.
307. Murkin JM, Martzke JS, Buchan AM, et al. A randomized study of the influence of perfusion technique and pH management strategy in 316 patients undergoing coronary artery bypass surgery: II. Neurologic and cognitive outcomes. *J Thorac Cardiovasc Surg* 1995;110:349.
308. Skaryak LA, Chai PJ, Kern FH, et al. Blood gas management and degree of cooling: effects of cerebral metabolism before and after circulatory arrest. *J Thorac Cardiovasc Surg* 1995;110:1649.
309. Watanabe T, Miura M, Inui K, et al. Blood and brain tissue gaseous strategy for profoundly hypothermic total circulatory arrest. *J Thorac Cardiovasc Surg* 1991;102:497.
310. Aoki M, Nomura F, Stromski ME, et al. Effects of pH on brain energetics after hypothermic circulatory arrest. *Ann Thorac Surg* 1993;55:1093.
311. Hiramatsu T, Miura T, Forbess JM, et al. pH strategies and cerebral energetics before and after circulatory arrest. *J Thorac Cardiovasc Surg* 1995;109:948.
312. Aoki M, Nomura F, Stromski ME, et al. Effects of pH on brain energetics after hypothermic circulatory arrest. *Ann Thorac Surg* 1993;55:1093.
313. Kawata H, Fackler JC, Aoki M, et al. Recovery of cerebral blood flow and energy state in piglets after hypothermic circulatory arrest versus recovery after low-flow bypass. *J Thorac Cardiovasc Surg* 1993;106:671.
314. Robbins RC, Balaban RS, Swain JA. Intermittent hypothermic asanguineous cerebral perfusion (cerebroplegia) protects the brain during prolonged circulatory arrest. *J Thorac Cardiovasc Surg* 1990;99:878.
315. Coles JG, Taylor MJ, Pearce JM, et al. Cerebral monitoring of somotosensory evoked potentials during profoundly hypothermic circulatory arrest. *Circulation* 1984;70[Suppl]: I96.
316. Kirshbom PM, Skaryak LR, DiBernardo LR, et al. pH-stat cooling improves cerebral metabolic recovery after circulation arrest in a piglet model of aortopulmonary collaterals. *J Thorac Cardiovasc Surg* 1996;111:147; discussion 156.
317. Wong PC, Barlow CF, Hickey PR, et al. Factors associated with choreoathetosis after cardiopulmonary bypass in children with congential heart disease. *Circulation* 1992;86[Suppl II]: II-118.
318. Jonas RA, Bellinger DC, Rappaport LA, et al. Relation of pH strategy and developmental outcome after hypothermic circulatory arrest. *J Thorac Cardiovasc Surg* 1993;106:362.
319. Bellinger DC, Wernovsky G, Rappaport LA, et al. Cognitive development following repair as neonates of transposition of the great arteries using deep hypothermic circulatory arrest. *Pediatrics* 1991;87:701.
320. Hindman BJ, Dexter F, Cutkomp J, et al. pH-Stat mamagement reduces cerebral metabolic rate for oxygen CMR_{O2} during profound hypothermia (17°C): a study during cardiopulmonary bypass in rabbits. *Anesthesiology* 1995;82:983.
321. Hindman BJ, Dexter F, Cutkomp J, et al. pH-Stat management reduces the cerebral metabolic rate for oxygen during profound hypothermia (17°C). A study during cardiopulmonary bypass in rabbits. *Anesthesiology*. 1995;82:983; discussion 24A.
322. Murkin JM, Farrar JK, Tweed A, et al. Cerebral autoregulation and flow/metabolism coupling during cardiopulmonary bypass: the influence of Pa_{CO2}. *Anesth Analg* 1987;66:825.
323. Hindman BJ, Dexter F, Cutkomp J, et al. Cerebral blood flow and metabolism do not decrease at stable brain temperature during cardiopulmonary bypass in rabbits. *Anesthesiology* 1992; 77:342.
324. Taylor RH, Burrows FA, Bissonnette B. Cerebral pressure-flow velocity relationship during hypothermic cardiopulmonary bypass in neonates and infants. *Anesth Analg* 1992;74:636.
325. Buijs J, Van Bel F, Nandorff A, et al. Cerebral blood flow pattern and autoregulation during open-heart surgery in infants and young children: a transcranial, Doppler ultrasound study. *Crit Care Med* 1992;20:771.
326. Swain JA, McDonald TJ, Robbins RC, et al. Relationship of cerebral and myocardial intracellular pH to blood pH during hypothermia. *Am J Physiol* 1991;260:H1640.
327. Swain JA, McDonald TJ, Balaban RS, et al. Metabolism of the heart and brain during hypothermic cardiopulmonary bypass. *Ann Thorac Surg* 1991;51:105.
328. Aoki M, Nomura F, Stromski ME, et al. Effects of pH on brain energetics after hypothermic circulatory arrest. *Ann Thorac Surg* 1993;55:1093.
329. Currin RT, Gores GJ, Thurman RG, et al. Protection by acidotic pH against anoxic cell killing in perfused rat liver: evidence for a pH paradox. *FASEB J* 1991;5:207.
330. Nayler WG, Panagiotopoulos S, Elz JS, Daly MJ. Calcium-mediated damage during postischemic reperfusion. *J Mol Cell Cardiol* 1988;20[Suppl 2]:41.
331. Matsuda N, Kuroda H, Mori T. Beneficial actions of acidotic initial reperfusate in stunned myocardium of rat hearts. *Basic Res Cardiol* 1991;86:317.
332. Bonventre JV, Cheung JY. Effects of metabolic acidosis on viability of cells exposed to anoxia. *Am J Physiol* 1985;294:C149.
333. Giffard RG, Monyer H, Christine CW, et al. Acidosis reduces NMDA receptor activation, glutamate neurotoxity, and oxygen-glucose deprivation neuronal injury in cortical cultures. *Brain Res* 1990;506:339.
334. Tombaugh GC, Sapolsky RM. Mild acidosis protects hipocampal neurons from injury induced by oxygen and glucose deprivation. *Brain Res* 1990;506:343.
335. Crawford ES, Rubio PA. Reappraisal of adjuncts to avoid ischemia in the treatment of aneurysms of the descending thoracic aorta. *J Thorac Cardiovasc Surg* 1973;66:693.
336. O'Connor CJ, Rothenberg DM. Anesthetic considerations for descending thoracic aortic surgery: part 1. *J Cardiothorac Vasc Anesth* 1995;9:581.
337. Stenseth R, Myhre HO. Anaesthesia in surgery for aneurysm of the descending thoracic or thoracoabdominal aorta. *Acta Chir Scand* 1988;154:147.
338. Benumof JL. One-lung ventilation: which lung should be PEEP-ed? *Anesthesiology* 1982;56:161.
339. Katz JA, Laverne RG, Fairley BF, et al. Pulmonary oxygen exchange during endobronchial anesthesia: effect of tidal volume and PEEP. *Anesthesiology* 1982;56:164.
340. Benumof JL. Physiology of the open chest and one-lung ventilation. In: Kaplan JA, ed. *Thoracic anesthesia*. New York: Churchill Livingstone, 1983:278.
341. Rogers SN, Benumof JL. Halothane and isoflurane do not decrease PaO_2 during one-lung ventilation in intravenously anesthetized patients. *Anesth Analg* 1985;64:946.
342. Nugent M, Kaye MP, McGoon DC. Effects of nitroprusside on aortic and intraspinal pressures during thoracic aortic cross-clamping. *Anesthesiology* 1984;61:A68.

343. Roberts AJ, Nora JD, Hughes WA, et al. Cardiac and renal responses to cross-clamping of the descending thoracic aorta. *J Thorac Cardiovasc Surg* 1983;86:732.
344. Gelman S, Reves JG, Fowler K, et al. Regional blood flow during cross-clamping of the thoracic aorta and infusion of sodium nitroprusside. *J Thorac Cardiovasc Surg* 1983;85:287.
345. Stokland O, Miller MM, Ilebekk A. Mechanism of hemodynamic responses to occlusion of the descending thoracic aorta. *Am J Physiol* 1980;238:H423.
346. Pagani M, Pizzinelli P, Bergamaschi M, et al. A positive feedback sympathetic pressor reflex during stretch of the thoracic aorta in conscious dogs. *Circ Res* 1982;50:125.
347. Roizen MF, Beaupre PN, Alpert RA, et al. Monitoring with two-dimensional transesophageal echocardiography: comparison of myocardial function in patients undergoing supraceliac, suprarenal-infraceliac, or infrerenal aortic occlusion. *J Vasc Surg* 1984;1:300.
348. Schurlknight S, Beattie C, O'Rourke K, et al. Metabolic changes during high aortic cross-clamp surgery. *Abstracts of the Eighth Annual Meeting of the Society of Cardiovascular Anesthesiologists,* Richmond, VA, 1986:72.
349. Beattie C, Frank SM. Anesthesia for major vascular surgery. In: Rogers MC, Tinker JH, Covino BG, et al., eds. *Principles and practice of anesthesiology.* St. Louis: CV Mosby, 1993:1931.
350. O'Rourke K, Beattie C, Walman AT, et al. Acidosis during high cross-clamp surgery. *Anesthesiology* 1985;65:266.
351. Saleh SA, Crawford ES, Bamberger RA. Intraoperative acid-base management for the resection of thoracoabdominal aortic aneurysms: a comparison of continuous infusion of sodium bicarbonate versus the bolus. *Anesth Analg* 1982;61:213(abst).
352. Shenaq SA, Chelly JE, Kalberg H, et al. Use of nitroprusside during surgery for thoracoabdominal aortic aneurysm. *Circulation* 1984;70[Suppl I]:7.
353. Shenaq SA. Anesthesia for resection of abdominal aortic aneurysm: one approach at Baylor College of Medicine. In: Roizen MF, ed. *Anesthesia for vascular surgery.* New York: Churchill Livingstone, 1990.
354. Gelman S, McDowell H, Varner PD, et al. The reason for cardiac output reduction after aortic cross-clamping. *Am J Surg* 1988;155:578.
355. Lampe GH, Managano DT. Anesthetic management for abdominal aortic reconstruction. In: Roizen MF, ed. *Anesthesia for vascular surgery.* New York: Churchill Livingstone, 1990.
356. Godet G, Bertrand M, Coriat P, et al. Comparison of isoflurane with sodium nitroprusside for controlling hypertension during thoracic aortic cross-clamping. *J Cardiothorac Anesth* 1990;4:177.
357. Roizen MF, Beaupre PN, Alpert RA, et al. Monitoring with two dimensional transesophageal echocardiography. *J Vasc Surg* 1984;1:300.
358. Najafi H. Descending aortic aneurysmectomy without adjuncts to avoid ischemia: 1993 update. *Ann Thorac Surg* 1993;55:1042.
359. Biglioli P, Spirito R, Pompilio G, et al. Descending thoracic aorta aneurysmectomy: left-left centrifugal pump versus simple clamping technique. *Cardiovasc Surg* 1995;3:511.
360. Livesay JJ, Cooley DA, Ventemiglia RA, et al. Surgical experience in descending thoracic aneurysmectomy with and without adjuncts to avoid ischemia. *Ann Thorac Surg* 1985;39:37.
361. Svensson LG, Crawford ES, Hess KR, et al. Experience with 1509 patients undergoing thoracoabdominal aortic operations. *J Vasc Surg* 1993;17:357.
362. Cooley DA. Further experience with exsanguination for descending thoracic aneurysms. *J Card Surg* 1994;9:625.
363. Schepens MA, Defauw JJ, Hamerlijnck RP, et al. Use of left heart bypass in the surgical repair of thoracoabdominal aortic aneurysms. *Ann Vasc Surg* 1995;9:327.
364. Crawford ES, Walker HS III, Saleh SA, et al. Graft replacement of aneurysm in descending thoracic aorta: results without bypass or shunting. *Surgery* 1981;89:73.
365. Svensson LG, Crawford ES. Aortic dissection and aortic aneurysm surgery: clinical observations, experimental investigations, and statistical analyses. Part III. *Curr Probl Surg* 1993;30:10.
366. Najafi H. Descending aortic aneurysmectomy without adjuncts to avoid ischemia: 1993 update. *Ann Thorac Surg* 1993;55:1042.
367. Verdant A, Page A, Cossette R, et al. Surgery of the descending thoracic aorta: spinal cord protection with the Gott shunt. *Ann Thorac Surg* 1988;46:147.
368. Verdant A. Descending thoracic aortic aneurysms: surgical treatment with the Gott shunt. *Can J Surg* 1992;35:493.
369. von Segesser LK, Killer I, Jenni R, et al. Improved distal circulatory support for repair of descending thoracic aortic aneurysms. *Ann Thorac Surg* 1993;56:1373.
370. Cunningham JN, Laschinger JC, Spencer FC. Monitoring of somatosensory evoked potentials during surgical procedures on the thoracoabdominal aorta: IV. Clinical observations and results. *J Thorac Cardiovasc Surg* 1987;94:275.
371. Janusz MT. Experience with thoracoabdominal aortic aneurysm resection. *Am J Surg* 1994;167:501.
372. Najafi H, Javid H, Hunter J, et al. Descending aortic aneurysmectomy without adjuncts to avoid ischemia. *Ann Thorac Surg* 1980;30:326.
373. Bickerstaff LK, Pairolero PC, Hollier LH, et al. Thoracic aortic aneurysms: a population-based study. *Surgery* 1982;92:1103.
374. Molina JE, Cogordan J, Einzig S, et al. Adequacy of ascending aorta descending aorta shunt during cross-clamping of the thoracic aorta for prevention of spinal cord ischemia. *J Thorac Cardiovasc Surg* 1985;90:126.
375. Svensson LG, Antunes MJ, Kinsley RH. Traumatic rupture of the thoracic aorta: a report of 14 cases and a review of the literature. *S Afr Med J* 1985;67:853.
376. Svensson LG, Richard E, Couell A, et al. Relationship of spinal cord blood flow to vascular anatomy during thoracic aortic cross-clamping and shunting. *J Thorac Cardiovasc Surg* 1986;91:71.
377. Reed CC, Statford TB. *Cardiopulmonary bypass.* Houston, TX: Surgimedics, 1989:452.
378. Verdant A. Surgery of the descending thoracic aorta. Spinal cord protection with the Gott shunt. [1988, updated in 1995.] *Ann Thorac Surg* 1995;60:1151.
379. Lee Y, Jihayel A. Thoracic aortic aneurysm repair: hemodynamic changes and complications. In: Casthely PA, Bregman D, eds. *Cardiopulmonary bypass: physiology, related complications, and pharmacology.* New York: Futura, 1991:489.
380. Laschinger JC, Cunningham JN, Catinella FP, et al. Detection and prevention of intraoperative spinal cord ischemia after cross-clamping of the thoracic aorta: use of somatosensory evoked potentials. *Surgery* 1982;92:1109.
381. Katz NM, Blackstone EH, Kirklin JW, et al. Incremental risk factors for spinal cord injury following operations for acutely traumatic aortic transection. *J Thorac Cardiovasc Surg* 1981;81:669.
382. Cartier R, Orszulak TA, Pairolero PC, et al. Circulatory support during aortic crossclamping of the descending thoracic aorta: evidence of improved organ perfusion. *J Thorac Cardiovasc Surg* 1990;99:1038.
383. Svensson LG, Crawford ES, Hess KR, et al. Variables predictive of outcome in 832 patients undergoing repairs of the descending thoracic aorta. *Chest* 1993;104:1248.
384. Kazui T, Komatsu S, Yokoyama H. Surgical treatment of aneu-

rysms of the thoracic aorta with the aid of partial cardiopulmonary bypass: an analysis of 95 patients. *Ann Thorac Surg* 1987; 43:622.
385. Messick JM Jr, Newberg LA, Nugent M, et al. Principles of neuroanesthesia for the nonneurosurgical patient with CNS pathophysiology. *Anesth Analg* 1985;64:143.
386. Vacanti FX, Ames A III. Mild hypothermia and MG^{++} protect against irreversible damage during CNS ischemia. *Stroke* 1984; 15:695.
387. Kouchoukos NT, Daily BB, Rokkas CK, et al. Hypothermic bypass and circulatory arrest for operations on the descending thoracic and thoracoabdominal aorta. *Ann Thorac Surg* 1995; 60:67.
388. Crawford ES, Crawford JL, Safi HJ, et al. Thoracoabdominal aortic aneurysms: preoperative and intraoperative factors determining immediate and long-term results of operations in 605 patients. *J Vasc Surg* 1986;3:389.
389. O'Connor CJ, Rothenberg DM. Anesthetic considerations for descending thoracic aortic surgery: part II. *J Cardiothorac Vasc Anesth* 1995;9:734.
390. Hollier LH, Symmonds JB, Pairolero PC, et al. Thoracoabdominal aortic aneurysm repair: analysis of postoperative morbidity. *Arch Surg* 1988;123:871.
391. Golden MA, Donaldson MC, Wittemore AD, et al. Evolving experience with thoracoabdominal aortic aneurysm repair at a single institution. *J Vasc Surg* 1991;13:792.
392. Cox GS, O'Hara PJ, Hertzer NR, et al. Thoracoabdominal aneurysm repair: a representative experience. *J Vasc Surg* 1992; 15:780.
393. Hollier LH, Money SR, Naslund TC, et al. The risk of spinal cord dysfunction 150 consecutive patients undergoing thoracoabdominal aortic replacement. *Am J Surg* 1992;164:210.
394. Svensson LG, Coselli JC, Safi HJ, et al. Appraisal of adjuncts to prevent acute renal failure after surgery on the thoracic or thoracoabdominal aorta. *J Vasc Surg* 1989;10:230.
395. Ostri P, Mouritsen L, Jorgensen B, et al. Renal function following aneurysmectomy of the abdominal aorta. *J Cardiovasc Surg* 1986;27:714.
396. Janusz MT. Experience with thoracoabdominal aortic aneurysm resection. *Am J Surg* 1994;167:501.
397. Gloviczki P, Bower TC. Visceral and spinal cord protection during thoracoabdominal aortic reconstructions. *Semin Vasc Surg* 1992;5:163.
398. Bush HL, Huse JB, Johnson WL, et al. Prevention of renal insufficiency after abdominal aortic aneurysm resection by optimal volume loading. *Arch Surg* 1981;116:1517.
399. Anto HR, Chou SY, Porush JG, et al. Infusion intravenous pyelography and renal function: effects of hypertonic mannitol in patients with chronic renal insufficiency. *Arch Intern Med* 1981;141:1652.
400. Alpert RA, Roizen MF, Hamilton WK, et al. Intraoperative urinary output does not predict postoperative renal function in patients undergoing abdominal aortic revascularization. *Surgery* 1984;95:707.
401. Abbott JACC. Renal surface cooling: a method for preservation of renal function in prolonged renal ischemia. In: Wickham JEA, ed. *Intra-renal surgery.* London: Churchill Livingstone, 1984:83.
402. Collins GM, Green RD, Boyer D, et al. Protection of kidneys from warm ischemic injury: dosage and timing of mannitol administration. *Transplantation* 1980;29:83.
403. Bandy KDF. Preoperative imaging of aortic aneurysms. *Surg Clin North Am* 1989;69:721.
404. Svensson LG, Crawford ES, Hess KR, et al. Thoracoabdominal aortic aneurysms associated with celiac, superior mesenteric and renal artery occlusive disease: methods and analysis of results in 271 patients. *J Vasc Surg* 1992;16:378.
405. Hertzer NR, Bevan EG, Young JR, et al. Coronary artery disease in peripheral vascular patients: a classification of 1000 coronary angiograms and results of surgical management. *Ann Surg* 1984; 199:223.
406. Pass LJ, Eberhart RC, Brown JC, et al. The effect of mannitol and dopamine on the renal response to thoracic aortic cross-clamping. *J Thorac Cardiovasc Surg* 1988;95:608.
407. Nicholson ML, Baker DM, Hopkinson BR, et al. Randomized controlled trial of the effect of mannitol on renal reperfusion injury during aortic aneurysm surgery. *Br J Surg* 1996;83:1230.
408. Hanley MJ, Davidson K. Prior mannitol and furosemide infusion in a model of ischemic acute renal failure. *Am J Physiol* 1981;241:F556.
409. Sinsteden TD, O'Neil TJ, Hill S, et al. The role of high energy phosphate in norepinephrine-induced acute renal failure in the dog. *Circ Res* 1986;59:93.
410. Brown CB, Ogg CS, Cameron JS. High dose furosemide in acute renal failure: a controlled trial. *Clin Nephrol* 1981;15:90.
411. Grodin W, Scantlebury V, Warminton N. Dopmainergic stimulation of renal blood flow and renal function after transplantation. *Anesthesiology* 1984;61:A129(abst).
412. Davis RF, Lappas DG, Kirklin JK, et al. Acute oliguria after cardiopulmonary bypass: renal functional improvement with low-dose dopamine infusion. *Crit Care Med* 1982;10:852.
413. Polson RJ, Park GR, Lindop MJ, et al. The prevention of renal impairment in patients undergoing orthotopic liver grafting by infusion of low-dose dopamine. *Anaesthesia* 1987;42:15.
414. Elliott WJ, Weber RR, Nelson KS, et al. Renal and hemodynamic effects of intravenous fenoldopam versus nitroprusside in severe hypertension. *Circulation* 1990;81:970.
415. Russell JD, Churchill DN. Calcium antagonists and acute renal failure. *Am J Med* 1989;87:306.
416. Jacobsen WK, Gingrich GA, Wolley JL, et al. The effect of the calcium entry blocker verapamil on renal ischemia. *Anesthesiology* 1985;A114(abst).
417. Tataranni G, Malacarne F, Farinelli R, et al. Beneficial effects of verapamil in renal-risk surgical patients. *Ren Fail* 1994;16: 383.
418. Lelcuk S, Alexander F, Kobzik L, et al. Prostacyclin and thromboxane A2 moderate postischemic renal failure. *Surgery* 1985; 98:207.
419. Kaufman RP, Klauser JM, Anner H, et al. Inhibition of thromboxane (TX) synthesis by free radical scavengers. *J Trauma* 1988;28:458.
420. Lindner A, Cutler RE, Bell AJ. Attenuation of nephrotoxic acute renal failure in the dog with angiotensin-converting enzyme inhibitor (SQ-20,881). *Circ Res* 1982;51:216.
421. Joob AW, Harman PK, Kaiser DL, et al. There effect of renin-angiotensin system blockade on visceral blood flow during and after thoracic aortic cross-clamping. *J Thorac Cardiovasc Surg* 1986;91:411.
422. Koelz AM, Bertschin S, HermLavee M, et al. the angiotensin-converting enzyme inhibitor enalapril in acute ischemic renal failure in rats. *Experientia* 1988;44:172.
423. Horton JW. Alterations in intestinal permeability and blood flow in a new model of mesenteric ischemia. *Circ Shock* 1992; 36:134.
424. Bourchier RG, Gloviczki P, Larson MV, et al. The mechanisms and prevention of intravascular fluid loss following occlusion of the supraceliac aorta in dogs. *J Vasc Surg* 1991;13:637.
425. Cohen JR, Angus L, Asher A, et al. Disseminated intravascular coagulation as a result of supraceliac clamping: implications for thoracoabdominal aneurysm repair. *Ann Vasc Surg* 1987;1:552.
426. Elmore JR, Gloviczki P, Harper CM Jr, et al. Spinal cord injury

in experimental thoracic aortic occlusion: investigation of combined methods of protection. *J Vasc Surg* 1992;15:789.
427. Boros M, Kaszaki J, Nagy S. Oxygen free-radial-induced histamine release during intestinal ischemia and reperfusion. *Eur Surg Res* 1989;21:297.
428. Kazmers A, Zwolak R, Appleman HD, et al. Pharmacologic interventions in acute mesenteric ischemia: improved survival with intravenous glucagon, methylprednisolone, and prostacyclin. *J Vasc Surg* 1984;1:472.
429. Sardella GL, Bech FR, Cronewett JL. Hemodynamic effects of glucagon after acute mesenteric ischemia in rats. *J Surg Res* 1990; 49:354.
430. Costello TG, Fisher A. Neurological complications following aortic surgery. *Anaesthesia* 1983;38:230.
431. Wadouh F, Lindemann E, Arndt CF, et al. The arteria radicularis magna anterior as a decisive factor influencing spinal cord and damage during aortic occlusion. *J Thorac Cardiovasc Surg* 1984;88:1.
432. Svensson LG, Von Ritter CM, Groeneveld HT, et al. Cross-clamping of the thoracic aorta: influence of aortic shunts, papaverine, calcium channel blocker, allopurinol, and superoxide dismutase on spinal cord blood flow and paraplegia in baboons. *Ann Surg* 1986;204:38.
433. Laschinger JC, Cunningham JN Jr, Baumann FG, et al. Monitoring of somatosensory evoked potentials during surgical procedures on the thoracoabdominal aorta: II. Use of somatosensory evoked potentials to assess adequacy of distal aortic bypass and perfusion following thoracic aortic cross-clamping. *J Thorac Cardiovasc Surg* 1987;94:266.
434. Kleffer E, Thierry R, Chiras J, et al. Preoperative spinal cord arteriography in aneurysmal disease of the descending thoracic and thoracoabdominal aorta: preliminary results in 45 patients. *Ann Vasc Surg* 1989;3:34.
435. Piano G, Gewertz BL. Mechanism of increased cerebrospinal fluid pressure with thoracic aortic occlusion. *J Vasc Surg* 1990; 11:695.
436. Miyamoto K, Ueno A, Wada T, et al. A new and simple method of preventing spinal cord injury after simple and double aortic cross-clamping. *J Thorac Cardiovasc Surg* 1986;92:121.
437. Choi DW, Rothman SM. The role of glutamate neurotoxicity in hypoxic-ischemic neuronal death. *Annu Rev Neurosci* 1990; 13:171.
438. Choi DW. Methods of antagonizing glutamate. *Cerebrovasc Brain Metab Rev* 1990;2:105.
439. Kouchoukos NT, Rokkas CK. Descending thoracic and thoracoabdominal aortic surgery for aneurysm or dissection: how do we minimize the risk of spinal cord injury? *Semin Thorac Cardiovasc Surg* 1993;5:47.
440. Jex RK, Schaff HV, Piehler JM, et al. Early and late results following repair of dissections of the descnding thoracic aorta. *J Vasc Surg* 1986;3:226.
441. Olivier HF, Maher TD, Liebler GA, et al. Use of the BioMedicus centrifugal pump in traumatic tears of the thoracic aorta. *Ann Thorac Surg* 1984;38:586.
442. Frank SM, Parker S, Gorman R, et al. Thoracoabdominal aortic aneurysm repair with deep hypothermic circulatory arrest and selective upper and lower body function perfusion. *Anesthesiology* 1993;79:A152.
443. Laschinger JC, Cunningham JN, Nathan IM, et al. Experimental and clinical assessment of the adequacy of partial bypass in maintenance of spinal cord blood flow during operations on the thoracic aorta. *Ann Thorac Surg* 1983;36:417.
444. Kaplan BJ, Friedman WA, Alexander JA, et al. Somatosensory evoked potential monitoring of spinal cord ischemia during aortic operations. *Neurosurgery* 1986;19:82.
445. Laschinger JC, Cunningham JN, Cooper MM, et al. Monitoring of somatosensory evoked potentials during surgical procedures on the thoracoabdominal aorta: part I. *J Thorac Cardiovasc Surg* 1987;94:260.
446. Jex RK, Schaff HV, Piehler JM, et al. Early and late results following repair of dissections of the descending thoracic aorta. *J Vasc Surg* 1986;3:226.
447. Crawford ES. Thoracoabdominal aortic aneurysm: surgical techniques. In: Bergan JJ, Yao JST, eds. *Techniques in arterial surgery.* Philadelphia: WB Saunders Co, 1990:88.
448. Carlson DE, Kapr RB, Konchoukos NT. Surgical treatment of aneurysms of the descending thoracic aorta: an analysis of 85 patients. *Ann Thorac Surg* 1983;35:58.
449. Crawford ES, Mizrahi EM, Hess KR, et al. The impact of distal aortic perfusion and SEP monitoring on prevention of paraplegia following aortic aneurysm operations. *J Thorac Cardiovasc Surg* 1988;95:357.
450. Vacanti FX, Ames A III. Mild hypothermia and Mg^{++} protect against irreversible damage during CNS ischemia. *Stroke* 1984; 15:695.
451. Wisselink W, Becker MO, Nguyen JH, et al. Protecting the ischemic spinal cord during aortic clamping: the influence of selective hypothermia and spinal cord perfusion pressure. *J Vasc Surg* 1994;19:788.
452. Tabayashi K, Niibori K, Konno H, et al. Protection from postischemic spinal cord injury by perfusion cooling of the epidural space. *Ann Thorac Surg* 1993;56:494.
453. Marsala M, Vanicky I, Yaksh TL. Effect of graded hypothermia (27 degrees to 34 degrees C) on behavioral function, histopathology, and spinal blood flow after spinal ischemia in rat. *Stroke* 1994;25:2038.
454. Coles JG, Wilson GJ, Sima AF, et al. Intraoperative management of the thoracic aortic aneurysm: experimental evaluation of perfusion cooling of the spinal cord. *J Thorac Cardiovasc Surg* 1983;85:292.
455. Kouchoukos NT, Wareing TH, Izumoto H, et al. Elective hypothermic cardiopulmonary bypass and circulatory arrest for spinal cord protection during operations on the thoracoabdominal aorta. *J Thorac Cardiovasc Surg* 1990;99:659.
456. Berguer R, Porto J, Fedoronko B, et al. Selective deep hypothermia of the spinal cord prevents paraplegia after aortic cross-clamping in the dog model. *J Vasc Surg* 1992;15:62.
457. Davison JK, Cambria RP, Vierra DJ, et al. Epidural cooling for regional spinal cord hypothermia during thoracoabdominal aneurysm repair. *J Vasc Surg* 1994;20:304.
458. Murray MJ, Bower TC, Oliver WC Jr, et al. Effects of cerebrospinal fluid drainage in patients undergoing thoracic and thoracoabdominal aortic surgery. *J Cardiothorac Vasc Anesth* 1993; 7:266.
459. Grocott HP, Mutch WA. Epidural aneshtesia and acutely increased intracranial pressure: lumbar epidural anesthesia and acutely increased intracranial pressure. Lumbar epidural space hydrodynamics in a porcine model. *Anesthesiology* 1996;85: 1086.
460. Crawford ES, Coselli JS, Safi HJ. Partial cardiopulmonary bypass hypothermic circulatory arrest, and posterolateral exposure for thoracic aortic aneurysm operation. *J Thorac Cardiovasc Surg* 1987;94:824.
461. Hollier LH. Protecting the brain and spinal cord. *J Vasc Surg* 1987;5:524.
462. Nugent M: Pro: cerebrospinal fluid drainage prevents paraplegia. *J Cardiothorac Vasc Anesth* 1992;6:366.
463. Oka Y, Miyamoto T. Prevention of spinal cord injury after cross-clamping of the thoracic aorta. *Jpn J Surg* 1984;14:159.
464. McCullough JL, Hollier LH, Nugent M. Paraplegia after thoracic aortic occlusion: influence of cerebrospinal fluid drainage. *J Vasc Surg* 1988;7:153.

465. Bower TC, Murray MJ, Gloviczki P, et al. Effects of thoracic aortic occlusion and cerebrospinal fluid drainage on regional spinal cord blood flow in dogs: correlation with neurologic outcome. *J Vasc Surg* 1988;9:135.
466. Dasmahapatra HK, Coles JG, Wilson GJ, et al. Relationship between cerebrospinal fluid dynamics and reversible spinal cord ischemia during experimental thoracic aortic occlusion. *J Thorac Cardiovasc Surg* 1988;95:920.
467. Crawford ES, Svensson LG, Hess KR, et al. A prospective randomized study of cerebrospinal fluid drainage to prevent paraplegia after high-risk surgery on the thoracoabdominal aorta. *J Vasc Surg* 1990;13:36.
468. Schoenwald P, Gottlieb A, Lewis B, et al. Cerebrospinal fluid pressure (CSFP) during aortic cross-clamp (XC) as a predictor of neurologic outcome during thoracoabdominal aneurysm repair. *Anesthesiology* 1992;77:A71.
469. Hollier LH, Money SR, Naslund TC, et al. Risk of spinal cord dysfunction in patients undergoing thoracoabdominal aortic replacement. *Am J Surg* 1992;164:210.
470. Woloszyn T, Corrado P, Marini P, et al. Cerebrospinal fluid drainage does not counteract the negative effect of sodium nitroprusside on spinal cord perfusion pressure during aortic cross-clamping. *Curr Surg* 1989;46:489.
471. Svensson LG, Stewart RW, Cosgrove DM, et al. Intrathecal papaverine for the prevention of paraplegia after operation of the thoracic or thoracoabdominal aorta. *J Thorac Cardiovasc Surg* 1988;96:823.
472. Svensson LG, Grum DF, Bernarski M, et al. Appraisal of cerebrospinal fluid alterations during aortic surgery with intrathecal papaverine administration and cerebrospinal fluid drainage. *J Vasc Surg* 1990;11:243.
473. Breckwoldt WL, Genco CM, Connolly RJ, et al. Spinal cord protection during aortic occlusion: efficacy of intrathecal tetracaine. *Ann Thorac Surg* 1991;51:959.
474. Woloszyn TT, Marini CP, Coons MS, et al. Cerebrospinal fluid drainage and steroids provide better spinal cord protection during aortic cross-clamping than does either treatment alone. *Ann Thorac Surg* 1990;49:78.
475. Acher CW, Wynn MM, Archibald J. Naloxone and spinal fluid drainage as adjuncts in the surgical treatment of thoracoabdominal and thoracic aneurysms. *Surgery* 1990;108:755.
476. Wynn MM, Acher CW, Popic PM, et al. Combined use of spinal fluid drainage and naloxone reduces the risk of neurologic deficit in thoracoabdominal aneurysm repair. *Anesthesiology* 1993;79:A165.
477. Woloszyn TT, Marini CP, Coons MS, et al. Cerebrospinal fluid drainage and steroids provide better spinal cord protection during aortic cross-clamping than does either treatment alone. *Ann Thorac Surg* 1990;49:79.
478. DelRossi AJ, Cernaianu AC, Cilley JH, et al. Preventive effect of Fluosol-DA for paraplegia encountered after surgical treatment of the thoracic aorta: preliminary results in a dog model. *J Thorac Cardiovasc Surg* 1990;99:665.
479. Svensson LG, Patel V, Robinson MF, et al. Influence of preservation or perfusion of intraoperatively identified spinal cord blood supply on spinal motor evoked potentials and paraplegia after aortic surgery. *J Vasc Surg* 1991;13:355.
480. Svensson LG, Patel V, Coselli JS, et al. Preliminary report of localization of spinal cord blood supply by hydrogen during aortic operations. *Ann Thorac Surg* 1990;49:528.
481. Cunningham JN, Laschinger JC, Merkin BA, et al. Measurement of spinal cord ischemia during operations upon the thoracic aorta: initial experience. *Ann Surg* 1982;196:285.
482. Mizrahi EM, Crawford ES. Somatosensory evoked potentials during reversible spinal cord ischemia in man. *Electroencephalogr Clin Neurophysiol* 1984;58:120.
483. Coles JG, Wilson GJ, Sima AF. Intraoperative detection of spinal cord ischemia using somatosensory evoked potentials during thoracic occlusion. *Ann Thorac Surg* 1980;34:299.
484. Lesser RP, Raudzens P, Luders H, et al. Postoperative neurological deficits may occur despite unchanged intraoperative somatosensory evoked potentials. *Ann Neurol* 1986;19:22.
485. Grundy BL. Intraoperative monitoring of sensory evoked potentials. *Anesthesiology* 1983;58:72.
486. Takaki O, Okumura F. Application and limitation of somatosensory evoked potential monitoring during thoracic aortic aneurysm surgery: a case report. *Anesthesiology* 1985;65:700.
487. Schepens MA, Boezeman EH, Hamerlijnck RP, et al. Somatosensory evoked potentials during exclusion and reperfusion of critical aortic segments in thoracoabdominal aortic aneurysm surgery. *J Card Surg* 1994;9:692.
488. McPherson RW, Mahla M, Johnson R, et al. Effects of enflurane, isoflurane, and nitrous oxide on somatosensory evoked potentials during fentanyl anesthesia. *Anesthesiology* 1985;62:626.
489. Elmore JR, Gloviczki P, Harper CM, et al. Failure of motor evoked potentials to predict neurologic outcome in experimental thoracic aortic occlusion. *J Vasc Surg* 1991;14:131.
490. Wadouh F, Arndt CF, Metzger H, et al. Direct measurement of oxygen tension on the spinal cord surface of pigs after occlusion of the descending aorta. *J Thorac Cardiovasc Surg* 1985; 89:787.
491. Allen BT, Doblas M, Owen J, et al. Cerebrospinal fluid pressure, somatosensory and motor evoked potentials in spinal cord ischemia after lumbar artery ligation. *Surg Forum* 1991;42:262.
492. Laschinger JC, Owen J, Rosenbloom M, et al. Detrimental effects of sodium nitroprusside on spinal cord motor tract perfusion during thoracic aortic cross-clamping. *Surg Forum* 1987; 38:195
493. Coles JG, Wilson GJ, Sima AF, et al. Intraoperative detection of spinal cord ischemia using somatosensory cortical evoked potentials during thoracic aortic occlusion. *Ann Thorac Surg* 1982;34:299.
494. North RB, Drenger B, Beattie C, et al. Monitoring of spinal cord stimulation evoked potentials during thoracoabdominal aneurysm surgery. *Neurosurgery* 1991;28:325.
495. Mongan PD, Peterson RE, Williams D. Spinal evoked potentials are predictive of neurologic function in a porcine model of aortic occlusion. *Anesth Analg* 1994;78:257.
496. Williams GM, Perler BA, Burdick JF, et al. Angiographic localization of spinal cord blood supply and its relationship to postoperative paraplegia. *J Vasc Surg* 1991;13:23.
497. Robertson CS, Foltz R, Grossman RG, et al. Protection against experimental ischemic spinal cord injury. *J Neurosurg* 1986;64: 633.
498. Nylander WA, Plunkett RJ, Hammon JW, et al. Thiopental modification of ischemic spinal cord injury in the dog. *Ann Thorac Surg* 1982;33:64.
499. Laschinger JC, Cunningham JN, Cooper MM, et al. Prevention of ischemic spinal cord injury following aortic cross-clamping: use of corticosteroids. *Ann Thorac Surg* 1984;38:500.
500. Braughler JM, Hall ED. Correlation of methylprednisolone levels in cat spinal cord with its effects on $(N^+ + K^+)$-ATPase, lipid peroxidation and alpha motor neuron function. *J Neurosurg* 1982;56:838.
501. Faden AI, Jacobs TP, Smith MT. Evaluation of the calcium channel antagonist nimodipine in experimental spinal cord ischemia. *J Neurosurg* 1984;60:796.
502. Gelbfish JS, Phillips T, Rose DM, et al. Acute spinal cord ischemia: prevention of paraplegia with verapamil. *Circulation* 1986;74:5
503. Guha A, Tator CH, Piper I. Increase in rat spinal cord blood

flow with the calcium channel blocker, nimodipine. *J Neurosurg* 1985;63:250.
504. Benthuysen JL. Naloxone therapy in spinal trauma: anesthetic effects. *Anesthesiology* 1987;66:238.
505. Faden AI, Jacobs TP, Holaday JW. Opiate antagonist improves neurologic recovery after spinal injury. *Science* 1981;211:493.
506. Lim KH, Connolly M, Rose D, et al. Prevention of reperfusion injury of the ischemic spinal cord: use of recombinant superoxide dimutase. *Ann Thorac Surg* 1986;42:282.
507. Grabitz K, Freye E, Prior R, et al. Does prostaglandin E 1 and superoxide dismutase prevent ischaemic spinal cord injury after thoracic aortic cross-clamping? *Eur J Vasc Surg* 1990;4:19.
508. Granke K, Hollier LH, Zdrahal P, et al. Longitudinal study of cerebral spinal fluid drainage in polyethylene glycol-conjugated superoxide dismutase in paraplegia associated with thoracic aortic cross-clamping. *J Vasc Surg* 1991;13:615.
509. Oxyurt E, Graham DI, Woodruff GN, et al. Protective effect of the glutamate antagonist, MK-801 in focal cerebral ischemia in the cat. *J Cereb Blood Flow Metab* 1988;8:138.
510. Kochhlar A, Zivin JA, Lyden PD, et al. Glutamate antagonist therapy reduces neurologic deficits produced by focal central nervous system ischemia. *Arch Neurol* 1988;45:148.
511. Altura BT, Altura BM. Interactions of magnesium and potassium on cerebral vessels-aspects in view of stroke. *Magnesium* 1984;3:195.
512. Simpson JI, Eide TR, Koski G, et al. Intrathecal magnesium protects against the spinal cord ischemia seen with thoracic aortic cross clamping. *Proceedings of the 16th Annual Meeting of the Society of Cardiovascular Anesthesiologists,* Montreal, Canada, April 1994:240.
513. Geisler FH, Dorsey FC, Coleman WP. Recovery of motor function after spinal-cord injury: a randomized, placebo-controlled trial with GM-1 ganglioside. *N Engl J Med* 1991;324:1829.
514. Mezrow CK, Mazzani M, Wolfe D, et al. Poloxamer 188 improves neurologic outcome after hypothermic circulatory arrest. *J Thorac Cardiovasc Surg* 1992;103:1143.
515. Drummond JC, Moore SS, Zivin JA, et al. The effect of hyperglycemia on neurologic outcome following spinal cord ischemia in the rabbit. *Anesth Analg* 1978;66:S43.
516. LeMay DR, Neal S, et al. Paraplegia in the rat induced by aortic cross-clamping: model characterization and glucose exacerbation of neurologic deficit. *J Vasc Surg* 1987;6:383.
517. Lundy EF, Ball TD, Mandell MA, et al. Dextrose administration increases sensory/motor impairment and paraplegia after intrarenal aortic occlusion in the rabbit. *Surgery* 1987;102:737.
518. Lanier WL, Strangland KJ, Scheithauer BW, et al. The effects of dextrose infusion and head position on neurologic outcome after complete cerebral ischemia in primates: examination of a model. *Anesthesiology* 1987;66:39.
519. Moore WS, Vescera CL. Repair of abdominal aortic aneurysm by transfemoral endovascular graft placement. *Ann Surg* 1994; 220:331.
520. Moore WS. The role of endovascular grafting technique in the treatment of infrarenal abdominal aortic aneurysm. *Cardiovasc Surg* 1995;3:109.
521. Dake MD, Miller DC, Semba CP, et al. Transluminal placement of endovascular stent-grafts for the treatment of descending thoracic aortic aneurysms. *N Engl J Med* 1994;331:1729.
522. Balm R, Eikelboom BC, May J, et al. Early experience with transfemoral endovascular aneurysm management (TEAM) in the treatment of aortic aneurysms. *Eur J Vasc Endovasc Surg* 1996;11:214.
523. Katzen BT, Becker GJ, Benenati JF, et al. Treatment of abdominal aortic aneurysms with the Endovascular Technologies tube and bifurcating Endovascular Grafting System: technical aspects. *Tech Vasc Intervent Radiol* 1998;1:9.
524. Kahn RA, Moskowitz DM, Manspeizer H, et al. Endovascular aortic repair is associated with greater hemodynamic stability compared with open aortic reconstruction. *J Cardiothorac Vasc Anesth* 1999;13:42.
525. Baxendale BR, Baker DM, Hutchinson A, et al. Haemodynamic and metabolic response to endovascular repair of infra-renal aortic aneurysms. *Br J Anaesth* 1996;77:581.
526. Norgren L, Albrechtsson U, Swartbol P. Side-effect of endovascular grafting to treat aortic aneurysm. *Br J Surg* 1996;83:520.
527. Schoenwald PK, Sprung J, Sullivan T. Anesthetic considerations for treatment of abdominal aortic aneurysm (AAA) with an endovascular graft. *Anesth Analg* 1998;86:S99.
528. Schoenwald PK, Sprung J. Anesthesia for endovascular aortic aneurysm stent-graft repair. In: Dolmatch BL, Blum U, eds. *Stent-grafts current clinical practice.* New York: Thieme, 2000: 69.
529. Baker AB, Lloyd G, Bookallil MJ, et al. Retrospective review of 100 cases of endoluminal aortic stent-graft surgery from an anaesthetic perspective. *Anaesth Intensive Care* 1997;25:378.
530. Blum U, Voshage G, Lammer J, et al. Endoluminal stent-grafts for infrarenal abdominal aortic aneurysms. *N Engl J Med* 1997; 336:13.
531. Machan L, Fry P. Abdominal aortic aneurysm repair using the World Medical Talent prosthesis. *Tech Vasc Intervent Radiol* 1998;1:25.
532. Tanito Y, Endou M, Koide Y, et al. ATP-induced ventricular asystole and hypotension during endovascular stenting surgery. *Can J Anaesth* 1998;45:491.
533. Baker AB, Bookallil MJ, Lloyd G. Intentional asystole during endoluminal thoracic aortic surgery without cardiopulmonary bypass. *Br J Anaesth* 1997;78:444.
534. Ritchie JL, ACC/AHA Task Force. ACC/AHA guidelines for perioperative cardiovascular evaluation for non-cardiac surgery. *Circulation* 1996;93:1280.
535. Mangano DT, Layug EL, Wallace A, et al. Effect of atenolol on mortality and cardiovascular morbidity after noncardiac surgery. *N Engl J Med* 1996;335:1713.
536. Wallace A, Layug B, Tateo I, et al. Prophylactic atenolol reduces postoperative myocardial ischemia. *Anesthesiology* 1998;88:7.
537. Landesberg G, Einav S, Christopherson R, et al. Perioperative ischemia and cardiac complications in major vascular surgery: importance of the preoperative twelve-lead electrocardiogram. *J Vasc Surg* 1997;26:570.
538. Mangano DT. Perioperative cardiac morbidity. *Anesthesiology* 1987;72:153.
539. Tuman KJ, McCarthy RJ, March RJ, et al. Effects of epidural anesthesia and analgesia on coagulation and outcome after major vascular surgery. *Anesth Analg* 1991;73:696.
540. Christopherson R, Beattie C, Frank SM, et al. Perioperative morbidity in patients randomized to epidural or general anesthesia for lower extremity vascular surgery. *Anesthesiology* 1993;79: 422.
541. Drake MD, Miller DC, Mitchell RS, et al. The "first generation" of endovascular stent-grafts for patients with aneurysms of the descending thoracic aorta. *J Thorac Cardiovasc Surg* 1998; 116:689.
542. Newman RJ, Jones IS. A prospective study of 413 consecutive car occupants with chest injuries. *J Trauma* 1984;24:129.
543. Cohn PF, Braunwald E. Traumatic heart disease. In: Braunwald E, ed. *Heart disease: a textbook of cardiovascular medicine.* Philadelphia: WB Saunders Co, 1988;1535.
544. Holcroft JW, Blaisdell FW. Trauma to the torso. In: Wilmore DW, Brennan MF, Harken AH, et al., eds. *American College of Surgeons: care of the surgical patient.* New York: Scientific American, 1989:sect IV, ch 1:1.
545. Gerlock AAJ, Muhletaler CA, Coulam CM, et al. Traumatic

aortic aneurysm: validity of esophageal tube displacement sign. *AJR Am J Roentgenol* 1980;135:713.

546. Pate JW, Fabian TC, Walker WA. Acute traumatic rupture of the aortic isthmus: repair with cardiopulmonary bypass. *Ann Thorac Surg* 1995;59:90.
547. Olivier HF Jr, Maher TD, Liebler GA, et al. Use of the Biomedicus centrifugal pump in traumatic tears of the thoracic aorta. *Ann Thorac Surg* 1984;38:586.
548. Higgins RS, Sanchez JA, DeGuidis L, et al. Mechanical circulatory support decreases neurologic complications in the treatment of traumatic injuries of the thoracic aorta. *Arch Surg* 1992; 127:516.
549. Hess PJ, Howe HR, Ribicsek F, et al. Traumatic tears of the thoracic aorta: improved results using the Biomedicus pump. *Ann Thorac Surg* 1989;48:6.
550. Nocolosi AC, Almassi GH, Bousamra M, et al. Mortality and neurologic morbidity after repair of traumatic aortic disruption. *Ann Thorac Surg* 1996;61:875.
551. Katz NM, Blackstone EH, Kirklin JW, et al. Incremental risk factors for spinal cord injury following operation for acute traumatic aortic transection. *J Thorac Cardiovasc Surg* 1981;81:669.
552. Astrup J, Skovsted P, Gjerris F, et al. Increase in extracellular potassium in the brain during circulatory arrest: effects of hypothermia, lidocaine, and thiopental. *Anesthesiology* 1981;55:256.
553. Sturm JT, Billiar TR, Luxeberg MG, et al. Risk factors for the development of renal failure following the surgical treatment of traumatic aortic rupture. *Ann Thorac Surg* 1987;43:425.
554. Cernainu AC, Cilley JH, Baldino WA, et al. Determinants of outcome in lesions of the thoracic aorta in patient with multiorgan system system trauma. *Chest* 1992;101:331.
555. Conte S, Lacour-Gayet F, Serraff A, et al. Surgical management of neonatal coarctation. *J Thorac Cardiovasc Surg* 1995;109: 663.
556. Zehr KJ, Gillinov AM, Redmond JM, et al. Repair of coarctation of the aorta in neonates and infants: a thirty-year experience. *Ann Thorac Surg* 1995;59:33.
557. Rothman A. Coarctation of the aorta: an update. *Curr Probl Pediatr* 1998;28:37.
558. Allan LD, Chita SK, Handerson RH, et al. Coarctation of the aorta in prenatal life: an echocardiographic, anatomical and functional study. *Br Heart J* 1988;59:356.
559. McNamara DG. Coarctation of the aorta: difficulties in clinical recognition. *Heart Dis Stroke* 1992;1:202.
560. Carvalho JS, Redington AN, Shinebourne EA, et al. Continuous wave Doppler echocardiography and coarctation of the aorta: gradients and flow patterns in the assessment of severity. *Br Heart J* 1990;64:133.
561. Simpson IA, Soho DJ, Valdez-Cruz LM, et al. Color Doppler flow mapping in patients with coarctation of the aorta: new observations and improved evaluation with color flow diameter and proximal acceleration as predictors of severity. *Circulation* 1988;77:736.
562. Ramaciotti C, Chin AJ. Noninvasive diagnosis of coarctation of the aorta in the presence of a patent ductus arteriosus. *Am Heart J.* 1993;125:179.
563. Sharma S, Anand R, Kanter KR, et al. The usefulness of echocardiography in the surgical management of infants with congenital heart disease. *Clin Cardiol* 1992;15:891.
564. Mohiaddin RH, Kilner PJ, Rees S, et al. Magnetic resonance volume flow and jet velocity mapping in aortic coarctation. *J Am Coll Cardiol* 1993;22:1515.
565. Simpson IA, Chung HJ, Glass RF, et al. Cine magnetic resonance imaging for evaluation of anatomy and flow relations in infants and children with coarctation of the aorta. *Circulation* 1988;78:142.
566. Santoro G, di Carlo D, Carotti A, et al. Origin of both coronary arteries from the pulmonary artery and aortic coarctation. *Ann Thorac Surg* 1995;60:706.
567. Brouwer RMHJ, Erasmus ME, Ebels T, et al. Influence of age on survival, late hypertension, and recoarctation in elective aortic coarctation repair. *J Thorac Cardiovasc Surg* 1994;108:525.
568. van Son JA, van Asten WN, van Lier HJ, et al. Detrimental sequelae on the hemodynamics of the upper left limb after subclavian flap angioplasty in infancy. *Circulation* 1990;81:996.
569. Parks WJ, Ngo TD, Plauth WH, et al. Incidence of aneurysm formation after Dacron patch aortoplasty repair for coarctation of the aorta: long-term results and assessment utilizing magnetic resonance angiography with three-dimensional surface rendering. *J Am Coll Cardiol* 1995;26:266.
570. Huggon IC, Qureshi SA, Baker EJ, et al. Effect of introducing balloon dilation of native aortic coarctation on overall outcome in infants and children. *Am J Cardiol* 1994;73:799.
571. Ovaert C, Benson LN, Nykanen D, et al. Transcatheter treatment of coarctation of the aorta: a review. *Pediatr Cardiol* 1998; 19:27.
572. Shaddy RE, Boucek MM, Sturtevant JE, et al. Comparison of angioplasty and surgery for unoperated coarctation of the aorta. *Circulation* 1993;87:793.
573. Vermilion RP, Snider AR, Bengur AR, et al. Doppler evaluation of femoral arteries in children after aortic balloon valvuloplasty or coarctation balloon angioplasty. *Pediatr Cardiol* 1993;14:13.
574. DeGroff CG, Rice MJ, Reller MD, et al. Intravascular ultrasound can assist angiographic assessment of coarctation of the aorta. *Am Heart J* 1994;128:836.
575. Rosenthal E, Qureshi SA, Tynan M. Stent implantation for aortic recoarctation. *Am Heart J* 1995;129:1220.
576. Suarez de Lezo J, Pan M, Romero M, et al. Balloon-expandable stent repair of severe coarctation of aorta. *Am Heart J* 1995; 129:1002.
577. Bennett MWR, Cheema SPS, Entress AH, et al. The use of thoracic epidural anesthesia I repair of an aortic coarctation. *J Cardiothorac Vasc Anesth* 1995;9:174.
578. Watterson KG, Dhasmana JP, O'Higgins JW, et al. Distal aortic pressure during coarctation operation. *Ann Thorac Surg* 1990; 49:978.
579. Crawford FA, Sade RM. Spinal cord injury associated with hyperthermia during aortic coarctation repair. *J Thorac Cardiovasc Surg* 1984;87:616.
580. Park SC, Neches WH. The neurologic complications of congenital heart disease. *Neurol Clin* 1993;11:441.
581. Leandro J, Williamson Balfe J, Smallhorn JF, et al. Coarctation of the aorta and hypertension. *Child Nephrol Urol* 1992;12:124.
582. Stewart JM, Gewitz MH, Woolf PK, et al. Elevated arginine vasopressin and lowered atrial natriuretic factor associate with hypertension in coarctation of the aorta. *J Thorac Cardiovasc Surg* 1995;110:900.
583. Malan JE, Benatar A, Levin SE. Long-term follow-up of coarctation of the aorta repaired by patch angioplasty. *Int J Cardiol* 1991;30:23.
584. Choy M, Rocchini AP, Beekman RH, et al. Paradoxical hypertension after repair of coarctation of the aorta in children: balloon angioplasty versus surgical repair. *Circulation* 1987;75: 1186.
585. Kimball TR, Reynolds JM, Mays WA, et al. Persistent hyperdynamic cardiovascular state at rest and during exercise in children after successful repair of coarctation of the aorta. *J Am Coll Cardiol* 1994;24:194.
586. Krogmann ON, Rammos S, Jakob M, et al. Left ventricular diastolic dysfunction late after coarctation repair in childhood: influence of left ventricular hypertrophy. *J Am Coll Cardiol* 1993;21:1454.
587. Gardiner HM, Celermajer DS, Sorensen KE, et al. Arterial reac-

tivity is significantly impaired in normotensive young adults after successful repair of aortic coarctation in childhood. *Circulation* 1994;89:1745.

588. Sciolaro C, Copeland J, Cork R, et al. Long-term follow-up comparing subclavian flap angioplasty to resection with modified oblique end to end anastomosis. *J Thorac Cardiovasc Surg* 1991;101:1.
589. Morrow RW. Aortic arch and pulmonary artery abnormalities. In: Oski FA, DeAngelis CD, Feigin RD, et al., eds. *Principles and practice of pediatrics.* Philadelphia: JB Lippincott; 1990: 1450.
590. Azarow KS, Pearl RH, Hoffman MA, et al. Vascular ring: does magnetic resonance imaging replace angiography? *Ann Thorac Surg* 1992;53:882.
591. Schlesinger AE, Mendeloff E, Sharkey AM, et al. MR of right aortic arch with mirror-image branching and a left ligamentum arteriosum: an unusual cause of a vascular ring. *Pediatr Radiol* 1995;25:455.
592. Burke RP, Rosenfeld HM, Wernovsky G, et al. Video-assisted thoracoscopic vascular ring division in infants and children. *J Am Coll Cardiol* 1995;25:943.
593. Becker CI, Ibawi MN, Idriss FS, et al. Vascular anomalies causing tracheoesophageal compression. *J Thorac Cardiovasc Surg* 1989;97:725.

Cardiac Anesthesia: Principles and Clinical Practice, Second Edition, edited by Fawzy G. Estafanous, Paul G. Barash, and J.G. Reves. Lippincott Williams & Wilkins, Philadelphia © 2001.

28

EMERGENCY SITUATIONS

DOUGLAS V. BROWN
CHRISTOPHER J. O'CONNOR
KENNETH J. TUMAN

Advances in the knowledge and skill of cardiologists, anesthesiologists, and cardiac surgeons who care for patients with severe cardiac disease have paralleled the growing frequency with which cardiac anesthesiologists are confronted with emergency situations. These advances include a deeper understanding of the etiology and pathophysiology of acquired cardiovascular disease and improvements in diagnostic and therapeutic methods. Emergency situations in cardiac anesthesia present challenges even beyond those encountered in the high-risk patient who presents for elective surgery. The patient's survival often mandates that a focused, organized, and efficient approach to anesthetic management be expeditiously instituted. This chapter presents the pathophysiology, goals of medical and surgical management, and clinical priorities that are necessary to effectively manage a variety of emergency situations.

EMERGENCIES ASSOCIATED WITH CARDIAC CATHETERIZATION

Complications of Routine Cardiac Catheterization

During the 1960s and 1970s, cardiac catheterization was developed as a diagnostic tool for evaluating hemodynamics, ventricular dynamics, coronary anatomy, and valvular function. The invasive character of cardiac catheterization has led to various complications that may present as emergency situations for anesthesiologists and their surgical colleagues (1,2). Complications of cardiac catheterization may broadly be classified into five categories: allergic, arrhythmic, ischemic, neurologic, and peripheral vascular events.

Allergic Events

Allergic events may be associated with the use of radiocontrast material, protamine, or any other drug administered during the course of the procedure. True anaphylactoid reactions to standard hyperosmolar radiocontrast dye occur in 0.2% of exposed patients. Reactions often occur on first administration and are dose dependent. Individuals with previous dye reactions, as well as those who are atopic or have asthma, are more susceptible to dye-induced anaphylactoid reactions. Premedication with glucocorticosteroids and antihistamines modestly decreases anaphylactoid reactions in these "at-risk" patients. Although low-osmolality contrast dye is a more expensive alternative to hyperosmolar radiocontrast, it is associated with a much lower (0.04%) incidence rate of anaphylactoid reactions (3,4). When a severe reaction occurs in the cardiac catheterization laboratory, many patients lack adequate cardiopulmonary reserves and require prompt aggressive intervention to manage circulation and ventilation. Anesthesiologists may be called upon for airway management, endotracheal intubation, and assistance with hemodynamic support.

Contrast dye can also cause less severe side effects. Mild hypotension, attributable to dye-induced vasodilation, and nausea and vomiting occur in 5% of patients after dye injection. Transient bradycardia can also occur. These events, like anaphylactoid reactions, are most commonly precipitated by hyperosmolar contrast dye. Finally, hyperosmolar radiocontrast acts as a diuretic and can cause hypovolemia and possibly postcatheterization renal dysfunction, particularly in patients with diabetes or preexisting renal insufficiency.

Arrhythmias

A frequent complication of routine cardiac catheterization is precipitation of various arrhythmias related to mechanical effects of intraventricular catheters, development of ischemia, or vasovagal effects related to stimulation of the Bezold-Jarisch reflex (5). Ventricular ectopic activity, bundle-branch blocks, and bradyarrhythmias generally are benign events, but they may precipitate significant hypotension in certain patients with advanced heart disease such as critical aortic stenosis, left main or triple-vessel coronary

D. V. Brown, C. J. O'Connor, and K. J. Tuman: Department of Anesthesiology, Rush-Presbyterian—St. Luke's Medical Center, Chicago, Illinois 60612

artery disease, low ejection fraction, and myocardial failure. These arrhythmias account for most rhythm disturbances seen during routine catheterizations. More serious arrhythmias such as ventricular tachycardia, supraventricular tachydysrhythmias, and asystole occur in less than 0.5% of catheterizations and may require countershock, pacemaker insertion, or pharmacotherapy (1).

Pacing, if required, can be quickly established by passing a pacing wire into the left ventricle through the existing arterial sheath or more traditionally, into the right ventricle if central venous access has been established (6). Alternatively, transcutaneous pacemakers permit rapid institution of cardiac pacing, and some cardiac catheterization laboratories routinely apply these electrodes to the skin in high-risk patients. Transcutaneous pacing electrodes typically have a large surface area and may also be used for defibrillation. When patients with these devices in place must be transported to the operating room from the catheterization suite, the appropriate direct-current power source plus electrocardiographic (ECG) and hemodynamic monitoring must be employed.

Ischemic, Neurologic, and Peripheral Vascular Events

Patients with acute ischemic syndromes, a prior history of significant arrhythmias, severe aortic stenosis, or other evidence of advanced heart disease are at greatest risk of cardiac arrest secondary to arrhythmias during routine cardiac catheterization. Precipitation or exacerbation of preexisting myocardial ischemia during coronary artery injections is commonly associated with arrhythmogenesis and may progress to gross mechanical dysfunction of the heart if the ischemia is prolonged or severe. Vascular injury (including arterial dissection) of the coronary vessels or ostia is unusual during diagnostic cardiac catheterization, but if it occurs, it may be associated with acute coronary occlusions necessitating thrombolytic therapy or emergency coronary artery surgery. Embolization of atheromatous material is possible during coronary-ostial cannulation or intracoronary injections. It may be associated with acute ischemic syndromes that require both pharmacologic and mechanical support of systemic perfusion while the patient is awaiting urgent or emergent coronary revascularization. Precipitation of acute ischemic syndromes during cardiac catheterization is the most frequent reason for emergent surgical intervention.

Embolization of atherosclerotic debris during cardiac catheterization may also be associated with neurologic injury involving any of the cerebral vessels. The occurrence of microemboli during cardiac catheterization is well documented, and transcranial Doppler ultrasonography demonstrates frequent cerebral microembolism during routine cardiac catheterization and angioplasty (7). Although most embolic events are related to solution injection and likely represent cavitation bubbles, 30% of these emboli are related to wire and catheter manipulation around the aortic arch (7). These later embolic events tend to be more common in patients with the most severe aortic atheroma and likely represent embolization of atherosclerotic debris. Fortunately, the incidence of acute neurologic injury after left-sided heart catheterization is low, between 0.03% and 0.3%, and most of these neurologic deficits are temporary. Risk factors for neurologic events include female gender, left ventricular hypertrophy, depressed ejection fraction, and severe coronary artery disease (1,8).

Because of the use of flexible and minimally traumatic catheters, cardiac perforation occurs very infrequently during routine diagnostic catheterizations. Vascular injury at the site of arterial cannulation, however, occurs more commonly and is related to arterial sheath size, the presence of peripheral vascular disease, and the use of anticoagulants. Older age, smaller body surface area, and smaller body weight are also associated with injury (9). The incidence of vascular injury after routine cardiac catheterization is approximately 1% (10,11). The femoral artery is most commonly cannulated, and the brachial artery is frequently used when puncture of the femoral artery is contraindicated or not feasible. The overall incidence of local vascular complications is similar when femoral or brachial arteries are cannulated, although thrombosis and arterial dissection are more common when using the brachial artery, and hemorrhage, arteriovenous fistula, and pseudoaneurysm are more prevalent after a femoral approach (1).

Vascular injuries may be associated with significant hematoma formation and may even require transfusion in some patients. The administration of systemic heparinization or thrombolytic therapy before and/or after catheterization, as well as the widespread concomitant use of antiplatelet therapy, increases the risk of significant hematoma formation. Emergent surgical repair of the femoral (or occasionally brachial) artery is occasionally required to maintain adequate limb perfusion and to prevent further blood loss. After femoral artery catheter removal, external pressure should be applied to the suprainguinal and inguinal areas for 20 to 30 minutes to reduce the incidence of hematoma formation. When the femoral vessels are punctured above the inguinal ligament, significant bleeding may occur retroperitoneally without obvious hematoma formation in the femoral area. In this case, pressure applied to the skin entry site (commonly below the inguinal ligament) can exacerbate bleeding, because distal flow is occluded without tamponade of a suprainguinal vessel puncture site. If hematoma formation and vascular injury are limited, most surgical repairs of femoral vessels can be performed under local anesthesia. Local anesthesia supplemented with intravenous sedation may be less satisfactory for the management of large hematomas, major arterial or venous lacerations, or pseudoaneurysms, in which vascular control often necessitates greater dissection, and the hematoma makes it difficult to effectively apply local anesthetics. Regional anesthesia may be contraindicated in some of these patients because of hypovolemia or profound anticoagulation initiated before or during cardiac catheterization procedures, particularly in patients with acute myocardial ischemia.

Mortality

The overall mortality rate associated with routine diagnostic cardiac catheterization is low, even though greater numbers of increasingly aged and acutely ill and unstable patients are being studied (1,2,12). However, routine diagnostic catheterization is associated with greater intrinsic risk in patients with unstable and global myocardial ischemia and in patients with significant left main coronary artery disease (12). As for patients undergoing therapeutic cardiac catheterization, minimization of mortality risk in these high-risk patients requires facility in managing profound circulatory collapse and access to emergent surgical intervention. The anesthesiologist may be called upon for resuscitative skills in the cardiac catheterization laboratory or may not encounter these complications until patients arrive emergently in the operating room. Anesthetic and critical care management of these patients is intrinsically similar to that for patients with complications of interventional catheterization (described later in this chapter).

Although cardiac insult is responsible for many of the complications of diagnostic and interventional catheterization, respiratory depression may also occur as a result of anxiolytic and analgesic agents given during cardiac catheterization. Oversedation, resulting in airway obstruction or apnea and hypoxemia may require resuscitation by the anesthesiologist.

Complications of Therapeutic Cardiac Catheterization

Percutaneous Transluminal Coronary Angioplasty

Therapeutic cardiac catheterization involves interventional techniques, such as percutaneous transluminal coronary angioplasty (PTCA) and percutaneous balloon valvuloplasty for the treatment of cardiovascular disease. Therapeutic catheterization procedures are associated with more (and more frequent) complications than purely diagnostic catheterizations. Since its introduction in 1977, PTCA has grown at a phenomenal rate. In the United States, PTCA is currently a more common procedure than coronary artery bypass surgery (13). The indications for PTCA have expanded from single-vessel coronary artery disease involving a single, concentric subtotal stenosis with well-preserved left ventricular function and stable but medically refractory angina to significantly more severe and complex coronary artery disease. Improved technology has facilitated nonsurgical revascularization in increasing numbers of high-risk patients, including those with unstable ischemic syndromes, multivessel coronary disease, stenotic coronary artery bypass grafts, and sometimes severely impaired left ventricular function, cardiogenic shock, or acute myocardial infarction. Although the indications for PTCA are expanding to include more seriously ill patients with complex coronary anatomy, PTCA is also being performed in patients with less severe coronary disease. Refractoriness to a combination of antianginal agents is no longer a prerequisite for PTCA, and it is now being performed on smaller, more distal vessels as well as on coronary arteries with angiographically less significant stenosis (14,15). PTCA has continued to gain popularity, despite the limited documentation that outcome is superior to that of alternative treatments (coronary artery surgery or medical therapy) and the persistent problem of restenosis, which occurs in 30% to 50% of lesions 6 months after the procedure. The reduced cost and low incidence of important noncardiac (particularly central nervous system) complications associated with shorter hospital stays makes PTCA particularly appealing. The risk of death associated with PTCA is approximately 1%, and the mortality rate is greater in the presence of older age, female gender, multivessel coronary disease, PTCA of the proximal left anterior descending coronary artery, and emergent patient status (16).

Vascular complications occur in 3% to 6% of patients and are much more common after percutaneous interventional cardiac catheterization than after diagnostic cardiac catheterization (1,10). The large-diameter vascular catheters necessary for introduction of therapeutic devices, particularly in patients with peripheral vascular disease, are the primary cause of the increased risk of vascular complications. The prolonged duration of arterial catheter presence and the more liberal use of anticoagulants also contribute to the higher incidence of vascular injury associated with interventional cardiac catheterization procedures.

Adverse cardiac outcomes are typically due to temporary coronary occlusions induced by balloon inflations, which place an intolerable ischemic burden on marginally compensated myocardium and lead to hemodynamic collapse. In patients with markedly impaired left ventricular systolic function, severe myocardial ischemia and myocardial infarction may be caused by acute coronary occlusions resulting from balloon inflation, large dissections of the arterial intima or media, or thrombus formation—particularly if substantial collateral circulation is absent. Coronary air embolism may occur during PTCA and manifest as a spectrum of responses, depending on the amount of air and the mass of myocardium jeopardized. Although most cases of coronary air embolism result in varying degrees of ischemia, arrhythmias, and transient hypotension, air embolism to the coronary circulation during PTCA may have more serious consequences that require immediate institution of cardiopulmonary resuscitation, temporary pacing, intraaortic balloon counterpulsation, defibrillation, and airway control.

The air lock usually clears spontaneously within minutes, but aggressive pressure and flow support are critical because hypotension and low-flow states may place previously dilated sites at risk of reocclusion. High pressure and flow also facilitate the spontaneous resolution of the coronary artery air lock. Aspiration of coronary air with a balloon angioplasty catheter as well as intracoronary verapamil administration have been reported to improve coronary blood flow after air embolism (17). Despite these risks, PTCA may be a therapeutic option for some patients who are deemed poor candidates for coronary artery surgery because of impaired left ventricular function, poor target vessels, or noncardiac contraindications.

Urgent or emergent coronary artery surgery for failed PTCA has decreased drastically. Although emergent surgery was previously required in more than 5% of all PTCA procedures, the current incidence is approximately 1% (18,19). Several factors have contributed to the decreased frequency of emergent surgical intervention. Acute coronary occlusions and dissections once requiring cardiac revascularization are often now successfully reopened and reperfused in the catheterization laboratory by placement of an intracoronary stent. The indications for PTCA have expanded since its introduction into clinical medicine and include patients with distal vessel stenosis. Irreversible occlusion of a small, distal coronary artery does not justify emergent surgical bypass, as only a small amount of myocardium is jeopardized. Finally, the threshold for surgical intervention is higher than it was previously because now we know that the risk of emergent bypass is greater than that of more conservative management of failed PTCA. This altered threshold for performing coronary bypass means that patients presenting for emergent surgery are now more critically ill:(20) 20% are in cardiogenic shock and 5% require cardiopulmonary resuscitation upon arrival to the operating room. Still, aggressive measures to salvage myocardium can result in satisfactory in-hospital and long-term outcomes, even in cases of failed PTCA with unstable coronary and systemic circulation (21–23).

Several pharmacologic and mechanical techniques have been developed to improve tolerance to transient coronary artery occlusion during PTCA and to maintain systemic perfusion in the event of acute vessel closure. Intravenous and intracoronary infusions of nitroglycerin, β-adrenergic antagonists, and calcium channel blockers may postpone the onset of angina or ECG evidence of ischemia during balloon inflation (24,25). In addition, transcatheter coronary perfusion with an oxygen-carrying perfluorochemical emulsion has been shown to alleviate intraprocedural ischemia during PTCA (26). Nonetheless, the response to pharmacologic agents in this setting is not entirely predictable, and the significance of the interruption of coronary blood flow during balloon inflation depends largely on the extent of myocardium jeopardized and the quality of the ventricular muscle. Patients with limited contractile reserves or with large regions of myocardium at risk during PTCA of proximal coronary lesions may experience hemodynamic and electrical instability during balloon occlusion (27). Prompt resuscitative measures typically are successful but may necessitate mechanical support devices.

Mechanical Support During Coronary Angioplasty

Several devices may be employed to diminish myocardial ischemia during PTCA. These may be used prophylactically, particularly in high-risk patients, before the initiation of angioplasty. Mechanical support is also used after a failed PTCA with coronary artery occlusion or threatened occlusion with the goal of either avoiding emergent cardiac surgery or stabilizing the patient until surgery can be performed.

Intraaortic balloon counterpulsation is the most common method of mechanical support used in association with PTCA. Intraaortic counterpulsation decreases myocardial oxygen demand, may augment coronary blood flow in patent vessels, and provides modest augmentation of cardiac output as long as a stable cardiac rhythm is present. By these means, intraaortic counterpulsation may prevent or treat myocardial ischemia. The role of routine use of intraaortic balloon counterpulsation during high-risk PTCA is not clearly defined. Although some studies demonstrate improved outcome when implemented before PTCA (28), a multicenter trial in acute infarct patients who were stratified to a high-risk group based on clinical and angiographic variables did not find beneficial impact of prophylactic intraaortic balloon counterpulsation use (29). In this study, intraaortic balloon counterpulsation conferred modest benefits in reducing recurrent ischemia but did not reduce the rate of infarct-related artery reocclusion, reinfarction or mortality, and was associated with a higher incidence of stroke (29). After failed PTCA, intraaortic balloon counterpulsation may stabilize the patient and allow for further interventional catheterization maneuvers or may provide an effective bridge to anesthetic induction and cardiac surgery. Significant reductions in the incidence of Q-wave myocardial infarction after emergent coronary artery surgery have been reported when intraaortic counterpulsation is used after failed PTCA with myocardial ischemia, compared with similar circumstances in which counterpulsation is not used (30). Still, when intraaortic balloon counterpulsation is used in patients with cardiogenic shock or cardiac arrest after PTCA, the mortality rate is high (31,32).

When patients experience coronary artery dissection or abrupt closure during PTCA, distal anterograde coronary perfusion and circulatory stability may be maintained before bypass surgery by coronary autoperfusion with a "bailout" catheter or by active transcatheter infusion of blood or oxygenated perfluorocarbon (26). Placement of an autoperfusion catheter provides distal coronary flow and allows for additional prolonged angioplasty that may reopen the vessel lumen. During balloon inflation, blood enters side holes in the catheter that are proximal to the balloon, and it exits side holes distal to the balloon, providing coronary flow. If repeated angioplasty or other cardiac catheterization procedures such as intracoronary stent placement are not effective in correcting the closure, cardiac surgery is required. In this case, distal anterograde coronary perfusion and circulatory stability may still be maintained by leaving the autoperfusion or bailout catheter in place until surgical intervention. Autoperfusion catheters provide passive flow across a stented coronary stenosis and can allow for more controlled anesthetic induction and surgical revascularization. They also have permitted greater utilization of the internal mammary artery as a bypass graft and are associated with a reduction in Q-wave infarction compared to intraaortic balloon counterpulsation or no mechanical intervention (33,34). The prophylactic use of perfusion balloon catheters is recommended in high-risk patients in danger of hemodynamic collapse during balloon inflation, including patients with poor myocardial function and those in whom angioplasty is to be performed on a vessel responsible for supplying blood to a large portion of myocardium. Both bailout and perfusion balloon catheters may be difficult to place in tortuous, small, or diffusely diseased vessels and may not be effective in preventing ischemia in the distribution of side branches crossed by the stenosis or angioplasty balloon. Furthermore, because the lumen of the autoperfusion catheter is smaller than that of the native stenotic coronary vessel, this device does not maintain pre-PTCA coronary blood flow, and myocardial ischemia may occur for this reason (35). With conventional passive autoperfusion catheters, transcatheter blood flow varies linearly with proximal arterial perfusion pressure (36). Thus, distal coronary perfusion decreases with hypotension. Active autoperfusion catheters actively pump blood through the catheter. Because the pump pressurizes blood above aortic pressures, greater transluminal flow is achieved (36,37). Alternatively, blood flow through reperfusion catheters may be augmented and intracatheter thrombosis reduced by using intraaortic counterpulsation (33). Patients who arrive in the operating room with autoperfusion devices in situ may require heparin or streptokinase flushes through the catheter lumen to reduce the formation of thrombus resulting from low-flow velocities. Reperfusion catheters are typically withdrawn (at the femoral artery puncture site) after the first dose of cardioplegic solution is administered via the aortic root. This allows cardioplegic solution to flow past the obstruction into the distal coronary circulation and initially to achieve greater myocardial protection. Removal of the aortic crossclamp is generally not required to allow the catheter to be withdrawn. Care must be exercised to avoid dislodging these catheters during transport of the patient to the operating room and transfer to the operating table.

Synchronized coronary sinus retroperfusion has been applied as an adjunct to reduce ischemia and circulatory instability in high-risk PTCA (38). Delivery of retroperfused blood in a pulsatile manner via a nonocclusive coronary sinus catheter during diastole allows for normal coronary venous drainage during systole. Retroperfusion appears to benefit coronary perfusion in some patients undergoing PTCA of the left anterior descending coronary artery, the distribution of which drains into the great cardiac vein. It is unclear how well retroperfusion protects against ischemia during PTCA involving the right or circumflex coronary arteries, which may not be perfused by a coronary sinus catheter advanced into the great cardiac vein. The complexity of the apparatus and incompleteness of protection from ischemia currently limit the use of synchronized coronary sinus retroperfusion for support of the failed or failing angioplasty.

Another mechanical option for management of failed PTCA is placement of an intracoronary stent. The Food and Drug Administration approved the first coronary stent in 1993 for acute or threatened vessel closure during coronary interventions. Since their introduction into clinical medicine, the indications for stent placement have broadened and stent use has increased dramatically, although their ultimate role has yet to be defined. The rational for using intracoronary stents as a bailout technique in acute or threatened occlusion is based on their capacity to stent open the vessel, thereby reapproximating the dissection flap to the native vessel. The stent resists vascular recoil and constriction. The success rate in reestablishing coronary blood flow after failed angioplasty is more than 90%, which compares favorably to the 40% to 70% success rate using autoperfusion catheters (39,40). Consequently, intracoronary stents have decreased the need for emergent cardiac surgery after failed PTCA. Although 30% to 40% of patients who sustain abrupt vessel closure after PTCA required emergent surgery when autoperfusion balloon angioplasty was used, less than 10% of those managed with stents needed urgent surgical revascularization (40,41). Intracoronary stenting has thus emerged as the preferred approach for the treatment of acute and threatened closure after PTCA. Despite a high procedural success rate, the early experience with stenting was associated with an unacceptably high rate of stent thrombosis. Changes in stent placement technique, including the use of enhanced antiplatelet agents and balloon expansion of stents, have significantly decreased the thrombosis rate. Although now an uncommon occurrence, acute stent thrombosis contributes to the need for emergent cardiac surgery. Another complication that may require urgent surgical revascularization is myocardial ischemia from obstruction by an intracoronary stent placed across a branch point in the coronary circulation. Finally, stent placement followed by high-pressure balloon deployment to expand the stent can rupture the coronary artery and may cause both myocardial ischemia and pericardial tamponade. Coronary artery perforation complicates up to 2.5% of stent procedures. In this instance, emergent surgical intervention is often required and is associated with a 30% mortality rate (42).

None of the previously mentioned methods of supporting coronary and systemic circulation provides total circulatory support during the period between failure of PTCA and catastrophic perturbations of rhythm or cardiac output and the institution of standard cardiopulmonary bypass in the cardiac surgical operating room. Until recently, total circulatory support was possible only with traditional cardiopulmonary bypass requiring direct right atrial and central aortic cannulation or surgical cutdown of the femoral vessels. With the development of thin-walled large-bore catheters, percutaneous initiation of cardiopulmonary bypass has become possible and has been applied as a salvage technique to support circulation in patients who have developed cardiogenic shock, refractory ventricular dysrhythmias, and cardiac arrest during PTCA (43).

To date, no study has had sufficient numbers of patients to define precisely the utility of emergency percutaneous cardiopulmonary bypass in this setting. Its limitations include difficulty in placing arterial cannulas into atherosclerotic or tortuous vessels, time delay before instituting support (vessels cannulated and pump set up), bleeding because of high-dose heparinization, and creation of a bypass-dependent state in patients who may not be surgical candidates. The latter limitation is associated with not only ethical but also logistic problems. In one series, in-hospital mortality was high when emergent percutaneous cardiopulmonary bypass was instituted in previously hemodynamically stable patients undergoing various procedures in the cardiac catheterization laboratory. None of the patients with cardiac arrest refractory to resuscitation survived to hospital discharge. Cardiopulmonary bypass stabilized those patients who developed cardiogenic shock by increasing blood flow and blood pressure and allowed further surgical or cardiac catheterization interventions. These interventions, however, were life saving in only 26% of patients (43).

Prophylactic cardiopulmonary bypass support may be of value for certain PTCA patients, such as those with a target vessel supplying a large mass of residual viable myocardium in whom balloon inflation may result in hemodynamic deterioration or rapid demise in the event of abrupt coronary closure. Percutaneous bypass may also benefit patients with diminished left ventricular function. When instituted prophylactically in high-risk PTCA patients, use of percutaneous cardiopulmonary bypass increased the success rate of angioplasty when compared to intraaortic balloon counterpulsation (44). However, the incidence of myocardial infarction, emergent surgery, and death did not differ between the two groups. Further investigations are needed to define the use of prophylactic percutaneous cardiopulmonary bypass for supported angioplasty.

With abrupt vessel closure during PTCA, initial therapy is aimed at restoring coronary perfusion and hemodynamic stability. Cardiologists may employ intravenous nitroglycerin, prolonged angioplasty balloon inflations, endoluminal coronary stents, laser angioplasty, coronary perfusion catheters, and an intraaortic balloon counterpulsation device to relieve myocardial ischemia before alerting the anesthesia and surgery staff of the need for urgent or emergent surgery. If myocardial ischemia is relieved by these methods before the patient arrives in the operating room, a more favorable outcome may be expected (45). When ischemia persists and is associated with severe left ventricular dysfunction and hemodynamic collapse, time is a crucial variable in determining myocardial and patient salvage. Percutaneous support devices may have their greatest impact on survival if they are in situ in such high-risk patients and can be instituted immediately at the onset of a catastrophe to serve as a bridge from the angioplasty suite to the operating room.

Anticoagulation and Thrombolysis in Acute Ischemic Syndromes

The application of PTCA in acute ischemic syndromes involves many of the same issues that can complicate angioplasty in the setting of chronic, stable coronary artery disease. Pathologic studies, angiography, and angioscopy have documented the central role of atherosclerotic plaque rupture with superimposed coronary artery thrombus in the genesis of acute myocardial ischemic syndromes (46). Ample evidence suggests that thrombus formation is the event immediately responsible for reduction of coronary blood flow during unstable ischemic events. Of the many factors implicated in the genesis of unstable angina, in situ hypercoagulability is recognized as a leading etiologic mechanism (47). These factors have major implications for the management of PTCA in acute ischemic syndromes, primarily because of the increased risks of thrombotic occlusion during vessel dilation. Increased use of antiplatelet agents and heparin before, during, and after PTCA is now common. Thrombolytic therapy is occasionally used for PTCA if a large coronary artery thrombus is present. This approach may decrease the incidence of acute vessel closure during PTCA in patients who have acute ischemic syndromes, but additional studies are needed to define the precise role of these strategies.

In the 1980s, a number of randomized trials provided fundamental information on the role of intravenous thrombolytic therapy in acute myocardial infarction (48). These trials demonstrated that thrombolysis can be achieved with streptokinase, urokinase, recombinant tissue plasminogen activator, and other fibrinolytic agents. Streptokinase and urokinase are indirect activators of the conversion of plasminogen to plasmin, the primary human fibrinolytic enzyme. The latter two agents are nonspecific and activate both circulating and fibrin-bound plasminogen to produce a generalized fibrinolytic state. Tissue plasminogen activator is a serine protease, which requires adsorption to the surface of the fibrin clot to achieve activation of plasminogen and theoretically results in "localized" thrombolysis with less systemic fibrinolysis. Pharmacologic plasminogen conversion can also be achieved with anistreplase, which is an *in vitro*–manufactured plasminogen activator complex of human lysoplasminogen and streptokinase, modified chemically to preserve the fibrin-binding sites of the plasminogen moiety and inactivated by an anisoyl group placed at the catalytic site of plasminogen activation. Theoretically, therefore, this agent should also be associated with increased fibrin specificity, decreased plasminogen consumption, and decreased systemic fibrinogenolysis, although this advantage has not been realized in clinical practice.

Despite the impressive reductions in immediate mortality rates with the major thrombolytic agents after acute myocardial infarction, this therapy has significant limitations. Reperfusion does not occur in 15% to 40% of patients, and there is a reocclusion rate of 5% to 10% (49, 50). There has been considerable controversy regarding the efficacy of various thrombolytic agents. Accelerated administration of tissue plasminogen activator, a relatively fibrin-specific agent, achieves a higher patency rate 90 minutes after administration compared with the nonspecific agent streptokinase, but these differences in patency rates diminish or disappear within 180 minutes. This eventual equivalence in patency rates reflects late opening of arteries with nonspecific agents, and both agents are associated with similar reocclusion rates when heparin is administered after thrombolysis. Achieving coronary patency more quickly may be important in salvaging ischemic myocardium because a trend toward an improved survival rate was observed in patients administered tissue plasminogen activator (49, 50). Regardless of which thrombolytic regimen is employed, the resistance to reperfusion remains a limitation, even with combination thrombolytic therapy. The etiology of this resistance to early patency is not yet clear, but it may be explained by complex plaque architecture with intraplaque hemorrhage, the presence of platelet-rich thrombi, inadequate thrombolytic drug delivery because of limited flow to the affected vessel(s), and the presence of plasminogen activator inhibitors. Two patient groups in whom thrombolysis is particularly ineffective are those with prior bypass surgery or cardiogenic shock. It is speculated that failure of thrombolysis in saphenous vein grafts is due to their extensive clot burden and slow runoff, and poor perfusion limits the effectiveness of thrombolytics in cardiogenic shock (51). More potent thrombolytic therapy might theoretically improve the chance of reperfusion under such circumstances.

Most studies demonstrate the lack of major differences in global left ventricular function after early reperfusion in acute myocardial infarction. This finding is predictable because the zones of myocardium remote from the infarction typically become hypercontractile during the acute phase. Despite major salvage of jeopardized myocardium, overall ventricular function may show minimal or no change, because regional improvement in the function of the jeopardized region will allow the hyperdynamic compensation to return to normal while maintaining an adequate cardiac output. Regional myocardial function, however, is improved by thrombolysis, and earlier vessel patency established with tissue plasminogen activator demonstrated significantly less depression of regional wall motion of myocardium in the distribution of the culprit artery than when streptokinase was administered (48). More rapid reestablishment of coronary blood flow may salvage more at-risk myocardium and limit infarction size.

Tissue plasminogen activator was originally touted as having major advantages over streptokinase and urokinase because of relative fibrin clot selectivity, fibrinogen-sparing properties, and a shorter half-life, which would reduce the risk of clinical hemorrhagic events. However, the rate of bleeding complications with the "fibrin-specific" tissue plasminogen activator is higher than anticipated. In fact, the use of tissue plasminogen activator rather than streptokinase has been associated with a greater incidence of postinfusion intracranial hemorrhage (52,53). Furthermore, the production of fibrin(ogen)-degradation products is associated with a reduction in reocclusion rates in patients treated with tissue plasminogen activator, perhaps because fibrin (ogen)-degradation products serve as receptor blockers, occupying the platelet glycoprotein IIb/IIIa receptors and inhibiting platelet aggregation (54). Streptokinase, with greater fibrinogenolytic action, intrinsically elevates the activated partial thromboplastin time to a greater extent than does tissue plasminogen activator. Perhaps because of this, the use of intravenous heparin is essential in preventing reocclusion when tissue plasminogen activator is administered but less important after streptokinase. Because of the above shortcomings of current thrombolytic agents (bleeding, incomplete or failed reperfusion), new thrombolytic agents and strategies for adjunctive anticoagulant therapy as well as altered methods of delivery of current agents are under investigation.

Patients who have cardiovascular conditions mimicking acute myocardial infarction are at risk of unnecessary bleeding complications or catastrophic exacerbation of the underlying condition if they are treated inappropriately with thrombolytic agents (55). Symptoms and ECG abnormalities mimicking acute myocardial infarction may be caused by noncoronary syndromes such as aortic dissection or acute pericarditis. In patients in whom the diagnosis is not entirely clear after the initial ECG is obtained, emergent angiography or echocardiography may demonstrate evidence of ischemic disease or lead to diagnosis of other syndromes responsible for chest pain. Thrombolytic therapy carries the risk of producing rapid hemorrhagic cardiac tamponade with catastrophic consequences in patients with conditions such as aortic dissection or acute pericarditis, which can mimic acute myocardial infarction. The anesthesiologist should anticipate great blood loss and continued hemorrhage in patients who develop these complications and require operative intervention.

An alternative and perhaps superior treatment for acute myocardial infarction is emergent PTCA. The success rate in reestablishing coronary blood flow after acute coronary occlusion is approximately 90%, similar to the success rate of routine angioplasty and superior to the 60% to 85% success rate of thrombolytic therapy (56,57). Not only is early patency greater after PTCA, but complete reperfusion is greater and residual coronary stenosis is less (57). In-hospital and 6-month mortality rates are less in patients after PTCA than after thrombolysis (56,58). In addition, PTCA-treated patients had a lower incidence of positive stress test results and need for surgical revascularization 6 months after the intervention (58). PTCA may be particularly useful for patients with acute myocardial infarction in whom thrombolysis is contraindicated, such as those who have an active bleeding disorder, a history of recent cerebrovascular infarction, recent surgery, or sustained hypertension (diastolic blood pressure of more than 120 mm Hg). For most patients, however, PTCA will not replace thrombolytic therapy for acute myocardial infarction. Thrombolytics can be administered soon after presentation to medical personnel, often by paramedics while in route to the emergency room. PTCA, on the other hand, requires skilled personnel and equipment available in only a limited number of medical centers, and logistically, PTCA is delayed until both physician and patient arrive to the cardiac catheterization suite. Trials comparing the two modalities of acute infarct management performed outside of the tertiary care setting do not uniformly demonstrate an advantage with PTCA, and the delay intrinsic to PTCA compared to thrombolysis may be responsible for the reported equivocal outcomes.

After successful thrombolysis, the routine use of PTCA has not been shown to exert additional beneficial effects in terms of myocardial salvage (59,60). The combination therapy results in a greater rate of coronary artery reocclusion and subsequent reinfarction, an increased need for emergent coronary surgery, and an increased mortality rate (56). All of the following contribute to increased morbidity: intraplaque hemorrhage, platelet activation by thrombolytic therapy with enhanced platelet aggregation on the injured coronary endothelium after PTCA, and intramural hemorrhage and hematoma formation disrupting the vessel wall and resulting in plaque fissure or spontaneous dissection. As expected, the incidence of bleeding requiring blood transfusion is increased when PTCA accompanies thrombolytic therapy (56,60).

In contrast to a routine adjunctive strategy, rescue PTCA (PTCA after failed thrombolysis for acute infarction) may offer significant benefit in selected patients. Rescue PTCA is 85% successful in restoring coronary blood flow; it improves regional left ventricular function and may improve mortality rates compared to conservative management (56,61,62). Rescue angioplasty implemented after failure of thrombolytic therapy is associated with several risks, depending on the clinical setting. When PTCA is performed without thrombolysis after acute myocardial infarction, it is not associated with an excessive risk of bleeding and has complication rates similar to those reported for PTCA in patients undergoing elective procedures for stable ischemic syndromes (60). Intravenous thrombolysis alone is associated with less than a 10% risk of minor bleeding and less than a 0.5% risk of intracranial bleeding, but rescue PTCA after failed thrombolytic therapy may significantly increase the risk of major bleeding at the vascular entry site. This risk of hemorrhagic complications is compounded by clinical factors such as advanced age, female gender, and low fibrinogen levels (63). Rescue PTCA after failed thrombolysis is particularly hazardous in patients with right (compared with left) coronary artery occlusion. Significantly greater rates of periprocedural complications such as serious arrhythmias, cardiac arrest, and subsequent reocclusion have been noted in patients with right coronary artery occlusions requiring rescue PTCA. The exact etiology of these events is unclear but may involve reperfusion injury, an exaggerated Bezold-Jarisch reflex, or embolization of intraluminal fibrin. The patient population that has failed both thrombolysis and rescue PTCA is often in extremis with an 80% incidence of cardiogenic shock or recurrent acute myocardial infarction and a 30% mortality rate (62,64).

Patients who receive thrombolytic therapy just before emergent revascularization are likely to experience excessive mediastinal bleeding, particularly when undergoing reoperative coronary artery surgery (65). Although ϵ-aminocaproic acid and tranexamic acid—the lysine analog antifibrinolytic agents—have traditionally been used as an antidote for thrombolytic drugs, aprotinin has also successfully prevented postbypass bleeding after thrombolysis (66). *In vitro,* aprotinin and the lysine analogs are equally effective in countering the effects of thrombolytic agents (67). Aprotinin is a serine protease inhibitor, which significantly reduces perioperative bleeding via multiple mechanisms. In addition to antifibrinolytic activity, aprotinin preserves coagulation factors and platelet function (68). Ongoing fibrinolysis can deplete fibrinogen levels, and transfusion with cryoprecipitate or other blood products, such as fresh-frozen plasma, may be necessary to achieve effective hemostasis. Significant fibrinolytic activity requiring aggressive therapy after cardiopulmonary bypass has also been reported after intracoronary administration of thrombolytics (69).

Nonthrombolytic Anticoagulants Used During PTCA

Patients presenting for emergency cardiac surgery after failed PTCA have almost invariably received antiplatelet and anticoagulant agents. These agents may contribute to increased perioperative bleeding and may require blood component transfusion. Heparin, 5,000 to 20,000 U, is routinely administered during PTCA. In addition to unfractionated heparin, low-molecular-weight heparin agents are occasionally administered. Rather than inhibiting thrombin, these agents act primarily by inhibiting factor Xa. The activated clotting time does not accurately monitor anticoagulant activity in this setting. Additionally, protamine does not effectively reverse the effects of low-molecular-weight heparin agents. Their procoagulant effect is particularly notable in the postoperative period because their half-life is 3 to 4 hours, longer than that of conventional unfractionated heparin.

Angioplasty exposes the prothrombotic surface of arterial plaques to circulating platelets, and heparin alone has little effect on platelet activation. Antiplatelet therapy is, therefore, routine in PTCA patients. Aspirin (acetylsalicylic acid) is most commonly used and inhibits thromboxane A_2 by blocking cyclooxygenase. Other platelet inhibitors act to block the platelet glycoprotein IIb/IIIa receptor. This platelet receptor normally binds circulating fibrinogen and cross-links platelets as the final common pathway to platelet aggregation. Ticlopidine acts to selectively antagonize adenosine diphosphate (ADP)–induced platelet aggregation by blocking the platelet glycoprotein IIb/IIIa receptor specific for ADP. Used during coronary stenting procedures, ticlopidine decreases the thrombosis rate. Abciximab (ReoPro) is one of a new generation of antiplatelet agents whose activity results from binding of the platelet glycoprotein IIb/IIIa receptor. Abciximab consists of antigen-binding fragments of monoclonal immunoglobulin G derived from immunization of mice with human platelets. Clinical trials of abciximab in patients undergoing PTCA have demonstrated a reduction in thrombotic complications in both high- and low-risk patients, with the beneficial effects of abciximab still evident 6 months after the procedure (70–73). It is particularly beneficial in high-risk patients, and the benefits are additive to those achieved with coronary stenting. For these reasons, abciximab has become widely used during PTCA, particularly in high-risk patients. The serum half-life of abciximab is short, but the effect on platelet function is prolonged. After administration of abciximab, intense platelet inhibition occurs for 2 to 4 hours, partial inhibition is observed for 12 hours, and platelet function (measured by routine tests of platelet activity) is restored to within a normal range 24 to 36 hours after treatment (74). Still, low levels of glycoprotein IIb/IIIa receptor blockade occur up to 2 weeks after abciximab treatment, and this prolonged activity likely contributes to improved PTCA results. Major bleeding complications after PTCA are greater with abciximab use. Local vascular bleeding is responsible for most of these bleeding complications, although increased heparin doses, female gender, and the prolonged presence of vascular sheaths further contribute to bleeding complications (73).

Although clinical outcome after coronary artery bypass surgery is not adversely affected by abciximab treatment, bleeding diathesis and increased blood transfusion requirements are reported in emergent surgical patients receiving abciximab. Although there is no specific reversal agent for abciximab, platelet transfusion rapidly restores hemostatic function. This is probably a result of partial redistribution of abciximab from platelets with complete glycoprotein IIb/IIIa receptor blockade to newly transfused platelets, yielding a greater number of platelets with only partial glycoprotein IIb/IIIa receptor blockade (74). When surgery is delayed for 12 hours after abciximab administration, the risk of excessive bleeding is minimal and platelet transfusion is usually not required (75). Occasionally, profound thrombocytopenia can result from exposure to abciximab. This is fortunately a rare event occurring in less than 1% of patients. In contrast to patients with heparin-induced thrombocytopenia, abciximab-induced thrombocytopenia develops rapidly (within 24 hours) and is effectively treated with platelet transfusion. It is interesting that the extent of thrombocytopenia after cardiopulmonary bypass may be decreased with abciximab administration compared with untreated patients. Perhaps this is due to the prevention of platelet binding to components of the cardiopulmonary bypass circuit.

Percutaneous Balloon Valvuloplasty

Because of the success of percutaneous coronary (and peripheral) artery dilation and the advent of new balloon technology, interest in nonsurgical catheter balloon valvuloplasty has increased. Depending on the etiology of the stenotic lesion and the pathology of the specific valve, balloon valvuloplasty increases valve area by various means, including leaflet tearing, separation of commissural fusion, calcific nodular fracture, and annular and leaflet stretching (76). Catheter balloon valvuloplasty appears to be well established for conservative treatment of severe pulmonary valve stenosis in all patient age groups. Limited long-term follow-up data suggest that good intermediate results are obtainable with pulmonary valvuloplasty and that serious complications, including significant pulmonary insufficiency, are uncommon (77). Systemic hypotension and arrhythmias during balloon inflation are usually transient. Interest in percutaneous valvuloplasty for aortic valve stenosis in the elderly is declining because significant residual stenosis usually persists, even after optimum balloon inflation, and because aortic valvuloplasty is accompanied by a high incidence of major complications, including death, cardiac tamponade, acute increases in aortic regurgitation, aortic rupture, vascular damage, and systemic embolization. Furthermore, long-term survival for adults after balloon aortic valvuloplasty is similar to that of untreated severe aortic stenosis (78). Even with a good initial result, restenosis occurs in most patients within 6 months (78). This procedure may, however, have a role in selected patients with extremely severe disease, because it may allow them to subsequently undergo anesthesia and surgery at a lower risk than before development of this technique. Outcome data must be collected to determine whether these potential benefits can be realized.

Mitral stenosis may also be treated with percutaneous balloon valvuloplasty, most commonly performed using transseptal catheterization. The success of mitral valvuloplasty depends on the anatomy of the mitral valve, with calcification and thickening of the valve and subvalvular apparatus portending less favorable results. After successful mitral valvuloplasty, functional improvement is typical and the need for secondary surgery is infrequent. Mitral valvuloplasty is a particularly attractive treatment option in the pregnant patient, as the adverse effects of cardiopulmonary bypass on the fetus are avoided. It is also useful in patients with favorable mitral valvuloplasty characteristics but who are at high surgical risk. Although many patients are left with an atrial septal defect as a consequence of a transseptal approach to the mitral valve, the resultant shunt is usually small and does not require surgical correction. Severe mitral regurgitation after mitral valvuloplasty occurs in 5% of procedures and often requires acute surgical intervention (79). Hemopericardium resulting from wire puncture of the free wall of the myocardium is the other serious complication that presents for urgent surgical repair.

As catheter and balloon technology improve and further experience is gained, the results of percutaneous balloon valvuloplasty may improve and potential indications may expand. Anesthesiologists will likely encounter more patients undergoing these procedures who require resuscitation or airway management because of associated serious, acute complications. This is because these procedures will probably be limited to high-risk patients (those with poor ventricular function, severe coronary artery disease, or other medical illness), those of advanced age, or those who require temporary stabilization of an unstable state to improve their surgical risk.

Anesthetic Management of Operative Emergencies after Cardiac Catheterization or Coronary Angioplasty

Anesthetic management of complications related to cardiac catheterization and coronary angioplasty most commonly involves patients who have disruption of their basal coronary blood flow. Patients presenting for emergent coronary revascularization after failed PTCA with acute myocardial ischemia have a higher perioperative mortality rate than patients undergoing routine coronary artery bypass (45). When refractory ischemia is not present, however, surgical risk is similar in emergent and elective coronary bypass surgery patients. Left ventricular dysfunction, the need for inotropic support, and age are independent predictors of operative mortality in emergent surgical patients (80). Although the incidence of PTCA requiring emergent surgery has decreased in the past decade, an increased proportion of these patients present in a state of severe hemodynamic compromise and have a higher mortality (20).

Whether coronary arterial damage and impairment of myocardial blood flow are related to selective coronary angiography or are directly attributable to PTCA or other coronary instrumentation, initial management ideally begins in the catheterization laboratory. Rapid assessment of hemodynamic stability as well as degree of myocardial ischemia is necessary to plan anesthetic management (Fig. 28-1).

Hemodynamically Stable, Nonischemic Patient

In the stable nonischemic patient, a complete history, physical examination, and chart review in preparation for anesthesia and surgery are possible. Insertion of monitoring devices and anesthetic induction may proceed as in elective cases. When balloon dilation fails but no vascular damage results, a complete patient evaluation by the cardiac surgical and anesthesiology teams is appropriate and urgent revascularization is generally neither required nor indicated. Surgical revascularization can proceed electively under these circumstances without any unique anesthetic concerns. However, if PTCA fails and is associated with arterial damage but no evidence of ischemia, the risk of thrombus formation at the site of endothelial disruption often dictates urgent revascularization. In this instance, if the patient has recently ingested food or drink, sufficient time may be given for the stomach to empty before urgent surgical intervention proceeds.

Hemodynamically Stable, Ischemic Patient

The hemodynamically stable but ischemic patient requires more rapid assessment than the nonischemic patient. The ischemic, hypotensive patient is in imminent danger of cardiac arrest and must be stabilized and quickly moved to the operating room. Prompt restoration of myocardial blood flow during the early phases of myocardial infarction precipitated by diagnostic or therapeutic cardiac catheterization—when substantial amounts of nonfunctioning myocardium are still viable—remains the most rational and effective therapy for reducing morbidity and mortality rates. Patient evaluation is therefore limited to essential history, physical examination, and laboratory data, and it should be performed simultaneously with efforts to stabilize and transport the patient to the operating room for emergency revascularization. The amount of myocardium in jeopardy, the condition of collateral flow, and the nature and site of the vessel injured during PTCA all contribute to the likely clinical course. Large areas of ventricular muscle supplied by the injured vessel but a lack of significant amounts of distal collateral flow generally mean that the patient has little reserve and a high likelihood of cardiac arrest before

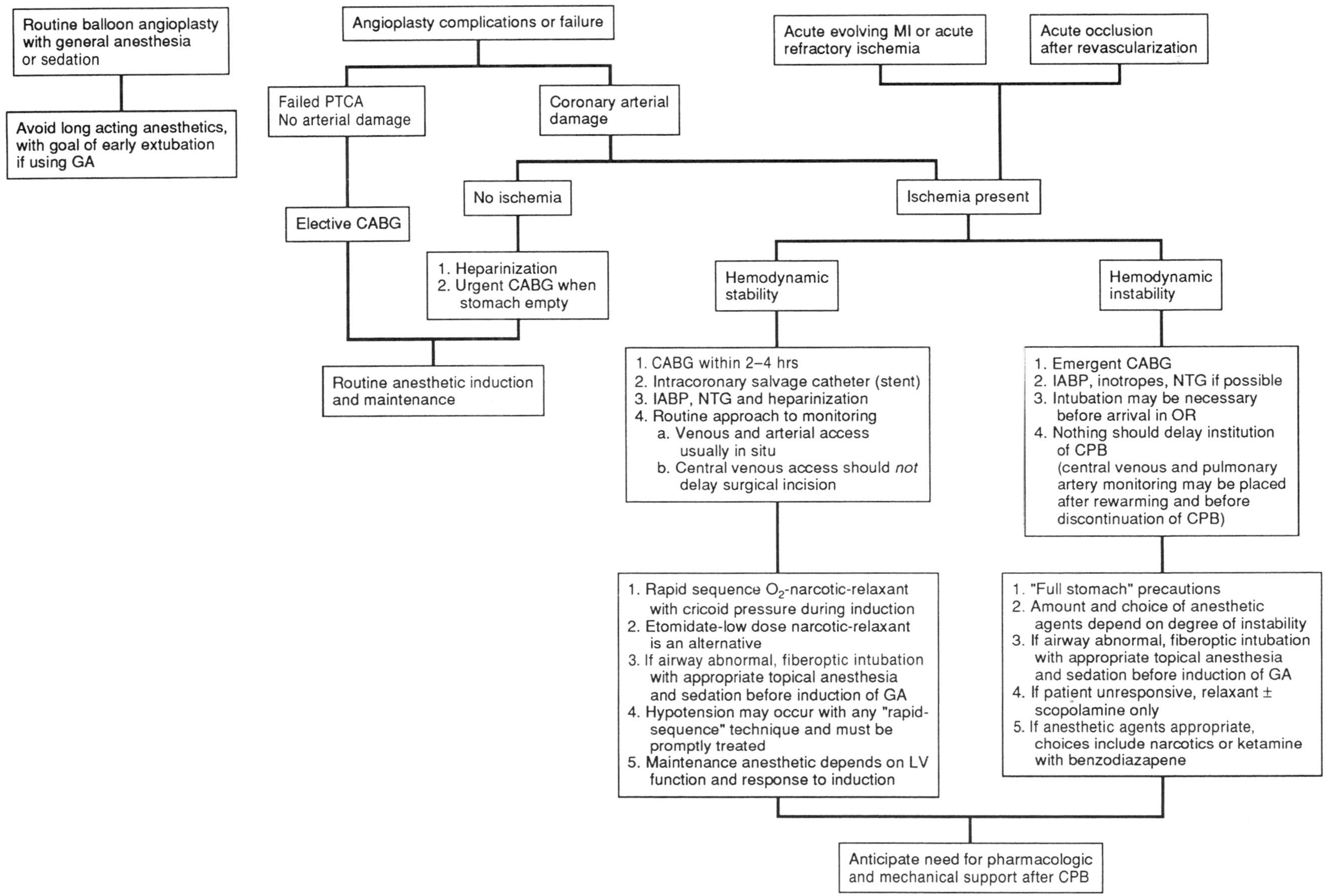

FIGURE 28-1. Anesthetic management for urgent or emergent coronary revascularization. (PTCA, percutaneous transluminal coronary angioplasty; CABG, coronary artery bypass grafting; IABP, intraaortic balloon pump; NTG, nitroglycerin; CPB, cardiopulmonary bypass; IV, intravenous.)

emergent revascularization. Intraluminal stents, perfusion catheters, and anticoagulation with heparin, antiplatelet drugs, or thrombolytic agents may be utilized in patients who are at increased risk of ischemic injury and infarction if vessel closure occurs. In some cases, these bailout methods allow use of internal mammary artery grafting, whereas a more urgent ischemic syndrome would necessitate the less time-consuming saphenous vein bypass procedure. Most of these patients have intraaortic counterpulsation devices in situ before they are transported to the operating room.

Extra care must be exercised in placing intravascular monitoring catheters when patients are anticoagulated. This is most important when nonspecific thrombolytic agents, such as streptokinase or urokinase, have been administered. Under these circumstances, catheters (particularly arterial) should be placed by experienced personnel, preferentially using vessels that are externally compressible. The external jugular vein may be safer than the internal jugular or subclavian vein for central cannulation in anticoagulated patients. Venous placement should be verified with a small-gauge catheter (18 gauge) and routine transduction of intravascular pressure (augmented by blood gas tension analysis if necessary) before any large-bore sheath device is placed. Additionally, in an effort to minimize inadvertent arterial puncture, safe cannulation of internal jugular or subclavian veins may be facilitated by ultrasound guidance, which allows for accurate visualization of veins and arteries before needle insertion.

Logistics of Surgical Revascularization after Failed Angioplasty

When myocardial ischemia accompanies vascular damage and failure of angioplasty, the objectives of emergency coronary revascularization are to support the acutely ischemic myocardium with the rapid institution of cardiopulmonary bypass and to alleviate the process that provoked the acute ischemia. These objectives apply not only to patients undergoing emergency surgical revascularization arising from complications of cardiac catheterization or PTCA, but also to patients with unstable angina or acute evolving myocardial infarction. During the 1980s, emergency surgical coronary revascularization was advocated for salvage of myocardial function when performed within 4 to 6 hours of symptoms of acute myocardial infarction (81). However, most centers currently reserve early operative intervention for patients with complicated myocardial infarction (i.e., threatened myocardial power failure or threatened extension of infarction indicated by persistent or recurrent pain or ECG changes). Patients with uncomplicated myocardial infarction commonly do not arrive at the hospital soon enough; delays often result in completion of diagnostic workup outside the 4- to 6-hour period during which surgical revascularization can potentially salvage myocardium. Prospective randomized trials with large numbers of patients have not yet defined the optimal application of medical therapy with thrombolysis or PTCA versus emergent surgical revascularization to patients with acute myocardial infarction. Because this is a heterogeneous disease, comparisons of alternative therapies must be made with caution. Metaanalysis of randomized clinical trials comparing thrombolytic therapy with primary PTCA suggests that PTCA decreases short-term mortality and the incidence of reinfarction (82). Anesthesiologists will likely continue to be involved in the care of patients with acute myocardial infarction undergoing emergency coronary artery revascularization either as primary therapy or after failed PTCA or thrombolysis. The same principles of anesthetic management apply to all of these situations.

Ischemia before, during, and after PTCA implies threatened or evolving myocardial infarction with all the problems inherent in acute coronary insufficiency. In this situation, intraaortic counterpulsation is often employed in combination with pharmacologic antianginal therapy, and revascularization should be achieved in a rapid but organized fashion (Fig. 28-1). With ongoing ischemia, the time before progression to infarction varies. Therefore, additional time should not be spent establishing vascular access before anesthetic induction if intravenous and arterial cannulas remain in place from cardiac catheterization. Appropriate additional invasive hemodynamic monitoring devices may be inserted simultaneously with surgical preparation and draping, but it should not delay induction of anesthesia or commencement of operation. If the patient's condition does not allow for preoperative pulmonary artery catheter placement, cardiac function and cardiac loading conditions can alternatively be assessed intraoperatively by transesophageal echocardiography. If hemodynamic instability exists when the patient arrives in the operating room, nothing should interfere with achieving cardiopulmonary bypass as rapidly as possible. The most crucial factors in successful emergency coronary revascularization after catheterization laboratory disasters are prompt restoration of myocardial perfusion and a coordinated effort among skilled cardiologists, anesthesiologists, and surgical teams.

Emergency surgical revascularization after acute failure of PTCA occurs sporadically and often unpredictably. These characteristics mandate that PTCA should be performed in facilities with the personnel and equipment required for rapid surgical support. An American College of Cardiology/American Heart Association Task Force report stated that an experienced cardiovascular surgical team should be available within the institution for emergency surgery for all angioplasty procedures (13). This standard has recently been challenged, and angioplasty is being performed outside of the United States without nearby surgical revascularization capabilities. With the advent of coronary stenting, advances in antiplatelet therapy, and improved technical competence, cardiologists can salvage many of the failed angioplasties that previously required surgery. This, in combination with selection of patients at low risk for surgical intervention (those with a coronary lesion that appears technically easy to angioplasty and involving a vessel not supplying blood to a large portion of myocardium and patients with normal or near normal cardiac function), provides the rational for performing low-risk PTCA without surgical standby. Within the United States, a major issue is the level of standby required for routine PTCA procedures. For patients who have preexisting conditions (e.g., poor left ventricular function, planned complex dilation) that place them at high risk of complications during PTCA, it may be appropriate to have a complete cardiac surgical, anesthesia, and perfusion team prepared for surgical intervention and an operating room in full readiness. For lower risk PTCA, however, less readiness seems appropriate.

Regardless of the exact system employed, several logistic details must be addressed for efficient triage of the patient during a PTCA-related emergency. An organized resuscitation cart and emergency equipment must be readily available in the cardiac catheterization and angioplasty suite. In addition, standard compatible monitoring lines and transducers should be used in the catheterization laboratory to facilitate expeditious transfer of patients without interruption of continuous monitoring. Availability of extracorporeal perfusion devices and personnel should be planned, because these elements are often the primary limitation to providing standby coverage for failed PTCA, rather than the lack of anesthesia, surgical personnel, or empty operating room.

Evaluation of Cardiopulmonary Function Before Surgical Revascularization

Evaluation of cardiopulmonary function is a major task for the anesthesiologist called upon to assist with preparation for emergency coronary revascularization. Myocardial ischemia in these patients is often associated with significant pain, anxiety, increased catecholamine levels, or reduced arterial oxygenation, which may adversely effect the balance of myocardial oxygen supply and demand. These events can often increase the difficulty and risk of performing cardiac catheterization and coronary angioplasty in the critically ill patient immediately after an acute myocardial infarction. General anesthesia has been shown to be feasible in patients undergoing interventional cardiac catheterization during acute myocardial infarction when pain, anxiety, or agitation does not respond to conventional measures (83). The adequacy of arterial oxygenation should be assessed immediately upon encountering the patient because sedation, hypoventilation, and underlying respiratory impairment are common under these circumstances. At the minimum, supplemental oxygen must be administered, and some patients require assisted or controlled ventilation, even before transport to the operating room. Confusion and combativeness in this situation are often signs of cerebral hypoperfusion and/or hypoxemia. In addition to observation of hemodynamic data (blood pressure, heart rate, and sometimes pulmonary artery pressures), the state of sympathetic tone, vasoconstriction, and adequacy of peripheral perfusion can usually be rapidly assessed by physical examination.

Cardiopulmonary Support Before Surgical Revascularization

If the anesthesiologist provides cardiopulmonary support with management of hemodynamics, arrhythmias, sedation, analgesia, oxygenation, and ventilation, the cardiologist is free to concentrate on the technically demanding aspects of maintaining coronary perfusion after vessel injury during PTCA. Coronary perfusion pressure must be maintained when additional mechanical obstruction of coronary blood flow occurs because of angioplasty devices, bailout catheters, or elevated intimal flaps after coronary artery dissection. Hypotension can result when myocardial ischemia or infarction involves enough myocardium to cause decreased stroke volume. Hypotension causes a further decrease in coronary blood flow and further myocardial dysfunction. As the left ventricle fails, increased left ventricular diastolic pressure and left ventricular dilation occur, further contributing to myocardial ischemia. A vicious cycle is established, which can rapidly progress to cardiogenic shock. Maintenance of systemic blood pressure is therefore critical and is particularly important in patients with right coronary artery lesions and right ventricular dysfunction, because a significant proportion of right coronary artery perfusion occurs during ventricular systole. If hypotension occurs but intraaortic counterpulsation has not yet been initiated, pharmacologic support of systemic pressure and flow must be employed. When cardiac output is low and hypotension is present, therapy with a combined β-adrenergic and α-adrenergic agonist drug may be necessary.

When ischemia is precipitated during diagnostic or therapeutic cardiac catheterization, nitroglycerin is often initiated early in an effort to dilate coronary vessels and limit or treat left ventricular distension. If cardiac output is adequate but vasodilation results in insufficient coronary driving pressure, an α-adrenergic agonist may be used. If coronary vasospasm has occurred during the catheterization or angioplasty procedure, α-adrenergic agonists must be used with caution or not at all. If large amounts of coronary vasodilators such as nifedipine or nicardipine have been administered during the course of PTCA, patients are often quite vasodilated systemically and may require significant pharmacologic support to maintain coronary perfusion pressure, particularly during anesthetic induction.

During transfer of the patient to the operating room, extreme care must be taken to prevent dislodgment or malpositioning of any coronary perfusion catheter and to avoid iatrogenic creation of a total coronary occlusion by the bailout catheter itself. One person must therefore be designated to hold the bailout catheter in position during transport and until cardiopulmonary bypass is instituted. If cardiac rhythm has become pacer dependent during the course of PTCA, care must also be exercised with transvenous or transcutaneous pacing devices during patient transport to avoid the adverse hemodynamic consequences associated with abrupt loss of cardiac rhythm.

Cardiopulmonary Arrest During Cardiac Catheterization or PTCA

The patient who develops cardiopulmonary arrest during the course of PTCA or diagnostic cardiac catheterization requires resuscitation with conventional basic and advanced cardiopulmonary support techniques followed by immediate institution of hypothermic cardiopulmonary bypass. Chest compressions should not be interrupted for more than 15 to 20 seconds and should be continued during skin preparation and draping (until the time of skin incision) by using sterile gloves. Central nervous system complications are very common in those who survive immediate operation after cardiac arrest during PTCA. Although etiologies of postoperative stroke are multifactorial, cardiopulmonary resuscitation must be aggressively maintained, because inadequate global cerebral perfusion probably contributes to this complication in many cases. Intraaortic counterpulsation and/or rapid institution of percutaneous cardiopulmonary bypass in the catheterization laboratory may improve neurologic outcome in patients with circulatory arrest, but outcome data that adequately address this issue are not yet available. After sternotomy, internal cardiac compressions should be continued while efforts are made to institute hypothermic cardiopulmonary bypass rapidly. Emergency coronary bypass in patients with previous cardiac surgery requires cannulation of the femoral vessels to facilitate rapid institution of cardiopulmonary bypass. Mediastinal dissection can safely commence once cardiopulmonary bypass is successfully achieved (84).

Despite prompt emergency surgical revascularization after complications of diagnostic or therapeutic cardiac catheterization, there is a high incidence of perioperative myocardial infarction and hospital mortality, particularly in high-risk patients undergoing aggressive, multivessel angioplasty (23,45,80,85,86). Not surprisingly, the need for cardiac massage before emergent cardiac revascularization after failed PTCA is the most significant risk factor for perioperative mortality; mortality rates approach 50% for such patients (86,87). Other risk factors for operative death after emergency coronary revascularization for failed angioplasty include previous myocardial infarction, cardiogenic shock, compromised ventricular function, multivessel coronary artery disease, advanced age, and previous coronary artery surgery. Recent data indicate that approximately 25% of patients with PTCA-related vessel injury experience acute left ventricular dysfunction (pulmonary edema) or cardiogenic shock (20,87). Despite aggressive use of mechanical circulatory assist devices and coronary reperfusion devices, cardiogenic shock increases the operative mortality rate of emergency surgical coronary revascularization five-fold (from 3% to 15%) after failed PTCA. Patients with previous coronary artery surgery who develop cardiogenic shock after failed PTCA have even greater operative risks.

Perioperative myocardial infarction is more likely to occur in patients who have failed PTCA and require emergency coronary artery surgery for ongoing ischemia, compared with those who have surgery without ischemia (21,45, 85). Not surprisingly, the overall incidence of perioperative myocardial infarction after surgical revascularization for failed PTCA is 10% to 40% and as high as 50% to 70% if failed PTCA is accompanied by preoperative cardiogenic shock (88). Because there appears to be a scientific foundation for the belief that the effectiveness of coronary reperfusion partially depends on the interval from the onset of occlusion to treatment (89), prompt surgical reperfusion is necessary. This is particularly true for patients with compromised myocardial perfusion who have spent long periods in the catheterization laboratory and for whom the "grace period" has been partially exhausted. Nonetheless, some investigators have found no correlation between the injury-to-reperfusion interval and perioperative myocardial infarction after emergency surgical revascularization for failed angioplasty (90). These findings may be explained by confounding factors, such as the amount of collateral coronary blood flow and the numerous and subtle pharmacologic and mechanical interventions used in these patients. Variability of these factors can significantly effect the length of the grace period during which reperfusion can restore function and viability of myocardium.

Anesthetic Management of the Patient with PTCA-Related Ischemia

When patients arrive in the operating room with PTCA-related ischemia, clinical experience suggests that there are relatively few options for choice of anesthesia, particularly when hemodynamic instability is present (Fig. 28-1). The goals of anesthetic induction and maintenance for these patients are to prevent hyperdynamic responses to intubation and surgical stimulation and to avoid excessive myocardial depression or peripheral vasodilation that could reduce coronary perfusion pressure and cause or aggravate myocardial ischemia. When the patient is hemodynamically stable, standard cardiac induction techniques are employed. Moderate doses of an opioid, such as fentanyl or sufentanil, in combination with benzodiazepines and volatile anesthetic agents, are often used for the induction and maintenance of anesthesia. Etomidate is also commonly used in this setting. Small doses of a nondepolarizing neuromuscular blocking drug should be administered before opioids are given to prevent chest wall rigidity and to optimize ventilation. Careful titration with reduced doses of sedative-hypnotic agents and opioids, along with the avoidance of potent volatile anesthetics, are indicated for hemodynamically unstable patients.

Patients who arrive in the operating room unresponsive from cerebral hypoperfusion and who are receiving cardiopulmonary resuscitation will require only oxygen, relaxant, and an amnestic such as scopolamine until systemic perfusion is improved or cardiopulmonary bypass is instituted. Anesthetic agents may then be cautiously added if appropriate; small doses of opioids, or ketamine with a benzodiazepine, may be used. Addition of benzodiazepines to opioids may produce additional hypotension resulting from vasodilation (91). This may be particularly likely in patients receiving large doses of nitroglycerin, in those who may be hypovolemic because of bleeding from arterial puncture sites, and in those whose perfusion pressure is maintained primarily with sympathetically mediated vasoconstriction. In these types of patients, administering the smallest amount of any anesthetic agent may decrease sympathetic tone and reduce coronary perfusion pressure. Addition of exogenous catecholamines or other sympathomimetic agents to maintain coronary perfusion pressure should be anticipated under these circumstances.

In the presence of a normal airway, a rapid-sequence induction of anesthesia using the agents just mentioned and cricoid pressure constitute the preferred technique if "full-stomach" precautions are indicated. Hypotension may occur with any rapid-sequence technique, and prompt treatment is required to maintain adequate coronary perfusion pressure. Rapid-sequence induction may also cause a hyperdynamic cardiac response manifest by hypertension and tachycardia. Like hypotension, hypertension and tachycardia may also aggravate myocardial ischemia. Rapidly acting agents to lower the blood pressure and heart rate, such as nitroglycerin and esmolol, should therefore be available during rapid-sequence inductions. While the patient is still in the catheterization suite or intensive care unit, the administration of 30 mL of 0.3 M sodium citrate to increase gastric pH in the patient with a full stomach who has undergone failed thrombolysis or angioplasty and now requires emergent surgical revascularization may reduce the risk of pulmonary injury if aspiration should occur. Metoclopramide (10 to 20 mg intravenously) may also help reduce gastric volume by improving gastric motility and emptying. Under postprandial conditions, the slow onset of action of H_2-blockers such as famotidine may limit effectiveness in reducing gastric volume and acidity. In addition, ranitidine can produce significant bradyarrhythmias after intravenous or oral administration (92).

When abnormal airway anatomy is present, fiberoptic intubation with appropriate topical anesthesia and carefully titrated intravenous sedation may be required before induction of general anesthesia. When this is deemed necessary, judicious pharmacologic manipulation of systemic hemodynamics using rapid-acting agents that are easily titrated, such as intravenous nitroglycerin and/or esmolol, may be necessary—particularly when there is significant cardiovascular reserve—to avoid excessive hemodynamic stress when intubation precedes the induction of general anesthesia. Optimally, sufficient personnel are available to allow one member of the anesthesia team to focus on airway management while others strive for hemodynamic stability and minimize sympathetic responses to airway manipulation, which could exacerbate underlying ischemia. There are no outcome data to support the selection (or avoidance) of any particular agents for maintenance of anesthesia in this setting, although clinical experience indicates that ventricular function and the response to induction of anesthesia will be the primary determinants in choosing anesthetic agents.

Emergence from Cardiopulmonary Bypass

Patients undergoing emergency coronary artery surgery for acute ischemia related to PTCA are likely to experience reperfusion injury during emergence from cardiopulmonary bypass. The need for pharmacologic or mechanical circulatory support as well as for antiarrhythmic therapy should be anticipated whenever incomplete revascularization, persistent ischemia after revascularization, poor preoperative ventricular function, definite myocardial infarction within 12 hours of induction of anesthesia, preoperative hemodynamic instability, or prolonged duration of aortic cross-clamping are present. Tolerance of cardioplegic arrest is markedly impaired in patients with acute myocardial infarction who require emergency myocardial revascularization as evidenced by the markedly greater frequency of inotropic support required to separate from bypass, compared with elective patients (65). The routine administration of cardioplegia via the aortic root does not protect the myocardium supplied by the acutely occluded coronary artery. Retrograde cardioplegia (i.e., cardioplegia administered into the coronary sinus) and combined antegrade/retrograde cardioplegia have been demonstrated to increase cardioplegia delivery and improve myocardial protection in areas of myocardium previously perfused by the acutely occluded vessel (93,94). Because much of the right coronary blood flow does not drain into the coronary sinus, cardioplegia is delivered less well to the right ventricle when administered in retrograde rather than antegrade fashion. Thus, retrograde cardioplegia may be inadequate in the territory of ischemic myocardium when the right coronary artery is occluded. The effect of retrograde cardioplegia on the incidence of myocardial infarction, the extent of infarcted tissue, and the mortality rate are unknown. Although retrograde cardioplegia is intuitively attractive, outcome data are needed before this technique can be definitively recommended for emergent coronary artery bypass surgery after failed PTCA. After aortic declamping in the warmed patient, adequate blood pressure must be maintained to provide perfusion of the coronary arteries. Coronary microvascular resistance steadily rises for some time after release of the aortic cross-clamp, so reperfusion of the myocardium—particularly the subendocardium—may be inhomogenous if coronary driving pressure is inadequate (95). This effect may delay functional recovery, produce scattered areas of cell death, and result in prolonged ventricular electrical instability. After cardiopulmonary bypass is discontinued, pharmacologic manipulation should be optimized to increase coronary perfusion and minimize myocardial metabolic demands without excessive myocardial depression.

Hypomagnesemia is common in patients after acute myocardial infarction and also after cardiopulmonary bypass (96). In acute infarction patients, early magnesium administration reduces infarct size and the mortality rate (97). In cardiac surgical patients, magnesium decreases postoperative dysrhythmias and improves immediate postoperative cardiac function (98). Patients with failed PTCA may suffer an acute infarction and may also require emergent surgery. Although serum magnesium concentrations can be monitored to guide magnesium administration, serum magnesium concentration does not accurately reflect intracellular magnesium stores (96). Additionally, laboratory determination of serum magnesium levels delays timely drug administration. Thus, empiric dosing of magnesium (e.g., 2 g magnesium sulfate intravenously) has been suggested in emergent cardiac surgical patients without renal dysfunction. If reperfusion injury is suspected after revascularization of the acutely ischemic heart, excessive calcium administration should be avoided after emergence from cardiopulmonary bypass, and calcium administration should probably be guided by measuring serum ionized calcium concentration. Recent studies on animals (99) and humans (100,101) strongly suggest that calcium administration inhibits the cardiotonic actions of β-adrenergic agonists such as epinephrine, probably by suppressing the intracellular production of cyclic adenosine monophosphate via interference with signal transduction through the β-adrenergic receptor complex. This is consistent with the finding that in patients recovering from aortocoronary bypass surgery, concomitant calcium administration impaired cardiac output increases that were due to dobutamine, but not those due to amrinone, a phosphodiesterase inhibitor (102).

Adherence to the principles of anesthetic management as outlined should maximize the probability of salvaging myocardium before the occurrence of irreversible injury, if emergency revascularization can be accomplished early enough. Future advances in techniques to maintain coronary and systemic perfusion in the interventional cardiology laboratory as well as improved methods of anticoagulation and thrombolysis should further improve patient outcome and reduce myocardial injury in this setting.

COMPLICATIONS OF ACUTE MYOCARDIAL INFARCTION

Postinfarction Ventricular Dysfunction

The most frequent complications of acute myocardial infarction that require surgical treatment are persistent ischemia and severe left ventricular dysfunction or cardiogenic shock with or without an acute mechanical defect. The pathophysiology and management of persistent or recurrent ischemia have been described. The magnitude of ventricular dysfunction after acute myocardial infarction may range from total circulatory collapse and cardiogenic shock to mild dysfunction requiring pharmacologic maintenance of tissue perfusion. The degree of cardiac dysfunction may be categorized into four hemodynamic classes by a hemodynamic model using the relation between preload (pulmonary wedge pressure) and left ventricular stroke work index ([mean blood pressure minus pulmonary wedge pressure] times stroke index) (Fig. 28-2). A patient in hemodynamic class I has clinically satisfactory tissue perfusion (Killip class I) (103), whereas a patient in hemodynamic class IV has hypotension, extremities that are cool to the touch, oliguria, and pulmonary congestion. The pathophysiologic basis of severe postinfarction left ventricular dysfunction and cardiogenic shock is generally involvement of more than 40% of ventricular mass in the process of ischemia, infarction, or necrosis (104). Patients with this degree of ventricular dysfunction are generally in hemodynamic class III or IV and typically exhibit sustained or intermittent pulmonary edema and inadequate tissue perfusion. Although ventricular dysfunction is the most common cause of pump failure after acute myocardial infarction, accounting for 80% of such occurrences, other mechanical causes may also contribute to this hemodynamic state and share many common pathophysiologic features (Fig. 28-3).

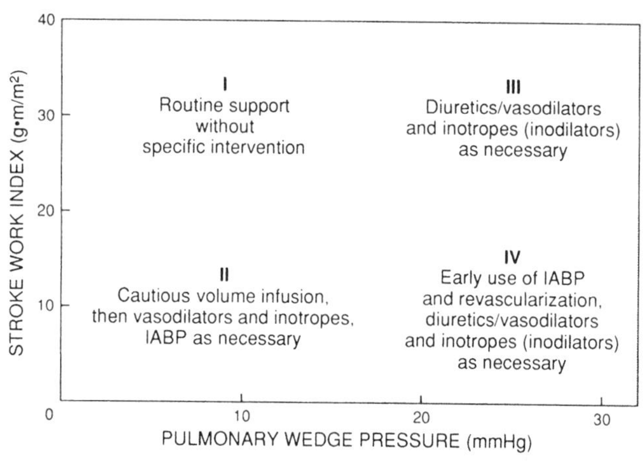

FIGURE 28-2. Stratification of therapy by hemodynamic subsets after acute myocardial infarction.

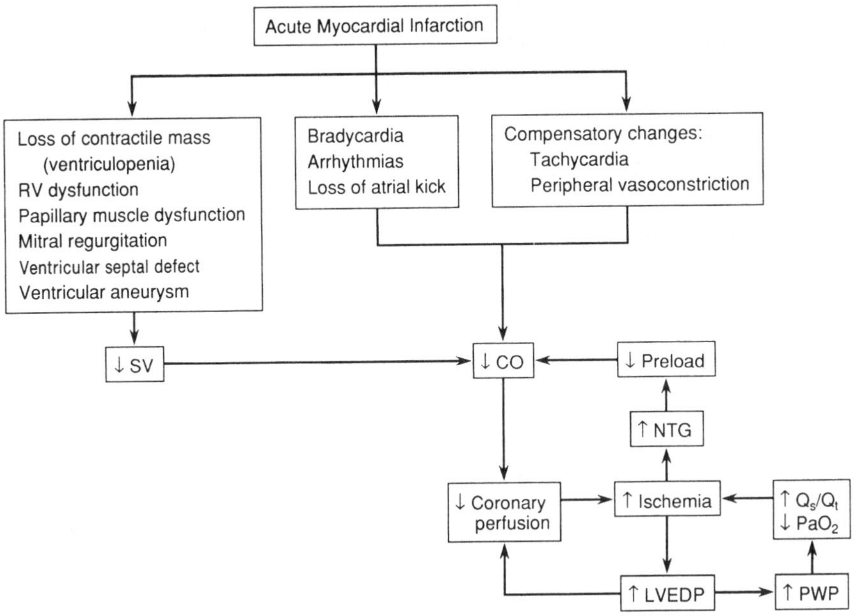

FIGURE 28-3. Pathogenesis of pump failure after acute myocardial infarction. (Q_s/Q_t, right-to-left shunt ratio; Pa_{O_2}, partial pressure of arterial oxygen.)

The importance of ventricular dysfunction as the chief determinant of short-term and long-term outcome after acute myocardial infarction is well established and depends primarily on infarct size and less so on abnormalities of compliance, residual contractile function, or mechanical disruption of infarcted structures (105). Several compensatory mechanisms are activated to attenuate the hemodynamic consequences of diminished contractile function after acute myocardial infarction. These include increased sympathoadrenal activity, left ventricular dilation with utilization of the Frank-Starling mechanism to generate preload recruitable stroke work, and hyperfunction of normally perfused myocardial segments that are remote from the site of infarction. The characterization of ventricular function into subsets on the basis of clinical and hemodynamic data not only helps prognostically but also facilitates rational therapeutic interventions.

After acute myocardial infarction, approximately 8% of patients exhibit tissue hypoperfusion with pulmonary congestion (class IV) and have an associated hospital mortality rate of 75% (106). Old age, anterior infarction, prior myocardial infarction, and perhaps diabetes mellitus are risk factors for the development of postinfarction cardiogenic shock (104). Therapy for patients in this hemodynamic subset must be aggressive with early use of aortic counterpulsation and revascularization. Combinations of vasodilators and inotropes to optimize forward flow and decrease pulmonary congestion are usually required. Applied in this setting, vasodilators produce their beneficial effects by reducing left ventricular filling pressure, which not only diminishes pulmonary congestion but also may reduce left ventricular volume, wall tension, and myocardial oxygen demand while facilitating subendocardial perfusion. Intravenous furosemide may have a venodilator action that precedes the diuretic effect. Phosphodiesterase inhibitors, including amrinone, milrinone, and enoximone, are inodilator agents. These may be particularly valuable in this subset of patients to increase myocardial contractility and reduce ventricular afterload. Potential advantages of phosphodiesterase inhibitors over conventional sympathomimetic agents include the absence of tachycardia, which may promote further myocardial ischemia, and a mechanism of action that is independent of β-receptors, which may be down-regulated during congestive heart failure.

When pulmonary congestion exists without a low-output state (class III), judicious administration of small doses of diuretics or vasodilators such as nitrates and sodium nitroprusside, or angiotensin-converting enzyme inhibitors such as enalaprilat may be used, particularly when pulmonary congestion is accompanied by evidence of mitral regurgitation or systemic hypertension. Vasodilation decreases left ventricular afterload, reducing mitral regurgitation and the degree of left-to-right shunting across a ventricular septal defect. Furthermore, it unloads the right ventricle, and because of interventricular dependence, it directly improves left ventricular compliance. All these mechanisms may contribute to control of pulmonary congestion. Small doses of intravenous morphine not only help calm the agitated patient but also contribute to venodilation.

A major principle of therapy for patients with pulmonary congestion after acute myocardial infarction involves maintenance of adequate respiratory gas exchange. In addition to reduction of pulmonary venous pressures, high concentrations of supplemental oxygen are generally required with analysis of arterial blood gas tensions to define adequacy of oxygenation and ventilation. Endotracheal intubation and controlled ventilation (with or without positive end-expiratory pressure [PEEP]) may be required in moribund patients. This is particularly true for those in cardiogenic shock who require paralysis and ventilation to reduce the excessive work of breathing, which may be experienced by patients who have impending respiratory failure. Patients who have only mild perfusion defects may be managed with continuous positive airway pressure (CPAP) delivered via a tight-fitting mask (as long as rising CO_2, falling pH, and poor mental status are absent). Hemodynamic monitoring coupled with arterial blood gas tension analysis is valuable for determining the effects of PEEP/CPAP on tissue oxygen delivery and for selecting appropriate levels of PEEP and CPAP.

After experiencing acute myocardial infarction, less than one quarter of patients present with low cardiac index and hypotension but no evidence of pulmonary congestion (class II). This clinical syndrome may result from hypovolemia, right ventricular myocardial infarction, bradyarrhythmias, and associated complications such as pulmonary embolism or systemic sepsis. Invasive hemodynamic monitoring or echocardiography may demonstrate evidence of hypovolemia, which may be compounded by diuretic or vasodilator administration, exacerbated by excessive vomiting or diaphoresis during evolution of acute myocardial infarction, or aggravated by high concentrations of α-adrenergic catecholamines, which increase capillary hydrostatic pressure and cause fluid extravasation.

Patients in hemodynamic subset II may be treated with cautious intravascular volume infusion under close clinical and hemodynamic observation. Intravenous fluid administration provides an increase in preload (end-diastolic fiber length) to improve stroke volume and is less costly in terms of myocardial oxygen extraction than pharmacologic options. It has been reported that the optimal range for left ventricular filling pressure after an acute myocardial infarction is between 15 and 25 mm Hg (107,108). These recommended filling pressures are greater than normal pulmonary wedge pressure of 6 to 12 mm Hg. A reduction in left ventricular compliance occurs with acute ischemia and infarction. Thus, higher filling pressures are required to achieve normal left ventricular end-diastolic volumes, a more physiologic measurement of left ventricular preload. Most clinicians prefer to administer fluid until the pulmonary wedge pressure is acutely elevated to a maximum of 20 mm Hg. Further acute volume infusion may precipitate pulmonary congestion or edema and should probably be avoided, particularly if crystalloid infusions are used and result in a significant reduction of intracapillary oncotic pressure from dilutional hypoalbuminemia. Absolute levels of filling pressure may not be optimal in any given patient,

TABLE 28-1. METHOD OF ADMINISTERING A FLUID CHALLENGE IN PATIENTS WITH ACUTE MYOCARDIAL ISCHEMIA OR INFARCTION

	PWP (mm Hg)	Fluid Administration Rate
Observe PWP for 5 min	<12	200 mL over 10 min
	<16	100 mL over 10 min
	≥ 16	50 mL over 10 min
Change in PWP during infusion	>7	Stop
Change in PWP immediately after 10-min infusion	≤ 3	Continue infusion
	>3, <7	Wait 5 min
Change in PWP after 5-min observation	≥ 3	Measure cardiac output, blood pressure, heart rate, venous oxygen saturation
	<3	Repeat fluid challenge

Note: PWP, pulmonary wedge pressure.
Source: From Weil MH, Henning RJ. New concepts in diagnosis and fluid treatment in circulatory shock. *Anesth Analg* 1979;58:124, with permission.

and the pulmonary wedge pressure and cardiac output should be carefully monitored during fluid administration. Fluid challenges in this setting may be guided by the response of the pulmonary wedge pressure (Table 28-1). Within this framework, the fluid challenge is continued as long as the cardiac output increases. Alternatively, fluid infusion can be guided by echocardiography. Echocardiography has the advantage of measuring intracardiac volumes rather than pressures, providing for more direct assessment of preload. Echocardiographic image acquisition and interpretation requires the involvement of skilled personnel, such as cardiologists or anesthesiologists and echocardiography technicians while pulmonary wedge pressure is usually easily obtained by intensive care nursing staff. Continuous or prolonged monitoring by echocardiography is therefore impractical, but this modality may be helpful in determining optimal ventricular loading conditions in the hypotensive patient after myocardial infarction. Patients whose pump function fails to improve despite treatment of bradyarrhythmias and hypovolemia generally have severely impaired ventricular diastolic and systolic function, and augmentation of contractility and perfusion pressure with sympathomimetic agents is generally required under these conditions.

Although isolated infarction of the right ventricle is rare, approximately one quarter of patients with acute inferior or posterior left ventricular myocardial infarctions have concomitant ischemia and infarction of the right ventricle because these areas share a common blood supply (109). Infarction of the posterior portion of the interventricular septum is commonly coexistent for similar reasons. One third of these patients exhibit a hypotensive, low cardiac output syndrome similar to that of classic cardiogenic shock, which is seen with a primary left ventriculopenic state. Elevation of right atrial and right ventricular end-diastolic pressures, the presence of a Kussmaul sign, and tricuspid regurgitation are suggestive of the diagnosis of right ventricular infarction. However, a wide spectrum of hemodynamic abnormalities may be observed, and right ventricular infarction may be clinically silent in 30% to 40% of cases. The ECG often shows evidence of acute inferoposterior injury as well as ST-segment elevation in right-sided precordial leads (V_3R to V_4R). Nonetheless, the clinical diagnosis of right ventricular infarction can be elusive and is often first suggested when a low-output hypotensive syndrome is produced without evidence of significant left ventricular dysfunction. In the absence of bradyarrhythmias (including atrioventricular dissociation), which are commonly observed with inferior ischemia and infarction, low cardiac output in the setting of right ventricular infarction and ischemia is predominantly due to impairment of left ventricular filling and low left ventricular end-diastolic volume. This reduction of left ventricular volume has multiple etiologies, which include right ventricular systolic dysfunction with a subsequent decrease in pulmonary blood flow and left ventricular inflow, as well as right ventricular dilation with increased intrapericardial pressure and leftward diastolic bulging of the ventricular septum (reverse Bernheim effect). As with other causes of low cardiac output syndrome not associated with pulmonary congestion, volume loading alone is rarely successful in improving the hemodynamic or clinical state in patients with right ventricular infarction (110). When left ventricular compliance is decreased, volume loading may elevate pulmonary wedge pressure but not provide any significant increase in left ventricular preload. Inotropic or other vasoactive drug therapy is generally necessary in these patients. Prognosis is extremely poor if severe left ventricular dysfunction or either papillary muscle or ventricular septal rupture coexists with right ventricular infarction (110). Rarely, emergency surgical intervention is attempted in patients with right ventricular infarction to treat shock if severe tricuspid regurgitation or if papillary muscle, free-wall, or ventricular septal rupture occurs.

Acute Ventricular Septal Defect

Acute ventricular septal rupture occurs in 0.5% to 2% of patients within an average of 2 to 6 days after onset of acute myocardial infarction, although it may occur any time within about the first 2 weeks after an acute infarction (111). Ventricular septal rupture is responsible for 1% to 5% of all infarction-related deaths. This complication is usually associated with total occlusion of a single coronary artery, occurs with both anterior and inferior or posterior infarction, and is secondary to infarction of the interventricular septum as well as a variable extent of the contiguous left or right ventricular myocardium. Septal rupture is most common in patients experiencing their first transmural myocardial infarction in whom collateral flow to the septum is limited or absent.

Clinical Features

Clinically, acute septal rupture is associated with sudden hemodynamic deterioration that frequently progresses to cardiogenic shock (112,113). Rupture of the ventricular septum results in a left-to-right interventricular shunt producing right ventricular volume overload, increased pulmonary blood flow, biventricular failure, and reduced systemic blood flow (Fig. 28-4). Systemic hypotension exacerbates myocardial hypoperfusion in the presence of associated coronary artery disease and may contribute to additional myocardial dysfunction and damage. The ratio of pulmonary-to-systemic vascular resistance and the degree of flow restriction conferred by the defect itself largely determine the severity of the shunt. Reduction in systemic blood flow results in a low-output hypotensive syndrome that often rapidly progresses to cardiogenic shock. Patients with intact mental status commonly complain of worsened chest pain and dyspnea, and physical examination reveals a new, harsh holosystolic precordial murmur, which is heard loudest along the lower left sternal border, and which may be accompanied by a precordial thrill in about one half of the cases. Right ventricular volume overload secondary to the intracardiac shunt in association with right ventricular ischemic dysfunction, and occasionally compounded by tricuspid regurgitation, sometimes results in signs of systemic venous congestion disproportional to the degree of pulmonary venous congestion that is present.

The sudden onset of pulmonary edema may herald the diagnosis, which can often be established by bedside catheterization of the right side of the heart; this is done by using a fiberoptic pulmonary artery catheter for venous oxygen saturation or by using cooximetered blood samples, which should show a step-up of blood oxygen saturation (more than 10%) from the right atrium to the right ventricle or proximal pulmonary artery. Alternatively, echocardiography can rapidly demonstrate the presence of a septal rupture and is both highly sensitive and specific for differentiating between septal rupture and acute mitral regurgitation (114). Color flow Doppler and two-dimensional (2D) imaging are complementary means of assessing for a ventricular septal defect. Color flow Doppler imaging can detect small lesions that may be missed with 2D assessment. Large defects are easily visible with conventional imaging while equalization of left and right ventricular pressures may limit interventricular flow and hence make detection by color flow Doppler imaging less apparent. Echocardiography not only accurately demonstrates the presence of a ventricular septal defect, but it also allows for the quantitative assessment of the defect. The absolute size of the ventricular septal defect, the

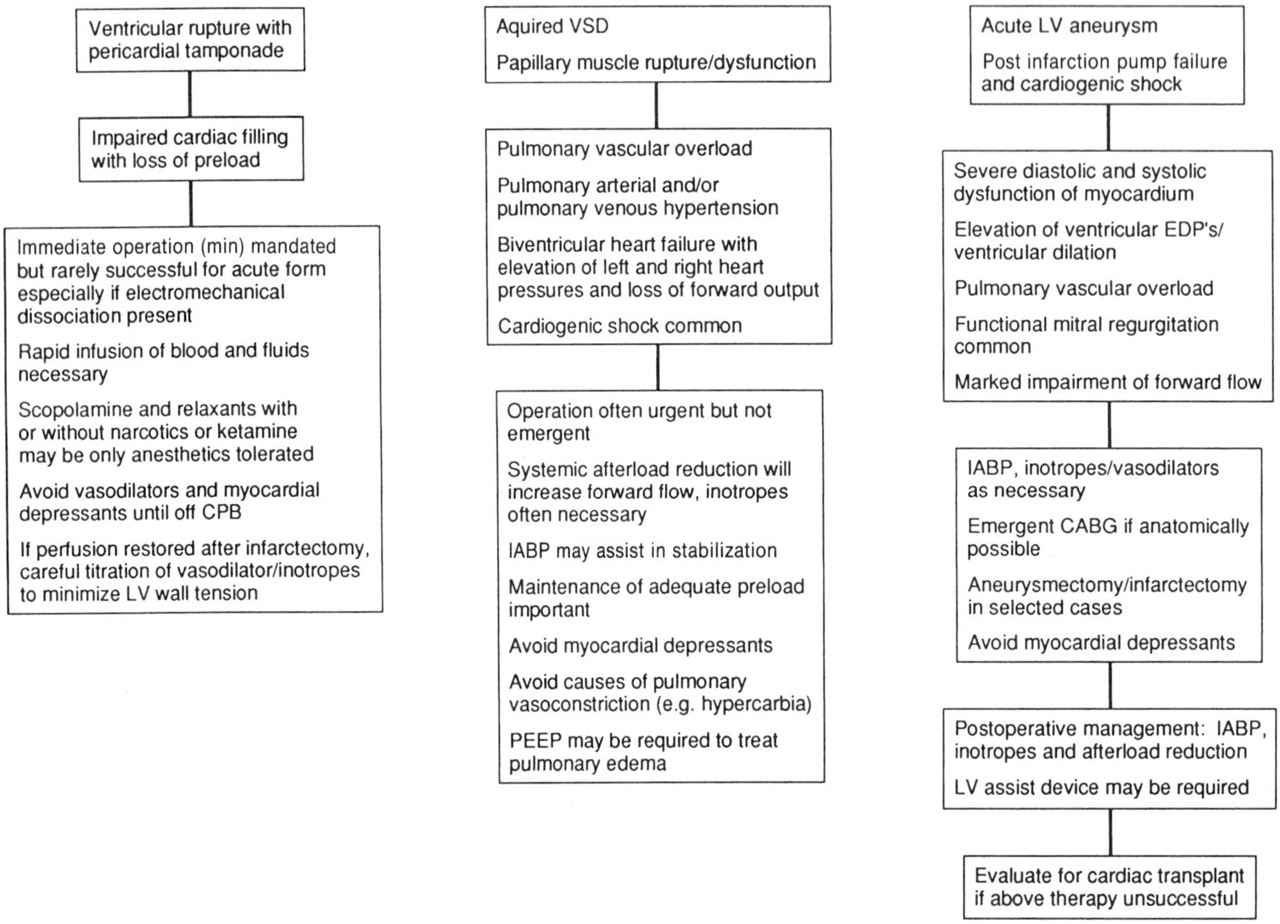

FIGURE 28-4. Mechanical complications of acute myocardial infarction. (CPB, cardiopulmonary bypass; IABP, intraaortic balloon pump; PEEP, positive end-expiratory pressure; CABG, coronary artery bypass grafting; LV, left ventricular; EDPs, end-diastolic pressures.)

pressure gradient between the two ventricles, and an estimate of the ratio of pulmonic to systemic blood flow can all be determined by echocardiography. Ventriculography is the definitive diagnostic test required if echocardiographic findings are equivocal and a strong clinical suspicion of the diagnosis remains. This study is not always necessary if definitive echocardiographic assessment is obtained or if the patient is moribund, and death is imminent without prompt surgical intervention.

In patients who can be stabilized with the support of systemic perfusion by intraaortic counterpulsation and pharmacologic intervention, coronary angiography is often performed before surgical closure of the defect because myocardial revascularization is needed in more than one third of these patients and incomplete coronary revascularization at time of septal rupture surgery is associated with an increased mortality rate (115). Assessment of left ventricular function by ejection fraction measurements must be done with caution in these patients, because the unloading effect of the left-to-right shunt may result in a left ventricular ejection fraction that does not reflect the extent of myocardial necrosis. Patients with concomitant right ventricular ischemia or infarction may have a depressed right ventricular ejection fraction because of right ventricular afterload mismatch resulting from increased pulmonary arterial pressures, as well as a right ventricular volume overload.

Management

Without operation, the clinical course of septal rupture is ominous: About one quarter of the patients die within 24 hours, one half die within 1 week, and three quarters of all patients die within 2 months (116). Conservative medical therapy of septal rupture is generally ineffective, but its principles of management are important for the preoperative stabilization of patients who develop acute myocardial infarction. A small fraction of patients who are stable (have no multisystem organ dysfunction and no evidence of worsening acidosis, hypoxemia, or renal failure) generally have a small septal defect and may be managed medically to allow

TABLE 28-2. CONSIDERATIONS IN ANESTHESIA FOR ACQUIRED CARDIAC DISEASE REQUIRING EMERGENCY SURGERY

	Heart rate	Preload	Afterload	Contractility	Anesthetic Choice
Acute cardiac tamponade[a]	Increase (80–110 beats/min)	Increase	Maintain	Increase	Local anesthetic, ketamine, narcotics, etomidate; avoid vasodilators and depressants
Acute mitral insufficiency[b]	Normal to slight increase	Maintain	Reduce	Maintain or increase	Any anesthetic that avoids increases in afterload and profound myocardial depression; often requires intra-aortic balloon pump
Acute aortic insufficiency[c]	Normal to slight increase	Maintain or slight increase	Reduce	Maintain or increase	Balanced with inhaled agent or opioid with pancuronium; avoid increases in afterload
Critical aortic stenosis[d]	Normal (70–80 beats/min) (avoid tachycardia and bradycardia) Sinus rhythm essential	Increase or maintain	Maintain (do not increase or decrease)	Maintain	Any anesthetic that will not markedly alter heart rate, preload or afterload, or perfusion pressure (e.g., narcotic-relaxant)
Acute tricuspid insufficiency[e]	Depends on associated valve lesions; if none, slight increase	Maintain	Reduce (unless associated aortic stenosis)	Maintain	Usually dictated by associated mitral or aortic valve disease
Acute ventricular septal rupture[f]	Maintain	Maintain	Reduce, but maintain perfusion	Maintain or increase	Avoid myocardial depression; avoid ↓ Pa_{CO_2} or ↑↑Pa_{O_2} (may produce right-to-left shunt); avoid increases in afterload (↑left-to-right shunt)

Notes: Pa_{CO_2}, partial pressure of arterial carbon dioxide; Pa_{O_2}, partial pressure of arterial oxygen.
[a] Secondary to cardiac trauma, perforation during catheterization, free wall rupture in acute myocardial infarction, post–cardiac surgery bleeding.
[b] Secondary to endocarditis, papillary muscle rupture, or dysfunction.
[c] Secondary to aortic dissection, infective endocarditis.
[d] Usually with concomitant coronary artery disease, crescendo angina, or discovered at catheterization.
[e] Usually secondary to endocarditis, rarely right ventricular infarction.
[f] Secondary to acute myocardial infarction.

recovery from acute myocardial infarction. Vasodilators are often used for reduction of systemic pressure and afterload to decrease the magnitude of left-to-right shunt and increase the forward stroke volume (Table 28-2). Simultaneous reduction in pulmonary vascular resistance often occurs and may negate some of the beneficial effects of systemic afterload reduction on intracardiac shunting. In addition, preexisting hypotension often precludes the aggressive use and benefits of vasodilator therapy. Inotropic and vasopressor therapies are often necessary to sustain adequate systemic and coronary collateral perfusion pressure and flow but potentially may increase left-to-right shunting if vasoconstriction becomes excessive. Intraaortic counterpulsation, in combination with vasodilator and inotropic therapy, is often a stabilizing intervention. However, it is generally considered to be a temporary measure that may allow performance of some diagnostic studies to define coronary anatomy and determine valvular competence before emergent operative intervention. In most patients, the severity of the left-to-right shunting determines how rapidly operative intervention should be carried out. Prompt surgical repair of the septal defect is necessary if any signs of regional or global hypoperfusion are present.

Current evidence suggests a 25% perioperative mortality rate for surgical repair of postinfarction ventricular septal defects (117). Preoperative hemodynamic status, location of the myocardial infarction, and the interval between infarction and surgery are factors influencing early perioperative mortality. The presence of cardiogenic shock increases the mortality rate to 33% to 50% (113,117) while persistence of class IV cardiogenic shock beyond the operation is associated with 100% mortality rate (118–120). Posterior location of the defect also increases the mortality rate, probably because it is often associated with right ventricular infarction and mitral regurgitation (113). Anterior septal defects are the most common and are associated with a better outcome than posterior lesions while the less common apical septal ruptures are associated with the highest survival rate because they are more often associated with a small-size acute myocardial infarction (112). When surgical repair is performed early, less than 1 week after an acute myocardial infarction, operative mortality rate also increases (113,121). Compared to that with medical management, however, the survival rate may increase with early surgery, particularly in patients with cardiogenic shock.

In addition to preoperative afterload reduction and maintenance of coronary and systemic flow, anesthetic management of patients with septal rupture involves several other principles. Factors that can decrease pulmonary vascular resistance (such as hypocarbia, alkalosis, and marked hyperoxia) should be avoided because reductions in pulmonary vascular resistance could increase shunting and impair systemic cardiopulmonary function. Maintenance of adequate preload, avoidance of myocardial depressants, and preservation of normocarbia are necessary to optimize systemic perfusion before surgical repair. Thermodilution cardiac output measurements do not accurately reflect systemic perfusion in the presence of intracardiac shunting, and the presence of a ventricular septal defect itself is a relative contraindication to placement of a pulmonary artery catheter because of the risk of paradoxical air or thrombotic embolism. If a flow-directed pulmonary artery catheter is used in the presence of a ventricular septal defect, consideration should be given to inflating the balloon with carbon dioxide or saline, rather than air. Intraoperative transesophageal echocardiography is useful not only in determining the location and severity of the septal rupture, but also in assessing adequacy of the surgical repair. Additionally, measurement of the aortic cross-sectional area, as well as the velocity-time integral of blood flow through the aorta, allows for calculation of left ventricular forward stroke volume and cardiac output. After the patient is separated from cardiopulmonary bypass, afterload reduction should be maintained to limit intraventricular pressures.

Mitral Regurgitation Due to Papillary Muscle Rupture or Dysfunction

Because of the delicate balance of geometry and function that is necessary for normal competent function of the mitral valve apparatus, minor disturbances of this equilibrium can result in variable degrees of valvular malfunction and regurgitation. Acute mitral regurgitation may result from ischemia or necrosis of the left ventricular papillary muscles and the portion of the left ventricular myocardium contiguous with the papillary muscles (papillary muscle dysfunction), from rupture of the tip or trunk of the papillary muscle itself, or least commonly from rupture of the chordae tendineae. The high tendency of papillary muscles to develop ischemia or infarction is partly related to a relatively high degree of tension developing during systole with an attendant high metabolic oxygen cost, coupled with a disadvantaged blood supply because of their innermost location at the end of the coronary arterial circulation. The anterolateral and posteromedial papillary muscles receive their blood supplies from different branches of the coronary arterial tree. The anterolateral papillary muscle receives its blood supply from the left anterior descending coronary artery or its diagonal branches as well as from the marginal branch of the left circumflex coronary artery. The posteromedial papillary muscle is supplied predominantly from the posterior descending branch of the angiographically dominant coronary artery (most commonly the right coronary artery) with a minor contribution from the nondominant artery. Posteromedial papillary muscle ischemia, infarction, or rupture is 5 to 10 times more common than that of the anterolateral papillary muscle, presumably because the blood supply of the former muscle arises predominantly from a single artery without the benefit of significant collateral flow.

Compromise of coronary blood flow with ischemia or infarction of a single papillary muscle alone is usually not sufficient to cause severe mitral regurgitation, unless it is associated with abnormal contractile function of the ventricular myocardium adjacent to the base of the affected papillary muscle. Most cases of mitral regurgitation that results from papillary muscle dysfunction are secondary to a lack of contraction or contraction of the papillary muscle occurring along a distorted axis (shifted by concomitant ventricular dilation and/or dyskinesia), which causes an inability of the mitral leaflets to coapt appropriately during systole. Dysfunction of the adjacent left ventricular wall may be due to recurrent or progressive myocardial ischemia after acute myocardial infarction has occurred. Ischemia or infarct-related papillary muscle dysfunction usually involves restricted leaflet motion, resulting in inability of the mitral valve leaflets to reach the level of the mitral annulus and coapt during systole (122). Because of the papillary muscle anatomy, the anterior leaflet almost always demonstrates restricted motion during ischemia-related mitral regurgitation, but this is rarely seen with the posterior leaflet (122). Actual rupture of the left ventricular papillary muscle (most commonly the posteromedial muscle, as already described) can occur, and about 50% of ruptures are associated with relatively small or subendocardial myocardial infarction, a similar proportion having single-vessel coronary artery disease (123,124). Acute mitral regurgitation secondary to papillary muscle rupture tends to occur in the first week after acute myocardial infarction and accounts for about 5% of infarctions resulting in death (123,124). The most common form of papillary muscle rupture involves one of the smaller heads of the muscle, whereas rupture of the main trunk of the papillary muscle occurs less frequently but is a more serious complication and when medically treated is associated with only brief survival.

Clinical Features

Recognition of mitral regurgitation secondary to papillary muscle dysfunction that complicates acute myocardial infarction requires a high degree of clinical suspicion. Mitral regurgitation can be either intermittent or persistent, and it is typically associated with a new systolic apical murmur of variable intensity, duration, and radiation. The murmur can be holosystolic or mid-systolic because of rapid equilibration of left ventricular and left atrial pressures during late systole. It may even be absent despite severe mitral regurgitation (125). In contrast to acute ventricular septal rupture, a palpable thrill is rare with papillary muscle rupture.

The clinical presentation depends on the severity of left ventricular dysfunction and the degree of acute valvular incompetence. In contrast to chronic mitral insufficiency (in which there is typically a large, compliant left atrium), when acute mitral regurgitation develops, there is usually a small, noncompliant left atrium, which results in significantly higher atrial and pulmonary artery pressures than in the chronic situation. Severe pulmonary hypertension is often associated with right ventricular failure. Patients with papillary muscle dysfunction and particularly those with papillary muscle rupture typically develop clinical manifestations of persistent or intermittent pulmonary congestion, pulmonary edema, hypotension, or occasionally cardiogenic shock related to diversion of significant portions of left ventricular forward flow to the left atrium (Fig. 28-4).

Unlike with acute ventricular septal rupture, the chest radiograph may demonstrate pulmonary congestion or edema that is preferentially distributed to the upper lobes, particularly the right upper lobe, occasionally mimicking parenchymal infiltrates. Isolated right upper-lobe edema is found radiographically in approximately 10% of patients with pulmonary edema associated with mitral regurgitation (126). These radiographic findings may be related to the mitral regurgitant jet being directed toward the orifice of the right upper-lobe pulmonary veins. Patients may demonstrate disproportionately large V waves on pulmonary wedge pressure tracings, although the size of the V wave does not correlate well with the degree of regurgitation and is more dependent on left atrial compliance (127). Precordial or transesophageal echocardiography and Doppler flow technology make it relatively easy to diagnose and assess the severity of mitral regurgitation at the patient's bedside. 2D imaging reveals the mitral valve anatomy and can distinguish between regurgitation caused by restricted valve leaflet motion, a prolapsing valve leaflet, and a flail leaflet secondary to papillary muscle rupture. Color flow Doppler imaging shows the regurgitant jet in the left atrium and provides an easily recognizable echocardiographic finding in mitral regurgitation. Mitral regurgitation severity is graded most commonly by color flow Doppler regurgitant jet length and area, but the pulmonary venous inflow pattern, the volume of regurgitant blood, and the regurgitant orifice area are also helpful in this determination. The size of the color flow Doppler jet in the left atrium as well as the pulmonary venous flow pattern are highly dependent upon afterload. A decreased blood pressure significantly decreases regurgitant jet area, increases systolic pulmonary flow velocity, and frequently results in an underestimation of mitral regurgitation severity (128). Regurgitant jets that are eccentric and travel along the side of the left atrial wall display smaller color flow Doppler images. Thus, using area of the jet to determine the severity of mitral regurgitation in this setting may also underestimate the true extent of regurgitation. Ejection fraction measured by echocardiography or ventriculography may be normal or supranormal, because almost 50% of patients with papillary muscle rupture demonstrate only a relatively small or subendocardial infarction (123) and because acute mitral regurgitation is associated with an effective ventricular afterload reduction. When echocardiography demonstrates hyperdynamic left ventricular wall motion in a postinfarction patient with pulmonary edema and shock, the diagnosis of papillary muscle rupture or dysfunction should be considered even if the characteristic echocardiographic findings of a flail, prolapsing, or restricted valve leaflet motion are not observed.

Management

Patients with severe mitral regurgitation and clinical deterioration should undergo prompt cardiac catheterization followed by surgical repair or replacement of the mitral valve, as well as coronary revascularization when indicated. Papillary muscle rupture is one of the few causes of pulmonary edema or cardiogenic shock complicating acute myocardial infarction in which aggressive and prompt surgical intervention can improve short-term and long-term survival, compared with the natural history of this condition with medical treatment. These improvements can be achieved only if the patients receive intensive stabilization before catheterization and surgery, with the aggressive use of intravenous vasodilating agents, diuretics, inotropic agents, and mechanical circulatory assist devices (balloon counterpulsation). These interventions are often necessary because compensatory peripheral vasoconstriction to maintain blood pressure contributes to a large increase in afterload and exacerbates mitral regurgitation while diminishing forward flow. There are reports of patients with ischemia-induced paroxysmal mitral regurgitation causing pulmonary edema who were treated successfully with PTCA that resulted in prompt resolution of mitral regurgitation and pulmonary edema; these reports suggest that this treatment modality can be successfully employed in selected unstable patients who have significant papillary muscle dysfunction related to myocardial ischemia (129). In addition to the mainstays of hemodynamic management (afterload reduction and pharmacologic or mechanical circulatory support) for patients with acute mitral regurgitation, intraoperative management of patients who have acute mitral insufficiency related to ischemia or infarction involves several other principles (Table 28-2). Determinants of the quantity of regurgitant flow include the effective size of the regurgitant orifice and the magnitude of the pressure gradient across it. During acute mitral regurgitation, changes in ventricular cavity size are reflected in the mitral orifice size. Therefore, it is generally desirable to maintain a normal or slightly increased heart rate in patients who have mitral regurgitation, because increases in rate tend to decrease the duration of diastole with a subsequent decline in end-diastolic pressure and volume. Some patients who have acute mitral regurgitation complicating myocardial infarction also have unstable ischemic syndromes; in these instances, increases in heart rate should be avoided when possible. Although definite myocardial ischemia usually receives top priority, maneuvers designed to prevent ischemia may sometimes need to be superseded by other goals. For example, if cardiac output and systemic perfusion become unacceptably low, increases in heart rate related to inotropic drug use may be unavoidable. An intraaortic counterpulsation device should be considered in the early stages of management of patients with acute mitral regurgitation, concurrent myocardial ischemia, and inadequate systemic perfusion.

Assessment of preload in these patients is necessary not only to minimize the occurrence and severity of pulmonary edema but also because volume loading can increase the regurgitant volume without any change in the ventriculoatrial pressure gradient, primarily on the basis of an increase in mitral valve orifice area (130). Although pulmonary artery catheterization permits measurement of systemic flow, calculation of systemic and pulmonary vascular resistance, and assessment of the degree of potential right heart stress, acute mitral regurgitation is associated with limitations in the interpretation of pulmonary wedge pressure tracings, which prevent accurate assessment of preload (131). Intraoperative transesophageal echocardiography may be beneficial not only for assessment of valvular and overall cardiac function but also for preload assessment in patients who have acute mitral regurgitation. Transesophageal echocardiography and Doppler color flow imaging have been shown to be beneficial in patients undergoing cardiac valve surgery (132). Postbypass echocardiographic findings may allow patients at risk of an adverse outcome to be identified while still in the operating room (132). This suggests that intraoperative echocardiography can be valuable in formulating the surgical plan, evaluating immediate operative results, and directing potential corrective action in the operating room in selected emergency patients at high risk of postoperative complications related to residual mitral regurgitation or valvular pathology.

Although the choice of anesthetic agents must be individualized, most patients requiring emergent mitral valve replacement are critically ill and often require induction of anesthesia with small doses of opioid combined with oxygen and relaxant. Concomitant administration of benzodiazepines or N_2O, or large doses of opioids are often poorly tolerated at the time of anesthetic induction. The presence of an intraaortic counterpulsation device generally provides more stable hemodynamics during induction of anesthesia, compared with the absence of mechanical support employed preoperatively.

Separation from Cardiopulmonary Bypass

The underlying, relatively small size of the infarcted area and the fact that mitral valvular surgery does not involve the area of necrosis contribute to a low (less than 10%) perioperative mortality rate. The major cause of postoperative morbidity in patients with postinfarct mitral regurgitation is cardiogenic shock. These patients have a mortality rate of more than 50% (133,134). Separating the patient from cardiopulmonary bypass after surgery to correct acute mitral regurgitation can occasionally present some unique difficulties. Left ventricular failure is not uncommon after separation from bypass in patients with chronic mitral valve regurgitation; however, it may also be observed in patients who have abnormal preoperative ventricular function and undergo mitral valve replacement for acute mitral regurgitation, because of a significantly greater left ventricular afterload, compared with that found before replacement of the acutely incompetent mitral apparatus. In these patients, pharmacologic therapy should be designed to reduce afterload and increase contractility. This can usually be accomplished with vasodilators and positive inotropic drugs, particularly catecholamines such as dobutamine or phosphodiesterase inhibitors such as milrinone. In addition, mitral valve repair rather than replacement is gaining popularity and has been employed in selected patients as part of the emergent surgical management of acute mitral regurgitation.

Dynamic outflow obstruction with hemodynamic characteristics similar to those seen with hypertrophic cardiomyopathy have been observed after mitral valvuloplasty (135, 136). Outflow obstruction in this situation is probably associated with systolic anterior motion of the anterior mitral valve leaflet, which is induced by surgically related changes in the left ventricular, chordal, or mitral geometry. Normally, the anterior part of the annulus moves posteriorly, together with the base of the anterior mitral leaflet. The backward motion of the anterior leaflet increases the size of the left ventricular outflow tract and prevents its narrowing during systole. Outflow obstruction after mitral valve repair is most common where a semirigid valvuloplasty ring is inserted, because the backward excursion is diminished. This may result in a narrower left ventricular outflow tract, which in turn may produce systolic anterior motion of the anterior mitral leaflet by the Bernoulli or Venturi effect. The left ventricular outflow gradient may be worsened by the reduction in the left ventricular volume that is common after correction of mitral regurgitation. This entity may become manifest on separation from cardiopulmonary bypass, and its diagnosis requires a high degree of suspicion. Clinical suspicion must be raised when inotropic therapy fails or is associated with worsened systemic perfusion, when loss of preload (including that contributed by coordinated atrial contraction) results in precipitous hypotension, or when a low-flow state is present after otherwise unremarkable surgical repair in a patient who had adequate preoperative ventricular function. The intraoperative diagnosis of dynamic outflow obstruction with systolic anterior motion of the anterior mitral leaflet is quickly and reliably confirmed with transesophageal echocardiography and should be routinely evaluated after separation from cardiopulmonary bypass. When dynamic subaortic obstruction occurs as a result of mitral valve repair, maintenance of sinus rhythm and adequate ventricular preload are important. Positive inotropes should be avoided, and direct-acting vasopressors, if necessary, should be used judiciously to maintain perfusion pressure.

Ventricular Free-Wall Rupture After Myocardial Infarction

Ventricular free-wall rupture (cardiorrhexis) remains a frequent cause of deaths (10% to 20%) related to acute myocardial infarction (137,138). Thrombolytic therapy has been demonstrated to slightly decrease the occurrence of free wall rupture (138,139). The timing of rupture, however, is altered with thrombolysis; early rupture is increased while late rupture is decreased (137). The peak incidence of rupture is in the first 24 hours after infarction when treated with thrombolytic therapy and is 2 to 7 days after infarction without thrombolysis (137). Rupture typically arises at the junction of normal myocardium and a large transmural infarction, and infarct expansion is common before rupture. The infarct-related coronary artery is invariably completely occluded with a thrombus and the collateral circulation is inadequate or absent. These characteristics are consistent with the observation that rupture generally occurs in patients who do not have a previous history of symptomatic coronary artery disease, so long-standing severely stenotic coronary atherosclerosis with collateralization is uncommon. Free-wall ruptures occur mainly in the left ventricle and can be seen with extensive anterior, lateral, or inferior infarctions that are associated with ST-segment elevation or signs of Q-wave formation while rupture of the right ventricle or atria are rare. Lateral wall ruptures may be more common because of an increase in the shearing forces associated with the action of the papillary muscles (116).

Left ventricular rupture may appear in several clinical forms. In its acute form, sudden rupture into the pericardial cavity is associated with a catastrophic clinical syndrome characterized by sudden intense pain followed rapidly by hypotension, jugular venous distention, cardiac tamponade, electromechanical dissociation, and sudden death. When acute free-wall rupture presents in this manner, prompt and heroic measures are required for patient survival, although immediate pericardiocentesis, emergency thoracotomy, and surgical repair are rarely successful (119,140). The diagnosis of free-wall rupture is rarely made before death in these patients, and even with a high index of suspicion, patients presenting with the acute form of rupture are rarely encountered in the operating room. A more subacute form of left ventricular rupture occurs in one third of cases and is associated with slow leakage of blood into the pericardial space over hours or days (141). Progressively worsening signs of cardiac tamponade may be detected in this situation only when a high index of suspicion is present. Ventricular failure with cardiogenic shock must be carefully differentiated from hypotension accompanied by the paradoxical pulse and increased venous pressure specific to cardiac tamponade. In addition to these classic signs of cardiac tamponade, patients with ventricular rupture may also present with bradycardia, nausea, emesis, or chest pain (111,142). Prompt investigation, diagnosis, and cardiopulmonary support enable emergency surgical intervention to occur, which can lead to gratifying long-term results in the subset of patients who develop the subacute form of free-wall rupture (116,119, 141). Intraaortic counterpulsation as a supportive preoperative measure for subacute cardiorrhexis is controversial and may only delay surgical treatment without yielding any significant clinical benefits (143,144). Prompt recognition of myocardial free-wall rupture coupled with improved capabilities for emergency resuscitation and transport into the operating room will have the largest impact on outcome for these patients.

Less commonly, hemopericardium that develops after free-wall rupture of the left ventricle is contained between adherent layers of the pericardium and epicardium, resulting in the pathologic formation of a false aneurysm or pseudoaneurysm. Such pseudoaneurysms typically contain a thrombus and communicate with the left ventricular cavity through a narrow aperture (Fig. 28-5). In contrast to a true ventricular aneurysm, the walls of a pseudoaneurysm are composed of pericardium and adhesions but are devoid of myocardial tissue. These characteristics predispose pseudoaneurysms to free rupture, in contrast to true ventricular aneurysms, which have a low risk of free rupture. Clinical features imitate those of acute ventricular aneurysm, with an increased cardiothoracic ratio and an abnormal bulge on chest radiography, congestive heart failure, recurrent ventricular arrhythmias, and persistent elevation of the ST segment on the ECG. Echocardiography and left ventriculography can be used to differentiate between true and false ventricular aneurysms. The typical narrow neck of the pseudoaneurysm is distinguished from the wide base of a true aneurysm, which is usually the true aneurysm's widest point

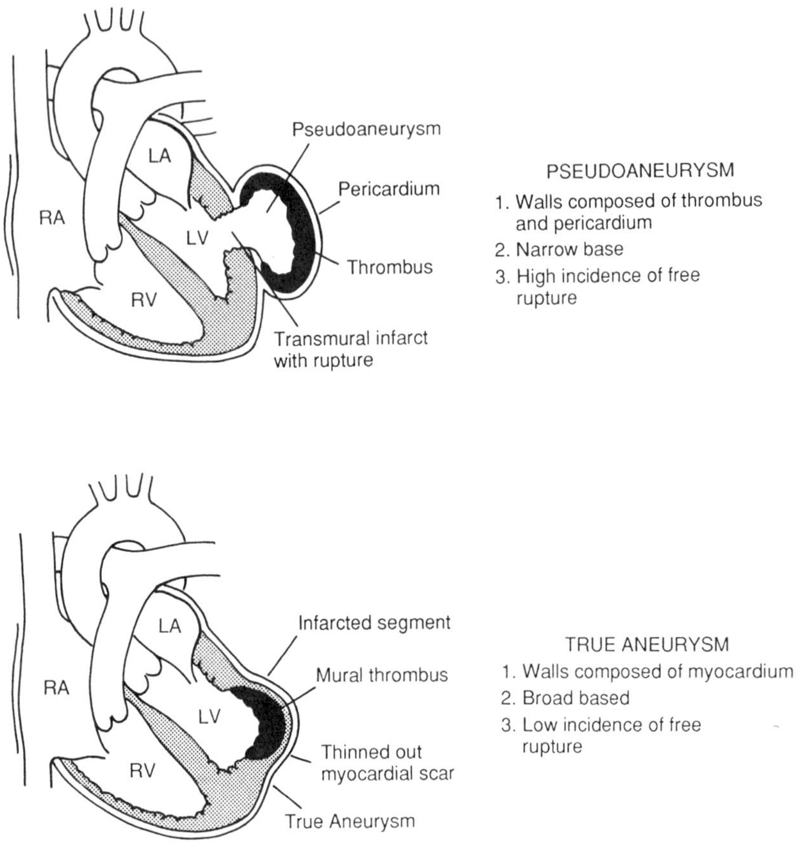

FIGURE 28-5. Ventricular aneurysms after acute myocardial infarction. (LA, left atrium; LV, left ventricle; RA, right atrium; RV, right ventricle.)

(145). Also, the neck of a pseudoaneurysm typically produces an abrupt interruption in the ventricular wall. This is in contrast to a true aneurysm in which the myocardial wall gradually tapers into the aneurysm wall. Because of the high risk of fatal rupture, urgent surgical intervention to repair a pseudoaneurysm is warranted, regardless of the amount of time that has passed since an acute myocardial infarction.

Anesthetic management of patients with ventricular rupture is usually based on the pathophysiology of cardiac tamponade. The key to successful management therefore includes augmentation of preload with blood and fluids administered as required and pharmacologic agents that avoid excessive vasodilation and myocardial depression while maintaining adequate coronary artery perfusion pressure (Table 28-2 and Fig. 28-4). Scopolamine and neuromuscular relaxants with small doses of ketamine or opioids may be the only anesthetics that are hemodynamically tolerable. Even small doses of anesthetic drugs may contribute to cardiovascular collapse in this situation, and if any anesthetic drugs (other than neuromuscular blocking drugs and oxygen) are to be given, they generally should not be administered until the patient is surgically draped and the surgeon is ready to begin. Although adequate venous access is essential for the patient with ventricular rupture, insertion of large-bore venous catheters should not delay swift transport to the operating room and initiation of cardiopulmonary bypass with prompt myocardial arrest.

Separation from cardiopulmonary bypass may be difficult after repair of ventricular rupture. It depends largely on the extent of preoperative left ventricular dysfunction, the presence of cardiogenic shock before operation, and the degree of preservation of function in the viable ventricular mass remaining after infarctectomy. Low cardiac output syndrome may require left ventricular support with inotropic medication, intraaortic counterpulsation, or ventricular assist devices. Inotropic and vasodilator drugs require careful titration after the patient's separation from cardiopulmonary bypass to minimize left ventricular wall tension (to avoid endangering the repair, which often involves residual infarcted tissue) while achieving adequate systemic perfusion. Postoperative complications after repair of ventricular rupture are usually related to the development of cardiogenic shock and inadequate perfusion of distal organs either preoperatively or during the postbypass period. Although neurologic impairment and renal dysfunction often occur after such procedures, long-term survival with partial or complete recovery has been reported and justifies an aggressive approach to an entity that is uniformly fatal when managed medically (116,119).

ACQUIRED CARDIAC DISEASE (WITHOUT MYOCARDIAL INFARCTION) REQUIRING EMERGENCY SURGERY

Acute Aortic Valve Insufficiency

Acute aortic valve insufficiency is almost uniformly an acquired cardiac disease, which is most commonly related to active infective endocarditis or dissection of the thoracic aorta. Although acute aortic insufficiency is typically an isolated major cardiovascular disturbance when secondary to infective endocarditis, aortic insufficiency due to proximal aortic dissection may be complicated by hemopericardium with tamponade, myocardial infarction from coronary artery dissection, or aortic rupture. Acute aortic insufficiency from either cause is associated with a pathophysiology and a clinical presentation different from those of chronic aortic insufficiency. Chronic aortic insufficiency has multiple etiologies, including aortic root disease, intrinsic valvular disease, and subvalvular causes. Chronic insufficiency produces left ventricular volume overload with a resulting increase in myocardial fiber length and an initial maintenance of ventricular function. Left ventricular wall tension and mass increase over time, whereas ventricular diastolic compliance and systolic function decline. Ultimately, increases in left ventricular diastolic pressure are associated with raised left atrial pressure and volume and the development of signs and symptoms of pulmonary venous hypertension. In contrast to chronic aortic insufficiency, patients with acute aortic insufficiency tolerate this lesion poorly. With acute insufficiency, a left ventricle of normal size and compliance is suddenly exposed to the same excessive diastolic overload seen in chronic aortic insufficiency. Rapidly rising left ventricular diastolic pressures in conjunction with the mechanical constraint of an acutely distended pericardium limit the otherwise massive increases in left ventricular end-diastolic volume that would occur with acute aortic regurgitation. The restriction to enlargement of left ventricular end-diastolic cavity size limits the Frank-Starling mechanism (which maintains effective forward stroke volume until late in the course of chronic aortic regurgitation) and results in a left ventricle that cannot effectively maintain forward stroke volume in acute aortic insufficiency. Systolic arterial pressure is maintained by increases in systemic vascular resistance, and because the aortic diastolic pressure cannot fall below the level of the elevated left ventricular end-diastolic pressure, a narrow pulse pressure is typically seen with acute aortic insufficiency. Thus, the classic physical signs of chronic aortic insufficiency that are attributable to a wide pulse pressure, such as a Quincke pulse, are not seen with acute aortic insufficiency. Further confounding the diagnosis, the diastolic murmur may be brief secondary to rapid equalization of left ventricular and aortic pressures. 2D and color flow Doppler echocardiographic imaging are a simple and reliable method to confirm the diagnosis of acute aortic insufficiency.

Initially, the rate at which the left ventricular diastolic pressure increases may be so rapid that premature closure of the mitral valve may prevent the large rise in left ventricular end-diastolic pressure from being transmitted to a pulmonary wedge pressure trace (146). However, the echocardiographic demonstration of premature mitral valve closure suggests overwhelming aortic regurgitation and usually occurs only in patients requiring urgent valve repair (146). The increased left ventricular diastolic pressure causes not only early mitral valve closure but also diastolic mitral regurgitation in some instances. Additionally, the sudden ventricular distension seen with acute aortic insufficiency commonly results in mitral annular enlargement and systolic mitral regurgitation. Thus, with acute aortic insufficiency, the pulmonary venous and arterial pressures can be elevated precipitously, and the right ventricle often cannot accommodate the sudden increase in work. If functional mitral insufficiency occurs, fulminant pulmonary edema that is refractory to medical therapy often develops.

Congestive heart failure secondary to acute aortic regurgitation is currently the leading cause of death from infective endocarditis. Serious conduction disturbances, including high-degree atrioventricular block due to myocardial abscess of the conduction system, can be seen with acute aortic valve disease. Surgical risk is far greater in patients with acute aortic insufficiency than in patients with chronic insufficiency not only because of the severity of the acute hemodynamic derangements but also because of the seriousness of the underlying medical conditions (e.g., infective endocarditis, dissecting aneurysm). Nonetheless, emergency surgical intervention can be the only lifesaving therapy for the patient with acute aortic regurgitation. Delaying surgical repair of acute aortic regurgitation after the onset of intractable cardiac failure resulting from disruption of valve leaflets or their supporting structures may contribute to adverse outcome, even when the surgical procedure itself has been entirely successful.

Patients who have acute aortic insufficiency and arrive in the operating room for emergency replacement of the valve are gravely ill. Patients who require urgent or emergent aortic valve surgery and have active infective endocarditis involving a fungal infection or persistent bacteremia typically have hemodynamic compromise, severe heart failure, an unstable prosthesis, or evidence of intracardiac extension of infection, such as rupture of the sinus of Valsalva or ventricular septum, conduction disturbances, or demonstration of an abscess by echocardiography or catheterization (147). Urgent surgical intervention is indicated, particularly in patients with large dehiscences of a prosthetic valve and acute valvular insufficiency, because the serious hemodynamic consequences of valvular dysfunction often progress rapidly in this situation. In addition to hemodynamic problems, patients with acute infective endocarditis involving the left heart structures often demonstrate signs of systemic embolization before and after surgical intervention. The most common sites of embolization are coronary vessels, spleen, kidneys, and brain, although almost every tissue and organ may be involved. The incidence of embolization of larger arteries is increasing because of intravenous drug addiction, which introduces a greater frequency of fungal colonization and infection. These characteristics explain the high mortality rate of 50% to 90% after medical therapy in patients who have native valvular endocarditis and develop significant hemodynamic impairment (148). Survival associated with surgical intervention is superior. A 28% to 33% mortality rate is seen in patients undergoing emergent aortic valve replacement for acute endocarditis with coexisting severe congestive heart failure, infection of a prosthetic aortic valve, or staphylococcal or fungal infection while a 7% to 10% perioperative mortality rate is observed in patients without these risk factors (147).

Anesthetic considerations for these critically ill patients are based on simple hemodynamic principles. Because the amount of regurgitant volume is determined largely by the duration of diastole and the pressure gradient between the left ventricle and the aorta, maintaining the heart rate in the normal range, 80 to 90 beats/minute, and slightly decreasing afterload usually will augment stroke volume and forward flow while reducing left ventricular size (Table 28-2). Bradycardia tends to result in left ventricular distension and increased orifice size of the regurgitant valve, with a greater degree of associated regurgitant flow as well as increased wall tension, myocardial oxygen cost, predisposition to ventricular arrhythmias, and ischemic damage. Although avoidance of increases in afterload (hypertension) is perhaps the most crucial aspect of the anesthetic management, afterload reduction must be attempted cautiously to avert excessive reductions in coronary perfusion pressure. Preload should be maintained at normal or slightly raised levels to promote forward filling of the ventricle during diastole. However, a narrow window exists for the optimal level of preload in patients who already have cardiac failure with pulmonary venous volume and pressure overload. Intraaortic counterpulsation is contraindicated in patients who have acute aortic insufficiency, even when hemodynamic collapse is present, because it only augments regurgitant diastolic flow. Prompt aortic valve replacement is the definitive therapy in such cases. Transportation to the operating room and preinduction activities should be conducted to minimize the period during which further hemodynamic deterioration can occur.

High doses of opioids, such as fentanyl or sufentanil, with oxygen and a muscle relaxant often are well tolerated by patients in these situations. Diazepam with ketamine has been shown to produce hemodynamic changes similar to those produced by opiate-based anesthesia in patients undergoing aortic valve replacement (149,150). For any of these techniques, intraoperative increases in systemic vascular resistance can be controlled with systemic vasodilators. When a balanced (both venous and arteriolar) vasodilator such as nitroprusside is used, decreases in both afterload and preload are seen if continuous pulmonary artery catheter monitoring is employed. Preload augmentation can subsequently result in significant increases in forward cardiac output. As noted, the pulmonary wedge pressure can significantly underestimate left ventricular preload when acute aortic insufficiency prompts early mitral valve closure. When ventricular function is preserved, a balanced anesthetic technique with a volatile anesthetic can provide adequate control of increases in afterload. However, patients with any degree of cardiac failure may not tolerate volatile anesthetics. When acute aortic insufficiency is secondary to aortic dissection, positive inotropic drugs should be used cautiously, if at all, because augmented ventricular contractility could increase the shear forces on the disrupted aortic wall. After cardiopulmonary bypass, patients with preoperative left or right ventricular dysfunction may require combinations of inotropes and vasodilators to maintain adequate systemic perfusion.

Blunt or Penetrating Cardiac Trauma

Trauma is the most common cause of death in young adults in the United States, with cardiovascular mortality a major contributor. Although there are a wide range of injuries and varying severity of injury seen in chest trauma patients, the two major life-threatening cardiac events are exsanguinating hemorrhage and cardiac tamponade. Both have a high mortality rate and require immediate surgical intervention, often in the emergency room.

Penetrating trauma can injure any cardiac structure, including the myocardial free walls, intracardiac septi, valvular and subvalvular structures, and coronary vessels. In penetrating injury, those without signs of life at the accident scene rarely benefit from aggressive treatment. Aggressive resuscitation, however, is often effective for patients in extremis but with some spontaneous perfusion on arrival to the emergency room. Emergency room thoracotomy is indicated in these patients to relieve tamponade and to control hemorrhage before transfer to the operating room for definitive care (151). In patients with moderate hemodynamic compromise, emergent exploratory thoracotomy is typically performed in the operating room, and in patients with penetrating injury who are hemodynamically stable, radiographic testing and echocardiographic examination can be performed to determine whether surgical treatment is necessary.

Similar to rapid exsanguination, traumatic pericardial tamponade is usually immediately lethal. Because the epicardial sac is acutely nondistensible, rapid accumulation of small volumes of fluid (as little as 50 to 100 mL) may increase intrapericardial pressure and reduce effective transmural diastolic filling pressure and ventricular filling, with a resultant decrease in stroke volume, cardiac output, and systemic arterial pressure. Nonetheless, the presence of cardiac tamponade in cardiac trauma patients is a favorable predictor of outcome, perhaps because it prevents exsanguination (151). Jugular venous distension may not occur in traumatic cardiac tamponade because hypovolemia is often present. Gunshot wounds (as opposed to stab wounds), multichamber injuries, lacerated coronary arteries, and coexistent noncardiac injuries significantly increase the mortality rate of penetrating cardiac trauma (151,152).

A high index of suspicion for cardiac injury is required after blunt chest trauma, and significant cardiac injury can occur without clinically apparent skeletal injury to the thorax. Rupture of a cardiac chamber is a common finding in patients with fatal nonpenetrating cardiac injuries. The right cardiac chambers are more likely to rupture than the left chambers, although any chamber can be affected (153). Myocardial rupture causes sudden death in most patients. For those alive on presentation, rapid recognition and emergent thoracotomy can be lifesaving. Emergency thoracotomy for hemodynamic instability after blunt trauma, however, is not as successful when performed after penetrating trauma (151). Aortic rupture is also common after blunt chest trauma. Diagnosis and management of great vessel injury is described fully elsewhere in Chapter 27. Myocardial contusion should be suspected in blunt chest trauma and may cause increases in cardiac enzymes and ECG changes similar to myocardial infarction, as well as abnormalities of wall motion (154). Dysrhythmias, including atrial fibrillation, are also common. Although myocardial contusion is not an indication for cardiac surgery, it may coexist with surgical injuries and act to decrease myocardial reserve. Additionally, it must be differentiated from coronary laceration, a potentially correctable cause of myocardial ischemia and infarction.

Adherence to a series of treatment priorities allows patient evaluation, diagnosis, and therapy to be conducted in an orderly fashion during a time when chaos may prevail. Appropriate airway management and intravenous catheter placement is essential. Those with blunt trauma are at risk for cervical spine fracture and manual in-line neck stabilization may be necessary during tracheal intubation. Large-bore venous access is ideally obtained both above and below the diaphragm to allow effective fluid administration in the event of great vein injury. Pulmonary injury often accompanies cardiac injury. The presence of flail chest injury, tension pneumothorax, and tracheobronchial disruption should be searched for with a brief but careful physical examination and a review of the chest radiograph. If any of these entities are present, prompt control of ventilation and thoracostomy tube(s) insertion are indicated. If major vessel disruption is suspected and chest radiography reveals a complete hemothorax, resuscitation efforts should continue. If the patient is not in cardiac arrest, decompression of the chest should take place in the operating room to avoid emergency room thoracotomy with rapid exsanguination from a previously tamponaded pleural space. Pulmonary contusion is often present and can significantly impair gas exchange. Large tidal volumes or PEEP used to improve oxygenation will often compromise venous return and systemic perfusion until bleeding is controlled and intravascular volume replenished. When pulmonary parenchymal hemorrhage is unilateral and hemodynamics are approaching or have achieved stability, endobronchial intubation and placement of the patient in the lateral decubitus position may be attempted to prevent contralateral pulmonary soilage. These maneuvers may not be possible in some patients with thoracic trauma, primarily because of ongoing intraoperative cardiopulmonary instability. Arterial or venous air embolism occurs more frequently than is generally appreciated, particularly in patients who have injuries caused by high-velocity missiles that result in lung parenchymal injury (155). Positive-pressure ventilation can force air from an injured bronchus into an adjacent pulmonary vein and produce systemic air embolization. This mechanism probably accounts for sudden arrhythmias and postoperative neurologic deficits occasionally observed after penetrating chest trauma in young patients with no episodes of cardiac arrest.

Anesthetic care is based on vigorous support of preload with blood and fluids and administration of pharmacologic agents that avoid excessive vasodilation and myocardial depression while maintaining adequate coronary artery perfusion pressure (Table 28-2). Additional details of the management of patients with acute traumatic tamponade are essentially identical to those described for patients with free-wall rupture after acute myocardial infarction. Most trauma-induced cardiac injuries can be treated without cardiopulmonary bypass. Certain lesions, such as penetrating injuries of the ascending aorta, may not benefit from the efforts required to institute cardiopulmonary bypass, and direct attempts to control the site of bleeding may have more positive effects on cerebral and overall outcome. Suboptimal outcomes can be related to a prolonged time interval until final control of bleeding and to the potential for a significant proportion of total cardiopulmonary bypass pump flow to move in a path between the cardiotomy suction, oxygenator, and femoral artery, only to reexit the injury site in the ascending aorta. This may also be observed with iatrogenic injuries occurring during sternotomy for reoperations; cerebral perfusion can be grossly inadequate despite acceptable total pump flow returning via the femoral artery. Other more common pitfalls in the management of penetrating cardiac trauma are summarized in Table 28-3. Although most patients with penetrating cardiac trauma and blunt cardiac rupture die before arrival at the hospital, those who arrive with vital signs have a good chance of survival if transport to the operating room is rapid, resuscitation is aggressive, and surgical repair is prompt (151,152).

TABLE 28-3. MANAGEMENT OF PENETRATING CARDIAC TRAUMA

Pitfalls	Treatment Prioritiies
Failure to infuse adequate fluids	If no jugular venous distention or evidence of heart failure, infuse at least 2 L of balanced salt solution over 15–20 min, use lower extremity vein if suspect superior vena caval injury
Failure to perform early endotracheal intubation	If severe shock or marginal ventilation or oxygenation, intubation should be performed in emergency department
Delay in moving patient to operating room	Prompt transport operating room while stabilizing patient
Failure to diagnose cardiac or great vessel injury in patient with penetrating chest wound	High index of suspicion of cardiac injury if shock develops after penetrating chest injury
Failure to recognize concomitant associated life-threatening injury	High index of suspicion for injuries such as pneumothorax, spinal cord injury, or tracheal injury
Delay in performing emergency department thoracotomy if patient has cardiac arrest before transfer to operating room	Prompt thoracotomy with pericardiotomy, open cardiac massage, control of bleeding, clamping descending aorta, and institution of cardiopulmonary bypass, if necessary
Failure to prevent pulmonary soilage when hemoptysis is unilateral	Use of endobronchial intubation and lateral decubitus position when possible if unilateral hemoptysis is present
Use of excessive ventilatory pressures during hand-bagging, increasing intrathoracic pressures and further decreasing venous return and potentially increasing incidence and severity of pulmonary venous air emboli	Avoid large tidal volumes and positive end-expiratory pressure to minimize compromise of marginal venous return; avoid respiratory alkalosis, which causes ionized hypocalcemia

EMERGENCY SITUATIONS AFTER CARDIAC SURGERY

Postoperative Hemorrhage and Cardiac Tamponade

Excessive mediastinal bleeding after cardiopulmonary bypass is a serious complication of cardiac surgery and is associated with an increased frequency of postoperative hypotension, shock, cardiac failure, arrhythmias, mediastinal infection, and renal failure (156). Mediastinal bleeding requiring surgical exploration also increases perioperative mortality (157). Despite technical improvements in procedures and equipment, postoperative hemorrhage remains a major cause of morbidity after cardiopulmonary bypass, necessitating surgical reexploration of the chest in approximately 6% of patients who have undergone cardiac operations (156). Reexploration for persistent bleeding is required more frequently after valvular or a second cardiac surgery than it is after first-time coronary artery bypass surgery (157). The hemorrhagic tendency after cardiopulmonary bypass is often a complex reflection of multiple hemostatic defects related to the duration of cardiopulmonary bypass as well as to hemodilution. Surgical trauma increases the bleeding tendency, particularly in the reoperated-on patient who often has significant amounts of well-vascularized adhesions that serve as bleeding sites postoperatively. Among patients reexplored for bleeding, two thirds have an identifiable source of bleeding (157). The most common bleeding sites are bypass graft anastomoses and graft side branches, the sternum, and the aortic cannulation site. Of note, half of explored patients demonstrate a concurrent coagulopathy contributing to mediastinal bleeding. Thus, the etiology of excessive chest drainage in many patients is related to both surgical bleeding and a persistent coagulopathy. A detailed discussion of the preoperative and early postoperative hematologic factors, the hemostatic changes associated with extracorporeal circulation, and the diagnosis and hemotherapy of these disorders is found in Chapter 11.

Evaluation of mediastinal bleeding in the postoperative period requires evaluation of chest tube drainage, hemodynamics, and hemostatic parameters. This discussion focuses on the diagnosis and therapy of surgically treatable causes of postoperative bleeding. Excessive chest tube drainage is considered to be present when the amount of drainage exceeds 250 to 300 mL/hour for the first 2 hours after operation or subsequently is greater than 100 to 150 mL/hour (158,159). An exception to these findings is the sudden drainage of a large amount of blood when the patient is repositioned immediately after surgery (e.g., to obtain a portable chest radiograph), which does not continue and represents prior blood loss that occurred at a slower rate and that accumulated in a location previously not drainable by the chest tubes. When bleeding occurs at rates faster than those just noted, surgically correctable bleeding is most often responsible, and surgical exploration is appropriate to prevent or treat cardiac tamponade and hemorrhagic shock (158, 159). Patients with excessive mediastinal bleeding and systemic arterial hypotension may have low filling pressures and depressed cardiac output with a clinical picture of hemorrhagic shock. Without concurrent blood component transfusion, substantial declines in hemoglobin concentration, and decreased platelet and coagulation factor levels may be observed, particularly if fluid resuscitation with colloid or crystalloid has ensued.

Excessive mediastinal bleeding also predisposes post-cardiac surgical patients to the development of cardiac tamponade. Cardiac tamponade can occur after cardiac surgery with minimal chest tube drainage because of clotted blood within the drainage tubes or mediastinum or because of adhesions or loculations around bleeding sites that prevent adequate mediastinal drainage. Unlike noncardiac surgery–related cardiac tamponade in which effusions typically extend circumferentially around the heart, most pericardial effusions after cardiac surgery are loculated and localized, most commonly posterior to the heart (160,161). A small effusion, when localized, can produce high intrapericardial pressures and tamponade physiology. Cardiac tamponade typically presents with elevation of intravascular filling pressures and low cardiac output. Because of the localized nature of the tamponade, the traditional signs of cardiac tamponade, including equalization of diastolic intracardiac pressures, pulsus paradoxus, and jugular venous distension, are frequently absent, potentially delaying the diagnosis (160). When mediastinal bleeding is present, chest radiography often shows an enlarged cardiac silhouette compared with previous films. This is not a sensitive marker, however, because a small loculated effusion may not cause an enlarged cardiac silhouette. Echocardiographic recognition of tamponade may be difficult in patients after cardiac surgery. A small localized effusion is technically more difficult to appreciate than a large circumferential effusion. In noncardiac surgical patients, the usual echocardiographic signs of cardiac tamponade are right atrial and right ventricular diastolic collapse. These signs unreliably predict tamponade when the effusion is loculated, and left ventricular compression is more common in surgical patients with tamponade (160). Precordial echocardiography often provides inadequate cardiac imaging during the early postoperative period because of the presence of mediastinal air, the location of chest drainage tubes, and the presence of surgical dressings that interfere with transducer positioning and cardiac image generation. For these reasons, and because of the proximity of the esophagus to the posterior mediastinum, transesophageal echocardiography may prove superior in this situation.

Cardiac tamponade is not uncommon postoperatively and is estimated to account for 10% of cases of persistent hypotension after cardiac surgery (162). When chest tube output is not excessive and loculated tamponade is present, clinical acumen is required in the early postoperative period to differentiate the clinical picture from right ventricular dysfunction or infarction, biventricular failure, or tricuspid regurgitation. Because of the occasional difficulties in distinguishing cardiac tamponade from other causes of a low-flow state in the immediate postoperative period, empiric inotropic and vasopressor therapy and mechanical support are common. As in situations of excessive mediastinal bleeding, prompt reexploration is indicated for cardiac tamponade. When patients who have excessive bleeding and systemic arterial hypotension arrive in the operating room, surgical relief of tamponade and control of bleeding should be achieved as quickly as possible. Most of these patients will have an absolute or a relative hypovolemia in addition to some degree of impairment of underlying ventricular function immediately after cardiopulmonary bypass and cardioplegic arrest. Oxygen, muscle relaxants, and scopolamine may be the only anesthetic drugs tolerated until hemodynamics are improved by blood volume replacement and relief of tamponade. When the patient's hemodynamics allow, small titrated doses of ketamine, opioids, or other agents may be administered. Maintenance of body temperature is necessary in bleeding patients with little cardiac reserve to avoid further impairment of hemodynamic stability as well as platelet function, and measures to prevent hypothermia (including warming of infused intravascular volume replacement) should be employed.

Myocardial Rupture After Cardiac Surgery

Ventricular rupture after cardiac surgery is exceedingly rare and is one of the most dreaded complications associated with mitral valve replacement (163,164). Survival rates are low, probably because the diagnosis is often delayed, because rupture occurs early in the postoperative period, when mediastinal hemorrhage is attributed to other more common causes. The pathophysiology of transverse midventricular rupture is probably related to abnormalities of the posterior left ventricular wall. Most commonly, patients who develop this complication after mitral valve replacement have had long-standing rheumatic disease or acute ischemic mitral incompetence. Even if the left ventricle has been protected from high pressures in the presence of chronic mitral stenosis, the gradually failing ventricle is often affected by the underlying degenerative rheumatic process, and clinical experience with patients who have postoperative ventricular rupture indicates that they often have a very thin, almost friable, posterior ventricular wall. These patients also commonly have a very large, sometimes calcified, friable left atrium. Patients with acute ischemic mitral regurgitation usually have much smaller atria but require much greater surgical retraction to expose the mitral valve apparatus. When the posteromedial papillary muscle is involved with ischemia or infarction of the posterior ventricular wall, the risk of postoperative rupture is increased. Suboptimal placement of the mitral valve suture ring or excessive excision of the old mitral valve may contribute to increased risk of rupture in some instances.

Excessive administration of inotropes, vasopressors, and fluid to facilitate separation from cardiopulmonary bypass after mitral valve replacement can adversely increase intraventricular pressure, produce ventricular distention, and elevate wall stress. This type of hyperdynamic state not only may occur because of exogenously administered catecholamines but can also be observed when patients are awakening from cardiac surgery in the intensive care unit. In this setting, appropriate administration of opioids and sedative drugs may need to be supplemented with vasodilators to reduce ventricular wall stress in patients who have recently (within 24 hours) undergone mitral valve replacement and who are believed to be at risk of rupture because of a very thin or recently infarcted posterior ventricular wall. The prophylactic use of intraaortic balloon counterpulsation is also advocated to further unload the left ventricle (164). When this complication is recognized or suspected, immediate sternotomy with manual posterior compression of the rupture is necessary but rarely successful in affecting ultimate outcome, even in the hands of an experienced cardiac surgeon. The principles of intraoperative management outlined for patients with ventricular free-wall rupture after acute myocardial infarction also apply when surgical repair of this injury is possible. Most important, systemic arterial pressure and cardiac filling pressure should be kept at values as low as are compatible with adequate systemic perfusion of vital organs. Chest compression during cardiopulmonary resuscitation after cardiac surgery is reported to cause acute hemorrhage secondary to mechanically induced rupture of myocardial and vascular sutures (165). Defibrillation is suggested as the preferred initial management before chest compression in cardiac surgical patients with an unstable rhythm.

REFERENCES

1. de Bono D. Complications of diagnostic cardiac catheterization: results from 34,041 patients in the United Kingdom confidential inquiry into cardiac catheter complications. *Br Heart J* 1993; 70:297.
2. Noto TJ, Johnson LW, Krone R, et al. Cardiac catheterization 1990: a report of the Registry of the Society for Cardiac Angiography and Interventions (SCA&I). *Cathet Cardiovasc Diagn* 1991;24:75.
3. Stellato C, Adkinson NF. Pathophysiology of contrast media anaphylactoid reactions: new perspectives on an old problem. *Allergy* 1998;53:1111.
4. Lieberman P. Anaphylactoid reactions to radiocontrast material. *Ann Allergy* 1991;67:91.
5. Mark AL. The Bezold-Jarisch reflex revisited: clinical implication of inhibitory reflexes originating in the heart. *J Am Coll Cardiol* 1983;1:90.
6. de la Serna F, Meier B, Pande AK, et al. Coronary and left ventricular pacing as standby in invasive cardiology. *Cathet Cardiovasc Diagn* 1992;25:285.
7. Bladin CF, Bingham L, Grigg L, et al. Transcranial doppler detection of microemboli during percutaneous transluminal coronary angioplasty. *Stroke* 1998;29:2367.
8. Lazar JM, Uretsky BF, Denys BG, et al. Predisposing risk factors and natural history of acute neurologic complications of left-sided catheterization. *Am J Cardiol* 1995;75:1056.
9. McCann RL, Schwartz LB, Pieper KS. Vascular complications of cardiac catheterization. *J Vasc Surg* 1991;14:375.
10. Muller DWM, Shamir KJ, Ellis SG, et al. Peripheral vascular complications after conventional and complex percutaneous coronary interventional procedures. *Am J Cardiol* 1992;69:63.
11. Ricci MA, Trevisani GT, Pilcher DB. Vascular complications of cardiac catheterization. *Am J Surg* 1994;167:375.
12. Morton BC, Higginson LAJ, Beanlands DS. Death in a catheterization laboratory. *Can Med Assoc J* 1993;149:165.
13. Ryan TJ, Bauman WB, Kennedy JW, et al. Guidelines for percutaneous transluminal coronary angioplasty: a report of the American College of Cardiology/American Heart Association Task Force on assessment of diagnostic and therapeutic cardiovascular procedures. *J Am Coll Cardiol* 1993;22:2033.
14. Topol EJ, Ellis SG, Cosgrove DM, et al. Analysis of coronary angioplasty practice in the United States with an insurance-claims data base. *Circulation* 1993;87:1489.
15. Pande AK, Meier B, Rutishauser W. Implications of coronary angiography in patients with suspected or known coronary artery disease. *Int J Cardiol* 1993;38:159.
16. Malenka DJ, O'Rourke D, Miler MA, et al. Cause of in-hospital death in 12,232 consecutive patients undergoing percutaneous transluminal coronary angioplasty. *Am Heart J* 1999;137:632.
17. Antonellis IP, Patsilinakos SP, Pamboukas CA, et al. Successful management of right coronary air embolus after intracoronary administration of verapamil. *Int J Cardiol* 1998;66:319.
18. Altmann DB, Racz M, Battleman DS, et al. Reduction in angioplasty complications after the introduction of coronary stents: results from a consecutive series of 2242 patients. *Am Heart J* 1996;132:503.
19. Ellis SG, Cowley MJ, Whitlow PL, et al. Prospective case-control comparison of percutaneous transluminal coronary revascularization in patients with multivessel disease treated in 1986-1987 versus 1991: improved in-hospital and 12-month results. *J Am Coll Cardiol* 1995;25:1137.
20. Boylan MJ, Lytle BW, Taylor PC, et al. Have PTCA failures requiring emergent bypass operation changed? *Ann Thorac Surg* 1995;59:283.
21. Talley JD, Weintraub WS, Roubin GS, et al. Failed elective percutaneous transluminal angioplasty requiring coronary artery bypass surgery: in-hospital and late clinical outcome at 5 years. *Circulation* 1990;82:1203.
22. Tuzcu M, Simpfendorfer C, Dorosti K, et al. Long-term outcome of unsuccessful percutaneous transluminal coronary angioplasty. *Am Heart J* 1990;119:1991.
23. Stark KS, Satler LF, Krucoff MW, et al. Myocardial salvage after failed coronary angioplasty. *J Am Coll Cardiol* 1990;15: 78.
24. Zalewski A, Savage M, Goldberg S. Protection of the ischemic myocardium during percutaneous transluminal coronary angioplasty. *Am J Cardiol* 1988;61:54.
25. Saito K, Nonogi H, Goto Y, et al. Antiischemic effect of intracoronary diltiazem on myocardial ischemia during PTCA. *Heart Vessels* 1996;11:92.
26. Kent KM, Cleman MW, Crowley MJ, et al. Reduction of myocardial ischemia during percutaneous transluminal coronary angioplasty with oxygenated fluosol. *Am J Cardiol* 1990;66:279.
27. Wohlgelernter D, Cleman M, Highman HA, et al. Regional myocardial dysfunction during coronary angioplasty: evaluation of 2-dimensional echocardiography and 12-lead electrocardiography. *J Am Coll Cardiol* 1986;7:1245.
28. Aguirre FV, Kern MJ, Bach R, et al. Intraaortic balloon pump support during high-risk coronary angioplasty. *Cardiology* 1994; 84:175.
29. Stone GW, Marsalese D, Brodie BR, et al. A prospective, randomized evaluation of prophylactic intra-aortic balloon counterpulsation in high risk patients with acute myocardial infarction treated with primary angioplasty. *J Am Coll Cardiol* 1997; 29:1459.
30. Murphy DA, Craver JM, Jones EL, et al. Surgical management of acute myocardial ischemia following percutaneous transluminal coronary angioplasty. *J Thorac Cardiovasc Surg* 1984;87: 332.
31. Alcan KE, Stentzer SH, Wallsh E, et al. The role of intra-aortic

balloon counterpulsation in patients undergoing percutaneous transluminal coronary angioplasty. *Am Heart J* 1983;105:527.
32. Phillips SJ. Percutaneous cardiopulmonary bypass and innovations in clinical counterpulsation. *Crit Care Clin* 1986;2:297.
33. Sundram P, Harvey JR, Johnson RG, et al. Benefit of the perfusion catheter for emergency coronary artery grafting after failed percutaneous transluminal coronary angioplasty. *Am J Cardiol* 1989;63:282.
34. Heikkinen L, Virtanen K, Heikkila J, et al. Surgical treatment of acute myocardial ischaemia related to coronary angioplasty with special reference to use of perfusion balloon catheter and long-term outcome. *J Cardiovasc Surg* 1997;38:101.
35. Ferrari M, Werner GS, von zur Muhlen F, et al. Coronary flow analysis during autoperfusion angioplasty. *Coronary Artery Dis* 1997;8:697.
36. Voelker W, Kerkhoffs W, Schmitz B, et al. Comparison of passive and active perfusion catheters: an in vitro study in a pulsatile coronary flow model. *Cathet Cardiovasc Diagn* 1996; 38:421.
37. de Muinck ED, den Heijer P, van Dijk RB, et al. Distal coronary hemoperfusion during percutaneous transluminal coronary angioplasty. *Cathet Cardiovasc Diagn* 1996;37:233.
38. Corday E, Kar S, Drury JK, et al. Coronary venous retroperfusion for support of ischemic myocardium. *Cardiovasc Rev Rep* 1990;9:50.
39. Foley JB, Pilon C, Brown RIG, et al. Experience of immediate stenting, perfusion balloon and secondary stenting in failed angioplasty. *Can J Cardiol* 1995;11:317.
40. de Muinck ED, den Heijer P, van Dijk RB, et al. Autoperfusion balloon versus stent for acute or threatened closure during percutaneous transluminal coronary angioplasty. *Am J Cardiol* 1994;74:1002.
41. de Feyter PJ, de Jaegere PPT, Serruys PW. Incidence, predictors, and management of acute coronary occlusion after coronary angioplasty. *Am Heart J* 1994;127:643.
42. Benzuly KH, Glazier S, Grines CL, et al. Coronary perforation: an unreported complication after intracoronary stent implantation. *J Am Coll Cardiol* 1996;29:975(abst).
43. Grambow DW, Deeb GM, Pavlides GS, et al. Emergent percutaneous cardiopulmonary bypass in patients having cardiovascular collapse in the cardiac catheterization laboratory. *Am J Cardiol* 1994;73:872.
44. Schreiber TL, Kodali UR, O'Neill WW, et al. Comparison of acute results of prophylactic intra-aortic balloon pumping with cardiopulmonary support for percutaneous transluminal coronary angioplasty (PTCA). *Cathet Cardiovasc Diagn* 1998;45: 115.
45. Craver JM, Weintraub WS, Jones EL, et al. Emergency coronary artery bypass surgery for failed percutaneous coronary angioplasty. A 10-year experience. *Ann Surg* 1992;215:425.
46. Falk E. Coronary Thrombosis: pathogenesis and clinical manifestations. *Am J Cardiol* 1991;68:28B.
47. Tofler GH, Brezinski DA, Schafer AI, et al. Concurrent morning increase in platelet aggregability and the risk of myocardial infarction and sudden cardiac death. *N Engl J Med* 1987;316: 1514.
48. Granger CB, Califf RM, Topol EJ. Thrombolytic Therapy for Acute Myocardial Infarction. *Drugs* 1992;44(3):293.
49. Cannon CP, McCabe CH, Diver DJ, et al. Comparison of front-loaded recombinant tissue-type plasminogen activator, anistreplase and combination thrombolytic therapy for acute myocardial infarction: results of the thrombolysis in myocardial infarction (TIMI) 4 trial. *J Am Coll Cardiol* 1994;24:1602.
50. The GUSTO Angiographic Investigators. The effects of tissue plasminogen activator, streptokinase, or both on coronary-artery patency, ventricular function, and survival after acute myocardial infarction. *N Engl J Med* 1993;329:1615.
51. Gruppo Italiano per lo Studio della Streptochinasi nell' Infarto Miocardico (GISSI). Effectiveness of intravenous thrombolytic treatment in acute myocardial infarction. *Lancet* 1986;1:397.
52. The GUSTO Investigators. An international randomized trial comparing four thrombolytic strategies for acute myocardial infarction. *N Engl J Med* 1993;329:674.
53. Neuhaus KL. More on thrombolysis and hemorrhagic stroke. *Circulation* 1995;92:2794.
54. Stump DC, Califf RM, Topol EJ, et al. Pharmacodynamics of thrombolysis with recombinant tissue-type plasminogen activator. *Circulation* 1989;80:1222.
55. Blankenship JC, Almquist AK. Cardiovascular complications of thrombolytic therapy in patients with a mistaken diagnosis of acute myocardial infarction. *J Am Coll Cardiol* 1989;14:1579.
56. Michels KB, Yusuf S. Does PTCA in acute myocardial infarction affect mortality and reinfarction rates? A quantitative overview (meta-analysis) of randomized clinical trials. *Circulation* 1995;91:476.
57. Zijlstra F, de Boer MJ, Hoorntje JCA, et al. A comparison of immediate coronary angioplasty with intravenous streptokinase in acute myocardial infarction. *N Engl J Med* 1993;328:680.
58. Garcia E, Elizaga J, Perez-Castellano N, et al. Primary angioplasty versus systemic thrombolysis in anterior myocardial infarction. *J Am Coll Cardiol* 1999;33:605.
59. Simoons ML, Arnold AE, Betriu A, et al. Thrombolysis with tissue plasminogen activator in acute myocardial infarction: no additional benefit for immediate percutaneous coronary angioplasty. *Lancet* 1988;1:197.
60. Rogers WJ, Baim DS, Gore JM, et al. Comparison of immediate invasive, delayed invasive, and conservative strategies after tissue-type plasminogen activator. Results of the thrombolysis in myocardial infarction (TIMI) Phase II-A Trial. *Circulation* 1990;81:1457.
61. Ellis SG, da Silva ER, Heyndrickx G, et al. Randomized comparison of rescue angioplasty with conservative management of patients with early failure of thrombolysis for acute anterior myocardial infarction. *Circulation* 1994;90:2280.
62. Ross AM, Lundergan CF, Rohrbeck SC, et al. Rescue angioplasty after failed thrombolysis: technical and clinical outcomes in a large thrombolysis trial. *J Am Coll Cardiol* 1998;31:1511.
63. Faxon DP. The risk of reperfusion strategies in the treatment of patients with acute myocardial infarction. *J Am Coll Cardiol* 1988;12:52A.
64. Gibson CM, Cannon CP, Greene RM, et al. Rescue angioplasty in the thrombolysis in myocardial infarction (TIMI) 4 trial. *Am J Cardiol* 1997;80:21.
65. Hill RF, Kates RA, Davis D, et al. Anesthetic implications for the management of patients with acute myocardial infarction: a matched cohort study of patients undergoing emergency myocardial revascularization. *J Cardiothorac Anesth* 1988;2:23.
66. Akhtar TM, Goodchild CS, Boylan MKG. Reversal of streptokinase-induced bleeding with aprotinin for emergency cardiac surgery. *Anaesthesia* 1992;47:226.
67. Hoffman JJ, Vijgen M. Prevention of in vitro fibrinogenolysis during laboratory monitoring of thrombolytic therapy with streptokinase or APSAC. *Blood Coagul Fibrinolysis* 1991;2:279.
68. Royston D. Aprotinin prevents bleeding and has effects on platelets and fibrinolysis. *J Cardiothorac Vasc Anesth* 1991; 5[Suppl 1]:18.
69. Goldberg M, Colonna-Romano P, Babins NA, et al. Emergency coronary artery bypass surgery following intracoronary streptokinase. *Anesthesiology* 1984;61:601.
70. EPIC Investigators. Use of a monoclonal antibody directed

against the platelet glycoprotein IIb/IIIa receptor in high-risk coronary angioplasty. *N Engl J Med.* 1994;330: 956.
71. Topol EJ, Byzova TV, Plow EF. Platelet GPIIb-IIIa blockers. *Lancet* 1999;353:227.
72. Genetta TB, Mauro VF. Abciximab: a new antiaggregant used in angioplasty. *Ann Pharmacother* 1996;30:251.
73. Foster RH, Wiseman LR. Abciximab. An updated review of its use in ischaemic heart disease. *Drugs* 1998;56:629.
74. Mascelli MA, Lance ET, Damaraju L, et al. Pharmacodynamic profile of short-term abciximab treatment demonstrates prolonged platelet inhibition with gradual recovery from GP IIb/IIIa receptor blockade. *Circulation* 1998;97:1680.
75. Gammie JS, Zenati M, Kormos RL. Abciximab and excessive bleeding in patients undergoing emergency cardiac operations. *Ann Thorac Surg* 1998;65:465.
76. Hill JA, Kleaveland JP. Valvuloplasty. In: Pepine CJ, Hill JA, Lambert CR, eds. *Diagnostic and therapeutic cardiac catheterization.* Baltimore: Williams & Wilkins, 1989:267.
77. O'Connor BK, Beekman RH, Lindauer A, et al. Intermediate-term outcome after pulmonary balloon valvuloplasty: comparison with a matched surgical control group. *J Am Coll Cardiol* 1992;20:169.
78. Wang A, Harrison JK, Bashore TM. Balloon aortic valvuloplasty. *Prog Cardiovasc Dis* 1997;40:27.
79. McCredie RM, Hill AT, Allan RM, et al. Percutaneous transseptal mitral valvotomy—progress report. *Aust NZ J Med* 1998;28:805.
80. Borkon AM, Failing TL, Piehler JM, et al. Risk analysis of operative intervention for failed coronary angioplasty. *Ann Thorac Surg* 1992;54:884.
81. VanHaeke J, Flameng W, Sergeant P, et al. Emergency bypass surgery: late effects on size of infarction and ventricular function. *Circulation* 1985;72[Suppl 2]:179.
82. Weaver WD, Simes RJ, Betriu A, et al. Comparison of primary coronary angioplasty and intravenous thrombolytic therapy for acute myocardial infarction: a quantitative review. *JAMA* 1997; 278:2093.
83. de Bruijn NP, Hlatky MA, Jacobs JR, et al. General anesthesia during PTCA for acute myocardial infarction: results of a randomized controlled clinical trial. *Anesth Analg* 1989;68:201.
84. Kahn JK, Rutherford BD, McConahay DR, et al. Outcome following emergency coronary artery bypass grafting for failed elective balloon coronary angioplasty in patients with prior coronary bypass. *Am J Cardiol* 1990;66:285.
85. Naunheim KS, Fiore AC, Fagan DC, et al. Emergency coronary artery bypass grafting for failed angioplasty: risk factors and outcome. *Ann Thorac Surg* 1989;47:816.
86. Carey JA, Davies SW, Bacon R, et al. Emergency surgical revascularisation for coronary angioplasty complications. *Br Heart J* 1994;72:428.
87. Hochberg MS, Gregory JJ, McCullough J, et al. Early emergent coronary bypass after failed angioplasty. *NJ Med* 1993;90:385.
88. Satter P, Krause E, Skupin M. Mortality trends in cases of elective and emergency aortocoronary bypass after percutaneous transluminal coronary angioplasty. *Thorac Cardiovasc Surg* 1987;35:2.
89. Tinker JH. The scientific foundations for reperfusion of the acutely ischemic myocardium. In: Reves JG, ed. *Acute revascularization of the infarcted heart.* Orlando, FL: Grune & Stratton, 1987:1.
90. Murphy DA, Craver JM, Jones EL, et al. Surgical management of acute myocardial ischemia following percutaneous transluminal coronary angioplasty. Role of the intra-aortic balloon pump. *J Thorac Cardiovasc Surg* 1984;87:332.
91. Tomicheck RC, Rosow CE, Philbin DM, et al. Diazepam-fentanyl interaction: hemodynamic and hormonal effects in coronary artery surgery. *Anesth Analg* 1983;62:881.
92. Hinrichsen H, Halabi A, Kirch W. Clinical aspects of cardiovascular effects of H_2-receptor antagonists. *J Clin Pharmacol* 1995; 35:107.
93. Kaukoranta PK, Lepojarvi MV, Kiviluoma KT, et al. Myocardial protection during antegrade versus retrograde cardioplegia. *Ann Thorac Surg* 1998;66:755.
94. Gates RN, Laks H. Retrograde cardioplegia. *Adv Cardiac Surg* 1998;10:115.
95. Digerness SB, Kirklin JW, Naftel DC, et al. Coronary and systemic vascular resistance during reperfusion after global myocardial ischemia. *Ann Thorac Surg* 1988;46:447.
96. Haigney MCP, Silver B, Tanglao E, et al. Noninvasive measurement of tissue magnesium and correlation with cardiac levels. *Circulation* 1995;92:2190.
97. Teo KK, Yusuf S. Role of magnesium in reducing mortality in acute myocardial infarction. *Drugs* 1993;46:347.
98. England MR, Gordon G, Salem M, et al. Magnesium administration and dysrhythmias after cardiac surgery. A placebo-controlled, double-blind, randomized trial. *JAMA* 1992;268:2395.
99. Zaloga GP, Willey S, Malcolm D, et al. Hypercalcemia attenuates blood pressure response to epinephrine. *J Pharmacol Exp Ther* 1988;247:949.
100. Zaloga GP, Strickland RA, Butterworth JF IV, et al. Calcium attenuates epinephrine's beta-adrenergic effects in postoperative heart surgery patients. *Circulation* 1990;81:196.
101. Royster RL, Butterworth JF IV, Prielipp RC, et al. A randomized, blinded, placebo-controlled evaluation of calcium chloride and epinephrine for inotropic support after emergence from cardiopulmonary bypass. *Anesth Analg* 1992;74:3.
102. Butterworth JF IV, Zaloga GP, Prielipp RC, et al. Calcium inhibits the cardiac stimulating properties of dobutamine but not of amrinone. *Chest* 1992;101:174.
103. Killip T III, Kimball JT. Treatment of myocardial infarction in a coronary care unit: a two year experience with 250 patients. *Am J Cardiol* 1967;20:457.
104. Califf RM, Bengtson JR. Cardiogenic shock. *N Engl J Med* 1994;330:1724.
105. Volpi A, De Vita C, Franzosi MG, et al. Determinants of 6-month mortality in survivors of myocardial infarction after thrombolysis. Results of the GISSI-2 data base. *Circulation* 1993;88:416.
106. Goldberg RJ, Gore JM, Alpert JS, et al. Cardiogenic shock after acute myocardial infarction. Incidence and mortality from a community-wide perspective, 1975–1988. *N Engl J Med* 1991; 325:1117.
107. Crexells C, Chatterjee K, Forrester JS, et al. Optimal level of filling pressure in the left side of the heart in acute myocardial infarction. *N Engl J Med* 1973;289:1263.
108. Russell RO, Rackey CE, Pombo J, et al. Effects of increasing left ventricular filling pressure in patients with acute myocardial infarction. *J Clin Invest* 1970;49:1539.
109. Isner JM, Roberts WC. Right ventricular infarction complicating left ventricular infarction complicating coronary artery disease. *Am J Cardiol* 1978;42:885.
110. Shah PK, Maddahi J, Berman DS, et al. Scintigraphically detected predominant right ventricular dysfunction in acute myocardial infarction: clinical, hemodynamic correlates and implications for therapy and prognosis. *J Am Coll Cardiol* 1985;6:1264.
111. Reeder GS. Identification and treatment of complications of myocardial infarction. *Mayo Clin Proc* 1995;70:880.
112. Cox FF, Morshuis WJ, Plokker HWT, et al. Early mortality

after surgical repair of postinfarction ventricular septal rupture: importance of rupture location. *Ann Thorac Surg* 1996;61:1752.
113. Bouchart F, Bessou JP, Tabley A, et al. Urgent surgical repair of postinfarction ventricular septal rupture: early and late outcome. *J Cardiac Surg* 1998;13:104.
114. Smyllie JH, Sutherland GR, Geuskens R, et al. Doppler color flow mapping in the diagnosis of ventricular septal rupture and acute mitral regurgitation after myocardial infarction. *J Am Coll Cardiol* 1990;15:1449.
115. Cox FF, Plokker HW, Morshuis WJ, et al. Importance of coronary revascularization for late survival after postinfarction ventricular septal rupture. A reason to perform coronary angiography prior to surgery. *Eur Heart J* 1996;17:1841.
116. Gray RJ, Sethna D, Matloff JM. The role of cardiac surgery in acute myocardial infarction with mechanical complications. *Am Heart J* 1983;106:723.
117. Lowe JE, Gall SA. Correlates of survival in patients with postinfarction ventricular septal defect. *Ann Thorac Surg* 1997;63:1508.
118. Scanlon PJ, Montoya A, Johnson SA, et al. Urgent surgery for ventricular septal rupture complicating acute myocardial infarction. *Circulation* 1985;72[Suppl 2]:185.
119. Bolooki H. Emergency cardiac procedures in patients in cardiogenic shock due to complications of coronary artery disease. *Circulation* 1989;70[Suppl 1):137.
120. Kay GN, Wagner GS. Hemodynamic abnormalities in acute myocardial infarction. *Dis Mon* 1986;32:445.
121. DiSumma M, Actis Dato GM, Centofanti P, et al. Ventricular septal rupture after a myocardial infarction: clinical features and long term survival. *J Cardiovasc Surg* 1997;38:589.
122. Godley RW, Wann LS, Rogers EW, et al. Incomplete mitral leaflet closure in patients with papillary muscle dysfunction. *Circulation* 1981;63:565.
123. Wei JY, Hutchins GM, Bulkley BH. Papillary muscle rupture in fatal acute myocardial infarction: a potentially treatable form of cardiogenic shock. *Ann Intern Med* 1979;90:149.
124. Nishimura RA, Schaff HV, Shuh C, et al. Papillary muscle rupture complicating acute myocardial infarction: analysis of 17 patients. *Am J Cardiol* 1983;51:373.
125. Samman B, Korr KS, Katz AS, et al. Pitfalls in the diagnosis and management of papillary muscle rupture: a study of four cases and review of the literature. *Clin Cardiol* 1995;18:591.
126. Schnyder PA, Sarraj AM, Duvoisin BE, et al. Pulmonary edema associated with mitral regurgitation: prevalence of predominant involvement of the right upper lobe. *Am J Roentgenol* 1993;161:33.
127. Fuchs RM, Heuser RR, Yin FCP, et al. Limitations of pulmonary wedge V waves in diagnosing mitral regurgitation. *Am J Cardiol* 1982;49:849.
128. Konstadt SN, Louie EK, Shore-Lesserson L, et al. The effects of loading changes on intraoperative Doppler assessment of mitral regurgitation. *J Cardiothorac Vasc Anesth* 1994;8:19.
129. LeFeuvre C, Metzger JP, Lachurie ML, et al. Treatment of severe mitral regurgitation caused by ischemic papillary muscle dysfunction: indications for coronary angioplasty. *Am Heart J* 1992;123:860.
130. Borkenhagen DM, Serur JR, Gorlin R, et al. The effect of left ventricular load or contractility on mitral regurgitant orifice size and flow in the dog. *Circulation* 1977;56:106.
131. Tuman KJ, Carroll GC, Ivankovich AD. Pitfalls in interpretation of pulmonary artery catheter data. Review. *J Cardiothorac Anesth* 1989;3:625.
132. Grimm RA, Stewart WJ. The role of intraoperative echocardiography in valve surgery. *Cardiac Clin* 1998;16:477.
133. Kishon Y, Oh JK, Schaff HV, et al. Mitral valve operation in postinfarction rupture of a papillary muscle: immediate results and long-term follow-up of 22 patients. *Mayo Clin Proc* 1992;67:1023.
134. Hochman JS, Boland J, Sleeper LA, et al. Current spectrum of cardiogenic shock and effect of early revascularisation on mortality. *Circulation* 1995;91:873.
135. Stewart WJ, Currie PJ, Salcedo EE, et al. Intraoperative Doppler color flow mapping for decision-making in valve repair for mitral regurgitation. Technique and results in 100 patients. *Circulation* 1990;81:556.
136. Odell JA, Orszulak TA. Surgical repair and reconstruction of valvular lesions. *Curr Opin Cardiol* 1995;10:135.
137. Becker RC, Charlesworth A, Wilcox RG, et al. Cardiac rupture associated with thrombolytic therapy: impact of time to treatment in the late assessment of thrombolytic efficacy (LATE) study. *J Am Coll Cardiol* 1995;25:1063.
138. Becker RC, Gore JM, Lambrew C, et al. A composite view of cardiac rupture in the United States National Registry of Myocardial Infarction. *J Am Coll Cardiol* 1996;27:1321.
139. Second International Study of Infarct Survival) Collaborative Group. Randomized trial of intravenous streptokinase, oral aspirin, both, or neither among 17,187 cases of suspected acute myocardial infarction. *Lancet* 1988;2:349.
140. Feneley MP, Chang VP, O'Rourke MF. Myocardial rupture after acute myocardial infarction: ten year review. *Br Heart J* 1983;49:550.
141. Lopez-Sendon J, Gonzalez A, Lopez de Sa E, et al. Diagnosis of subacute ventricular wall rupture after acute myocardial infarction: Sensitivity and specificity of clinical, hemodynamic and echocardiographic criteria. *J Am Coll Cardiol* 1992;19:1145.
142. Oliva PB, Hammill SC, Edwards WD. Cardiac rupture, a clinically predictable complication of acute myocardial infarction: report of 70 cases with clinicopathologic correlations. *J Am Coll Cardiol* 1993;22:720.
143. Hochreiter C, Goldstein J, Borer JS, et al. Myocardial free-wall rupture after acute infarction: survival aided by percutaneous intra-aortic balloon counterpulsation. *Circulation* 1982;65:1279.
144. Windsor HM, Chang VP, Shanahan MX. Postinfarction cardiac rupture. *J Thorac Cardiovasc Surg* 1982;84:755.
145. Catherwood E, Mintz GS, Kotler MN, et al. Two-dimensional echocardiographic recognition of left ventricular pseudoaneurysm. *Circulation* 1980;62:294.
146. Mann T, McLaurin LP, Grossman W, et al. Assessing the hemodynamic severity of acute aortic regurgitation due to infective endocarditis. *N Engl J Med* 1975;293:108.
147. Cohn LH, Birjiniuk V. Therapy of acute aortic regurgitation. *Cardiac Clin* 1991;9:339.
148. Rapaport E. The changing role of surgery in the management of infective endocarditis [Editorial]. *Circulation* 1978;58:598.
149. Dhadphale PR, Jackson APF, Alseri S. Comparison of anesthesia with diazepam and ketamine vs morphine in patients undergoing heart-valve replacement. *Anesthesiology* 1979;51:200.
150. Tuman KJ, Keane DM, Spiess BD, et al. Effects of high-dose fentanyl on fluid and vasopressor requirements after cardiac surgery. *J Cardiothorac Anesth* 1988;2:419.
151. Kavoius J, Golocovsky M, Champion HR. Predictors of outcome in patients who have sustained trauma and who undergo emergency thoracotomy. *Arch Surg* 1993;128:1158.
152. Mittal V, McAleese P, Young S, et al. Penetrating cardiac injuries. *Am Surg* 1999;65:444.
153. Kato K, Kushimoto S, Mashiko K, et al. Blunt traumatic rupture of the heart: an experience in Tokyo. *J Trauma* 1994;36:859.
154. Tenzer ML. The spectrum of myocardial contusion: a review. *J Trauma* 1985;25:620.

155. Ho AMH, Ling E. Systemic air embolism after lung trauma. *Anesthesiology* 1999;90:564.
156. Czer LSC. Mediastinal bleeding after cardiac surgery: etiologies, diagnostic considerations, and blood conservation methods. *J Cardiothorac Anesth* 1989;3:760.
157. Unsworth-White MJ, Herriot A, Valencia O, et al. Resternotomy for bleeding after cardiac operation: a marker for increased morbidity and mortality. *Ann Thorac Surg* 1995;59:664.
158. Michelson EL, Torosian M, Morganroth J, et al. Early recognition of surgically correctable causes of excessive mediastinal bleeding after coronary artery bypass surgery. *Am J Surg* 1980; 139:313.
159. Hartstein G, Jannssens M. Treatment of excessive mediastinal bleeding after cardiopulmonary bypass. *Ann Thorac Surg* 1996; 62:1951.
160. Russo AM, O'Connor WH, Waxman HL. Atypical presentations and echocardiographic findings in patients with cardiac tamponade occurring early and late after cardiac surgery. *Chest* 1993;104:71.
161. Chuttani K, Pandian NG, Mohanty PK, et al. Left ventricular diastolic collapse. An echocardiographic sign of regional cardiac tamponade. *Circulation* 1991;83:1999.
162. Reichert CLA, Visser CA, Koolen JJ, et al. Transesophageal echocardiography in hypotensive patients after cardiac operations. *J Thorac Cardiovasc Surg* 1992;104:321.
163. Reardon MJ, Letsou GV, Reardon PR, et al. Left ventricular rupture following mitral valve replacement. *J Heart Valve Dis* 1996;5:10.
164. Yoshida K, Ohshima H, Murakami F, et al. Left ventricular free wall rupture following mitral valve replacement. *Ann Thorac Cardiovasc Surg* 1998;4:336.
165. Bohrer H, Gust R, Bottiger BW. Cardiopulmonary resuscitation after cardiac surgery. *J Cardiothorac Vasc Anesth* 1995;9: 352.

Cardiac Anesthesia: Principles and Clinical Practice, Second Edition, edited by Fawzy G. Estafanous, Paul G. Barash, and J.G. Reves. Lippincott Williams & Wilkins, Philadelphia © 2001.

PART

VI

THE CARDIAC PATIENT AND ANESTHESIA FOR NONCARDIAC SURGERY

29

ANESTHESIA FOR CARDIAC SURGERY IN THE PREGNANT PATIENT

RUTH LANDAU
RICHARD M. SMILEY

The presence of significant cardiac disease has traditionally been one of the great contraindications to pregnancy. For the pregnant woman with cardiac disease, regardless of whether previously diagnosed, the potential inability of the maternal cardiovascular system to contend with normal pregnancy-induced physiologic changes may produce deleterious effects on both mother and fetus. Maternal functional status may deteriorate during pregnancy, as evidenced by the fact that 44% of women with cardiac disease first develop pulmonary edema (or class IV status) in the third trimester of pregnancy (1).

In the past few decades, much progress has been made in the counseling and management of the obstetric patient with cardiac disease, leading to a progressive decline in maternal mortality from cardiovascular causes (Fig. 29-1). The maternal mortality rate in the 1990s was less than 1% in patients with mild to moderate cardiac disease. The reasons for this improved outcome include the decrease in rheumatic heart disease, the availability of surgical correction for many serious congenital and acquired cardiac diseases, and improved medical therapy for arrhythmias, heart failure, and so on. However, this progress has also allowed more women with significant cardiac pathology to attempt pregnancy and may result in some presenting for cardiac surgery during their pregnancy, when deterioration occurs. The mortality rate for pregnant women with more severe cardiac pathologies (New York Heart Association class III or IV) is higher (reported to be 5% to 15%), and the fetal mortality approaches 30% in this population of women. The risk of maternal mortality depends on the specific cardiac defect and the functional status before or early in pregnancy (Table 29-1) (2). In the presence of severe diseases such as pulmonary hypertension, coarctation of the aorta with involvement of the aortic root, or Marfan syndrome with aortic involvement, family planning and prepregnancy counseling to avoid pregnancy are appropriate, and first-trimester abortions should be considered when acceptable.

This chapter discusses the management of the somewhat unusual situation of the pregnant woman who presents for cardiac surgery. For the anesthesiologist, appropriate management has to take into account the usual anesthetic implications of pregnancy, the maternal cardiovascular adaptations to pregnancy with progressive increase of stresses on the abnormal heart, and some specific maternal-fetal issues related to cardiopulmonary bypass (CPB) during pregnancy. In addition, two issues are briefly discussed that are not specific to cardiac surgery during pregnancy but should be of some interest to cardiac anesthesiologists: myocardial infarction (MI) during pregnancy, and pregnancy in the heart transplant recipient.

CARDIOVASCULAR CHANGES DURING PREGNANCY

The development of the uteroplacental circulation induces major modifications in the cardiovascular physiology of the pregnant woman. Uterine blood flow (UBF) is approximately 3% of the total cardiac output during the first trimester and increases to 10% to 15% of cardiac output during the third trimester. The UBF is not autoregulated; it is directly proportional to the mean perfusion pressure and inversely proportional to uterine vascular resistance (UVR). α-Adrenergic stimulation increase UVR and therefore potentially decreases UBF and may increase uterine tone. β-Adrenergic stimulation has a minimal effect on UVR and UBF, because the uterine vasculature is maximally dilated during pregnancy. β-Adrenergic stimulation decreases uterine tone via a cyclic adenosine monophosphate–mediated mechanism.

R. Landau: Department of Anesthesiology, University Hospital of Geneva, Geneva 1211 Switzerland

R. M. Smiley: Department of Anesthesiology, Columbia University and Department of Obstetric Anesthesia, New York Presbyterian Hospital, New York, New York 10032

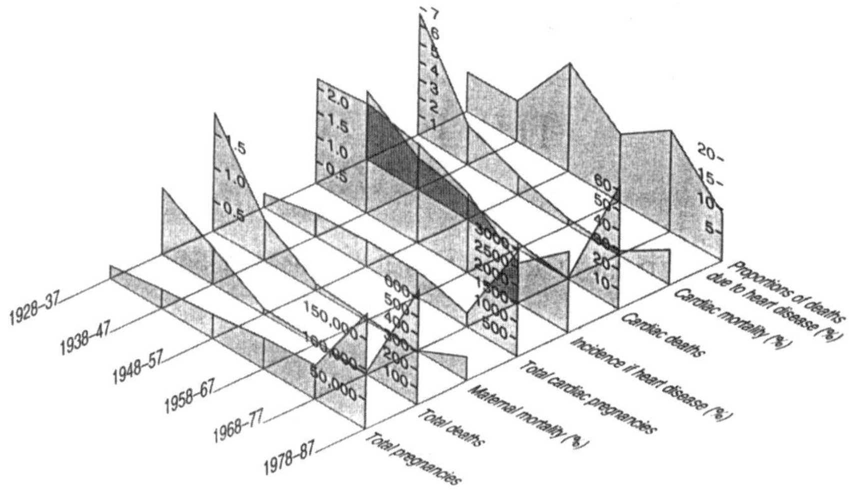

FIGURE 29-1. Heart disease, pregnancy, and cardiac mortality over six decades (1928–1987). (From Wooley CF, Sparks EH: Congenital heart disease, heritable cardiovascular disease and pregnancy. *Prog Cardiovasc Dis* 1992;35:41, with permission.)

Intravascular Volume

It is well established that the intravascular volume increases by 35% to 50% during pregnancy (3–5). The magnitude of the increase in red blood cell mass (20% to 30%) is not as great as the increase in plasma volume (50%), which results in a physiologic anemia of pregnancy (3,6). Many potential explanations for this volume expansion have been offered, all of which probably contribute to various degrees. Increased estrogen and progesterone production during pregnancy may increase blood volume by increasing the activity of the renin-angiotensin system (7,8). Enhanced activity of the renin-angiotensin system promotes sodium retention and volume expansion by stimulating the release of aldosterone and antidiuretic hormone. In addition, increased circulating levels of prostaglandin E_2 (PGE_2) and prostacyclin (PGI_2) may cause vasodilation with compensatory fluid retention to maintain apparent intravascular volume. These prostaglandins may also contribute to the decreased sensitivity exhibited by the maternal vasculature to the vasoconstricting effects of angiotensin II during pregnancy, allowing increased intravascular volume to be maintained at normal blood pressures (9,10). Teleologically, this volume expansion maximizes uteroplacental perfusion, protects the fetus during times of moderate maternal dehydration, and allows the obligate blood loss that will occur at delivery. However, it is this volume expansion and related effects that often result in hemodynamic deterioration in women with preexisting cardiac pathology.

TABLE 29-1. CARDIAC DISEASES AND MATERNAL MORTALITY RATE DURING PREGNANCY

<1%	5% to 15%	25% to 50%
Mitral stenosis, NYHA class I or II	Mitral stenosis, NYHA class III or IV	Pulmonary hypertension
Atrial or ventricular septal defect	Aortic stenosis or coarctation	Aortic coarctation with valvular involvement
Patent ductus arteriosus	Previous myocardial infarction	Marfan syndrome with aortic arch enlargement
Corrected tetralogy of Fallot	Uncorrected tetralogy of fallot	
Pulmonic/ tricuspid disease	Marfan syndrome with normal aortic arch	
Bioprosthetic valve	Mechanical valve	

Note: NYHA, New York Health Association.
Source: Data adapted from ACOG Technical Bulletin #168, Cardiac disease in pregnancy. *Int J Gynecol Obstet* 1993;41:298(reference 2).

Blood Pressure

Studies looking at changes in maternal blood pressure have produced conflicting results, with some studies showing a small decrease in mean arterial pressure and others not documenting any significant change (11–13). Confounding factors such as age and parity may mask blood pressure changes during pregnancy, because advancing age and parity appear to increase both systolic and diastolic blood pressures (14). In general, it is accepted that during pregnancy most women exhibit a widened pulse pressure, produced by a small fall in systolic pressure accompanied by a more significant fall in diastolic pressure. This becomes evident during the first trimester, becomes more pronounced during the second trimester, and may diminish at term, with blood pressures occasionally returning to prepregnancy values (14).

Heart Rate and Cardiac Output

The maternal heart rate increases by 10% to 20% during normal pregnancy (11,15–17). Cardiac output increases by as much as 40% to 50% (15,17–19). The early increase in cardiac output, which peaks between the 24th and 28th week, occurs sooner than the progressive increase in oxygen consumption noted throughout pregnancy (20–22). The relatively large increase in cardiac output observed early in gestation, coupled with the smaller increase in oxygen consumption, leads to a decreased arterial-venous oxygen difference in the first trimester.

A large percentage of the total change in cardiovascular parameters occurs by 8 weeks of gestation (11,22). This early appearance suggests a predominantly hormonal mechanism. The rate of increase in cardiac output is greatest in the first trimester, is slower in the second trimester, and peaks at approximately 24 to 28 weeks of gestation. In early pregnancy, the increase in cardiac output is secondary to an increase in stroke volume, achieved via a Frank-Starling mechanism. As a consequence, left ventricular end-diastolic volume increases, and this correlates with the expanded intravascular volume. As pregnancy progresses, the increase in heart rate assumes a greater role in the rising cardiac output. Oxygen consumption, a correlate of metabolic rate, also progressively increases throughout pregnancy, with 125% to 130% of nonpregnant values achieved at term, before labor and delivery (11,22). The obligate rise in cardiac output and heart rate is the factor most likely to result in cardiovascular decompensation in the gravida with significant cardiac disease, especially valvular stenosis or pulmonary hypertension.

Clark et al. (23) compared central hemodynamic data obtained by pulmonary artery catheterization of 10 healthy third-trimester patients with values recorded 11 to 13 weeks postpartum. There was no significant increase in left ventricular contractility as assessed by the left ventricular stroke work index. Pulmonary and central venous pressures were unchanged from nonpregnant values. In other studies (15, 16), ejection fraction was unchanged, supporting the observations that a hyperdynamic left ventricular function is not normally present and that the increased cardiac output is secondary to rises in stroke volume and heart rate.

Supine Hypotensive Syndrome

The compressive effect of the gravid uterus on the great vessels has been known for many years. Almost all women who are at or near term exhibit some degree of aortocaval compression by the gravid uterus when in the supine position (24,25). Caval compression by the uterus compromises venous return and ventricular filling, leading to a fall in cardiac output. A baroreceptor-mediated compensatory increase in sympathetic tone increases peripheral resistance and heart rate to maintain blood pressure in most women, so most pregnant women in the supine position do not become overtly hypotensive. However, about 10% of pregnant patients develop symptoms of hypotension when supine. This syndrome has been termed the "supine hypotensive syndrome of pregnancy" (26). It has been proposed that susceptible patients do not fully develop a paravertebral collateral circulation to overcome the caval occlusion or that these women are prone to vasovagal episodes, as evidenced by the fact that some patients become bradycardic when supine (24,26). By displacing the uterus to the left, the compressive effects of the uterus on the inferior vena cava can be minimized. This is particularly critical when the compensatory mechanism of sympathetic activation is compromised by drug therapy, cardiovascular disease, or regional or general anesthesia.

Cardiovascular Changes during the Postpartum Period

After delivery, the exact time for pregnancy-induced cardiovascular changes to revert to the prepregnancy state is unknown. Echocardiographic data obtained from 13 breast-feeding women 6 and 12 weeks postpartum, compared with their prepregnancy measurements, suggest that hemodynamic parameters may not be equivalent to prepregnancy measures even at 12 weeks postpartum (11). Stroke volume, end-diastolic volume, and cardiac output may remain increased and systemic vascular resistance decreased for several months after delivery. Postpartum values for both left ventricular wall thickness and mass have been shown to be increased when compared with those of a nonpregnant control group (16). An increase in aortic and pulmonary valve areas was reported in postpartum patients compared with nonpregnant controls, and in multiparous patients compared with primiparous patients (18,27). Therefore, at least in terms of the cardiovascular system, the postpartum woman is still, in the classic phrase, "a little bit pregnant." It is during this period that some women who have decompensated during labor and delivery, particularly those with mitral or aortic stenosis, may present for cardiac surgical repair.

DIAGNOSTIC STUDIES DURING PREGNANCY

There have been many reports of electrocardiographic (ECG) findings during pregnancy that would be viewed as abnormal in the nonpregnant woman. These include right-axis deviation and ST-segment abnormalities. ECG changes suggesting myocardial ischemia have been reported in as many as 37% of parturients undergoing cesarean section (28,29). These alterations have been attributed to hyperdynamic states (anxiety or imbalance of the autonomic system) promoting tachycardia or to the use of epidural epinephrine. These findings, although not directly relevant to the cardiac surgical patient, illustrate the potential problems in interpreting some "pregnant ECGs."

Some investigators have reported changes on chest radiographs in pregnancy that falsely indicate cardiac pathology. Normal pregnancy has been reported to result in enlargement of the left and right atria, pulmonary vessels, and the heart itself (30). In a later study of 200 routine chest radiographs in pregnant patients, however, no characteristic changes indicative of pregnancy were noted (31). The inconsistency in the radiographic findings may be attributable to the relatively small magnitude of the changes (typically less than 5 mm), which is on the order of the resolution of the radiographs. Turner suggested that the chest x-ray films of pregnant patients be interpreted with the same criteria used to interpret those of nonpregnant patients (31). Echocardiographic studies of normal human pregnancy show progressive left ventricular enlargement with a significant increase in total left ventricular mass. Left atrial and aortic root dimensions also increase with pregnancy (15,23,33).

More advanced diagnostic or therapeutic imaging studies may be required in pregnant women with significant heart disease. These may include use of radioactive materials or ionizing radiation, or both. Radionuclide ventriculography using technetium 99m and myocardial perfusion scanning with thallium 210 or ^{99m}technetium are expected to expose the fetus to less than 0.01 Gy. Cardiac catheterization and interventional procedures may also result in fetal exposure to 0.01 Gy. However, difficult procedures requiring longer fluoroscopy time could yield a fetal radiation exposure of 0.05 to 0.1 Gy. Termination of pregnancy is not generally recommended for fetal doses of radiation less than 0.05 Gy.

CARDIAC SURGERY DURING PREGNANCY

The first reported case of cardiac surgery during pregnancy was performed in 1956 by Daley et al. and published in 1957. Pulmonary commissurotomy without CPB was performed in a pregnant woman (3 months of gestation) who then delivered a normal baby at term (34). The first published case of cardiac surgery during pregnancy with CPB was performed by Leyse et al. in 1958 and reported in 1961. Aortic commissurotomy at 16 weeks of pregnancy resulted in good maternal outcome but fetal loss (35).

In a review of CPB during pregnancy over the period from 1958 to 1992, Pomini et al. (36) reported a maternal mortality rate of 2.9% and an embryo-fetal mortality rate of 20.2%. In a systematic review of all surgical cardiovascular cases occurring from 1984 to 1996 during pregnancy or immediately after delivery, Weiss et al. (37) reported 161 cases of surgery (137 with and 24 without CPB). Indications for surgery were native valve disease (58 cases), aortic-arterial dissection (32 cases), prosthetic valve dysfunction (23 cases), aortic-arterial aneurysm (17 cases), congenital anomaly (11 cases), pulmonary embolism (9 cases), heart tumor (7 cases), and coronary artery disease (4 cases); heart transplantations performed after delivery for peripartum cardiomyopathy or severe heart failure after coronary artery dissection were not included in the analysis. The most frequent surgical indications included rheumatic mitral stenosis, congenital aortic stenosis, dysfunction of a biologic prosthesis (it is common for prosthetic valves to degenerate during pregnancy) (38), thrombosis of a mechanical valve (despite heparin anticoagulation), and endocarditis. Endocarditis was the main indication for surgery to be postponed until after delivery and the main cause of death among valvular cases. Maternal outcome was worse when hospitalization occurred late in pregnancy and when surgery was performed immediately after delivery or postponed until later in the postpartum period. The global maternal mortality rate for the patients operated on during pregnancy was 6%, and the neonatal mortality rate was 30%. When surgery was performed immediately after delivery, maternal outcome was worse, with a mortality rate of 12% (5 cases) and a neonatal mortality rate of 5%. When surgery was postponed until some time after delivery, maternal mortality was even higher (14%). Neonatal outcome correlated with neither the gestational age at the time of surgery nor the duration and temperature of CPB. Not surprisingly, the highest maternal mortality rate was found among patients with aortic-arterial dissection repair and pulmonary embolectomy. The timing of operation and extremely emergent surgery were significant predictive factors of maternal and neonatal outcome. In the native valve surgery cases, 93% were performed with CPB and 7% in an emergency situation; the mortality rate was 9% (5 cases). In the prosthetic valvular group, all cases were done with CPB and 39% of them were emergent; the mortality rate was also 9% (2 cases) (37). This mortality rate is higher than the expected risk for valvular surgery; in a study of aortic valve replacement in a nonpregnant population of women of child-bearing age, the mortality rate was 2% (39). This suggests that pregnancy and the postpartum period increase the risk of valvular surgery two- to four-fold.

The most common preexisting cardiac disease manifested during pregnancy is mitral stenosis. However, with the decreasing incidence of rheumatic fever, it is seen much less frequently now than a few decades ago. As many as 25% of women with mitral stenosis are asymptomatic until they become pregnant, presenting when the hyperdynamic state associated with pregnancy accentuates murmurs and increases flow across the valve (1). Symptoms of pulmonary congestion usually appear by the midpoint of gestation and do not worsen after the 30th week of pregnancy. Labor may exacerbate cardiac symptoms secondary to the increased metabolic demand and tachycardia. Rapid volume shifts are dangerous and may account for sudden deaths reported in pregnant women with mitral stenosis. As with all patients with mitral stenosis, atrial fibrillation may occur acutely and lead to significant hemodynamic instability. The usual medical therapies (e.g., digitalization, verapamil) are appropriate in pregnancy, but electrical direct-current cardioversion should be performed promptly in many cases. There is little, if any, fetal risk of external cardioversion (40). Born et al. documented a maternal mortality rate of 13% and a neonatal mortality rate of 33% in a review of 30 women with rheumatic valvular disease operated on during pregnancy in the period from 1981 to 1992. Outcome in this series was influenced by prolonged cross-clamping and bleeding, but not by hypothermic CPB or gestational age at surgery (41).

Maternal mortality rates as high as 17% and fetal mortality rates as high as 32% have been reported in patients with aortic stenosis who become pregnant (42), although the severity of the lesion must be taken into account when risk is assessed. The increased cardiac output and left ventricular work demand of pregnancy frequently exacerbate symptoms. Acutely, any factor that decreases preload or venous return (e.g., caval compression by the enlarging uterus) will decrease the cardiac output in these patients, leading to a rapidly deteriorating course. A pulmonary autograft (Ross procedure) has been proposed as the procedure of choice in young women who require aortic valve replacement, because no valve-related complications were found in a series of 14 subsequent pregnancies in these patients (43).

In patients of child-bearing age, aortic insufficiency may manifest as an isolated lesion or in association with systemic vasculitis (e.g., rheumatoid arthritis, systemic lupus erythematosus, Marfan syndrome). The initial symptom of aortic regurgitation is usually fatigue, which is almost universally present in normal pregnant patients and prevents early diagnosis. Syncope, chest pain, and dyspnea on exertion are much more serious symptoms which develop later in the disease process. Aortic regurgitation is usually well tolerated in pregnancy, as might be expected from the hemodynamic profile, but when it results from active endocarditis surgery should be considered, because the mortality rate with medical therapy is high.

One of the most important decisions in the surgical/anesthetic management of these patients may be deciding *when* to perform the surgery. The timing of the surgery has been shown to be a major factor in determining maternal and fetal mortality. Many authors (44) suggest that the late second trimester or early third trimester (before the 30th week of gestation) is optimal. This timing avoids fetal drug exposure during organogenesis and allows surgery to be performed before the increased cardiovascular demands that occur later in the third trimester. If delivery becomes necessary, a neonate of almost 30 weeks' gestation has a reasonable chance of a good outcome. In most series, the overall fetal mortality rate is 20% to 30%. Parry et al., in 1996, suggested delaying surgery until near the end of the third trimester and performing a combined cesarean section with cardiac surgery (45). The cesarean section is done after heparinization but before cannulation, and the abdomen is left open during the valve operation to allow continuous assessment of uterine bleeding. When cardiac surgery is performed immediately after vaginal delivery maternal mortality has been shown to be as high as 12%, and even higher (14%) if surgery is performed in the postpartum period, compared with 6% when done during pregnancy (37). This may be a result of the increased cardiovascular demands of the postpartum period, or it may simply be a reflection of the fact that those patients presenting for cardiac surgery at this time may undergo surgery because they are *in extremis* after decompensation during labor and delivery.

MANAGEMENT OF CARDIOPULMONARY BYPASS AND ANESTHESIA

Heart surgery with CPB involves certain pathophysiologic effects, such as hypothermia, hemodilution, inhibition of coagulation, hemolysis, complement activation, and nonpulsatile flow, as well as acid-base changes that affect the uteroplacental circulation and the fetus. Nevertheless, multiple reports have demonstrated the relative safety of performing heart surgery with CPB during pregnancy (37,38, 45,46). However, because of the pregnancy-induced increases in cardiac output and oxygen consumption, alterations of routine CPB may be necessary to provide adequate perfusion and oxygenation to both mother and fetus. The major issues and controversies regarding CPB during pregnancy concern perfusion rate, pulsatile versus nonpulsatile flow, normothermic versus hypothermic management, and the impact of CPB on uterine tone and the fetal heart rate (FHR) tracing (bradycardia, loss of beat-to-beat variability).

Several studies have examined the quality (continuous versus pulsatile) and quantity (flow rate) of CPB while measuring the umbilical artery flow velocity with by transvaginal Doppler ultrasound. The first report of the use of Doppler ultrasonography during CPB in pregnancy was in 1989 during CPB for open mitral commissurotomy at 23 weeks' gestation (47). The authors reported that continuous, nonpulsatile CPB could maintain a pulsatile uterine flow. This conclusion has been questioned, with the suggestion that a pump artifact may have contributed to the observations (46). Both maternal and fetal outcome were favorable in the presence of high blood flow during CPB with a relatively high mean arterial pressure (85 to 95 mm Hg) and a normal FHR tracing. In a report in 1995 involving mitral valve replacement at 15 weeks of gestation with continuous CPB at high flow (4.7 L/minute) and hypothermia (29°C) and Doppler velocimetry, Goldstein et al. (48) described absent diastolic flow 10 minutes after initiation of CPB which persisted for 40 minutes and reappeared during the rewarming phase. In 1996, Khandelwal et al. (49) examined nonpulsatile CPB at normothermia during an aortic valve replacement at 19 weeks of gestation. Blood velocity waveforms were recorded with Doppler ultrasound at the level of the maternal main uterine artery and fetal vessels (49). A flat, nonpulsatile pattern in the uterine artery during CPB was noted. After unclamping of the aorta with continued extracorporeal circulation, a blunted pulsatile waveform was noted. As illustrated in Fig. 29-2B, a decrease in the FHR occurred immediately after maternal aortic clamping. Sustained bradycardia was noted throughout CPB, despite high pump flow rates, maintenance of normothermia, high mean arterial pressures, and hyperoxygenation. Transient fetal tachycardia was noted when normal circulation was resumed. The pulsatility indices of the fetal umbilical artery, middle cerebral artery, and descending aorta are reported in Fig. 29-2A.

Despite some suggestions described previously and later in this chapter, there are no firm scientific or clinical data supporting the superiority of a pulsating flow over a continuous flow in terms of uteroplacental flow and neonatal outcome. The use of pulsatile flow during CPB has been shown in sheep to preserve placental flow by prostaglandin production and/or inhibition of nitric oxide (NO) (50,51). It does appear that oxygen delivery to peripheral muscle is reduced with continuous flow and that the same phenomenon might occur in the fetus (52,53). In order to preserve placental flow and avoid hypotension-induced increased vascular resistance in the placenta, it is important to maintain a high flow rate and high perfusion pressure. Some investigators have found a direct correlation between pump flow and FHR pattern, suggesting that high flow with high maternal mean arterial pressure might improve placental flow and oxygen delivery to the fetus (54–56). There have been only a few case reports of the use of pulsatile CPB during pregnancy. Tripp et al., in 1999, described the use of a pulsatile perfusion for an aortic valve replacement at 14 weeks of gestation with a favorable maternal and fetal outcome (57). Oxygen delivery to the fetus is obviously crucial; however, there is not enough evidence in the literature to determine whether different priming solutions and severe hemodilution can adversely influence fetal outcome.

Hypothermia has been thought to be deleterious to the fetus through increasing uterine tone and thereby reducing UBF (58–62). The cause of the commonly seen uterine contractions during CPB is unknown but could be related to the presence of prostaglandins or other inflammatory factors known to be released during CPB, or to dilution of

A

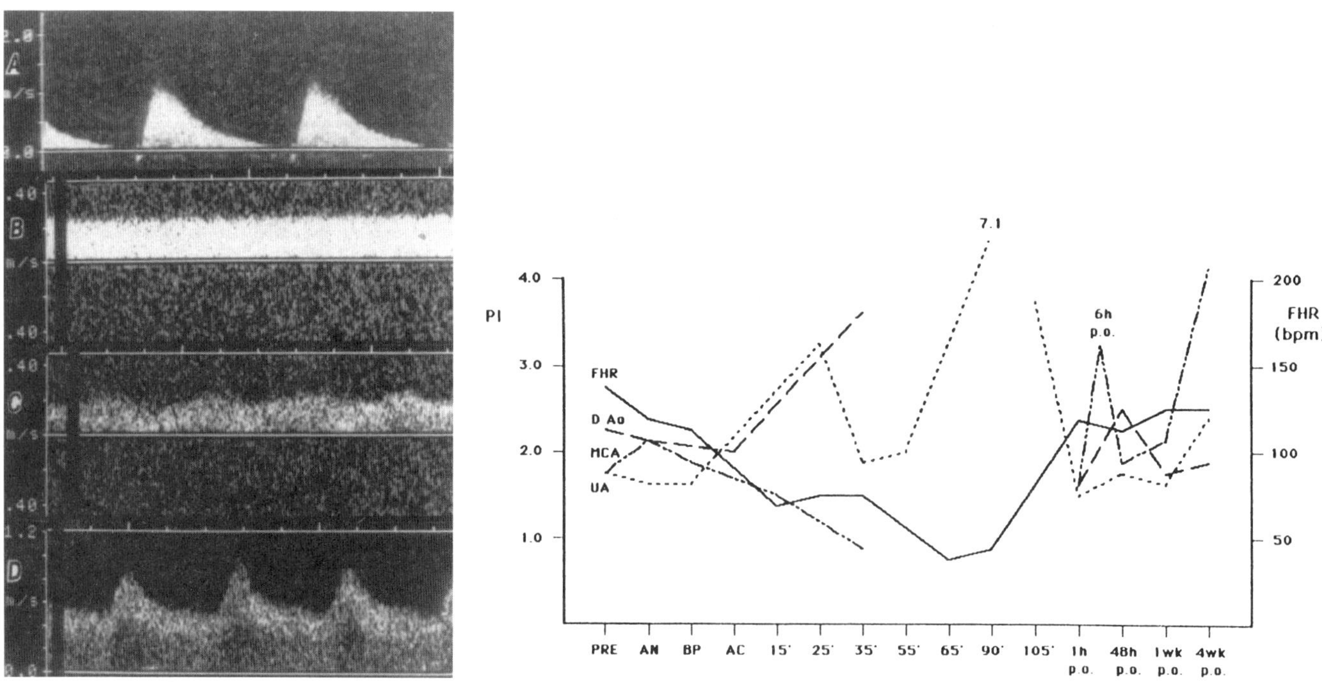

B

FIGURE 29-2. **A:** Blood velocity waveform pattern of the main uterine artery: *A*, before surgery; *B*, during cardiopulmonary bypass (CPB) with aortic clamp on; *C*, during CPB with aortic clamp off; *D*, postoperatively. **B:** Fetal heart rate (*FHR*) and pulsatility indices (*PI*) of fetal descending aorta (*Dao*), middle cerebral artery (*MCA*), and umbilical artery (*UA*) during and after CPB surgery. PRE, preoperative; AN, during general anesthesia before CPB; BP, beginning of CPB; AC, during bypass with aortic clamping; 15′–105′, respective minutes after initiation of CPB; p.o., postoperative; bpm, beats per minute. (From: Khandelwal M, Rasanen J, Ludormirski A, et al. Evaluation of fetal and uterine hemodynamics during maternal cardiopulmonary bypass. *Obstet Gynecol* 1996;88:667, with permission.)

progesterone and its inhibitory properties (63). Autoregulation of the FHR seems to be impaired when the temperature is reduced below 35°C. The placenta has been shown to be a poor oxygenator when placed in hypothermia (64). However, Buffolo et al., in 1994, reported the successful use of deep hypothermic circulatory arrest for an aortic arch aneurysm ruptured at 21 weeks of gestational age (65). The aortic aneurysm, secondary to Takayasu arteritis, was repaired with nonpulsatile CPB flow (mean flow rate, 2.4 L/minute/m^2) with 37 minutes of circulatory arrest at 19°C. Maternal and fetal outcomes were good.

In his series of 69 cases of CPB during pregnancy, Pomini specifically noted cases in which uterine contractility and FHR tracings were described (36). An important event during CPB is the initial hypotension that can compromise the fetal circulation. Almost all cases in which FHR was monitored reported fetal bradycardia on initiation of CPB. In some cases this bradycardia responded to an increase in pump flow (54–56). Loss of fetal beat-to-beat variability was frequently described, suggesting fetal stress, although such a finding is also common in the presence of certain drugs (e.g., opioids), so no definitive diagnosis can be made simply from loss of variability. Almost all cases reported a (presumably) compensatory fetal tachycardia once CPB was discontinued and normal maternal circulation was restored (36). In six cases, uterine contractions during CPB were observed, associated with FHR decelerations; serious decelerations disappeared despite the contractions as soon as normal maternal circulation was restored. One report, by Burke et al. in 1990, of a mitral valve replacement at normothermia (37°C) performed at 24 weeks' gestation, described a sinusoidal FHR pattern with oscillations between 120 and 150 beats/minute, returning to baseline with reduced variability for several hours at the end of CPB (66). Phenylephrine was used during CPB to raise the blood pressure to a mean of 50 mm Hg with no obvious positive or negative effect.

Maternal hyperventilation, often inadvertent, before or during bypass can result in alkalosis, further decreasing uteroplacental blood flow, and should be avoided. No maternal mortality or morbidity, nor instances of placental disruption, have been reported as a result of heparinization during CPB. Lamarra et al. reported in 1991 the use of aprotinin in an attempt to minimize bleeding in a reoperation for mitral valve replacement 2 hours after a cesarean section, with a positive maternal outcome (67).

There is no evidence for preferring any particular anesthetic strategy or drug regimen for surgery during pregnancy, and little or no information at all about anesthetic management in the case reports and series that comprise the clinical literature in the area of cardiac surgery during pregnancy. The choice of anesthetic technique and particular drugs should be based mostly on the usual criteria of patient pathophysiology, hemodynamics, and the surgical and postoperative plan. There are some controversies in the anesthetic management of pregnant women during noncardiac surgery, which would apply as well to surgery involving CPB. There is debate about the use of nitrous oxide because of its potential effect on methionine synthetase and DNA synthesis (68–71). Despite this theoretic concern, there is no evidence that clinical use of nitrous oxide in pregnant women should be avoided (72–74). Nitrous oxide is rarely part of most "cardiac anesthetics" in any case. Neither volatile agents nor barbiturates have been shown to be teratogenic in humans, although the number of studied anesthetic exposures during the vulnerable period of pregnancy has been small (75,76). It had been suggested that the use of benzodiazepines during the first trimester was associated with an increased incidence of cleft palate, which led to a contraindication for their use during pregnancy. This association has more recently been questioned (77). Although the evidence is weak, it would appear prudent to avoid benzodiazepines in early pregnancy if alternatives are readily available and appropriate. All opioids appear to be safe for use in anesthesia and postoperative analgesia during pregnancy. A summary of anesthetic and adjuvant drugs and some pregnancy-related effects is given in Table 29-2.

It is possible, perhaps likely, that some kind of pharmacologic hemodynamic support will be needed by the pregnant woman undergoing cardiac surgery. There is little scientific or clinical evidence for selecting one agent over another. The choice of inotropic or vasoactive drug should be based predominantly on the underlying pathology and hemodynamic goals, but several issues specific to pregnancy should be kept in mind. There is evidence that pregnancy is associated with a degree of resistance to vasoconstricting agents such as α-adrenergic agents and angiotensin II (9,10), and to β-adrenergic drugs (10,78–81). A recent human study did not detect this resistance to norepinephrine in the first and second trimester (82). The mechanism for the tolerance is unclear but may involve both pharmacokinetic and pharmacodynamic alterations. Higher doses of these drugs or infusions may be needed to achieve the desired hemodynamic effects. In practice, most of these agents are titrated to effect, so moderate alterations in sensitivity may be of more academic than clinical significance. Long clinical experience with the treatment of hypotension and decreased cardiac output from regional anesthetic-induced sympathetic blockade during cesarean section supports the safety of ephedrine as a first-line drug for "routine" hypotension and cardiac depression. The safety and utility of ephedrine has always been attributed to its being both a β- and mild α-adrenergic drug. The treatment of hypotension during pregnancy with drugs possessing a predominantly α-adrenergic mechanism (e.g., phenylephrine, perhaps norepinephrine) has been relatively contraindicated, based on data which suggested that although maternal blood pressure could be restored toward normal, UBF was further compromised. More recent studies during cesarean section have indicated

TABLE 29-2. ANESTHETIC AND CARDIOVASCULAR DRUGS: SPECIFIC CONSIDERATIONS RELEVANT TO PREGNANCY

Medication	Pregnancy Category[a]	Uterine Blood Flow	Uterine Tone	Comments	References
Induction agents					
Thiopental	C	↓ (40%)	—	—	111
Ketamine	D	↔	↑	—	112
		When not in labor: ↑ When in labor: ↓	↓ when in labor	—	113
Etomidate	C	—	—	—	—
Propofol	B	↔	—	—	111
Diazepam	D	↔	—	↑ risk of cleft lip (?)	—
Midazolam	D	↔	—	Teratogenic first trimester (?)	—
Inhalational agents[b]					
Nitrous oxide	—	—	—	Inhibition of DNA synthesis Safe at <50%	—
Halothane	—	↑ (22%) at 0.5%	Dose-dependent ↓ (1% relaxes uterus, 1.6% blocks oxytocics)	—	111
		↔ at 1.5 MAC ↓ at 2 MAC	—	—	114
Isoflurane	—	↔ at 1.5 MAC	Dose-dependent ↓ (1.5%: oxytocics not blocked)	—	111
		↓ (25%) at 1% + 50% N_2O			
Narcotics					
Fentanyl/sulfentanil	C	—	↔	↓ FH beat-to-beat variability Can mask fetal distress Neonatal chest rigidity	—
Muscle relaxants[c]					
Succinylcholine	C	—	↔	No placental transfer	—
Vecuronium	C	—	—	—	—
Pancuronium	C	—	↔	Used safely in fetal surgery	—
Atracurium	C	—	—	No placental transfer	—
Curare	—	—	—	Teratogenic in chick embryos	—
Inotropic and vasoactive drugs					
Ephedrine	C	↔ (when BP ↑ 50%)	—	↑ FH beat-to-beat variability	115
Phenylephrine	C	↓ UBF, ↑ UVR (when BP ↑ 20%)	—	25–50 μg safe for ↓ BP	83–86,116,117
Dopamine (conflicting data)	C	↑ at >5 μg/kg/min	—	↑ BP, ↑ CO	118
		↓ at >10 μg/kg/min, ↑↑ UVR	—	↑ BP, ↑ CO	119
				Fetal acidosis at high doses Variable changes in MHR	
Dobutamine	C	↓ UBF, ↑ UVR	—	↑ MHR, BP	120
Epinephrine	C	↓	↓ with low doses ↑ with high doses	—	—
Norepinephrine	C	↓ at >0.5 μg/kg/min	—	↑ BP, ↓ MHR	117,121
Amrinone	C	↔ at <40 μg/kg/min	—	↔ BP, ↔ MHR	120
Digoxin	C	—	—	↑ doses during pregnancy (↑ GFR) Used to treat fetal arrhythmias	122,123
β-Blockers[d]					
Esmolol	C	—	—	↓ FBP (12%), ↓ FHR (7%) ↔ fetal acid-base status	124
Labetolol	C	—	—	Safe	—
Propranolol	C	—	—	—	—

TABLE 29-2. ***Continued.***

Medication	Pregnancy Category[a]	Uterine Blood Flow	Uterine Tone	Comments	References
Vasodilators					
Nitroglycerin	C	↑	Uterine relaxation	—	125,126
Sodium nitroprusside	C	↔	—	Cyanide toxicity at high doses Safe at <3 μg/kg/min	127
Hydralazine	C	↑	—	Maternal reflex tachycardia	—
ACE inhibitors	D	—	—	Contraindicated because of fetal abnormalities	—
Magnesium sulfate	A	↑	Potent tocolytic	—	128
Calcium channel blockers					
Verapamil	C	↓	—	↑ PR interval in the fetus Used to treat fetal arrhythmias ↔ fetaL BP and acid-bases status	129 123,130
Nifedipine	C	No significant ↓	—	↓ BP, ↑ MHR	131
Nicardipine	C	↓	—	↑ MHR, ↑ CO	131
Antiarrhythmics					
Lidocaine	B	↔	—	First choice of ventricular arrhythmia	132
Procainamide	C	—	—	Used to treat fetal arrhythmia	133
Bretylium	C	—	—	Fetal safety not established	—
Anticholinergics					
Atropine	C	—	—	FHR and variability not affected	134
Glycopyrrolate	B	—	—	FHR and variability not affected	—
Diuretics					
Mannitol	C	—	—	Fetal diuresis, well tolerated	—
Furosemide	C	—	—	Fetal diuresis	135
Anticoagulants					
Heparin	C	—	—	Safe, no placental transfer	—
Warfarin	X	—	—	Fetal deformity, hemorrhage or death	—
Protamine	C	—	—	—	—
Gastrointestinal agents					
Sodium citrate	—	—	—	Used routinely in pregnancy	—
Cimetidine	B	—	—	—	—
Ranitidine	B	—	—	Used routinely in pregnancy	—
Metoclopramide	B	—	—	Used routinely in pregnancy	—
Analgesics					
Acetylsalicilic acid	—	—	—	Premature closure of fetus ductus arteriosus Possible pulmonary hypertension, small fetus ↑ risk of kernicterus, platelet dysfunction, ↓ factor XII	—
NSAIDs[e]	B/B/D	—	—	Premature closure of fetus ductus arteriosus Possible pulmonary hypertension	—

Note: ↔, no change; ↑, increase; ↓, decrease; ACE, angiotensin-converting enzyme; BP, blood pressure; CO, cardiac output; FBP, fetal blood pressure; FHR, fetal heart rate; GFR, glomerular filtration note; MHC, minimum alveolar concentration; MBP, maternal blood pressure; MHR, maternal heart rate; N_2O, nitrous oxide; NSAIDs, nonsteroidal antiinflammatory drugs; UBF uterine blood flow; UVR uterine vascular resistance.

[a] Pregnancy category:
A—Controlled studies in pregnant women show no risk to the fetus.
B—No evidence of risk in humans because animal studies are positive but human studies are negative, or because animal studies are negative and humans are not adequately studied.
C—Risk to the human fetus cannot be ruled out because animal studies are lacking or are positive for fetal risk; benefits may outweigh risks.
D—There is positive evidence of fetal risk, but benefits may still outweigh risks.
X—Contraindicated in pregnancy.

[b] ↓ MAC during pregnancy: 25%–40%.

[c] ↓ plasma pseudocholine esterase levels during pregnancy with no clinical significance.

[d] Potential increase in uterine tone with nonselective β-blockers.

[e] NSAIDs is pregnancy risk category B in first and second trimesters, D during third trimester.

that moderate doses (40- to 100-μg boluses) of phenylephrine are as safe and effective as ephedrine in restoring maternal blood pressure while allowing adequate UBF. This work supports the use of α-adrenergic agents when hemodynamically indicated (83–86). Ephedrine, phenylephrine, dobutamine, dopamine, epinephrine, and norepinephrine have all been utilized in pregnant women undergoing cardiac surgery. FHR monitoring is obviously necessary, and deterioration of the FHR in the face of potential uterine artery vasoconstriction should prompt reconsideration of the indication and need for such therapy.

CARDIOPULMONARY RESUSCITATION

Should the need for cardiopulmonary resuscitation (CPR) arise, there are a few special considerations during pregnancy (87). These include increased oxygen requirements, decreased functional residual capacity, and reduction of venous return if compression of the vena cava occurs. This can lead to severe and rapid hypoxia during periods of cardiac arrest. In addition to these physiologic changes, chest compressions are less effective secondary to an increase in the anterior-posterior diameter of the chest and engorgement of the breasts, which may also prevent adequate conduction of defibrillating doses of electrical energy. The apical lead of the defibrillator should be placed more laterally than is customary for nonpregnant patients. The fetal myocardial fibrillatory threshold exceeds that in adults, so there is little danger of harming the fetus with attempts at maternal defibrillation. A case report in which severe hypotension secondary to massive hemoptysis occurred in a woman at 36 weeks of gestation illustrates the dramatic effect of the "supine hypotensive syndrome" on the outcome of CPR in late gestation (88). Despite endotracheal intubation, closed-chest massage, and vigorous fluid and electrolyte therapy, adequate circulation was not restored until cesarean delivery of the baby. To optimize maternal and fetal survival, Katz et al. suggested that only 4 minutes elapse between onset of cardiopulmonary arrest and delivery of the infant by cesarean section ("perimortem" cesarean section) (89), a recommendation echoed by others (90). The potential to "crash" onto bypass in the cardiac operating room might suggest some modification of this rule in specific circumstances, especially if the underlying cardiac pathology (e.g., mitral stenosis), makes successful CPR unlikely even after delivery. Drug therapy should not be different than in the nonpregnant patient. In particular, epinephrine should be given early in "resuscitation" doses (500 μg to 1 mg), because its deleterious effects on UBF should be of no concern in the face of a cardiac arrest. The approach to CPR during pregnancy varies according to the gestational age and is summarized in the algorithm in Fig. 29-3. After 20 weeks of gestation, in addition to standard CPR techniques, the uterus must be displaced from the abdominal and pelvic veins by tilting to the left (91).

MYOCARDIAL INFARCTION DURING PREGNANCY

The estimated incidence of MI during pregnancy is 1 : 10,000, with a preponderance of anterior versus inferior infarctions and with most being transmural (92). MIs typi-

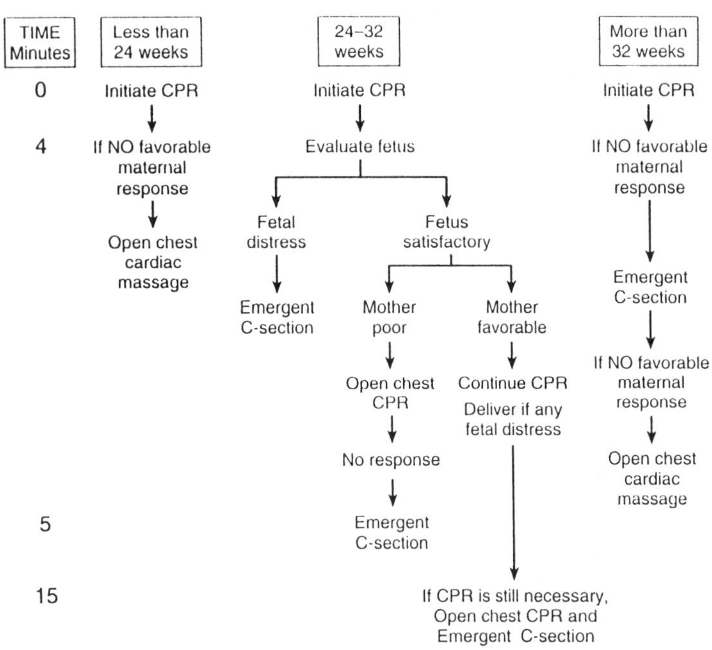

FIGURE 29-3. Management of cardiopulmonary arrest in pregnant women. (From: Lee RV, Medrazzi FC: Cardiopulmonary resuscitation of pregnant women. In: Elkayam U, Gleicher N, eds. *Cardiac problems in pregnancy: diagnosis and management of maternal and fetal disease,* 2nd ed. New York: Alan R. Liss, 1990:307. Copyright © Alan R. Liss, 1990. Reprinted by permission of [Wiley-Liss, Inc., a subsidiary of] John Wiley & Sons, Inc.)

cally occur antepartum in multiparous females and postpartum in primiparous patients. The latter finding is probably consequent to the increased incidence of preeclampsia in primiparous women. The overall mortality rate is higher in the younger population, with 48% for women younger than 35 years of age and 34% for older women. The highest mortality rate appears to be associated with MI in the third trimester or if delivery occurs within 2 weeks of an acute MI. Fetal mortality appears to be associated with maternal outcome, because 15 of 23 deaths occurred simultaneously with maternal death in the cases reviewed by Hankins et al. (93).

In a review of 105 cases of acute MI in pregnancy, Roth et al. reported that atherosclerotic disease was found in fewer than 50% of pregnant women in whom coronary anatomy was investigated (94). Other causes of MI may include thrombosis, coronary artery spasm (spontaneous, or induced by bromocryptine mesylate, coronary artery dissection, or collagen vascular disease), Kawasaki disease, cocaine use, aortic stenosis, aortic prosthetic valve thrombosis, sickle cell disease, and pheochromocytoma. It is well established that pregnancy is a hypercoagulable state due to the decreased release of tissue plasminogen activator (t-PA), increased fast-acting t-PA inhibitor, and a reduction in functional protein S levels. Transient coronary spasm in pregnancy might result in acute coronary thrombosis. At the time of separation of the placenta, hypercoagulability is further promoted, because the placenta is a major source of t-PA inhibitor. In pregnancy-induced hypertension and preeclampsia, enhanced vascular reactivity to angiotensin II and norepinephrine as well as endothelial dysfunction may also induce coronary constriction.

Coronary arterial dissections have been reported to occur during and after pregnancy, with most cases in the postpartum period. The first case was described by Pretty in 1931 (95). Advanced maternal age and multiparity may increase the risk. The majority of the cases reported involve the proximal or mid-left anterior descending coronary artery (94). The dissection may be hormonally mediated, resulting from an excess of progesterone during pregnancy that induces structural abnormalities in coronary vessel walls, loss of normal corrugation in elastic fibers, fragmentation of reticular fibers, and marked transformation of muscular arteries. Klutstein et al., in a report of three cases, suggested stent implantation, because the arterial wall is very friable and angioplasty alone does not prevent propagation of the dissection (96). In their series, two women were treated by primary stenting and the third by coronary artery bypass grafting without CPB at 20 weeks of pregnancy, with a favorable maternal and fetal outcome. Curiel reported a case in which a 33-year-old woman had a massive MI 4 days after delivery and was referred for heart transplantation (97).

Cardiac enzyme changes in the pregnant patient may not be diagnostic for MI. Numerous authors have shown that an elevation of the creatine kinase MB isoenzyme (CK-MB) fraction can result from sources other than the heart (98). Placental CK normally contains a 1% MB fraction (99). In normal pregnancy, the serum MB fraction may be elevated almost 100% from that of the nonpregnant state (2.1 versus 1.1 units/L). Although the exact source of the elevated MB fraction remains unknown, most of the CK elevation seen after delivery is from the MM fraction secondary to skeletal muscle damage during labor; some patients are also positive for the BB fraction, because the uterus contains only CK-BB. It is postulated that the elevated CK-MB may come from cord blood or from some small amount of myocardial damage associated with normal pregnancy (100).

Treatment of acute infarction in pregnancy is similar to that in nonpregnant patients, with several additional considerations. β-Adrenergic antagonists may be useful although, they may be associated with premature labor (101,102). Cardioselective β-blockers are preferred. Systemic thrombolytic therapy is relatively contraindicated in pregnancy because of the potential increased risk of both maternal and fetal hemorrhage. If fibrinolytic agents are used before 14 weeks of gestation, there may be significant effects on the placenta and its implantation; later use has resulted in pregnancy loss (103). Circulating plasminogen activated by thrombolytics may be responsible for the onset of premature labor.

There are several case reports of percutaneous transluminal coronary angioplasty during pregnancy, with or without intracoronary thrombolysis. The risks of angioplasty in pregnancy are similar to those in the nonpregnant population and include arrhythmias, arterial embolization, contrast agent toxicity, and vascular injury at the catheter site, as well as fetal radiation exposure. Catheterization should be avoided in the first trimester because of the radiation risks to the fetus. The risks to the fetus should maternal arrest or prolonged arrhythmia occur during the procedure need to be considered. Only a few cases of intracoronary thrombolysis during pregnancy have been reported (104–106). Urokinase is the preferred agent because it is a human protein, so there are fewer allergic, febrile, and hypotensive reactions than with streptokinase, and there is less systemic lytic effect as measured by serum fibrinogen levels. The effective dose of urokinase in pregnancy may be increased because of the inhibitors secreted by the placenta. Weiss et al. (37) reported only four cases of coronary artery bypass grafting performed for coronary artery disease, with a maternal morbidity rate of 75% and no fatal cases.

CARDIAC TRANSPLANTATION

There have not been any reports of cardiac transplantation during pregnancy. However, cardiac transplantation has been a therapy for postpartum cardiomyopathy and other acute postpartum decompensation (97,107). In addition, the cardiac anesthesiologist might well be consulted about the obstetric and anesthetic management of the pregnant woman who has previously undergone cardiac transplantation. The first case of a successful pregnancy after heart transplantation was reported by Lowenstein et al. in 1988. The literature reports more than 30 such pregnancies. Three classes of maternal risk are associated with pregnancy after cardiac transplantation: cardiovascular, immunologic (rejection), and infectious.

A transplanted heart is denervated and responds to pregnancy-related hemodynamic changes without the autonomic nervous system. However, through adaptive mechanisms involving an increase in stroke volume in response to increased central venous pressure and volume (Frank-Starling mechanism), as well as an increased response to the circulating catecholamines resulting in an increased contractility, a transplanted heart should tolerate the hemodynamic changes induced by pregnancy and delivery. Rejection, however, may result in systolic and diastolic dysfunction leading to an inability of the transplanted heart to increase the stroke volume in response to increased venous return. Fetal risks are mostly related to the immunosuppressive therapy. There may be a higher incidence of spontaneous abortions, stillbirth, congenital malformations, prematurity, low birth weight, and infection (mostly viral). Cyclosporine crosses the placenta and can be found in cord blood, amniotic fluid, and breast milk at high concentrations; however, no teratogenic or lethal effects have been associated with therapeutic doses. Azathioprine induces bone marrow suppression, and metabolites of the drug cross the placenta. Nevertheless, azathioprine appears to be safe and is not associated with an increased risk of congenital abnormalities. In a review of 22 pregnancies among heart transplant recipients, Morini et al. (108) reported that pregnancy outcome did not seem to correlate with time since transplantation, which ranged from 3 to 72 months. The course and outcome of pregnancy were influenced by the woman's clinical condition and cardiovascular function. The most frequent complications were hypertension (36%), infections (27%), and preeclampsia (13%). The spontaneous abortion rate was not higher than in the general population, which is estimated to be 15% to 20%. Preterm birth occurred in 41% of cases. Scott et al. (109) reported similar findings in a series of 30 pregnancies after cardiac transplantation, and Wagoner et al. (110) described the immunosuppressive therapy, management, and outcome of heart transplant recipients during pregnancy in a review of 32 cases. Although all of these reports showed an increased incidence of complications, pregnancy seemed to be fairly well tolerated by heart transplant recipients. Heart transplantation is not in itself an indication for cesarean section. Morini reported a vaginal delivery rate of 62.5%, mostly performed under regional anesthesia.

SUMMARY

Despite 40 years of CPB during cardiac surgery in pregnant women, only about 200 cases have been reported. Few of these reports even mention anesthesia care outside of CPB management. In the era of evidence-based medicine, this provides little support for firm recommendations regarding anesthetic strategy. The anesthetic and surgical management of a pregnant woman undergoing cardiac surgery is likely to be stressful for all concerned. In the context of this unusual circumstance, it is important not to forget the basics of anesthetic care in pregnancy. Left uterine displacement, aspiration prophylaxis, and rapid-sequence induction with cricoid pressure are indicated for any anesthesia in a pregnant woman after approximately 18 weeks of gestation. FHR monitoring and uterine tocodynamometry should be used, given the known effects of CPB. Relatively high pressures and flows should probably be used during CPB. The anesthesiologist and perfusionist must be prepared to treat alterations in the FHR with increases in perfusion pressure or flow and to use tocolytic drugs (volatile agents, β-adrenergic agonists, nitroglycerin, magnesium sulfate) for uterine hypertonicity or contractions. Hyperventilation should be avoided. There is some evidence that pulsatile bypass is preferable, but this has not been clearly demonstrated. Although hypothermia has been used successfully, we recommend avoiding it unless it is strongly indicated. Consultation with an obstetrician/perinatologist is obviously mandatory preoperatively. The obstetrician must be available intraoperatively and postoperatively in the event that a decision must be made regarding urgent or emergent delivery. Facilities for resuscitation and care of the neonate are essential.

REFERENCES

1. Szekely P, Turner R, Snaith L. Pregnancy and the changing pattern of rheumatic heart disease. *Br Heart J* 1973;35:1293.
2. Anonymous. ACOG Technical Bulletin. Cardiac disease in pregnancy. *Int J Gynecol Obstet* 1993;41:298.
3. Pritchard. Changes in the blood volume during pregnancy and delivery. *Anesthesiology* 1965;26:393.
4. Pirani BB, Campbell DM, MacGillivray I. Plasma volume in normal first pregnancy. *J Obstet Gynaecol Br Commonw* 1973; 80:884.
5. Hytten FE, Paintin DP. Increase in plasma volume in normal first pregnancy. *J Obstet Gynaecol Br Commonw* 1963;70:407.
6. Chesley LC. Plasma and red cell volumes during pregnancy. *Am J Obstet Gynecol* 1972;112:440.
7. Walters WA, Lim YL. Cardiovascular dynamics in women receiving oral contraceptive therapy. *Lancet* 1969;2:881.
8. Little B. Water and electrolyte balance during pregnancy. *Anesthesiology* 1965;26:408.
9. Gant NF, Daley GL, Chand S, et al. A study of angiotensin II pressor response throughout primigravid pregnancy. *J Clin Invest* 1973;52:2682.
10. Gant NF, Worley RJ, Everett RB, et al. Control of vascular

responsiveness during human pregnancy. *Kidney Int* 1980;18: 253.
11. Capeless EL, Clapp JF. Cardiovascular changes in early phase of pregnancy. *Am J Obstet Gynecol* 1989;161:1449.
12. Andros G. Blood pressure in normal pregnancy. *Am J Obstet Gynecol* 1945;50:305.
13. MacGillivray I, Rose GA, Rowe B. Blood pressure survey in pregnancy. *Clin Sci* 1969;37:395.
14. Christianson RE. Studies on blood pressure during pregnancy. I: influence of parity and age. *Am J Obstet Gynecol* 1976;125: 509.
15. Katz R, Karliner JS, Resnik R. Effects of a natural volume overload state (pregnancy) on left ventricular performance in normal human subjects. *Circulation* 1978;58:434.
16. Robson SC, Hunter S, Moore M, et al. Haemodynamic changes during the puerperium: a Doppler and M-mode echocardiographic study. *Br J Obstet Gynaecol* 1987;94:1028.
17. Ueland K, Novy MJ, Peterson EN, et al. Maternal cardiovascular dynamics: IV. The influence of gestational age on the maternal cardiovascular response to posture and exercise. *Am J Obstet Gynecol* 1969;104:856.
18. Robson SC, Dunlop W, Moore M, et al. Combined Doppler and echocardiographic measurement of cardiac output: theory and application in pregnancy. *Br J Obstet Gynaecol* 1987;94: 1014.
19. Clark SL, Southwick J, Pivarnik JM, et al. A comparison of cardiac index in normal term pregnancy using thoracic electrical bio-impedance and oxygen extraction (Fick) techniques. *Obstet Gynecol* 1994;83:669.
20. Pernoll ML, Metcalfe J, Schlenker TL, et al. Oxygen consumption at rest and during exercise in pregnancy. *Respir Physiol* 1975;25:285.
21. Prowse CM GE. Respiratory and acid-base changes during pregnancy. *Anesthesiology* 1965;26:392.
22. Clapp JF, Seaward BL, Sleamaker RH, et al. Maternal physiologic adaptations to early human pregnancy. *Am J Obstet Gynecol* 1988;159:1456.
23. Clark SL, Cotton DB, Lee W, et al. Central hemodynamic assessment of normal term pregnancy. *Am J Obstet Gynecol* 1989;161:1439.
24. Kerr MG, Scott DB, Samuel E. Studies of the inferior vena cava in late pregnancy. *Br Med J* 1964;1:533.
25. Bieniarz J, Yoshida T, Romero-Salinas G, et al. Aortocaval compression by the uterus in late human pregnancy: IV. Circulatory homeostasis by preferential perfusion of the placenta. *Am J Obstet Gynecol* 1969;103:19.
26. Holmes F. The supine hypotensive syndrome. *Anaesthesia* 1995; 50:972.
27. Hart MV, Morton MJ, Hosenpud JD, et al. Aortic function during normal human pregnancy. *Am J Obstet Gynecol* 1986; 154:887.
28. Palmer CM, Norris MC, Giudici MC, et al. Incidence of electrocardiographic changes during cesarean delivery under regional anesthesia [see comments]. *Anesth Analg* 1990;70:36.
29. Palmer CM. What do electrocardiographic and echocardiographic changes during cesarean delivery mean? [Letter; comment]. *Anesth Analg* 1993;76:457.
30. Keats TE. Some innocent, but misleading variations in cardiac contour. *Med Times* 1968;96:337.
31. Turner AF. The chest radiograph in pregnancy. *Clin Obstet Gynecol* 1975;18:65.
32. Robson SC, Hunter S, Dunlop W. Left atrial dimension during early puerperium [Letter]. *Lancet* 1987;2:111.
33. Rubler S, Damani PM, Pinto ER. Cardiac size and performance during pregnancy estimated with echocardiography. *Am J Cardiol* 1977;40:534.
34. Daley R, Harrison GK, McMillan IKR. Direct vision pulmonary valvotomy during pregnancy. *Lancet* 1957;273:875.
35. Leyse R, Ofstun M, Dillard DH, et al. Congenital aortic stenosis in pregnancy, corrected by extracorporeal circulation. *JAMA* 1961;176:1009.
36. Pomini F, Mercogliano D, Cavalletti C, et al. Cardiopulmonary bypass in pregnancy. *Ann Thorac Surg* 1996;61:259.
37. Weiss BM, von Segesser LK, Alon E, et al. Outcome of cardiovascular surgery and pregnancy: a systematic review of the period 1984–1996. *Am J Obstet Gynecol* 1998;179:1643.
38. Sullivan HJ. Valvular heart surgery during pregnancy. *Surg Clin North Am* 1995;75:59.
39. von Segesser LK, Schwaller A, Amman FW. Initial follow-up results of aortic valve replacement with the CarboMedics bileaflet prosthesis. *Helv Chir Acta* 1993;60:457.
40. Curry JJ, Quintana FJ. Myocardial infarction with ventricular fibrillation during pregnancy treated by direct current defibrillation with fetal survival. *Chest* 1970;58:82.
41. Born D, Martinez EE, Almeida PA, et al. Pregnancy in patients with prosthetic heart valves: the effects of anticoagulation on mother, fetus, and neonate. *Am Heart J* 1992;124:413.
42. Arias F, Pineda J. Aortic stenosis and pregnancy. *J Reprod Med* 1978;20:229.
43. Ross D. Replacement of the aortic valve with a pulmonary autograft: the "switch" operation. *Ann Thorac Surg* 1991;52:1346.
44. Johnson MD, Saltzman DH. Cardiac disease. In: Datta S, ed. *Anesthetic and obstetric management of high-risk pregnancy.* St. Louis: Mosby, 1996:210.
45. Parry AJ, Westaby S. Cardiopulmonary bypass during pregnancy. *Ann Thorac Surg* 1996;61:1865.
46. Strickland RA, Oliver WC Jr, Chantigian RC, et al. Anesthesia, cardiopulmonary bypass, and the pregnant patient. *Mayo Clin Proc* 1991;66:411.
47. Farmakides G, Schulman H, Mohtashemi M, et al. Uterine-umbilical velocimetry in open heart surgery. *Am J Obstet Gynecol* 1987;156:1221.
48. Goldstein I, Jakobi P, Gutterman E, et al. Umbilical artery flow velocity during maternal cardiopulmonary bypass. *Ann Thorac Surg* 1995;60:1116.
49. Khandelwal M, Rasanen J, Ludormirski A, et al. Evaluation of fetal and uterine hemodynamics during maternal cardiopulmonary bypass. *Obstet Gynecol* 1996;88:667.
50. Champsaur G, Parisot P, Martinot S, et al. Pulsatility improves hemodynamics during fetal bypass: experimental comparative study of pulsatile versus steady flow. *Circulation* 1994;90:II47.
51. Sabik JF, Heinemann MK, Assad RS, et al. High-dose steroids prevent placental dysfunction after fetal cardiac bypass. *J Thorac Cardiovasc Surg* 1994;107:116.
52. Trimakas AP, Maxwell KD, Berkay S, et al. Fetal monitoring during cardiopulmonary bypass for removal of a left atrial myxoma during pregnancy. *Johns Hopkins Med J* 1979;144:156.
53. Page PA, Toung T. A new probe for measurement of muscle pO2 and its use during cardiopulmonary bypass. *Surg Gynecol Obstet* 1975;141:579.
54. Werch A, Lambert HM, Cooley D, et al. Fetal monitoring and maternal open heart surgery [Letter]. *South Med J* 1977;70: 1024.
55. Koh KS, Friesen RM, Livingstone RA, et al. Fetal monitoring during maternal cardiac surgery with cardiopulmonary bypass. *Can Med Assoc J* 1975;112:1102.
56. Bahary CM, Ninio A, Gorodesky IG, et al. Tococardiography

in pregnancy during extracorporeal bypass for mitral valve replacement. *Isr J Med Sci* 1980;16:395.

57. Tripp HF, Stiegel RM, Coyle JP. The use of pulsatile perfusion during aortic valve replacement in pregnancy. *Ann Thorac Surg* 1999;67:1169.
58. Hess OW, Davis CD. Electronic evaluation of the fetal and maternal rate during hypothermia in a pregnant woman. *Am J Obstet Gynecol* 1964;89:801.
59. Jadhon ME, Main EK. Fetal bradycardia associated with maternal hypothermia. *Obstet Gynecol* 1988;72:496.
60. Richter RC, Slate RK, Rudolph AM. Fetal blood flow during hypothermic cardiopulmonary by-pass in utero. *J Cardiovasc Surg* 1985;26:86.
61. Utley JR. Pathophysiology of cardiopulmonary bypass: current issues. *J Card Surg* 1990;5:177.
62. Vandewater SL, Paul VM. Observation on the fetus during experimental hypothermia. *Can Anaesth Soc J* 1960;7:44.
63. Korsten HH, Van Zundert AA, Mooij PN, et al. Emergency aortic valve replacement in the 24th-week of pregnancy. *Acta Anaesthesiol Belg* 1989;40:201.
64. Hawkins JA, Paape KL, Adkins TP, et al. Extracorporeal circulation in the fetal lamb: effects of hypothermia and perfusion rate. *J Cardiovasc Surg (Torino)* 1991;32:295.
65. Buffolo E, Palma JH, Gomes WJ, et al. Successful use of deep hypothermic circulatory arrest in pregnancy. *Ann Thorac Surg* 1994;58:1532.
66. Burke AB, Hur D, Bolan JC, et al. Sinusoidal fetal heart rate pattern during cardiopulmonary bypass. *Am J Obstet Gynecol* 1990;163:17.
67. Lamarra M, Azzu AA, Kulatilake EN. Cardiopulmonary bypass in the early puerperium: possible new role for aprotinin. *Ann Thorac Surg* 1992;54:361.
68. Rowland AS, Baird DD, Shore DL, et al. Nitrous oxide and spontaneous abortion in female dental assistants. *Am J Epidemiol* 1995;141:531.
69. Reitz M, Antoninirumpf E, Lanz E. DNA single strand breaks in peripheral human lymphocytes after anesthesia with isoflurane–nitrous oxide–oxygen. *Arzneimittelforschung* 1993;43-2:1258.
70. Fujinaga M, Baden JM, Yhap EO, et al. Reproductive and teratogenic effects of nitrous oxide, isoflurane, and their combination in Sprague-Dawley rats. *Anesthesiology* 1987;67:960.
71. Mazze RI, Fujinaga M, Rice SA, et al. Reproductive and teratogenic effects of nitrous oxide, halothane, isoflurane, and enflurane in Sprague-Dawley rats. *Anesthesiology* 1986;64:339.
72. Mazze RI. Nitrous oxide during pregnancy [Editorial]. *Anaesthesia* 1986;41:897.
73. Crawford JS, Lewis M. Nitrous oxide in early human pregnancy. *Anaesthesia* 1986;41:900.
74. Aldridge LM, Tunstall ME. Nitrous oxide and the fetus: a review and the results of a retrospective study of 175 cases of anaesthesia for insertion of Shirodkar suture. *Br J Anaesth* 1986;58:1348.
75. Mazze RI, Källén B. Reproductive outcome after anesthesia and operation during pregnancy: a registry study of 5405 cases. *Am J Obstet Gynecol* 1989;161:1178.
76. Duncan PG, Pope WDB, Cohen MM, et al. Fetal risk of anesthesia and surgery during pregnancy. *Anesthesiology* 1986;64:790.
77. Rosenberg L, Mitchell AA, Parsells JL, et al. Lack of relation of oral clefts to diazepam use during pregnancy. *N Engl J Med* 1983;309:1282.
78. Nisell H, Martinsson A, Hjemdahl P. Reduced β_2-adrenoceptor sensitivity in normal pregnancy but not in pregnancy-induced hypertension. *Gynecol Obstet Invest* 1988;25:262.
79. Nisell H, Hjemdahl P, Linde B. Cardiovascular responses to circulating catecholamines in normal pregnancy and in pregnancy-induced hypertension. *Clin Physiol* 1985;5:479.
80. DeSimone CA, Leighton BL, Norris MC, et al. The chronotropic effect of isoproterenol is reduced in term pregnant women. *Anesthesiology* 1988;69:626.
81. Weiner CP, Martinez E, Chestnut DH, et al. Effect of pregnancy on uterine and carotid artery response to norepinephrine, epinephrine, and phenylephrine in vessels with documented functional endothelium. *Am J Obstet Gynecol* 1989;161:1605.
82. Ramsay MM, Broughton Pipkin F, Rubin PC. Pressor, heart rate and plasma catecholamine responses to noradrenaline in pregnant and nonpregnant women. *Br J Obstet Gynaecol* 1993;100:170.
83. Moran D, Perillo M, LaPorta R, et al. Phenylephrine in the prevention of hypotension following spinal anesthesia for cesarean delivery. *J Clin Anesth* 1991;3:301.
84. Hall PA, Bennett A, Wilkes MP, et al. Spinal anaesthesia for caesarean section: comparison of infusions of phenylephrine and ephedrine. *Br J Anaesth* 1994;73:471.
85. Ramanathan S, Grant GJ. Vasopressor therapy for hypotension due to epidural anesthesia for cesarean section. *Acta Anaesthesiol Scand* 1988;32:559.
86. Thomas DG, Robson SC, Redfern N, et al. Randomized trial of bolus phenylephrine or ephedrine for maintenance of arterial pressure during spinal anaesthesia for caesarean section. *Br J Anaesth* 1996;76:61.
87. Emergency Cardiac Care Committee and Subcommittees, American Heart Association. Guidelines for cardiopulmonary resuscitation and emergency cardiac care: part IV. Special resuscitation situations. *JAMA* 1992;268:2242.
88. DePace NL, Betesh JS, Kotler MN. "Postmortem" cesarean section with recovery of both mother and offspring. *JAMA* 1982;248:971.
89. Katz VL, Dotters DJ, Droegemueller W. Perimortem cesarean delivery. *Obstet Gynecol* 1986;68:571.
90. Lopez-Zeno JA, Carlo WA, O'Grady JP, et al. Infant survival following delayed portmortem cesarean delivery. *Obstet Gynecol* 1990;76:991.
91. Rees GA, Willis BA. Resuscitation in late pregnancy. *Anaesthesia* 1988;43:347.
92. Ginz B. Myocardial infarction in pregnancy. *J Obstet Gynaecol Br Commonw* 1970;77:610.
93. Hankins GD, Wendel GD Jr, Leveno KJ, et al. Myocardial infarction during pregnancy: a review. *Obstet Gynecol* 1985;65:139.
94. Roth A, Elkayam U. Acute myocardial infarction associated with pregnancy. *Ann Intern Med* 1996;125:751.
95. Pretty HC. Dissecting aneurysm of coronary artery in a woman aged 42. *Br Med J* 1931;1:667.
96. Klutstein MW, Tzivoni D, Bitran D, et al. Treatment of spontaneous coronary artery dissection: report of three cases [see comments]. *Cathet Cardiovasc Diagn* 1997;40:372.
97. Curiel P, Spinelli G, Petrella A, et al. Postpartum coronary artery dissection followed by heart transplantation. *Am J Obstet Gynecol* 1990;163:538.
98. Tsung SH. Several conditions causing elevation of serum CK-MB and CK-BB. *Am J Clin Pathol* 1981;75:711.
99. Laboda HM, Britton VJ. Creatine kinase isoenzyme activity in human placenta and in serum of women in labor. *Clin Chem* 1977;23:1329.
100. McNeely MD, Baerris B, Papsin FR, et al. Creatine kinase and its isoenzymes in the serum of women during pregnancy and the peripartum period. *Clin Chem* 1977;23:1878.
101. Rubin PC. Current concepts: beta-blockers in pregnancy. *N Engl J Med* 1981;305:1323.
102. Rotmensch HH, Rotmensch S, Elkayam U. Management of

cardiac arrhythmias during pregnancy: current concepts. *Drugs* 1987;33:623.
103. Turrentine MA, Braems G, Ramirez MM. Use of thrombolytics for the treatment of thromboembolic disease during pregnancy. *Obstet Gynecol Surv* 1995;50:534.
104. Webber MD, Halligan RE, Schumacher JA. Acute infarction, intracoronary thrombolysis, and primary PTCA in pregnancy. *Cathet Cardiovasc Diagn* 1997;42:38.
105. Sanchez-Ramos L, Chami YG, Bass TA, et al. Myocardial infarction during pregnancy: management with transluminal coronary angioplasty and metallic intracoronary stents. *Am J Obstet Gynecol* 1994;171:1392.
106. Glazier JJ, Eldin AM, Hirst JA, et al. Primary angioplasty using a urokinase-coated hydrogel balloon in acute myocardial infarction during pregnancy. *Cathet Cardiovasc Diagn* 1995;36:216.
107. Joseph SG. Peripartum cardiomyopathy: successful treatment with cardiac transplantation. *West J Med* 1987;146:230.
108. Morini A, Spina V, Aleandri V, et al. Pregnancy after heart transplant: update and case report. *Hum Reprod* 1998;13:749.
109. Scott JR, Wagoner LE, Olsen SL, et al. Pregnancy in heart transplant recipients: management and outcome. *Obstet Gynecol* 1993;82:324.
110. Wagoner LE, Taylor DO, Olsen SL, et al. Immunosuppressive therapy, management, and outcome of heart transplant recipients during pregnancy [published erratum appears in *J Heart Lung Transplant* 1994 Mar-Apr;13(2):342]. *J Heart Lung Transplant* 1993;12:993.
111. Alon E, Rosen MA, Schnider SM. Maternal and fetal effects of propofol anesthesia in the ewe. *Anesthesiology* 1991;75:A1077.
112. Craft JB Jr, Coaldrake LA, Yonekura ML, et al. Ketamine, catecholamines, and uterine tone in pregnant ewes. *Am J Obstet Gynecol* 1983;146:429.
113. Cosmi EV, Marx GF. The effect of anesthesia on the acid-base status of the fetus. *Anesthesiology* 1969;30:238.
114. Palahniuk RJ, Shnider SM. Maternal and fetal cardiovascular and acid-base changes during halothane and isoflurane anesthesia in the pregnant ewe. *Anesthesiology* 1974;41:462.
115. Ralston DH, Shnider SM, DeLormimier AA. Effects of equipotent ephedrine, metariminol, mephenteramine and methoxamine on uterine blood flow in the pregnant ewe. *Anesthesiology* 1974;40:354.
116. Ring G, Krames E, Shnider SM, et al. Comparison of nitroprusside and hydralazine in hypertensive pregnant ewes. *Obstet Gynecol* 1977;50:598.
117. Greiss FC Jr, Van Wilkes D. Effects of sympathomimetic drugs and angiotensin on the uterine vascular bed. *Obstet Gynecol* 1964;23:925.
118. Blanchard K, Dandavino A, Nuwayhid B, et al. Systemic and uterine hemodynamic responses to dopamine in pregnant and nonpregnant sheep. *Am J Obstet Gynecol* 1978;130:669.
119. Callender K, Levinson G, Shnider SM, et al. Dopamine administration in the normotensive pregnant ewe. *Obstet Gynecol* 1978;51:586.
120. Fishburne JI, Meis PJ, Urban RB, et al. Vascular and uterine responses to dobutamine and dopamine in the gravid ewe. *Am J Obstet Gynecol* 1980;137:944.
121. Wheeler AS, James FMd, Meis PJ, et al. Effects of nitroglycerin and nitroprusside on the uterine vasculature of gravid ewes. *Anesthesiology* 1980;52:390.
122. Kerenyi TD, Gleicher N, Meller J, et al. Transplancental cardioversion of intrauterine supraventricular tachycardia with digitalis. *Lancet* 1980;2:393.
123. Owen J, Colvin EV, Davis RO. Fetal death after successful conversion of fetal supraventricular tachycardia with digoxin and verapamil. *Am J Obstet Gynecol* 1988;158:1169.
124. Ostman PL, Chestnut DH, Robillard JE, et al. Transplacental passage and hemodynamic effects of esmolol in the gravid ewe. *Anesthesiology* 1988;69:738.
125. Peng AT, Gorman RS, Shulman SM, et al. Intravenous nitroglycerin for uterine relaxation in the postpartum patient with retained placenta [Letter]. *Anesthesiology* 1989;71:172.
126. DeSimone CA, Norris MC, Leighton BL. Intravenous nitroglycerin aids manual extraction of a retained placenta [Letter]. *Anesthesiology* 1990;73:787.
127. Stempel JE, O'Grady JP, Morton MJ, et al. Use of sodium nitroprusside in complications of gestational hypertension. *Obstet Gynecol* 1982;60:533.
128. Dandavino A, Woods JR. Circulatory effects of magnesium sulfate in normotensive and renal hypertensive pregnant sheep. *Am J Obstet Gynecol* 1977;127:769.
129. Murad SHN, Tabsh KMA. Effects of verapamil on uterine blood flow and maternal cardiovascular function in the awake pregnancy ewe. *Anesth Anal* 1985;64:7.
130. Wolff F, Breuker KH, Schlensker KH, Bolte A. Prenatal diagnosis and therapy of fetal heart rate anomalies: with a contribution on the placental transfer of verapamil. *J Perinat Med* 1980;8:203.
131. Veille JC, Bissonnette JM, Hohimer AR. The effect of a calcium channel blocker (nifedipine) on uterine blood flow in the pregnant goat. *Am J Obstet Gynecol* 1986;154:1160.
132. Biehl D, Shnider SM, Levinson G, et al. The direct effects of circulating lidocaine on uterine blood flow and foetal well-being in the pregnant ewe. *Can Anaesth Soc J* 1977;24:445.
133. Dumesic DA, Silverman NH, Tobias S, et al. Transplacental cardioversion of fetal supraventricular tachycardia with procainamide. *N Engl J Med* 1982;307:1128.
134. Abboud T, Raya J, Sadri S, et al. Fetal and maternal cardiovascular effects of atropine and glycopyrrolate. *Anesth Analg* 1983;62:426.
135. Wladimiroff JW. Effect of frusemide on fetal urine production. *Br J Obstet Gynaecol* 1975;82:221.

30

THE ADULT NONCARDIAC PATIENT

LEE A. FLEISHER
PAUL G. BARASH

INTRODUCTION

The adult patient with cardiovascular disease undergoing noncardiac surgery is a constantly evolving topic with regard to both preoperative evaluation and perioperative management. Although the focus of much of the 1980s and early 1990s was on identification of the patient with significant cardiovascular disease and potential preoperative interventions, much of the recent research has focused on intraoperative and postoperative interventions to reduce risk. These studies, many of which are randomized or include large administrative data sets, have helped better define the absolute risk and risk reduction associated with particular techniques or care systems. This chapter attempts to highlight these advances with respect to perioperative management.

Preoperative Cardiovascular Evaluation

Until recent years, it was traditionally considered appropriate to obtain a complete database with respect to a patient's cardiovascular status before undergoing noncardiac surgery. With the strong economic pressures to reduce inappropriate testing and additional research identifying the lack of value when testing is applied indiscriminately, the more recent focus has been to use history and directed testing in those patients in whom the results would lead to changes in perioperative management. Additionally, studies evaluating the beneficial effect of perioperative β-blocker usage have questioned the utility of any diagnostic testing if perioperative morbidity and mortality is greatly reduced (1). The next several years will be important in that generalizability of these study findings to routine care will be required to determine whether virtually all testing for preoperative evaluation is unnecessary.

There have been numerous reviews and two recent guidelines published to address the preoperative cardiovascular evaluation. The American Heart Association/American College of Cardiology (AHA/ACC) published a consensus-based document backed by available evidence in 1996 and plans to publish an update in 2001 (2). The American College of Physicians also published (1997) an evidence-based guideline to identify the utility of preoperative testing. Both guidelines highlight the importance of limiting testing to those circumstances in which perioperative management would change (3). Additionally, both assert that coronary interventions before noncardiac surgery should be limited to those patients in whom the intervention would be contemplated independent of the planned noncardiac procedure.

L. A. Fleisher: Department of Anesthesiology and Critical Care Medicine, Johns Hopkins Medical Institutions, Baltimore, Maryland 21287

P. G. Barash: Department of Anesthesiology, Yale University School of Medicine, New Haven, Connecticut 06510

Approach to the Patient

Although numerous risk indices have been published to define patients who are at increased risk for perioperative complications, this approach has limited utility to the anesthesiologist. Risk indices such as the original Cardiac Risk Index, Revised Cardiac Risk Index, and Detsky Index use a weighted or simple additive scale for specific risk factors (4–6) (Fig. 30-1). The approach can establish a prior probability of significant cardiovascular disease, whereby the primary care doctors or others can determine the value of additional diagnostic testing, but it does not provide the anesthesiologist with specific information to change perioperative management. For this purpose, information with respect to cardiovascular function and reserve and ischemic potential is important, and good communication between the primary care physician or specialist and the anesthesia provider is required.

CLINICAL RISK FACTORS

Congestive Heart Failure

The impact of congestive heart failure (CHF) on perioperative morbidity and mortality is often minimized. In virtually

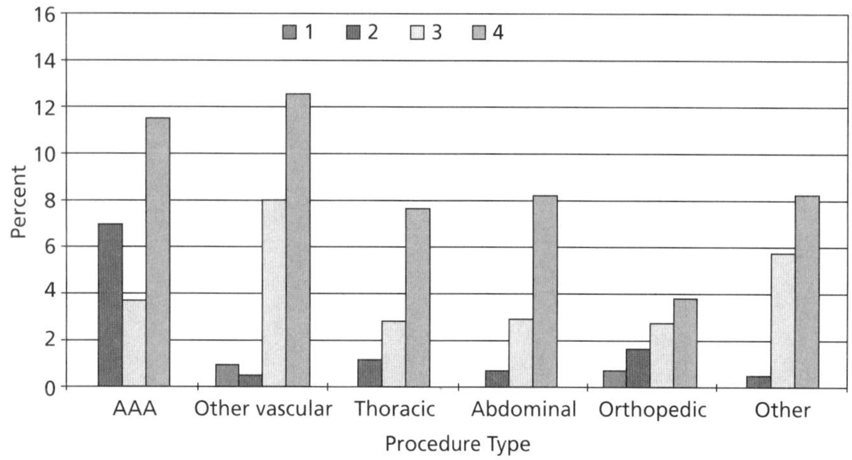

FIGURE 30-1. *Bars* represent rate of major cardiac complications in entire patient population (both derivation and validation cohorts combined) for patients in Revised Cardiac Risk Index classes according to type of procedure performed. Note that, by definition, patients undergoing abdominal aortic aneurysm (AAA), thoracic, and abdominal procedures were excluded from class I. In all subsets except patients undergoing AAA, there was a statistically significant trend toward greater risk with higher risk class. (From Lee TH, Marcantonio ER, Mangione CM, et al. Derivation and prospective validation of a simple index for prediction of cardiac risk of major noncardiac surgery. *Circulation* 1999;100:1043, with permission.)

all studies, the presence of active CHF is associated with the highest perioperative risk. Approximately 2.3 million Americans currently have CHF, with an additional 400,000 being added each year. The incidence of CHF doubles with each decade of age between 45 and 75 years, and CHF is the number one diagnostic related group (DRG) diagnosis in the elderly. Various diagnostic schemes have been used to define CHF clinically. The Boston criteria rely on three categories: history, physical examination, and chest radiograph. The Framingham criteria use both major clinical factors (e.g., rales, cardiomegaly) and minor factors (e.g., dyspnea on exertion, decreased vital capacity). The physiologic hallmarks of CHF include (a) decreased cardiac output, (b) increased ventricular filling pressures, (c) increased systemic vascular resistance, and (d) acidosis. Dysrhythmias are an important component of the disease process and its associated mortality.

In patients with CHF, a designation of New York Health Association functional class IV conferred a significantly greater risk than designation of a better functional class. In a study by Rao et al. of patients with prior myocardial infarctions (MIs), 12.5% of those with preoperative CHF sustained a perioperative MI (7). From the perspective of the anesthesiologist, it is important to define the cause of CHF. Patients who have CHF from a nonischemic origin are at risk for perioperative CHF but rarely sustain myocardial necrosis. In contrast, the patient who has ischemic cardiomyopathy is at high risk for perioperative MI and ventricular dysfunction. Physical examination and a chest radiograph help determine whether the patient is well compensated. In some instances, an arterial blood gas analysis should be obtained to further determine patient status.

Coronary Artery Disease

Time elapsed since a prior MI has traditionally been an important predictor of perioperative risk (7–9). The more recent the MI, particularly within the previous 3 to 6 months, the greater the perioperative risk. However, advances in the management of acute MI make the older data less valid (10). The AHA/ACC guidelines advocate the use of 30 days as the acute period, with high risk continuing for up to 6 to 8 weeks (2). After that time, a prior MI places the patient at moderate risk, and further evaluation depends on other clinical symptoms.

The presence of angina has not consistently been a risk factor in the various studies. However, the presence of unstable angina was associated with a 28% incidence of perioperative MI (11). Such patients would benefit from the delay of surgery and more intensive medical therapy. For those patients with chronic stable angina, exercise tolerance appears to be a good method of assessing risk. Patients who develop chest pain with minimal exercise and have associated shortness of breath are at high risk for perioperative ischemia and left ventricular dysfunction. In contrast, patients who can play three sets of tennis before the onset of angina appear to at much lower risk.

Cardiovascular Risk Factors

Diabetes has been associated with a high incidence of perioperative cardiac morbidity in several studies, particularly those involving patients undergoing vascular surgery (12). Diabetics have a high incidence of both silent ischemia and silent MI (13). The presence of autonomic dysfunction has been associated with a higher incidence of silent cardiovascular disease (14).

Of all the forms of cardiovascular disease, hypertension is the most prevalent, affecting more than 59 million people. Hypertension is also an important marker as a risk factor for CHF and ischemic heart disease. Hypertension results in (a) an increased systemic vascular resistance, (b) decreased intravascular volume, (c) exaggerated pressor response, and (d) edema. Most hypertension is essential; however, in cer-

TABLE 30-1. HYPERTENSION

Category	Systolic (mm Hg)	Diastolic (mm Hg)
Normal	<130	<85
High-normal	130–139	85–89
Hypertension		
Stage 1 (mild)	140–159	90–99
Stage 2 (moderate)	160–179	100–109
Stage 3 (severe)	180–209	110–119
Stage 4 (very severe)	≥210	≥120

Adapted from Fifth report of the Joint National Committee on Detection, Evaluation, and Treatment of High Blood Pressure. *Arch Intern Med* 1993;153:1254.

tain patients, as indicated by history, physical examination, and baseline laboratory data, a more extensive workup may reveal a primary and treatable cause of hypertension (e.g., renal artery stenosis).

Blood pressure (BP) values should be obtained with the use of an appropriately sized cuff (covering two-thirds of the length of the arm) and with the patient in a relaxed setting. Frank et al. demonstrated marked discrepancies in preoperative BP measurements in vascular surgery patients depending on which arm the measurement was obtained from (14a). For patients older than 18 years of age, hypertension is defined as BP higher than 140/90 mm Hg (15) (Table 30-1). Although most interventional trials have used reduction of diastolic BP as an end point, reanalysis of these trials suggests that elevation of systolic BP is at least as important as a determinant of long-range morbidity and mortality (16).

Future cardiovascular complications appear to correlate better with the mean 24-hour BP than with isolated measurements (17). This may be a primary relationship, or it may reflect the increased left ventricular mass in these patients. Left ventricular hypertrophy can lead to an increased risk for development of myocardial ischemia from imbalances of supply and demand or reserve regardless of the anatomic status of the coronary circulation. One investigator proposed that the strain pattern seen in some patients with left ventricular hypertrophy represents a chronic ischemic state (18). Therefore, in patients with hypertension, even in the absence of left ventricular hypertrophy or coronary artery disease (CAD), the anesthesiologist must be at increased vigilance for myocardial ischemia (19).

IMPORTANCE OF SURGICAL PROCEDURE

The surgical procedure influences the extent of the preoperative evaluation required by determining the potential range of changes in perioperative management. For example, use of a pulmonary artery (PA) catheter or transesophageal echocardiography (TEE) may be appropriate for a patient

TABLE 30-2. CARDIAC RISK[a] STRATIFICATION FOR NONCARDIAC SURGICAL PROCEDURES

Risk Level	Examples
High (often >5%)	Emergent major operations, particularly in the elderly Aortic and other major vascular procedures Peripheral vascular surgery Anticipated prolonged surgical procedures associated with large fluid shifts and/or blood loss
Intermediate (generally <5%)	Carotid endarterectomy Head and neck procedures Intraperitoneal and intrathoracic procedures Orthopedic surgery Prostate surgery
Low[b] (generally <1%)	Endoscopic procedures Superficial procedures Cataract surgery Breast surgery

[a] Combined incidence of cardiac death and nonfatal myocardial infarction.
[b] Do not generally require further preoperative cardiac testing.
Source: Eagle K, Brundage B, Chaitman B, et al. Guidelines for perioperative cardiovascular evaluation of the noncardiac surgery: a report of the American Heart Association/American College of Cardiology Task Force on Assessment of Diagnostic and Therapeutic Cardiovascular Procedures. *Circulation* 1996;93:1278.

undergoing major abdominal or vascular surgery but would not be considered appropriate for ambulatory surgery. Similarly, coronary revascularization may be beneficial for procedures associated with a high incidence of morbidity and mortality, but not those associated with a low incidence, as described later. There is little hard data to define the surgery-specific incidence of complications. It is known that peripheral procedures, such as those included in a study of ambulatory surgery completed at the Mayo Clinic, are associated with an extremely low incidence of morbidity and mortality (20). Similarly, major vascular procedures are associated with some of the highest incidence rates for complications, as are infrainguinal and aortic surgery (21). Eagle et al. published data on the incidence of perioperative MI and mortality by procedure for patients enrolled in the Coronary Artery Surgery Study (CASS) (22). High-risk procedures include major vascular, abdominal, thoracic, and orthopedic surgery (Table 30-2).

IMPORTANCE OF EXERCISE TOLERANCE

Exercise tolerance is one of the most important determinants of perioperative risk and the need for invasive moni-

TABLE 30-3. ESTIMATED ENERGY REQUIREMENT FOR VARIOUS ACTIVITIES

No. Metabolic Equivalents	Questions
1	Can you take care of yourself? Eat, dress, or use the toilet? Can you walk indoors around the house? Can you walk a block or two on level ground at 2–3 mph or 3.2–4.8 km/hr? Can you do light work around the house such as dusting or washing dishes?
4	Can you climb a flight of stairs or walk up a hill? Can you walk on level ground at 4 mph or 6.4 km/hr? Can you run a short distance? Can you do heavy work around the house such as scrubbing floors or lifting or moving heavy furniture? Can you participate in moderate recreational activities such as golf, bowling, dancing, doubles tennis, or throwing a baseball or football?
>10	Can you participate in strenuous sports such as swimming, singles tennis, football, basketball, or skiing?

Source: Eagle K, Brundage B, Chaitman B, et al. Guidelines for perioperative cardiovascular evaluation of the noncardiac surgery: a report of the American Heart Association/American College of Cardiology Task Force on Assessment of Diagnostic and Therapeutic Cardiovascular Procedures. *Circulation* 1996;93:1278.

toring (23). An excellent exercise tolerance, even in a patient with stable angina, suggests that the myocardium can be stressed without becoming dysfunctional. If a patient can walk a mile without becoming short of breath, than the probability of extensive CAD is small. Alternatively, if patients become dyspneic with associated chest pain during minimal exertion, then the probability of extensive CAD is high. A greater degree of CAD has been associated with a higher perioperative risk (24). Additionally, these patients are at risk for development of hypotension with ischemia and therefore may benefit from more extensive monitoring or coronary revascularization. Exercise tolerance can be assessed with formal treadmill testing or with a questionnaire that assesses activities of daily living (2) (Table 30-3).

Reilly et al. evaluated the predictive value of self-reported exercise tolerance for serious perioperative complications and demonstrated that a poor exercise tolerance (inability to walk four blocks and climb two flights of stairs) independently predicted a complication with an odds ratio of 1.94 (25). The likelihood of a serious adverse event was inversely related to the number of blocks that could be walked. Therefore, there is good evidence to suggest that minimal additional testing is necessary if the patient is able to relate a good exercise tolerance.

DECISION-MAKING ALGORITHMS

As mentioned earlier, numerous guidelines and review articles have been published that incorporate algorithms to define the optimal strategy for determining which patients should undergo further diagnostic testing. One such algorithm has been published by the AHA/ACC Task Force on Guidelines on Perioperative Evaluation of the Cardiac Patient undergoing Noncardiac Surgery based on the available evidence and expert opinion. The approach advocated integrates clinical history (Table 30-4), surgery-specific risk, and exercise tolerance (Fig. 30-2) (2). First, the clinician must evaluate the urgency of the surgery and the appropriateness of a formal preoperative assessment. Next, the physician determines whether the patient has undergone a previous revascularization procedure or coronary evaluation.

TABLE 30-4. CLINICAL PREDICTORS OF INCREASED PERIOPERATIVE CARDIOVASCULAR RISK (MYOCARDIAL INFARCTION, CONGESTIVE HEART FAILURE, DEATH)

- Major
  - Unstable coronary syndrome
    - Recent myocardial infarction[a] with evidence of important ischemic risk with clinical symptoms or noninvasive study
    - Unstable or severe[b] angina (Canadian class III or IV)[c]
  - Decompensated congestive heart failure
  - Significant arrhythmia
    - High-grade atrioventricular block
    - Symptomatic ventricular arrhythmia in the presence of underlying heart disease
    - Supraventricular arrhythmia with uncontrolled ventricular rate
  - Severe valvular disease
- Intermediate
  - Mild angina pectoris (Canadian class I or II)
  - Prior myocardial infarction by history or pathologic Q waves
  - Compensated or prior congestive heart failure
  - Diabetes mellitus
- Minor
  - Advanced age
  - Abnormal ECG (left ventricular hypertrophy, left bundle branch block, ST-T abnormalities)
  - Rhythm other than sinus (e.g., atrial fibrillation)
  - Low functional capacity (e.g., inability to climb one flight of stairs with a bag of groceries)
  - History of stroke
  - Uncontrolled systemic hypertension

Note: ECG, electrocardiogram.
[a] The American College of Cardiology National Database Library defines recent myocardial infarction as >7 days but ≤1 month (30 days).
[b] May include "stable" angina in patients who are unusually sedentary.
[c] Campeau L. Grading of angina pectoris. Circulation 1976;54:522.
Source: Eagle K, Brundage B, Chaitman B, et al. Guidelines for perioperative cardiovascular evaluation of the noncardiac surgery: a report of the American Heart Association/American College of Cardiology Task Force on Assessment of Diagnostic and Therapeutic Cardiovascular Procedures. *Circulation* 1996;93:1278.

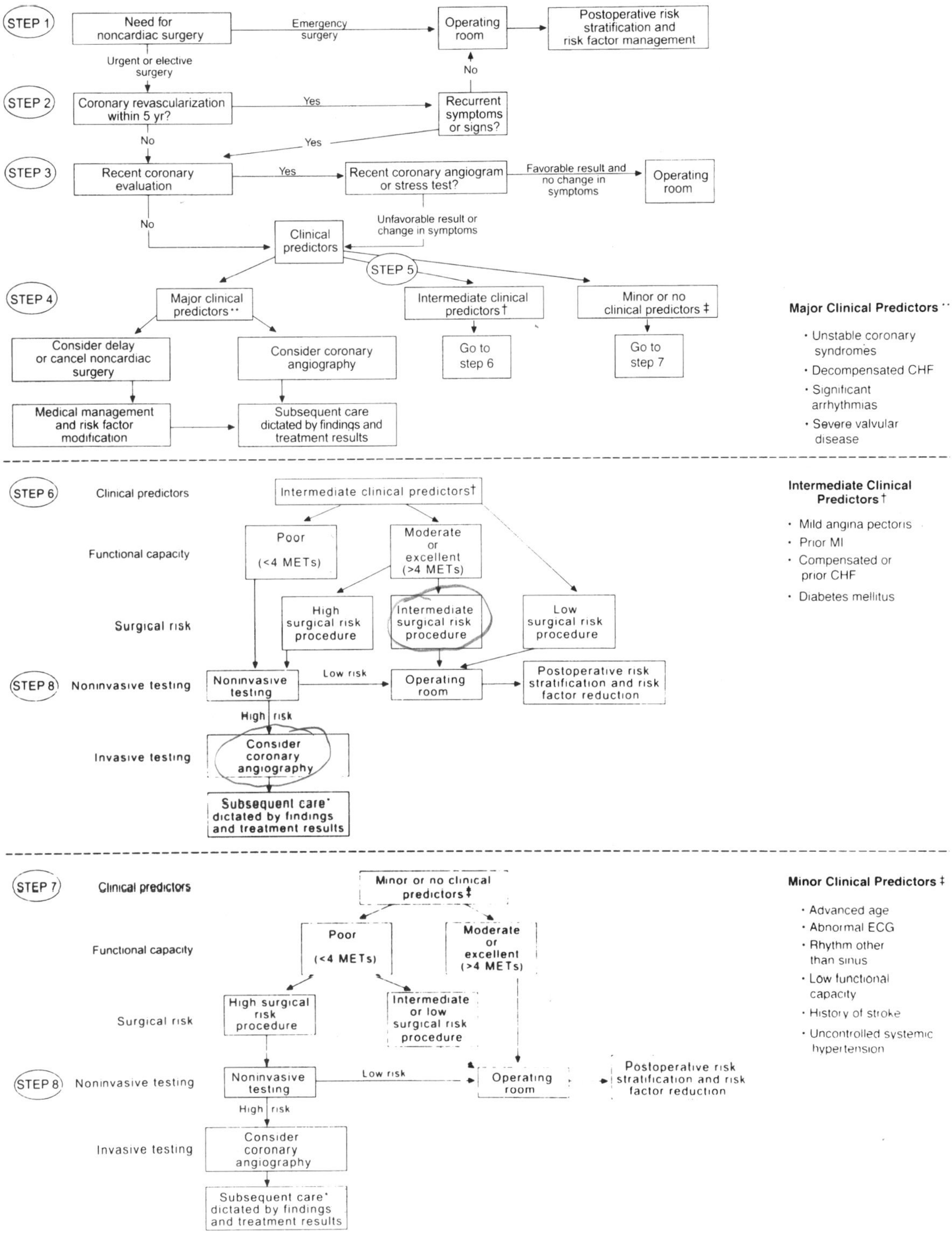

FIGURE 30-2. The American Heart Association/American College of Cardiology Task Force on Perioperative Evaluation of Cardiac Patients undergoing Noncardiac Surgery has proposed an algorithm for decisions regarding the need for further evaluation. This represents one of many algorithms proposed in the literature. It is based on expert opinion and incorporates six steps. First, the clinician must evaluate the urgency of the surgery and the appropriateness of a formal preoperative assessment. Next, the physician must determine whether the patient has had a previous revascularization procedure or coronary evaluation. Those patients with unstable coronary syndromes should be identified, and appropriate treatment should be instituted. The decision to have further testing depends on the interaction of the clinical risk factors, surgery-specific risk, and functional capacity. (Adapted from Eagle K, Brundage B, Chaitman B, et al. Guidelines for perioperative cardiovascular evaluation of the noncardiac surgery: a report of the American Heart Association/American College of Cardiology Task Force on Assessment of Diagnostic and Therapeutic Cardiovascular Procedures. *Circulation* 1996;93:1278, with permission.)

Those patients with unstable coronary syndromes should be identified, and appropriate treatment instituted. Finally, the decision to undergo further testing depends on the interaction of the clinical risk factors, surgery-specific risk, and functional capacity. For patients at intermediate clinical risk, both the exercise tolerance and the extent of the surgery are taken into account with regard to the need for further testing. Importantly, no preoperative cardiovascular testing should be performed if the results will not change perioperative management.

The American College of Physicians guidelines attempt to apply the evidence-based approach to preoperative testing (3). The initial decision point is the assessment of risk using the Detsky modification of the Cardiac Risk Index (6). If the patient is in class II or III, he or she is considered to be at high risk. If the patient is in class I, the presence of other clinical factors, according to work by Eagle et al. (2) or Vanzetto et al. (26) is used to further stratify risk. Those who have multiple markers for cardiovascular disease according to these risk indices and are undergoing major vascular surgery are considered appropriate subjects for further diagnostic testing by either dipyridamole imaging or dobutamine stress echocardiography. The guidelines suggest that there is insufficient evidence to recommend diagnostic testing for patients undergoing nonvascular surgery.

CORONARY REVASCULARIZATION

Before cardiovascular testing is performed, it is important to determine whether the results will affect perioperative management. Among the various interventions, several investigators have proposed coronary revascularization before noncardiac surgery as a means of reducing perioperative risk. There are no randomized trials to address this issue, and such a trial would require a very large sample size and have multiple confounding issues (27). However, there are several large cohort studies suggesting that, among patients who survive coronary artery bypass grafting (CABG), the risk with subsequent noncardiac surgery is low (22,29). Although there is little evidence to support the notion of coronary revascularization solely for the purpose of improving perioperative outcome, it is true that for specific patient subsets long-term survival may be enhanced by revascularization. Rihal et al. analyzed the CASS database and found that CABG significantly improved survival among those patients with both peripheral vascular disease and triple-vessel CAD, especially the group with depressed ventricular function (30).

The value of percutaneous transluminal coronary angioplasty (PTCA) is less well established. In several series, a low incidence of cardiovascular complications was observed among patients undergoing "prophylactic" PTCA before vascular surgery, but it was difficult to determine the expected complication rate in a comparison group with single- or double-vessel disease (31). Posner et al. used data from Washington state in a case-controlled study to demonstrate that individuals who had PTCA before noncardiac surgery had a significantly reduced incidence of perioperative morbidity compared with matched controls (32). Importantly, no improvement in outcome was demonstrated if the PTCA was performed within 90 days of the noncardiac surgery, suggesting that acute interventions for single- or double-vessel disease may not affect outcome. For those perioperative MIs that result from plaque rupture and coronary thrombosis in noncritical lesions, as seen in the ambulatory setting, single-vessel PTCA of more critical stenoses would theoretically have minimal benefit (33). Ellis et al. studied 21 patients who underwent coronary angiography before major vascular surgery and sustained a perioperative cardiac event (34). None of the MIs occurred in areas distal to a critical stenosis, whereas approximately one-third occurred distal to noncritical stenoses. Therefore, the current evidence does not support the use of PTCA beyond established indications for nonoperative patients.

Risks Versus Benefits of Coronary Revascularization

An alternative approach to determining the optimal strategy for medical care in the absence of clinical trials is construction of a decision analysis. Three decision analyses have been published on the issue of cardiovascular testing before major vascular surgery (35–37) (Fig. 30-3). They all assumed that patients with significant CAD would undergo CABG before noncardiac surgery. The models found that the optimal decision was sensitive to local morbidity and mortality rates within the clinically observed range. These models suggest that preoperative testing for the purpose of coronary revascularization is not the optimal strategy if perioperative morbidity and mortality are low. However, in the one model by Glance that included a long-term perspective, selective testing was found to be cost-effective in the appropriate age group (37).

Importantly, the primary cost (both in dollars and morbidity) of preoperative testing and revascularization is the revascularization procedure itself. Therefore, the indications for revascularization, and consequently the frequency of its use, have a significant impact on the model. Secondly, potential long-term benefits of coronary revascularization in this population were not included in all analyses, potentially biasing against the revascularization arm. If long-term survival is included in the models, then coronary revascularization may lead to improved overall outcome and may be a cost-effective intervention. However, a patient's age should be included in the equation. For example, an 80-year-old diabetic patient with significant comorbid diseases may gain little additional life years and may actually have a decrease

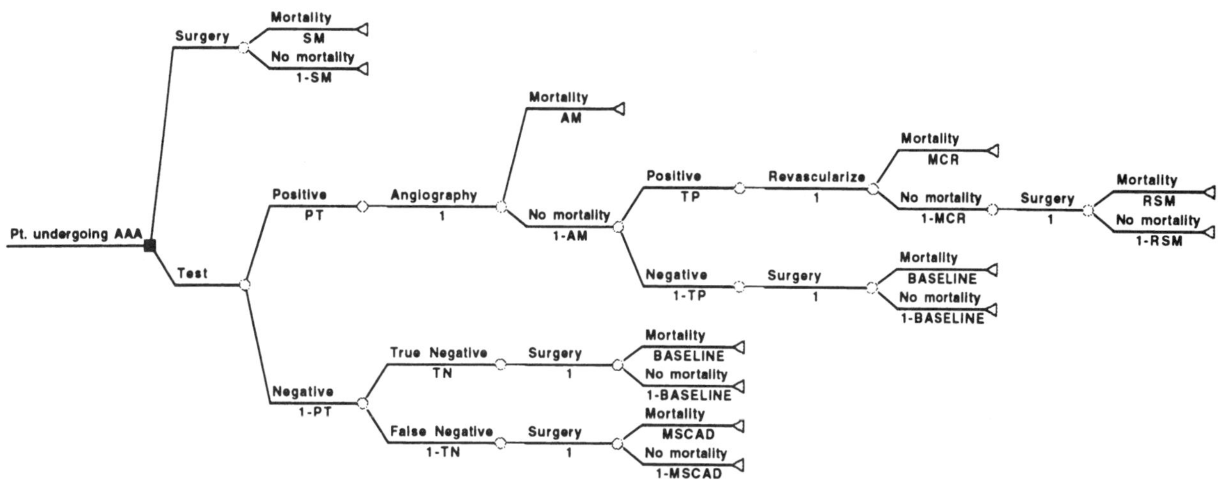

FIGURE 30-3. A decision algorithm evaluating vascular surgery alone versus coronary artery revascularization before vascular surgery. There are currently no randomized trials to address the optimal strategy. By outlining the multiple decision points at which a patient can sustain mortality by choosing to undergo coronary revascularization first, the optimal strategy for preoperative evaluation can be demonstrated. Specifically, variation in mortality rates at each decision point can change the optimal strategy. (From Fleisher LA, Skolnick ED, Holroyd KJ, et al. Coronary artery revascularization before abdominal aortic aneurysm surgery: a decision analytic approach. *Anesth Analg* 1994;79:661, with permission.)

in the quality of their final years by undergoing coronary revascularization. In contrast, a 55-year-old man with an abdominal aortic aneurysm who is found to have occult left main CAD would have a substantial increase in both the length and the quality of his life from preoperative cardiovascular testing and coronary revascularization. Therefore, appropriate patients with diffuse disease or a significant left main coronary artery stenosis amenable to surgery who have an acceptable risk should undergo CABG before noncardiac surgery. In this instance, the procedure is justified based on long-term benefit, and performing it before noncardiac surgery reduces the risk of a fatal or nonfatal perioperative MI.

CHOICE OF DIAGNOSTIC TEST

Many tests have been proposed to further refine the presence and extent of CAD (Table 30-5). Exercise electrocardiography (ECG) is a useful test to diagnose CAD but is rarely indicated preoperatively because it requires the patient to have a good exercise capacity (and such a patient would not require testing). Ambulatory ECG has been shown to predict perioperative cardiac events, but the majority of patients at highest risk have ECG findings that prohibit the accurate diagnosis of silent ischemia and the test cannot be accurately quantified (24,38). Both dipyridamole imaging and dobutamine stress echocardiography have been advocated for patients who are unable to exercise, particularly those undergoing major vascular surgery (39,40). The value of dipyridamole imaging has been questioned, but a blinded study by Vanzetto et al. demonstrated high predictive value if the test is reserved for patients with multiple risk factors who are undergoing major vascular surgery (26,41). Importantly, those patients at greatest risk have larger areas of reversible defect or increased lung uptake on thallium imaging. Dobutamine stress echocardiography has also received a great deal of attention, because its positive and negative predictive values are among the best of any preoperative diagnostic test. This test may most closely mimic the hyperdynamic state seen during the perioperative period. Those patients who are at greatest risk develop new regional wall motion abnormalities at lower heart rates. In two metaanalyses, dobutamine stress echocardiography had the best pre-

TABLE 30-5. SENSITIVITY AND SPECIFICITY OF VARIOUS DIAGNOSTIC TESTS FOR DETECTING CORONARY ARTERY DISEASE

Test	Sensitivity (%)	Specificity (%)
Exercise electrocardiography	81	66
Exercise thallium imaging		
Qualitative planar	84	87
Quantitative planar	89	89
Single photon emission computed tomography (SPECT)	94	82
Dipyridamole thallium imaging	85	90
Stress echocardiography	80–90	80–90
Stress radionuclide angiography	70–80	70–80

dictive value, but there was a great deal of overlap with dipyridamole imaging (42,43). Finally, echocardiography is frequently performed before surgery, but the Guidelines are unable to define additive value for this test beyond clinical assessment. In summary, pharmacologic stress testing is of value but should be reserved for those patients who are at highest clinical risk. This specific choice of diagnostic test depends on local institutional factors.

CHOICE OF ANESTHETIC TECHNIQUE AND AGENT

There are many different approaches to the anesthetic care of the patient with CAD. The specific choice of anesthetic technique and intraoperative monitors depends on the integration of patient and surgery-specific factors. There have been several issues regarding the safety of the inhalational agents in patients with CAD. Isoflurane, because of its vasodilating properties, was shown to cause a coronary artery steal phenomenon leading to myocardial ischemia in an animal model (44). There are also case reports of myocardial ischemia associated with isoflurane use (45). This led to an editorial suggesting that isoflurane should not be used in patients with CAD (46). However, several large-scale randomized and nonrandomized studies in patients undergoing CABG did not demonstrated any increased incidence of myocardial ischemia or infarction in patients receiving isoflurane compared with other inhalation agents or narcotic-based techniques (47–49). In a subsequent analysis of one of the randomized trials, those patients who demonstrated steal-prone anatomy on coronary angiography did not have a higher incidence of myocardial ischemia with isoflurane than with other inhalational agents (49). Based on the accumulated data from human studies, most anesthesiologists do not believe that coronary steal presents a major threat of using isoflurane, and it has become the most widely used anesthetic, including for those patients with CAD.

There are theoretic concerns regarding the safety of desflurane. Desflurane was shown to be associated with airway irritability leading to tachycardia in volunteer studies (50). In a large-scale study comparing a narcotic-based anesthetic with a desflurane-based anesthetic, the desflurane group had a significantly higher incidence of myocardial ischemia but no difference in MI incidence (51). By including narcotic with desflurane, this tachycardia can frequently be ablated. Studies are ongoing to determine the safety profile of desflurane in patients undergoing major vascular surgery.

Sevoflurane was compared with isoflurane in one randomized trial in patients at high risk for cardiovascular disease. No differences in the incidence of myocardial ischemia was observed; however, the incidence of MI was too low to detect any difference (52). Overall, there appears to be no one best inhalation anesthetic for patient with CAD.

High-dose narcotic techniques offer the advantages of hemodynamic stability and lack of myocardial depression. In the early 1980s, Lowenstein et al. proposed a high-dose narcotic technique for patients undergoing CABG (53). Narcotic-based anesthetics were frequently considered the "cardiac anesthesia" and advocated for use in all high-risk patients, including those undergoing noncardiac surgery. The disadvantage of these traditional high-dose narcotic techniques is the requirement for postoperative ventilation. Despite the theoretic advantages of a high-dose narcotic technique, several large-scale trials in patients undergoing CAB showed no difference in survival or major morbidity compared with the inhalation-based technique (47,48). This has in part led to the abandonment of high-dose narcotics in much of cardiac surgery and to the trend toward early extubation.

An ultrashort-acting narcotic (remifentanil) has been introduced into clinical practice that allows the delivery of high doses of narcotics without the requirement for prolonged postoperative ventilation. It has been suggested as an ideal agent in patients undergoing cardiac surgery to facilitate early extubation (54). At present, it is unknown whether the unique properties of remifentanil offer advantages for the high-risk patient undergoing noncardiac surgery.

Current evidence supports the contention that there is no one best general anesthetic technique for patients with CAD undergoing noncardiac surgery and has led to the abandonment of the concept of a "cardiac anesthetic."

Regional Anesthesia

A great deal of research has focused on comparisons of regional versus general anesthesia for patients with CAD, particularly for those patients undergoing infrainguinal bypass surgery (Table 30-6). Yeager et al. demonstrated improved outcome with a combined regional and general anesthesia versus general anesthesia alone in a mixed population of patients undergoing intraabdominal and thoracic surgery; however, there were many flaws in this study, leading other investigators to design more rigorously controlled trials (55). Three major trials have been published involving patients undergoing infrainguinal surgery. Tuman et al. evaluated a combined general plus regional anesthesia versus general anesthesia alone and noted a decreased incidence of all-cause cardiac morbidity with no difference in acute MI or cardiac death (56). Importantly, the group that included regional anesthesia demonstrated a decreased hypercoagulable state by thromboelastography, compared with the general anesthesia group. Christopherson et al. randomly assigned 100 patients to epidural anesthesia plus epidural analgesia versus general anesthesia plus postoperative intravenous patient-controlled analgesia (57). They noted no difference in cardiac morbidity, although the regional anesthesia group did demonstrate a significantly reduced incidence of graft thrombosis and reoperation. This was associ-

TABLE 30-6. CARDIAC AND VASCULAR OUTCOMES IN STUDIES OF REGIONAL VERSUS GENERAL ANESTHESIA IN PATIENTS UNDERGOING VASCULAR SURGERY

		Congestive Heart Failure (%)		Myocardial Infarction (%)		Death (%)		Vascular Graft Occlusion (%)	
Author	n	RA	GA	RA	GA	RA	GA	RA	GA
Tuman et al.	80	5	10	0	8	0	0	3	20
Baron et al.	173	6	8	6	6	3	5	—	—
Christopherson et al.	100	—	—	4	4	2	2	4	20
Bode et al.	423	8	6	6	3	3	2	6	4
Bois et al.	124	5	0	4	8	0	0	—	—

Note: GA, general anesthesia; RA, regional anesthesia.
Source: Data from Norris EJ, Frank SM. Anesthesia for vascular surgery. In: Miller RD, ed. *Anesthesia,* 5th edition, vol 2. New York: Churchill Livingstone, 1999:1876.

ated with an increase in markers of thrombosis in the general anesthesia group. Bode et al. randomly assigned such patients to receive epidural, spinal, or general anesthesia and found no difference in cardiac outcome or graft thrombosis (58). Importantly, those patients who had a failed regional technique had the highest incidence of cardiac morbidity. In an accompanying editorial, an informal metaanalysis suggest that no difference in cardiac morbidity could be detected between regional and general anesthesia unless the effect was extremely small (59).

Several groups have also evaluated the benefit of regional anesthesia in patients undergoing aortic surgery. Baron et al. compared general anesthesia with regional plus general anesthesia for aortic surgery and was also unable to find a difference in cardiac morbidity (60). Bois et al. demonstrated improved postoperative analgesia without an effect on the rate of myocardial ischemia in patients undergoing aortic surgery with postoperative epidural analgesia compared with intravenous patient-controlled morphine analgesia (61). Norris et al. randomly assigned 240 patients to four groups: intraoperative general anesthesia with or without intraoperative and postoperative epidural analgesia. There was no difference in outcome among the four groups (E. Norris, *personal communication, 2000*). One of the issues with all of the studies involving regional anesthesia is that under ideal conditions some of the advantages of regional anesthesia may not become apparent. Therefore, it is important for anesthesiologists to do what they do best.

Monitored anesthesia care (MAC) was frequently considered optimal in appropriate high-risk patients as a means of avoiding general anesthesia. However, in a large-scale epidemiologic study, MAC was associated with increased 30-day mortality rate, compared with inhalational techniques in a univariate analysis, although the difference did not remain significant in multivariate analysis (62). The major issue with MAC is the ability to adequately block the stress response, because inadequate analgesia associated with tachycardia may be worse than the potential hemodynamic effects of general or regional anesthesia. Although MAC can supplement analgesia, the ability to provide good local anesthesia is important. However, with the newer short-acting intravenous agents, essentially general anesthesia can be administered without an endotracheal tube. This allows the anesthesiologist to provide intense anesthesia for short or peripheral procedures without the potential effects of endotracheal intubation and extubation.

GENERAL PRINCIPLES OF MANAGEMENT

In high-risk patients undergoing noncardiac surgery, multiple studies have demonstrated the association of perioperative myocardial ischemia with cardiac morbidity. Importantly, intraoperative ischemia has the poorest association with perioperative cardiac morbidity, and postoperative ischemia has the strongest relationship (63). It also appears that the duration of postoperative ischemia may be a critical determinant of morbidity. Landesberg et al. demonstrated that a cumulative duration of postoperative ST-segment depression greater than 2 hours was the best predictor of MI or cardiac death (64). Fleisher et al. demonstrated a relationship between a continuous episode of 30 minutes of ST-segment changes and postoperative cardiac morbidity (65) (Fig. 30-4). The accumulated evidence has led most anesthesiologists and postoperative caregivers to target their management to reducing perioperative ischemia in the absence of trials with sufficient numbers of patients to demonstrate differences in overt outcome.

Over the past decade numerous studies have attempted to evaluate the relationship between hemodynamics and perioperative ischemia and MI (Fig. 30-5). Since the pioneering work of Slogoff and Keats (66), tachycardia has been shown to be the strongest predictor of perioperative ischemia. Although traditionally a heart rate greater than 100 beats/minute has been defined as the lower limit for tachycardia, slower heart rates may result in myocardial ischemia. Frank et al. reported on a vascular patient who demonstrated marked ST depression preoperatively and

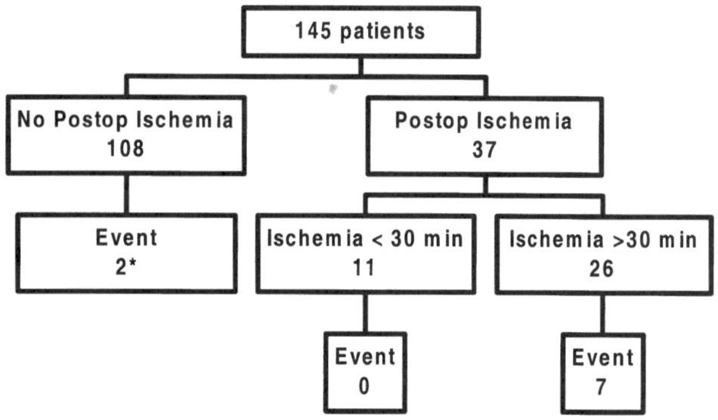

FIGURE 30-4. Pattern of perioperative ischemic changes and postoperative myocardial infarction (MI) in a cohort of high-risk patients undergoing noncardiac surgery. Of those patients who sustained a perioperative MI during the period in which they were monitored, all demonstrated at least 30 minutes of continuous ST-segment changes. In the two patients who sustained a perioperative MI without ischemia (denoted by *), the event occurred after the period of monitoring. (From Fleisher LA, Nelson AH, Rosenbaum SH. Postoperative myocardial ischemia: etiology of cardiac morbidity or manifestation of underlying disease. *J Clin Anesth* 1995;7:97, with permission.)

postoperatively at heart rates lower than 100 beats/minute, which resolved intraoperatively with heart rates lower than 70 beats/minute (67). In noncardiac surgery patients, Mangano et al. were unable to demonstrate a relationship between acute increases in heart rate and myocardial ischemia, although there was a generalized tachycardia in the postoperative period (68,69). This may predispose the patient to develop myocardial ischemia with small decreases in supply.

Although there has been concern about hypotension in patients with CAD, there is no evidence to support such a contention. In two studies involving patients undergoing CABG, the vast majority of episodes of intraoperative ischemia were not associated with any hemodynamic changes (70,71). In the absence of tachycardia, hypotension has not been shown to be associated with myocardial ischemia.

Hypothermia has also been associated with an increased incidence of myocardial ischemia in vascular surgery patients. In a randomized trial involving patients either undergoing vascular surgery or with known risk factors for CAD, use of forced air warming to maintain normothermia was associated with a significant reduction in cardiac morbidity and myocardial ischemia for the first 24 hours (72). Therefore, there is strong evidence that maintenance of normothermia should be a goal of intraoperative management.

Anemia has also been associated with an increased incidence of myocardial ischemia. In a small retrospective study of patients undergoing infrainguinal bypass surgery, hematocrit less than 27% was associated with a significantly increased risk of postoperative MI (73). Hogue et al. performed Holter monitoring of patients undergoing radical prostatectomy and also demonstrated an increased incidence of ischemia in anemic patients (74). Until definitive randomized trials are conducted to determine the value of transfusions for low hematocrit, it would seem prudent to maintain hematocrit greater than 27% for high-risk patients.

There has been recent interest in decreasing the perioperative hypercoagulable state in patients with CAD. An autopsy study of patients who sustained fatal perioperative MIs demonstrated a high proportion of patients with severe triple-vessel disease with plaque rupture and acute thrombosis (75). As described earlier, regional anesthesia and analgesia were associated with a decreased thrombotic state and a lower incidence of cardiac complications in one study (56). Additionally, the angiographic study by Ellis described previously also supported the notion that many of the acute major events are the result of thrombosis superimposed on a small stenosis (34). Future research will most likely focus

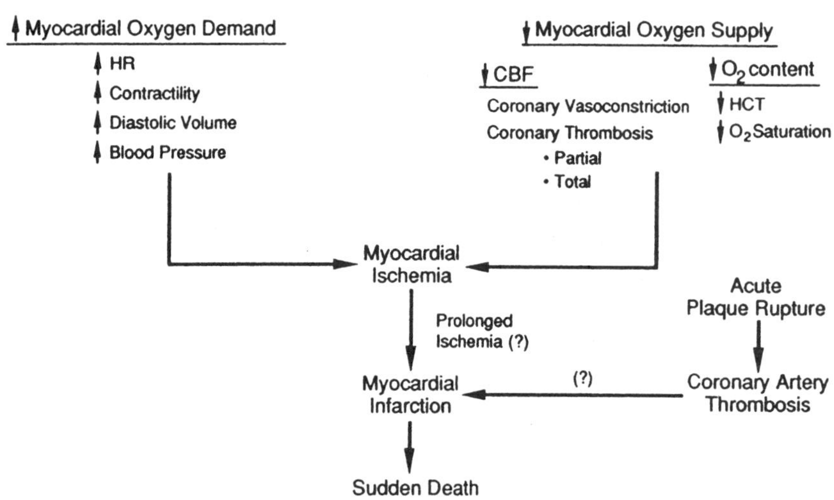

FIGURE 30-5. Pathophysiology of acute coronary syndromes during the perioperative period. The perioperative period is associated with acute changes in myocardial oxygen supply and demand that can lead to myocardial ischemia. If the ischemia is prolonged, there is evidence to suggest that it can lead to a myocardial infarction. Alternatively, an acute thrombosis may be the cause of perioperative myocardial infarction, and ischemia may simply be the manifestation of the underlying disease. (From Beattie C, Fleisher LA. Preface: Perioperative myocardial ischemia and infarction. *Int Anesth Clin* 1992;30, with permission.)

on pharmacologic manipulation of the clotting mechanism that can reduce the likelihood of coronary thrombosis without increased bleeding at the surgical site.

PERIOPERATIVE PHARMACOLOGIC MANAGEMENT

Many trials have investigated the value of intraoperative and postoperative use of pharmacologic agents to decrease perioperative cardiac morbidity. Nitroglycerin has been a mainstay of antiischemic therapy, but its value during the perioperative period is controversial. Two randomized clinical trials have focused on high-risk noncardiac surgery patients. Coriat et al. studied a cohort of patients undergoing carotid endarterectomy using a high-dose narcotic technique (76). They demonstrated a significantly reduced incidence of myocardial ischemia with 1.0 μg/kg/minute of nitroglycerin, compared with 0.5 μg/kg/minute. However, there were no patients who sustained a perioperative MI. Dodds et al. compared nitroglycerin at 1.0 μg/kg/minute with placebo using a balanced anesthetic technique in high-risk patients undergoing a diverse group of noncardiac surgeries and demonstrated no difference in perioperative myocardial ischemia or infarction (77). Many of the effects of nitroglycerin are mimicked by the anesthetic agents, minimizing nitroglycerin's potential beneficial effects and potentially leading to more profound hypotension. Therefore, the evidence does not support the routine prophylactic use of this agent.

β-Adrenergic blockade has been shown to reduce perioperative morbidity in several trials. Mangano et al. randomly assigned high-risk patients to receive 7 days of atenolol or placebo (78). Although there was no difference in perioperative mortality, the atenolol group had a significantly improved 6-month survival rate (79). There were differences in long-term treatment between the two groups that might have influenced survival, and approximately 40% of the patients were unable to tolerate the full atenolol dose. Poldermans et al. published a study on the use of bisoprolol in high-risk vascular patients (1). They screened patients and performed dobutamine echocardiography in the subset of patients with risk factors. Patients with positive scans were randomly assigned to receive either placebo or preoperative treatment plus 30-days of postoperative treatment of bisoprobl; a significantly lower incidence of fatal and nonfatal MIs was reported in the treatment group. An accompanying editorial suggested that such a strategy may obviate the need for extensive preoperative testing; however, patients with extensive cardiovascular disease on echocardiography were excluded from the study (80). Therefore, the use of β-blockade in patients with known but not extensive CAD is associated with improved outcome.

α_2-Agonists have received a great deal of attention as adjuvants to the anesthetic management. Ellis et al. randomly assigned high-risk noncardiac surgery patients to receive either clonidine or placebo and demonstrated a significantly decreased incidence of intraoperative but not postoperative ischemia (81). Stuhmeier et al. randomly assigned 297 elective vascular surgery patients and demonstrated a significantly reduced incidence of perioperative myocardial ischemia with fewer nonfatal MIs compared to the placebo group (82). Perioperative administration of mivazerol, a new intravenous α_2-agonist, was associated with a significantly reduced incidence of myocardial ischemia with no difference in cardiac events (83). In a large-scale study of 2,854 patients, 1,897 of whom with CAD and the remainder with risk factors, no benefit was demonstrated in the rate of cardiac complications (84). Importantly, in a predefined subgroup of 904 patients with known CAD who were undergoing vascular surgery, the use of mivazerol was associated with a relative risk of 0.66 of sustaining a cardiac event, compared with placebo. At the current time, there are no plans to continue development of this compound.

MONITORING

The choice of perioperative monitoring modality (Fig. 30-6) depends on the interaction of patient-specific risk, surgical procedure to be performed, and location of care. Many studies have demonstrated the predictive value and association between perioperative ST-segment changes and major cardiac events, as described previously (63–65,85). Furthermore, the duration, either cumulative or continuous, of perioperative ST changes has been shown to be the strongest predictor of poor outcomes (64,65). Therefore, ST-segment monitoring is becoming a standard during the intraoperative period for high-risk patients. However, patients at low to moderate risk may also develop ST-segment changes. These changes may not reflect true myocardial ischemia, as suggested a recent case series (86).

The value of ST-segment monitoring during the postoperative period is controversial. Most currently installed intensive care unit monitors do not include ST-segment monitoring, although virtually all of the new machines do have it available. The period of greatest risk may be the time when the patient is on the ward and unmonitored. Many of the monitoring companies have developed ST telemetry monitors, but they have not been tested in the perioperative period. The issue is whether early treatment of prolonged ST-segment changes leads to improved outcome. Until such studies are completed, the efficacy of such monitors is debatable.

There have been numerous articles devoted to the value of PA monitoring, but few randomized clinical trials. Traditionally, changes in pulmonary capillary wedge pressure have been considered a sensitive marker for myocardial ischemia. However, several studies have documented the poor

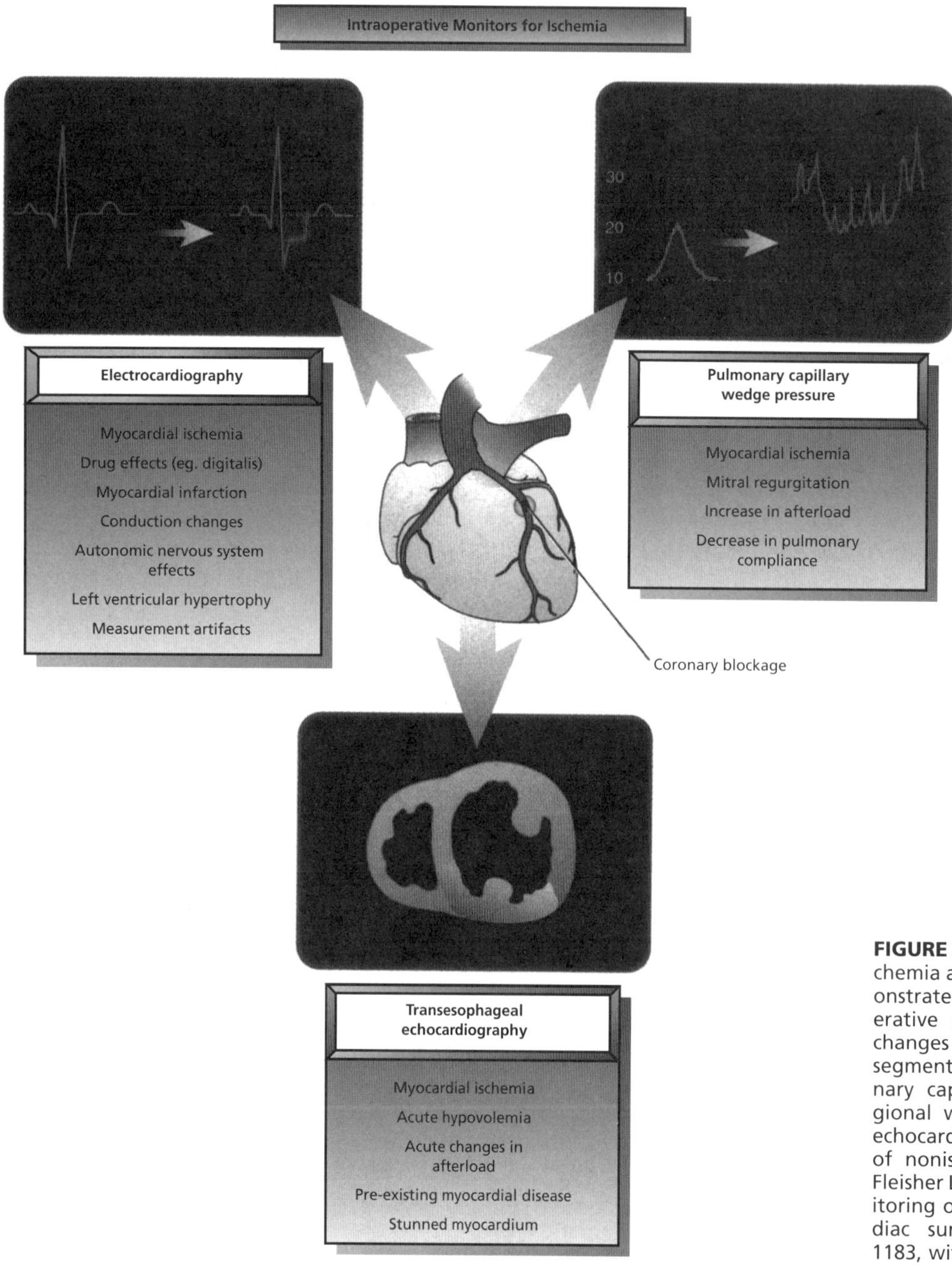

FIGURE 30-6. Monitors for myocardial ischemia and ventricular function and demonstrated changes associated with perioperative myocardial ischemia. Significant changes on each of the monitors (the ST segment of the electrocardiogram, pulmonary capillary wedge pressure, and regional wall motion on transesophageal echocardiogram) may also be the result of nonischemic causes, as listed. (From Fleisher LA. Real-time intraoperative monitoring of myocardial ischemia in noncardiac surgery. *Anesthesiology* 2000;92: 1183, with permission.)

sensitivity (33%) and specificity of such changes for myocardial ischemia (87).

The value of PA catheter monitoring has come under close scrutiny since publication of an article by Connors et al. and an accompanying editorial in the *Journal of the American Medical Association* (88,89). Using a variation of a case-controlled design to match patients enrolled in a study of end-of-life decisions among patients admitted to an intensive care unit who had an anticipated 50% mortality rate within 6 months, they demonstrated increased mortality among those patients who received a PA catheter. In the accompanying editorial, the authors suggested that a randomized, controlled trial be performed or a moratorium placed on the use of the catheter (89). This led the National Institutes of Health and the Food and Drug Administration to convene a panel and plan several large-scale, randomized trials. From a perioperative perspective, the patients in the Connors study were not similar to those seen for elective surgery and the results may not be generalizable, although they are provocative.

Several randomized trials have attempted to address issues of outcome in vascular surgery patients with respect to the use of a PA catheter. For patients undergoing aortic surgery, a PA catheter was not associated with improved outcomes, compared with use of a central venous pressure catheter, if the ejection fraction was greater than 50% in one small study, or if the patient had a negative cardiovascular workup or prior coronary intervention in a second study (90,91). In contrast, Berlauk et al. randomly assigned unselected patients undergoing infrainguinal bypass surgery to receive (a) a PA catheter placed preoperatively with optimization of hemodynamics, (b) a PA catheter placed immediately before surgery, or (c) a PA catheter only if indicated (92). Those patients who had a PA catheter placed had a lower incidence of postoperative graft thrombosis but no difference in major cardiac morbidity. In fact, two patients in the cohort who had preoperative PA catheter placement and hemodynamic optimization had a preoperative MI. Bender et al. randomly assigned 104 consecutive patients to receive a PA catheter either routinely on the morning of surgery or only if indicated intraoperatively or postoperatively (93). There was no overall difference in the incidence of cardiac complications or surgical intensive care unit stay.

The American Society of Anesthesiologists has published Guidelines on the use of the PA catheter (94). Based on a review of the available literature (1993), they advocate reserving the PA catheter for those circumstances in which a high-risk patient is undergoing a high-risk surgery in a setting in which the PA catheter will make a difference in management. For example, if there is a high probability of significant fluid shifts and the patient has signs of left ventricular dysfunction, then the PA catheter may provide important information for treatment.

Alternative means of assessing cardiac output have been developed using transesophageal M-mode and pulse Doppler ultrasonography and analysis of end-tidal carbon dioxide. The accuracy of these devices is improved compared with previously developed technology. There are currently no published studies addressing the value of this noninvasive assessment of cardiac output for high-risk patients.

TEE is an extremely sensitive noninvasive tool for detection of intraoperative wall motion abnormalities and fluid status. In patients undergoing aortic cross-clamping, TEE proved to have a significantly better sensitivity for detection of intraoperative ischemia compared to electrocardiography (95). In a large-scale technology assessment study, TEE detected significantly more episodes of intraoperative myocardial ischemia than did either 2- or 12-lead ECG (96) (Fig. 30-2). However, the additive value of TEE for major postoperative morbidity was extremely small. Importantly, this monitoring modality cannot be used during the period of greatest risk (i.e., the postoperative period). TEE is rarely used for noncardiac surgery except in selected institutions.

POSTOPERATIVE SURVEILLANCE FOR A PERIOPERATIVE MYOCARDIAL INFARCTION

The optimal and most cost-effective strategy for monitoring high-risk patients for major morbidity after noncardiac surgery is unknown. Instances of myocardial ischemia and MI that occur postoperatively are usually silent, most likely because of the confounding effects of analgesics and surgical pain. Creatine kinase (CK-MB) is also less specific for myocardial necrosis postoperatively, since it has been shown to be released during aortic surgery and after mesenteric ischemia (97,98). Further confounding the issue is the fact that most perioperative MIs are non–Q wave in nature, and nonspecific ST-T wave changes are common (64,65). Therefore, the diagnosis of perioperative MI is particularly difficult with these traditional tests. In one older study of diabetic and hypertensive patients, Charlson et al. determined the best combination of these three tests for detecting a perioperative event and demonstrated that daily ECGs plus symptom-directed CK-MB isoenzyme determinations yielded the best sensitivity and specificity (99).

Detection of a perioperative MI has been simplified by the approval of troponin T and troponin I. Adams et al. studied 108 patients undergoing high-risk surgery and obtained measurements of CK-MB, total CK, and cardiac troponin I, daily ECGs, and preoperative and postoperative echocardiograms (100). Eight vascular surgery patients sustained a perioperative MI, as confirmed by the presence of new segmental wall motion abnormalities. All eight patients had elevations of cardiac troponin I, and six had elevated CK-MB. Troponin I had a specificity of 99%, whereas CK-MB had a specificity of 81%. Lee et al. measured levels of CK-MB and troponin T in 1,175 patients and created receiver operating characteristic curves (101). They found that troponin T had a similar performance for diagnosing an MI and a significantly better correlation for major cardiac complications with an acute MI. Metzler et al. examined the sensitivity of defining a positive test as 0.6 ng/mL and demonstrated a positive predictive value of 87.5% and a negative predictive value of 98% (102). Both troponin I and troponin T hold great promise as a sensitive and specific marker of perioperative myocardial injury.

The implications of a perioperative MI are controversial. Traditionally, perioperative MIs were associated with a 30% to 50% short-term mortality rate. With the improved sensitivity of the assays and perioperative surveillance protocols, asymptomatic MIs are being detected. Recent series have reported incidences of fatal perioperative MI of less than 20% (64,103). There also appears to be a shift in the timing of a perioperative MI. Studies from the 1980s suggested that the second and third postoperative days included the peak incidence (7). Badner et al., using troponin T as a marker for MI, suggested that the immediate and first postoperative days had the highest incidence (103) (Fig. 30-7).

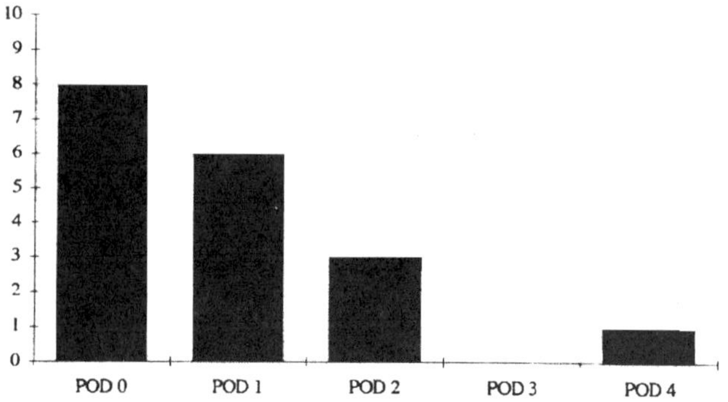

FIGURE 30-7. Rates of perioperative myocardial infarction (MI) by postoperative day in a cohort of high-risk noncardiac surgery patients. A diagnosis of perioperative MI was made if the total creatine kinase (CK) was greater than 174 U/L and in the presence of two of the following: (a) CK-2/CK (mass or activity) greater than 5%; (b) new Q waves lasting 0.04 seconds or longer and 1 mm deep in at least two contiguous leads; (c) troponin T concentration greater than 0.2 μg/L; and (d) a positive result on pyrophosphate scan. The perioperative MIs occurred on the day of operation in eight patients, on day 1 in six, on day 2 in three, and on day 4 in one patient, demonstrating that the MI was an early event. (From Badner NH, Knill RL, Brown JE, et al. Myocardial infarction after noncardiac surgery. *Anesthesiology* 1998;88:572, with permission.)

The question that remains is the long-term implications of a perioperative MI. Mangano et al. demonstrated significantly worse survival among those patients who sustained a cardiac event, compared with those who did not (104). Yeager et al. used a case-controlled method to retrospectively compare their cohort of patients who underwent major vascular surgery (105). Survival was significantly reduced for those patients who had symptomatic MIs. In contrast, MIs that were diagnosed by elevated CK-MB without cardiovascular signs or symptoms were not associated with worse survival when patients were matched with those who had similar degrees of CAD. Lopez-Jimenez et al. found that abnormal troponin T levels were associated with an increased incidence of cardiovascular complications within 6 months after surgery (106). Further research will be required to determine the implications of elevated postoperative cardiac enzymes or nonspecific ECG changes.

POSTOPERATIVE ANALGESIA

There is interest in the value of postoperative analgesia regimens for reduction of perioperative cardiac morbidity. The value of postoperative analgesia has been reviewed elsewhere (107). If postoperative tachycardia and catecholamine surges are one of the causes of perioperative cardiac morbidity, then more intense analgesia regimens may reduce these changes. Additionally, there is growing interest in the role of postoperative analgesia in reducing the hypercoagulable state. Several studies comparing general versus regional anesthesia have demonstrated reduced platelet aggregability with epidural anesthesia (56,108,109). It is unclear whether this finding is related to intraoperative or postoperative management. Future research will focus on how best to deliver postoperative analgesia to maximize the potential benefits in reducing complications.

POSTOPERATIVE INTENSIVE CARE UNIT

Since the study by Rao et al. which demonstrated reduced risk of reinfarction in a cohort of patients who had 3 days of postoperative ICU management compared with historical controls, clinicians have suggested that postoperative care can affect outcome (7). Pronovost et al. analyzed hospital discharge data for 2,987 patients in nonfederal acute care hospitals in Maryland who had undergone abdominal aortic surgery from January 1994 through December 1996 (110). In a multivariate analysis adjusted for patient demographics, comorbid disease, severity of illness, hospital and surgeon volume, and hospital characteristics, not having daily rounds by an ICU physician was associated with a threefold increase of in-hospital mortality. Furthermore, not having daily rounds by an ICU physician was associated with an increased risk of cardiac arrest. The authors concluded that organizational structure of the ICU can have a profound impact on outcomes.

ANESTHESIA FOR PATIENTS WITH HEART TRANSPLANTS

Patients with heart transplants present for noncardiac surgery much more frequently than patients who have undergone nontransplant cardiac surgery (111). The majority of these operations are emergent with resultant perioperative mortality. Long-term immunosuppression often leads to intraabdominal processes. Pancreatitis, cholecystitis, peptic ulcer disease, and gastrointestinal bleeding are common. Steroid therapy also results in an increased incidence of lymphomas and neoplasms.

To best manage the patient with a heart transplant, the anesthesiologist should understand the physiologic changes that are present. The transplanted heart is devoid of nervous system innervation and appears to undergo autonomic reinnervation with time, with sympathetic effects greater than parasympathetic effects (112). Therefore, aside from intrinsic control mechanisms, cardiovascular responsiveness depends predominantly on circulating factors, with some autonomic effects recovering over time. This results in a blunted response to stress and exercise, with the increase in heart rate not occurring for several minutes. Control of cardiac output depends on changes in ventricular volumes and the Frank-Starling mechanism. The denervated heart is prone to dysrhythmias and may require a pacemaker for bradycardia.

Management of noncardiac surgery in the patient with a heart transplant has been reviewed elsewhere (113). During the preoperative evaluation, it is important to determine the presence of rejection, hypertension, heart failure, dysrhythmia, and/or CAD. A careful history and physical examination should discern any signs of pulmonary infection. Premedication should avoid myocardial depressants. Stress doses of steroid should be administered.

The goal of intraoperative management is maintenance of adequate filling pressures and ventricular function. The use of invasive monitors must be weighed against the risk of infection in an immunocompromised host. Myocardial depressants should be avoided whenever possible. Changes in heart rate will only occur in response to catecholamines; therefore, direct-acting vasoactive agents should be used. Cyclosporine has been associated with an increased sensitivity to barbiturates and opioids in mice, without a clinical effect observed in humans (113,114). However, narcotics may not result in the decrease in heart rate that is mediated through vagal mechanisms. Additionally, standard monitoring for myocardial ischemia should be employed in these patients.

ANESTHESIA FOR PATIENTS WITH PRIOR CORONARY ARTERY BYPASS GRAFTS

As discussed previously, the patient with a prior CABG is at lower cardiac risk than similar patients who were treated medically. There has been little evidence related to the optimal period that should elapse between CABG and elective noncardiac surgery. The one study to address this issue was published in the 1980s. The authors reported that in 121 patients after CABG the risk of cardiac complications was very high during the first month and did decrease to normal values until after 6 months (115). A CABG may be particularly beneficial to the patient who has hibernating myocardium, which improves with time after revascularization. Therefore, in most elective cases, it would be prudent to delay noncardiac surgery for a minimum of 1 month.

The optimal period between PTCA and noncardiac surgery is even more controversial. There have been no investigations to address this issue. In a letter to the editor, Buffington and Smith reviewed the natural history of PTCA and suggested that the optimal time for elective surgery begins 2 to 4 weeks after angioplasty and extends to approximately 4 weeks (116). Whether these data also apply to patients who undergo intracoronary stent placement is unknown. In addition to issues related to restenosis, a coronary stent presents a nidus for thrombosis and may present a greater risk than balloon angioplasty (117).

There are also pathophysiologic concerns regarding the potential benefit of PTCA. The critical stenosis, particularly if collateral circulation exists, may not be etiologically involved in many infarcts. Ellis et al. identified a cohort of patients who underwent coronary angiography preoperatively and sustained a fatal or nonfatal postoperative MI (34). Of the 21 patients identified, 7 had no culprit stenosis, 6 had only a moderate stenosis, and 8 had a critical stenosis without adequate collaterals in the distribution of subsequent necrosis. There were no infarctions distal to critical stenoses with adequate collaterals. This work suggests that many infarcts may not be prevented by angioplasty of critical stenoses, except those with inadequate collaterals. This work is supported by the results from Posner et al. in which angioplasty less than 90 days before noncardiac surgery was not associated with improved outcome, compared with controls (32).

ANESTHESIA FOR PATIENTS WITH VALVULAR REPLACEMENT

In the patient with a functioning prosthetic heart valve, the major issues are antibiotic prophylaxis and anticoagulation. All patients with prosthetic valves who are undergoing procedures that could cause transient bacteremia should receive prophylaxis (118).

The common practice for patients undergoing noncardiac surgery with a prosthetic valve in place is cessation of anticoagulants 3 days before surgery. This allows the prothrombin time to fall to within 20% of normal. The oral anticoagulants can then be resumed on postoperative day 2. Using a similar protocol, Katholi et al. had no perioperative episodes of thromboembolism or hemorrhage in 25 patients (119). An alternative approach in patients at high risk for thromboembolism is conversion to heparin during the perioperative period. The heparin can be discontinued 4 to 6 hours before surgery and resumed shortly thereafter. Current prosthetic valves may have a lower incidence of thrombosis, and it may not be cost-effective to administer heparin in a hospital setting (120).

REFERENCES

1. Poldermans D, Boersma E, Bax JJ, et al. The effect of bisoprolol on perioperative mortality and myocardial infarction in high-risk patients undergoing vascular surgery. Dutch Echocardiographic Cardiac Risk Evaluation Applying Stress Echocardiography Study Group. *N Engl J Med* 1999;341:1789.
2. Eagle K, Brundage B, Chaitman B, et al. Guidelines for perioperative cardiovascular evaluation of the noncardiac surgery: a report of the American Heart Association/American College of Cardiology Task Force on Assessment of Diagnostic and Therapeutic Cardiovascular Procedures. *Circulation* 1996;93:1278.
3. Palda VA, Detsky AS. Perioperative assessment and management of risk from coronary artery disease. *Ann Intern Med* 1997; 127:313.

4. Goldman L, Caldera DL, Nussbaum SR, et al. Multifactorial index of cardiac risk in noncardiac surgical procedures. *N Engl J Med* 1977;297:845.
5. Lee TH, Marcantonio ER, Mangione CM, et al. Derivation and prospective validation of a simple index for prediction of cardiac risk of major noncardiac surgery. *Circulation* 1999;100:1043.
6. Detsky A, Abrams H, McLaughlin J, et al. Predicting cardiac complications in patients undergoing non-cardiac surgery. *J Gen Intern Med* 1986;1:211.
7. Rao TL, Jacobs KH, El-Etr AA. Reinfarction after anesthesia in patients with myocardial infarction. *Anesthesiology* 1983;59:499.
8. Tarhan S, Moffitt EA, Taylor WF, et al. Myocardial infarction after general anesthesia. *JAMA* 1972;220:1451.
9. Shah KB, Kleinman BS, Sami H, et al. Reevaluation of perioperative myocardial infarction in patients with prior myocardial infarction undergoing noncardiac operations. *Anesth Analg* 1990;71:231.
10. Ryan TJ, Anderson JL, Antman EM, et al. ACC/AHA Guidelines for the Management of Patients with Acute Myocardial Infarction: executive summary. A report of the American College of Cardiology/American Heart Association Task Force on Practice Guidelines (Committee on Management of Acute Myocardial Infarction). *Circulation* 1996;94:2341.
11. Shah KB, Kleinman BS, Rao T, et al. Angina and other risk factors in patients with cardiac diseases undergoing noncardiac operations. *Anesth Analg* 1990;70:240.
12. Eagle KA, Coley CM, Newell JB, et al. Combining clinical and thallium data optimizes preoperative assessment of cardiac risk before major vascular surgery. *Ann Intern Med* 1989;110:859.
13. Kannel W, Abbott R. Incidence and prognosis of unrecognized myocardial infarction: an update on the Framingham Study. *N Engl J Med* 1984;311:1144.
14. Acharya DU, Shekhar YC, Aggarwal A, et al. Lack of pain during myocardial infarction in diabetics: is autonomic dysfunction responsible? *Am J Cardiol* 1991;68:793.
14a. Frank SM, Norris EJ, Christopherson R, et al. Right- and-left-arm blood pressure discrepancies in vascular surgery patients. *Anesthesiology* 1991;75:457.
15. The sixth report of the Joint National Committee on prevention, detection, evaluation, and treatment of high blood pressure. *Arch Intern Med* 1997;157:2413.
16. Kannel WB. Historic perspectives on the relative contributions of diastolic and systolic blood pressure elevation to cardiovascular risk profile. *Am Heart J* 1999;138:205.
17. Parati G, Pomidossi G, Albini F, et al. Relationship of 24-hour blood pressure mean and variability to severity of target-organ damage in hypertension. *J Hypertension* 1987;5:93.
18. Pringle SD, MacFarlane PW, McKillop JH, et al. Pathophysiologic assessment of left ventricular hypertrophy and strain in asymptomatic patients with essential hypertension. *J Am Coll Cardiol* 1989;13:1377.
19. Hollenberg M, Mangano DT, Browner WS, et al. Predictors of postoperative myocardial ischemia in patients undergoing noncardiac surgery. The Study of Perioperative Ischemia Research Group. *JAMA* 1992;268:205.
20. Warner MA, Shields SE, Chute CG. Major morbidity and mortality within 1 month of ambulatory surgery and anesthesia. *JAMA* 1993;270:1437.
21. Krupski WC, Layug EL, Reilly LM, et al. Comparison of cardiac morbidity between aortic and infrainguinal operations. Study of Perioperative Ischemia (SPI) Research Group. *J Vasc Surg* 1992;15:354.
22. Eagle KA, Rihal CS, Mickel MC, et al. Cardiac risk of noncardiac surgery: influence of coronary disease and type of surgery in 3368 operations. CASS Investigators and University of Michigan Heart Care Program. Coronary Artery Surgery Study. *Circulation* 1997;96:1882.
23. McPhail N, Calvin JE, Shariatmadar A, et al. The use of preoperative exercise testing to predict cardiac complications after arterial reconstruction. *J Vasc Surg* 1988;7:60.
24. Fleisher LA, Rosenbaum SH, Nelson AH, et al. Preoperative dipyridamole thallium imaging and Holter monitoring as a predictor of perioperative cardiac events and long tem outcome. *Anesthesiology* 1995;83:906.
25. Reilly DF, McNeely MJ, Doerner D, et al. Self-reported exercise tolerance and the risk of serious perioperative complications. *Arch Intern Med* 1999;159:2185.
26. Vanzetto G, Machecourt J, Blendea D, et al. Additive value of thallium single-photon emission computed tomography myocardial imaging for prediction of perioperative events in clinically selected high cardiac risk patients having abdominal aortic surgery. *Am J Cardiol* 1996;77:143.
27. Cohen MC, McKenna C, Lewis SM, et al. Requirements for controlled clinical trials of preoperative cardiovascular risk reduction. *Control Clin Trials* 1995;16:89.
28. Reference deleted in page proofs.
29. Huber KC, Evans MA, Bresnahan JF, et al. Outcome of noncardiac operations in patients with severe coronary artery disease successfully treated preoperatively with coronary angioplasty. *Mayo Clin Proc* 1992;67:15.
30. Rihal CS, Eagle KA, Mickel MC, et al. Surgical therapy for coronary artery disease among patients with combined coronary artery and peripheral vascular disease. *Circulation* 1995;91:46.
31. Gottlieb A, Banous M, Sprung J, et al. Perioperative cardiovascular morbidity in patients with coronary artery disease undergoing vascular surgery after percutaneous transluminal coronary angioplasty. *J Cardiothor Vasc Anesth* 1998;12:501.
32. Posner KL, Van Norman GA, Chan V. Adverse cardiac outcomes after noncardiac surgery in patients with prior percutaneous transluminal coronary angioplasty. *Anesth Analg* 1999;89:553.
33. Ambrose JA, Tannenbaum MA, Alexopoulos D, et al. Angiographic progression of coronary artery disease and the development of myocardial infarction. *J Am Coll Cardiol* 1988;12:56.
34. Ellis SG, Hertzer NR, Young JR, et al. Angiographic correlates of cardiac death and myocardial infarction complicating major nonthoracic vascular surgery. *Am J Cardiol* 1996;77:1126.
35. Fleisher LA, Skolnick ED, Holroyd KJ, et al. Coronary artery revascularization before abdominal aortic aneurysm surgery: a decision analytic approach. *Anesth Analg* 1994;79:661.
36. Mason JJ, Owens DK, Harris RA, et al. The role of coronary angiography and coronary revascularization before noncardiac surgery. *JAMA* 1995;273:1919.
37. Glance LG. Selective preoperative cardiac screening improves five-year survival in patients undergoing major vascular surgery: a cost-effectiveness analysis. *J Cardiothorac Vasc Anesth* 1999;13:265.
38. Raby KE, Goldman L, Creager MA, et al. Correlation between perioperative ischemia and major cardiac events after peripheral vascular surgery. *N Engl J Med* 1989;321:1296.
39. Boucher CA, Brewster DC, Darling RC, et al. Determination of cardiac risk by dipyridamole-thallium imaging before peripheral vascular surgery. *N Engl J Med* 1985;312:389.
40. Poldermans D, Arnese M, Fioretti PM, et al. Improved cardiac risk stratification in major vascular surgery with dobutamine-atropine stress echocardiography. *J Am Coll Cardiol* 1995;26:648.
41. Baron JF, Mundler O, Bertrand M, et al. Dipyridamole-thal-

lium scintigraphy and gated radionuclide angiography to assess cardiac risk before abdominal aortic surgery. *N Engl J Med* 1994; 330:663.
42. Mantha S, Roizen MF, Barnard J, et al. Relative effectiveness of four preoperative tests for predicting adverse cardiac outcomes after vascular surgery: a meta-analysis. *Anesth Analg* 1994; 79:422.
43. Shaw LJ, Eagle KA, Gersh BJ, et al. Meta-analysis of intravenous dipyridamole-thallium-201 imaging (1985 to 1994) and dobutamine echocardiography (1991 to 1994) for risk stratification before vascular surgery. *J Am Coll Cardiol* 1996;27:787.
44. Buffington CW, Romson JL, Levine A, et al. Isoflurane induces coronary steal in a canine model of chronic coronary occlusion. *Anesthesiology* 1987;66:280.
45. Sigurdsson GH, Brouwer RP, Thomson D. Repeated episodes of myocardial ischaemia during combined thoracic epidural-isoflurane anaesthesia. *Acta Anaesthesiol Scand* 1994;38:521.
46. Becker LC. Is isoflurane dangerous for the patient with coronary artery disease? [Editorial]. *Anesthesiology* 1987;66:259.
47. Leung JM, Goehner P, O'Kelly BF, et al. Isoflurane anesthesia and myocardial ischemia: comparative risk versus sufentanil anesthesia in patients undergoing coronary artery bypass graft surgery. The Study of Perioperative Ischemia (SPI) Research Group. *Anesthesiology* 1991;74:838.
48. Slogoff S, Keats AS. Randomized trial of primary anesthetic agents on outcome of coronary artery bypass operations. *Anesthesiology* 1989;70:179.
49. Slogoff S, Keats AS, Dear WE, et al. Steal-prone coronary anatomy and myocardial ischemia associated with four primary anesthetic agents in humans. *Anesth Analg* 1991;72:22.
50. Ebert TJ, Muzi M. Sympathetic hyperactivity during desflurane anesthesia in healthy volunteers: a comparison with isoflurane. *Anesthesiology* 1993;79:444.
51. Helman JD, Leung JM, Bellows WH, et al. The risk of myocardial ischemia in patients receiving desflurane versus sufentanil anesthesia for coronary artery bypass graft surgery. The Study of Perioperative Ischemia (SPI) Research Group. *Anesthesiology* 1992;77:47.
52. Ebert TJ, Kharasch ED, Rooke GA, et al. Myocardial ischemia and adverse cardiac outcomes in cardiac patients undergoing noncardiac surgery with sevoflurane and isoflurane. Sevoflurane Ischemia Study Group. *Anesth Analg* 1997;85:993.
53. Lowenstein E, Hallowell P, Levine FH, et al. Cardiovascular response to large doses of intravenous morphine in man. *N Engl J Med* 1969;281:1389.
54. Royston D. Patient selection and anesthetic management for early extubation and hospital discharge: CABG. *J Cardiothorac Vasc Anesth* 1998;12:11.
55. Yeager MP, Glass DD, Neff RK, et al. Epidural anesthesia and analgesia in high-risk surgical patients. *Anesthesiology* 1987;66: 729.
56. Tuman KJ, McCarthy RJ, March RJ, et al. Effects of epidural anesthesia and analgesia on coagulation and outcome after major vascular surgery. *Anesth Analg* 1991;73:696.
57. Christopherson R, Beattie C, Frank SM, et al. Perioperative morbidity in patients randomized to epidural or general anesthesia for lower extremity vascular surgery. Perioperative Ischemia Randomized Anesthesia Trial Study Group. *Anesthesiology* 1993;79:422.
58. Bode RH Jr, Lewis KP, Zarich SW, et al. Cardiac outcome after peripheral vascular surgery: comparison of general and regional anesthesia. *Anesthesiology* 1996;84:3.
59. Go AS, Browner WS. Cardiac outcomes after regional or general anesthesia: do we have the answer? [Editorial; comment]. *Anesthesiology* 1996;84:1.
60. Baron JF, Bertrand M, Barre E, et al. Combined epidural and general anesthesia versus general anesthesia for abdominal aortic surgery. *Anesthesiology* 1991;75:611.
61. Bois S, Couture P, Boudreault D, et al. Epidural analgesia and intravenous patient-controlled analgesia result in similar rates of postoperative myocardial ischemia after aortic surgery. *Anesth Analg* 1997;85:1233.
62. Cohen M, Duncan PG, Tate RB. Does anesthesia contribute to operative mortality? *JAMA* 1988;260:2859.
63. Mangano DT, Browner WS, Hollenberg M, et al. Association of perioperative myocardial ischemia with cardiac morbidity and mortality in men undergoing noncardiac surgery. *N Engl J Med* 1990;323:1781.
64. Landesberg G, Luria MH, Cotev S, et al. Importance of long-duration postoperative ST-segment depression in cardiac morbidity after vascular surgery. *Lancet* 1993;341:715.
65. Fleisher LA, Nelson AH, Rosenbaum SH. Postoperative myocardial ischemia: etiology of cardiac morbidity or manifestation of underlying disease. *J Clin Anesth* 1995;7:97.
66. Slogoff S, Keats AS. Does perioperative myocardial ischemia lead to postoperative myocardial infarction? *Anesthesiology* 1985; 62:107.
67. Frank SM, Beattie C, Christopherson R, et al. Perioperative rate-related silent myocardial ischemia and postoperative death. *J Clin Anesth* 1990;2:326.
68. Mangano DT, Wong MG, London MJ, et al. Perioperative myocardial ischemia in patients undergoing noncardiac surgery: II. Incidence and severity during the 1st week after surgery. The Study of Perioperative Ischemia (SPI) Research Group. *J Am Coll Cardiol* 1991;17:851.
69. Mangano DT, Hollenberg M, Fegert G, et al. Perioperative myocardial ischemia in patients undergoing noncardiac surgery: I. Incidence and severity during the 4 day perioperative period. The Study of Perioperative Ischemia (SPI) Research Group. *J Am Coll Cardiol* 1991;17:843.
70. Leung JM, O'Kelly BF, Mangano DT, et al. Relationship of regional wall motion abnormalities to hemodynamic indices of myocardial oxygen supply and demand in patients undergoing CABG surgery. *Anesthesiology* 1990;73:802.
71. Gordon MA, Urban MK, O'Connor T, et al. Is the pressure rate quotient a predictor or indicator of myocardial ischemia as measured by ST-segment changes in patients undergoing coronary artery bypass surgery. *Anesthesiology* 1991;74:848.
72. Frank SM, Fleisher LA, Breslow MJ, et al. Perioperative maintenance of normothermia reduces the incidence of morbid cardiac events: a randomized clinical trial. *JAMA* 1997;277:1127.
73. Nelson AH, Fleisher LA, Rosenbaum SH. Relationship between postoperative anemia and cardiac morbidity in high-risk vascular patients in the intensive care unit. *Crit Care Med* 1993;21: 860.
74. Hogue CW Jr, Goodnough LT, Monk TG. Perioperative myocardial ischemic episodes are related to hematocrit level in patients undergoing radical prostatectomy. *Transfusion* 1998;38: 924.
75. Dawood MM, Gutpa DK, Southern J, et al. Pathology of fatal perioperative myocardial infarction: implications regarding pathophysiology and prevention. *Int J Cardiol* 1996;57:37.
76. Coriat P, Daloz M, Bousseau D, et al. Prevention of intraoperative myocardial ischemia during noncardiac surgery with intravenous nitroglycerin. *Anesthesiology* 1984;61:193.
77. Dodds TM, Stone JG, Coromilas J, et al. Prophylactic nitroglycerin infusion during noncardiac surgery does not reduce perioperative ischemia. *Anesth Analg* 1993;76:705.
78. Mangano DT, Layug EL, Wallace A, et al. Effect of atenolol on mortality and cardiovascular morbidity after noncardiac surgery.

Multicenter Study of Perioperative Ischemia Research Group. *N Engl J Med* 1996;335:1713.

79. Wallace A, Layug B, Tateo I, et al. Prophylactic atenolol reduces postoperative myocardial ischemia. McSPI Research Group. *Anesthesiology* 1998;88:7.
80. Lee TH. Reducing cardiac risk in noncardiac surgery [Editorial; comment]. *N Engl J Med* 1999;341:1838.
81. Ellis JE, Drijvers G, Pedlow S, et al. Premedication with oral and transdermal clonidine provides safe and efficacious postoperative sympatholysis. *Anesth Analg* 1994;79:1133.
82. Stuhmeier KD, Mainzer B, Cierpka J, et al. Small, oral dose of clonidine reduces the incidence of intraoperative myocardial ischemia in patients having vascular surgery. *Anesthesiology* 1996;85:706.
83. Anonymous. Perioperative sympatholysis: beneficial effects of the alpha 2-adrenoceptor agonist mivazerol on hemodynamic stability and myocardial ischemia. McSPI—Europe Research Group. *Anesthesiology* 1997;86:346.
84. Oliver MF, Goldman L, Julian DG, et al. Effect of mivazerol on perioperative cardiac complications during non-cardiac surgery in patients with coronary heart disease: the European Mivazerol Trial (EMIT). *Anesthesiology* 1999;91:951.
85. Raby KE, Barry J, Creager MA, et al. Detection and significance of intraoperative and postoperative myocardial ischemia in peripheral vascular surgery. *JAMA* 1992;268:222.
86. Fleisher LA, Zielski MM, Schulman SP. Perioperative ST-segment depression is rare and may not indicate myocardial ischemia in moderate-risk patients undergoing noncardiac surgery. *J Cardiothorac Vasc Anesth* 1997;11:155.
87. van Daele ME, Sutherland GR, Mitchell MM, et al. Do changes in pulmonary capillary wedge pressure adequately reflect myocardial ischemia during anesthesia? A correlative preoperative hemodynamic, electrocardiographic, and transesophageal echocardiographic study. *Circulation* 1990;81:865.
88. Connors AF Jr, Speroff T, Dawson NV, et al. The effectiveness of right heart catheterization in the initial care of critically ill patients. SUPPORT Investigators. *JAMA* 1996;276:889.
89. Dalen JE, Bone RC. Is it time to pull the pulmonary artery catheter? [Editorial]. *JAMA* 1996;276:916.
90. Isaacson IJ, Lowdon JD, Berry AJ, et al. The value of pulmonary artery and central venous monitoring in patients undergoing abdominal aortic reconstructive surgery: a comparative study of two selected, randomized groups. *J Vasc Surg* 1990;12:754.
91. Joyce WP, Provan JL, Ameli FM, et al. The role of central haemodynamic monitoring in abdominal aortic surgery: a prospective randomized study. *Eur J Vasc Surg* 1990;4:633.
92. Berlauk JF, Abrams JH, Gilmour IJ, et al. Preoperative optimization of cardiovascular hemodynamics improves outcome in peripheral vascular surgery: a prospective, randomized clinical trial. *Ann Surg* 1991;214:289.
93. Bender J, Smith-Meek M, Jones C. Routine pulmonary artery catheterization does not reduce morbidity and mortality of elective vascular surgery: results of a prospective, randomized trial. *Ann Surg* 1997;226:229.
94. Anonymous. Practice guidelines for pulmonary artery catheterization: a report by the American Society of Anesthesiologists Task Force on Pulmonary Artery Catheterization. *Anesthesiology* 1993;78:380.
95. Roizen MF, Beaupre PN, Alpert RA, et al. Monitoring with two-dimensional transesophageal echocardiography: comparison of myocardial function in patients undergoing supraceliac, suprarenal-infraceliac, or infrarenal aortic occlusion. *J Vasc Surg* 1984;1:300.
96. Eisenberg MJ, London MJ, Leung JM, et al. Monitoring for myocardial ischemia during noncardiac surgery: a technology assessment of transesophageal echocardiography and 12-lead electrocardiography. The Study of Perioperative Ischemia Research Group. *JAMA* 1992;268:210.
97. Andersen PT, Nielsen LK, Moller-Pettersen J, et al. Non-cardiac creatine kinase-B activity in serum after abdominal aortic bypass surgery. *Acta Chir Scand* 1988;154:359.
98. Graeber GM, Clagett GP, Wolf RE, et al. Alterations in serum kinase and lactate dehydrogenase: association with abdominal aortic surgery, myocardial infarction and bowel necrosis. *Chest* 1990;97:521.
99. Charlson ME, MacKenzie CR, Ales K, et al. Surveillance for postoperative myocardial infarction after noncardiac operations. *Surg Gyn Obstet* 1988;167:407.
100. Adams JE 3rd, Sicard GA, Allen BT, et al. Diagnosis of perioperative myocardial infarction with measurement of cardiac troponin I. *N Engl J Med* 1994;330:670.
101. Lee TH, Thomas EJ, Ludwig LE, et al. Troponin T as a marker for myocardial ischemia in patients undergoing major noncardiac surgery. *Am J Cardiol* 1996;77:1031.
102. Metzler H, Gries M, Rehak P, et al. Perioperative myocardial cell injury: the role of troponins. *Br J Anaesth* 1997;78:386.
103. Badner NH, Knill RL, Brown JE, et al. Myocardial infarction after noncardiac surgery. *Anesthesiology* 1998;88:572.
104. Mangano DT, Browner WS, Hollenberg M, et al. Long-term cardiac prognosis following noncardiac surgery. The Study of Perioperative Ischemia Research Group. *JAMA* 1992;268:233.
105. Yeager RA, Moneta GL, Edwards JM, et al. Late survival after perioperative myocardial infarction complicating vascular surgery. *J Vasc Surg* 1994;20:598.
106. Lopez-Jimenez F, Goldman L, Sacks DB, et al. Prognostic value of cardiac troponin T after noncardiac surgery: 6-month follow-up data. *J Am Coll Cardiol* 1997;29:1241.
107. Liu S, Carpenter RL, Neal JM. Epidural anesthesia and analgesia: their role in postoperative outcome. *Anesthesiology* 1995;82:1474.
108. Tuman KJ, McCarthy FJ, Spiess BD. Epidural anaesthesia and analgesia decreases postoperative hypercoagulability in high-risk vascular patients. *Anesth Analg* 1990;70:S414.
109. Rosenfeld BA, Beattie C, Christopherson R, et al. The effects of different anesthetic regimens on fibrinolysis and the development of postoperative arterial thrombosis. Perioperative Ischemia Randomized Anesthesia Trial Study Group. *Anesthesiology* 1993;79:435.
110. Pronovost PJ, Jenckes MW, Dorman T, et al. Organizational characteristics of intensive care units related to outcomes of abdominal aortic surgery. *JAMA* 1999;281:1310.
111. Jones MT, Menkis AH, Kostuk WJ, et al. Management of general surgical problems after cardiac transplantation. *Can J Surg* 1988;31:259.
112. Brunner-La Rocca HP, Weilenmann D, Bracht C, et al. Relative frequency of functional sympathetic and parasympathetic reinnervation after heart transplantation. *J Heart Lung Transplant* 1998;17:725.
113. Melendez JA, Delphin E, Lamb J, et al. Noncardiac surgery in heart transplant recipients in the cyclosporine era. *J Cardiothorac Vasc Anesth* 1991;5:218.
114. Cirella VN, Pantuck CB, Lee YJ, et al. Effects of cyclosporine on anesthetic action. *Anesth Analg* 1987;66:703.
115. Cruchley P, Kaplan J, Hug C, et al. Non-cardiac surgery in patients with prior myocardial revascularization. *Can Anesth J* 1983;30:629.

116. Buffington CW, Smith AJ. Timing of elective surgery after coronary angioplasty [Letter]. *Anesthesiology* 1995;82:1544.
117. Gandhi MM, Dawkins KD. Fortnightly review: intracoronary stents. *BMJ* 1999;318:650.
118. Dajani A, Taubert K, Wilson W, et al. Prevention of bacterial endocarditis: recommendations by the American Heart Association. *JAMA* 1997;277:1794.
119. Katholi RE, Nolan SP, McGuire LB. The management of anticoagulation during noncardiac operations in patients with prosthetic heart valves: a prospective study. *Am Heart J* 1978;96:163.
120. Eckman MH, Beshansky JR, Durand-Zaleski I, et al. Anticoagulation for noncardiac procedures in patients with prosthetic heart valves: does low risk mean high cost? *JAMA* 1990;263: 1513.

Cardiac Anesthesia: Principles and Clinical Practice, Second Edition, edited by Fawzy G. Estafanous, Paul G. Barash, and J.G. Reves. Lippincott Williams & Wilkins, Philadelphia © 2001.

31

PEDIATRIC NONCARDIAC ANESTHESIA

RAAFAT S. HANNALLAH
SUSAN T. VERGHESE

It has been estimated that 0.8% of children born in the United States will be diagnosed to have some form of congenital heart disease (Table 31-1) (1). Many of these children will require surgery for noncardiac conditions that are commonly encountered during childhood (e.g., inguinal hernia, dental caries, or chronic tonsillitis). Moreover, many children with congenital heart disease have other associated noncardiac (e.g., orthopedic or genitourinary) congenital anomalies that require surgical repair (Table 31-2) (2). Many of these procedures are performed in general hospitals by noncardiac anesthesiologists. It is therefore essential that the anesthesiologist be knowledgeable not only of the basics of pediatric anesthesia but also of the pathophysiology of the cardiac lesions.

The factors that most influence the choice of anesthetic technique, agents, and monitoring in the cardiac patient undergoing noncardiac surgery are the degree of cardiac and pulmonary impairment caused by the congenital cardiac defect and the magnitude of the surgical procedure. This chapter describes the preoperative evaluation of children with congenital heart disease with a special emphasis on the implications of the primary lesion and prior medical or surgical treatment on the choice of anesthetic agents and techniques.

PATHOPHYSIOLOGY OF CONGENITAL CARDIAC LESIONS

Although knowledge of the exact anatomic defect in children with congenital heart disease is essential for planning surgical repair, a simple, workable classification can be based primarily on pathophysiology (Table 31-3) (3). This classification separates congenital heart lesions into the following three groups:

1. Lesions that cause pulmonary blood flow to increase as a result of left-to-right shunting (i.e., ventricular septal defect). Left uncorrected, these lesions will result in a volume and/or pressure overload to the pulmonary circulation and congestive heart failure.
2. Lesions that cause pulmonary blood flow to decrease as a result of right-to-left shunting (i.e., tetralogy of Fallot). These result in a relative inability to oxygenate blood, which may eventually lead to cyanosis. Cyanosis may also develop as a result of mixing of systemic and pulmonary venous return, a phenomenon that may occur in patients with a single ventricle or transposition of great arteries.
3. Lesions that primarily obstruct blood flow. These anomalies result in reduced blood flow distal to the obstructive lesion, as well as increased cardiac workload, and in some cases, congestive heart failure.

A knowledge of the physiologic consequences of shunting or obstruction is essential to understanding the hemodynamic consequences of any congenital heart deformity. Application of these physiologic concepts permits the anesthesiologist to design a rational management plan for the child with congenital heart disease.

The physiology of shunting of or obstruction to blood flow is explained by the relationship: $Q = P/R$, where Q equals blood flow, P equals pressure gradient, and R equals resistance to blood flow. Shunting of blood between the systemic and pulmonary circulations in the presence of a communicating defect depends on the pressure difference between the two sides of the circulation. The quality and direction of shunt flow may be further influenced by an outflow tract obstruction in either side of the heart. A detailed description of the hemodynamic changes of all congenital heart lesions is beyond the scope of this chapter; some representative examples of commonly encountered lesions are presented in Chapter 21.

FUNCTIONAL ASSESSMENT

A thorough history and physical examination are essential to evaluate the significance of the heart disease and its potential

R. S. Hannallah and S. T. Verghese: Department of Anesthesiology and Pediatrics, George Washington University Medical Center and Department of Anesthesiology, Children's National Medical Center, Washington, D.C. 20010

TABLE 31-1. THE TEN MOST COMMON CONGENITAL HEART DEFECTS

Defect	Percentage of Total Defects
Ventricular septal defect	28
Secundum atrial septal defect	10
Patent ductus arteriosus	10
Tetralogy of Fallot	10
Pulmonary stenosis	10
Aortic stenosis	7
Coarctation of the aorta	5
Transposition of the great arteries	5
Primum atrial septal defect	3
Total anomalous pulmonary venous return	1

implications on anesthetic management (Table 31-4) (1). Review of available cardiac data (e.g., electrocardiogram, chest x-ray film, echocardiography, and cardiac catheterization) is a part of the preanesthetic workup of these patients, regardless of the planned surgical procedure. A complete written cardiac evaluation from the treating cardiologist is necessary in patients with complex lesions.

Based on the findings, the cardiac lesion can be classified into one of the following categories:

1. No cardiac disease, in spite of a "cardiac" finding (e.g., an innocent heart murmur).
2. A known cardiac lesion with minimal or no symptoms or physical findings (e.g., a small atrial or ventricular septal defect). Although no special anesthetic agents or

TABLE 31-3. FLOW CHARACTERISTICS OF VARIOUS CONGENITAL CARDIAC LESIONS

Increased pulmonary blood flow lesions
- Atrial septal defect
- Ventricular septal defect
- Patent ductus arteriosus
- Endocardial cushion defect (atrioventricular canal abnormality)
- Anomalous origin of coronary arteries
- Transposition of the great arteries[a]
- Anomalous pulmonary venous drainage[a]
- Truncus arteriosus[a]
- Single ventricle[a]

Decreased pulmonary blood flow lesions
- Tetralogy of Fallot
- Pulmonary atresia
- Tricuspid atresia
- Ebstein anomaly
- Truncus arteriosus[a]
- Transposition of the great arteries[a]
- Single ventricle[a]

Obstructive lesions
- Aortic stenosis
- Pulmonary stenosis
- Coarctation of the aorta
- Asymmetric septal hypertrophy

[a] Systemic hypoxemia occurs as a result of the mixing of systemic and pulmonary venous returns. Classification as an increased or decreased pulmonary blood flow lesion depends on the absence or presence within the anatomic variation of obstruction to pulmonary blood flow.
Source: From Conahan TJ III. *Cardiac anesthesia.* Menlo Park, CA: Addison Wesley, 1982, with permission.

TABLE 31-2. CHROMOSOMAL SYNDROMES ASSOCIATED WITH CARDIOVASCULAR MALFORMATION IN INFANTS

Syndrome	No. of Patients	No. and Diagnosis of CHD
21 trisomy (Down)	63	32 ECD; 6 VSD; 6 TOF; 4 PDA; 2 ASD; 2 VSD and ASD; 2 Cor. Pul.; 2 TAPVR; 1 TA; 1 MA; 1 NSHD; 1 SV; 1 MR; 1 VSD and PDA; 1 ASD primum
E trisomy (Edwards)	7	3 VSD and PDA, 2 Dextro and CHD, 1 VSD, 1 VSD and ASD
D trisomy (Patau)	5	1 TOF; 1 AoAtres; 1 PDA; 1 CoAo and PDA; 1 ASD secundum
Turner (XO)	5	1 severe CoAo; 1 AoAtres; 1 Levoc-Asplen; 1 TGA and IVs; 1 Truncus
Klinefelter (XXY)	1	1 VSD
Cat eye (Trisomy extrasmall chromosome)	1	1 TA and TAPVR
XYY	1	1 TGA and IVS
A translocation	1	1 PDA
C translocation	2	1 TOF; 1 systemic hypertension
C deletion	2	1 VSD; 1 VSD and ASD
G translocation	1	1 TAPVR

Note: ECD, endocardial cushion defect; VSD, ventricular septal defect; TOF, tetralogy of Fallot; PDA, patent ductus arteriosus; ASD, atrial septal defect; Cor. Pul., cor pulmonale; TAPVR, total anomalous pulmonary venous return; TA, tricuspid atresia; MA, mitral atresia; NSHD, no significant heart disease; SV, single ventricle; MR, mitral regurgitation; Dextro, CHD, dextrocardia with heart disease; AoAtres, aortic atresia; CoAo, coarctation of the aorta; Levoc-Asplen, levocardia, asplenia syndrome; TGA, transposition of the great arteries; Truncus, truncus arteriosus; IVs, intact ventricular septum.
Source: From Greenwood RD. Extracardiac abnormalities in infants with congenital heart disease. *Pediatrics* 1975; 55:485, with permission.

TABLE 31-4. PREOPERATIVE EVALUATION OF THE PEDIATRIC CARDIAC PATIENT

History
1. Exercise tolerance
2. Drugs (e.g., digoxin and diuretics)
3. Disease complications

Physical findings
Laboratory data
1. Blood count
2. Electrolytes, calcium, glucose, blood urea nitrogen
3. Clotting variables
4. Urinalysis

Results of chest radiography
Electrocardiography
Echocardiogram
Cardiac catheterization data
1. Oxygen saturations
2. Shunt magnitude
3. Variation from expected anatomy

Cardiology consultation review
Discussion with patient and family

techniques are indicated in these children, strict antiembolization precautions must be observed and the need for antibiotic prophylaxis considered.

3. A known, uncorrected cardiac lesion with significant symptomatology (e.g., congestive heart failure, cyanosis, or outflow tract obstruction).
4. A known cardiac lesion that has undergone palliative surgery.
5. A known cardiac lesion that has undergone corrective surgery.

The physiologic abnormalities causing cardiovascular impairment, including congestive heart failure, cyanosis, dysrhythmias, ventricular outflow obstruction, and shunting, will be discussed after a brief review of the significance of murmurs.

Heart Murmurs

A common problem in pediatric anesthesia is that of a child in whom a previously undiagnosed cardiac murmur is first heard during the preanesthetic examination. Even if the child appears healthy and shows no signs of cardiac disease, the cause of the murmur must be correctly diagnosed before anesthesia and surgery. The key to the proper preoperative evaluation of such a child is to determine whether the murmur is innocent, in which case there is no need to change the standard anesthetic management in any way or to administer antibiotic prophylaxis against subacute bacterial endocarditis, or whether it is an organic or a functional murmur, in which case the choice of anesthetic agents and techniques may be modified and subacute bacterial endocarditis prophylaxis may be indicated. Table 31-5 lists the types of murmurs (4).

TABLE 31-5. DIFFERENTIAL DIAGNOSIS OF HEART MURMURS

Type of Murmur	Anatomic Defect	Physiologic Defect
Organic	Yes	Yes
Functional	No	Yes
Innocent	No	No

Organic Murmur

An *organic murmur* is a murmur that is associated with an organic heart disease. An anatomic defect is present, resulting in physiologic abnormalities such as increased blood flow to the lungs or congestive heart failure. The defect may be valvular, in the form of stenosis or regurgitation, or it may be characterized by an abnormal communication such as an atrial or a ventricular septal defect.

Functional Murmur

A murmur that is associated with a disturbance in function in the absence of an anatomic defect is termed a *functional murmur*. Functional murmurs are typically seen in patients with high–cardiac output disorder such as anemia, fever, and thyrotoxicosis. These conditions result in an increase in blood flow and turbulence across the valves, which causes the murmur to be heard.

Innocent Murmur

An *innocent murmur*, by contrast, is heard in the absence of anatomic or physiologic defects. Intracardiac phonocardiographic recordings as well as echocardiographic and Doppler studies have demonstrated that innocent murmurs can originate from the right or the left side of the heart. They result from turbulence at the base of the pulmonary artery or the aorta where these vessels take off from respective ventricles. Turbulence is usually accompanied by vibrations in a frequency detectable by the human ear and is therefore heard as a murmur. These murmurs are heard more readily in children than in adults because of their thinner chest and the proximity of the heart to the chest wall. Indeed, innocent murmurs are so common in children that cardiologists may hear them in more than half of all pediatric patients at some time between infancy and adolescence.

TABLE 31-6. DIAGNOSIS OF "OCCULT" HEART DISEASE

- History
  - Prematurity (PDA?)
  - Small for gestational age (congenital heart disease common)
  - Other congenital problems or identifiable syndromes (e.g., Down syndrome) known to have a high association with cardiac disease (see also Table 31-2)
  - Growth pattern, failure to thrive
  - Feeding difficulty
  - Frequent "chest colds," pneumonia, or wheezing (may result from left-to-right shunting and increase pulmonary blood flow)
- Physical examination
  - General
    - Signs of increased cardiac output (may cause a functional murmur)
      - Pallor (? anemia)
      - Large thyroid (? thyrotoxicosis)
    - Peripheral pulses (rule out coarctation)
    - Erythema of finger tips (may indicate mild hypoxia)
  - Cardia
    - Heart size
    - Cardiac impulse; feel for a thrill at xiphoid or apical areas
    - Auscultation
      - First heart sound (intensity, variability, localization)
      - Second heart sound (splitting; variability with respiration; is P_2 loud?)
      - Third heart sound?
      - Characteristics of the murmur
        - Location
        - Transmission
        - Timing
        - Loudness
        - Quality
        - Pitch
        - Changes with position, respiration, or exercise
- Diagnostic tests
  - Chest x-ray
  - Electrocardiography
  - Echocardiography

Diagnosis of an Innocent Murmur

Innocent murmur is a specific diagnosis that should be made based on the specific features of the murmur as well as the absence of any evidence of cardiac disease. More often than not, the "guilt" or "innocence" of the murmur will be based on features other than the murmur itself. A complete cardiovascular history and physical examination must, therefore, be an integral part of the evaluation process for any murmur. The goal is to rule out the presence of occult or subtle manifestations of otherwise minimally symptomatic heart disease that may be responsible for the murmur (Table 31-6).

The most common types of innocent murmurs in children are a Still murmur, innocent pulmonic systolic murmur, and cervical venous hum (Tables 31-7–31.9). Although each individually named murmur has specific features that differentiate it from the others, all innocent murmurs share certain characteristics that differentiate them from organic murmurs (Table 31-10).

Many believe that most innocent murmurs should be recognized by physical examination alone (4,5), although in some cases, an electrocardiogram, a chest x-ray film, or an echocardiography may be needed to confirm the diagnosis.

The qualifications of the examiner, however, have a major bearing on the power of discrimination between innocent and organic murmurs in children (5,6). When a qualified pediatric cardiologist makes the diagnosis of "no

TABLE 31-7. STILL MURMUR

- Left sternal border
- 3rd and 4th spaces
- Musical "groaning"
- Normal splitting of S_2
- Rule out
  - Atrial septal defect
  - Ventricular septal defect
  - Mitral regurgitation
  - Subaortic stenosis

TABLE 31-8. INNOCENT PULMONIC SYSTOLIC MURMUR

- Left sternal border
- 2nd space
- Coarse
- Best heard in supine position
- Normal splitting of S_2
- Rule out
  - Atrial septal defect
  - Pulmonic stenosis

TABLE 31-9. CERVICAL VENOUS HUM

- Low anterior neck
- Continuous, roaring, loud
- Diastolic accentuation
- Transmitted below clavicle
- Disappears in supine position
- Rule out
  - Patent ductus arteriosus

TABLE 31-10. CLINICAL FEATURES OF ALL INNOCENT MURMURS

- Low intensity
- Early systole
- Short duration
- Crescendo-decrescendo
- Poorly transmitted
- No cardiovascular abnormalities

TABLE 31-11. DIAGNOSIS OF A HEART MURMUR

	Clinical Diagnosis			
By Whom?	No Heart Disease	Possible Heart Disease		Definite Heart Disease
Anesthesiologist	Yes	Yes	No	Yes
Pediatrician	Yes	No	Yes	Yes
Cardiology consult?	No	Yes		Yes

Source: From Hannallah RS. The pediatric patient. In: Wetchler BV, ed. *Anesthesia for ambulatory surgery,* 2nd ed. Philadelphia: Lippincott Williams & Wilkins, 1991:140, with permission.

heart disease" or "definite heart disease" on the basis of a patient's history and physical examination alone, diagnostic tests provide little useful additional information concerning the significance of the murmur (5,7).

This experience, however, cannot be generalized to examinations performed by physicians less skilled in pediatric cardiology including many pediatricians and probably most anesthesiologists. At Children's National Medical Center, the grid shown in Table 31-11 serves as a guide as to when a cardiology consultation is needed before proceeding with surgery in a child with a previously undiagnosed heart murmur.

Congestive Heart Failure

Congestive heart failure is not a disease but a symptom complex caused by an underlying cardiac condition. The clinical diagnosis of congestive heart failure rests upon the identification of its four cardinal signs: tachycardia, tachypnea, cardiomegaly, and hepatomegaly. Other symptoms and signs are listed in Table 31-12. The classic radiologic findings of cardiac failure are increased cardiac size and pulmonary congestion. Echocardiography is ideal as a noninvasive tool to measure cardiac chamber sizes, ejection fraction, and circumferential fiber-shortening rate. Exercise tolerance (including feeding tolerance in infants) is the simplest and most informative method of estimating cardiac reserve in patients with congenital heart disease. Heart failure must be controlled before any elective noncardiac surgery is scheduled. Control of congestive heart failure improves pulmonary function and reduces the possibility of perioperative hypoxemia and respiratory failure. Digoxin remains the therapy of choice for treatment of heart failure in infants and children. It is often used in combination with diuretics such as furosemide or spironolactone or chlorothiazide. Preoperative evaluation in these patients should include digoxin level measurements and serum electrolyte determinations (Table 31-4).

TABLE 31-12. SIGNS AND SYMPTOMS OF CONGESTIVE HEART FAILURE IN INFANTS AND CHILDREN

Grunting respirations
Nasal flaring
Tachypnea
Intercostal and substernal retractions
Tachycardia
Pallor
Hepatomegaly
Irritability
Difficult feeding
Sweating
Failure to thrive

In children whose congestive heart failure is caused by lesions that increase pulmonary blood flow (e.g., ventricular septal defect), the anesthesiologist must attempt to reduce the shunt and increase systemic perfusion. The goal is to increase the ratio of right heart pressures to left heart pressures. This can be accomplished by manipulating the impedance to outflow of the respective ventricles. Increasing the ratio of pulmonary vascular resistance (PVR) to systemic vascular resistance (SVR) results in less blood being shunted into the lung. Avoiding hypocarbia and the use of high mean airway pressures (including positive end-expiratory pressure) during ventilation are commonly used to maintain PVR (3). Generalized vasoconstriction resulting from a high sympathetic tone due to light anesthesia or vasopressor administration may have little or no effect on the PVR/SVR ratio. Worsening cardiac failure during anesthesia can be recognized by systemic hypotension, diminished heart tone, decreased oxygen saturation, poor skin perfusion, decreased urine output, and the development of metabolic acidosis. Therapy should start with optimizing the determinant of myocardial performance (cardiac rhythm, preload, contractility, afterload) that is most impaired.

Cyanosis

Any child with a cardiac lesion that causes right-to-left shunting from obstructed pulmonary blood flow, venous admixture to the systemic circulation, or both may ultimately develop cyanosis (Table 31-3). Detection of cyanosis depends on hemoglobin concentration, oxygen saturation, and cutaneous perfusion. Severe chronic hypoxemia results in polycythemia, with an increase in blood volume and viscosity, neovascularization, alveolar hyperventilation, and coagulopathy. Coagulation abnormalities include thrombocytopenia, platelet dysfunction, hypofibrinogenemia, and accelerated fibrinolysis and factor deficiency. Bleeding time may be prolonged. The increased sympathetic tone due to chronic hypoxemia leads to down-regulation of β-receptors in the myocardium, leading to global ventricular dysfunction. Increased blood viscosity increases the cardiac workload by elevating the SVR. If the hematocrit level is high (60% or more), clotting of existing shunts (e.g., Blalock-

Taussig) as well as cerebral and/or renal thrombosis may occur. In children with cyanotic heart disease, hyperviscosity is associated with thrombosis of intracranial veins and sinuses—sometimes resulting in stroke. Children younger than 5 years are at increased risk, particularly during periods of dehydration and fever. Because of the risk of hemoconcentration, preoperative fasting (nothing per os [NPO]) times should be held to a minimum in cyanotic children or the patient should be hydrated intravenously (8). Scheduling these patients early in the morning will not only avoid prolonged fasting but also provide a longer postoperative observation period during recovery.

Anesthetic manipulations in cyanotic children should be designed to avoid further increases in right-to-left shunting and the consequent reductions in pulmonary blood flow (3). Right-to-left shunting may be decreased by reducing PVR/SVR ratio and by relieving the degree of right-sided heart obstruction. Reductions in PVR are accomplished by hyperventilation with a high inspired O_2 concentration and avoidance of high mean airway pressure. Shunting of blood into the lungs can usually be improved by elevating the SVR. Maintaining only a light level of anesthesia and administering α-adrenergic agonists may be effective. For example, infusion of phenylephrine into children with tetralogy of Fallot will increase SVR, reduce intracardiac shunting, and result in decreased cyanosis (3). Decreasing SVR, by contrast, promotes shunting of blood from the lungs and can create or intensify cyanosis. For that reason, vasodilators and deep levels of anesthesia should be avoided in cyanotic children. Anesthetic agents such as isoflurane and propofol decrease SVR, allowing blood to flow from the lungs to the systemic circulation and aggravate hypoxemia. If a child with congenital heart disease that is obstructing pulmonary blood flow becomes hypovolemic, and systemic hypotension develops, both the right-to-left shunt and the cyanosis are intensified. Coronary artery perfusion may also be compromised. If left untreated, this physiologic sequence can lead to shock and cardiovascular collapse. Aggressive treatment with fluid resuscitation and vasopressors are essential (3).

Dysrhythmias

Dysrhythmias are the result of either altered cardiac impulse generation or altered cardiac impulse conduction. In patients with congenital heart disease, disorders of the conduction system—both congenital and acquired—are more common than disorders of impulse generation. The etiologies for conduction system disturbance that produce dysrhythmias include the following:

1. Injury occurring at the time of surgery (status post) ventricular septal defect, transposition of the great arteries, atrioventricular canal, tetralogy of Fallot, Fontan repair).
2. Intrinsic anatomic or physiologic abnormalities.
3. Damage resulting from chronic hypoxia or hemodynamic stress.
4. Combination of all three.

Ventricular Outflow Obstruction

Pulmonic stenosis in children is usually the result of valvular obstruction, although supravalvular, infundibular, or peripheral arterial stenosis also occur (1). Obstruction to right ventricular outflow leads to pressure overload of the right ventricle.

The most common variety of aortic stenosis in children is valvular. This results in left ventricular hypertrophy and increased diastolic volume. In severe cases, relative coronary insufficiency may be present. Significant symptoms of angina and/or syncope is seen in less than 10% of patients (1).

A major concern for the anesthesiologist is that right or left ventricular outflow obstruction can be present in children in the absence of significant symptoms or exercise intolerance. The first indication of any cardiac dysfunction may be a precipitous drop in arterial blood pressure when potent inhalation anesthetics are used in an affected child. Newborns undergoing general anesthesia for congenital cataract surgery may not have clinical evidence yet of significant ventricular outflow obstruction. Careful history and physical examination are essential to detect these lesions in their early asymptomatic stages.

Shunting

A shunt-producing defect is nonrestrictive if there is no pressure gradient across the defect, and it is restrictive if there is a significant resistance across it, producing a pressure gradient between the two chambers.

The obvious sequelae of intracardiac shunts include arterial desaturation (right to left), paradoxical embolization, pulmonary circulatory overload with associated vascular changes (left to right), volume overload of right ventricle, and ventilatory changes.

Eisenmenger syndrome occurs in patients with increasing pulmonary hypertension due to prolonged left-to-right shunting, resulting in shunt reversal, cor pulmonale, and worsening cyanosis. Excessive pulmonary blood flow and pressure contribute to the development of pulmonary vascular obstructive disease. Anesthetic management in these patients should include avoidance of hypovolemia and SVR decrease by anesthetic agents or an increase in PVR due to cold, acidosis, hypercarbia, hypoxia, and catecholamines.

Prior Surgical Intervention

A child's cardiac lesion may be virgin or in some stage of surgical repair (either palliated or corrected). By definition, palliative surgery neither creates a normal anatomic relationship between the cardiovascular structures nor establishes normal blood flow pathway; it simply replaces a sequence of abnormal relationship with another more functional system. Corrective cardiac surgery, on the other hand, is designed to normalize the relationships between cardiovascular structures and create a normal route for blood flow. The true result of corrective surgery is, more often than not, merely reparative; cardiovascular problems associated with the original anomaly quite often remain, and ironically, new difficulties may develop (Table 31-13) (3). In one survey (9), only individuals with surgery for atrial septal defect, pulmonic stenosis, and patent ductus arteriosus came close to being considered cured. Arrhythmias, congestive heart failure, and pulmonic hypertension often develop after surgery for tetralogy of Fallot, ventricular septal defect, coarctation of the aorta, aortic stenosis, and transposition of great vessels (9). The cardiovascular physiology after correction of complex defects may pose a challenge for the anesthesiologist, as evident in patients who undergo Fontan repair or cardiac transplantation.

S/P Fontan Repair

The Fontan procedure is a surgical technique used for correction of tricuspid atresia, pulmonary atresia, and any single ventricle, and it is used as part of the Norwood procedure for repair of hypoplastic left-sided heart syndrome. The procedure is based on the concept that central venous pressure is sufficient to drive blood through the pulmonary circulation if pulmonary hypertension is not present. Since its first introduction in 1971 by Fontan and Baudet, the Fontan procedure has undergone many modifications. It has been applied to single-ventricle hearts and to malformations in which a biventricular repair is not possible because of an underdeveloped ventricle. Currently, this technique involves total caval-to-pulmonary artery anastomosis. First, the superior vena cava is connected end-to-side to the superior aspect of the right pulmonary artery (alone, this would be a bidirectional Glenn shunt). In a subsequent procedure, the inferior vena cava is tunneled through the right atrial free wall to the inferior surface of the right pulmonary artery. A defect is purposefully left in this baffle to decompress the right side of the heart, leading to a mild systemic arterial oxygen desaturation. This baffle defect can be closed later by means of a transcatheter device or surgically. Complications of the Fontan procedure include pleural effusion, ascites, chylothorax, renal failure, low cardiac output, obstruction or deterioration of conduits or valves, cirrhosis, atrioventricular valve insufficiency, and cardiomyopathy.

Patients who have had a Fontan procedure are dependent on the central venous pressure to drive pulmonary blood flow, because they do not have a subpulmonic ventricle. Anesthetic management should aim at maintenance of relatively high central venous pressure by maintaining preload (driving force) and a low PVR. High positive airway pressure with mechanical ventilation can decrease systemic venous return and be detrimental. Factors that increase PVR such as hypoxemia, hypercarbia, metabolic acidosis, endogenous or exogenous catecholamines, and myocardial depressants must be avoided. If a patient is undergoing extensive noncardiac surgery, postoperative ventilation in the intensive care unit, which allows for a slow and controlled emergence from general anesthesia with adequate analgesia, may be beneficial. In patients with a Fontan procedure or a Glenn anastomosis, cannulation of the superior vena cava via the right internal jugular vein should be avoided because of the risk of thrombosis of the superior vena cava.

S/P Cardiac Transplantation

Pediatric patients with complex cardiac defects not amenable to surgical repair and those with dilated cardiomyopathy frequently undergo cardiac transplantation. There is a high perioperative mortality and rejection rate in these patients.

Those with successful transplants receive prolonged steroid therapy, which produces growth retardation and osteoporosis. Long-term use of cyclosporine results in coronary vascular disease, renal dysfunction, and hypertension.

Because the transplanted heart is a denervated heart, the resting heart rate is determined by the donor's sinuatrial node. Heart rate is unresponsive to drugs (e.g., atropine, pancuronium, or fentanyl) and physiologic compensatory mechanisms (e.g., carotid sinus massage). During exercise and periods of physiologic stress, cardiac output increases due to increased venous return and increased circulatory catecholamines. Management of these patients, therefore, requires maintenance of adequate venous return. If vasopressor therapy is indicated, direct-acting chronotropic and inotropic agents such as isoproterenol, dopamine, and epinephrine should be selected. Regional techniques (spinal and epidural) that can reduce venous return should be used cautiously in patients after Fontan procedure or after cardiac transplantation. Strict asepsis during vascular catheter placement and tracheal intubation should be maintained.

PREANESTHETIC MEDICATION

The decision to use preanesthetic medication as well as the selection of a drug or drugs is based on the child's age, psychological status, and cardiovascular function. The purpose of premedication is to alleviate psychological and cardiovascular stress before and during anesthetic induction. It decreases the likelihood of excitement and sympathetic stimulation that may predispose the child to various types of cardiovascular compromise that may eventually result in cyanosis or congestive heart failure (3). Children with compensated congenital heart disease can receive a standard dose of most commonly used agents (e.g., oral midazolam 0.5 mg/kg). To reduce the risk of hypercyanotic episode, one

TABLE 31-13. RESIDUAL CARDIOVASCULAR DEFECTS AFTER SURGICAL REPAIR OF CONGENITAL HEART LESIONS

Lesions	Operations	Residual Defects
Palliative procedures		
VSD, AVC, SV	PA banding	Inadequate PBF → hypoxemia, or excessive PBF → CHF
TOF, PAtr, TAtr	Blalock-Taussig shunt (subclavian artery → PA) Waterston shunt (ascending Ao → PA) Potts shunt (descending Ao → PA)	Inadequate PBF → hypoxemia, or excessive PBF → CHF
	Glenn shunt (SVC → PA) Fontan procedure (RA → PA)	Inadequate PBF → hypoxemia
TGA, SV, TAtr MAtr	Blalock-Hanlon atrial septectomy Balloon atrial septostomy	Inadequate mixing → hypoxemia = CHF
Corrective procedures		
Coarctation of aorta	Coarctation resection	Systemic ↑ BP Residual coarctation Aortic and cerebral aneurysms AV and MV abnormalities LV dysfunction
ASD	ASD closure	Residual ASD RV dysfunction
VSD	VSD closure	Residual VSD LV dysfunction Conduction disturbances Pulmonary ↑ BP
AVC	ASD and/or VSD closure TV and/or MV repair	Residual ASD or VSD TR, MR, MV prolapse RV and/or LV dysfunction Conduction disturbances Pulmonary ↑ BP
TOF, PAtr	VSD closure + RVOT repair Rastelli procedure	Residual VSD Ventricular dysfunction Conduction disturbances PS or PI
PS	Pulmonary valvulotomy Subvalvular resection	Residual stenosis RV dysfunction PI
AS	Aortic valvulotomy Subvalvular resection	Residual stenosis LV dysfunction AI
TGA	Mustard, Senning procedures (intraatrial baffles)	Residual ASD RV dysfunction Conduction disturbances Caval ± pulmonary venous obstruction TR
	Arterial switch procedure	LV dysfunction LVOT, RVOT obstruction AI Coronary insufficiency

AI, aortic insufficiency; Ao, aorta; AS, aortic stenosis; ASD, atrial septal defect; AV, aortic valve; AVC, atrioventricular canal; ↑ BP, hypertension; CHF, congestive heart failure; LV, left ventricle; LVOT, left ventricular outflow tract; MAtr, mitral atresia; MR, mitral regurgitation; MV, mitral valve; PA, pulmonary artery; PAtr, pulmonary atresia; PBF, pulmonary blood flow; PI, pulmonary insufficiency; PS, pulmonic stenosis; RA, right atrium; RV, right ventricle; RVOT, right ventricular outflow tract; SV, single ventricle; SVC, superior vena cava; TAtr, tricuspid atresia; TGA, transposition of the great arteries; TOF, tetralogy of Fallot; TR, tricuspid regurgitation; TV, tricuspid valve; VSD, ventricular septal defect.

Source: From Campbell FW, Schwartz AS. Anesthesia for noncardiac surgery in the pediatric patient with congenital heart disease. ASA refresher courses in anesthesiology. Philadelphia: Lippincott Williams & Wilkins, 1986:75, with permission.

should give cyanotic children more substantial premedication than noncyanotic children (3). This is particularly useful if the child has a history of worsening hypoxemia when excited or agitated. Close observation and oxygen saturation monitoring may be required in the latter group. Supplemental oxygen should be available to maintain oxygen saturation at the baseline level if needed.

ANTIBIOTIC PROPHYLAXIS

Bacterial endocarditis is an infrequent but severe complication of congenital heart disease.

Patients undergoing surgical and dental procedures or instrumentations involving mucosal surfaces or contaminated tissues commonly suffer from transient bacteremia (10). Bloodborne bacteria may lodge in damaged or abnormal valves or on the endothelium near congenital anatomic defects, leading to bacterial endocarditis.

Certain cardiac conditions are more often associated with endocarditis than others (Tables 31-14 and 31-15) (10). Patients with lesions associated with jet formation and vortex shedding (e.g., aortic stenosis) are at greater risk than those with low-pressure, high-flow conditions such as isolated secundum atrial septal defects. Furthermore, certain dental and surgical procedures are much more likely to initiate the bacteremia that results in endocarditis than others (Tables 31-16 and 31-17) (10).

Because it is impossible to predict which patients will develop this infection or which particular procedures will be responsible, prophylactic antibiotics are recommended for all patients at risk for developing endocarditis who are undergoing those procedures most likely to produce bacter-

TABLE 31-14. SELECTED CARDIAC CONDITIONS IN WHICH ENDOCARDITIS PROPHYLAXIS IS RECOMMENDED BY THE AMERICAN HEART ASSOCIATION

- High-risk category
  - Prosthetic cardiac valves, including bioprosthetic and homograft valves
  - Previous bacterial endocarditis
  - Complex cyanotic congenial heart disease (e.g., single ventricle states, transposition of the great arteries, tetralogy of Fallot)
  - Surgically constructed systemic pulmonary shunts or conduits
- Moderate-risk category
  - Most other congenital cardiac malformations (other than above and below)
  - Acquired valvar dysfunction (e.g., rheumatic heart disease)
  - Hypertrophic cardiomyopathy
  - Mitral valve prolapse with valvar regurgitation and/or thickened leaflets

Source: From Danjani AS, Taubert KA, Wilson W, et al. Prevention of bacterial endocarditis—recommendations by the American Heart Association. *JAMA* 1997;277:1794, with permission.

TABLE 31-15. CARDIAC CONDITIONS IN WHICH ENDOCARDITIS PROPHYLAXIS IS NOT RECOMMENDED BY THE AMERICAN HEART ASSOCIATION

- Negligible-risk category (no greater risk than the general population)
  - Isolation secundum atrial septal defect
  - Surgical repair of atrial septal defect, ventricular septal defect, or patent ductus arteriosus (without residua beyond 6 mo)
  - Previous coronary artery bypass graft surgery
  - Mitral valve prolapse without valvar regurgitation
  - Physiologic, functional, or innocent heart murmurs
  - Previous Kawasaki disease without valvar dysfunction
  - Previous rheumatic fever without valvar dysfunction
  - Cardiac pacemakers (intravascular and epicardial) and implanted defibrillators

Source: From Danjani AS, Taubert KA, Wilson W, et al. Prevention of bacterial endocarditis—recommendations by the American Heart Association. *JAMA* 1997;277:1794, with permission.

TABLE 31-16. SELECTED PROCEDURES IN WHICH ENDOCARDITIS PROPHYLAXIS IS RECOMMENDED BY THE AMERICAN HEART ASSOCIATION[a]

- Dental
  - Dental extractions
  - Periodontal procedures including surgery, scaling and root planing, probing, and recall maintenance
  - Dental implant placement and reimplantation of avulsed teeth
  - Endodontic (root canal) instrumentation or surgery only beyond the apex
  - Subgingival placement of antibiotic fibers or strips
  - Initial placement of orthodontic bands but not brackets
  - Intraligamentary local anesthetic injections
  - Prophylactic cleaning of teeth or implants where bleeding is anticipated
- Others
  - Respiratory tract
    - Tonsillectomy and/or adenoidectomy
    - Surgical operations that involve respiratory mucosa
    - Bronchoscopy with a rigid bronchoscope
  - Gastrointestinal tract[b]
    - Sclerotherapy for esophageal varices
    - Esophageal stricture dilation
    - Endoscopic retrograde cholangiography with biliary obstruction
    - Biliary tract surgery
    - Surgery operations that involve intestinal mucosa
  - Genitourinary tract
    - Prostatic surgery
    - Cystoscopy
    - Urethral dilation

[a] Prophylaxis is recommended for patients with high- and moderate-risk cardiac conditions.
[b] Prophylaxis is recommended for high-risk patients; optional for medium-risk patients.
Source: From Danjani AS, Taubert KA, Wilson W, et al. Prevention of bacterial endocarditis—recommendations by the American Heart Association. *JAMA* 1997;277:1794, with permission.

TABLE 31-17. ENDOCARDITIS PROPHYLAXIS IS NOT RECOMMENDED BY THE AMERICAN HEART ASSOCIATION

Dental
- Restorative dentistry[a] (operative and prosthodontic) with or without retraction cord[b]
- Local anesthetic injections (nonintraligamentary)
- Intracanal endodontic treatment; postplacement and buildup
- Placement of rubber dams
- Postoperative suture removal
- Placement of removable prosthodontic or orthodontic appliances
- Taking of oral radiographs
- Fluoride treatments
- Taking of oral radiographs
- Orthodontic appliance adjustment
- Shedding of primary teeth

Others
- Respiratory tract
  - Endotracheal intubation
  - Bronchoscopy with a flexible bronchoscope, with or without biopsy[c]
  - Tympanostomy tube insertion
- Gastrointestinal tract
  - Transesophageal echocardiography[c]
  - Endoscopy with or without gastrointestinal biopsy[c]
- Genitourinary tract
  - Vaginal hysterectomy[c]
  - Vaginal delivery
  - Cesarean section
  - In uninfected tissue
    - Urethral catheterization
    - Uterine dilatation and curettage
    - Therapeutic abortion
    - Sterilization procedures
    - Insertion or removal of intrauterine devices
- Other
  - Cardiac catheterization, including balloon angioplasty
  - Implanted cardiac pacemakers, implanted defibrillators, and coronary stents
  - Incision or biopsy of surgically scrubbed skin
  - Circumcision

[a] This indicates restoration of decayed teeth (filling cavities) and replacement of missing teeth.
[b] Clinical judgment may indicate antibiotic use in selected circumstances that may create significant bleeding.
[c] Prophylaxis is optional for high-risk patients.
Source: From Danjani AS, Taubert KA, Wilson W, et al. Prevention of bacterial endocarditis—recommendations by the American Heart Association. *JAMA* 1997;277:1794, with permission.

emia with organisms that commonly cause endocarditis (10). In patients with mitral valve prolapse, prophylaxis is recommended if there is mitral regurgitation. The clinical approach to patients with suspected mitral valve prolapse is shown in Fig. 31-1.

The Committee on Rheumatic Fever and Bacterial Endocarditis of the American Heart Association has recently updated its recommendations for antibiotic prophylaxis (10). Risk levels have been stratified, a two-dose antibiotic

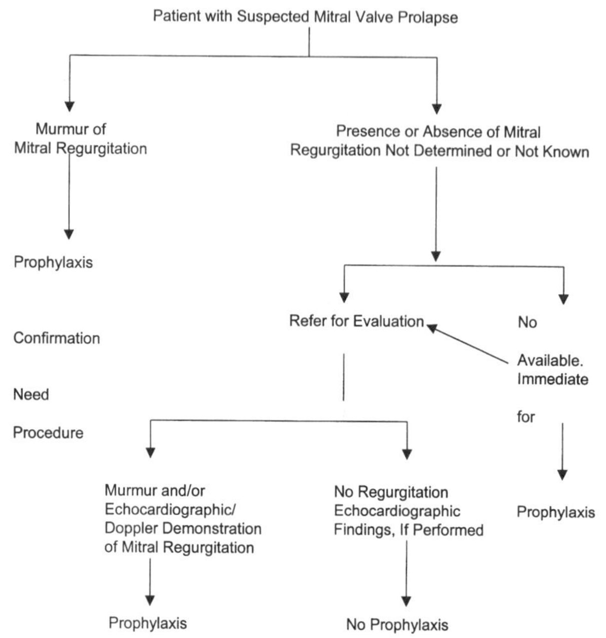

FIGURE 31-1. Approach to patient with suspected mitral valve prolapse. (From Danjani AS, Taubert KA, Wilson W, et al. Prevention of bacterial endocarditis—recommendations by the American Heart Association. *JAMA* 1997;277:1794, with permission.)

TABLE 31-18. PROPHYLACTIC REGIMENS FOR DENTAL, ORAL, RESPIRATORY TRACT, OR ESOPHAGEAL PROCEDURES

Situation	Agent	Regimen
Standard general prophylaxis	Amoxicillin	Children: 50 mg/kg orally 1 hr before procedure
Unable to take oral medications	Ampicillin	Children: 50 mg/kg IM or IV within 30 min before procedure[b]
Allergic to penicillin	Clindamycin ***or***	Children: 20 mg/kg orally 1 hr before procedure
	Cephalexin[a] ***or*** Cefadroxil[a] ***or***	Children: 50 mg/kg orally 1 hr before procedure
	Azithromycin ***or*** Clarithromycin	Children: 15 mg/kg orally 1 hr before procedure
Allergic to penicillin and unable to take oral medications	Clindamycin ***or***	Children: 20 mg/kg IV within 30 min before procedure[b]
	Cefazolin[a]	Children: 25/mg IM or IV within 30 min before procedure[b]

Note: IV, intravenously; IM, intramuscularly.
[a] Cephalosporins should not be used in individuals with immediate-type hypersensitivity reaction (urticaria, angioedema, or anaphylaxis) to penicillins.
[b] At the Children's National Medical Center the drugs are given IV as soon as an IV catheter is inserted after induction but *before* airway or surgical manipulation.

TABLE 31-19. PROPHYLACTIC REGIMENS FOR GENITOURINARY GASTROINTESTINAL (EXCLUDING ESOPHAGEAL) PROCEDURES

Situation	Agents	Regimen[a]
High-risk patients	Ampicillin plus gentamicin	Children: ampicillin 50 mg/kg IM or IV (not to exceed 2.0 g) plus gentamicin 1.5 mg/kg within 30 min of starting the procedure;[b] 6 hr later, ampicillin 25 mg/kg IM/IV or amoxicillin 25 mg/kg orally
High-risk patients allergic to ampicillin/amoxicillin	Vancomycin plus gentamicin	Children: vancomycin 20 mg/kg IV over 1–2 hr plus gentamicin 1.5 mg/kg IV/IM; complete injection/infusion within 30 min of starting the procedure[b]
Moderate-risk patients	Amoxicillin *or* ampicillin	Children: amoxicillin 50 mg/kg orally 1 hr before procedure, or ampicillin 50 mg/kg IM/IV within 30 min of starting the procedure[b]
Moderate-risk patients allergic to ampicillin/amoxicillin	Vancomycin	Children: vancomycin 20 mg/kg IV over 1–2 hr; complete infusion within 30 min of starting the procedure[b]

Note: IV, intravenously; IM, intramuscularly.
[a] No second dose of vancomycin or gentamicin is recommended.
[b] At the Children's National Medical Center the drugs are given IV as soon as an IV catheter is inserted after induction but *before* airway or surgical manipulation.

regimen has been suggested, and the relative risk of bacteremia in clinical circumstances has been clarified. Tables 31-18 and 31-19 show a summary of the recommended standard, as well as an alternative regimen for pediatric patients.

MONITORING

Children with congenital heart disease who are undergoing noncardiac surgical procedures in which major blood loss or fluid translocation is not anticipated should be monitored in the same way as any other pediatric patient undergoing a similar procedure. This includes a precordial or esophageal stethoscope, electrocardiogram for monitoring heart rate and detecting dysrhythmias, noninvasive blood pressure monitor, temperature probe, inspired O_2 concentration monitor, continuous-pulse oximetry, and end-tidal CO_2 measurement. Monitoring of arterial O_2 saturation by pulse oximetry is of particular value in the child with cyanotic congenital heart disease because of the possibility that anesthesia and surgical manipulation may further reduce pulmonary blood flow and intensify hypoxemia (3). Use of bispectral monitoring in children undergoing noncardiac surgery can be helpful in titrating appropriate agents that will ensure adequate depth of anesthesia without circulatory depression.

Several special considerations govern these monitoring procedures. The site of blood pressure measurement may be limited by previous cardiac surgery. For example, previous Blalock-Taussig shunt or subclavian flap angioplasty repair of coarctation of the aorta prohibits the use of the affected arm for accurate blood pressure determination (3).

The decision to use invasive monitoring is dependent on the magnitude of the operative procedure and the severity of the cardiac dysfunction. Arterial catheter and central venous catheters are very helpful in monitoring patients with poor cardiac reserve and in guiding the use of intravenous fluids or vasopressors. Cannulation at the dorsalis pedis or posterior tibial arteries is preferable to that at the radial arteries in patients awaiting definitive repair.

When interpreting the readings of end-tidal carbon dioxide monitoring in children with congenital heart disease, one must take into account the effect of shunting on the arterial carbon dioxide–to–end-tidal carbon dioxide difference ($PaETCO_2$). That difference is generally stable in children with acyanotic shunting, although children with mixing congenital heart lesions may demonstrate large individual variations (11). In children with cyanotic shunting, on the other hand, the $PaETCO_2$ is not always constant, and the $PETCO_2$ cannot be used during surgery to estimate reliably the $PaCO_2$.

More extensive monitoring is warranted if the child's cardiovascular function, the extent of the anesthetic and surgical manipulations, or both pose the risk of circulatory instability. The hemodynamic consequences of surgery, rather than the nature of the lesion *per se,* are of primary importance in assessing the need for invasive monitoring in most cases.

INTRAVENOUS ACCESS AND EMBOLIZATION PRECAUTIONS

The need for prolonged fasting before elective surgery in healthy pediatric patients has been challenged. Studies have shown that children who are allowed to drink clear liquids until 2 hours of anesthesia induction do not manifest an increase in gastric volume or acidity, compared with those who fast overnight. Although there is still no uniform fasting practice for children before elective surgery in the United States and Canada, most pediatric anesthesiologists have now liberalized preoperative fasting requirements for otherwise healthy outpatients (12). Solid food is still not allowed on the day of surgery. Children may drink clear liquids until 2 hours of the scheduled surgical time. Breast-fed infants are allowed to nurse up to 4 hours preoperatively. Possible

TABLE 31-20. AIR BUBBLE PRECAUTIONS

Remove all bubbles from the IV tubing.
Connect the IV tubing to the venous cannula while there is free-flowing IV fluid and blood.
Eject small amounts of solution from syringe to clear air from the needle and hub before IV injection.
Aspirate injection port before injection to clear any air.
Hold the syringe upright to keep bubbles at the plunger end.
Do not inject the last milliliter from the syringe.
Do not leave a central line open to air.

Note: IV, intravenous.

benefits of shorter fasting times include minimizing thirst and discomfort while awaiting surgery, less hypovolemia-induced hypotension during induction, avoidance of the danger of excessive hemoconcentration in cyanotic children, and less concern about hypoglycemia. It is important to note that the new guidelines apply only to clear liquids (not solids) and to children who are reasonably healthy.

Even after a short NPO period, most anesthesiologists still consider that establishing intravenous access is a wise precaution in children with congenital heart disease during noncardiac surgery. This permits adequate hydration, pharmacologic manipulation of hemodynamics, administration of antibiotic prophylaxis, and rapid administration of resuscitation medications if they become necessary (3).

The introduction of air bubbles or particulate matter into the vasculature of a child with a right-to-left shunting lesion may lead to systemic embolization. Even shunts that are predominantly left to right may be bidirectional at the level of the lesion and allow air to cross from the right side to the left side. Rigorous precautions are therefore essential during the establishment of intravenous access and administration of intravenous agents. Meticulous prophylaxis is the best safeguard against venous-to-arterial embolization (Table 31-20) (3). All intravenous equipment—tubing, connection sites, injection ports, and stopcocks—must be carefully checked to ensure it is air-free immediately before being connected to the patient. During injection into an intravenous or arterial catheter, great care must be taken not to introduce air or particulate matter. Some anesthesiologists choose not to administer N_2O after induction in children with congenital heart disease lesions with right-to-left shunting or systemic and pulmonary venous mixing to avoid increasing the size of air bubbles that may have inadvertently been introduced into the intravenous line (3).

CHOICE OF ANESTHETICS

The choice of anesthetic agents for the child with congenital heart disease depends on the type of operation to be performed, the anticipated duration of surgery, the preference of the anesthesiologist, and the patient's cardiovascular status (3). Although no anesthetic techniques have proven especially superior for specific anomalies, a classification of lesions according to alterations in blood flow and clinical presentation suggests general hemodynamic objectives that will promote or maintain the child's circulation (Table 31-21) (13).

The choice of anesthetic induction technique depends on the child's age, psychological preparedness, cardiovascular status, and whether an intravenous catheter is present. The recognized cardiovascular effects of the anesthetic agents must also be taken into consideration. Anesthetic induction also may be influenced by factors that alter the uptake and distribution of inhalation or intravenous agents.

The speed of induction of an inhalation anesthetic is determined by the rates of anesthetic inflow into the lungs, transfer of the agent from the lungs to the arterial blood, and anesthetic transfer from the arterial blood. Anesthetic equilibration between the alveoli and arterial blood, and in turn the brain, usually is rapid. Under most circumstances, the speed of induction depends on those factors that determine the rate of rise of alveolar anesthetic level (3). In children with congenital heart disease with diminished pulmonary blood flow, the transfer of the agent from the lungs to the arterial blood is slowed. Inhalation induction in a patient with a right-to-left shunt can be prolonged because the shunted blood decreases or dilutes the partial pressure

TABLE 31-21. CARDIAC GRID FOR COMMON CONGENITAL HEART DISEASE (DESIRED HEMODYNAMIC CHANGES)

	Preload	PVR	SVR	HR	Contractility
ASD	↑	↑	↓	N	N
VSD (R→L)	N	↓	↑	N	N
VSD (L→R)	↑	↑	↓	N	N
IHSS	↑	N	N-↑	*↓	*↓
PDA	↑	↑	↓	N	N
Coarctation	↑	N	↓	N	N
Valvular					
Pulmonary stenosis	↑	↓	N	↓	↑
Infundibular					
Pulmonary stenosis	↑	↓	N	↓	*↓
AS	↑	N	*↑	*↓	N-↑
MS	↑	N-↓	N	*↑	N-↑
AR	↑	N	↓	N-↑	N-↑
MR	↑	N-↓	↓	N-↑	N-↑

Note: ASD, atrial septal defect; VSD, ventricular septal defect; IHSS, idiopathic hypertrophic subaortic stenosis; PDA, patient ductus arteriosus; AS, aortic stenosis; MS, mitral stenosis; AR, aortic regurgitation; MR, mitral regurgitation; PVR, pulmonary vascular resistance; SVR, systemic vascular resistance; *, an overriding consideration.

Source: From Moore RA. Anesthesia for the pediatric congenital heart patient for noncardiac surgery. *Anesthesiol Rev* 1981;8(12):23, with permission.

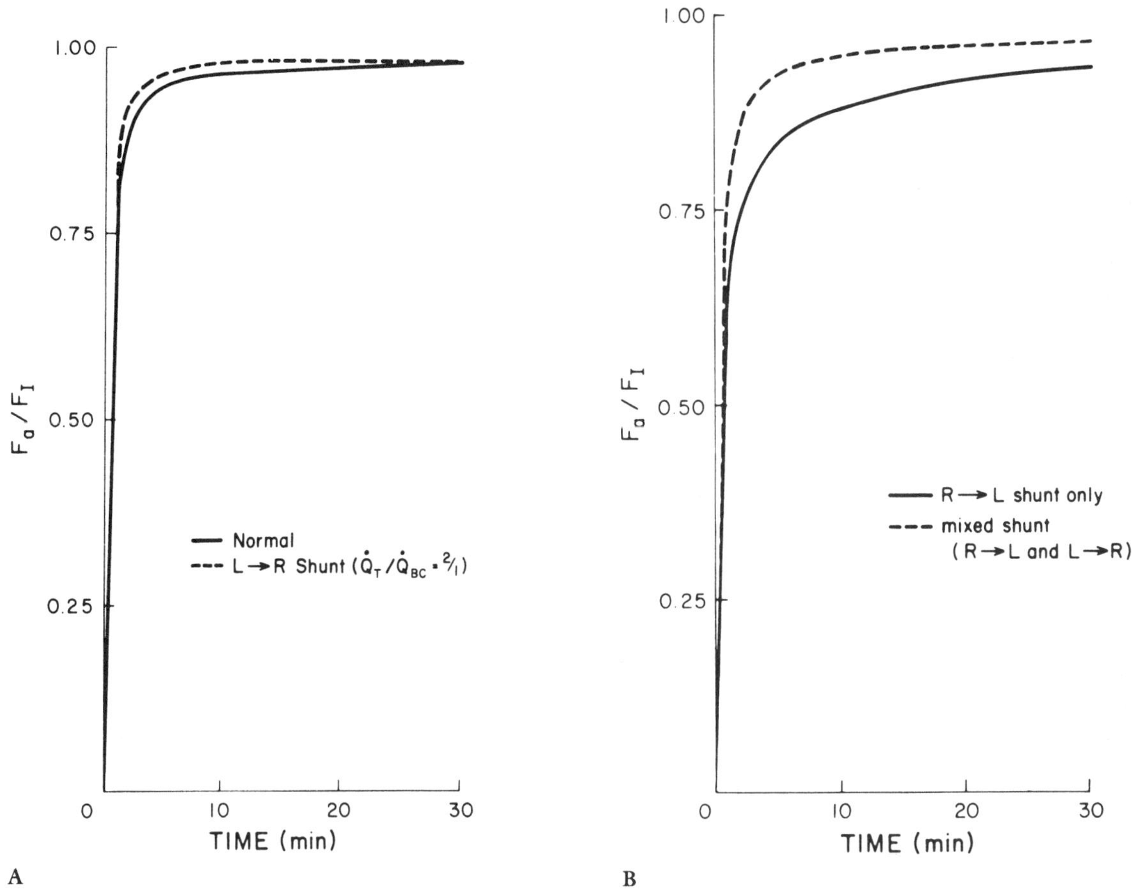

FIGURE 31-2. Arterial-to-inspired (Fa/Fi) concentration ratio for nitrous oxide modeled with **(A)** left-to-right and **(B)** right-to-left, and mixed shunting. The normal Fa/Fi ratio without shunting is represented by the solid line. (From Tanner GE, Angers DG, Barash PG, et al. Effect of left-to-right, mixed left-to-right, and right-to-left shunts on inhalational anesthetic induction in children: a computer model. *Anesth Analg* 1985;64:101, with permission.)

of the anesthetic in the blood that is reaching the brain, compared with the partial pressure in the blood leaving the lungs (Fig. 31-2). A high inspired concentration of soluble anesthetic agents, combined with augmented ventilation, can be used to counteract this effect.

In patients with left-to-right shunting, the speed of inhalation induction is unchanged. Recirculation through the lungs of left-to-right shunt blood, which already carries a high concentration of anesthetic, reduces anesthetic uptake from the alveoli and promotes a more rapid rise in alveolar partial pressure. The augmented pulmonary blood flow, however, increases anesthetic uptake from the alveoli, thereby delaying the rise in alveolar anesthetic levels. So although a left-to-right shunt increases pulmonary blood flow, it does not substantially alter the rate of anesthetic induction.

There are, however, two exceptions to this rule. First, when systemic cardiac output is not maintained, the reduction in systemic venous return to the lungs results in a more rapid rise in alveolar anesthetic level. Second, in patients with a large right-to-left shunt that by itself will slow the speed of induction, the coexistence of a left-to-right shunt will speed the rate of induction, thereby counteracting the initial delay. The effects of shunting on the speed of inhalation inductions is more pronounced for N_2O than for the more soluble volatile anesthetics (Fig. 31-3).

The pharmacokinetics of intravenous agents may also be affected by shunting of blood, as can be readily seen by examining cardiac output curves in children with congenital heart disease (Fig. 31-4) (3). In patients whose lesions are characterized by left-to-right shunting and increased pulmonary blood flow, an intravenous bolus of a given drug reaches the brain at the same time as if no shunt existed. Its initial peak concentration is lower, however, and its effect is prolonged. In lesions with right-to-left shunting, in which systemic venous blood bypasses the pulmonary circulation, the bolus reaches the brain sooner than predicted. Both anesthetic effects and cardiovascular toxicity may, therefore,

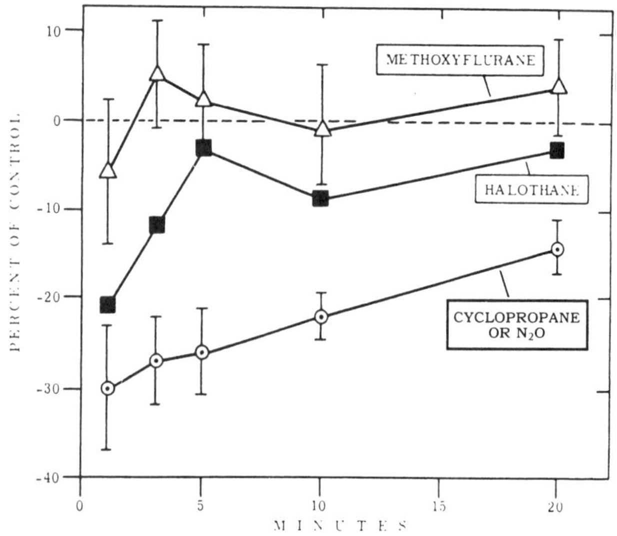

FIGURE 31-3. The rate of rise in alveolar concentration of inhalation anesthetic is prolonged in patients with right-to-left shunting. A greater impact is seen with less soluble anesthetics such as cyclopropane (and nitrous oxide) than with highly soluble agents such as methoxyflurane. The rate of rise of alveolar halothane concentration lies between that of nitrous oxide of methoxyflurane. The curves for enflurane and isoflurane (not shown) should lie between halothane and nitrous oxide. (From Stoelting RK, Longnecker DE. The effect of right-to-left shunting on the rate of increase of arterial anesthetic concentration. *Anesthesiology* 1972;36:352, with permission.)

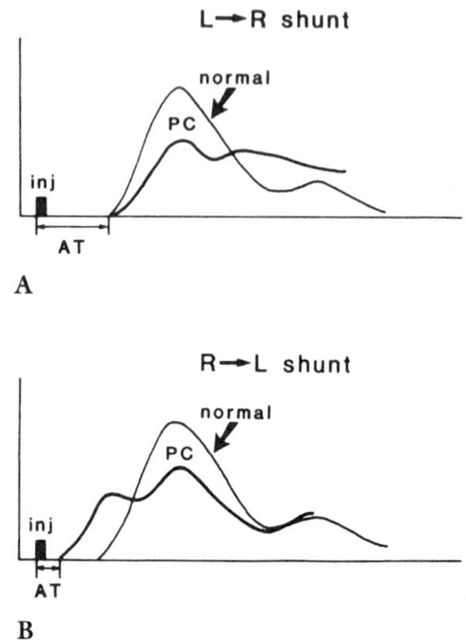

FIGURE 31-4. Effect of intracardiac shunting on the pharmacokinetics of intravenous agents. In patients with left-to-right shunts, the appearance time of the drug in the systemic circulation is within the reference range, but its initial peak concentration is lower and its total effect is prolonged. In this case, the pulmonary recirculation of the drug delays its entrance into the systemic circulation, and consequently an intravenous anesthesia induction would be delayed. In patients with right-to-left shunts, the appearance time of a drug in the systemic circulation is shortened because blood bypasses the pulmonary circulation. In this situation, intravenous anesthetic induction would be more rapid than usual. (From Campbell FW, Schwartz AJ. Anesthesia for noncardiac surgery in the patient with congenital heart disease. *ASA refresher courses in anesthesiology* 1986;14(6):75, with permission.)

appear more rapidly after intravenous administration of intravenous agents in these patients.

N_2O is often used as the carrier gas with other volatile anesthetics to facilitate inhalation induction in children. Of concern, however, is the potential hazard of air bubble enlargement in children with shunting lesions, and the fact that the use of N_2O may preclude the administration of high concentrations of inspired O_2. N_2O may also cause increases in PVR in noncyanotic children.

Volatile anesthetic agents are widely used during cardiac and noncardiac surgery in children with congenital heart disease. Mask induction with sevoflurane (and to a lesser degree, halothane) is associated with minimal struggle and is often selected when intravenous catheters are not already placed. The use of volatile anesthetics permits the delivery of high oxygen concentration when appropriate. Although all of the volatile agents are myocardial depressants, the actual effect on cardiac output and arterial blood pressure is modified by other factors such as the effect on SVR. Both halothane and isoflurane may cause a dose-dependent decrease in arterial blood pressure; the mechanism is different in each case (14). The decrease in blood pressure associated with the use of halothane is mainly due to a reduction in cardiac output. SVR remains largely unchanged. The decrease in blood pressure with isoflurane, on the other hand, is due to a decrease in SVR while cardiac output remains within the reference range (Figs. 31-5 and 31-6). The difference in the effect of these two commonly used agents on SVR is important to recognize in children with balanced shunts, in whom a drop in systemic resistance can result in an increase in right-to-left shunting and hypoxia. It is important to recognize that these circulatory effects of the volatile agents are dose related, titratable, and well tolerated by most children with congenital heart disease. Sevoflurane is associated with less bradycardia or dysrhythmias than halothane. Cardiovascular changes at equipotent concentrations of sevoflurane and halothane in healthy children have been measured by echocardiography. Sevoflurane resulted in a lesser decrease in cardiac output than halothane. Halothane caused a greater decrease in heart rate and cardiac index at all concentrations than sevoflurane (15).

The potential hazards of volatile anesthetics are generally related to relative anesthetic overdose. Myocardial depression resulting from an anesthetic overdose will decrease cardiac output and result in systemic hypotension in patients with severe aortic stenosis. In children with severe pulmonic stenosis, halothane may decrease pulmonary blood flow and compromise oxygenation (3). The hemodynamic effects of these drugs, on the other hand, may be desirable in some

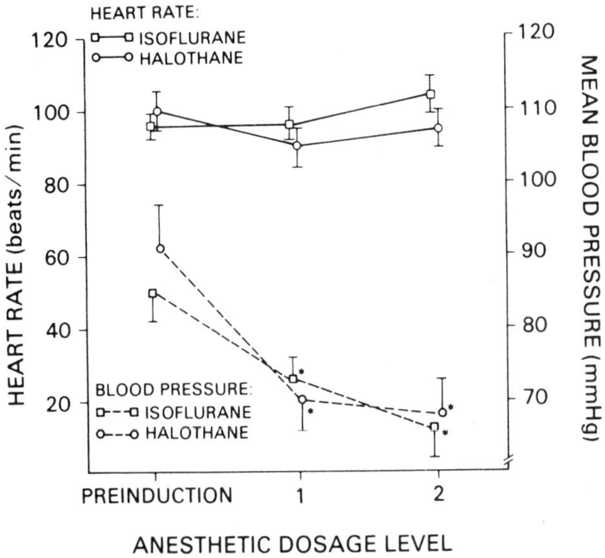

FIGURE 31-5. Changes in heart rate (*solid line*) and mean blood pressure (*dashed line*) with increasing concentrations of isoflurane (□) or halothane (○). Values and mean ± standard error of the mean. Significant changes within each group from preinduction are noted (*, $P < .05$).

children. For example, the negative chronotropic and inotropic actions of halothane may reduce the degree of outflow obstruction and promote forward cardiac output in patients with subvalvular aortic stenosis, or increase pulmonary blood flow in patients with pulmonic stenosis or tetralogy of Fallot.

The effect of volatile anesthetics on the heart rate is also dose dependent. Barash et al. (16) reported a dose-dependent depression of ventricular function in children during halothane anesthesia that produced a significant decrease in cardiac output, heart rate, and blood pressure. The administration of atropine resulted in a rapid improvement in cardiac output and blood pressure (Fig. 31-7).

The use of opioids in anesthesia for children with congenital heart disease is associated with excellent hemodynamic stability. High-dose narcotic techniques can be used in children undergoing major surgical procedures who will need postoperative ventilatory support. Both fentanyl (25 to 75 μg/kg) and sufentanil (5 to 20 μg/kg) can be used in very sick infants and children with all forms of congenital heart disease, as both agents produce minimal pulmonary and systemic hemodynamic changes. Remifentanil can be used even in children undergoing short surgical procedures without prolongation of recovery. Pancuronium, or specific vagolytic agents, is often combined with opioids in these children because it tends to prevent excessive slowing of the heart rate, which would result otherwise. Low doses of narcotics may be used to supplement a reduced volatile anesthetic concentration in children undergoing less extensive procedures. They also can be combined with muscle

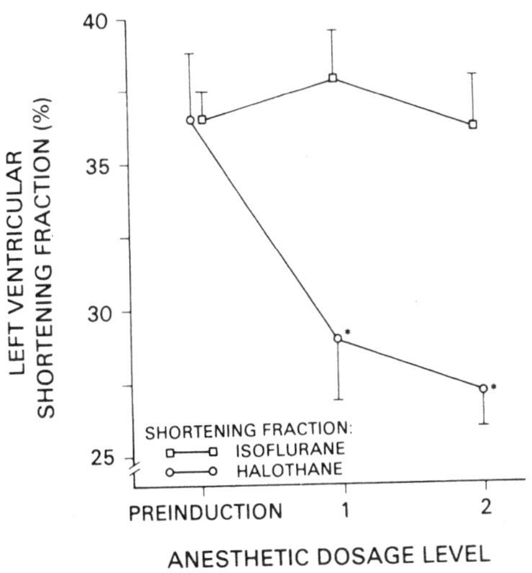

FIGURE 31-6. Changes in left ventricular shortening fraction during isoflurane (□) or halothane (○) administration. Values are mean ± standard error of the mean. Significant changes from preinduction are noted (*, $P < .05$).

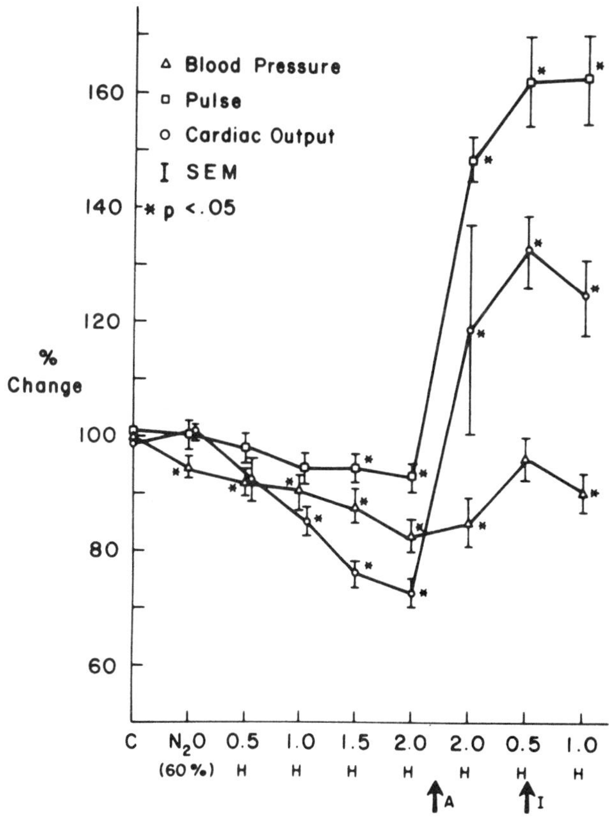

FIGURE 31-7. Changes in blood pressure, pulse, and cardiac output with increasing concentrations of halothane (*H*). (A, atropine; I, intubation.) (From Barash PG, Glanz S, Katz JD, et al. Ventricular function in children during halothane anesthesia: an echocardiographic evaluation. *Anesthesiology* 1978;49:79, with permission.)

relaxants and N_2O in a balanced intravenous technique. "Light" anesthetic techniques maintain sympathetic tone, cardiac output, and SVR (3), the latter two of which may be desirable in children with severe valvular stenosis or ventricular failure. Most children with decreased pulmonary blood flow lesions tolerate balanced anesthetic techniques, provided that excessive sympathetic tone does not cause PVR to rise.

Ketamine can be administered intramuscularly to induce anesthesia (4 to 8 mg/kg) or sedation (2 to 3 mg/kg) in an uncooperative child with congenital heart disease. The sympathomimetic effects of ketamine maintain contractility and SVR. In the absence of hypoventilation, a ketamine dose of 2 mg/kg intravenously does not increase PVR in children with congenital heart disease, including those with pulmonary vascular disease.

Thiopental (4 to 6 mg/kg intravenously) is well tolerated in normovolemic children with compensated congenital heart disease. Reduced doses must be used in children whose circulatory function is compromised. The hemodynamic effects of propofol in children with congenital heart disease are similar to those of thiopental. Rectal methohexital may be used in children with congenital heart disease as long as the child is carefully monitored for possible hypoxia or hypoventilation during induction.

The choice of specific neuromuscular blocking agents in children with congenital heart disease is usually made on the basis of the drugs' predicted cardiovascular effects as well as their duration of action. Pancuronium is a popular choice in major cases because its vagolytic effect supports heart rate and cardiac output, particularly in children who receive high-dose opioids. If tachycardia is not desirable, or for shorter procedures, mivacurium, atracurium, vecuronium, rocuronium, or rapacuronium can be used with minimal effects on hemodynamic functions.

Intravenous succinylcholine can produce bradycardia or sinus arrest in children. Its use should be preceded by, or combined with, atropine.

POSTOPERATIVE MANAGEMENT AND ANALGESIA

The postoperative management plan depends on the cardiac status of the child as well as the extent of surgical intervention. Children with well-compensated heart disease scheduled for minor surgical procedures can be appropriate candidates for ambulatory surgery. They can be discharged like any other child when appropriate criteria are met (17). Children with cyanotic heart disease, on the other hand, may require overnight hospitalization to ensure adequate intravenous hydration after even minor procedures such as dental surgery if oral intake is not rapidly resumed postoperatively. Prevention and/or treatment of postoperative nausea and vomiting is essential to ensure adequate oral intake and good hydration. Patients who have undergone extensive surgery and/or whose cardiac status is uncompensated may require postoperative intensive care.

The need for analgesics after surgery depends on the nature of the procedure and the pain threshold of the patient. Postoperative pain or discomfort can be managed by one or a combination of the following methods (17).

Mild Analgesics

Acetaminophen is the most commonly used mild analgesic for pediatric patients. For young children, the initial dose is often administered rectally (up to 45 mg/kg) before awakening from anesthesia (18). Supplemental doses are given orally (10 to 20 mg/kg) every 4 to 6 hours (not when necessary) to maintain adequate blood level and therefore effective analgesia. The maximum daily dose of acetaminophen should not exceed 100 mg/kg. Acetaminophen can be combined with codeine for more effective control of moderately severe pain and/or discomfort. Acetaminophen with codeine elixir contains 120 milligrams of acetaminophen and 12 milligrams of codeine per 5 milliliters. The usual dose is 5 mL for children 3 to 6 years, and 10 mL for the 7-to-12 year age-group.

Nonsteroidal Antiinflammatory Drugs

Nonsteroidal antiinflammatory drugs (NSAIDs) such as ketorolac have proven effective in relieving postoperative pain after minor operations in children. Ketorolac is an efficacious NSAID. Early administration immediately after induction seems to provide optimal postoperative analgesia. Several studies have demonstrated the analgesic and opioid-sparing effects of ketorolac, which may reduce the incidence of opioid-related adverse effects such as respiratory depression, nausea, and vomiting. Ketorolac, however, like many other NSAIDs, has some troubling side effects, with reported instances of decreased bone repair after osteotomy, bronchospasm, acute renal failure, and possibly increased surgical bleeding secondary to altered platelet function (19). Several recent articles reported an increased incidence of postoperative hemorrhage in patients who received ketorolac. Some, however, did not find increased bleeding when ketorolac was given at the end of the procedure. More studies are required to determine the optimal dose and route of administration of ketorolac, as well as its efficacy as an analgesic after more painful outpatient surgical procedures in children. It is expected that newer NSAIDs will soon be available that will selectively block pain receptors with minimal side effects. These should be extremely valuable in pediatric outpatients.

Potent Narcotic Analgesics

When narcotics are indicated in the recovery period, a short-acting drug should be chosen. Intravenous use allows more accurate titration of the dose and avoids the use of "standard" dosages based on weight, which may lead to a relative overdose. If remifentanil is used intraoperatively, planning for postoperative analgesia must be started before the patient awakes. Fentanyl, up to a dose of 2.0 μg/kg, is our drug of choice for intravenous use. Meperidine (0.5 mg/kg) and codeine (1.0 to 1.5 mg/kg) can be used intramuscularly if an intravenous route is not established. Intramuscularly administered codeine tends to result in less vomiting than other opioids, particularly morphine.

Regional Analgesia

Regional anesthesia can be combined with light general anesthesia to provide excellent postoperative pain relief, with minimal or no need for narcotics. By placing the block before surgery starts but after the child is asleep, one can reduce the requirement for general anesthetic agents during surgery, which in turn may result in better hemodynamic stability, a more rapid recovery, earlier ambulation and discharge, more rapid return of appetite, and less nausea and vomiting.

The types of blocks that can be used safely in the pediatric cardiac patient are limited only by the skill and interest of the anesthesiologist. The technique chosen should be simple to perform, should have minimal effects on PVR, and should not interfere with motor function and early ambulation. Simple infiltration of the operative area with local anesthetics provides postoperative pain relief after such procedures as dental extractions and surgical excision of superficial lesions.

Ilioinguinal and Iliohypogastric Nerve Block

Ilioinguinal and iliohypogastric nerve block can be performed by infiltration of 0.25% bupivacaine solution (in doses up to 2 mg/kg) in the region medial to the anterior superior iliac spine. This block has been used to provide excellent postoperative analgesia for pediatric outpatients after elective inguinal herniotomy or orchiopexy.

Dorsal Nerve Block of the Penis

Dorsal nerve block of the penis can be performed by simple injection of 1 to 4 mL of 0.25% of bupivacaine without epinephrine deep to the Buck fascia 1 cm from the midline. This has been shown to provide more than 6 hours of analgesia after circumcision with no complications. Alternate approaches to penile block are a midline injection or subcutaneous infiltration, which presumably blocks the nerve after it has ramified into the subcutaneous tissue. Topical application of lidocaine on the incision site at the conclusion of surgery has also been shown to be effective.

Caudal Block

Caudal block provides excellent and reproducible postoperative analgesia after a wide variety of surgical procedures such as circumcision, hypospadias repair, orchiopexy, and herniotomy. By using bupivacaine, 0.25% solution in a dose of 0.5 to 0.7 mL/kg, no motor paralysis is produced. Hypotension secondary to sympathetic blockade is rare in children younger than 6 years (20). Analgesia (as measured by subsequent need for a mild oral analgesic) lasts 4 to 6 hours with this technique.

REFERENCES

1. Watson SP, Watson DC. Anatomy, physiology and hemodynamics of congenital heart disease. In: Ream AK, Fogdall RP, eds. *Acute cardiovascular management.* Philadelphia: JB Lippincott Co, 1982:571.
2. Greenwood RD, Rosenthal A, Parisi L, et al. Extra-cardiac abnormalities in infants with congenital heart disease. *Pediatrics* 1975; 55:485.
3. Campbell FW, Schwartz AJ. Anesthesia for noncardiac surgery in the pediatric patient with congenital heart disease. In: Barash PG, ed. *ASA refresher courses in anesthesiology.* 1986;14:75.
4. Perry LW. The innocent murmur in children. *Med Today* 1969; 3:1.
5. Smythe JF, Teixeira OHP, Vlad P, et al. Initial evaluation of heart murmurs: are laboratory tests necessary? *Pediatrics* 1990; 86:497.
6. Miller RA, Stamler J, Smith JM, et al. The detection of heart disease in children: results of mass field trials with use of tape recorded heart sounds II. The Michigan City study. *Circulation* 1965;32:956.
7. Newburger JW, Rosenthal A, Williams RG, et al. Noninvasive tests in the initial evaluation of heart murmurs in children. *N Engl J Med* 1983;308:61.
8. Hollinger I. Anesthesia for non-cardiac surgery in infants and children with congenital heart disease. *Prog Anesthesiol* 1989; 3(10):1.
9. Morris CD, Menashe VD. 25-year mortality after surgical repair of congenital heart defect in childhood: a population-based cohort study. *JAMA* 1991;266:3447.
10. Dajani AS, Taubert KA, Wilson W, et al. Prevention of bacterial endocarditis—recommendations by the American Heart Association. *JAMA* 1997;277:1794.
11. Lazzell VA, Burrows FA. Stability of the intraoperative arterial to end-tidal carbon dioxide pressure difference in children with congenital heart disease. *Can J Anaesth* 1991;38:859.
12. Practice guideline for preoperative fasting and the use of pharmacologic agents to reduce the risk of pulmonary aspiration: application to healthy patients undergoing elective procedures. *Anesthesiology* 1999;90:896.
13. Moore RA. Anesthesia for the pediatric congenital heart patient for noncardiac surgery. *Anesthesiol Rev* 1981;8(12):23.
14. Wolf WJ, Neal MB, Peterson MD. The hemodynamic and cardiovascular effects of isoflurane and halothane anesthesia in children. *Anesthesiology* 1986;64:328.
15. Wodey E, Pladys P, Copin C, et al. Comparative hemodynamic depression of sevoflurane versus halothane in infants—an echocardiographic study. *Anesthesiology* 1997;87:795.
16. Barash PG, Glanz S, Katz JD, et al. Ventricular function in children during halothane anesthesia: an echocardiographic evaluation. *Anesthesiology* 1978;49:79.

17. Hannallah RS, Epstein BS. The pediatric patient. In: Wetchler BV, ed. *Anesthesia for ambulatory surgery,* 2nd ed. Philadelphia: JB Lippincott Co, 1991:173.
18. Anderson BJ, Holford NH, Woollard GA, et al. Perioperative pharmacodynamics of acetaminophen analgesia in children. *Anesthesiology* 1999;90:411.
19. Gillis JC, Brogden RN. Ketorolac: a reappraisal of its pharmacodynamic and pharmacokinetic properties and therapeutic use in pain management. *Drugs* 1997;53:139.
20. Dohi S, Naito H, Takahashi T. Age-related changes in blood pressure and duration of motor block in spinal anesthesia. *Anesthesiology* 1979;50:319.

PART

VII

THE ANESTHESIOLOGIST AND CARDIAC SURGERY

32

PRACTICE MANAGEMENT: QUALITY ASPECTS

MICHAEL G. LICINA
MARGARET ROBERTS-BROWN
NORMAN J. STARR

What is quality? Each of us recognizes and appreciates quality. Yet providing a universal definition for *quality* as a concept is difficult. Perhaps W. E. Deming, a recognized leader and pioneer in the automotive continuous quality improvement (QI) process, stated it best. "Quality is a never-ending cycle of continuous improvement."

Practice management is the continuum of processes, often unique for each practice, that impact the provision of patient care. These processes include staffing, operating room scheduling, billing, and QI practices. In this chapter, we focus on the QI aspects of practice management (quality management). The goal of quality management is to accomplish this task by not only improving the individuals in the department but also improving the systems or processes in our practice.

The evolution of health care into this millennium mirrors that of the American automobile industry in the 1980s. As such, each health care provider's goal is very similar to that of the autoworker's. This goal is to move the patient (product) through the hospital (factory) efficiently and with documentable high-quality perioperative care. Even health care and industrial commercial advertisement slogans are similar: "We provide quality care" versus "Quality is job number one." It is not surprising that the QI programs established in industry are now being used in hospitals, essentially because they are currently part of the Joint Commission on Accreditation of Healthcare Organization (JCAHO) survey process.

When quality measurements were introduced to the health care industry in the 1980s, hospitals adopted quality assurance (QA). A QA program concentrates on identifying poor providers, rather than defective processes. Action in the QA program is only taken when a variable passes a predetermined threshold (Fig. 32-1, *upper graph*). Our current morbidity and mortality conferences are examples of QA. Today in the health care industry, QA has dimensions of a larger scale. QA now represents documentation of patient care. Hospitals use this documentation to ensure customers (e.g., the public and insurance companies) that they are receiving quality care. Thus, when we discuss QA, we must determine which process we are discussing, bad outcomes/outliers (medical QI process) versus a statement/documentation of overall patient care quality.

As QA became accepted, the next step in the evolution of medical quality management was variously known as QI, continuous QI (CQI), or total quality management. Through these processes, not only are outliers identified but the processes associated with the outliers can be continuously monitored and perhaps improved. The improvement is accomplished in two ways. The first reduces the variability of the process that is being monitored. The second shifts the process in the desired direction. The use of benchmarking is an example of CQI (Fig. 32-1, *lower graph*).

The most recent advance in medical practice management is also derived from the nonhealth industry. The process used is called statistical process control (SPC). SPC is an extension of the CQI program. Walter A. Shewhart developed the theory of SPC in the 1920s to improve processes at AT&T (Bell Laboratories). SPC was also used during World War II to help improve war production quality but was largely ignored by American industry after the war. W. E. Deming (a Shewhart student) introduced the principles of SPC to the Japanese automobile industry in the 1950s, and it is well documented that the Japanese automobile industry was improved thanks to SPC. In fact, as Toyota, for example, became a leader in the automotive industry, the American automobile industry suffered. This was particularly true in late 1970s and the early 1980s. A portrait of Deming currently hangs in the corporate headquarters of Toyota, as a testament of SPC. SPC was reintroduced into American industry in the late 1980s with excellent re-

M. G. Licina, M. Roberts-Brown, and N. J. Starr: Department of Cardiothoracic Anesthesiology, The Cleveland Clinic Foundation, Cleveland, Ohio 44195.

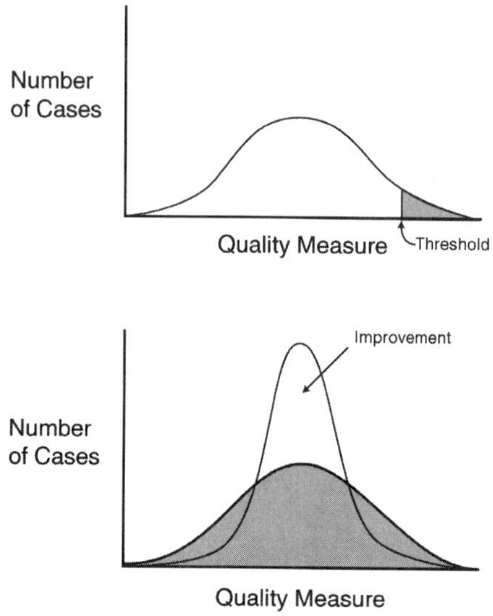

FIGURE 32-1. Quality assurance approach (*upper graph*). Quality improvement approach (*lower graph*).

sults, particularly in the automotive industry. Advertisements from the auto industry included "Quality is job one!" and "It's the benchmark for quality!" SPC was introduced into the health care industry in the 1990s. Beginning in the year 2000, JCAHO will look for hospitals to use SPC to support reaccreditation.

For illustrative purposes, the following chapter will focus on the quality management process in the Department of Cardiothoracic Anesthesia (CTA) at the Cleveland Clinic Foundation (CCF), a location the authors are most familiar with.

OVERVIEW OF THE CCF CTA DEPARTMENT

This superspecialized department is large and complex, as reflected in its organization. The department is responsible for nearly 4,000 adult cardiac operations, 1,500 thoracic operations, and 500 congenital cardiac operations a year. Cardiac anesthesiologists and cardiologists perform more than 2,200 intraoperative transesophageal echocardiograms per year. Intensivists working in the department's Section of Critical Care are responsible for the postoperative management of adult cardiac and thoracic patients. The geographical area where services are provided includes 15 anesthetizing locations in three different areas of the hospital plus a 54-bed cardiovascular intensive care unit (CVICU). The department is also responsible for several ancillary teams who support both the operating rooms and the CVICU. They include CRNAs, clinical engineers, anesthesia equipment specialists, respiratory therapists, and the cardiothoracic anesthesia database team. There are more than 100 participants including residents, fellows, and student nurse anesthetists. Our CQI program monitors each of the aforementioned areas and includes all departmental groups and employees. Quality management involves interdepartmental groups as well, including cardiothoracic staff surgeons, staff cardiologists, operating room and intensive care nurses, perfusionists, blood bank personnel, and various medical subspecialties (e.g., infectious disease, neurology, and nephrology). All these interactions are coordinated via the institution's office of quality management. The departmental quality management team consists of the departmental leadership, administrator, CQI coordinator, and representatives from the various departmental groups. Thus, with such a large and diverse representation, the quality management programs are quite complex and will be reviewed in the following section.

DEPARTMENTAL QUALITY MANAGEMENT

Critical Indicators in the CQI process

A key element of the department's quality management process is the identification of *critical indicators.* As each patient enters the operating room, the QI process is initiated. This consists of entering data on the following two forms, the Cardiothoracic Anesthesia Continuous Quality Improvement Incident Reporting Form (CACQIIRF) and Critical Incident Review Form (CIRF). The first form (Fig. 32-2) lists 36 indicators that relate to anesthetic practice. The last indicator, "Other (specify)," is used to capture unspecified indicators or unusual events. The 36 variables not only relate to common anesthetic practice but also are tailored specifically to the cardiothoracic arena. This is very similar to the approach outlined by Macario et al. (1). Macario et al. sent questionnaires to anesthesiologists associated with ambulatory surgery. The questionnaire required the anesthesiologists to correlate the importance of 33 clinical anesthesia outcome variables, ranging from nausea to death, to the frequency of their occurrence. Although death was an important occurrence in the ambulatory surgery study, fortunately it occurred extremely infrequently, whereas in comparison, death is an event of higher frequency within the cardiac surgery patient population. Nausea (high frequency of occurrence, moderate importance) was a valuable and important critical indicator in ambulatory anesthesia. In cardiac anesthesia, nausea (low frequency, low importance) is not a valuable critical indicator. The department's CACQIIRF reflects the same thought process as that in the paper by Macario et al., except that our indicators were arrived at by consensus of the CTA physicians as well as American Society of Anesthesiologist's (ASA) guidelines.

These CQI critical indicators are captured in the operating rooms, CVICU, or the nursing floors. Although any person involved with the care of the patient can record the critical event, it is the primary duty of database assistants to record these isolated events on the CACQIIRF.

Cardiothoracic Anesthesia Continuous Quality Improvement Incident Reporting Form

Patient Name, Clinic No., & Surgeon

Date of Operation ☐

Where there are boxes, check the box corresponding to where the incident was first observed.

Date of Incident	OR	ICU	Floor	
☐	☐	☐	☐	Aspiration at intubation
☐		☐	☐	Brachial plexus
☐	☐	☐	☐	Carotid hematoma/injury
☐	•			Death in O.R.
☐		☐	☐	Death within 48 hours
☐		•		Died without awakening
☐	☐	☐		Double lumen tube comp
☐	☐	☐	☐	Epidural wet tap
☐	☐	☐		Epistaxis requiring packing
☐	☐	☐	☐	Esophageal rupture due to TEE
☐	☐	☐		Failed regional
☐		☐	☐	Leg neuropathy
☐	☐	☐	☐	Lip or dental injury
☐	☐	☐	☐	Malignant arrhythmia
☐	☐	☐	☐	Mean arterial line injury
☐	☐	☐	☐	Ocular injury
☐	•			On CPB unexpectedly
☐	☐	☐	☐	PA rupture
☐		☐	☐	Peripheral nerve injury
☐		☐	☐	Postdural headache

Date of Incident	OR	ICU	Floor	
☐	☐	☐		Prolonged hypoxemia during 1 lung vent
☐	•			Protamine reaction with return to bypass
☐	•			Pulmonary edema in O.R.
☐	☐	☐	☐	Pulse oximetry injury
☐		☐	☐	Recall
☐	•			Respiratory arrest in O.R.
☐	☐	☐		Seizure due to anesthetic toxicity
☐	☐	☐	☐	Self extubation
☐	•			Total spinal
☐	☐	☐	☐	Transfusion reaction
☐		☐	☐	Ulnar neuropathy
☐	☐	☐	☐	Unable to intubate
☐	•			Unplanned circulatory arrest
☐	☐	☐	☐	Vocal cord paralysis
☐		☐	☐	Wound dehiscence
☐	☐	☐	☐	Other (specify): ________

☐ NO INCIDENTS TO REPORT

Form CTA–QI (Revised 2/19/96)

Anesthesia Staff ________
Resident ________
CRNA ________

Chart ordered? ◯ yes ◯ no
Date ordered ☐
Reviewer ________

FIGURE 32-2. Cardiothoracic Anesthesia Continuous Quality Improvement Incident Reporting Form.

From these critical indicators, sentinel events are identified. JCAHO defines a *sentinel event* as "an unexpected occurrence or variation involving death or serious physical or psychological injury, or risk thereof. The event is called 'sentinel' because it sends a signal or sounds a warning that requires immediate attention." This definition states that the unexpected occurrence includes those that lead to "unanticipated death or permanent loss of function . . . is associated with significant deviation from the usual process[es] . . . ; or has undermined, or has the potential for undermining, the public's confidence in the hospital."(2) Thus, a sentinel event could represent a substandard anesthetic practice. In situations in which a sentinel event has occurred, immediate corrective action is necessary. For example, erroneous administration of type A blood to a blood type B patient will incur a blood transfusion reaction and possibly death. This is a sentinel event requiring immediate action. Although JCAHO suspended mandatory reporting of sentinel events in March 1998, in this specific example, the occurrence must be reported to other national organizations such as the American Red Cross and the National Association of Blood Banking. In contrast, death in the cardiac surgery operating room, or within 48 hours, may or may not be a sentinel event, as the patient's serious disease process may be the reason for the poor outcome. Even though this case must be investigated, it may not be recorded as a sentinel event in the department's quality management reports.

Per our protocol, once a CQI indicator has been noted, the CQI secretary will complete a second form, the CIRF (Fig. 32-3) and assign the case to be reviewed by an unbiased staff anesthesiologist, one who was not involved with the case. This staff anesthesiologist performs a chart review and questions all appropriate personnel involved with the case. The reviewing physician then summarizes the events that occurred, makes a recommendation regarding the etiology of the event, and recommends any potential action. The departmental CQI coordinator reviews the summarized results. The case is presented by the responsible anesthesia personnel at a monthly departmental conference where the management is reviewed and discussed. This focused review of events may lead to a required change of practice, either

QUALITY IMPROVEMENT INCIDENT REVIEW FORM

QA Tracking Number:
Indicator Identified:
Name of Patient: **Clinic No.:**
Reviewer: **Date of Occurrence:**
Surgeon: **Date:**
Anesthesiologist:
Assistant (CRNA, Resident, Fellow):
Indicator/occurrence noted on:
only on database only on anesthesia record database and record

Brief Description:

FIGURE 32-3. Quality Improvement Incident Review Form.

individually or departmentally. The results of this process are then summarized on the CIRF, including any "follow-up" action that is necessary. A monthly summary is sent to the departmental chairperson for review, possible action, and inclusion in the monthly staff minutes. Should the results of the process indicate a problem in another department, the CQI coordinator and department chairperson forward the summarized results to the appropriate departmental personnel as well as the institutional office of quality management

One of the recent improvements in this aspect of QI has been the expansion of the responsibility of chart reviews to include all staff physicians. Each staff physician may be required to review one patient's chart each month. The CQI coordinator's secretary randomly chooses this case, although staff physicians are not permitted to review their own records for obvious reasons.

The inclusion of all staff physicians in the initial review is important for several reasons. First, it is an educational tool, as they can see problems in reconstructing events based on hospital chartings. This experience has led to better documentation of patient care. Secondly, no one can "control" the overall focused review process; it is extremely unbiased and it eliminates the "they're out to get me" attitude. Thirdly, the reviewer will have the opportunity to learn from alternative modes of patient care, as the department's 22 staff physicians will certainly have differing ideas and methods of intraoperative management. Additionally the staff physicians must review the literature regarding the indicator, enhancing the educational aspect of the process. This, by intent, will lead to better patient management and patient care. As described, this process of reviewing cases as signaled by critical indicators is the equivalent of the old QA program and is part of the current CQI program.

Education

The critical indicator review program was expanded to become part of the departmental education. Each month, one of the education conferences is dedicated to a review of one of the critical indicators from a case that was reviewed. In advance of the conference, appropriate papers about the topic are distributed to the audience as an educational tool. The discussion is in an American Board of Anesthesiology oral examination format (3). Residents and fellows are questioned on this and associated subject matter for preparation of the American Board of Anesthesiology oral examination and to ensure trainee reading compliance. At each monthly CQI meeting, an anesthesia malpractice journal (4) is reviewed and the articles discussed. It is hoped that by reviewing and discussing these litigated cases, the quality management in our department will be positively influenced. In addition, the residents and fellows have an opportunity to experience the problems of anesthetic practice in "the real world."

Annually, the following three areas are reviewed at the CQI monthly meeting: (a) a review of difficult airways (5), including the ASA algorithm, hands-on intubation practice on mannequins with light wands, intubating laryngeal mask airways, and retrograde wire techniques with accompanying review of the department's two difficult airway carts, (b) latex allergy, and (c) malignant hyperthermia, including the corresponding carts. Incorporating education into the CQI process is vital whether or not the practice incorporates residency training.

Finally, there are institutionally mandated compulsory annual meetings required of all departmental personnel, which deal with electrical and fire safety, hazardous material handling, infectious control and prevention, hospital disaster plans, and awareness for domestic violence. This information is also considered as part of the departmental CQI program.

Quality Improvement, Continuous Quality Improvement, Benchmarking

The second phase of practice management is QI or continuous QI (6). For us, CQI also begins upon the patient's entry into the operating room. Each patient has data collected and entered into a computerized database. Data collected include demographics, preoperative history and physical examination results, and intraoperative and postoperative information. Additional data are captured either electronically through downloads from other hospital systems or manually. Manual data collection is performed by our database assistants, who with the exception of the collection of preoperative information collect the information prospectively at the patient's bedside. This information is recorded on the cardiac or thoracic database forms (Appendixes 32-1 and 32-2). Two departmentally developed preoperative and ICU admission severity scoring systems, pertinent for coronary artery bypass graft surgery, are programmed into the database; using these scores, outcome or incidence of morbidity may be stratified by severity and risk for patient groups as well as individual patients (7,8). These scoring systems are well correlated with mortality, significant major morbidities, hospital length of stay, and financial costs. Although not stratified by risk scoring, the similar comparisons are available through the database on other procedures, such as valvular repairs, transplants, or ventricular assist devices. Patient information may be further enhanced by linking with other institutional databases. Preselected outcome measures are used to generate the department's outcomes report that *benchmarks* performance against historical controls. This is an example of risk management practice.

Benchmarks track a certain practice parameter over time and establish an incidence or threshold. This may be a percentage or an absolute number of occurrences. Upper and lower limits are determined as 2 standard deviations from the baseline's year's mean. Benchmarks are evaluated and updated, as determined by performance improvement. If the trend lines are such that the majority of the new data points are below the center line (reflecting the mean of the data points) then new benchmarks are established for that particular field. In the last 5 years, new benchmarks have been twice established. Figures 32-4 and 32-5 show the benchmarking for initial postsurgical intubation time after all coronary artery bypass graft surgeries for the years 1997 and 1998, respectively. The upper bar graphs in each table compare the intubation hours within the patient groups designated through the Cleveland Clinic Preoperative Severity Scoring system. The lower graphs show the benchmarking of the intubation times for the last eight quarters. In each of these graphs, there is a trend downward. Comparison of the mean lines for these graphs also reveals a shift downward (1997 mean line y-axis intercept 24 hours versus 1998 mean line y-axis intercept 21 hours). Thus, there has been an improvement in the process, but what influenced the improvement? Figure 32-6 plots the initial intubation times as a percentage of the patients on the y-axis versus years divided into quarters on the x-axis. The intubation times are divided into more than 24 hours (blue), 8 to 24 hours (yellow), 4 to 8 hours (red), and less than 4 hours (purple). On this graph, arrows reveal a change in recovery or weaning protocols and the corresponding effect on the intubation times. The modification of the last two weaning protocols had no apparent effect on the process. At that time, the various anesthetic management techniques by the staff were addressed (see last arrow). Although results of this intervention are pending, initial review of the raw data

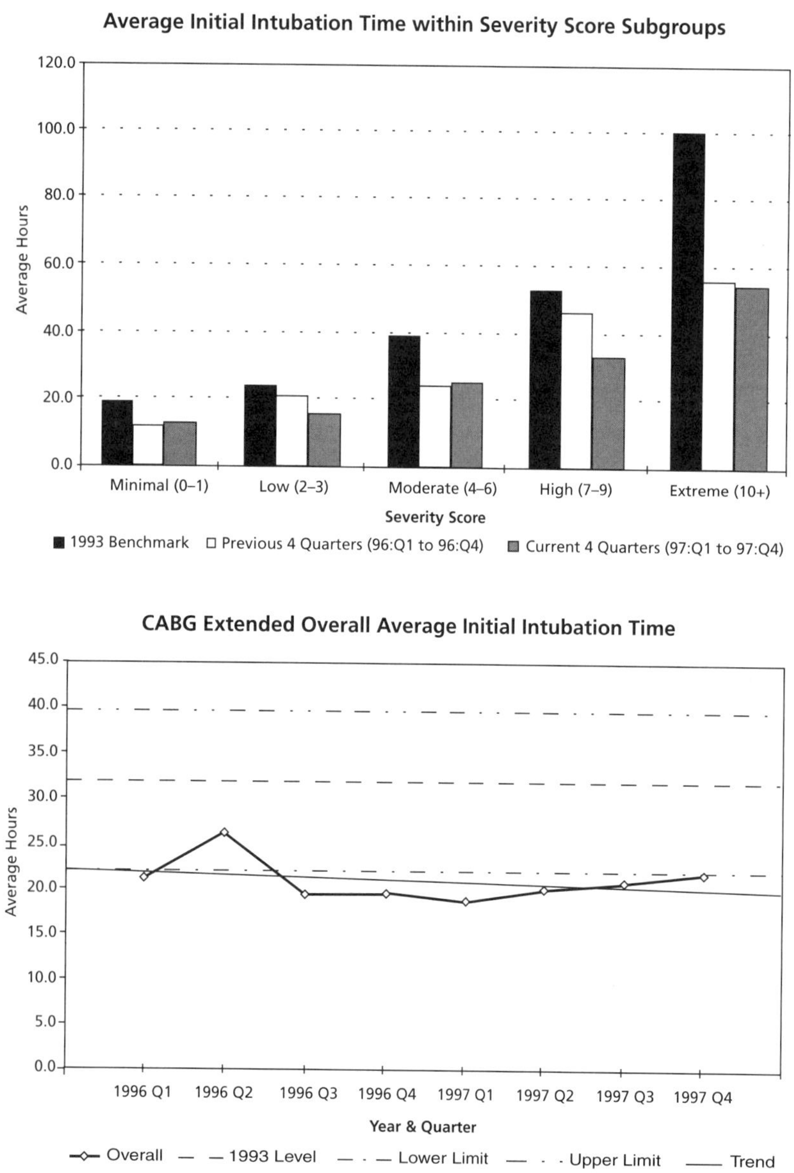

FIGURE 32-4. Cardiothoracic anesthesia quarterly cardiac database report charts for coronary artery bypass grafting extended cases for 1997.

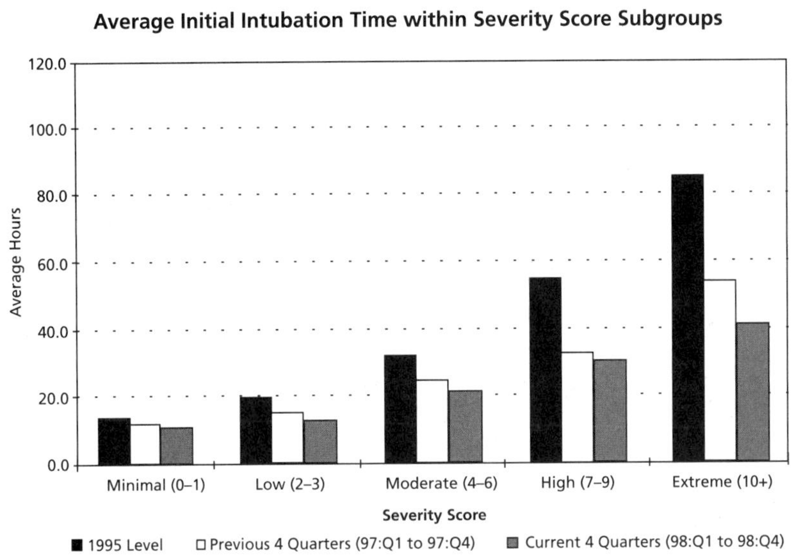

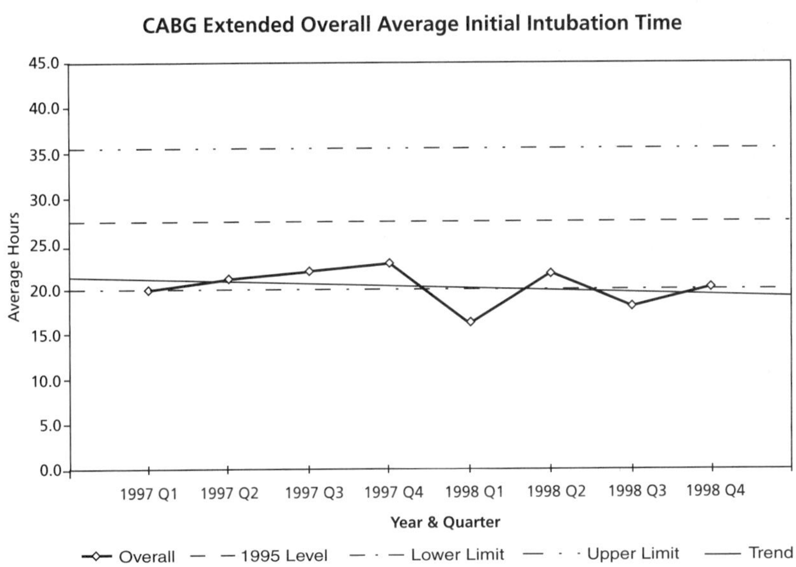

FIGURE 32-5. Cardiothoracic anesthesia quarterly cardiac database report charts for coronary artery bypass grafting extended cases for 1998.

indicates that more than 50% of the cardiac surgical patients are extubated in less than 8 hours. Information, as illustrated by this example, is monitored quarterly, and reports (Appendix 32-3) are distributed for analysis by the department. Based on these reports, new interventions or changes in protocols are made and reported in the next quarterly report. If the trend lines are increasing or most of the data points are above the center line, there is a problem that must be addressed by the quality management team. The team would review the process and the patient's records to look for any common denominator that could explain the problem. For instance, if an area of concern happens to be major infections, such as sternal wound infections, and it is discovered that a certain ICU area is associated with most of the occurrences, the team can narrow its focus to events or personnel in that ICU area. For example, perhaps there is an employee who works directly with the patients and it has been documented that this employee does not follow proper hand-washing protocol. The employee relearns this technique and the CQI process continues to monitor sternal wound infections to indicate whether the wound rate trends back to baseline.

As noted previously, the database information, with benchmarking, can be combined with institutional financial databases to measure financial performance, as it is related to severity of illness and outcome. This benchmarking is then included in quarterly and annual quality management reports.

The introduction of *transesophageal echocardiography* (TEE) in the operating room brought another area of re-

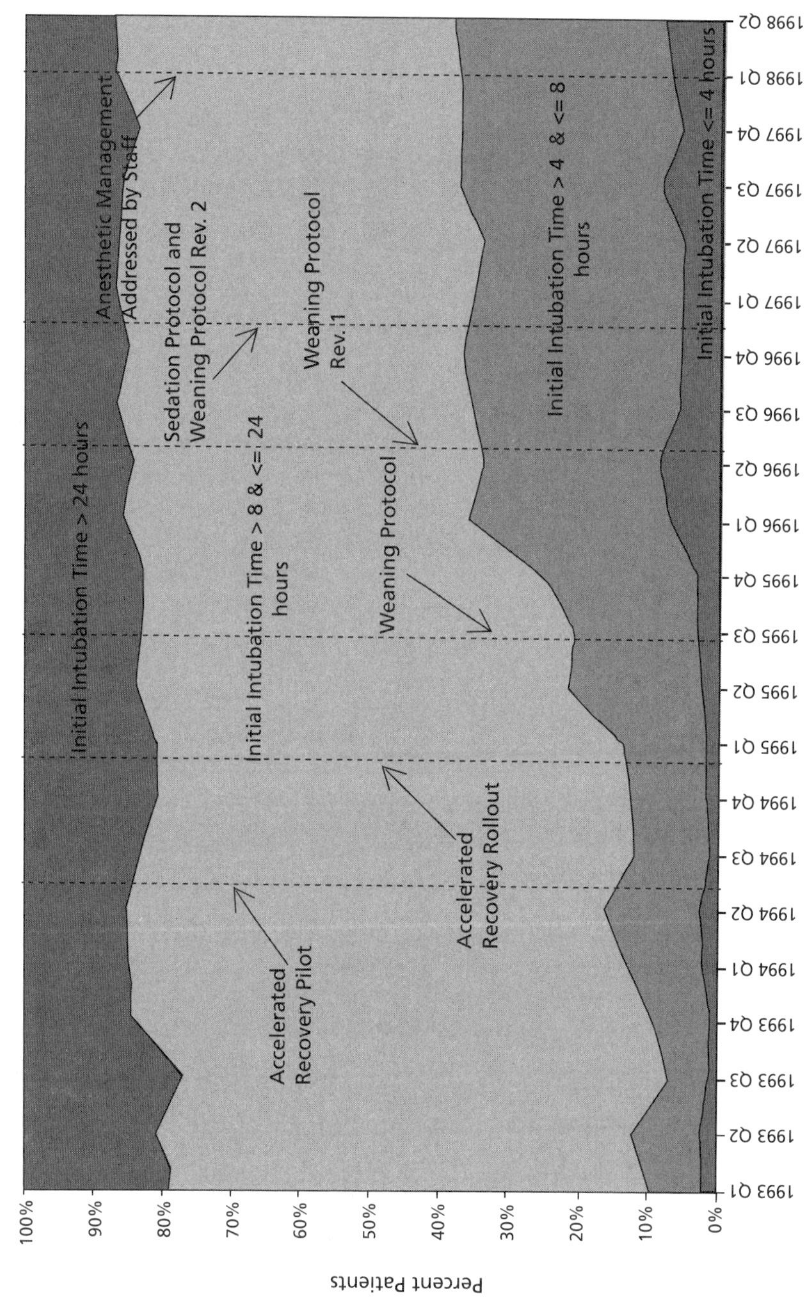

FIGURE 32-6. Initial intubation times for cardiac patients.

sponsibility to the cardiac anesthesia quality management team. The processes of QA and CQI were incorporated in the intraoperative echocardiographic service, in conjunction with the cardiology's quality management team.

The following is a historical perspective for the development of CQI in the intraoperative echocardiography service. Rafferty et al. (9) reported on the use of TEE in 846 consecutive procedures and reported on complications of TEE, record keeping, quality of images, and an audit of the QA system for echocardiography. Rafferty and colleagues suggested a need to formalize QA for intraoperative TEE, both for the anesthesiologists and for the reviewing cardiologists. This was an early attempt at QI in this area.

The American Society of Echocardiography (ASE) has published a supplement to its journal entitled *Recommendations for Continuous Quality Improvement in Echocardiography* (10) in response to the questions raised by Rafferty and others. Our CTA and cardiology departments follow the ASE guidelines. Both departments have practice management groups that interact to ensure compliance of these principles.

There are eight principal ASE guidelines:

1. There must be *adequate primary training* of the sonographers and physicians. The anesthesiologists in our institution are required to have 1 year of echocardiography training including 2 months of transthoracic echocardiography, 1 month of outpatient TEE, 3 months of intraoperative TEE (functions as a cardiology fellow), and 6 months of proctorship in which the anesthesiologist provides anesthesia care but performs the TEE on his or her specific cases while supervised by a credentialed staff (11).
2. *Maintenance of technical skills.* Each physician is required to maintain a case volume in order to maintain his or her skills and competency. In the operating room theater, all echocardiographic studies are entered in a computer, which prints reports on the number of studies done by each staff over a time period. The case volume required by our practice management group is 50 echocardiographic studies per year per physician. The national requirement is 600 intraoperative echocardiograms per year per service (collectively).
3. *Physician-sonographer relationships.* This is not an issue in the operating room, as a trained echocardiography physician performs all the transesophageal and epicardial examinations. However, the recommendation is that whenever a study is performed by a sonographer, the supervising physician should be available and trained at an ASE level 3 (600 studies a year, 50 studies a month).
4. *Periodic review.* The review is unbiased and focuses on study performance and interpretation. The ASE recommendations for performance review can be accomplished by either of two methods. These methods are (a) *prospective review* once a month, in which the study is repeated by another individual or (b) *retrospective review* of randomly selected digital clips or videotapes. The interpretation review consists of five cases randomly reviewed per month or 15 cases per quarter.

   These elements are incorporated into our review process with the following four additional mechanisms: (a) direct observation by a senior cardiologist while the anesthesiologist is performing the echocardiographic study; (b) cardiologist review of digital loops recorded by the anesthesiologist in the operating room; the cardiologist, with the anesthesiologist present, then repeats the study; (c) retrospective review of digital clips or videotapes by the cardiologist compared with the dictated anesthesiologist's echocardiographic report; (d) the anesthesiologist requests assistance from the cardiologist in performance or interpretation of the study.

   All these mechanisms provide continuing improvement as well as education.

   Echocardiographic equipment also falls under periodic review. The equipment must be calibrated every 6 months with a test phantom. Routine cleaning of the exterior of the equipment with an aseptic solution plus filter cleaning is required. The TEE probes should be checked for electrical current leakage every 3 months. Monthly calibration of all the equipment for image acquisition devices and off-line measurement systems is required. Manufacturer's maintenance schedule should be followed. All electrical systems should be regularly checked for safety according to local standards.
5. *Continuing education.* The ASE requires each physician to have at least 50 hours of category 1 CME credits dedicated to echocardiography over a period of 3 years. The ASE requires each echocardiographic service to have at least two service conferences twice a month. There is a mandatory annual requirement to attend two thirds of the conferences by each physician and sonographer. This is for a level III service. The difference for a level III versus a level II service is the number of studies done. The ASE has established a level II service for small practices and those who cannot comply with the ASE level III requirements. For level II service, the requirements can be found in the ASE journal supplement (11). The echocardiography staff is encouraged to attend and teach at formal meetings on echocardiography. These meetings can be resident conferences, plus local, regional, and national meetings. The echocardiography staff is encouraged to pass the Perioperative Transesophageal Echocardiography Examination of the National Board of Echocardiography.
6. *Utilization review* is another aspect of the CQI process where periodic review of indications for the procedure. The review should occur at monthly meetings attended by physicians and sonographers. Five randomly chosen cases should be reviewed and discussed regarding the following questions.

Was the study ordered for a recognized indication?

Was the proper test performed?

Was the study designed to answer the question at hand?

Was the study interpreted and the report generated in a timely fashion?

7. *Processing of the information* involves the need for standards for interpretive review and final report generation. In all the echocardiography service areas, whether in the operating room or the echocardiography lab, a handwritten note is placed on the patient's chart. In the operating room, this note is written by the echocardiography staff, but in the outpatient lab, it is written by the sonographer and must be reviewed by the echocardiography staff. The echocardiography staff via computer approves the final report. Timeliness is important in the age of electronic charting, because no echocardiography report will appear in an electronic chart until it is approved. Patient care may be compromised if approval is not done in a timely manner. This approval should be done within 24 hours. If it is an emergency, echocardiography staff should review it within 30 minutes. This last case scenario can occur in the cardiac anesthesia arena. For example, an emergency echocardiography is done in the cardiovascular intensive care unit by a sonographer, and the videotape is brought to the operating room for review by the anesthesia echocardiography staff.
8. *Documentation of the CQI process* is important. This document is required by accrediting organizations such as JCAHO or may be needed by other organizations at the local to national levels. It should be included in the department's practice management reports. This area overlaps with the critical indicators previously discussed in that complications resulting from the TEE probe need focused peer review (12–16). In our hospital, this focused review is incorporated in both cardiology's and cardiac anesthesia's practice management files.

One area that has recently been resolved is what constitutes a complete echocardiographic study and standard nomenclature for archiving a study using the multiplane TEE probe. A task force from the ASE and the Society of Cardiovascular Anesthesiologists, recently published guidelines addressing this issue (17). These guidelines will help strengthen the ASE CQI principles and improve patient care.

Echocardiography, as it is integrated into the cardiothoracic anesthesia department's quality management team, is a very time-consuming process due to the numerous requirements. Perhaps by using SPC (discussed in the next section), this aspect of the quality management program can be strengthened.

An area that the department has not featured but that holds a lot of promise is electronic operating room charting (18). There have been studies in which electronic operating room chart data were transferred into a database. Such information collected at these hospitals was combined to look at predictors of mortality, stroke, and myocardial infarction after coronary artery bypass graft surgery (19). This article was accompanied by an editorial by Fleisher et al. (20). The editorial discussed the use of electronic operating room charting in databases and the potential for outcome research. The electronic charting should allow for more consistent, accurate data collection to be analyzed in a constructive manner. One of the major problems with handwritten charting is the potential for retrieving inaccurate information, for much of the record keeping is done after the event has occurred and is subject to interpretation. The use of electronic operating room charting opens the way for consistent accurate information to be used in the CQI process.

Statistical Process Control

SPC is an extension of the CQI program previously discussed. SPC is a method of measuring process improvement using statistically validated methods as control charts (21, 22). Why use SPC? Outcome research may lead to erroneous conclusions in measuring process improvement. This may occur when outcome research uses aggregate measures (before-and-after results placed in a bar graph). The following example from Levett et al. (23) looks at typical outcome research versus using SPC. In this article, coronary artery bypass grafting mortality rates were compared before and after a new protocol was instituted in January 1995. The bar graph in Fig. 32-7 shows the overall mortality rate was decreased from 5% in 1994 to 4% in 1995. Did the new protocol lead to a change in this mortality rate? Unfortunately, some of us may believe that it did. To correctly look at this problem, a control chart should be constructed with percent mortality on the vertical y-axis versus time in months on the horizontal x-axis (Fig. 32-8). Two observations are notable. The first is the lack of stability in the data points in 1994. The points appear random. Focus on the data points for 1994: Four points are above the upper con-

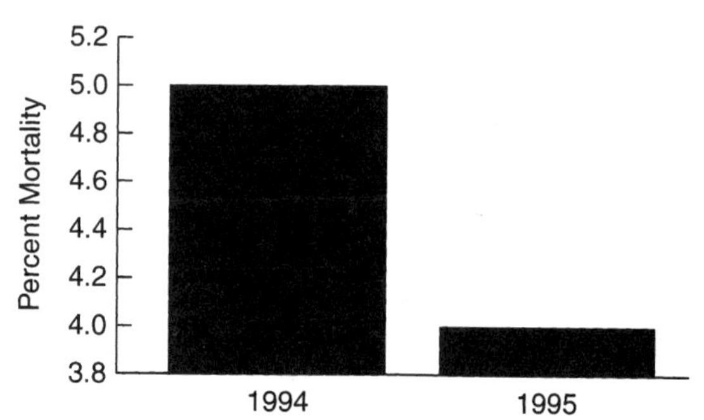

FIGURE 32-7. Bar graph comparing coronary artery bypass grafting mortality rates before and after the new protocol was instituted.

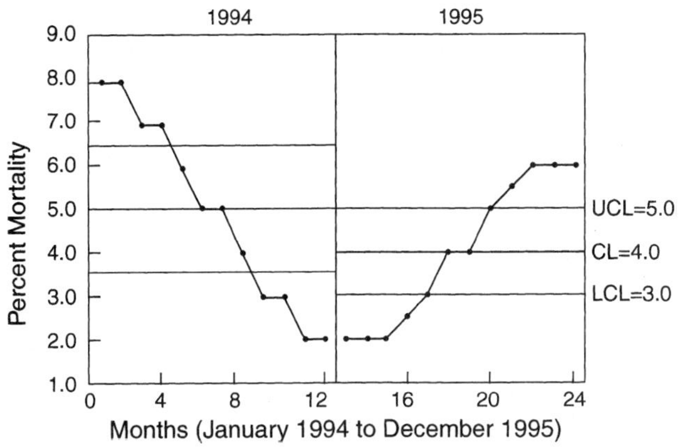

FIGURE 32-8. Control chart constructed with percent mortality on the vertical y-axis versus time in months on the horizontal x-axis.

trol limit line and four points are below the lower control limit line. This by definition of stability (explanation in the variance section) demonstrates the process (% mortality) is not stable. In fact, one might say there was a general trend for a reduced mortality rate before implementation of the new protocol, and that after protocol implementation, the mortality trend worsened even though the aggregate mortality rate in 1995 was lower. Thus, it is extremely important that before initiating new protocols for process improvement, one must observe that the process is stable, unlike this situation. This is an excellent example in which bar charting can be misleading. The control chart used plots (data points) versus time. This concept called *time-series design* is useful, as it provides a way to easily look at, think about, and analyze a process. In addition, it is easy to (a) note when the process change was made, (b) follow the results to determine whether there was process improvement, and (c) monitor the improvement over time.

Organization of the SPC Process

Because SPC is new to most of us and will be used in the JCAHO accreditation, a brief explanation of the theory is warranted. The first step is to *identify an area or process* that may need improvement (Fig. 32-9). The next step is to *organize a team* to look at this problem. The team should consist of persons familiar with and responsible for all aspects of the process that you want to improve. Initially, the team should develop a *flowchart* of the current process. Team members share information and diagram the process to determine whether a special cause of variation exists. A process is standardized when there is no special cause of variation (explanation in the variance section). The lack of standardization will lead to erroneous results, as in the prior example (Fig. 32-7). *Identifying the customer* is the next step. The customer, for example, may be the patient, the cardiac surgeon, other hospital services, insurance companies, or the government. The customer identifies which aspects of the process are important. These aspects are called *quality characteristics* (QC). The team will sort through the QCs and determine the *key quality characteristic* (KQC). This KQC is the primary focus of the team's effort. The KQC is selected on the basis of the Pareto analysis (later discussion). Once the KQC is selected, the team selects an operational definition of the KQC and develops a *data collection plan.* The operational definition is a clear and concise definition of the KQC. This is important so the team members do not have different thoughts on the KQC. For example, if

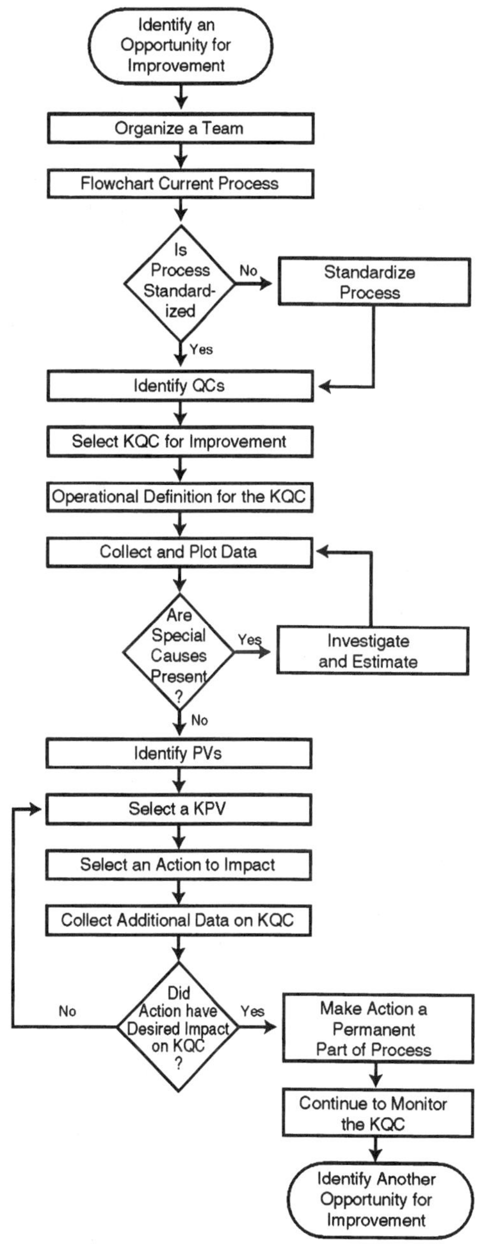

FIGURE 32-9. An algorithm helps to identify an area or process that needs improvement.

the KQC is a myocardial infarction, how is myocardial infarction defined? There are many ways of defining myocardial infarction such as electrocardiographic changes or a combination of lactate dehydrogenase, creatine kinase-MB, troponin levels, or new wall motion abnormalities on echocardiograms. The team must decide which or all of these variables to include in the operational definition. Once the team agrees on an operational definition, it will be used throughout the project. The data are then used to construct either a *run* or a *control chart.* These charts are analyzed for any *special causes of variation.* The team starts to formulate an improvement strategy when the process exhibits only common cause variation. The development of an improvement strategy begins by identifying *process variables* (PVs). The PVs are the variables that have the greatest impact on the KQC. From all the PVs, one *key process variable* (KPV) is selected and an improvement strategy is formulated around this variable. The strategy improvement related to the KPV is implemented, more data are collected and the impact of the KPV on the KQC is evaluated. Data are collected and another control chart is made. If this KPV did not have the desired effect on the KQC, then another KPV is selected and the process is repeated. Once the KPV effect is desirable, monitoring by control charts on an ongoing basis ensures the improvements are maintained.

Pareto analysis is useful in determining process characteristics to be considered. Vilfredo Pareto was an Italian economist who observed that only a small portion of the Italian population owned the majority of land and wealth. In fact, 20% of the population owned 80% of the wealth. Dr. Joseph Juran applied the Pareto principle to the CQI theory, to help determine which of the many opportunities in a process should be looked at first. This has been known as "separating the vital few from the trivial many." The Pareto analysis states that in any group of characteristics that contribute to a common effect, only a few will contribute to most of the effect. To do this in the CQI format, a Pareto diagram can be made and a Pareto analysis can be accomplished with computer software. For example, what are the factors contributing to delayed extubation in the ICU? The team finds that there are seven reasons or characteristics for this. Each reason occurs a certain percentage of the time. One reason occurs 50% of the time and each of the rest less than 8% of the time. Which characteristic would you look at first?—via the Pareto analysis, the one characteristic that occurs more than 50% of the time, instead of the six characteristics that collectively occur less than 50% of the time.

The concept of *variation* is important in the SPC process. Variation is a major part of our lives; for example, no two physicians are exactly alike, no two surgeries are exactly alike, and two golf games by the same individual are not alike. Thus, throughout all the processes that we look at through CQI, there will be an underlying variation associated with the process. This underlying variation in a process is called *common cause variation* (*random variation*). For example, in golf, you are a 36-stroke handicapper. This indicates you have a lot of room for improvement. So your common cause variation is that you will shoot approximately 36 strokes over par on the average. Now you take a lesson (new protocol) and change your swing (KQC), and after this lesson, your scores improve to where you are now, a 20-stroke handicapper. In this situation, you have improved your golf game (process) by decreasing the common cause variability (golf swing) associated with it. A medical example of common cause variation is surgeon X does a mitral valve repair operation in about 4 hours. If you would plot the operating room times for each of surgeons X's mitral valve repairs, you would have a range of operating room times from 2.5 hours to 5 hours. This is the common cause variation of surgeon X's mitral valve repair times.

There is another cause of variation called *special cause variation* (*nonrandom variation*). For example, you are now playing golf as a 20 handicapper and routinely shoot a score in the 90s, but you notice one day your score was 130. If this is plotted on a control chart, it is special cause variation. In this situation, you want to find out what happened and if there is anything you can do to eliminate this. If you investigate the bad round of golf, you realize you were on duty all night caring for a cardiac patient. Thus, by discovering that you shouldn't stay up all night working before a golf match, the special cause of variation in your golf game can be eliminated. Using the medical example of surgeon X and mitral valve repair times, a control chart is constructed of mitral valve repair times versus days of the month. On the control chart, you discover three mitral valve repair operating room times of 7, 7.5, and 8 hours each in the last 3 months, whereas the rest of the times were between 2.5 and 5 hours. These three long times are special causes of variation and must be investigated. Upon investigation, it is discovered that the surgeon was not available to perform these operations due to "important meetings." Thus, waiting for the surgeon due to meetings was a special cause variation. This special cause variation must be eliminated before any protocol attempting to improve operating room times can be implemented.

Common cause variation is an inherent part of every process. It is important to shift common cause variation to a lower level to improve the process. Special cause variation is an abnormal or irregular cause in a process that is not inherent to that process. This special cause variation must be eliminated before process improvement can be implemented when you are evaluating whether a process is standardized.

The basic ideas of Shewhart and Deming regarding variation can be summarized as follows:

1. All processes have variation.
2. Processes that contain only common cause variation are predictable and can be looked at statistically.

3. Special causes of variation are bad and must be identified and eliminated.
4. If you don't eliminate special causes of variation, any improvement process will not be valid—wasting both time and resources.
5. Eliminate the special cause variation before attempting process improvement.

There are two ways of depicting variation—either statically or dynamically. The static display is a bar graph, table, or histogram. A dynamic display can be a run or a control chart.

The following section discusses run charting versus control charting.

Run Charts. A run chart is a dynamic display of data shown or run over time. The advantage of a run chart is that it is easy to construct and to interpret.

Mechanics of a Run Chart. The data to be measured are plotted along the y-axis (vertical) versus time, the x-axis (horizontal). To construct a run chart, you need at least 15 data points (the number 15 was determined statistically (24). The data points are connected via a line. After the line is constructed, you need to determine the *median.* The easiest way to determine the median is to determine the *median position.* The median position is calculated by adding the total number of data points plus 1 and dividing this number by 2. For example, you have 18 data points, 18 + 1 = 19. 19 / 2 = 9.5. Therefore, 9.5 is the median position. The *median line,* which is different than the median position, will be where one half of the data points will be above the line and one half will be below the line. In this case, there will be nine points above and nine points below the median line. The median line is constructed between the ninth and tenth data point because the median position is 9.5. This line is horizontal and parallel to the x-axis. The *median value* is obtained by noting where the median line crosses the y-axis.

The first step in analyzing a run chart is determining a run. A *run* is defined as one or more consecutive data points on the same side of the median (data points lying on the median are to be ignored). In the following example (Fig. 32-10, control chart example), there are six runs. Tests for analyzing run charts for a source of variation are included in Appendix 32-4. If one of these four tests is positive for a special cause of variation, you must investigate this special cause of variation. As mentioned in the previous section, any special cause of variation identified by one of these tests requires investigation and elimination before process improvement.

The run charts are simple to use and understand but are not sensitive in detecting special causes as with control charts.

Control Charts. Special cause variation may not be detected when using a run chart and plotting. The statistical basis for control charting was developed by Walter A. Shewhart in the 1920s and was published in his book *Economic Control of Quality of Manufactured Product* (24). This book is the foundation for SPC.

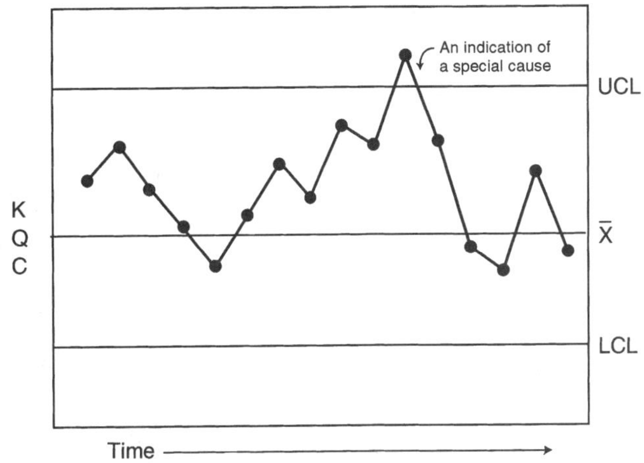

FIGURE 32-10. A control chart showing how the control limits are used to determine the capability of the process and to identify special causes of variation.

Control charting is set up very similar to run charting with a few differences. The y-axis plots the data from the KQC and the x-axis plots time exactly like a run chart. However, the center line is not the median but the mean, ($\bar{x}$ or x-bar), and upper control limits and lower control limits are established. The control limits are used in determining the capability of the process and to identify special causes of variation (Fig. 32-10).

The upper control limit and lower control limit are determined for a bell-shaped distribution curve (Fig. 32-11) and are set at 3 standard deviations or 3 sigmas from the mean or x-bar. The 3-sigma value was chosen to balance the risk from tampering versus undercontrolling. Tampering (type I error) refers to detection of special cause variation when the process is stable but in fact there is no special cause variation. Undercontrolling (type II error) refers to presence of special cause variation, which is hidden in the process because the control limits are too wide to recognize it. Type II errors occur when you conclude that no special cause variation exists when it does. Any data point that lies outside of the upper or lower control limit is a special cause variation. The control chart can be set up in six zones (three zones above the x-bar and three zones below the x-bar). These zones are each 1-sigma wide (Fig. 32-12). Zone A is located next to the upper and lower control limits, and zone C is located near the mean line. Tests for special cause of variation are listed in Appendix 32-5. If your control chart has a positive test for special cause variation, it must be investigated.

Control charts must take into account the type of data you are collecting. There are basically two types of data;

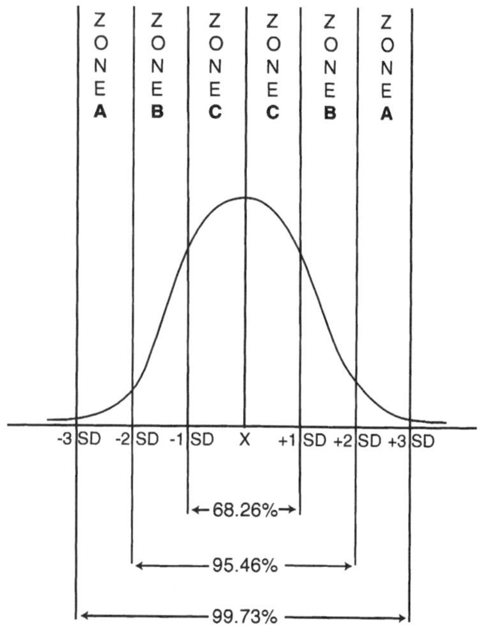

FIGURE 32-11. The upper control limit and lower control limit are determined for a bell-shaped distribution curve and are set at 3 standard deviations or 3 sigmas from the mean or x-bar.

discrete (attributes) data and continuous (variables) data. Discrete data are data such as smoker versus nonsmoker, yes versus no, black versus white. Continuous data are data that can take on different values on a continuous scale. Examples of continuous data include hematocrit levels, time, and temperature.

Once the control chart variable is determined, the control chart tree (Fig. 32-13) can be used to decide which control chart (there are currently seven) you should use for the process you are investigating. The explanation for this chart is beyond the scope of this chapter, but more details can be found in *Economic Control of Quality of Manufactured Product* and *Measuring Quality Improvement in Healthcare* (24,25).

How do you determine whether the control chart shows process improvement? If the new protocol had a beneficial effect on the process then the upper control limit, the lower control limit, and the mean line will be shifted downward from the preprotocol change control chart to the postprotocol change control chart (Fig. 32-14). Comparison of the old control chart to the new one will identify special cause variation in the new chart. Thus, this special cause of variation reflects improvement in the process. There was a nonrandom (special cause variation) change (the new protocol) that improved the process.

	Zone A	+3 SD
	Zone B	+2 SD
	Zone C	+1 SD
-1 SD	Zone C	
-2 SD	Zone B	
-3 SD	Zone A	

FIGURE 32-12. Six zones, 1-sigma wide each, are drawn on the control chart. Three zones should be placed above the x-bar and three zones should fall below the x-bar.

The last use of the control charts is to monitor the processes.

Control charts are used in SPC for (a) *preprotocol review* to look for standardization; (b) *postprotocol review* to look for improvement; and (c) *monitoring* to make sure the process improvement is maintained.

In Fig. 32-14, the control chart is reproduced from raw Cleveland Clinic data submitted in abstract form. The goal of the study was to improve the number of preoperative patients "cleared for surgery." The KQC is the number of patients not cleared for surgery from the anesthesia preoperative center. The intervention was the Internal Medicine Preoperative Assessment, Consultation and Treatment Center (IMPACT Center), where patients are processed before proceeding to the anesthesia preoperative center. The IMPACT Center ensures medical preparation of the patients preoperatively before anesthesia clearance. The control charts show that after the protocol change, the mean line was shifted downward and the new chart (after IMPACT Center) revealed a special cause of variation compared to the old control chart (before IMPACT Center). The test used to determine the special cause of variation was eight successive points in zone C on the same side of the center line (Appendix 32-5). Thus, the IMPACT Center had a positive effect on the KQC (not cleared yet) and the process (anesthesia clearance for surgery) was improved. With the improvement in the process, the common cause variation was reduced, as seen in the after IMPACT Center control chart.

Boggs et al. (16) used the SPC process in examining peak expiratory flow rate (PEFR) control charts in asthmatics. PEFR home monitoring of pulmonary function is a simple, inexpensive method to monitor asthmatics. The current national and international guidelines recommend monitoring of PEFRs via the use of run charts. Boggs and colleagues found that the use of control charts in SPC process provided "clinical insights, practical knowledge, and opportunities unavailable to patients and physicians via traditional PEFR charting."

In another study, Shahian et al. (27) used SPC to look at common adverse outcomes after cardiac surgery. The common adverse outcomes were death, myocardial infarction, stroke, and atrial fibrillation. These outcomes were plotted on control charts in 1,131 patients over a 17-quarter time period. The author's concluded that " statistical quality control may be a valuable method to analyze the variability of these adverse postoperative events over time, with the

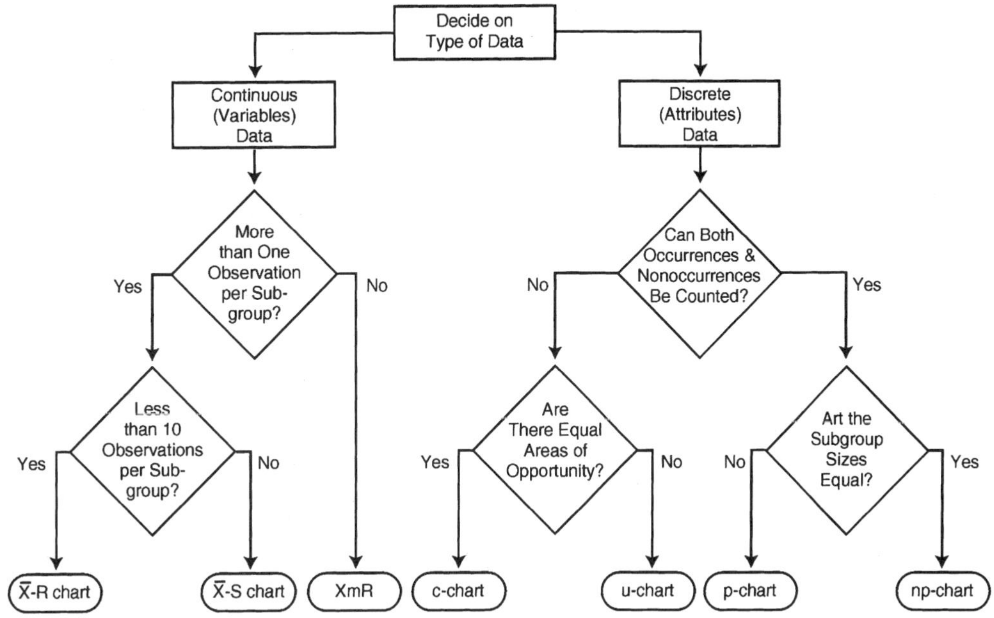

FIGURE 32-13. Algorithm used to decide which control chart should be used for the process being investigated.

ultimate goal of reducing that variability and producing better outcomes."

SPC may be useful in optimizing operating room personnel management patterns. For example, Posner et al. (28) evaluated the quality of anesthetic care and productivity associated with alternating staffing patterns. The results of the study were conflicting. When staffing was at higher concurrent and productivity levels, there were lower patient injury rates (actual events) but increased critical incidents (potential events). This would be an area in which the SPC process would be helpful. If the results were due to a lack of standardization and thus had a special cause of variation, the SPC process would identify it. The use of the SPC process in this situation could lead to clarification of this valuable information.

Patient survey reports, like patient satisfaction surveys, are fraught with problems. SPC can be used in developing an accurate patient survey system (29). In this article, the authors explain the issues with conducting sound patient surveys and how to avoid pitfalls that will lead to inaccurate or inconclusive results. The survey process should include the following criteria: psychometrically sound questionnaire, avoidance of data collection bias, and whether the study is enumerative or analytic. A psychometrically sound

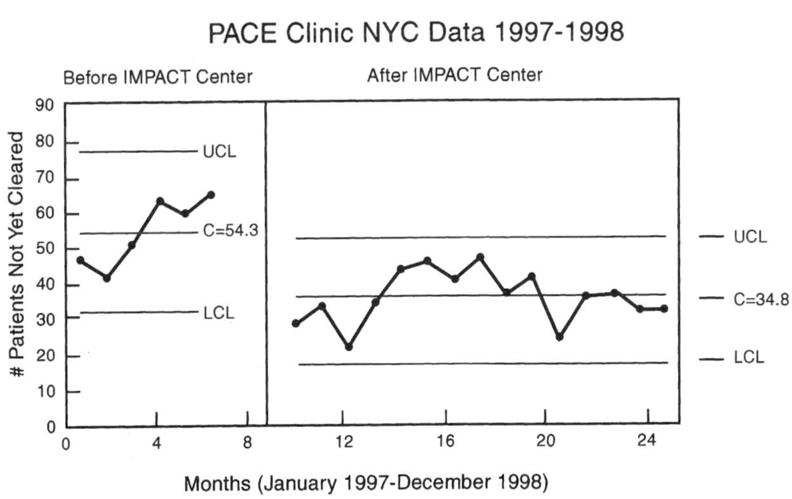

FIGURE 32-14. Chart showing a beneficial effect. The upper control limit, the lower control limit, and the mean line shifted downward from the preprotocol change control chart to the postprotocol change control chart.

questionnaire is one which the degree of accuracy is determined by its degree of reliability and validity. Avoidance in data collection bias is accomplished by observing whether the survey's construction will have interviewer bias or nonresponse bias. An enumerative study is done on a static population for a given period and/or location to describe outcomes. An analytic study examines a process over time evaluating why the outcomes were observed and whether any process improvement protocols changed the process by SPC. Thus, SPC is a useful tool in developing and conducting patient satisfaction surveys.

SUMMARY

The methods of improving patient care have changed dramatically over the last 20 years. The quality management process has evolved from a QA approach only, in which the process had to exceed above a threshold before the QA program acted to CQI with benchmarking. QA is still a part of our quality management process, as with sentinel events. Benchmarking occurs both internally at an institutional level and externally through to the nation level with all the associated problems (30). Gabel (30), in a recent ASA newsletter article, looked at performance measurement initiatives by the American Medical Association and the ASA and the government's interaction with these initiatives.

The standard CQI format has problems, including (a) the failure to standardize the process, (b) failure to separate special cause variation from common cause variation (type I versus type II errors), (c) benchmarking is limited by the validity of the data, and (d) risk adjustment of outcomes encounters problems with nonhomogeneous populations and variability with time. This has led to the incorporation of SPC into the established CQI program.

With external pressures from insurance providers and government to improve patient care and decrease costs, patient management guidelines have been introduced. These guidelines are supposed to standardize medical processes to improve patient care but have not been widely accepted by physicians (31). SPC would be ideal to be used for proving the utility of patient management guidelines.

SPC has the ability to be useful in all types of quality management. SPC, as an extension of the current CQI program, will be the method of improving quality in medicine in this millennium.

APPENDIX 32-1.

A sample cardiac database form from the Cleveland Clinic Foundation.

Clinic Number
Patient Name

Cardiac Database
The Cleveland Clinic Foundation

Room #'s

○ CCF
○ Kaiser

Notes

Form CTDB (cardiac7.pm5) Revised 6/2/99

Pre-Op History & Physical

Birthdate (yy/mm/dd): ☐☐/☐☐/☐☐

Race: ○ Black ○ White ○ Other

☐ Jehovah Witness
☐ COPD / Asthma
☐ Lung Surgery
☐ Pulmonary Hypertension
☐ Smoking – Current or Ever
☐ History of Congestive Heart Failure
☐ Hypertension

○ No Myoc. Infarc.
○ MI ≤ 1 week
○ MI > 1 wk. & < 3 mos.
○ MI 3 to 6 mos.
○ MI > 6 mos.

○ No Diabetes
○ IDDM
○ NIDDM
○ Diet Control

☐ History of Dysrhythmia
☐ A Fib
☐ A Flutter
☐ V Tach
☐ V Fib
☐ Junctional
☐ ETOH

☐ Stroke
☐ Vasc Surg/Dilat
☐ Vascular Disease
☐ Carotid Surgery
☐ Carotid Disease
☐ Dialysis

Cath Report

LVF — EF%: ☐

Source________________

○ Normal ○ Mild ○ Mild–Mod
○ Mod ○ Mod–Sev ○ Severe

☐ *Check if above LVF is derived*

☐ Left Main ≥ 70% – LMT%: ☐

AV Insufficiency
○ None ○ 1+ ○ 2+ ○ 3+ ○ 4+

☐ AV Stenosis — Gradient ☐
Area ☐

MV Insufficiency
○ None ○ 1+ ○ 2+ ○ 3+ ○ 4+

☐ MV Stenosis — Gradient ☐
Area ☐

Progress Notes

☐ Cardiogenic Shock
☐ Endocarditis
☐ Preop IABP ☐ Preop ECMO
☐ Preop Asst. Vent. ☐ Preop VAD

Lab Report

	Value	
HCT	☐	
Bun	☐	☐ *Check if derived*
Creat	☐	☐ *Check if derived*
Albumin	☐	
Bilirubin	☐	

Pre-Op Medications ☐ None

#1 ☐ #4 ☐
#2 ☐ #5 ☐
#3 ☐ #6 ☐

Intra-Op Operative Notes

Operation Date (or Nonsurg Admit Date) (yy/mm/dd): ☐☐/☐☐/☐☐

# of Redos: ☐ Nonsurg Admit Tm ☐ :

Admit Date (yy/mm/dd) ☐ Discharge Date (yy/mm/dd) ☐

Procedure ☐

☐ LIMA ☐ Heartmate
☐ RIMA ☐ Novacor
☐ Inferior Epigast ☐ Thoratec
☐ Gastro ☐ Abiomed
☐ SVG ☐ ECMO
☐ Radial Artery ☐ Cardiomyoplas.
☐ LVAD ☐ RVAD ☐ Congenital

☐ Mini Invasive ☐ Converted Mini
☐ Heartport

☐ Left Vent Remodeling ☐ DOR
☐ Transmyocardial Revascularization

ORIS

☐ IABP Post Bypass
☐ AV Replace
☐ AV Repair
☐ MV Replace
☐ MV Repair
☐ PV Replace/Repair
☐ TV Replace/Repair
☐ Aorta Surgery
☐ Stent
☐ Heart Transplant
☐ Heart/Lung Transplant
☐ Myomectomy
☐ IVC Repair
☐ Bypass Ablation/Maze Procedure
☐ VA Repair
☐ Carotid Repair
☐ AICD Implant/Explant
☐ PA Repair
☐ Sternal Work
☐ Tracheostomy
☐ Post MI VSD
☐ Unlisted

OR Prior/Return

	Date (yy/mm/dd)	R#1	R#2	RBC Units
#1	☐	☐	☐	☐
#2	☐	☐	☐	☐
#3	☐	☐	☐	☐
#4	☐	☐	☐	☐
#5	☐	☐	☐	☐

Additional Number of Returns ☐

Reasons for OR Prior/Return

1. LVAD I/R
2. RVAD I/R
3. Heartmate I/R
4. IABP I/R
5. Bleeding
6. Tamponade
7. Bronchoscopy
8. Cardiac Arrest
9. Cysto
10. GI Procedure
11. Revision Main
12. Sternal Work
13. Tracheostomy
14. Vascular
15. Cancel
16. ECMO I/R
17. Transplant
18. Other

APPENDIX 32-1. *Continued*

Discharge Summary

	Date (yy/mm/dd)	Time (hh:mm)	R#1	R#2
Init Dischg				
1st Re-ad				
1st Dischg				
2nd Re-ad				
2nd Dischg				
3rd Re-ad				
3rd Dischg				
4th Re-ad				
4th Dischg				
5th Re-ad				
5th Dischg				

Add'l # of Reads ☐ Add'l Hours ☐

Reasons for Readmission
1. Pulmonary
2. Cardiac
3. Infection
4. Neuro
5. Renal
6. GI
7. Other

Anesthesia Record

☐ Emergency

Weight (kg) [Value] Height (cm) [Value]

	Value
PCO_2	
Heart Rate	
MAP	
PA Sys	
PA Dia	
PA Mean	
CVP	
CO	

	No. of Units
FFP	
Platelets	
RBC	
Cryo	

Urine Output [Value]

Page 2 (Revised 6/2/99)

Anesthetics

- ☐ Alfentanil (N)
- ☐ Diazapam (S)
- ☐ Enflurane (I)
- ☐ Etomidate (S)
- ☐ Fentanyl (N)
- ☐ Halothane (I)
- ☐ Isoflurane (I)
- ☐ Ketamine (S)
- ☐ Midazolam (S)
- ☐ Morphine (N)
- ☐ Propofol (S)
- ☐ Sufentanil (N)
- ☐ Infusion OR
- ☐ Infusion cont. to ICU

Drugs

- ☐ Inotropes/Pressors – Induction/Bypass
- ☐ Amicar
- ☐ Aminophylline
- ☐ Amrinone (I)
- ☐ Dobutamine (I)
- ☐ Dopamine (I)
- ☐ Epinephrine (I)
- ☐ Isuprel (I)
- ☐ Lidocaine (A)
- ☐ Norepinephrine (P)
- ☐ NTG (D)
- ☐ Nitroprusside (D)
- ☐ Phenylephrine (P)
- ☐ Procainamide (A)
- ☐ Milrinone (I)
- ☐ Esmolol
- ☐ Insulin
- ☐ Aprotinin
- ☐ Cardizem
- ☐ Amiodarone
- ☐ Vasopressin
- ☐ Other: ____________

Post-Op Resp Ther Chart

Mode: ☐ SIMV ☐ AC ☐ PCV ☐ PRVC ☐ Other__________

☐ Arrived Extubated

	Value		Value
Vent Rate		pH	
Tidal Vol		PCO_2	
FIO_2		PO_2	
PEEP		HCO_3	

Intubation Summary

	Date (yy/mm/dd)	Time (hh:mm)	R#1	R#2
Init Extub				
1st Reint				
1st Extub				
2nd Reint				
2nd Extub				
3rd Reint				
3rd Extub				
4th Reint				
4th Extub				
5th Reint				
5th Extub				

Add'l # of Retubes ☐ Add'l Hours ☐

Reasons for Reintubation
1. Pulmonary
2. Airway/Aspiration
3. Cardiac/CHF
4. Infection/Pneumonia
5. Neuro
6. Renal
7. GI
8. Surgery
9. Self Extubation
10. Other

Perfusion Record

☐ No Bypass ☐ No X Clamp ☐ VAVD ☐ RCP ☐ Spinal Cooling

	Time #1 (hh:mm)	Time #2	Time #3	Time #4	Time #5
Start CPB					
X Clamp On					
X Clamp Off					
Off CPB					
Circ Arrrest Start					
Circ Arrest Stop					

APPENDIX 32-1. *Continued*

Nurses Notes – Admission

	Value
Core Temp	☐
Heart Rate	☐
MAP	☐
CVP	☐
PA Sys	☐
PA Dia	☐
CO	☐

	Date (yy/mm/dd)	Time (hh:mm)
RTC	☐	☐

☐ Awake Only

Drugs	DOS	POD 1
Aminophylline	☐	☐
Amiodarone (A)	☐	☐
Amrinone (I)	☐	☐
Calcium Block	☐	☐
Dobutamine (I)	☐	☐
Dopamine (I)	☐	☐
Epinephrine (I)	☐	☐
Fentanyl	☐	☐
Insulin Drip	☐	☐
Isuprel (I)	☐	☐
Lidocaine (A)	☐	☐
Other Antiarr (A)	☐	☐
Muscle Relax	☐	☐
Nor Epineph (P)	☐	☐
Nitroprusside (D)	☐	☐
NTG (D)	☐	☐
Phenylephrine (P)	☐	☐
Propofol	☐	☐
PCA Pump	☐	☐
Milrinone (I)	☐	☐
Amicar	☐	☐
Esmolol	☐	☐
Lanoxin	☐	☐
Vasopressin	☐	☐

	Date
Adverse Drug Reaction	☐
Agitation Requiring Rx	☐

DIC Date (yy/mm/dd) ☐

RBC ○ 1 ○ 2 ○ 3 ○ 4 ○ ≥ 5

Auto Trans (ml) ☐

	Date
Major Transfusion	☐

ICU Events

Cardiac	Date
Asystole	☐
Atrial Arrythmia	☐
VT/VF	☐
Low CO	☐
IABP	☐
ECMO	☐
Open Chest	☐
Perm Pacer	☐
Heart Block	☐

Neuro	Date
Shiver Req Rx	☐
Focal Deficit	☐
Global Deficit	☐
Seizure	☐
Encephalopathy	☐
ETOH	☐
Spinal Cord Injury	☐

Renal	Date
Dialysis Start	☐
Anuria	☐

GI/Hepatic	Date
TPN Start	☐
TPN End	☐
Enteral Feed	☐

Infections	Date
Fungemia	☐
Bacteremia	☐
Line Sepsis	☐
Sepsis Syndrome	☐
Septic Shock	☐
Empyema	☐
Endocarditis	☐
Mediastinitis	☐
Sternal Wound	☐
Wound	☐
Pneumonia	☐
Urinary	☐

Pulmonary	Date
ARDS	☐
Aspir Pneu	☐
Atelectasis	☐
Bronchospasms	☐
Bronchoscopy	☐
CHF	☐
Diaph Paraly	☐
Effusion	☐
Pneumothorax	☐
Pulm Edema	☐
Pulm Embolus	☐
Resp Insuff/Distress	☐
Resp Failure	☐
Tracheobronchitis	☐

GI/Hepatic Complications	Date
Cholecystitis	☐
Hepatitis	☐
GI Bleed	☐
Ileus Post 2 Days	☐
Pancreatitis	☐

	Date
MSOF	☐

	Date
DNR Order	☐

Death Date (yy/mm/dd) ☐

Time of Death (hh:mm) ☐

Place: ○ OR ○ ICU ○ Floor

	Reason Code
Cause of Death	☐

Page 3 (Revised 6/2/99)

APPENDIX 32-1. *Continued*

Labs

First ICU Value

	Value
HCT	
K	
Glucose	

Cardiac	DOS	POD 1	POD 2
CPK			
MB			
AST			

Renal

SCR POD 1	
SCR POD 2	
SCR POD 3	
High SCR	
High SCR Date	

Infection

First WBC	
First WBC Date	
High WBC	
High WBC Date	

GI/Hepatic

High Bili	
High Bili Date	
High Lactic Acid	
High LA Date	
Low Transferrin	
Low Trans Date	

Blood

Low Platelet	
Low Plat Date	
High D-Dimer	
High D-D Date	
Low HCT	
Low HCT Date	

QA Complications

- ☐ Aspiration at Intubation
- ☐ Brachial Plexus
- ☐ Carotid Hematoma/Injury
- ☐ Death within 48 hours
- ☐ Died w/o Awakening
- ☐ Double Lumen Tube Complication
- ☐ Epidural Wet Tap
- ☐ Epistaxis
- ☐ Esophageal Rupture TEE
- ☐ Failed Regional
- ☐ Leg Neuropathy
- ☐ Lip/Dental Injury
- ☐ Malignant Arrhythmia
- ☐ Mean Arterial Line Injury
- ☐ Ocular Injury
- ☐ On CPB Unexpectedly
- ☐ PA Rupture
- ☐ Peripheral Nerve Injury
- ☐ Postdural Headache
- ☐ Prolonged Hypoxemia
- ☐ Protamine Rx
- ☐ Pulmonary Edema in OR
- ☐ Pulse Oximetry Injury
- ☐ Recall
- ☐ Respiratory Arrest in OR
- ☐ Seizure due to Anes Toxicity
- ☐ Self Extubation
- ☐ Total Spinal
- ☐ Transfusion Rx
- ☐ Ulnar Neuropathy
- ☐ Unable to Intubate
- ☐ Unplanned Circulatory Arrest
- ☐ Vocal Cord Paralysis
- ☐ Wound Dehiscence
- ☐ Other:____________________

Page 4 (Revised 6/2/99)

APPENDIX 32-2.

A sample thoracic database form from the Cleveland Clinic Foundation.

Thoracic Database
The Cleveland Clinic Foundation

••• Followed? •••
○ Yes ○ No

○ ICU
○ PACU
○ Other

○ CCF
○ Kais

Clinic Number
Patient Name

Notes

Room #'s

Pre-Op History & Physical

Birthdate (yy/mm/dd):

☐☐ / ☐☐ / ☐☐

Race: ○ Black ○ White ○ Other

- ☐ Jehovah Witness
- ☐ COPD / Asthma
- ☐ Cystic Fibrosis
- ☐ Pulmonary Hypertension
- ☐ Smoking – Current or Ever
- ☐ History of Congestive Heart Failure
- ☐ Hypertension

○ No Myoc. Infarc.
- ○ MI ≤ 1 week
- ○ MI > 1 wk. & < 3 mos.
- ○ MI 3 to 6 mos.
- ○ MI > 6 mos.

○ No Diabetes
- ○ IDDM
- ○ NIDDM
- ○ Diet Control

- ☐ History of Dysrhythmia
- ☐ Stroke
- ☐ Vascular Surgery/Dilatations
- ☐ Vascular Disease
- ☐ Carotid Surgery
- ☐ Carotid Disease
- ☐ Dialysis
- ☐ Valvular Heart Disease
- ☐ Angina/CAD

Documented Cancer:
☐ Lung ☐ Esoph ☐ Chest Wall
☐ Other________________

Pulmonary Function

☐ None Charted

PFT's	Measured	% Predicted
FVC		
FEV_1		
D_LCO		

	Left %	Right %
V/Q Scan		

Preop ABG's	Value
FiO_2	
pH	
PCO_2	
PO_2	
HCO_3	
O_2 Sat	

Progress Notes

- ☐ Preop Ventilation
- ☐ Preop Tracheostomy
- ☐ Preop ECMO

Lab Report

	Value	
HCT		
Bun		☐ *Check if derived*
Creat		☐ *Check if derived*
Albumin		
Bilirubin		

Pre-Op Medications ☐ None

#1
#2
#3
#4
#5
#6

OR Prior/Return

	Date (yy/mm/dd)	R#1	R#2	RBC Units
#1				
#2				
#3				
#4				
#5				

Intra-Op Operative Notes

Operation Date (yy/mm/dd):

☐☐ / ☐☐ / ☐☐

Nonsurg Admit Tm
:

Admit Date (yy/mm/dd) Discharge Date (yy/mm/dd)

of Prior Cardiac Operations ☐
of Prior Lung Operations ☐
of Prior Esophageal Operations ☐

(each preceded by "#")

Procedures
#1
#2
#3
#4
#5
#6

Admitting Diagnoses
#1
#2
#3
#4
#5
#6

○ Vol Reduction – Full Sternotomy
○ Vol Reduction – Mini Invasive

Additional Number of Returns ☐

Reasons for OR Prior/Return

1. Bleeding	8. Sternal Work
2. Tamponade	9. Tracheostomy
3. Bronchoscopy	10. Vascular
4. Cardiac Arrest	11. Cancel
5. Cysto	12. ECMO I/R
6. GI Procedure	13. Bronchopleural Fistula
7. Revision Main	14. Other

Form THDB (thorac6.pm5) Revised 8/4/99

APPENDIX 32-2. *Continued*

Anesthesia Record

☐ Emergency

	Value
Weight (kg)	
Height (cm)	

	Value
PCO2	
Heart Rate	
MAP	
CVP	

	No. of Units
FFP	
Platelets	
RBC	
Cryo	

	Value
Urine Output	

Discharge Summary

	Date (yy/mm/dd)	R#1	R#2
Init Dischg			
1st Re-ad			
1st Dischg			
2nd Re-ad			
2nd Dischg			
3rd Re-ad			
3rd Dischg			
4th Re-ad			
4th Dischg			
5th Re-ad			
5th Dischg			

Add'l # of Reads ☐ Add'l Days ☐

Reasons for Readmission

1. Pulmonary	5. Renal
2. Cardiac	6. GI
3. Infection	7. Other
4. Neuro	

Anesthetics

- ☐ Alfentanil (N)
- ☐ Diazapam (S)
- ☐ Enflurane (I)
- ☐ Etomidate (S)
- ☐ Fentanyl (N)
- ☐ Halothane (I)
- ☐ Isoflurane (I)
- ☐ Ketamine (S)
- ☐ Midazolam (S)
- ☐ Morphine (N)
- ☐ Propofol (S)
- ☐ Sufentanil (N)
- ☐ Infusion OR
- ☐ Infusion cont. to ICU

Drugs in OR

- ☐ Induction/Bypass
- ☐ Aminophylline
- ☐ Amrinone (I)
- ☐ Dobutamine (I)
- ☐ Dopamine (I)
- ☐ Epinephrine (I)
- ☐ Isuprel (I)
- ☐ Lidocaine (A)
- ☐ Norepinephrine (P)
- ☐ NTG (D)
- ☐ Nitroprusside (D)
- ☐ Phenylephrine (P)
- ☐ Procainamide (A)
- ☐ Milrinone (I)
- ☐ Esmolol
- ☐ Inhaled Bronchodilators
- ☐ Cardizem
- ☐ Ketorolac
- ☐ Vasopressin
- ☐ Other____________________

Post-Op Resp Ther Chart

Mode: ☐ SIMV ☐ AC ☐ PCV ☐ PRVC
☐ HFV/Jet Ventilator
☐ Other____________________

☐ Dble Lumen Tube ☐ Arrived Extubated

	Value		Value
Vent Rate		pH	
Tidal Vol		PCO_2	
FIO_2		PO_2	
PEEP		HCO_3	
		Sat. on Arrival	

Intubation Summary

	Date (yy/mm/dd)	Time (hh:mm)	R#1	R#2
Init Extub				
1st Reint				
1st Extub				
2nd Reint				
2nd Extub				
3rd Reint				
3rd Extub				
4th Reint				
4th Extub				
5th Reint				
5th Extub				

Add'l # of Retubes ☐ Add'l Hours ☐

Reasons for Reintubation

1. Pulmonary	6. Renal
2. Airway/Aspiration	7. GI
3. Cardiac/CHF	8. Surgery
4. Infection/Pneumonia	9. Self Extubation
5. Neuro	10. Other

Intraoperative Management

One Lung Ventilation
- ○ Right Double Lumen
- ○ Left Double Lumen
- ○ Bronchial Blocker

- ☐ HFV/Jet Ventilation
- ☐ Pleural Catheter
- ☐ Intercostal Nerve Block

- ☐ Spinal
- ☐ Thoracic Epidural
- ☐ Lumbar Epidural

Drug(s)

☐ Bupivicaine	☐ Lidocaine
☐ Epinephrine	☐ Marcaine
☐ Fentanyl	☐ Morphine

☐ Other:____________________

Page 2 (Revised 8/4/99)

APPENDIX 32-2. *Continued*

Nurses Notes – Admission

	Value
Core Temp	☐
Heart Rate	☐
MAP	☐
CVP	☐

	Date (yy/mm/dd)	Time (hh:mm)
RTC	☐	☐

☐ Awake Only

Drugs	DOS	POD 1
Aminophylline	☐	☐
Amrinone (I)	☐	☐
Dobutamine (I)	☐	☐
Dopamine (I)	☐	☐
Epinephrine (I)	☐	☐
Isuprel (I)	☐	☐
Lidocaine (A)	☐	☐
Other Antiarr (A)	☐	☐
Muscle Relax	☐	☐
Nor Epineph (P)	☐	☐
Nitroprusside (D)	☐	☐
NTG (D)	☐	☐
Phenylephrine (P)	☐	☐
Propofol	☐	☐
Milrinone (I)	☐	☐
Esmolol	☐	☐
Narcotics	☐	☐
Ketorolac	☐	☐
IV PCA	☐	☐
Epidural	☐	☐
Epidural Infusion	☐	☐
Epidural PCA	☐	☐
Lanoxin	☐	☐
Vasopressin	☐	☐

	Date
Adverse Drug Reaction	☐
Agitation Requiring Rx	☐

DIC Date (yy/mm/dd) ☐

RBC ○ 1 ○ 2 ○ 3 ○ 4 ○ ≥ 5

	Date
Major Transfusion	☐

ICU Events

Cardiac	Date
Asystole	☐
Atrial Arrythmia	☐
VT/VF	☐
Low CO	☐
IABP	☐
ECMO	☐
Open Chest	☐
Perm Pacer	☐
Heart Block	☐

Neuro	Date
Shiver Req Rx	☐
Focal Deficit	☐
Global Deficit	☐
Seizure	☐
Encephalopathy	☐

Renal	Date
Dialysis Start	☐
Anuria	☐

GI/Hepatic	Date
TPN Start	☐
TPN End	☐
Enternal Feed	☐

Infections	Date
Fungemia	☐
Bacteremia	☐
Line Sepsis	☐
Sepsis Syndrome	☐
Septic Shock	☐
Empyema	☐
Endocarditis	☐
Mediastinitis	☐
Wound	☐
Pneumonia	☐
Urinary	☐

Pulmonary	Date
ARDS	☐
Aspir Pneu	☐
Atelect (Bronched)	☐
Bronchopleural Fistula	☐
CHF	☐
Diaph Paralysis	☐
Effusion (Tapped)	☐
Chylothorax	☐
Hemothorax	☐
Pneumothorax	☐
Pulm Edema	☐
Pulm Embolus	☐
Pulm Hemorrhage	☐
Resp Insuff/Distress	☐
Resp Failure	☐
Tracheobronchitis	☐

GI/Hepatic Complications	Date
Cholecystitis	☐
Hepatitis	☐
GI Bleed	☐
Ileus Post 2 Days	☐
Pancreatitis	☐
Esoph Fistula	☐

	Date
MSOF	☐

	Date
DNR Order	☐
Death Date (yy/mm/dd)	☐
Time of Death (hh:mm)	☐

Place: ○ OR ○ ICU ○ Floor

	Reason Code
Cause of Death	☐

☐ Post MI Enzymes

APPENDIX 32-2. *Continued*

Labs

☐ No Labs

First ICU Value	Value
HCT	
K	
Glucose	
Renal	
SCR POD 1	
SCR POD 2	
SCR POD 3	
High SCR	
High SCR Date	
Infection	
First WBC	
First WBC Date	
High WBC	
High WBC Date	
GI/Hepatic	
High Bili	
High Bili Date	
High Lactic Acid	
High LA Date	
Low Transferrin	
Low Trans Date	
Blood	
Low Platelet	
Low Plat Date	
High D-Dimer	
High D-D Date	
Low HCT	
Low HCT Date	

QA Complications

- ☐ Aspiration at Intubation
- ☐ Brachial Plexus
- ☐ Carotid Hematoma/Injury
- ☐ Death within 48 hours
- ☐ Died w/o Awakening
- ☐ Double Lumen Tube Complication
- ☐ Epidural Wet Tap
- ☐ Epistaxis
- ☐ Esophageal Rupture TEE
- ☐ Failed Regional
- ☐ Leg Neuropathy
- ☐ Lip/Dental Injury
- ☐ Malignant Arrhythmia
- ☐ Mean Arterial Line Injury
- ☐ Ocular Injury
- ☐ On CPB Unexpectedly
- ☐ PA Rupture
- ☐ Peripheral Nerve Injury
- ☐ Postdural Headache
- ☐ Prolonged Hypoxemia
- ☐ Protamine Rx
- ☐ Pulmonary Edema in OR
- ☐ Pulse Oximetry Injury
- ☐ Recall
- ☐ Respiratory Arrest in OR
- ☐ Seizure due to Anes Toxicity
- ☐ Self Extubation
- ☐ Total Spinal
- ☐ Transfusion Rx
- ☐ Ulnar Neuropathy
- ☐ Unable to Intubate
- ☐ Unplanned Circulatory Arrest
- ☐ Vocal Cord Paralysis
- ☐ Wound Dehiscence
- ☐ Other__________________

Page 4 (Revised 8/4/99)

APPENDIX 32-3.

Cardiothoracic anesthesia quarterly thoracic database report.

	Year Quarter										1995	Expected Range	
Indicator	1999 Q1		1999 Q2		1999 Q3		1999 Q4		Grand Total		Level	Lower	Upper
Cases in ORIS with at least one Thoracic Procedure performed													
Cases in ORIS by Procedure													
Abdominal/Peritoneum/Omentum/Loparotomy													
Bronchoscopy													
Cardiac/Pericardial Window/Vascular													
Chest Wall Resection/Repair/Pectus													
Debridement													
Decortication													
Diaphram/Hiatal Hernia													
Thoracic Duct													
Esophagoscopy/Dilitation/Endoscopy													
Esophageal Repair													
Esophagus Excision/Esophagectomy													
Esophagus Incision/Heller Myotomy													
Larynx/Vocal Cord													
Single Lung Transplant													
Double Lung Transplant													
Mediastinoscopy													
Open Lung Biopsy													
Pleural													
Pulmonary Resection													
Rib/Clavicle													
Thoracoscopy													
Thoracotomy													
Thymus													
Tracheal													
Tracheo/Bronchial													
Zenker's Diverticulum													
Non-Thoracic Related Procedure													
Cases Followed													
Cases Not Followed													

APPENDIX 32-3. *Continued*

	Year Quarter										1995	Expected Range	
Indicator	1999 Q1		1999 Q2		1999 Q3		1999 Q4		Grand Total		Level	Lower	Upper
Cases Followed													
Cases Followed by Procedure													
Abdominal/Peritoneum/Omentum/Loparotomy													
Bronchoscopy													
Cardiac/Pericardial Window/Vascular													
Chest Wall Resection/Repair/Pectus													
Debridement													
Decortication													
Diaphram/Hiatal Hernia													
Thoracic Duct													
Esophagoscopy/Dilitation/Endoscopy													
Esophageal Repair													
Esophagus Excision/Esophagectomy													
Esophagus Incision/Heller Myotomy													
Larynx/Vocal Cord													
Single Lung Transplant													
Double Lung Transplant													
Mediastinoscopy													
Open Lung Biopsy													
Pleural													
Pulmonary Resection													
Rib/Clavicle													
Thoracoscopy													
Thoracotomy													
Thymus													
Tracheal													
Tracheo/Bronchial													
Zenker's Diverticulum													
Non-Thoracic Related Procedure													

APPENDIX 32-3. *Continued*

	Year Quarter										1995	Expected Range	
Indicator	1999 Q1		1999 Q2		1999 Q3		1999 Q4		Grand Total		Level	Lower	Upper
Cases Not Followed													
Cases Not Followed by Procedure													
Abdominal/Peritoneum/Omentum/Loparotomy													
Bronchoscopy													
Cardiac/Pericardial Window/Vascular													
Chest Wall Resection/Repair/Pectus													
Debridement													
Decortication													
Diaphram/Hiatal Hernia													
Thoracic Duct													
Esophagoscopy/Dilitation/Endoscopy													
Esophageal Repair													
Esophagus Excision/Esophagectomy													
Esophagus Incision/Heller Myotomy													
Larynx/Vocal Cord													
Single Lung Transplant													
Double Lung Transplant													
Mediastinoscopy													
Open Lung Biopsy													
Pleural													
Pulmonary Resection													
Rib/Clavicle													
Thoracoscopy													
Thoracotomy													
Thymus													
Tracheal													
Tracheo/Bronchial													
Zenker's Diverticulum													
Non-Thoracic Related Procedure													

APPENDIX 32-3. *Continued*

(Followed Cases Only)

	Year Quarter										1995	Expected Range	
Indicator	1999 Q1		1999 Q2		1999 Q3		1999 Q4		Grand Total		Level	Lower	Upper
Cases Followed													
Mortality													
Morbidity - MI													
Morbidity - Pulmonary													
Morbidity - Renal Failure													
Morbidity - Neurologic													
Morbidity - Serious Infection													
- Pneumonia													
Overall Morbidty													
# of OR Priors/Returns													
Average # of OR Priors/Returns per 100 Cases													
Cases with at least one OR Prior/Return													
OR Prior/Returns - Bleeding													
OR Prior/Returns - Tamponade													
OR Prior/Returns - Cardiac Arrest													
OR Prior/Returns - Revision Main													
OR Prior/Returns - Sternal Work													
OR Prior/Returns - ECMO Insert/Removal													
OR Prior/Returns - Bronchopleural Fistula													
Average Initial ICU Intubation Time in hours													
Median Initial ICU Intubation Time in hours													
Initial ICU Intubation Time < = 4 hours													
Initial ICU Intubation Time > 4 & < = 8 hours													
Initial ICU Intubation Time > 8 & < = 24 hours													
Initial ICU Intubation Time > 24 hours													
Average Total OR + ICU Intubation Time in hours													
Median Total OR + ICU Intubation Time in hours													

APPENDIX 32-3. *Continued*

(Followed Cases Only)

	Year Quarter										1995	Expected Range	
Indicator	1999 Q1		1999 Q2		1999 Q3		1999 Q4		Grand Total		Level	Lower	Upper
# of Reintubations													
Average # of Reintubations per 100 Cases													
Cases Reintubated at least once													
Cases Reint. within 24 hrs. of Initial Extubation													
Cases Reintubated - Pulmonary													
Cases Reintubated - Airway/Aspiration													
Cases Reintubated - Cardiac/CHF													
Cases Reintubated - Infection/Pneumonia													
Cases Reintubated - Neurologic													
Cases Reintubated - Renal													
Cases Reintubated - GI													
Cases Reintuibated - Self-Extubation													
Average Initial ICU LOS in days													
Median Initial ICU LOS in days													
Average Total ICU LOS in days													
Median Total ICU LOS in days													
Total ICU LOS < = 1 day													
Total ICU LOS = 2 days													
Total ICU LOS = 3 days													
Total ICU LOS > = 4 days													
# of Readmissions													
Average # of Readmissions per 100 Cases													
Cases Readmitted at least once													
Cases Read. on Init. ICU Disch. or day after													
Cases Readmitted - Pulmonary													
Cases Readmitted - Cardiac													
Cases Readmitted - Infection													
Cases Readmitted - Neurologic													
Cases Readmitted - Renal													
Cases Readmitted - GI													

APPENDIX 32-3. *Continued*

(Followed Cases Only)

	Year Quarter										1995	Expected Range	
Indicator	1999 Q1		1999 Q2		1999 Q3		1999 Q4		Grand Total		Level	Lower	Upper
Incidence of QA Complications													
Aspiration at Intubation													
Brachial Plexus													
Carotic Hematoma/Injury													
Death within 48 Hours													
Died w/o Awakening													
Double Lumen Tube Complication													
Epidural Wet Tap													
Epistaxis													
Esophageal Rupture TEE													
Failed Regional													
Leg Neuropathy													
Lip/Dental Injury													
Malignant Arrhythmia													
Mean Arterial Line Injury													
Ocular Injury													
On CPB Unexpectedly													
PA Rupture													
Peripheral Nerve Injury													
Postdural Headache													
Prolonged Hypoxemia													
Protamine Reaction													
Pulmonary Edema in OR													
Pulse Oximetry Injury													
Recall													
Respiratory Arrest in OR													
Seizure due to Anes. Toxicity													
Self Extubation													
Total Spinal													
Transfusion Reaction													
Ulnar Neuropathy													
Unable to Intubate													
Unplanned Circulatory Arrest													
Vocal Cord Paralysis													
Wound Dehiscence													
Other Complication													

APPENDIX 32-4.

Test 1: Too Few or Too Many Runs in the Data

Calculate the number of useful observations. Useful observations are determined by subtracting the number of data points lying on the median line from the total number of data points. Then look at the table below. Compare your number of useful observations in column 1, then look at the number in column 2, which is the lower limit of the number of runs you should have for the number of useful observations. Then look in column 3: This number will be the maximum number of runs you should have in the run chart. If the number of runs falls outside these limits, you have a special cause of variation that needs to be evaluated.

Useful Observations	*Lower Limit*	*Upper Limit*
15	4	12
16	5	12
17	5	13
18	6	13
19	6	14
20	6	15
21	7	15
22	7	16
23	8	16
24	8	17
25	9	17
26	9	18
27	9	19
28	10	19
29	10	20
30	11	20
31	11	21
32	11	22
33	11	22
34	12	23
35	13	23
36	13	24
37	13	25
38	14	25
39	14	26
40	15	26

Test 2: The Long Run

A special cause of variation can exist if a run contains too many data points. If you have 20 or more useful observations, then a run of 8 or more data points indicates a special cause of variation. If you have less than 20 useful observations, then a run of 7 or more data points indicates a special cause.

Test 3: Statistical Trend

In this test, a trend is defined as a consecutive increase or decrease in data points, in which you count points on the median.

Number of Data Points	*Number of Consecutive Ascending or Descending Points*
5–8	5 or more
9–20	6 or more
21–100	7 or more

Then if you have 18 data points and 6 or more are consecutively ascending or descending, then you have a special cause of variation.

Test 4: Saw-Tooth Pattern

Another test for special cause variation is the saw-tooth pattern or 14 or more consecutive points forming a zigzag pattern (alternating up, down, up, down, and so on).

APPENDIX 32-5.

Test for Special Causes in Control Charts

Entire Chart Tests (Both Sides of the Mean Line)

1. Seven or more consecutive points steadily increasing or decreasing indicates a trend when the data set has 21 or more data points (6 points indicate a trend if you have less than 21 data points).
2. Saw-tooth pattern of alternating 14 points.
3. Fifteen consecutive points in zone C.

Tests to Each Side of the Center Line

1. One point outside the 3-sigma limit.
2. Two out of three successive points in zone A or beyond.
3. Four out of five successive points in zone B or beyond.
4. Eight successive points in zone C or beyond on the same side of the center line.

REFERENCES

1. Macario A, Weinger M, Truong P, et al. Which clinical anesthesia outcomes are both common and important to avoid? The perspective of a panel of expert anesthesiologists. *Anesth Analg* 1999; 88:1085.
2. Gilbert HC. Choosing the best outcomes measurement tool for your practice. *ASA Newsletter* 1998;62(6):19.
3. *Handbook for associate examiners of the American Board of Anesthesiology,* March, 1997.
4. Macready N, ed. *Anesth malpract prev.* Philadelphia: Lippincott Williams & Wilkins, 2000;5(1).
5. Rosenberg H. Improving quality for airway emergencies: the airway team. *Am J Anesth,* 1999;26:423.
6. Kritchevsky SB, Simmons BP. Continuous quality improvement.

Concepts and applications for physician care. *JAMA* 1991; 266(13):1817.
7. Higgins TL, Estafanous FG, Loop FD, et al. Stratification of morbidity and mortality outcome by preoperative risk factors in coronary artery bypass patients. A clinical severity score. *JAMA* 1992;267(17):2344.
8. Higgins TL, Estafanous FG, Loop FD, et al. ICU admission score for predicting morbidity and mortality risk after coronary artery bypass grafting. *Ann Thorac Surg* 1997;64:1050.
9. Rafferty T, LaMantia KR, Davis E, et al. Quality assurance for intraoperative transesophageal echocardiography monitoring: a report of 846 procedures. *Anesth Analg* 1993;76:228.
10. Savage RM, Licina MG, Koch CG, et al. Educational program for intraoperative transesophageal echocardiography. *Anesth Analg* 1995;81:399.
11. Recommendations for continuous quality improvement in echocardiography. American Society of Echocardiography. *J Am Soc Echocardiogr,* 1995;8[Suppl, Pt 2]:1.
12. Spahn DR, Schmid S, Carrel T, et al. Hypopharynx perforation by a transesophageal echocardiography probe. *Anesthesiology* 1995;82(2):581.
13. Latham P, Hodgins LR. A gastric laceration after transesophageal echocardiography in a patient undergoing aortic valve replacement. *Anesth Analg* 1995;81:641.
14. Kharasch ED, Sivarajan M. Gastroesophageal perforation after intraoperative transesophageal echocardiography. *Anesthesiology* 1996;85(2):426.
15. Chow MS, Taylor MA, Hanson CW III. Splenic laceration associated with transesophageal echocardiography. *J Cardiothorac Vasc Anesth* 1998;12(3):314.
16. Daniel WG, Erbel R, Kasper W, et al. Safety of transesophageal echocardiography. A multicenter survey of 10,419 examinations. *Circulation* 1991;83:817.
17. Shanewise JS, Cheung AT, Aronson S, et al. ASE/SCA guidelines for performing a comprehensive intraoperative multiplane transesophageal echocardiography examination: recommendations of the American Society of Echocardiography Council for Intraoperative Echocardiography and the Society of Cardiovascular Anesthesiologists Task Force for Certification in Perioperative Transesophageal Echocardiography. *Anesth Analg* 1999;89:870.
18. Koch JF. Becoming an information-driven organization. *ASA Newsletter* 1999;63(4):18.
19. Reich DL, Bodian CA, Krol M, et al. Intraoperative hemodynamic predictors of mortality, stroke, and myocardial infarction after coronary artery bypass surgery. *Anesth Analg* 1999;89:814.
20. Fleisher LA, Barash PG. Governmental databases, hospital information systems, and clinical outcomes: big brother or big help? *Anesth Analg* 1999;89:811.
21. Larkin H. Redefining business quality. 'Total quality management' and 'continuous quality improvement' promise to improve medicine. But what do the terms really mean? *American Medical News* 1992 Oct 26:11.
22. Solberg LI, Mosser G, McDonald S. The three faces of performance measurement: improvement, accountability, and research. *J Quality Improvement* 1997;23(3):135.
23. Levett JM, Carey RG. Measuring for improvement: from Toyota to thoracic surgery. *Ann Thorac Surg* 1999;68:353.
24. Shewhart WA. *Economic control of quality of manufactured product.* New York: Van Nostrand, 1931.
25. Carey RG, Lloyd RC. *Measuring quality improvement in healthcare. A guide to statistical process control applications.* New York: Quality Resources, 1995.
26. Boggs PB, Hayati F, Washburne WF, et al. Using statistical process control charts for the continual improvement of asthma care. *J Quality Improvement* 1999;25(4):163.
27. Shahian DM, Williamson WA, Svensson LG, et al. Applications of statistical quality control to cardiac surgery. *Ann Thorac Surg* 1996;62:1351.
28. Posner KL, Freund PR. Trends in quality of anesthesia care associated with changing staffing patterns, productivity, and concurrency of case supervision in a teaching hospital. *Anesthesiology* 1999;91(3):839.
29. Carey RG. How to choose a patient survey system. *J Quality Improvement* 1999;25(1):20.
30. Gabel RA. Performance measurement: providing objective data for improved care. *ASA Newsletter* 1999;63(11):22.
31. Cabana MD, Rand CS, Powe NR, et al. Why don't physicians follow clinical practice guidelines? A framework for improvement. *JAMA* 1999;282(15):1458.

33

EDUCATION IN CARDIOTHORACIC ANESTHESIA

KATHERINE P. GRICHNIK
RANDALL M. SCHELL
J.G. REVES

"Teaching anesthesia demands the more urgent consideration since scientific progress is the future obligation of the student of today."—E. A. Rovenstein (1)

SCOPE OF THE FIELD

The field of cardiac anesthesiology is broad and encompasses the physiology and pharmacology of many organ systems, primarily those in the thorax and the systemic circulation. It also requires an in-depth understanding of coagulation, immunology, and central and peripheral nervous systems. Moreover, it is presumed that the cardiac anesthesiologist is a board-certified anesthesiologist and knowledgeable about the entire field of anesthesiology. This chapter, like excellent predecessors (2,3), exclusively addresses the education of the cardiac anesthesiologist, leaving others to communicate the concerns for education in the broader field of anesthesiology (4).

Chapters in this book contain the information that constitutes what we believe to be the knowledge base (curriculum) for the education of the cardiac anesthesiologist. This chapter focuses primarily on goals, objectives, and recommendations for the education process. Much of this chapter represents our philosophy but also included is some information on the emerging philosophy of teaching principles. However, until a consensus curriculum and an external examination for accreditation of the cardiac anesthesiologist is created, educational recommendations will remain parochial, that is, related to each program's experience and teaching philosophy.

K. P. Grichnik and J. G. Reves: Department of Anesthesiology, Duke University Medical Center, Durham, North Carolina 27710

R. M. Schell: Department of Anesthesiology, Loma Linda University and Loma Linda University Medical Center, Loma Linda, California 92354

ELEMENTS OF THE EDUCATIONAL PROGRAM

Goals

The goals of educating the cardiac anesthesiologist are (a) mastery of the knowledge, skills, and techniques required to practice cardiac anesthesiology, (b) a working knowledge of the principles and concepts that underlie the practice, and (c) to acquire judgment, expertise, and the ability to be a consultant to those who seek advice outside and inside the discipline of anesthesiology. The student must also learn how to solve unforeseen problems and to answer important questions, in addition to mastering the technical skills and acquiring the available knowledge.

Most educators agree that it is crucial to distinguish teaching facts and skills from how to learn and to answer an unanticipated question. Some would argue (2,5) (including ourselves) that it is more valuable to learn how to learn than simply to learn facts. In this regard, Stead (5) distinguished between training and education; training is aimed at the formation of habits so ingrained by repetition that only minimal thought or concentration is required for performance, whereas education is the solution of problems by the use of knowledge that requires thought. Our objective is not to train students but to educate them.

From a teaching perspective, there are three areas of learning: (a) cognitive, (b) psychomotor, and (c) affective (3). It is very useful to conceptualize teaching and learning cardiothoracic anesthesiology using this type of classification. *Cognitive* learning centers on the knowledge base. As in many educational endeavors, knowledge is well defined. Agreement on what constitutes the *psychomotor domain* of learning, however, is often poorly defined or nonexistent. A clear, written definition of the psychomotor skills that must be mastered when learning cardiothoracic anesthesiology is not available. Many psychomotor skills that are essential for learning cardiothoracic anesthesiology are obvious. Intraarterial and pulmonary artery monitoring, for example, are techniques that must be learned by the student of cardiothoracic anesthesiology. The last category for learning is the *affective domain.* The word affective refers to the "emotional" aspect of education. Specifically, the affective domain covers those aspects of learning that enable the student to interact with others and understand relationships. The goal is to enable the learner to understand his or her personal values and those of others in order to develop interactions that will be most efficient and effective (3).

Learning will be enhanced if the faculty is interested in teaching and if the environment is one in which the gathering of new knowledge is exciting for teachers and faculty. The creation of such an environment is not easy, nor are the techniques for accomplishing it. The paramount requirement of the faculty is that they determine what constitutes excellence and how to demand it—no small task.

What must be done to reach these goals? The words of Sir William Osler answer that question.

> It seems a bounden duty on such an occasion to be honest and frank so I propose to tell you the secret of life as I have seen the game played and as I have tried to play it myself. Not only has it been the touchstone of progress, but also it is the measure of success in everyday life. And the master word is "work."(6).

Objectives

Successful education begins with clear objectives. Educational objectives for cardiac anesthesia are to educate the resident or fellow to (a) be a skilled clinician, (b) be an informed consultant, and (c) learn how to answer important questions. To meet these objectives, one must accomplish three fundamental tasks: (a) definition of educational objectives based on a consensus among educators and faculty in the field, (b) designation of the curriculum and appropriate learning activities, and (c) development of tests and other assessment procedures to measure progress and competence (4).

Curriculum

The Joint Council on In-Training Examinations of the American Board of Anesthesiology (ABA) and the American Society of Anesthesiologists (ASA) has created an outline listing topical areas that define content of resident learning in cardiothoracic anesthesiology (7) (Appendix 33-1). An outline of the content of knowledge categories that should be contained in a cardiac anesthesiology curriculum is shown in Table 33-1. In addition to traditional studies of physiology, pharmacology, and anatomy, there are topics particularly germane to this field that involve technical skills as well as equipment and instrumentation. For example, an understanding of the complex physiology and the technical aspects of extracorporeal circulation are clearly important for cardiac procedures as is a firm understanding of the physiology of one-lung anesthesia for thoracic procedures.

TABLE 33-1. ONE PROPOSED CURRICULUM FOR CARDIAC ANESTHESIA FELLOWSHIP TRAINING

- Year 1
  - Educational
    - Lecture and case presentations
    - Instruction in writing and grant preparation
    - ? Instruction in public speaking
  - Echocardiography
    - Transthoracic echocardiography
    - Transesophageal echocardiography
  - Cardiac Intensive Care
    - Adult
    - Pediatric
  - Complex Clinical Cases
    - Adult
    - Pediatric
    - Transplant
    - Emerging technologies
  - Research
    - Clinical
    - Basic science
    - Information systems and database inquiries
  - Electives
    - Cardiology catheterization laboratory
    - Perfusion
- Year 2
  - Clinical and/or basic science research
    - Execution of research project
    - Presentation of research and manuscript
    - Statistical methods training
    - Study design training
      - Master of clinical trials degree
    - Introduction of research funding and grants
    - Instruction in writing and grant preparation
    - Instruction in the ethics of research

The teaching of effective psychosocial skills should be included in the curriculum. These skills may not be highly valued by faculty when residency competency is assessed, but it is imperative that students learn the requisite skills of building effective teamwork in the complex setting of the cardiac operating room (8). This is best learned when the faculty role model espouses the philosophy that the patient is of supreme importance and that nurses, technicians, perfusionists, surgeons, and anesthesiologists are all key players on the health care team. Each has a role that should be clearly defined long before the patient enters the operating room. The efficient and effective performance of the team depends on mutual understanding of each player's role and respect for each. Close communication among team members is always necessary (9).

The cardiac anesthesiologist and his or her assistant must not be hidden from the surgical field by the drapes because continuous communication and coordination between the anesthesiologist and the surgeon is vitally important. Potentially dangerous situations can be handled more quickly and efficiently when these two most experienced of the team act in unison (10). The behavior of the attending anesthesiologist and surgeon toward each other and other individuals in the operating room is a model that others will adopt. The operating room behavior of these two role models must be exemplary in order for the patient to receive optimal care and for the other workers to learn effective psychosocial skills.

Participants

The participants in the education of cardiac anesthesiologists are teachers and students. We readily acknowledge that the faculty cardiac anesthesiologist may also be learning and that there are many other learners as well: surgeons, cardiologists, medical students, certified registered nurse anesthetists, perfusionists, nurses, and technicians. However, the focus of education must be on the primary learner, not the teacher (4).

Students

The pupil is the anesthesiology resident or cardiothoracic anesthesiology fellow. The fellows are giving up potential income to stay in the formal educational process. By our society's standards, this sacrifice almost assuredly reflects a keen interest in the educational offerings. The ideal student has a desire to learn and to work; education proceeds well if the student has these two attributes (almost regardless of the quality of the faculty) (5).

Faculty

Teachers or mentors must have a grasp of the field and must be committed to educating students. It is their responsibility to teach the skills and facts as well as to open the students' minds to the methods and techniques of scientific inquiry. Unfortunately, physician teachers are seldom, if ever, schooled in the art and science of education. Only recently has attention been focused in our literature on characterizing the attributes of a good teacher (11–13).

The traditional assumption that "if you know your field, you should be able to teach it" has been challenged (13–15). Learning to effectively teach is a complex process, which evolves over time. First, teachers must have an adequate knowledge base. Expert teachers have a rich, tightly connected subject matter knowledge with detailed plans organized for how to teach that content (15). Second, one must understand the background of the learner including what typical errors learners make and what is normal development for a student in a given educational situation. Third, general teaching principles apply, which may be selectively used in various learning situations (Table 33-2). Traits of effective clinical teachers, some of which are not easily adapted to the cardiac surgical operating room, are also listed in Table 33-2. This list is a useful reminder of qualities we seek in effective teachers.

TABLE 33-2. CLINICAL TEACHING ATTRIBUTES

General teaching principles
Actively involve learners
Meet individual needs
Be practical and relevant
Be selective and realistic
Provide feedback and evaluation
Capture attention and have fun
Instructional effectiveness depends on
Allocating time for teaching
Creating a teaching/learning environment of trust
Demonstrating clinical credibility
A complete educational experience requires
An initial orientation
A final evaluation
Overall education is facilitated when
Learners are able to present a case
Teachers manage the case presentation
Didactic sessions are used to enhance clinical case material
Teaching takes place at the bedside, allowing students to learn physician-patient relationships
Teachers and students discuss psychosocial issues
Maintained teaching effectiveness occurs when
Attention is paid to transferring the teaching responsibility

Source: From Mattern WD, Weinholtz D, Friedman CP. The attending physician as teacher. *N Engl J Med* 1980;308:1129, and from Irby DM. What clinical teachers in medicine need to know. *Acad Med* 1994;69(5):333, with permission.

Excellent clinicians serve as role models for education in clinical practice while other faculty members may teach and conduct research; it is often difficult to find one faculty person who is excellent in these three areas. Therefore, a faculty must consist of a group of physicians who excel in one or more of the following areas: clinical care, teaching, and/or research activities. We believe that cardiac anesthesia education is the responsibility of a dedicated faculty of one or more individuals who have earned the "title" of a cardiac anesthesiologist in their own education, practice, and/or research. This title denotes an individual who has one and preferably more of the following credentials: has a fellowship in cardiac anesthesia, specializes in the practice of cardiac anesthesia, and/or conducts clinical or basic science investigation in the field.

Resources

Education, like all activities, requires the commitment of adequate resources to be successful. Money must be available for salaries of faculty and to purchase materials and make technology available for modern teaching methods. There must be time for both faculty and students to prepare and participate in the educational mission. Faculty need nonclinical time to prepare for education, and students need time to read and to attend conferences. Access to a comprehensive medical library and adequate computer support with intranet/Internet access is important. The final re-

TABLE 33-3. RESIDENCY REVIEW COMMITTEE REQUIREMENTS FOR RESIDENCY EDUCATION IN CARDIOTHORACIC ANESTHESIOLOGY

1. Anesthesia for 20 patients undergoing surgical procedures involving cardiopulmonary bypass
2. Twenty other major vascular cases
3. Twenty intrathoracic (thoracotomy, thoracoscopy) noncardiac cases
4. Significant experience with certain specialized techniques for airway management (such as fiberoptic intubation, double-lumen endotracheal tube placement, and laryngeal mask airway management), central vein catheter placement, pulmonary artery catheter placement, and peripheral artery cannulation
5. Structured postanesthesia care experience including responsibilities for management of hemodynamic changes in the intensive care unit and postanesthesia care unit
6. Critical care rotation, to include active participation in patient care by anesthesia residents beyond ventilatory management

source required in clinical education is clinical material. In resident education, the Residency Review Committee (RRC) has specified the minimal number of clinical cases required for residency programs to retain accreditation (7) (Table 33-3). No number or type of cases has been specified as constituting a minimally acceptable clinical experience for cardiothoracic anesthesiology fellows. However, learners must have adequate exposure to achieve competence and consultant status in the field. The number and complexity of cases should be greater than that required for residents. This cannot happen when there are too few cases to allow each learner to participate singularly in the care of patients.

METHODS OF EDUCATION

Educational Techniques

A large number of educational methods and study aids are available to the student and teacher. None are effective if the educational goals are not clearly delineated. Here, we outline the methods that we employ in educating cardiac anesthesiologists, although realizing that many other successful methods exist. Teachers should select the best techniques to ensure that the necessary knowledge, concepts, skills, and attitudes are achieved (16).

Case Management

Case management is the mainstay of clinical education. Its objective is to use the case to teach about pathology, pharmacology, physiology, technical skills, and psychosocial interactions. The most effective faculty members say, "I learn from every case no matter how many I have done"; this should be true for the student as well. Case management teaching begins with preoperative assessment of the patient, includes the perioperative period, and ideally ends with appropriate postoperative follow-up. During each of the many steps in the patient's progress through the hospital course, there is the opportunity to learn much of the material and many skills required to become a cardiac anesthesiologist. This teaching technique is optimal if the faculty has informed the student, on the preceding day, of particular learning objectives for a given day (e.g., the natural course of aortic stenosis if the patient has this pathology or alternative approaches to the internal jugular vein). To avoid repetition, some have recommended that each student keep a list of educational objectives and be responsible for covering this material during the rotation. The teacher must be satisfied that the student has mastered the knowledge and skills or recommend remedial measures.

Questions posed to students during clinical cases must be properly asked. One can categorize questions into two types: closed and open (4). Closed questions are designed merely to elicit facts, whereas open questions require thinking and problem solving. For example, it is clear that the closed and open questions, respectively, that follow are different: "What are the determinants of oxygen supply and demand?" "What might explain the ST-segment changes observed on the electrocardiogram?" Open questions are the preferred teaching method.

It is presumed that many of the skills required for the practice of anesthesiology (e.g., tracheal intubation) will already be mastered before clinical rotations on cardiothoracic anesthesiology as a resident or fellow. The skill and techniques that must be learned during cardiac anesthesia education are invasive hemodynamic monitoring, basic cardiopulmonary perfusion, analysis and interpretation of tests of the coagulation system, electrocardiographic interpretation, principles and methods of cardiac pacing, and at least an introduction into methods of echocardiography. Elemental steps ensure the proper mastery of skills (4,17).

1. Analyze and separate the skill into its component parts, and determine which aspects of the skill are most difficult to perform.
2. Sequentially arrange critical steps for success.
3. Provide students with a model of the skill they are expected to perform, demonstrate it effectively in its entirety, and explain the rationale for each of the steps.
4. Make provisions for students to practice until the skill is achieved.
5. Provide continuing supervision and evaluation to offset tendencies to lose skills.

Clinical practitioners are often judged by their skill (or lack thereof), rather than by their knowledge; thus, the perfection and maintenance of optimal skills is essential for the successful education of the cardiac anesthesiologist.

An advantage of case management teaching is that it occurs in the real environment of practice. Nothing is simulated, and the conditions of the actual operating room will contribute the various stresses, distractions, and frustrations that prepare the learner for real experiences to be encountered when formal instruction and education are completed.

Another important component for the teacher is adequate feedback. Evaluation of the teacher by the student is critical to improvement and success of the teacher. A sample faculty evaluation form is in Appendix 33-2.

Reading

The development of a scholarly approach to learning absolutely depends on the ability to assimilate facts and concepts into knowledge by reading. In an ideal educational program, the student learns to read critically. The teacher is responsible for providing guidance in this activity, because it is impossible to read all the material available. The faculty should make recommendations for required reading according to the level of the learner. One reading assignment method is to give residents who first rotate on the cardiac anesthesia service a list of key papers, primarily of the review classification, and a list of pertinent chapters in textbooks devoted to cardiac anesthesiology. A notebook distributed before the rotation containing learning objectives, resource material, and anesthetic protocols for the usual operations performed by the particular cardiac anesthesiology service is often helpful. Although some dismiss protocols as cookbook learning, we find it useful for new residents to know the orderly progression of events that are expected during normal case management. An example of a protocol for giving anesthesia for a coronary artery bypass graft operation is shown in Table 33-4. Protocols may be more or less detailed depending on a particular educational setting. Whereas the junior resident needs material synthesized in review articles and book chapters, the senior resident and fellow are expected to become familiar with original scientific papers and concepts published in the literature, which form the scientific and conceptual foundation of the practice of cardiac anesthesia.

TABLE 33-4. CARDIAC ANESTHESIA PATIENT MANAGEMENT PROTOCOL

Preoperative steps
1. Evaluate and visit the patient
2. Discuss the patient and anesthetic plan with attending (before operation)
3. Adequately premedicate, assess which chronic medications need to be continued on the day of surgery and order anticipated supportive drips

Operative steps
4. Place monitoring devices and catheters
5. Induce and maintain anesthesia
6. Anticoagulate the patient after communication with the "team"
7. Establish adequate anticoagulation
8. Commence cardiopulmonary bypass (CPB) after communication with the team
9. Communicate pharmacologic interventions (including anticoagulation) with the perfusionists
10. Measure and communicate coagulation status, hemoglobin, and electrolyte formation regularly (about every 30–45 min during CPB)
11. Anticipate and plan any drug or assist-device needs before discontinuation of CPB
12. Discontinue CPB when the team is prepared and the patient is warm, has a stable rhythm, acceptable cardiac function, and acceptable hematocrit and electrolytes
13. Major pharmacologic and blood product interventions must be communicated to the team
14. Decisions regarding assist devices should be made conjointly with the surgeons
15. Report to intensive care unit personnel should be complete

Postoperative steps
16. Postoperative visits should be thorough and informative for the patient and the anesthesia team

Lectures

Lectures are a traditional method of teaching and are used in cardiac anesthesiology education. A series of well-planned lectures that address primary topics and have clear objectives are an integral part of the curriculum. Lectures that discuss diseases, pertinent pharmacology, and physiology are generally given by the faculty as part of a general anesthesiology curriculum or a rotation on the cardiac anesthesia service. Other recommended topics include cardiopulmonary bypass, ventricular assist technology, coagulation, interpretation of cardiac diagnostic information, operative risk assessment, anesthesia principles for cardiac operations, relevant monitoring techniques, and emerging technologies. A successful lecture presentation has clear objectives, useful visual aids, and directions for obtaining information not available within the framework of a lecture. A summary at the end ensures that the lecturer accomplished the stated goals. Lectures are an effective way of highlighting carefully synthesized knowledge. Lectures are never intended to be comprehensive treatments of a subject. This remains in the province of reading materials. Lectures also can epitomize the worst learning situation, in which the student is completely passive. Learning requires active participation, and this occurs during a lecture only when the student is actively listening and thinking about what is presented. Similarly, lecture preparation and presentation by the resident in a formal setting is also a valuable educational tool.

Conferences

Conferences should be designed to address principles and to provoke questioning of the soundness of ideas on which we base our practices (15,18). The seminar format is an effective way to teach and learn. The potential improvement of this method over the didactic lecture is that the student actively participates by presenting material, by asking questions of the teacher, and by having questions posed to him or her. However, conferences, like other methods of education, should have clearly established educational goals. Topics that lend themselves to this method of teaching are clinical management and research. Both subjects require open discussion by experts as well as learners to challenge those in attendance to think about the issues. Often in this setting, fresh ideas are brought to a particular topic, and everyone—both faculty and students—learns. The format encourages the discussion of ideas rather than retention of facts. We have designed a weekly cardiac anesthesia conference that lasts about 1 hour (15). The first half involves the discussion of an interesting case, during which the residents call on faculty to comment on various aspects of case management based on their experience and knowledge of the literature. The purpose of this exercise is for the students to learn from the experienced clinicians about case management. The second half of the conference focuses on a well-defined research problem or on new developments in the field. Its purpose is to stretch the imagination of students and faculty. If it is to succeed, the topics must be provocative and those in attendance must participate. This type of conference has "something for everyone" and should be a rewarding weekly experience for members of the cardiac anesthesia division as well as others in the department of anesthesia. In some settings, it is possible to have a case conference in seminar style that involves cardiologists, cardiac surgeons, and cardiac anesthesiologists. This type of seminar is very worthwhile and should be a part of the educational program, if feasible. The creation of heart centers and heart institutes fosters this type of interdepartmental educational collaboration (19). As medical centers begin to organize these programmatic initiatives, education will clearly benefit. We predict that the medical centers of the future will adopt an approach that is more disease and/or organ system–based, with less departmental emphasis (14). Thus, cardiac anesthesiology will find its home in the Heart Center or Heart Institute.

Multimedia Instruction

There are now many modes of instruction that are complementary to hands-on instruction and that make an excellent addition to a well-rounded education. Multimedia can be used effectively to teach new, complex, and rapidly developing anesthetic and surgical techniques (20). Video and CD-ROM instruction are particularly effective. Most video equipment and CD-ROM disks are portable and relatively inexpensive; tapes or disks can be used at work or in the home, bringing a new versatility to this audiovisual medium of teaching. Teaching a technique such as how to cannulate the radial or pulmonary artery lends itself to this form of instruction. Each step can be carefully and systematically illustrated—usually with a real patient. Repetition of steps, essential for teaching, can be easily accomplished. Playbacks can ensure that all points can be revisited and emphasized. Extensive libraries of videotapes and CD-ROM disks are available to institutions for this purpose. Additionally, access to wide-ranging information is available on the Internet for those with easy access, particularly in the work setting. Internet Web sites have been established that allow medical questions to be posed and answered by the founders of a particular site. However, the quality and accuracy of such information must be assessed. In Appendix 33-3, a list of the useful Web sites are listed as compiled by the Society for Cardiovascular Anesthesia (SCA).

Simulators

Simulators are the logical extension of electronic learning. Many of the real-life experiences a cardiac anesthesiologist is likely to confront, particularly with regard to hemodynamics and arrhythmias, are relatively easily simulated. Simulators in anesthesia take the form of a variety of devices, ranging from a simple computer screen to a theater-type simulator in which most of the operating room setting can be reproduced (21,22). An advantage of a simulator is that it permits a learner to "crash," that is, to make a series of errors that result in disaster without harm. The errors can be pointed out by the teacher, and on subsequent training sessions, the trainee will be able to avoid previous mistakes. Not only can errors of commission be made, but errors of omission and speed of response can be studied and improved upon with this type of instruction. Simulators can also be used for teaching such skills as cardiopulmonary resuscitation and fiberoptic intubation. An important aspect of simulator use is also to learn to accurately report the occurrence and outcome of a critical incident (23). Simulators are very expensive and as such tend to be located within regions of the country for many hospitals and anesthetic programs to share. An increasing role for simulators in the education of the cardiac anesthesiologist is predicted.

Specialized Outrotations

Specialized outrotations are often arranged by the faculty to supplement learning experiences within a department or division. These educational experiences can be very rewarding as long as the objectives are clear and the faculty and facilities permit the realization of the goals. Examples of rotations useful in the training of cardiac anesthesiologists are experiences with cardiologists in cardiac catheterization laboratories, in cardiac surgical intensive care to learn management of cardiac and thoracic surgical patients, and in the cardiology echocardiography laboratory. These supplemental educational opportunities and others like them depend on the availability of high-quality learning settings and the particular needs, goals, and level of education of the pupil.

Meetings

Meetings represent the final method of teaching and learning. There are a wide variety of educational meetings, and the teacher has a responsibility to aid the student in the appropriate selection of these opportunities. Instruction may include didactic lectures, scientific presentations, and interactive panels or workshops. The value of meetings is enhanced by the social interaction with others who share one's interest in a field, but come from different places of work or education. These meetings are crucial for the development of ideas and exchange of information. A student, with the teacher's guidance, should select the meetings most appropriate to that individual's educational needs.

Assessment of Learning

The quality and competence of instruction and learning must be assessed. Traditionally, this is achieved by examination and/or periodic evaluation. In evaluating the performance of faculty or residents, one should establish four levels for each category of evaluation; for example, these levels might be labeled "frequently fails," "occasionally fails," "meets expectations," and "exceeds criteria."(24) These categories lend themselves to numeric analysis, in case one wants to mathematically grade faculty or resident performance. Factors considered important in faculty evaluation by the student are availability/presence, personal attributes (role model), case-related teaching ability, didactic teaching ability, and overall contribution to resident education (2). (See Appendix 33-2 for a sample faculty evaluation form.) Another method of evaluating faculty is by the quality of the product of their work, namely the success of their pupils in examinations and in their subsequent careers. Evaluation of the effectiveness of faculty teaching has become important, as it may contribute to the promotion of a faculty member; alternative promotion tracks toward tenure are being at least evaluated in most academic centers. Under one such scheme, a faculty member may be promoted in a clinical educator track, which would require evidence of effective teaching.

Testing is one effective method of determining how well learning has taken place. A danger of testing is that it predefines the information (facts) to be learned and therefore is educationally confining (25). One interesting finding in our field is that skills are perfected earlier in the educational process than knowledge, and there is a poor correlation between skills achievement and information acquisition (18). This may explain why the occasional resident is considered excellent on clinical competence evaluations but does surprisingly poorly on examinations. Faculty evaluation of clinical competence should address specific items in patient care management, knowledge, personal qualities, and technical skills. Noncognitive skills also predict overall performance: conscientiousness and composure predict two thirds of variability in critical incident scores (26); it seems prudent for faculty to develop and assess these characteristics in trainees. The ABA recognizes these attributes as crucial and as such require a biannual assessment of noncognitive characteristics in a student of anesthesiology (incorporated into Table 33-5).

TABLE 33-5. CLINICAL COMPETENCE OF CARDIAC ANESTHESIA RESIDENTS

Knowledge development
Attitude and character
Scholarship
Continuing education
Skill acquisition
Disciplines of medical field
Technical skills and correct use
Monitoring capabilities
Pediatric and adult care capabilities
Delivery of care
Judgment
Risk evaluation and assessment
Planning and execution
Follow-up
Noncognitive essential characteristics
Honest and ethical
Reliable, conscientious, responsible
Reacts to stressful situations in an appropriate manner
Has no documented abuse of alcohol or illegal use of drugs
Has no physical, sensory or motor impairment that precludes individual responsibility for any aspect of anesthesiology care
Extension of basics
Research
Teaching and writing
Community health objectives

Source: From Flynn M, Fogdall R. Education and training of the cardiac anesthesiologist. In: Ream AK, Fogdall R, eds. *Acute cardiovascular management.* Philadelphia: JB Lippincott, 1982:877, and ABA Clinical Competence Committee Report.

Testing brings up a number of issues: (a) the method of testing, (b) the grading of tests, (c) the periodicity of testing, and (d) what to do with the testing information. There are few data on the value of types of tests or even testing in general to guide the teacher in the cardiac anesthesia field. It is recommended that anesthesia residents be given a set of educational objectives when they begin a rotation on the cardiac anesthesia service and an examination at the end of the rotation to see that the residents perform at a satisfactory level. The examination can be written and/or oral. If the examination is written, the faculty must vary it sufficiently that resident networking does not make it well known to all and therefore of little value in measuring information learned. An oral examination at the end of the 2-month rotation on cardiac anesthesia may be preferable. The purpose of the examination is to test the resident's knowledge and judgment. The oral examination also prepares the resident for oral examination to receive board certification in anesthesiology. It is assumed that the individual's skills have been tested and clinical competence assessed each day (Table 33-6). Although there is little information on how to guide the faculty in the task of determining clinical competence, when it is evaluated, faculty tend to be more concerned that students meet a minimum level of competence than that they achieve excellence (8). We believe that this is a mistake. Of several possible factors that weigh in the decisions regarding competence, preoperative evaluation and anesthetic management are considered essential by faculty. Some have suggested that it is ideal to give written examinations before an elective rotation as well as after so the student and teacher can measure progress in the individual. The arguments against this are the paucity of testing instruments and the lack of interest by the faculty to ensure that it is done well.

TABLE 33-6. RESIDENT/FELLOW EVALUATION: DAILY CHECKLIST: CARDIAC ANESTHESIA SERVICE

Name of trainee:	Date:
Training status: R[ ], F[ ], Other[ ]	
Case type and age:	
Preoperative	
Evaluation	
Presentation	
Preparation	
Notes	
Line placement	
Preparation	
Rapport with patient	
Technical skills	
Management	
Prebypass:	
OR preparation	
Induction	
Intubation	
Management	
Pre-CPB preparations	
Bypass:	
Transition	
Management	
Evaluations (lab, etc.)	
Infusion drug preparations	
Blood/coag preparations	
Post-CPB	
Transition management:	
Cardiovascular	
Respiratory	
Volume	
Blood/coagulation	
Preparations for ICU	
ICU:	
Transportation	
Change over	
Patient status	
Postop note	
General	
Anesthesia record	
"Style"	
Understanding concepts	
Working with attending	
Working with surgeons	
Working with nurses	
Complications	

Source: From Flynn M, Fogdall R. Education and training of the cardiac anesthesiologist. In Ream AK, Fogdall R, eds. *Acute cardiovascular management.* Philadelphia: JB Lippincott, 1982:877, with permission.
Note: R, residency; F, fellowship; OR, operating room; CPB, cardiopulmonary bypass; ICU, intensive care unit.

EDUCATING THE RESIDENT

Objectives of Resident Education

There are different objectives for residents, which are dependent on their educational level and institution of training. We have the following educational objectives for residents who rotate on the cardiac anesthesia service.

Clinical Anesthesia Year 2

The clinical anesthesia year 2 (CA2) resident must acquire a thorough understanding of the common cardiac and thoracic diseases. These include atherosclerotic heart and vascular disease, valvular heart disease, electrophysiologic disturbances that produce arrhythmias, adult congenital diseases, and acquired cardiomyopathies. The residents should learn pharmacology related to the use of cardiovascular drugs and the cardiovascular properties of anesthetic drugs and techniques. CA2 residents are expected to become proficient in the technical aspects of invasive monitoring, as well as understand the indications for and interpretation of physiologic and other types of monitoring used in the care of cardiac surgical patients. Principles of cardiopulmonary bypass and other means of cardiac support should be learned. The CA2 rotation may be combined with experience in vascular and/or thoracic anesthesia. As such, the resident would be expected to acquire knowledge about primary vascular and thoracic disease states as well as learn techniques and procedures unique to vascular and/or thoracic surgery. Because many CA2 residents may not elect to repeat a rotation on cardiac anesthesia, they must have enough knowledge and experience to meet the requirements for certification as an anesthesiologist as set forth by the ABA (27).

Clinical Anesthesia Year 3

The clinical anesthesia year 3 (CA3) resident may elect to spend additional time during a year to gain either advanced clinical training or subspecialty education. The time spent during the CA3 year varies (*vide infra*), but there are similar expectations for these students. The CA3 resident will be expected to attain the objectives of the CA2 resident (*vide supra*) plus acquire additional knowledge and experience. The knowledge should include current developments and research in this rapidly progressing field. The CA3 resident should also gain experience with more sophisticated monitoring modalities, such as transesophageal echocardiography (TEE) and electrophysiologic monitoring. Whereas the CA2 resident must be familiar with the common adult cardiac pathology, the CA3 resident should learn about the more rare forms of heart and lung disease and the more complicated management cases (e.g., combined carotid and coronary artery bypass surgical procedures). The CA3 resident might be expected to participate in pediatric congenital patient management if a sufficiently long experience is elected. The ultimate objective of the CA3 resident is board certification and consultant status as an anesthesiologist. The goal of the CA3 resident who elects to spend 9 to 12 months in cardiac anesthesia is to be a subspecialist in cardiac anesthesiology. This CA3 resident must be a consultant in the subspecialty, expert in the skills and techniques of monitoring, and knowledgeable about the current and new directions in which this field is moving. It is difficult in our opinion to see how a CA3 resident can meet these great expectations in 9 to 12 months, and we recommend that the subspecialist resident spend 2 years in this subspecialty educational track.

Structure of Resident Education

In subspecialty education, the achievement of skills and knowledge should be emphasized, not the time or route taken to reach these ends (28). Although there is no absolute agreement on the time in which residents are first exposed to cardiac anesthesia, they should have learned the fundamentals of anesthesia skills and medical management before the cardiac rotation. According to one survey, two thirds of anesthesia programs report that the first cardiac resident rotation is in the CA2 year for a 2-month period (2). However, no consensus has been developed on the number of cases or on the length of the cardiac anesthesia rotation.

The academic year of 1988/89 was the first to require that all anesthesia residents spend a third (CA3) year in an approved residency program to be eligible for certification according to the ABA. This change in the curriculum continuum of education in anesthesiology has had an effect on the time that residents elect to spend in anesthesia subspecialties (3,14,29). Residents can now obtain additional education in cardiac anesthesia during the CA3 year in several ways. They may elect to take the cardiac anesthesia subspecialty track (6 to 12 months), advanced clinical track (less than 6 months), or the clinical scientist track and spend as much as 6 months in cardiac anesthesia, and perhaps more if the research were in cardiac anesthesia. Nobody has agreed on a curriculum for cardiac anesthesia training during the anesthesia residency, and an anesthesia resident may finish an approved training program with a varied exposure to cardiac anesthesia (3,29).

EDUCATING THE CARDIAC ANESTHESIOLOGY FELLOW

Fellowship programs exist because the knowledge, judgment, and skills necessary to act as a consultant cardiac anesthesiologist cannot be obtained during the 3-year residency. We believe 2 years should be dedicated to the education of the cardiac anesthesia fellow. This education may begin with a CA3 (postgraduate year 4) subspecialty track and extend through or beyond the postgraduate year 5 or may be commenced after a full 3-year residency (postgraduate years 5 and 6). The goal of subspecialty training is to teach the fellows a clinical practice, complete with requisite skills as well as a body of knowledge that can be found in the literature: general anesthesia textbooks, general anesthesia literature, subspecialty anesthesia journals, and medical specialty journals (14,29). The fellowship should provide an emphasis on the scientific foundations of the subspecialty. The model cardiac anesthesia subspecialist would then not only expertly perform the technical aspects of cardiac anesthesia but also be a consultant capable of clinically applying knowledge of cardiac and pulmonary anatomy, physiology, pathophysiology, and pharmacology to the perioperative care. The individual would identify important questions, formulate hypotheses, test the hypotheses scientifically, and apply this new knowledge, thereby establishing new standards of care and advancing the field of anesthesiology to affect patient outcome.

Education Goals

If the fellowship program is to develop the fellow into the consultant and clinical subspecialty role of cardiac anesthesiologist, the educational and training objectives should be designed to fulfill this goal. Clinical and academic objectives should be developed for each institution and fellow.

Educational Objectives

There are several educational objectives in different realms that the fellow strives to accomplish.

Clinical

The clinical objective is to provide the knowledge and skills required for expertise in clinical cardiac anesthesiology, which requires proficiency in the following areas:

1. Assessment of the patient's cardiovascular disease process on the basis of the history and physical examination as well as by interpreting the results of technical invasive and noninvasive studies performed by the cardiologist.
2. Evaluation of the patient's therapeutic medical regimen, specifically to determine whether it has minimized the

upcoming anesthetic risks or requires recommendations for further therapeutic interventions before surgery.
3. Prescription of appropriate perioperative monitoring and therapy for the cardiac surgical patient. This includes the following: (a) a properly conducted preoperative patient consultation; (b) the prescription of immediate preoperative cardiac medications and sedatives; (c) the determination of specific cardiovascular monitoring requirements and expertise with invasive and noninvasive (e.g., TEE) monitoring techniques; (d) the design and administration of anesthetic medications specifically tailored to the patient's disease process and the surgical procedure; (e) an understanding of the principles of extracorporeal circulation; (f) an understanding of myocardial preservation and cardioplegia; and (g) recommendations, consultation, and participation in postoperative intensive care.

Research

The research objective is to provide the experience required to understand and contribute to the science of cardiovascular biology as it relates to anesthesiology. This necessitates experience with cardiovascular anesthesia research, which includes the following:

1. The ability to ascertain and formulate clinically relevant problems in cardiac anesthesiology.
2. Designing, setting up, and executing clinical and/or laboratory studies that are structured to answer specific questions according to the scientific method.
3. An introduction to and an understanding of statistical analytic techniques.
4. Preparation of effective presentations for scientific meetings.
5. An introduction to research funding and grants.
6. The ability to critically evaluate the research of other investigators.

Teaching

This objective is to provide teaching experience in residency education by fellow participation in the following:

1. Lecture preparation and presentation.
2. Clinical teaching during intraoperative cardiac anesthesia.
3. Evaluation of methods of assessment of faculty and trainees in clinical care, supervision, and teaching.

Curriculum

Presently there is no specific curriculum, prescribed training time for minimal competence, or certification process for cardiac anesthesiology fellowship training. The training program may consist of 1 year of research or clinical activities exclusively, 1 year of clinical, and 1 year of research, or some other combination.

Many believe that the educational standard would be enhanced if an accreditation mechanism were developed for cardiothoracic anesthesiology training programs. To this end, the SCA, the largest organization in the world representing practitioners of this subspecialty, has launched an initiative to develop a proposal for accreditation of training programs in cardiothoracic anesthesiology. This proposal will ultimately be reviewed by the RRC and if supported, submitted for approval by the American Board of Medical Specialties, the parent organization for all accrediting medical specialty boards.

To be most effective, the program, like the educational goals, should be personalized according to the institutional and individual objectives (e.g., private practice, academic anesthesia), the educational background of the fellow, and the career goals of the individual. The triad of patient care, research, and teaching can form the framework for this program (2).

Clinical Training

The program should provide for developing competence in the management of complex clinical problems in cardiac anesthesiology. This education may begin during the CA3 year. We believe that a full year of clinical experience is essential for the development of the cardiac anesthesia fellow. One suggested curriculum for clinical training in cardiac anesthesia is in Table 33-7.

TABLE 33-7. SUGGESTED CURRICULUM FOR CLINICAL TRAINING OF THE CARDIAC ANESTHESIA FELLOWSHIP

Clinical training	Time estimated
1. Orientation lectures	1 week
ACLS training (if not already certified)	
Provide educational materials	
2. Primary management of adult cardiac anesthesia	4–8 months
Patients (graded responsibility)	
Coronary and valvular surgery	
Transplantation	
Adult congenital	
Other	
3. Pediatric cardiac anesthesia	3 months
Congenital heart surgery	
Catheterization laboratory	
Intensive care	
Echocardiography	
Attend combined anesthesia, cardiac surgery, and pediatric cardiology conferences	
4. Special training	
Transesophageal echocardiography	6–12 weeks
Cardiac intensive care	4 weeks
Cardiac diagnostic laboratory	Elective
Experience in cardiopulmonary bypass perfusion	Elective

If the trainee is not ACLS certified, time and appropriate classes should be made available to obtain certification. The initial responsibility and experience of the fellow may involve preoperative assessment and intraoperative management of the adult cardiac surgical patient. The cardiac anesthesia faculty then provides direct supervision. This allows the fellow time to become familiar with the cardiac surgical team, attain proficiency in perioperative patient management, and complete designated reading in selected cardiac anesthesia textbooks and journals. The optimal number of cases for competency has not been defined, although it is usual for a fellow to anesthetize one patient per day. More important than the number of cases is that the fellow be exposed to increasingly difficult clinical cases and more clinical responsibility in patient management. Increasing responsibility may include the opportunity to supervise others in the conduct of a cardiac anesthetic. However, this is dependent on the number of years of postgraduate training, the board status of the fellow, and hospital privilege rules. If a fellow meets the necessary criteria, he or she may be eligible to participate in the supervision of residents and/or nurse anesthetists as a junior faculty member.

Clinical training in pediatric cardiac anesthesia depends on the institution's experience. Pediatric cardiac anesthesia differs greatly from adult cardiac anesthesia, but it may be the least well taught area of cardiac fellowship training. At Duke University, fellows spend 3 months on this service, which includes anesthesia for congenital heart surgery, the cardiac catheterization laboratory, and arrhythmia surgery. The fellow has the option of concentrating clinical work in the field of pediatric cardiac anesthesia, including training in intraoperative echocardiography and pediatric cardiac intensive care. Participation in pediatric cardiology, pediatric cardiac anesthesia, and cardiac surgery conferences during the rotation will enhance the experience.

Special Clinical Training

Transesophageal Echocardiography

The clinical use of TEE has grown explosively, crossing interspecialty boundaries and involving anesthesiologists in the mid-1980s. The indications for TEE are numerous, and it is the definitive diagnostic modality for many perioperative cardiovascular disorders. TEE is valuable for assessing biventricular function, native and prosthetic valve function, assessing the suitability and outcome of valvular repairs, diagnosing diseases of the aorta (dissection, atherosclerosis), and assessing atrial pathology and congenital abnormalities, among other purposes. Because the cardiologist cannot be in the operating room continuously monitoring the patient, it is recommended that the cardiac anesthesiologist understand the principles of echocardiography (30). Fellowship training in cardiac anesthesiology should include training in TEE.

The American Society of Echocardiography (ASE) established the initial guidelines for the training of physicians who are responsible for the performance and interpretation of echocardiographic studies in 1987 (31). These recommendations, entitled *Optimal Physician Training in Echocardiography,* apply to transthoracic echocardiography and not specifically to TEE. They recognize three levels of training. If independent responsibility for echocardiography studies is assumed, the second level of training should be reached. This includes approximately 300 two-dimensional and M-mode studies and 225 Doppler examinations performed over approximately 6 months, during which the physician is primarily studying echocardiography.

The ASE then published *Guidelines for Physician Training in Transesophageal Echocardiography* (32). These outline the technical and cognitive skills required and make recommendations on the training components desirable for those performing and interpreting TEE (Table 33-8). It is recommended that after level II training in general echocardiography, at least 50 TEE examinations should be performed with supervision before independent examinations. In its recommendations, the ASE recognized that anesthesiologists frequently use TEE for monitoring global and regional myocardial function and left ventricular volume. However, the ASE emphasized the importance of a collaborative relationship with cardiology when important diagnostic issues arise that require intraoperative evaluation.

Recognizing that, in many institutions, the realities of clinical practice preclude full-time posting in the echocardiography laboratory, alternative pathways for training of anesthesiologists have been sought. Cahalan et al. (33) have suggested that TEE can be safely and effectively learned "on the job" provided an expert or mentor is available to ensure that essential information is not missed (33). A formalized echocardiography training program for anesthesiologists has not been established, and guidelines are evolving. An example of TEE training for the cardiac anesthesiologist may be to spend 4 to 8 weeks in an echocardiography laboratory learning the principles of echocardiography followed by supervised experience performing intraoperative TEE. A minimum of 100 TEE examinations may be required.

Two levels of training were recognized and recom-

TABLE 33-8. A SAMPLE TRAINING PROGRAM FOR THOSE PERFORMING AND INTERPRETING TEE

Component	Duration	Number of Studies Done
Basic echocardiography		
Laboratory experience	1–6 months	100–300
TEE examinations under close supervision	Variable	50–100
Continuing education	Annual	50–100

Note: TEE, transesophageal echocardiography.

mended by a combined ASA and SCA task force examining practice parameters for the use of TEE in the perioperative period. Anesthesiologists with basic training in TEE were deemed able to use TEE for indications that lie within the customary practice of anesthesiology (e.g., ischemia diagnosis and assessment of ventricular function) (34). Anesthesiologists with more advanced training would be able to use TEE to its greatest potential to diagnose problems in the perioperative period.

The task force did not provide national recommendations for credentialing in TEE, as this is deemed a hospital-specific responsibility. However, the ASE and the SCA have created a perioperative TEE certification examination. There are no requirements to document training in order to take the examination and the examination is given annually. Credentialing in TEE may therefore consist of demonstration of a relevant training in TEE (such as part of a cardiac fellowship), evidence of current competence, and having a passing score on the perioperative TEE certification examination.

All intraoperative echocardiography programs must develop a close collaborative working relationship with cardiologists who have expertise in intraoperative TEE and who are available for immediate consultation to assist in difficult intraoperative decisions. The fellow in cardiac anesthesia is expected to learn when it is appropriate to consult with these cardiologists. Improvements in multimedia electronic links may make it possible for a cardiologist to assist with the interoperation of an intraoperative TEE on-line while the TEE is being performed.

Intensive Care

Many cardiac fellowship programs have a formal rotation in intensive care, whereas others allow the fellow to elect to participate in the postoperative cardiac intensive care unit as a 1- or 2-month rotation. An intensive care rotation provides for increased interaction and a closer relationship with the cardiac surgeons. It also allows the fellow to observe and manage the postoperative complications related to cardiac anesthesia and surgery. Managing postoperative fluid, hemodynamic, and coagulation problems, among others, will make the cardiac anesthesia fellow more aware of postoperative concerns that may have been caused by intraoperative events and care decisions. Although most training is in the adult cardiac intensive care unit, if time is available, these recommendations also apply to the pediatric cardiac intensive care.

Cardiac Diagnostic Laboratory

The cardiac anesthesiologist preoperatively evaluates written cardiac catheterization data on most pediatric or adult patients before cardiac surgery. Catheterization data provide an assessment of ventricular function, type and extent of valvular lesions, location and extent of coronary lesions, location and quantification of intracardiac shunts, and diagnosis of congenital cardiac lesions. These data may determine the appropriate hemodynamic monitoring and anesthetic technique and predict postoperative status.

Despite the importance of understanding this information, few cardiac anesthesiologists have any formal training in interpreting cardiac catheterization data and rely on written reports. Cardiac fellows should be provided elective training time in the cardiac diagnostic laboratory. It is unfortunate if the fellow finishes training and does not understand catheterization data and the principles of myocardial function tests (e.g., radionucleotide) and perfusion (e.g., stress thallium).

Cardiopulmonary Perfusion

The cardiac anesthesiologist works closely with the perfusion team and cardiac surgeon to successfully commence, maintain, and wean from cardiopulmonary bypass during cardiac surgery. Although the physiology of cardiopulmonary bypass should be very familiar to all cardiac anesthesiologists, the mechanics and technical aspects may be less so. It is useful to provide elective time for the cardiac fellow to associate with the perfusion team to learn how to establish and maintain a cardiopulmonary bypass circuit, to manage an intraaortic balloon pump, and to understand the principles of ventricular assist devices and extracorporeal membrane oxygenation. With this knowledge, the cardiac anesthesiologist can assist the perfusionist and surgeon in diagnosing and managing problems associated with extracorporeal circulation.

Research

> "I have never seen anybody improve in the art and technique of inquiry by any means other than engaging in inquiry."—Pasteur

Research is an education in critical and scientific inquiry. It does not necessarily mean writing papers or laboratory investigation. Minimally, a cardiac anesthesia fellowship should teach principles and conduct of investigation. The goal is not quantity of publications to promote academic advancement, but rather to develop career-long skills of scientific inquiry and the ability to scrutinize critically the work of others (35). There is little proof that "success" in research endeavors correlates with clinical skills (36). Rather, the objective of research training is to develop curiosity, teach critical inquiry, and impart the motivation to set standards of excellence. If this is the definition and objective of research endeavors, all should participate and become proficient in it.

There is a lack of formal training in anesthesia research (14,29,37,38). Because only 6 months may be spent in the clinical scientist track during the CA3 year and few choose to enter a CA4 year, with even fewer choosing research, the problem of exposure to and education in research persists. Critical questions are when and how will subspecialists learn

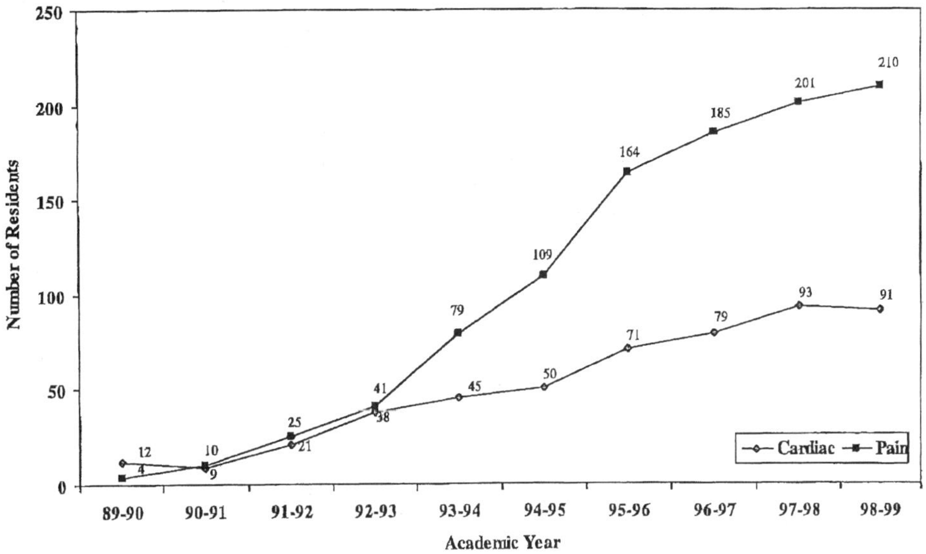

FIGURE 33-1. Past-graduate year 5 (clinical anesthesia year 4) residents in 12-month cardiac and pain subspecialties.

this aspect of training, so vital to the development of academic physicians, and how will they expand the role of anesthesiologists in the medical community (39,40)? The critical issue of subspecialty training and certification persists. Creation of sanctioned subspecialty fellowships in critical care and pain management has resulted in growth of those subspecialties in both numbers of residents choosing additional training in these subspecialties (Fig. 33-1). Thus, certification of cardiac anesthesiology as a subspecialty may result in increased numbers of residents choosing to do a CA4 year and thus be exposed to opportunities for an education in research.

Because research is so important to the subspecialty trainee, supervised opportunities for academic development should be available. For the cardiac subspecialist to have an adequate exposure to clinical research that will enable independent clinical research, a minimum of 1 year may be required. Basic science or "bench research" would require yet another year of basic science investigation. The duration of subspecialty training therefore depends on the objectives. One year may be adequate in many instances while as many as 3 years may be required for others. If this investment is not made, the future of basic science creation by physician scientists in cardiothoracic anesthesiology is jeopardized (14). Suggestions that may increase the likelihood of a productive period of research training include the following:

1. Seek a mentor (cardiac anesthesiologist or otherwise) actively investigating and successfully publishing in an area of interest to the fellow. Every effort should be made to integrate laboratory and clinical interests. The mentor should be committed to assisting the fellow's research education.
2. Design the proposed research project in advance with assistance from the mentor, and obtain appropriate hospital Internal Review Board or Animal Care Committee approval.
3. Proposed project should already be funded by the anesthesia department or by a research grant, and necessary equipment should be available at the time the project is initiated.
4. Required support staff should be readily available (e.g., research technicians, statisticians, and secretarial help to assist in manuscript searches and retrievals).
5. A personal computer and necessary software should be accessible, and appropriate computer literacy training accomplished.
6. Development classes in study design, statistics, writing skills, speech training, and grantmanship should be encouraged.
7. Adequate funding should be made available for attending scientific meetings to present results of research and develop new areas of interest.
8. Preservation of "protected" (nonclinical) time to conduct the research.

These suggestions may increase the prospect that the cardiac subspecialty fellow will successfully complete the part of the educational objectives previously described. Specifically, the fellow will acquire the ability to ascertain and formulate clinically relevant problems in cardiac anesthesiology; will design, set up, and execute clinical and/or laboratory studies that are structured to answer specific questions according to the scientific method; will have a basic understanding of statistical analytic techniques; will prepare effective scientific presentations; will have an understanding of research funding and grants; and will be able to critically evaluate the research of other investigators.

Independent of the number of publications, the research training is successful if the cardiac fellow has developed intellectual curiosity, has learned to apply the methods of critical injury, has set personal standards of excellence, and understands that the aim of medical research is to provide relevant knowledge that may lead to better patient care.

Teaching

Teaching is the third component of a well-designed anesthesia education program (41). The cardiac anesthesia fellow should actively participate in the organization and presentation of appropriate conferences and meetings. Examples of these meetings include the following:

1. Lectures on cardiac anesthesia to the anesthesia residents: initially learn lecture preparation and presentation skills.
2. Direct Cardiac Anesthesia Journal Club: learn critical analysis of scientific papers.
3. Cardiac Anesthesia Conference: learn to interact with visiting lecturers; learn to present information in a more formal environment.
4. Interdepartmental conferences: interaction with all areas of medicine (e.g., cardiology, cardiac surgery, medicine, physiology, pharmacology, pediatrics); advance the image of the cardiac anesthesiologist as a consultant specialist.

The fellowship training period is a valuable time to learn lecture preparation and presentation skills. Writing and public speaking classes may improve the presentations. Proper skills in preparation of slides, computerized projections, and overhead projections are invaluable. Constructive critique of a fellow's lectures by the cardiac faculty that focus on the content, delivery, and audience interest in the presentation are also important and greatly enhance additional lecture performances. Teaching is not always optimally accomplished in a lecturer-audience format. The operating room offers an excellent opportunity for fellows to learn instructional skills on a personal level. Residents who have been instructed by the fellow can critique that individual's effectiveness.

Whether the goal of the cardiac anesthesiology fellow is to become an academician or private practitioner, the teaching skills acquired during fellowship training will enhance communication with both medical and nonmedical personnel.

Evaluation-Fellowship Achievements

Evaluation of the fellow's progress at regular intervals is suggested. A standard evaluation form covering patient care areas (e.g., clinical skills), knowledge areas (e.g., integrative ability), and personal qualities (e.g., attitude, communication) should be completed by the fellowship training faculty every 1 to 3 months. There should also be a format by which one can evaluate the individual teaching faculty, the overall training program, and one's own progress in the attainment of individual goals with the fellowship program director.

TABLE 33-9. FELLOWSHIP ACHIEVEMENTS CRITERIA FOR COMPLETION OF A CARDIAC ANESTHESIOLOGY FELLOWSHIP

There is faculty evaluation and consensus that the fellow has met the *individual program objectives.*[a]
The fellow can safely and skillfully manage complicated cardiac surgical patients.
The fellow has become an integral member of the cardiac surgical team.
The fellow has participated in educational endeavors, including both didactic lecture presentation and clinical supervision if possible.
If non–board certified, the fellow has taken steps to obtain American Board of Anesthesiology certification.
ACLS certified.

[a] The major criteria for satisfactory completion of the cardiac anesthesiology fellowship.

Although examinations (oral and written) can be utilized to assess the academic progress of the trainee and the strengths and weaknesses of the training program, it is recommended that the major criteria for satisfactory completion of the fellowship training be faculty evaluation and consensus that the fellow has met the individual program objectives (Table 33-9).

Certification

Cardiovascular anesthesia subspecialty education, like other anesthesia subspecialties (excluding critical care medicine and pain management), lacks an ABA-sanctioned certification. It is time for educators in cardiovascular anesthesia to formulate curricula, establish training guidelines, and plan subspecialty certification requirements (29,38,42). We believe, as did Flynn et al. (2) and editorialists (3,29,42,43), that with changes in the overall anesthesia educational continuum, subspecialty certification is inevitable and desirable. As this occurs, concrete educational goals as well as competency examinations will help define the educational program more precisely and with widespread consensus.

However, several questions remain: Should subspecialty cardiac certification be mandatory? How many cardiac patients undergoing a given procedure should the cardiac anesthesia fellow anesthetize during training, and over what period of time? What weight should be placed on the individual educational components of patient care, teaching, or research? What body of knowledge should be grasped, and what criteria and evaluation process should be used for satisfactory completion of a formal education program in cardiac anesthesiology?

Unlike general anesthesiology, in which a series of examinations as well as competency evaluation lead to certification by the ABA, there is no parallel certification process in cardiac anesthesia. The certification process and outlined curricula should stimulate subspecialty education in cardiac anesthesia. We need a clear definition of educational objectives, a curriculum for educating the cardiac anesthesiologist, an examination system, a certification process, and a well-considered study of the number of cardiac anesthesiologists required to provide clinical care, conduct the research, and educate other cardiac anesthesiologists. In the United States, this planning is being done in concert with the ABA, the graduate medical education council, the Society of Cardiac Anesthesiologists, the ASA, and the Society of Academic Chairman.

SUMMARY

The education of cardiac anesthesiologists is essential for the development of the field. We have emphasized the elements and organization of an educational program and raised some of the issues that face students and teachers of this discipline. The remainder of this book addresses the body of knowledge that we believe constitutes the core curriculum of this subject.

APPENDIX 33-1.

Content Outline (Abridged-to include cardiothoracic anesthesiology topics)
Joint Council on In-Training Examinations
American Board of Anesthesiology
American Society of Anesthesiologists

Revised January 1996

- I. Physiologic Sciences
  - A. Physiology
    - 1. Respiration
      - Lung volumes
      - Lung mechanics
      - Ventilation-perfusion
      - Diffusion
      - Blood gas transport
      - Regulation of ventilation
      - Nonrespiratory functions of lungs
    - 2. Cardiovascular
      - Cardiac cycle
      - Ventricular function
      - Venous return
      - Blood pressure
      - Microcirculation
      - Organ perfusion
      - Regulation of circulation and blood volume
    - 3. Central and peripheral nervous system
      - Autonomic nervous system
    - 4. Hepatic function
    - 5. Renal function
    - 6. Endocrine function
    - 7. Temperature regulation
  - B. Pharmacology
    - 1. General concepts
    - 2. Anesthetics: gases and vapors
    - 3. Anesthetics: intravenous
    - 4. Anesthetics: local
    - 5. Muscle relaxants
    - 6. Autonomic drugs
    - 7. Cardiovascular drugs
    - 8. Diuretics
    - 9. Drug interactions
- II. Physical Sciences
  - A. Anatomy
    - 1. Topographical anatomy as landmarks
    - 2. Radiologic anatomy
    - 3. Respiratory system
    - 4. Cardiovascular system
  - B. Biochemistry
    - 1. Normal body metabolism
    - 2. Acid-base regulation
    - 3. Water and electrolytes
  - C. Physics
    - 1. Mechanics
    - 2. Flow velocity
    - 3. Uptake and distribution of inhalation anesthetics
    - 4. Physics of breathing systems
    - 5. Monitoring methods
    - 6. Instrumentation
    - 7. Ventilators
    - 8. Defibrillators
    - 9. Pacemakers
- III. A. Anesthesia procedures, methods and techniques
    - 1. Evaluation of the patient and preoperative preparation
    - 2. Intravenous fluid therapy during anesthesia
    - 3. Complications
      - Trauma
      - Temperature
      - Bronchospasm, laryngospasm
    - 4. Special techniques
      - Controlled hypotension
      - Controlled hypothermia
  - B. Disease states: clinical problems and their management
    - 1. Respiratory
      - Obstructive disease
      - Restrictive disease
      - Management of the patient with respiratory disease
    - 2. Cardiovascular
      - Ischemic heart disease
      - Valvular heart disease
      - Rhythm disorders and conduction defects
      - Heart failure and cardiomyopathy
      - Cardiac tamponade and constrictive pericarditis
      - Circulatory assist

Myocardial preservation
Pulmonary embolism
Hypertension
Peripheral circulatory failure
Vascular diseases
Cardiopulmonary resuscitation

3. Other entities

Pediatric anesthesia
Neonatal physiology
Congenital heart disease
Emergencies in the newborn

4. Special problems in

Laparoscopic surgery
Thoracoscopy

APPENDIX 33-2.

Sample Faculty Evaluation Form

Faculty Name______________________________ Date of Evaluation__________

Are you a: CA1 CA2 CA3 CA4 ? (please circle)

Number of times worked with attending (please circle): 1-3 3-5 5 or more

Other (call, OB, etc.)__________

Areas of Evaluation

A) Availability: ______________

B) Clinical Teaching: ______________

C) Responsiveness: ______________

D) Interaction: ______________

E) Professional Characteristics: ______________

F) Adequate feedback on daily performance: ______________

G) Ability to stimulate your reading: ______________

H) Overall Effectiveness: ______________

COMMENTS:

Key	
1.	Always meets and often surpasses these expectations.
2.	Usually meets these expectations.
3.	Sometimes meets these expectations but improvement is needed.
4.	Often does not meet these expectations.
5.	Too little contact for adequate evaluation.

APPENDIX 33-3.

Useful Web Sites as Compiled by the Society for Cardiovascular Anesthesia

Anesthesia Society Links
- SPA home page: http://www.pedsanesthesia.org/
- ASRA home page: http://www.asra.com/
- ASA home page: http://www.asahq.org/
- IARS home page: http://www.iars.org/
- Canadian Anaesthesiologists Society: http://www.cas.ca/
- EACTA: http://www.eacta.org
- Australian Anaesthesia Web site: http://www.usyd.edu.au/su/anaes/anaes.html

Journal links
- *Anesthesia and Analgesia:* http://www.iars.org/journal.html
- *Journal of Cardiothoracic and Vascular Anesthesia:* http://www.jcardioanesthesia.com/
- *Anesthesiology:* http://www.anesthesiology.org/
- *JTCVS:* http://www.ctsnet.org/section/jtcs
- *Annals of Thoracic Surgery:* http://www.sts.org/annals/
- *Journal of the American College of Cardiology:* http://www.cardiosource.com/jacc.html
- *Circulation:* http://circ.ahajournals.org/
- *Circulation Research:* http://circres.ahajournals.org/
- *New England Journal of Medicine:* http://www.nejm.org/content/index.asp
- *JAMA:* http://www.ama-assn.org/public/journals/jama/toc.htm

On-line CT surgery text
- *Cardiac Surgery in the Adult.* L. Henry Edmunds: http://www.ctsnet.org/book/edmunds/
- AATS: http://ctdigest.com

Search engines and literature search
- Yahoo Anesthesiology: http://www.yahoo.com/Health/Medicine/Anesthesiology/
- Medline: http://www.nlm.nih.gov/medlineplus/

Cardiothoracic surgery links
- Cardiothoracic Surgery Network: http://www.ctsnet.org/
- The Society of Thoracic Surgeons: http://sts.org/
- Heart Surgery Forum: http://www.hsforum.com/

Cardiology links
- American Heart Association: http://www.americanheart.org
- American College of Cardiology: http://www.acc.org/login/index.taf

Echocardiography links
- American Society of Echocardiography: http://asecho.org/
- Acuson Home Page: http://www.acuson.com/
- Echocardiography Online Journal: http://www2.umdnj.edu/~shindler/index.html
- GASNET TEE Tutorial Terry Rafferty: http://groucho.med.yale.edu/education/reference/echomanual/
- Martin London's TEE website: http://members.xoom.com/ml22ml/TEE/

Perfusion links
- The Perfusion Home Page: http://www.perfusion.com

Practice guidelines
- ASA TEE Practice Parameters: http://www.asahq.org/practice/tee/tee.html
- ASA PAC Practice Parameters: http://www.asahq.org/practice/pulm/pulm artery.html

General Anesthesiology Web sites
- GASNET: http://gasnet.med.yale.edu/
- Critical Care Medicine on the Internet: http://www.invivo.net/bg/index2.html
- The Virtual Anaesthesia Textbook: http://www.usyd.edu.au/su/anes/VAT/VAT.html

REFERENCES

1. Rovenstine EA. Anesthesia: organization for teaching. *Anesth Analg* 1937;Nov/Dec:318.
2. Flynn M, Fogdall R. Education and training of the cardiac anesthesiologist. In: Ream AK, Fogdall R, eds. *Acute cardiovascular management.* Philadelphia: JB Lippincott Co, 1982:877.
3. Schwartz AJ. Learning cardiothoracic anesthesia. In: Thys DM, ed, *Textbook of cardiothoracic anesthesiology.* New York: McGraw-Hill, 2001 (*in press*).
4. Schwartz A. Teaching anesthesia. In: Miller R, ed. *Anesthesia.* New York: Churchill Livingstone, 1990:2371.
5. Stead E. Anesthesiologists come of age. *Anesthesiology* 1985;62:774.
6. Osler W. *The master word in medicine. Aequanimitas and other addresses.* Philadelphia: Blaskiston and Co, 1904.
7. ABA-ASA. *Content outline. Joint council on in-training examinations.* Park Ridge, IL: American Board of Anesthesiology–American Society of Anesthesiologists, 1996.
8. Orkin F, Greenhow D. A study of decision making: how faculty define competence. *Anesthesiology* 1978;48:267.
9. Papper E. Anesthesiology comes of age. *JAMA* 1989;62:1225.
10. Kirklin JW, Barratt-Boyers BG. *Cardiac surgery.* New York: John Wiley and Sons, 1986:61.
11. Cleave-Hogg D, Benedict C. Characteristics of good anesthesia teachers. *Can J Anaesth* 1997;44:587.
12. Shysh AJ, Eagle CJ. The characteristics of excellent clinical teachers. *Can J Anaesth* 1997;44(6):577.
13. Greene NM. *Anesthesiology and the university.* Philadelphia: JB Lippincott Co, 1975.
14. Reves JG, Greene NM. Anesthesiology and the academic medical center: place and promise at the start of the new millennium. *Int Anesthesiol Clin* 2000;38:1.
15. Irby DM. What clinical teachers in medicine need to know. *Acad Med* 1994;69(5):333.
16. Norman J. Learning and teaching in anaesthesia. *Br J Anaesth* 1977;49:197.
17. Sivarajan M, Miller E, Hardy C, et al. Objective evaluation of clinical performance and correlation with knowledge. *Anesth Analg* 1984;63:603.
18. Dripps R. Graduate training in anesthesiology. *Surgery* 1972;72:525.
19. Reves JG. Remarks to the new cardiac subspecialty residents. *Anesthesiol Rep* 1988;1:147.
20. Ortega RA, Arkoff H, Havel RC. The use of multimedia to teach new cardiac anesthesia procedures. *J Cardiothorac Anesth* 1998;12:695

21. Gaba D. Improving anesthesiologists' performance by simulating reality. *Anesthesiology* 1992;76:491.
22. Schwid H, O'Donnell D. Anesthesiologists' management of simulated critical incidents. *Anesthesiology* 1992;76:495.
23. Spence AA. The expanding role of simulators in risk management. *Br J Anaesth* 1997;78(6):633.
24. Viets J, Foster S. A clinical evaluation system for anesthesiology residents. *J Med Educ* 1988;63:463.
25. Dreosti A, Sando M. The influence of examinations on anaesthetic training. *Anesth Intensive Care* 1976;4:326.
26. Rhoton MF, Barnes A, Flashburg M, et al. Influence of anesthesiology residents' noncognitive skill on the occurrence of critical incidents and the residents' overall clinical performances. *Acad Med* 1991;66:359.
27. American Board of Anesthesiology. Booklet of information. Raleigh, NC: Office of the Board, 1999.
28. Safar P, Grenvik A. Organization and physician education in critical care medicine. *Anesthesiology* 1977;47:82.
29. Reves JG, Nugent M. New directions in anesthesia subspecialty training. *Anesth Analg* 1989;69:1.
30. Clements FM. The evolution of the anesthesiologist-echocardiographer. In: de Bruijn NP, Clements FM, eds. *Intraoperative use of echocardiography.* Philadelphia: JB Lippincott Co, 1991:1.
31. Pearlman AS, Gardin JM, Martin RP, et al. Guidelines for optimal physician training in echocardiography: recommendations of the American Society of Echocardiography Committee for Physician Training in Echocardiography. *Am J Cardiol* 1987;60:158.
32. Pearlman AS, Gardin JM, Martin RP, et al. Guidelines for physician training in transesophageal echocardiography. Recommendations of the American Society of Echocardiography Committee for Physician Training in Echocardiography. *J Am Soc Echocardiogr* 1992;5:187.
33. Cahalan M, Foster E. Training in transesophageal echocardiography: in the lab or on the job? *Anesth Analg* 1995;81:217.
34. Thys DM. Training, certification and credentialing in transesophageal echocardiography. *J Cardiothorac Vasc Anesth* 1996;10:309.
35. Gaylard DG, Lamberty JM. The attitudes of junior anaesthetists to research: a survey. *Anaesthesia* 1989;44:681.
36. Skinner AC. Fraud in medicine. *Br Med J* 1988;296:574.
37. Aitkenhead AR. Does anaesthetics research need training? *Br J Hosp Med* 1986;May:287.
38. Rogers M. Anesthesiology—the road not yet taken. *Anesthesiology* 1985;63:575.
39. Reyes JG, Newfield P, Striker TW, et al. The effect of the extended (3-year) anesthesia curriculum on anesthesia subspecialty education. *J Cardiothorac Vasc Anesth* 1992;6:392.
40. Hornbein Thomas F. The 28th Rovenstine lecture: lessons from on high. *Anesthesiology* 1991;74:772.
41. Landers DF, Becker GL, Newland MC, et al. Lecture practices in United States anesthesiology residencies. *Anesth Analg* 1992;74:112.
42. Reves JG. Pro: the CA-3 year as presently constructed is detrimental to anesthesia training. *J Cardiothorac Anesth* 1990;4:757.
43. Albrecht RF, Soder WG. Con: the CA-3 year as presently constructed is very beneficial for anesthesia training. *J Cardiothorac Anesth* 1990;4:760.

Cardiac Anesthesia: Principles and Clinical Practice, Second Edition, edited by Fawzy G. Estafanous, Paul G. Barash, and J.G. Reves. Lippincott Williams & Wilkins, Philadelphia © 2001.

INDEX

Page numbers followed by *f* indicate figures; page numbers followed by *t* indicate tables

C

I

M

Q

R

T

W

X

Z